Molecular Pathology in Clinical Practice

Debra G.B. Leonard
Editor

Molecular Pathology in Clinical Practice

Second Edition

Springer

Editor
Debra G.B. Leonard, M.D., Ph.D.
Professor and Chair
Department of Pathology and Laboratory Medicine
University of Vermont College of Medicine and University of Vermont Medical Center
Burlington, VT, USA

ISBN 978-3-319-79285-9 ISBN 978-3-319-19674-9 (eBook)
DOI 10.1007/978-3-319-19674-9

Springer Cham Heidelberg New York Dordrecht London

Softcover re-print of the Hardcover 2nd edition 2016

Printed on acid-free paper

Springer International Publishing AG Switzerland is part of Springer Science+Business Media (www.springer.com)

To Greg
With love and thanks

Preface

Today, molecular and genomic information is informing the patient care decisions in many, if not most, areas of healthcare. Clearly, cancer diagnosis, prognosis, and treatment are driven largely by the molecular variants that drive the cancer and are the targets for new therapies. Medical genetics is moving beyond the classic single gene genetic disorders as we understand the genetic risk factors that drive the common chronic diseases that are costly to our healthcare system. While the clinical relevance of all areas of the human genome is not yet understood, our knowledge is growing rapidly and expanding well beyond the protein-coding genes to include many regulatory-coding regions, such as microRNAs and long noncoding RNAs (lncRNAs), in regions of the genome which used to be considered "junk." For infectious diseases, we are beginning to understand not only the well-known and emerging infectious agents, but that health and disease also relates to the symbiotic relationship of each patient with their microbiomes. Finally, the technologies available to the clinical molecular laboratory have advanced so the genome of individual patients can be analyzed for clinical care, even resulting in the definition of genomic critical values, which are recommended to be reported any time an exome or genome is sequenced for clinical purposes.

Molecular Pathology in Clinical Practice addresses all areas of clinical molecular pathology practice in a single textbook. This second edition has 12 new chapters, in addition to updates on the chapters from the first edition. The new chapters cover diseases not included in the first edition, plus two chapters on next-generation sequencing applications in genetics and cancer, and a proteomics chapter. The purpose of this textbook remains to provide a comprehensive reference for the practicing molecular pathologist as well as a resource for pathologists in any area of practice. The book also will continue to be used by training programs, both for Anatomic and Clinical Pathology and for Molecular Genetic Pathology trainees. This book is not meant to be a recipe book for clinical molecular tests, simply because the specifics of testing change quite rapidly in molecular pathology as new technologies emerge and are integrated into clinical molecular practice. Instead, the emphasis remains the molecular variants being detected for clinical purposes, the clinical usefulness of molecular test results, and the clinical and laboratory issues that require special attention. While this textbook focuses on molecular and genomic testing, with only a single chapter covering proteomics, the reader must understand that the genome does not drive all disease and health, but works in concert with the environment, the metabolome, the methylome, and other determinants of disease and health.

As we move toward genomic medicine, the molecular pathologist and all pathologists will play a significant role in the proper utilization of molecular and genomic tests to improve patient outcomes and the cost-effectiveness of the care we deliver. In the era of US healthcare reform, the promise of genomic medicine aligns almost perfectly with the healthcare reform goals of improving individual patient outcomes, improving the health of populations, and reducing the cost of healthcare. While much of genomic research focuses on the clinical significance of pathogen and patient genomic variants for diagnosis and therapy, evidence of the value of genomics in clinical care also is needed, especially as we move toward population health management and global payment models.

My hope is that you apply the information in *Molecular Pathology in Clinical Practice* to the care you provide for your patients.

Burlington, VT, USA Debra G.B. Leonard

Contents

Contributors

Archana Agarwal, M.D. Department of Pathology, University of Utah, Salt Lake City, UT, USA

Dara L. Aisner, M.D., Ph.D. Department of Pathology, University of Colorado, Aurora, CO, USA

Kevin Alby, Ph.D. Department of Pathology and Laboratory Medicine, Perelman School of Medicine, University of Pennsylvania, Philadelphia, PA, USA

Robert W. Allen, Ph.D. School of Forensic Sciences, Center for Health Sciences, Oklahoma State University, Tulsa, OK, USA

Daniel A. Arber, M.D. Department of Pathology, Stanford University Medical Center, Stanford, CA, USA

Aneel A. Ashrani, M.D., M.S. Division of Hematology, Department of Internal Medicine, Mayo Clinic College of Medicine, Rochester, MN, USA; Special Coagulation Laboratory, Mayo Comprehensive Hemophilia Center, Rochester, MN, USA; Department of Laboratory Medicine and Pathology, Division of Hematopathology and Laboratory Genetics, Mayo Clinic Rochester, Rochester, MN, USA

Renkui Bai, M.D., Ph.D., F.A.C.M.G. Genetic Testing for Mitochondrial Disorders, GeneDx, Gaithersburg, MD, USA

Monica J. Basehore, Ph.D. Greenwood Genetic Center, Greenwood, SC, USA

Samantha M. Baxter, M.S., C.G.C. Laboratory for Molecular Medicine, Partners HealthCare, Cambridge, MA, USA

Lora J.H. Bean, Ph.D., F.A.C.M.G. Department of Human Genetics, Emory Genetics Laboratory, Emory University, Atlanta, GA, USA

Rachel Beeri, Ph.D. Medical Genetics Institute, Shaare Zedek Medical Center, Jerusalem, Israel

Kathryn C. Behling, M.D., Ph.D. Department of Biomedical Sciences, Cooper Medical School of Rowan University, Camden, NJ, USA; Department of Pathology, Cooper University Hospital, Camden, NJ, USA

Daniel B. Bellissimo, Ph.D. Obstetrics, Gynecology and Reproductive Sciences, University of Pittsburgh School of Medicine, Pittsburgh, PA, USA; Magee-Womens Hospital, Pittsburgh, PA, USA

Dani Bercovich, Ph.D. GGA–Galil Genetic Analysis, Biotechnology Program, Tel Hai College, Kazerin, Israel

D. Hunter Best, Ph.D. Department of Pathology, University of Utah School of Medicine, Salt Lake City, UT, USA; ARUP Institute for Clinical and Experimental Pathology, Salt Lake City, UT, USA

Dario de Biase, B.Sc., Ph.D. Anatomic Pathology, Ospedale Bellaria, Bologna University School of Medicine, Bologna, Italy

Andrea Biondi, M.D. Department of Pediatrics, University of Milano-Bicocca, Monza, Italy

Jon D. Blumenfeld, M.D. The Susan R. Knafel Polycystic Kidney Disease Center, The Rogosin Institute, New York, NY, USA; Clinical Medicine, Nephrology and Hypertension, Weill Cornell Medical College, New York, NY, USA

Gregary Bocsi, D.O. Department of Pathology, University of Colorado School of Medicine, Aurora, CO, USA

Rita M. Braziel, M.D. Division of Hematopathology, Department of Pathology, Oregon Health & Science University, Portland, OR, USA

Eileen M. Burd, Ph.D. Pathology and Laboratory Medicine, Microbiology Emory University, Atlanta, GA, USA

Angela M. Caliendo, M.D., Ph.D. Department of Medicine, Alpert Medical School of Brown University, Providence, RI, USA; Rhode Island Hospital, Providence, RI, USA

Giovanni Cazzaniga, Ph.D. Pediatrics, Centro Ricerca Tettamanti, Università di Milano Bicocca, Monza, Italy

Kristen J. Champion, Ph.D., F.A.C.M.G. Med Fusion Laboratories, Lewisville, TX, USA

Zhao Chen, Ph.D. Department of Genetics, Perelman School of Medicine, University of Pennsylvania, Philadelphia, PA, USA

Christin D. Collins, Ph.D., F.A.C.M.G. Emory Genetics Laboratory, Department of Human Genetics, Emory University, Decatur, GA, USA

Emily M. Coonrod, Ph.D. Program in Personalized Health, Dean's Office Research Unit, University of Utah, Salt Lake City, UT, USA

Shale A. Dames, M.S. ARUP Institute for Clinical and Experimental Pathology, Salt Lake City, UT, USA

Vivianna M. Van Deerlin, M.D., Ph.D. Pathology and Laboratory Medicine, Molecular Pathology Laboratory, Perelman School of Medicine at the University of Pennsylvania, Philadelphia, PA, USA

Robert C. Doebele, M.D., Ph.D. Division of Medical Oncology, University of Colorado Denver, Aurora, CO, USA

Jennifer B. Dunlap, M.D. Division of Hematopathology, Oregon Health & Sciences University, Portland, OR, USA

Jacob D. Durtschi, B.S. Bioinformatics, Institute for Clinical and Experimental Pathology, Salt Lake City, UT, USA

Lisa Edelmann, Ph.D. Department of Genetics and Genomic Sciences, Icahn School of Medicine, Mount Sinai Medical Center, New York, NY, USA

Kojo S.J. Elenitoba-Johnson, M.D. Department of Pathology and Laboratory Medicine, Perelman School of Medicine at the University of Pennsylvania, Philadelphia, Stellar-Chance Laboratories, PA, USA

Robert W. Eppsteiner, M.D. Department of Otolaryngology—Head and Neck Surgery, University of Iowa Hospitals and Clinics, Iowa City, IA, USA

Guang Fan, M.D., Ph.D. Division of Hematopathology, Department of Pathology, Oregon Health and Science University, Portland, OR, USA

Daniel H. Farkas, Ph.D. Obstetrics, Gynecology and Reproductive Medicine, Michigan State University, Grand Rapids, MI, USA

Helen Fernandes, Ph.D. Department of Pathology and Laboratory Medicine, Weill Cornell Medical College, New York, NY, USA

David R. Foran, Ph.D. Forensic Science Program, School of Criminal Justice, Michigan State University, East Lansing, MI, USA

Betty A. Forbes, Ph.D. Division of Clinical Pathology, Pathology Department, Virginia Commonwealth University Medical Center, Richmond, VA, USA

Wilbur A. Franklin, M.D. Department of Pathology, University of Colorado Denver, Aurora, CO, USA

Michael J. Friez, Ph.D. Med Fusion Laboratories, Lewisville, TX, USA

Birgit H. Funke, Ph.D., F.A.C.M.G. Department of Pathology, Harvard Medical School, Cambridge, MA, USA

Arupa Ganguly, Ph.D. Department of Genetics, Perelman School of Medicine, University of Pennsylvania, Philadelphia, PA, USA

Christine C. Ginocchio, Ph.D., M.T.(A.S.C.P.) Department of Pathology and Laboratory Medicine, Hofstra North Shore-LIJ School of Medicine, Hempstead, NY, USA; Scientific and Medical Affairs, BioMerieux, Durham, NC, USA; Scientific and Medical Affairs, BioFire Diagnostics, Salt Lake City, UT, USA

Eliahu Golomb, M.D., Ph.D. Department of Pathology, Shaare Zedek Medical Center, Medical Genetics Institute, Jerusalem, Israel

James P. Grenert, M.D., Ph.D. University of California San Francisco, San Francisco, CA, USA

David Grimwade, Ph.D., F.R.C.Path. Department of Medical and Molecular Genetics, Cancer Genetics Laboratory, King's College London, Faculty of Life Sciences and Medicine, London, UK

Guangyu Gu, M.D. Pathology Department, ARUP Laboratories, University of Utah, Salt Lake City, UT, USA

Kevin C. Halling, M.D., Ph.D. Department of Laboratory Medicine and Pathology, Division of Laboratory Genetics, Mayo Clinic, Rochester, MN, USA

Randall T. Hayden, M.D. Department of Pathology, St. Jude Children's Research Hospital, Memphis, TN, USA

Madhuri R. Hegde, Ph.D. Department of Human Genetics, Emory University School of Medicine, Emory University, Atlanta, GA, USA

Jaimie D. Higgs, M.S., C.G.C. GeneDx, Gaithersburg, MD, USA

David R. Hillyard, M.D. Department of Pathology, School of Medicine, University of Utah, Salt Lake City, UT, USA; Molecular Infectious Disease Testing and Infectious Disease Sequencing Core, ARUP Laboratories, Salt Lake City, UT, USA

Benjamin H. Hinrichs Pathology and Laboratory Medicine, Gastrointestinal Pathology, Emory University, Atlanta, GA, USA

Albert K. Ho, M.D., Ph.D. Quest Diagnostics, Nichols Institute, Chantilly, VA, USA

Jill A. Hollenbach, Ph.D., M.P.H. Center for Genetics, Children's Hospital Oakland Research Institute, Oakland, CA, USA

Pei Hui, M.D., Ph.D. Department of Pathology, Yale University School of Medicine, New Haven, CT, USA

Daniel M. Jones, M.D., Ph.D. School of Health Professions, University of Texas MD Anderson Cancer Center, Houston, TX, USA

Melanie A. Jones, Ph.D. Department of Human Genetics, Emory University School of Medicine, Emory University, Atlanta, GA, USA

Jeanne A. Jordan, Ph.D. Epidemiology and Biostatistics, School of Public Health and Health Services, The George Washington University, Washington DC, USA

Malek Kamoun, M.D., Ph.D. Pathology and Laboratory Medicine, Penn Medicine, Philadelphia, PA, USA

Karen Kaul, M.D., Ph.D. Pathology and Laboratory Medicine, North Shore University Health System, Evanston, IL, USA

Inbal Kedar, M.S. Cancer Genetics, The Raphael Recanati Genetics Institute, Rabin Medical Center, Beilinson Hospital, Petah Tikva, Israel

Michelle L. Kluge, M.S., C.G.C. Department of Laboratory Medicine and Pathology, Division of Hematopathology and Laboratory Genetics, Mayo Clinic College of Medicine, Rochester, MN, USA; Mayo Comprehensive Hemophilia Center, Mayo Clinic Rochester, Rochester, MN, USA

Steven Knapper, D.M., B.M.B.Ch., F.R.C.Path. Department of Haematology, Cardiff University, Cardiff, UK

Ruth Kornreich, Ph.D. Department of Genetics and Genomic Sciences, Mount Sinai School of Medicine, New York, NY, USA

Colleen S. Kraft, M.D., M.Sc. Pathology and Laboratory Medicine, Medicine, Infectious Diseases, Emory University, Atlanta, GA, USA

Patti Krautscheid, M.S., L.C.G.C. ARUP Laboratories, Salt Lake City, UT, USA

Danielle LaGrave, M.S., L.C.G.C. ARUP Laboratories, Salt Lake City, UT, USA

Priti Lal, M.D. Pathology and Laboratory Medicine, Anatomic Pathology, University of Pennsylvania, Philadelphia, PA, USA

Ehud Lavi, M.D. Anatomic Pathology, Pathology and Laboratory Medicine, Weill Cornell Medical College, New York, NY, USA

Nicky Leeborg, M.D. Division of Hematopathology, Department of Pathology, Oregon Health and Science University, Portland, OR, USA

Debra G.B. Leonard, M.D., Ph.D. Department of Pathology and Laboratory Medicine, University of Vermont College of Medicine and University of Vermont Medical Center, Burlington, VT, USA

Ephrat Levy-Lahad, M.D. Medical Genetics Institute, Shaare Zedek Medical Center, Hebrew University Medical School, Jerusalem, Israel

Tracey Lewis, Ph.D. ARUP Institute for Clinical and Experimental Pathology, Salt Lake City, UT, USA

Fang-Yuan Li, M.D., Ph.D. Department of Molecular and Human Genetics, Baylor Miraca Genetics Laboratory, Baylor College of Medicine, Houston, TX, USA

Elaine Lyon, Ph.D. Department of Pathology, University of Utah School of Medicine, Salt Lake City, UT, USA; Molecular Genetics and Genomics, ARUP Laboratories, Salt Lake City, UT, USA

Deqin Ma, M.D., Ph.D. Department of Pathology, University of Iowa Hospitals and Clinics, Iowa City, IA, USA

Steven J. Mack, Ph.D. Children's Hospital Oakland Research Institute, Oakland, CA, USA

Rong Mao, M.D. Department of Pathology, University of Utah School of Medicine, Salt Lake City, UT, USA; ARUP Institute for Clinical and Experimental Pathology, Salt Lake City, UT, USA

Rebecca L. Margraf, Ph.D. ARUP Laboratories, Institute for Clinical and Experimental Pathology, Salt Lake City, UT, USA

Maria Martinez-Lage, M.D. Pathology and Laboratory Medicine, Neuropathology, Perelman School of Medicine at the University of Pennsylvania, Philadelphia, PA, USA

Jason D. Merker, M.D., Ph.D. Department of Pathology, Stanford University School of Medicine, Stanford, CA, USA

Rachel Michaelson-Cohen, M.D. Medical Genetics Institute, Shaare Zedek Medical Center, Hebrew University Medical School, Jerusalem, Israel

Carolyn Mies, M.D. Genomic Health Inc., Redwood City, CA, USA

Christine E. Miller, M.S., C.L.G.C. ARUP Laboratories, Salt Lake City, UT, USA

Melissa B. Miller, Ph.D. Department of Pathology and Laboratory Medicine, University of North Carolina School of Medicine, Chapel Hill, NC, USA

Krzysztof Mrózek, M.D., Ph.D. Comprehensive Cancer Center, The Ohio State University, Columbus, OH, USA

Duane W. Newton, Ph.D., D.(A.B.M.M.) Clinical Microbiology Laboratory, Division of Clinical Pathology, University of Michigan, Ann Arbor, MI, USA

Yuri E. Nikiforov, M.D., Ph.D. Department of Pathology and Laboratory Medicine, Division of Molecular and Genomic Pathology, University of Pittsburgh Medical Center, Pittsburgh, PA, USA

Marina N. Nikiforova, M.D. Department of Pathology and Laboratory Medicine, Division of Molecular and Genomic Pathology, University of Pittsburgh Medical Center, Pittsburgh, PA, USA

Frederick S. Nolte, Ph.D. Molecular Pathology, Pathology and Laboratory Medicine, Medical University of South Carolina, Charleston, SC, USA

Shuji Ogino, M.D., Ph.D., M.S. Department of Pathology, Harvard Medical School, Brigham and Women's Hospital, Boston, MA, USA; Department of Medical Oncology, Dana-Farber Cancer Institute, Boston, MA, USA; Department of Epidemiology, Harvard T.H. Chan School of Public Health, Boston, MA, USA

Nirali M. Patel, M.D. Department of Pathology and Laboratory Medicine, Lineberger Comprehensive Cancer Center, University of North Carolina at Chapel Hill, Chapel Hill, NC, USA; Molecular Genetics Laboratory, UNC Hospitals, Chapel Hill, NC, USA

Deborah Ann Payne, Ph.D. Molecular Services, American Pathology Partners, Inc., Denver, CO, USA

John D. Pfeifer, M.D., Ph.D. Department of Pathology, Washington University School of Medicine, St. Louis, MO, USA

Herbert F. Polesky, M.D. In Memoriam

V.M. Pratt, Ph.D., F.A.C.M.G. Pharmacogenomics Laboratory, Department of Medical and Molecular Genetics, Indiana University School of Medicine, Indianapolis, IN, USA

Thomas W. Prior, Ph.D. Department of Pathology, Ohio State University Medical Center, Columbus, OH, USA

Rajiv K. Pruthi, M.B.B.S. Division of Hematology, Department of Internal Medicine, Mayo Clinic Rochester, Rochester, MN, USA

Raymund R. Razonable, M.D., F.I.D.S.A. Division of Infectious Diseases, Department of Internal Medicine, Mayo Clinic, Rochester, MN, USA

Hanna Rennert, Ph.D., F.A.C.M.G. Department of Pathology and Laboratory Medicine, Weill Cornell Medical College, New York Presbyterian Hospital, New York, NY, USA

Ran Reshef, M.D. Department of Medicine, Hematology and Oncology Division, Perelman School of Medicine at the University of Pennsylvania, Philadelphia, PA, USA

Andrew Ricci, M.D. Department of Pathology, Hartford Hospital, Hartford, CT, USA

Delphine Rolland, Pharm.D., Ph.D. Department of Pathology, University of Michigan Medical School, Ann Arbor, MI, USA

Kandelaria M. Rumilla, M.D. Department of Laboratory Medicine and Pathology, Laboratory Genetics, Mayo Clinic, Rochester, MN, USA

Iris Schrijver, M.D. Pathology Department, Stanford University, Stanford, CA, USA

Stuart A. Scott, Ph.D. Department of Genetics and Genomic Sciences, Icahn School of Medicine at Mount Sinai, New York, NY, USA; Mount Sinai Genetic Testing Laboratory, New York, NY, USA

Carlos Alberto Scrideli, M.D., Ph.D. Pediatrics, Pediatric Oncology and Hematology, Ribeirão Preto Medical School, University of Sao Paulo, Ribeirão Preto, Sao Paulo, Brazil

Antonia R. Sepulveda, M.D., Ph.D. Department of Pathology and Cell Biology, Columbia University Medical Center, New York, NY, USA

A. Eliot Shearer, B.Sc. Department of Otolaryngology—Head and Neck Surgery, University of Iowa Hospitals and Clinics, Iowa City, IA, USA

Patricia R. Slev, Ph.D., D.(A.B.C.C) Department of Pathology, School of Medicine, University of Utah, Salt Lake City, UT, USA; Serologic Hepatitis and Retrovirus Laboratory, Immunology Core Laboratory, ARUP Laboratories, Salt Lake City, UT, USA

Richard J.H. Smith, M.D. Department of Otolaryngology—Head and Neck Surgery, University of Iowa Hospitals and Clinics, Iowa City, IA, USA

Sarah T. South, Ph.D. Pathology Department, ARUP Laboratories, University of Utah, Salt Lake City, UT, USA; Department of Pediatrics, ARUP Laboratories, University of Utah, Salt Lake City, UT, USA

Elaine Spector, Ph.D., F.A.C.M.G. Department of Pediatrics, Denver Genetics Laboratories, Children's Hospital Colorado, Aurora, CO, USA

Steven Sperber, M.S., Ph.D., F.A.C.M.G. Department of Genetic and Genomic Sciences, Mount Sinai Genetic Testing Laboratory, Icahn School of Medicine at Mount Sinai, New York, NY, USA

Catherine A. Stolle, Ph.D. Department of Pathology and Laboratory Medicine, The Children's Hospital of Philadelphia, Philadelphia, PA, USA

Kelli L. Sumner, B.S. ARUP Institute for Clinical and Experimental Pathology, Salt Lake City, UT, USA

Giovanni Tallini, M.D. Anatomic Pathology, Ospedale Bellaria, Bologna University School of Medicine, Bologna, Italy

Adrian Y. Tan, Ph.D. Department of Pathology, Weill Cornell Medical College, New York, NY, USA

Reha Toydemir, M.D., Ph.D. Pathology Department, ARUP Laboratories, University of Utah, Salt Lake City, UT, USA

Gregory J. Tsongalis, Ph.D. Department of Pathology, Geisel School of Medicine at Dartmouth, Lebanon, NH, USA; Norris Cotton Cancer Center, Lebanon, NH, USA

Marileila Varella-Garcia, Ph.D. Division of Medical Oncology, University of Colorado Denver, Aurora, CO, USA

Cecily P. Vaughn, M.S. ARUP Institute for Clinical and Experimental Pathology, Salt Lake City, UT, USA

Karl V. Voelkerding, M.D. Department of Pathology, ARUP Institute for Clinical and Experimental Pathology, University of Utah, Salt Lake City, UT, USA

Victor W. Weedn, M.D., J.D. Department of Forensic Sciences, George Washington University, Washington, DC, USA

Thomas M. Williams, M.D. In Memoriam

Robert B. Wilson, M.D., Ph.D. Department of Pathology and Laboratory Medicine, Perelman School of Medicine at the University of Pennsylvania, Philadelphia, PA, USA

Lee-Jun C. Wong, Ph.D., F.A.C.M.G. Department of Molecular and Human Genetics, Baylor Miraca Genetics Laboratory, Baylor College of Medicine, Houston, TX, USA

Whitney Wooderchak-Donahue, Ph.D. ARUP Institute for Clinical and Experimental Pathology, Salt Lake City, UT, USA

Amy C. Yang, M.D. Department of Genetics and Genomic Sciences, Division of Medical Genetics, Mount Sinai School of Medicine, New York, NY, USA

Yaping Yang, Ph.D. Department of Molecular and Human Genetics, Medical Genetics Laboratory and Whole Genome Laboratory, Baylor College of Medicine, Houston, TX, USA

Barbara A. Zehnbauer, Ph.D., F.A.C.M.G., F.A.C.B. Centers for Disease Control and Prevention, Atlanta, GA, USA

Basics of Molecular Biology

1

Deborah Ann Payne

Abstract

Molecular biology entails the analysis and study of the chemical organization of the cell. Molecules comprise the smallest chemical component capable of performing all the activities (structural or catalytic) of a substance. One or more atoms constitute each molecule. Many molecules comprise the various cellular and subcellular components of an organism. Molecules form not only the physical structure of the organism but communicate information between the various compartments of the cell. This communication can be the transfer of information from DNA to RNA and finally to protein or the subtle regulation of the cell's internal homeostatic processes. This communication relies on the interaction of various molecules to insure the fidelity of the message or cellular regulation. This chapter describes the physical organization of cells, cellular organelles, and molecules important in cell division, inheritance, and protein synthesis and describes how genetic information is communicated within the cell.

Keywords

Molecular biology • Genetic • Gene • Nucleic acids • DNA • RNA • Protein • Nucleotides • Amino acids • Codon • Transcription • Translation • Replication • Chromatin • Chromosomes • Complementary • Cell cycle • Hybridization • Denaturation • Mitochondria • Mutation • Ribosome • Polymerase • Exon • Intron

Introduction

Molecular biology entails the analysis and study of the chemical organization of the cell. Molecules comprise the smallest chemical component capable of performing all the activities (structural or catalytic) of a substance. One or more atoms constitute each molecule. Many molecules comprise the various cellular and subcellular components of an organism. Molecules form not only the physical structure of the organism but communicate information between the various compartments of the cell. This communication can be the transfer of information from DNA to RNA and finally to protein or the subtle regulation of the cell's internal homeostatic processes. This communication relies on the interaction of various molecules to insure the fidelity of the message or cellular regulation. This chapter describes the physical organization of cells, cellular organelles, and molecules important in cell division, inheritance, and protein synthesis and describes how genetic information is communicated within the cell.

Organization of the Cell

The cell is a mass of protoplasm surrounded by a semipermeable membrane [1]. Cells constitute the smallest element of living matter capable of functioning independently; however, within complex organisms, cells may require interaction with other cells. To function independently, cells must produce nucleic acids, proteins, lipids, and energy. In complex

D.A. Payne, Ph.D. (✉)
Molecular Services, American Pathology Partners, Inc.,
6116 East Warren Avenue, Denver, CO 80222, USA
e-mail: dpayne@unipathdx.com

D.G.B. Leonard (ed.), *Molecular Pathology in Clinical Practice*, DOI 10.1007/978-3-319-19674-9_1

organisms, these organic processes form and maintain tissues and the organism as a whole.

Genes consist of discrete regions of nucleic acids that encode proteins, and control the function of the cell. Deoxyribonucleic acid (DNA) and ribonucleic acid (RNA) comprise the two types of nucleic acids found in all cells. Chromosomes, made up of double-stranded DNA complexed with proteins, contain all the genes required for the cell to live and function.

Prokaryotic Cells

Prokaryotic cells are simple organisms lacking subcellular compartments, such as bacteria. The majority of prokaryotic nucleic acids form circular strands comprising approximately 1×10^6 base pairs (bp) (Table 1.1) [2]. Additional extrachromosomal genetic elements consist of circular plasmids also known as episomes and linear mobile genetic elements called transposable elements or transposons. Plasmids range in size from 2,686 to 500,000 bp and first gained notoriety in the 1950s by being associated with antibiotic resistance in bacteria [3, 4]. Transposons also may confer antibiotic resistance on the host bacteria. All these genetic elements exist in direct contact with the bacteria's cytoplasm.

Eukaryotic Cells

Cytoplasm

In contrast to prokaryotic cells, eukaryotic cells are complex, highly compartmentalized structures. The cytoplasm contains multiple membrane-bound compartments known as organelles. The cellular membrane separates the cellular cytoplasm from the external environment. The membranes consist of hydrophobic lipid bilayers. The lipid bilayer contains proteins that serve as receptors and channels.

Nucleus and Nucleolus

The nucleus of the cell contains the cell's linear chromosomes and serves as the primary locus of inherited genetic material. Inner- and outer-pore-containing membranes define the nucleus and separate the chromosomes from the surrounding cytoplasm. Further partitioning occurs within the nucleus to generate the nucleolus, which functions as the ribosome-generating factory of the cell. Instead of additional membranes, fibrous protein complexes separate the nucleolus from the rest of the nucleus. In this structure, the nucleolus organizer (a specific part of a chromosome containing the genes that encode ribosomal RNAs) interacts with other molecules to form immature large and small ribosomal subunits. Following processing, immature subunits depart the nucleolus and enter the nucleus. Eventually, mature ribosomal subunits and other molecules exit the nucleolus through the nuclear pores and enter the cytoplasm.

Table 1.1 Comparison of sizes (in base pairs) of various genetic elements [2–5]

Genetic element	Size in base pairs
Human chromosome	3.3×10^9
Bacterial chromosome	$1–4 \times 10^6$
Mitochondrial chromosome	16,569
Bacteriophage	39,000
CAM plasmid	500,000
pUC19 plasmid (engineered plasmid)	2,686
Retrotransposon (i.e., SINE to LINE 1)	75–7,000
Long intergenic noncoding RNA (lincRNA)	>200
Transcribed ultraconserved regions (T-UCR)	>200
Telomeric repeat containing RNAs (TERRA)	>200
Small nucleolar RNA (snoRNA)	60–300
Promoter upstream transcripts (PROMPTs)	<200
Promoter-associated small RNAs (PASR)	22–200
Transcription start site-associated RNA (TSSa-RNA)	20–90
PIWI-interacting RNA (piRNA)	26–31
microRNA (miRNA)	22
Transcription initiation RNA (tiRNA)	17–18

Mitochondria

Mitochondria are membrane-bound organelles within the cytoplasm of cells that have several cellular functions. Inheritable genetic material, independent from the nuclear chromosomes, resides in mitochondria. These maternally derived organelles contain their own circular chromosome (16,569 bp) and replicate independently from the cell and one another. As a result, not all mitochondria in a given cell have the same mitochondrial DNA (mtDNA) sequence. The genetic diversity of these organelles within and between different cells of the same organism is known as heteroplasmy. A range (approximately 39–1,283) of mitochondrial genomes are present per cell, and this number may vary with different disease states [6, 7]. Mitochondrial genes encode mitochondria-specific transfer RNA molecules (tRNA). In addition, the mtDNA contains genes that encode proteins used in oxidative phosphorylation, including subunits of the cytochrome c oxidase, cytochrome b complex, some of the ATPase complex, and various subunits of NAD dehydrogenase. Other components of the oxidative phosphorylation pathway are encoded by nuclear genes. For this reason, not all mitochondrial genetic diseases demonstrate maternal transmission. Mutations associated with mitochondrial diseases can be found at MITOMAP (http://www.mitomap.org/MITOMAP). The higher copy number per cell of mtDNA compared with genomic DNA (i.e., approximately 100 to 1) enables the detection and characterization of mtDNA from severely degraded samples and scant samples. For this reason, mtDNA is suitable for paleontological, medical, and forensic genetic investigations. Analysis of mtDNA has applications for diagnosis of mitochondrial-inherited genetic diseases, disease prognosis, as well as forensic identification of severely decomposed bodies [6–9].

Other Cellular Organelles

Membranes not only segregate heritable genetic molecules into the nucleus and mitochondria, but also separate various cellular functions into distinct areas of the cell. The compartmentalization of cellular functions (such as molecular synthesis, modification, and catabolism) increases the local concentration of reactive molecules and improves the biochemical efficiency of the cell. This partitioning also protects inappropriate molecules from becoming substrates for these processes. One example of this segregation is the endoplasmic reticulum (ER), which consists of a complex of membranous compartments where proteins are synthesized. Glycoproteins are synthesized by ribosome-ER complexes known as rough ER (RER), while lipids are produced in the smooth ER. The Golgi apparatus possesses numerous membrane-bound sacs where molecules generated in the ER become modified for transportation out of the cell. In addition, peroxisomes and lysosomes segregate digestive and reactive molecules from the remainder of the cellular contents to prevent damage to the cell's internal molecules and infrastructure. The pathologic accumulation of large molecules within lysosomes occurs when enzymes cannot chemically cleave or modify the large molecules. Lysosomal storage and mucopolysaccharide storage diseases are associated with a variety of genetic variants and mutations. Similarly, peroxisomal diseases are associated with genetic defects in the peroxisomal enzyme pathway [1].

Biological Molecules

Carbon can covalently bond to several biologically important atoms (i.e., oxygen, hydrogen, and nitrogen) and forms the scaffold for all biomolecules. Basic subunit biomolecules can combine to form more complex molecules such as carbohydrates, nucleic acids, and amino acids.

Carbohydrates

Carbohydrates serve as energy reservoirs and are a component of nucleic acids. In addition, carbohydrates also attach to lipids and proteins. The basic unit of a carbohydrate consists of the simple sugars or monosaccharides. These molecules have carbon, oxygen, and hydroxyl groups that most commonly form ringed structures. The oxygen can react with the hydroxyl group of another simple sugar to form a chain. As a result, the formula for a simple sugar is $(CH_2O)^n$, where n represents various numbers of these linked building block units.

Two pentose sugars, deoxyribose and ribose, comprise the sugar element of DNA and RNA molecules, respectively. As the name indicates, deoxyribose ("de-," a prefix meaning "off" and "oxy," meaning "oxygen") lacks one hydroxyl (OH) group compared with ribose.

Nucleic Acids

Nucleic acids are composed of chains of nucleotides. Each nucleotide is composed of a sugar (either ribose or deoxyribose), a phosphate ($-PO_4$) group, and a purine or pyrimidine base. The nucleotides are joined into a DNA or RNA strand by a sugar-phosphate-linked backbone with the bases attached to and extending from the first carbon of the sugar group. The purine and pyrimidine bases are weakly basic ring molecules, which form N-glycosidic bonds with ribose or deoxyribose sugar. Purines are comprised of two rings, a six-member ring and a five-member ring ($C_5H_4N_4$), while pyrimidines consist of a single six-member ring ($C_4H_2N_2$). Purines (guanine, G, and adenine, A) pair with pyrimidines (cytosine, C, and thymine, T) via hydrogen bonds between two DNA molecules (Fig. 1.1). The additional hydrogen bond that forms between G and C base pairing (i.e., three hydrogen bonds) dramatically enhances the strength of this interaction compared to the two hydrogen bonds present between A and T nucleotides. This hydrogen-bonding capacity between G:C and A:T forms a pivotal molecular interaction for all nucleic acids and assures the passage of genetic information during DNA replication, RNA synthesis from DNA (transcription), and the transfer of genetic information from nucleic acids to the amino acids of proteins.

Numerous types of base modifications increase the number of nucleotides beyond the classic four types (i.e., A, T, G, and C). Although these modifications do not alter the base's hydrogen bonding characteristics, modified nucleotides serve various functions in the cell including (1) regulating gene function, (2) suppressing endoparasitic sequence reactivation, (3) identifying DNA damage, and (4) facilitating translation. Modifications such as 5-methylcytosine, 5-hydroxymethylcytosine, 5-formylcytosine, and 5-carboxylcytosine influence gene expression. Most endoparasitic sequences such as retrotransposons (e.g., long interspersed nucleotide elements [LINE 1]) are hypermethylated in normal tissue but hypomethylated in cancer tissue [10].

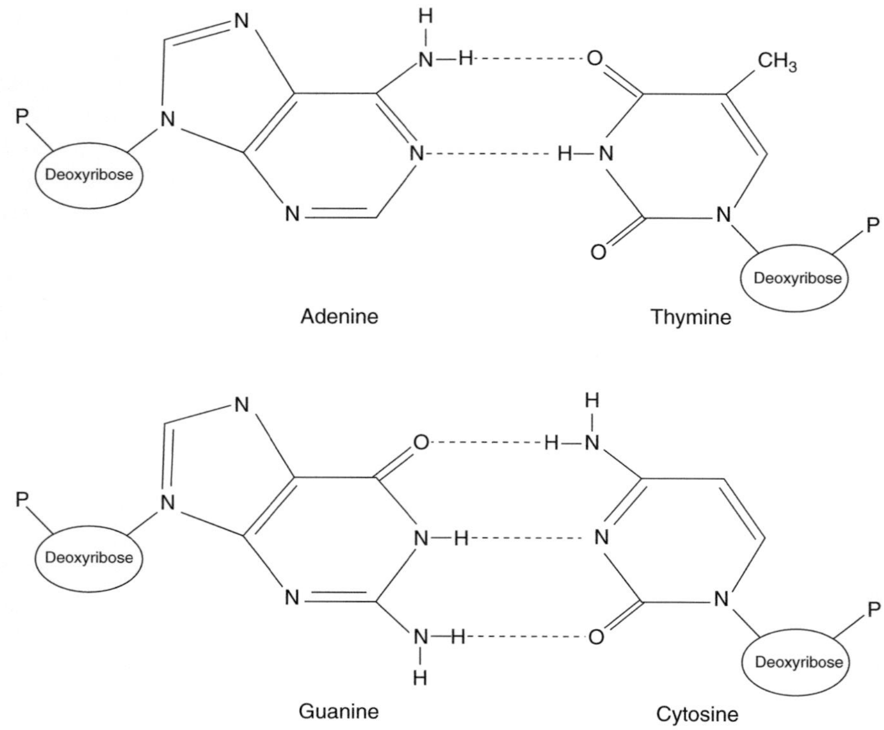

Figure 1.1 DNA base pairing. DNA nucleotides are composed of three moieties (e.g., sugar, base, and phosphate groups). The bases are either purine (adenine and guanine) or pyrimidine (thymine and cytosine). Note the difference in hydrogen bonds between adenine and thymine base pairs, with two hydrogen bonds, compared to cytosine and guanine base pairs, with three hydrogen bonds. Reprinted with permission from Leonard D. Diagnostic Molecular Pathology. 2003:1–13. Copyright Elsevier (2003)

Presumably the hypermethylation of the LINE 1 sequences prevents various insults to the host genome by inactivating the ability of these elements to transpose themselves. Methylation also regulates the phenomenon of imprinting. Methylation mechanisms include P-element-induced wimpy testis (in *Drosophila*, PIWI) proteins and PIWI-interacting noncoding RNAs (specifically, piRNA) [11]. Additionally, certain modifications such as 8-oxoguanine and 8-oxoadenine are associated with DNA damage. Base pair modifications are not limited to DNA but also influence the function of tRNAs [12]. Some of these modifications include 5-formylcytidine, queuosine, 5-taurinomethyluridine, and 5-taurinomethyl-2-thiouridine. Certain tRNA modification defects result in mitochondrial disease [13]. Modifications of rRNA include 2′-O-methylation and pseudouridylation and enable rRNA folding and stability. Such modifications result from interactions of the bases with small nucleolar ribonucleoproteins and noncoding small nucleolar RNAs [5]. With the advent of methodologies that simplify the detection of modified bases, the role of modified bases in human disease may become better understood [14].

Amino Acids

Amino acids are the building blocks of proteins. Amino acids linked together via peptide bonds form large, complex molecules. Amino acids consist of an amino group (NH_3), a carboxyl group (COO–), an R group, and a central carbon atom. The R group can be a simple hydrogen, as found in glycine, or as complex as an imidazole ring, as found in histidine. Twenty different R groups exist (Table 1.2), and determine whether an amino acid has a neutral, basic, or acidic charge. The amino group of a polypeptide is considered the beginning of the protein (N-terminus), while the carboxyl group is at the opposite end, providing directionality to the protein.

Genetic Molecules

Nucleic acids encode genetic information but also participate in additional physiological processes ranging from metabolism to energy transfer. Nucleotides constitute the monomeric units of nucleic acids (Fig. 1.1). Nucleosides consist of two components (ribose or deoxyribose in RNA and DNA, respectively, and either a purine or pyrimidine base). A nucleotide is produced from a nucleoside by the addition of one to three phosphate groups through a covalent bond with the hydroxyl group of the 5′ carbon of the nucleoside's sugar ring.

Nucleic acids consist of chains of nucleotides linked by phosphodiester bonds between the 3′ carbon of the first nucleotide's sugar ring and the 5′ carbon of the adjacent nucleotide's sugar ring. The phosphodiester linkages cause nucleic acids to have a 5′ to 3′ directionality. The alternating

Table 1.2 Amino acids

Amino acid	Amino acid symbols: Three letter	Single letter	Linear structure
Alanine	ala	A	CH_3–CH(NH_2)–COOH
Arginine	arg	R	HN=C(NH_2)–NH–(CH_2)$_3$–CH(NH_2)–COOH
Asparagine	asn	N	H_2N–CO–CH_2–CH(NH_2)–COOH
Aspartic acid	asp	D	HOOC–CH_2–CH(NH_2)–COOH
Cysteine	cys	C	HS–CH_2–CH(NH_2)–COOH
Glutamic acid	glu	E	HOOC–(CH_2)$_2$–CH(NH_2)–COOH
Glutamine	gln	Q	H_2N–CO–(CH_2)$_2$–CH(NH_2)–COOH
Glycine	gly	G	NH_2–CH_2–COOH
Histidine	his	H	**NH**–CH=N–CH=**C**–CH_2–CH(NH_2)–COOH
Isoleucine	ile	I	CH_3–CH_2–CH(CH_3)–CH(NH_2)–COOH
Leucine	leu	L	(CH_3)$_2$–CH–CH_2–CH(NH_2)–COOH
Lysine	lys	K	H_2N–(CH_2)$_4$–CH(NH_2)–COOH
Methionine	met	M	CH_3–S–(CH_2)$_2$–CH(NH_2)–COOH
Phenylalanine	phe	F	Ph–CH_2–CH(NH_2)–COOH
Proline	pro	P	**NH**–(CH_2)$_3$–**CH**–COOH
Serine	ser	S	HO–CH_2–CH(NH_2)–COOH
Threonine	thr	T	CH_3–CH(OH)–CH(NH_2)–COOH
Tryptophan	trp	W	**Ph**–NH–CH=**C**–CH_2–CH(NH_2)–COOH
Tyrosine	tyr	Y	HO–Ph–CH_2–CH(NH_2)–COOH
Valine	val	V	(CH_3)$_2$–CH–CH(NH_2)–COOH

The two bolded atoms in each of histidine (N–C), proline (N–C), and tryptophan (Ph–C) are covalently bonded to each other. Ph is a phenyl ring.

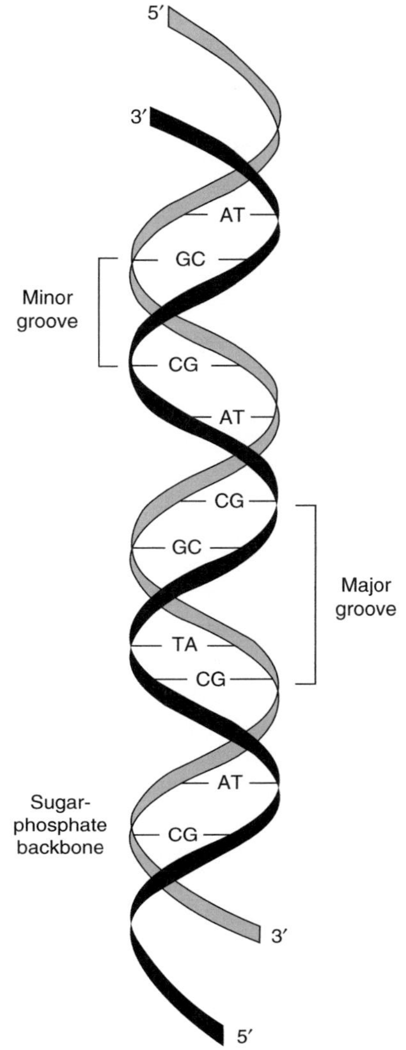

Figure 1.2 Double-stranded DNA. The two DNA strands are oriented in an antiparallel relationship, with asymmetric base pairing of two DNA strands that generates the minor and major grooves of the DNA double helix. Reprinted with permission from Leonard D. Diagnostic Molecular Pathology. 2003:1–13. Copyright Elsevier (2003)

sugar-phosphate chain forms a continuous molecule with bases extending from the 1′ carbon of each sugar. For this reason, the sugar-phosphate chain is referred to as the backbone of nucleic acids (Fig. 1.2). The phosphate groups give nucleic acids a negative charge that imparts important physiochemical properties to nucleic acids. The negative charge of DNA facilitates the binding of mammalian DNA to various proteins and allows separation of nucleic acid molecules by charge and size during gel or capillary electrophoresis.

Structure

In double-stranded DNA, the two DNA strands are held together by exact A:T and G:C hydrogen bonding between the bases of the two strands, in which case the two strands are said to be complementary. The two strands are oriented in opposite 5′ to 3′ directions, such that one strand is oriented 5′ to 3′ and the complementary strand is oriented 3′ to 5′ in an antiparallel fashion (see Fig. 1.2). In this case, "anti-" refers to the head (or 5′ end) of one DNA strand being adjacent to the tail (or 3′ end) of the opposite strand.

The molecular curves of the two DNA strands form antiparallel helices known as the DNA double helix. This double-helix form (the B form) has ten nucleotide base pairs per turn, occupying 3.4 nm. Because the bonds between the sugar and the base are not perfectly symmetrical, the strands curve slightly. The slight curve of the offset glycosidic bonds results in major and minor grooves characteristic of the B form of the double helix [15]. Many clinical molecular tests target the minor groove of DNA with sequence-specific probes known as minor groove-binding (MGB) probes. Two other forms of DNA exist as the Z and A forms. The Z form acquires a zigzag shape, while the A form has very shallow and very deep grooves.

Thermodynamics of Nucleotide Base Pairing

Thermodynamics plays a major role in the structure and stability of nucleic acid molecules. The core mechanism of nucleic acid thermodynamics centers on the hydrogen-bonding capabilities of the nucleotides. The stability of these interactions not only influences the formation and stability of duplex (or double-stranded) nucleic acids but also impacts the structure and catalytic characteristics of single-stranded nucleic acids through intramolecular base pairing. In addition to these physiological functions, the phenomenon of complementary base pairing profoundly impacts clinical diagnostic test development. Prior to the advent of clinical molecular testing, many clinical tests required a target-specific antibody to identify or detect a target protein. The procedures for generating and validating diagnostic antibodies require extensive time and expense. The application of techniques utilizing the capability of two molecules to base pair as the basis for detection and characterization of target nucleic acids has greatly facilitated clinical molecular test development. The formation of hydrogen bonding between two pieces of nucleic acid is called hybridization, or annealing, and the disruption of the hydrogen bonds holding two nucleic acid molecules together is called denaturation, or melting. The fact that clinical molecular tests use hybridization techniques based on A:T and G:C base pairing underscores the necessity for understanding the thermodynamics of the hydrogen base pairing of nucleic acids.

Short pieces of DNA or RNA called probes, or primers, that contain a specific sequence complementary to a disease-related region of DNA or RNA from a clinical specimen are frequently used for clinical molecular tests. To achieve hybridization of a DNA or RNA probe to genomic DNA for a clinical molecular test, the two genomic DNA strands must be separated, or denatured, prior to probe hybridization. Increasing the temperature of a DNA molecule is one mechanism for disrupting the hydrogen bonds between the DNA base pairs and denaturing double-stranded DNA into single-stranded form. The temperature at which 50 % of the double-stranded DNA molecules separate into single-stranded form constitutes the melting temperature (T_m). The shorter the two complementary DNA molecules are, the easier it is to calculate the T_m. This primarily results from the decreased likelihood of nonspecific intramolecular annealing or base pairing compared to inter- and intramolecular base pairing. The simplest and least accurate formula for determining the T_m for short double-stranded DNA multiplies the sum of the G:C base pairs by 4 and multiplies the sum of the A:T base pairs by 2 and then adds these numbers together:

$$T_m = [4(\mathrm{G:C})] + [2(\mathrm{A:T})]$$

Although this is the least accurate method for calculation of the T_m of a double-stranded DNA molecule, it mathematically illustrates that G:C bonds are roughly twice the strength of A:T bonds. This formula works fairly well for short DNA molecules (i.e., <18 bp); however, as the length of the DNA molecule increases to 100 bp, the nearest neighbor T_m calculation for DNA and RNA is more accurate [16, 17]:

$$T_m = \frac{\Delta H}{\Delta S + R\ln(\mathrm{Ct})} - 273.15$$

where

ΔH = enthalpy of the nucleic acid fragment
ΔS = entropy of the nucleic acid fragment
$R = 1.987\ \mathrm{cal K^{-1}\ mol^{-1}}$
Ct = total strand concentration

For longer sequences (>100 bp), the most accurate formula for calculation of T_m is as follows [18]:

$$T_m = 81.5°\mathrm{C} + 16.6(\log_{10}[\mathrm{Na^+}]) + 0.41[\%\mathrm{GC}] \\ -0.65(\%\,\mathrm{formamide}) - 675/\mathrm{length} - \%\mathrm{mismatch}$$

Table 1.3 demonstrates the effect of increasing the relative amounts of G:C base pairs on the T_m using these formulas.

Intramolecular base pairing also generates complex three-dimensional forms within single-stranded nucleic acid molecules. As a result, the single-stranded nature of eukaryotic RNA molecules affords great structural diversity via intramolecular base pairing. These conformations strain the linear RNA molecule and produce chemically reactive RNA forms. Catalytic RNA molecules play pivotal roles in cellular functions and in gene-targeting therapies.

Intra- and intermolecular base pairing can negatively affect hybridizations. Dimers, bulge loops, and hairpin loops exemplify some of these interactions. Hairpins inhibit plasmid replication and attenuate bacterial gene expression [2].

Table 1.3 Melting temperature calculations for short oligomers

Total length	Number of G:C	Number of A:T	T_m^a	%G:C[b]	A:T+G:C[c]
30	30	0	106.2	100.0	100.0
30	25	5	101.2	93.2	100.0
30	20	10	89.5	79.5	90.0
30	10	20	83.4	72.7	80.0
30	0	30	71.6	59.0	60.0
20	20	0	90.4	88.8	80.0
20	10	10	72.7	65.1	60.0
20	0	20	55.9	47.8	40.0

[a]Nearest-neighbor calculation of T_m [16]
[b]T_m method for sequences over 100 bases [18]
[c]4(G+C)+2(A+T) formula

These detrimental effects also may include initiation of spurious nonspecific polymerization, steric hindrance of hybridization of short stretches of nucleic acids (i.e., 10–30 base pieces of single-stranded nucleic acids, known as oligomers or primers), and depletion of probes or primers away from the specific target by either primer dimerization or other mechanisms. These interactions can result in poor sensitivity or specificity for clinical molecular tests.

Topology

The DNA and RNA molecules assume various geometric shapes or topologies that are independent of base pair interactions. Eukaryotic nucleic acids take on linear forms, in contrast to the circular forms of mitochondrial and bacterial chromosomal DNA. Transposable elements within the human genome also have a linear topology. Viral genomes occur as different forms, ranging from segmented linear to circular, and can be present in the nucleus, cytoplasm, or integrated within the human genome. Although the conformation of RNA molecules can be complex via intramolecular base pairing, the topology of messenger RNA (mRNA) molecules is primarily linear. An organism's genomic topology influences the biochemical mechanisms used during replication and the number of replication cycles a given chromosome can undertake. In contrast to circular genomes, linear genomes limit the total number of possible replication cycles due to progressive shortening of the linear chromosome. In order to mitigate the shortening of the linear chromosomes, the ends of the chromosome contain tandem guanine base-rich repeats known as telomeres.

Mammalian Chromosomal Organization

The human genome contains approximately 3.3×10^9 base pairs of DNA. At least 2.94 % of the genome encodes genes according to the GENCODE reference gene set [19]. However, more protein-encoding genes may be identified if the bioinformatic definition of a gene changes [20]. Approximately, 80.4 % of the genome engages in at least one RNA- and/or chromatin-based activity with many of these bases being located in regions possessing repeated sequences. Most of the repeated sequences are retrotransposons, including long interspersed repeat sequences 1 (LINE 1), short interspersed repeat sequences (SINE, including Alu sequences), retrotransposable element 1 (RTE-1), endogenous retroviruses, a chimeric element (SVA) composed of "SINE-R," and variable number of tandom repeats (VNTRs). The ability of retrotransposons to duplicate and insert within the genome (i.e., either autonomously or with the help of autonomous elements) has been associated with various types of genetic mutations. Mechanisms for mutations include insertional mutagenesis, unequal homologous recombination resulting in the loss of genomic sequences, and generation of novel genes. More than 100 different reports associate retrotransposons with various genetic disorders ranging from hemophilia to breast cancer [21, 22]. Retrotransposons influence transcription of microRNAs (discussed later in this chapter). Because transposable elements can replicate and cause genetic deletions with the human genome, the number of human base pairs is not static. However in germline cells, piRNAs stabilize the genome by cleaving transposable element transcripts [5].

The total DNA is contained in 46 double-stranded DNA pieces complexed with proteins to form chromosomes. The diploid human cell possesses 46 chromosomes: two of each of the 22 autosomal chromosomes, plus either two X chromosomes in females, or one X and one Y chromosome in males. Since the length of each helical turn of a double-stranded DNA molecule is 3.4 nm and consists of ten bases, the length of the total genomic DNA in each cell measures approximately 1 m in length.

For each cell to contain these long DNA molecules, the double-stranded DNA must be compressed. A complex of eight basic histones (two copies each of histone 2 [H2], H3, H4, and H5) package the DNA [23]. The histone complex contains positively-charged amino acids that bind to 146 bases of negatively-charged DNA. Histones fold the DNA either partially or tightly, resulting in compression of the DNA strand. Tight folding of the DNA condenses the DNA into heterochromatin. Following packaging and condensation, the nucleic acid strand widens from 2 to 1,400 nm, with extensive overall shortening of the nucleic acid in the metaphase chromosome. Light microscopy easily permits the visualization of condensed metaphase chromosomes.

Hypersensitivity to DNase I identifies approximately 2.9 million sites with less condensed DNA in the genome [24]. Less condensed DNA binds histone 1 (H1) proteins or other sequence-specific DNA-binding molecules. Some of these DNA-binding molecules regulate gene expression (discussed later in this chapter). In contrast, tightly condensed chromosomes lack the "open spaces" for binding of regulatory proteins and prevent gene expression from highly condensed DNA regions. These proteins also may prevent access to nucleic acid probes or primers for clinical molecular tests. Some tissue fixation methods can create covalent links between the nucleic acid and these proteins that can cause molecular testing artifacts (e.g., false-negative results). As a result, many DNA extraction protocols include a protein-digestion step to liberate the DNA from the DNA-binding proteins. Removal of the proteins facilitates hybridization with short pieces of nucleic acid, such as primers or probes.

DNA Replication

Eukaryotic DNA Replication

The replication of DNA is a complex process requiring specific physiological temperatures and a host of proteins. As mentioned previously, clinical molecular testing methods rely on the ability to denature or melt a double-stranded DNA template. Using chemical or physical conditions, separation of DNA strands can be accomplished with alkaline conditions or high temperatures (i.e., 95 °C). Under physiological conditions, dissociation of DNA strands for replication is accomplished by numerous enzymes, such as helicases and topoisomerases. The region of transition from double-stranded to separated single-stranded DNA is called the replication fork. The replication fork moves along the double-stranded DNA molecule as replication proceeds. At the replication fork, various primases, initiating proteins, and polymerases bind to the original or parental DNA strands and generate two new daughter strands. Known collectively as a replisome, these enzymatic activities generate two new nucleic acid strands that are complementary to and base paired with each of the original two template or parent DNA strands. This replication process is known as semiconservative because each resulting double-stranded DNA molecule consists of one new and one old DNA strand (Fig. 1.3).

Polymerases function to synthesize new nucleic acid molecules from nucleotide building blocks. The sequence of the new strand is based on the sequence of an existing nucleic acid molecule, and the polymerase adds nucleotides according to the order of the bases of the parent strand, using G:C and A:T pairing. The new strand is antiparallel to the parent strand and is synthesized in a 5′ to 3′ direction. Of the two parent strands of genomic DNA, one strand (called the leading strand) can be read continuously in a 3′ to 5′ direction by the polymerase, with the new strand generated in a continuous 5′ to 3′ direction. In contrast, the opposite strand (known as the lagging strand) cannot be read continuously by the polymerase. The replication fork moves along the lagging strand in a 5′ to 3′ direction, and the polymerase synthesizes only by reading the parent strand in a 3′ to 5′ direction while synthesizing the new strand in a 5′ to 3′ direction. Therefore, synthesis cannot proceed continuously along the lagging strand, which must be copied in short stretches primed from RNA primers and forming short DNA fragments known as Okazaki fragments. The new strand complementary to the lagging strand is formed by removal of the RNA primer regions and ligation of the short DNA fragments into a continuous daughter strand complementary to the lagging strand.

Discontinuous 3′ to 5′ replication results in the progressive loss of ends of the chromosomes known as telomeres in normal cells. The guanine-rich telomeres form secondary structures (or caps) that prevent chemical processes that can damage the chromosome. Apoptosis occurs when the number of uncapped telomeres reaches a critical threshold that triggers cell death. Telomerase reverse transcriptase (hTERT) and telomeric repeat containing RNAs (TERRAs) contribute to telomere homeostasis by adding bases to the 3′ end. Mutations in the hTERT and/or the telomerase RNA template (hTERC) decrease telomerase activity and are associated with dyskeratosis congenital, bone marrow failure, and pulmonary fibrosis [25–27]. Telomerase activity varies with cell type with lymphocytes experiencing more telomere length shortening than granulocytes. Telomeres shorten with age with the most prominent shortening occurring between birth and the first year of age, followed by childhood and after puberty or adulthood [28]. In contrast to these age-related changes, some malignant cells retain telomerase activity that permits the addition of these terminal telomeric sequences to the chromosomes, prolonging the life of the cell.

While replication requires many proteins, the polymerase determines the speed and accuracy of new strand synthesis. The rate that the four nucleotides are polymerized into a nucleic acid chain defines the processivity of the enzyme. The processivity of most polymerases approximates 1,000 bases per minute.

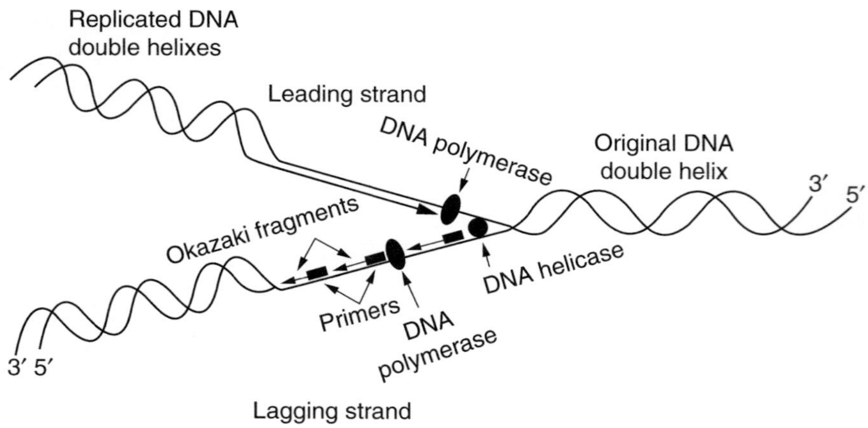

Figure 1.3 DNA replication. Replication fork depicting the leading and lagging strands and the numerous proteins and Okazaki fragments involved with replication. Reprinted with permission from Leonard D. Diagnostic Molecular Pathology. 2003:1–13. Copyright Elsevier (2003)

Table 1.4 Fidelity of various polymerases

Polymerase	Error rate ($\times 10^{-6}$)
pol a[a]	250
pol beta[a]	666
pol gamma[a]	100
Pfu[b]	1
VentR[b]	3
Taq[b]	8
Klenow fragment DNA polymerase 1	8
HIV reverse transcriptase[c]	600

[a]Detectable phenotypic change and heteroduplex expression studies [29]
[b]Forward mutation assay [30]
[c]M13mp2-based fidelity assays [31]

The fidelity of the polymerase refers to the accuracy of the enzyme to incorporate the correct complementary bases in the newly synthesized DNA. Incorporation of incorrect bases or other replication errors can result in cell death or oncogenesis. The error rate of polymerases varies widely from 1 in 1,500 to 1 in 1,000,000 bases (Table 1.4). DNA is susceptible to base pair changes while in the single-stranded form due to the activity of various deaminating enzymes. Many of these enzymes are induced during inflammation and have been associated with somatic hypermutation of rearranged immunoglobulin genes [32].

This DNA editing process may be a mechanism to protect the host genome from viruses replicating within the nucleus [33, 34]. To correct the erroneous incorporation of bases or other replication errors, protein complexes proofread and correct synthesis errors. In normal cells, the cell cycle pauses to facilitate error repair in the G2 phase of the cell cycle (Fig. 1.4). Malignant cells may not pause to allow for error correction, resulting in the accumulation of damaged or mutated DNA.

The complexity of the biochemical reactions necessary for replicating eukaryotic nuclear DNA demonstrates a high degree of regulation for generating two strands from one replication fork. In addition to these complexities, replication in eukaryotic cells occurs at multiple origins. These multiple sites grow progressively until the newly generated strands join to form complete chromosomal-length DNA.

Bacterial and Mitochondrial Replication

The relatively small chromosomes of bacteria (approximately 10^6 base pairs) are replicated by a simpler mechanism compared with eukaryotic chromosome replication. A single origin of replication initiates the duplication of the bacterial chromosome, and replication occurs simultaneously on both strands in opposite directions from the origin of replication.

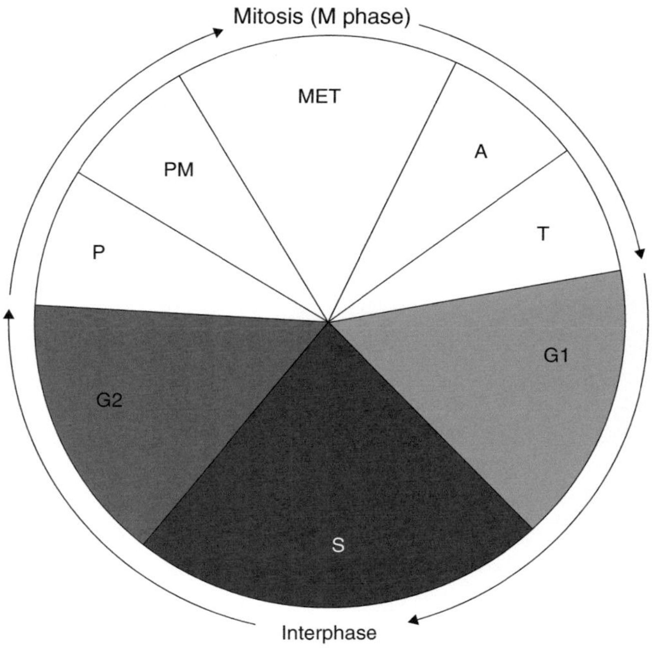

Figure 1.4 Cell cycle. The *clear panels* are the ordered phases of mitosis (M phase), while the *gray* and *black panels* are the ordered stages of interphase. *A* anaphase, *G1* gap 1, *G2* gap 2, *MET* metaphase, *P* prophase, *PM* prometaphase, *S* DNA synthesis, *T* telophase

This efficient replication process depends on the circular topology of the bacterial genome.

Another unique feature of prokaryotic chromosomal replication is the mechanism by which bacterial chromosomes are protected. The lack of a protective nuclear membrane in bacteria makes the chromosome susceptible to attack by viruses (i.e., bacteriophages). As a result, many bacteria produce restriction enzymes that degrade foreign nucleic acids. These restriction enzymes recognize specific short sequences and cleave the bacteriophage DNA at those sites. However, methylation of the recognition sequences in the bacterial chromosomal DNA prevents most restriction enzymes from digesting the chromosomal DNA of the bacteria. Following replication, methylating enzymes add methyl groups to the new bacterial chromosomal DNA, preventing chromosomal degradation by the restriction enzymes. This methylation and restriction process functions as a primitive immune system by destroying foreign bacteriophage DNA before it can usurp the bacteria's replication system. Bacterial restriction enzymes are used to specifically cleave DNA in clinical molecular tests and can be used to identify genetic variations.

Additional types of replication occur in some viruses and bacteria. The rolling-circle mechanism of replication proceeds with an initial single-strand cut or nick in double-stranded circular genomes, followed by replication proceeding from the nick in a 5′ to 3′ direction. The new strand displaces the old strand as replication proceeds. RNA viral genomes use the enzyme transcriptase for replication. In the case of retroviruses, a reverse transcriptase generates an intermediate DNA molecule, which integrates into the host chromosome and then is used for generation of progeny RNA molecules. The high error rate of human immunodeficiency virus (HIV) reverse transcriptase produces numerous mutations in the HIV viral genome during replication [31]. Some of these mutations confer resistance to antiretroviral therapies and can be identified by clinical molecular tests.

Cell Division and Cell Cycle

In eukaryotic cells, the cell cycle refers to the entire process of generating two daughter cells from one original cell, with chromosomal replication as one of the steps. The two parts of the cell cycle are called interphase and mitosis. DNA synthesis occurs during interphase and consists of three stages: gap 1 (G1), synthesis (S), and gap 2 (G2) (Fig. 1.4). Regulation of cell division depends on specific cell-cycle-dependent proteins known as cyclins and growth factors. Some of these factors cause the cycle to progress while others stop the cycle at certain stages. Checkpoints, or times when the cycle may be paused, exist at the G1/S and G2/mitosis (M) interfaces and allow the cell time to repair any DNA damage that may be present before and after replication of the DNA, respectively.

Growth factors initiate the G1 phase via cell surface receptors. Several molecular events such as the dephosphorylation of the retinoblastoma protein and cyclin binding to cyclin-dependent kinases (Cdk) transition the cell toward the G1/S checkpoint. The amount of cellular P53 protein determines whether the cell progresses beyond this checkpoint, with higher levels preventing cell cycle progression. Because various DNA-damaging events, such as ultraviolet light, radiation, carcinogens, and double-stranded DNA breaks, induce production of P53 protein, this molecule serves as a sentinel for mutated DNA. The functional failure of P53 removes this sentinel pause in the cell cycle process and results in the accumulation of genetic errors. Alternatively, downregulation of P53 pathway genes may occur through interaction with the promoter of long intergenic noncoding RNAs (specifically lincRNA-p21) [35]. Therefore, inactivation of P53 facilitates oncogenesis.

Once DNA repairs have taken place during G1 prior to replication of the DNA, the cell proceeds to S phase. DNA synthesis to create a second complete set of chromosomes occurs in the S phase, followed by the G2 phase. Replication errors occurring during the S phase are corrected in the G2 phase, called the G2/M checkpoint. This final checkpoint marks the end of interphase.

Mitosis, the process of physical division of the parent cell into two daughter cells, occurs during mitosis or M phase of the cell cycle. During mitosis, the duplicated chromosomes are physically separated so that each daughter cell receives the correct number of chromosomes. Mitosis consists of five phases: prophase, prometaphase, metaphase, anaphase, and telophase. The duplicated chromosomes condense during prophase. A structural element known as the mitotic spindle originates from two structures called centrioles, which move to opposite sides or poles of the cell and the spindle forms between the centrioles. The nuclear membrane dissipates, proteins form kinetochores on the chromosomes, and microtubules attach to the kinetochores during prometaphase. The duplicated chromosome pairs attach at central points along the spindles. The arrangement of the highly condensed chromosome pairs along an equatorial cell plane denotes metaphase. As previously discussed, highly condensed chromosomes cannot bind proteins necessary for gene expression. As a result, the cell's internal machinery focuses solely on cell division during metaphase. The centriole-derived spindle guidelines pull the duplicate chromosomes apart and drag them toward each centriole during anaphase. With the separation of the daughter chromosomes (chromatids) into opposite poles of the cell and the reformation of nuclear membranes around the two daughter sets of chromosomes, telophase begins.

Cytokinesis, or the division of the cytoplasm, is the last step in cell division. During cytokinesis, the mitochondria are randomly and potentially unevenly distributed in the daughter cells. The cell cycle can then be reinitiated by one or both of the daughter cells to generate additional cells. Alternatively, some cells become quiescent in a G0 phase (between telephase and G1) and either have a prolonged delay before initiating replication again or no longer divide.

Cell division to generate gametes (eggs and sperm) is called meiosis and consists of two divisions, meiosis I and meiosis II. Like mitosis, this process begins with the duplication of chromosomes in prophase I. During metaphase I, the maternal and paternal homologous chromosomes pair (i.e., pairing occurs between each of the pairs of the 22 autosomal chromosomes, the two X chromosomes in females and the X and Y chromosomes in males). Each pair attaches to the spindle apparatus along the equatorial plane of the cell spindle. DNA may be exchanged between the paired chromosomes by either crossing-over or recombination mechanisms during this pairing stage of meiosis I. During anaphase I, homologous chromosomes separate into daughter cells, resulting in 23 duplicated chromosomes of assorted maternal and/or paternal origin in each daughter cell. A second cell-division cycle, meiosis II, separates the duplicated chromosomes, resulting in haploid cells (eggs or sperm) containing only one copy of each of the 22 chromosomes plus an X (egg or sperm) or Y (only sperm) chromosome.

From Gene to Protein

The genomic DNA content is the same in all cells of the same person, unless mosaicism or cell-type specific gene rearrangements are present, and encodes all the genetic information for cellular function, in combination with the mtDNA-encoded products. Encoded in the DNA are the blueprints for the RNA and protein molecules present in any type of cell. Different parts of the genetic information are used by different types of cells to accomplish each cell's specific function. DNA is used to produce RNA which in turn can be used to produce proteins by processes called transcription and translation, respectively. The regions of DNA that encode RNA for production of proteins are called genes.

Replication requires an increase in building materials for the duplicated daughter cells. Highly condensed metaphase chromatin cannot produce gene products because proteins that initiate gene expression cannot bind to the chromosomes at this phase of replication. Regulation of such processes involves some long noncoding RNAs (lncRNA) that mediate chromatin remodeling and X chromosome inactivation [36, 37]. In contrast, partially condensed or unfolded chromatin permits the binding of specific proteins (e.g., RNA polymerases) that synthesize mRNA and tRNA, which ultimately facilitate the production of gene products, specifically proteins.

Some RNA molecules function as the mediators between DNA and protein, while others have a regulatory function (discussed later in the chapter). RNA essentially is in the same language as DNA because, as nucleic acids, RNA can base pair with complementary DNA sequences. Like transferring spoken language to a written form, this process of copying information from DNA to RNA is referred to as transcription. The transcription complex, composed of proteins, must unwind the double-stranded DNA at the specific gene site to be copied into RNA, locate the polymerase binding site on one of the DNA strands, and generate a primary (1°) transcript, which is one component of heterogeneous nuclear RNA (hnRNA) by reading the DNA strand in a 3′ to 5′ direction, with RNA synthesis proceeding in a 5′ to 3′ direction. The 1° RNA transcript is processed into mRNA, and finally the DNA in the region of the gene becomes double-stranded again. Numerous DNA sequences bind RNA and proteins that regulate and coordinate gene expression. These sequences can be used to identify the locations of genes within the entire human genome sequence. Since the generation of the first draft of the human genome, the interest in understanding gene structure has increased with the goal of identifying disease-associated genes [38–40].

Gene Structure

Promoting Transcription

Processed and primary transcripts cover 62.1 % and 74.7 % of the human genome, respectively [20]. Not all transcribed sequences produce functional proteins. In fact, most transcripts serve regulatory functions with many of these being lncRNAs (http://www.lncrnadb.org/). According to the Gencode annotation v7, the genome possesses 20,687 protein encoding genes, 8,801 small RNAs (miRNA, piwiRNA, PASRs, TSSa-RNA, PROMPTs, and tiRNA [see Table 1.1]), 9,640 lncRNAs (linRNA, T-UCR and TERRAs), and 863 transcriptionally active pseudogenes from a total of 11,224 total pseudogenes. Some sequences that bind RNA polymerases in combination with transcription factors to drive and regulate the production of 1° RNA transcripts are listed in Table 1.5. Proteins and transcription factors bind to sequences located 5′, or upstream, of the gene to be expressed which

Table 1.5 Examples of nucleic acid motifs

Name	Sequence
AP1-binding site	TGASTCAG
AP2-binding site	$GCCN_{3/4}GGC$
AP3-binding site	GGGTGTGGAAAG
AP4-binding site	YCAGCTGYGG
C/EBP	TGTGGAAAG
CCAAT box	CCAAT
CP1-binding site	YN(6)RRCCAATCA
CP2-binding site	YAGYN(3)RRCCAATC
CREB	TGACGTCA
CTF/NF1-binding sites	GCCAAT
GCN4 target site	ATGASTCAT
Glucocorticoid receptor	GGTACAN(3)TGTTCT
Homeobox protein-binding site	TCAATTAAAT
HSTF	CNNGAANNTTCNNG
INF-stimulated response	RGGAANNGAAACT
Lariat consensus sequence	YNYTRAY
MALT box	GGAKGGA
NF-1	TTGGMN(5)GCCAAT
Octamer sequence	ATTTGCAT
Poly A signal	AATAAA
Splice acceptor	Y(11)NYAGG
Splice donor	MAGGTRAGT
TATA box	TATA
Translational initiation sequence	RNNMTGG

R=A or G; Y=C or T; M=C or A; W=A or T; S = G or C; N=A, T, C or G are collectively called the promoter region of a gene. Negative numbering denotes the location of these sequences upstream of the first protein-coding codon of the gene. The promoter sequence initiates (or promotes) transcription of the downstream gene and harbors conserved sequences that are recognized by the transcription complex of enzymes.

The complexity and organization of the transcription regulatory sequences of genes differ between prokaryotic and eukaryotic cells. Prokaryotes contain a simple gene structure with sequences for polymerase binding occurring at −35 and −10 for each gene. The −10 sequence contains a consensus sequence of TATAAT, while the −35 region consists of TTGACA. Variations of these sequences as well as the sequences located adjacent to the gene determine the strength of the promoter's transcriptional activity. For example, small differences such as having a TATATA sequence rather than the consensus sequence at the −10 position will decrease the promoter binding to the RNA polymerase and result in decreased production of mRNA for that gene. In bacteria, operons regulate expression of multiple genes with related functions from the same promoter.

In eukaryotic genes, various promoter sequences bind multiple proteins and/or regulatory RNA molecules, which catalytically modify and activate other bound proteins. Enhancer sequences increase the production of mRNA but are far removed from the gene. One of the pivotal proximally located sequences comprises a TATA box (TATAAA) located at −25 (Fig. 1.5). These bases initiate binding of a TATA-binding protein (TBP) within the transcription factor D complex. Following this binding, transcription factors B, H, and E bind to and open the DNA strands downstream from the promoter. Finally, transcription factor F and RNA polymerase II bind to the transcription complex. The close proximity of these proteins to RNA polymerase II permits phosphorylation of the polymerase and initiation of transcription.

In eukaryotic cells, variations in the recognition sequences alter the efficiency of transcription. These variations may be base pair changes or base modifications. As previously mentioned, consensus sequences enable the polymerase to bind and initiate transcription. The strength of the binding is determined by how closely the promoter-binding sites resemble the prototypical consensus sequence. Additionally, the presence of modified bases near or distant from the promoter region also can influence the efficiency of transcription. The two main locations for methylcytosine are CpG dinucleotide islands and regions known as CpG shores that are located approximately 2,000 bp away from the islands. Typically, hypermethylation in CpG dinucleotide islands and CpG island shores downregulate gene expression [41]. Methylation of bases in non-CpG islands and island shores also has been described and is associated with CHG and CHH sites (i.e., H indicates either A, C, or T at the position) [42]. As a result, a gene may appear to be unaltered or intact but may be transcriptionally silent due to methylated bases near to or within the promoter region. In contrast, increased transcriptional activity occurs with gene-body methylation. The proposed mechanism of enhanced methylated gene-body associated transcriptional activity suggests that elongation efficiency and prevention of spurious initiations result from genes methylated in this manner [43]. These are just a few mechanisms used to control gene expression. Additional regulatory mechanisms involve the next steps of gene expression.

Elongation and Termination of the mRNA

Once the RNA polymerase binds to the promoter, transcription begins at position +1 of the gene sequence. The polymerase reads the DNA in a 3′ to 5′ direction, while synthesis of the 1° RNA transcript proceeds in a 5′ to 3′ direction. In bacteria, the complete transcript serves as the template for translation. Transcription ends with a termination process. The mRNA must be terminated in bacteria; termination of the transcript can result from attenuation or the formation of hairpin structures. Termination occurs at several sites beyond the polyadenylation signal in eukaryotic cells and is dependent on bases near the stop codon [44]. Because the eukary-

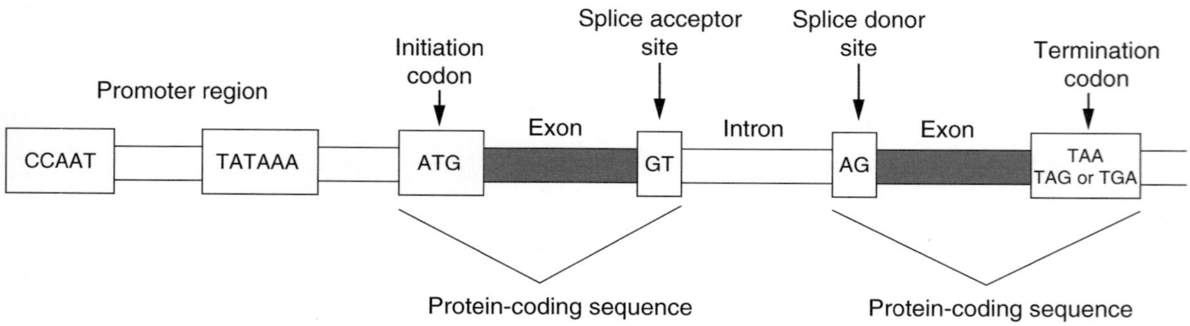

Figure 1.5 Gene structure. Gene structure depicting coding and noncoding regions of the eukaryotic gene. Reprinted with permission from Leonard D. Diagnostic Molecular Pathology. 2003:1–13. Copyright Elsevier (2003)

otic cell transcripts are polyadenylated, termination of transcription by a process similar to attenuation is not necessary to regulate gene expression.

In eukaryotic cells, once the 1° RNA transcript has been produced in the nucleus, this transcript is processed to form an mRNA by splicing to remove the non-protein coding introns (intervening sequences) and join together the protein-coding exons. Introns are located between sequences called exons, which encode the protein sequence and are translated from RNA to amino acids during protein synthesis. Splicing involves a complex of ribonucleoproteins known as a spliceosome, which recognizes consensus sequences at the 5′ and 3′ ends of the intron. Genetic changes to these splice donor (A/C AG G U A/G AGU) and splice acceptor ($[U/C]_u$ N C/U AG G/A) consensus sequences may prevent the spliceosome from recognizing and catalyzing the splicing event [45, 46]. Autoantibodies directed to or alterations in the steady-state level of the spliceosome may play a role in some diseases [47, 48]. Alternate splicing may generate multiple distinct transcripts from a single gene. That is, some exons may be spliced out in one mRNA molecule but retained in another. As a result, alternate splicing generates different RNAs and proteins from the same gene and 1° RNA transcript [49, 50].

An additional mechanism of generating diversity from 1° RNA transcripts entails *trans*-splicing (initially identified in *Drosophila* cells). Essentially, two separate, unrelated transcripts form a hybrid molecule by using the splice donor from one transcript and the splice acceptor from the second transcript. Complementary intronic sequences in both transcripts facilitate the generation of the chimeric mRNA. When the process is used for gene therapy applications, normal gene function has been restored from defective genes using *trans*-splicing [51, 52]. Other therapeutic applications for catalytic RNA molecules involve innovative treatments for HIV-infected patients. In this application, synthetic ribozymes cleave drug-resistant variants of HIV [53–55]. RNA editing involving adenosine deaminases acting on tRNAs (ADATs) changes transcripts that will ultimately produce different polypeptides (i.e., by converting adenosine into inosine which can base pair with A, C, or U). For example, intestinal APOBEC1 deaminases edit a specific residue in human apolipoprotein B (apoB) by introducing a stop codon resulting in a smaller protein in the intestine compared with the liver [56].

Additional modifications of the 1° RNA eukaryotic transcript enhance the stability and transport of the mRNA. One such modification occurs immediately after the generation of the 1° transcript and involves addition of a 7-methyl guanosine linked in an unusual 5′ to 5′ linkage to the triphosphate at the 5′ end of the transcript, also known as the 5′ cap. This cap protects the transcript from degradation. Another 1° transcript modification is cleavage at a polyadenylation signal (AAUAA) near the 3′ end of the transcript, followed by the addition of 100–200 adenosine residues (poly-A tail) by polyadenylate polymerase. Mutations in the polyadenylation signal have been associated with altered transcriptional stability. In the case of the prothrombin G20210A [F2 AF478696.1:g.21538G>A(c.*97G>A)] variant, the change results in a more stable mRNA resulting in a gain of function [57]. The poly-A tail facilitates transportation of the mature mRNA into the cytoplasm and protection of the transcript from degradation by exonucleases. A given gene may have several polyadenylation signals, providing another level of variation for a single gene [58–60].

After the completion of a full-length mRNA, posttranscriptional regulation influences whether the message will proceed to translation. RNA interference (iRNA) is mediated by short interfering RNAs (siRNAs) and microRNAs (miRNAs). While functionally similar, miRNAs differ from siRNAs in that miRNAs are transcribed from a primary miRNA (pri-miRNA). Many miRNA promoters are found in Alu sequences [61, 62]. The 70–100-nucleotide pri-RNA transcript forms a double-stranded hairpin structure which is cleaved in the nucleus by the RNase III protein Drosha resulting in a double-stranded hairpin pre-miRNA molecule. Exportin 5 transports the pre-miRNA molecule to the cytoplasma where the dicer protein further digests the pre-miRNA into a 21–25 nucleotide double-stranded molecule. The RNase III protein Dicer removes the hairpin but its activity is influenced by the size of the hairpin loop. Dicer also acts on siRNA molecules derived from externally introduced double-stranded RNA. At this point, both siRNA and miRNA bind to the RNA-induced silencing complex (RISC). The miRNA-RISC complex aligns with the target mRNA and either translationally represses or cleaves the mRNA. The siRNA-RISC complex binds to and degrades the mRNA [63]. Changes in miRNA expression profiles are associated with the initiation and progression of oncogenesis [64]. In addition, miRNAs also are regulated by epigenetic modifications [65].

Translation

Translation is the next step in using information from the DNA gene to produce a functional protein. This process changes the genetic information from a nucleic-acid-based language into an amino-acid-based language of polypeptides and proteins. For these reasons, the term “translation” describes this complex cascade of events.

Following transportation of the mRNA into the cytoplasm, translation begins with the mRNA binding to a ribosome and requires additional nucleic acids, specifically protein-associated RNA molecules (Fig. 1.6). A ribosome is a complex of about 50 different proteins associated with

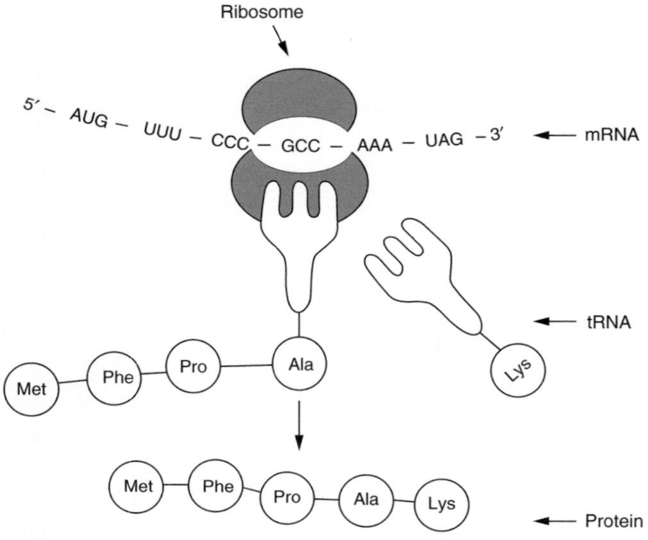

Figure 1.6 RNA translation. RNA is translated through binding events between the mRNA, a ribosome, tRNA, and amino acids, resulting in the production of a protein polypeptide chain. Reprinted with permission from Leonard D. Diagnostic Molecular Pathology. 2003:1–13. Copyright Elsevier (2003)

several ribosomal RNA (rRNA) molecules. Prokaryotic ribosomes consist of 30S and 50S subunits. Svedberg (S) units are the sedimentation rate of a particle. In bacteria, one class of small RNAs (i.e., sRNAs) produce catalytic RNAs, such as RNase P, that process tRNAs and rRNAs [66]. In eukaryotes, rRNA molecules associate with proteins in the nucleolus to form 40S and 60S subunits. Recognition of the 5′ cap of the eukaryotic mRNA by a ribosome initiates the process of translation.

Each amino acid is encoded by one or more three-nucleotide sequences, which are collectively known as the genetic code (Table 1.6). Each set of three nucleotides of an mRNA that encodes an amino acid is called a codon. As seen in Table 1.6, the first and second nucleotide positions largely determine which amino acid is encoded by the mRNA codon, while the third base has less effect on which amino acid will be incorporated. In addition to encoding amino acids, certain mRNA codons are used to initiate (START) or terminate (STOP) translation. The genetic code differs slightly between organisms and between mtDNA and eukaryotic DNA (Table 1.7). Thus, while one mRNA encodes only one protein sequence, a protein sequence can be encoded by several different mRNA sequences. This is referred to as the degeneracy of the genetic code.

Synthesis of the encoded protein begins at the initiation codon of the mRNA, the first AUG codon after the promoter, which encodes a methionine amino acid. This methionine codon establishes the reading frame of the mRNA. The next step in the translation process uses RNA molecules to bridge the information from the sequential three-nucleotide mRNA codons to the encoded amino acid in the growing polypeptide chain of the protein. Another set of RNA molecules, transfer RNAs (tRNAs), contain a sequence complementary to each mRNA codon known as the anticodon. The 3′ end of each type of tRNA binds the specific amino acid corresponding to its anticodon sequence. Base pairing of mRNA codons with complementary tRNA anticodons permits sequential alignment of each new amino acid (attached to the opposite end of the tRNA from the anticodon sequence) with the growing polypeptide chain and occurs in the small subunit of the ribosome. The large subunit of the ribosome catalyzes the covalent bonds linking each sequential amino acid to the growing polypeptide chain.

Translation ceases when the ribosome encounters a stop codon (UAA, UAG, or UGA). Release factors bound to the stop codon catalyze the addition of a water molecule rather than an amino acid, resulting in a COOH terminus to the completed polypeptide chain [67, 68]. Some factors bound to the 3′ untranslated portion of the gene also affect termination. In bacteria, small non-coding RNA (sRNA) molecules serve a quality control role. One group of sRNA are referred to as tmRNAs as they have properties common to both tRNA and mRNA. When translation stalls before reaching a termination codon (e.g., due to a rare codon), the tmRNA provides a C terminal tag which facilitates clearing of abnormal polypeptides and enables the ribosome to be released and recycled back to functional translation [69]. Additionally, some sRNA molecules regulate mRNA utilization through an antisense mechanism [66].

Structure of Proteins

Just as nucleic acids form various structures via intra- and intermolecular base pairing, proteins also assume various structures depending on the types and locations of amino acids. The primary structure of a protein is the sequence of amino acids from amino terminus (NH) to carboxy terminus (COOH) of the protein. The secondary structure refers to how amino acid groups interact with neighboring amino acids to form structures called an alpha helix or a beta sheet. The tertiary structure of a protein is created by amino acids sequentially distant from one another creating intramolecular interactions. The quaternary structure of a protein defines the three-dimensional and functional conformation of the protein. The shape that is ultimately assumed by the protein depends on the arrangement of the different charged, uncharged, polar, and nonpolar amino acids.

Table 1.6 The human genetic code

First base of codon	Second base of codon			
	U	*C*	*A*	*G*
U	***UUU***	***UCU***	***UAU***	***UGU***
	Phenylalanine (Phe/F)	Serine (Ser/S)	Tyrosine (Tyr/Y)	Cysteine (Cys/C)
	UUC	***UCC***	***UAC***	***UGC***
	Phenylalanine (Phe/F)	Serine (Ser/S)	Tyrosine (Tyr/Y)	Cysteine (Cys/C)
	UUA	***UCA***	***UAA***	***UGA***
	Leucine (Leu/L)	Serine (Ser/S)	*STOP*	*STOP*
	UUG	***UCG***	***UAG***	***UGG***
	Leucine (Leu/L)	Serine (Ser/S)	*STOP*	Tryptophan (Trp/W)
C	***CUU***	***CCU***	***CAU***	***CGU***
	Leucine (Leu/L)	Proline (Pro/P)	Histidine (His/H)	Arginine (Arg/R)
	CUC	***CCC***	***CAC***	***CGC***
	Leucine (Leu/L)	Proline (Pro/P)	Histidine (His/H)	Arginine (Arg/R)
	CUA	***CCA***	***CAA***	***CGA***
	Leucine (Leu/L)	Proline (Pro/P)	Glutamine (Gln/Q)	Arginine (Arg/R)
	CUG	***CCG***	***CAG***	***CGG***
	Leucine (Leu/L)	Proline (Pro/P)	Glutamine (Gln/Q)	Arginine (Arg/R)
A	***AUU***	***ACU***	***AAU***	***AGU***
	Isoleucine (Ile/I)	Threonine (Thr/T)	Asparagine (Asn/N)	Serine (Ser/S)
	AUC	***ACC***	***AAC***	***AGC***
	Isoleucine (Ile/I)	Threonine (Thr/T)	Asparagine (Asn/N)	Serine (Ser/S)
	AUA	***ACA***	***AAA***	***AGA***
	Isoleucine (Ile/I)	Threonine (Thr/T)	Lysine (Lys/K)	Arginine (Arg/R)
	AUG START	***ACG***	***AAG***	***AGG***
	Methionine (Met/M)	Threonine (Thr/T)	Lysine (Lys/K)	Arginine (Arg/R)
G	***GUU***	***GCU***	***GAU***	***GGU***
	Valine (Val/V)	Alanine (Ala/A)	Aspartic acid (Asp/D)	Glycine (Gly/G)
	GUC	***GCC***	***GAC***	***GGC***
	Valine (Val/V)	Alanine (Ala/A)	Aspartic acid (Asp/D)	Glycine (Gly/G)
	GUA	***GCA***	***GAA***	***GGA***
	Valine (Val/V)	Alanine (Ala/A)	Glutamic acid (Glu/E)	Glycine (Gly/G)
	GUG	***GCG***	***GAG***	***GGG***
	Valine (Val/V)	Alanine (Ala/A)	Glutamic acid (Glu/E)	Glycine (Gly/G)

Table 1.7 Exceptions to the universal code in mammals

Codon	Nuclear code	Mitochondrial code
UGA	Stop	Trp
AUA	Ile	Met
AGA	Arg	Stop
AGG	Arg	Stop

Posttranslational Modifications

After generation of the polypeptide chain of amino acids, additional enzymatic changes may diversify the function of the protein. These changes are termed posttranslational modifications and can include proteolytic cleavage, glycosylation, phosphorylation, acylation, sulfation, prenylation, and vitamin C- and vitamin K-mediated modifications. In addition, selenium may be added to form selenocysteine. The seleno-cysteinyl-tRNA recognizes the UGA stop codon and adds this unusual amino acid.

Mutations: Genotype vs Phenotype

Genetic information exists in the form of nucleic acids known as the genotype. In contrast, the encoded proteins function to create a phenotype, an outwardly observable characteristic. Genotypic alterations may or may not cause phenotypic alterations. Some genotype changes are called synonymous mutations because the change in the codon does not change the amino acid. Sometimes these synonymous mutations are called "silent"; however, protein function can be altered by a synonymous mutation. Some of the mechanisms associated with deleterious synonymous mutations include exon skipping or alteration of the conformation of the protein by using codons encoding rare anticodons [70]. The mechanisms by which synonymous mutations create phenotypic changes are not clearly understood and make clinical interpretation of these mutations difficult.

Missense mutations refer to genetic changes that result in the incorporation of a different amino acid at a specific codon location. These changes may not dramatically alter the protein if the replacement amino acid is similar in size and charge to the original amino acid (for example, a hydrophobic amino acid replaces another hydrophobic amino acid). However, replacement of an amino acid with a different type of amino acid may significantly change the conformation of the protein and, thus, change its function. For example, in sickle cell anemia, a valine replaces a glutamic acid at a single position and permits the polymerization of the beta globin molecules to cause stiffening and sickling of the red blood cell under low-oxygen conditions. Different forms of proteins (known as conformers) provide the mechanism for diseases ranging from Creutzfeldt-Jacob disease to Huntington disease.

Nonsense mutations describe base changes that replace an amino-acid-encoding codon with a stop codon, which causes premature termination of translation and results in a truncated protein [71]. Truncation may result from the addition or deletion of one or two nucleotide bases, resulting in a shift in the translational reading frame. Frameshifts often result in premature termination when stop codons are formed downstream from the mutation. Alterations in splice donor or acceptor sites may either erroneously generate or prevent appropriate splicing of the 1° transcript, resulting in a frameshift mutation [72]. Genetic changes in the untranslated portions of the gene affecting the promoter, enhancer, or polyadenylation signals may affect the expression of the gene product and result in a phenotypic change. Not all genotypic changes affect the phenotype. Genetic changes affecting the third base of the codon rarely alter the gene code and, therefore, would be less likely to cause incorporation of a different amino acid.

With the sequencing of the human genome, numerous single-nucleotide variants and other types of variants have been identified, demonstrating the individual nature of human beings. Numerous studies currently target correlating genotype variations to disease phenotypes. These efforts, in combination with improved understanding of gene structure and function, promise continued improvement for diagnosis, treatment, and patient outcomes in the future.

References

1. Passarge E. Color atlas of genetics. 3rd ed. Stuttgart: Thieme; 2007.
2. Willets N. Plasmids. In: Scaife DLJ, Galizzi A, editors. Genetics of bacteria. London: Academic; 1985. p. 165–95.
3. Hewitt WL. Penicillin-historical impact on infection control. Ann N Y Acad Sci. 1967;145:212–5.
4. Livermore DM. Antibiotic resistance in staphylococci. Int J Antimicrob Agents. 2000;16 Suppl 1:S3–S10.5.
5. Esteller M. Non-coding RNAs in human disease. Nat Rev. 2011;12:861–74.
6. Virtamo J, Albanes D, Rothman N, Lan Q, Lim U, Liu C-S, Weinstein SJ, Chanock S, Bonner MR. A prospective study of mitochondrial DNA copy number and risk non-Hodgkin of lymphoma. Blood. 2008;112:4247–9.
7. Wen Q, Hu Y, Ji F, Qian G. Mitochondrial DNA alterations of peripheral lymphocytes in acute lymphoblastic leukemia patients undergoing total body irradiation therapy. Radiat Oncol. 2011;6(133):1–7.
8. MtDNA population database http://empop.org/
9. http://nij.gov/topics/forensics/evidence/dna/research/mitochondrial.htm
10. Wilson A, Power B, Molloy P. DNA hypomethylation and human diseases. Biochim Biophys Acta. 1775;2007:138–62.
11. Watanabe T, Tomizawa S, Mitsuya K, Totoki Y, Yamamoto Y, Kuramochi-Miyagawa S, et al. Role for piRNA and noncoding RNA in de novo DNA methylation of the imprinted mouse Rasgrf1 locus. Science. 2011;332:848–52.
12. Phelps S, Malkiewicz A, Agris P, Joseph S. Modified nucleotides in $tRNA^{Lys}$ and $tRNA^{Val}$ are important for translocation. J Mol Biol. 2004;338:439–44.
13. Suzuki T, Nagao A, Suzuki T. Human mitochondrial diseases caused by lack of taurine modification in mitochondrial tRNAs. Wiley Interdiscip Rev RNA. 2011;2(3):376–86.
14. Clark T, Murray I, Morgan R, Kislyuk A, Spittle K, Boitano M, Formenkov A, Roberts R, Korlach J. Characterization of DNA methyltransferase specificities using single molecule real time DNA sequencing. Nucleic Acids Res. 2012;40:1–12.
15. Crick JWJF. A structure for deoxyribonucleic acid. Nature. 1953;171:737.
16. Breslauer KJ, Frank R, Blocker H, Marky LA. Predicting DNA duplex stability from the base sequence. Proc Natl Acad Sci U S A. 1986;83:3746–50.
17. Freier SM, Kierzek R, Jaeger JA, et al. Improved free-energy parameters for predictions of RNA duplex stability. Proc Natl Acad Sci U S A. 1986;83:9373–7.
18. Lewis ME, Arentzen R, Baldino Jr F. Rapid, high-resolution *in situ* hybridization histochemistry with radioiodinated synthetic oligonucleotides. J Neurosci Res. 1986;16:117–24.
19. The ENCODE Project Consortium. An integrated encyclopedia of DNA elements in the human genome. Nature. 2012;489:57–74.
20. Djebali S, Davis CA, Merkel A, Dobin A, Lassmann T, Mortazavi A, et al. Landscape of transcription in human cells. Nature. 2012;489:101–8.
21. Roy-Engel A, Belancio V. Retrotransposons and human disease. In: Cooper D, editor. Encyclopedia of life sciences. Chichester: Wiley; 2011. doi:10.1002/9780470015902.a0005492.pub2.
22. Belancio VP, Hedges DJ, Deininger P. Mammalian non-LTR retrotransposons: for better or worse, in sickness and in health. Genome Res. 2008;18:343–58.
23. Felsenfeld G, Groudine M. Controlling the double helix. Nature. 2003;421:448–53.
24. Thurman RE, Rynes E, Humbert R, Vierstra J, Maurano MT, Haugen E, et al. The accessible chromatin landscape of the human genome. Nature. 2012;489:75–82.
25. Clado RT, Young NS. Telomere diseases. N Engl J Med. 2009;361:2353–65.
26. Kirwan M, Dokal I. Dyskeratosis congenita: a genetic disorder of many faces. Clin Genet. 2008;73:103–12.
27. Armanios MY, Chen JJ, Cogan JD, Alder JK, Ingersoll RG, et al. Telomerase mutations in families with idiopathic pulmonary fibrosis. N Engl J Med. 2007;356:1317–26.
28. Aubert G, Baerlocher GM, Vulto I, Poon SS, Lansdorp PM. Collapse of telomere homeostasis in hematopoietic cells by heterozygous mutations in telomerase genes. PLoS Genet. 2012;8(5):e1002696.

29. Kunkel TA, Alexander PS. The base substitution fidelity of eucaryotic DNA polymerases. Mispairing frequencies, site preferences, insertion preferences and base substitutions by dislocation. J Biol Chem. 1986;261(1):160–6.
30. Cline J, Braman JC, Hogrefe HH. PCR fidelity of Pfu DNA polymerase and other thermostable polymerases. Nucleic Acids Res. 1996;24:3546.
31. Roberts JD, Bebenek K, Kunkel TA. The accuracy of reverse transcriptase from HIV-1. Science. 1988;242:1171–3.
32. Di Noia JM, Neuberger MS. Molecular mechanisms of antibody somatic hypermutation. Annu Rev Biochem. 2007;76:1–22.
33. Suspene R, Aynaud M-M, Koch S, Pasdeloup D, Labetoule M, Gaertner B, Vartanian J-P, Meyerhans A, Wain-Hobson S. Genetic editing of Herpes simplex virus 1 and Epstein-Barr Herpesvirus genomes by human APOBEC3 cytidine deaminases in culture and in vivo. J Virol. 2011;85:7594–602.
34. Vartanian JP, et al. Massive APOBE3G editing of hepatitis B viral DNA in cirrhosis. PLoS Pathog. 2010;6:e1000928.
35. Huarte M, et al. A large intergenic noncoding RNA induced by p53 mediates global gene repression in the p53 response. Cell. 2010;142:409–19.
36. Navarro P, Page DR, Avner P, Rouggeulle C. Tsix-mediated epigenetic switch of a CTCF-flanked region of the Xist promoter determines the Xist transcription program. Genes Dev. 2006;20:2787–92.
37. Plath K, Fang J, Mlynarczyk-Evans SK, Cao R, Worringer KA, Wang H, et al. Role of histone H3 lysine 27 methylation in X inactivation. Science. 2003;300:131–13538.
38. Kochetov AV, Ischenko IV, Vorobiev DG, et al. Eukaryotic mRNAs encoding abundant and scarce proteins are statistically dissimilar in many structural features. FEBS Lett. 1998;440:351–5.
39. Gotoh O. Homology-based gene structure prediction: simplified matching algorithm using a translated codon (tron) and improved accuracy by allowing for long gaps. Bioinformatics. 2000;16:190–202.
40. Olivier M, Aggarwal A, Allen J, et al. A high-resolution radiation hybrid map of the human genome draft sequence. Science. 2001;291:1298–302.
41. Doi A. Differential methylation of tissue and cancer-specific CpG island shores distinguishes human induced pluripotent stem cells, embryonic stem cells and fibroblasts. Nat Genet. 2009;41:1350–3.
42. Esteller M. Cancer epigenetics: DNA methylomes and histone-modified maps. Nat Rev Genet. 2007;8:286–98.
43. Hellman A, Chess A. Gene body-specific methylation on the active X chromosome. Science. 2007;315:1141–3.
44. McCaughan KK, Brown CM, Dalphin ME, Berry MJ, Tate WP. Translational termination efficiency in mammals is influenced by the base following the stop codon. Proc Natl Acad Sci U S A. 1995;92:5431–5.
45. Bruno C, Lofberg M, Tamburino L, et al. Molecular characterization of McArdle's disease in two large Finnish families. J Neurol Sci. 1999;165:121–5.
46. Hou VC, Conboy JG. Regulation of alternative pre-mRNA splicing during erythroid differentiation. Curr Opin Hematol. 2001;8:74–9.
47. Lipes J, Skamene E, Newkirk MM. The genotype of mice influences the autoimmune response to spliceosome proteins induced by cytomegalovirus gB immunization. Clin Exp Immunol. 2002;129:19–26.
48. Seidl R, Labudova O, Krapfenbauer K, et al. Deficient brain snRNP70K in patients with Down syndrome. Electrophoresis. 2001;22:43–8.
49. Garzon D, Yu G, Fahnestock M. A new brain-derived neurotrophic factor transcript and decrease in brain-derived neurotrophic factor transcripts 1,2 and 3 in Alzheimer's disease parietal cortex. J Neurochem. 2002;82:1058–64.
50. Sakata N, Yamazaki K, Kogure T, Mukai T. Alternative splicing of Rh blood group polypeptide mRNA produces a novel transcript containing a short nucleotide insertion on human erythroleukemia K562 cells. Cell Biol Int. 2001;25:697–703.
51. Liu X, et al. Partial correction of endogenous DeltaF508 CFTR in human cystic fibrosis airway epithelia by spliceosome-mediated RNA trans-splicing. Nat Biotechnol. 2002;20:47–52.
52. Phylactou LA, Darrah C, Wood MJ. Ribozyme-mediated trans-splicing of a trinucleotide repeat. Nat Genet. 1998;18:378–81.
53. Phylactou LA, Kilpatrick MW, Wood MJ. Ribozymes as therapeutic tools for genetic disease. Hum Mol Genet. 1998;7:1649–53.
54. Lan N, Howrey RP, Lee SW, Smith CA, Sullenger BA. Ribozyme-mediated repair of sickle beta-globin mRNAs in erythrocyte precursors. Science. 1998;280:1593–6.
55. Mansfield SG, Kole J, Puttaraju M, et al. Repair of CFTR mRNA by spliceosome-mediated RNA trans-splicing. Gene Ther. 2000;7:1885–95.
56. Petit V, Vartanian J-P, Wain-Hobson S. Powerful mutators lurking in the genome. Philos Trans R Soc B. 2009;364:705–15.
57. Ceelie H, Spaargaren-van Riel CC, Bertina RM, Vos HL. G20210A is a functional mutation in the prothrombin gene; effect on protein levels and 3′-end formation. J Thromb Haemost. 2004;2:119–27. doi:10.1111/j.1538-7836.2003.00493.x.
58. Urano Y, Watanabe K, Sakai M, Tamaoki T. The human albumin gene. Characterization of the 5′ and 3′ flanking regions and the polymorphic gene transcripts. J Biol Chem. 1986;261:3244–51.
59. Lin B, Rommens JM, Graham RK, et al. Differential 3′ polyadenylation of the Huntington disease gene results in two mRNA species with variable tissue expression. Hum Mol Genet. 1993;2:1541–5.
60. Boyd CD, Mariani TJ, Kim Y, Csiszar K. The size heterogeneity of human lysyl oxidase mRNA is due to alternate polyadenylation site and not alternate exon usage. Mol Biol Rep. 1995;21:95–103.
61. Zhang R, Wang YQ, Su B. Molecular evolution of a primate specific microRNA family. Mol Biol Evol. 2008;25(7):1493–502.
62. Lehnert S, Van Loo P, Thilakarathne PJ, Marynen P, Bebeke G, Schuit FC. Evidence of co-evolution between human micro RNAs and Alu-repeats. PLoS One. 2009;4(2):e4456.
63. He L, Hannon GJ. MicroRNAs: small RNAs with a big role in gene regulation. Nat Rev. 2004;5:522–31.
64. Calin GA, Croce CM. MicroRNA signatures in human cancers. Nat Rev. 2006;6:857–66.
65. Agirre X, Martinez-Climent JA, Odero MD, Prosper F. Epigenetic regulation of miRNA genes in acute leukemia. Leukemia. 2012;26:395–403.
66. Gottesman S. The small RNA regulators of Escherichia coli: roles and mechanisms. Annu Rev Microbiol. 2004;58:303–28.
67. Gallie DR. Protein-protein interactions required during translation. Plant Mol Biol. 2002;50:949–70.
68. Chavatte L, Frolova L, Kisselev L, Favre A. The polypeptide chain release factor eRF1 specifically contacts the s(4)UGA stop codon located in the A site of eukaryotic ribosomes. Eur J Biochem. 2001;268:2896–904.
69. Barends S, Kraal B, van Wezel GP. The tmRNA-tagging mechanism and the control of gene expression: a review. Wiley Interdiscip Rev RNA. 2011;2(2):233–46. doi:10.1002/wrna.48. Epub 2010; Sep 27. Review.
70. Sauna ZE, Kimchi-Sarfaty C. Understanding the contribution of synonymous mutations to human disease. Nat Rev Genet. 2011;12(10):683–91.
71. Stratakis CA. Mutations of the gene encoding the protein kinase A type I-alpha regulatory subunit (PRKAR1A) in patients with the "complex of spotty skin pigmentation, myxomas, endocrine overactivity, and schwannomas" (Carney complex). Ann N Y Acad Sci. 2002;968:3–21.
72. Valentine CR. The association of nonsense codons with exon skipping. Mutat Res. 1998;411:87–117.

Molecular Pathology Methods

2

D. Hunter Best, Shale A. Dames, Whitney Wooderchak-Donahue, Tracey Lewis, Kelli L. Sumner, Cecily P. Vaughn, Rong Mao, and Daniel H. Farkas

Abstract

Molecular pathology is based on the principles, techniques, and tools of molecular biology as they are applied to diagnostic medicine in the clinical laboratory. Molecular biology methods were used to elucidate the genetic and molecular basis of many diseases, and these discoveries ultimately led to the field of molecular pathology. As molecular research identifies the most fundamental causes and markers of disease, clinical testing of human and pathogen genetic material has become routine in laboratory medicine. Underlying mutations responsible for genetic diseases, including cancers, are being discovered and used in clinical molecular tests. In this chapter, fundamental and more advanced molecular biology techniques, as practiced in the molecular pathology laboratory, are reviewed.

Keywords

Molecular pathology • PCR • Polymerase chain reaction • Sequencing • Primers • Probes • Nucleic acid • Polymerase • Microarrays • DNA • RNA • Electrophoresis • Capillary electrophoresis • Hybridization • Denaturation • Southern blot • Northern blot • FISH • Amplification • Cytogenetics • Ligation • Melt curve

Introduction

Molecular pathology is based on the principles, techniques, and tools of molecular biology as they are applied to medical practice in the clinical laboratory. These tools were developed in the research setting and perfected throughout the second half of the twentieth century, long before the Human Genome Project (HGP) was conceived. Molecular biology methods were used to elucidate the genetic and molecular basis of many diseases, and these discoveries ultimately led to the field of molecular pathology. Eventually the insights these tools provided for laboratory medicine were so valuable to the armamentarium of the pathologist that they were incorporated into pathology practice. Today, clinical molecular testing continues to grow rapidly as in vitro diagnostic companies develop new kits for the marketplace and as the insights into disease that have been gained as a result of the HGP develop into clinical laboratory tests.

Molecular pathology is a natural extension of anatomic and clinical pathology. As molecular research identifies the

D.H. Best, Ph.D. (✉) • R. Mao, M.D.
Department of Pathology, University of Utah School of Medicine, Salt Lake City, UT USA

ARUP Institute for Clinical and Experimental Pathology, Salt Lake City, UT, USA
e-mail: Hunter.best@aruplab.com

S.A. Dames, M.S. • W. Wooderchak-Donahue, Ph.D.
K.L. Sumner, B.S. • C.P. Vaughn, M.S. • T. Lewis, Ph.D.
ARUP Institute for Clinical and Experimental Pathology, Salt Lake City, UT USA

D.H. Farkas, Ph.D.
Obstetrics, Gynecology and Reproductive Medicine, Michigan State University, Grand Rapids, MI, USA

D.G.B. Leonard (ed.), *Molecular Pathology in Clinical Practice*, DOI 10.1007/978-3-319-19674-9_2

most fundamental causes and markers of disease, clinical testing of human and pathogen genetic material has become routine in laboratory medicine. Underlying sequences and variations responsible for genetic diseases, cancers and infectious diseases are being discovered and used in clinical molecular tests. Some have become routine tests in molecular pathology and are described in detail elsewhere in this book.

In this chapter, fundamental and more advanced molecular biology techniques, as practiced in the molecular pathology laboratory, are reviewed. The entire field of molecular pathology is relatively new, having begun in the 1980s and matured through the 1990s. The new century has brought important advances in automated nucleic acid preparation [1–3], polymerase chain reaction (PCR), real-time PCR, deoxyribonucleic acid (DNA) sequencing, genomic microarrays, and, most recently, massively parallel sequencing of large portions of the genome. More and more, the underlying biochemistry occurring in laboratory instruments may be invisible to the user. The goal of this chapter is to describe the principles of these methods so that practitioners have adequate information for instrument troubleshooting and test interpretation.

Gene products, such as proteins and polypeptides, are molecules and could technically be classified within "molecular pathology." This chapter focuses on nucleic acid methods, including investigation of DNA and ribonucleic acid (RNA). The field will eventually move beyond genomics to proteomics. Proteomics is not addressed in this chapter since clinical proteomics is in extremely limited practice in molecular pathology today (see Chap. 61).

Basic Science Discoveries: The Foundation

Molecular pathology techniques are rooted in fundamental molecular biology discoveries of the 1940s–1980s [4]. The clinical laboratory application of molecular biology techniques would not be possible without the discovery by Griffith and Avery that nucleic acid is the genetic material. The foundation of work by Chargaff and Franklin was capitalized on by Watson and Crick, who elucidated the structure of DNA. Understanding DNA structure is seminal to understanding nucleic acid hybridization, which is central to almost all molecular methods used in the clinical molecular pathology laboratory. Additionally, work by Nirenberg (unraveling the genetic code), Wilcox, Smith, Nathans, and others (use of restriction endonucleases for DNA manipulation), Baltimore and Temin (discovery of RNA-dependent DNA polymerase or reverse transcriptase), Britten and Davis (hybridization kinetics), Kornberg and Okazaki (work on DNA polymerases and DNA replication, respectively), Southern (development of solid-phase DNA hybridization, i.e., the Southern blot), Sanger, Maxam, and Gilbert (development of DNA sequencing), Mullis (discovery of PCR for in vitro nucleic acid amplification), and their scientific collaborators and competitors led to a refined understanding of how DNA may be manipulated in vitro for research and ultimately clinical molecular testing purposes.

General Methods

Nucleic Acid Isolation

The first step of most molecular pathology tests is isolation of DNA or RNA from a patient specimen, by either manual or automated methods. Nucleic acid purification begins with lysis of the cells in the sample. Cell lysis liberates cellular macromolecules including proteins, lipids, and nucleic acids. Cell lysis can be accomplished using a detergent solution to break cell membranes and remove lipids. Proteins are enzymatically degraded with protease or selectively precipitated. Protein digestion is performed at about 56 °C which permanently denatures many proteins but does not affect nucleic acids. This process is followed by selective nucleic acid extraction that takes advantage of the physical and chemical differences between nucleic acids and other cellular molecules, forming the basis for their isolation. The nucleic acid is then purified from the soluble contaminants produced in the extraction method by precipitation in an ethanol–salt solution. Variations on this theme that combine extraction and purification are the selective adsorption of nucleic acids to silica columns under chaotropic salt conditions or magnetic bead chemistry. The isolated nucleic acid is resuspended in a dilute salt buffer, for example, 10 mM Tris/1 or 0.1 mM EDTA pH 7.6–8.0 (TE buffer).

The initial lysis step is modified according to the specimen. If the specimen is fresh or frozen solid tissue, the tissue is first homogenized in an appropriate buffer (often TE buffer). If the specimen is formalin-fixed, paraffin-embedded (FFPE) tissue, the paraffin is removed with an organic solvent such as xylenes, followed by rehydration through an alcohol series to a dilute salt buffer before protease digestion. FFPE tissue also is heated during the prolonged protease digestion step to reverse formalin cross-linking between proteins (primarily histones) and nucleic acids. Although this reduces the degree of nucleic acid shearing in subsequent vortexing or centrifugation steps, DNA longer than that packaged into a nucleosome (about 200 base pairs [bp]) is difficult to recover from FFPE tissue. Whole blood specimens may require Ficoll separation and a centrifugation step to separate the DNA-containing white blood cells (WBCs) from the erythrocytes prior to recovery of nucleic acids from WBCs because of the inhibition of PCR by hemoglobin. This blood fractionation step generally is not performed in automated nucleic acid extraction instruments.

Organic (Phenol) Extraction

Nucleic acids have a strong net negative charge because of the phosphate groups in the sugar–phosphate backbone, and thus are highly soluble in an aqueous environment. By contrast, proteins, lipids, and carbohydrates contain varying proportions of charged and uncharged domains producing hydrophobic and hydrophilic regions. This difference makes proteins entirely soluble in organic solutions or confines them to the interface between the organic and aqueous phases during an organic extraction. This characteristic forms the basis for phenol–chloroform extraction, in which phenol is added to an aqueous solution containing cellular constituents, mixed, and then centrifuged to separate the aqueous and organic phases. If the pH of the extraction is near neutral, both DNA and RNA stay in the aqueous phase, while proteins are in the phenol–chloroform phase or aqueous-phenol interface. If the pH is acidic, the phosphate groups of DNA are preferentially neutralized, driving DNA into the organic phase (or interface) and allowing RNA to be selectively extracted. This method produces high-quality nucleic acids but is relatively labor-intensive, employs hazardous chemicals, and produces liquid organic waste.

Ethanol–Salt Precipitation

Nucleic acids can be precipitated in an aqueous solution by the addition of concentrated ethanol and salt. Ethanol makes the solution hydrophobic, while salt increases the ionic strength of the solution, thereby reducing the repulsion of the negatively charged sugar–phosphate backbone of nucleic acids. Centrifugation allows the nucleic acid precipitate to be collected and resuspended in a dilute salt buffer (TE buffer).

Chaotropic Salt-Silica Column Extraction

Chaotropic salts, such as sodium iodide (NaI) or guanidinium isothiocyanate (GITC), disrupt the structure of water, promoting the solubility of nonpolar substances, such as proteins, in polar solvents, such as water. Saturated chaotropic salts also promote the adsorption of nucleic acids to glass or silica columns. Nucleic acids are purified by a series of washing steps including reducing agents, such as sodium azide, to further remove contaminants and inhibit remaining enzymes. The nucleic acids are eluted from the column with a dilute, nonchaotropic salt buffer. Since the method is simple, fast, offered in commercial kits by several manufacturers and adaptable to high-throughput robotic nucleic acid isolation, this method is widely used by clinical molecular laboratories.

Magnetic Bead Extraction

Another solid phase extraction method uses ligand-coated magnetic beads to capture nucleic acids. After cell lysis, DNA molecules are attracted to the ligands on the magnetic beads. The beads are immobilized by a magnet, allowing multiple washings of the bound nucleic acids to remove proteins and other contaminants. The nucleic acids then are eluted from the ligands on the magnetic particles with an elution buffer. Magnetic bead extraction chemistries are widely available commercially, and ideal for automation and use in high test volume settings.

RNA vs DNA Isolation

DNA is the repository of genetic information, which is then transcribed into RNA. RNA is the major constituent of ribosomes (ribosomal RNA or rRNA), forms transfer RNA (tRNA) and messenger RNA (mRNA) which are central in protein translation, and plays a regulatory role in gene expression as microRNA (miRNA) and long-noncoding RNA (lncRNA). DNA is a hardy molecule present at stable cellular levels (with the exceptions of gene amplification and deletion in tumor cells). In contrast, the level of RNA corresponding to a gene can fluctuate dramatically within a very short time in response to changes in a cell's microenvironment and functional needs. This fluctuation results from changes in both the rate of transcription and degradation of RNA species.

DNA is relatively easy to isolate and store because deoxyribonucleases (DNases) are easily denatured by heating or inhibited by sequestration of divalent cations needed for their function. RNA, by contrast, is rapidly degraded by a variety of ribonuclease (RNase) enzymes that are replete within the cell and on the skin surface. While this is necessary for cellular homeostasis, the ubiquity of RNases is problematic for the molecular analysis of RNA. RNases are very stable, active in virtually any aqueous environment, and can regain their activity after denaturation. As a result, RNA is subject to rapid degradation by RNases in most laboratory settings, making RNA a notoriously labile molecule. In addition, RNA is inherently chemically unstable under physiological conditions, primarily due to the spontaneous cleavage of the backbone phosphodiester linkages by intramolecular transesterification reactions involving the 2′-hydroxyl group of the ribose. This contrasts with DNA which lacks the reactive hydroxyl group in its deoxyribose sugar group, resulting in an inherently greater stability. The rate of degradation varies among RNA species, leading to further analytical complexity for the clinical molecular laboratory.

RNA analysis depends on successful RNA isolation and preservation. The overall techniques are similar to those described above for DNA isolation, but with the mandatory addition of steps to inhibit or degrade cellular RNases and prevent their reintroduction into the isolated RNA. RNA isolation must be performed promptly after specimen collection, particularly if RNA quantitation is desired. If RNA isolation is delayed, the sample should be stored at −80 °C, or at an intermediary isolation point in a stable buffer with RNase inhibitors. Scrupulously clean laboratory technique is required, including careful cleansing of laboratory equipment with bleach, autoclaving of glassware, preparation of reagents with nuclease-free water, and wearing and frequently changing gloves. Addition of GITC or β-mercaptoethanol to the RNA isolation reagents inhibits or denatures RNases present in the sample. The isolated RNA is rehydrated in water or TE buffer that is nuclease free, and stored at −80 °C to further inhibit the activity of any residual RNases.

Despite these difficulties, RNA is valuable in the clinical molecular laboratory for several reasons. Many clinically significant viruses, such as human immunodeficiency virus (HIV) and hepatitis C virus (HCV), have RNA genomes. Quantitation of RNA provides an important measure of gene expression, which can be used in the diagnosis or monitoring of disease. In addition, mRNA does not contain introns, which is an advantage when analyzing neoplastic translocations with variable intronic breakpoints such as *BCR–ABL* [5]. An advancement is the availability of blood collection tubes containing a preservative solution that increases RNA stability at room temperature (PAXgene, Qiagen Valencia, CA), allowing a longer timeframe from collection to purification without RNA degradation.

Nucleic Acid Measurement for Quantity and Quality

Nucleic acid quantitation is optional for many protocols that utilize in vitro nucleic acid amplification. Some methods, however, require use of accurate quantities of nucleic acid necessitating assessment of the yield and concentration of purified nucleic acids, which is typically done using ultraviolet (UV) spectrophotometry. The absorbance of a nucleic acid solution is measured at several wavelengths. The maximal absorbance for nucleotides is at 260 nm of UV light (A_{260}), while for proteins the maximal absorbance is at 280 nm (A_{280}). Nucleic acids can therefore be quantified by the A_{260} measurement, while the A_{260}/A_{280} ratio provides an estimate of the purity of the sample. Pure DNA has an A_{260} of 1.0 at a concentration of 50 μg/ml and an A_{260}/A_{280} ratio of 1.8, while pure RNA has an A_{260} of 1.0 at a concentration of 40 μg/ml and an A_{260}/A_{280} ratio of 2.0. Lower A_{260}/A_{280} ratios indicate the presence of protein in the solution. Other contaminants can be detected by their absorbance at other wavelengths, such as phenol at A_{270} and guanidinium at A_{230}.

Ethidium bromide (EtBr) intercalates into DNA strands, causing DNA to fluoresce upon illumination with UV light. The fluorescence intensity of EtBr correlates with the number of base pairs of DNA in which the EtBr is intercalated, which is a function of both the size (length) and quantity of the DNA fragment. Therefore, by staining sample DNA with EtBr in an electrophoresis gel and comparing the brightness to mass standards in adjacent lanes, the quantity of DNA can be estimated. This provides a convenient system for estimation of post-PCR DNA quantity prior to sequencing. More importantly, the image of the EtBr-stained sample DNA can be used to assess DNA quality. High-quality, substantially intact genomic DNA forms a single band close to the well which serves as the origin of electrophoresis. In contrast, DNA degradation is apparent as a smear of EtBr-stained DNA extending downward from the well. EtBr is mutagenic and produces light background staining and, therefore, largely has been replaced in the clinical laboratory by other intercalating dyes such as SYBR Green.

Electrophoresis

In electrophoresis, an electric field is used to separate charged molecules by differential mobility in a sieving matrix that can be either liquid or solid (gel). The differential mobility is determined by the size of the molecule and its conformation, the net charge of the molecule (as modified by pH), temperature, and the pore size of the matrix. DNA, being negatively charged, migrates towards the anode (+) when an electric field is applied to an electrolyte solution. The size of DNA can be modified by restriction endonuclease digestion (see below), rendering DNA fragments small enough to be mobile in the matrix. Nucleic acid conformation can be modified with denaturing conditions prior to or during electrophoresis. Nucleic acids usually are electrophoresed at a slightly alkaline pH to ionize all phosphate groups in the backbone of the molecule, enhancing the negative charge which allows nucleic acids to be moved in the electrophoretic field.

The pore size of the matrix is determined by the composition and concentration of the polymer. For any given pore size, the mobility of a molecule through the matrix is inversely proportional to the log of its size. Therefore, for a given size difference between two molecules, the difference in the rate of migration will be substantially less if both molecules are large. The limiting mobility is defined as the rate of migration through the gel at which large molecules can no longer be separated for any given pore size. This may be related to the tendency of sections of long DNA fragments to "snake" through different pores in the gel, retarding the mobility of the fragment. The limiting mobility of gels can be overcome by using pulsed field gel electrophoresis (PFGE), in which the voltage gradient is periodically reoriented.

Polyacrylamide Gels

In clinical molecular laboratories, the matrices used most commonly are acrylamide and agarose. Polyacrylamide gels are formed by cross-linking acrylamide monomers with bisacrylamide in the same salt buffer used for electrophoresis and pouring the solution in a thin space between two glass plates. A comb is inserted at one edge between the plates to form wells for sample insertion. After the gel has formed, the plates are mounted in a vertical electrophoresis unit such that the gel forms a bridge between two buffer chambers. Samples, controls, and sizing standards are mixed with a loading buffer containing a dye to track the progress of electrophoresis and glycerol to increase the density of the aqueous samples so the samples sink to the bottom of the wells, then loaded into the wells. Electrodes are attached to the buffer chambers and connected to a power supply providing constant voltage. After electrophoresis, the glass plates are separated and the gel is soaked in EtBr (or another intercalating agent) solution. DNA is visualized by EtBr staining under UV light. Polyacrylamide forms very small pores and is useful for high resolution of DNA fragments from 100 to 1,000 bp. However, polyacrylamide gels are thin and fragile, the glass plates are cumbersome to work with, and nonpolymerized acrylamide is a lung irritant and neurotoxin; therefore, alternatives to polyacrylamide gel electrophoresis are desirable in the clinical laboratory. Although more costly, precast acrylamide gels are commerically available to circumvent the biohazards of nonpolymerized acrylamide.

Agarose Gels

Agarose gels are formed by boiling an agarose gel powder until the agarose has completely dissolved in the same buffer used for electrophoresis, optionally adding EtBr (or another intercalating agent), then pouring the solution into a horizontal casting tray. One or more gel combs can be used to form rows of wells in the agarose. After cooling and polymerization, the gel is loaded in a horizontal electrophoresis apparatus and covered with buffer in a single chamber. DNA is mixed with a loading buffer, as described above for acrylamide gels, wells are loaded and electrophoresis performed as described above. Agarose gels have a larger pore size than acrylamide gels. Agarose gels with a concentration of 1 % are used to separate DNA fragments of 1–20 kilobases (kb), while higher concentration gels are useful to separate smaller DNA fragments. Agarose gels are thicker and more stable than polyacrylamide gels but do not provide the same degree of resolution. Agarose is safer than acrylamide but still must be handled and disposed of with care if the gel contains EtBr. Other modified agarose compounds are available that can be mixed in various ratios with standard agarose to increase the resolution of agarose gels. Like acrylamide gels, precast agarose gels are commerically available.

Capillary Electrophoresis

Capillary electrophoresis (CE) is a widely used separation technology for analysis of proteins, peptides, chemicals, natural products, pharmaceuticals, and DNA. CE systems are commercially available and generally provide more consistent and standardized results with less time and effort than gel electrophoresis. Using CE, DNA fragments are rapidly separated with a high-voltage gradient, because the capillary dissipates heat quickly. Therefore, one CE run takes approximately half an hour or less, and if 8, 16, or more capillaries are run simultaneously, the process reduces the time from standard electrophoresis, which requires 3–4 h. This is a significant time savings in the clinical laboratory for applications such as DNA sequencing. CE enables more standardized results, maximization of workforce efficiency, increased productivity and throughput, and the potential for error reduction. CE also uses smaller sample volumes. As such, CE has become the method of choice for most clinical molecular laboratories.

In CE, electrophoretic separation takes place in a capillary tube ranging in length from 25 to 100 cm and approximately 50–75 μm in diameter. Most capillary tubes are made of glass (silica) walls that often are covered with an external polyimide coating. Acid silanol groups impart a negative charge on the internal wall of the capillary. A low-viscosity acrylamide-based flowable polymer acts as the electrolyte solution and sieving matrix within the silica capillary, and is responsible for the conductivity of current through the capillary. Polymer concentration affects the pore size and movement characteristics of the DNA through the capillary.

A small section of the capillary coating is removed at one end of the capillary to create a detection window. The detection window is optically aligned with the detection system of the instrument. The detection system often includes either a diode or argon laser combined with a charge-coupled device (CCD) camera or filter wheel and photomultiplier tube. The opposite end of the capillary and electrode is used for sample injection by electrokinesis. In electrokinetic injection, the capillary and electrode are moved into the sample well. The sample enters the capillary when a voltage of 2–5 kV is applied for approximately 5–15 s. The voltage causes sample ions including DNA to migrate electrophoretically into the capillary in a flat flow profile. Electrokinetic injection produces increased resolution compared to hydrodynamic injection, which produces a laminar (curved) flow profile. After the injection, the capillary and electrode are returned to a buffer reservoir for the separation. The DNA fragments separate by size and charge during migration through the capillary (smaller fragments moving more quickly than larger fragments) and are detected through the window at the far end of the capillary.

In the clinical molecular laboratory, DNA sequencing and DNA fragment sizing and/or quantitation are the most common applications performed on CE instruments. One negative aspect of CE as opposed to older polyacrylamide gel technology is that CE is more sensitive to contaminants and DNA concentration. DNA, being negatively charged, migrates into the capillary when voltage is applied. If there are any other charged particles in the sample, they also are injected into the capillary. For example, salt is an ionic competitor. If salt is present, the fluorescent signal intensity of the sample will be greatly reduced because of ionic competition during the brief injection. Proper sample preparation is therefore a key to successful CE.

After a post-reaction purification step, if needed for the specific CE application, DNA samples are resuspended in a sample loading solution. High-quality deionized formamide often is used as the sample loading solution. If DNA is denatured prior to CE, the formamide maintains the denatured state of DNA and provides a very stable environment for fluorescent dyes. Following the post-reaction purification and resuspension of products, the samples are ready for analysis on the CE instrument. The fragments are injected into the capillary and detected by laser-induced fluorescence, and data are generated for analysis using software supplied by the manufacturer for different CE applications.

Restriction Endonucleases

Restriction endonucleases (REs) cleave DNA at specific nucleotide recognition sequences. Restriction endonucleases are naturally occurring proteins produced by and purified from bacteria. Each bacterial species contains one or more REs, each recognizing a unique sequence of base pairs in double-stranded DNA, called recognition sites (most commonly 4–8 bp long). The natural function of REs within bacteria is to digest and inactivate foreign DNA (such as bacteriophage DNA). The frequency of recognition sites in target DNA for any given RE is inversely proportional to the size of the recognition site. Some REs do not cleave DNA when their recognition sites are methylated; this can be useful in certain clinical laboratory applications such as detection of imprinted genes in genetic diseases or promoter hypermethylation in tumors. Some mutations occur at RE recognition sites and can be detected by a change in the RE digestion pattern of a PCR product or genomic DNA. Unique DNA restriction fragment patterns are generated by digestion with different REs, creating a range of DNA restriction fragment sizes, which can be fractionated and detected using agarose gel electrophoresis. Restriction endonuclease digestion is commonly used as a component of clinical molecular tests.

Specific Methods

DNA Sequencing

The ability to sequence DNA has been essential to the field of molecular pathology because sequence information is a prerequisite for PCR, PCR alternatives, and hybridization with probes necessary for successful Southern blot analysis. The method for DNA sequencing developed by Sanger, Nicklen, and Coulson [6] is the basis for most DNA sequencing performed both in clinical laboratories and for the HGP.

The Sanger sequencing reaction uses a single DNA primer and DNA polymerase resulting in linear, rather than the exponential, PCR amplification (see below). Components essential to the Sanger sequencing reaction include: (1) DNA template that is purified and quantitated; (2) sequence-specific primers, complementary to the opposite strands and ends of the DNA region to be sequenced, which is desalted and usually purified by high-performance liquid chromatography (HPLC); (3) small proportions of dideoxynucleoside triphosphates (ddNTPs) in addition to the conventional deoxyribonucleoside triphosphates (dNTPs) used in DNA sequencing reaction; and (4) an electrophoresis technique capable of clearly distinguishing single nucleotide length differences in DNA strands dozens or hundreds of nucleotides in length. Dideoxynucleotides differ from deoxynucleotides by having a hydrogen atom attached to the 3′ carbon rather than an hydroxyl (-OH) group, which is present on the deoxynucleotide. Because the ddNTPs lack a 3′-OH group, elongation of the newly polymerized DNA chain cannot occur once a ddNTP has been incorporated (arabinonucleosides also can be used as inhibitors of elongation). The end result is a set of newly synthesized DNA chains that are complementary to the template DNA but that vary in length, with the length determined by the point at which the ddNTP was incorporated into the 3′ end of the chain.

In the original paper, four reactions were performed for each template, with the addition of a single inhibitor to each, ddGTP, ddATP, ddTTP, or araCTP [6]. The DNA chains were separated by polyacrylamide gel electrophoresis under denaturing conditions and visualized using (α-^{32}P)-dATP on a radio-autograph. The four reactions were run in consecutive lanes of the gel, and the complementary DNA sequence was determined by manual inspection based on the size of each chain, and the specific ddNTP in the reaction. As sequencing techniques evolved, radioactive labeling was replaced by fluorescent labeling. Two major categories of fluorescent labeling are used for sequencing. In dye-primer labeling, the sequencing primer is labeled, and the sequencing reaction requires four tubes differing only in the incorporation of the specific ddNTP. In dye-terminator labeling, the sequencing primer is unlabeled and instead each ddNTP is labeled with a different fluorophore, thus enabling the entire sequencing reaction to be performed in a single tube. Dye-primer labeling may be used in fragment analysis for detection of microsatellite instability, loss of heterozygosity, forensic identification, or allogeneic bone marrow transplantation monitoring using short tandem repeat polymorphisms. Automated sequencers recognize both the size of the DNA chain and the fluorescent color of the chain to assign the nucleotide sequence, and also function as precise detectors for fragment analysis [7].

Conventional DNA sequencing with polyacrylamide gel electrophoresis (whether using manual or automated sequence detection) is time-consuming and labor-intensive. The introduction of CE facilitated the use of sequencing and fragment analysis by the clinical laboratory [8]. The sequencing reaction products are purified by ethanol precipitation or a chaotropic salt-silica column technique before injection into the CE unit to remove excess salts, dyes, and unincorporated primers that would compete for injection into the capillary. Numerous protocols and commercial kits are available for the post-reaction purification. After the post-reaction purification step, samples are resuspended in a sample loading solution containing high-quality deionized formamide to denature the DNA. Formamide also provides a very stable environment for fluorescent dyes. The fragments are injected into the capillary, detected by laser-induced fluorescence, and rendered into sequence by the analysis software. An electropherogram of the DNA sequence is generated by the detection software by correlating the fluorescent intensity of each dye wavelength corresponding to a specific ddNTP as a function of migration time.

Examples of Applications of DNA Sequencing

1. *CFTR* mutation analysis for cystic fibrosis
2. *BRCA1* mutation analysis for breast/ovarian cancer
3. *CEBPA* mutation analysis for acute myeloid leukemia (AML)
4. High-resolution human leukocyte antigen (HLA) typing for allogeneic bone marrow transplantation

Southern Blot

The Southern blot was developed by E.M. Southern in 1975 and was the first molecular biology tool to have a major impact on clinical molecular pathology. The Southern blot is in limited use, having been largely replaced by amplification methods. Development of the Southern blotting was based on prior knowledge of nucleic acid isolation, gel electrophoresis, RE digestion, and nucleic acid probe labeling for detection of DNA sequences of interest.

The Southern blot is a labor-intensive, time-consuming clinical laboratory method [9]. High-quality DNA is isolated from a patient specimen, subjected to RE digestion, and then separated by size (fractionated) by agarose gel electrophoresis. "Blotting" is the transfer of the fractionated DNA from the gel to a solid support such as a nylon membrane. A small piece of DNA complementary to the sequence of interest for the test being performed is labeled in one of a variety of ways and called a probe. The probe is hybridized to the fractionated DNA on the membrane, and then the location of the probe (and the DNA fragments relevant to the test) is detected using the probe label. This detection step allows the gene of interest to stand out from the vast background of DNA present in the sample. If the banding pattern visualized on the membrane is different from the normal pattern, this may be indicative of a mutation in the targeted sequence. As examples, a more intense probe signal indicates sequence amplification, lack of a signal indicates sequence deletion, and a shift in the band size indicates a change in a RE recognition site.

Because no amplification of target DNA occurs, Southern blot analysis requires a large mass of DNA. Because the banding pattern depends on the specific cuts made by the RE and not just random DNA breaks, the DNA must be largely intact and of high molecular weight. Therefore, electrophoresis of the isolated DNA to be used for a Southern blot test prior to analysis is important for assessing the integrity of the DNA, since only a small degree of DNA degradation is tolerable. Degraded DNA may produce false-negative results if a signal from high-molecular-weight DNA is expected, while false-positive results may occur if partially degraded DNA results in unusually sized bands. Fortunately, most tests in the clinical molecular laboratory today are based on PCR, which is less affected by DNA degradation. Polymorphisms within RE recognition sites also change banding patterns, a principle used to advantage in other molecular tests.

The physical movement of the DNA from the gel to the membrane may be accomplished by manual capillary transfer, automated vacuum transfer, or electrotransfer. DNA in the gel first is "conditioned": depurination with dilute HCl and subsequent denaturation with NaOH. Dilute and brief acid treatment causes hydrolysis of the DNA phosphodiester backbone to occur spontaneously at the sites of depurination. This acid-induced fragmentation facilitates efficient transfer of the highest-molecular-weight DNA species from the gel to the membrane, but does not alter the original size fractionation achieved by RE digestion and electrophoresis. Alkali treatment denatures double-stranded DNA (dsDNA) to single-stranded DNA (ssDNA), essential for subsequent nucleic acid hybridization with a labeled ssDNA probe. The DNA is permanently fixed to the membrane by thoroughly drying the blot in an oven or by exposing the blot to a precise amount of UV irradiation.

DNA probes are labeled before use in hybridization assays to permit visualization of probe–target binding. Note that in reverse hybridization assays, described below, unlabeled probes are immobilized and the target is labeled during the amplification step that precedes hybridization. Probe labels may be isotopic or nonisotopic. High-specific-activity DNA probes may be generated by in vitro biochemical reactions that synthesize new DNA from dNTPs, using the probe as a template. One type of the dNTPs is labeled with a reporter molecule such as ^{32}P, biotin, or digoxigenin. When incorporated into the newly synthesized DNA, the labeled dNTP, even though it is only one of the four dNTPs in the DNA probe, is sufficient to label the entire probe for detection. The probe is used in vast molar excess relative to the target DNA in nucleic acid hybridization to drive the hybridization reaction to occur as quickly as possible.

The blot is immersed in prehybridization buffer to prepare the DNA on the blot for hybridization with a probe. Prehybridization buffer contains blocking agents included to minimize unwanted nonspecific DNA probe binding that would otherwise contribute to high background on the final image of the Southern blot used to view the results and make diagnostic conclusions. The prehybridization step equilibrates the membrane and blocks sites on the nylon membrane without DNA to prevent the probe from binding nonspecifically and increasing background nonspecific signal. A large volume of blocking agent is therefore advantageous. Addition of the labeled probe to the blot begins the hybridization phase of the Southern blot process. A small volume of buffer is used to facilitate probe and target specifically finding each other, thereby promoting hybridization. Hybridization takes several hours to overnight at an appropriate temperature determined by multiple variables: concentrations of the two species; time permitted for hybridization; complexities of the nucleic acids involved; length of the probe and its target and their complementarity to each other (or degree of mismatch); pH; temperature; and ionic strength of the buffer used.

After hybridization, the blot is washed with buffers containing sodium chloride and detergent to remove excess probe and reduce background nonspecific hybridization of the probe. Sodium chloride concentration and stringency are inversely related: the lower the sodium chloride concentration, the more stringent the wash condition. Increasingly stringent washes remove more nonspecifically bound probe. The temperature of the wash buffer and stringency are directly related: high-temperature washes are more stringent than low-temperature washes and further contribute to hybridization specificity. When appropriately stringent washing of the blot is complete, only the specific hybrids of interest should remain. Visualization of these specific hybrids, which appear as bands, is achieved by autoradiography for radioactive probes or by luminography for chemiluminescent probes. Biotinylated probes are visualized by chemical reactions, resulting in insoluble colored precipitates at the site of hybridization on the blot itself that serve as the endpoint (this is also the detection scheme used in the line probe assay; see below). Simple visual inspection of the blot or the radiograph is used for both isotopic and nonisotopic Southern blots to determine the position where the labeled probe hybridized to its target patient DNA. That position, relative to detection of appropriate controls and the distance of migration from the gel wells, allows interpretation.

Northern blotting is an extension of Southern blotting that uses RNA instead of DNA as the target of investigation. Northern blotting is as labor intensive as Southern blotting but even more problematic due to the highly labile nature of RNA. While northern blotting has been very useful in the research setting to demonstrate the selective expression of genes in various organs, tissues, or cells, it has not become a routine tool in the clinical molecular laboratory.

Examples of Applications of Southern Blotting
1. Fragile X syndrome diagnosis
2. Myotonic dystrophy diagnosis

Polymerase Chain Reaction

In the mid-1980s, Mullis and coworkers developed a method, the polymerase chain reaction (PCR), to amplify target sequences of DNA exponentially [10]. As the name suggests, the method is a DNA polymerase-mediated cyclical reaction resulting in amplification of specific nucleic acid sequences. Arguably, PCR is the single most important "invention" leading to the development of a new discipline in clinical laboratory medicine, that is, molecular pathology. Both PCR and the Southern blot are techniques used to investigate specific genomic targets. However, PCR is orders of magnitude more sensitive and rapid, permitting turnaround times from specimen receipt to report generation of 24 h or less. PCR lends itself to much higher test volumes than Southern blotting, a crucial point in its adoption in the clinical laboratory setting. Opportunity for high test volumes, excellent specificity and sensitivity, and the rapid turnaround times of PCR are the principal reasons this technology is used so widely in clinical molecular laboratories.

In PCR, a unique sequence of the nucleic acid of interest, e.g., oncogene, invading pathogen DNA, gene mutation, is chosen as the target for amplification. The inherent specificity of the ensuing reaction is provided by two short oligonucleotides (see Fig. 2.1) that serve as primers for DNA polymerase-mediated DNA synthesis using denatured target DNA as a template. The two primers are complementary to opposite strands and opposite ends of the targeted DNA template region. Usually the primers bracket the area of interest, but one type of PCR (allele-specific PCR; see below) uses primers that overlap the area of interest. Successful PCR depends on temperature cycling, and in the first step of PCR the reaction temperature is raised to 95–98 °C to denature the target DNA, and thus is called the denaturation step. After 10–60 s at this high temperature, the temperature is reduced

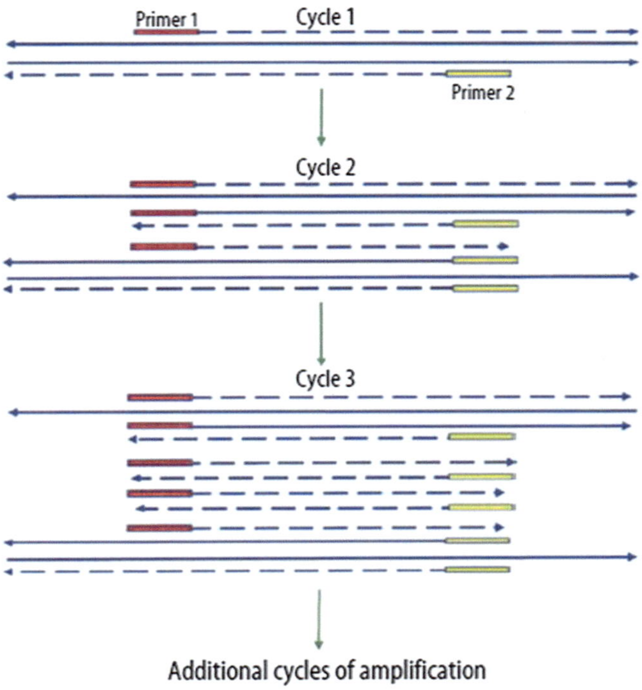

Figure 2.1 The polymerase chain reaction

to 50–70 °C, depending on the specific protocol, and held there for usually 10–60 s. This facilitates hybridization (annealing) between the denatured target DNA and the PCR primers, and is called the annealing step. This hybridization event is favored over target DNA reannealing because the PCR primers are small and present in vast molar excess, and move more rapidly in solution than larger DNA molecules.

The hybridized PCR primers form local areas of double strandedness with the template DNA, thereby serving as sites for DNA polymerase to bind and synthesize a new strand of DNA, using the target DNA as a template and dNTPS present in the reaction solution. Subsequent to the initial discovery of PCR, the opportunity for automating the temperature cycling was realized by using DNA polymerase from hot-spring living bacteria, *Thermus aquaticus* (hence the term "*Taq* polymerase"). *T. aquaticus* thrives at very high temperatures, and so its proteins do not denature at the high temperatures needed to denature DNA in the first step of PCR. Catalysis by *Taq* polymerase of a new strand of DNA proceeds at a temperature intermediate to the near-boiling temperature used for denaturation and the relatively lower temperature used for annealing. DNA polymerization occurs during this extension step, typically at 65–75 °C. Taken together, these three steps (denaturation, annealing, and extension) define one PCR cycle.

Temperature cycling is automated through the use of an instrument called a thermal cycler. Thermal cyclers hold small capped tubes (or 96- or 384-well microtiter plates for larger volume testing) containing the reagents needed for PCR, and cycle among the temperatures needed for the different steps of the PCR [11]. A single PCR tube contains template DNA (<1 ng to 1 μg), *Taq* DNA polymerase, two PCR primers (15–30 nucleotides long), all four dNTPs, Mg^{2+}, and buffer to maintain an elevated pH (8.4) optimal for *Taq* polymerase activity.

The repetition of the cycles generates exponential amplification of the target DNA because each double-stranded target DNA molecule, theoretically even if there is only one, is replicated after one PCR cycle. Both the original and replicated DNA molecules can function as templates for cycle 2, in true "chain reaction" style, generating another doubling, or four copies of the original target. Cycle 3 ends with eight molecules, and doubling continues with completion of each new cycle. This doubling plateaus in later cycles since reagents, usually dNTPs, become limiting. Additionally, the enzyme may not function at 100 % efficiency, and so true exponential amplification is theoretical, although there is a true exponential phase of amplification.

Greater than one billion copies of the original target DNA region are generated after 32 cycles of PCR: 2^{32} or more than four billion, the difference owing to the fact that unit-length amplicons are not generated until the end of the second cycle of PCR. Amplicons (PCR products) are defined as replicated target molecules created by PCR. Unit-length amplicons are those whose ends are defined by the primers. During the first cycle, the primers are extended by *Taq* polymerase using template DNA. The termination of this extension is undefined and a function of how far the polymerase moves down the template during the time allotted by the temperature cycle. The enzyme, therefore, moves beyond the ends of the primer-binding site on the complementary strand. After completion of the first cycle, therefore, the newly synthesized DNA molecules are greater in length than the sequence bracketed on each strand by the primers. In the second cycle, DNA molecules are synthesized from the products of the first cycle whose ends are defined by the two primers, thus generating unit-length or specific amplicons. While all of the above is true, the practical clinical laboratory difference between one- and four billion-fold amplification is irrelevant because either number is sufficient for detection of the target, e.g., by electrophoresis with SYBR green or EtBr used as an intercalating agent for visualization.

Several factors affect PCR specificity and sensitivity. The production of specific PCR amplicons is a function of both the complementarity of the primers to the target DNA and the annealing temperature of the PCR cycle. Heating denatures the primer and target DNA. The temperature at which a primer melts from the target DNA varies directly with the length of the primer and the guanine–cytosine (GC) content of the primer, and inversely with the degree of mismatch between the primer and the target DNA. The melting temperature (T_m)

of the primer is the temperature at which 50 % of the primer is denatured from the target DNA. If the thermal cycler is programmed to reach an annealing temperature higher than the primer T_m, the efficiency of PCR is compromised and sensitivity decreased. In contrast, if the annealing temperature is substantially less than the primer T_m, the primer can bind to both complementary and noncomplementary DNA, resulting in reduced PCR specificity as nontarget DNA is amplified (and potentially decreased sensitivity as reaction components are used nonspecifically). Therefore, the ideal annealing temperature is slightly less than the Tm of both primers, and the primers should be designed to have a very similar T_m. The annealing temperature can be decreased with subsequent cycles during PCR in a process called "touchdown" PCR. This allows the initial cycles to produce specific products at high annealing temperatures, while later cycles amplify previously generated amplicons more efficiently using lower annealing temperatures, thereby increasing sensitivity (see below the use of touchdown PCR in multiplex PCR).

Taq polymerase is very sensitive to mismatches between the primer and the target DNA at the 3′ end of the primer but can withstand considerable noncomplementarity at the 5′ end of the primer. Numerous PCR variations have been designed to take advantage of both these facts. *Taq* polymerase also requires Mg^{2+} as a cofactor for stabilization of primer annealing. Insufficient Mg^{2+} decreases PCR efficiency, while too much Mg^{2+} stabilizes nonspecific primer annealing. Primers with a high GC content may show a narrow range of tolerance for variation from ideal PCR conditions, leading to decreased amplification or nonspecific products. This may be alleviated by using PCR additives such as dimethyl sulfoxide (DMSO), betaine or glycerol, but the success and amount of these additives may need to be determined empirically for different primer pairs. Another strategy to improve specificity is the use of "hot-start" PCR, in which a crucial PCR reactant such as *Taq* is either physically or chemically sequestered from other PCR reagents until denaturation begins. This prevents the generation of nonspecific amplification products by inhibiting the activity of *Taq* at lower temperatures and until after the initial PCR denaturation step.

PCR is more sensitive than Southern blot hybridization because of the amplification of the target sequence. However, the specificity of the amplified PCR product(s) must be verified. Simple agarose gel electrophoresis coupled with intercalating agent staining may be used to observe the PCR product(s). When a clinical PCR protocol is established, such gels may be subjected the first time to blot hybridization with a specific probe complementary to the internal, non-primer sequence of the amplicon(s). This exercise proves that the PCR-generated band not only is the correct size and highly likely to be the correct target, but also is a DNA fragment that has high or perfect homology with a known probe or the correct target sequence. For example, hybridization of a particular 302 bp PCR product band detectable on an agarose gel with a defined cytomegalovirus (CMV) DNA probe confirms that the oligonucleotide primers synthesized based on the CMV sequence and used in the PCR are recognizing CMV-specific DNA and that the PCR is indeed specific for CMV sequence. An alternative method to validate the specificity of the PCR product is to sequence the PCR product. Following this one-time validation analysis, electrophoresis alone may be the assay endpoint, as opposed to blot hybridization or sequencing.

There have been significant commercial endeavors to automate or semiautomate high-volume PCR-based clinical tests. For example, denatured aliquots of completed PCRs can be added to microtiter plates with wells to which specific DNA probes are bound. In the presence of amplicon, if the patient is infected with the pathogen of interest or a specific mutation is present, the amplicons hybridize to the bound probe and are retained in the well during subsequent washing steps. Biochemical reactions are used to detect labeled moieties in the amplicons ("built in" to the PCR components), facilitating colorimetric detection of a positive patient reaction by an automated plate reader. Absence of colored product in a well indicates a negative result for that patient specimen, provided that all positive and negative controls are within tolerance limits. This scheme has gained US Food and Drug Administration (FDA) approval or clearance for clinical PCR-based detection kits for *Chlamydia trachomatis*, *Neisseria gonorrhoeae*, HCV (qualitative), and HIV [12]. (For a complete list of FDA-approved or -cleared tests, go to http://www.fda.gov/MedicalDevices/ProductsandMedicalProcedures/InVitroDiagnostics/ucm330711.htm). Subsequent generations of PCR instrumentation are available that completely automate the amplification and detection processes [13].

Another aspect of PCR that is attractive for the clinical molecular laboratory is the ability to use relatively crude DNA extractions from patient specimens rather than highly purified DNA. Cell lysis and subsequent DNA liberation accomplished by boiling or treatment with detergent may be sufficient to process a specimen in preparation for PCR [14]. Conventional PCR-based tests may be completed with turnaround times of as short as 2–4 h, while real-time PCR can be completed in 30 min, making this technique attractive for rapid clinical testing.

Examples of Applications of PCR

1. Detection of the diagnostic *BCL2–IGH* gene rearrangement in follicular lymphoma
2. Detection of *Chlamydia trachomatis* in urine

PCR Variations

PCR-Restriction Fragment Length Polymorphism Analysis

Polymorphisms are inherited differences found among the individuals in a population at a frequency >1 % of that population. The term "polymorphism" is not synonymous with the term "mutation" which is used for germline variations that are pathogenic and found less frequently in a population, or are nongermline changes in a tumor cell (somatic mutations). In the case of restriction fragment length polymorphisms (RFLP), DNA sequence differences alter RE recognition sites, manifested either as obliteration or creation of a restriction site. With obliteration of a RE site, the DNA of individuals with an RFLP exhibits a larger restriction fragment of DNA than those without the polymorphism. With creation of a new RE site, RE digestion results in two smaller fragments relative to the individual without the polymorphism. In either case, the polymorphism is detectable by creation of a new restriction fragment pattern, that is, a restriction fragment length polymorphism. In PCR-RFLP, the PCR products are digested by one or a combination of REs and electrophoresed to detect polymorphisms or mutations which are seen as changes in the DNA fragment sizes reflected by changes in the band pattern on the gel (or chromatogram).

Examples of Applications of PCR-RFLP Analysis
1. Detection of sickle-cell hemoglobin (HbS) gene mutation
2. Detection of the *Mnl*I restriction enzyme polymorphism created by the Factor V Leiden mutation [15]

Restriction-Site Generating PCR

Some DNA sequence variants create or abolish RE recognition sites and can easily be detected by PCR-RFLP. Unfortunately, most variants do not alter a RE recognition site. In restriction-site generating PCR (RG-PCR) (and a related research technique called PCR-mediated site-directed mutagenesis [PSDM]), an artificial RE recognition site is generated during PCR using a specially designed PCR primer [16, 17]. The primer contains a base mismatch to the template DNA adjacent to the variable base of the variant that creates a RE recognition site in the PCR product. The mismatched base in the primer is located near or at the 3′ end of the primer, which is near or adjacent to the variable base of the variant, and together they create a novel restriction site within either the variant or non-variant amplicon. The presence or absence of the RE recognition site is determined from the pattern of digested PCR product fragments by gel electrophoresis. Not all sequences are amenable to the generation of a restriction site, and the amplification efficiency is often decreased due to destabilization of the primer with the mismatch.

Examples of Applications of RG-PCR
1. Identification of mutations in the *CTFR* gene in cystic fibrosis
2. Identification of mutations in the *ATM* gene in ataxia–telangiectasis

Multiplex PCR

Multiplex PCR is a technique used for amplification of several discrete genetic loci with multiple PCR primer pairs in a single reaction. Multiplex PCR simultaneously answers several related questions about a specimen without the need for multiple individual PCR reactions. Multiplex PCR is commonly used for verification that amplifiable nucleic acid is present in the sample, for example, amplification of a housekeeping gene in addition to the gene sequence(s) of interest, and to check for the presence of PCR inhibitors that can prevent amplification of target nucleic acid, for example, coamplification of an exogenously added internal control. Multiplex PCR often requires painstaking optimization of PCR conditions and careful design of the multiple primer pairs to match PCR efficiencies and to prevent the generation of primer-dimers (PCR products generated by the primers alone due to complementarity between primer regions) and other nonspecific PCR products that may interfere with the amplification of specific products. Touchdown PCR can be used with multiplex PCR if the primer pairs have different annealing temperatures. Concentrations of individual primer pairs may need to be optimized to account for different amplification efficiencies and competition between the primer pairs.

Examples of Applications of Multiplex PCR
1. Detection of enterovirus and herpes simplex virus (HSV) nucleic acids in cerebrospinal fluid (CSF)
2. Detection of pathogenic enteric bacteria in stool
3. Analysis of multiple *BRCA1* loci in a breast cancer patient [18]
4. Identification of different bacteria in a respiratory infection specimen [19]
5. Amplification of multiple microsatellite loci for bone marrow engraftment analysis

Single Nucleotide Extension

Another method for a multiplexed assay is single nucleotide extension (SNE) or single base extension (SBE). In this method, either a single long-range PCR or a multiplexed PCR is used to amplify the region(s) of interest. This is followed by a multiplexed set of extension primers of differing lengths that hybridize one base upstream to the variant(s) of interest. A second, linear amplification, similar to Sanger sequencing, adds the next nucleotide (at the variant position) using ddNTPs, with each type labeled with a different fluorophore. The products are separated by CE or mass spectrometry, and the specific fluorescent signal of the incorporated base indicates which base was added, and whether the variant is present or not. This method can be used to genotype up to approximately 20 mutations at once. SNE and SBE can be considered sequencing, but of just one base.

Examples of Applications of SNE

1. Analysis of common mutations in *GALT* for galactosemia [20]
2. Analysis of common mutations in *BTD* for biotinidase deficiency
3. Analysis of multiple mutations in the *CFTR* gene for cystic fibrosis [21]

Nested PCR

For nested PCR, two pairs of PCR primers with one set internal to the other (nested) are used to sequentially amplify a single locus. The first pair is used to amplify the locus as in any PCR assay. A dilution of the first PCR reaction then is amplified with the nested primers. Alternatively, semi-nested PCR is performed using one of the original PCR primers and one new internal primer in a second round of amplification. Both nested and semi-nested PCR generate a second PCR product that is shorter than the first one [22]. The logic behind this strategy is that if the wrong locus was amplified incorrectly or nonspecifically, the probability is very low that it would be amplified a second time by a second pair of primers. Thus, nested PCR enhances specificity while also increasing sensitivity. The problem with nested PCR is the high risk of amplicon contamination when the first-round PCR products are used to set up the second round of PCR with the nested primers (see Amplicon Carryover Contamination section below for information on PCR contamination control). For this reason, many clinical laboratories do not use nested PCR procedures.

Allele-Specific PCR

Allele-specific PCR (AS-PCR) also is referred to as amplification refractory mutation system (ARMS), PCR amplification of specific alleles (PASA) and PCR amplification with sequence-specific primers (PCR-SSP). AS-PCR is based on the principle that a 3′ mismatch between a PCR primer and the template DNA prevents PCR amplification [23]. AS-PCR is especially useful for detection of single nucleotide polymorphisms (SNPs) or mutations. For AS-PCR, target DNA is amplified in two separate and simultaneous reactions. Each reaction contains an allele-specific primer (either non-variant or variant) and a second primer common to both reactions. PCR is performed under stringent conditions, to prevent PCR amplification if a mismatch is present. Genotype is based on amplification in either one of the reactions alone (homozygous non-variant or variant) or both reactions (heterozygous). Detection of the amplicon is either by gel electrophoresis or real-time PCR technology (see below). A disadvantage of AS-PCR is that unsuspected nucleotide variants located in the DNA template at or adjacent to the 3′ binding site of the primer would prevent amplification, leading to incorrect genotyping.

AS-PCR can detect one variant allele in the presence of 40 copies of the non-variant allele. In addition, AS-PCR can be combined with multiplex PCR using multiple allele-specific primers in the same reaction tube. This technique is known as multiplex ARMS, a useful method when a single disease is caused by different mutations in one or more genes. Multiplex PCR-SSP also is commonly used in low-resolution HLA typing, in which multiple primer pairs for HLA loci are used along with control primers that amplify a housekeeping gene to verify that amplifiable DNA is present in each reaction tube.

Examples of Applications of AS-PCR

1. Detection of multiple cystic fibrosis *CFTR* mutations
2. Detection of common α-1 antitrypsin deficiency mutations
3. Detection of common phenylketonuria mutations

Allele-Specific Oligonucleotide Hybridization

Allele-specific oligonucleotide hybridization (ASOH), also known as dot-blot analysis, is used for genotyping of highly polymorphic regions of DNA. ASOH can be thought of as a variation of the Southern blot, in that patient DNA amplified by PCR is bound to a membrane and hybridized with labeled allele-specific oligonucleotide probes [24]. Reverse dot-blot analysis differs from ASOH in that unlabeled allele-specific oligonucleotide probes are spotted onto different membrane locations and hybridized with labeled PCR amplicons.

For ASOH, the PCR products are denatured and a small amount of denatured (single stranded) amplicon is spotted onto a nylon or nitrocellulose membrane. The amplicon is permanently bound to the membrane by baking under vacuum or UV cross-linking. Amplicons from different specimens can be spotted at different locations to interrogate the genotype of multiple specimens simultaneously. Duplicate membranes are made for each probe type. Each membrane is hybridized with two different labeled oligonucleotide probes (one complementary to the variant sequence and another to the non-variant sequence of the same DNA region). The membranes are washed to remove nonspecifically bound probe. Samples that hybridize strongly to only one probe indicate homozygosity for the non-variant or variant allele; those that hybridize with both probes are heterozygous. The oligonucleotide probes are labeled and detected by radioactivity (often avoided in clinical molecular laboratories), fluorescence, colorimetry, chemiluminescence or mass spectrometry. One drawback of ASOH is the potentially ambiguous discrimination of a positive compared to a negative signal. Optimization of the assay and the use of both positive and negative controls help to define and score ASOH results.

Example of Application of ASOH
1. Low-resolution HLA typing

Oligonucleotide Ligation Assay

Oligonucleotide ligation assay (OLA) is a highly specific method for detecting well-defined alleles that differ by a single base [25, 26]. The target sequence is initially amplified using PCR and then denatured. A pair of allele-specific oligonucleotide (ASO) probes (one specific for the non-variant allele and the other specific for the variant allele), a common reporter probe (complementary to a sequence common to both alleles), and DNA ligase are added to the denatured PCR products. The ASO probes are designed to differ from one another only at the terminal 3′ base. The common reporter probe is positioned immediately adjacent to the 3′ terminal end of the ASO probes. If the ASO is complementary to the amplicon, DNA ligase can covalently join the adjacent ASO and reporter probes. If the ASO is not a perfect match to the amplicon, the 3′ base does not anneal with the template DNA, and DNA ligase cannot join the ASO and reporter probes. The ligation products are analyzed by electrophoresis. Alternatively, one of the probes can be biotinylated at the 5′ end and the other probe tagged at the 3′ end with a reporter molecule such as fluorescein or digoxigenin. If ligation occurs, the ligation product is biotinylated at one end, facilitating capture onto a streptavidin-coated microtiter plate. The opposite end contains the reporter label. Washing removes unbound label and the reporter molecule is detected.

Example of Application of OLA
1. Detection of multiple *CFTR* mutations for cystic fibrosis

High-Resolution Melting Curve Analysis

Melting curve analysis takes advantage of the principle that DNA sequences that are a perfect match will melt at a higher temperature than those that contain either a heterozygous or homozygous nucleotide variant. Typically, in genotyping by high-resolution melting curve analysis, an area of interest (approximately 50 bases, including primers) is amplified in the presence of a double-stranded DNA-intercalating fluorophore or double-stranded DNA-intercalating dye. After amplification, the temperature is decreased to the point that the DNA will reanneal. The temperature then gradually is increased while the fluorescence is monitored. Variants are identified by a change in melting curve shape as compared to a non-variant control. While the typical use of melting curve analysis is to identify single nucleotide variants of interest, it can also be used as a rapid scanning method to detect potential sequence variants in a gene of interest. Melting curve analysis can be affected by factors such as salt concentration and DNA quantity, so all samples and controls must be prepared and amplified in an identical manner to exclude this as a possible confounding factor.

Examples of Applications of Melting Curve Analysis
1. Factor V Leiden genotyping
2. *HFE*-associated hereditary hemochromatosis genotyping

Pyrosequencing

Pyrosequencing is a useful method for variant detection when analytical sensitivity (limit of detection) or quantitation is important. In pyrosequencing, amplified targets are sequenced by adding and detecting incorporation of nucleotides one at a time. First, a target region is amplified and PCR products are captured through use of a biotinylated primer, which has been included in the PCR, along with a streptavidin-coated bead. Capture of the product onto the bead via the incorporated biotin group allows purification of the specific PCR product, followed by denaturation to create a single-stranded target. A sequencing primer close to the region of interest is then annealed to the captured single-stranded DNA amplicon. Deoxynucleotides are added one at a time in the presence of four enzymes: polymerase, sulfurylase, luciferase, and apyrase. Incorporation of the nucleotide releases pyrophosphate which participates in a chain reaction with luciferin, facilitated by sulfurylase and luciferase, to generate light. The amount of light released is directly proportional to the quantity of nucleotide incorporated. Apyrase removes unincorporated nucleotides. If the complementary base is not on the strand being sequenced, then no incorporation occurs and no light is released. The next nucleotide is then added to the pyrosequencing reaction and the steps are repeated. Nucleotides may be added in cyclic fashion (ACGTACGT…) or in an order specific to the target sequence, with allowance for anticipated variants.

Compared to other methodologies, pyrosequencing is particularly useful when analytical sensitivity is of particular concern, such as in detection of somatic mutations in tumor specimens which yield both non-variant and variant DNA. Analytical sensitivity of 5 % can be achieved with pyrosequencing, as compared to approximately 20 % for Sanger sequencing and approximately 10 % for melting

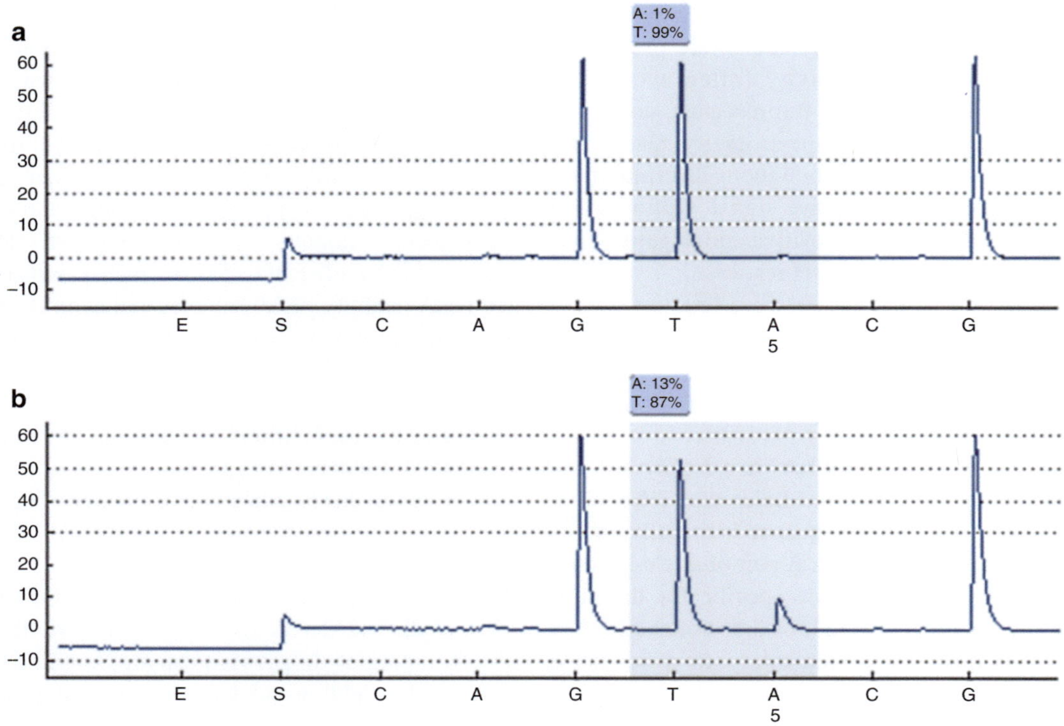

Figure 2.2 Pyrosequencing graphs for *BRAF* codon 600. Nucleotides were dispensed in the following order: CAGTACG. (**a**) Results for a non-variant sample showing the sequence GTG for codon 600. (**b**) Results for a variant sample (V600E), which has alleles with the sequence GAG, in addition to alleles harboring the normal sequence. Variant (V600E) alleles are present in this sample at 13 %.

curve analysis [27]. Quantification of mutant alleles also is provided by pyrosequencing results. Pyrosequencing is best suited for detection of variants within a targeted region. As compared to scanning methodologies, the region of interrogation may be somewhat smaller (under 100 bases, typically just multiple codons), but variants are both detected and characterized. An example of pyrosequencing results for codon 600 of *BRAF* is shown in Fig. 2.2.

Examples of Applications of Pyrosequencing

1. *KRAS* mutation detection in multiple tumor types
2. *BRAF* mutation detection in multiple tumor types
3. LINE-1 methylation

Reverse Transcription-Polymerase Chain Reaction

Reverse transcription-polymerase chain reaction (RT-PCR) may be thought of as RNA-based PCR. RT-PCR was made possible by the discovery in the early 1970s of retroviral reverse transcriptase (RT), an RNA-dependent DNA polymerase, by Baltimore and Temin [28], for which they shared the Nobel Prize in 1975. Reverse transcriptase catalyzes DNA synthesis using RNA as the template, producing a DNA strand complementary to the RNA template, called complementary DNA (cDNA). Complementary DNA is far more stable than the corresponding RNA because it is not subject to degradation by RNase. Complementary DNA can be treated like any other DNA target in subsequent PCR. Logistically, RT-PCR is trivially more time-consuming than PCR due to the extra enzymatic step of reverse transcription, but there are enzymes that combine reverse transcription and DNA polymerase activities, facilitating the use of RT-PCR in the clinical molecular laboratory. With the introduction of techniques to successfully isolate and protect RNA from ubiquitous RNases, to synthesize cDNA by reverse transcription and with the discovery of PCR, RNA analysis is virtually as rapid and sensitive as PCR-based DNA investigation. RT-PCR is a high-volume test method for the clinical molecular laboratory as used for the diagnosis and quantification of RNA viruses in human specimens, principally HIV and HCV.

Examples of Applications of RT-PCR

1. HIV and HCV viral load determinations
2. Detection of *BCR–ABL* translocation diagnostic of chronic myelogenous leukemia

Real-Time (Quantitative) PCR

Real-time (quantitative) PCR is based on the generation of a fluorescent signal by the PCR process, which is detected during PCR cycling, i.e., in real time, and reflects the amount of PCR product synthesized [29–31]. Different real-time PCR methods use alternative ways to generate a fluorescent signal during PCR. These include an intercalating dye such as SYBR Green that binds the minor groove of DNA, or an oligonucleotide used as a primer or probe and labeled with a fluorogenic dye. Instruments that combine in vitro nucleic acid amplification and real-time detection of the PCR product dramatically increased testing options for oncology, infectious diseases and genetics because of the wide range of readily available amplification primers and detection schemes, rapid turnaround time, and reduced risk of PCR amplicon contamination.

Real-time PCR is different from conventional PCR in several ways. Amplicon generation, temperature profiles and melting curves are monitored in real time, reducing the time required for post-PCR analysis. In most applications, post-amplification processing of the PCR products by gel electrophoresis or other method is eliminated. Because the reaction tubes remain closed after PCR starts, risk of amplicon carryover contamination within the laboratory is reduced. Results are more reproducible between runs since quantitation of target is based on amplification cycle threshold in the log-linear phase of amplification rather than traditional endpoint analysis in the PCR plateau phase. Real-time PCR methods have a wide dynamic range, up to 10 logs. Real-time PCR systems with intercalating dye or fluorogenic probes can be used to perform melting curve analysis, adding a check for the specificity of amplification or potentially the detection of unknown sequence variants (see below).

The simplest real-time PCR method uses intercalating dyes that insert into the stacked bases of DNA PCR products, allowing detection of amplification in real time. These dyes, for example, SYBR Green and ethidium bromide (EtBr), are nonsequence-specific dyes that increase in fluorescence when bound to double-stranded DNA. Intercalating dyes are used for melting curve analysis, qualitative and semiquantitative PCR, product discrimination and purity, and determination of primer and probe melting T_m. Intercalating dyes can be used for quantitative PCR. Results, however, are more specific and accurate with a sequence-specific probe for real time monitoring of amplicon production since fluorescence is directly proportional to the amount of specific amplicon produced which reduces the background contributed by primer-dimers or nonspecific PCR products. Intercalating dye fluorescence represents all double-stranded DNA, including primer-dimers and other nonspecific products that can be visualized with an endpoint melting curve analysis.

Most fluorogenic oligonucleotide techniques take advantage of the principle of fluorescent resonance energy transfer (FRET), in which the energy from one dye molecule (the donor) is transferred without the emission of a photon to an acceptor dye molecule when the two are in close proximity. If the acceptor is a fluorophore, a photon is emitted at a characteristic wavelength. However, if the acceptor does not emit a photon, the energy is dissipated and fluorescence from the donor is quenched. The reporter dye can be either the donor (if no FRET takes place) or the acceptor (if FRET does take place) and is defined as the one whose fluorescence correlates with the quantity of desired PCR amplicon. Several fluorogenic techniques are described below.

TaqMan

The TaqMan technique uses a short probe complementary to a non-primer internal sequence of the PCR product. The probe is labeled at the 5′ end with a reporter donor dye and at the 3′ end with an acceptor dye that quenches the reporter when the probe is intact. During the extension phase of PCR, probe bound to an amplicon is cleaved by the 5′ endonuclease activity of *Taq* polymerase, freeing the reporter dye from the quencher and resulting in fluorescence. The fluorescent signal increases proportionally to the number of amplicons generated during the log-linear phase of amplification. To ensure that hydrolysis of the probe occurs, a two-step PCR can be used with annealing and extension taking place at the same temperature (approximately 60 °C). Ideally, the TaqMan probe binding site is located near one primer and the size of the amplicon is no longer than 200–300 bases. One negative aspect of this method is that once the probe is hydrolyzed, it is unavailable for subsequent reactions or melting curve analysis, thus requiring an excess amount of probe in the reaction mix with the potential to decrease the PCR efficiency.

Molecular Beacon

A molecular beacon is a probe with a 5′ reporter dye and 3′ quencher dye, which forms a hairpin loop structure when not bound to target DNA, thereby juxtaposing the reporter and quencher dyes with quenching of fluorescence. The loop sequence is complementary to the non-primer amplicon sequence. When the loop of the molecular beacon probe hybridizes to the amplicon during the annealing step of real-time PCR, the reporter dye is separated from the quencher, resulting in fluorescence. For the molecular beacon probe to anneal to the amplicon, the amplicon-probe hybrid must be more stable than the internal base-pairing stem of the hairpin so that a fluorescent signal is generated. Generally, DABCYL is the nonfluorescent universal quencher and the other dye is a reporter fluorophore such as FAM, Cy3, TET, TAMRA, Texas Red, ROX, or Cy5.

Hybridization

Hybridization is typically a two-probe system in which one probe contains a donor dye and the other contains the reporter acceptor dye. The probes are designed to anneal to one strand of the PCR product adjacent to one another and internal to the primers. This juxtaposes the dyes, allowing FRET to occur. This probe format works well with the traditional three-step PCR with annealing at approximately 55 °C (primer specific) and extension at 72 °C, the optimal temperature for *Taq* polymerase activity. When DNA polymerase encounters the probes, they are displaced from the target strand rather than hydrolyzed and thus are available for the next round of amplification as well as endpoint melting curve analysis. In a variation of this method, a single unlabeled probe may be used in conjunction with an intercalating dye.

Uniprimer (Amplifluor, Sunrise)

Like molecular beacon probes, the uniprimer system uses a hairpin structure in the probe to quench fluorescence. The 3′ region of the fluorogenic probe is identical to a nonbinding region at the 5′ end of the reverse PCR primer. This allows the fluorogenic probe to become a primer for the newly formed amplicon by the third round of PCR. The probe is then opened in the fourth and subsequent rounds of PCR by the polymerase action of *Taq*, allowing fluorescence to occur. The advantage of this system is that the same fluorogenic probe sequence can be used in any PCR reaction (universal fluorogenic primer).

Scorpion

Scorpion also uses a hairpin structure in the probe to quench fluorescence. The fluorogenic probe is part of the reverse primer, and the nucleotides in the hairpin are complementary to the PCR amplicon sequence between the primers. The Scorpion probe unfolds and anneals to the PCR amplicon, allowing fluorescence to take place beginning in the first round of PCR.

Lux

Lux is a variation of real-time PCR that uses a single fluorophore in a primer with a hairpin loop structure. The fluorophore is quenched by the complementary structure of nucleotides in the stem of the hairpin. When the primer is incorporated into double-stranded DNA, thus opening the hairpin, fluorescence is maximal. The advantage of this system is lower production costs with the use of only one fluorophore.

The following concepts are important for understanding the use of real-time PCR in a clinical molecular laboratory. When optimizing real-time PCR, the amplification curve of the fluorescent signal vs the number of PCR cycles should be monitored to determine when optimal conditions have been achieved. The amplification curve should be sigmoidal (S shaped) with three phases: baseline (background signal or lag phase), log-linear (exponential amplification phase), and plateau. For each phase, several characteristics should be assessed. The baseline phase of the curve represents initial cycles of amplification in which accumulation of the specific signal has not yet exceeded the background signal. The fluorescent signal in this phase is from unbound probe or autofluorescing components in the reaction. The log-linear phase of the curve represents exponential amplification of the target and provides useful information about the reaction. The curve can be described by the following equation: $Tn = T_0(E)n$, where Tn is the amount of target sequence at cycle n, T_0 is the initial amount of target sequence at cycle 0, and E is the amplification efficiency of the target sequence. The crossing point represents the number of PCR cycles at which the amplification curve enters the log-linear phase. There is an inverse linear relationship between the crossing-point cycle number and the number of template copies present in a reaction.

The slope of the log-linear phase is a reflection of amplification efficiency, and the efficiency of the reaction can be determined by identifying the crossing points of known standards and plotting a line of linear regression (Fig. 2.3). The efficiency can then be determined using the following equation: $E = 10^{-1/\text{slope}}$, where E is efficiency and slope is the slope of the standard curve. Using this equation, the slope should be between -3 and -4, with -3.3 indicative of efficiency close to or at 2. The inflection point of the amplification curve is the point at which the log-linear amplification curve goes from positive to negative and begins to enter the plateau phase. If there is no inflection point, the curve may represent not amplification of DNA, but rather signal drift. Drift is characterized by gradual increase or decrease in fluorescence without amplification of product.

Plateau is defined as the phase of amplification when critical components of the PCR become rate limiting and amplicon accumulation is minimized or stops. The plateau is also the point at which incremental increase in fluorescent signal stops. As the rate of accumulation slows and enters the plateau phase, the curve levels. Since endpoint measurements often are made in conventional PCR when reaction components are limited, minor sample variations can have a relatively major effect on endpoint product production. The plateau phase can be shortened by decreasing the number of PCR cycles for reduced nonspecific amplicon production.

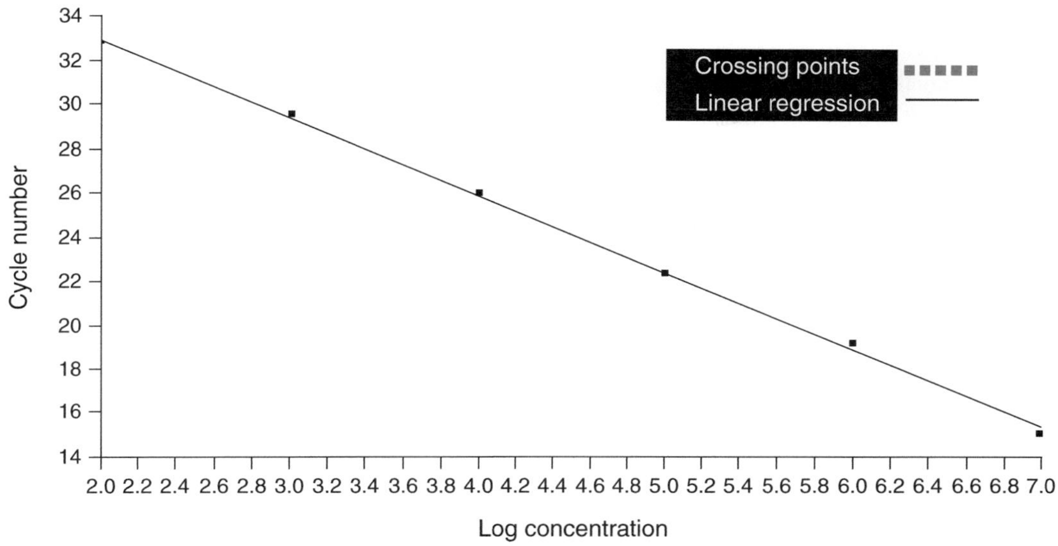

Figure 2.3 Standard curve generated from results of real-time PCR of a tenfold dilution series of a known standard

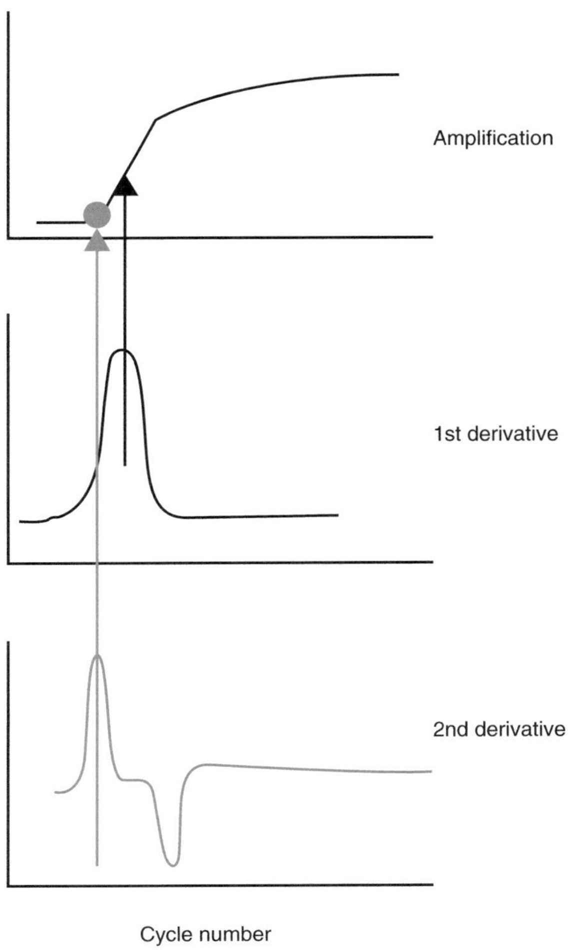

Figure 2.4 Graphical depiction of the second derivative maximum method used to identify the crossing point (*Y* axis is fluorescence value)

Several factors contribute to the plateau phase: PCR product reannealing vs primer annealing, enzyme or dNTPs becoming limiting, and amplicon buildup with resultant reaction inhibition.

In real-time PCR, the log-linear phase of the amplification curve is used for data analysis and provides a more accurate measurement than endpoint analysis. The cycle at which the curve crosses a specified threshold is called the cycle threshold (C_t), or crossing point (C_p). The C_t value can be used for qualitative or quantitative analysis. A qualitative analysis uses the defined C_t as a pass/fail measurement. A quantitative assay uses the C_t of defined standards of known template concentration to generate a standard curve. Then, the C_t values for unknown samples are used to extrapolate the concentration(s) in the unknown samples from the standard curve. Some commercial real-time PCR software allows determination of the C_t by a mathematical analysis of the amplification curve, rather than crossing at a set fluorescent signal threshold. Plotting the second derivative of the amplification curve generates a peak that corresponds to a point near the baseline of the growth curve (see Fig. 2.4). The cycle at which this peak occurs is designated as the C_t or C_P. This analysis method can provide better run-to-run reproducibility than manually setting the C_t using the primary signal.

DNA Methylation and Methylation-Specific PCR

DNA methylation is a mechanism by which the cell regulates gene expression. Methylation is an enzyme-mediated modification that adds a methyl (-CH_3) group at a selected site on

DNA or RNA. In humans, methylation occurs only at cytosine (C) bases adjacent to a guanine (G) base, known as CpG dinucleotides. CpG dinucleotides are prone to spontaneous mutation and have been selectively depleted from the mammalian genome. However, some regions of DNA contain CpG dinucleotides and are referred to as CpG islands. CpG islands are found primarily in the 5′ region of expressed genes, often in association with promoters. When the promoter CpG island is methylated, the corresponding gene is silenced and transcription does not occur. This is one method of silencing imprinted genes, as the methylation pattern and resulting transcription repression is passed on through cell divisions. Aberrant CpG island methylation of tumor-suppressor genes is frequent in cancer and appears to be an important mechanism of neoplastic transformation.

Methylated DNA can be distinguished from unmethylated DNA using sodium bisulfite treatment of DNA, which converts unmethylated C to uracil (U) but leaves methylated C intact [32]. This in vitro treatment can be assessed by one of several methods to distinguish C from U, including restriction endonuclease digestion with methylation-sensitive enzymes, sequencing, or methylation-specific PCR (MSP) [33]. In MSP of bisulfite-treated DNA, primer pairs that specifically identify either methylated or unmethylated DNA are used. The primers are designed to hybridize to regions containing one to three CpG sites concentrated in the 3′ region of the primer to increase amplification specificity, and enough non-CpG cytosines to ensure that unmodified DNA is not amplified. Gel electrophoresis is used to detect the presence or absence of the amplicon in each of the two reactions, indicating the presence of unmethylated or methylated alleles or both. A modification of quantitative MSP combines MSP with real-time PCR to distinguish the high-level CpG methylation in neoplasia from low-level methylation that can occur with aging or in nonneoplastic conditions such as metaplasia [34].

Examples of Applications of Methylation-Specific PCR

1. Analysis of imprinted genes in Prader–Willi and Angelman Syndromes
2. Clonality assessment based on X chromosome inactivation
3. Abnormal methylation in neoplasia

Mass Spectrometry

Mass spectrometry (MS) is a flexible platform for variant and target detection for clinical laboratory applications. In preparation for MS-based detection, a variety of PCR methods such as SNE can be adopted. PCR is performed to amplify the region(s) of interest, then products are enzymatically treated, diluted and/or cleaned to remove unincorporated dNTPs and reduce salts which could interfere with analysis. During MS analysis of the PCR products, samples are ionized, then separated based on their mass-to-charge ratios. The ions are detected after laser desorption with a nitrogen laser. Mass spectra of PCR products are obtained by detecting positive ions of the nucleic acids. Differences in mass due to nucleotide base changes can be detected [21]. Mass spectrometry can detect low levels of sequence variations useful for detecting mosaicism, somatic changes in a normal background and heteroplasmy in mitochondrial DNA.

Example of Application of Mass Spectrometry

1. Cystic fibrosis carrier testing

Multiplex Ligation-Dependent Probe Amplification (MLPA)

Deletions and duplications of single or multiple exons in specific genes are associated with many human diseases (reviewed in ref. 35). Although partial gene deletions or duplications account for less than 10 % of all disease-causing mutations for most hereditary conditions, some disorders can have deletion or duplication rates of 10–30 % or higher [36–44]. Multiplex Ligation-dependent Probe Amplification (MLPA, MRC Holland, Amsterdam, The Netherlands) is a semi-quantitative method used to detect abnormal copy numbers at an exon level resolution and has a high multiplexing capability [45]. The inclusion of MLPA in the clinical molecular laboratory can significantly increase the detection rate of many genetic disorders. Typically, MLPA kits contain a mixture of exon-specific probes targeted to the gene of interest and control probes that hybridize to other genomic areas.

In MLPA, DNA is denatured and incubated overnight with a mixture of probes that consist of two immediately adjacent oligonucleotides per target exon, each containing one of the PCR primer sequences (Fig. 2.5a). After hybridization, probes are ligated and the fragments are amplified by PCR using dye-tagged universal primers. Probes that are not ligated contain only one primer sequence and cannot be amplified to generate a signal. Amplification products that are typically between 130 and 480 bp in length, are separated by size using CE (Fig. 2.5a). The number of probe ligation products directly correlates to the number of target sequences in the sample. Deletions and duplications of the targeted regions are detected when the height ratios of the fluorescent peaks are lower or higher than the normal height ratio range of 0.7–1.4, respectively. An example of a large gene deletion where the deleted probes fall below the lower normal peak height ratio range of 0.7 is shown in Fig. 2.5b.

Several variations on the traditional MLPA procedure have been developed. One example is reverse transcriptase

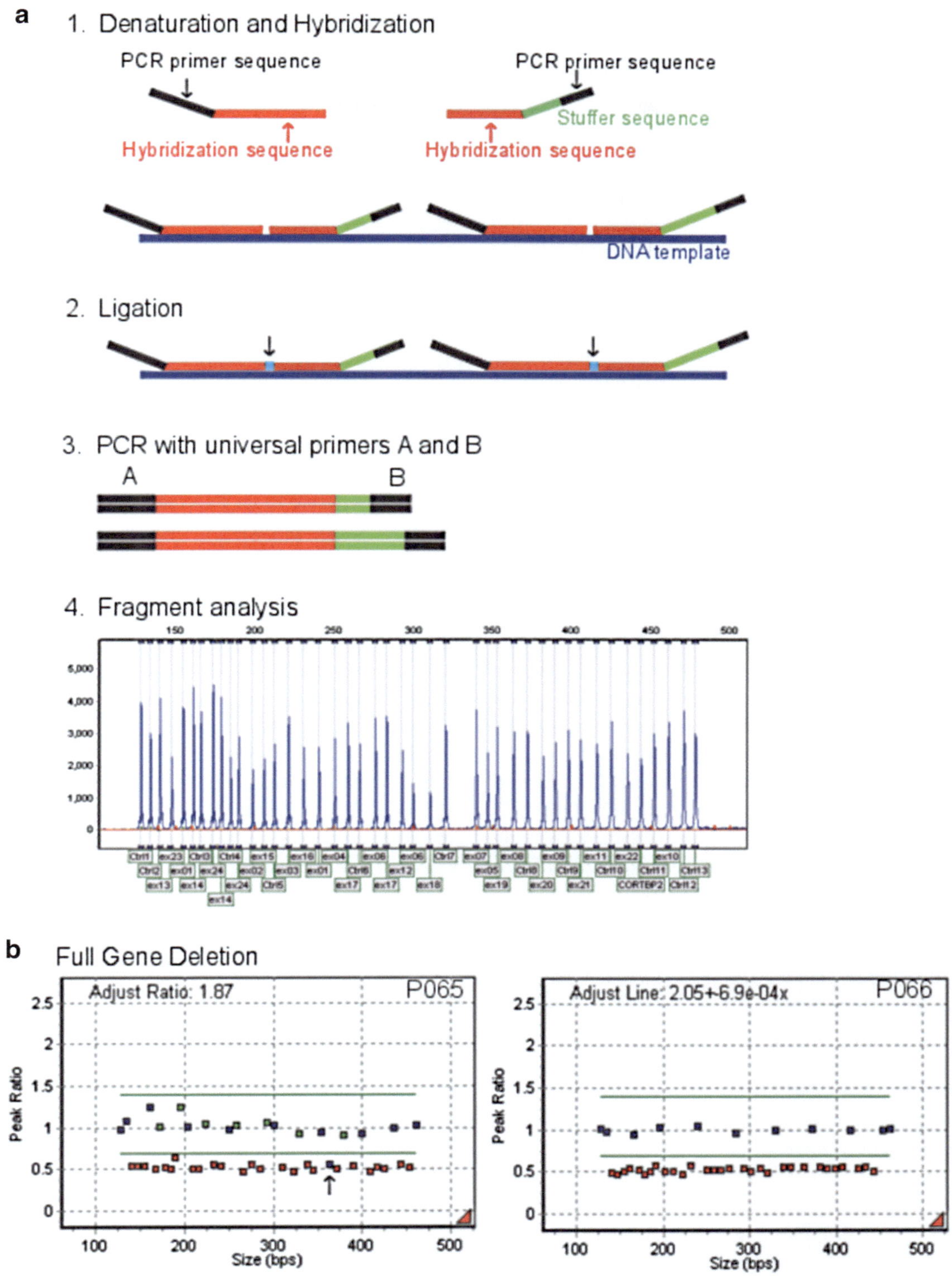

Figure 2.5 Multiplex Ligation-Dependent Probe Amplification (MLPA). In (**a**), the process of MLPA is shown. First, DNA template (*blue*) is denatured and then allowed to hybridize to exon specific probe hybridization sequences (*red*) which are targeted to the gene of interest. Adjacent probes are ligated together, and only ligated probes are amplified using universal primers A and B. Fragment analysis is used to separate the amplified fragments by size whereby the hybridization and stuffer sequences for each MLPA probe set determine the length of the amplified product. In (**b**), MLPA results of a large gene deletion are shown. Two MLPA kits (P065 and P066) were used to test for large *FBN1* gene deletions and duplications that cause Marfan syndrome. An additional control probe (*black arrow*) located 301 Kb upstream from *FBN1* exon 1 on the *DUT* (*deoxyuridine triphosphatase*) gene on chromosome 15q15-q21.1 also was deleted in this sample

MLPA (RT-MLPA) which can be used for mRNA profiling [46]. The only difference between traditional MLPA and RT-MLPA is that RT-MLPA begins with the reverse transcription of mRNA into cDNA before continuing with the typical MLPA reaction; the ligase enzyme cannot ligate probes which are bound to RNA. Methylation-Specific MLPA (MS-MLPA) is another variation that can be used to detect both copy number changes as well as the methylation status of the DNA target [47]. MS-MLPA is useful for imprinting disease testing [48–50] and the analysis of methylation aberrations in tumor samples [51, 52].

PCR Variations for Unknown Sequence Variants

Most of the techniques discussed above are used to screen for sequence variants (both mutations and polymorphisms) based on previous knowledge of the variant i.e., the sequence of the variant is either known or defined by previous scientific reports. In contrast, both research and clinical molecular pathology need methods to identify sequence variants without prior knowledge of their existence i.e., the sequence of the variant is unknown. Sequencing is the ultimate screening technique, but is costly and labor-intensive. The goal of the scanning techniques described below (denaturing gradient gel electrophoresis [DDGE], temperature gradient gel electrophoresis [TGGE], heteroduplex analysis [HA], single-strand conformation polymorphism [SSCP], denaturing high-performance liquid chromatography [DHPLC], protein truncation test [PTT], and variant screening by high-resolution melting [HRM] curve analysis) is to select DNA regions with possible variant sequences for follow up confirmation, thereby reducing costs relative to sequencing. Should an unknown variant be detected, for example by a shift in the mobility of the PCR product on a gel or capillary, the PCR product with altered mobility may be isolated and sequenced.

Denaturing Gradient Gel Electrophoresis and Temperature Gradient Gel Electrophoresis

Denaturing gradient gel electrophoresis (DGGE) [53, 54] and temperature gradient gel electrophoresis (TGGE) [55, 56] are similar methods for separating DNA fragments with similar lengths but different sequences and depends upon different mobilities within a linear gradient of increasingly denaturing conditions. In DGGE, the gradient is created with a mixture of urea and formamide, and in TGGE with a combination of water baths at different temperatures and a cooling plate under the gel. Both DGGE and TGGE exploit the markedly decreased mobility of partially melted dsDNA compared to either fully annealed dsDNA or ssDNA. Melting within a dsDNA fragment occurs within stretches of base pairs called melting domains. The point at which a domain begins to denature is referred to as the melting temperature (T_m), whether melting was induced by temperature or denaturing chemicals. In general, GC-rich sequences are more resistant to denaturation because of the three hydrogen bonds holding a GC pair together, as opposed to the two hydrogen bonds in an AT base pair. During electrophoresis, once a dsDNA fragment reaches the point at which the melting domain with the lowest T_m begins to denature, mobility of the fragment through the gel nearly ceases. Fragments that melt early in the gel can therefore be separated from those that melt later. Complete denaturation of the dsDNA can be prevented by adding a GC-rich region to the 5′ end of one of the primers (GC clamp), increasing the sensitivity for detection of sequence variants.

For DGGE and TGGE, the denaturing conditions and the time of electrophoresis are optimized such that non-variant sequences migrate to an intermediate position in the gel by the end of electrophoresis, allowing sequence variants creating either a higher or lower T_m to be identified. The denaturing gradient may be perpendicular or parallel to the electric field. Perpendicular gradient gels covering a broad range of denaturing conditions are loaded with the non-variant sequence in all lanes to find the optimal, narrower denaturing gradient (chemical or temperature) for later use in parallel gradient gels. Parallel gradients are used to assess patient samples but also to optimize the time of electrophoresis by loading the non-variant sequence in different lanes at different times. Double-gradient DGGE adds a sieving gradient, for example, 6–12 % polyacrylamide, colinear with the denaturing gradient in the gel matrix, further improving band resolution.

Both DGGE and TGGE work best with DNA fragments less than 500 bp in length. When GC-clamped fragments are analyzed, the sensitivity of detecting a SNP is close to 99 %. Following electrophoresis, specific bands can be isolated from the gel and sequenced. DNA fragments with a high GC content are not easily analyzed by DGGE, since all fragments are more resistant to melting.

Examples of Applications of DGGE or TGGE

1. *APC* gene mutation analysis for familial adenomatous polyposis [57]
2. *CTFR* gene mutation analysis for cystic fibrosis [58]
3. *TCRγ* gene rearrangements for lymphoma [59]

Heteroduplex Analysis

Heteroduplex formation results when non-variant and variant alleles are coamplified, denatured, and allowed to reanneal in a post-PCR annealing step [60]. Some of the strands pair with the complementary strand from the same allele and form homoduplexes. However, some strands pair with a strand from the other allele and form heteroduplexes. Because the heteroduplexes have mismatched base pairs between strands, they form a partially open dsDNA sequence that migrates more slowly during electrophoresis than the fully annealed homoduplexes.

Two types of heteroduplex structures can be formed [61]. When the mismatch consists of one or more single-base mutations, small open areas of dsDNA called "bubble-type" heteroduplexes are formed. When the mismatch is formed by insertions or deletions between the two alleles, a pronounced bending of the dsDNA is produced and referred to as a "bulge-type" heteroduplex. Bulge-type heteroduplexes markedly affect the mobility of the dsDNA, whereas bubble-type heteroduplexes may be difficult to detect electrophoretically. Detection of single base-pair bubble-type mismatches can be enhanced in two ways. Electrophoresis can be performed with mutation detection enhancement (MDE) gels, an altered form of polyacrylamide used for improved resolution. Alternatively, the post-PCR introduction of a known sequence with a short deletion to form a bulge-type heteroduplex enhances the separation of sequences with base-pair mismatches in a process known as universal heteroduplex generation.

Examples of Applications of Heteroduplex Analysis

1. *HIV* subtyping
2. *CFTR* gene mutation analysis for cystic fibrosis
3. *NF1* gene mutation analysis for neurofibromatosis type 1

Single-Strand Conformation Polymorphism

The principle of single-strand conformation polymorphism (SSCP) is the differential gel electrophoretic separation of ssDNA that folds into a specific secondary structure based on its sequence [62–64]. For SSCP, the region of interest is amplified and the resulting amplicons are denatured using heat or a denaturation buffer, or both, prior to gel or capillary electrophoresis. Amplicons with different sequences will assume different folding conformations upon denaturation. Conformational differences reflecting sequence changes are detected as differences in electrophoretic mobility of the ssDNA in a nondenaturing polyacrylamide matrix. In general, a non-variant sample generates two bands, one for each of the two strands of the dsDNA product. Bands of variant ssDNA migrate to positions different from those of the non-variant ssDNA. A homozygous variant sample generates two bands, but with different migration patterns from the two non-variant bands. If a heterozygous variant is present, four bands are generated: two with non-variant mobility and two with variant mobility. Mutations also may change the conformation of only one strand but not the other in heterozygous specimens, resulting in three bands. DNA may be purified from the gel, allowing even rare somatic mutations in tumors to be sequenced.

Temperature, ionic environment and pH affect nucleic acid conformation and therefore must be held constant throughout the SSCP electrophoresis. Accurate temperature control during SSCP increases reliability and is an easily modifiable parameter in repeatable, nonisotopic tests that may increase sensitivity. SSCP is adversely affected if unincorporated primers are allowed to bind to the ssDNA during denaturing and cooling prior to electrophoresis, or if nonspecific bands are produced by low-fidelity PCR. In SSCP, electrophoretic mobility patterns of variant alleles can be difficult to distinguish from non-variant alleles. Another disadvantage of SSCP is that multiple test conditions are required for 100 % sensitivity for detection of all sequence variants.

SSCP is most sensitive when the DNA amplicon is less than 200 bp in length. Sensitivity decreases as the fragment length increases. This can be overcome by RE digestion of larger PCR products prior to electrophoresis. When RE digestion is used, the procedure is referred to as restriction endonuclease fingerprinting-single-strand conformation polymorphism (REF-SSCP). Additionally, SSCP is relatively less sensitive for G to C mutation detection; however, addition of glycerol enhances mutation detection in this circumstance.

Variations of SSCP include RNA-SSCP (rSSCP), dideoxy fingerprinting (ddF), bidirectional ddF (bi-ddF), and SSCP detection of virtually all mutations. RNA adopts more conformational structures than does ssDNA, allowing enhanced detection using rSSCP. RNA-SSCP is not widely used because of the relative difficulty in obtaining intact RNA for analysis. Dideoxy fingerprinting involves a dideoxy Sanger single-primer termination reaction (cycle-sequencing reaction; for additional information on the Sanger reaction, see the section on sequencing, above) followed by nondenaturing electrophoresis. A fingerprint bandshift is indicative of sequence changes. In bi-ddF, the dideoxy Sanger termination reaction is performed with two opposing primers in the same well or tube.

The detection of an altered SSCP pattern does not identify the exact sequence variation present in the analyzed DNA. Therefore, positive SSCP results require DNA sequence analysis to confirm and identify the sequence variation.

Examples of Applications of SSCP

1. Screening for mutations in the adenomatous polyposis coli (*APC*) gene
2. Mutation analysis of the *ATP7B* gene for Wilson disease
3. Mutation analysis in *BRCA1* for familial breast cancer
4. Pathogen identification [65]

Denaturing High-Performance Liquid Chromatography

Denaturing high-performance liquid chromatography (DHPLC) is an ion-paired, reversed-phase, liquid chromatography method used to identify variants, including SNPs and small insertions or deletions, by distinguishing between heteroduplex and homoduplex DNA [66]. DHPLC is conceptually similar to heteroduplex analysis (HA; see above). Conventional HA makes use of a gel matrix to separate homoduplex and heteroduplex species in a non-denaturing environment, whereas DHPLC uses partially denaturing conditions in a liquid chromatography column to exaggerate the separation between the two species.

For DHPLC, the gene to be tested is amplified using high-fidelity PCR to prevent the production of PCR artifacts (pseudoalleles) that could produce false-positive results. The optimal amplicon length is between 100 and 500 bp. PCR product purification usually is not necessary, as unincorporated primers, nucleotides, and genomic DNA do not interfere with the analysis. DHPLC requires heteroduplex formation, accomplished by heating and slow cooling of the PCR products. Therefore, for conditions in which only one variant allele type may be present (such as recessive diseases, X-linked conditions in males, or small tumor samples with loss of heterozygosity in all cells), PCR products from non-variant control samples and patient samples are mixed in equal proportions before heating and cooling to produce heteroduplex DNA and distinguish from homozygous non-variant alleles. The addition of non-variant PCR amplicons is not required when using DHPLC to test PCR products from heterozygous individuals, which naturally form heteroduplexes when denatured and slowly cooled.

The duplexes are injected into a DHPLC column, and the DNA binds to the stationary matrix. Binding is aided by triethylammonium acetate. Because the stability of the binding depends on the temperature, the column is optimally held at the T_m of the PCR fragment. The T_m can be calculated using a variety of proprietary or free software programs. The DNA is next eluted from the matrix using acetonitrile and DNA absorbency is measured at 260 nm. The linear gradient of acetonitrile established in the column allows separation of DNA fragments based on size or the presence of heteroduplexes, or both. All DNA fragments impart a characteristic profile when the absorbance is plotted against elution time. The peak of maximum absorbance is the retention time of that DNA sample at a given acetonitrile concentration. Heteroduplexes are less stable and thus have a lower affinity for the column. The concentration of acetonitrile required to separate heteroduplexes from the column is therefore lower, so heteroduplexes elute from the column earlier than homoduplexes.

The column temperature and gradient conditions can be optimized for the separation of any heteroduplex-homoduplex mixture. Some DNA fragments have more than one melting domain and the analysis may be performed at more than one temperature. One advantage of DHPLC is that reinjection of the same sample at different temperatures is possible. Other advantages include high detection rates of variants, rapid separation times per sample, a high degree of automation, and the ability to collect elution fractions and sequence each eluted fragment. Disadvantages of DHPLC include the need for expensive equipment and columns, high-fidelity PCR, and optimization of each reaction required to achieve the highest sensitivity of mutation detection.

Examples of Applications of DHPLC

1. *RET* and *CFTR* mutation detection [67]
2. *BRCA1* and *BRCA2* mutation analysis [68]

Protein Truncation Test

The protein truncation test (PTT) is used to identify mutations that result in premature termination of translation. Although initially developed for Duchenne muscular dystrophy testing, PTT has been applied widely [69], since protein-truncating mutations are associated with multiple types of hereditary cancer syndromes, including cancers of the breast, ovary, and colon.

In PTT, the gene segment of interest is amplified by PCR. The amplicons are used for in vitro transcription and translation in a coupled reaction. The resulting proteins are separated using sodium dodecyl sulfate (SDS) polyacrylamide gel electrophoresis. The presence of a premature termination codon is demonstrated by the visualization of a lower-molecular-weight protein band than for the non-truncated protein. Relatively large gene fragments (2–4 kb) can be analyzed using PTT.

Examples of Applications of PTT

1. Duchenne muscular dystrophy diagnosis
2. *BRCA1* and *BRCA2* mutation detection for breast cancer [70]
3. *APC* mutations for colorectal cancer [71]

Variant Scanning by High-Resolution Melting Curve Analysis

High-resolution melting curve analysis (described in detail above) can be used for variant scanning of many genes. In this method, a large region of a gene, e.g., an exon or any region that is ≤500 bp, is amplified and then melted in the presence of a non-variant control DNA. A deviant melt indicates a base change within the region and sequencing of that region must be performed in order to determine the clinical significance of the detected variant. This method is useful for investigating genetic causes for suspected biochemical disorders found during newborn screening.

Examples of Applications of Variant Scanning by High-Resolution Melting Curve Analysis

1. Screening for Medium Chain Acyl-CoA Dehydrogenase (MCAD) deficiency mutations [72]
2. Screening for Ornithine Transcarbamylase (OTC) deficiency mutations

Other Nucleic Acid Amplification Methods

PCR is widely used in the clinical laboratory. The proprietary nature of PCR prompted the development of alternative methods for nucleic acid amplification. Several are described here: ligase chain reaction (LCR); transcription mediated amplification (TMA), strand displacement amplification (SDA), and nucleic acid sequence-based amplification (NASBA).

Ligase Chain Reaction

Ligase chain reaction (LCR) [73, 74] is initiated when a mixture of target DNA, thermostable DNA ligase, four oligonucleotide probes, and NAD^+ or ATP is heated to denature dsDNA (both target and complementary probes) in the reaction mixture. Two pairs of complementary probes are used, and, of necessity, their correct design requires knowledge of the sequence of the DNA target. After denaturation and subsequent reaction cooling, the four probes in the reaction mixture hybridize to their complementary sequences on each target DNA sister strand. The two probes that hybridize to one sister strand and the two probes that bind to the other sister strand are designed such that when hybridized, the 3′ hydroxyl end of the upstream probe is immediately adjacent to the 5′ phosphate end of the downstream probe. Thermostable DNA ligase enzymatically ligates the two bound probes, thus achieving a "doubling" of the mass of target DNA in the reaction. As the temperature cycling proceeds, a theoretical exponential amplification of the mass of target DNA in the original reaction occurs because the resultant ligated amplicons also serve as targets for probe hybridizations and ligations. In practice, amplification is less than exponential, but sufficient to achieve target DNA amplification and assessment by various methods.

Target-independent blunt-end ligation of the probes in the reaction can occur in LCR, which can cause unacceptably high levels of background signal, limiting the sensitivity and specificity of the method. This problem has been solved by use of gap LCR (G-LCR). In G-LCR, the probes are designed such that they cannot be ligated in a target-independent manner because they are not blunt ended. When G-LCR probes hybridize to target DNA, a gap of one or more bases exists between the probes hybridized to the same target strand. T his gap is then biochemically "filled" in the reaction, thus providing a suitable substrate for target-dependent ligation by DNA ligase.

Examples of Applications of LCR

1. *Chlamydia trachomatis* detection
2. *Neisseria gonorrhoeae* detection

Transcription-Mediated Amplification

Transcription-mediated amplification (TMA) uses RNA as the template, two primers, and two enzymes: reverse transcriptase (RT) and RNA polymerase. One primer contains a promoter sequence that binds RNA polymerase. As the amplification process begins, the promoter-containing primer hybridizes to the target RNA at a complementary site. Reverse transcriptase then synthesizes a cDNA copy of the target RNA template by extension of the 3′ end of the promoter-primer. The result is an RNA–DNA duplex. The RNA component is degraded by the RNase H activity inherent in RT. The other primer in the reaction mixture hybridizes to the DNA copy, and a new DNA strand is synthesized from the end of the primer by reverse transcriptase, generating a dsDNA molecule. The other enzyme in the mixture, RNA polymerase, binds the promoter sequence in the DNA template and initiates transcription. Each of the resulting newly synthesized RNA amplicons reenters the TMA cycle, serving as a template for a new round of replication and exponential expansion of the RNA target. Each DNA template can generate 10^2–10^3 copies of RNA amplicon, with the potential for 10^8- to 10^9-fold amplification in less than 1 h. The process is autocatalytic and isothermal. Acridinium ester-labeled DNA probes are added after completion of the reaction to initiate detection and quantitation based on chemiluminescence.

Examples of Applications of TMA

1. *Chlamydia trachomatis* detection [75]
2. *Neisseria gonorrhoeae* detection
3. HCV detection (qualitative) [76]

Strand Displacement Amplification

Strand displacement amplification (SDA) is an isothermal in vitro nucleic acid amplification technique [77]. Hemimodified DNA is polymerized by using three conventional dNTPs and one containing a 5′-[α-thio]triphosphate. The primer(s) is designed with an RE recognition site in the 5′

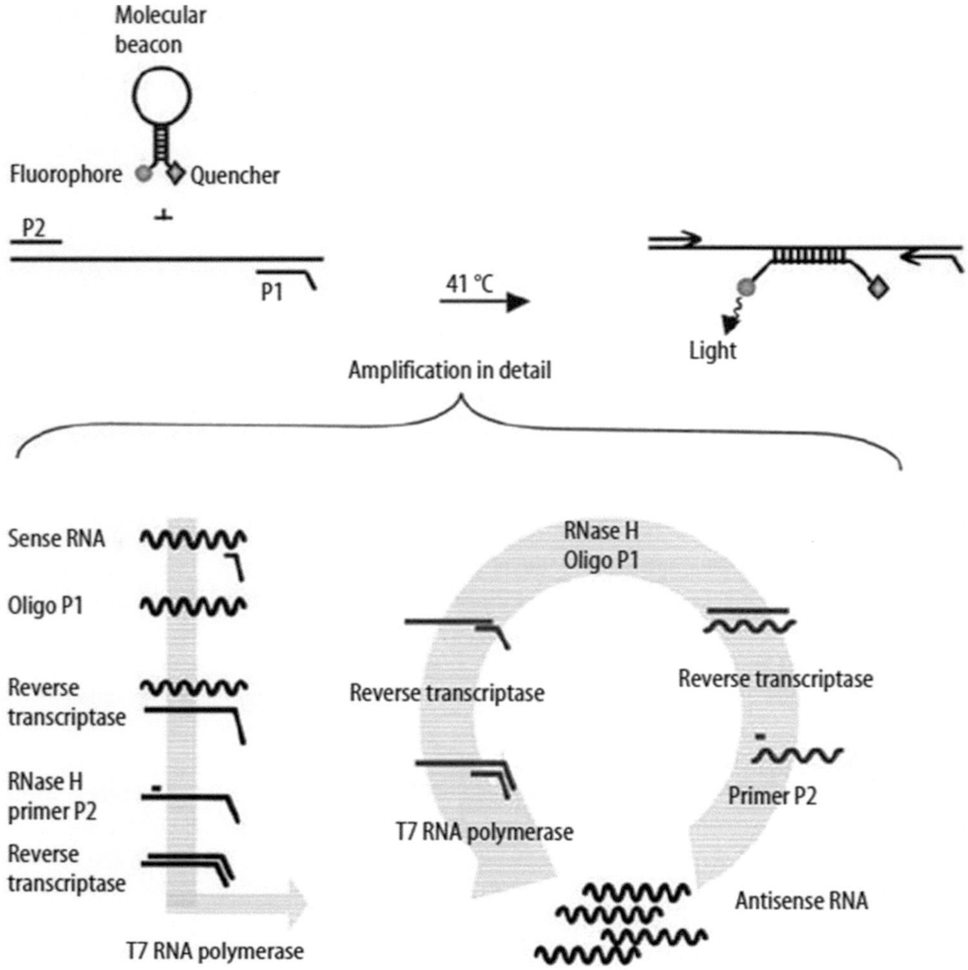

Figure 2.6 Schematic of NASBA Method. Two primers are used: P1 (antisense) and P2 (sense). The P1 overhang is a T7 RNA polymerase recognition sequence. A molecular beacon (with fluorophore and quencher, by definition) serving as probe with reporter molecules coupled to NASBA generates a real-time detection system.

overhang end. The recognition site is specific for an RE that can nick the unmodified DNA strand at a double-stranded hemiphosphorothioate recognition site, that is, when the newly synthesized strand incorporates the 5′-[α-thio]triphosphate nucleotide in the recognition sequence. DNA polymerase lacking 5′ to 3′ exonuclease activity is used to extend the 3′ end at the nick and displace the downstream strand. DNA nicking and polymerization with re-formation of the hemiphosphorothioate recognition site continuously cycle, generating complementary copies of the DNA target. Linear amplification (called target-generation SDA) occurs when a single primer is used. Exponential amplification (exponential SDA) is achieved by using two primers complementary to opposite DNA strands, with both primers containing RE recognition sites in the 5′ overhang end. Strand displacement amplification has been used in a microarray format [78].

Examples of Applications of SDA

1. *Chlamydia trachomatis* detection
2. *Neisseria gonorrhoeae* detection

Nucleic Acid Sequence-Based Amplification

Nucleic acid sequence-based amplification (NASBA) is an isothermal method for amplifying nucleic acids using two sequence-specific primers (P1, antisense, and P2, sense; see Fig. 2.6), and the coordinated activities of three enzymes: avian myeloblastosis virus reverse transcriptase (AMV-RT), RNase H, and T7 RNA polymerase [79]. A primer with a T7 RNA polymerase recognition sequence at its 5′ end is used by AMV-RT to transcribe cDNA from the RNA template. The RNA template is destroyed by RNase H. AMV-RT then extends the second primer to synthesize dsDNA. The T7 RNA polymerase binds to the recognition sequence in the dsDNA and synthesizes multiple antisense RNA transcripts, and the cycle is repeated. Generally, amplification is approximately 10^{12}-fold in 1–2 h.

In NASBA, nucleic acids serve as amplification templates only if they are single stranded and contain primer-binding regions. NASBA is performed isothermally at 41 °C, so RNA is preferentially amplified, because at this temperature genomic DNA remains double stranded and does not bind primers, allowing RNA detection in the presence of genomic DNA without false-positive results. NASBA can be used for specific DNA amplification by introducing a DNA denaturation step before amplification.

Quantitative detection of target nucleic acids is achieved by use of an internal calibrator added during RNA isolation. The calibrator is included at a known concentration, is coamplified during the NASBA process, and is subsequently identified along with the target RNA. Quantification is based on the analysis of signals generated in real time (one color for calibrator and another for target).

Examples of Applications of NASBA

1. HIV quantitation
2. CMV detection

Amplicon Carryover Contamination

Vast numbers of target DNA copies are generated when PCR and other in vitro nucleic acid amplification methods are used. By contrast, signal amplification methods (see below) do not generate vast quantities of amplicon and do not create the potential for amplicon carryover contamination of the laboratory workspace. Amplicons from previous reactions inadvertently introduced into new amplification reactions for the same amplicon are suitable substrates for amplification. Clinical molecular laboratories therefore take precautions to prevent generation of false-positive results from amplicon carryover contamination.

Amplicon contamination and false-positive results are prevented by using physical barriers and chemical and UV light techniques to destroy amplicons or make them unsuitable for amplification. The physical barriers include performance of nucleic acid isolation, PCR setup, thermal cycling, and post-PCR analysis in separate areas of the laboratory (different rooms are ideal). Air flow is controlled such that air pressure is positive, that is, flows out of the room, in the isolation and PCR setup rooms, and is negative in the thermal cycling and post-PCR analysis rooms. Hoods are another way of providing physical separation of the different steps of amplification-based tests. Other physical separation techniques include the use of barrier pipette tips, frequent glove changes, designated laboratory coats for the pre- or post-PCR areas of the laboratory, and PCR tube openers or careful, slow opening of tubes and microtiter plates to prevent aerosolization of contents. Real-time PCR reduces the chances of amplicon contamination since the PCR product is detected and quantified without opening the real-time PCR reaction vessel.

Chemical techniques to prevent amplicon contamination include thorough cleansing with bleach of work areas and instruments before and after use. UV lights frequently are placed in hoods and work areas. UV light creates thymine dimers within amplicons, rendering the amplicons unsuitable as substrates for further amplification. The introduction of isopsoralens in PCR reactions allows DNA cross-linking of amplicons by UV light, also rendering them unsuitable for further amplification. Deoxyuridine may be used in lieu of thymidine in the reaction mixture. Use of deoxyuridine has minimal effect on amplification or product detection, but amplicons with uracil are substrates for uracil-N-glycosylase (UNG). UNG has no effect on DNA that contains only thymidine residues (new patient DNA in subsequent reactions), but digests the uracil-containing amplicons, allowing removal of contaminating amplicons before a new PCR proceeds [80]. So-called UNG sterilization is performed prior to PCR cycling to rid the reaction of any amplicon contaminants that may be present.

Signal Amplification Methods

Branched DNA Method

The branched DNA method (bDNA) [81, 82] begins with the addition of a lysis buffer to a small volume of serum, plasma, or culture supernatant containing cells or virus. The lysis reagent contains detergent to release target nucleic acid, inhibitors to prevent target degradation, and multiple capture extenders (oligonucleotides) that hybridize to specific areas of the target RNA or DNA. In the case of the HIV bDNA test, the capture extenders hybridize to multiple sequences in the viral *pol* gene. A common sequence on the capture extenders interacts with capture probes immobilized on the surface of 96-microwell plates, thereby anchoring the target nucleic acid to the plate.

Multiple target probes are added to each well that hybridize to different, conserved sequences on the target nucleic acid. In the HIV bDNA assay, more than 80 target probes covering a large portion of the 3,000 bp of the *pol* gene are used. The target probes contain key sequences that form the foundation for signal amplification, accomplished via the sequential addition of preamplifier (complementary to a region of the target probes), amplifier (complementary to a region of the preamplifier molecule), and alkaline-phosphatase-modified label probes (complementary to portions of the amplifier molecule).

Preamplifier, amplifier and label probes, as well as the preamplifier region of the binding probes, contain the non-natural nucleotides 5-methyl-2′-deoxyisocytidine (iso^{Me}C) and 2′-deoxyisoguanosine (isoG). These isomers of natural bases can participate in Watson–Crick base pairing with each other but not with cytosine or guanine residues in probes or in natural DNA or RNA sequences. Incorporation of non-natural bases into the synthetic probe molecules increases the specificity of hybridization by decreasing nonspecific probe interactions, and increases the sensitivity of the assay since higher concentrations of probes can be used.

The series of probes results in formation of large hybridization complexes on the target RNA or DNA. For example, if each hybridization step was 100 % efficient in the HIV bDNA assay, each target molecule would be labeled with more than 10,000 alkaline phosphatase molecules. Addition of dioxetane substrate for the alkaline phosphatase results in steady-state chemiluminescent signal. The signal is proportional to the amount of target RNA or DNA present in the sample. The amount of target RNA or DNA in a specimen may be calculated by interpolation from a standard curve generated by signals produced from calibrators that contain known concentrations of the specific viral, bacterial, or cellular RNA or DNA.

Examples of Applications of bDNA method
1. HIV quantitation [83, 84]
2. Hepatitis B virus (HBV) quantitation [85–88]
3. HCV quantitation [89, 90]

Hybrid Capture

Hybrid capture (HC) is a signal amplification system based on antibody binding of RNA–DNA hybrids. The first step of HC is the hybridization of unlabeled RNA probes with denatured target DNA. The resulting RNA–DNA hybrids are captured to the surface of microplate wells by an immobilized antibody that recognizes RNA–DNA hybrids. A second anti-RNA–DNA monoclonal antibody conjugated to alkaline phosphatase is added next. Many secondary antibodies bind to each RNA–DNA hybrid. Dioxetane-based substrate is added, which is cleaved by the alkaline phosphatase, producing a chemiluminescent signal. The signal is measured using a microplate luminometer and is proportional to the amount of target DNA in the specimen [91]. The sensitivity of HC can be increased by using a precipitation buffer and high-speed centrifugation.

Examples of Applications of HC
1. Human papilloma virus detection [92]
2. CMV quantitation [93]
3. *Chlamydia trachomatis* and *Neisseria gonorrhoeae* detection [94]
4. HBV quantitation [95]

Fluorescence In Situ Hybridization

In fluorescence in situ hybridization (FISH), fluorescently tagged DNA or RNA probes are used to identify genomic sequences of interest [96, 97]. The major advantages of FISH are the utility for testing of FFPE tissue sections, correlation of probe hybridization with tissue morphology, and the increased resolution provided by FISH for identification of specific abnormalities when partnered with conventional cytogenetics. The number and location of the fluorescent signal(s) can identify chromosomal abnormalities including gene amplification, gene deletion or structural rearrangements such as translocations.

FISH is performed by sequential steps of denaturation, hybridization, and washing. Slides are prepared in the cytogenetic or histology laboratory. Fluorescently labeled probe(s) are then applied to the slide along with a nuclear counterstain and reagents to enhance denaturation and reduce background. The slides are sealed and incubated (usually overnight) in a humid environment at high temperature. These conditions denature the probe and patient DNA, allowing hybridization to occur between the probe and its complementary DNA sequence in the specimen without binding to nonspecific sites. Excess nonspecifically bound probe is washed away, and the pattern of fluorescence is observed with fluorescence microscopy. The fluorescent signal(s) can be enhanced by the use of a digital imaging system and computer software.

The specificity of FISH is largely based on probe selection. Ideally, the probe is complementary to the gene of interest; however, if the disease gene is unknown, satellite probes that identify a chromosomal region linked to the disease may be used. Labeled bacterial or yeast artificial chromosomes (BAC or YAC, respectively) are typically used as FISH probes, but short oligonucleotides also can be used with signal amplification techniques. Probes that identify individual whole chromosomes or chromosomal arms are often called "painting probes" due to the colorful patterns generated. Other probes that hybridize to a specific gene can be used for the detection of deletions or duplications and are called single-copy gene probes. Probes that hybridize to the α-satellite regions near centromeres are used in clinical cytogenetics to identify and count individual chromosomes. Probes that hybridize to the subtelomeric portions of chromosomes are used to identify cryptic telomeric abnormalities such as translocations.

Dual-color FISH (dFISH) employs two probes with different fluorescence wavelengths to identify structural chromosomal rearrangements. Each probe generates a characteristic color by itself (split signal) and a third color when the two probes are juxtaposed (fusion signal). A fusion signal indicating chromosomal rearrangement is used to identify disease-causing mutations that predictably involve only two partner genes, for example, *BCR* and *ABL*. However, when a particular gene with multiple potential translocation partners is tested, it is more efficient to have both probes bind to the 5′ and 3′ ends of the particular gene such that the non-rearranged allele shows the fusion signal and the rearranged allele shows two split signals (so-called "break apart" probes). This is the technique used for *MLL* gene detection, which is rearranged with over 30 different partner genes in various types of leukemia.

Spectral karyotyping (SKY) and multiplex FISH (M-FISH) are modifications of conventional FISH that utilize multiple fluorochromes, specialized optics, and image analysis that can simultaneously identify all chromosomes [98]. Array-based comparative genomic hybridization (aCGH, described below), also called "copy number karyotyping," is a variation of FISH that detects relative gains or losses of the genome [99]. Array-based CGH is used to compare the ratios of patient specimen DNA, labeled with one fluorochrome, to that of control non-variant DNA, labeled with a different fluorochrome when hybridized to control chromosomes. Colorimetric probes are used in chromogenic in situ hybridization (CISH), which has the advantage that the signal does not fade with time or require fluorescence microscopy for analysis.

Examples of Applications of FISH

1. Detection of *BCR–ABL* in chronic myelogenous leukemia
2. Detection of *HER2* gene amplification for breast cancer diagnosis and prognosis
3. Detection of *MYCN* amplification in neuroblastoma [100]

DNA Arrays

In DNA arrays, the word "array" is jargon for an orderly distribution of molecules on solid supports ranging from nylon membranes to printed circuit boards to glass slides to silicon surfaces. There are macroscopic arrays, for example, reverse line blots on nylon membranes, and microarrays, for example, DNA chips. Synonyms for microarrays include gene chip, DNA chip, genome chip, biochip, gene array, DNA array, and DNA microarray. Forms of arrays currently utilized in the clinical molecular laboratory include (but are not limited to): aCGH, SNP arrays, and expression arrays.

Comparative Genomic Hybridization Arrays

First described by Kallioniemi in 1992, array-based comparative genomic hybridization (aCGH) is a technique developed for genome-wide characterization of copy number changes [101]. In its original form, differentially labeled test and reference genomic DNA were co-hybridized to normal metaphase chromosomes. The relative fluorescence ratio along the length of the chromosomes represented the relative DNA copy number. Array CGH (aCGH) is an advancement of CGH technology that uses clones, most commonly BACs or oligonucleotides, arrayed along a physical surface as the hybridization target, rather than metaphase chromosomes. The arrayed surfaces are commonly called microarrays, and the surface may hold millions of unique sequences as the hybridization targets. Much like the original CGH process, test and reference genomic DNAs are labeled with different fluorescent dyes, denatured, and then hybridized with the arrayed clones on the surface of the chip. The relative fluorescence ratios of the reference and test signals at the arrayed DNA elements provide a locus by locus measure of DNA copy number variation. In aCGH, the targets can be nonoverlapping clones evenly spaced across the genome, overlapping clones densely packed only in areas of interest, or a combination of the two approaches.

The uses of aCGH include gene discovery, cancer classification, and diagnostic assays. Analysis of DNA from mantle cell lymphomas by aCGH revealed homozygous deletions at 2q13 in 3 of the 29 samples leading to the discovery of the tumor suppressor gene BIM [102]. Since aCGH has a much higher resolution than conventional karyotyping, its use has led to the recognition of new microdeletion and microduplication syndromes such as that at 17q21.31 [103, 104]. Such discoveries are indicative of the role of aCGH in gene discovery and the development diagnostic tests.

The patterns of copy number variations detected by aCGH have led to diagnostically significant subgroup classifications of cancers. One example is that of differentiating diffuse large B-cell lymphoma types into subtypes based on copy number patterns [105]. The ABC subtype is genomically characterized by gain of 3q, 18q, and 19q and loss of 6q and 9p21, whereas the GCB subtype is genomically characterized by gain of 1q, 2p, 7q, and 12q. The subtypes have disparate biology and clinical outcomes.

As the number of unique targets on an array increases, so does the resolution. In 2005, a targeted array capable of detecting exonic level copy number variations was used to screen 162 exons of 5 genes [106]. In 2008, three groups showed the utility of CGH to detect exonic level copy number variation in the dystrophin gene [107–109]. The ability of custom-designed aCGH to detect exon copy number changes provides new opportunities for research and diagnosis.

Within the past decade, aCGH has emerged as a diagnostic tool in the clinical laboratory. Occasionally referred to as molecular karyotyping, the International Standard Cytogenomic Array Consortium recommended in 2010 genome-wide aCGH as the first-tier clinical diagnostic test for individuals with multiple congenital anomalies and developmental delays [110]. As a result, targeted arrays are increasingly being used in the clinical laboratory for both cancer and congenital conditions.

SNP Arrays

The basic principle of the SNP array is the same as the DNA microarray. DNA is fluorescently labeled, hybridized with arrayed DNA probes, imaged, and interpreted. The difference is that for SNP arrays, the target probes are designed around single-nucleotide polymorphisms (SNPs) distributed throughout the genome. Signal intensity following hybridization is dependent on both the amount of target DNA as well as the affinity to the target. Thus, interrogating the SNP targets provides both copy number and SNP allelic information. The resolution of SNP arrays is limited by the distribution of SNPs in the human genome. The highest density SNP chips now have over four million SNP targets (Illumina Human Omnio5-Quad Bead Chip). Applications of SNP arrays include genome-wide association studies (GWAS), determination of heterozygosity, and molecular karyotyping of clinical samples.

Expression Arrays

Gene expression arrays are a powerful tool for comparing complex RNA populations. RNA is isolated from a test sample, converted to fluorescently labeled cDNA, and hybridized to a microarray. The fluorescence at each DNA element is then quantified, providing a measure of the abundance of the RNA molecules in the test sample. Detection limits are as low as 1–10 copies of mRNA per cell depending on the technology and cell type. As a means of candidate gene discovery, genome-wide expression microarrays with large densities are appropriate for analysis of differential patterns of gene expression between normal and diseased tissues while high-density, targeted expression arrays can identify novel exon skipping events and alternative splicing events [111, 112]. Expression arrays have gained acceptance in the clinical laboratory as a means of defining clinical subtypes of cancer [113]. Such arrays have demonstrated gene expression patterns which have been correlated with clinical outcomes and therapy response. Currently, five gene expression arrays are offered clinically for prognostic testing for breast cancer: Mammaprint, MapQuant Dx, OncotypeDx, PAM50 Breast Cancer Intrinsic Subtype Classifier, and Theros Breast Cancer Index.

Massively Parallel Sequencing

Massively parallel sequencing, also known as next-generation sequencing (NGS), has been widely adopted by the basic research community [114, 115]. Until recently, the use of NGS for clinical diagnostics was hindered by the relatively high cost of instruments, assay development and sequencing, as well as the bioinformatics infrastructure and expertise required for analysis. Since its introduction, advances in NGS platforms and sequencing chemistries have improved workflow, base qualities, read lengths, and total bases of sequence per experiment, all while reducing the cost per base sequenced [116]. Advances in enrichment and capture technologies have enabled the development of cost effective gene panels or exome sequencing for inherited disorders. NGS assays developed or under development include gene panels for autism, cardiomyopathies, X-linked mental retardation, the RAS pathway, among others, as well as the introduction of exome and genome sequencing in laboratories accredited by CMS under the Clinical Laboratory Improvement Act of 1988 (CLIA) [117–119]. The use of NGS for inherited disorders will supplant sequencing strategies such as Sanger sequencing or array-based genotyping when it is cost-effective and diagnostically viable. At this time bioinformatic analysis is still cumbersome and Sanger verification of putative variants of significance remains commonplace. However, improvements and standardization of bioinformatic analysis should ultimately reduce confirmatory Sanger verification and permit a high degree of certainty and reproducibility when detecting and reporting variants. (See Chap. 62 for a full discussion of NGS.)

Next Generation Sequencing Methods

The principles of NGS sequencing methodologies include sequencing by synthesis and sequencing by ligation. All platforms require the incorporation of adapters to target DNA and subsequent PCR-based generation of clonally amplified and clustered DNA. The two strategies primarily used for colony/cluster generation include in-solution emulsion PCR (emPCR) and surface bridge amplification. Once the DNA has been clonally enriched, sequencing chemistries differ depending upon platform [114, 115]. Illumina sequencing takes advantage of reversible dye-labeled terminators. Each dye terminator representing A, T, C, or G is sequentially introduced to the DNA molecule being synthesized and the surface of the flow cell is imaged. Once the complementary base has been incorporated into the extending DNA molecule, no further extension can occur until the dye is cleaved, resulting in an extendable deoxyribonucleotide triphosphate (dNTP), such that a single base is added during each cycle [114]. Technology from Roche relies upon the sequential introduction of the different dNTP bases, except the method of detection is pyrosequencing. The incorporation of a given base to the DNA being synthesized results in the release of a pyrophosphate and subsequent luciferase luminescence [120]. Since the reaction uses dNTP, single base extension does not always result, as homopolymer extension may occur during a single cycle. Technology from Life Technologies does not rely on DNA polymerase extension, rather sequencing by ligation is used. The process involves the use of multiple primers offset by one base at the 3′ end of the adapter. Fluorescently labeled interrogation probes representing two adjacent nucleotides are ligated to the primer. Once the ligation reaction has occurred and imaging is completed, the dye is cleaved off the interrogation probe, and a subsequent ligation can be performed [121]. Other methods of polymerase-mediated NGS include measuring the charge associated with nucleotide extension and the visual detection of dye-labeled nucleotide extension.

High throughput NGS platforms have made sequencing of an individual human genome in a reasonable timeframe a reality. Genome sequencing for clinical purposes is not commonplace at this time and is pursued mostly for gene discovery. Paradoxically genome sequencing is the simplest application of NGS and the most bioinformatically intensive. Because of the ease of set up, lack of need for specific assay design, and the costs associated with target-specific enrichment, genome sequencing will ultimately be performed for clinical purposes in the future [122]. However, a number of bioinformatic, regulatory, and ethical issues will need to be addressed before genome sequencing for clinical purposes will be commonplace.

Exome sequencing is a method that holds significant promise for clinical molecular laboratories. Exome sequencing can be used for gene discovery and in certain instances can be used for gene panel or pathway analysis. Because the human exome is roughly 1.5 % of the human genome, bioinformatic analysis is not as daunting as genome analysis, yielding roughly 30,000–50,000 variants [123]. Exomes from different patients can be differentially labeled using unique short sequence tags, multiplexed and sequenced in the same sequencing run, which reduces sequencing costs.

While high-throughput NGS platforms can be used to sequence genomes or multiple exomes in a single test, these instruments may not always be optimal for NGS of smaller gene panels. The use of barcodes or indexes enables pooling of multiple samples to leverage sequencing throughput, but the time required for sequencing can take days. Recently, a number of platforms have been introduced with lower throughput and faster turnaround times that facilitate the sequencing of smaller gene panels or exomes. This advancement has permitted the introduction of time-sensitive NGS-based clinical tests that are less expensive than Sanger sequencing tests, with a similar turnaround time.

Bioinformatics and Data Analysis

A typical NGS test may yield from 1 to 600 gigabytes (Gb) of sequence data. Conventional analysis pipelines and software programs developed for Sanger sequencing are totally inadequate for analysis of the large volumes of NGS data. A number of commercial and freeware software applications are available that align and perform variant calling. The steps of data analysis involve assessing the quality of the sequencing data, aligning the sequence fastq files to a reference sequence, determining the differences between the reference sequence and the patient's sequence, and collecting the data [124]. These sequence variants are bioinformatically processed to ensure the quality and accuracy of the alignment. Once the data have been processed and filtered, annotation of the variants is performed, and subsequent post-annotation filtering allows for the selection of a subset of variants of interest [116, 123, 125]. The process from raw sequence data to final variant reporting is bioinformatically intensive.

Development of bioinformatics and statistical workflows for NGS are not universal; different purposes for NGS testing require different metrics for alignment and data reporting. Public and private databases are used for annotation purposes to help determine what variants should be examined further. It is important that internal databases be developed that track areas of reproducible misalignments, miscalls, and variant frequencies to supplement public, nonclinical, and sometimes inaccurate, research-derived databases. Because of the vast amount of data associated with one test, it is not feasible to manually verify data for each variant. Tests may yield from a few to over three million variants. A paradigm shift is required for clinical laboratorians and clinicians who are accustomed to manually analyzing all variants that are reported. While graphical user interfaces are available to examine variants (should one wish to do so) clinical laboratorians and clinicians will have to rely upon the tools and pipelines developed by bioinformaticians. It is extremely important that all stakeholders are involved in pipeline development and validation to ensure that everyone involved with test interpretation understands the process and that the data reporting is accurate and useful.

Clinical Applications of Next-Generation Sequencing

NGS technologies permit sequencing of entire individual patient genomes. As the cost of NGS decreases, genome sequencing is likely to become increasingly popular as a strategy for identifying the genetic basis of diseases as it offers the potential of finding mutations in the noncoding regions, such as regulatory elements or noncoding RNAs, and the ability to detect large gene rearrangements [126, 127]. However, at present, the expense of NGS reagents and the high demand in bioinformatics makes the targeting of a subset of genome more appealing at the present time. The subset of a genome often focuses on a set of genes at different chromosomal loci which are important in a specific disease [119]. Two examples are provided by an X-Linked intellectual disability 92-gene NGS panel and a cardiomyopathy panel of 46 genes [117, 118]. This use of NGS is the logical extension of Sanger sequencing of a panel of selected genes associated with a particular phenotype.

Exome sequencing uses a targeted selection approach to capture the majority of the protein-coding exons of genes, microRNAs and noncoding RNAs in the human genome, followed by NGS sequencing. Because the exome represents only approximately 1.5 % of the genome and contains 85 % of known disease causing mutations, exome sequencing is considered the most cost-effective method for identifying the causative mutation in rare diseases [126]. However, with a massive amount of variants detected by exome sequencing, data analysis is complicated, especially when putative causative mutations such as missense mutations are identified. Family history and pedigree segregation studies are useful to determine the causality of the mutations [128].

Conclusion

The molecular methods used in the clinical laboratory will continue to evolve and develop as researchers and instrument manufacturers develop new methods that improve on the sensitivity, specificity, cost and speed of current methods. Drivers for adoption of new technologies in the clinical laboratory include but are not limited to reduced technologist hands-on time, reduced cost, shortened turnaround time, interfacing of results to information systems to reduce human transcription errors, and improvements in the detection of analytes with clinical significance. Molecular pathology will continue to be at the leading edge of methods development, resulting in a constant stream of new test and method validations with all the required steps new tests require from a regulatory compliance perspective. While this is challenging for the molecular pathology laboratory leadership and staff, this innovation also is one of the exciting aspects of molecular pathology practice.

References

1. Fiebelkorn KR, Lee BG, Hill CE, Caliendo AM, Nolte FS. Clinical evaluation of an automated nucleic acid isolation system. Clin Chem. 2002;48(9):1613–5.
2. Kessler HH, Muhlbauer G, Stelzl E, Daghofer E, Santner BI, Marth E. Fully automated nucleic acid extraction: MagNA Pure LC. Clin Chem. 2001;47(6):1124–6.
3. Williams SM, Meadows CA, Lyon E. Automated DNA extraction for real-time PCR. Clin Chem. 2002;48(9):1629–30.
4. Davies J, Reznikoff WS, editors. Milestones in biotechnology: classic papers on genetic engineering. Boston: Butterworth-Heinemann; 1992.
5. Lm W. A nested reverse-transcriptase polymerase chain reaction assay to detect BCR/ABL. In: Kileen AA, editor. Methods in molecular medicine molecular pathology protocols. Totowa, NJ: Humana Press; 2001. p. 105–14.
6. Sanger F, Nicklen S, Coulson AR. DNA sequencing with chain-terminating inhibitors. Proc Natl Acad Sci U S A. 1977;74(12):5463–7.
7. Esch RK. Basic nucleic acid procedures. In: Coleman WB, Tsongalis GJ, editors. Molecular diagnostics for the clinical laboratorian. Totowa, NJ: Humana Press; 1997. p. 55–8.
8. Schmalzing D, Koutny L, Salas-Solano O, Adourian A, Matsudaira P, Ehrlich D. Recent developments in DNA sequencing by capillary and microdevice electrophoresis. Electrophoresis. 1999;20(15–16):3066–77. doi:10.1002/(SICI)1522-2683(19991001)20:15/16<3066::AID-ELPS3066>3.0.CO;2-X.
9. Farkas DH. Specimen procurement, processing, tracking, and testing by the Southern blot. In: Farkas DH, editor. Molecular biology and pathology: a guidebook for quality control. San Diego: Academic; 1993. p. 51–75.
10. Mullis K, Faloona F, Scharf S, Saiki R, Horn G, Erlich H. Specific enzymatic amplification of DNA in vitro: the polymerase chain reaction. 1986. Biotechnology. 1992;24:17–27.
11. Farkas DH. Thermal Cyclers. In: Laboratory instrument evaluation, verification, and maintenance manual. Koenig AS (Editor). Northfield, IL: College of American Pathologists; 1998. p.130–3.
12. Loeffelholz MJ, Lewinski CA, Silver SR, Purohit AP, Herman SA, Buonagurio DA, Dragon EA. Detection of Chlamydia trachomatis in endocervical specimens by polymerase chain reaction. J Clin Microbiol. 1992;30(11):2847–51.
13. DiDomenico N, Link H, Knobel R, Caratsch T, Weschler W, Loewy ZG, Rosenstraus M. COBAS AMPLICOR: fully automated RNA and DNA amplification and detection system for routine diagnostic PCR. Clin Chem. 1996;42(12):1915–23.
14. Greenfield L, White TJ. Sample preparation methods. In: Persing DH, Smith TF, Tenover FC, White TJ, editors. Diagnostics molecular microbiology principles and applications. Washington, DC: American Society for Microbiology; 1993. p. 126–7.
15. Liu XY, Nelson D, Grant C, Morthland V, Goodnight SH, Press RD. Molecular detection of a common mutation in coagulation factor V causing thrombosis via hereditary resistance to activated protein C. Diagn Mol Pathol. 1995;4(3):191–7.
16. Lindeman R, Hu SP, Volpato F, Trent RJ. Polymerase chain reaction (PCR) mutagenesis enabling rapid non-radioactive detection of common beta-thalassaemia mutations in Mediterraneans. Br J Haematol. 1991;78(1):100–4.
17. Sorscher EJ, Huang Z. Diagnosis of genetic disease by primer-specified restriction map modification, with application to cystic fibrosis and retinitis pigmentosa. Lancet. 1991;337(8750):1115–8. doi:0140-6736(91)92785-Z [pii].
18. Khanna M, Park P, Zirvi M, Cao W, Picon A, Day J, Paty P, Barany F. Multiplex PCR/LDR for detection of K-ras mutations in primary colon tumors. Oncogene. 1999;18(1):27–38. doi:10.1038/sj.onc.1202291.
19. McMillin DE, Muldrow LL, Laggette SJ. Simultaneous detection of toxin A and toxin B genetic determinants of Clostridium difficile using the multiplex polymerase chain reaction. Can J Microbiol. 1992;38(1):81–3.
20. Jama M, Nelson L, Pont-Kingdon G, Mao R, Lyon E. Simultaneous amplification, detection, and analysis of common mutations in the galactose-1-phosphate uridyl transferase gene. J Mol Diagn. 2007;9(5):618–23. doi:10.2353/jmoldx.2007.070027.
21. Farkas DH, Miltgen NE, Stoerker J, van den Boom D, Highsmith WE, Cagasan L, McCullough R, Mueller R, Tang L, Tynan J, Tate C, Bombard A. The suitability of matrix assisted laser desorption/ionization time of flight mass spectrometry in a laboratory developed test using cystic fibrosis carrier screening as a model. J Mol Diagn. 2010;12(5):611–9. doi:10.2353/jmoldx.2010.090233.
22. Sugita T, Nakajima M, Ikeda R, Niki Y, Matsushima T, Shinoda T. A nested PCR assay to detect DNA in sera for the diagnosis of

deep-seated trichosporonosis. Microbiol Immunol. 2001;45(2):143–8.
23. Ferrie RM, Schwarz MJ, Robertson NH, Vaudin S, Super M, Malone G, Little S. Development, multiplexing, and application of ARMS tests for common mutations in the CFTR gene. Am J Hum Genet. 1992;51(2):251–62.
24. Bugawan TL, Begovich AB, Erlich HA. Rapid HLA-DPB typing using enzymatically amplified DNA and nonradioactive sequence-specific oligonucleotide probes. Immunogenetics. 1991;34(6):413.
25. Jarvius J, Nilsson M, Landegren U. Oligonucleotide ligation assay. Methods Mol Biol. 2003;212:215–28.
26. Nickerson DA, Kaiser R, Lappin S, Stewart J, Hood L, Landegren U. Automated DNA diagnostics using an ELISA-based oligonucleotide ligation assay. Proc Natl Acad Sci U S A. 1990;87(22):8923–7.
27. Tsiatis AC, Norris-Kirby A, Rich RG, Hafez MJ, Gocke CD, Eshleman JR, Murphy KM. Comparison of Sanger sequencing, pyrosequencing, and melting curve analysis for the detection of KRAS mutations: diagnostic and clinical implications. J Mol Diagn. 2010;12(4):425–32. doi:10.2353/jmoldx.2010.090188.
28. Baltimore D. RNA-dependent DNA polymerase in virions of RNA tumour viruses. Nature. 1970;226(5252):1209–11.
29. Bernard PS, Wittwer CT. Real-time PCR technology for cancer diagnostics. Clin Chem. 2002;48(8):1178–85.
30. Bustin SA. Absolute quantification of mRNA using real-time reverse transcription polymerase chain reaction assays. J Mol Endocrinol. 2000;25(2):169–93. doi:JME00927 [pii].
31. Lay MJ, Wittwer CT. Real-time fluorescence genotyping of factor V Leiden during rapid-cycle PCR. Clin Chem. 1997; 43(12):2262–7.
32. Olek A, Oswald J, Walter J. A modified and improved method for bisulphite based cytosine methylation analysis. Nucleic Acids Res. 1996;24(24):5064–6. doi:l60209 [pii].
33. Herman JG, Graff JR, Myohanen S, Nelkin BD, Baylin SB. Methylation-specific PCR: a novel PCR assay for methylation status of CpG islands. Proc Natl Acad Sci U S A. 1996;93(18):9821–6.
34. Lo YM, Wong IH, Zhang J, Tein MS, Ng MH, Hjelm NM. Quantitative analysis of aberrant p16 methylation using real-time quantitative methylation-specific polymerase chain reaction. Cancer Res. 1999;59(16):3899–903.
35. Emanuel BS, Shaikh TH. Segmental duplications: an 'expanding' role in genomic instability and disease. Nat Rev Genet. 2001;2(10):791–800. doi:10.1038/35093500.
36. Aldred MA, Vijayakrishnan J, James V, Soubrier F, Gomez-Sanchez MA, Martensson G, Galie N, Manes A, Corris P, Simonneau G, Humbert M, Morrell NW, Trembath RC. BMPR2 gene rearrangements account for a significant proportion of mutations in familial and idiopathic pulmonary arterial hypertension. Hum Mutat. 2006;27(2):212–3. doi:10.1002/humu.9398.
37. Aretz S, Stienen D, Uhlhaas S, Stolte M, Entius MM, Loff S, Back W, Kaufmann A, Keller KM, Blaas SH, Siebert R, Vogt S, Spranger S, Holinski-Feder E, Sunde L, Propping P, Friedl W. High proportion of large genomic deletions and a genotype phenotype update in 80 unrelated families with juvenile polyposis syndrome. J Med Genet. 2007;44(11):702–9. doi:10.1136/jmg.2007.052506.
38. Beetz C, Nygren AO, Schickel J, Auer-Grumbach M, Burk K, Heide G, Kassubek J, Klimpe S, Klopstock T, Kreuz F, Otto S, Schule R, Schols L, Sperfeld AD, Witte OW, Deufel T. High frequency of partial SPAST deletions in autosomal dominant hereditary spastic paraplegia. Neurology. 2006;67(11):1926–30. doi:10.1212/01.wnl.0000244413.49258.f5.
39. Depienne C, Fedirko E, Forlani S, Cazeneuve C, Ribai P, Feki I, Tallaksen C, Nguyen K, Stankoff B, Ruberg M, Stevanin G, Durr A, Brice A. Exon deletions of SPG4 are a frequent cause of hereditary spastic paraplegia. J Med Genet. 2007;44(4):281–4. doi:10.1136/jmg.2006.046425.
40. Kanno J, Hutchin T, Kamada F, Narisawa A, Aoki Y, Matsubara Y, Kure S. Genomic deletion within GLDC is a major cause of non-ketotic hyperglycinaemia. J Med Genet. 2007;44(3):e69. doi:10.1136/jmg.2006.043448.
41. Kluwe L, Nygren AO, Errami A, Heinrich B, Matthies C, Tatagiba M, Mautner V. Screening for large mutations of the NF2 gene. Genes Chromosomes Cancer. 2005;42(4):384–91. doi:10.1002/gcc.20138.
42. Michils G, Tejpar S, Thoelen R, van Cutsem E, Vermeesch JR, Fryns JP, Legius E, Matthijs G. Large deletions of the APC gene in 15% of mutation-negative patients with classical polyposis (FAP): a Belgian study. Hum Mutat. 2005;25(2):125–34. doi:10.1002/humu.20122.
43. Redeker EJ, de Visser AS, Bergen AA, Mannens MM. Multiplex ligation-dependent probe amplification (MLPA) enhances the molecular diagnosis of aniridia and related disorders. Mol Vis. 2008;14:836–40.
44. Taylor CF, Charlton RS, Burn J, Sheridan E, Taylor GR. Genomic deletions in MSH2 or MLH1 are a frequent cause of hereditary non-polyposis colorectal cancer: identification of novel and recurrent deletions by MLPA. Hum Mutat. 2003;22(6):428–33. doi:10.1002/humu.10291.
45. Schouten JP, McElgunn CJ, Waaijer R, Zwijnenburg D, Diepvens F, Pals G. Relative quantification of 40 nucleic acid sequences by multiplex ligation-dependent probe amplification. Nucleic Acids Res. 2002;30(12):e57.
46. Eldering E, Spek CA, Aberson HL, Grummels A, Derks IA, de Vos AF, McElgunn CJ, Schouten JP. Expression profiling via novel multiplex assay allows rapid assessment of gene regulation in defined signalling pathways. Nucleic Acids Res. 2003;31(23):e153.
47. Nygren AO, Ameziane N, Duarte HM, Vijzelaar RN, Waisfisz Q, Hess CJ, Schouten JP, Errami A. Methylation-specific MLPA (MS-MLPA): simultaneous detection of CpG methylation and copy number changes of up to 40 sequences. Nucleic Acids Res. 2005;33(14):e128. doi:10.1093/nar/gni127.
48. Bittel DC, Kibiryeva N, Butler MG. Methylation-specific multiplex ligation-dependent probe amplification analysis of subjects with chromosome 15 abnormalities. Genet Test. 2007;11(4):467–75. doi:10.1089/gte.2007.0061.
49. Dikow N, Nygren AO, Schouten JP, Hartmann C, Kramer N, Janssen B, Zschocke J. Quantification of the methylation status of the PWS/AS imprinted region: comparison of two approaches based on bisulfite sequencing and methylation-sensitive MLPA. Mol Cell Probes. 2007;21(3):208–15. doi:10.1016/j.mcp.2006.12.002.
50. Procter M, Chou LS, Tang W, Jama M, Mao R. Molecular diagnosis of Prader-Willi and Angelman syndromes by methylation-specific melting analysis and methylation-specific multiplex ligation-dependent probe amplification. Clin Chem. 2006;52(7):1276–83. doi:10.1373/clinchem.2006.067603.
51. Hess CJ, Errami A, Berkhof J, Denkers F, Ossenkoppele GJ, Nygren AO, Schuurhuis GJ, Waisfisz Q. Concurrent methylation of promoters from tumor associated genes predicts outcome in acute myeloid leukemia. Leuk Lymphoma. 2008;49(6):1132–41. doi:10.1080/10428190802035990.
52. Jeuken J, Cornelissen S, Boots-Sprenger S, Gijsen S, Wesseling P. Multiplex ligation-dependent probe amplification: a diagnostic tool for simultaneous identification of different genetic markers in glial tumors. J Mol Diagn. 2006;8(4):433–43. doi:10.2353/jmoldx.2006.060012.
53. Fodde R, Losekoot M. Mutation detection by denaturing gradient gel electrophoresis (DGGE). Hum Mutat. 1994;3(2):83–94. doi:10.1002/humu.1380030202.

54. Lerman LS, Beldjord C. Comprehensive mutation detection with denaturing gradient gel electrophoresis. In: Cotton RGH, Edkins E, Forrest S, editors. Mutation detection: a practical approach. Oxford: Oxford University Press; 1998. p. 35–9.
55. Riesner D, Steger G, Zimmat R, Owens RA, Wagenhofer M, Hillen W, Vollbach S, Henco K. Temperature-gradient gel electrophoresis of nucleic acids: analysis of conformational transitions, sequence variations, and protein-nucleic acid interactions. Electrophoresis. 1989;10(5–6):377–89. doi:10.1002/elps.1150100516.
56. Rosenbaum V, Riesner D. Temperature-gradient gel electrophoresis. Thermodynamic analysis of nucleic acids and proteins in purified form and in cellular extracts. Biophys Chem. 1987;26(2–3):235–46. doi:0301-4622(87)80026-1 [pii].
57. van der Luijt RB, Khan PM, Vasen HF, Tops CM, van Leeuwen-Cornelisse IS, Wijnen JT, van der Klift HM, Plug RJ, Griffioen G, Fodde R. Molecular analysis of the APC gene in 105 Dutch kindreds with familial adenomatous polyposis: 67 germline mutations identified by DGGE, PTT, and southern analysis. Hum Mutat. 1997;9(1):7–16. doi:10.1002/(SICI)1098-1004(1997)9:1<7::AID-HUMU2>3.0.CO;2-8 [pii] 10.1002/(SICI)1098-1004(1997)9:1<7::AID-HUMU2>3.0.CO;2-8.
58. De Braekeleer M, Mari C, Verlingue C, Allard C, Leblanc JP, Simard F, Aubin G, Ferec C. Complete identification of cystic fibrosis transmembrane conductance regulator mutations in the CF population of Saguenay Lac-Saint-Jean (Quebec, Canada). Clin Genet. 1998;53(1):44–6.
59. Alkan S, Cosar E, Ergin M, Hsi E. Detection of T-cell receptor-gamma gene rearrangement in lymphoproliferative disorders by temperature gradient gel electrophoresis. Arch Pathol Lab Med. 2001;125(2):202–7. doi:10.1043/0003-9985(2001)125<0202:DOTCRG>2.0.CO;2.
60. Nagamine CM, Chan K, Lau YF. A PCR artifact: generation of heteroduplexes. Am J Hum Genet. 1989;45(2):337–9.
61. Bhattacharyya A, Lilley DM. The contrasting structures of mismatched DNA sequences containing looped-out bases (bulges) and multiple mismatches (bubbles). Nucleic Acids Res. 1989;17(17):6821–40.
62. Hayashi K. PCR-SSCP: a simple and sensitive method for detection of mutations in the genomic DNA. PCR Methods Appl. 1991;1(1):34–8.
63. Liu Q, Feng J, Buzin C, Wen C, Nozari G, Mengos A, Nguyen V, Liu J, Crawford L, Fujimura FK, Sommer SS. Detection of virtually all mutations-SSCP (DOVAM-S): a rapid method for mutation scanning with virtually 100% sensitivity. Biotechniques. 1999;26(5):932. 936–8, 940–2.
64. Orita M, Iwahana H, Kanazawa H, Hayashi K, Sekiya T. Detection of polymorphisms of human DNA by gel electrophoresis as single-strand conformation polymorphisms. Proc Natl Acad Sci U S A. 1989;86(8):2766–70.
65. Widjojoatmodjo MN, Fluit AC, Verhoef J. Molecular identification of bacteria by fluorescence-based PCR-single-strand conformation polymorphism analysis of the 16S rRNA gene. J Clin Microbiol. 1995;33(10):2601–6.
66. Liu W, Smith DI, Rechtzigel KJ, Thibodeau SN, James CD. Denaturing high performance liquid chromatography (DHPLC) used in the detection of germline and somatic mutations. Nucleic Acids Res. 1998;26(6):1396–400. doi:gkb270 [pii].
67. O'Donovan MC, Oefner PJ, Roberts SC, Austin J, Hoogendoorn B, Guy C, Speight G, Upadhyaya M, Sommer SS, McGuffin P. Blind analysis of denaturing high-performance liquid chromatography as a tool for mutation detection. Genomics. 1998;52(1):44–9. doi:10.1006/geno.1998.5411. S0888-7543(98)95411-8 [pii].
68. Wagner T, Stoppa-Lyonnet D, Fleischmann E, Muhr D, Pages S, Sandberg T, Caux V, Moeslinger R, Langbauer G, Borg A, Oefner P. Denaturing high-performance liquid chromatography detects reliably BRCA1 and BRCA2 mutations. Genomics. 1999;62(3):369–76. doi:10.1006/geno.1999.6026. S0888-7543(99)96026-3 [pii].
69. Roest PA, Roberts RG, Sugino S, van Ommen GJ, den Dunnen JT. Protein truncation test (PTT) for rapid detection of translation-terminating mutations. Hum Mol Genet. 1993;2(10):1719–21.
70. Pohlreich P, Stribrna J, Kleibl Z, Zikan M, Kalbacova R, Petruzelka L, Konopasek B. Mutations of the BRCA1 gene in hereditary breast and ovarian cancer in the Czech Republic. Med Princ Pract. 2003;12(1):23–9. doi:10.1159/00006816368163 [pii].
71. Zajac V, Kovac M, Kirchhoff T, Stevurkova V, Tomka M. The most frequent APC mutations among Slovak familial adenomatous polyposis patients. Adenomatous polyposis coli. Neoplasma. 2002;49(6):356–61.
72. McKinney JT, Longo N, Hahn SH, Matern D, Rinaldo P, Strauss AW, Dobrowolski SF. Rapid, comprehensive screening of the human medium chain acyl-CoA dehydrogenase gene. Mol Genet Metab. 2004;82(2):112–20. doi:10.1016/j.ymgme.2004.04.004.
73. Burczak JD, Ching S, Hu H-Y, Lee HH. Ligase chain reaction for the detection of infectious agents. In: Wiedbrauk DL, Farkas DH, editors. Molecular methods for virus detection. San Diego: Academic; 1995. p. 315–28.
74. Laffler TG, Carrino JJ, Marshall RL. The ligase chain reaction in DNA-based diagnosis. Ann Biol Clin (Paris). 1993;51(9):821–6.
75. Mahony J, Chong S, Jang D, Luinstra K, Faught M, Dalby D, Sellors J, Chernesky M. Urine specimens from pregnant and non-pregnant women inhibitory to amplification of Chlamydia trachomatis nucleic acid by PCR, ligase chain reaction, and transcription-mediated amplification: identification of urinary substances associated with inhibition and removal of inhibitory activity. J Clin Microbiol. 1998;36(11):3122–6.
76. Gorrin G, Friesenhahn M, Lin P, Sanders M, Pollner R, Eguchi B, Pham J, Roma G, Spidle J, Nicol S, Wong C, Bhade S, Comanor L. Performance evaluation of the VERSANT HCV RNA qualitative assay by using transcription-mediated amplification. J Clin Microbiol. 2003;41(1):310–7.
77. Walker GT, Little MC, Nadeau JG, Shank DD. Isothermal in vitro amplification of DNA by a restriction enzyme/DNA polymerase system. Proc Natl Acad Sci U S A. 1992;89(1):392–6.
78. Westin L, Xu X, Miller C, Wang L, Edman CF, Nerenberg M. Anchored multiplex amplification on a microelectronic chip array. Nat Biotechnol. 2000;18(2):199–204. doi:10.1038/72658.
79. Sooknanan R, van Gemen B, Malek LT. Nucleic acid sequence-based amplification. In: Wiedbrauk DL, Farkas DH, editors. Molecular methods for virus detection. San Diego: Academic; 1995. p. 261–85.
80. Spadoro JP, Dragon EA. Quality control of the polymerase chase reaction. In: Farkas DH, editor. Molecular biology and pathology: a guidebook for quality control. San Diego: Academic; 1993. p. 149–58.
81. Nolte FS. Branched DNA signal amplification for direct quantitation of nucleic acid sequences in clinical specimens. Adv Clin Chem. 1998;33:201–35.
82. Wilber JC. Branched DNA for quantification of viral load. Immunol Invest. 1997;26(1–2):9–13.
83. Elbeik T, Alvord WG, Trichavaroj R, de Souza M, Dewar R, Brown A, Chernoff D, Michael NL, Nassos P, Hadley K, Ng VL. Comparative analysis of HIV-1 viral load assays on subtype quantification: Bayer Versant HIV-1 RNA 3.0 versus Roche Amplicor HIV-1 Monitor version 1.5. J Acquir Immune Defic Syndr. 2002;29(4):330–9.
84. Gleaves CA, Welle J, Campbell M, Elbeik T, Ng V, Taylor PE, Kuramoto K, Aceituno S, Lewalski E, Joppa B, Sawyer L, Schaper C, McNairn D, Quinn T. Multicenter evaluation of the Bayer

VERSANT HIV-1 RNA 3.0 assay: analytical and clinical performance. J Clin Virol. 2002;25(2):205–16.

85. Hann HW, Fontana RJ, Wright T, Everson G, Baker A, Schiff ER, Riely C, Anschuetz G, Gardner SD, Brown N, Griffiths D, United States Lamivudine Compassionate Use Study Group. A United States compassionate use study of lamivudine treatment in nontransplantation candidates with decompensated hepatitis B virus-related cirrhosis. Liver Transpl. 2003;9(1):49–56. doi:10.1053/jlts.2003.50005.
86. Hendricks DA, Stowe BJ, Hoo BS, Kolberg J, Irvine BD, Neuwald PD, Urdea MS, Perrillo RP. Quantitation of HBV DNA in human serum using a branched DNA (bDNA) signal amplification assay. Am J Clin Pathol. 1995;104(5):537–46.
87. Martinot-Peignoux M, Boyer N, Colombat M, Akremi R, Pham BN, Ollivier S, Castelnau C, Valla D, Degott C, Marcellin P. Serum hepatitis B virus DNA levels and liver histology in inactive HBsAg carriers. J Hepatol. 2002;36(4):543–6.
88. Pawlotsky JM, Bastie A, Hezode C, Lonjon I, Darthuy F, Remire J, Dhumeaux D. Routine detection and quantification of hepatitis B virus DNA in clinical laboratories: performance of three commercial assays. J Virol Methods. 2000;85(1–2):11–21.
89. Beld M, Sentjens R, Rebers S, Weegink C, Weel J, Sol C, Boom R. Performance of the New Bayer VERSANT HCV RNA 3.0 assay for quantitation of hepatitis C virus RNA in plasma and serum: conversion to international units and comparison with the Roche COBAS Amplicor HCV Monitor, Version 2.0, assay. J Clin Microbiol. 2002;40(3):788–93.
90. Trimoulet P, Halfon P, Pohier E, Khiri H, Chene G, Fleury H. Evaluation of the VERSANT HCV RNA 3.0 assay for quantification of hepatitis C virus RNA in serum. J Clin Microbiol. 2002;40(6):2031–6.
91. Lorincz A, Anthony J. Hybrid capture: a system for nucelic acid detection by signal amplification technology. In: Van Dyke C, Woodfork K, editors. Luminescence biotechnology: instruments and applications. Boca Raton, FL: CRC Press; 2002. p. 149–58.
92. Lorincz AT. Hybrid Capture method for detection of human papillomavirus DNA in clinical specimens: a tool for clinical management of equivocal Pap smears and for population screening. J Obstet Gynaecol Res. 1996;22(6):629–36.
93. Mazzulli T, Drew LW, Yen-Lieberman B, Jekic-McMullen D, Kohn DJ, Isada C, Moussa G, Chua R, Walmsley S. Multicenter comparison of the digene hybrid capture CMV DNA assay (version 2.0), the pp 65 antigenemia assay, and cell culture for detection of cytomegalovirus viremia. J Clin Microbiol. 1999;37(4):958–63.
94. Schachter J, Hook 3rd EW, McCormack WM, Quinn TC, Chernesky M, Chong S, Girdner JI, Dixon PB, DeMeo L, Williams E, Cullen A, Lorincz A. Ability of the digene hybrid capture II test to identify Chlamydia trachomatis and Neisseria gonorrhoeae in cervical specimens. J Clin Microbiol. 1999;37(11):3668–71.
95. Kessler HH, Pierer K, Dragon E, Lackner H, Santner B, Stunzner D, Stelzl E, Waitzl B, Marth E. Evaluation of a new assay for HBV DNA quantitation in patients with chronic hepatitis B. Clin Diagn Virol. 1998;9(1):37–43.
96. Dyanov HM, Dzitoeva SG. Method for attachment of microscopic preparations on glass for in situ hybridization, PRINS and in situ PCR studies. Biotechniques. 1995;18(5):822–4. 826.
97. Guan XY, Zhang H, Bittner M, Jiang Y, Meltzer P, Trent J. Chromosome arm painting probes. Nat Genet. 1996;12(1):10–1. doi:10.1038/ng0196-10.
98. Schrock E, du Manoir S, Veldman T, Schoell B, Wienberg J, Ferguson-Smith MA, Ning Y, Ledbetter DH, Bar-Am I, Soenksen D, Garini Y, Ried T. Multicolor spectral karyotyping of human chromosomes. Science. 1996;273(5274):494–7.
99. du Manoir S, Speicher MR, Joos S, Schrock E, Popp S, Dohner H, Kovacs G, Robert-Nicoud M, Lichter P, Cremer T. Detection of complete and partial chromosome gains and losses by comparative genomic in situ hybridization. Hum Genet. 1993;90(6):590–610.
100. Hachitanda Y, Toyoshima S, Akazawa K, Tsuneyoshi M. N-myc gene amplification in rhabdomyosarcoma detected by fluorescence in situ hybridization: its correlation with histologic features. Mod Pathol. 1998;11(12):1222–7.
101. Kallioniemi A, Kallioniemi OP, Sudar D, Rutovitz D, Gray JW, Waldman F, Pinkel D. Comparative genomic hybridization for molecular cytogenetic analysis of solid tumors. Science. 1992;258(5083):818–21.
102. Tagawa H, Karnan S, Suzuki R, Matsuo K, Zhang X, Ota A, Morishima Y, Nakamura S, Seto M. Genome-wide array-based CGH for mantle cell lymphoma: identification of homozygous deletions of the proapoptotic gene BIM. Oncogene. 2005;24(8):1348–58. doi:10.1038/sj.onc.1208300.
103. Sharp AJ, Hansen S, Selzer RR, Cheng Z, Regan R, Hurst JA, Stewart H, Price SM, Blair E, Hennekam RC, Fitzpatrick CA, Segraves R, Richmond TA, Guiver C, Albertson DG, Pinkel D, Eis PS, Schwartz S, Knight SJ, Eichler EE. Discovery of previously unidentified genomic disorders from the duplication architecture of the human genome. Nat Genet. 2006;38(9):1038–42. doi:10.1038/ng1862.
104. Shaw-Smith C, Pittman AM, Willatt L, Martin H, Rickman L, Gribble S, Curley R, Cumming S, Dunn C, Kalaitzopoulos D, Porter K, Prigmore E, Krepischi-Santos AC, Varela MC, Koiffmann CP, Lees AJ, Rosenberg C, Firth HV, de Silva R, Carter NP. Microdeletion encompassing MAPT at chromosome 17q21.3 is associated with developmental delay and learning disability. Nat Genet. 2006;38(9):1032–7. doi:10.1038/ng1858.
105. Tagawa H, Suguro M, Tsuzuki S, Matsuo K, Karnan S, Ohshima K, Okamoto M, Morishima Y, Nakamura S, Seto M. Comparison of genome profiles for identification of distinct subgroups of diffuse large B-cell lymphoma. Blood. 2005;106(5):1770–7. doi:10.1182/blood-2005-02-0542.
106. Dhami P, Coffey AJ, Abbs S, Vermeesch JR, Dumanski JP, Woodward KJ, Andrews RM, Langford C, Vetrie D. Exon array CGH: detection of copy-number changes at the resolution of individual exons in the human genome. Am J Hum Genet. 2005;76(5):750–62. doi:10.1086/429588.
107. Bovolenta M, Neri M, Fini S, Fabris M, Trabanelli C, Venturoli A, Martoni E, Bassi E, Spitali P, Brioschi S, Falzarano MS, Rimessi P, Ciccone R, Ashton E, McCauley J, Yau S, Abbs S, Muntoni F, Merlini L, Gualandi F, Ferlini A. A novel custom high density-comparative genomic hybridization array detects common rearrangements as well as deep intronic mutations in dystrophinopathies. BMC Genomics. 2008;9:572. doi:10.1186/1471-2164-9-572.
108. del Gaudio D, Yang Y, Boggs BA, Schmitt ES, Lee JA, Sahoo T, Pham HT, Wiszniewska J, Chinault AC, Beaudet al, Eng CM. Molecular diagnosis of Duchenne/Becker muscular dystrophy: enhanced detection of dystrophin gene rearrangements by oligonucleotide array-comparative genomic hybridization. Hum Mutat. 2008;29(9):1100–7. doi:10.1002/humu.20841.
109. Hegde MR, Chin EL, Mulle JG, Okou DT, Warren ST, Zwick ME. Microarray-based mutation detection in the dystrophin gene. Hum Mutat. 2008;29(9):1091–9. doi:10.1002/humu.20831.
110. Miller DT, Adam MP, Aradhya S, Biesecker LG, Brothman AR, Carter NP, Church DM, Crolla JA, Eichler EE, Epstein CJ, Faucett WA, Feuk L, Friedman JM, Hamosh A, Jackson L, Kaminsky EB, Kok K, Krantz ID, Kuhn RM, Lee C, Ostell JM, Rosenberg C, Scherer SW, Spinner NB, Stavropoulos DJ, Tepperberg JH, Thorland EC, Vermeesch JR, Waggoner DJ, Watson MS, Martin CL, Ledbetter DH. Consensus statement: chromosomal microarray is a first-tier clinical diagnostic test for individuals with developmental disabilities or congenital anomalies. Am J Hum Genet. 2010;86(5):749–64. doi:10.1016/j.ajhg.2010.04.006.

111. Chen P, Lepikhova T, Hu Y, Monni O, Hautaniemi S. Comprehensive exon array data processing method for quantitative analysis of alternative spliced variants. Nucleic Acids Res. 2011;39(18):e123. doi:10.1093/nar/gkr513.
112. Schutte M, Elstrodt F, Bralten LB, Nagel JH, Duijm E, Hollestelle A, Vuerhard MJ, Wasielewski M, Peeters JK, van der Spek P, Sillevis Smitt PA, French PJ. Exon expression arrays as a tool to identify new cancer genes. PLoS One. 2008;3(8):e3007. doi:10.1371/journal.pone.0003007.
113. Wesolowski R, Ramaswamy B. Gene expression profiling: changing face of breast cancer classification and management. Gene Expr. 2011;15(3):105–15.
114. Holt RA, Jones SJ. The new paradigm of flow cell sequencing. Genome Res. 2008;18(6):839–46. doi:10.1101/gr.073262.107.
115. Marguerat S, Wilhelm BT, Bahler J. Next-generation sequencing: applications beyond genomes. Biochem Soc Trans. 2008;36(Pt 5):1091–6. doi:10.1042/BST0361091.
116. Tucker T, Marra M, Friedman JM. Massively parallel sequencing: the next big thing in genetic medicine. Am J Hum Genet. 2009;85(2):142–54. doi:10.1016/j.ajhg.2009.06.022.
117. Meder B, Haas J, Keller A, Heid C, Just S, Borries A, Boisguerin V, Scharfenberger-Schmeer M, Stahler P, Beier M, Weichenhan D, Strom TM, Pfeufer A, Korn B, Katus HA, Rottbauer W. Targeted next-generation sequencing for the molecular genetic diagnostics of cardiomyopathies. Circ Cardiovasc Genet. 2011;4(2):110–22. doi:10.1161/CIRCGENETICS.110.958322.
118. Hu H, Wrogemann K, Kalscheuer V, Tzschach A, Richard H, Haas SA, Menzel C, Bienek M, Froyen G, Raynaud M, Van Bokhoven H, Chelly J, Ropers H, Chen W. Mutation screening in 86 known X-linked mental retardation genes by droplet-based multiplex PCR and massive parallel sequencing. Hugo J. 2009;3(1–4):41–9. doi:10.1007/s11568-010-9137-y.
119. Raffan E, Semple RK. Next generation sequencing–implications for clinical practice. Br Med Bull. 2011;99:53–71. doi:10.1093/bmb/ldr029.
120. Margulies M, Egholm M, Altman WE, Attiya S, Bader JS, Bemben LA, Berka J, Braverman MS, Chen YJ, Chen Z, Dewell SB, Du L, Fierro JM, Gomes XV, Godwin BC, He W, Helgesen S, Ho CH, Irzyk GP, Jando SC, Alenquer ML, Jarvie TP, Jirage KB, Kim JB, Knight JR, Lanza JR, Leamon JH, Lefkowitz SM, Lei M, Li J, Lohman KL, Lu H, Makhijani VB, McDade KE, McKenna MP, Myers EW, Nickerson E, Nobile JR, Plant R, Puc BP, Ronan MT, Roth GT, Sarkis GJ, Simons JF, Simpson JW, Srinivasan M, Tartaro KR, Tomasz A, Vogt KA, Volkmer GA, Wang SH, Wang Y, Weiner MP, Yu P, Begley RF, Rothberg JM. Genome sequencing in microfabricated high-density picolitre reactors. Nature. 2005;437(7057):376–80. doi:10.1038/nature03959.
121. Mir KU, Qi H, Salata O, Scozzafava G. Sequencing by Cyclic Ligation and Cleavage (CycLiC) directly on a microarray captured template. Nucleic Acids Res. 2009;37(1):e5. doi:10.1093/nar/gkn906.
122. Mamanova L, Coffey AJ, Scott CE, Kozarewa I, Turner EH, Kumar A, Howard E, Shendure J, Turner DJ. Target-enrichment strategies for next-generation sequencing. Nat Methods. 2010;7(2):111–8. doi:10.1038/nmeth.1419.
123. Ng SB, Bigham AW, Buckingham KJ, Hannibal MC, McMillin MJ, Gildersleeve HI, Beck AE, Tabor HK, Cooper GM, Mefford HC, Lee C, Turner EH, Smith JD, Rieder MJ, Yoshiura K, Matsumoto N, Ohta T, Niikawa N, Nickerson DA, Bamshad MJ, Shendure J. Exome sequencing identifies MLL2 mutations as a cause of Kabuki syndrome. Nat Genet. 2010;42(9):790–3. doi:10.1038/ng.646.
124. Mao C, Evans C, Jensen RV, Sobral BW. Identification of new genes in Sinorhizobium meliloti using the Genome Sequencer FLX system. BMC Microbiol. 2008;8:72. doi:10.1186/1471-2180-8-72.
125. Fujimoto A, Nakagawa H, Hosono N, Nakano K, Abe T, Boroevich KA, Nagasaki M, Yamaguchi R, Shibuya T, Kubo M, Miyano S, Nakamura Y, Tsunoda T. Whole-genome sequencing and comprehensive variant analysis of a Japanese individual using massively parallel sequencing. Nat Genet. 2010;42(11):931–6. doi:10.1038/ng.691.
126. Drmanac R. The advent of personal genome sequencing. Genet Med. 2011;13(3):188–90. doi:10.1097/GIM.0b013e31820f16e6.
127. Green ED, Guyer MS, National Human Genome Research Institute. Charting a course for genomic medicine from base pairs to bedside. Nature. 2011;470(7333):204–13. doi:10.1038/nature09764.
128. Haas J, Katus HA, Meder B. Next-generation sequencing entering the clinical arena. Mol Cell Probes. 2011;25(5–6):206–11. doi:10.1016/j.mcp.2011.08.005.

Section I

Genetics

Section Editor: Elaine Lyon

Genetic Counseling

3

Christine E. Miller

Abstract

Genetic counseling is a relatively new profession that began four decades ago. Genetic counselors are master level-trained individuals who have specialized knowledge in medical genetics and counseling. About 83 % work directly with patients on a daily basis, while approximately 17 % work in laboratories or other non-patient contact areas. Genetic counselors are trained to be nondirective and advocate for patient autonomy and informed consent. The genetic counseling process involves drawing a family medical pedigree, reviewing medical records, performing risk assessments, explaining medical and scientific information, discussing disease management, treatment and surveillance options, reviewing testing options, and facilitating the decision-making process. Genetic counselors believe that patients will make the best choice for themselves if their decision is made in the context of their belief systems and past experiences. Genetic counseling positions and subspecialties are rapidly evolving to meet patients' needs. Given the speed of gene discovery, genetic counselors must work to keep abreast of knowledge of specific diseases, innovative testing methods, and new disease treatments and surveillance options.

Keywords

Genetic counseling • Genetics • Informed consent • Risks • Benefits • Screening • Testing • Patient • Family • Proband • Family history • Autosomal • Dominant • Recessive • X-linked • Carrier • Ethnicity

Genetic Counseling: The Discipline and the Provider

Genetic counseling is a relatively new healthcare profession rooted in a combination of medical genetics and counseling theory. The first program to train master-level genetic counselors was Sarah Lawrence College (New York) graduating its first class of eight students in 1971 [1]. Due to the increasing demand for genetic counseling services in the era of genomic medicine, by 2012, there were a total of 31 master-level genetic counseling training programs in the USA and over 2,500 practicing genetic counselors [2]. The American Board of Genetic Counseling (ABGC) provides accreditation for genetic counseling programs that meet specific educational criteria and it administers a national certification examination for genetic counselors. Thirteen states now regulate the profession of genetic counseling requiring genetic counselors to obtain licensure prior to providing this service to citizens of their state. Of the genetic counselors who provide direct patient counseling, approximately 32 % are employed in prenatal genetics, 22 % in cancer genetics, and 14 % in pediatric genetic settings. Thirty-two percent of genetic counselors have expanded into other subspecialties, including artificial reproductive technology (ART), neurology,

C.E. Miller, M.S., C.L.G.C. (✉)
ARUP Laboratories, 500 Chipeta Way, MS D-115, Salt Lake City, UT 84108, USA
e-mail: MILLERC@aruplab.com

D.G.B. Leonard (ed.), *Molecular Pathology in Clinical Practice*, DOI 10.1007/978-3-319-19674-9_3

Table 3.1 Process of genetic counseling

Precounseling assessment	Construct medical pedigree, review pertinent medical records, and perform clinical assessment
Risk assessment	Calculate risk for occurrence using medical pedigree, test results, medical literature, and Bayesian analysis
Counsel patient, couple, or family	Explain medical and scientific information, discuss disease management, treatment and surveillance options, review various testing options, facilitate decision-making process and order appropriate genetic test(s)
Follow up	Summarize discussion in written form for referring healthcare provider and consultant(s), share information about support groups or patient-friendly information on the Internet, provide referrals to psychotherapists or family therapists, as necessary

psychiatry, cardiology, ophthalmology, and genomic and laboratory medicine. Approximately 9 % of genetic counselors work in diagnostic laboratories providing education and support to the patients and physicians who request help with genetic test selection and result interpretation [3]. Genetic counseling is a profession that actively responds to the changing landscape of medicine and matches the trends and needs in the healthcare marketplace.

Physicians with a subspecialty in genetics also provide genetic counseling services. Physician geneticists have a background in various disciplines such as obstetrics, pediatrics, and internal medicine have obtained specialty training in medical genetics and are board certified by the American Board of Medical Genetics (ABMG). As genomic medicine evolves into mainstream healthcare, all providers will need some genetic training to be able to order appropriate tests for their patients and understand the clinical significance of molecular and genomic test results.

Genetic counseling is a process whereby a genetic counselor (1) elicits a family history to construct a medical family pedigree, (2) obtains necessary records to confirm reported diagnoses, (3) determines the risk for occurrence or recurrence of a specific disorder(s), (4) communicates the natural history of the disorder(s) and risk for recurrence, and (5) explains screening, testing, or treatment options to the patient/family in a nondirective manner helping them make the best possible adjustment to the condition(s). Table 3.1 summarizes the key stages of the genetic counseling process. In 2007, the National Society of Genetic Counseling (NSGC) released an expanded scope of practice which included genetic counselors' ability to order genetic tests and perform clinical assessments in accordance with state and federal regulations [4]. The scope of practice will need continual reassessment to meet patients' needs in this rapidly evolving profession.

Clinical Genetic Counseling

Prenatal Setting

Women are referred for prenatal (and less commonly preconception) genetic counseling and prenatal diagnosis for numerous reasons including advanced maternal age (>34 years), abnormal screening test results, abnormal ultrasound findings, family history of an inherited condition, consanguinity, teratogen exposure, and multiple miscarriages or stillbirths. Although all women are at risk to have a child with a chromosome abnormality, this risk increases with maternal age. Thus, advanced maternal age remains one of the most common reasons a woman is referred for prenatal genetic counseling. In 2007, the American College of Obstetrics and Gynecology (ACOG) recommended all women be offered first- and second-trimester maternal serum screening (MSS) for Down syndrome, trisomy 18, and open neural tube defects [5]. ACOG stated that women of all ages should have the option of invasive diagnostic testing. This is a large departure from when prenatal diagnosis was mainly offered to women 35 years and older in the 1970s and early 1980s.

Amniocentesis remains the most common prenatal diagnostic technique. The procedure involves guiding a needle through the abdominal wall into the uterus and withdrawing 20 cc of amniotic fluid, which contains fetal cells, for cytogenetic and molecular analysis. Optimally, amniocentesis is performed under ultrasound guidance between 14 and 18 weeks of gestation, but can be performed safely throughout the remainder of pregnancy as well. It has been reported to be associated with a fetal loss rate of 1 in 770 by experienced practitioners [6]. Another diagnostic procedure, called chorionic villus sampling (CVS), involves removal of a small amount of chorionic villi from the placenta, either transcervically or transabdominally, to obtain fetal cells for testing. Although the miscarriage risk associated with CVS is greater than that of amniocentesis at most centers, the advantage is that CVS can be performed in the first trimester of pregnancy at 10–13 weeks of gestation [7]. A new screening test for Down syndrome, performed by isolating cell-free fetal DNA in the maternal circulation, may significantly reduce the number of invasive diagnostic procedures performed. Early publications indicate the sensitivity of this maternal blood test for Down syndrome is >98 % with a specificity of 99.8 %, which compares highly favorably to traditional maternal serum screening for Down syndrome with a sensitivity of 60–93 % and specificity of 1–5 % [8].

Given the increasing sophistication of ultrasonography equipment and its routine use in pregnancy, most fetal anomalies such as neural tube defects, holoprosencephaly, abdominal wall defects, or severe cardiac abnormalities are detected prenatally and rarely present unexpectedly in the

Table 3.2 Disorders recommended for routine screening in specific ethnic groups

Ethnicity	Disease	Carrier frequency	Recommended by
African, Mediterranean, Southeast Asian, Middle Eastern	Alpha thalassemia	1 in 3 Africans	ACOG
African, Mediterranean, Middle Eastern, Asian Indian	Sickle cell anemia	1 in 12 African Americans	ACOG
Northern African, Southern European, Asian Indian	Beta thalassemia	1 in 12 Southern Europeans	ACOG
Ashkenazi Jewish	Tay-Sachs	1 in 30	ACMG, ACOG
	Canavan	1 in 50	ACMG, ACOG
	Familial dysautonomia	1 in 32	ACMG, ACOG
	Bloom syndrome	1 in 100	ACMG
	Fanconi anemia (type C)	1 in 89	ACMG
	Gaucher	1 in 15	ACMG
	Niemann-Pick (type A)	1 in 90	ACMG
	Mucolipidosis IV	1 in 127	ACMG
All ethnicities	Cystic fibrosis	1 in 25 Caucasians	ACMG, ACOG
All ethnicities	Spinal muscular atrophy	1 in 35 Caucasians	ACMG

delivery room. Thus, prenatal genetic counselors often find themselves providing crisis counseling for individuals who have just been informed about a significant birth defect following a "routine ultrasound examination to confirm the pregnancy's dates." In fetal abnormality cases, when CVS or amniocentesis is performed, consideration is given to ordering comparative genomic hybridization (CGH) instead of just chromosome analysis since CGH can detect relatively small regions of deleted or duplicated genetic material compared with standard chromosome analysis [9].

Screening tests for single-gene disorders are recommended for expectant individuals or those planning a pregnancy in "high-risk ethnic groups" (see Table 3.2). The specific criteria used to select tests for population screening is based on a number of factors such as incidence in the population to be screened, medical knowledge of the disorder, and sensitivity and specificity of testing methods. In 2001, screening for cystic fibrosis (CF) was recommended but was controversial for the following three reasons: (1) the majority of expectant individuals would need to be offered screening; (2) the screening panel would not detect all carriers and would have variable detection rates depending on ethnicity; and (3) insufficient numbers of genetic counselors were available to provide informed consent [10]. Nevertheless, cystic fibrosis screening was successfully implemented by obstetricians and other primary care providers and couples who screened positive were referred to a genetic counselor.

In 2011, in dramatic divergence from ACOG and the American College of Medical Genetics (ACMG) testing guidelines, several direct to consumer marketing companies began promoting carrier screening tests for expectant couples for hundreds of exceedingly rare conditions, many of which were unfamiliar for most healthcare providers. Thus, providing proper informed consent for such prenatal panels was and remains difficult, at best. Furthermore, when a woman learns she is a carrier for a rare condition, a gene sequencing test may need to be offered to her reproductive partner since many of the mutations targeted on such panels represent a small percentage of the causative mutations for the specific condition. This may present two additional problems: (1) there may not be a clinical laboratory specifically performing sequence analysis for the rare genetic disorder in question, and (2) even if one succeeds in finding such a laboratory to perform sequencing, the reproductive partner may be found to have a variant of uncertain significance. This uncertainty may lead to confusion and high anxiety for a couple who thought that they were undergoing routine prenatal screening and would receive clear and clinically interpretable results.

Preimplantation genetic diagnosis (PGD) offers an alternative to prenatal testing for couples who are at risk of having a child with a genetic condition. Through in vitro fertilization (IVF), a single cell is removed from each embryo, usually on day 3 at the 8-cell stage, and tested for the specific genetic condition or familial mutation; then, the unaffected embryos are transferred back to the mother. PGD was first successfully performed in 1990 and is presently being offered for many monogenic disorders and chromosome abnormalities [11]. However, PGD is not yet routine as there are still many obstacles in the process related to the highly technical nature of the procedures and the difficulties in performing cytogenetic or molecular analysis on a single cell. The rate of pregnancy among patients undergoing IVF and PGD varies, but rarely exceeds about one third. Genetic counseling for couples considering PGD is imperative. Couples need to understand the risks and benefits of these complex procedures and the likelihood of a successful pregnancy. Couples need to weigh these factors against those of standard prenatal diagnosis procedures. IVF and PGD are very expensive, approximately $15,000 per cycle, and are not covered by most insurance providers.

Prenatal genetic counselors explain the risks for various genetic conditions, present patients with prenatal diagnostic testing choices, and discuss management and outcome options. They help patients make informed and autonomous choices by encouraging exploration of personal, spiritual, and cultural beliefs that affect decision making [12, 13]. Genetic counselors support patients who choose to continue affected pregnancies by arranging appointments with pediatric specialists, fetal and pediatric surgeons, and neonatal intensive care physicians to help the family prepare for the delivery and offer to arrange contact with other families who have had a baby with the same condition. Genetic counselors also support patients who choose to terminate affected pregnancies by making the necessary referrals for the procedure, encouraging autopsy when the diagnosis is still in question, and providing referrals to support groups for individuals who have had a therapeutic abortion.

Pediatric and Adult Setting

Genetic conditions can occur with unique symptoms at all stages of life, from birth defects in a newborn to cognitive changes in an older adult. When a baby is born with birth defects or an individual at any age develops symptoms, the first step in clinical care is establishing an accurate diagnosis. Often medical geneticists are consulted by physicians caring for babies born with birth defects or other clinical symptoms to determine if there is one unifying syndrome or diagnosis that provides an explanation. Providing a diagnosis is helpful as it enables one to predict if the condition is associated with other problems that may develop over time, such as learning problems, behavioral disorders, cancers, or other medical conditions that are not present at the time of the examination. This may allow for early intervention, therapy and medical screening to reduce the impact of, or risk associated with, the conditions. Early diagnosis also may provide an explanation for likely causes of the condition and, therefore, potential recurrence risk for siblings or offspring of the affected individual. Up until 2010, chromosome analysis was a first line test in the evaluation of developmental disabilities, autism or multiple congenital anomalies. CGH should be the initial test for these conditions because the detection of causative deletions or duplications at 15–20 % is much higher than with chromosome analysis (3 %) [14].

Some individuals are affected with what appears to be a genetic condition, yet even after undergoing many tests, the diagnosis remains elusive. Exome sequencing has been conducted for such individuals on a research basis with a 25 % success rate in determining a diagnosis [15]. In 2012, exome sequencing also began to be offered on a clinical basis. Usually, in addition to sequencing the exome of the affected child, the exomes of the parents also are sequenced to determine if the child has de novo mutations or recessive mutations in the same gene from each parent. Analyzing such a large amount of data is very complex and requires an experienced bioinformatics specialist. Genetic counselors often are involved with developing the consent forms for exome sequencing as well as consenting the family members participating in exome sequencing research or clinical testing. Genetic counseling for exome sequencing is very time consuming because the genetic counselor, the patient, and their family members must consider what types of genetic variant information they are interested in learning about and are prepared to hear. For instance, in addition to the variants identified that may be causative for the disease in question, mutations predisposing to other conditions such as cancer, heart disease, and dementia may be detected.

When newborn screening for phenylketonuria was first available in the mid-1960s, the criteria developed to determine if a disorder should be considered for newborn screening included the following: (1) an acceptable treatment protocol is in place that changes the outcome for patients diagnosed early, (2) the condition's natural history is understood, (3) there is an understanding about who will require treatment, and (4) testing is reliable for both affected and unaffected patients and is acceptable to the public [16]. Many states screened for only a few conditions up until the late 1990s when tandem mass spectrometry (MSMS) technology was developed for newborn screening; then the number of conditions screened expanded dramatically. Now, most states screen for at least the 29 rare, mostly metabolic, conditions recommended by ACMG in 2005 [17]. Many of the new conditions being screened do not satisfy all of the criteria originally used for inclusion in newborn screening protocols. Genetic counselors often coordinate, or are heavily involved with, state newborn screening programs and provide valuable information to pediatricians or other healthcare providers caring for newborns who have a positive screen for one or more of these rare disorders.

The increasing access to and availability of genetic testing has improved the diagnostic capabilities for many disorders. Diagnosis of a genetic condition brings emotional, social, and financial burden for the patient and the family. Unlike many other areas of medicine, genetics has medical implications beyond the patient, extending to the entire family. Whether a diagnosis is made during the neonatal, pediatric, or adult years, the importance of genetic counseling remains. The goals of genetic counseling for the patient and

Table 3.3 Elements of pretest predictive genetic counseling [20]

Obtain family history and confirm diagnoses
Review natural history and inheritance of condition, as well as a priori risk
Discuss the benefits, limitations, and risks of testing, and the confidentiality of test results
Discuss motives for testing, anticipated result, psychosocial preparedness, and support system
Present alternatives to testing and assure that testing is voluntary and informed consent is provided

the family following the diagnosis of a genetic condition include: education about the natural history of the condition and medical implications; explanation of the genetic cause, mechanism of inheritance, and recurrence risks; identification of appropriate social and emotional resources; attentiveness to the patient's and the family's reactions to the diagnosis and their coping strategies; promotion of the best possible emotional adjustment for the patient and family; and facilitation of access to necessary medical and social services [18].

Genetic testing for diagnostic purposes is occurring more frequently without pretest counseling when ordered by a primary care provider or a specialist; however, once a positive test result is disclosed, patients are referred for genetic counseling to assist them with understanding the meaning and implications of the test result.

Predictive genetic testing can inform individuals, prior to the onset of symptoms, that they will develop or are at increased risk to develop a hereditary disorder. Experience with predictive genetic testing for adult-onset conditions such as Huntington disease and hereditary cancer syndromes has led to the development and strong endorsement of a multidisciplinary approach to predictive genetic testing that includes pretest and posttest genetic counseling protocols [19, 20]. This approach allows the patient to explore his or her motives for testing, expectations for testing, the risks and benefits of testing, and coping strategies prior to testing. Use of this recommended counseling process is especially important when no treatment or medical intervention is available for the disorder. Most predictive testing protocols require at least two pretest counseling visits (see Table 3.3) to allow the patient time to consider the benefits and risks of testing, develop a support network during the testing process, and ensure voluntary participation in testing. Experiences with Huntington disease testing have shown that patients are at risk for adverse outcomes after the disclosure of predictive genetic test results, whether the result is positive or negative [21]. Result disclosure should be done in person by a genetic counselor or healthcare professional knowledgeable about the disorder and the implications of the test result. Also, a support person for the patient should be present at the pre- and posttest counseling visits.

Cancer Setting

Cancer genetic counseling, which developed in the early 1990s, is now the second most common area of specialization for master level-trained genetic counselors. Genetic testing for inherited cancer syndromes can be useful for diagnosis and medical management for individuals with a tumor or cancer symptoms. For instance, women with breast cancer who have an inherited mutation in *BRCA1*, a tumor-suppressor gene, may be counseled by their oncologist to consider mastectomy and chemotherapy instead of lumpectomy and radiation. Furthermore, other at-risk family members could have targeted testing for the familial mutation and those who test positive may consider undergoing risk-reducing prophylactic mastectomy and oophorectomy. Chapters 22–30 highlight the various issues related to molecular testing for hereditary cancer syndromes, which include variable clinical utility, complex medical management options, dilemmas with molecular testing approaches, and testing in the research setting or during early transition of a test to the clinical laboratory. The potential risks and benefits associated with testing vary based on the specific hereditary cancer syndrome, as well as the patient and family history. The American Society of Clinical Oncology recommends pre- and posttest counseling for individuals referred for cancer genetic testing [22]. The genetic counselor discusses the details of the genetic testing (detection rate, clinical utility, recurrence risk, etc.), as well as early detection and prevention options for individuals with a positive test result. Often, hereditary cancer syndromes increase an individual's risk for cancer in multiple organ systems, which makes medical management, screening, and early detection more complex. For example, some individuals at risk for von Hippel-Lindau syndrome need at least annual screening for brain and spine hemangioblastomas, retinal angiomas, pheochromocytoma, renal cell carcinoma, and other tumors.

Informed Consent

In the healthcare setting, the process of informed consent is a protection for patients. Prior to diagnostic testing or therapeutic intervention, the provider explains the procedure to the patient, along with the risks, benefits, and alternatives, so that the patient can voluntarily make informed decisions about diagnostic and treatment options [23]. Depending on state law and laboratory standards, variation in informed consent requirements for genetic testing exist. Position statements and guidelines for informed consent for genetic testing are available for a growing number of conditions or groups of conditions. The majority of guidelines address issues related to predictive genetic testing. The NSGC recommends

Table 3.4 Key elements of informed consent for genetic testing

Discussion of purpose of the test and risks of procedures involved in obtaining a sample for testing
Clinical utility of the test and interpretation of all possible test results (positive, negative, uncertain, test failure)
Discussion of risks, benefits, and limitations of testing (including psychosocial, cultural, and financial)
Presentation of alternatives to genetic testing
Description of the procedure for communication of results
Confidentiality of test results
Voluntary nature of informed consent

obtaining informed consent prior to predictive genetic testing for adult-onset conditions. Guidelines for informed consent prior to genetic testing stress that this is more than having a patient read and sign a piece of paper. Informed consent should be a communication process that fosters autonomous and informed decision making by the patient [24, 25]. Presentation of the key elements of informed consent (Table 3.4) needs to be tailored to the individual patient's learning style, educational and cultural background, and family situation to optimize the usefulness of informed consent for the patient and their family. This is a time-intensive process that cannot be done by primary care physicians during a routine office visit. The informed consent process also applies to collection of tissue or body fluids for genetic or other research purposes [26].

Genetic Testing for Children and Adolescents

The benefits and harms of genetic testing need to be carefully evaluated before proceeding with testing in children who may not be able to appreciate the implications of such results. When genetic testing directly impacts medical management or treatment for a child with symptoms or clinical features of a condition, the benefits of testing are clear and the well-being of the child is being promoted. However, when genetic testing does not impact medical management, or the condition in question will occur in adulthood, the implications of testing become more complex and the benefits become less clear. The ACMG and the American Society of Human Genetics wrote "Points to Consider: Ethical, Legal and Psychosocial Implications of Genetic Testing in Children and Adolescents" [27]. The recommendations are the following:

1. Timely medical benefit to the child should be the primary justification for genetic testing.
2. Substantial psychological benefits to the competent adolescent also may be a justification for genetic testing.
3. If the medical or psychological benefits of a genetic test will not accrue until adulthood, as in the case of carrier status or adult-onset diseases, genetic testing should be deferred.
4. If the balance of benefits and harms is uncertain, the provider should respect the decision of the competent adolescent and his or her family.
5. Testing should be discouraged when the provider determines that the potential harms of genetic testing in children and adolescents outweigh the potential benefits.

Education and counseling for the parents and the child, at an appropriate level, should be provided. The benefits and harms related to medical issues, psychosocial issues, and reproductive issues need to be presented and discussed. Children and certainly adolescents have decision-making capacity. The child's competence and wishes should be assessed prior to genetic testing and carefully balanced with parental authority. This is especially true for adolescents who can articulate a specific opinion that differs from that of his or her parents [27]. Assent from the child or adolescent should be obtained in addition to informed consent from the parents.

Legal Protection

In the past decade, there was great concern about the risk for health insurance discrimination related to testing for predisposition to various familial cancer syndromes and adult onset conditions such as Huntington disease. With the passage of the Genetic Information Nondiscrimination Act (GINA) in 2008, a federal law that protects Americans from being treated unfairly because of differences in their DNA that may affect their health, this concern has largely been put to rest as GINA provides protection against health insurance and employment discrimination. Even so, GINA does not provide protection against life insurance, disability insurance, or long-term care insurance discrimination [28]. Furthermore, GINA does not provide protection for federal employees or those who are employed by companies with less than 15 individuals. Genetic counselors need to explore whether their patients are protected from health and employment discrimination and incorporate this into the discussion of risks and benefits of genetic testing.

Other Roles for Genetic Counselors

Research Testing

Genetic counseling can be valuable to individuals who are participating in research genetic testing. Research participants may have difficulty understanding the purpose, risks, and benefits of the study. In addition, many participants have expectations of receiving research testing results and do not appreciate the limitations of reporting results in the research setting. Therefore, consent forms created by genetic counselors in language understandable to the general public are a critical component of genetic research. Disclosure of genetic research results to participants is optimally done by a professional able to provide genetic counseling. For many rare conditions, clinical testing is not available; therefore, research testing is the only option for families. When genetic testing is transitioning from research to the clinical setting, a genetic counselor can be a liaison between the participant and the laboratory and be responsible for informed consent and disclosure of results.

Genetic Counselors Working in the Laboratory

Genetic tests differ in many ways from other laboratory tests. One difference is the necessity for the laboratory to receive clinical information, including the patient's symptoms and family history, for proper interpretation of test results. Genetic counselors understand the clinical information needed by molecular laboratories to interpret specific genetic tests. Additionally, genetic counselors can review the clinical information provided to determine whether the test ordered is the most appropriate and cost-effective test given the patient's symptoms and family history. One study of genetic counselors who reviewed thousands of genetic test orders for a laboratory over a 10-month period revealed that greater than one-third of complex genetic tests were misordered [29]. Oftentimes, other healthcare providers do not understand the importance of obtaining medical records documenting a familial condition. For example, if a patient requests testing for spinocerebellar ataxia (SCA) because this condition has been diagnosed in a sibling, the specific type of SCA must be determined, as there are currently 17 causative genes and commercial testing is available for only about 9 of the 17 genes. If the individual requesting the test does not know the specific SCA type, one could order testing for all of the commercially available types; however, a negative result would not eliminate the individual's risk because the proband may have one of the SCAs not included in the testing. A genetic counselor can work with an at-risk individual to obtain the necessary family history information and documentation so that the most accurate and efficient approach to testing can be used and the interpretation of the results will be more informative. An accurate and comprehensive family history is a valuable tool in a diagnostic evaluation as it can be used as a medical screening tool, establish a pattern of inheritance, identify individuals at risk, and determine strategies for genetic testing.

Understanding the clinical validity of a genetic test result can be difficult for both healthcare providers and patients. However, the sensitivity and specificity of the test method used by the testing laboratory are paramount to the interpretation of the results [12]. Many molecular, biochemical, and cytogenetic laboratories have genetic counselors on staff who can be a useful resource for other healthcare providers and the public. They are able to provide the necessary education and information to determine the appropriate approach to genetic testing, facilitate the details of ordering a test, and help interpret and communicate test results (Table 3.5).

Table 3.5 Genetic counselors working in the laboratory

Obtain test-specific clinical information and family history to ensure that the most appropriate test is performed
Facilitate or document the informed consent process to assure that the patient's autonomy is protected
Assist referring physicians and patients with understanding the test results and implications for the patient and family members
Facilitate collection of appropriate family samples for clarifying the significance of variants of uncertain significance

Summary

The goals of genetic counseling are to address the informational and emotional needs of patients and their families [13]. For example, the explanation of risks and benefits associated with a genetic test that is tailored to a patient's educational needs as well as their family, social, and cultural background facilitates informed decision making by promoting patient autonomy and informed consent. The key goals of genetic counseling for most patient encounters include the following:

- Obtain and interpret family medical history information.
- Educate patients so that they understand the medical and genetic information (inheritance and recurrence risks) needed to make health-management decisions and understand their condition.
- Promote informed decision making and informed consent.
- Be aware of nontechnical factors (social, cultural, financial, and emotional factors) that influence patients in the decision-making process.
- Foster genetic competence in patients and families.
- Identify social and professional resources for patients.

As genetic testing expands and is incorporated into mainstream healthcare, especially for disease prevention and treatment (pharmacogenetics) for common disorders, pre- and posttest genetic counseling for every test will not be feasible. However, genetic counseling services need to be available to assist healthcare providers and patients with education and support facilitating safety in genetic testing.

References

1. Sarah Lawrence College Graduate Programs; History. http://www.slc.edu/graduate/programs/human-genetics/character/history/index.html. Accessed 20 Jan 2012.
2. Genetic counseling Programs-US; Accreditation of Training; Programs; http://www.abgc.net/Training_Program_Accreditation/US_Accredited_Programs.asp. Accessed 18 Jan 2012.
3. 2010 Professional Status Survey: Executive Summary; Primary Specialty Area. http://www.nsgc.org/Portals/0/Publications/PSS%202010%20Executive%20Summary%20FINAL.pdf. Accessed 18 Jan 2012.
4. Resta R, Biesecker BB, Bennett RL, et al. A new definition of Genetic Counseling: National Society of Genetic Counselors' Task Force report. J Genet Couns. 2006;15(2):77–83.
5. ACOG Practice Bulletin. Clinical Management Guidelines for Obstetrician—Gynecologists. Number 77, Jan 2007.
6. Odibo AO et al. Revisiting the fetal loss rate after second-trimester genetic amniocentesis: a single center's 16 year experience. Obstet Gynecol. 2008;111:589–95.
7. Shulman LP, Elias S. Amniocentesis and chorionic villus sampling in fetal medicine. West J Med. 1993;159(special issue): 260–8.
8. Palomaki GE, Kloza EM, Lambert-Messerlian GM, et al. DNA sequencing of maternal plasma to detect Down syndrome: an international clinical validation study. Genet Med. 2011;13(11): 913–20.
9. Fiorentino F, Caiazzo F, Napolitano S, et al. Introducing array comparative genomic hybridization into routine prenatal diagnosis practice: a prospective study on over 1000 consecutive clinical cases. Prenat Diagn. 2011;31(13):1270–82.
10. National Institutes of Health Consensus Development Conference Statement on genetic testing for cystic fibrosis. Arch Intern Med. 1999;159:1529–39.
11. Kanavakis E, Traeger-Synodinos J. Preimplantation genetic diagnosis in clinical practice. J Med Genet. 2002;39:6–11.
12. Burke W. Genomic medicine: genetic testing. N Engl J Med. 2002;347:1867–75.
13. Weil J. Genetic counseling in the era of genomic medicine: as we move towards personalized medicine, it becomes more important to help patients understand genetic tests and make complex decisions about their health. EMBO Rep. 2002;3:590–3.
14. Miller DT, Adam MP, Swaroop A, et al. Consensus statement: chromosomal microarray is a first-tier clinical diagnostic test for individuals with developmental disabilities or congenital anomalies. Am J Hum Genet. 2010;86:749–64.
15. Gahl WA, Markello TC, Toro C, et al. The National Institutes of Health Undiagnosed Diseases Program: insights into rare diseases. Genet Med. 2012;14(1):51–9.
16. Ross LF. Screening for conditions that do not meet the Wilson and Jungner criteria: the case of Duchenne muscular dystrophy. Am J Med Genet. 2006;140A(8):914–22.
17. Natowicz M. Newborn screening—setting evidence-based policy for protection. N Engl J Med. 2005;353:867–70.
18. Walker AP. The practice of genetic counseling. In: Baker DL, Schulette JL, Uhlmann WR, editors. A guide to genetic counseling. New York: Wiley-Liss; 1998. p. 1–20.
19. Almqvist EW, Bloch M, Brinkman R, Craufurd D, Hayden MR. A worldwide assessment of the frequency of suicide, suicide attempts, or psychiatric hospitalization after predictive testing for Huntington disease. Am J Hum Genet. 1999;64:1289–92.
20. International Huntington Association and World Federation of Neurology. Guidelines for the molecular genetic predictive test in Huntington's disease. J Med Genet. 1994;31:555–9.
21. McKinnon WC, Baty BJ, Bennett RL, et al. Predisposition genetic testing for late-onset disorders in adults: a position paper of the National Society of Genetic Counselors. JAMA. 1997;278:1217–20.
22. American Society of Clinical Oncology (ASCO). Policy statement update: genetic testing for cancer susceptibility. J Clin Oncol. 2003; 21:2397–406.
23. Andrews LB. Compromised consent: deficiencies in the consent process for genetic testing. JAMA. 1997;52:39–44.
24. Geller G, Botkin JR, Green MJ, et al. Genetic testing for susceptibility to adult-onset cancer: the process and content of informed consent. JAMA. 1997;277:1467–74.
25. Sharpe NF. Informed consent and Huntington disease: a model for communication. Am J Med Genet. 1994;50:239–46.
26. American Society of Human Genetics (ASHG) Report. Statement on informed consent for genetic research. Am J Hum Genet. 1996;59:471–4.
27. American College of Medical Genetics/ASHG. Points to consider: ethical, legal and psychosocial implications of genetic testing in children and adolescents. Am J Hum Genet. 1995;57:1233–41.
28. Clifton JM, VanBeuge SS, Mladenka C, et al. The Genetic Information Nondiscrimination Act 2008: what clinicians should understand. J Am Acad Nurse Pract. 2010;22(5):246–9.
29. Miller C. Value of genetic counselors in the laboratory. Adv Med Lab Prof http://laboratorian.advanceweb.com/features/articles/value-of-genetic-counselors-in-the-laboratory.aspx?CP=2.

Pedigree Analysis and Risk Assessment

4

Patti Krautscheid and Danielle LaGrave

Abstract

The genetic family history, or pedigree, is a valuable tool for assessment of disease risk. Use of standardized symbols and nomenclature in pedigrees is recommended to ensure accurate communication of information to end users. There are common questions which should always be asked during collection of a family health history; however, questioning is often tailored for the condition under evaluation. Pedigrees may also help assess disease transmission patterns in the family which may be Mendelian (autosomal recessive, autosomal dominant, X-linked recessive, X-linked dominant, Y-linked), chromosomal, mitochondrial, or multifactorial. When atypical patterns of inheritance are seen, consideration should be given to other factors which can influence transmission including, imprinting, uniparental disomy, unstable DNA, gene-environment interactions, mosaicism, and synergistic heterozygosity. Recognition of the mode of inheritance within a family can be useful for estimating disease risk for family members or offspring. Risk assessment also may be confounded by logistical factors, such as family dynamics and limited information, or processes such as variable expression of disease, penetrance, heterogeneity, mosaicism, lyonization, or consanguinity. Many different laboratory methods are used for direct detection of genetic mutations associated with disease. When direct mutation analysis is not feasible, gene discovery or assessing risk for disease may be facilitated by linkage analysis or genome/exome sequencing. Bayesian analysis is a statistical construct that allows for the combination of incremental contributors to risk to determine an individual's risk of developing or transmitting a disorder.

Keywords

Family history • Pedigree • Genetics • Relationships • Risk • Inheritance • Traits • Diagnosis • Maternal • Paternal • Mutations • Genotype • Phenotype • Probability • Dominant • Recessive • X-linked • Carrier • Ethnicity • Transmission

The Genetic Family History

The personal and family medical pedigree has evolved from its earliest ancestors in the fifteenth century to its current form and has become an essential tool in many aspects of the clinical genetics evaluation. Originally used primarily to display relationship information, the pedigree was used for the first time to demonstrate inheritance of traits in the mid-nineteenth century when Pliney Earl published on inheritance

P. Krautscheid, M.S., L.C.G.C. (✉) • D. LaGrave, M.S., L.C.G.C.
ARUP Laboratories, 500 Chipeta Way, Salt Lake City, UT 84108, USA
e-mail: patti.krautscheid@aruplab.com

D.G.B. Leonard (ed.), *Molecular Pathology in Clinical Practice*, DOI 10.1007/978-3-319-19674-9_4

of color blindness and Francis Galton described inheritance of artistic ability and genius [1].

Symbols used to document pedigree information have varied, often depending on personal, professional, or national preferences. The key to functionality for pedigrees, however, is the degree to which they are able to communicate information uniformly to all users. In 1993, a National Society of Genetic Counselors (NSGC) task force surveyed genetic counselors regarding interpretation of pedigree symbols and conformity of usage. Numerous different symbols were being used for very common scenarios, such as pregnancy and miscarriage, and it became evident that standardization was needed. The group established a recommended nomenclature for pedigrees, which has become the widely accepted standard for recording a family health history [2].

The currently recommended methods for documenting pedigree information including symbols, spatial relationships, and nomenclature for clinical/investigative status are detailed in Figs. 4.1, 4.2, 4.3, and 4.4. These standards allow recording of traditional relationships, as well as those nontraditional relationships which are developing as new technologies are applied, in a manner that meets medical-legal requirements and protects patient confidentiality. Because pedigrees contain sensitive information and may be accessed by many individuals, especially if part of the electronic medical record, care should be taken in considering what information to include in a pedigree. To ensure compliance with the Health Insurance Portability and Accountability Act (HIPAA) standards in the USA, the pedigree standardization guidelines recommend including less identifying information on the pedigree [2]. For example, for pedigrees not intended for publication, designating family members using initials or first names (instead of complete names) and listing ages or the year of birth/death (instead of exact dates of birth or death) are preferred. The current standards also serve as a baseline for future additions or modifications as the field continues to evolve.

Pedigrees now form the cornerstone for determination of diagnosis, pattern of inheritance, and recurrence risk. Visually recording elements of family and medical history in the form of a pedigree serves many purposes including: user orientation (to family relationships, source of the information included and reason for pedigree construction), improved readability, risk assessment, validation of information included, compliance with medical documentation standards, communication, and patient education. Well-constructed pedigrees also may result in cost savings by describing evaluations already performed to avoid duplicate testing, and documenting familial mutations necessary for the most cost-effective testing of family members. In addition, collection of family medical information has aided in the understanding of many unique features of hereditary disorders, including natural history, variability, and gene-gene or gene-environment interactions.

Collection of a family pedigree represents an opportunity to build a relationship with the patient and family and to learn about how the family functions. As the genetic counselor or other healthcare provider explains the purpose of obtaining family history, an atmosphere of open communication and respect can be established. This process provides a window to the social relationships and psychosocial and educational needs of patients and families. In the social sciences, genograms are used to graphically depict family dynamics that influence individual behaviors [3]. This information also is essential for successful counseling of patients in the clinical genetics setting, and while not always recorded in the same fashion, family dynamics are a vital part of the process of pedigree gathering. Observations about coping mechanisms, assumptions about disease causation, family hierarchy, key life experiences, stress levels, body language, and religious and ethnic influences all are integrated into consideration about the most effective ways to communicate information about a diagnosis, prognosis, or management plan to patients and families.

Ideally, the pedigree is collected in a face-to-face session. This is usually done prior to or at the beginning of the clinical genetics evaluation, but may be done later, particularly when evaluating a pregnancy or a newborn with an unanticipated, newly diagnosed condition. Advance notice to patients and their families about the nature of information to be collected can facilitate the accuracy and completeness of the information provided by the family. In addition, electronic tools such as the US Surgeon General's Family Health Portrait tool (http://www.hhs.gov/familyhistory) are available to engage patients in collecting their family health information.

At a minimum, a three-generation pedigree should be collected, including all first-degree relatives (parents, children, full siblings), second-degree relatives (grandparents, aunts, uncles, nieces and nephews, half-siblings, grandchildren), and, as pertinent, many third-degree relatives (cousins, great-aunts, great-uncles, great-grandparents). This group can be expanded or condensed, depending on the nature of the referral and patient responses to preliminary questioning about features relevant to the reason for referral. For example, genetic evaluations for hereditary cancer syndromes may necessitate a more extended family pedigree, while a brief, focused pedigree may suffice when discussing cystic fibrosis carrier testing.

Information that should be collected about each individual in the pedigree is listed in Table 4.1. Modifications may be needed depending on the nature of the diagnosis under investigation; recommendations from the NSGC detail additional questions appropriate for individuals being evaluated for hereditary cancer syndromes [4]. Because family medical histories change over time, pedigrees should be updated as new information is learned.

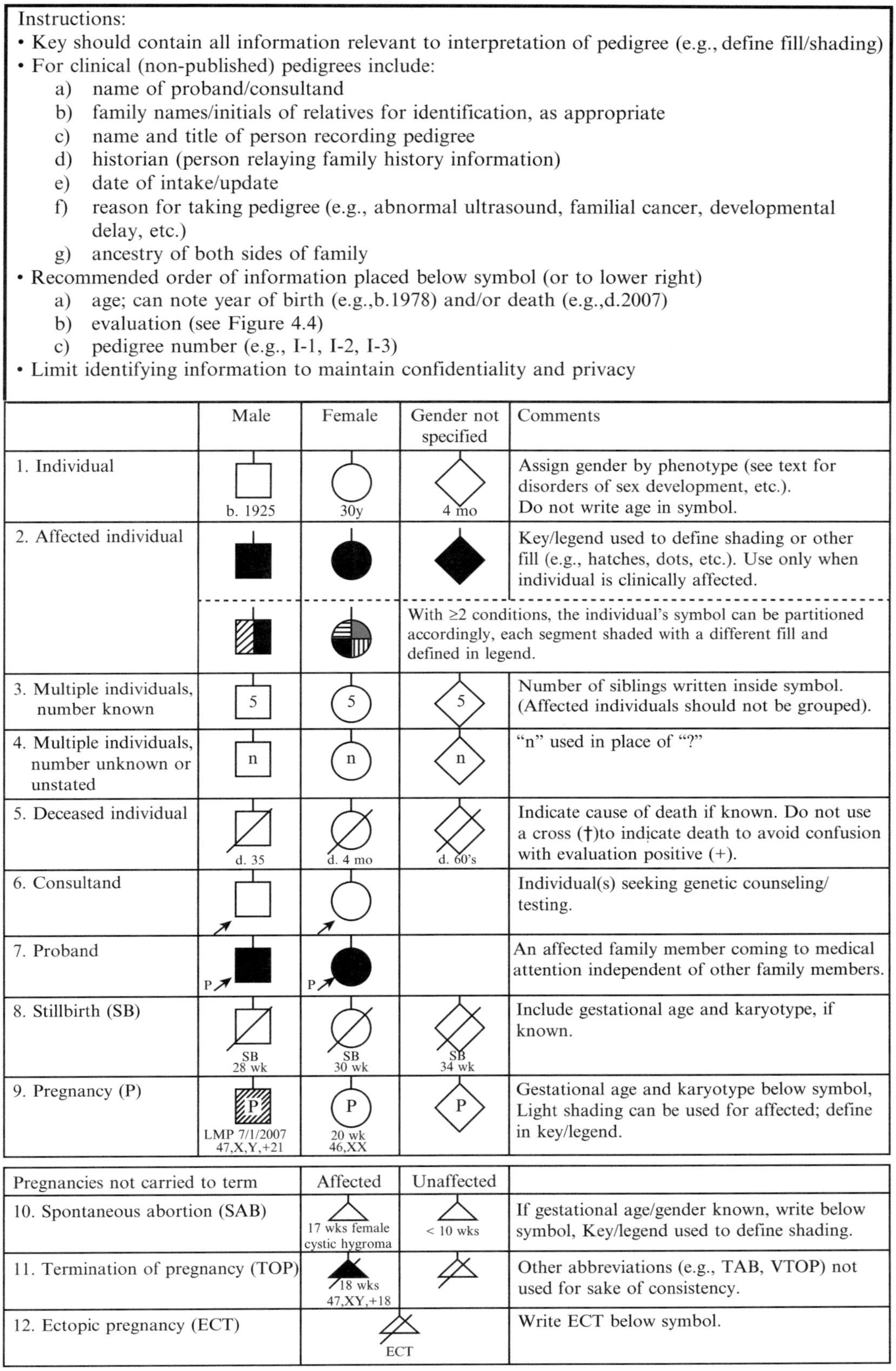

Figure 4.1 Common pedigree symbols, definitions, and abbreviations. From Bennett R, French K, Resta R, Doyle D. Standardized human pedigree nomenclature: update and assessment of the recommendations of the national society of genetic counselors. J Genet Couns. 17;2008:424–33 [2]. Reprinted with permission from Springer.

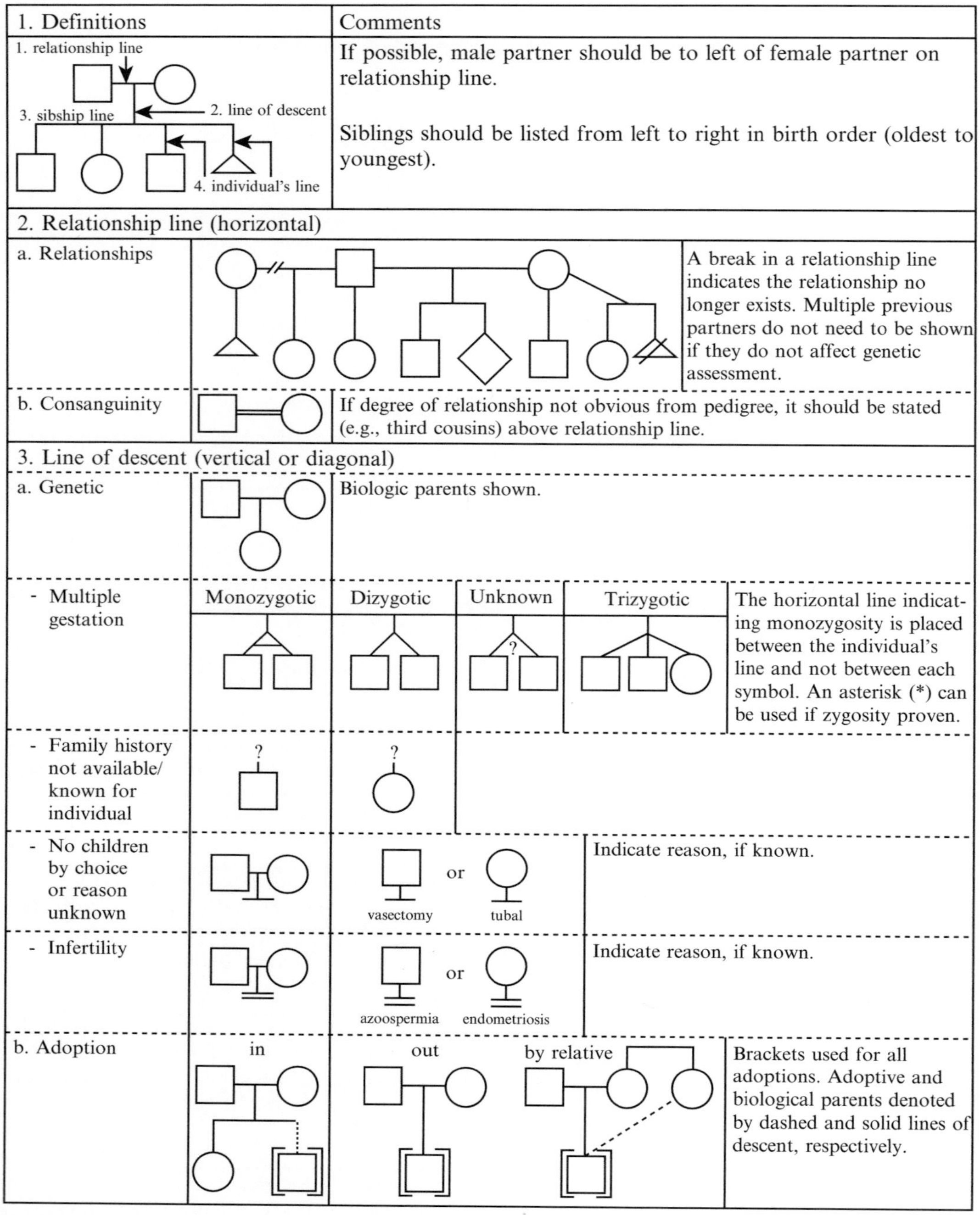

Figure 4.2 Pedigree line definitions. From Bennett R, French K, Resta R, Doyle D. Standardized human pedigree nomenclature: update and assessment of the recommendations of the national society of genetic counselors. J Genet Couns. 17;2008:424–33 [2]. Reprinted with permission from Springer

Ethnicity, consanguinity, and unique biological relationships should be recorded using standard notation. All reported diagnoses or conditions ideally should be confirmed through authorized request and review of medical records. Key records to obtain include pathology reports, test results (particularly for any genetic testing that has been performed), imaging reports, and autopsy reports. In the absence of these documents, family genealogies or death certificates may provide some degree of verification of reported information.

An important issue in the use of pedigrees for clinical evaluations and research is the issue of individual confidentiality [5]. Each member of the family has a right to expect that medical information will remain confidential.

Instructions:
- D represents egg or sperm donor
- S represents surrogate (gestational carrier)
- If the woman is both the ovum donor and a surrogate, in the interest of genetic assessment, she will only be referred to as a donor (e.g., 4 and 5)); the pregnancy symbol and its line of descent are positioned below the woman who is carrying the pregnancy
- Available family history should be noted on the gamete donor and/or gestational carrier

Possible Reproductive Scenarios		Comments
1. Sperm donor	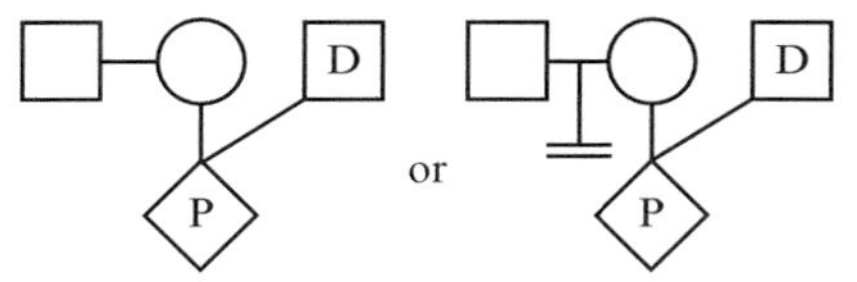	Couple in which woman is carrying pregnancy using donor sperm. No relationship line is shown between the woman carrying the pregnancy and the sperm donor.
2. Ovum donor	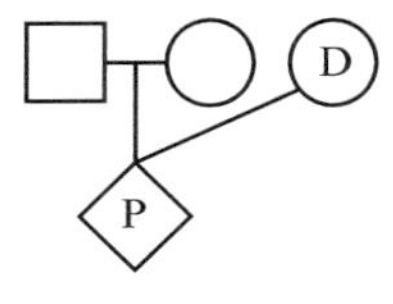	Couple in which woman is carrying pregnancy using a donor egg and partner's sperm. The line of descent from the birth mother is solid because there is a biologic relationship that may affect the fetus (e.g., teratogens).
3. Surrogate only	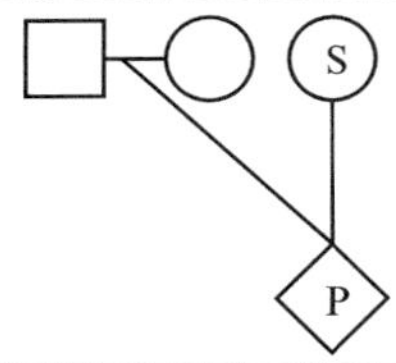	Couple whose gametes are used to impregnate a woman (surrogate) who carries the pregnancy. The line of descent from the surrogate is solid because there is a biological relationship that may affect the fetus (e.g., teratogens).
4. Surrogate ovum donor	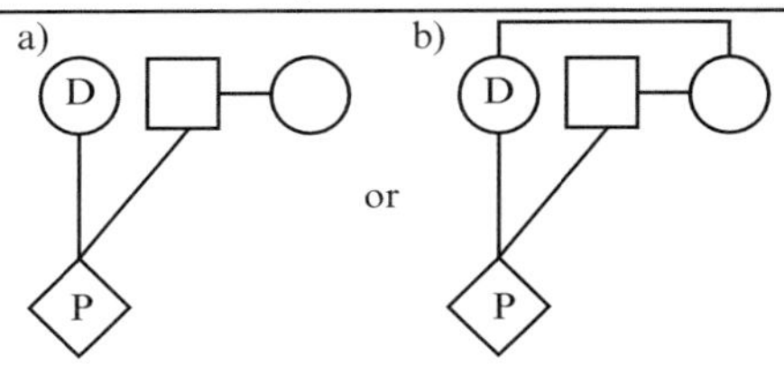	Couple in which male partner's sperm is used to inseminate a) an unrelated woman or b) a sister who is carrying the pregnancy for the couple.
5. Planned adoption	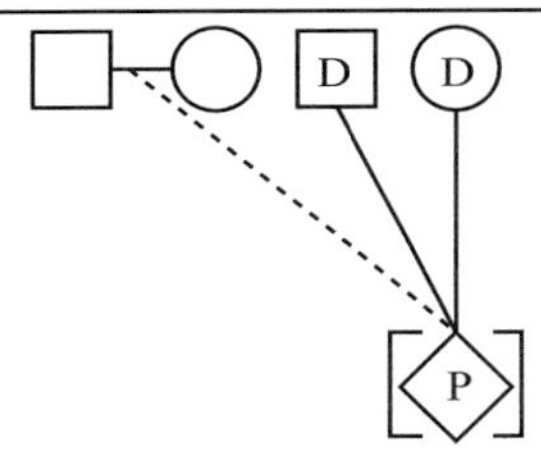	Couple contracts with a woman to carry a pregnancy using ovum of the woman carrying the pregnancy and donor sperm.

Figure 4.3 Assisted reproductive technology symbols and definitions. From Bennett R, French K, Resta R, Doyle D. Standardized human pedigree nomenclature: update and assessment of the recommendations of the national society of genetic counselors. J Genet Couns. 17;2008:424–33 [2]. Reprinted with permission from Springer

This becomes complicated when one considers the pedigree that may contain both reported ("hearsay") and confirmed information for numerous individuals. Those people may have willingly shared information with the patient but may not want it shared with other family members. If subsequent to an evaluation a patient requests release of his or her pedigree to another family member, a provider should carefully consider the question of ownership of the pedigree information and be attuned to the potential consequences of releasing the (identifiable) information about other family members. Current interpretation of regulations outlined by HIPAA and other medical records privacy legislation may influence how such information is shared. Professional organizations including the American Society of Human Genetics also have developed position statements on this issue [6].

Patterns of Inheritance

One key use of the carefully collected and verified pedigree is determination of the most likely mode of inheritance of a condition in a family. This will have relevance to assessing recurrence risks, approaches to testing, and in some cases even

Instructions:
- E is used for evaluation to represent clinical and/or test information on the pedigree
  a. E is to be defined in key/legend
  b. If more than one evaluation, use subscript (E1, E2, E3) and define in key
  c. Test results should be put in parentheses or defined in key/legend
- A symbol is shaded only when an individual is clinically symptomatic
- For linkage studies, haplotype information is written below the individual. The haplotype of interest should be on left and appropriately highlighted
- Repetitive sequences, trinucleotides and expansion numbers are written with affected allele first and placed in parentheses
- If mutation known, identify in parentheses

Definition	Symbol	Scenario	
1. Documented evaluation (*) Use only if examined/evaluated by you or your research/clinical team or if the outside evaluation has been reviewed and verified.	*	Woman with negative echocardiogram.	* E– (echo)
2. Carrier–not likely to manifest disease regardless of inheritance pattern		Male carrier of Tay-Sachs disease by patient report (* not used because results not verified).	
3. Asymptomatic/presymptomatic carrier–clinically unaffected at this time but could later exhibit symptoms		Woman age 25 with negative mammogram and positive BRCA1 DNA test.	* 25y E_1–(mammogram) E_2+(5385insC BRCA1)
4. Uninformative study (u)	Eu	Man age 25 with normal physical exam and uninformative DNA test for Huntington disease (E2).	* 25y E_1–(physical exam) E_2u(36n/18n)
5. Affected individual with positive evaluation (E+)	E+	Individual with cystic fibrosis and positive mutation study; only one mutation has currently been identified.	E+(ΔF508) Eu * E+(ΔF508/u)
		10 week male fetus with a trisomy 18 karyotype.	P * 10wk E+(CVS) 47,XY,+18

Figure 4.4 Pedigree symbols of genetic evaluation/testing information. From Bennett R, French K, Resta R, Doyle D. Standardized human pedigree nomenclature: update and assessment of the recommendations of the national society of genetic counselors. J Genet Couns. 17;2008:424–33 [2]. Reprinted with permission from Springer

prognosis. The concept of patterns of inheritance extends from the seventeenth-century work of Gregor Mendel, who described transmission of traits associated with single genetic loci. Transmission of human genetic conditions and traits has proven to be more complex, involving not only the single-gene patterns first described by Mendel but also chromosomal inheritance, mitochondrial inheritance, and multifactorial inheritance. Other genetic factors which can influence transmission of disease include imprinting, uniparental disomy, unstable DNA, gene-environment interactions, mosaicism, and synergistic heterozygosity. Undoubtedly, additional factors influencing transmission and expression of inherited traits will be elucidated as our understanding of the human genome expands. As of January 2012, the Online Mendelian Inheritance in Man (OMIM), a continuously updated catalog of human genes and genetic phenotypes, listed 13,775 identified genes and 4,520 genetic disorders for which the molecular basis is known [7]. Identified genetic disorders with known patterns of inheritance are commonly inherited as autosomal, X-linked, or mitochondrial.

Table 4.1 Collection of family medical history: what to ask?

For all family members
Current age; year of birth
Exact relationship to the proband
General physical and mental health status
History of major acute or chronic illness, hospitalizations, and surgeries
History of learning problems, diagnosed disabilities, or intellectual disability
Highest grade level completed (when relevant)
Employment (when relevant)
Reproductive history, including pregnancies, miscarriages, elective terminations, infertility, and choice not to have children
Gestational age and last menstrual period for ongoing pregnancies
Consanguinity
Ethnicity
Targeted questions relevant to the reason for evaluation, for example, key symptoms or features of the condition in question, pertinent evaluations
Age at death; year of death; cause of death
For family member known to be affected by the condition in question
Diagnosis
Age at diagnosis or disease onset
Method of diagnosis
Evaluations and testing completed
Symptoms
Information about ongoing treatment or management plan
Availability of medical records for review

Mendelian Inheritance Patterns

For a summary of Mendelian inheritance patterns, see Table 4.2.

Autosomal Dominant Inheritance

In classic autosomal dominant inheritance, an affected individual has one non-functional or mutant allele at a particular locus, the presence of which causes disease. Each affected individual in a pedigree has a 50 % chance of passing the disease-associated mutation to each of his or her offspring. Additional genetic and non-genetic factors may influence the occurrence of these conditions in families. A key feature of autosomal dominant inheritance is the observance of male-to-male transmission of the condition or trait. Transmission from fathers to sons is not seen in X-linked dominant inheritance, which can be confused with autosomal dominant inheritance on first analysis. Table 4.2 lists additional features of autosomal dominant inheritance, and an example pedigree is shown in Fig. 4.5.

Table 4.2 Features of Mendelian patterns of inheritance

Autosomal dominant
Male-to-male transmission occurs; both sexes can transmit to offspring
Affected family members in multiple generations; "vertical transmission" typically showing affected descendants of affected individuals and unaffected descendants of unaffected individuals
Males and females affected, typically to comparable extent
Variability of clinical findings
Later/adult onset in some disorders
Homozygotes may be more severely affected than heterozygotes
Homozygosity may be lethal
Occurrence of new mutations
Nonpenetrance; apparent "skipping" of generations
Germline mosaicism reported
Autosomal recessive
Affected family members are usually in one generation; "horizontal" inheritance
Males and females equally likely to be affected; parental consanguinity or a small mating pool may influence disease occurrence
Disease severity is usually consistent among affected family members
Early onset of symptoms more typical
New mutations rare
May see higher frequency of disease in certain ethnic groups
X-linked dominant
No male-to-male transmission
Affected females usually have milder symptoms than affected males
Affected males have no affected sons, but all daughters will be affected
May mimic autosomal dominant inheritance
May be lethal in affected males; reflected by a paucity of males or overrepresentation of females in the pedigree
Increased occurrence of miscarriage may be observed
X-linked recessive
No male-to-male transmission
Males more frequently affected
Carrier females usually unaffected but may have mild symptoms
Affected males in a family are related through females
Y-linked
Male-to-male transmission only
Association with increased rates of male infertility
Discrepancy between chromosomal and phenotypic sex

Autosomal Recessive Inheritance

In autosomal recessive inheritance, an affected individual has two non-functional or mutant alleles at a particular locus. Carriers of autosomal recessive conditions have one nonfunctional allele at the gene locus, but usually have no symptoms as they also have one normal, functional copy of the gene. If both partners of a couple are carriers of the same autosomal recessive condition, with each pregnancy there is a one in four (25 %) chance of having an affected child, a two-in-four

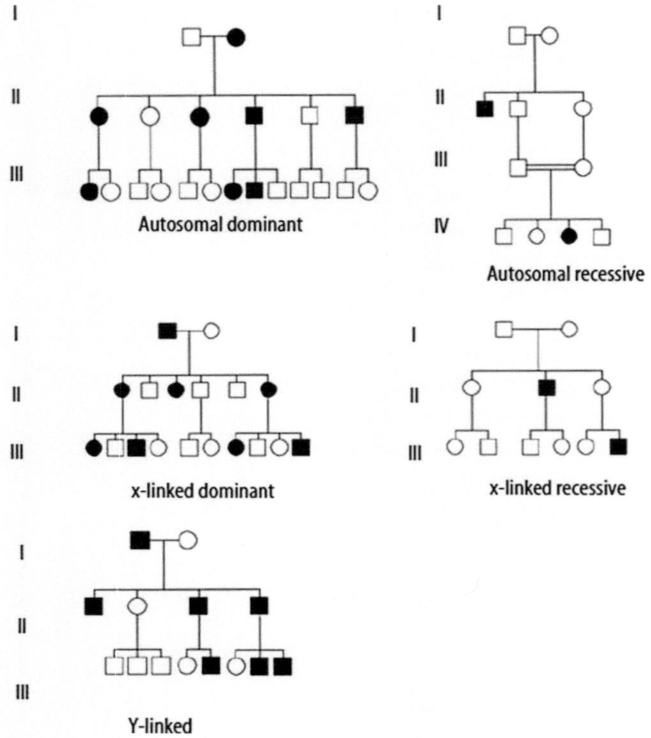

Figure 4.5 Example pedigrees for Mendelian patterns of inheritance

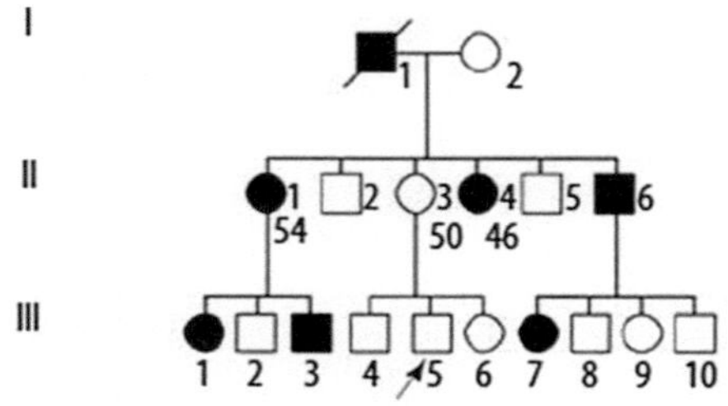

For II.3	Gene present	Gene not present
Prior probability	1/2	1/2
Conditional probability	1/4	1
Joint probability	$\frac{1/8}{1/8+1/2}$	$\frac{1/2}{1/8+1/2}$
Posterior probability	1/5 =20%	4/5 =80%
For III.5	1/5x1/2=1/10=10%	

Figure 4.6 Bayesian analysis for risk assessment in an autosomal dominant, adult-onset hereditary cancer disorder. Ages of selected individuals in generation II are shown below the pedigree symbols

(50 %) chance that a child will be a carrier and a one in four (25 %) chance a child will be neither a carrier nor affected. After birth, if a child of a carrier couple is not affected by the condition in question, he or she has a two-in-three chance of being a carrier. Risk to future offspring of a known carrier depends on the likelihood that his or her partner is also a carrier. This is influenced by the frequency of the disease, which may vary among different ethnic groups or populations. Features of autosomal recessive inheritance are listed in Table 4.2, and an example pedigree is shown in Fig. 4.5.

X-Linked Dominant Inheritance

In X-linked dominant inheritance, an affected individual has one nonfunctional or mutant allele at a locus on an X-chromosome. X-linked dominant conditions can occur in either males or females. Risk for offspring of an affected female is 50 %, regardless of the sex of the offspring. Risk to offspring of affected males is sex dependent, with all daughters but no sons inheriting the gene mutation. Many of these conditions, however, are lethal in males, so pedigrees may show overrepresentation of females or increased frequency of miscarriages, presumably of affected male fetuses (see Table 4.2 and Fig. 4.6).

X-Linked Recessive Inheritance

Traditional X-linked recessive inheritance is characterized by occurrence of the condition in males having a non-functional or mutant allele for a gene on the X-chromosome. Affected males in the family will be related to each other through females. (See the pedigree in Fig. 4.5, and Table 4.2 for additional features.) Typically, carrier females are unaffected; however, due to lyonization (random inactivation of one X chromosome in each somatic cell in a female), carrier females may have mild symptoms. This occurs when, by chance, the X chromosome with the non-functional allele remains active in a majority of the cells within the critical tissue(s) for the disorder. The likelihood of symptoms in carrier females varies considerably among disorders. Risk to offspring of carrier females is 25 % overall, or 50 % for affected status if the fetus/offspring is male. Fifty percent of the female offspring of carrier females will also be carriers. Offspring of affected males will not be classically affected, but all daughters will be carriers.

Y-Linked Inheritance

In rare cases, a mutation can occur in one of a limited number of genes on the Y chromosome. This can result in disparity between chromosomal and phenotypic sex if the SRY region is involved, or can be associated with hereditary forms of male infertility. This may be identified more frequently as reproductive technologies such as intracytoplasmic sperm injection (ICSI) are used to aid in achieving pregnancies for previously infertile males, due to Y-chromosome deletions, for example (see Table 4.2 and Fig. 4.5).

Codominant Inheritance

In codominant inheritance, two different alleles of the gene of interest are present and each is expressed. Therefore, the resulting phenotype is influenced by expression of both alleles. Traits inherited in this fashion include the ABO blood group and alpha-1-antitrypsin deficiency.

Non-Mendelian Inheritance Patterns

For a summary of non-Mendelian inheritance patterns, see Table 4.3.

Chromosomal Disorders

Chromosome abnormalities can occur sporadically or can be caused by familial transmission of duplications, deletions, or rearrangements that can result in imbalance of genetic material in the offspring. Chromosomal disorders caused by changes in the number of chromosomes (e.g., Down syndrome) occur most often due to random events during meiosis, and are typically not inherited. Copy number variants (CNVs), small deletions, or duplications of chromosomal material may be benign or disease causing, and may be inherited or de novo. Chromosomal rearrangements, such as translocations (the exchange of parts of nonhomologous chromosomes) and inversions (the breakage and reversal of a single chromosome segment), usually are deleterious when unbalanced. Unbalanced rearrangements are commonly inherited from a parent who carries a balanced version of the rearrangement. Chromosome abnormalities commonly are associated with multiple phenotypic effects as they usually cause deletion and/or duplication of many genes on the chromosomal segment(s) involved.

Table 4.3 Features of non-Mendelian patterns of inheritance

Chromosomal
Occurrence of congenital anomalies involving two or more organ systems
Occurrence of intellectual disability with dysmorphism or congenital anomalies
Multiple pregnancy losses or infertility in carriers of balanced translocations
Many occur as sporadic conditions with negative family history
Mitochondrial
Extreme variability of clinical symptoms; multiple organ systems involved
Degenerative/neuromuscular disorders predominate
Maternal transmission (fathers do not transmit disease)
Multiple generations affected (matrilineal)
Males and females equally likely to be affected
Environmental factors may influence symptoms
Multifactorial inheritance
Implicated in common adult-onset disorders
Males and females affected
The number and sex of affected relatives influence recurrence risk
Degree of relationship to affected relatives influences recurrence risk

The classic microdeletion syndromes (e.g., DiGeorge syndrome, Williams syndrome) are clinically recognizable disorders resulting from the loss of many adjacent genes along a defined segment of a chromosome and usually result from a de novo event. The mechanism responsible for common microdeletion/microduplication syndromes is homologous recombination between stretches of nearly identical sequence that either remove or duplicate the unique intervening sequence [8]. Microdeletion/duplication syndromes are most reliably detected using array comparative genomic hybridization (aCGH) or fluorescence in situ hybridization (FISH) because the abnormalities are usually not detectable using standard cytogenetics.

Risks to offspring of individuals with chromosomal rearrangements or CNVs depend on the specific chromosome region(s) involved, size of the abnormality, and sometimes the sex of the transmitting parent. In apparently sporadic cases of unbalanced chromosomal rearrangements or disease-associated CNVs, parental testing with respect to the chromosomal abnormality should be performed to assess recurrence risk. Absence of a parental chromosome abnormality in such cases reduces the risk to future offspring. It is important to note that novel CNVs identified in an affected individual and in an unaffected parent should not be assumed to be benign; such CNVs may be disease causing but exhibit variable expressivity or reduced penetrance [9].

Mitochondrial Disorders

The mitochondrial (mt) genome is a 16.5 kb circular strand of DNA located within the mitochondria. Unlike nuclear genes, the mt genome has a very high mutation rate due to lack of DNA repair mechanisms. In general, large deletions in the mtDNA arise as new mutations and confer low risk to relatives, while point mutations and duplications are commonly maternally transmitted [10]. Individuals inherit essentially all their mitochondrial DNA from their mothers; thus, transmission of mtDNA mutations is maternal. Affected males do not transmit mtDNA mutations to offspring. In each cell, including egg cell progenitors, there may be up to 1,000 mitochondria. If a mutation occurs in one of these mitochondria, as the mitochondrion divides over time, the mutation becomes present in a percentage of the overall mitochondrial population in the cell. When the cell divides, the mitochondria are distributed stochastically to the daughter cells. The daughter cells may inherit only mutant mtDNA or no mutant mtDNA (homoplasmy), or a mix of mutant and nonmutant mtDNA (heteroplasmy). When the proportion of mutant mtDNA exceeds a critical threshold in the cell, mitochondrial dysfunction results. As the degree of heteroplasmy may differ among individuals in a family, predicting risk to offspring of affected females is difficult. The level of heteroplasmy may differ in cell populations of different organs or tissues of an affected individual; therefore, conditions caused by mtDNA mutations often result in phenotypes affecting multiple organ systems and exhibit highly variable expression. Mutations in nuclear genes which affect mitochondrial function also can result in mitochondrial diseases. Such disorders are inherited in either an autosomal or X-linked fashion and tend to have expression that more closely resembles other Mendelian disorders.

Table 4.4 Genetic factors influencing transmission

Genomic imprinting
Gender of transmitting parent modifies gene/disease expression (parent-of-origin effects)
May appear to skip generations
Uniparental disomy
Single/isolated case in a family
Documentation of only one carrier parent in individuals with an autosomal recessive disease
X-linked recessive disorders occurring in 46,XX females
Unstable DNA
Anticipation (increasing severity with subsequent generations)
Gender of the transmitting parent may influence disease likelihood and severity
Synergistic heterozygosity
Unaffected, unrelated parents have multiple affected offspring
Described for genes with autosomal recessive inheritance
Implicated genes act in the same biological pathway or their proteins form complexes

Multifactorial Disorders

Multifactorial disorders are the result of the interaction or additive effect of multiple genetic and environmental factors. The likelihood of expression of a trait or disease is based on the relative contributions of each of the factors involved. With a relatively low concentration of contributing factors, no effect will be seen. Above a critical cutoff of accumulated factors, the condition occurs. Risk to relatives of affected individuals increases as more family members are affected, presumably reflecting the presence of a higher "dose" of critical factors in the family or shared environmental factors. For multifactorial disorders that are more common in one sex, such as pyloric stenosis or neural tube defects, the risk for recurrence is higher for relatives when the affected individual is of the less commonly affected sex. Empiric risk figures for multifactorial disorders may be used for genetic counseling, but should be modified based on individual factors including number of affected relatives, relationship of affected family members to the counselee, severity of disease, and sex.

Genetic Mechanisms Influencing Transmission

For a summary of several known genetic factors which influence transmission, see Table 4.4.

Genomic Imprinting

Imprinting refers to differential expression of genes depending on the parent of origin. The process is reversible, as it affects the action of the gene but not the gene structure; genes that are passed from a male (imprinted as male) to a female are then reimprinted as female before being transmitted to the next generation, and so on. Genomic imprinting is thought to occur early in development, most likely in the germ cells [11]. Imprinting errors have been described in a number of disorders including about 3 % of individuals with Angelman syndrome and an estimated 1 % of patients with Prader-Willi syndrome. If an affected individual has a mutation in an imprinting control center, which controls gene expression by regulating methylation, recurrence risks may be as high as 50 %.

Uniparental Disomy

Uniparental disomy (UPD) is defined as both copies of a chromosome or chromosome segment being derived from the same parent. The frequency of this phenomenon is unknown. UPD can occur as heterodisomy (the presence of both copies of a chromosome from one parent) or isodisomy (two copies of the same parental chromosome). This becomes clinically relevant when males and females differentially imprint the chromosomal segment in question, or when the parent who transmits the disomic region carries a mutation for a recessive disorder in that region [11]. Some disorders which can be caused by UPD include Beckwith-Wiedemann syndrome, Angelman syndrome, and Prader-Willi syndrome. UPD has been reported as a rare cause of autosomal recessive disorders, including cystic fibrosis and sickle cell anemia, and should be considered as a mechanism for autosomal recessive disease when only one parent can be confirmed as a carrier. In addition, X-linked recessive disorders occurring in 46,XX females may be caused by UPD.

Unstable DNA

Most classic hereditary disorders are caused by static or stable mutations in one or a few genes. For trinucleotide repeat disorders (e.g., fragile X syndrome, Huntington disease, myotonic dystrophy) the causative gene alterations are unstable and consist of a variable number of copies of a tandemly repeated three-nucleotide sequence. Trinucleotide repeats are stable and usually inherited without alteration when the repeat size falls with a specific range, which is gene specific. DNA replication of the repetitive sequence may result in errors leading to expansion (additional copies of the trinucleotide sequence) or contraction (loss of copies of the trinucleotide sequence) of the number of repeat copies. With expansion, the gene segment becomes less stable and thus more likely to expand further. Intermediate lengths of expanded trinucleotide repeats are called pre-mutations, which are extremely unstable and highly likely to undergo further expansion. Individuals who carry pre-mutations typically do not have classic symptoms of the associated disorder but may show mild signs or develop associated symptoms at later ages.

If the trinucleotide repeat expands into the disease-associated size range, gene function is disrupted and symptoms occur in the individual. Disease severity typically correlates with the size of the repeated segment, with earlier age of onset and more severe symptoms with increasing repeat size. The clinical phenomenon of anticipation (earlier onset and more severe disease in subsequent generations) is explained mechanistically by the progressive expansion of the trinucleotide repeat region from one generation to the next. Sex of the transmitting parent also can influence the likelihood and degree of expansion, and is gene specific (the significant parent of origin varies by disease). Many common trinucleotide repeat disorders are associated with neurological phenotypes.

Synergistic Heterozygosity

This phenomenon can be described as the interaction of genes at multiple loci needed to express a phenotype. Heterozygous mutations in two or more distinct genes may lead to an overall decrease in function if the gene products form a complex or participate in the same developmental or metabolic pathway [12]. Examples of disorders resulting from synergistic processes include non-syndromic hearing loss resulting from heterozygous mutations in both the *GJB2* gene (encoding Connexin26) and the *GJB6* gene (encoding Connexin30). The connexins co-localize in the inner ear tissues to form gap junctions which are important for cellular communications. The presence of a heterozygous large deletion within the *GJB6* gene results in the loss of expression of *GJB2* on the same chromosome by removing a cis-acting regulatory element [13]. Thus, individuals carrying a *GJB2* mutation on one chromosome and a *GJB6* mutation on their other chromosome present with non-syndromic hearing loss. Digenic inheritance, or heterozygosity for a recessive mutation at two distinct loci, has been reported for inherited disorders including severe insulin resistance, primary congenital glaucoma, and retinitis pigmentosa. Recurrence risks for conditions resulting from synergistic heterozygosity depend on the number of loci involved, the specific genes implicated, genetic linkage of the loci, and the degree of decreased function conferred by each mutation. For classic digenic inheritance of recessive gene mutations which are not linked, risk for recurrence is expected to be 25 %.

Other Factors Affecting Risk and Risk Assessment

Understanding modes of inheritance provides a framework for risk assessment for close relatives of individuals affected by hereditary disorders; however, many factors influence the ability to clearly define patterns of inheritance in families. From a logistical perspective, family members may not know details about medical conditions in distant relatives, or relatives may not wish to share those details by providing medical records. For some, there may be stigma or guilt attached to discussion of hereditary conditions in themselves or their children. Mechanistically, there are a number of processes that may confound pedigree interpretation (Table 4.5). Variable expressivity and pleiotropy relate, respectively, to the presence of different degrees of severity of symptoms and the presence of varying phenotypic features in affected individuals. These could lead to misclassification of affected status, or failure to recognize the presence of a single clinical entity in affected family members. Further, gaps in an otherwise

Table 4.5 Factors affecting risk and risk assessment

Variable expressivity/pleiotropy
Typical age of disease onset
Penetrance
Heterogeneity
Phenocopies
Sex-influenced expression (sex-limited vs sex-influenced)
Family size/paucity of at-risk sex
Nonpaternity
Consanguinity/inbreeding
Lyonization
New mutation
Mosaicism (somatic or germline)
Modifying genes
Environmental and lifestyle effects

classic pedigree can occur due to variability in age of onset, particularly with adult-onset disease due to penetrance, or likelihood that an individual who carries the gene mutation(s) for a condition will show signs or symptoms. Some conditions show genetic heterogeneity, that is, can be caused by mutations in a number of different genes or by multiple distinct mutations at the same loci. Phenocopies, similar conditions with different genetic or nongenetic etiologies or both, also may occur within a family and lead to misinterpretations of patterns of inheritance and, thus, of risk to family members. Small family size or relatively low frequency of the at-risk sex in sex-influenced disorders (sex-limited vs sex-influenced expression) may result in failure to recognize a hereditary disorder and underestimation of risk.

Accurate reporting of relationships within a pedigree is critical. Nonpaternity, estimated at 3 % in Western industrialized nations [14], may explain transmission patterns that seem to deviate from the expected. Consanguinity, or sharing of common ancestors, is particularly important when considering transmission of autosomal recessive traits. In a consanguineous union, there is an increased chance that a gene mutation present in a common ancestor and associated with an autosomal recessive condition may be transmitted through both sides of the family and occur in the homozygous state in offspring. In general, the risk for congenital malformations or adverse medical outcomes in the offspring of consanguineous unions is increased over the general population and varies depending on the degree of relatedness of the couple [15].

Risk assessment for disorders caused by mutations in X-linked genes or for chromosomal rearrangements involving the X chromosome may be influenced by lyonization. Female carriers of X-linked recessive disorders may be symptomatic if the affected X chromosome is preferentially active while female carriers of X-linked dominant disorders may be asymptomatic if the affected X chromosome is preferentially inactivated. Spontaneous new mutations, which are not inherited from either parent but may be transmitted to offspring, are a common cause for some autosomal dominant or X-linked conditions. Parental testing may be necessary to determine if a mutation occurred sporadically and can be helpful in clarifying recurrence risk and establishing risk to family members. Somatic mosaicism, or the presence of at least two populations of cells with different genetic makeup in the same individual, may result in an atypical or mild disease phenotype depending on the type and percentage of cells affected. Mosaicism which is restricted to the egg or sperm cells (germline mosaicism) can lead to unrecognized or indefinable risk to future offspring because such individuals are asymptomatic and it is difficult to estimate the percentage of germ cells affected.

Finally, factors outside of the critical gene can influence expression of traits and thus the assessment of risk. Expression of some genes is influenced by variant forms of other so-called modifying genes. Polymorphisms or mutations in these modifying genes can change gene-gene or protein-protein interactions to affect the expression of the condition. Similarly, environmental or lifestyle factors such as dietary habits, medical screening practices and specific exposures (medications, radiation, smoke, etc.) may positively or negatively affect gene function and expression of clinical symptoms.

Each of these factors must be carefully considered in the overall diagnostic and risk assessment, initially based on collection of a family pedigree and continued through clinical evaluation, including physical examination and indicated diagnostic testing.

Direct and Indirect Mutation Analysis

The ability to directly interrogate mutations or gene regions associated with disease often provides a more definitive answer about individual risk than pedigree evaluation. Currently, there are clinical or research tests offered for over 2,500 different genetic diseases (http://www.ncbi.nlm.nih.gov/, accessed on 17 January 2012), and this list will continue to increase as additional genes are implicated in disease. Molecular methods of gene analysis vary and technologies selected by clinical molecular laboratories may be influenced by numerous factors including the number of gene(s) and sample(s) to be analyzed, size of the gene(s), gene structure, and the number and type of gene mutations to be interrogated. Sanger sequencing is considered the gold standard for DNA sequencing and is frequently used in clinical testing. Mutation scanning techniques such as conformation-sensitive gel electrophoresis (CSGE), denaturing gradient gel electrophoresis (DGGE), denaturing high-performance liquid chromatography (DHPLC), single-strand conformation polymorphism (SSCP), and high-resolution melting (Wittwer) are commonly utilized for genes which may contain a variety of disease-causing sequence alterations [16, 17]. If a sequence alteration is suspected by a scanning method, sequencing to confirm the presence of the variant can be targeted only to the suspicious gene region which makes scanning technologies economical. For analysis of a small number of defined mutations within a gene, including small insertions, deletion rearrangements, or changes in the number of repeats, polymerase chain reaction (PCR) and fragment analysis may be used [16]. For detection of defined, disease-causing single-nucleotide polymorphisms (SNPs), allele-specific PCR and fluorescent monitoring, single-nucleotide extension (SNE), or oligonucleotide ligation assays (OLA) may be used. Southern blot analysis, multiplex ligation-dependent probe amplification (MLPA), or array hybridization techniques may be utilized to identify loss or gain of entire genes or gene segments. Southern blot analysis also may be used to identify large trinucleotide repeats.

New high-throughput sequencing technologies, collectively referred to as next-generation sequencing (NGS), use DNA synthesis or ligation processes for massively parallel sequencing of numerous DNA templates. NGS technologies have improved sequencing speed and accuracy and lowered costs of testing multiple genes for a single disease dramatically [18]. By targeting regions of the genome or genes of interest, NGS technologies are being applied to clinical molecular testing. Panels of genes associated with a particular disease phenotype (e.g., cardiomyopathy or X-linked intellectual disability) can be assembled for analysis by NGS, which is especially cost effective for diseases demonstrating genetic heterogeneity. Exome sequencing targets only the protein-encoding regions of the genome, which harbor the majority of identified disease-causing mutations, yet represent only 1 % of the entire genome. Exome sequencing is being used to identify causative mutations for Mendelian disorders difficult to identify by targeted sequencing of specific genes [19]. Genome sequencing also is being applied in clinical settings to identify rare Mendelian disorders [20]. A detailed discussion of molecular methods is provided in Chap. 2 and NGS technologies in Chap. 59 and 60.

Direct methods of identifying mutations are invaluable when the disease-associated gene is known; however, historically and even today, for many conditions the causative gene has not been identified or is not characterized adequately to allow for mutation-specific testing. The classic method for determining the causative gene for a Mendelian disorder is linkage analysis. Linkage analysis uses polymorphic genetic markers near the genomic locus of interest to assess association with the disease phenotype in the family. As linkage analysis requires samples from multiple family members, both affected and unaffected, this type of indirect mutation analysis may not be feasible for genetic assessment of very rare Mendelian disorders, sporadic cases, or unrelated cases. In addition, linkage analysis may not be an ideal method of gene discovery for conditions demonstrating diverse clinical phenotypes, those resulting from mutations in more than one gene or influenced by gene-environment interactions. Integration of exome or genome sequencing with linkage and homozygosity data can help elucidate previously unidentified causative mutations or candidate genes [19].

Bayesian Analysis Used in Risk Modification

Numerous factors, some listed above, influence the likelihood that a given individual in the family may be affected by, or a carrier of, the presenting condition. When it is not possible to do direct diagnostic testing for the condition (e.g., if the causative gene is unknown, when the affected relative is not available for testing, or for complex traits), it is possible to combine incremental contributors to risk by utilizing Bayesian analysis. Bayesian analysis is a statistical construct that uses information about the likelihood of occurrence of past events or conditions, and the current status of those events or conditions for the individual, to predict the likelihood of a future event or condition, in this case, the presence or absence of a particular gene mutation or genetic condition [12]. Some factors that may be considered in genetic risk assessment using Bayesian analysis include ethnicity, degree of relationship to affected family members, inheritance pattern, laboratory results, incidence of the disease, and natural history of the condition. The probability assigned based on past events is called the prior probability. The probability based on current information or observations is called the conditional probability. The calculated probability for each possible outcome of an event or condition is the joint probability, and the final probability of one outcome as a percentage of all possible outcomes is the posterior probability. Calculations often utilize data from multiple generations and are usually done in tabular form. The example pedigree in Fig. 4.6 demonstrates an autosomal dominant cancer predisposition syndrome affecting males and females equally. Based on Mendelian inheritance alone, the risk that individual III.5 carries the disease-causing mutation is 25 %. However, knowing that 75 % of gene carriers have been diagnosed with cancer by age 50, risk can be recalculated as demonstrated. (See Chap. 5 for a complete discussion of Bayesian analysis.)

References

1. Resta R. The crane's foot: the rise of the pedigree in human genetics. J Genet Couns. 1993;2:235–60.
2. Bennett RL, French KS, Resta RG, Doyle DL. Standardized human pedigree nomenclature: update and assessment of the recommendations of the National Society of Genetic Counselors. J Genet Couns. 2008;17(5):424–33.
3. Daly M, Farmer J, Harrop-Stein C, et al. Exploring family relationships in cancer risk counseling using the genogram. Cancer Epidemiol Biomarkers Prev. 1999;8(4 Pt 2):393–8.
4. Riley BD, Culver JO, Skrzynia C, et al. Essential elements of genetic cancer risk assessment, counseling, and testing: updated recommendations of the National Society of Genetic Counselors. J Genet Couns. 2012;21(2):151–61.
5. Botkin J. Protecting the privacy of family members in survey and pedigree research. JAMA. 2001;285(2):207–11.
6. ASHG Statement. Professional disclosure of familial genetic information. The American Society of Human Genetics Social Issues Subcommittee on Familial Disclosure. Am J Hum Genet. 1998; 62(2):474–83.
7. McKusick-Nathans Institute for Genetic Medicine JHU. Online Mendelian Inheritance in Man, OMIM®. http://omim.org. Accessed 15 Jan 2011.
8. Deak KL, Horn SR, Rehder CW. The evolving picture of microdeletion/microduplication syndromes in the age of microarray analysis: variable expressivity and genomic complexity. Clin Lab Med. 2011;31(4):543–64.

9. Sharp AJ. Emerging themes and new challenges in defining the role of structural variation in human disease. Hum Mutat. 2009;30(2):135–44.
10. Chinnery P. GeneReviews: mitochondrial disorders overview. National Center for Biotechnology Information; 2011.
11. Nussbaum R, McInnes R, Willard H. Thompson & Thompson genetics in medicine. Philadelphia, PA, USA: W.B. Saunders; 2001.
12. Young I. Introduction to risk calculation in genetic counseling. 3rd ed. Oxford: Oxford University Press; 2007.
13. Lerer I, Sagi M, Ben-Neriah Z, Wang T, Levi H, Abeliovich D. A deletion mutation in GJB6 cooperating with a GJB2 mutation in trans in non-syndromic deafness: a novel founder mutation in Ashkenazi Jews. Hum Mutat. 2001;18(5):460.
14. Voracek M, Haubner T, Fisher ML. Recent decline in nonpaternity rates: a cross-temporal meta-analysis. Psychol Rep. 2008;103(3):799–811.
15. Bennett R, Motulsky A, Bittles A, et al. Genetic counseling and screening of consanguineous couples and their offspring: recommendations of the National Society of Genetic Counselors. J Genet Couns. 2002;11:97–120.
16. Bruns D, Ashwood E, Burtis C. Fundamentals of molecular diagnosis. St. Louis: Saunders; 2007.
17. Montgomery JL, Sanford LN, Wittwer CT. High-resolution DNA melting analysis in clinical research and diagnostics. Expert Rev Mol Diagn. 2010;10(2):219–40.
18. Zhang J, Chiodini R, Badr A, Zhang G. The impact of next-generation sequencing on genomics. J Genet Genomics. 2011;38(3):95–109.
19. Ku CS, Naidoo N, Pawitan Y. Revisiting Mendelian disorders through exome sequencing. Hum Genet. 2011;129(4):351–70.
20. Bick D, Dimmock D. Whole exome and whole genome sequencing. Curr Opin Pediatr. 2011;23(6):594–600.

Bayesian Analysis

5

Robert B. Wilson and Shuji Ogino

Abstract

The purpose of this chapter is to describe basic and general principles of Bayesian analysis for molecular pathologists. Analyses based on Bayes' theorem are routinely applied to calculate probabilities in a wide variety of circumstances, not limited to medicine or genetics. In molecular pathology, Bayesian analysis is commonly used to calculate genetic risk, incorporating population data, pedigree information, and genetic testing results. Bayesian analysis is introduced with two simple, concrete examples. In subsequent sections, the general principles illustrated by these examples are discussed and applied to more complex scenarios. Although the technologies for genetic testing will continue to change, Bayesian analysis and genetic risk assessment will remain fundamental aspects of genetic testing and genetic counseling.

Keywords

Bayesian analysis • Genetics • Risk • Calculation • Carriers • Affected • Relationship • Prior risk • Probability • Ethnicity • Frequencies • Pedigree • Family history • Consultand

Introduction

The purpose of this chapter is to describe basic and general principles of Bayesian analysis for molecular pathologists. Thomas Bayes first described the theorem named after him in an essay on 'the doctrine of chances,' published posthumously in 1763, and republished in 1958 [1]. Analyses based on Bayes' theorem are routinely applied to calculate probabilities in a wide variety of circumstances, not limited to medicine or genetics. In molecular pathology, Bayesian analysis is commonly used to calculate genetic risk, incorporating population data, pedigree information, and genetic testing results. First, Bayesian analysis will be introduced with two simple, concrete examples. In subsequent sections, the general principles illustrated by these examples are discussed and applied to more complex scenarios. For more in-depth treatments, the reader is referred to "Introduction to Risk Calculation in Genetic Counseling" by Young [2] and "The Calculation of Genetic Risks" by Bridge [3], as well as several articles on genetic risk assessment that include advanced Bayesian analyses, particularly for spinal muscular

R.B. Wilson, M.D., Ph.D.
Department of Pathology and Laboratory Medicine, Perelman School of Medicine at the University of Pennsylvania, Philadelphia, PA, USA

S. Ogino, M.D., Ph.D., M.S. (✉)
Department of Pathology, Harvard Medical School, Brigham and Women's Hospital, 450 Brookline Ave., Room JF-215C, Boston, MA 02215, USA

Department of Medical Oncology, Dana-Farber Cancer Institute, 450 Brookline Ave., Room JF-215C, Boston, MA 02215, USA

Department of Epidemiology, Harvard T.H. Chan School of Public Health, Boston, MA 02115, USA
e-mail: shuji_ogino@dfci.harvard.edu

D.G.B. Leonard (ed.), *Molecular Pathology in Clinical Practice*, DOI 10.1007/978-3-319-19674-9_5

atrophy (SMA) [4, 5], cystic fibrosis (CF) [6–9], and autosomal dominant disorders [10].

Bayesian Analysis Using Pedigree Information

In the pedigree shown in Fig. 5.1a, the two brothers of the consultand (indicated by the arrow) have Kennedy disease (X-linked spinal and bulbar muscular atrophy, OMIM #300377), which is caused by a CAG trinucleotide repeat expansion in the androgen receptor (*AR*) gene (OMIM #310200). Because both of the consultand's brothers are affected, we can assume that the consultand's mother is an obligate carrier. Before taking into account the consultand's three unaffected sons, her carrier risk is 1/2, since there is a 1/2 chance that she inherited the mutant X chromosome from her mother. If we take into account that the consultand has three unaffected sons, how does her carrier risk change?

Bayesian analysis starts with mutually exclusive hypotheses. In this example, there are two: that the consultand is a carrier, and that the consultand is a non-carrier. Setting up a table with separate columns for each hypothesis facilitates Bayesian analyses, as shown in Fig. 5.1b for this case. The first row of the table comprises the "prior" probability for each hypothesis. In this example, the prior probabilities are the probability that the consultand is a carrier (1/2), and the probability that she is a non-carrier (also 1/2), *prior* to taking into account the subsequent information that she has three unaffected sons.

The second row of the table comprises the "conditional" probability for each hypothesis. The conditional probability for each hypothesis is the probability that the subsequent information would occur if we assume that each hypothesis is true. In this example, the subsequent information is that the consultand has three unaffected sons. Thus, the conditional probabilities are the probability that the consultand would have three unaffected sons under the assumption (or "condition") that she is a carrier, and the probability that she would have three unaffected sons under the assumption (or "condition") that she is a non-carrier. If we assume that she is a carrier, the probability that she would have three unaffected sons is 1/2 × 1/2 × 1/2 = 1/8. This is because she would have to have passed the normal X chromosome three times in succession, each time with a probability of 1/2. If we assume that she is a non-carrier, the probability that she would have three unaffected sons approximates 1, since only in the event of a rare de novo mutation would a non-carrier have an affected son. Thus, the conditional probabilities in this example are 1/8 for carrier and 1 for non-carrier (Fig. 5.1b).

The third row of the table comprises the "joint" probability for each hypothesis, which is the product of the prior and conditional probabilities for each hypothesis. For the first hypothesis in this example, that the consultand is a carrier, the joint probability is the prior probability that she is a carrier, times the conditional probability that a carrier would have three normal sons, which in this case is 1/2 × 1/8 = 1/16 (Fig. 5.1b). For the second hypothesis in this example, that the consultand is a non-carrier, the joint probability is the prior probability that she is a non-carrier, times the conditional probability that a non-carrier would have three normal sons, which in this case is 1/2 × 1 = 1/2 (Fig. 5.1b).

The fourth row of the table comprises the "posterior" probability for each hypothesis. The posterior probability for each hypothesis is the probability that each hypothesis is true after (or "posterior" to) taking into account both prior and

a

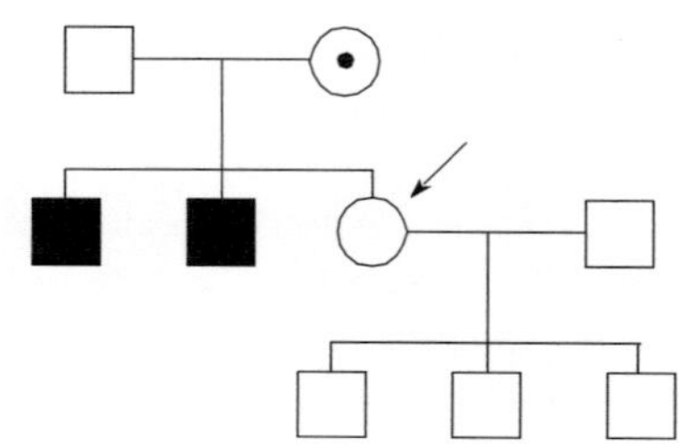

b

	Hypothesis	
	Carrier	Non-carrier
Prior Probability	1/2	1/2
Conditional Probability (of three normal sons)	1/8	~1
Joint Probability	1/16	1/2
Posterior Probability	(1/16) / (1/16 + 1/2) = 1/9	(1/2) / (1/16 + 1/2) = 8/9

c

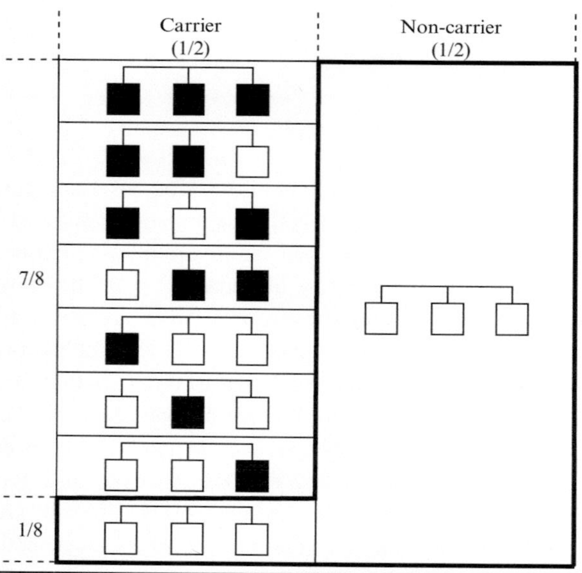

Figure 5.1 (**a**) Pedigree of a family with individuals affected with Kennedy disease (see text). (**b**) Bayesian analysis for the consultand in **a**. (**c**) Schematic representation of the Bayesian analysis of **b**. Pedigrees shown in the *boxes* represent all possible disease status outcomes for the third generation of the pedigree in **a**, given the carrier or non-carrier status of the consultand. Each *small box* to the *left* represents 1/16 of the total area. (See text for full description.)

subsequent information. The posterior probability for each hypothesis is calculated by dividing the joint probability for that hypothesis by the sum of all the joint probabilities. In this example, the posterior probability that the consultand is a carrier is the joint probability for the first hypothesis (1/16), divided by the sum of the joint probabilities for both hypotheses (1/16 + 1/2 = 9/16), or 1/16 ÷ 9/16 = 1/9. The posterior probability that the consultand is a non-carrier is the joint probability for the second hypothesis (1/2 = 8/16), divided by the sum of the joint probabilities for both hypotheses (1/16 + 1/2 = 9/16), or 8/16 ÷ 9/16 = 8/9. Thus, taking into account the prior family history, and the subsequent information that she has three unaffected sons, the probability that the consultand is a carrier is 1/9 (Fig. 5.1b).

The preceding example is illustrated graphically in Fig. 5.1c. The total area represents the total prior probabilities. The left half represents the prior probability that the consultand is a carrier (1/2), and the right half represents the prior probability that she is a non-carrier (also 1/2). Under the hypothesis that the consultand is a carrier, there are eight possibilities, comprising all the permutations of zero, one, two, or three affected sons. The area of the small rectangle that contains three unshaded squares (for three unaffected sons) comprises 1/8 of the left half and represents the conditional probability of three normal sons under the hypothesis that the consultand is a carrier. The area of this small rectangle is 1/16 of the total area and therefore also represents the joint probability that the consultand is a carrier (1/2), and that as a carrier she would have three normal sons (1/8), or 1/2 × 1/8 = 1/16.

Under the hypothesis that the consultand is a non-carrier, there is essentially only one possibility, which is that all three sons are unaffected. The area of the larger rectangle that contains the pedigree with three unshaded squares (for three unaffected sons) comprises all of the non-carrier half and represents the conditional probability of three normal sons under the hypothesis that the consultand is a non-carrier. The area of this larger rectangle is 1/2 of the total area and therefore also represents the joint probability that the consultand is a non-carrier (1/2), and that as a non-carrier she would have three normal sons (~1), or 1/2 × 1 = 1/2. The "reverse-L-shaped" box, which is demarcated by a bold line, represents the sum of the joint probabilities, or 9/16 of the total area.

Because the consultand has three unaffected sons, the area of the reversed-L-shaped box represents the only component of the prior probabilities needed to determine the posterior probability that the consultand is a carrier. Taking into account that all three of the consultand's sons are unaffected, Bayesian analysis allows us to *exclude* 7/16 of the prior probabilities, those that include one or more affected sons, from consideration. (Note that this explains why the joint probabilities sum to less than 1.) The posterior probability that the consultand is a carrier is therefore the area of the small rectangle with three unshaded squares (for three unaffected sons) divided by the area of the entire reversed-L-shaped box, which represents the only probabilities relevant to the consultand's risk, or 1/16 ÷ 9/16 = 1/9. Likewise, the posterior probability that the consultand is a non-carrier is the area of the larger rectangle with three unshaded squares (for three unaffected sons) divided by the area of the entire reversed-L-shaped box, or 8/16 ÷ 9/16 = 8/9.

Bayesian Analysis Using Genetic Test Results

In the second example, information from a test result modifies the prior risk. In the pedigree shown in Fig. 5.2a, the consultand is pregnant with her first child and has a family history of cystic fibrosis (CF; OMIM #219700). CF is caused by mutations in the cystic fibrosis transmembrane conductance regulator gene (*CFTR*; OMIM #602421). The consultand is an unaffected European Caucasian and her brother died years earlier of complications of CF. She undergoes carrier testing for the 23 mutations recommended by the American College of Medical Genetics (ACMG) CF screening guidelines [11–13], which detects approximately 90 % of disease alleles in European Caucasians. The consultand tests negative for all 23 mutations. What is her carrier risk after testing?

As in the first example, the two hypotheses are that the consultand is a carrier and that she is a non-carrier. The prior probability that she is a carrier is 2/3. Because the consultand is unaffected, she could not have inherited disease alleles from both parents. Thus, she either inherited a disease allele from her mother or father, or she inherited only normal alleles; in two of these three scenarios she would be a carrier (shown in Fig. 5.2b). The prior probability that the consultand is a non-carrier is 1/3 (Fig. 5.2c).

As in the first example, the conditional probability for each hypothesis is the probability that the subsequent information would occur if we assume that each hypothesis is true. In this example, the subsequent information is that the consultand tests negative for all 23 mutations. Thus, the conditional probabilities are the probability that the consultand would test negative under the assumption (or "condition") that she is a carrier, and the probability that she would test negative under the assumption (or "condition") that she is a non-carrier. If we assume that she is a carrier, the probability that she would test negative is 1/10, since the test detects 90 % of European Caucasian disease alleles or carriers. If we assume that she is a non-carrier, the probability that she would test negative approximates 1. Thus, the conditional probabilities in this example are 1/10 and 1 for the carrier and non-carrier hypotheses, respectively (Fig. 5.2c).

a

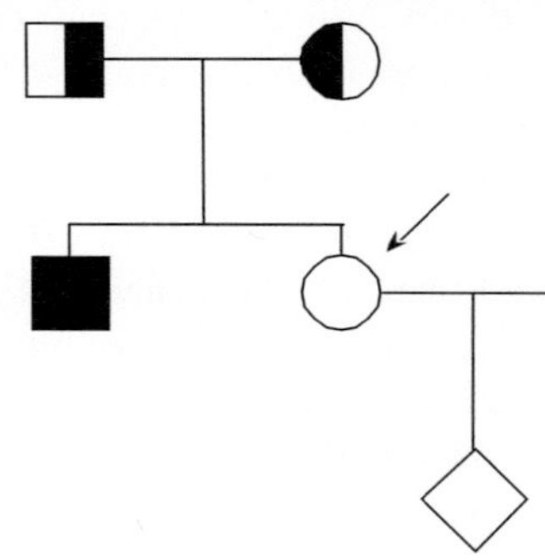

b

		Maternal Allele	
		mt	N
Paternal Allele	mt	(mt/mt)	**mt/N**
	N	**N/mt**	N/N

c

	Hypothesis	
	Carrier	Non-carrier
Prior Probability	2/3	1/3
Conditional Probability (of a negative test result)	1/10	1
Joint Probability	1/15	1/3
Posterior Probability	(1/15) / (1/15 + 1/3) = 1/6	(1/3) / (1/15 + 1/3) = 5/6

d

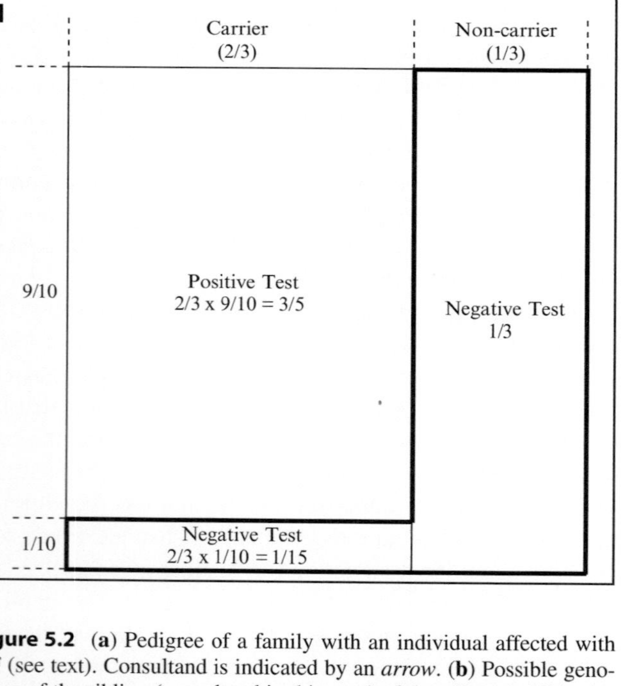

Figure 5.2 (**a**) Pedigree of a family with an individual affected with CF (see text). Consultand is indicated by an *arrow*. (**b**) Possible genotypes of the sibling (consultand in this case) of the affected child prior to genetic testing. The mt/mt genotype (in *parentheses*) is excluded based on the fact that the consultand is unaffected. Abbreviations: *mt* mutant, *N* normal. (**c**) Bayesian analysis for the consultand in **a**. (**d**) Schematic representation of the Bayesian analysis of **c** (see text)

As in the first case, the joint probability for each hypothesis is the product of the prior and conditional probabilities for that hypothesis. For the first hypothesis in this example, that the consultand is a carrier, the joint probability is the prior probability that she is a carrier (2/3) multiplied by the conditional probability that a carrier of European Caucasian ancestry would test negative (1/10), or $2/3 \times 1/10 = 1/15$ (Fig. 5.2c). For the second hypothesis in this example, that the consultand is a non-carrier, the joint probability is the prior probability that she is a non-carrier (1/3) multiplied by the conditional probability that a non-carrier would test negative (1), or $1/3 \times 1 = 1/3$ (Fig. 5.2c).

Finally, the posterior probability is calculated for each hypothesis by dividing the joint probability for that hypothesis by the sum of all the joint probabilities. In this example, the posterior probability that the consultand is a carrier and tests negative for 23 CF mutations is the joint probability for the first hypothesis (1/15) divided by the sum of the joint probabilities for both hypotheses ($1/15 + 1/3 = 2/5$), or $1/15 \div 2/5 = 1/6$ (Fig. 5.2c). The posterior probability that the consultand is a non-carrier and tests negative for 23 CF mutations is the joint probability for the second hypothesis (1/3) divided by the sum of the joint probabilities for both hypotheses (2/5), or $1/3 \div 2/5 = 5/6$ (Fig. 5.2c).

The preceding example is illustrated graphically in Fig. 5.2d. The total area represents the total prior probabilities. The left 2/3 represents the prior probability that the consultand is a carrier, and the right 1/3 represents the prior probability that the consultand is a non-carrier. Under the hypothesis that the consultand is a carrier, there are two possibilities for the test result: positive or negative. The area of the small rectangle on the lower left comprises 1/10 of the 2/3 carrier region and represents the conditional probability of a normal test result under the hypothesis that the consultand is a carrier. The area of this small rectangle is $1/10 \times 2/3 = 1/15$ of the total probabilities area and therefore also represents the joint probability that the consultand is a carrier (2/3) and that as a European-Caucasian carrier she would test negative for all 23 mutations (1/10), or $2/3 \times 1/10 = 1/15$ (Fig. 5.2d).

Under the hypothesis that the consultand is a non-carrier, there is essentially only one possibility for the test result, which is negative. The area of the rectangle that comprises all of the 1/3 non-carrier region represents the conditional probability of a negative test result under the hypothesis that the consultand is a non-carrier. The area of this rectangle is 1/3 of the total area and therefore also represents the joint probability that the consultand is a non-carrier (1/3), and that as a non-carrier she would test negative (~1), or $1/3 \times 1 = 1/3$. The "reverse-L-shaped" box, which is demarcated by a bold line, represents the sum of the joint probabilities, or 2/5 ($=1/3 + 1/15$) of the total area.

Because the consultand tested negative, the area of the reverse-L-shaped box represents the only component of the prior probabilities needed to determine the posterior probability that the consultand is a carrier. Taking into account that she tested negative, Bayesian analysis allows us to *exclude* 3/5 of the prior probability, that portion comprising a positive test result, from consideration. (Note, again, that this explains why the joint probabilities sum to less than 1.) The posterior probability that the consultand is a carrier is therefore the area of the small rectangle at the lower left divided by the area of the reverse-L-shaped box, which represents the only probabilities relevant to the consultand's risk, or $1/15 \div 2/5 = 1/6$. Likewise, the posterior probability that the consultand is a non-carrier is the area of the larger rectangle on the right divided by the area of the reverse-L-shaped box, or $1/3 \div 2/5 = 5/6$.

Simple Bayesian Analyses Generalized: Carrier vs Non-carrier

The preceding Bayesian analyses can be generalized as in Table 5.1. Note that if the correct prior and conditional probabilities can be determined, the rest is simple calculation. Setting up a spreadsheet, as in Table 5.1, facilitates clinical Bayesian analyses.

A very common application of Bayesian analysis in molecular pathology is to calculate carrier risk after a negative test result, as in the second example above. The need to calculate carrier risk in this scenario stems from the fact that the sensitivity of most carrier tests is, at present, less than 100 %; therefore, a negative test result decreases, but does not eliminate, carrier risk. Hypothesis 1 in this scenario is that the consultand is a carrier, and Hypothesis 2 is that the consultand is a non-carrier (Table 5.1). The prior carrier probability ("A" in Table 5.1) depends on whether there is a family history, and if so, the relationship of the consultand to the affected family member as shown by the family pedigree. In the absence of a family history, the prior carrier probability is the population carrier risk for that disease. In the case of cystic fibrosis (CF) and some other diseases, the appropriate population risk depends on the ethnicity of the consultand. The conditional probabilities ("C" and "D" in Table 5.1) are one minus the test sensitivity for the carrier hypothesis, and the test specificity for the non-carrier hypothesis, respectively. The remainder of the table is completed through calculation, with the posterior probabilities ("G" and "H" in Table 5.1) representing one minus the negative predictive value, and the negative predictive value, respectively. This is shown schematically in Fig. 5.3.

For illustration, suppose in the second example above (Fig. 5.2) that the consultand's husband is Ashkenazi Jewish, that he has no family history of CF, and that he tests negative for all 23 mutations in the ACMG screening guidelines panel. What is his carrier risk? The carrier risk in Ashkenazi Jewish populations, and therefore the husband's prior carrier risk in the absence of a family history, is approximately 1/25 ("A" in Table 5.1). Thus, his prior probability of being a non-carrier is 24/25 ("B" in Table 5.1). The ACMG screening guidelines panel of 23 mutations detects 94 % of CF mutations in Ashkenazi Jewish populations [11–13], so the conditional probability of a negative test, under the hypothesis that he is a carrier, is 6 % = 3/50 ("C" in Table 5.1). Under the hypothesis that he is a non-carrier, the conditional probability of a negative test approximates 1 ("D" in Table 5.1). (This is generally the case in genetic testing, since non-carriers by definition lack mutations in the relevant disease gene and hence, unless there are technical problems, essentially always should test negative.) The Bayesian analysis table for this example is shown in Table 5.2. The joint probabilities ("E" and "F" in Table 5.1) are the products of the prior and conditional probabilities, and the posterior probabilities ("G" and "H" in Table 5.1) derive from each joint probability

Table 5.1 Simple Bayesian analyses generalized

	Hypothesis	
	1	2
Prior probability	A	B = 1 − A
Conditional probability	C	D
Joint probability	E = AC	F = BD
Posterior probability	G = E/(E + F)	H = F/(E + F)

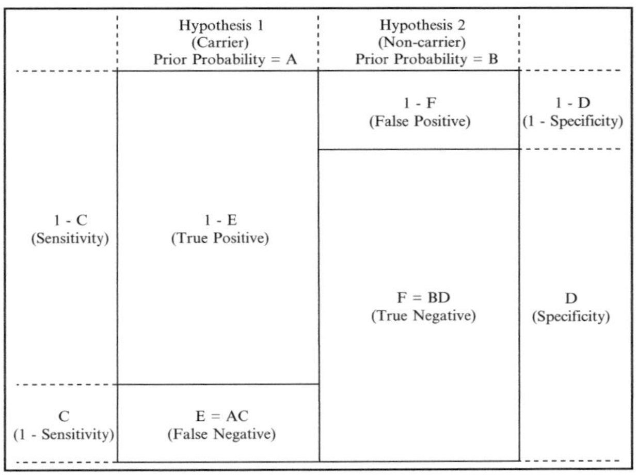

Figure 5.3 Schematic representation of the generalized Bayesian analysis shown in Table 5.1, for the case of a negative carrier test. The *small boxes* represent true positive, false positive, true negative, and false negative rates for a particular consultand, i.e., the prior probabilities are influenced by factors such as family history or signs and symptoms, and the sensitivity and specificity of the test are influenced by factors such as ethnicity. For a negative carrier test, the posterior carrier probability (one minus the negative predictive value) is the false negative rate divided by the sum of the false and true negative rates, or E/(E + F).

Table 5.2 Bayesian analysis for an Ashkenazi Jewish individual without a family history of CF who tests negative for the ACMG screening guidelines panel of 23 *CFTR* mutations

	Hypothesis	
	Carrier	**Non-carrier**
Prior probability	1/25	24/25
Conditional probability (of negative test result)	3/50	1
Joint probability	3/1,250	24/25
Posterior probability	(3/1,250)/ (3/1,250 + 24/25) = 1/401	(24/25)/ (3/1,250 + 24/25) = 400/401

Table 5.3 Bayesian analysis for the consultand in Fig. 5.2a after testing of the parents (see text)

	Hypothesis	
	Carrier	**Non-carrier**
Prior probability	2/3	1/3
Conditional probability (of negative test result)	1/2	1
Joint probability	1/3	1/3
Posterior probability	(1/3)/ (1/3 + 1/3) = 1/2	(1/3)/ (1/3 + 1/3) = 1/2

Table 5.4 Alternative Bayesian analysis for the consultand in Fig. 5.2a after testing of the parents (see text)

	Hypothesis		
	Carrier		
	Carrier with paternal (detectable) mutation	**Carrier with maternal (undetectable) mutation**	**Non-carrier**
Prior probability	1/3	1/3	1/3
Conditional probability (of negative test result)	0	1	1
Joint probability	0	1/3	1/3
Posterior probability	0	1/2	1/2

divided by the sum of the joint probabilities. The husband's posterior carrier risk after the negative test result is 1/401.

What is the risk that the fetus of the mother (consultand) in Fig. 5.2 and the father from Table 5.2 is affected with CF? Prior to testing, the risk was the prior probability that the mother was a carrier (2/3), times the prior probability that the father was a carrier (1/25), times the probability that the fetus would inherit two disease alleles (1/4), or $2/3 \times 1/25 \times 1/4 = 1/150$. After testing, the risk is the posterior probability that the mother is a carrier (1/6), times the posterior probability that the father is a carrier (1/401), times the probability that the fetus would inherit two disease alleles (1/4), or $1/6 \times 1/401 \times 1/4 \cong 1/9{,}600$.

Often, testing is performed on additional family members and genetic risks need to be modified accordingly. In the example above, testing of both parents of the mother (consultand) would affect her carrier risk calculations. Detection of mutations in both parents using the same mutation test panel would essentially rule out carrier status for the mother, since we would then know that the sensitivity of the test for the mutations she is at risk of carrying is essentially 100 %. Alternatively, if the test results for the mother's parents only are positive for one of her parents (for example, her father) and negative for the other parent (her mother), then the sensitivity of the test for the mutations she is at risk of carrying is essentially 50 %. The Bayesian analysis for the mother, modified from Fig. 5.2c, is shown in Table 5.3. The conditional probability of a negative test under the hypothesis that she is a carrier has changed from 1/10 to 1/2, which increases the posterior probability that she is a carrier to 1/2. Taken together with her husband's carrier risk of 1/401 (Table 5.2), the risk that the fetus is affected with CF can be modified to $1/2 \times 1/401 \times 1/4 \cong 1/3{,}200$.

Another way of conceptualizing the Bayesian analysis described above is to separate the carrier hypothesis into two sub-hypotheses as shown in Table 5.4. (See also Sect. "Bayesian Analyses with More Than Two Hypotheses" below.) The two sub-hypotheses are (1) that the consultand is a carrier with a paternal (detectable) mutation and (2) that she is a carrier with a maternal (undetectable) mutation. The prior probability of each hypothesis is 1/3; i.e., half of 2/3. The conditional probability of a negative test result, under the sub-hypothesis that she is a carrier of a detectable paternal mutation, is 0. The conditional probability of a negative test result, under the sub-hypothesis that she is a carrier of an undetectable maternal mutation, is 1. As in the generalized Bayesian analysis shown in Table 5.1, the joint probability for each hypothesis is the product of the prior and conditional probabilities for that hypothesis, and the posterior probability for each hypothesis is the joint probability for that hypothesis divided by the sum of all the joint probabilities. The posterior probability that she has a detectable paternal mutation is 0, and the posterior probability that she has an undetectable maternal mutation is 1/2 (Table 5.4).

Simple Bayesian Analyses Generalized: Affected vs Unaffected

Another common application of Bayesian analysis in molecular pathology is to calculate the risk that a patient is affected with a particular disease after a negative test result. Again, the need to calculate risk in this scenario stems from the fact that the sensitivities of many genetic tests are less than

Table 5.5 Bayesian analysis for a child with clinically typical type III SMA who tests negative for homozygous deletions of the *SMN1* gene

	Hypothesis	
	Affected	Unaffected
Prior probability	0.87	0.13
Conditional probability (of negative test result)	0.06	~1
Joint probability	0.052	0.13
Posterior probability	0.29	0.71

Table 5.6 Bayesian analysis for a child with clinically typical type III SMA who has one copy of the *SMN1* gene by dosage analysis

	Hypothesis	
	Affected	Unaffected
Prior probability	0.87	0.13
Conditional probability (of one-copy test result)	0.06	0.021
Joint probability	0.052	0.0027
Posterior probability	0.95	0.05

100 %. Hypothesis 1 (in Table 5.1 and Fig. 5.3) in this scenario is that the patient is affected, and Hypothesis 2 is that the patient is unaffected. The prior probability ("A" in Table 5.1 and Fig. 5.3) usually derives mostly from signs and symptoms, but also may depend on aspects of the patient's history, including family history in diseases with a genetic component. As in the CF example above, the conditional probabilities ("C" and "D" in Table 5.1 and Fig. 5.3) are one minus the test sensitivity for the affected hypothesis, and the test specificity for the unaffected hypothesis, respectively. The remainder of the analysis is accomplished by calculation, with the posterior probabilities ("G" and "H" in Table 5.1) representing one minus the negative predictive value, and the negative predictive value, respectively.

For example, suppose that a Caucasian child with clinically typical type III spinal muscular atrophy (type III SMA; Kugelberg-Welander disease; OMIM #253400) tests negative for the homozygous deletion of the *SMN1* gene found in most affected individuals. What is the probability that the child is affected with *SMN1*-linked SMA? The Bayesian analysis for this scenario is shown in Table 5.5. Wirth et al. found that 17 of 131 individuals with clinically typical type III SMA lacked mutations in both *SMN1* alleles (and therefore were considered to have diseases unrelated to *SMN1*) [14]; hence the prior probability that the child is affected with *SMN1*-linked type III SMA is 114/131 or 0.87. Approximately 6 % of individuals with *SMN1*-linked type III SMA have a deletion of one *SMN1* allele and a subtle mutation, undetectable by simple PCR testing for a homozygous deletion, in the other *SMN1* allele [15]; hence, the conditional probability of a negative test result under the hypothesis that the child is affected is 6/100 or 0.06. Homozygous deletions of *SMN1*, when present, are highly specific for *SMN1*-linked SMA; hence the conditional probability of a negative test result under the hypothesis that the child is unaffected with *SMN1*-linked SMA approximates 1. Following the simple calculation rules in Table 5.1, the posterior probability that the child is affected with *SMN1*-linked type III SMA is approximately 0.29 (Table 5.5).

Suppose that *SMN1* dosage analysis is performed on the child's DNA (i.e., the SMA carrier test), and the result is that the child has one copy of the *SMN1* gene. What is the probability that he or she is affected with *SMN1*-linked SMA? The Bayesian analysis for this scenario is shown in Table 5.6. Again, the prior probability that the child is affected with *SMN1*-linked type III SMA is 0.87. Because approximately 6 % of individuals with *SMN1*-linked type III SMA have a deletion of one *SMN1* allele and a subtle mutation in the other *SMN1* allele that is detectable as a single copy by dosage analysis [15], the conditional probability of a one-copy test result under the hypothesis that the child is affected is again 0.06. However, the carrier frequency for SMA in the Caucasian population is approximately 1/47 [16]; hence, in this scenario, the conditional probability of a single-copy test result under the hypothesis that the child is unaffected with *SMN1*-linked SMA is 1/47 or 0.021. Following the simple calculation rules in Table 5.1, the posterior probability that the child is affected with *SMN1*-linked type III SMA is approximately 0.95 (Table 5.6).

Suppose instead that the result of the *SMN1* dosage analysis is that the child has two copies of the *SMN1* gene. What is the probability that the child is affected with *SMN1*-linked SMA? The Bayesian analysis for this scenario is shown in Table 5.7. Again, the prior probability that the child is affected with *SMN1*-linked type III SMA is 0.87. Only approximately 9 in 10,000 individuals with *SMN1*-linked type III SMA would be expected to have two subtle, non-deletion mutations, detectable as two copies by dosage analysis [15]; hence, the conditional probability of a two-copy test result under the hypothesis that the child is affected is approximately 0.0009. Because approximately 6.9 % of unaffected Caucasian individuals have three copies of the *SMN1* gene, and approximately 2.1 % of unaffected Caucasian individuals have one copy of the *SMN1* gene, for a total of 9 % of unaffected Caucasian individuals without two copies of *SMN1* [16], the conditional probability of a two-copy test result under the hypothesis that the child is unaffected with *SMN1*-linked SMA is 91/100 or approximately 0.9. Following the simple calculation rules in Table 5.1, the posterior probability that the child is affected with *SMN1*-linked type III SMA is only approximately 0.006 (Table 5.7).

Profiling by proteomics, RNA microarrays, and/or analysis of single-nucleotide polymorphisms (SNPs) is likely to play an important role in molecular pathology, and clinical test results will be reported, in many cases, as probabilities or

Table 5.7 Bayesian analysis for a child with clinically typical type III SMA who has two copies of the *SMN1* gene by dosage analysis

	Hypothesis	
	Affected	**Unaffected**
Prior probability	0.87	0.13
Conditional probability (of two-copy test result)	0.0009	0.9
Joint probability	0.00078	0.12
Posterior probability	0.006	0.994

Table 5.8 Bayesian analysis for a consultand with a 20 % lifetime risk of developing a disease and a proteomic profile 16 times more common in those who develop the disease than in those who do not

	Hypothesis	
	Affected eventually	**Never affected**
Prior probability	0.2	0.8
Conditional probability (of profiling result)	16	1
Joint probability	3.2	0.8
Posterior probability	0.8	0.2

relative risks. For example, suppose that a consultand has a 20 % lifetime risk of developing a particular disease (based on family history, physical examination, and/or clinical laboratory test results) and that his or her proteomic profile is 16 times more common in those who go on to develop the disease than in those who do not. What is his or her lifetime risk of developing the disease? The Bayesian analysis for this scenario is shown in Table 5.8. Hypothesis 1 (from Table 5.1) is that the consultand will develop the disease, and Hypothesis 2 is that the consultand will not develop the disease. The prior probabilities are 0.2 and 0.8 for Hypotheses 1 and 2, respectively. Because the conditional probability of the proteomic profiling result is 16 times more likely in those who develop the disease than in those who do not, the conditional probabilities ("C" and "D" in Table 5.1) are 16 and 1, respectively. Following the simple calculation rules in Table 5.1, the posterior probability that the consultand will develop the disease is 0.8 (Table 5.8).

Note that because posterior probabilities are normalized joint probabilities, the absolute values of the conditional probabilities are unimportant, as long as the ratio (i.e., the odds ratio) between them is correct. This also is true of prior probabilities. For example, in the scenario above, prior probabilities of 1 and 4 can be substituted for 0.2 and 0.8 and the same answer is obtained. Likewise, in the first example of this chapter (Fig. 5.1a), prior probabilities of 1 and 1 can be substituted for 1/2 and 1/2, and conditional probabilities of 1 and 8 can be substituted for 1/8 and 1, and the same answer is obtained. Hence, relative risks are easily incorporated into Bayesian analyses.

Bayesian Analyses with More Than One Conditional Probability

Often there is more than one test result, and/or pedigree information, that can be incorporated as conditional probabilities in a single Bayesian analysis. For example, consider the pedigree in Fig. 5.4a, in which the two maternal great uncles of the consultand were affected with Duchenne muscular dystrophy (DMD; OMIM #310200), a severe X-linked recessive disease caused by mutations in the *DMD* gene (OMIM

a

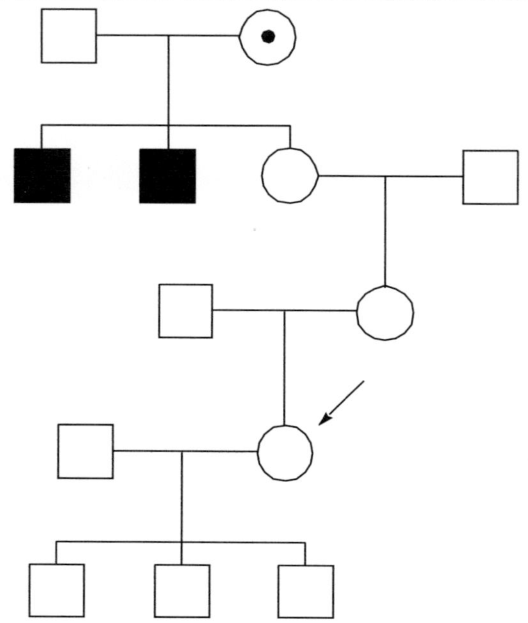

b

	Hypothesis	
	Carrier	Non-carrier
Prior Probability	1/8	7/8
Conditional probability (of negative genetic test result)	1/3	1
Conditional Probability (of normal CPK result)	1/3	19/20
Conditional Probability (of three normal sons)	1/8	1
Joint Probability	1/576	133/160
Posterior Probability	0.002	0.998

Figure 5.4 (**a**) Pedigree of a family with individuals affected with DMD (see text). (**b**) Bayesian analysis for the consultand in **a**, taking into account her normal carrier test result, her normal CPK test result, and her three normal sons

#300377). Her maternal grandmother's carrier risk was 1/2, her mother's carrier risk was 1/4, and therefore her prior carrier risk is 1/8. Suppose that her carrier testing is negative using a highly specific test (an analysis for heterozygous deletions in the *DMD* gene) that detects 2/3 of carriers. Suppose also that her serum creatine phosphokinase (CPK), which is elevated in 2/3 of carriers, is within normal limits. Taking into account her prior probability of 1/8, her normal molecular and CPK test results, and, in addition, her three normal sons, what is the probability that she is a carrier?

The Bayesian analysis for this scenario is shown in Fig. 5.4b. Each conditional probability is given its own line. Because the genetic test detects 2/3 of carriers and is highly specific, the conditional probabilities of a negative genetic test result under the hypotheses that she is a carrier and non-carrier are 1/3 and 1, respectively. Because serum CPK is elevated in 2/3 of carriers, the conditional probability of a normal serum CPK for the hypothesis that she is a carrier is 1/3. Because 5 % of non-carrier women have an abnormal serum CPK (i.e., the normal range is defined as comprising 95 % of normal individuals), the conditional probability of a normal serum CPK under the hypothesis that she is a non-carrier is 95 % or 19/20. Finally, as in Fig. 5.1b, the conditional probabilities of three normal sons under the hypotheses that she is a carrier and non-carrier are 1/8 and 1, respectively. The joint probabilities for each hypothesis are the products of the prior probability, and all conditional probabilities, for each hypothesis (Fig. 5.4b). Calculation of posterior probabilities then proceeds exactly as in Table 5.1. In this scenario, taking into account her normal test results and her three normal sons, the consultand's carrier risk is lowered from 1/8 to 0.002, or approximately 1/500.

Bayesian Analyses with More Than Two Hypotheses

In some Bayesian analyses, more than two hypotheses must be considered. For example, consider the pedigree in Fig. 5.5a, in which a child with clinically typical type I spinal muscular atrophy (type I SMA; Werdnig–Hoffmann disease; OMIM #253300) lacks both copies of the *SMN1* gene. By dosage analysis, the child's (unaffected) mother has one copy of the *SMN1* gene and, therefore, carries one copy of the *SMN1* gene on one chromosome 5, and zero copies of the *SMN1* gene on the other chromosome 5, called the "1+0" genotype. However, the child's (unaffected) father has two copies of the *SMN1* gene and therefore could have one of three possible genotypes: (1) two copies of the *SMN1* gene on one chromosome 5 and zero copies of the *SMN1* gene on the other chromosome 5 (the "2+0" genotype), (2) one copy of the *SMN1* gene on one chromosome 5 and a subtle mutation in the *SMN1* gene on the other chromosome 5 (the "$1+1^D$" genotype, where "1^D" stands for a "one-copy-disease" allele), or (3) one copy of the *SMN1* gene on each chromosome 5 (the "1+1" non-carrier genotype), in which case he passed a *de novo* deletion of the *SMN1* gene to his affected child. The relative frequencies of the various *SMN1* alleles in several major ethnic groups are known [16], which allows the corresponding genotype frequencies to be calculated [15]. The paternal and maternal de novo deletion rates are also known ($\mu_p = 2.11 \times 10^{-4}$ and $\mu_m = 4.15 \times 10^{-5}$, respectively) [15]; thus, the probability that the father is a carrier can be calculated, which obviously has important implications for recurrence risk.

Assuming Asian ethnicity for the father, the Bayesian analysis for the father's carrier risk is shown in Fig. 5.5b. There are three hypotheses for the father's genotype: 2+0, 1+1, and $1+1^D$. The prior probabilities are the relative frequencies for these genotypes in Asian populations [16]. The conditional probabilities are the probabilities that the father passes a 0-copy allele to his child under each hypothesis. For the 2+0 genotype, the conditional probability of passing a 0-copy allele is 0.5, whereas for the 1+1 and $1+1^D$ genotypes, the conditional probability of passing a 0-copy allele is the de novo deletion rate of μ_p. As in the generalized Bayesian analysis shown in Table 5.1, the joint probability for each hypothesis is the product of the prior and conditional probabilities for that hypothesis, and the posterior probability for each hypothesis is the joint probability for

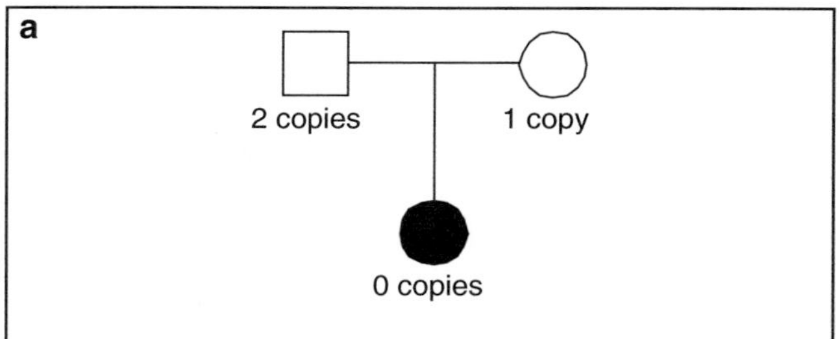

b

	Hypothesis (Father's Genotype)		
	2 + 0	1 + 1	$1 + 1^D$
Prior Probability (relative probability)	7.86×10^{-4}	8.92×10^{-1}	3.78×10^{-4}
Conditional Probability (of passing a 0-copy allele)	0.5	μ_p	μ_p
Joint Probability	3.93×10^{-4}	1.88×10^{-4}	7.97×10^{-8}
Posterior Probability	0.68	0.32	0.00014

Figure 5.5 (**a**) Pedigree of a family with an individual affected with type I SMA, with the SMA carrier test results indicated below each individual (see text). (**b**) Bayesian analysis for the father of the affected child in **a**, assuming Asian ethnicity

that hypothesis divided by the sum of all the joint probabilities. The father's carrier risk is the sum of the posterior probabilities of the first (2+0) and third ($1+1^D$) columns, or approximately 0.68. The third column contributes little to the carrier risk because the frequency of the $1+1^D$ genotype is low and the conditional probability of a de novo deletion is also low. In contrast, although the frequency of the 2+0 genotype is much lower than that of the 1+1 genotype, this is counterbalanced by the higher conditional probability of passing a 0-copy allele under the former hypothesis.

Suppose that the father's parents, the paternal grandfather and grandmother of the affected child, are tested and found to have three copies and one copy of the *SMN1* gene, respectively (Fig. 5.6a). What is the father's carrier risk? The Bayesian analysis for this scenario is shown in Fig. 5.6b. Again, there are three hypotheses for the father's genotype: 2+0, 1+1, and $1+1^D$. However, in this scenario, the father's prior probabilities derive from the prior and conditional probabilities of his parents. Because the grandfather has three copies of the *SMN1* gene, his genotype is either 2+1 (columns A and C) or $2+1^D$ (columns B and D), and his prior probabilities are the relative frequencies for these genotypes in Asian populations [16]. Because the (unaffected) grandmother has one copy of the *SMN1* gene, her genotype is 1+0, and her prior probability is the relative population frequency of the 1+0 genotype for type I SMA in Asian populations, which is the carrier frequency of 1/64 (1.57×10^{-2}) [15]. (Note that because the grandmother must have a 1+0 genotype, simply a prior probability of 1 could be used; as noted above, the absolute values of the conditional probabilities are unimportant, as long as the ratio between them is correct.) The four columns (A through D) show the four possible permutations of grandparental genotypes (prior probabilities) with passage of particular alleles to the father (conditional probabilities) so that he would have a two-copy SMA carrier test result. Under the hypothesis that the father has a 2+0 genotype, he could have inherited a two-copy "allele" (two copies of *SMN1* on one chromosome 5) from the grandfather (2+1) at a probability of 0.5 and a 0-copy allele from the grandmother (1+0) at a probability of 0.5 (column A), or he could have inherited a two-copy allele from the grandfather ($2+1^D$) at a probability of 0.5 and a 0-copy allele the grandmother (1+0) at a probability of 0.5 (column B). Under the hypothesis that the father has a 1+1 genotype, he could have inherited a one-copy allele from the grandfather (2+1) at a probability of 0.5 and a one-copy allele the grandmother (1+0) at a probability of 0.5 (column C). Under the hypothesis that the father has a $1+1^D$ genotype, he could have inherited a 1^D allele from the grandfather ($2+1^D$) at a probability of 0.5 and a one-copy allele the grandmother (1+0) at a probability of 0.5 (column D).

The father's prior probabilities are the products of the prior and conditional probabilities for the grandparents for each column/permutation. Under the hypothesis that the father is 2+0, the conditional probability of passing a 0-copy allele to his child is 0.5 (columns A and B), whereas under the hypothesis that the father has a 1+1 or $1+1^D$ genotype, the conditional probability of passing a 0-copy allele to his child is the de novo deletion rate of μ_p (columns C and D). As in the generalized Bayesian analysis shown in Table 5.1, the joint probability for each column is the product of the prior and conditional probabilities for that column, and the posterior probability for each column is the joint probability for that column divided by the sum of all the joint probabilities. The father's carrier risk is the sum of the posterior probabilities of columns A (2+0), B (2+0), and D ($1+1^D$), or approximately 0.999. The father's increased carrier risk in this scenario derives almost entirely from the probability that he has the 2+0 genotype; this is unsurprising since the grandfather's three-copy test result demonstrates the presence of a two-copy allele in the family. (Note that because the grand-

a

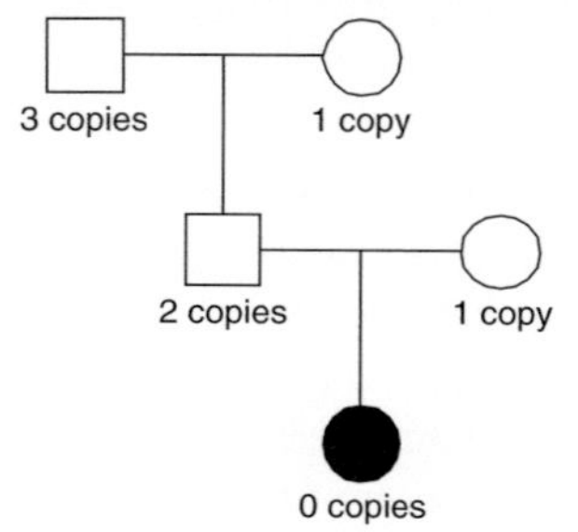

b

	Hypothesis (Father's Genotype)			
	2 + 0		1 + 1	$1+1^D$
	A	B	C	D
Grandfather's Genotype	2 + 1	$2+1^D$	2 + 1	$2+1^D$
Prior probability (relative probability)	8.95×10^{-2}	1.90×10^{-5}	8.95×10^{-2}	1.90×10^{-5}
Conditional probability (of passing a 2-copy allele)	0.5	0.5	--	--
Conditional probability (of passing a 1 or 1^D allele)	--	--	0.5	0.5
Grandmother's Genotype	1 + 0	1 + 0	1 + 0	1 + 0
Prior probability	1.57×10^{-2}	1.57×10^{-2}	1.57×10^{-2}	1.57×10^{-2}
Conditional probability (of passing a 0-copy allele)	0.5	0.5	--	--
Conditional probability (of passing a 1-copy allele)	--	--	0.5	0.5
Father's Genotype	2 + 0		1 + 1	$1+1^D$
Conditional probability (of passing a 0-copy allele)	0.5	0.5	μ_p	μ_p
Joint Probability	1.75×10^{-4}	3.71×10^{-8}	7.40×10^{-8}	1.57×10^{-11}
Posterior Probability	0.999	0.00021	0.00042	0.000000089

Figure 5.6 (**a**) Pedigree of a family with an individual affected with type I SMA (see text). (**b**) Bayesian analysis for the father of the affected child in **a**, assuming Asian ethnicity

mother's prior and conditional probabilities are the same in every column, excluding her data from the analysis will not change the result.)

Suppose instead that the father's parents, the paternal grandfather and grandmother of the affected child, are tested and both are found to have two copies of the *SMN1* gene (Fig. 5.7a). What is the father's carrier risk? The Bayesian analysis for this scenario is shown in Fig. 5.7b, again assuming Asian ethnicity. Again, there are three hypotheses for the father's genotype: 2+0, 1+1, and $1+1^D$. However, in this scenario, the number of possible permutations of grandparental genotypes (prior probabilities) with passage of particular alleles to the father (conditional probabilities) is dramatically increased. This is because each grandparent could have either a 2+0, 1+1, or $1+1^D$ genotype, and the father could have received a two-copy allele, a 0-copy allele, a one-copy allele, or a 1^D allele from either grandparent, in most cases by direct Mendelian inheritance and in some cases from de novo deletions. The organization of the Bayesian analysis in Fig. 5.7b is guided by the possible genotypes of the father, which determine the grandparental genotype permutations that need to be considered. Under the hypothesis that the father has the 2+0 genotype, he could have received a two-copy allele from one [2+0] grandparent and a 0-copy allele from the other [2+0] grandparent, both by direct inheritance (columns A and B), or he could have

a

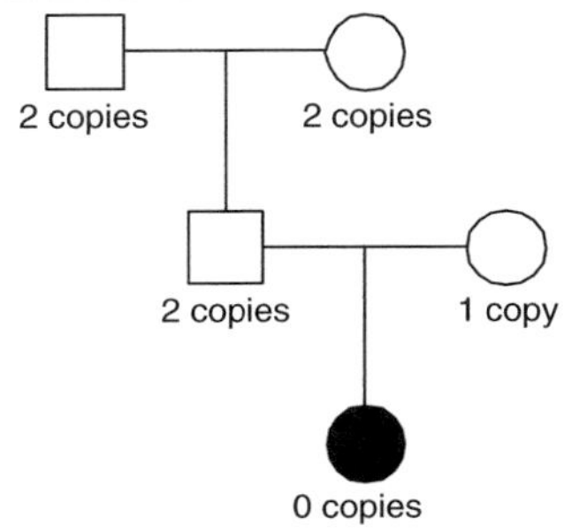

b

	Hypothesis (Father's Genotype)													
	2 + 0						1 + 1				$1 + 1^D$			
	A	B	C	D	E	F	G	H	I	J	K	L	M	N
Grandfather's Genotype	2 + 0	2 + 0	2 + 0	2 + 0	1 + 1	$1 + 1^D$	1 + 1	1 + 1	$1 + 1^D$	$1 + 1^D$	1 + 1	$1 + 1^D$	$1 + 1^D$	$1 + 1^D$
Prior Probability	7.9×10^{-4}	7.9×10^{-4}	7.9×10^{-4}	7.9×10^{-4}	0.89	3.8×10^{-4}	0.89	0.89	3.8×10^{-4}	3.8×10^{-4}	0.89	3.8×10^{-4}	3.8×10^{-4}	3.8×10^{-4}
Conditional Probability (of passing a 2-copy allele)	0.5	--	0.5	0.5	--	--	--	--	--	--	--	--	--	--
Conditional Probability (of passing a 0-copy allele)	--	0.5	--	--	2.1×10^{-4}	2.1×10^{-4}	--	--	--	--	--	--	--	--
Conditional Probability (of passing a 1-copy allele)	--	--	--	--	--	--	1	1	0.5	0.5	1	--	--	0.5
Conditional Probability (of passing a 1^D allele)	--	--	--	--	--	--	--	--	--	--	--	0.5	0.5	--
Grandmother's Genotype	2 + 0	2 + 0	1 + 1	$1 + 1^D$	2 + 0	2 + 0	1 + 1	$1 + 1^D$	1 + 1	$1 + 1^D$	$1 + 1^D$	1 + 1	$1 + 1^D$	$1 + 1^D$
Prior Probability	7.9×10^{-4}	7.9×10^{-4}	0.89	3.8×10^{-4}	7.9×10^{-4}	7.9×10^{-4}	0.89	3.8×10^{-4}	0.89	3.8×10^{-4}	3.8×10^{-4}	0.89	3.8×10^{-4}	3.8×10^{-4}
Conditional Probability (of passing a 2-copy allele)	--	0.5	--	--	0.5	0.5	--	--	--	--	--	--	--	--
Conditional Probability (of passing a 0-copy allele)	0.5	--	4.2×10^{-5}	4.2×10^{-5}	--	--	--	--	--	--	--	--	--	--
Conditional Probability (of passing a 1-copy allele)	--	--	--	--	--	--	1	0.5	1	0.5	--	1	0.5	--
Conditional Probability (of passing a 1^D allele)	--	--	--	--	--	--	--	--	--	--	0.5	--	--	0.5
Father's Genotype	2+0						1+1				$1 + 1^D$			
Conditional Probability (of passing a 0-copy allele)	0.5	0.5	0.5	0.5	0.5	0.5	2.1 x	2.1 x	2.1×10^{-4}	2.1×10^{-4}	2.1×10^{-4}	2.1×10^{-4}	2.1×10^{-4}	2.1×10^{-4}
Joint Probability	7.7×10^{-8}	7.7×10^{-8}	7.3×10^{-9}	3.1×10^{-1}	3.7×10^{-8}	1.6×10^{-11}	1.7×10^{-4}	3.6×10^{-8}	3.6×10^{-8}	7.5×10^{-12}	3.6×10^{-8}	3.6×10^{-8}	7.5×10^{-12}	7.5×10^{-12}
Posterior Probability	4.6×10^{-4}	4.6×10^{-4}	4.3×10^{-5}	1.8×10^{-8}	2.2×10^{-4}	9.3×10^{-8}	0.998	2.1×10^{-4}	2.1×10^{-4}	4.5×10^{-8}	2.1×10^{-4}	2.1×10^{-4}	4.5×10^{-8}	4.5×10^{-8}

Figure 5.7 (**a**) Pedigree of a family with an individual affected with type I SMA (see text). (**b**) Bayesian analysis for the father of the affected child in **a**, assuming Asian ethnicity. (**c**) Bayesian analysis for the father of the affected child in **a**, assuming African-American ethnicity. (In the interest of space, only two significant digits are shown)

c	Hypothesis (Father's Genotype)													
	2 + 0						**1 + 1**				**$1+1^D$**			
	A	B	C	D	E	F	G	H	I	J	K	L	M	N
Grandfather's Genotype	2 + 0	2 + 0	2 + 0	2 + 0	1 + 1	$1+1^D$	1 + 1	1 + 1	$1+1^D$	$1+1^D$	1 + 1	$1+1^D$	$1+1^D$	$1+1^D$
Prior Probability	3.7×10^{-3}	3.7×10^{-3}	3.7×10^{-3}	3.7×10^{-3}	0.52	2.9×10^{-4}	0.52	0.52	2.9×10^{-4}	2.9×10^{-4}	0.52	2.9×10^{-4}	2.9×10^{-4}	2.9×10^{-4}
Conditional Probability (of passing a 2-copy allele)	0.5	--	0.5	0.5	--	--	--	--	--	--	--	--	--	--
Conditional Probability (of passing a 0-copy allele)	--	0.5	--	--	2.1×10^{-4}	2.1×10^{-4}	--	--	--	--	--	--	--	--
Conditional Probability (of passing a 1-copy allele)	--	--	--	--	--	--	1	1	0.5	0.5	1	--	--	0.5
Conditional Probability (of passing a 1^D allele)	--	--	--	--	--	--	--	--	--	--	--	0.5	0.5	--
Grandmother's Genotype	2 + 0	2 + 0	1 + 1	$1+1^D$	2 + 0	2 + 0	1 + 1	$1+1^D$	1 + 1	$1+1^D$	$1+1^D$	1 + 1	$1+1^D$	$1+1^D$
Prior Probability	3.7×10^{-3}	3.7×10^{-3}	0.52	2.9×10^{-4}	3.7×10^{-4}	3.7×10^{-3}	0.52	2.9×10^{-4}	0.90	2.9×10^{-4}	2.9×10^{-4}	0.52	2.9×10^{-4}	2.9×10^{-4}
Conditional Probability (of passing a 2-copy allele)	--	0.5	--	--	0.5	0.5	--	--	--	--	--	--	--	--
Conditional Probability (of passing a 0-copy allele)	0.5	--	4.2×10^{-5}	4.2×10^{-5}	--	--	--	--	--	--	--	--	--	--
Conditional Probability (of passing a 1-copy allele)	--	--	--	--	--	--	1	0.5	1	0.5	--	1	0.5	--
Conditional Probability (of passing a 1^D allele)	--	--	--	--	--	--	--	--	--	--	0.5	--	--	0.5
Father's Genotype	2 + 0						1 + 1			$1+1^D$				
Conditional Probability (of passing a 0-copy allele)	0.5	0.5	0.5	0.5	0.5	0.5	2.1×10^{-4}	2.1×10^{-4}	2.1×10^{-4}	2.1×10^{-4}	2.1×10^{-4}	2.1×10^{-4}	2.1×10^{-4}	2.1×10^{-4}
Joint Probability	1.7×10^{-6}	1.7×10^{-6}	2.0×10^{-8}	1.1×10^{-11}	1.0×10^{-7}	5.7×10^{-11}	5.6×10^{-5}	1.6×10^{-8}	1.6×10^{-8}	4.3×10^{-12}	1.6×10^{-8}	1.6×10^{-8}	4.3×10^{-12}	4.3×10^{-12}
Posterior Probability	2.9×10^{-2}	2.9×10^{-2}	3.3×10^{-4}	1.9×10^{-7}	1.7×10^{-3}	9.5×10^{-7}	0.938	2.6×10^{-4}	2.6×10^{-4}	7.3×10^{-8}	2.6×10^{-4}	2.6×10^{-4}	7.3×10^{-8}	7.3×10^{-8}

Figure 5.7 (continued)

received a two-copy allele from one [2+0] grandparent by direct inheritance and a de novo deletion allele from the other [1+1 or $1+1^D$] grandparent (columns C, D, E, and F). Under the hypothesis that the father has the 1+1 genotype, he must have received a one-copy allele from each [1+1 or $1+1^D$] grandparent (columns G, H, I, and J). Under the hypothesis that the father has the $1+1^D$ genotype, he must have received a one-copy allele from one [1+1 or $1+1^D$] grandparent and a 1^D allele from the other [1+1 or $1+1^D$] grandparent (columns K, L, M, and N).

More specifically, under the hypothesis that the father has the 2+0 genotype, column A shows the prior probability that the grandfather has a 2+0 genotype (7.87×10^{-4}), the conditional probability that he passes a two-copy allele to the father (0.5), the prior probability that the grandmother has a 2+0 genotype (7.87×10^{-4}), and the conditional probability that she passes a 0-copy allele to the father (0.5). Under the hypothesis that the father has the 1+1 genotype, column G shows the prior probability that the grandfather has a 1+1 genotype (0.89), the conditional probability that he passes a one-copy allele to the father (1), the prior probability that the grandmother has a 1+1 genotype (0.89), and the conditional probability that she passes a one-copy allele to the father (1). Under the hypothesis that the father has the $1+1^D$ genotype, column K shows the prior probability that the grandfather has a 1+1 genotype (0.89), the conditional probability that he passes a one-copy allele to the father (1), the prior probability that the grandmother has a $1+1^D$ genotype (3.78×10^{-4}), and the conditional probability that she passes a 1^D allele to the father (0.5).

Again, the father's prior probabilities are the products of the prior and conditional probabilities for the grandparents for each column/permutation. Under the hypothesis that the father has a 2+0 genotype, the conditional probability of passing a 0-copy allele to his child is 0.5 (columns A through F), whereas under the hypothesis that the father has a 1+1 or $1+1^D$ genotype, the conditional probability of passing a 0-copy allele to his child is the de novo deletion rate of μ_p (columns G through L). As in the generalized Bayesian analysis shown in Table 5.1, the joint probability for each column is the product of the prior and conditional probabilities for that column, and the posterior probability for each column is the joint probability for that column divided by the sum of all the joint probabilities. The father's carrier risk is the sum of the posterior probabilities of columns A through F (2+0), and K through N ($1+1^D$), or approximately 1/622. Relative to the previous scenario (Fig. 5.6), in which the father also had two copies of *SMN1* but the grandparents had different *SMN1* copy numbers, the father's dramatically decreased carrier risk in this scenario derives from the much lower probability that a two-copy allele is present in his family, and illustrates the importance of integrating all available genetic testing information into risk assessment calculations.

The use of one comprehensive Bayesian analysis table incorporating all necessary information allows simultaneous calculations of the carrier risks of the father, grandfather, and grandmother. Such a comprehensive approach is necessary because the two-copy test results for the grandparents influence the carrier risk of the father, and the two-copy test result for the father influences the carrier risks of the grandparents. Using Fig. 5.7b, the posterior carrier risk of the grandfather is the sum of the posterior probabilities of columns A through D, F, I, J, and L through N, or approximately 0.0014 (1/720), and the carrier risk of the grandmother is the sum of the posterior probabilities of columns A, B, D through F, H, J, K, M, and N, or approximately 0.0016 (1/640). The posterior probability that all three of them are carriers is the sum of the posterior probabilities of columns A, B, D, F, M, and N, or approximately 0.00092 (1/1,085).

From carrier testing more than 72,000 individuals for SMA, Sugarman et al. showed that SMA allele frequencies differ significantly by ethnicity; in particular, they found that 27.5 % of alleles in the African-American population are two-copy, which is dramatically higher than in other ethnic groups [16]. If we repeat the Bayesian analysis shown in Fig. 5.7b, assuming African American, rather than Asian, ethnicity, the result is very different (Fig. 5.7c); specifically, the father's carrier risk (again, the sum of the posterior probabilities of columns A through F [2+0], and K through N [$1+1^D$]) is approximately 1/16. The reason the carrier risk is so much higher in this case is that, because of the higher two-copy allele frequency in the African-American population compared to Asian populations, the prior probability that the grandparents are 2+0, rather than 1+1 or $1+1^D$, is many fold higher. Thus, as in the case of CF, the appropriate population risk depends on the ethnicity of the consultand, and the consultand's family, and must be taken into account in genetic risk assessment for SMA.

Concluding Remarks

Bayesian analysis plays a central role in genetic risk assessment, and those who offer genetic testing should be proficient. Genetic risk should be assessed as accurately as possible, using all available information at a particular point in time, including the most up-to-date estimates of carrier and allele frequencies, information from the pedigree, and results of laboratory testing. Although the technologies for genetic testing will continue to change, Bayesian analysis and genetic risk assessment will remain fundamental aspects of genetic testing and genetic counseling.

References

1. Bayes T. An essay towards solving a problem in the doctrine of chances. Biometrika. 1958;45:296–315.
2. Young I. Introduction to risk calculation in genetic counseling. 3rd ed. Oxford: Oxford University Press; 2006.
3. Bridge P. The calculation of genetic risks: worked examples in DNA diagnostics. Baltimore, MD: The Johns Hopkins University Press; 1997.
4. Ogino S, Leonard DGB, Rennert H, Gao S, Wilson RB. Heteroduplex formation in SMN gene dosage analysis. J Mol Diagn. 2001;3(4):150–7.
5. Ogino S, Wilson RB. Genetic testing and risk assessment for spinal muscular atrophy (SMA). Hum Genet. 2002;111:477–500.
6. Ogino S, Wilson RB. Bayesian analysis and risk assessment in genetic counseling and testing. J Mol Diagn. 2004;6:1–9.
7. Ogino S, Wilson RB, Gold B, Hawley P, Grody WW. Bayesian analysis for cystic fibrosis risks in prenatal and carrier screening. Genet Med. 2004;6:439–49.
8. Ogino S, Wilson RB, Grody WW. Bayesian risk assessment for autosomal recessive diseases: fetal echogenic bowel with one or no detectable CFTR mutation. J Med Genet. 2004;41:e70.
9. Ogino S, Flodman P, Wilson RB, Gold B, Grody WW. Risk calculations for cystic fibrosis in neonatal screening by immunoreactive trypsinogen and CFTR mutation tests. Genet Med. 2005;7:317–27.
10. Ogino S, Wilson RB, Gold B, Flodman P. Bayesian risk assessment in genetic testing for autosomal dominant disorders with age-dependent penetrance. J Genet Couns. 2007;16:29–39.
11. Grody WW, Cutting GR, Klinger KW, Richards CS, Watson MS, Desnick RJ. Laboratory standards and guidelines for population-based cystic fibrosis carrier screening. Genet Med. 2001;3:149–54.
12. Richards CS, Bradley LA, Amos J, et al. Standards and guidelines for CFTR mutation testing. Genet Med. 2002;4:379–91.
13. Watson MS, Cutting GR, Desnick RJ, et al. Cystic fibrosis population carrier screening: 2004 revision of American College of Medical Genetics mutation panel. Genet Med. 2004;6:387–91.
14. Wirth B, Herz M, Wetter A, et al. Quantitative analysis of survival motor neuron copies: identification of subtle SMN1 mutations in patients with spinal muscular atrophy, genotype-phenotype correlation, and implications for genetic counseling. Am J Hum Genet. 1999;64:1340–56.
15. Ogino S, Wilson RB, Gold B. New insights on the evolution of the SMN1 and SMN2 region: simulation and meta-analysis for allele and haplotype frequency calculations. Eur J Hum Genet. 2004;12:1015–23.
16. Sugarman EA, Nagan N, Zhu H, et al. Pan-ethnic carrier screening and prenatal diagnosis for spinal muscular atrophy: clinical laboratory analysis of >72,400 specimens. Eur J Hum Genet. 2012;20:27–32.

6 Intellectual Disability and Developmental Delay: Cytogenetic Testing

Guangyu Gu, Reha Toydemir, and Sarah T. South

Abstract

Intellectual disability/developmental delay (ID/DD) is not a specific diagnosis, but a description of certain conditions in which intellectual functioning shows significant limitations when compared to the expected level for age. This chapter discusses the methods for evaluating an individual for ID/DD. In addition, advantages, limitations, and interpretation challenges are discussed.

Keywords

Intellectual disability • Developmental delay • Comparative genomic hybridization • Array • Chromosomes • Copy number variants • Deletions • Cytogenetic • Microdeletion • Microduplication • Microarray

Introduction

Intellectual disability and developmental delay (ID/DD) is not a specific diagnosis. It is rather a description of certain conditions in which intellectual functioning or at least two areas of adaptive performance show significant limitations when compared to the expected level for age. The adaptive areas include gross or fine motor skills, speech or language, cognition, social or personal, and activities related to daily living. A significant delay is described as two or more standard deviations from the age and cultural norms. The prevalence of ID/DD is approximately 3 % [1] with some studies suggesting up to 16 % of children referred to pediatric clinics have some developmental problems [2].

G. Gu, M.D. • R. Toydemir, M.D., Ph.D.
Pathology Department, ARUP Laboratories, University of Utah, 500 Chipeta Way, MS 391, Salt Lake City, UT, USA

S.T. South, Ph.D. (✉)
Pathology Department, ARUP Laboratories, University of Utah, 500 Chipeta Way, MS 391, Salt Lake City, UT, USA

Department of Pediatrics, ARUP Laboratories, University of Utah, Salt Lake City, UT, USA
e-mail: sarah.south@aruplab.com

Clinical Utility

Early identification of the underlying etiology of ID/DD is critical for treatment planning, prognosis, and family planning. Although fairly common, the cause of ID/DD remains mostly unknown. This is due in part to the highly heterogeneous etiology of ID/DD. Both genetic causes and environmental factors affect the development of the brain. The development of the brain requires the orchestrated action of many genes. In fact, 86 % of human genes are involved in the formation and differentiation of the human brain [3]. As chromosomal aberrations are considered a major cause of non-syndromic ID/DD [4, 5], cytogenetic studies are recommended for all children with ID/DD when an etiology has not been determined [6, 7].

Available Assays

Over the past few decades, many exciting advances in cytogenetics and molecular cytogenetics have allowed the identification of genomic imbalances related to ID/DD in an increasing number of both mild and severe cases. Conventional cytogenetics techniques, such as G-banding, have been widely used to detect numerical and structural chromosomal

D.G.B. Leonard (ed.), *Molecular Pathology in Clinical Practice*, DOI 10.1007/978-3-319-19674-9_6

abnormalities, including deletions, duplications, and translocations. The development of fluorescence in situ hybridization (FISH) methods has enabled the identification of many microdeletion and microduplication syndromes and subtelomere rearrangements that are generally undetectable by conventional banding techniques [8, 9]. Most recently, chromosomal microarray analysis (CMA), including array-based comparative genomic hybridization (aCGH) and single-nucleotide polymorphism (SNP) arrays, has become a standard cytogenetic diagnostic test for the identification of copy number variations (CNVs) in patients with DD [10, 11].

G-Banded Karyotyping

In cases of DD with and without dysmorphic features, G-banded karyotyping is still a valuable technique that allows for analysis of chromosomes from a tissue of interest to identify large-scale genomic aberrations. This conventional cytogenetic approach may detect aneuploidy, chromosomal mosaicism, and many other structural abnormalities (Fig. 6.1). The limit of resolution of G-banding is between 5 and 10 Mb and depends on the region of the genome and the length of chromosomes. The rearrangements of chromosome segments smaller than 5 Mb cannot reliably be detected. Likewise, the chromosomal origin of a small marker chromosome may not be identified by G-banded karyotyping.

Fluorescence In Situ Hybridization

FISH approaches were first described in 1986 [12] and have become essential for many comprehensive cytogenetic analyses. Most any DNA segment can be used as a FISH probe. For clinical use, most probes are between 100 and 500 kb. This provides a resolution far greater than that of G-banding for the identification of deletions, insertions and translocation breakpoints. The types of probes include (1) painting probes, which are used to identify the chromosomal origin of a DNA segment and are useful for distinguishing translocations; (2) centromere probes that hybridize to alpha-satellite DNA located at the centromere of each chromosome, which are used to identify aneuploidy of specific chromosomes or to identify the chromosomal origin of marker chromosomes; (3) beta-satellite probes, which are used to

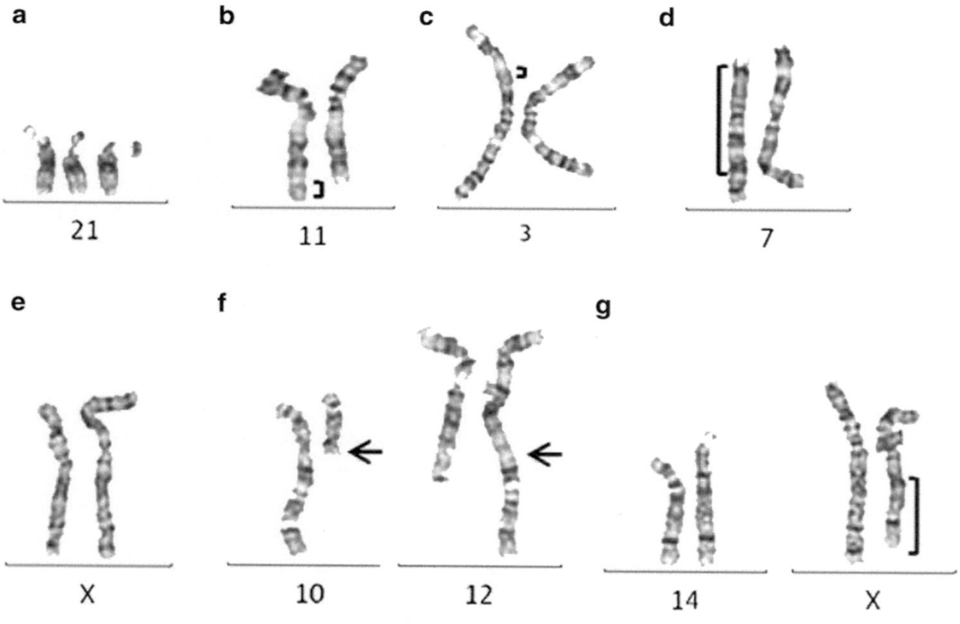

Figure 6.1 Common types of chromosome abnormalities detected by standard chromosome analysis (G-banded karyotyping). (**a**) Aneuploidy, defined as the loss or gain of an entire chromosome, shown as trisomy 21. (**b**) Terminal deletion, shown as a deletion of distal 11q (normal chromosome 11 on *left*, with deleted region *bracketed*, and deleted 11 on *right*). (**c**) Interstitial deletion, shown within 3p (normal chromosome 3 on *left*, with deleted region *bracketed*, and deleted 3 on *right*). (**d**) Inversion, shown as a pericentric inversion of chromosome 7 (normal chromosome 7 on *left* with inverted region *bracketed*, and inverted 7 on *right*). (**e**) Isochromosome, defined as the loss of one chromosome arm with duplication and mirror image of other arm, shown as isochromosome Xq (normal X on *left* and isochromosome Xq on *right*). (**f**) Balanced translocation, shown between 10q and 12q (with normal 10 and 12 on *left* of each pair and translocated 10 and 12 on *right with arrows* marking breakpoints of the translocation). (**g**) Unbalanced translocation, shown between 14q and Xq with two normal 14 chromosomes, one normal X, and one X with a deletion of part of Xq and replacement with gain of 14q region bracketed, leading to partial 14q trisomy and partial Xq monosomy.

identify beta-satellite regions on the short arm of acrocentric chromosomes; (4) subtelomeric probes, which are used to detect subtelomeric rearrangements of chromosome arms; and (5) locus-specific probes, which hybridize to unique gene sequences and are used to identify contiguous gene syndromes and other microdeletion or microduplication syndromes (Fig. 6.2).

FISH allows the determination of the frequency and location of specific DNA sequences in cells in any state of the cell cycle and in archived formalin-fixed, paraffin-embedded tissues. However, FISH can only detect deletions, duplications, and rearrangements of the chromosomal region complementary to the probe. Clinically, suspicion of a syndrome with known cytogenetic etiology is normally required to run a FISH study. Also, the number of probes that can be mixed and used in a single FISH assay is limited and depends on the number of fluorochromes available for probe labeling; in most clinical applications, this is limited to three unique regions probed per hybridization.

Chromosomal Microarray Analysis

Chromosomal Microarray Methodology

CMA allows for the detection of loss or gain at multiple loci at a much higher resolution than either conventional chromosome analysis or FISH. For CMA testing using aCGH, the patient's genomic DNA and control genomic DNA are labeled with different fluorochromes and co-hybridized onto DNA substrates immobilized on a solid support (Fig. 6.3). Several aCGH platforms have been developed for diagnostic purposes. Initially, bacterial artificial chromosomes (BACs, between 80 and 200 kb) were used as array targets (Fig. 6.4) [13]. Oligonucleotide arrays (25–85 bp) were subsequently constructed to allow for higher resolution [14, 15].

Arrays that target clinically meaningful regions of the genome have been used for postnatal and prenatal cases with normal chromosome analysis results and for general screening purposes [16–20]. The whole genome designed array

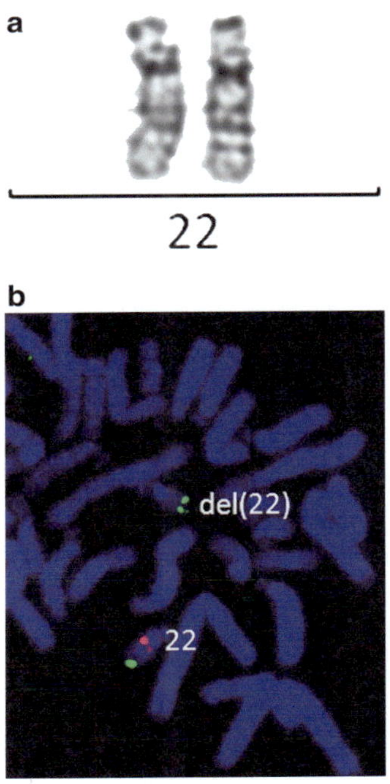

Figure 6.2 Chromosomally cryptic 22q11.2 deletion detected by FISH, but not by G-banded karyotyping. (**a**) Normal banding pattern for each chromosome 22. (**b**) FISH with a specific probe to the *TUPLE1* gene in *red* and control probe in *green* show a deletion of one copy of this gene on one chromosome 22

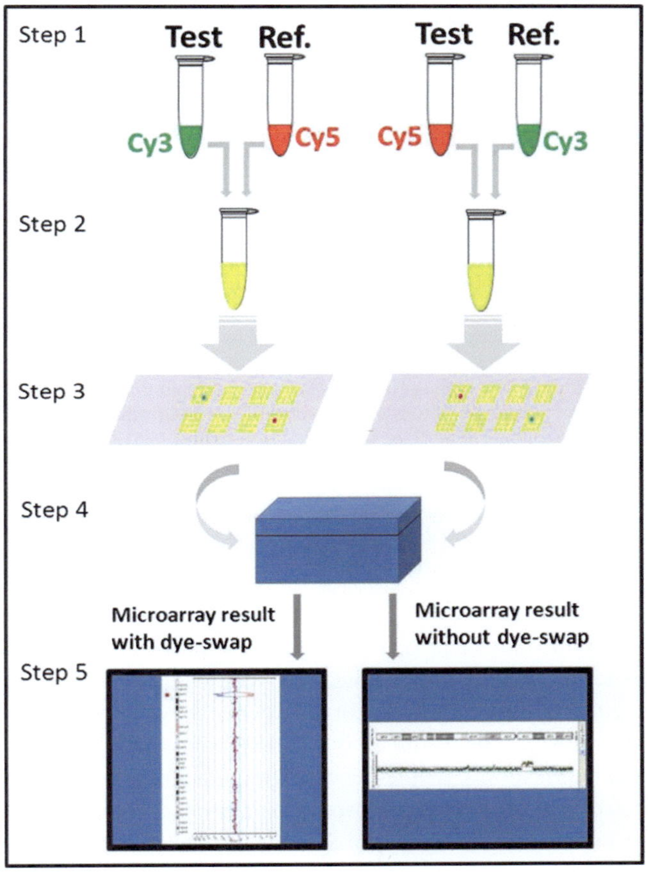

Figure 6.3 Steps in aCGH procedure. *Step 1*: Test and reference DNA are fragmented and labeled with fluorescent dyes, Cy3 and Cy5. *Step 2*: Equal amounts of labeled test and reference DNAs are mixed together. *Step 3*: The combined labeled test and reference DNAs are applied to the microarray and compete to hybridize to the target DNA (segments of the human genome) on the microarray. *Step 4*: Fluorescent signals are measured in the microarray scanner. *Step 5*: Analysis software generates data linking signal to relative copy number of test DNA compared to reference DNA for each probe on the microarray. To confirm the result, this process is repeated with the fluorochromes switched between the test and reference DNAs (called a dye-swap), so that a true loss or gain would have the opposite fluorescent signal in the repeat test. In lieu of a dye-swap repeat, multiple independent probes adjacent in the genome but separate on the microarray showing a contiguous loss or gain increases confidence in the accuracy of result.

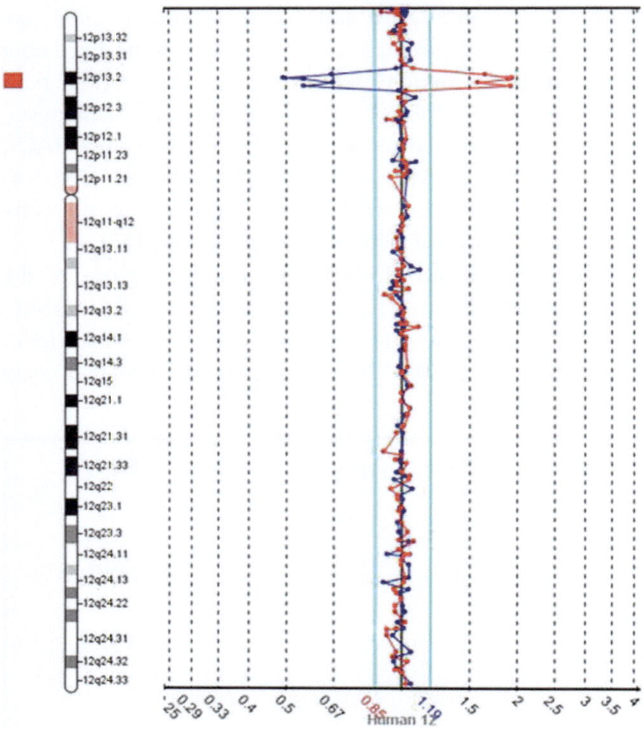

Figure 6.4 Example of a deletion detected by the original aCGH with the dye-swap repeat using BAC-based targets. Data from chromosome 12 with each dot representing a BAC probe mapping approximately every one megabase across chromosome 12. In both runs, less of the labeled test DNA hybridized to the BACs in region 12p13 when compared to the reference DNA, as represented by the reciprocal deviation from the *central black line* (representing zero) on the *Y*-axis and the *red bar to the left* of the schematic chromosome 12 (for this software, when equal hybridization of test and reference DNAs occurs, the *dots map* within the *aqua lines* near the *central black line*)

offers full coverage of the genome as the technology and genomic architecture allows. The copy number of some regions of the genome cannot be accurately evaluated by this technology, notably repetitive regions and small deletions and duplications. Whole-genome design is important for the discovery of new chromosomal syndromes [21, 22] and detection of recently discovered syndromes that may have occurred since the design of a targeted array. Many platforms in clinical use are currently a combination of both whole-genome coverage and enrichment of targets at known clinically relevant regions.

The SNP array is another type of oligonucleotide array. SNPs are DNA sequence variations in which a single nucleotide in the sequence of the oligonucleotide differs between individuals or between paired chromosomes in an individual. Similar to aCGH, SNP arrays contain probes that can detect imbalances at thousands of loci in the genome. In contrast to aCGH, SNP arrays also can be used for detecting long contiguous stretches of homozygosity, which may be caused by either consanguinity or uniparental disomy (UPD) of a genomic interval (Fig. 6.5). Both consanguinity and UPD increase the risk of autosomal recessive conditions. In addition, UPD of specific chromosomal regions is associated with imprinting defects, such as UPD of chromosome 15 in patients with Prader-Willi syndrome and Angelman syndrome.

Advantages of CMA Testing

Compared with G-banded karyotyping, CMA analyzes chromosomes for genomic gains and losses at a much higher resolution, which allows the detection of smaller or cryptic abnormalities (Figs. 6.6 and 6.7) and provides better definition of cytogenetic abnormalities (Fig. 6.8). The detection of abnormalities by CMA is usually more detailed, automatable, and less subjective than G-banded karyotyping. Furthermore, archived or non-growing tissue can be used for CMA, but not G-banded karyotyping. CMA also may provide information on the mechanism of the genetic aberration. For example, depending on the observed pattern of imbalance in the proband and the parents, the proband may be predicted to have an unbalanced segregation of a translocation or inversion which is present in a balanced form in either parent. Also, analysis of the flanking regions of the imbalance allows determination of whether the rearrangement is mediated by non-allelic homologous recombination [25]. Information about the likely mechanism then informs the likelihood of recurrence in subsequent pregnancies.

The diagnostic yield of a G-banded karyotype in individuals with ID/DD is approximately 3 %. FISH analysis of subtelomeric regions may provide a diagnosis in another 2–3 % of cases [26]. Several large cohort studies have shown that CMA has the highest yield as a single diagnostic test for individuals with ID/DD [5, 11, 27–29]. The detection rate varies between studies, likely due to differences in platform design, populations studied, and interpretation methods (see below); however, these studies still demonstrated between a 10 and 28.9 % detection rate for pathogenic aberrations in patients with ID/DD, and less than 0.6 % of cases with probable disease-causing balanced de novo aberrations remained undetectable. Thus, CMA has been recommended as a "first-line test" in the initial evaluation of patients with nonsyndromic ID/DD by the American College of Medical Genetics (ACMG) Practice Guidelines [10].

Limitations of CMA Testing

CMA alone cannot detect balanced rearrangements (such as translocations, inversions, and point mutations) and some cases of mosaicism (depending on the platform, size, direction, and percentage of mosaicism of imbalance [30–32]). Also, arrays will not detect CNVs in the regions of the genome that are not on the array platform, and, therefore, the resolution of the array is dependent both on the design and the genomic architecture. The array will not identify the

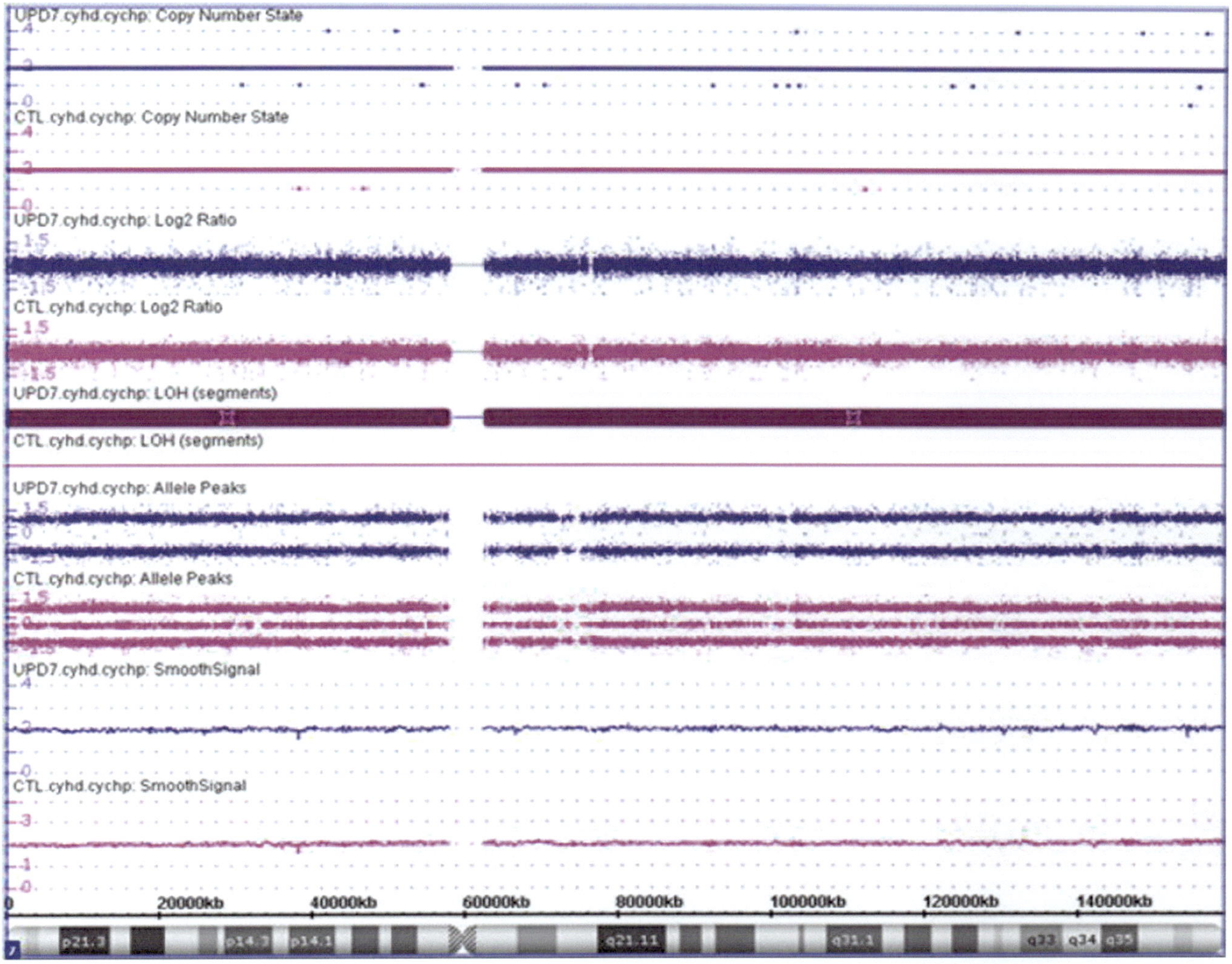

Figure 6.5 CMA finding consistent with uniparental isodisomy of chromosome 7. UPD7 case shown in *purple* and a normal case shown in *pink* for comparison. (**a**) The copy number state is determined to be 2 (normal diploid) across the vast majority of the chromosome both for the UPD7 and normal cases (CTL). (**b**) Estimation of the copy number state based on the log2 ratio of the hybridization of the patient DNA to the control DNA, with signal centered at zero. (**c**) Loss of heterozygosity is noted across the entire chromosome for the UPD7 case (*maroon bar*) due to the allele peak pattern which shows only values at 1.0 and −1.0; whereas the normal case shows normal heterozygosity (*no maroon bar*) with values at 1.0, 0, and −1.0. These values are determined by assigning each allele a value of 0.5 and then plotting A–B. Therefore a locus with AA is (0.5+0.5)−0=1; a locus with AB is 0.5−0.5=0; and a locus with BB is 0−(0.5+0.5)=−1. (**d**) For the UPD7 case, all of chromosome 7 shows no evidence of any AB loci, suggestive that both chromosome 7 s are 100 % identical. Maternal UPD7 is associated with Russell-Silver syndrome; whereas paternal UPD7 has not been associated with a specific clinical consequence. Additionally, recessive disorders mapping to chromosome 7, such as cystic fibrosis, should be considered for this child. Although this example shows isodisomy for all of chromosome 7, also note that UPD may have parts of the affected chromosome showing isodisomy whereas other parts of the same chromosome still show heterodisomy due to crossing over between the homologous chromosomes.

genomic location of gained material and this may be relevant as duplications with a single breakpoint within a gene may or may not disrupt the open reading frame of that one copy of the gene, depending on the orientation and location of the duplicated material.

Finally, the detection of CNVs of unknown clinical significance is challenging for interpretation due the current lack of published data on these variations (Fig. 6.9). This is an expanding field and reevaluation of the clinically uncertain findings at a later date may result in the reclassification of some of these results.

CMA Interpretation for Patients with ID/DD

ACMG published guidelines for the interpretation and reporting of CNVs detected in the postnatal and constitutional setting [34]. Some of the major points are summarized here,

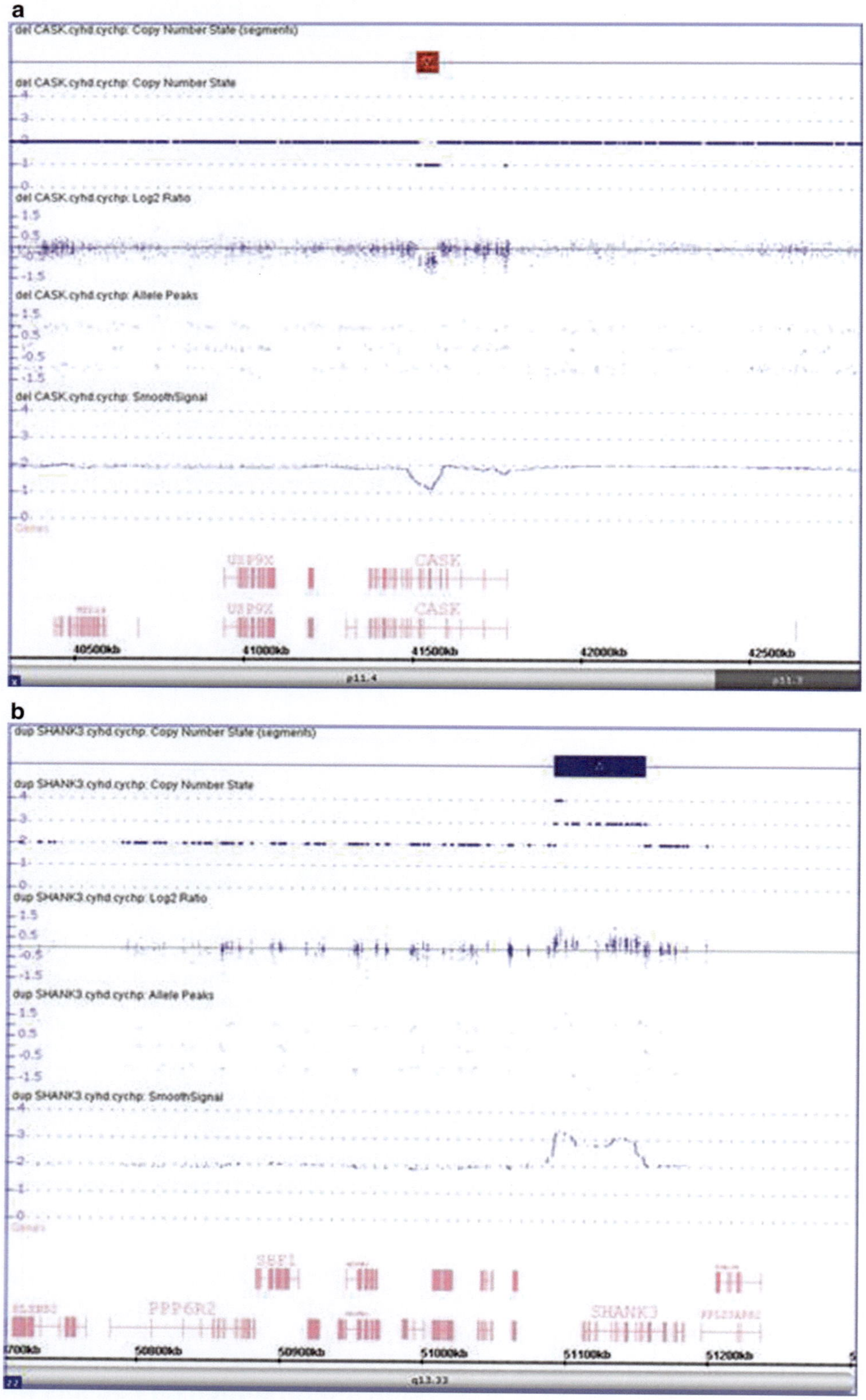

Figure 6.6 Detection of intragenic loss and small gain using CMA. (**a**) The CMA shows a 63 kb deletion within Xp11.4 in a female patient (region *highlighted by red bar at top*). This deletion involves three exons of the gene *CASK*. Deletions of *CASK* have been found in female and male patients with X-linked cognitive disability, optic atrophy, brainstem and cerebellar hypoplasia, microcephaly, and dysmorphic facial features [23]. (**b**) The CMA shows a 64 kb gain within 22q13.33, indicating trisomy for this region (region *highlighted by blue bar at top*). This duplication has a breakpoint within the *SHANK3* gene. Disruption of *SHANK3* has been reported in patients with global developmental delay [24].

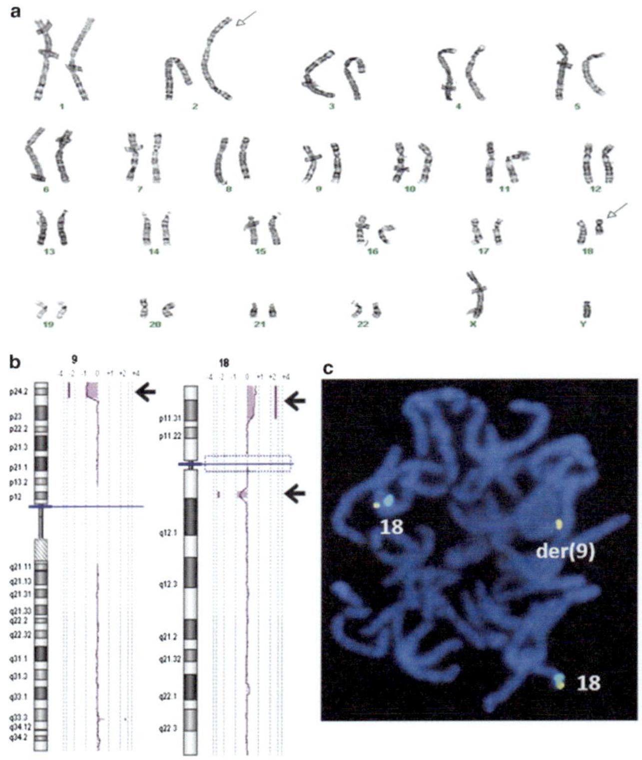

Figure 6.7 Identification of cryptic abnormality by CMA in addition to a visible chromosome abnormality by G-banded karyotype. (**a**) Chromosome G-banding shows a translocation between 2q and 18q (*arrows*). (**b**) Genomic microarray shows a 1.2 Mb interstitial deletion at the 18q breakpoint, but also a 5.9 Mb terminal deletion of 9p and a 6.0 Mb terminal duplication of 18p (*arrows*). (**c**) FISH with the 18p subtelomere probe (fusion signal) shows additional signal is on the derivative 9, consistent with an unbalanced translocation not detected in chromosome analysis

though the guideline provides more comprehensive recommendations. Many detected CNVs already may be described in the medical literature and their pathogenic or benign nature be well understood; however, many other detected changes may represent rare variations. Assessing the clinical significance of an identified CNV can be challenging due to the presence of benign CNVs within the genome, the potential for incomplete penetrance and variable expressivity, and the continual discovery of new associations of clinical conditions with genetic alterations.

A number of databases are available to assist with the interpretation of CMA results including PubMed, OMIM (currently at http://www.omim.org), GeneReviews (currently at http://www.ncbi.nlm.nih.gov/sites/GeneTests/), DECIPHER [35], the International Standard Cytogenetic Array Consortium (ISCA) database housed by dbVar (currently available at http://www.ncbi.nlm.nih.gov/dbvar/studies/nstd37/), and the Database of Genomic Variants [36]. New microdeletion and microduplication syndromes are identified regularly. The pathogenic nature of some recurrent microdeletion and microduplication regions may not yet be clear; therefore, frequent literature reviews are important to assess newly defined phenotypic associations.

A primary consideration for interpretation of results is the functions and density of the genes within the variant interval. For example, regions with very few genes, or primarily containing repetitive elements or pseudogenes, may be less likely of clinical significance than similar regions that are very gene rich. When assessing the gene content, the impact of gene dosage on the function of the genes in the interval should be considered. Factors to consider include gene dosage in control populations, the focal nature of the alterations in the literature, the associated phenotype, other reported findings in the described patient(s) that may contribute to the phenotype, the molecular mechanism of the mutation (i.e., loss of function vs gain of function vs unknown), and the inheritance pattern (i.e., dominant vs recessive effect and issues of penetrance). For deletions, primary consideration will be on the evidence for the phenotypic effect of haploinsufficiency of the region. For duplications, primary consideration will be on the triplosensitivity of the region; however duplication breakpoints within a gene may or may not disrupt the function of the gene.

Additional considerations for identified CNVs within a gene will be the exonic vs intronic nature of the alteration as well as if the gene exists in multiple isoforms, and whether the CNV in question does or does not involve all isoforms. Comparison of the identified CNV to control and patient populations is of significant value in predicting the pathogenicity of the variant. Finally, investigation of the established contiguous gene syndromes and microdeletion or microduplication syndromes associated with the interval is important because these may not be identified simply by a literature search focused on the genes within the interval.

Laboratory Issues

Based upon the technical performance and probe density of the microarray platform being used for clinical testing, size restrictions may be established for copy number calls, which can differ based on the type of variation. Different thresholds may be established for deletions, duplications, for regions of the genome well associated with clinical conditions, and for uncharacterized regions of the genome. Such size thresholds should not be set based on assumptions regarding an association between size and clinical significance because relatively large copy number changes can be benign and relatively small copy number changes can be clinically significant.

Parental studies may be considered as part of the interpretation of an identified CNV; however, due to issues of incomplete penetrance and variable expressivity, the finding of a

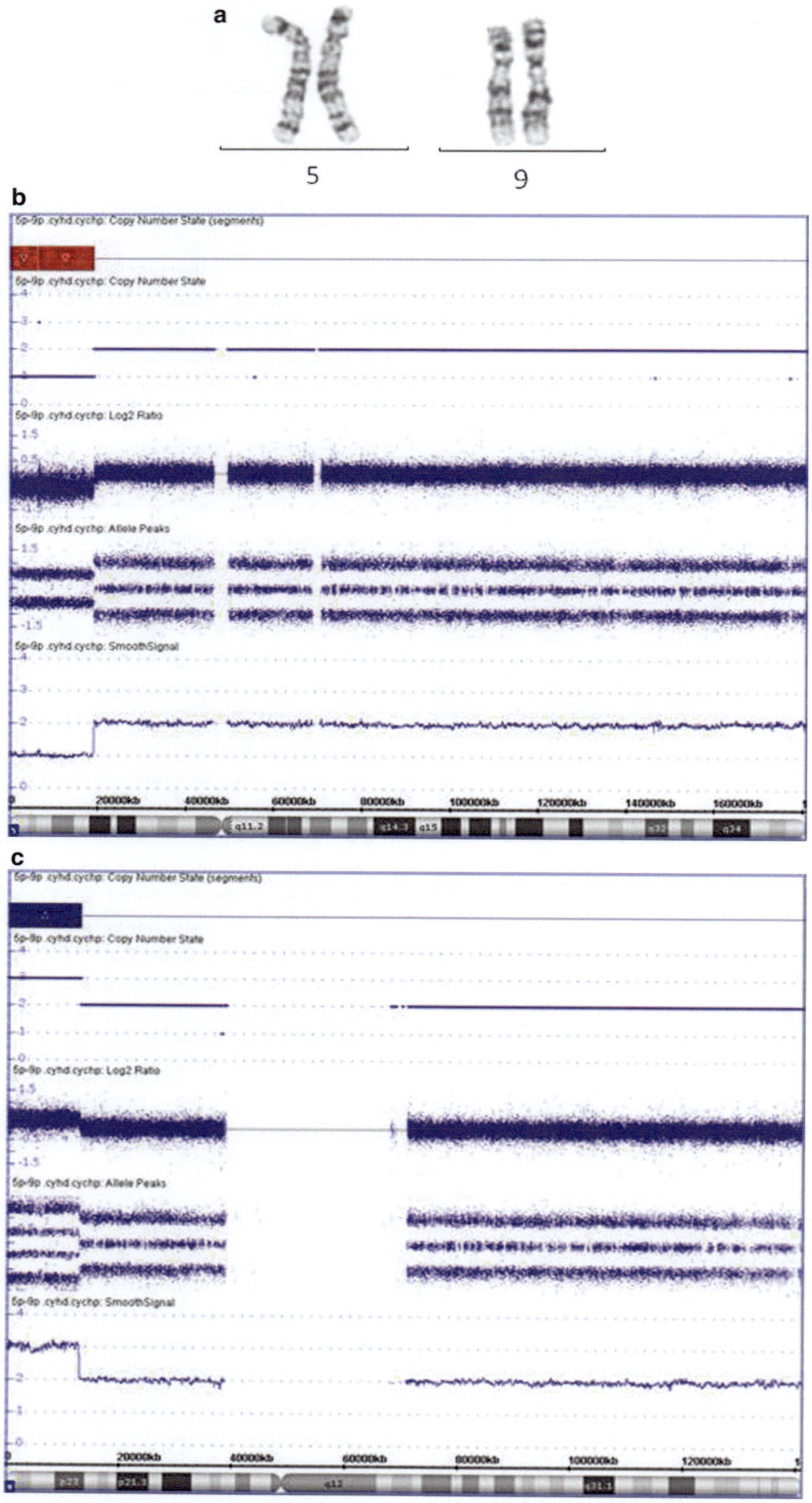

Figure 6.8 CMA often provides a better definition of a chromosome abnormality, leading to better genotype-phenotype correlation and recurrence risk estimation. (**a**) Chromosome analysis shows a terminal deletion on the short arm of chromosome 5 (abnormal chromosome on *right*) with two normal appearing chromosome 9 s. (**b** and **c**) The CMA analysis indicates that there is a 19.0 Mb terminal deletion of 5p (**b**), and a 12.8 Mb terminal duplication of 9p (**c**), suggesting an unbalanced translocation involving 5p and 9p. This abnormality is associated with the Cri-du-Chat syndrome and 9p duplication syndrome separately, so this patient is likely to have a clinical phenotype with features of both syndromes. In addition, there is a higher probability of a parent carrying a balanced rearrangement of 5p and 9p then if this was only a 5p deletion. This increases the urgency for parental testing for recurrence risk determination.

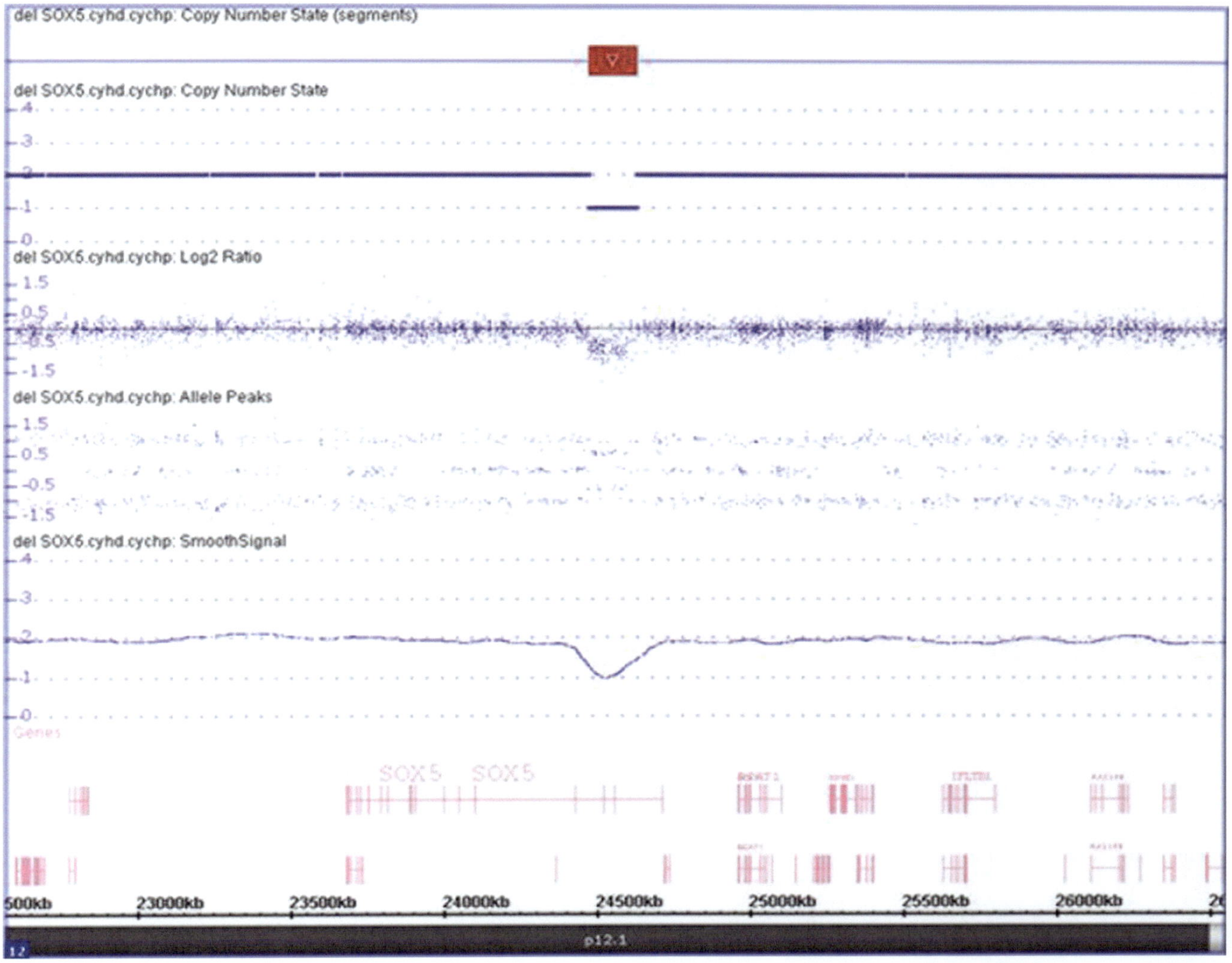

Figure 6.9 CMA detection of an abnormality of unknown clinical significance. CMA result from a 16-year-old female with behavior/conduct disorder, epilepsy, hydrocephaly, multiple congenital anomalies, and gait abnormalities. The CMA shows a 156 Kb deletion involving 12p12.1 (indicated by *red bar at top*). This deletion is within the gene *SOX5* and includes two untranslated exons in the 5′ untranslated region of one of the *SOX5* transcripts. Due to absence at the time of the patient's test results of publications associating disruption of *SOX5* with human disease, this deletion was reported as an abnormality of unknown clinical significance. Subsequently, a study showed that haploinsufficiency of *SOX5* at 12p12.1 is associated with speech delay, intellectual disability, behavior abnormalities, and dysmorphic features [33], allowing reclassification of this finding as likely pathogenic.

CNV in a clinically normal parent may not rule out a causal relationship between the alteration and the phenotype of the patient [37, 38].

Conclusions and Future Directions

ID/DD is a common medical condition, and determining the etiology can be challenging. Even though it is still an evolving field, the diagnostic success of cytogenomic microarray technology has exceeded that of conventional cytogenetic techniques. As more medical specialists utilize this technology, understanding of the pathogenesis of ID/DD will improve.

References

1. Shevell M, Ashwal S, Donley D, et al. Practice parameter: evaluation of the child with global developmental delay: report of the Quality Standards Subcommittee of the American Academy of Neurology and The Practice Committee of the Child Neurology Society. Neurology. 2003;60:367–80.
2. Rydz D, Srour M, Oskoui M, et al. Screening for developmental delay in the setting of a community pediatric clinic: a prospective assessment of parent-report questionnaires. Pediatrics. 2006;118:e1178–86.
3. Kang HJ, Kawasawa YI, Cheng F, et al. Spatio-temporal transcriptome of the human brain. Nature. 2011;478:483–9.
4. van Karnebeek CD, Jansweijer MC, Leenders AG, et al. Diagnostic investigations in individuals with mental retardation: a systematic literature review of their usefulness. Eur J Hum Genet. 2005;13:6–25.

5. Rauch A, Hoyer J, Guth S, et al. Diagnostic yield of various genetic approaches in patients with unexplained developmental delay or mental retardation. Am J Med Genet A. 2006;140:2063–74.
6. van Karnebeek CD, Koevoets C, Sluijter S, et al. Prospective screening for subtelomeric rearrangements in children with mental retardation of unknown aetiology: the Amsterdam experience. J Med Genet. 2002;39:546–53.
7. Moeschler JB, Shevell M. Clinical genetic evaluation of the child with mental retardation or developmental delays. Pediatrics. 2006;117:2304–16.
8. Knight SJ, Horsley SW, Regan R, et al. Development and clinical application of an innovative fluorescence in situ hybridization technique which detects submicroscopic rearrangements involving telomeres. Eur J Hum Genet. 1997;5:1–8.
9. Ligon AH, Beaudet al, Shaffer LG. Simultaneous, multilocus FISH analysis for detection of microdeletions in the diagnostic evaluation of developmental delay and mental retardation. Am J Hum Genet. 1997;61:51–9.
10. Manning M, Hudgins L. Array-based technology and recommendations for utilization in medical genetics practice for detection of chromosomal abnormalities. Genet Med. 2010;12:742–5.
11. Miller DT, Adam MP, Aradhya S, et al. Consensus statement: chromosomal microarray is a first-tier clinical diagnostic test for individuals with developmental disabilities or congenital anomalies. Am J Hum Genet. 2010;86:749–64.
12. Pinkel D, Straume T, Gray JW. Cytogenetic analysis using quantitative, high-sensitivity, fluorescence hybridization. Proc Natl Acad Sci U S A. 1986;83:2934–8.
13. Bejjani BA, Saleki R, Ballif BC, et al. Use of targeted array-based CGH for the clinical diagnosis of chromosomal imbalance: is less more? Am J Med Genet A. 2005;134:259–67.
14. Lucito R, Healy J, Alexander J, et al. Representational oligonucleotide microarray analysis: a high-resolution method to detect genome copy number variation. Genome Res. 2003;13:2291–305.
15. Ylstra B, van den Ijssel P, Carvalho B, et al. BAC to the future! or oligonucleotides: a perspective for micro array comparative genomic hybridization (array CGH). Nucleic Acids Res. 2006;34:445–50.
16. Le Caignec C, Boceno M, Saugier-Veber P, et al. Detection of genomic imbalances by array based comparative genomic hybridisation in fetuses with multiple malformations. J Med Genet. 2005;42:121–8.
17. Bejjani BA, Shaffer LG. Application of array-based comparative genomic hybridization to clinical diagnostics. J Mol Diagn. 2006;8:528–33.
18. Sahoo T, Cheung SW, Ward P, et al. Prenatal diagnosis of chromosomal abnormalities using array-based comparative genomic hybridization. Genet Med. 2006;8:719–27.
19. Shaffer LG, Kashork CD, Saleki R, et al. Targeted genomic microarray analysis for identification of chromosome abnormalities in 1500 consecutive clinical cases. J Pediatr. 2006;149:98–102.
20. Baldwin EL, Lee JY, Blake DM, et al. Enhanced detection of clinically relevant genomic imbalances using a targeted plus whole genome oligonucleotide microarray. Genet Med. 2008;10:415–29.
21. Vissers LE, de Vries BB, Osoegawa K, et al. Array-based comparative genomic hybridization for the genome-wide detection of submicroscopic chromosomal abnormalities. Am J Hum Genet. 2003;73:1261–70.
22. Ishkanian AS, Malloff CA, Watson SK, et al. A tiling resolution DNA microarray with complete coverage of the human genome. Nat Genet. 2004;36:299–303.
23. Hayashi S, Okamoto N, Chinen Y, et al. Novel intragenic duplications and mutations of CASK in patients with mental retardation and microcephaly with pontine and cerebellar hypoplasia (MICPCH). Hum Genet. 2012;131:99–110.
24. Durand CM, Betancur C, Boeckers TM, et al. Mutations in the gene encoding the synaptic scaffolding protein SHANK3 are associated with autism spectrum disorders. Nat Genet. 2007;39:25–7.
25. South ST. Chromosomal structural rearrangements: detection and elucidation of mechanisms using cytogenomic technologies. Clin Lab Med. 2011;31:513–24.
26. Ravnan JB, Tepperberg JH, Papenhausen P, et al. Subtelomere FISH analysis of 11 688 cases: an evaluation of the frequency and pattern of subtelomere rearrangements in individuals with developmental disabilities. J Med Genet. 2006;43:478–89.
27. Pickering DL, Eudy JD, Olney AH, et al. Array-based comparative genomic hybridization analysis of 1176 consecutive clinical genetics investigations. Genet Med. 2008;10:262–6.
28. Hochstenbach R, van Binsbergen E, Engelen J, et al. Array analysis and karyotyping: workflow consequences based on a retrospective study of 36,325 patients with idiopathic developmental delay in the Netherlands. Eur J Med Genet. 2009;52:161–9.
29. Sagoo GS, Butterworth AS, Sanderson S, et al. Array CGH in patients with learning disability (mental retardation) and congenital anomalies: updated systematic review and meta-analysis of 19 studies and 13,926 subjects. Genet Med. 2009;11:139–46.
30. Lu X, Shaw CA, Patel A, et al. Clinical implementation of chromosomal microarray analysis: summary of 2513 postnatal cases. PLoS One. 2007;2, e327.
31. Stankiewicz P, Beaudet al. Use of array CGH in the evaluation of dysmorphology, malformations, developmental delay, and idiopathic mental retardation. Curr Opin Genet Dev. 2007;17:182–92.
32. Xiang B, Li A, Valentin D, et al. Analytical and clinical validity of whole-genome oligonucleotide array comparative genomic hybridization for pediatric patients with mental retardation and developmental delay. Am J Med Genet A. 2008;146A:1942–54.
33. Lamb AN, Rosenfeld JA, Neill NJ, et al. Haploinsufficiency of SOX5 at 12p12.1 is associated with developmental delays with prominent language delay, behavior problems, and mild dysmorphic features. Hum Mutat. 2012. doi:10.1002/humu.22037.
34. Kearney HM, Thorland EC, Brown KK, et al. American College of Medical Genetics standards and guidelines for interpretation and reporting of postnatal constitutional copy number variants. Genet Med. 2011;13:680–5.
35. Firth HV, Richards SM, Bevan AP, et al. DECIPHER: database of chromosomal imbalance and phenotype in humans using Ensembl resources. Am J Hum Genet. 2009;84:524–33.
36. Zhang J, Feuk L, Duggan GE, et al. Development of bioinformatics resources for display and analysis of copy number and other structural variants in the human genome. Cytogenet Genome Res. 2006;115:205–14.
37. Sharp AJ. Emerging themes and new challenges in defining the role of structural variation in human disease. Hum Mutat. 2009;30:135–44.
38. Girirajan S, Eichler EE. Phenotypic variability and genetic susceptibility to genomic disorders. Hum Mol Genet. 2010;19:R176–87.

Developmental Delay: Gene Testing

7

Christin D. Collins, Monica J. Basehore,
Kristen J. Champion, and Michael J. Friez

Abstract

Although the classic childhood phenotypes of many developmental disorders have been established for some time, only recently have the genetic etiologies of some of these disorders been identified. Understanding the genetic basis of these disorders allows for molecular confirmation of the clinical diagnosis in an individual which can then be utilized for risk counseling and prenatal testing. This chapter reviews the molecular basis, clinical utility, testing strategy, and interpretation of clinical molecular tests for single-gene causes of developmental delay, which include fragile X syndrome, Angelman syndrome, Rett syndrome, Noonan spectrum disorders, and X-linked intellectual disability.

Keywords

Developmental delay • Fragile X syndrome • Angelman syndrome • Prader-Willi syndrome • Uniparental disomy • Rett syndrome • X-linked intellectual disability • Noonan syndrome • Mosaicism • De novo • Permutation • Trinucleotide repeat expansion

Introduction

Although the classic childhood phenotypes of many developmental disorders have been established for some time, only recently have the genetic etiologies of some of these disorders been identified. Investigations of the molecular basis of these conditions have resulted in the identification of new genes, leading to insights into the function of new proteins and biochemical pathways. This chapter reviews the molecular basis and testing strategy of single-gene causes of developmental delay (DD) and/or intellectual disability (ID), which include fragile X syndrome, Angelman syndrome, Rett syndrome, Noonan spectrum disorders, and X-linked intellectual disability.

C.D. Collins, Ph.D., F.A.C.M.G. (✉)
Emory Genetics Laboratory, Department of Human Genetics, Emory University, 2165 North Decatur Road, Decatur, GA 30033, USA
e-mail: christin.d.collins@emory.edu

M.J. Basehore, Ph.D.
Greenwood Genetic Center, 101 Gregor Mendel Circle, Greenwood, SC 29646, USA
e-mail: mbasehore@ggc.org

K.J. Champion, Ph.D., F.A.C.M.G. • M.J. Friez, Ph.D.
Med Fusion Laboratories, 2501 South State Highway 121, Suite 1100 Lewisville, TX 75067, USA
e-mail: kchampion@medfusionsvs.com; friez@ggc.org

Fragile X Syndrome

Molecular Basis

Named for its association with a chromosomal fragile site observed in many patients (*FRAXA* chromosomal locus Xq27.3), fragile X syndrome (FXS) is the most common cause of inherited ID. FXS results from loss or severe reduction of the protein FMRP, encoded by the *FMR1* (fragile X mental retardation) gene [1]. All patients with FXS have mutations in *FMR1*, as no mutations leading to FXS have been identified in other genes. Both males and females may

D.G.B. Leonard (ed.), *Molecular Pathology in Clinical Practice*, DOI 10.1007/978-3-319-19674-9_7

be affected with FXS, but females are typically less severely affected. Thus, FXS is considered to be X-linked dominant with reduced penetrance in females [2].

The *FMR1* gene encompasses 38 kilobases (kb) of genomic DNA and has 17 exons [3]. The major *FMR1* messenger RNA produced in most tissues is approximately 4 kb, although several protein isoforms are generated by alternative splicing toward the 3′ end of the mRNA in some tissues. While FMRP can be detected in the nucleus, the majority of the protein associates with translating ribosomes in the cytoplasm, functioning as a negative translational regulator. FMRP also has a role in neuronal synapse maturation and plasticity. Autopsy samples from FXS patients have shown failure of dendritic spines to assume a normal mature size, shape, and distribution.

The molecular genetics of *FMR1* are complex given the presence of a trinucleotide repeat region in the 5′ untranslated region of exon 1. This repeat sequence is composed primarily of CGG repeats and ends 69 base pairs upstream of the translational ATG start codon. The *FMR1* repeat region is naturally polymorphic, with variation of the CGG repeats in normal (i.e., stably inherited) alleles ranging from 5 to 44 repeats, with the vast majority of individuals in the general population having 20–40 repeats. Intermediate alleles containing 45–54 repeats occasionally have minor variations of a few repeats when transmitted from parent to child, producing no clinical consequences. However, in rare instances, transmission of intermediate alleles may result in expansion of the CGG repeat to form pathological alleles. *FMR1* alleles with 55 repeats up to 200 repeats are considered to be premutations because of their potential instability. Individuals with a premutation allele do not have typical characteristics associated with FXS; however, they are at risk of repeat expansion when maternally transmitted and are associated with a later onset fragile X tremor/ataxia syndrome characterized by progressive intention tremor and cognitive decline [4]. Primary ovarian insufficiency is another phenotype that presents in approximately 20 % of females that carry an *FMR1* premutation allele [5].

Almost all mutations (>99 %) that cause FXS occur as a result of instability of the trinucleotide repeat causing dramatic expansion of the repeat segment (>200 to a few thousand CGG repeats). Rarely, deletions and point mutations in *FMR1* account for the remaining mutations found in patients with FXS. The mechanism of repeat instability in *FMR1* is believed to be DNA polymerase slippage during DNA replication. AGG repeats, spaced at about ten repeat intervals within the CGG repeat segment, may mitigate potential repeat instability through disruption of higher order molecular structures formed during DNA replication. These secondary structures contribute to polymerase slippage, and alleles that lack interrupting AGG repeats are at higher risk of expansion. Since FXS occurs strictly through maternal inheritance, individuals with full mutations (>200 CGG repeats) may inherit a similarly sized allele from their mothers or, alternatively, their mothers may have a premutation-sized allele. With repeat expansion to a full mutation, hypermethylation of the CpG dinucleotides within the *FMR1* promoter region almost always occurs, resulting in decreased or completely absent transcription and the concomitant loss of FMRP. Patients with partial methylation of a full mutation (methylation mosaics) may have some FMRP expression, resulting in a less severe phenotype. In addition, patients with a mixture of cells having either a premutation or full mutation (premutation/full mutation size mosaics) frequently are identified during molecular testing. These patients usually have ID but may perform at the lower end of normal intellect (IQ >70). Because methylation is not an all-or-none phenomenon within *FMR1*, the FXS phenotype may encompass a spectrum of possible affectations from mild to severe. Table 7.1 summarizes the classification of *FMR1* alleles.

Table 7.1 Normal and pathological *FMR1* allele types

Allele type	Repeat range	Methylation status
Normal	5–44	Not methylated
Intermediate/gray zone	45–54	Not methylated
Premutation	55–200	Not methylated
Full mutation	>200	Methylated
Methylation mosaic	>200	Variable methylation
Premutation/ full-mutation mosaic (repeat size mosaic)	Mixed premutation and full mutation	Full mutation may be methylated

Clinical Utility of Testing

Due to the presence of unrecognized *FMR1* alterations in unaffected carrier mothers, the first indication of FXS within a family is usually the diagnosis of an affected child. Unfortunately, many families do not learn the FXS diagnosis for long periods after first concerns about their child's development or behavior, and many have subsequent pregnancies before diagnosis for their first child. Such situations highlight the importance of diagnosing FXS so that children and families can receive the benefits of genetic counseling and early intervention services. Other than the infrequent deletion or point mutation, which often are spontaneous and not inherited from a parent, mothers of *all* FXS patients are either premutation or full mutation carriers. In turn, at least one of the mother's parents has an *FMR1* alteration. Consequently, *FMR1* mutations may be present in siblings of an affected individual as well as other extended family members. It is important to remember that each daughter of unaffected males with a premutation (transmitting males) is an obligate carrier of a premutation, and that their offspring are at risk for FXS. Many extended families have been documented in which an *FMR1* mutation has been transmitted through numerous generations and into family branches unknown to one another.

For DD children, *FMR1* molecular testing is diagnostic, as FXS affects development from infancy; however, the nonspecific nature of FXS during early development makes the testing approach one of ruling out FXS in most situations. The hallmark finding in almost all patients with FXS is ID, but the physical and behavioral features of males with FXS are variable prior to puberty. Physical features not readily recognizable in preschool-age boys and become more obvious with age: long face, prominent forehead, large ears, prominent jaw, and enlarged testicles (macroorchidism). Motor milestones and speech are frequently delayed, and temperament often is affected (e.g., hyperactivity, hand flapping, hand biting, temper tantrums, and occasionally autism). Females with FXS usually have milder manifestations and as a result are more difficult to diagnose clinically. FXS always should be suspected in males with mild to moderate ID and females with mild ID until shown otherwise by negative *FMR1* analysis.

Women who are full-mutation or premutation carriers have a 50 % risk of transmitting their abnormal allele in each pregnancy. While transmission of a full mutation always leads to a child with a full mutation, the risk of a premutation transmission resulting in an affected offspring with a full mutation is proportional to the maternal allele size. Empirically, the 50 % risk of a female carrier producing an affected male child is reduced to 7 % if the premutation contains 56–59 repeats, 10 % for 60–69 repeats, 29 % for 70–79 repeats, 36 % for 80–89 repeats, and 47 % for 90–99 repeats; it reaches the maximum, 50 %, when a premutation has >100 and up to 200 repeats. Because females have approximately 50 % penetrance, the risk of having an affected female child is half that of having an affected male child in any premutation repeat interval category.

Prenatal testing for *FMR1* mutations is available in some clinical molecular laboratories. Genomic DNA isolated from amniocytes obtained during amniocentesis at 16–18-week gestation or from chorionic villus sampling (CVS) at 10–12-week gestation can be used for testing. Prenatal molecular analysis proceeds in much the same fashion as that performed on DNA obtained from adult peripheral blood. However, the DNA analysis of CVS may be more complex, as chorionic villi are extraembryonic. Hypermethylation in CVS may be incomplete and not representative of the true *FMR1* methylation status in fetal tissues; therefore, a follow-up amniocentesis occasionally may be required to resolve ambiguous CVS test results.

General population screening for *FMR1* mutations has been proposed but remains controversial. In comparison to most disorders already screened for in the newborn period, FXS is more prevalent and testing is highly reliable; however, before population screening is practical for newborns and women of reproductive age, the relatively high costs and the technical complexities of testing must be resolved. Several recent studies demonstrate that higher throughput testing for population-screening purposes is becoming increasingly possible, both from a cost and a time perspective [6, 7]. Protein testing of FMRP may also be useful for screening populations with ID.

Available Assays

Routine clinical testing for *FMR1* mutations includes molecular assessment of both the trinucleotide repeat number and the *FMR1* methylation status. Traditional approaches to this testing include two concurrent analyses: (1) double-digest Southern blot analysis using a methylation-sensitive restriction enzyme such as *Eag*I, *Bss*HII, or *Nru*I along with a methylation-insensitive restriction enzyme such as *Eco*RI or *Hind*III [8]; and (2) polymerase chain reaction (PCR) assays specific for the CGG repeat segment of *FMR1* (Fig. 7.1) [9]. When used in conjunction with PCR, Southern blot analysis provides a more complete inspection of the trinucleotide repeat region by detecting multiple possible molecular events, including repeat expansion, DNA methylation, and the relatively rare *FMR1* deletions. Specialized fragile X chromosome cytogenetic analysis, using special culture techniques to induce fragile sites, is no longer used for diagnosis of FXS due to low sensitivity. While only a very few FXS patients with point mutations in *FMR1* have been identified, clinical molecular testing does not routinely investigate this gene for point mutations, deletions, insertions, or inversions downstream of the repeat segment.

In most clinical laboratories, PCR is used to size normal and smaller premutation-sized alleles with a typical sensitivity of up to approximately 120 repeats. PCR product yield is inversely proportional to the number of trinucleotide repeats such that with traditional PCR methods, little or no product can be obtained when larger repeats are present. Since the inception of diagnostic testing for FXS, different testing strategies to facilitate the transition away from Southern blots have been met with limited success. Although some PCR-based testing protocols have higher sensitivity regarding detection of larger repeats, most laboratories have been reluctant to adopt these practices due to technical difficulties. The ability to rapidly identify trinucleotide expansions in an efficient and cost-effective manner has been revisited in recent years and several very similar protocols to address this challenge have been developed [6, 10–13]. Each of these new methods relies on a triplet repeat-primed PCR reaction to separate alleles with apparent CGG expansions from those without expansions. Typically, this is based on a threshold of

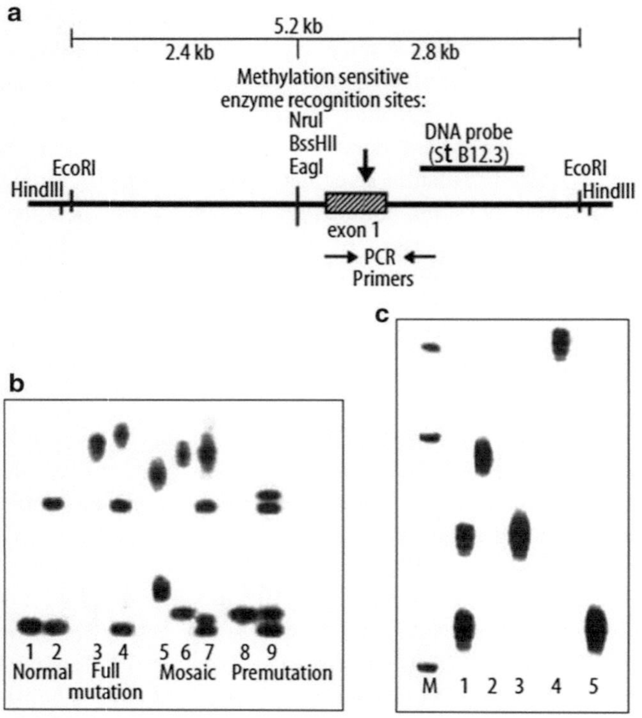

Figure 7.1 Repeat expansion and methylation in *FMR1*. (**a**) Restriction enzyme map of *FMR1*, with locations of restriction enzyme sites, DNA probe, and PCR primers used in molecular testing. *Top line* indicates DNA fragments generated using *Eco*RI and *Eag*I as depicted in the Southern blot analysis in **b** (2.8 kb and 5.2 kb fragments are detected by the DNA probe StB12.3). The *vertical arrow* indicates the location of the CGG repeat in exon 1. (**b**) Southern blot analysis of *FMR1*. Only the 2.8 kb fragment is detected in normal males (*lane 1*), while both the 2.8 kb and 5.2 kb fragments are detected in normal females (*lane 2*) due to methylation associated with normal X-inactivation that prevents cutting of the inactivated methylated allele with the methylation-sensitive restriction enzyme *Eag*I, *Bss*HII, or *Nru*I. Completely methylated full mutations are depicted in *lane 3* (affected male with full mutation) and *lane 4* (affected female with full mutation contained on one of her X chromosomes; normal allele on her other X chromosome). Smeary signals occur due to variable repeat expansion within peripheral lymphocytes used for DNA isolation. Mosaic patterns are illustrated in *lane 5* (male with partial methylation of full mutation), *lane 6* (male with premutation/full-mutation mosaicism), and *lane 7* (female with premutation/full-mutation mosaicism). *Lane 8* illustrates a transmitting male with a premutation and *lane 9* illustrates a female with a premutation. Both premutations contain approximately 75 repeats. (**c**) PCR analysis of *FMR1* repeats from five individuals separated on a 6 % polyacrylamide gel. *Lane 1* contains PCR products from a female with 20 and 30 repeats, respectively, contained within her two normal alleles. *Lanes 2, 3*, and *5* are males with normal repeat alleles (40, 30, and 20 repeats, respectively), while *lane 4* illustrates a male with a 65-repeat premutation allele. Smeary signals result from DNA polymerase stuttering during the PCR amplification.

55 trinucleotide repeats; however, the threshold can be adjusted according to the needs of the user (Fig. 7.2). Patients with expanded alleles detected by this PCR screening test then can be reflex tested by Southern blot analysis for further evaluation of expansion size and methylation status. This considerable advancement in testing allows the opportunity to significantly reduce the number of Southern blots needed, thereby significantly decreasing the turnaround time for most samples tested. Although only routinely performed in a few clinical laboratories, protein-based testing for FMRP can be utilized. Since severity of the FXS phenotype appears to inversely correlate with FMRP expression, assessment of FMRP production in patients with methylation mosaicism may be a useful prognostic indicator of disease severity [14].

Interpretation of Test Results

Because *FMR1* appears to be the only disease-causing gene for FXS, test specificity is 100 %. Using both Southern blot analysis and PCR specific for the *FMR1* locus, test sensitivity for repeat expansion can be estimated to be nearly 99 %, as only rare point mutations, small deletions/insertions remote from the repeat segment, or gene inversions would be missed. Non-repeat expansion molecular alterations may be under-ascertained in *FMR1* since gene regions downstream of the repeat segment in exon 1 are rarely investigated. When identified, the presence of cellular mosaicism, in either repeat size or methylation status, presents potential problems for the prediction of FXS severity. Essentially all patients with mutations resulting in reduction of FMRP are impaired, but expression of variable amounts of FMRP may allow some individuals to function at a higher level than expected; therefore, these individuals may occasionally have higher intelligence quotients (IQ>70). Prognostication of severity based on testing of a young child should be predicated with great caution during genetic counseling, because no long-term study exists following the development of individuals with methylation mosaicism.

Laboratory Issues

If the etiology of ID in an individual is unknown, DNA analysis for FXS should be performed as part of a comprehensive genetic evaluation that includes routine cytogenetic analysis (see Chap. 6), since cytogenetic abnormalities have been identified at least as frequently as *FMR1* mutations in individuals with ID. In addition, the use of Southern blotting on DNA isolated from amniocytes for prenatal *FMR1* analysis, with typical 2- to 3-week turnaround times, may lead to stressful situations on occasion regarding the timing of possible pregnancy termination. Utilization of CVS specimens provides additional time for possible pregnancy termination, but equivocal results sometimes occur due to incomplete methylation when a full mutation is present, requiring follow-up amniocentesis.

PCR-based kits used to estimate repeat copy number are available through some commercial vendors but not widely utilized. Many laboratories use laboratory-developed methods for both *FMR1* Southern blot analysis and PCR. Patient

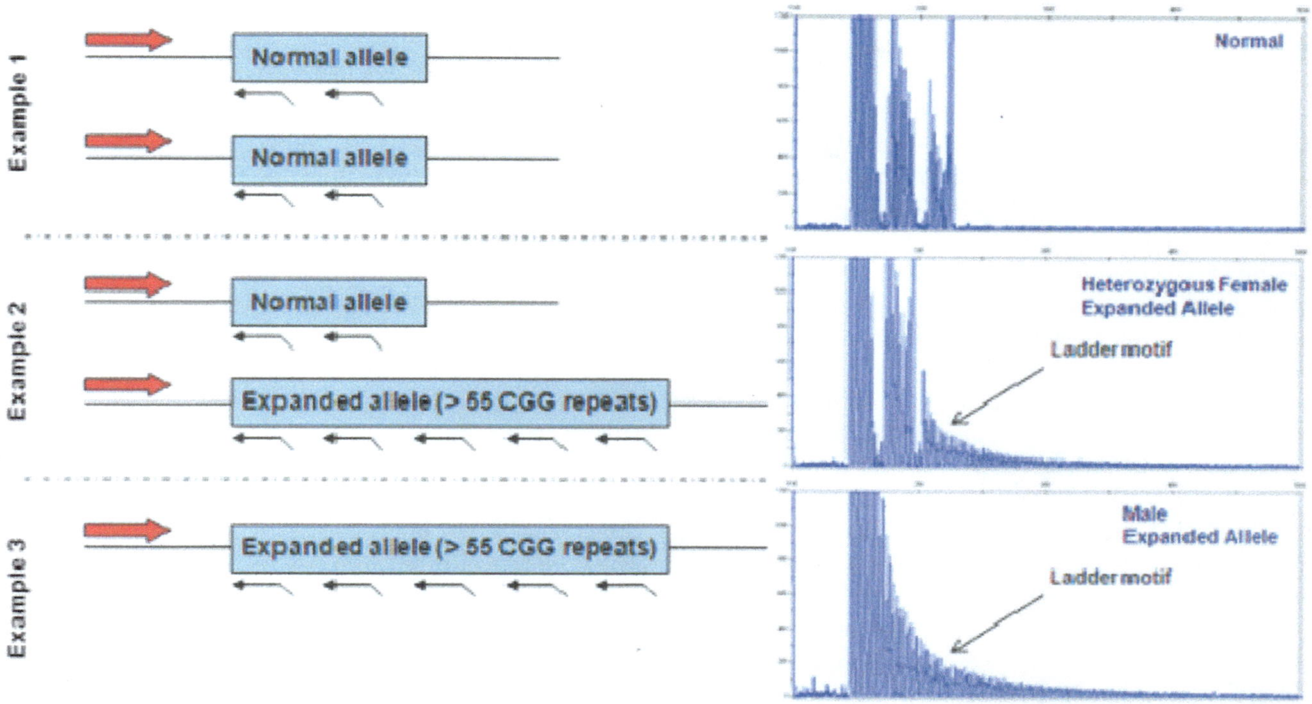

Figure 7.2 Triplet repeat-primed *FMR1* PCR screening test for fragile X alleles. The forward PCR primer is located upstream of the *FMR1* CGG region while the fluorescently-labeled reverse primer randomly binds inside the *FMR1* CGG repeat region. These PCR primers generate different sized amplicons depending on the size of the CGG repeat region present. The presence or absence of a trinucleotide "ladder" can be easily identified and a threshold of 55 CGG repeats typically is used to define expanded *FMR1* alleles. Example 1 shows the trace for a female with two normal alleles, neither of which results in the characteristic ladder motif present for expanded alleles. Example 2 illustrates the typical pattern for a female with one normal allele and one expanded allele while Example 3 illustrates the typical pattern for a male with an expansion at the *FMR1* locus. From Basehore MJ, Marlowe NM, Jones JR, Behlendorf DE, Laver TA, Friez MJ. Validation of a screening tool for the rapid and reliable detection of CGG trinucleotide repeat expansions in FMR1. Genet Test Mol Biomarkers. 2012 Jun;16(6):465–70. doi: 10.1089/gtmb.2011.0134. Epub 2012 Jan 6. Reprinted with permission from Mary Ann Liebert, Inc.

control cell lines may be purchased from the Coriell Institute (http://coriell.umdnj.edu/). Testing for FXS is routinely included in proficiency tests administered by the College of American Pathologists.

Angelman Syndrome and Prader-Willi Syndrome

Molecular Basis

Angelman syndrome (AS) is a neurodevelopmental disorder characterized by severe DD/ID, gait ataxia, microcephaly, seizures, and a happy demeanor that includes frequent laughing, smiling, and excitability [15]. AS is caused by deficient expression of the maternally inherited copy of the *UBE3A* (ubiquitin-protein ligase E3A) gene which can result from one of several different genetic abnormalities involving the proximal part of the long arm of chromosome 15 (15q11–q13). This two megabase (Mb) region of chromosome 15 contains multiple imprinted genes, meaning that their expression is dependent on the parent of origin. Within this region of chromosome 15, the *MKRN3*, *MAGEL2*, *NECDIN*, and *SNURF–SNRPN* genes, as well as a cluster of C/D box small nucleolar RNAs (snoRNAs) are paternally expressed, while the *UBE3A* and *ATP10C* genes are maternally expressed. Imprinting of genes in this domain is coordinately controlled by a bipartite imprinting center (IC) which overlaps the *SNRPN* promoter and extends approximately 35 kb upstream. Flanking this imprinted region are several low-copy repeats that predispose the region to chromosomal rearrangement by unequal crossing over.

Imprinted *UBE3A* expression is tissue specific, displaying predominantly maternal expression in the human fetal brain and adult frontal cortex but biparental expression in other tissues. *UBE3A* encodes a protein that is involved in the ubiquitination pathway which targets certain proteins for degradation [16]. Four known genetic mechanisms cause loss of *UBE3A* expression, and explain 85–90 % of AS cases [17]. A 4 Mb deletion of the maternal chromosome 15q11–q13 region occurs sporadically in 65–70 % of cases and is due to unequal crossing over. Paternal uniparental disomy

(UPD) of chromosome 15 is detected in about 7 % of cases and is likely to be postzygotic in origin. Approximately 3 % of AS cases involve an imprinting defect caused by microdeletions of the IC and result in lack of expression of the maternally inherited *UBE3A* gene in the brain. Point mutations within *UBE3A* (mostly truncating mutations) are found in approximately 11 % of cases [17]. Currently, approximately 10 % of patients with a clinical diagnosis of AS have no identifiable chromosomal or molecular abnormality, most likely due to an undetected abnormality affecting the *UBE3A* gene or a mutation in another gene within the ubiquitination pathway.

While the AS phenotype results from loss of expression of maternally expressed *UBE3A*, another developmental disorder, Prader-Willi syndrome (PWS), is due to loss of expression of *paternally* expressed genes within this 15q11–q13 region. PWS is characterized by infantile hypotonia, hypogonadism, dysmorphic appearance, small hands and feet, hyperphagia and obesity, DD, and ID. Approximately 70 % of PWS cases involve a 4 Mb deletion of the paternal chromosome 15q11–13, while 20 % of PWS cases are due to maternal UPD of chromosome 15. Another 1–5 % of cases are thought to be due to an imprinting defect. Recent evidence suggests that loss of expression of one or more of the C/D box snoRNAs, including SNORD116, encoded within the *SNRPN* locus may cause the PWS phenotype [18, 19]. The following section reviews the available diagnostic testing for AS, as well as PWS, since the primary testing method used to diagnose AS also will diagnose PWS.

Clinical Utility of Testing

Infants with AS commonly present with non-specific findings such as DD and/or seizures. These findings may result in a broad differential diagnosis, which can include inborn errors of metabolism, mitochondrial encephalopathy, cerebral palsy, and other neurodevelopmental syndromes including Rett syndrome, Christianson syndrome, and Pitt-Hopkins syndrome, which will be reviewed later in this chapter. Analysis of parent-specific DNA methylation imprints in the 15q11–q13 chromosome region is typically the first test that is ordered as it will detect approximately 80 % of individuals with AS, including those with a deletion, paternal UPD, or an IC defect. This analysis also is used to diagnose PWS and will detect nearly 100 % of those cases. Methylation analysis for AS/PWS typically investigates the methylation status of CpG dinucleotide sites within the promoter region of the *SNRPN* gene. Once the diagnosis of AS (or PWS) is established through an abnormal DNA methylation pattern, the specific genetic mechanism involved can be investigated for the purposes of genetic counseling. Fluorescent in situ hybridization (FISH) or array-based comparative genomic hybridization (aCGH) analysis can be used to detect a deletion, while DNA microsatellite analysis can be performed to investigate the presence of UPD. For patients with an AS phenotype but normal DNA methylation, sequence analysis of the *UBE3A* gene can be used for further evaluation of the diagnosis. Collectively, molecular testing for AS through DNA methylation studies and sequencing of *UBE3A* will identify an alteration in approximately 90 % of individuals with clinical AS/PWS.

The recurrence risk for AS in a family and the type of prenatal testing that is available will vary according to the chromosome or molecular defect that is ultimately detected in the proband. For this reason, prenatal diagnosis should be undertaken only after the specific genetic mechanism in the proband has been determined and the parents have received genetic counseling. In cases where de novo deletions or UPD have been demonstrated, recurrence risk will be low, although prenatal testing may be offered for reassurance purposes. For cases of IC and *UBE3A* mutations, recurrence risk can be as high as 50 %. Since germline mosaicism has been reported in mothers of AS patients with *UBE3A* mutations, prenatal testing should be offered even if a mutation is not identified in the mother. Because methylation status within the promoter region of the *SNRPN* gene is established in early embryonic development, DNA methylation analysis on cells obtained from CVS is theoretically possible; however, most clinical molecular laboratories currently performing prenatal methylation testing prefer to use amniocytes for testing due to the relative hypomethylation of cells derived from the placenta [15]. Prenatal testing is appropriate for families without a previous child with AS if a deletion of chromosome 15q11–q13 is suspected on chromosome analysis of CVS or amniotic fluid, or if trisomy 15 is noted on CVS but a normal karyotype is found on amniotic fluid, which would suggest that a trisomy rescue event may have occurred (possibly resulting in UPD). Prenatal testing also would be indicated if either a de novo chromosome 15 translocation or a supernumerary marker chromosome is found by karyotype analysis.

Parents of patients with deletions, specifically the mothers of AS patients, should be tested by chromosome and FISH analysis to determine if they carry balanced chromosome rearrangements or deletions which are not expressed as an abnormal phenotype in that parent. Chromosome analysis is appropriate for parents of patients with UPD combined with a Robertsonian translocation to determine whether the translocation is inherited or de novo. Parents also should be tested for mutations that are identified in the proband, such as IC deletions or *UBE3A* mutations. If a parent of an AS patient is found to be a carrier of a mutation or a chromosomal translocation, then the siblings of that parent should be offered testing.

Available Assays

DNA Methylation Analysis

Standard molecular techniques for the methylation analysis of CpG sites within the *SNRPN* gene promoter region include (1) double-digest Southern blot analysis using a methylation-sensitive enzyme such as *Not*I along with a methylation-insensitive enzyme such as *Xba*I [20]; (2) PCR amplification of the *SNRPN* promoter region following either *Not*I or mcrBC digestion; and (3) methylation-specific PCR (MS-PCR) which is based on modifying DNA with bisulfite, which converts unmethylated cytosine (C) to uracil (U), followed by amplification using primers specific for the unmethylated and methylated alleles [21].

Methylation-specific multiplex ligation-dependent probe amplification (MS-MLPA) provides a method to simultaneously semiquantitatively analyze copy number changes and DNA methylation status at numerous sites across the 15q11–q13 region. Oligonucleotide probes specific to the *SNRPN* gene are utilized, of which a subset contain a *Hha*I restriction site. After hybridization and ligation, the methylation-sensitive restriction enzyme *Hha*I is used to digest the unmethylated DNA. PCR amplification using a universal primer is performed, followed by separation of the amplification products by capillary electrophoresis. If the site is not methylated, the *Hha*I digestion will prevent amplification of the MS-MLPA probe. If the CpG sites are methylated, the *Hha*I enzyme is unable to digest the DNA, and PCR products are generated and detected. Individuals with AS will have two unmethylated (maternal) alleles and accordingly no MS-MLPA signal will be present. Individuals with no methylation abnormality will show a 50 % reduction in the MS-MLPA signal due to the presence of both a methylated and an unmethylated allele. Individuals with PWS will have two methylated (paternal) alleles and will show a 50 % increase in the MS-MLPA signal compared to normal controls.

Pyrosequencing is a quantitative method available to assess the CpG methylation status of the *SNRPN* gene [22]. As in MS-PCR, the genomic DNA is treated with bisulfite to convert unmethylated C to U, whereas methylated cytosine (^{m}C) will remain unchanged. During PCR amplification of the bisulfite-treated DNA, the U will be amplified as thymine (T) and the ^{m}C will be amplified as C. Pyrosequencing, which is a "sequencing-by-synthesis" method based on the luminometric detection of a pyrophosphate release that occurs upon the incorporation of nucleotides into the sequence, is then utilized to discriminate C and ^{m}C by the presence of a T or C at each CpG site analyzed, respectively. This information is used to determine the percent methylation at each CpG site, which will be approximately 50 % for normal individuals who have both a methylated (paternal) and unmethylated (maternal) allele. Individuals with AS will have 0 % methylation at each site, and individuals with PWS will have 100 % methylation at each site.

Uniparental Disomy Analysis

For individuals who exhibit methylation abnormalities but are negative for a deletion by FISH or aCGH, DNA microsatellite analysis to test for whole or segmental UPD of chromosome 15 is available for further evaluation of the diagnosis. UPD analysis requires DNA from the proband as well as both parents. Polymorphic repetitive regions (microsatellites) along chromosome 15 are analyzed to determine if the proband's genetic constitution reflects contribution from both parents at all loci tested (biparental) or from only one parent (UPD). Paternal UPD of chromosome 15 is consistent with AS while maternal UPD of chromosome 15 is consistent with PWS. Alternatively, SNP-based arrays can be used to detect segmental and whole chromosome UPD, but may not identify all cases of UPD, because the segment of UPD may be too small to be detected by SNPs designed to evaluate UPD of larger chromosomal regions. Abnormal methylation studies and biparental inheritance of chromosome 15 is suggestive of an imprinting center defect.

Targeted *UBE3A* Analysis

When DNA methylation testing is normal, *UBE3A* sequence analysis should be considered. The majority of mutations identified in the *UBE3A* gene are protein truncating mutations [23, 24]. These mutations must be present on the maternal allele in order to be pathogenic since *UBE3A* expression occurs only from the maternal allele. In some cases, small intragenic deletions of *UBE3A* have been detected, so gene-specific deletion and duplication testing should be considered for individuals who test negative for *UBE3A* gene sequencing [25, 26].

Interpretation of Test Results

If the methylation pattern or methylation-specific amplification is characteristic of only paternal inheritance in the individual tested, then a diagnosis of AS is confirmed (Fig. 7.3, lane 8). Conversely, a methylation pattern characteristic of only maternal inheritance is diagnostic for PWS (Fig. 7.3, lane 7). Methylation assays detect virtually all cases of PWS and AS that are caused by large deletions, UPD, and IC defects; however, they will not detect rare small deletions that do not involve the *SNRPN* locus or sequence alterations within the *UBE3A* gene. Therefore, methylation analysis will detect approximately 80 % of AS cases. Sequencing of the *UBE3A* gene will detect another 11 % of cases. Approximately 10 % of AS cases will not be detected with the currently available tests.

Laboratory Issues

If the etiology of DD in a patient is unknown, DNA analysis should be performed as part of a comprehensive genetic evaluation that includes assessment of single gene disorders

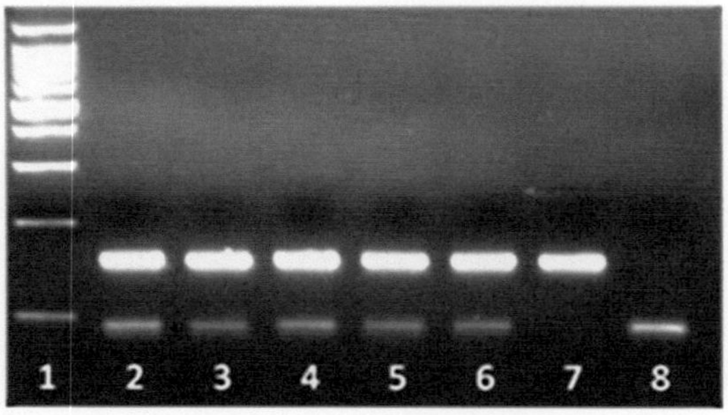

Figure 7.3 Methylation-sensitive PCR (MS-PCR) analysis of *SNRPN* DNA of patient samples referred to a clinical molecular laboratory. PCR products are amplified from the methylated and unmethylated alleles of the *SNRPN* locus. Normal individuals exhibit a biparental inheritance pattern (both upper methylated and lower unmethylated allele PCR products present; *lanes 2–6*), whereas patients with PWS show a pattern of only maternal inheritance (only upper methylated allele PCR product present; *lane 7*) and patients with AS show a pattern of only paternal inheritance (only lower unmethylated allele PCR product present; *lane 8*). Molecular weight ladder present in *lane 1*.

by molecular and cytogenetic approaches. Although every laboratory does not need to provide all testing methods, a smooth progression through the various tests may be necessary to determine the genetic mechanism causing AS. Testing is facilitated by a clinical molecular laboratory that is able to offer DNA methylation, FISH, UPD analysis and sequencing of the *UBE3A* gene, as well as gene-specific deletion/duplication testing. Mutation analysis of the IC is available only on a research basis.

The *SNRPN* probe for Southern blot analysis is available from American Type Culture Collection (http://www.atcc.org). Caution should be exercised when interpreting MS-PCR results, as allele dropout has been reported [27]. Because of the risk of allele dropout, multiple MS-PCR primer sets should be considered to minimize the possibility of a false-positive result. An MS-MLPA kit is available from MRC-Holland (http://www.mrc-holland.com). A pyrosequencing kit to evaluate methylation status of the AS/PWS critical region is available from Qiagen (http://www.qiagen.com). There are many microsatellite markers available for testing of the 15q11–q13 region, but caution should be exercised because some previously used markers are now considered problematic, such as *DS15S113* and *D15S817* [28, 29].

Rett Syndrome and Other *MECP2*-Related Disorders

Molecular Basis

Rett syndrome is an X-linked neurodevelopmental disorder that almost exclusively affects females. In the classic form of the disease, affected girls appear to develop normally until the age of 6–18 months followed by a characteristic pattern of regression, which includes deceleration of head growth leading to acquired microcephaly, autistic features, loss of speech and purposeful hand use, irregular breathing patterns, stereotypical hand wringing, and seizures [30]. There are well-documented criteria for the clinical diagnosis of Rett syndrome which include the clinical features that are considered as either necessary or supportive for the diagnosis [31]. The frequency of classic Rett syndrome is approximately 1 in 10,000 females [32]. In 1999, mutations in the methyl-CpG-binding protein 2 (*MECP2*) gene located at Xq28 were reported to be the underlying cause for Rett syndrome [33]. Since that time, a broader range of clinical phenotypes have also been associated with mutations in *MECP2* [34]. This section focuses on *MECP2* variants causing Rett and atypical-Rett syndromes which are X-linked dominant conditions. The other *MECP2*-related phenotypes primarily affect males and are considered to be X-linked recessive disorders.

Since being associated with *MECP2*, the field of Rett syndrome research has focused attention on determining the function of the MECP2 protein to better understand the underlying pathophysiology of the condition. The current perspective of MECP2 function is complex and is based on its apparent involvement as both a transcriptional repressor and activator [35]. MECP2 binds preferentially to methylated DNA via its methyl-CpG-binding domain, and silences transcription by recruiting corepressor complexes through its transcriptional repression domain. More recent studies have demonstrated that loss of MECP2 leads to reduced expression of numerous genes, implying a role in upregulating gene expression, although the mechanisms involved are not well understood [36]. This is an area of great interest given that Rett syndrome is not associated with any sort of gross anatomic abnormalities of the brain. MECP2 clearly affects transcriptional regulation more dramatically in certain regions of the brain than other regions. The physiologic significance of these differences needs to be understood in order for individuals affected by Rett syndrome to benefit from promising new therapeutic options in the future.

Clinical Utility of Testing

Independent studies have confirmed *MECP2* as the major causative gene for Rett syndrome by the identification of pathogenic mutations in approximately 95 % of classic cases. Approximately 85 % of classic Rett patients have either point mutations or small insertions/deletions within the *MECP2* coding region, while larger deletions have been identified in approximately 10 % of classic cases [37]. Nearly 50 % of Rett patients have one of eight recurrent point mutations, while most of the remainder has one of the many other described pathogenic alterations. It should be noted that greater than 99 % of mutations in individuals with classic Rett syndrome are de novo, with the large majority occurring on the paternally inherited allele [38]. Mutations also have been found in atypical mild variant cases and in severe early-onset cases of Rett syndrome. In addition, *MECP2* mutations have been documented in patients with an Angelman-like presentation and in individuals with autistic phenotypes. Affected males with variable phenotypes ranging from lethal neonatal encephalopathy to uncharacterized ID have been shown to be caused by *MECP2* mutations. The presentation of Rett syndrome also has been documented in males with Klinefelter (47, XXY) syndrome, as well as those with mosaic *MECP2* mutations [39]. Definitive genotype-phenotype correlations have not been consistent, although several findings related to specific mutations appear to be reproducible [40]. Some studies have investigated multiple individuals with the same mutation but variable degrees of clinical severity, demonstrating that additional factors beyond the specific *MECP2* alteration play significant roles in the presentation of Rett syndrome [41]. In males, larger duplications of Xq28 that include *MECP2* have a consistent set of clinical features that include hypotonia, severe ID, absence of speech, seizures, and recurrent respiratory infections that often lead to death at an early age [42]. Given the spectrum of neurodevelopmental phenotypes associated with *MECP2* mutations, the clinical utility of molecular testing is significant.

Available Assays

The *MECP2* gene is composed of four exons, which give rise to two distinct MECP2 isoforms [43]. Diagnostic testing for Rett syndrome should begin with DNA sequence analysis of the entire *MECP2* coding region given the profile of known mutations. In the past, mutation scanning using denaturing high performance liquid chromatography (DHPLC) was used, but very few laboratories still utilize this method given the relative ease of sequencing *MECP2*. Sanger sequencing with capillary electrophoresis continues to be considered the gold standard for point mutation detection. Approximately 85 % of classic Rett syndrome patients have mutations that are detectable by sequencing of *MECP2*, which is performed by numerous clinical molecular laboratories (http://www.genetests.org/).

To increase the overall mutation detection for the *MECP2* gene, additional testing is available for larger *MECP2* dosage alterations, present in approximately 10 % of classic Rett patients. Deletions and duplications involving all or part of the gene have been identified by dosage-sensitive testing methods such as multiplex ligation-dependent probe amplification (MLPA), quantitative real-time PCR analysis, and targeted aCGH.

Interpretation of Test Results

Rett syndrome is commonly considered in females with DD, making the volume of *MECP2* testing performed worldwide significant. Molecular confirmation of Rett syndrome is straightforward when one of the eight common *MECP2* mutations is present. Interpreting other less common alterations can be assisted by use of available mutation databases. RettBASE, the database dedicated to *MECP2* (http://mecp2.chw.edu.au/), and the Human Gene Mutation Database (HGMD) are currently the most comprehensive resources. Some of the changes reported in the databases are not clinically correlated, leaving their pathogenicity uncertain. When other novel variants are identified, evaluation of additional family members to determine the segregation pattern may allow the clinical significance of an alteration to be interpreted with greater certainty. For females with variants of unknown clinical significance, the most common strategy is to test both parents. Alterations that are shown to be de novo are normally accepted as pathogenic mutations. In some rare cases, two de novo alterations are present with uncertainty which change is pathogenic, or whether their collective impact on protein function is causative of the symptoms. A variant of unknown significance inherited from the father is interpreted as not being clinically significant given the expectation that the variant would have an even greater phenotypic consequence in a male with a single X chromosome. When variants are inherited from the mother, the interpretation becomes more challenging and typically requires additional testing which often includes both X-inactivation testing of the mother and variant analysis of additional family members. If the proband and her mother carry the same alteration and both have normal/random X-inactivation patterns, the variant typically is interpreted as a benign variant with no clinical significance. Testing of extended family members has the potential to identify the change in a phenotypically normal male which also confirms that the change is not clinically relevant. When testing males, the interpretation issues change to some degree and the strategy for these will be discussed later in the X-linked intellectual disability section of this chapter.

Laboratory Issues

One of the issues encountered in sequence-based clinical testing is the interpretation of novel sequence variations, particularly alleles of uncertain pathogenic significance. A valuable resource for laboratories and referring clinicians is provided by the American College of Medical Genetics, which has issued updated recommended standards and guidelines for interpretation of sequence variations [44]; the recommendations are available at http://www.acmg.net. Another current issue pertaining to molecular testing for Rett syndrome is the value of two-tier testing (sequencing followed by dosage analysis) to provide comprehensive mutation analysis of *MECP2*. Identification of the mutation in the proband facilitates prenatal testing in subsequent pregnancies, although the majority of *MECP2* point mutations are de novo and of paternal origin, with extremely low rates of recurrence. Prenatal testing should be offered to females who are known to carry a point mutation or large rearrangement in *MECP2*. In cases where the mother is not a carrier, prenatal testing may be sought for parental reassurance due to rare reports of germline mosaicism [45]. The current focus on point mutation analysis within the coding region by sequence analysis does not rule out potential mutations in regulatory elements or other important noncoding regions of *MECP2*. Equally important to consider are the other conditions that phenotypically overlap with Rett syndrome and should be given further consideration when clinical testing for *MECP2* is negative. Several of these syndromes and their respective gene associations are discussed in the following section.

Angelman/Rett Syndrome Second-Tier Testing

Molecular Basis

AS and Rett syndromes are clinically similar conditions that often present with numerous overlapping phenotypic features. Clinicians with significant clinical experience typically can distinguish the two conditions, but in many cases clinical diagnosis can be challenging. As discussed earlier, AS and Rett syndromes are caused by disruption or loss of normal gene function of the *UBE3A* and *MECP2* genes, respectively. Testing for these conditions is common given their prevalence and the number of individuals with DD suggestive of one or both of these diagnoses. Accordingly, many patients have clinical presentations that mimic AS and Rett syndrome and have normal clinical test results for both disorders. In these instances, additional testing of genes causing diseases with overlapping phenotypes may provide the molecular diagnosis needed. Some of the most common conditions that should be considered in the differential diagnosis for AS and Rett syndrome for which diagnostic testing is available are discussed in this section. The syndromes detailed in this section are not meant to be an all-inclusive list, but rather as a starting point for second tier testing for patients with features in this clinical spectrum of ID/DD.

Clinical Utility of Testing

The molecular confirmation of a clinical diagnosis allows the physician to provide recurrence risks and genetic counseling, as well as prenatal diagnosis, to the proband and additional family members. Once the presence of a causative mutation has been established in an individual, targeted analysis of fetal samples is available for prenatal testing, as well as for other family members.

Molecular Genetic Testing

CDKL5 Gene

Mutations in the *CDKL5* (cyclin-dependent kinase-like 5) gene have been identified in individuals with early-onset infantile spasms and clinical features that overlap other neurodevelopmental disorders, such as AS and Rett syndromes [46]. Subsequently, mutations in *CDKL5* (also known as Serine Threonine Kinase 9 or *STK9*) have been associated with an atypical variant of Rett syndrome, which includes ID and other severe neurological symptoms including severe early-onset seizures, regression of communication and skills, and global developmental delay. Rett-like stereotypies such as hand-wringing have been identified in individuals with *CDKL5* mutations, further indicating a shared clinical differential.

Mutations identified in *CDKL5* show haploinsufficiency, including missense and splicing mutations, small deletions and insertions, as well as nonsense mutations. De novo mutations and evidence of germline mosaicism have been reported, suggesting that the presence of an affected proband in a family is sufficient to consider prenatal diagnosis. Large deletions have also been detected, thus deletion and duplication testing should be considered if an individual tests negative for sequence mutations.

FOXG1 Gene

Point mutations and deletions in the *FOXG1* (forkhead box G1) gene are associated with a developmental disorder known as the congenital variant of Rett syndrome. This disorder exhibits features of classic Rett syndrome, but with an earlier onset within the first months of life. Reports of individuals with mutations in the *FOXG1* gene show a clinical profile consisting of postnatal microcephaly, apraxia, absent language, stereotypical hand and mouth movements, seizures, poor sleep, and hypoplasia of the corpus callosum with decreased white matter volume [47–49]. Unlike Rett syndrome, individuals with a *FOXG1* mutation do not have periods of normal development; thus regression is not usually a feature.

In addition to sequence mutations, deletions and duplications have been reported in the *FOXG1* gene. Deletions have been identified in a cohort of patients with severe mental retardation, microcephaly, absent language, and/or brain anomalies [50]. Duplications have been associated with epilepsy, mental retardation, and speech impairment [51]. For patients suspected to have the congenital variant of Rett syndrome, sequence analysis is recommended as the first step in mutation identification. For patients in whom mutations are not identified by gene sequencing, deletion/duplication testing is appropriate.

SLC9A6 Gene

Mutations in the *SLC9A6* (solute carrier family 9, member 6) gene are found in Christianson syndrome, an X-linked condition associated with ID, microcephaly, seizures, ataxia, and absent speech [52]. Individuals with *SLC9A6* mutations may exhibit an apparently happy disposition, with laughter and excessive smiling, that is reminiscent of AS [53]. Additional reports suggest that individuals have deceleration of head growth in the first year of life, epilepsy, and a thin body habitus [52]. The clinical spectrum caused by mutations in SLC9A6 resembles AS in younger individuals and should be considered as part of the differential. The clinical spectrum of carrier females can range from ID to absence of symptoms [52, 54].

TCF4 Gene

Mutations in the *TCF4* (transcription factor 4) gene are found in Pitt-Hopkins syndrome. Haploinsufficiency mutations are causative of disease, which also include deletions of the *TCF4* gene [55]. In cases where parental samples were available, de novo occurrence of the mutation was established [56, 57]. Pitt-Hopkins syndrome is characterized by ID, intermittent hyperventilation and apnea, and a characteristic facial gestalt that includes a wide mouth [58]. Additional clinical features seen in individuals with Pitt-Hopkins may include clubbing of the fingers and toes, thick lips, prominent nose, and epilepsy.

Available Assays

Sequence-based tests are considered the gold standard for point mutation detection, with deletion/duplication testing increasing the yield of identifiable mutations. Standard sequencing protocols and custom primer designs are utilized for gene-specific analysis. Targeted aCGH and MLPA assays can be designed for interrogation of deletions and duplications. With the implementation of next-generation sequencing (NGS) in the clinical molecular laboratory setting, testing for multiple genes causative of disorders with similar phenotypes is increasingly available. Testing for single gene disorders that share a clinical presentation feature, such as DD, may be offered as a single test panel inclusive of the many genes associated or with a DD or ID phenotype. Additional comments regarding NGS and targeted gene panels can be found in the XLID section later in this chapter and in Chap. 59.

Interpretation of Test Results

The identification of sequence alterations is standard in many clinical laboratories. The interpretation of the clinical significance of identified variants is dependent upon the identification of the change in individuals with disease, familial segregation of the variant with the disease phenotype, clinical suspicion, conservation, protein prediction, presence in the general population, and functional evidence that the change is disease causing.

Laboratory Issues

Large deletions and duplications, mutations in the promoter region, mutations in some regulatory regions, as well as deep intronic mutations will likely not be detected by traditional Sanger sequencing methods. Deletion/duplication testing for the gene of interest may be appropriate to identify larger dosage alterations not detected by traditional sequencing methods.

Noonan Syndrome and Related Disorders

Molecular Basis

Noonan syndrome (NS) is a clinically and genetically heterogeneous congenital disorder with an estimated prevalence of 1 in 1,000–2,500 live births [59]. First described by the pediatric cardiologist, Jacqueline Noonan in 1968 [60], NS is characterized by distinctive facial features, short stature, congenital heart defects, variable cognitive deficits, and an increased risk of specific cancers [60, 61]. Until recently, the diagnosis of NS was based solely on clinical findings; however, genetic mutations now are identifiable in approximately 60–80 % of patients with a clinical diagnosis of NS.

NS is a Mendelian trait transmitted in an autosomal dominant manner with a significant but unclear percentage of cases due to de novo mutations. In 1994, linkage analysis of a large NS family was used to definitively establish the first NS locus in the chromosome 12q22-qter interval which led to the subsequent identification of the first causative gene, protein tyrosine phosphatase nonreceptor type 11 (*PTPN11*) [62–64]. There are currently nine genes (*PTPN11*, *SOS1*, *RAF1*, *KRAS*, *BRAF*, *SHOC2*, *NRAS*, *MAP2K1*, and *CBL*) that have been causally related to NS and more are likely to be discovered (Table 7.2) [64–74]. Interestingly, all of these genes encode components of the same molecular pathway, the RAS-mitogen activated protein kinase (RAS-MAPK) signal transduction pathway, which mediates many diverse cellular functions including proliferation, migration, survival, cell fate determination, differentiation, and senescence. In addition to NS, there are several other clinically related disorders also linked to germline mutations within the RAS-MAPK pathway (Table 7.2) [70, 75–81]. These disorders include LEOPARD syndrome, Costello syndrome, cardiofaciocutaneous (CFC) syndrome, neurofibromatosis

Table 7.2 Genetic syndromes of the RAS-MAPK pathway

Syndrome	Gene	Chromosome location	Protein
Noonan	*PTPN11*	12q24.1	SHP2
	SOS1	2p22.1	SOS1
	RAF1	3p25.1	CRAF
	KRAS	12p12.1	KRAS
	BRAF	7q34	BRAF
	SHOC2	10q25	SHOC2
	NRAS	1p15.2	NRAS
	MAP2K1	15q22.31	MEK1
	CBL	11q23.3	CBL
LEOPARD	*PTPN11*	12q24.1	SHP2
	RAF1	3p25.1	CRAF
	BRAF	7q34	BRAF
Costello	*HRAS*	11p15.5	HRAS
Cardiofaciocutaneous	*BRAF*	7q34	BRAF
	MAP2K1	15q22.31	MEK1
	MAP2K2	19p13.3	MEK2
	KRAS	12p12.1	KRAS
Neurofibromatosis 1	*NF1*	17q11.2	Neuro-fibromin
Legius	*SPRED1*	15q14	SPRED1

type 1 and Legius syndrome. Collectively, this group of developmental disorders has come to be referred to as the RASopathies or alternatively, the neurocardiofacialcutaneous syndrome (NCFCS) family.

The RAS-MAPK pathway is activated in response to cytokine, hormone, and growth factor stimulation, and is a major mediator of early and late developmental processes, including morphology determination, organogenesis, synaptic plasticity, and growth. Dysregulation of the RAS-MAPK pathway, specifically enhanced activation, has been well established as one of the primary causes of many types of cancer. RAS-MAPK pathway genes are found to be somatically mutated in approximately 20 % of all malignancies [82]. Only relatively recently has this pathway also come to be known for its role in developmental disorders such as NS. Similar to the somatic mutations that are involved in cancer, germline mutations responsible for NS and related disorders are almost exclusively gain-of-function missense mutations.

Functionally, these mutations have been demonstrated to result in increased signal transduction through the RAS-MAPK pathway leading to the clinical manifestations of NS and other disorders, although the exact cellular mechanism remains unclear. Given the role of the RAS-MAPK pathway in oncogenesis, it is not surprising that, the NCFCS family of disorders share an increased risk of malignancy, with the exception of CFC syndrome. In general, the germline mutations that cause these developmental disorders are distinct from the somatic mutations observed in cancer, and it has been hypothesized that the mutations capable of surviving in the germline may be less strongly activating than those involved in cancer [83].

Clinical Utility of Testing

Due to variability in the phenotypic manifestations of NS, as well as significant clinical overlap with other disorders, establishing a diagnosis of NS by clinical examination alone can be difficult. Therefore, diagnostic testing is increasingly being used to confirm or establish a diagnosis of NS, especially in patients presenting without a prior family history. The disorders that have considerable clinical overlap with NS include not only other conditions within the NCFCS family, but also Turner syndrome, Aarskog syndrome, fetal alcohol syndrome, mosaic trisomy 22, and Baraitser-Winter syndrome, among others. A molecular diagnosis of NS is established through the detection of a pathogenic mutation in one of the nine known NS genes. Identifying the disease-causing mutation not only provides the patient with a definitive diagnosis of NS, but also allows the clinician to provide the family with an accurate recurrence risk. If the mutation was inherited from an affected parent, then the couple has a 50 % chance of having another child affected with NS. However, if the mutation is determined to be de novo in the proband, then the recurrence risk for the couple would be <1 %, allowing for the rare possibility of germline mosaicism. Furthermore, identification of the causative mutation allows the couple the option of having prenatal or preimplantation genetic diagnosis (PGD) for subsequent pregnancies. Prenatal testing for NS may be warranted even without prior identification of a disease-causing mutation in the family, based on abnormal ultrasound findings. Though not specific for NS, prenatal features associated with NS that may be detected on ultrasound examination include polyhydramnios, cardiac defects, cystic hygroma, and increased nuchal translucency. Of fetuses with normal chromosomes, 1–3 % of cases with nuchal edema detected in the first trimester and 10 % of second-trimester fetuses with a cystic hygroma will be diagnosed with NS [84, 85]. Lastly, establishing a definitive diagnosis of NS through molecular testing is important to provide the patient and their family with accurate information regarding prognosis, cancer risk, and potential therapeutic options, because this information varies considerably depending on the specific disorder.

Available Assays

When NS is clinically suspected, a karyotype and/or aCGH should be performed to rule out Turner syndrome, mosaic trisomy 22, or other chromosomal alterations. Provided the patient has a normal karyotype, molecular analysis of the nine genes known to cause NS should be performed. The order in which these genes are tested and the molecular technology used to detect mutations within these genes may vary. As gain-of-function missense mutations are the primary type of mutation associated with NS, Sanger sequencing of the entire coding region of each gene is typically considered the standard testing approach. Genotype/phenotype correlations have been reported in NS and may be used to determine the specific order in which the NS genes should be tested. For patients with a classic NS presentation, a sequential approach typically is taken, starting with sequencing of the *PTPN11* gene followed by sequencing of the remaining eight genes in the following order: *SOS1*, *RAF1*, *KRAS*, *SHOC2* (targeted analysis for the recurrent p.S2G mutation), *BRAF*, *MAP2K1*, *NRAS*, and *CBL*. This approach will identify a disease-causing mutation in approximately 60–80 % of individuals with a clinical diagnosis of NS. Mutations in the *PTPN11* gene are detected in approximately 50 % of individuals with NS and are more common in familial cases. *PTPN11* mutations are more common in patients with a classic facial presentation and pulmonary valve stenosis or atrial septal defect, and are less common in patients with hypertrophic cardiomyopathy (HCM) [86]. Importantly, patients with *PTPN11* mutations are at an increased risk for bleeding diathesis and juvenile myelomonocytic leukemia. Individuals with *SOS1* mutations (10–13 % of individuals with a clinical diagnosis of NS) are more likely to have ectodermal features including keratosis pilaris, sparse hair, curly hair, or sparse eyebrows, and are less likely to have short stature or cognitive deficits [66]. The majority of individuals with *RAF1* mutations have HCM, and the *SHOC2* p.S2G recurrent mutation has been associated with a distinctive hair phenotype called loose anagen hair in which the hair is extremely fine in texture, grows very slowly and can be easily plucked from the scalp [67, 68, 71].

As an alternative to sequential testing, simultaneous testing of all nine NS genes can be performed using Sanger sequencing, microarray-based sequencing, or NGS. A simultaneous approach may allow for faster test results and may or may not offer a potential cost reduction compared to sequential testing. Currently, the clinical utility of copy number analysis of the NS genes is unclear, since deletion/duplication of these genes is not a commonly observed disease mechanism; although gene duplications involving the *PTPN11* gene have been reported in individuals with clinical NS [87, 88].

Laboratory Issues

As with other sequence-based molecular testing, the major potential laboratory issue associated with molecular testing for NS is the detection of variants of unknown or uncertain clinical significance. When a sequence variant is unable to be classified as benign or pathogenic, testing of the proband's parents and/or other family members can be used to further assess the pathogenicity of the variant. Because disease-causing mutations associated with NS are almost invariably missense mutations, intronic sequence variants or variants of other mutation classes generally are considered less likely to be pathogenic. Additionally, the results of laboratory testing should be interpreted in the context of the patient's clinical features to ensure that the appropriate clinical diagnosis is ultimately made because other conditions are known to be allelic with NS (i.e., LEOPARD syndrome and CFC syndrome). Another important issue to consider when testing for NS is that negative testing of the known NS genes cannot rule out a clinical diagnosis of NS. Approximately 20–40 % of NS patients will not have a pathogenic mutation identified with currently available testing. Presumably this percentage will decrease as more genes causative of NS are identified.

X-Linked Intellectual Disability

Molecular Basis

Conditions that present with ID as the predominant phenotypic feature and are caused by defects of an X-linked gene are collectively referred to as X-linked intellectual disability (XLID). Although the primary clinical feature is ID, other serious and complicated physical, neurological and muscular features may also be present in patients with XLID [89–91]. As of early 2012, approximately 100 X-linked genes have been associated with ID and therefore are considered to be authenticated XLID genes. Even though the current number of genes is significant, many additional XLID genes likely exist because there are families with multiple affected males and a clearly X-linked pattern of inheritance that cannot be explained by mutations in the current list of associated genes [92]. Recently, new molecular technologies have accelerated the pace of genotype-phenotype discoveries and continued progress in the field of XLID is expected in the years ahead.

Beyond the unifying presentation of ID, individuals with one of the many XLID conditions can have a diverse array of additional clinical features. For classification purposes, XLID is divided into two general categories: syndromal and nonsyndromal. Syndromal XLID encompasses those conditions that present with additional phenotypic features that allow them to be differentiated from one another clinically. The majority of the syndromal XLID conditions have consistent clinical presentations that can include dysmorphic features, neurodevelopmental delays and possibly other physical manifestations. While an experienced clinician can identify some of these syndromes by their presentation, many of the

XLID syndromes have features that overlap to such a degree that they are difficult to differentiate. In some cases, the associated phenotype is known to evolve over time, potentially making the diagnosis more problematic in adults than in children. Adding interest to syndromal XLID conditions is the fact that some genes display phenotypic heterogeneity and are associated with more than one clearly defined syndromal presentation.

In contrast, individuals with a nonsyndromal form of XLID have no additional consistent clinical findings beyond ID, making diagnosis much more complicated at the molecular level. Roughly two-thirds of XLID is believed to be nonsyndromal, which reinforces the importance of having testing options that adequately address this XLID group. Both nonsyndromal and syndromal presentations have been attributed to the same gene, further complicating XLID molecular diagnosis. Furthermore, for many of the XLID genes, only a small number of families with mutations have been identified, making genotype-phenotype correlations difficult. On the other hand, a number of well-described XLID syndromes have been diagnosed in many patients throughout the world, allowing these conditions to be more distinct and recognizable [93].

Correlating with the broad spectrum of phenotypic presentations associated with XLID, the known genes causative of XLID have a wide range of functions and are not simply intermediates of a particular signaling, biochemical, or functional pathway, as noted with the RASopathies in the previous section. The following cellular activities are interrupted by mutations in at least one XLID gene: regulation of transcription, enzymatic function, energy production, myelination, cellular structure, lysosomal function, regulation of cell cycle activities, RNA binding, neuronal migration, cell adhesion, peroxisomal transport, phosphatase activity, kinase signaling, ion channel/exchange function, deacetylase activity, ubiquitin-related activity, nonsense-mediated decay, vesicular transport, and protease activity. A complete list of XLID conditions organized by the year of gene discovery, gene function and method used for discovery is available at http://www.ggc.org/images/documents/genes-involved-in-xlmr.pdf. As stated earlier, advances in molecular methods available to the clinical molecular laboratory, such as NGS, will continue to improve the diagnostic testing available for XLID [94].

Clinical Utility of Testing

FXS is the most common XLID condition, and the clinical utility of testing for this disorder, as discussed earlier in this chapter, applies in general to the entirety of XLID [95]. There are caveats that make FXS unique in some regards due to the trinucleotide repeat expansion that underlies nearly all cases of this condition. Details of FXS and *FMR1* testing will not be reiterated here; however, another XLID condition caused by a trinucleotide expansion is much less common and known as FRAXE (or ID associated with fragile site FRAXE). FRAXE is caused by expansion of a CCG repeat in the 5′ untranslated region of *AFF2* (previously known as *FMR2*). For the remainder of the XLID conditions, more traditional Mendelian alterations, such as point mutations, small insertions/deletions, and other larger scale deletions and duplications, account for the mutational spectrum [96, 97]. For some genes, the mutational diversity is minimal, while for others, it is quite extensive with large numbers of pathogenic alterations documented in the literature and in the HGMD. In most clinical settings, FXS is one of the first genetic tests requested for individuals with ID/DD, given the relative prevalence of FXS and especially in younger children when the clinical presentation may not be fully developed. Once FXS and other cytogenetic rearrangements have been ruled out, a testing strategy appropriate for the affected individual is developed.

As therapeutic options are generally limited and related to early interventions, the benefit to affected individuals is limited at the present time. One of the greatest benefits to identifying the specific XLID gene and mutation is providing reproductive information for the extended family. In many cases, families have multiple affected males prior to reaching a confirmed XLID diagnosis, which emphasizes the need for earlier clinical diagnosis and testing. Females that are heterozygous for a pathogenic XLID mutation most often are phenotypically normal, making prediction of carrier status virtually impossible in the absence of molecular testing. This uncertainty can lead to great angst for properly counseled females who have a 50 % chance that each pregnancy will result in the transmission of the X chromosome that carries the pathogenic alteration. This translates to 50 % of male offspring inheriting the abnormal X chromosome and being affected, while 50 % of female offspring will be carriers. For some XLID conditions, carrier females can present with features that are clinically recognizable, albeit, less severe in comparison to classically affected males.

X-inactivation (XI) is another genetic mechanism that plays a role in XLID. Carrier females often exhibit preferential inactivation of the X chromosome that carries a pathogenic mutation which serves as a protective factor. Some XLID conditions almost always are associated with skewed or nonrandom XI in carrier females, while other conditions have not been linked to biased inactivation of the X chromosome. In some XLID families, some carrier females have random (i.e., normal) XI, while other females with the same change have completely skewed XI, suggesting that other factors play a role in this complex biological process.

Available Assays

Due the high prevalence of FXS as a cause of ID/DD, FXS is the only XLID condition for which testing is available in most clinical molecular laboratories. Given the frequency of ID/DD in the general population, FXS testing is a more frequently ordered test in comparison to most other molecular studies performed for inherited disorders. For the remainder of XLID conditions, clinical testing has historically targeted the most common syndromes and has been offered by a limited number of laboratories. More recently, the paradigm of single gene testing for conditions with genetic heterogeneity is being supplemented with newer testing options such as targeted gene panels performed by NGS. Targeted NGS requires that the genomic DNA first be enriched for the regions of interest using one of several different technologies that are based either on PCR that is multiplexed at high orders of magnitude or by in-solution hybridization methods that have been developed to complement the newest sequencing platforms. XLID became one of the first targeted applications of NGS to be offered diagnostically, making comprehensive testing for individuals with a suspected X-linked disorder a reality. Even though a targeted panel for known XLID genes represents a major advancement in the field, single gene testing likely will continue to be an important option, evolving to targeted gene panels, and eventual transition to exome or genome sequencing, as these options become practical and cost effective in the clinical laboratory setting.

In addition to investigating genes by sequencing, either single genes or a gene panel, the possibility of larger scale deletions or duplications not detected by sequencing should be considered. Deletions in X-linked genes should be detected in males by a loss of amplification (or enrichment) and subsequent lack of sequence data. Duplications are not typically detectable by sequencing, so other technologies are necessary for detection. MLPA and aCGH have been the two principal methods for assessing dosage, each with its own benefits and limitations (not discussed in detail here) [98].

Interpretation of Test Results

Whether interpreting results from single-gene studies or from larger XLID gene panels, common issues are encountered. Clearly pathogenic alterations (nonsense, frameshift, consensus splice site) are not difficult to interpret as being clinically significant. Other novel variants such as missense, synonymous and intronic changes can be more challenging to resolve [99]. The most helpful method for determining the pathogenicity of a variant of unknown clinical significance often comes in the form of further testing of appropriate family members. Confirming the carrier status of the proband's mother is the first priority, especially in cases where there may not be a definitive X-linked family history. De novo mutations in known XLID genes are expected to be pathogenic in nearly all cases, but some rare exceptions to this rule may exist. For variants that are proven to be maternally inherited, the next step is ascertaining the availability of additional family members for testing. In principle, this becomes an exercise of segregation testing of the maternally related males that are available and willing to participate. The presence of a variant of unknown significance in a phenotypically normal male allows the change to be interpreted as a benign variant. In larger pedigrees, clear segregation of the abnormal allele only in affected males and the normal allele in unaffected males increases the likelihood that the variant is pathogenic, although. In such families the alteration may be a benign variant that is in linkage disequilibrium with the genuine disease-causing mutation. For some of the XLID genes, there may be an enzymatic/functional assay or biomarker that can be utilized to help substantiate the pathogenicity of a change that appears to be clinically relevant. RNA analysis also can be very helpful in determining if certain changes lead to altered splicing that affects the final transcript for the gene, but in general this analysis is not a clinically available service. The interpretation of molecular XLID test results has a variety of recurring themes that always need to be considered in the context of the individual patient/family being tested.

Laboratory Issues

Many of the laboratory issues discussed earlier in this chapter also apply to XLID testing. The newest area of issues pertaining to XLID and other targeted panels relates to the use of the most recently developed technologies for enrichment and sequencing. Significant effort is required to develop and validate targeted NGS gene panels that are designed to address a specific clinical condition, and then updating these gene panel tests as new genes are identified. This will continue to be an ongoing issue for some time, but will likely be overcome as targeted panels are replaced by exome and/or genome sequencing. Another issue pertaining to NGS-based testing relates to the current common practice of confirming novel changes using Sanger sequencing. The need for this as a routine procedure will likely diminish as NGS technologies become more standardized. Another issue that may become more common is the identification of alterations that appear to be mosaic. NGS allows for lower levels of mosaicism to be detected compared to Sanger sequencing, thus making secondary confirmation by Sanger sequencing a potentially difficult challenge for clinical laboratories. Lastly, bioinformatics and data management are significant issues that require attention as clinical laboratories shift away from single-gene testing towards use of NGS for targeted panels and exome or genome sequencing.

Conclusions and Future Directions

Much progress has been made in identifying individual genes and causative mutations for ID/DD. Some tests, such as FXS repeat testing or methylation analysis for AS/PWS are widely available in clinical laboratories; however, testing genes for less prevalent syndromes is performed in only those laboratories which have sequencing capabilities and expertise. As the field moves towards NGS platforms, new genes will be discovered and shown to be associated with ID/DD and incorporated into clinical tests. Challenges will remain with interpretation of variants of uncertain clinical significance, but as testing becomes more widely available, understanding of the molecular basis for these disorders will increase.

References

1. Pieretti M, Zhang FP, Fu YH, Warren ST, Oostra BA, Caskey CT, Nelson DL. Absence of expression of the FMR-1 gene in fragile X syndrome. Cell. 1991;66(4):817–22.
2. Saul R, Tarleton J (updated 1/26/2012) Fragile X syndrome. GeneReviews at GeneTests: Medical Genetics Information Resource [database online]. http://www.ncbi.nlm.nih.gov/books/NBK1384/. Accessed January 2012
3. Eichler EE, Richards S, Gibbs RA, Nelson DL. Fine structure of the human FMR1 gene. Hum Mol Genet. 1993;2(8):1147–53.
4. Hagerman RJ, Leehey M, Heinrichs W, Tassone F, Wilson R, Hills J, Grigsby J, Gage B, Hagerman PJ. Intention tremor, parkinsonism, and generalized brain atrophy in male carriers of fragile X. Neurology. 2001;57(1):127–30.
5. Allingham-Hawkins DJ, Babul-Hirji R, Chitayat D, Holden JJ, Yang KT, Lee C, Hudson R, Gorwill H, Nolin SL, Glicksman A, Jenkins EC, Brown WT, Howard-Peebles PN, Becchi C, Cummings E, Fallon L, Seitz S, Black SH, Vianna-Morgante AM, Costa SS, Otto PA, Mingroni-Netto RC, Murray A, Webb J, Vieri F, et al. Fragile X premutation is a significant risk factor for premature ovarian failure: the International Collaborative POF in Fragile X study–preliminary data. Am J Med Genet. 1999;83(4):322–5.
6. Lyon E, Laver T, Yu P, Jama M, Young K, Zoccoli M, Marlowe N. A simple, high-throughput assay for Fragile X expanded alleles using triple repeat primed PCR and capillary electrophoresis. J Mol Diagn. 2010;12(4):505–11.
7. Basehore MJ, Marlowe NM, Jones JR, Behlendorf DE, Laver TA, Friez MJ. Validation of a screening tool for the rapid and reliable detection of CGG trinucleotide repeat expansions in FMR1. Genet Test Mol Biomarkers. 2012;16:465–70.
8. Rousseau F, Heitz D, Biancalana V, Blumenfeld S, Kretz C, Boue J, Tommerup N, Van Der Hagen C, DeLozier-Blanchet C, Croquette MF, et al. Direct diagnosis by DNA analysis of the fragile X syndrome of mental retardation. N Engl J Med. 1991;325(24):1673–81.
9. Fu YH, Kuhl DP, Pizzuti A, Pieretti M, Sutcliffe JS, Richards S, Verkerk AJ, Holden JJ, Fenwick Jr RG, Warren ST, et al. Variation of the CGG repeat at the fragile X site results in genetic instability: resolution of the Sherman paradox. Cell. 1991;67(6):1047–58.
10. Tassone F, Pan R, Amiri K, Taylor AK, Hagerman PJ. A rapid polymerase chain reaction-based screening method for identification of all expanded alleles of the fragile X (FMR1) gene in newborn and high-risk populations. J Mol Diagn. 2008;10(1):43–9.
11. Filipovic-Sadic S, Sah S, Chen L, Krosting J, Sekinger E, Zhang W, Hagerman PJ, Stenzel TT, Hadd AG, Latham GJ, Tassone F. A novel FMR1 PCR method for the routine detection of low abundance expanded alleles and full mutations in fragile X syndrome. Clin Chem. 2010;56(3):399–408.
12. Hantash FM, Goos DG, Tsao D, Quan F, Buller-Burckle A, Peng M, Jarvis M, Sun W, Strom CM. Qualitative assessment of FMR1 (CGG)n triplet repeat status in normal, intermediate, premutation, full mutation, and mosaic carriers in both sexes: implications for fragile X syndrome carrier and newborn screening. Genet Med. 2010;12(3):162–73.
13. Chen L, Hadd A, Sah S, Filipovic-Sadic S, Krosting J, Sekinger E, Pan R, Hagerman PJ, Stenzel TT, Tassone F, Latham GJ. An information-rich CGG repeat primed PCR that detects the full range of fragile X expanded alleles and minimizes the need for southern blot analysis. J Mol Diagn. 2010;12(5):589–600.
14. Tassone F, Hagerman RJ, Ikle DN, Dyer PN, Lampe M, Willemsen R, Oostra BA, Taylor AK. FMRP expression as a potential prognostic indicator in fragile X syndrome. Am J Med Genet. 1999;84(3):250–61.
15. Dagli A, Williams C (updated 6/16/2011) Angelman Syndrome. GeneReviews at GeneTests: Medical Genetics Information Resource [database online]. http://www.ncbi.nlm.nih.gov/books/NBK1144/. Accessed January 2012
16. Kishino T, Lalande M, Wagstaff J. UBE3A/E6-AP mutations cause Angelman syndrome. Nat Genet. 1997;15(1):70–3.
17. Williams CA, Driscoll DJ, Dagli AI. Clinical and genetic aspects of Angelman syndrome. Genet Med. 2010;12(7):385–95.
18. Gallagher RC, Pils B, Albalwi M, Francke U. Evidence for the role of PWCR1/HBII-85 C/D box small nucleolar RNAs in Prader-Willi syndrome. Am J Hum Genet. 2002;71(3):669–78.
19. Duker AL, Ballif BC, Bawle EV, Person RE, Mahadevan S, Alliman S, Thompson R, Traylor R, Bejjani BA, Shaffer LG, Rosenfeld JA, Lamb AN, Sahoo T. Paternally inherited microdeletion at 15q11.2 confirms a significant role for the SNORD116 C/D box snoRNA cluster in Prader-Willi syndrome. Eur J Hum Genet. 2010;18(11):1196–201.
20. Beuten J, Sutcliffe JS, Casey BM, Beaudet al, Hennekam RC, Willems PJ. Detection of imprinting mutations in Angelman syndrome using a probe for exon alpha of SNRPN. Am J Med Genet. 1996;63(2):414–5.
21. Kubota T, Das S, Christian SL, Baylin SB, Herman JG, Ledbetter DH. Methylation-specific PCR simplifies imprinting analysis. Nat Genet. 1997;16(1):16–7.
22. White HE, Durston VJ, Harvey JF, Cross NC. Quantitative analysis of SNRPN(correction of SRNPN) gene methylation by pyrosequencing as a diagnostic test for Prader-Willi syndrome and Angelman syndrome. Clin Chem. 2006;52(6):1005–13.
23. Fang P, Lev-Lehman E, Tsai TF, Matsuura T, Benton CS, Sutcliffe JS, Christian SL, Kubota T, Halley DJ, Meijers-Heijboer H, Langlois S, Graham Jr JM, Beuten J, Willems PJ, Ledbetter DH, Beaudet al. The spectrum of mutations in UBE3A causing Angelman syndrome. Hum Mol Genet. 1999;8(1):129–35.
24. Malzac P, Webber H, Moncla A, Graham JM, Kukolich M, Williams C, Pagon RA, Ramsdell LA, Kishino T, Wagstaff J. Mutation analysis of UBE3A in Angelman syndrome patients. Am J Hum Genet. 1998;62(6):1353–60.
25. Lawson-Yuen A, Wu BL, Lip V, Sahoo T, Kimonis V. Atypical cases of Angelman syndrome. Am J Med Genet A. 2006;140(21):2361–4.
26. Sato K, Iwakoshi M, Shimokawa O, Sakai H, Ohta T, Saitoh S, Miyake N, Niikawa N, Harada N, Saitsu H, Mizuguchi T, Matsumoto N. Angelman syndrome caused by an identical familial 1,487-kb deletion. Am J Med Genet A. 2007;143(1):98–101.
27. Hussain Askree S, Hjelm LN, Ali Pervaiz M, Adam M, Bean LJ, Hedge M, Coffee B. Allelic dropout can cause false-positive results

for Prader-Willi and Angelman syndrome testing. J Mol Diagn. 2011;13(1):108–12.
28. Beckmann JS, Tomfohrde J, Barnes RI, Williams M, Broux O, Richard I, Weissenbach J, Bowcock AM. A linkage map of human chromosome 15 with an average resolution of 2 cM and containing 55 polymorphic microsatellites. Hum Mol Genet. 1993;2(12):2019–30.
29. Ramsden SC, Clayton-Smith J, Birch R, Buiting K. Practice guidelines for the molecular analysis of Prader-Willi and Angelman syndromes. BMC Med Genet. 2010;11:70.
30. Samaco RC, Neul JL. Complexities of Rett syndrome and MeCP2. J Neurosci. 2011;31(22):7951–9.
31. Neul JL, Kaufmann WE, Glaze DG, Christodoulou J, Clarke AJ, Bahi-Buisson N, Leonard H, Bailey ME, Schanen NC, Zappella M, Renieri A, Huppke P, Percy AK. Rett syndrome: revised diagnostic criteria and nomenclature. Ann Neurol. 2010;68(6):944–50.
32. Christodoulou J, Ho G. MECP2-related disorders. GeneReviews at GeneTests: Medical Genetics Information Resource. 2009. (updated 5/02/2009) [database online] http://www.ncbi.nlm.nih.gov/books/NBK1497/. Accessed January 2012.
33. Amir RE, Van den Veyver IB, Wan M, Tran CQ, Francke U, Zoghbi HY. Rett syndrome is caused by mutations in X-linked MECP2, encoding methyl-CpG-binding protein 2. Nat Genet. 1999;23(2): 185–8.
34. Villard L. MECP2 mutations in males. J Med Genet. 2007;44(7): 417–23.
35. Chahrour M, Jung SY, Shaw C, Zhou X, Wong ST, Qin J, Zoghbi HY. MeCP2, a key contributor to neurological disease, activates and represses transcription. Science. 2008;320(5880):1224–9.
36. Skene PJ, Illingworth RS, Webb S, Kerr AR, James KD, Turner DJ, Andrews R, Bird AP. Neuronal MeCP2 is expressed at near histone-octamer levels and globally alters the chromatin state. Mol Cell. 2010;37(4):457–68.
37. Fang PJW, Glaze DG, Percy A, Zoghbi HY, Roa BB. MECP2 gene deletions account for ~10% of Rett syndrome cases. Am Soc Hum Genet. 2004;476:2652.
38. Trappe R, Laccone F, Cobilanschi J, Meins M, Huppke P, Hanefeld F, Engel W. MECP2 mutations in sporadic cases of Rett syndrome are almost exclusively of paternal origin. Am J Hum Genet. 2001;68(5):1093–101.
39. Topcu M, Akyerli C, Sayi A, Toruner GA, Kocoglu SR, Cimbis M, Ozcelik T. Somatic mosaicism for a MECP2 mutation associated with classic Rett syndrome in a boy. Eur J Hum Genet. 2002;10(1):77–81.
40. Neul JL, Fang P, Barrish J, Lane J, Caeg EB, Smith EO, Zoghbi H, Percy A, Glaze DG. Specific mutations in methyl-CpG-binding protein 2 confer different severity in Rett syndrome. Neurology. 2008;70(16):1313–21.
41. Shahbazian MD, Zoghbi HY. Rett syndrome and MeCP2: linking epigenetics and neuronal function. Am J Hum Genet. 2002;71(6): 1259–72.
42. Friez MJ, Jones JR, Clarkson K, Lubs H, Abuelo D, Bier JA, Pai S, Simensen R, Williams C, Giampietro PF, Schwartz CE, Stevenson RE. Recurrent infections, hypotonia, and mental retardation caused by duplication of MECP2 and adjacent region in Xq28. Pediatrics. 2006;118(6):e1687–1695.
43. Mnatzakanian GN, Lohi H, Munteanu I, Alfred SE, Yamada T, MacLeod PJ, Jones JR, Scherer SW, Schanen NC, Friez MJ, Vincent JB, Minassian BA. A previously unidentified MECP2 open reading frame defines a new protein isoform relevant to Rett syndrome. Nat Genet. 2004;36(4):339–41.
44. Richards CS, Bale S, Bellissimo DB, Das S, Grody WW, Hegde MR, Lyon E, Ward BE. ACMG recommendations for standards for interpretation and reporting of sequence variations: revisions 2007. Genet Med. 2008;10(4):294–300.
45. Venancio M, Santos M, Pereira SA, Maciel P, Saraiva JM. An explanation for another familial case of Rett syndrome: maternal germline mosaicism. Eur J Hum Genet. 2007;15(8):902–4.
46. Tao J, Van Esch H, Hagedorn-Greiwe M, Hoffmann K, Moser B, Raynaud M, Sperner J, Fryns JP, Schwinger E, Gecz J, Ropers HH, Kalscheuer VM. Mutations in the X-linked cyclin-dependent kinase-like 5 (CDKL5/STK9) gene are associated with severe neurodevelopmental retardation. Am J Hum Genet. 2004;75(6): 1149–54.
47. Ariani F, Hayek G, Rondinella D, Artuso R, Mencarelli MA, Spanhol-Rosseto A, Pollazzon M, Buoni S, Spiga O, Ricciardi S, Meloni I, Longo I, Mari F, Broccoli V, Zappella M, Renieri A. FOXG1 is responsible for the congenital variant of Rett syndrome. Am J Hum Genet. 2008;83(1):89–93.
48. Mencarelli MA, Spanhol-Rosseto A, Artuso R, Rondinella D, De Filippis R, Bahi-Buisson N, Nectoux J, Rubinsztajn R, Bienvenu T, Moncla A, Chabrol B, Villard L, Krumina Z, Armstrong J, Roche A, Pineda M, Gak E, Mari F, Ariani F, Renieri A. Novel FOXG1 mutations associated with the congenital variant of Rett syndrome. J Med Genet. 2010;47(1):49–53.
49. Philippe C, Amsallem D, Francannet C, Lambert L, Saunier A, Verneau F, Jonveaux P. Phenotypic variability in Rett syndrome associated with FOXG1 mutations in females. J Med Genet. 2010;47(1):59–65.
50. Kortum F, Das S, Flindt M, Morris-Rosendahl DJ, Stefanova I, Goldstein A, Horn D, Klopocki E, Kluger G, Martin P, Rauch A, Roumer A, Saitta S, Walsh LE, Wieczorek D, Uyanik G, Kutsche K, Dobyns WB. The core FOXG1 syndrome phenotype consists of postnatal microcephaly, severe mental retardation, absent language, dyskinesia, and corpus callosum hypogenesis. J Med Genet. 2011;48(6):396–406.
51. Brunetti-Pierri N, Paciorkowski AR, Ciccone R, Mina ED, Bonaglia MC, Borgatti R, Schaaf CP, Sutton VR, Xia Z, Jelluma N, Ruivenkamp C, Bertrand M, de Ravel TJ, Jayakar P, Belli S, Rocchetti K, Pantaleoni C, D'Arrigo S, Hughes J, Cheung SW, Zuffardi O, Stankiewicz P. Duplications of FOXG1 in 14q12 are associated with developmental epilepsy, mental retardation, and severe speech impairment. Eur J Hum Genet. 2011;19(1):102–7.
52. Gilfillan GD, Selmer KK, Roxrud I, Smith R, Kyllerman M, Eiklid K, Kroken M, Mattingsdal M, Egeland T, Stenmark H, Sjoholm H, Server A, Samuelsson L, Christianson A, Tarpey P, Whibley A, Stratton MR, Futreal PA, Teague J, Edkins S, Gecz J, Turner G, Raymond FL, Schwartz C, Stevenson RE, Undlien DE, Stromme P. SLC9A6 mutations cause X-linked mental retardation, microcephaly, epilepsy, and ataxia, a phenotype mimicking Angelman syndrome. Am J Hum Genet. 2008;82(4):1003–10.
53. Schroer RJ, Holden KR, Tarpey PS, Matheus MG, Griesemer DA, Friez MJ, Fan JZ, Simensen RJ, Stromme P, Stevenson RE, Stratton MR, Schwartz CE. Natural history of Christianson syndrome. Am J Med Genet A. 2010;152A(11):2775–83.
54. Christianson AL, Stevenson RE, van der Meyden CH, Pelser J, Theron FW, van Rensburg PL, Chandler M, Schwartz CE. X linked severe mental retardation, craniofacial dysmorphology, epilepsy, ophthalmoplegia, and cerebellar atrophy in a large South African kindred is localised to Xq24-q27. J Med Genet. 1999;36(10): 759–66.
55. Rosenfeld JA, Leppig K, Ballif BC, Thiese H, Erdie-Lalena C, Bawle E, Sastry S, Spence JE, Bandholz A, Surti U, Zonana J, Keller K, Meschino W, Bejjani BA, Torchia BS, Shaffer LG. Genotype-phenotype analysis of TCF4 mutations causing Pitt-Hopkins syndrome shows increased seizure activity with missense mutations. Genet Med. 2009;11(11):797–805.
56. Amiel J, Rio M, de Pontual L, Redon R, Malan V, Boddaert N, Plouin P, Carter NP, Lyonnet S, Munnich A, Colleaux L. Mutations in TCF4, encoding a class I basic helix-loop-helix transcription factor, are responsible for Pitt-Hopkins syndrome, a severe epileptic encephalopathy associated with autonomic dysfunction. Am J Hum Genet. 2007;80(5):988–93.
57. Zweier C, Sticht H, Bijlsma EK, Clayton-Smith J, Boonen SE, Fryer A, Greally MT, Hoffmann L, den Hollander NS, Jongmans M, Kant

SG, King MD, Lynch SA, McKee S, Midro AT, Park SM, Ricotti V, Tarantino E, Wessels M, Peippo M, Rauch A. Further delineation of Pitt-Hopkins syndrome: phenotypic and genotypic description of 16 novel patients. J Med Genet. 2008;45(11):738–44.
58. Pitt D, Hopkins I. A syndrome of mental retardation, wide mouth and intermittent overbreathing. Aust Paediatr J. 1978;14(3):182–4.
59. Nora JJ, Nora AH, Sinha AK, Spangler RD, Lubs HA. The Ullrich-Noonan syndrome (Turner phenotype). Am J Dis Child. 1974;127(1):48–55.
60. Noonan JA. Hypertelorism with Turner phenotype. A new syndrome with associated congenital heart disease. Am J Dis Child. 1968;116(4):373–80.
61. Romano AA, Allanson JE, Dahlgren J, Gelb BD, Hall B, Pierpont ME, Roberts AE, Robinson W, Takemoto CM, Noonan JA. Noonan syndrome: clinical features, diagnosis, and management guidelines. Pediatrics. 2010;126(4):746–59.
62. van der Burgt I, Berends E, Lommen E, van Beersum S, Hamel B, Mariman E. Clinical and molecular studies in a large Dutch family with Noonan syndrome. Am J Med Genet. 1994;53(2):187–91.
63. Jamieson CR, van der Burgt I, Brady AF, van Reen M, Elsawi MM, Hol F, Jeffery S, Patton MA, Mariman E. Mapping a gene for Noonan syndrome to the long arm of chromosome 12. Nat Genet. 1994;8(4):357–60.
64. Tartaglia M, Mehler EL, Goldberg R, Zampino G, Brunner HG, Kremer H, van der Burgt I, Crosby AH, Ion A, Jeffery S, Kalidas K, Patton MA, Kucherlapati RS, Gelb BD. Mutations in PTPN11, encoding the protein tyrosine phosphatase SHP-2, cause Noonan syndrome. Nat Genet. 2001;29(4):465–8.
65. Roberts AE, Araki T, Swanson KD, Montgomery KT, Schiripo TA, Joshi VA, Li L, Yassin Y, Tamburino AM, Neel BG, Kucherlapati RS. Germline gain-of-function mutations in SOS1 cause Noonan syndrome. Nat Genet. 2007;39(1):70–4.
66. Tartaglia M, Pennacchio LA, Zhao C, Yadav KK, Fodale V, Sarkozy A, Pandit B, Oishi K, Martinelli S, Schackwitz W, Ustaszewska A, Martin J, Bristow J, Carta C, Lepri F, Neri C, Vasta I, Gibson K, Curry CJ, Siguero JP, Digilio MC, Zampino G, Dallapiccola B, Bar-Sagi D, Gelb BD. Gain-of-function SOS1 mutations cause a distinctive form of Noonan syndrome. Nat Genet. 2007;39(1):75–9.
67. Pandit B, Sarkozy A, Pennacchio LA, Carta C, Oishi K, Martinelli S, Pogna EA, Schackwitz W, Ustaszewska A, Landstrom A, Bos JM, Ommen SR, Esposito G, Lepri F, Faul C, Mundel P, Lopez Siguero JP, Tenconi R, Selicorni A, Rossi C, Mazzanti L, Torrente I, Marino B, Digilio MC, Zampino G, Ackerman MJ, Dallapiccola B, Tartaglia M, Gelb BD. Gain-of-function RAF1 mutations cause Noonan and LEOPARD syndromes with hypertrophic cardiomyopathy. Nat Genet. 2007;39(8):1007–12.
68. Razzaque MA, Nishizawa T, Komoike Y, Yagi H, Furutani M, Amo R, Kamisago M, Momma K, Katayama H, Nakagawa M, Fujiwara Y, Matsushima M, Mizuno K, Tokuyama M, Hirota H, Muneuchi J, Higashinakagawa T, Matsuoka R. Germline gain-of-function mutations in RAF1 cause Noonan syndrome. Nat Genet. 2007;39(8):1013–7.
69. Schubbert S, Zenker M, Rowe SL, Boll S, Klein C, Bollag G, van der Burgt I, Musante L, Kalscheuer V, Wehner LE, Nguyen H, West B, Zhang KY, Sistermans E, Rauch A, Niemeyer CM, Shannon K, Kratz CP. Germline KRAS mutations cause Noonan syndrome. Nat Genet. 2006;38(3):331–6.
70. Sarkozy A, Carta C, Moretti S, Zampino G, Digilio MC, Pantaleoni F, Scioletti AP, Esposito G, Cordeddu V, Lepri F, Petrangeli V, Dentici ML, Mancini GM, Selicorni A, Rossi C, Mazzanti L, Marino B, Ferrero GB, Silengo MC, Memo L, Stanzial F, Faravelli F, Stuppia L, Puxeddu E, Gelb BD, Dallapiccola B, Tartaglia M. Germline BRAF mutations in Noonan, LEOPARD, and cardiofaciocutaneous syndromes: molecular diversity and associated phenotypic spectrum. Hum Mutat. 2009;30(4):695–702.
71. Cordeddu V, Di Schiavi E, Pennacchio LA, Ma'ayan A, Sarkozy A, Fodale V, Cecchetti S, Cardinale A, Martin J, Schackwitz W, Lipzen A, Zampino G, Mazzanti L, Digilio MC, Martinelli S, Flex E, Lepri F, Bartholdi D, Kutsche K, Ferrero GB, Anichini C, Selicorni A, Rossi C, Tenconi R, Zenker M, Merlo D, Dallapiccola B, Iyengar R, Bazzicalupo P, Gelb BD, Tartaglia M. Mutation of SHOC2 promotes aberrant protein N-myristoylation and causes Noonan-like syndrome with loose anagen hair. Nat Genet. 2009;41(9):1022–6.
72. Cirstea IC, Kutsche K, Dvorsky R, Gremer L, Carta C, Horn D, Roberts AE, Lepri F, Merbitz-Zahradnik T, Konig R, Kratz CP, Pantaleoni F, Dentici ML, Joshi VA, Kucherlapati RS, Mazzanti L, Mundlos S, Patton MA, Silengo MC, Rossi C, Zampino G, Digilio C, Stuppia L, Seemanova E, Pennacchio LA, Gelb BD, Dallapiccola B, Wittinghofer A, Ahmadian MR, Tartaglia M, Zenker M. A restricted spectrum of NRAS mutations causes Noonan syndrome. Nat Genet. 2010;42(1):27–9.
73. Nystrom AM, Ekvall S, Berglund E, Bjorkqvist M, Braathen G, Duchen K, Enell H, Holmberg E, Holmlund U, Olsson-Engman M, Anneren G, Bondeson ML. Noonan and cardio-facio-cutaneous syndromes: two clinically and genetically overlapping disorders. J Med Genet. 2008;45(8):500–6.
74. Martinelli S, De Luca A, Stellacci E, Rossi C, Checquolo S, Lepri F, Caputo V, Silvano M, Buscherini F, Consoli F, Ferrara G, Digilio MC, Cavaliere ML, van Hagen JM, Zampino G, van der Burgt I, Ferrero GB, Mazzanti L, Screpanti I, Yntema HG, Nillesen WM, Savarirayan R, Zenker M, Dallapiccola B, Gelb BD, Tartaglia M. Heterozygous germline mutations in the CBL tumor-suppressor gene cause a Noonan syndrome-like phenotype. Am J Hum Genet. 2010;87(2):250–7.
75. Sarkozy A, Obregon MG, Conti E, Esposito G, Mingarelli R, Pizzuti A, Dallapiccola B. A novel PTPN11 gene mutation bridges Noonan syndrome, multiple lentigines/LEOPARD syndrome and Noonan-like/multiple giant cell lesion syndrome. Eur J Hum Genet. 2004;12(12):1069–72.
76. Aoki Y, Niihori T, Kawame H, Kurosawa K, Ohashi H, Tanaka Y, Filocamo M, Kato K, Suzuki Y, Kure S, Matsubara Y. Germline mutations in HRAS proto-oncogene cause Costello syndrome. Nat Genet. 2005;37(10):1038–40.
77. Rodriguez-Viciana P, Tetsu O, Tidyman WE, Estep AL, Conger BA, Cruz MS, McCormick F, Rauen KA. Germline mutations in genes within the MAPK pathway cause cardio-facio-cutaneous syndrome. Science. 2006;311(5765):1287–90.
78. Niihori T, Aoki Y, Narumi Y, Neri G, Cave H, Verloes A, Okamoto N, Hennekam RC, Gillessen-Kaesbach G, Wieczorek D, Kavamura MI, Kurosawa K, Ohashi H, Wilson L, Heron D, Bonneau D, Corona G, Kaname T, Naritomi K, Baumann C, Matsumoto N, Kato K, Kure S, Matsubara Y. Germline KRAS and BRAF mutations in cardio-facio-cutaneous syndrome. Nat Genet. 2006;38(3):294–6.
79. Wallace MR, Marchuk DA, Andersen LB, Letcher R, Odeh HM, Saulino AM, Fountain JW, Brereton A, Nicholson J, Mitchell AL, et al. Type 1 neurofibromatosis gene: identification of a large transcript disrupted in three NF1 patients. Science. 1990;249(4965):181–6.
80. Brems H, Chmara M, Sahbatou M, Denayer E, Taniguchi K, Kato R, Somers R, Messiaen L, De Schepper S, Fryns JP, Cools J, Marynen P, Thomas G, Yoshimura A, Legius E. Germline loss-of-function mutations in SPRED1 cause a neurofibromatosis 1-like phenotype. Nat Genet. 2007;39(9):1120–6.
81. Digilio MC, Conti E, Sarkozy A, Mingarelli R, Dottorini T, Marino B, Pizzuti A, Dallapiccola B. Grouping of multiple-lentigines/LEOPARD and Noonan syndromes on the PTPN11 gene. Am J Hum Genet. 2002;71(2):389–94.
82. Bos JL. ras oncogenes in human cancer: a review. Cancer Res. 1989;49(17):4682–9.

83. Tidyman WE, Rauen KA. The RASopathies: developmental syndromes of Ras/MAPK pathway dysregulation. Curr Opin Genet Dev. 2009;19(3):230–6.
84. Hiippala A, Eronen M, Taipale P, Salonen R, Hiilesmaa V. Fetal nuchal translucency and normal chromosomes: a long-term follow-up study. Ultrasound Obstet Gynecol. 2001;18(1):18–22.
85. Lee KA, Williams B, Roza K, Ferguson H, David K, Eddleman K, Stone J, Edelmann L, Richard G, Gelb BD, Kornreich R. PTPN11 analysis for the prenatal diagnosis of Noonan syndrome in fetuses with abnormal ultrasound findings. Clin Genet. 2009;75(2):190–4.
86. Zenker M, Buheitel G, Rauch R, Koenig R, Bosse K, Kress W, Tietze HU, Doerr HG, Hofbeck M, Singer H, Reis A, Rauch A. Genotype-phenotype correlations in Noonan syndrome. J Pediatr. 2004;144(3):368–74.
87. Shchelochkov OA, Patel A, Weissenberger GM, Chinault AC, Wiszniewska J, Fernandes PH, Eng C, Kukolich MK, Sutton VR. Duplication of chromosome band 12q24.11q24.23 results in apparent Noonan syndrome. Am J Med Genet A. 2008;146A(8): 1042–8.
88. Graham Jr JM, Kramer N, Bejjani BA, Thiel CT, Carta C, Neri G, Tartaglia M, Zenker M. Genomic duplication of PTPN11 is an uncommon cause of Noonan syndrome. Am J Med Genet A. 2009;149A(10):2122–8.
89. Stevenson R, Schwartz C, Schroer R. Oxford monographs on medical genetics No. 39. Oxford: Oxford University Press; 2000.
90. Stevenson RE, Schwartz CE. X-linked intellectual disability: unique vulnerability of the male genome. Dev Disabil Res Rev. 2009;15(4):361–8.
91. Gecz J, Shoubridge C, Corbett M. The genetic landscape of intellectual disability arising from chromosome X. Trends Genet. 2009;25(7):308–16.
92. Chiurazzi P, Schwartz CE, Gecz J, Neri G. XLMR genes: update 2007. Eur J Hum Genet. 2008;16(4):422–34.
93. Rejeb I, Ben Jemaa L, Chaabouni H. X linked mental retardation. Tunis Med. 2009;87(5):311–8.
94. Hu H, Wrogemann K, Kalscheuer V, Tzschach A, Richard H, Haas SA, Menzel C, Bienek M, Froyen G, Raynaud M, Van Bokhoven H, Chelly J, Ropers H, Chen W. Mutation screening in 86 known X-linked mental retardation genes by droplet-based multiplex PCR and massive parallel sequencing. Hugo J. 2009;3(1-4):41–9.
95. Michelson DJ, Shevell MI, Sherr EH, Moeschler JB, Gropman AL, Ashwal S. Evidence report: Genetic and metabolic testing on children with global developmental delay: report of the Quality Standards Subcommittee of the American Academy of Neurology and the Practice Committee of the Child Neurology Society. Neurology. 2011;77(17):1629–35.
96. Tarpey PS, Smith R, Pleasance E, Whibley A, Edkins S, Hardy C, O'Meara S, Latimer C, Dicks E, Menzies A, Stephens P, Blow M, Greenman C, Xue Y, Tyler-Smith C, Thompson D, Gray K, Andrews J, Barthorpe S, Buck G, Cole J, Dunmore R, Jones D, Maddison M, Mironenko T, Turner R, Turrell K, Varian J, West S, Widaa S, Wray P, Teague J, Butler A, Jenkinson A, Jia M, Richardson D, Shepherd R, Wooster R, Tejada MI, Martinez F, Carvill G, Goliath R, de Brouwer AP, van Bokhoven H, Van Esch H, Chelly J, Raynaud M, Ropers HH, Abidi FE, Srivastava AK, Cox J, Luo Y, Mallya U, Moon J, Parnau J, Mohammed S, Tolmie JL, Shoubridge C, Corbett M, Gardner A, Haan E, Rujirabanjerd S, Shaw M, Vandeleur L, Fullston T, Easton DF, Boyle J, Partington M, Hackett A, Field M, Skinner C, Stevenson RE, Bobrow M, Turner G, Schwartz CE, Gecz J, Raymond FL, Futreal PA, Stratton MR. A systematic, large-scale resequencing screen of X-chromosome coding exons in mental retardation. Nat Genet. 2009;41(5):535–43.
97. Whibley AC, Plagnol V, Tarpey PS, Abidi F, Fullston T, Choma MK, Boucher CA, Shepherd L, Willatt L, Parkin G, Smith R, Futreal PA, Shaw M, Boyle J, Licata A, Skinner C, Stevenson RE, Turner G, Field M, Hackett A, Schwartz CE, Gecz J, Stratton MR, Raymond FL. Fine-scale survey of X chromosome copy number variants and indels underlying intellectual disability. Am J Hum Genet. 2010;87(2):173–88.
98. Bauters M, Weuts A, Vandewalle J, Nevelsteen J, Marynen P, Van Esch H, Froyen G. Detection and validation of copy number variation in X-linked mental retardation. Cytogenet Genome Res. 2008;123(1–4):44–53.
99. Raymond FL, Whibley A, Stratton MR, Gecz J. Lessons learnt from large-scale exon re-sequencing of the X chromosome. Hum Mol Genet. 2009;18(R1):R60–64.

Congenital Disorders of Glycosylation

8

Melanie A. Jones and Madhuri R. Hegde

Abstract

Glycosylation is the addition of sugars (glycans) to proteins and lipids and is the most frequent modification of both secreted and membrane-bound proteins. Defective synthesis, assembly or processing of glycans results in a group of disorders known as congenital disorders of glycosylation (CDG). Biochemical testing assesses the level of glycosylation on glycoproteins, such as transferrin, as well as the structure of *N*-linked or *O*-linked glycans released from glycoproteins. Molecular CDG single gene and gene panel testing is clinically available for more than 30 CDG-associated genes. An exome sequencing approach is being used to identify the gene defect in individuals with unknown types of CDG (CDG-Ix and CDG-IIx), and can lead to the identification of new CDG genes. Identification of the molecular mechanisms for new subtypes of CDG will provide important building blocks for the development of new treatments and therapies for individuals affected with CDG.

Keywords

Glycosylation • Congenital disorders • *N*-glycosylation • *O*-glycosylation • Lipids • Serum transferrin

Introduction

Glycosylation is the addition of sugars (glycans) to proteins and lipids and is the most frequent modification of both secreted and membrane-bound proteins [1]. Two types of protein glycosylation occur, *N*-linked and *O*-linked, which differ in the linkage of the oligosaccharide to protein.

Approximately 50 % of all proteins in the human genome are *N*-glycosylated [2]. In *N*-glycosylation, an oligosaccharide is assembled, beginning in the cytosol and continued in the endoplasmic reticulum (ER). The sugar chain precursor is assembled on a lipid dolichol pyrophosphate carrier in the ER membrane and consists of two *N*-acetylglucosamine residues, nine mannose residues, and three glucose residues. Once the assembly process is complete, the oligosaccharyltransferase complex transfers the oligosaccharide to specific asparagine residues on nascent polypeptide chains in the lumen of the ER. After linkage, modification of the glycan begins with the trimming of sugar chains in the ER, and further modification of these sugar chains takes place in the Golgi apparatus. This pathway is well described, and many enzymes are involved in both the assembly and the post-linkage processing of the glycan chain [3]. *N*-glycosylated proteins are important for a variety of biological processes, including intracellular targeting, cell-cell recognition, protein folding and stability, and immune response [1].

In contrast, *O*-linked-glycosylation occurs in the Golgi apparatus with sugars added sequentially to serine or threonine amino acids of proteins. *O*-glycosylated proteins provide a barrier against pathogens, serve as lubricants, provide cushioning and physical integrity to the extracellular matrix, and function as co-receptors for a number of growth factors [1].

M.A. Jones, Ph.D. • M.R. Hegde, Ph.D. (✉)
Department of Human Genetics, Emory University School of Medicine, Emory University, Whitehead Biomedical Research Building, 615 Michael Street, Suite 305A, Atlanta, GA 30322, USA
e-mail: mhegde@emory.edu

D.G.B. Leonard (ed.), *Molecular Pathology in Clinical Practice*, DOI 10.1007/978-3-319-19674-9_8

Glycosylation of lipids begins within the cytosol and continues in the ER and Golgi apparatus. Glycosylated lipids are involved in signaling, membrane diffusion, and sorting [4]. Hence, the proper development and functioning of multiple organ systems are dependent upon normal glycosylation of proteins and lipids.

Molecular Basis of Disease

An impaired *N*-glycosylation biosynthesis pathway, due to mutations in genes that encode proteins that function within this pathway or are involved in intracellular protein or nucleotide sugar trafficking between the endoplasmic reticulum and Golgi apparatus, affects multiple organ systems including the brain, heart, bone, endocrine system, immune system, liver, gastrointestinal tract, and vision [1]. Defects within the *O*-glycosylation pathway mainly affect muscle, bone, cartilage, and the extracellular matrix [1]. Defects in lipid glycosylation primarily affect the nervous system [5, 6].

Defective synthesis, assembly or processing of glycans results in a group of disorders known as congenital disorders of glycosylation (CDG) [1]. The majority of individuals with CDG have symptoms that began in infancy. These symptoms can include severe developmental delay, ataxia, seizures, liver fibrosis, cardiac dysfunction, retinopathy, skeletal abnormalities, and coagulopathies. The liver and intestine are most affected in CDG because these organs consume the most mannose for glycoprotein synthesis. Approximately 20 % of children do not survive beyond 5 years of age due to widespread organ dysfunction and severe infections. Worldwide occurrence of CDG has an estimated prevalence as high as 1 in 20,000. The great variability of symptoms and severity of disease across individuals with CDG makes the diagnosis of these disorders challenging to pediatric health care providers. The majority of CDG types are due to autosomal recessive inheritance. The exceptions include an X-linked *N*-glycosylation defect and two autosomal dominant *O*-glycosylation defects.

CDG patients are classified as having either Type I, Type II, or combined Type I and Type II defects, which is defined by serum transferrin analysis. This designation is based on whether the *N*-glycosylation defect results in either hypo- or mis-glycosylation [7]. Type I CDGs are caused by defects in genes that create the sugar chain precursors or in genes that attach these precursors to proteins and lipids. These defects result in a glycan structure that is partially or totally missing. Type II CDGs are caused by defects in genes that modify the sugar chains after they are attached to proteins and lipids. These defects result in a structurally altered glycan. Combined Type I and Type II defects have recently been reported, making an accurate diagnosis in these patients even more challenging. Most CDG subtypes have been described in only a few individuals; therefore, an understanding of phenotypes for these CDG subtypes is limited.

Currently, efficient treatment is only available for one subtype of CDG, MPI-CDG (CDG-Ib), caused by mutations in the phosphomannose-isomerase (*MPI*) gene [8]. The defect in MPI-CDG is the inability to convert fructose-6 phosphate to mannose-6-phosphate. The enzyme hexokinase can form mannose-6-phosphate from the administration of oral mannose, thereby bypassing the defect. Two other CDGs that can respond to treatment include SLC35C1-CDG (CDG-IIc) in which fucose is an effective treatment for recurrent infections with hyperleukocystosis, and PIGM-CDG in which butyrate upregulates PIGM transcription, thereby controlling seizures [9, 10]. Only supportive therapy and symptom-based treatment is available for all other CDG subtypes.

Clinical Utility of Testing

Due to the multisystem involvement of CDG, subtype diagnosis based on the clinical phenotype often is not possible. A combination of biochemical and molecular testing is used to identify the CDG subtype. Confirmation of the specific gene defect is important because some life-threatening phenotypes (i.e., cardiac dysfunction) have presented in only certain subtypes of CDG and may develop at any time. Confirmation of the defect allows for close monitoring of different organs for dysfunction and complications that may arise due to coagulation abnormalities. A growing number of individuals have a biochemical diagnosis of CDG without identification of a disease-causing mutation in a known CDG gene. Although molecular testing may miss some mutations in deep intronic or promoter regions of CDG-associated genes, many individuals with negative testing likely have mutations in genes not yet associated with CDG.

Genotype-phenotype correlations are not well described for many subtypes of CDG because only a few individuals have had mutations detected in the majority of CDG-associated genes [11]. Even in the most common CDG subtype, PMM2-CDG (CDG-Ia), individuals with the same mutation have variable severity of the clinical symptoms [12]. Identification of both disease-causing mutations in the affected individual allows carrier and prenatal testing of other family members.

Available Assays

Biochemical Assays

The standard screening for individuals with symptoms of CDG is biochemical testing to assess the level of glycosylation on glycoproteins, such as transferrin, and the structure of *N*-linked or *O*-linked glycans released from glycoproteins [13]. Transferrin is an iron-binding protein that is synthesized and metabolized mainly in the liver and is the most sensitive serum glycoprotein marker for CDG. Glycosylation of transferrin can be analyzed using isoelectric focusing (IEF), electrospray ionization mass spectrometry or matrix-assisted laser desorption/ionization–time-of-flight mass spectrometry. Transferrin contains two biantennary *N*-glycan chains with a total of four terminal sialic acid residues. A normal IEF profile of transferrin isomers consists predominantly of four sialic acids (tetrasialotransferrin). For type I CDG, an abnormal profile is observed with a decreased amount of tetrasialotransferrin and increased amounts of asialo- and disialotransferrin due to some transferrin molecules lacking either one or both *N*-glycan chains. For type II CDG, an abnormal profile consists of an increase of tri-, di-, mono-, or sometimes asialotransferrin due to a portion of the glycan chains being incomplete. Serum transferrin analysis is relatively of low cost and is available in many clinical laboratories. Transferrin testing is a rapid screen for CDG, but does not identify the specific gene defect.

Serum transferrin screening for CDG has limitations. Several CDG subtypes including MOGS-CDG (CDG-IIb), SLC35C1-CDG (CDG-IIc), and SLC35A1-CDG (CDG-IIf) present with a normal transferrin pattern [1]. Some patients with PMM2-CDG (CDG-Ia) may have a normal transferrin pattern later in life, and analysis of PMM2 enzyme activity may be needed to confirm the diagnosis [14]. These examples demonstrate that a normal transferrin pattern does not necessarily exclude an individual from having CDG, with approximately 25 % of CDG cases estimated to have a normal transferrin pattern [15]. False-positive results can be observed in individuals presenting with liver disease, other metabolic disorders including galactosemia and fructosemia, or alcoholism [16–18]. Transferrin analysis also is not accurate in children less than 6 months of age and may give false-negative results [7]. Transferrin analysis also is reported to have false-positive results in infants less than 3 weeks of age [19].

MALDI-TOF-MS can be used for analysis of *N*- and *O*-linked glycan structures. This technique protects glycans from fragmentation and allows for the structural detail of *N*- and *O*-linked glycans to be analyzed. This technique has been used to characterize a number of subtypes of CDG that could not be detected by IEF of transferrin and is particularly useful for characterizing Type II defects, combined Type I and Type II defects, and multiple glycosylation defects [20]. Caution needs to be exercised with interpretation of *O*-glycan MALDI-TOF-MS profiles from patients with cancer or diabetes because these conditions can alter *O*-glycans at the cellular level [21]. This analysis is available only in a few clinical laboratories.

Enzyme activities of phosphomannomutase (PMM) and phosphomannose isomerase are assessed in patient fibroblasts or leukocytes if the patient is suspected to have a Type I CDG [13]. This will diagnose or rule out two common CDGs, PMM2-CDG (CDG-Ia) (700 individuals worldwide), and MPI-CDG (CDG-Ib) (20 individuals worldwide). Analysis using leukocytes is preferred, especially for PMM enzyme activity, because rapidly dividing fibroblasts can give high PMM residual activity levels [22]. Enzyme activity assays are clinically available only for these two CDG subtypes, and performed by several laboratories worldwide.

Molecular Assays

Since serum transferrin analysis can only determine whether the patient has Type I or Type II CDG, follow up with molecular testing is needed to determine the specific gene defect and to direct testing of additional family members, as needed. If individuals have reduced PMM or MPI enzyme activity, PCR amplification and sequencing of the respective genes can be performed to determine the disease-causing mutations. Single gene testing is currently available for more than 30 genes associated with CDG (Table 8.1). Only a few laboratories provide molecular testing for the more rare CDG subtypes. A comprehensive clinical CDG next-generation sequencing panel is available for comprehensive mutation detection in 38 CDG-associated genes when it is unclear what defect an individual with CDG may have based on phenotype [23]. Array-based comparative genomic hybridization (aCGH) also can be used to detect exon and gene deletions and duplications in these CDG-associated genes.

For the most common CDG, PMM2-CDG (CDG-Ia), over 90 mutations have been identified [8]. The most common mutation is p.Arg141His that leads to almost complete inactivation of the enzyme [12]. This amino acid substitution is seen in about 40 % of compound heterozygous individuals. Another mutation, p.Phe119Leu, is frequently found in affected Northern Europeans with the compound heterozygote genotype (p.Arg141His and p.Phe119Leu), and represents 72 % of mutations in *PMM2*. Due to the limited number of individuals with defects in the other CDG genes, no common mutations have been identified across individuals.

Interpretation of Results

The majority of mutations identified in CDG patients are missense and nonsense mutations, and small insertions and deletions. Since only a few patients have been identified with defects in each of the CDG genes, the list of mutations in Human Gene Mutation Database is very limited for many

Table 8.1 Subtypes of congenital disorders of glycosylation

CDG subtype	Type of defect
PMM2-CDG (CDG-Ia)*	*N*-glycosylation
MPI-CDG (CDG-Ib)*	*N*-glycosylation
ALG6-CDG (CDG-Ic)*	*N*-glycosylation
ALG3-CDG (CDG-Id)*	*N*-glycosylation
ALG12-CDG (CDG-Ig)*	*N*-glycosylation
ALG8-CDG (CDG-Ih)*	*N*-glycosylation
ALG2-CDG (CDG-Ii)*	*N*-glycosylation
DPAGT1-CDG (CDG-Ij)*	*N*-glycosylation
ALG1-CDG (CDG-Ik)*	*N*-glycosylation
ALG9-CDG (CDG-IL)*	*N*-glycosylation
RFT1-CDG (CDG-In)*	*N*-glycosylation
DPM3-CDG (CDG-Io)*	*N*-glycosylation
ALG11-CDG (CDG-Ip)*	*N*-glycosylation
SRD5A3-CDG (CDG-Iq)*	*N*-glycosylation
DDOST-CDG (CDG-Ir)*	*N*-glycosylation
ALG13-CDG (CDG-Is)*	*N*-glycosylation
MAGT1-CDG*	*N*-glycosylation
TUSC3-CDG*	*N*-glycosylation
DHDDS-CDG*	*N*-glycosylation
MAN1B1-CDG	*N*-glycosylation
PGM1-CDG	*N*-glycosylation
ST3GAL3-CDG	*N*-glycosylation
MGAT2-CDG (CDG-IIa)*	*N*-glycosylation
MOGS-CDG (CDG-IIb)*	*N*-glycosylation
TMEM165-CDG (CDG-IIk)	*N*-glycosylation
DPM1-CDG (CDG-Ie)*	Multiple glycosylation
MPDU1-CDG (CDG-If)*	Multiple glycosylation
DOLK-CDG (CDG-Im)*	Multiple glycosylation
SLC35C1-CDG (CDG-IIc)*	Multiple glycosylation
B4GALT1-CDG (CDG-IId)*	Multiple glycosylation
COG7-CDG (CDG-IIe)*	Multiple glycosylation
SLC35A1-CDG (CDG-IIf)*	Multiple glycosylation
COG1-CDG (CDG-IIg)*	Multiple glycosylation
COG8-CDG (CDG-IIh)*	Multiple glycosylation
COG4-CDG*	Multiple glycosylation
COG5-CDG*	Multiple glycosylation
COG6-CDG*	Multiple glycosylation
SEC23B-CDG*	Multiple glycosylation
GNE-CDG*	Multiple glycosylation
ATP6V0A2-CDG*	Multiple glycosylation
POMT1–POMT2-CDG*	*O*-glycosylation
POMGNT1-CDG*	*O*-glycosylation
B3GALTL-CDG*	*O*-glycosylation
EXT1–EXT2-CDG	*O*-glycosylation
B4GALT7-CDG	*O*-glycosylation
GALNT3-CDG	*O*-glycosylation
SLC35D1-CDG	*O*-glycosylation
LFNG-CDG	*O*-glycosylation
CHST14-CDG	*O*-glycosylation
CHST3-CDG	*O*-glycosylation
CHST6-CDG	*O*-glycosylation
CHSY1-CDG	*O*-glycosylation
B3GAT3-CDG	*O*-glycosylation
FKTN-CDG	*O*-glycosylation
LARGE-CDG	*O*-glycosylation
FKRP-CDG	*O*-glycosylation
PIGA-CDG	Lipid glycosylation
PIGM-CDG	Lipid glycosylation
PIGO-CDG	Lipid glycosylation
PIGV-CDG	Lipid glycosylation
ST3GAL5-CDG	Lipid glycosylation
SIAT9-CDG	Lipid glycosylation

Subtypes with an asterisk indicate that clinical testing is available

CDGs; therefore, a conservative approach should be taken for novel variants identified in CDG genes that have not been previously reported. Interpretation of duplications identified by array CGH is difficult because the duplication may or may not disrupt the function of the encoded protein. The presence of one known disease-causing mutation in a specific CDG gene can assist with the interpretation of aCGH results. Parental studies can be useful in determining whether two variants identified in a single gene are on the same or opposite alleles.

Laboratory Issues

Serum transferrin analysis is prone to both false-positive and false-negative results; therefore, if a patient has a strong clinical indication of CDG, follow-up with additional biochemical or molecular testing is recommended. If biochemical testing indicates an individual has CDG, molecular testing is used to confirm the diagnosis and to identify the disease-causing mutations. Testing for the majority of CDGs is provided by only a few laboratories worldwide. A list of laboratories that test for each CDG subtype is provided on the GeneTests website (http://www.ncbi.nlm.nih.gov/sites/GeneTests/).

Conclusions and Future Directions

Due to the wide spectrum of symptoms and variable severity of CDG, pediatric physicians should be educated to consider glycosylation disorders in patients presenting with multi-organ dysfunction and symptoms that include developmental delay, failure to thrive, liver dysfunction, or neurological involvement. As testing for CDG continues, the number of patients that lack a molecular diagnosis will likely increase, highlighting the need for broader molecular testing to identify the causative gene in these patients. Greater than 40 % of CDG patients are estimated to have an unknown type of CDG (CDG-Ix or CDG-IIx) and lack a molecular diagnosis, with the majority of unsolved cases being CDG-IIx. Approximately, 250–500 genes are estimated to be involved in the process of glycosylation, with the likelihood that defects in a number of these genes will result in CDG. CDG is an ideal candidate syndrome for exome sequencing, and this approach already has successfully identified the gene defect in a previous CDG-Ix patient [24]. New CDG genes identified from exome or genome sequencing can be added to the clinical CDG next-generation sequencing panel to provide a more comprehensive test.

Improved molecular diagnosis of CDG will reduce the number of patients lacking genetic characterization, shorten a patient's time to diagnosis, facilitate genetic counseling, improve patient management, and facilitate carrier or prenatal testing for other family members. Molecular diagnosis of additional patients with CDG will provide an estimate of the prevalence of each subtype and a greater understanding of the spectrum of phenotypes associated with each subtype. The clinical outcome and natural course for each CDG subtype will also be elucidated. As more patients are identified, the study of genotype/phenotype correlations can be assessed. Identification of new genes also will provide insight into new pathways that are linked to glycosylation. Furthermore, identification of new genes associated with CDG will provide important building blocks for the development of new treatments and therapies for individuals afflicted with different subtypes of CDG.

References

1. Freeze HH. Genetic defects in the human glycome. Nat Rev Genet. 2006;7(7):537–51.
2. Schachter H, Freeze HH. Glycosylation diseases: quo vadis? Biochim Biophys Acta. 2009;1792(9):925–30.
3. Marquardt T, Denecke J. Congenital disorders of glycosylation: review of their molecular bases, clinical presentations and specific therapies. Eur J Pediatr. 2003;162(6):359–79.
4. Hancock JF. GPI-anchor synthesis: Ras takes charge. Dev Cell. 2004;6(6):743–5.
5. Krawitz PM, Schweiger MR, Rodelsperger C, Marcelis C, Kolsch U, Meisel C, et al. Identity-by-descent filtering of exome sequence data identifies PIGV mutations in hyperphosphatasia mental retardation syndrome. Nat Genet. 2010;42(10):827–9.
6. Simpson MA, Cross H, Proukakis C, Priestman DA, Neville DC, Reinkensmeier G, et al. Infantile-onset symptomatic epilepsy syndrome caused by a homozygous loss-of-function mutation of GM3 synthase. Nat Genet. 2004;36(11):1225–9.
7. Lefeber DJ, Morava E, Jaeken J. How to find and diagnose a CDG due to defective N-glycosylation. J Inherit Metab Dis. 2011;34(4):849–52. doi:10.1007/s10545-011-9370-0.
8. Jaeken J. Congenital disorders of glycosylation. Ann N Y Acad Sci. 2010;1214:190–8.
9. Gazit Y, Mory A, Etzioni A, Frydman M, Scheuerman O, Gershoni-Baruch R, et al. Leukocyte adhesion deficiency type II: long-term follow-up and review of the literature. J Clin Immunol. 2010; 30(2):308–13.
10. Almeida A, Layton M, Karadimitris A. Inherited glycosylphosphatidyl inositol deficiency: a treatable CDG. Biochim Biophys Acta. 2009;1792(9):874–80.
11. Vodopiutz J, Bodamer OA. Congenital disorders of glycosylation-a challenging group of IEMs. J Inherit Metab Dis. 2008;31(2):267–9.
12. Grunewald S. The clinical spectrum of phosphomannomutase 2 deficiency (CDG-Ia). Biochim Biophys Acta. 2009;1792(9): 827–34.
13. Marklova E, Albahri Z. Screening and diagnosis of congenital disorders of glycosylation. Clin Chim Acta. 2007;385(1-2):6–20.
14. Vermeer S, Kremer HP, Leijten QH, Scheffer H, Matthijs G, Wevers RA, et al. Cerebellar ataxia and congenital disorder of glycosylation Ia (CDG-Ia) with normal routine CDG screening. J Neurol. 2007;254(10):1356–8.
15. Jaeken J. Congenital disorders of glycosylation (CDG): it's (nearly) all in it! J Inherit Metab Dis. 2011;34(4):853–8.
16. Adamowicz M, Pronicka E. Carbohydrate deficient glycoprotein syndrome–like transferrin isoelectric focusing pattern in untreated fructosaemia. Eur J Pediatr. 1996;155(4):347–8.
17. Charlwood J, Clayton P, Keir G, Mian N, Winchester B. Defective galactosylation of serum transferrin in galactosemia. Glycobiology. 1998;8(4):351–7.
18. Stibler H, Borg S, Joustra M. Micro anion exchange chromatography of carbohydrate-deficient transferrin in serum in relation to alcohol consumption (Swedish Patent 8400587-5). Alcohol Clin Exp Res. 1986;10(5):535–44.
19. Clayton P, Winchester B, Di Tomaso E, Young E, Keir G, Rodeck C. Carbohydrate-deficient glycoprotein syndrome: normal glycosylation in the fetus. Lancet. 1993;341.
20. Faid V, Chirat F, Seta N, Foulquier F, Morelle W. A rapid mass spectrometric strategy for the characterization of N- and O-glycan chains in the diagnosis of defects in glycan biosynthesis. Proteomics. 2007;7(11):1800–13.
21. Ungar D. Golgi linked protein glycosylation and associated diseases. Semin Cell Dev Biol. 2009;20(7):762–9.
22. Grunewald S, Schollen E, Van Schaftingen E, Jaeken J, Matthijs G. High residual activity of PMM2 in patients' fibroblasts: possible pitfall in the diagnosis of CDG-Ia (phosphomannomutase deficiency). Am J Hum Genet. 2001;68(2):347–54.
23. Jones MA, Bhide S, Chin E, Ng BG, Rhodenizer D, Zhang VW, Sun JJ, Tanner A, Freeze HH, Hegde MR. Targeted polymerase chain reaction-based enrichment and next generation sequencing for diagnostic testing of congenital disorders of glycosylation. Genet Med. 2011;13(11):921–32.
24. Jones MA, Ng BG, Bhide S, Chin E, Rhodenizer D, He P, Losfeld ME, He M, Raymond K, Berry G, Freeze HH, Hegde MR. DDOST mutations identified by whole-exome sequencing are implicated in congenital disorders of glycosylation. Am J Hum Genet. 2012; 90(2):363–8.

Neuromuscular Diseases

9

Thomas W. Prior

Abstract

This chapter describes clinical manifestations, pathology, and the molecular diagnosis of selected neuromuscular disorders which are commonly tested for in the molecular pathology laboratory. Neuromuscular function can be impaired as a result of defects in the nervous system, muscle, or both. The disorders described are all heritable. However the disorders have different patterns of inheritance and are caused by different types of mutations. The molecular assay utilized is determined by the type of mutation to be identified. The molecular testing allows for more accurate diagnostic, carrier, predictive, and prenatal testing. The clinical utility, interpretation, and laboratory issues will be described for each disorder.

Keywords

Neuromuscular disease • Duchenne • Becker • Muscular dystrophy • X-linked • Myotonic dystrophy • Spinal muscular atrophy • SMA • Mitochondrial encephalomyopathies • Kearns-Sayre syndrome • Mitochondrial encephalomyopathy with lactic acidosis and stroke-like episodes • MELAS • Myoclonic epilepsy with ragged-red fibers • MERRF • Kennedy disease • Spinobulbar muscular dystrophy

Introduction

This chapter describes clinical manifestations, pathology, and the molecular diagnosis of selected neuromuscular disorders which are commonly tested for in the molecular pathology laboratory. Neuromuscular function can be impaired as a result of defects in the nervous system, muscle, or both. The disorders described in this chapter are all heritable. However the disorders often have different patterns of inheritance and are caused by different types of mutations. The molecular assay utilized is determined by the type of mutation to be identified. The molecular testing allows for more accurate diagnostic, carrier, predictive, and prenatal testing. Furthermore, by better understanding the pathogenesis of the disease, new therapeutic strategies will be developed in the future. The clinical utility, interpretation, and laboratory issues will be described for each disorder.

Duchenne and Becker Muscular Dystrophies

Molecular Basis of Disease

Duchenne and Becker muscular dystrophies (DMD and BMD) are X-linked, allelic, neuromuscular diseases characterized by progressive muscular weakness and degeneration of skeletal muscle. DMD is the most common X-linked recessive lethal disease, with an incidence of approximately 1 in 3,500 newborns, and approximately one-third of cases are the result of new mutations [1, 2]. Affected children are usually wheelchair bound by the age of 12 years. As the disease progresses, contractures increasingly develop, leading to asymmetrical spinal deformities. Most patients die at

T.W. Prior, Ph.D. (✉)
Department of Pathology, Ohio State University Medical Center, 125 Hamilton Hall, 1645 Neil Ave., Columbus, OH 43210, USA
e-mail: thomas.prior@osumc.edu

D.G.B. Leonard (ed.), *Molecular Pathology in Clinical Practice*, DOI 10.1007/978-3-319-19674-9_9

about 20 years of age due to pneumonia, related to chronic respiratory insufficiency. The allelic disorder BMD has a milder clinical course and slower disease progression. BMD occurs approximately one-tenth as frequently as DMD, with an incidence of about 1 in 35,000. The majority of patients with BMD initially experience difficulties between 5 and 15 years of age, although an onset in the third or fourth decade or even later can occur. By definition the affected patients remain ambulatory until 16 years of age or later, thus allowing clinical distinction from patients with DMD.

The *DMD* gene is the largest human gene isolated, spanning more than 2,000 kilobases (kb) of genomic DNA, and is composed of 79 exons that encode a 14 kb transcript, which is translated into a protein named dystrophin [3, 4]. Dystrophin is a 427 kilodalton (kDa) cytoskeletal protein consisting of four domains: (1) an amino terminus that associates with actin or an actin-like protein; (2) a rod domain consisting of long, flexible rows of 24 alpha helical repeats; (3) a cysteine-rich region; and (4) a unique carboxy terminus [5]. Dystrophin has been shown to be tightly associated with a large oligomeric complex of sarcolemmal glycoproteins through its cysteine-rich domain and carboxy terminus, while the amino-terminal domain interacts with actin or an actin-like protein.

By immunohistochemistry, dystrophin localizes to the cytoplasmic face of the muscle cell membrane and at post-synaptic membrane specializations in neurons. Dystrophin makes up only 0.002 % of total muscle protein but up to 5 % of the membrane skeleton. Dystrophin is found in skeletal muscle, smooth muscle, cardiac muscle, and brain. There are slightly different forms of dystrophin messenger RNA (mRNA) in different tissues due to different transcription start sites and alternative splicing. The function of dystrophin is not known for certain, but proposed functions include important roles for the organization and stabilization of the sarcolemma and in protection of muscle fibers from contraction-induced injury. Patients with DMD have very little or no detectable dystrophin, whereas BMD patients have an altered size and/or quantity of dystrophin [6]. However, the disease etiology may be more complex than a simple loss of dystrophin, because several of the dystrophin-associated proteins that interact with dystrophin also are absent. The dystrophin-associated proteins may be involved directly with the calcium flux in the dystrophic fibers. Thus, the loss of dystrophin may be the first of many steps that ultimately lead to muscular dystrophy.

Testing, utilizing complementary DNA (cDNA) probes derived from the 14 kb mRNA and multiplex polymerase chain reaction (PCR) analysis, has shown that approximately 65 % of the DMD/BMD cases are due to deletions in the dystrophin gene [7, 8]. The deletions are nonrandomly distributed and occur primarily in the center (~80 %) and less frequently near the 5′ end (~20 %) of the gene. The 200 kb region covering intron 44, exon 45, and intron 45 is the major deletion breakpoint region of the gene. The majority of the larger deletions initiate at the 5′ end of the gene.

The size or location of the deletion does not clearly correlate with the severity and progression of the disease. One of the largest deletions (35 exons) identified is in a mild BMD patient. Furthermore, sequences deleted in DMD patients often overlap with deletions in BMD patients. However, a theory was proposed that if a deletion disrupts the translational reading frame of the dystrophin mRNA triplet codons, then little or no dystrophin will be synthesized, most often resulting in the more severe disease, DMD [9]. In the milder disease, BMD, the deletion maintains the translational reading frame, and a partially functional protein is produced. The reading frame hypothesis explains the phenotypic differences observed in about 92 % of the DMD/BMD cases. One major exception to the reading frame hypothesis has been the identification of BMD patients with an out-of-frame deletion of exon 3 through exon 7. An alternate splicing mechanism or new cryptic translational start site may account for the production of an altered dystrophin protein and the milder phenotype in these patients. A small number of DMD patients with in-frame deletions also have been identified. The more severe phenotype in these patients may be due to the overall effect of the deletion on the protein conformation or may be the result of mRNA instability. Phenotypic variability even has been observed in several patients who share identical gene deletions. Deletion of exon 45, the most commonly observed DMD deletion, also has been associated with the BMD phenotype. Some genetic variability may be due to other molecules involved in destruction of damaged muscle fibers, in muscle regeneration, or in the cellular response to different hormones.

The large gene size, particularly of the introns, which average 35 kb, may account for part of the high deletion rate; however, in addition to size, other factors must be involved. The observed nonrandom deletion pattern may reflect domain-associated variation in chromosomal stability. For instance, complications related to the maintenance of replication, correct transcription, and proper splicing of such a large gene may play an extremely important role. Partial gene duplications have been identified in 5–8 % of patients. Unlike the deletion distribution, approximately 80 % of the duplications are located at the 5′ end of the gene and only 20 % in the central gene region. Out-of-frame duplications occur in DMD patients and in-frame duplications in BMD patients, thus suggesting that the reading-frame genotype-phenotype hypothesis also holds true for duplications.

Small mutations (point mutations and small deletions and duplications) in the dystrophin gene also have been identified in DMD patients [10]. The majority of these mutations have been unique to individual patients and have resulted in a truncated dystrophin protein lacking part or all of the C-terminus. The truncated proteins are presumably unstable, and little or no dystrophin is produced. Therefore, these types of mutations provide little information on structural/functional relationships in the dystrophin protein. The identification of DMD mutations that do not cause protein truncation may provide further insight into the function of dystrophin, as well as defining the essential regions and conformations necessary for dystrophin stability. A DMD missense mutation was found in the actin-binding domain [11]. The patient was shown to have correctly localized dystrophin, thus indicating that an intact actin-binding domain is essential for protein function and not just protein localization. The distribution of small mutations is fairly random throughout the gene sequence; however, whereas less than 5 % of the gene deletions are found upstream of exon 55, more than 40 % of the small mutations are located in this same region of the gene [12].

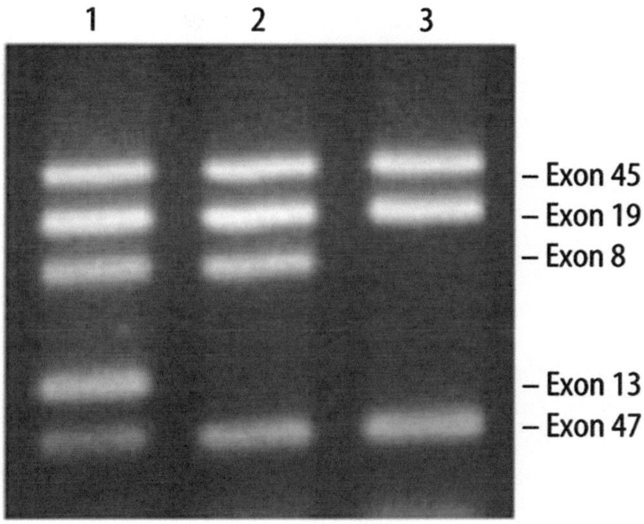

Figure 9.1 Multiplex DNA amplification of DMD exons 8, 13, 19, 45, and 47. *Lane 1*: normal control; *lane 2*: DMD patient with exon 13 deletion; *lane 3*: DMD patient with exon 8 and 13 deletions.

Clinical Utility of Testing and Available Testing

The most important impact of DNA testing for DMD/BMD has been on presymptomatic diagnosis and the correct diagnosis of patients with DMD/BMD-like symptoms, as well as for carrier detection and prenatal diagnosis. The western immunoblot is a sensitive protein test for the diagnosis of DMD or BMD, but requires a muscle biopsy from the patient. Proteins from the muscle biopsy specimen are separated by electrophoresis, transferred to a membrane, and incubated with antibodies against specific dystrophin domains. Dystrophin from unaffected patients is 427 kDa in size. The complete absence of dystrophin is very specific for the diagnosis of DMD, whereas the presence of an altered molecular weight form or reduced amount of dystrophin, or both, is consistent with BMD. It must be emphasized, however, that the clinical diagnosis and phenotype predictions should never be made exclusively on the basis of dystrophin western blot analysis. Patients with markedly reduced dystrophin levels may have the milder BMD phenotype. Furthermore, western blot analysis is generally not sensitive enough to detect female carriers. Lastly, a muscle biopsy, which some families may view as traumatic, is not necessary if a molecular diagnosis is secured first.

The genetic test methods commonly used to identify large rearrangements in the dystrophin gene are: Southern blot, multiplex PCR and multiplex ligation-dependent probe amplification (MLPA). Southern blot analysis using a full-length dystrophin cDNA clone as a probe detects deletions as well as gene duplications. The cDNA probes detect the site of the mutation, so meiotic recombination events are irrelevant. Therefore, the chance of diagnostic error is greatly reduced. Diagnostic strategies are based on initially identifying deletions/duplications in the affected patient [13]. The deletions are simply detected by examination of Southern blots for the presence or absence of each exon containing genomic restriction fragments, which hybridize to the cDNA probe, whereas duplications are detected as an increased intensity of the restriction fragment. From a practical perspective, Southern blot analysis requires the use of a radioisotope, is labor intensive, and is time consuming. Therefore most laboratories perform a deletion/duplication screen using either multiplex PCR [14] or MLPA [15].

Multiplex PCR simultaneously amplifies specific deletion prone exons within the *DMD* gene. Deletion of specific exons from a patient's sample results in absence of the corresponding ethidium bromide-stained amplification products by gel electrophoresis analysis (Fig. 9.1). Multiplex PCR, using primer sets for about 20–25 different exons, detects approximately 98 % of the deletions in the *DMD* gene. In contrast to Southern blot analysis, which may require several cDNA hybridizations and take several weeks to complete, multiplex PCR testing can be completed in one day. This makes the technique ideal for prenatal diagnosis, when time is critical. Additional refinements of the multiplex PCR assays have enabled the quantitative analysis of the DMD gene exons, allowing for the detection of duplications in males as well as deletions and duplications in carrier females.

Testing using MLPA has been utilized for both DMD deletion/duplication detection and carrier dosage determinations. The MLPA analysis has been shown to reproducibly generate each of the 79 DMD exons and their sizes should correspond to each probe pair. MLPA technology not only accurately detects deletions but also quantifies the copy number of each exon and therefore can be used for duplication and carrier determinations. Using capillary electrophoresis for analysis of the MLPA products, computer-aided scoring is a sensitive method to normalize the peak height or area of each PCR product to an endogenous two-copy control locus product. A heterozygous deletion should give a ratio of approximately 0.5 whereas an elevated copy number should give a reference value greater than 1.5. MLPA technology has been shown to exhibit a high degree of accuracy for the quantitative detection dystrophin exons, a high degree of reproducibility, and a capacity for testing a large number of samples simultaneously. One major limitation of MLPA technology is that DNA polymorphic sequence variants located under the probe-binding sites may interfere with probe hybridization and may result in false-positive results.

The identification of a deletion in a DMD patient not only confirms the diagnosis but also allows accurate carrier testing for other family members. Carrier status is determined by gene dosage analysis, which is used to assess whether a female at risk of being a carrier exhibits no reduction or 50 % reduction in band intensity for bands that are deleted in the affected male relative. A 50 % reduction (single-copy intensity) for the deleted band or bands indicates a deletion on one of her X chromosomes and confirms her carrier status. Southern blot, quantitative multiplex PCR, or MLPA can be used for gene dosage analysis. Dosage determinations permit direct carrier analysis and eliminate the inherent problems of linkage testing (recombinations, noninformative meioses, unavailability of family members, and spontaneous mutations). This is important since, unlike affected males, carrier females are generally asymptomatic, and creatine phosphokinase is elevated in only approximately two-thirds of known carriers.

As previously described, large genomic deletions and duplications have been identified in approximately two-thirds of the DMD/BMD population. The other mutations are due to smaller types of mutations within the dystrophin gene which require a sequence-based testing strategy. In most clinical molecular laboratories, these mutations have gone undetected because sequencing the entire gene is both expensive and labor intensive. With the advances in DNA sequencing technology, point mutation analysis of exons in the *DMD* gene is now feasible. The identification of these mutations is not only important for the confirmation of the diagnosis, but also important for the determination of carrier status. Due to the high mutation rate in the dystrophin gene, carrier testing based on indirect linkage results often is limited for extended family members of isolated cases of the disease. Knowledge of the exact causative mutation allows for the determination of the origin of the mutation in families with simplex cases of the disease.

Interpretation of Test Results

The analysis of gene mutations and protein determinations has greatly improved diagnosis, carrier detection, and prenatal counseling. Amplification techniques will confirm the clinical diagnosis in approximately 65 % of the DMD and BMD patients and should be performed as the initial molecular test due to the relatively common occurrence of deletions and duplications. If the patient tests negative by deletion/duplication analysis, gene sequencing of the coding regions and intron/exon boundaries should be performed. By gene sequencing, detection rates can be increased to greater than 90 %; however, even with sequencing, not all mutations are identified. Some of the undetected mutations may reside in the large dystrophin introns or in regulatory regions. Furthermore, genetic heterogeneity in the DMD phenotype may be another reason for less than 100 % sensitivity of testing. If there is any question of the diagnosis after negative results by molecular testing, western blot analysis of the dystrophin protein should be performed on a muscle biopsy specimen.

When gene dosage testing indicates that the mother does not have the deletion present in the affected child, she still has an uncertain risk of carrier status, due to the possibility of germline mosaicism [16]. Cases of germline mosaicism in DMD have been reported, in which a deletion is transmitted to more than one offspring by a mother who shows no evidence of the mutation in her somatic cells. Cases of germline mosaicism have important counseling implications. First and most obvious is the need to perform carrier studies on all female siblings of affected males, regardless of the outcome of testing for the mother. Furthermore, a negative deletion result in a mother does not rule out a recurrence risk for future pregnancies, and prenatal diagnosis still should be offered. The exact recurrence risk in germline female carriers is unknown because the risk is related to the percentage of the mutant clone in the mosaic mother. In these cases, the recurrence risk for subsequent pregnancies is significantly higher than a new mutation with a low recurrence risk. Mothers of apparently sporadic DMD cases have an estimated 15 % recurrence risk in future pregnancies.

Linkage analysis can provide valuable information but is limited by the possibility of recombination between the polymorphic marker and the unknown mutation, the presence of sporadic mutations, and unavailability of family members. The intragenic recombination rate over the entire length of the *DMD* gene is estimated to be as high as 12 %. The high recombinational error rate can be partially overcome by using microsatellite markers throughout the gene. Linkage analysis results often are extremely limited for extended family members of isolated cases of DMD/BMD, due to the possibility of the occurrence of a new mutation. Linkage analysis indicates only whether the female at risk inherited the same X chromosome as the affected male, not whether she is a carrier of a defective gene. Furthermore, since the gene mutation remains unidentified, a correct clinical diagnosis is essential. This is extremely important with patients presenting with the milder BMD phenotype, since this phenotype can overlap with other neuromuscular disorders.

Laboratory Issues

As a result of the discovery of the *DMD* gene and elucidation of the disease mutation spectrum, clinical diagnostic testing for DMD and BMD has significantly improved.

Until an effective treatment is found to cure or arrest the progression of the disease, prevention of new cases through accurate diagnosis, and carrier and prenatal testing is of the utmost importance. Furthermore, molecular therapies (such as antisense oligonucleotides, antibiotics, or chimeric RNA/DNA) are being applied according to the specific dystrophin mutation. This requires a comprehensive mutation analysis and identification of all types of dystrophin mutations. Although the majority of laboratories offer testing for dystrophin deletions and duplications, sequencing of the entire gene becomes necessary for all patients who are negative for the deletion/duplication screen. Proficiency testing for both *DMD* deletion/duplication testing and carrier testing is currently offered through the College of American Pathologists (CAP), and proficiency specimens are sent to participants twice per year.

Myotonic Dystrophy

Molecular Basis of Disease

Myotonic dystrophy type I (DM1) is the most common inherited form of muscular dystrophy affecting adults, with an incidence of approximately 1 in 8,000 individuals. DM1 is an autosomal dominant, multisystem disorder characterized by progressive muscle weakness, myotonia, intellectual impairment, cataracts, and cardiac arrhythmias. The diagnosis can be problematic because of the wide range and severity of symptoms. Often, affected individuals have children before they are diagnosed. A severe congenital form of DM results in mental retardation, respiratory distress, hypotonia, and in many cases death due to respiratory complications shortly after birth. Those that survive the neonatal period initially follow a static course, eventually learning to walk but with significant mental retardation. The congenital form is most often observed in the offspring of women who are themselves affected, although the disease in a mother may not be diagnosed until after the birth of a congenitally affected child [17].

The myotonic dystrophy protein kinase gene (*DMPK*) at chromosome 19q13.3 is the only known gene associated with DM1. The DM1 mutation involves an expanded CTG trinucleotide repeat, located at the 3′ untranslated region (UTR) of the *DMPK* gene [18–20]. The number of CTG triplets varies in the normal population from 5–34 repeats, and within this range the alleles are stably transmitted. Individuals with 35–49 repeats (premutation alleles) do not have symptoms but their children are at an increased risk of inheriting larger repeats and having symptoms. When the number of repeated CTGs exceeds 50 (in some patients up to several thousands), the allele becomes unstable and results in the DM1 phenotype. There is a significant correlation between the number of CTG repeats and the age of onset and clinical severity. Mildly affected patients have 50–100 repeats, and these patients may only have cataracts. More classically affected patients have 100–1,000 repeats and congenital cases often have 1,000–6,000 repeats. Somatic mosaicism of the CTG repeat occurs and results in patients with similar repeat sizes having different severity of symptoms, which calls for caution in genetic counseling. The trinucleotide repeat region is mitotically and meiotically unstable, with a bias towards length increase in the next generation, accounting for the clinical phenomenon of "anticipation" (increasing severity in successive generations of the same family, with earlier age of onset). Although repeat expansions occur through both maternal and paternal transmissions, the larger repeat expansions observed in congenital cases are almost exclusively due to maternal transmissions.

The CTG repeat is located within the 3′ UTR of the *DMPK* gene that encodes a protein kinase, named myotonin protein kinase. Since protein kinases are involved in signal transduction pathways in all cells in the body, a defective protein kinase was considered as a mechanism in which a single-gene defect could result in the diverse symptoms characteristic of DM1; however, since the repeat is not in the protein-coding region of *DMPK*, the molecular mechanism by which the mutation exerts its dominant expression is difficult to explain. One theory is that the myotonin kinase mRNA with long CUG repeats, and not the protein, results in a gain-of-function RNA pathogenesis [21, 22]. Novel RNA-binding proteins that specifically bind to CUG repeats may be depleted by excessive CUG repeats in the DM1 transcripts. Muscleblind-like protein (MBNL1) and CUG-binding protein (CUGBP1) are two RNA-binding proteins proposed to be involved in the pathogenesis. The depletion of these CUG-binding proteins causes splicing alterations of the chloride channel gene (*CLC1*) and the insulin receptor genes (*IR*), resulting in myotonia and insulin resistance, phenotypes that are related to the clinical features of DM1.

Clinical Utility of Testing and Available Testing

The majority of clinically significant mutations can be identified by Southern blot analysis; however, PCR is essential for the detection of smaller CTG expansions (<100 repeats). Although the PCR test is less expensive and faster than Southern blot analysis, longer repeats often are not reliably amplified. Southern blot analysis can be performed using *Hind*III restriction digestion and the probe pMDY1 [19], which spans the repeat region (Fig. 9.2). The probe pMDYI detects a *Hind*III polymorphism with normal alleles of 8.5 and 9.5 kb, the frequencies of which are approximately 0.6 and 0.4, respectively. The polymorphism is due to a 1 kb insertion telomeric to the CTG repeat, and is almost in complete linkage disequilibrium with the CTG repeat mutation in most populations [20]. The mutation is found on the larger 9.5 kb allele, suggesting that there were a limited number of

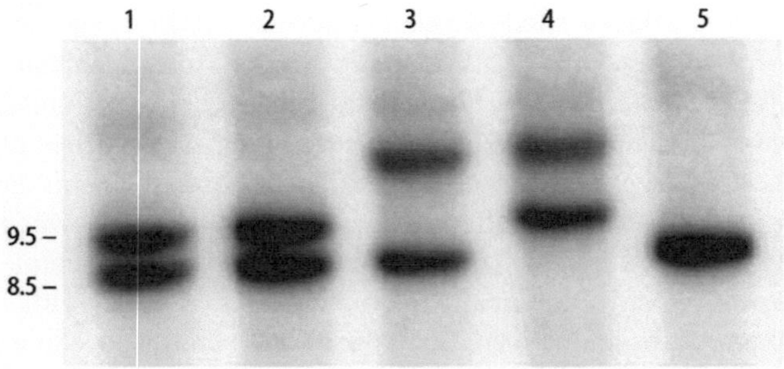

Figure 9.2 Autoradiogram of a Southern blot for myotonic dystrophy. Normal alleles are 8.5 and 9.5 kb. *Lanes 1, 2,* and *5*: unaffected individuals; *lanes 3* and *4*: expanded and normal alleles in DM patients with repeat expansions

ancestral mutations that occurred on a chromosome having the 1 kb insertion. Alternatively, the larger allele may be predisposed to DM1 mutations. Typical increases in the range of 1–4 kb are observed on Southern blots in the DM1 population. Many of the larger expansions are detected as smears, indicating somatic cell heterogeneity of the expanded alleles. Background signal may interfere with the detection of larger expanded alleles since expanded alleles often appear as diffuse smears due to the somatic instability of the mutation. The efficiency of the detection of these somatically variable expansions is increased by use of a restriction enzyme with a recognition sequence which occurs relatively infrequently in the human genome, which will generate a larger restriction fragment containing the expansion. (*Eco*RI creates a large 9–10 kb fragment.) The larger fragment lengths reduce the smearing effect of the somatic variability of the unstable repeats. Decreasing the electrophoretic migration also improves the detection of larger somatic mosaic expansions. Molecular testing can identify individuals who are asymptomatic or exhibit equivocal symptoms, such as cataracts. These smaller expansions are detected using alternate restriction enzymes which reduce the normal size fragment, such as *Bam*HI, or by PCR amplification across the repeat region. The most efficient approach for identifying expansions is a combination of different restriction enzymes and variation in electrophoretic duration. PCR amplification across the repeat region is used to exclude DM1 by demonstrating the presence of two different normal size alleles (8.5 and 9.5 kb). Since the heterozygosity frequency for the CTG repeats is approximately 75 % in the normal population, approximately 25 % of unaffected individuals will be homozygous for one normal allele. Therefore, the presence of a single PCR band does not confirm a diagnosis of DM1. All single bands require a Southern blot confirmation.

Several cases of reverse mutations have been reported in DM1, whereby there is a spontaneous correction of a deleterious expansion mutation upon transmission to an unaffected offspring. The mechanism for the DM1 reverse mutations remains unknown. A gene conversion mechanism, whereby the normal parental allele replaces the expanded allele, may best account for the reversion events in DM. The reversions may provide an explanation of the lack of penetrance observed in some DM families.

Interpretation of Test Results

PCR and/or Southern blot analysis for the *DMPK* CTG repeat region is used for symptomatic confirmatory diagnostic testing. Onset in adulthood typically presents with muscle weakness and myotonia. *DMPK* testing can be particularly useful in individuals for whom DM1 is part of a wider differential diagnosis, such as infants with muscular hypotonia. Prenatal problems, with congenital DM1, may be suspected when reduced fetal movements and polyhydramnios are observed on ultrasound. The testing also is helpful in identifying individuals who are asymptomatic or exhibit equivocal symptoms, such as cataracts. No new mutations have been described for DM1, which is consistent with the linkage disequilibrium data. To account for the maintenance of the mutation in the population, the theory developed that there is a high incidence of minimally expanded alleles in DM1 families which produce few symptoms and are stably transmitted over several generations [23]. For counseling purposes, testing can be used to identify the side of the family carrying the mutation, which is important for appropriate genetic counseling.

The triplet repeat size does correlate with muscular disability and is inversely related with the age of onset of the disease. However, there is a significant overlap of repeat size in patients with differing severity. When comparing unrelated affected individuals with small to moderate differences in repeat sizes, it is generally difficult to accurately predict the severity of the disease in each case. This is due to the overlap of triplet repeat size in patients with differing severity of the disease and the sometimes lack of a correlation between organ involvement and repeat size. As a result of the somatic heterogeneity observed in DM1, genotype/phenotype associations derived from leukocytes may not be as accurate as the measurement of the repeat size in the affected tissues (muscles, heart, others) [24]. Within a family, when a child has a significant increase in allele size compared to the parent, prediction of an earlier age of onset and more severe disease is more certain. Genetic counseling is very important not only for the affected patient, but also for other at-risk interested family members. DM1 testing can be used for prenatal diagnosis using either amniotic fluid cells or chorionic villus samples. Molecular testing has largely replaced muscle biopsy, muscle enzyme studies, and electromyography as the first diagnostic procedure.

Myotonic dystrophy type 2 (DM2, MIM 602668), previously termed proximal myotonic myopathy is due to a CCTG expansion located in intron 1 of the zinc finger protein 9 (*ZNF9*) gene on chromosome 3q21 [25]. Individuals affected with DM2 also have a complex clinical presentation that is similar to DM1, including myotonia, cardiac involvement, insulin insensitivity, and histological abnormalities in skeletal muscle. Patients with DM2 often can be distinguished from DM1 by more proximal muscle weakness and sparing of facial muscle involvement. Further distinguishing characteristic features of DM2 include muscle pain, the absence of congenital cases, and milder course of the disease without significant mental involvement.

Laboratory Issues

Many molecular pathology laboratories offer DNA testing for DM1. The majority of laboratories are using a combination of PCR and Southern blot testing. Although the PCR test is less expensive and faster than Southern blot, longer repeats are not reliably amplified. The availability of DNA testing has reduced the use of invasive (muscle biopsy) and noninvasive (electromyography) tests for the diagnosis of DM1. The combination of PCR and Southern blot analysis can detect all DM1 mutations. Proficiency testing is offered through the College of American Pathologists and proficiency specimens are sent to participants twice per year.

Spinal Muscular Atrophy

Molecular Basis of Disease

The autosomal recessive disorder proximal spinal muscular atrophy (SMA) is a severe neuromuscular disease characterized by degeneration of alpha motor neurons in the spinal cord, which results in progressive proximal muscle denervation and atrophy resulting in the symptoms of weakness and paralysis. SMA is the second-most common fatal autosomal recessive disorder after cystic fibrosis, with an estimated prevalence of 1 in 10,000 live births [26]. Childhood SMA is subdivided into clinical groups on the basis of age of onset and clinical course. Type I SMA (Werdnig-Hoffmann disease) is characterized by severe, generalized muscle weakness and hypotonia at birth or within the first 3 months after birth. Death from respiratory failure usually occurs within the first 2 years of life. Children affected with Type II SMA are able to sit, although they cannot stand or walk unaided, and survive beyond 4 years of age. Type III SMA (Kugelberg-Welander syndrome) is a milder form, with onset during infancy or youth, and patients may walk unaided. Type III SMA is further subdivided into two groups, type IIIa (onset before 3 years of age) and type IIIb (onset at age ≥3 years). Cases presenting with the first symptoms of the disease at the age of 20–30 years are classified as type IV, or proximal adult-type SMA. The described classification is based on age of onset and clinical course, although SMA demonstrates a continuous range of severity.

SMA is caused by mutations in the survival motor neuron (*SMN1*) gene which has nine exons [27]. Two almost identical *SMN* genes are present on 5q13: the telomeric *SMN1* gene that is the SMA-causing gene, and the centromeric *SMN2* gene. Exon 7 of the *SMN1* gene is deleted in approximately 95 % of affected patients, while small, more subtle mutations have been identified in the majority of the remaining affected patients. The genotypic explanation for the phenotypic variability results from variability in the number of *SMN2* gene copies, which influences the severity of the disease [28–30]. The number of *SMN2* gene copies varies from 0–3 copies in the normal population, with approximately 10 % of unaffected individuals having no gene copies of *SMN2*. However, milder patients with type II or III SMA on average have more gene copies of *SMN2* than do type I SMA patients. The extra *SMN2* gene copies are thought to arise through gene conversions, whereby the *SMN2* gene is copied either partially or totally into the telomeric *SMN1* locus.

SMA is caused by low levels of SMN protein rather than by a complete absence of the protein. Complete loss of SMN protein function results in loss of viability of a fetus and in utero death. SMA is possible because *SMN2* can partially replace the lost function of *SMN1*. Five base pair differences exist between *SMN1* and *SMN2* transcripts, and none of these differences change amino acids. The normal *SMN1* gene produces predominately a full-length transcript, whereas the *SMN2* gene produces predominately an alternate, exon-7-deleted product with only 10–20 % of transcripts being full-length. The inclusion of exon 7 in *SMN1* transcripts and exclusion of this exon in the majority of *SMN2* transcripts is caused by a single nucleotide difference at +6 in *SMN* exon 7, which alters splicing efficiency by disrupting an exonic splicing enhancer and results in absence of exon 7 in the majority of *SMN2* transcripts. The SMN exon 7 region encodes a highly conserved tyrosine-glycine (Y-G) dodecapeptide motif which is crucial for the oligomerization and function of the SMN protein [31]. SMA arises because the levels of full-length SMN protein from the *SMN1* gene are lost, and only partially rescued by the low number of full-length SMN protein from the *SMN2* gene. The *SMN2* gene cannot completely compensate for the lack of SMN protein; however, the small amounts of full-length transcript generated by *SMN2* are able to prevent in utero lethality. Additional copies of the *SMN2* gene result in greater amounts of full-length SMN protein and produce a milder type II or III phenotype.

SMN plays a role in small nuclear ribonucleoprotein (snRNP) biogenesis and function [32]. The SMN protein is required for pre-mRNA splicing. Immunofluorescence studies using a monoclonal antibody to the SMN protein demonstrate that the SMN protein is localized to novel nuclear structures called "gems," which display similarity to and possibly interact with coiled bodies, which are thought to play a role in the processing and metabolism of snRNAs. SnRNPs and possibly other splicing components require regeneration from inactivated to activated functional forms. SMN functions in the reassembly and regeneration of these splicing components. Mutant SMN, such as that present in SMA patients, lacks the splicing-regeneration activity of wild-type SMN. SMA may be the result of a genetic defect in spliceosomal snRNP biogenesis in motor neurons. Consequently, the motor neurons of SMA patients may be impaired in their capacity to produce specific mRNAs and as a result become deficient in proteins that are necessary for the growth and function of these cells. Possibly, the altered splicing of a unique set of premessenger RNAs results in deficient proteins, which are necessary for motor neuron growth and survival. In addition to its role in spliceosomal ribonucleoprotein assembly, SMN may have other functions in motor neurons. A subset of SMN complexes are located in axons and growth cones of motor neurons and may be involved in some aspects of axonal transport and localized translation of specific mRNAs.

Clinical Utility of Testing and Available Testing

The molecular diagnosis of SMA consists of the detection of the absence of exon 7 of the *SMN1* gene (Fig. 9.3). Although the gene region contains many repetitive elements and the centromeric *SMN2* copy is almost identical to the *SMN1* gene, an exonic base pair difference allows distinction of *SMN1* and *SMN2* PCR products using restriction-site generating PCR (RG-PCR) followed by restriction enzyme digestion. The absence of detectable *SMN1* exon 7 in SMA patients is utilized to diagnose SMA, with a sensitivity of approximately 95 %.

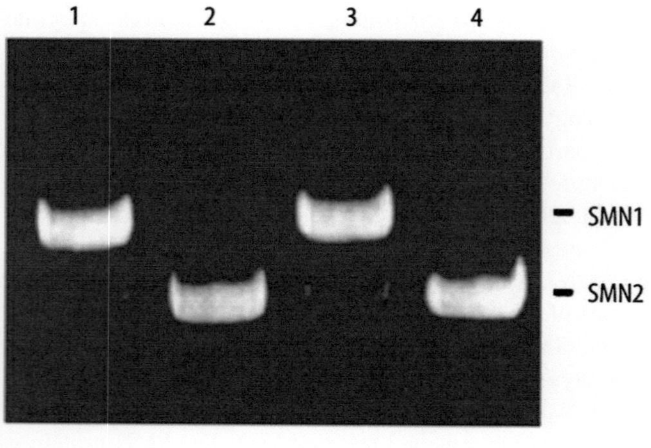

Figure 9.3 Restriction enzyme digestion of RG-PCR products distinguishes *SMN1* from *SMN2* exon 7 PCR products. *Lanes 1* and *3*: normal controls with *SMN1* present and *SMN2* deletion; *lanes 2* and *4*: SMA patients with *SMN1* deletion and *SMN2* present. *RG-PCR* restriction-site generating polymerase chain reaction.

Although the absence of both copies of exon 7 of the *SMN1* gene is a very reliable and sensitive test for SMA, about 5 % of affected patients have other types of mutations in the *SMN1* gene that will not be detected by homozygous exon 7 deletion testing. Due to the high deletion frequency, and according to the Hardy-Weinberg equilibrium, most of these patients will be compound heterozygotes, with one *SMN1* allele being deleted and the other allele containing a point mutation or other types of small mutations. Determination that a SMA patient has only a single copy of *SMN1* supports the diagnosis of SMA, with the possibility that the remaining *SMN1* gene contains a more subtle mutation, including nonsense mutations, missense mutations, splice site mutation insertions, and small deletions. These mutations have been essential in defining important structural and functional domains of the SMN protein. Many of the same intragenic mutations have been reported in unrelated patients [33, 34].

Since SMA is one of the most common lethal genetic disorders, with a carrier frequency of 1 in 40–60, carrier testing is useful to many families. *SMN1* dosage testing is used to determine the *SMN1* copy number and detect SMA carriers. Most carriers have one *SMN1* copy and most non-carriers will have two *SMN1* copies, or less frequently three *SMN1* copies. Carrier detection for the heterozygous state was initially shown to be more technically challenging because the SMA region is characterized by the presence of many repeated elements. In addition, the *SMN2* copy number varies with approximately 10–15 % of non-carriers lacking any *SMN2* copies, whereas many of the more mildly affected SMA patients have more *SMN2* copies. Thus, a straightforward dosage assay using the *SMN2* gene as the internal control would not be reliable. A number of techniques have been developed for the detection of SMA carriers. Quantitative PCR and MLPA assays are most often used for the identification of SMA carriers by determination of the number of copies of the *SMN1* gene as well as for the *SMN2* gene [35, 36].

Interpretation of Test Results

The presence of *SMN1* exon 7 does not entirely exclude a diagnosis of SMA. Although the absence of both copies of the *SMN1* gene is a very reliable and sensitive assay for the majority of SMA patients, about 5 % of affected patients have other types of mutations in the *SMN1* gene that will not be detected by PCR deletion testing. Most of these patients will be compound heterozygotes, with one *SMN1* allele deleted and the other allele with a point mutation or other small insertion or deletion. If the clinical suspicion remains high after a negative deletion test, then dosage carrier testing to determine whether there is a single copy of *SMN1* should be considered. If a patient with a SMA phenotype possesses only a single copy of *SMN1*, the remaining copy most likely contains a more subtle mutation, including nonsense mutations, missense mutations, splice site mutation insertions, and small deletions. A dosage testing result of two copies of the *SMN1* gene for a patient with an SMA phenotype greatly reduces the likelihood of SMA, although very rare cases of SMA can be due to two non-deletion mutations of *SMN1*.

The SMA carrier test has two limitations. First, approximately 2 % of SMA cases arise as the result of de novo mutation events, which is high compared to most autosomal recessive disorders [37]. The high rate of de novo mutations in *SMN1* may account for the high carrier frequency in the general population despite the genetic lethality of the type I disease. The large number of repeated sequences around the *SMN1* and *SMN2* locus likely predisposes this region to unequal crossovers and recombination events and results in the high de novo mutation rate. Second, the copy number of *SMN1* can vary on a chromosome; about 5 % of the normal population possess three copies of *SMN1* [28]. A carrier may have one chromosome 5 with two *SMN1* copies and the other chromosome 5 with zero *SMN1* copies, resulting in a two-copy carrier test result for a carrier. Using haploid conversion technique, which allows for single-chromosome analysis, Mailman et al. identified a parent of an affected child with two *SMN1* genes on one chromosome [38]. The finding of two *SMN1* genes on a single chromosome has serious genetic counseling implications, because a carrier with two *SMN1* genes on one chromosome and an *SMN1* deletion on the other chromosome will have the same dosage result as a non-carrier with one *SMN1* gene on each chromosome 5. Thus, the finding of normal two *SMN1* copy dosage significantly reduces the risk of being a carrier; however there is still a residual risk of being a carrier, and subsequently a small recurrence risk of future affected offspring for individuals with two *SMN1* gene copies. Risk assessment calculations using Bayesian analysis are essential for the proper genetic counseling of SMA families. A report has shown that there are significant differences among different ethnic groups in carrier frequencies and the two-copy chromosome genotypes [35]. The results from this study provide adjusted detection rates based on ethnicity, and thus allow for more accurate Bayesian risk estimates.

Laboratory Issues

Many molecular pathology laboratories offer testing for the homozygous deletion of *SMN1*. Most laboratories use PCR amplifications of exon 7 and exon 8 in two separate reactions, with restriction enzyme digestion to differentiate *SMN1* from *SMN2* PCR products, and report results for both *SMN1* exons 7 and 8. Some laboratories only test for exon 7 deletion. As a consequence of the *SMN1* gene being relatively small, and given the uniform spectrum of mutations, sequencing of the SMN1 gene is relatively straightforward and can identify mutations in patients who are negative for the diagnostic homozygous deletion test. However, it is necessary to verify that the intragenic mutation has occurred in the *SMN1* gene and not the *SMN2* gene. As an initial screen, primers that do not distinguish between *SMN1* and *SMN2* often are used to amplify each exon for direct DNA sequencing. If variants or mutations are identified, *SMN1*-specific long-range PCR amplification is followed by either direct DNA sequencing of that long-range product or nested PCR sequencing. Carrier testing is performed by a fewer number of clinical molecular laboratories. Proficiency testing for the homozygous *SMN1* deletion is offered by the CAP. These proficiency specimens are sent to participants twice per year. External proficiency testing is not available for carrier testing, so proficiency testing most often is achieved by specimen exchange between laboratories performing carrier testing.

Mitochondrial Encephalomyopathies

Molecular Basis of Disease

Mitochondria are semiautonomous replicating cellular organelles containing genetic material. Each mitochondrion contains multiple copies of the mitochondrial DNA genome (mtDNA), with replication, transcription, and translation machineries separate from these cellular functions. Human mtDNA encodes 13 polypeptides of the respiratory chain subunits, 28 ribosomal RNAs (rRNAs), and 22 transfer RNAs (tRNAs) in a circular double-stranded genome of approximately 16.5 kb.

Unlike nuclear DNA, in which each cell contains pairs of chromosomes, one of maternal and the other of paternal origin, mtDNA is inherited exclusively from the mother. This type of transmission is called maternal inheritance, since the sperm's mitochondria do not contribute to the zygote. Although both sexes are equally affected by mitochondrial diseases, inheritance of the disorder is from the mother. Mitochondrial mutations are often present in only some of the mtDNA molecules of a cell (heteroplasmy). Heteroplasmy occurs because mitochondria segregate randomly into daughter cells during mitosis, which results in cells containing both mutant and wild-type mtDNA. Thus, the proportion of heteroplasmic mutation may vary widely between different tissues or even between different cells of the same tissue. The proportion of mutant to wild-type mtDNA plays a role in determining the clinical variability and severity often observed in the mitochondrial disorders. The phenotype-genotype correlation in the mitochondrial disorders is complex and influenced by age, the type and extent of respiratory chain disruption caused by the mutation, and the tissue-specific threshold for the pathogenic effect.

The term "mitochondrial encephalomyopathies" is used to describe mitochondrial disorders in which both muscle and the central nervous system are affected. These disorders affect multiple systems, with diverse clinical features due to defects in the mitochondrial function. Mitochondrial diseases are individually uncommon, but collectively pose a significant burden to human health. This chapter is restricted to those disorders in which the mutation event involves mtDNA, in contrast to the many nuclear genetic disorders that result in mitochondrial pathology. This occurs when the nuclear encoded protein functions in the mitochondria, which are described in Chap. 10. This chapter discusses Kearns-Sayre syndrome (KSS), mitochondrial encephalomyopathy with lactic acidosis and stroke-like episodes (MELAS), and myoclonic epilepsy with ragged-red fibers (MERRF).

Kearns-Sayre Syndrome

The common features of KSS include progressive external ophthalmoplegia (PEO), pigmentary degeneration of the retina, and defects of cardiac conduction [39]. The typical affected patient presents before the age of 20 years with PEO and pitosis, followed by development of pigmentary retinal degeneration and cardiac conduction block. Other features of the disorder may include ataxia, deafness, dementia, and diabetes mellitus. The most common type of mutation found in KSS is a deletion in the mtDNA (Fig. 9.4), and almost of all these deletions occur sporadically [40]. Approximately one third of KSS cases are due to a common 4,977 bp deletion, which is associated with direct repeats at the deletion junction. The severity of KSS depends on the extent of heteroplasmy and the tissue distribution of structurally altered mtDNA. An extreme KSS phenotype occurs when the frequency of deleted mtDNA in muscle cells is greater than 85 %. In contrast, when lower levels of heteroplasmy for the deletion are present, then PEO may be the only symptom.

Mitochondrial Encephalomyopathy with Lactic Acidosis and Stroke-Like Episodes

Patients with MELAS are usually normal at birth but develop stunted growth, intermittent vomiting, seizures, and recurrent cerebral insults resembling strokes during the first years of life [41]. An episodic course follows, with recurrent stroke-like episodes, only partial recovery, and eventual deterioration, with death from respiratory failure often before 20 years of age. Milder adult-onset cases have been reported. Approximately 80 % of all MELAS cases are the result of an m.3243A>G point mutation in the mtDNA gene encoding mt-tRNA(Leu) [42]. The point mutation alters the normal structural conformation of the tRNA, thereby impairing protein synthesis. The m.3243A>G mutation occurs in the heteroplasmic state, with variation among different tissue types. When the mutation is present in greater than 90 % of the mtDNA of the muscle tissue, there is increased likelihood of recurrent strokes and classic MELAS manifestations. However, when the heteroplasmy of the mutation is less than 90 %, later onset and more moderate symptoms may occur.

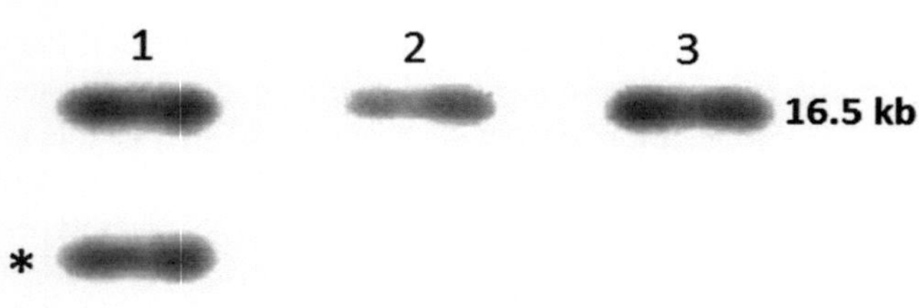

Figure 9.4 Autoradiogram of a Southern blot of muscle mitochondrial DNA. *Lane 1*: Kearns-Sayre patient with heteroplasmic deletion; *lanes 2* and *3*: unaffected individuals. The normal allele is 16.5 kb and the deleted allele fragment is indicated by the *asterisk*.

Myoclonic Epilepsy with Ragged-Red Fibers

MERRF is a rare mitochondrial disorder with symptoms including muscle weakness, myoclonus, generalized seizures, ataxia, and deafness [43]. The hallmark morphologic change seen in the muscle biopsy is the ragged-red fibers. The term "ragged-red fibers" refers to large clumps of abnormal mitochondria that accumulate beneath the sarcolemma and stain red with the Gomori trichome stain. The majority of MERRF cases are the result of a point mutation (m.8344A>G) in the mt-tRNA(Lys) gene. The MERRF mutation, like the MELAS mt-tRNA(Leu) mutation, diminishes overall mitochondrial protein synthesis. Similar to the other mitochondrial disorders, a more classic MERRF phenotype is observed when the mutation is present at higher levels in the muscle and nerve.

Clinical Utility of Testing and Available Testing

The symptoms of the mitochondrial disorders often are nonspecific and are common to many other neuromuscular diseases. The diversity of clinical syndromes allows mitochondrial disease to appear in the differential diagnosis of almost any neurological condition, from stroke to myopathy. As a result, the mitochondrial diseases often are considered only after many other diagnoses have been excluded. However, genetic testing for mitochondrial diseases is becoming increasingly available. Southern blot analysis or long-range PCR is used to detect the deletions observed in KSS, using DNA from a muscle biopsy. PCR-RFLP testing is used for the common tRNA point mutations found in MERRF and MELAS. Patients with MERRF have high levels of the mutant mtDNA in the blood, and therefore blood is an appropriate specimen for testing. In contrast, patients with the MELAS mutation often have low levels of the mutation in the blood, leading to false-negative results when blood is used for testing, such that DNA from a muscle biopsy is preferred for testing.

Interpretation of Test Results

If clinical suspicion is strong and the blood results are negative, then mtDNA from a muscle biopsy should be tested. Since the disorders are highly clinically heterogeneous and there is considerable phenotypic overlap, the classic MERRF and MELAS point mutations and the KSS deletions frequently are ordered together and tested as a mitochondrial test panel. The m.8344A>G MERRF mutation is associated with other phenotypes, including Leigh syndrome, myoclonus or myopathy with truncal lipomas, and proximal myopathy. The m.3243A>G MELAS mutation can result in milder phenotypes, including sensorineural deafness with diabetes. Furthermore, these mutations sometimes are found in asymptomatic relatives of the index case.

Laboratory Issues

If the common mtDNA mutations are not detected, more extensive testing for rarer mutations may be useful for diagnosis. Sequencing of the mtDNA is available from several clinical molecular laboratories, which may identify a novel mutation; however, since the mtDNA is very polymorphic, novel mutations must be verified for functional effects.

Kennedy Disease

Molecular Basis of Disease

Spinal and bulbar muscular atrophy (SBMA), or Kennedy disease, is a rare X-linked, slowly progressive, adult-onset motor neuropathy [44]. The age of onset is usually 30–50 years of age and is characterized by muscle cramps, proximal and bulbar weakness, and fasciculation. Endocrine abnormalities, including gynecomastia and testicular atrophy, are common. The disease is caused by a CAG trinucleotide repeat expansion in the coding region of the androgen receptor gene (*AR*) [45]. The CAG repeat found within the first exon of *AR* is polymorphic in normal populations, and ranges in length from 10–36 repeats. Patients with SBMA have a CAG repeat expansion that does not overlap with the normal population and ranges from 40–62 repeats. Similar to other trinucleotide repeat disorders, the number of CAG repeats correlates with disease severity and inversely with age of onset. Considerable variability in age of onset is seen among family members with similar CAG repeat lengths, suggesting that factors other than just the size of the repeat modulate the onset and severity of the disease. While CAG repeats in the unaffected range are stably transmitted, expanded CAG repeats are transmitted less stably and tend to increase in size by paternal transmission.

The pathogenic mechanism of SBMA expansion involves gain of a toxic function of the protein product. The mutant allele is both transcribed and translated, arguing against a loss of function mechanism. Individuals with mutations producing a loss of AR protein function have testicular feminization and do not have the motor neuropathy seen in SBMA patients. The exact mechanism by which the expanded polyglutamine tract in the AR protein produces the neuropathy of SBMA is uncertain.

Clinical Utility of Testing and Available Testing

Despite distinct clinical features, SBMA is often misdiagnosed due to the heterogeneity of manifestations and lack of full expression in some family members. Many of the cases are sporadic, and some patients have only mild signs of motor neuron disease and mild gynecomastia. Amyotrophic lateral sclerosis, type III SMA, hereditary motor and sensory neuropathy, limb-girdle muscular dystrophy, and facioscapulohumeral muscular dystrophy are included in the differential diagnosis for some patients affected with SBMA [46]. PCR amplification of the repeat sequence within the first exon of the *AR* gene accurately determines the number of CAG repeats and is used for the diagnosis of SBMA. In addition, carrier females and young asymptomatic males may be identified by molecular testing for a repeat expansion with implications for genetic counseling and potential early treatment.

Interpretation of Test Results

The definitive diagnosis of SBMA is by the analysis of the CAG repeat in the *AR* gene from a blood or buccal specimen without the need for a muscle biopsy. All patients with SBMA have a CAG repeat expansion, and no other related mutations in the *AR* gene have been identified. Some studies have described a correlation between repeat size and age of onset, but interfamilial and intrafamilial variation is large for any given repeat length [46].

Laboratory Issues

Several clinical molecular laboratories offer DNA testing for SBMA. The PCR test is accurate and requires only a blood sample. PCR with electrophoretic analysis of the PCR products allows for accurate assessment of the repeat size. External proficiency testing currently is not available for SBMA.

References

1. Emery AEH. Muscle histology and creatine kinase levels in the fetus in Duchenne muscular dystrophy. Nature. 1977;266:472–3.
2. Moser H. Duchenne muscular dystrophy: pathogenetic aspects and genetic prevention. Hum Genet. 1984;66:17–34.
3. Hoffman EP, Brown RH, Kunkel LM. Dystrophin: the protein product of the Duchenne muscular dystrophy locus. Cell. 1987;51:919–28.
4. Koenig M, Hoffman EP, Bertelson CJ, et al. Complete cloning of the Duchenne muscular dystrophy (DMD) cDNA and preliminary genomic organization of the DMD gene in normal and affected individuals. Cell. 1987;50:509–17.

5. Ahn AH, Kunkel LM. The structural and functional diversity of dystrophin. Nat Genet. 1993;3:283–7.
6. Hoffman EP, Fischbeck K, Brown RH, et al. Dystrophin characterization in muscle biopsies from Duchenne and Becker muscular dystrophy patients. N Engl J Med. 1988;318:1363–8.
7. Darras BT, Blattner P, Harper JF, et al. Intragenic deletions in 21 Duchenne muscular dystrophy (DMD)/Becker muscular dystrophy (BMD) families studied with the dystrophin cDNA: location of breakpoints on HindIII and BglII exon-containing fragment maps, meiotic and mitotic origin of mutations. Am J Hum Genet. 1988;43:620–9.
8. Forrest SM, Cross GS, Flint T, et al. Further studies of gene deletions that cause Duchenne and Becker muscular dystrophies. Genomics. 1988;2:109–17.
9. Monaco AP, Bertelson CJ, Liechti-Gallati S, et al. An explanation for the phenotypic differences between patients bearing partial deletions of the DMD locus. Genomics. 1988;2:90–5.
10. Roberts RG, Gardner RJ, Bobrow M. Searching for the 1 in 2,400,000: a review of dystrophin gene point mutations. Hum Mutat. 1994;4:1–11.
11. Prior TW, Papp AC, Snyder PJ, et al. A missense mutation in the dystrophin gene in a Duchenne muscular dystrophy patient. Nat Genet. 1993;4:357–61.
12. Prior TW, Bartolo C, Pearl DK, et al. Spectrum of small mutations in the dystrophin coding region. Am J Hum Genet. 1995;57:22–33.
13. Prior TW, Friedman KJ, Highsmith WE, et al. Molecular probe protocol for determining carrier status in Duchenne and Becker muscular dystrophies. Clin Chem. 1990;36:441–6.
14. Chamberlain JS, Gibbs RA, Ranier JE, et al. Deletion screening of the Duchenne muscular dystrophy locus via multiplex DNA amplification. Nucleic Acids Res. 1988;16:11141–56.
15. Lalic T, Vossen RH, Coffa J, et al. Deletion and duplication screening in the *DMD* gene using MLPA. Eur J Hum Genet. 2005;13:1231–4.
16. Bakker E, Van Broeckhoven C, Bonten EJ, et al. Germline mosaicism and Duchenne muscular dystrophy mutations. Nature. 1987;329:554–7.
17. Harper PS. Congenital myotonic dystrophy in Britain, II: genetic basis. Arch Dis Child. 1975;50:514–21.
18. Brook HG, McCurrach ME, Harley HG, et al. Molecular basis of myotonic dystrophy: expansion of a trinucleotide (CTG) repeat at the 3′ end of a transcript encoding a protein kinase family. Cell. 1992;68:799–808.
19. Fu YH, Pizzuti A, Fenwick R, et al. An unstable triplet repeat in a gene related to myotonic muscular dystrophy. Science. 1992;255:1256–8.
20. Mahadevan M, Tsilfidis C, Sabourin L, et al. Myotonic dystrophy mutation: an unstable CTG repeat in the 3′ untranslated region of the gene. Science. 1992;255:1253–5.
21. Ranum LP, Day JW. Myotonic dystrophy: RNA pathogenesis comes into focus. Am J Hum Genet. 2004;74:793–804.
22. Sabouri LA, Mahadevan MS, Narang M, et al. Effect of the myotonic dystrophy mutation on mRNA levels of the DM gene. Nat Genet. 1993;4:233–8.
23. Barcelo JM, Mahadevan MS, Tsilfidis C, et al. Intergenerational stability of the myotonic dystrophy protomutation. Hum Mol Genet. 1993;2:705–9.
24. Anvret M, Ahlberg G, Grandell U, et al. Larger expansions of the CTG repeat in muscle compared to lymphocytes from patients with myotonic dystrophy. Hum Mol Genet. 1993;2:1397–400.
25. Liquori C, Ricker K, Mosley M, et al. Myotonic dystrophy type 2 caused by a CCTG expansion in intron 1 of ZNF9. Science. 2001;293:864–7.
26. Pearn J. Incidence, prevalence, and gene frequency studies of chronic childhood spinal muscular atrophy. J Med Genet. 1978;15:409–13.
27. Lefebvre S, Burglen L, Reboullet S, et al. Identification and characterization of a spinal muscular atrophy-determining gene. Cell. 1995;80:155–65.
28. McAndrew PE, Parsons DW, Simard LR, et al. Identification of proximal spinal muscular atrophy carriers and patients by analysis of SMNT and SMNC gene copy number. Am J Hum Genet. 1997;60:1411–22.
29. Mailman MD, Heinz JW, Papp AC, et al. Molecular analysis of spinal muscular atrophy and modification of the phenotype by SMN2. Genet Med. 2002;4:20–6.
30. Velasco E, Valero C, Valero A, Moreno F, Hernandez-Chico C. Molecular analysis of the SMN and NAIP genes in Spanish spinal muscular atrophy (SMA) families and correlation between number of copies of cBCD 541 and SMA phenotype. Hum Mol Genet. 1996;5:257–63.
31. Talbot K, Ponting CP, Theodosiou AM, et al. Missense mutation clustering in the survival motor neuron gene: a role for a conserved tyrosine and glycine rich region of the protein RNA metabolism? Hum Mol Genet. 1997;6:497–501.
32. Liu Q, Dreyruss G. A novel nuclear structure containing the survival of motor neurons protein. EMBO J. 1996;15:3355–65.
33. Wirth B. An update of the mutation spectrum of the survival motor neuron gene (*SMN1*) in autosomal recessive spinal muscular atrophy. Hum Mutat. 2000;15:228–37.
34. Parsons DW, McAndrew PE, Iannaccone ST, et al. Intragenic telSMN mutations: frequency, distribution, evidence of a founder effect and modification of spinal muscular atrophy phenotype by cenSMN copy number. Am J Hum Genet. 1998;63:1712–23.
35. Hendrickson BC, Donohoe C, Akmaev VR, et al. Differences in *SMN1* allele frequencies among ethnic groups within North America. J Med Genet. 2009;46:641–4.
36. Huang C-H, Chang Y-Y, Chen C-H. Copy number analysis of survival motor neuron genes by multiplex ligation-dependent probe amplification. Genet Med. 2007;9:241–8.
37. Wirth B, Rudnik-Schoneborn S, Hahnen E, et al. Prenatal prediction in families with autosomal recessive proximal spinal muscular atrophy (5q11.2-q13.3): molecular genetics and clinical experience in 109 cases. Prenat Diagn. 1995;15:407–17.
38. Mailman MD, Hemingway T, Darsey RL, et al. Hybrids monosomal for human chromosome 5 reveal the presence of a spinal muscular atrophy (SMA) carrier with two *SMN1* copies on one chromosome. Hum Genet. 2001;108:109–15.
39. Berenberg R, Pellock J, DiMauro S, et al. Lumping or splitting? "Ophthalmopelgia-plus" or Kearns-Sayre syndrome? Ann Neurol. 1977;1:37–42.
40. Moraes CT, DiMauro S, Zeviani M, et al. Mitochondrial DNA deletions in progressive external ophthalmoplegia and Kearns-Sayre syndrome. N Engl J Med. 1989;320:1293–9.
41. Hirano M, Ricci E, Koenigsberger MR, et al. MELAS: an original case and clinical criteria for diagnosis. Neuromuscul Disord. 1992;2:125–35.
42. Goto Y, Nonaka I, Horai S. A mutation in the tRNALeu (UUR) gene associated with the MELAS subgroup of mitochondrial encephalomyopathies. Nature. 1990;348:651–3.
43. Silvestri G, Ciafaloni E, Santorelli FM, et al. Clinical features associated with the A>G transition at nucleotide 8344 of mtDNA ("MERRF mutation"). Neurology. 1993;43:1200–6.
44. Kennedy WR, Alter M, Sung JH. Progressive proximal spinal and bulbar muscular atrophy of late onset: a sex-linked recessive trait. Neurology. 1968;18:671–80.
45. La Spada AR, Wilson AR, Lubahn DB. Androgen receptor mutations in X-linked spinal muscular atrophy. Nature. 1991;353:77–9.
46. Amato AA, Prior TW, Barohn R, Snyder P, Papp A, Mendell JR. Kennedy's disease: a clinicopathologic correlation with mutations in the androgen receptor gene. Neurology. 1993;43:791–4.

Mitochondrial Disorders

10

Renkui Bai and Jaimie D. Higgs

Abstract

Mitochondrial disorders, also known as mitochondrial respiratory chain (RC) disorders, or oxidative phosphorylation (OXPHOS) disorders, are a heterogeneous group of disorders resulting from primary dysfunction of the mitochondrial respiratory chain or ATR synthesis. Mitochondrial disorders may affect a single organ, but many involve multiple organ systems particularly those that are highly dependent on aerobic metabolism (brain, skeletal muscle, heart, kidney, and endocrine system). This chapter describes mitochondrial diseases resulting from OXPHOS deficiency and genes directly and/or indirectly involved in the respiratory chain and ATP synthesis.

Keywords

Mitochondria • Oxidative phosphorylation • Leber Hereditary Optic Neuropathy, LHON • Kearns–Sayre syndrome • Chronic progressive external ophthalmoplegia, CPEO • Mitochondrial encephalomyopathy with lactic acidosis and stroke-like episodes, MELAS • Myoclonic epilepsy with ragged-red fibers, MERRF • Neurogenic weakness with ataxia and retinitis pigmentosa, NARP • Leigh syndrome • Mitochondrial neurogastrointestinal encephalopathy • MNGIE • Alpers syndrome

Introduction

Mitochondria are DNA-containing intracellular organelles with multiple functions. The major function of mitochondria is production of adenosine triphosphate (ATP) through oxidative phosphorylation (OXPHOS), which includes the oxygen-consuming respiratory chain (RC) and ATP synthesis that provides about 90 % of the energy needed by the cell. In addition, mitochondria also are home to many other metabolic pathways, including the tricarboxylic acid cycle, protein import, fatty acid and amino acid oxidation, apoptosis, and biosynthesis of ketone bodies, pyrimidines, heme, and urea. Mitochondrial disorders, also known as mitochondrial RC disorders, or OXPHOS disorders, are a heterogeneous group of disorders resulting from primary dysfunction of the mitochondrial RC or ATP synthesis. Mitochondrial disorders may affect a single organ, but many involve multiple organ systems, particularly those that are highly dependent on aerobic metabolism (brain, skeletal muscle, heart, kidney, and endocrine system). Patients may present at any age. Some affected individuals exhibit clinical features that fall into a discrete clinical syndrome, such as Leber Hereditary Optic Neuropathy (LHON), Kearns–Sayre syndrome (KSS), chronic progressive external ophthalmoplegia (CPEO), mitochondrial encephalomyopathy with lactic acidosis and stroke-like episodes (MELAS), myoclonic epilepsy with ragged-red fibers (MERRF), neurogenic weakness with ataxia and retinitis pigmentosa (NARP), Leigh syndrome (LS), mitochondrial neurogastrointestinal encephalopathy (MNGIE), or Alpers syndrome (progressive neuronal degeneration of

R. Bai, M.D., Ph.D., F.A.C.M.G. (✉)
Genetic Testing for Mitochondrial Disorders, GeneDx, 207 Perry Parkway, Gaithersburg, MD 20877, USA
e-mail: renkui@genedx.com

J.D. Higgs, M.S., C.G.C.
GeneDx, Gaithersburg, MD, USA

D.G.B. Leonard (ed.), *Molecular Pathology in Clinical Practice*, DOI 10.1007/978-3-319-19674-9_10

children with liver disease). However, often the clinical features are highly variable and nonspecific, and many affected individuals do not fit well into one particular category. Common features of mitochondrial disorders may include, but are not limited to, ptosis, external ophthalmoplegia, proximal myopathy, exercise intolerance, cardiomyopathy, gastrointestinal reflux, liver failure, sensorineural deafness, optic atrophy, pigmentary retinopathy, diabetes mellitus, encephalopathy, seizures, migraines, stroke-like episodes, ataxia, spasticity, chorea, and dementia. The prevalence of mitochondrial disorders has been estimated at 1 in 5,000 to 8,500 [1–4].

This chapter describes mitochondrial diseases resulting from OXPHOS deficiency and genes directly and/or indirectly involved in the RC and ATP synthesis. This chapter does not include other pathways in the mitochondria, such as pyruvate dehydrogenase metabolism, fatty acid beta-oxidation, the urea cycle, the methionine metabolism pathway, and other mitochondrial functions.

Molecular Basis of Mitochondrial Disorders

Mitochondrial disorders result from dysfunction of one or more of the OXPHOS complexes. The OXPHOS system consists of about 90 structural proteins (subunits) assembled into five multiprotein enzyme complexes (Complex I to V) embedded in the inner mitochondrial membrane. Thirteen of the structural protein subunits are encoded by the mitochondrial genome (referred to as mtDNA), and the rest are encoded by nuclear genes. Complex I (NADH dehydrogenase, also called NADH:ubiquinone oxidoreductase) consists of approximately 46 structural protein subunits, seven encoded by mtDNA and approximately 39 encoded by nuclear genes. Complex II (succinate dehydrogenase or SDH) consists of four protein subunits: SDHA, SDHB, SDHC, and SDHD, all encoded by nuclear genes. Complex III (cytochrome bc1 complex) consists of 11 subunits, 1 encoded by mtDNA and the rest encoded by nuclear genes. Complex IV (cytochrome c oxidase) consists of 13 protein subunits, three encoded by mtDNA and the rest encoded by nuclear genes. Complex V (ATP synthase) consists of approximately 18 subunits, two encoded by mtDNA and the rest encoded by nuclear genes. In addition to the structural subunits of the OXPHOS system, many nuclear gene-encoded proteins are involved in the biosynthesis, maintenance, transcription, and translation of mtDNA, and in the assembly of the OXPHOS complexes. The two ribosomal RNAs (rRNAs) (12S and 16S) and 22 transfer RNAs (tRNAs) encoded by mtDNA also are involved in the translation processes of the mitochondrial genome.

Mitochondrial disorders can be caused by mutations in mtDNA, as well as mutations in nuclear genes. Approximately 29 % of patients (approximately 15–20 % pediatric and approximately 40 % adult) with primary mitochondrial disorders are caused by mutations in mtDNA, and the remainders likely are caused by nuclear defects [5–8]. Most of the nuclear gene-encoded proteins are synthesized in the cytoplasm and imported into mitochondria. Although there are more than 1,000 proteins in the mitochondria, only approximately 77 nuclear gene-encoded proteins are structural subunits of the five OXPHOS complexes [9], and only 200–300 proteins are directly or indirectly involved in the buildup and primary function of the OXPHOS complexes [10]. The rest of the proteins, which are not involved in the composition or primary function of the OXPHOS system, are components of the numerous other mitochondrial pathways. Although mutations in genes encoding proteins not involved in the OXPHOS functions do not cause a primary mitochondrial OXPHOS disorder, the diseases caused by mutations in non-OXPHOS genes may have features that overlap with those of primary mitochondrial disorders, or may cause secondary dysfunction of the mitochondrial RC system [11–13]. Disorders due to nuclear gene mutations that affect mitochondrial function may be inherited in an autosomal dominant, autosomal recessive, or X-linked manner.

Mutations in the Mitochondrial Genome

Human mtDNA encodes for two rRNAs, 22 tRNAs, and 13 proteins that are part of the respiratory chain. Mutations in mtDNA are either maternally inherited or arise de novo. In most cases, mtDNA point mutations are inherited, whereas gross deletions arise de novo [14]. Each mitochondrion has multiple copies of mtDNA and there are hundreds to thousands of mitochondria per cell, which varies based on the cell type. Usually, mutations affect only a fraction of the mtDNA; the coexistence of normal and mutant mtDNA is called heteroplasmy. In general, the disease severity correlates with the level of mutant mtDNA. When the percentage of mutant mtDNA (mutation load) reaches a certain threshold that varies by tissue type, age, and specific mutation, the function of that tissue is impaired [14]. As the mutation load varies within and between tissues, the manifestation of mitochondrial disease may reflect tissue-specific mutation load [2]. In certain tissues, like blood, there may be selection against some of these mutations, so that cells with normal mtDNA are selectively retained. For some mutations, the mutation load in the peripheral blood may decrease with age. Mutations in mtDNA may only be identified in specific tissues, particularly those with a lower rate of cell division such as skeletal muscle, heart, and brain [14].

During oogenesis, only a small subset of mtDNA molecules from the mother is passed into the germ cells that will become the next generation (bottleneck effect): therefore, the inheritance of mitochondrial DNA disorders within families is difficult to predict. A mother can pass on a small proportion or a high proportion of mutant mtDNA to her children, making the difference between a child being born without disease and another having a very severe form of the disease, respectively. The types of mtDNA mutations include quality defects (point mutations, deletions, duplications, and complex rearrangements) and quantity defects (mtDNA copy number changes including depletion and over-replication). To date, more than 400 definitive or likely pathogenic point mutations and more than 120 single deletions/duplications or complex rearrangements have been reported in the mtDNA mutation database Mitomap (www.mitomap.org).

MtDNA Point Mutations

MtDNA point mutations account for approximately 80 % of patients with primary mtDNA disorders [1]. Of the over 400 point mutations with disease associations in the Mitomap database (www.mitomap.org), about 58 (or approximately 14 %) are recurrent, definitive mutations and account for 70–80 % of patients with mitochondrial disorders associated with primary mtDNA point mutations [1]. The rest either are seen in a single family or lack solid evidence of the pathogenicity of the mutation. Overall, these point mutations, either definitive or reported, can be divided into three major classes [15]: (1) mutations in the protein-coding genes associated with LHON; (2) mutations in the protein-coding genes associated with other phenotypes; and (3) mutations in tRNA and rRNA genes associated with various multisystem disorders.

The LHON mutations have been subclassified into two main categories [15]. The first category includes well characterized and causative mutations designated the primary LHON mutations. This group includes the three most common LHON mutations (m.3460G>A, m.11778G>A, and m.14484T>C) and accounts for approximately 95 % of LHON patients. The second category includes mutations that have been reported in a single family and thus require additional independent reports to confirm their causal association with LHON (www.mitomap.org). These mutations usually appear to be homoplasmic, although heteroplasmic mutations are seen in a small percentage of patients and family members [16]. LHON mutations usually are associated with reduced penetrance; only about 50 % of males and 10 % of females harboring a primary pathogenic mutation suffer visual loss, and the severity of visual loss among members of the same family is highly variable [17, 18]. This marked incomplete penetrance, gender bias, and intra-family variability could be due to the level of heteroplasmy of the mutation, additional mitochondrial and/or nuclear genetic factors modulating the phenotypic expression of LHON, or environmental factors contributing to the onset of visual failure [19].

Of the mtDNA mutations in the protein-coding genes associated with other phenotypes, the m.8993T>G and m.8993T>C mutations (in the *ATP6* gene) associated with maternally inherited Leigh syndrome (MILS) and NARP are the most common [20]. Approximately 10–20 % of individuals with LS have either the m.8993T>G or m.8993T>C *MT-ATP6* mutation, while approximately another 10–20 % of patients with LS have mutations in other mitochondrial genes, e.g., other mutations in the mitochondrial genes *MT-ATP6, MT-TL1, MT-TK, MT-TW, MT-TV, MT-ND1, MT-ND2, MT-ND3, MT-ND4, MT-ND5, MT-ND6* and *MT-CO3* [20]. Of individuals with NARP, greater than 50 % likely have a detectable mutation at m.8993T, with the m.8993T>G mutation being the most common although the m.8993T>C mutation has also been described. The m.9176T>G mutation in the *ATP6* gene and the m.13513G>A mutation in the *ND5* gene each accounts for 1–5 % of patients with LS. Mutations in this category usually are more deleterious to the function of their associated protein than are LHON mutations and can cause OXPHOS complex deficiency.

Mutations in the mitochondrial tRNAs and rRNAs affect protein synthesis. Commonly, a pathogenic tRNA mutation leads to a combined OXPHOS defect, in part through a decreased overall rate of mitochondrial protein synthesis. Depending on which tRNA is mutated and the percentage of the corresponding amino acid in the different electron transport chain (ETC) complex subunits, the effects on the individual ETC complexes could be different. Mutations in the tRNAs also have been reported to cause isolated OXPHOS complex deficiency [8, 21, 22]. Many different pathogenic mechanisms lead to defective translation caused by a tRNA mutation, including impaired transcription termination, impaired tRNA maturation, defective posttranscriptional modification of the tRNA, impaired tRNA folding and stability, reduced aminoacylation, decreased binding to the translation factor mtEFTu or the mitochondrial ribosome, and altered codon decoding [23, 24]. Among the more than 30 definitive mutations in mitochondrial tRNAs recorded in Mitomap (www.mitomap.org), m.3243A>G in the mitochondrial *tRNALeu* (*UUR*) gene (*MT-TL1*) and m.8344A>G in the mitochondrial *tRNALys* gene (*MT-TK*) are the most common. The m.3243A>G mutation is present in approximately 80 % of patients with MELAS [14], in approximately 2–7 % of patients with maternally inherited diabetes and deafness (MIDD) [25], in approximately 10 % of Finnish patients with hypertrophic cardiomyopathy [25], and in association with LS [14]. The m.8344A>G mutation is present in over 80 % of MERRF patients [26].

A list of 58 common mtDNA point mutations that account for approximately 60–70 % of mtDNA point mutation-associated primary mitochondrial disorders is summarized in Table 10.1.

Table 10.1 Common mitochondrial DNA mutations and their associated disorders

mtDNA mutations	Gene	Associated disorders
m.583G>A	*MT-TF*	MELAS, mitochondrial myopathy and exercise intolerance [27]
m.1494C>T	*MT-RNR1*	Maternally inherited deafness or aminoglycoside-induced deafness [27]
m.1555A>G	*MT-RNR1*	Account for majority of patients with mitochondrial non-syndromic hearing loss and aminoglycoside induced hearing loss [28]
m.1606G>A	*MT-TV*	Ataxia, myoclonus and deafness [27]
m.3243A>G	*MT-TL1*	MELAS (m.3243A>G present in ~80 % of cases) [14]; MIDD (m.3243A>G present in ~2–7 % of patients) [25]; LS [14]; Hypertrophic cardiomyopathy (m.3243A>G present in ~10 % of Finnish patients) [25]; Sensorineural hearing loss, focal segmental glomerulosclerosis, cardiac plus multi-organ dysfunction [27]
m.3271T>C	*MT-TL1*	MELAS (m.3271T>C present in ~7.5 % of cases) [29]
m.3256C>T	*MT-TL1*	MELAS [27]
m.3260A>G	*MT-TL1*	Maternal myopathy and cardiomyopathy [27]
m.3291 T>C	*MT-TL1*	MELAS, myopathy, deafness plus cognitive impairment [27]
m.3302A>G	*MT-TL1*	Mitochondrial myopathy [27]
m.3303C>T	*MT-TL1*	Maternal myopathy and cardiomyopathy [27]
m.3460G>A	*MT-ND1*	LHON (together m.3460G>A, m.11778G>A, and m.14484T>C account for 95 % of patients) [27, 30]
m.3635G>A	*MT-ND1*	LHON [27]
m.3697G>A	*MT-ND1*	MELAS/LS/LHON and dystonia [27]
m.3700G>A	*MT-ND1*	LHON [27]
m.3733G>A	*MT-ND1*	LHON [27]
m.3733G>C	*MT-ND1*	LHON [31]
m.3890G>A	*MT-ND1*	Progressive encephalomyopathy/LS/optic atrophy [27]
m.4171C>A	*MT-ND1*	LHON [27]
m.4298G>A	*MT-TI*	Chronic progressive external ophthalmoplegia/multiple sclerosis [27]
m.4300A>G	*MT-TI*	MICM [27, 30]
m.4308G>A	*MT-TI*	Chronic progressive external ophthalmoplegia [27]
m.4332G>A	*MT-TQ*	Encephalopathy/MELAS [27]
m.5537AinsT	*MT-TW*	LS [27]
m.5650G>A	*MT-TA*	Myopathy [27]
m.5703G>A	*MT-TN*	Chronic progressive external ophthalmoplegia/mitochondrial myopathy [27]
m.7445A>G	*MT-CO1*	Sensorineural hearing loss [27]
m.7472insC (=C7471CC)	*MT-TS1*	Progressive encephalopathy/ataxia, myoclonus and deafness/motor neuron disease-like [27]
m.7497G>A	*MT-TS1*	Mitochondrial myopathy/exercise intolerance [27]
m.7511T>C	*MT-TS1*	Sensorineural hearing loss [27]
m.8344A>G	*MT-TK*	MERRF (m.8344A>G present in over 80 % of patients) [26, 27]
m.8356T>C	*MT-TK*	MERRF [26, 27]
m.8363G>A	*MT-TK*	MERRF [26]; MICM [26, 27]
m.8993T>G	*MT-ATP6*	LS (~10–20 % of patients have either m.8993T>G or m.8993T>C) [20, 27]; NARP (mutation at nucleotide 8993 estimated to be present in 20 % to >50 % of patients. m.8993T>G is more common than m.8993T>C.) [20, 27]
m.8993T>C	*MT-ATP6*	LS (~10–20 % of patients have either m.8993T>C or m.8993T>G) [20]; NARP (mutation at nucleotide 8993 is estimated to be present in 20 % to >50 % of patients. m.8993T>C is less common than m.8993T>G.) [20, 27]
m.9176T>G	*MT-ATP6*	LS (present in ~1–5 % of patients) [20, 27]; NARP (present in ~1–5 % of patients) [20, 27]
m.9176T>C	*MT-ATP6*	LS (1–5 % of patients) [27, 32–34]
m.9185T>C	*MT-ATP6*	LS/ataxia syndromes/NARP-like disease [27]
m.10010T>C	*MT-TG*	Progressive encephalopathy [27]
m.10158T>C	*MT-ND3*	LS [27]
m.10191T>C	*MT-ND3*	LS/Leigh-like disease/epilepsy, strokes, optic atrophy and cognitive decline [27]
m.10197G>A	*MT-ND3*	LS/dystonia/stroke/LHON and dystonia [27]
m.10663T>C	*MT-ND4L*	LHON [27]

(continued)

Table 10.1 (continued)

mtDNA mutations	Gene	Associated disorders
m.11777C>A	*MT-ND4*	LS [27]
m.11778G>A	*MT-ND4*	LHON (together m.11778G>A, m.3460G>A and m.14484T>C account for 95 % of patients with LHON. Of the three m.11778G>A is the most common, present in ~70 % of Caucasian patients and 90 % of Asian patients [27, 30]; Progressive dystonia [27]
m.12147G>A	*MT-TH*	MERFF-MELAS/encephalopathy [27]
m.12315G>A	*MT-TL2*	Chronic progressive external ophthalmoplegia/Kearns–Sayre syndrome [27]
m.12706T>C	*MT-ND5*	LS [27]
m.13513G>A	*MT-ND5*	MELAS (rare) [35]; LS/MELAS/LHON-MELAS overlap syndrome [27]
m.13514A>G	*MT-ND5*	LS/MELAS [13]
m.14459G>A	*MT-ND6*	LHON (rare) [27, 36]
m.14482C>G	*MT-ND6*	LHON [27]
m.14482C>A	*MT-ND6*	LHON [27]
m.14484T>C	*MT-ND6*	LHON (Together m.14484T>C, m.3460G>A and m.11778G>A account for 95 % of patients with LHON [30]. m.14484T>C is the most common cause of LHON in French Canadians [27, 37]
m.14487T>C	*MT-ND6*	LS [27, 38, 39]
m.14495A>G	*MT-ND6*	LHON [27]
m.14568C>T	*MT-ND6*	LHON [27]
m.14674T>C	*MT-TE*	Reversible COX deficiency myopathy [27]
m.14709T>C	*MT-TE*	MIDD (present in ~7 % of patients) [27, 40]

LHON Leber hereditary optic neuropathy, *LS* Leigh syndrome, *MELAS* mitochondrial encephalomyopathy, lactic acidosis, and stroke-like episodes; *MERRF* myoclonic epilepsy and ragged red muscle fibers; *MICM* maternally inherited hypertrophic cardiomyopathy; *MIDD* maternally inherited diabetes and deafness; *NARP* neurogenic weakness with ataxia and retinitis pigmentosa.

Single Large-Scale Rearrangements

More than 120 single deletions, duplications and complex rearrangements associated with a primary mtDNA disorder have been published and recorded in the mtDNA mutation database, Mitomap (www.mitomap.org). The size of disease-causing mtDNA single deletions varies from several base pairs to 10 kb. The large-scale single deletions (>1 kb) are the most common rearrangements and account for approximately 97 % of the reported pathogenic deletions of the mtDNA and >99 % of patients with mtDNA deletion associated diseases. Greater than 80 % of deletions are associated with direct repeats of 3–13 bp in length (www.mitomap.org). The most common large-scale deletions are between a 13 bp direct repeat from m.8470 to m.8482 in the *ATPase8* gene and from m.13447 to m.13459 in the *ND5* gene. Large duplications of mtDNA almost always coexist with large-scale single deletions and have been observed in a subset of patients who harbor large-scale mtDNA single deletions [41–45]. MtDNA duplications alone are not disease causing, although they may have modifying effects on the phenotype caused by mtDNA deletions [42, 43]. In about 20 % of patients with primary mtDNA disorders, the disorder is caused by large-scale single deletions in mtDNA [1].

Patients with large-scale single deletions usually have one of the three mitochondrial DNA deletion syndromes: Pearson syndrome, KSS, or progressive external ophthalmoplegia (PEO). The clinical features of the major mtDNA deletion syndromes are described in Table 10.2. In Pearson syndrome, mtDNA deletions are usually more abundant in blood than in other tissues. In PEO, mtDNA deletions are confined to skeletal muscle. In KSS, approximately 90 % of patients have a large-scale (i.e., 1.1–10 kb) mtDNA deletion. Deletions are usually present in all tissues of individuals with KSS, and may be identified in blood leukocytes. However, in many cases, the level of heteroplasmy of the deletion is too low in blood cells to be detected, and a muscle biopsy may be necessary [41]. Pearson syndrome patients who survive infancy may develop KSS at a later age [46]. An individual may have a large-scale mtDNA deletion abundant in blood and undetectable in muscle at an early age and have Pearson syndrome. If this individual survives, the same deletion can be abundant in muscle and undetectable in blood at a later age and cause KSS.

Copy Number Changes (Depletion or Over-Replication)

Abnormal amounts of mtDNA, either decreases of copy number (depletion) or increases of copy number (over-replication), can be indicative of mitochondrial dysfunction. MtDNA depletion syndrome is a group of mitochondrial disorders characterized by a reduced amount of mitochondrial DNA in tissues. The disorders associated with mtDNA depletion syndrome generally involve neurological symptoms that occur during infancy or childhood. Symptoms may include muscle weakness, hypotonia, exercise intolerance, developmental delay, lactic acidosis, encephalopathy, hepa-

Table 10.2 Characteristics of mitochondrial DNA deletion syndromes [1, 41]

mtDNA deletion syndrome	Disease characteristics	Characteristics of mtDNA deletions
KSS	A triad of (1) onset <20 yo, (2) pigmentary retinopathy, and (3) PEO, plus at least one of the following: cardiac conduction block, cerebrospinal fluid protein concentration greater than 100 mg/dL, or cerebellar ataxia.	~90 % have a large-scale 1.1–10 kb deletion usually present in all tissues, but most abundant in muscle, and often undetectable in blood cells. A deletion of 4,977 bp is the most common. Over 120 deletions have been associated with KSS. Large-scale duplications have also been reported.
PEO	Ptosis, ophthalmoplegia, variably severe proximal limb weakness; relatively benign, may be the early sign of KSS.	Deletion/duplication analysis is estimated to identify a deletion in approximately 50 % of patients. Deletions are confined to skeletal muscle.
Pearson syndrome	Sideroblastic anemia, exocrine pancreas dysfunction, usually fatal in infancy. Children who survive the disease usually go on to develop KSS.	Deletions are usually more abundant in blood than other tissue types. Deletion load gradually decreases in blood and increases in muscle as it evolving to PEO and KSS.

KSS Kearns–Sayre syndrome, *PEO* progressive external ophthalmoplegia

topathy, or myopathy. MtDNA depletion syndrome is usually caused by mutations in the nuclear genes involved in mtDNA biosynthesis or maintenance, such *POLG*, *TYMP*, *C10ORF2*, *DGUOK*, *MPV17*, etc.

Mitochondrial over-replication can be a cellular response to mitochondrial dysfunction and is characterized by ragged red fibers in the affected muscle specimens of patients with mtDNA mutations in tRNA genes or with large-scale mtDNA deletions [47, 48]. Over-replication of mtDNA also has been reported in a later-onset, mild KSS patient with a high heteroplasmy (92 %) for a deletion in the mtDNA [49].

Mutations in the Nuclear Genes

Nuclear genes encode the structural protein subunits that are components of the mitochondrial OXPHOS complexes, as well as proteins involved in biosynthesis, maintenance, transcription and translation of the mitochondrial DNA, proteins involved in the assembly of the OXPHOS complexes, and cofactors of the electron transport chain that are indirectly involved in the primary function of the OXPHOS system. Proteins needed for the assembly of an OXPHOS complex, referred to as assembly factors, are not usually components of the final structure. Fewer than 100 nuclear genes have been associated with disease-causing mutations for a primary mitochondrial OXPHOS disorder. These nuclear genes encode proteins from all the above categories. Although most of these nuclear gene-encoded proteins are synthesized in the cell cytoplasm and imported into the mitochondria, some of these proteins have dual localization (located in both mitochondria and cytoplasm), such as ISCU and LRPPRC, and some are localized in the cytoplasm but not localized in mitochondria, such as the small subunit of P53-inducible ribonucleotide reductase encoded by the *RRM2B* gene and thymidine phosphorylase encoded by the *TYMP* gene. As mtDNA genes also are involved in the structure and/or function of mitochondria, relevant mtDNA genes are discussed with nuclear genes in this section.

Genes Encoding OXPHOS Complex Structural Subunits or Assembly Factors

Complex I (CI) deficiency is the most common cause of mitochondrial disorders and accounts for about one-third of patients with primary mitochondrial disorders [50, 51]. Mutations in the mtDNA account for about 29 % of patients with confirmed isolated CI deficiency, while the rest are considered to be due to nuclear gene defects [8]. Mutations have been identified in 17 of the 39 nuclear genes encoding the structural subunits and in 10 nuclear genes encoding the assembly factors for CI (see Table 10.3). Mutations in these genes have been seen in approximately 20 % of patients with isolated CI deficiency [8]. Each gene accounts for less than 5 % of patients with CI deficiency [52]. The diseases resulting from these mutations range from severe lethal infantile mitochondrial disease, congenital lactic acidosis, encephalocardiomyopathy, and LS to adult onset muscle weakness, exercise intolerance, liver dysfunction, ataxia, and progressive neurodegeneration [52, 53]. Some genes with mutations expected to cause combined (multiple) OXPHOS deficiency, such as *MT-TL1*, *MT-TS2*, and *MT-TW* in the mtDNA, and *POLG*, *SUCLA2*, *C10ORF2*, and *TAZ* in the nuclear genome, can be associated with an isolated complex deficiency (Table 10.3). In contrast, patients with mutation(s) in CI subunit genes (either mtDNA or nuclear), can present with combined Complex I and III deficiency [54, 55], likely due to supercomplex formation of the respiratory chain [56–58].

Although Complex II (CII) has four known genes (*SDHA*, *SDHB*, *SDHC* and *SDHD*) encoding the structural subunits and two known genes (*SDHAF1* and *SDHAF2*) encoding the assembly factors, only two genes, *SDHA* and *SDHAF1*, have

Table 10.3 Genes associated with isolated OXPHOS deficiency and associated diseases

Isolated OXPHOS complex deficiency	Genes	Diseases and clinical features	References
CI	mtDNA-genes encoding structural subunits: *ND1*; *ND2*; *ND3*; *ND4*; *ND4L*; *ND5*; *ND6*	LHON, LS, NARP, MELAS	(www.mitomap.org)
	nDNA-genes encoding structural subunits: *NDUFS1*; *NDUFS2*; *NDUFS3*; *NDUFS4*; *NDUFS6*; *NDUFS7*; *NDUFS8*; *NDUFV1*; *NDUFV2*; *NDUFA1*; *NDUFA2*; *NDUFA9*; *NDUFA10*; *NDUFA11*; *NDUFA12*; *NDUFB3*; *NDUFB9*	Progressive encephalomyopathy; leukoencephalopathy with macrocephaly; LS; LLS; leukoencephalopathy; LIMD; cardiomyopathy and encephalopathy; progressive cavitating leukoencephalopathy; hypertrophic cardiomyopathy and encephalomyopathy; progressive neurodegeneration	[69–73]
	nDNA-genes encoding assembly factors: *NDUFAF1*; *NDUFAF2*; *NDUFAF3* (*C3ORF60*); *NDUFAF4* (*C6orf66*); *NDUFAF5* (*C20orf7*); *NDUFAF6* (*C8ORF38*); *ACAD9*; *FOXRED1*; *NUBPL*	Exercise intolerance; hypertrophic cardiomyopathy; encephalopathy; progressive encephalopathy; LS; encephalomyopathy; lactic acidosis; encephalomyopathy with macrocephaly; leukoencephalopathy, Leigh-like syndrome	[74–77]
	Other genes in the mtDNA: *MT-TL1*; *MT-TS2*; *MT-TW*	MELAS; Mitochondrial Myopathy; Mitochondrial Encephalopathy	[8, 21, 22]
	Other nDNA-encoded genes: *POLG*; *SUCLA2*; *C10ORF2*	Liver involvement; encephalopathy; 3-methylglutaconic aciduria; epilepsy	[78–80]
CII	nDNA-genes encoding structural subunits: *SDHA*	LS; cardiomyopathy	[81–83]
	nDNA-genes encoding assembly factor: *SDHAF1*	Infantile leukoencephalopathy	[84]
CIII	mtDNA-genes encoding structural subunits: *MT-CYB*	LHON; encephalopathy; cardiomyopathy, myopathy	(www.mitomap.org)
	nDNA-genes encoding structural subunit: *UQCRB*; *UQCRC2*; *UQCRQ*; *CYC1*	Hypoglycemia; liver dysfunction; lactic acidosis; psychomotor retardation with extrapyramidal signs	[85–88]
	nDNA-genes encoding assembly factors: *BCS1L*; *TTC19*	Encephalopathy; liver failure; tubulopathy; GRACILE syndrome; Björnstad syndrome	[61, 89]
CIV	mtDNA-genes encoding structural subunits: *MT-CO1*, *MT-CO2*, *MT-CO3*	Encephalopathy; myopathy; sideroblastic anemia; myoglobinuria; MELAS	(www.mitomap.org)
	nDNA-genes encoding structural subunits: *COX6B1*; *COX4I2*	Infantile encephalomyopathy, or exocrine pancreatic insufficiency and anemia	[90]
	nDNA-genes encoding assembly factors: *SURF1*; *SCO1*; *SCO2*; *COX10*; *COX14* (*C12ORF62*); *COX15*; *COX20*; *LRPPRC*; *COA5* (*C2orf64*)	LS; French-Canadian LS; encephalopathy; cardiomyopathy; myopathy; liver failure; tubulopathy	[91–94]
	Other genes: *ETHE1*; *FASTKD2*; *PET100*; *TACO1*	Ethylmalonic encephalopathy; Encephalomyopathy; LS	[95–98]
CV	mtDNA-genes encoding structural subunits: *ATP6*; *ATP8*	LS; NARP; cardiomyopathy	(www.mitomap.org)
	nDNA-genes encoding structural subunits: *ATP5E*	3-methylglutaconic aciduria; lactic acidosis; mild mental retardation; peripheral neuropathy	[99]
	nDNA-encoded assembly factor: *ATPAF2* (*ATP12*); *TMEM70*	Encephalopathy, lactic acidosis, cardioencephalomyopathy	[100–102]
	Other genes: *SLC25A3* (*PHC*)	Lactic acidosis; hypertrophic cardiomyopathy; muscular hypotonia	[103]

CI Complex I, *CII* Complex II, *CIII* Complex III, *CIV* Complex IV, *CV* Complex V, *LHON* Leber hereditary optic neuropathy, *LS* Leigh syndrome, *MELAS* mitochondrial encephalomyopathy, lactic acidosis, and stroke-like episodes, *MERRF* myoclonic epilepsy and ragged red muscle fibers, *MICM* maternally inherited hypertrophic cardiomyopathy, *MIDD* maternally inherited diabetes and deafness, *mtDNA* mitochondrial DNA, *NARP* neurogenic weakness with ataxia and retinitis pigmentosa, *nDNA* nuclear DNA.

been associated with CII deficiency, and present as LS or mitochondrial encephalopathy (see Table 10.3). The rest of the genes, *SDHB*, *SDHC SDHD*, and *SDHAF2*, are considered tumor suppressor genes, with mutations associated with hereditary paraganglioma and pheochromocytoma syndromes only, suggesting that mutations in these genes are involved in tumorigenesis [59].

Complex III (CIII) deficiency is relatively rare and accounts for only about 7 % of patients with an OXPHOS complex deficiency [51, 60]. Of the 11 structural subunits of CIII, mutations have been reported in the only subunit encoded by the *MT-CYB* gene in the mtDNA and 4 (*UQCRB*, *UQCRC2*, *UQCRQ* and *CYC1*) of the 10 subunits encoded by nuclear genes (Table 10.3). More than 20 pathogenic mutations in the *MT-CYB* gene account for the vast majority of known pathogenic mutations in the CIII subunits and most of these mutations are located outside of the transmembrane domain of the protein [61]. The *UQCRB*, *UQCRQ* and *UQCRC2* genes each have one homozygous pathogenic mutation described in a single family and the *CYC1* gene has two different homozygous pathogenic mutations identified in two unrelated patients. In addition, mutations in two genes (*BCS1L* and *TTC19*) encoding CIII assembly factors are associated with primary mitochondrial disorders due to CIII deficiency (Table 10.3). More than 20 pathogenic mutations in the *BCS1L* gene are in the human gene mutation database (HGMD) (www.hgmd.org) and account for the majority of patients with CIII deficiency. Clinical features range from mild congenital sensorineural hearing loss and distorted hair (pili torti), the hallmarks of Björnstads syndrome, tubulopathy alone or combined with cholestasis, and/or encephalopathy to GRACILE syndrome (growth retardation, amino aciduria, cholestasis, iron overload, lactic acidosis, and early death) [62–64].

Complex IV (CIV; Cytochrome c oxidase or COX) is the terminal component of the respiratory chain catalyzing the reduction of molecular oxygen to water. COX is composed of three catalytic subunits encoded by mtDNA genes and ten accessory subunits encoded by nuclear genes. The accessory subunits are involved in structural stabilization, assembly of the complex, and modulation of COX catalytic activity. Disease-causing mutations occur in all three mtDNA genes (*MT-CO1*, *MT-CO2* and *MT-CO3*) encoding catalytic subunits of COX, but almost all the mutations were seen in a single family and are considered "private" mutations. Of the ten genes encoding accessory subunits of COX, only *COX6B1* and *COX4I2* (Table 10.3) have pathogenic mutations. In addition, mutations occur in nine nuclear genes (*SURF1*; *SCO1*; *SCO2*; *COX10*; *COX14* [*C12ORF62*]; *COX15*; *COX20*; *LRPPRC*; *COA5* [*C2orf64*]) encoding COX assembly factors that are not themselves components of the final COX structure, and account for the majority of patients with isolated COX deficiency (Table 10.3). The *SURF1* gene represents the most common gene accounting for 25–75 % of LS associated with COX deficiency [65]. Furthermore, mutations in *ETHE1*, *FASTKD2*, and *TACO1* also are associated COX deficiency (Table 10.3).

Complex V (ATP synthase) deficiency most commonly is caused by mutations in the mtDNA encoded ATP6 and ATP8 proteins, and as described earlier in this chapter, m.8993T>G and m.8993T>C are the most common mutations (Table 10.1). The severity of disease caused by these mutations depends on mutation load: a low mutation load is asymptomatic; an intermediate mutation load causes NARP; and a high mutation load causes MILS [66, 67]. Only two of the approximately 16 nuclear genes encoding the subunits of complex V (*ATP5E*) and two genes encoding the assembly factors, *ATPAF2* (*ATP12*) and *TMEM70*, have mutations which cause ATP synthase deficiency (Table 10.3). The presentation of patients with isolated ATP synthase deficiency caused by mutations in nuclear genes is remarkably homogeneous with neonatal onset, lactic acidosis, hypertrophic cardiomyopathy, psychomotor retardation, and, in most cases, 3-methyl-glutaconic aciduria. These patients usually have diminished content of ATP synthase and lack striatal brain involvement [68].

Genes Encoding Proteins Essential for MtDNA Biosynthesis and/or Maintenance

Although mtDNA resides in mitochondria, its biosynthesis (replication), maintenance, transcription, and translation are controlled by proteins encoded by nuclear genes, synthesized in the cytoplasm, and imported into mitochondria [171]. The mtDNA copy number is related to energy demand, i.e., tissues with the highest respiratory demand, such as muscle, liver, heart, and brain, have the greatest number of mtDNA copies per cell. Normal mtDNA replication and maintenance is important for both the quality and quantity of mtDNA and requires normal function of the mtDNA replisome as well as normal mitochondrial deoxynucleoside triphosphate (dNTP) pool maintenance. Major proteins or enzymes involved in mtDNA replication include DNA polymerase gamma (with its catalytic subunits encoded by the *POLG* gene and its accessory subunit encoded by the *POLG2* gene) and Twinkle helicase encoded by the *C10ORF2* gene (also known as *PEO1*). Major proteins involved in the maintenance of the large dNTP pool are encoded by genes including *TK2*, *TYMP*, *DGUOK*, *RRM2B*, *SUCLA2*, *SUCLG1*, etc [24]. Mutations in genes involved in mtDNA replication or dNTP pool maintenance may cause quality or quantity defects of mtDNA. To date, disease-causing mutations have been identified in many genes involved in mtDNA replication or dNTP pool maintenance (Table 10.4). Mutations in *POLG* are the most common and account for approximately 25 % of all patients with mitochondrial disease presentations [172, 173]. Mutations in *POLG*, *POLG2*, *ANT1*, *C10ORF2*, *RRM2B*, and *OPA1* have been reported to be associated with autosomal-dominant external ophthalmoplegia (adPEO) with multiple mtDNA deletions (Table 10.4). Mutations in

Table 10.4 Genes associated with combined/multiple OXPHOS deficiency and associated diseases

Combined OXPHOS complex deficiency	Genes	Diseases and clinical features
CI + CIII + CIV	**Genes involved in mtDNA replication**	
	POLG	Mitochondrial DNA depletion syndrome 4A (Alpers type), MTDPS4A [104]; Mitochondrial DNA depletion syndrome 4B (MNGIE type), MTDPS4B [105]; adPEO with multiple mtDNA deletions [106]; arPEO with multiple mtDNA deletions [107]; Mitochondrial recessive ataxia syndrome, includes sensory ataxic neuropathy, dysarthria, and ophthalmoparesis (SANDO) and spinocerebellar ataxia with epilepsy (SCAE) [108, 109]
	POLG2	adPEO mitochondrial DNA deletions [110]
	C10ORF2	Mitochondrial DNA depletion syndrome 7 (hepatocerebral type) [111]; adPEO with multiple mtDNA deletions [112]
	Genes involved in dNTP pool maintenance	
	DGUOK	Mitochondrial DNA depletion syndrome 3, MTDPS3 (hepatocerebral type) [113]
	TK2	Mitochondrial DNA depletion syndrome 2 (myopathic type), MTDPS2 [114]
	TYMP	Mitochondrial DNA depletion syndrome 1 (MNGIE type); MTDPS1 [115]
	RRM2B	Mitochondrial DNA depletion syndrome 8A (encephalomyopathic type with renal tubulopathy), MTDPS8A [116]; Mitochondrial DNA depletion syndrome 8B (MNGIE type), MTDPS8B [117] adPEO [118]; arPEO [118, 119]
	SLC25A4	adPEO with multiple mtDNA deletions [120]; Familial hypertrophic cardiomyopathy [121]
	SUCLG1	Mitochondrial DNA depletion syndrome 9 (encephalomyopathic type with methylmalonic aciduria), MTDPS9 [122, 123]
	SUCLA2	Mitochondrial DNA depletion syndrome 5 (encephalomyopathic with methylmalonic aciduria), MTDPS5 [124, 125]
	Other	
	OPA1	Optic atrophy 1 [126]; Optic atrophy with or without deafness, ophthalmoplegia, myopathy, ataxia, and neuropathy [127, 128]
	MPV17	Mitochondrial DNA depletion syndrome 6 (hepatocerebral type), MTDPS6 [127, 128]
CI + CIII/CIV (or + CV)	**Genes involved in tRNA modification**	
	PUS1	Mitochondrial myopathy; lactic acidosis; sideroblastic anemia 1 [129]
	TRMU	Liver failure, acute infantile [130]
	Elongation factors	
	GFM1	COXPD1 (OMIM#609060); Progressive hepatoencephalopathy [131]; fatal neonatal liver failure and lactic acidosis [132]
	TUFM	COXPD4 (OMIM#610678); Lactic acidosis; fatal encephalopathy; diffuse cystic leukodystrophy; micropolygyria [133]
	TSFM	COXPD3 (OMIM#610505); Progressive encephalomyopathy or concentric hypertrophic cardiomyopathy [134]
	Ribosomal protein	
	MRPL3	COXPD9 (OMIM#614582); Mitochondrial cardiomyopathy [135]
	MRPL44	COXPD15 (OMIM#615395); Hypertrophic cardiomyopathy [136]
	MRPS16	COXPD2 (OMIM#610678); Agenesis of the corpus callosum; dysmorphism; fatal neonatal lactic acidosis [137]
	MRPS22	COXPD5 (OMIM#611719); Microcephaly; dilated cardiomyopathy; dysmorphic features; tubulopathy; hypotonia [138, 139]
	Genes encoding aminoacyl-tRNA synthetase	
	AARS2	COXPD8 (OMIM#614096); Fatal infantile hypertrophic mitochondrial cardiomyopathy [140]
	DARS2	Leukoencephalopathy with brain stem and spinal cord involvement and lactate elevation [141]
	EARS2	COXPD12 (OMIM#614924) [142]
	FARS2	COXPD14 (OMIM#614946) [143]
	HARS2	Ovarian dysgenesis; sensorineural hearing loss [144]
	LARS2	Perrault syndrome 4 [145]
	MARS2	Spastic ataxia 3 [146]
	RARS2	Pontocerebellar hypoplasia, type 6; profound developmental delay; progressive severe microcephaly; hypotonia; cerebral, pontine, and cerebellar atrophy [147]
	SARS2	Hyperuricemia; pulmonary hypertension; renal failure; alkalosis [148]
	YARS2	Mitochondrial myopathy; lactic acidosis; sideroblastic anemia 2 [149]
	Genes encoding peptide release factor	
	C12orf65	COXPD7 (OMIM#613559); LS; optic atrophy; ophthalmoplegia [150]
	Other	
	ELAC2	COXPD17 (OMIM#615440) [151]
	MTFMT	COXPD15 (OMIM#614947) [152]
	MTO1	COXPD10 (OMIM#614702) [153]
	NDUFS4	Infantile encephalopathy; microcephaly; lactic academia [54]
	TAZ	Barth Syndrome [154]

(continued)

Table 10.4 (continued)

Combined OXPHOS complex deficiency	Genes	Diseases and clinical features
CI–III + CII–III	**MtDNA encoded genes with mutations causing CoQ10 deficiency**	
	MT-TL1	(Secondary) CoQ10 deficiency in MELAS [155]
	Nuclear genes with mutations causing CoQ10 deficiency	
	ADCK3 (*CABC1*)	CoQ10 deficiency and progressive cerebellar atrophy with cerebellar ataxia and seizures [156]
	APTX	(Secondary) CoQ10 deficiency with Ataxia, early-onset, with oculomotor apraxia and hypoalbuminemia [157, 158]
	BRAF	(Secondary) CoQ10 deficiency with multisystemic infantile presentation in one patient with cardiofaciocutaneous syndrome
	COQ2	CoQ10 deficiency with infantile encephalomyopathy, nephropathy [159, 160]
	COQ6	Steroid-resistant nephrotic syndrome (SRNS) with sensorineural deafness (SND) [161]
	PDSS1	CoQ10 deficiency and multisystem disease with early-onset deafness, encephaloneuropathy, obesity, livedo reticularis, and valvulopathy [162]
	PDSS2	CoQ10 deficiency with infantile onset fatal LS and nephrotic syndrome [163]
	COQ9	CoQ10 deficiency with neonatal lactic acidosis, and multisystem disease [164]
	ETFDH	(Secondary) Myopathic form of CoQ10 deficiency and multiple acyl-CoA deficiency [165]
CIII + CIV	*PNPT1*	COXPD13 (OMIM#614932) PubMed: [166]
CI + CII + CIV	*GFER*	Autosomal-recessive myopathy with cataract [167]
CI + CII + CIII	*ISCU*	Hereditary myopathy with lactic acidosis [168]
CI + CII + CIII	*BOLA3*	Multiple mitochondrial dysfunctions syndrome 2; fatal deficiency of multiple respiratory chain and 2-oxoacid dehydrogenase enzymes [169]
	NFU1	Multiple mitochondrial dysfunctions syndrome 1; fatal deficiency of multiple respiratory chain and 2-oxoacid dehydrogenase enzymes [169]
CI + CIII + CIV + CV	*RMND1*	COXPD11 (OMIM#614922) [170]
CI + CII + CIII + CIV + CV	*AIFM1*	COXPD6 (OMIM#300816) [76]

adPEO autosomal dominant external ophthalmoplegia, *arPEO* autosomal recessive progressive external ophthalmoplegia, *CI* Complex I, *CII* Complex II, *CIII* Complex III, *CIV* Complex IV, *CV* Complex V (ATP synthase), *COXPD* combined OXPHOS deficiency, *MELAS* mitochondrial encephalomyopathy, lactic acidosis, and stroke-like episodes, *mtDNA* mitochondrial DNA

POLG, *C10ORF2* (*PEO1*), *RRM2B*, and *SLC25A4* (*ANT1*) account for approximately 45 %, 15–35 %, 9 %, and 4–15 % of familial PEO with multiple deletions, respectively. Mutations in *POLG2* are rare and account for less than 2 % of adPEO [173, 174]. Mutations in *POLG* and *RRM2B* are associated with autosomal-recessive external ophthalmoplegia (arPEO) with multiple mtDNA deletions (Table 10.4). Mutations in *POLG*, *C10ORF2*, *RRM2B*, *DGUOK*, *MPV17*, *TK2*, *SUCLA2*, *SUCLG1*, and *TYMP* are associated with different types of mtDNA depletion syndromes (Table 10.4). Approximately 69 % of patients with myopathic mtDNA depletion syndrome and more than 84 % of patients with hepatocerebral mitochondrial DNA depletion syndrome harbor mutations in one of these nine genes [175]. Mutations in genes involved in mtDNA biosynthesis and maintenance account for approximately 40 % of patients with combined OXPHOS deficiency [176].

Genes Encoding Mitochondrial Translational Machinery

The 13 proteins encoded by mtDNA are synthesized in mitochondria using a nonuniversal genetic code as follows: UGA codes for tryptophan (W) instead of a stop (X) codon; AGA & AGG codes for a stop (X) codon instead of arginine (R); and AUA codes for methionine (M) instead of isoleucine (I). The mitochondrial translational machinery consists of two rRNAs and 22 tRNAs encoded by mtDNA and approximately 100 proteins encoded by nuclear genes, including initiation, elongation, and termination translation factors; up to 81 mitochondrial ribosomal proteins (MRPs); and approximately 19 mitochondrial aminoacyl-tRNA synthetases and methionyl-tRNA transformylase [177, 178]. Theoretically, mitochondrial protein synthesis deficiency can be caused by mutations in any of the components of the mitochondrial translational machinery and can result in OXPHOS deficiency affecting theoretically all complexes containing mtDNA-encoded subunits (CI, CIII, CIV, and CV).

To date, in addition to the two rRNAs and 22 tRNAs encoded by mtDNA with many disease-causing mutations reported to be associated with combined (multiple) complex deficiency (www.mitomap.org), pathogenic mutations associated with combined OXPHOS deficiency also have been reported in many nuclear genes encoding components of the mitochondrial translational machinery, including two genes involved in tRNA modification (*PUS1* and *TRMU*), three genes encoding elongation factors (*GFM1*, *TUFM*, and

TSFM), ten genes encoding aminoacyl-tRNA synthetase (*AARS2*, *DARS2*, *EARS2*, *FARS2*, *HARS2*, *LARS2*, *MARS2*, *RARS2*, *YARS2*, and *SARS2*), and one gene encoding peptide release factor (*C12orf65*) (Table 10.4). Of all the 81 human MRPs, mutations have been found in only four: *MRPS16*, *MRPS22*, *MRPL3* and *MRPL44* (see Table 10.4). Mutations in both *MRPS16* and *MRPS22* genes result in a marked decrease in the 12S rRNA transcript level, probably caused by impaired assembly of the mito-ribosomal small subunit, generating unincorporated and instable 12S rRNA [137, 138]. Similarly, mutations in both *MRPL3* and *MRPL44* genes result in a marked decrease in the 16S rRNA transcript level [135, 136].

Genes Involved in Mitochondrial Dynamics

Mitochondrial fusion and fission (collectively termed mitochondrial dynamics) are important for mitochondrial inheritance and for the maintenance of mitochondrial functions [179]. Three nuclear-gene encoded proteins are required for mitochondrial fusion: Mitofusins 1 and 2 (Mfn1 and Mfn2) for outer membrane fusion, and Opa1 for inner membrane fusion [180]. Dynamin-related protein Drp1 is required for mitochondrial division (fission) [181, 182]. *OPA1* mutations cause autosomal-dominant optic atrophy [183, 184]. In most cases, this disease specifically involves degeneration of retinal ganglion cells. However, more diverse *OPA1*-related phenotypes have been described recently, and they include disorders of mtDNA maintenance [180]. Mutations in the *MFN2* gene cause the autosomal-dominant Charcot–Marie–Tooth disease type 2A, which is a peripheral neuropathy caused by degeneration of axons in long sensory and motor nerves of the distal extremities [185]. A mutation in the *DNM1L* gene has been reported in a patient with lethal encephalopathy due to defective mitochondrial and peroxisomal fission. The patient presented in the first days of life with microcephaly, abnormal brain development, optic atrophy and hypoplasia, and lactic acidemia, and died at age 37 days. Overexpression of the mutant DNM1L from the patient in fibroblasts from control subjects induced aberrant mitochondrial and peroxisomal phenotypes, indicating that the mutation acted in a dominant-negative manner [186].

Genes Involved in CoQ10 Biosynthesis or Metabolism

Coenzyme Q10 (CoQ10), or ubiquinone, is a mobile lipophilic electron carrier critical for electron transfer by the mitochondrial inner membrane respiratory chain from Complex II and I to Complex III. Intracellular synthesis is the major source of CoQ10, although a small proportion is acquired through diet. CoQ10 is synthesized in the mitochondrial inner membrane. At least 12 genes are involved in COQ10 biosynthesis [187]. Primary CoQ10 deficiency is a rare, clinically heterogeneous autosomal recessive disorder with six major phenotypes [187, 188]: (1) an encephalomyopathic form with seizures and ataxia; (2) a multisystem infantile form with encephalopathy, cardiomyopathy, and renal failure; (3) a predominantly cerebellar form with ataxia and cerebellar atrophy; (4) LS with growth retardation; (5) an isolated myopathic form; and (6) nephrotic syndrome. Typical CoQ10 deficiency has relatively normal isolated Complex I, II, and III activity, but deficient I+III and II+III activity. Mutations in any of the genes involved in COQ10 biosynthesis may cause CoQ10 deficiency. To date, mutations in six nuclear genes, *COQ2*, *ADCK3* (*CABC1*, *COQ8*), *COQ6*, *COQ9*, *PDSS1*, and *PDSS2* have been reported to be associated with primary CoQ10 deficiency (Table 10.4). CoQ10 levels also can be affected by other genetic defects (such as mutations of mtDNA, *ETFDH*, *APTX*, and *BRAF* genes) that are not directly related to the CoQ10 biosynthetic process (see Table 10.4). CoQ10 deficiency can be treated by supplementation with CoQ10.

Genes Indirectly Affecting OXPHOS Function

Although not involved in the structure and assembly of the OXPHOS system, both *SLC25A4* (*ANT1*) and *SLC25A3* (*PHC*) are important for the major function of the OXPHOS system-ATP synthesis. The mitochondrial phosphate carrier (PHC), encoded by *SLC25A3*, transporting inorganic phosphate into the mitochondrial matrix, is essential for the aerobic synthesis of ATP. A homozygous *SLC25A3* mutation has been identified in two siblings with lactic acidosis, hypertrophic cardiomyopathy, and muscular hypotonia who died within the first year of life. Functional investigation of intact mitochondria showed a deficiency of ATP synthesis in muscle [99]. ANT1 encoded by the *SLC25A4* gene determines the rate of ADP/ATP flux between the mitochondrion and the cytosol and is an important regulator of oxidative energy metabolism. Mutations in the *SLC25A4* gene have been reported in patients with autosomal dominant progressive external ophthalmoplegia with mtDNA deletions, and in patients with familial hypertrophic cardiomyopathy (Table 10.4).

The *TIMM8A* gene, located on the X chromosome, encodes the mitochondrial import inner membrane translocase subunit Tim8 that acts in a complex together with the Tim13 protein in a chaperone-like manner to facilitate the import of nuclear-encoded precursor proteins into the mitochondrial inner membrane. Mutations in *TIMM8A* cause deafness-dystonia-optic neuropathy (DDON) syndrome (also known as Mohr-Tranebjaerg syndrome), a rare neurodegenerative disease with early-onset deafness, dystonia and other neurological abnormalities including cortical blindness, spasticity, dementia and mental retardation [189].

The mitochondrial iron-sulfur cluster assembly enzyme, ISCU, is important for normal mitochondrial function [190]. Mutations in the *ISCU* gene have been reported to be associated with hereditary myopathy with lactic acidosis, and combined OXPHOS deficiency (Table 10.4).

The mitochondrial disulfide relay system (DRS) drives the import of cysteine-rich proteins into the intermembrane space via an oxidative folding mechanism. Proven substrates of the DRS include many proteins relevant to COX biogenesis, thus connecting the DRS to the OXPHOS system. Mutations in the *GFER* gene, encoding the DRS protein, GFER, are associated with autosomal recessive progressive mitochondrial myopathy with cataract and combined respiratory chain deficiency (Table 10.4).

The *SPG7* gene encodes paraplegin, a component of the m-AAA protease. The m-AAA protease is an ATP-dependent proteolytic complex of the mitochondrial inner membrane that degrades misfolded proteins and regulates ribosome assembly [191]. Mutations in the *SPG7* gene are associated with autosomal recessive spastic paraplegia [192, 193]. Patients with *SPG7* mutations show typical signs of mitochondrial OXPHOS defects [194].

The *NFU1* and *BOLA3* genes each encode a protein that plays an essential role in the production of iron-sulfur (Fe-S) clusters for the normal maturation of ipoate-containing 2-oxoacid dehydrogenases and for the assembly of the mitochondrial RC complexes [169]. Mutations in *NFU1* and *BOLA3* are associated with an autosomal recessive fetal mitochondrial disease: multiple mitochondrial dysfunctions syndrome [169]. Patients with mutations in *NFU1* have abnormalities of the glycine-cleavage system, the branched-chain alpha-keto acid dehydrogenase, and a significant reduction in activity of mitochondrial respiratory chain complexes [195]. Patients with mutations in *BOLA3* have decreased activity of the pyruvate dehydrogenase complex, the branched-chain alpha-keto acid dehydrogenase, and the mitochondrial RC complexes [195]. The above data suggest that mitochondrial dysfunction can result from a multitude of mechanisms other than direct impairment of the components of the OXPHOS system.

Common Mitochondrial Diseases with Highly Heterogeneous Underlying Molecular Defects

Some affected individuals exhibit clinical features that fall into a discrete clinical syndrome with underlying molecular defects confined to a specific gene(s) in the mitochondrial genome, such as, LHON, KSS, MELAS, MERRF, NARP, and MILS. MNGIE is mostly caused by mutations in *TYMP* [196] or *POLG* [197]. For the majority of patients with a mitochondrial disorder, the causative mutation can be in the mtDNA or in one of the many nuclear genes important for normal mitochondrial function. Therefore, predicting the causative gene from the clinical presentation can be difficult.

Chronic Progressive External Ophthalmoplegia

CPEO is a disorder characterized by slowly progressive paralysis of the extraocular muscles. Patients usually experience bilateral, symmetrical, progressive ptosis, followed by ophthalmoparesis months to years later. Ciliary and iris muscles are not involved. CPEO can be caused by mtDNA rearrangements (1.1–10 kb large-scale single deletions and duplications) (www.mitomap.org); mtDNA point mutations (m.3243A>G, m.4274T>C); or mutation(s) in many different nuclear genes (*C10ORF2* [*PEO1*], *OPA1*, *POLG* [*POLG1*], *POLG2*, *RRM2B*, *SLC25A4* [*ANT1*], and *TYMP*).

Optic Atrophy

Hereditary optic atrophy is a generic term referring to a heterogeneous group of genetic disorders that affect retinal ganglion cells and the optic nerve, leading to impaired vision. The most common forms of these disorders are autosomal dominant optic atrophy (ADOA; MIM#165500) and LHON (MIM#53500). Almost all LHON patients have mutations in the mtDNA, which account for approximately 10 % of patients suspected of having a hereditary optic atrophy. The clinical features of LHON may overlap with those caused by mutations in the nuclear genes. Mutations in *OPA1* account for 30–40 % of patients with suspected hereditary optic atrophy and approximately 40–50 % of patients with hereditary optic atrophy due to mutations in the nuclear genes [198, 199]. Mutations in many other genes have also been reported to be associated with hereditary optic atrophy, including *AUH*, *C12ORF65*, *CISD2* (*WFS2*), *NDUFS1*, *OPA3*, *POLG* (*POLG1*), *SPG7*, *TIMM8A* (*DDP1*), *TMEM126A*, and *WFS1* (Table 10.5). Almost all of these genes are important for normal mitochondrial function.

Leigh Syndrome

LS is an early-onset progressive neurodegenerative disorder with a characteristic neuropathology consisting of focal, bilateral lesions in one or more areas of the central nervous system, including the brainstem, thalamus, basal ganglia, cerebellum, and spinal cord. The lesions are areas of demyelination, gliosis, necrosis, spongiosis, or capillary proliferation. Approximately 30–40 % of patients with LS are due to mutations in the mtDNA, while the rest are due to mutations in the nuclear genes. Mutations in about 50 nuclear genes have been reported to be associated with LS or Leigh-like syndrome (Table 10.5).

Table 10.5 Genes with pathogenic mutations for common mitochondrial disease syndromes or with overlapping clinical features

Disease or features	Associated genes with disease-causing mutations
Leigh (Leigh-like) syndrome	*ADCK3 (CABC1; COQ8); AIFM1; APTX; BCS1L; NDUFAF6 (C8ORF38); COQ2; COQ9; COX10; COX15; DLAT; DLD; ETFDH; FOXRED1; GFER; GFM1 (EFG1); LIPT1; LRPPRC; MTFMT; NDUFA1; NDUFA10; NDUFA2; NDUFA9; NDUFA10; NDUFA12; NDUFAF2; NDUFAF4 (C6ORF66); NDUFAF7 (C2ORF56); NDUFS1; NDUFS2; NDUFS3; NDUFS4; NDUFS7; NDUFS8; NDUFV1; PC; PDHA1; PDHB; PDHX; PDP1; PDSS1; PDSS2; SCO2; SDHA; SDHAF1; SERAC1; SLC19A3; SUCLA2; SURF1; TACO1; TIMM44; TPK1; TTC19; TUFM*
Mitochondrial encephalopathy	*ACAD9; ACO2; AFG3L2; APTX; ATPAF2 (ATP12); BCS1L; BOLA3; NDUFAF6 (C8ORF38); C10ORF2; COQ2; COX10; COX14 (C12ORF62); COX15; COX20 (FAM36A); COX6B1; DARS2; DGUOK; DLD; DNM1L; EARS2; ETHE1; FARS2; FASTKD2; FBXL4; FH; GFM1 (EFG1); GFM2; HLCS; HSPD1; LIAS; LRPPRC; MARS2; MFN2; MPV17; MRPL12; MTPAP; NDUFA1; NDUFA10; NDUFA11; NDUFAF2; NDUFAF4 (C6ORF66); NDUFS1; NDUFS2; NDUFS3; NDUFS4; NDUFS6; NDUFS7; NDUFS8; NDUFV1; NDUFV2; NFU1; PC; PDHA1; POLG; RARS2; RMND1; SCO1; SCO2; SDHA; SDHAF1; SERAC1; SLC19A3; SUCLA2; SUCLG1; SURF1; TK2; TMEM70; TPK1; TSFM; TTC19; TUFM; TYMP (ECGF1, TP)*
Lactic acidosis	*ACAD9; ADCK3 (CABC1; COQ8); AGK; ATPX; ATP5E; ATPAF2 (ATP12); BCS1L; BOLA3; C20ORF7 (NDUFAF5); C8ORF38 (NDUFAF6); COQ2; COQ9; COX10; COX14 (C12ORF62); COX15; COX6B1; DARS2; DGUOK; DLAT; DLD; DNM1L; EARS2; ETFA; ETFB; ETFDH; ETHE1; FARS2; FBP1; FH; FOXRED1; G6PC; GFM1 (EFG1); GYS2; ISCU; HLCS; LIAS; LRPPRC; MPC1 (BRP44L); MRPS16; MRPS22, MTO1; NDUFA9; NDUFA11; NDUFAF1; NDUFAF3 (C3ORF60); NDUFAF4 (C6ORF66); NDUFS1; NDUFS2; NDUFS3; NDUFS4; NDUFS6; NDUFS7; NDUFS8; NDUFV1; NFU1; PC; PDHA1; PDHB; PDHX; PDP1; PDSS1; PDSS2; POLG (POLG1); PUS1; RRM2B; SCO2; SERAC1; SLC25A3 (PHC); SLC25A4 (ANT1); SLC37A4; SUCLA2; SUCLG1; SURF1; TAZ; TIMM44; TK2; TMEM70; TPK1; TRMU; TSFM; TUFM; TYMP; UQCRB; YARS2*
Cardiomyopathy due to mitochondrial OXPHOS dysfunction	*AARS2; ACAD9; ATP5E; ATPAF2 (ATP12); COQ9; COX15; DNAJC19; MRPL3; MRPL44; MRPS22; NDUFA2; NDUFA10; NDUFA11; NDUFAF4 (C6ORF66); NDUFS2; NDUFS4; NDUFS7; NDUFS8; NDUFV2; OPA3; POLG; SCO2; SDHA; SLC25A3 (PHC); SLC25A4 (ANT1); TAZ; TMEM70; TSFM*

Mitochondrial Encephalopathy

The clinical features of mitochondrial encephalopathy may overlap that of LS. Mutations in more than 50 nuclear genes important for normal mitochondrial function have been reported to be associated with mitochondrial diseases with encephalopathy as one of the major clinical features (Table 10.5).

Lactic Acidosis

Lactic acidosis or elevated lactate in blood or cerebrospinal fluid is one of the clinical features in 50–87 % of patients with primary mitochondrial disorders [200, 201]. To date, mutations in more than 80 nuclear genes have been reported to be associated with mitochondrial disorders with lactic acidosis or elevated lactate levels (Table 10.5).

Cardiomyopathy Due to Mitochondrial OXPHOS Dysfunction

Up to 40 % of pediatric patients with mitochondrial disorders have cardiomyopathy as one of the major features [200, 202]. To date, many mutations in the mtDNA (www.mitomap.org) and mutations in more than 20 nuclear genes are associated with primary mitochondrial disorders with cardiomyopathy (Table 10.5).

Genotype and Phenotype Correlation of Mitochondrial Disorders

Mitochondrial disorders are clinically and genetically highly heterogeneous in a number of ways. The same disease syndrome can be caused by mutations in mtDNA, or mutations in different nuclear genes involved in the function of different mitochondrial complexes. Mutations in the same gene or even the same mutation can cause different disease syndromes. Mutation(s) in genes theoretically involved in a single OXPHOS complex may actually cause deficiency of multiple OXPHOS complexes. Mutation(s) in genes involved in multiple OXPHOS complexes may cause deficiency of a single OXPHOS complex. Finally, the phenotypes resulting from different complex deficiencies overlap with each other. Therefore, genotype–phenotype correlations for mitochondrial disorders are not well established.

Clinical Utility of Testing

While the diagnosis of mitochondrial disorders is usually suspected clinically [203], biochemical and/or molecular evaluations often are necessary to confirm a specific diagnosis. Since biochemical testing is not definitive and may not be reliable and reproducible [204], molecular genetic confirmation is important, when possible, to confirm the diagnosis, provide guidance on management and prognosis, and permit accurate recurrence risk counseling. For mitochondrial disorders that result from mutations in nuclear genes, identification of the specific familial mutation(s) facilitates prenatal testing.

Identification of a specific disease-causing mutation for mitochondrial diseases has several major clinical utilities. First, diagnostic testing confirms a clinical diagnosis of a specific mitochondrial disease syndrome, distinguishes between primary and secondary mitochondrial disorders, establishes the genetic cause of a primary mitochondrial disorder, and provides prognostic information. A specific diagnosis is used to guide selection of optimal treatment for the affected patient. Test results can inform genetic counseling, recurrence risk determination, and family planning. Predictive testing for asymptomatic family members of a proband with a known mitochondrial disease-causing mutation enables clinical monitoring, follow-up, and optimal treatment of family members with a positive result, and reduces anxiety and foregoing clinical monitoring for family members with a negative test result. Identification of known, pathogenic nuclear gene mutations can be used for prenatal testing of the fetus in at-risk pregnancies. An example of genetic test results used for therapeutic decision-making is patients with Alpers-Syndrome and other POLG-related disorders, due to homozygous or compound heterozygous mutations in the *POLG* gene, should avoid valproic acid which induces or accelerates liver disease in these patients. Another example is patients with CoQ10 deficiency due to mutations in genes involved in the biosynthesis of CoQ10 can be treated by supplementation of CoQ10.

Available Assays

Testing MtDNA

Testing Common MtDNA Point Mutations

To date, more than 50 definitive disease-causing point mutations of mtDNA have been reported (www.mitomap.org). These point mutations account for 70–80 % of patients with primary mtDNA disorders associated with mtDNA point mutations. Many testing methods are used for detection of common mtDNA point mutations including polymerase chain reaction-allele specific oligonucleotide hybridization (PCR-ASO), PCR-restriction fragment length polymorphism (PCR-RFLP), pyrosequencing, real-time amplification-refractory mutation system quantitative PCR (real-time ARMS-qPCR), Sanger sequencing, or next-generation sequencing (NGS). Each method has advantages and disadvantages compared to other methods. The lowest level of heteroplasmy detectable varies from 0.1–1 % by real-time ARMS-qPCR, to 20–25 % by Sanger sequencing (Table 10.6).

Deletion/Duplication Testing of MtDNA

Large-scale mtDNA single deletions can be detected by Southern blot analysis, array-based comparative genomic hybridization (aCGH), or long-range PCR. Both Southern blot analysis and aCGH can detect large-scale single deletions with heteroplasmy of about 15 % or higher [209]. Southern blot analysis may be able to detect multiple deletions of mtDNA, usually in muscle specimens [210]. Long-range PCR is more sensitive in detecting large-scale single deletions and multiple deletions; however, as mtDNA dele-

Table 10.6 Comparison of methods for mtDNA common point mutation analysis

Method	Advantages	Disadvantages	Lowest level of heteroplasmy detectable
PCR-RFLP	Roughly quantitative	Not sensitive; incomplete digestion may result in false positive or false negative results; the adjacent sequences may affect enzyme site.	5–10 % [205, 206]
PCR-ASO	Sensitive; not affected by the adjacent variants	Not quantitative; need radioactive isotope	2 % [205, 206]
Pyro sequencing	Roughly quantitative	Need specific instrument; reliability affected by the adjacent nucleotide sequences.	1–5 % [207]
ARMS-qPCR	Quantitative; sensitive; not affected by the adjacent variants	Need real-time PCR machine; accurate	0.1–1 % [208]
Sanger sequencing	Can detect many variants in a fragment simultaneously	Labor-intensive	20–25 %
Next-generation sequencing	Can analyze many genes and many variants simultaneously	Need expensive instrument	~2 %

ARMS amplification refractory mutation system, *ASO* allele-specific oligonucleotide hybridization, *PCR* polymerase chain reaction, *RFLP* restrictive fragment length polymorphism tions accumulate with age, false-positive results can occur because some low-level age-related deletions of mtDNA do not have clinical significance.

Sequence Analysis of Entire Mitochondrial Genome

Sequence analysis of the entire mitochondrial genome can be done by using Sanger sequencing of 24–50 overlapping PCR amplicons covering the entire mitochondrial genome or by using NGS. Sanger sequencing can detect mutation heteroplasmy of 20–25 % or higher. NGS can detect mutation heteroplasmy as low as 1–2 %. NGS can use either multiple over-lapping amplicons covering the mitochondrial genome, or two whole mitochondrial genome amplicons overlapping at the D-loop (noncoding) region (GeneDx unpublished data). The latter method also detects large-scale single deletions in the mtDNA which account for about 20 % of patients with a primary mitochondrial DNA disorder [1], in addition to point mutations and small insertions or deletions which account for about 80 % of patients with a primary mitochondrial DNA disorders. Although this method cannot detect large duplications of mtDNA, large duplications usually coexist with large-scale mtDNA single deletions and are seen in a subset of patients with KSS [42, 43]. NGS using two whole mitochondrial genome amplicons overlapping at the D-loop (noncoding) region can detect almost all of the primary disease-causing quality defects of mtDNA (see Table 10.7).

Real-Time PCR Analysis of mtDNA to Determine Depletion or Over-Replication

The mtDNA content in muscle or liver tissue can be quantified using real-time PCR for mtDNA and nuclear genes. By comparing the patient result with tissue- and age-matched controls, mtDNA depletion or over replication can be determined [211].

Testing Nuclear Genes

Sequence Analysis of Single Nuclear Genes

Currently, the majority of clinical molecular laboratories offer sequencing of individual nuclear genes. Because mutations in the *POLG* gene are considered to be responsible for

Table 10.7 Comparison of methods for testing entire mitochondrial genome

Disease-causing quality defects in mtDNA				Methods				
Type		Information and comments		Sanger sequencing	Southern blot	aCGH	NGS with multiple partial mtDNA amplicons	NGS with two whole mtDNA amplicons
		Primary or secondary mutations	% Primary mtDNA disorders					
Point mutations		Primary	~80 %	Y	N	N	Y	Y
Lowest heteroplasmy (point mutations) detectable		~10 % patients positive for some point mutations with <5 % mutant in blood, but ≥30 % in muscle; ≥25 % mutant could cause disease		≥25 %	NA	NA	~2 %	~2 %
Deletions	≤20 bp (rare)	Primary	~20 %	Y	N	N	Y	Y
	>20–1,000 bp (Rare)	Primary		Y	N	N	Some	Y
	1 kb (account for >99 % patients with MDS)	Primary		N	Y	Y	N	Y
Large duplications (seen only in a subset of KSS patients with LSDs)		Primary	Always coexist with LSDs	NA	Some	Y	N	N
Multiple deletions (due to mutations in nuclear genes)		Secondary	0 %	N	Some	N	N	Some
Lowest heteroplasmic LSDs detectable		~99 % of the LSDs are de novo; all reported disease-causing LSDs are >15 %		NA	~1 %	~15 %	NA	~15 %
% of patients with primary mtDNA disorders diagnosed				<80 %	~20 %	~20 %	~80 %	>99 %

aCGH array-based comparative genomic hybridization, *KSS* Kearns–Sayre syndrome, *LSD* large single deletion, *MDS* mtDNA deletion syndromes, *mtDNA* mitochondrial DNA, *N* no, *NA* not applicable, *NGS* next-generation sequencing, *Y* yes up to 25 % of patients with mitochondrial disorders, sequencing of this gene is often a good first testing option. Mutations in several other genes (*C10ORF2*, *DGUOK*, and *MPV17*) are known to be responsible for more than 50 % of patients with hepatocerebral mtDNA depletion syndrome, and therefore also are good candidates for single gene sequencing. For the vast majority of other genes, the positive detection rate is very low, and the overall cost of sequencing multiple single genes is very high.

Sequence Analysis of Multiple Genes

For patients with diseases that fall into a specific category, such as CI deficiency, or CIV deficiency, mutations in many different nuclear genes could be causal. For the more than 20 nuclear genes with known disease-causing mutations for CI deficiency, no single gene is responsible for more than 5 % of the patients [52]. Therefore, sequencing the multiple genes individually is neither time-efficient nor cost-effective. NGS can analyze many genes simultaneously at a cost that is often less than sequencing multiple single genes individually and is therefore more suitable for testing of diseases with many candidate genes, such as CI deficiency, CIV deficiency, LS, and other mitochondrial diseases (see Tables 10.3, 10.4, and 10.5). Multi-gene panels that sequence the majority of genes known to cause mitochondrial disease are the best testing approach at this time.

NGS is not optimal for detection of large deletions or duplications in the nuclear genome, and many laboratories rely on aCGH for clinical testing for these types of variants.

Interpretation of Results

Positive Result

A positive result indicates that a disease-causing mutation was identified that confirms the diagnosis of a particular type of mitochondrial disorder and provides valuable information to the physician and family members about treatment, prognosis, and recurrence risk. For mtDNA mutations, it is difficult to provide prognosis and recurrence risk for most of the patients because of the uncertainty of the degree of heteroplasmy by tissue type. For patients with disease-causing nuclear gene mutations, all first-degree relatives (e.g., children, siblings, and parents) can be offered predictive genetic testing with appropriate genetic counseling before and after the testing is performed. If a family member is found to be positive for the familial mutation(s), this individual is also at risk to develop the specific mitochondrial disorder or may be at risk to have children with the specific mitochondrial disorder. Of note for genetic counseling is the fact that mitochondrial diseases are highly variable in the symptoms, age of onset, severity, and response to therapeutic agents, even among members of the same family who have the same genetic mutation(s).

Negative Result

A negative result in an individual suspected of having a mitochondrial disorder does not rule out a genetically inherited mitochondrial disease. Possible reasons for a false-negative result are that the patient has a mutation in a gene not included in the testing panel, or located in a part of a mitochondrial disease gene not covered by the test. A true negative result is expected if the patient does not have a heritable type of mitochondrial disease. A negative result obtained by a specific genetic test for an individual with a definite mitochondrial disorder indicates that predictive testing of asymptomatic family members will not be informative and is not warranted. However, family members of a clinically affected individual with negative test results may still be at risk for mitochondrial disease and thus should be evaluated by a specialist in mitochondrial medicine, as indicated. If an asymptomatic individual is negative for a mutation identified in a family member with a definitive mitochondrial disorder, the result is considered a true negative. This indicates that the individual is not at increased genetic risk for the familial mitochondrial disorder and instead has the same risk as a person in the general population to develop a mitochondrial disorder. Specific clinical monitoring for the development of a mitochondrial disorder is not necessary in individuals with a true negative result.

Variant of Unknown Significance

One of the most difficult results to interpret is the finding of a variant of unknown clinical significance (VUS). This situation indicates that the pathogenic role of the variant cannot be clearly established. In some cases, testing of other family members may help clarify the clinical significance of a VUS. If other relatives with mitochondrial disease are found to have the same variant, it is more likely that the variant is disease causing. The greater the number of affected family members who carry the VUS, the greater is the likelihood that the VUS is pathogenic. Likewise, if an individual has an apparently sporadic mitochondrial disorder, the finding that a VUS is de novo (arose new in that individual and was not inherited from a parent) indicates that the variant is likely disease causing.

Test Sensitivity

Technical Sensitivity

As discussed above and in Table 10.6, for mtDNA point mutations, the lowest level of heteroplasmy of mutations detectable by different methods varies from 0.1–1 % by real-time ARMS-qPCR [208] to 20–25 % by Sanger sequencing. For large-scale single deletions, both Southern blot analysis and aCGH can detect large-scale single deletions with heteroplasmy of approximately 15 % or higher [209]. Sanger sequencing can detect point mutations, small deletions, and small insertions in both mtDNA and nuclear genes.

Clinical Sensitivity

Depending on the method used and how many genes are tested, the clinical sensitivity of genetic testing for different diseases varies significantly. See Tables 10.2, 10.3, 10.4, and 10.5 for details.

Laboratory Issues

Many laboratories offer molecular genetic testing for mitochondrial disorders. Most laboratories offer common mtDNA mutation testing by using PCR-ASO, PCR-RFLP, real-time ARMS-qPCR, pyrosequencing, Sanger sequencing, or other methods. A patient with a disease-causing mutation with heteroplasmy of <5 % in the blood may have >50 % heteroplasmy in the muscle tissue or other tissues. More than 10 % of patients positive for the m.3243A>G mutation have a level of heteroplasmy less than 5 % in the blood specimen [212]. Since blood samples are still the most common sample sent for clinical molecular testing for mitochondrial disorders, it is important to use a technology that is able to detect low heteroplasmic mtDNA mutations. For NGS testing of large numbers of nuclear genes, some laboratories use PCR-based sequence enrichment, while other laboratories use capture (hybridization)-based enrichment. Compared to capture based-enrichment, PCR-based enrichment is more sensitive, easier to use, and is highly reproducible for targeted NGS testing [213]. Approximately 25 % of human genes in the genome have pseudogenes (www.pseudogene.org). PCR-based sequence enrichment selectively amplifies only the genes of interest, thus avoiding many pseudogene/homologous sequence problems inherent to hybridization-based sequence enrichment (target capture) methods that can cause both false-positive and false-negative results.

References

1. Chinnery PF. (1993 updated 2010) GeneReviews [Internet]. Seattle (WA): University of Washington, Seattle; 1993.
2. Tarnopolsky MA, Raha S. Med Sci Sports Exerc. 2005;37:2086–93.
3. van Adel BA, Tarnopolsky MA. J Clin Neuromuscul Dis. 2009;10:97–121.
4. Zhu X, Peng X, Guan MX, Yan Q. Acta Biochim Biophys Sin (Shanghai). 2009;41:179–87.
5. Chinnery PF. Trends Genet. 2003;19:60–2.
6. Dimauro S, Davidzon G. Ann Med. 2005;37:222–32.
7. Jaksch M, Kleinle S, Scharfe C, Klopstock T, Pongratz D, Muller-Hocker J, Gerbitz KD, Liechti-Gallati S, Lochmuller H, Horvath R. J Med Genet. 2001;38:665–73.
8. Swalwell H, Kirby DM, Blakely EL, Mitchell A, Salemi R, Sugiana C, Compton AG, Tucker EJ, Ke BX, Lamont PJ, Turnbull DM, McFarland R, Taylor RW, Thorburn DR. Eur J Hum Genet. 2011;19:769–75.
9. DiMauro S, Schon EA. N Engl J Med. 2003;348:2656–68.
10. Calvo SE, Mootha VK. Annu Rev Genomics Hum Genet. 2010;11:25–44.
11. de Keyzer Y, Valayannopoulos V, Benoist JF, Batteux F, Lacaille F, Hubert L, Chretien D, Chadefeaux-Vekemans B, Niaudet P, Touati G, Munnich A, de Lonlay P. Pediatr Res. 2009;66:91–5.
12. Fragaki K, Cano A, Benoist JF, Rigal O, Chaussenot A, Rouzier C, Bannwarth S, Caruba C, Chabrol B, Paquis-Flucklinger V. Mitochondrion. 2011;11:533–6.
13. Hui J, Kirby DM, Thorburn DR, Boneh A. Dev Med Child Neurol. 2006;48:132–6.
14. Longo N. Neurol Clin. 2003;21:817–31.
15. Ruiz-Pesini E, Lott MT, Procaccio V, Poole JC, Brandon MC, Mishmar D, Yi C, Kreuziger J, Baldi P, Wallace DC. Nucleic Acids Res. 2007;35:D823–8.
16. Riordan-Eva P, Harding AE. J Med Genet. 1995;32:81–7.
17. Holt IJ, Miller DH, Harding AE. J Med Genet. 1989;26:739–43.
18. Isashiki Y, Nakagawa M. Jpn J Ophthalmol. 1991;35:259–67.
19. Man PY, Turnbull DM, Chinnery PF. J Med Genet. 2002;39:162–9.
20. Thorburn DR, Rahman S. (1993 updated 2011) GeneReviews [Internet]. Seattle (WA): University of Washington, Seattle; 1993.
21. Kirby DM, Crawford M, Cleary MA, Dahl HH, Dennett X, Thorburn DR. Neurology. 1999;52:1255–64.
22. Wong LJ, Yim D, Bai RK, Kwon H, Vacek MM, Zane J, Hoppel CL, Kerr DS. J Med Genet. 2006;43, e46.
23. Florentz C, Sohm B, Tryoen-Toth P, Putz J, Sissler M. Cell Mol Life Sci. 2003;60:1356–75.
24. Smits P, Smeitink J, van den Heuvel L. J Biomed Biotechnol. 2010;2010:737385.
25. Majamaa K, Moilanen JS, Uimonen S, Remes AM, Salmela PI, Karppa M, Majamaa-Voltti KA, Rusanen H, Sorri M, Peuhkurinen KJ, Hassinen IE. Am J Hum Genet. 1998;63:447–54.
26. DiMauro S, Hirano M. (1993 updated 2009) GeneReviews [Internet]. Seattle (WA): University of Washington, Seattle; 1993.
27. MITOMAP. updated 2013. www.mitomap.org.
28. Pandya A. (1993 Updated April 2011) GeneReviews [Internet]. Seattle (WA): University of Washington, Seattle; 1993–2015.
29. Goto Y, Nonaka I, Horai S. Biochim Biophys Acta. 1991;1097:238–40.
30. Mackey DA, Oostra RJ, Rosenberg T, Nikoskelainen E, Bronte-Stewart J, Poulton J, Harding AE, Govan G, Bolhuis PA, Norby S. Am J Hum Genet. 1996;59:481–5.
31. Achilli A, Iommarini L, Olivieri A, Pala M, Hooshiar Kashani B, Reynier P, La Morgia C, Valentino ML, Liguori R, Pizza F, Barboni P, Sadun F, De Negri AM, Zeviani M, Dollfus H, Moulignier A, Ducos G, Orssaud C, Bonneau D, Procaccio V, Leo-Kottler B, Fauser S, Wissinger B, Amati-Bonneau P, Torroni A, Carelli V. PLoS One. 2012;7, e42242.
32. Campos Y, Martin MA, Rubio JC, Solana LG, Garcia-Benayas C, Terradas JL, Arenas J. Neurology. 1997;49:595–7.
33. Makino M, Horai S, Goto Y, Nonaka I. Neuromuscul Disord. 1998;8:149–51.
34. Thyagarajan D, Shanske S, Vazquez-Memije M, De Vivo D, DiMauro S. Ann Neurol. 1995;38:468–72.
35. DiMauro S, Hirano M. (1993 updated 2010) GeneReviews [Internet]. Seattle (WA): University of Washington, Seattle; 1993.

36. Crispim D, Estivalet AA, Roisenberg I, Gross JL, Canani LH. Arq Bras Endocrinol Metabol. 2008;52:1228–35.
37. Macmillan C, Kirkham T, Fu K, Allison V, Andermann E, Chitayat D, Fortier D, Gans M, Hare H, Quercia N, Zackon D, Shoubridge EA. Neurology. 1998;50:417–22.
38. Lebon S, Chol M, Benit P, Mugnier C, Chretien D, Giurgea I, Kern I, Girardin E, Hertz-Pannier L, de Lonlay P, Rotig A, Rustin P, Munnich A. J Med Genet. 2003;40:896–9.
39. Ugalde C, Triepels RH, Coenen MJ, van den Heuvel LP, Smeets R, Uusimaa J, Briones P, Campistol J, Majamaa K, Smeitink JA, Nijtmans LG. Ann Neurol. 2003;54:665–9.
40. Sternberg D, Chatzoglou E, Laforet P, Fayet G, Jardel C, Blondy P, Fardeau M, Amselem S, Eymard B, Lombes A. Brain. 2001;124:984–94.
41. DiMauro S, Hirano M. (1993 updated 2011) GeneReviews [Internet]. Seattle (WA): University of Washington, Seattle; 1993.
42. Manfredi G, Vu T, Bonilla E, Schon EA, DiMauro S, Arnaudo E, Zhang L, Rowland LP, Hirano M. Ann Neurol. 1997;42:180–8.
43. Odoardi F, Rana M, Broccolini A, Mirabella M, Modoni A, D'Amico A, Papacci M, Tonali P, Servidei S, Silvestri G. Am J Med Genet A. 2003;118A:247–54.
44. Poulton J, Deadman ME, Gardiner RM. Lancet. 1989;1:236–40.
45. Poulton J, Morten KJ, Weber K, Brown GK, Bindoff L. Hum Mol Genet. 1994;3:947–51.
46. Schroder R, Vielhaber S, Wiedemann FR, Kornblum C, Papassotiropoulos A, Broich P, Zierz S, Elger CE, Reichmann H, Seibel P, Klockgether T, Kunz WS. J Neuropathol Exp Neurol. 2000;59:353–60.
47. Moslemi AR, Tulinius M, Holme E, Oldfors A. Neuromuscul Disord. 1998;8:345–9.
48. Tokunaga M, Mita S, Sakuta R, Nonaka I, Araki S. Ann Neurol. 1993;33:275–80.
49. Wong LJ, Perng CL, Hsu CH, Bai RK, Schelley S, Vladutiu GD, Vogel H, Enns GM. J Med Genet. 2003;40, e125.
50. Skladal D, Halliday J, Thorburn DR. Brain. 2003;126:1905–12.
51. von Kleist-Retzow JC, Cormier-Daire V, de Lonlay P, Parfait B, Chretien D, Rustin P, Feingold J, Rotig A, Munnich A. Am J Hum Genet. 1998;63:428–35.
52. Tucker EJ, Compton AG, Calvo SE, Thorburn DR. IUBMB Life. 2011;63(9):669–77.
53. Distelmaier F, Koopman WJ, van den Heuvel LP, Rodenburg RJ, Mayatepek E, Willems PH, Smeitink JA. Brain. 2009;132: 833–42.
54. Budde SM, van den Heuvel LP, Janssen AJ, Smeets RJ, Buskens CA, DeMeirleir L, Van Coster R, Baethmann M, Voit T, Trijbels JM, Smeitink JA. Biochem Biophys Res Commun. 2000;275: 63–8.
55. Saada A, Edvardson S, Shaag A, Chung WK, Segel R, Miller C, Jalas C, Elpeleg O. J Inherit Metab Dis. 2012;35:125–31.
56. Boekema EJ, Braun HP. J Biol Chem. 2007;282:1–4.
57. Dudkina NV, Sunderhaus S, Boekema EJ, Braun HP. J Bioenerg Biomembr. 2008;40:419–24.
58. Schagger H, de Coo R, Bauer MF, Hofmann S, Godinot C, Brandt U. J Biol Chem. 2004;279:36349–53.
59. Baysal BE. J Med Genet. 2008;45:689–94.
60. Rotig A. Diabetes Metab. 2010;36:97–107.
61. Benit P, Lebon S, Rustin P. Biochim Biophys Acta. 2009;1793: 181–5.
62. Hinson JT, Fantin VR, Schonberger J, Breivik N, Siem G, McDonough B, Sharma P, Keogh I, Godinho R, Santos F, Esparza A, Nicolau Y, Selvaag E, Cohen BH, Hoppel CL, Tranebjaerg L, Eavey RD, Seidman JG, Seidman CE. N Engl J Med. 2007;356:809–19.
63. Kotarsky H, Karikoski R, Morgelin M, Marjavaara S, Bergman P, Zhang DL, Smet J, van Coster R, Fellman V. Mitochondrion. 2010;10:497–509.
64. Visapaa I, Fellman V, Vesa J, Dasvarma A, Hutton JL, Kumar V, Payne GS, Makarow M, Van Coster R, Taylor RW, Turnbull DM, Suomalainen A, Peltonen L. Am J Hum Genet. 2002;71:863–76.
65. Sue CM, Karadimas C, Checcarelli N, Tanji K, Papadopoulou LC, Pallotti F, Guo FL, Shanske S, Hirano M, De Vivo DC, Van Coster R, Kaplan P, Bonilla E, DiMauro S. Ann Neurol. 2000;47: 589–95.
66. Carelli V, Baracca A, Barogi S, Pallotti F, Valentino ML, Montagna P, Zeviani M, Pini A, Lenaz G, Baruzzi A, Solaini G. Arch Neurol. 2002;59:264–70.
67. Houstek J, Pickova A, Vojtiskova A, Mracek T, Pecina P, Jesina P. Biochim Biophys Acta. 2006;1757:1400–5.
68. Sperl W, Jesina P, Zeman J, Mayr JA, Demeirleir L, VanCoster R, Pickova A, Hansikova H, Houst'kova H, Krejcik Z, Koch J, Smet J, Muss W, Holme E, Houstek J. Neuromuscul Disord. 2006;16:821–9.
69. Ostergaard E, Rodenburg RJ, van den Brand M, Thomsen LL, Duno M, Batbayli M, Wibrand F, Nijtmans L. J Med Genet. 2011;48(11):737–40.
70. Pagniez-Mammeri H, Loublier S, Legrand A, Benit P, Rustin P, Slama A. Mol Genet Metab. 2012;105:163–72.
71. van den Bosch BJ, Gerards M, Sluiter W, Stegmann AP, Jongen EL, Hellebrekers DM, Oegema R, Lambrichs EH, Prokisch H, Danhauser K, Schoonderwoerd K, de Coo IF, Smeets HJ. J Med Genet. 2011;49:10–5.
72. Calvo SE, Compton AG, Hershman SG, Lim SC, Lieber DS, Tucker EJ, Laskowski A, Garone C, Liu S, Jaffe DB, Christodoulou J, Fletcher JM, Bruno DL, Goldblatt J, Dimauro S, Thorburn DR, Mootha VK. Sci Transl Med. 2012;4(118):118ra110.
73. Haack TB, Madignier F, Herzer M, Lamantea E, Danhauser K, Invernizzi F, Koch J, Freitag M, Drost R, Hillier I, Haberberger B, Mayr JA, Ahting U, Tiranti V, Rotig A, Iuso A, Horvath R, Tesarova M, Baric I, Uziel G, Rolinski B, Sperl W, Meitinger T, Zeviani M, Freisinger P, Prokisch H. J Med Genet. 2012;49: 83–9.
74. Calvo SE, Tucker EJ, Compton AG, Kirby DM, Crawford G, Burtt NP, Rivas M, Guiducci C, Bruno DL, Goldberger OA, Redman MC, Wiltshire E, Wilson CJ, Altshuler D, Gabriel SB, Daly MJ, Thorburn DR, Mootha VK. Nat Genet. 2010;42:851–8.
75. Fassone E, Duncan AJ, Taanman JW, Pagnamenta AT, Sadowski MI, Holand T, Qasim W, Rutland P, Calvo SE, Mootha VK, Bitner-Glindzicz M, Rahman S. Hum Mol Genet. 2010;19:4837–47.
76. Ghezzi D, Sevrioukova I, Invernizzi F, Lamperti C, Mora M, D'Adamo P, Novara F, Zuffardi O, Uziel G, Zeviani M. Am J Hum Genet. 2010;86:639–49.
77. Pagniez-Mammeri H, Rak M, Legrand A, Benit P, Rustin P, Slama A. Mol Genet Metab. 2012;105:173–9.
78. Gauthier-Villars M, Landrieu P, Cormier-Daire V, Jacquemin E, Chretien D, Rotig A, Rustin P, Munnich A, de Lonlay P. Neuropediatrics. 2001;32:150–2.
79. Wortmann SB, Rodenburg RJ, Jonckheere A, de Vries MC, Huizing M, Heldt K, van den Heuvel LP, Wendel U, Kluijtmans LA, Engelke UF, Wevers RA, Smeitink JA, Morava E. Brain. 2009;132:136–46.
80. Hakonen AH, Goffart S, Marjavaara S, Paetau A, Cooper H, Mattila K, Lampinen M, Sajantila A, Lonnqvist T, Spelbrink JN, Suomalainen A. Hum Mol Genet. 2008;17:3822–35.
81. Bourgeron T, Rustin P, Chretien D, Birch-Machin M, Bourgeois M, Viegas-Pequignot E, Munnich A, Rotig A. Nat Genet. 1995;11:144–9.
82. Levitas A, Muhammad E, Harel G, Saada A, Caspi VC, Manor E, Beck JC, Sheffield V, Parvari R. Eur J Hum Genet. 2010;18:1160–5.
83. Parfait B, Chretien D, Rotig A, Marsac C, Munnich A, Rustin P. Hum Genet. 2000;106:236–43.

84. Ghezzi D, Goffrini P, Uziel G, Horvath R, Klopstock T, Lochmuller H, D'Adamo P, Gasparini P, Strom TM, Prokisch H, Invernizzi F, Ferrero I, Zeviani M. Nat Genet. 2009;41:654–6.
85. Barel O, Shorer Z, Flusser H, Ofir R, Narkis G, Finer G, Shalev H, Nasasra A, Saada A, Birk OS. Am J Hum Genet. 2008;82: 1211–6.
86. Haut S, Brivet M, Touati G, Rustin P, Lebon S, Garcia-Cazorla A, Saudubray JM, Boutron A, Legrand A, Slama A. Hum Genet. 2003;113:118–22.
87. Miyake N, Yano S, Sakai C, Hatakeyama H, Matsushima Y, Shiina M, Watanabe Y, Bartley J, Abdenur JE, Wang RY, Chang R, Tsurusaki Y, Doi H, Nakashima M, Saitsu H, Ogata K, Goto Y, Matsumoto N. Hum Mutat. 2013;34:446–52.
88. Gaignard P, Menezes M, Schiff M, Bayot A, Rak M, Ogier de Baulny H, Su CH, Gilleron M, Lombes A, Abida H, Tzagoloff A, Riley L, Cooper ST, Mina K, Sivadorai P, Davis MR, Allcock RJ, Kresoje N, Laing NG, Thorburn DR, Slama A, Christodoulou J, Rustin P. Am J Hum Genet. 2013;93:384–9.
89. Ghezzi D, Arzuffi P, Zordan M, Da Re C, Lamperti C, Benna C, D'Adamo P, Diodato D, Costa R, Mariotti C, Uziel G, Smiderle C, Zeviani M. Nat Genet. 2011;43:259–63.
90. Diaz F. Biochim Biophys Acta. 2010;1802:100–10.
91. Huigsloot M, Nijtmans LG, Szklarczyk R, Baars MJ, van den Brand MA, Hendriksfranssen MG, van den Heuvel LP, Smeitink JA, Huynen MA, Rodenburg RJ. Am J Hum Genet. 2011;88: 488–93.
92. Ylikallio E, Suomalainen A. Ann Med. 2012;44:41–59.
93. Weraarpachai W, Sasarman F, Nishimura T, Antonicka H, Aure K, Rotig A, Lombes A, Shoubridge EA. Am J Hum Genet. 2012;90:142–51.
94. Szklarczyk R, Wanschers BF, Nijtmans LG, Rodenburg RJ, Zschocke J, Dikow N, van den Brand MA, Hendriks-Franssen MG, Gilissen C, Veltman JA, Nooteboom M, Koopman WJ, Willems PH, Smeitink JA, Huynen MA, van den Heuvel LP. Hum Mol Genet. 2013;22:656–67.
95. Heberle LC, Al Tawari AA, Ramadan DG, Ibrahim JK. Brain Dev. 2006;28:329–31.
96. Ghezzi D, Saada A, D'Adamo P, Fernandez-Vizarra E, Gasparini P, Tiranti V, Elpeleg O, Zeviani M. Am J Hum Genet. 2008;83:415–23.
97. Lim SC, Smith KR, Stroud DA, Compton AG, Tucker EJ, Dasvarma A, Gandolfo LC, Marum JE, McKenzie M, Peters HL, Mowat D, Procopis PG, Wilcken B, Christodoulou J, Brown GK, Ryan MT, Bahlo M, Thorburn DR. Am J Hum Genet. 2014;94:209–22.
98. Weraarpachai W, Antonicka H, Sasarman F, Seeger J, Schrank B, Kolesar JE, Lochmuller H, Chevrette M, Kaufman BA, Horvath R, Shoubridge EA. Nat Genet. 2009;41:833–7.
99. Herzer M, Koch J, Prokisch H, Rodenburg R, Rauscher C, Radauer W, Forstner R, Pilz P, Rolinski B, Freisinger P, Mayr JA, Sperl W. Neuropediatrics. 2010;41:30–4.
100. Cizkova A, Stranecky V, Mayr JA, Tesarova M, Havlickova V, Paul J, Ivanek R, Kuss AW, Hansikova H, Kaplanova V, Vrbacky M, Hartmannova H, Noskova L, Honzik T, Drahota Z, Magner M, Hejzlarova K, Sperl W, Zeman J, Houstek J, Kmoch S. Nat Genet. 2008;40:1288–90.
101. De Meirleir L, Seneca S, Lissens W, De Clercq I, Eyskens F, Gerlo E, Smet J, Van Coster R. J Med Genet. 2004;41:120–4.
102. Spiegel R, Khayat M, Shalev SA, Horovitz Y, Mandel H, Hershkovitz E, Barghuti F, Shaag A, Saada A, Korman SH, Elpeleg O, Yatsiv I. J Med Genet. 2011;48:177–82.
103. Mayr JA, Merkel O, Kohlwein SD, Gebhardt BR, Bohles H, Fotschl U, Koch J, Jaksch M, Lochmuller H, Horvath R, Freisinger P, Sperl W. Am J Hum Genet. 2007;80:478–84.
104. Naviaux RK, Nguyen KV. Ann Neurol. 2004;55:706–12.
105. Vissing J, Ravn K, Danielsen ER, Duno M, Wibrand F, Wevers RA, Schwartz M. Neurology. 2002;59:926–9.
106. Mancuso M, Filosto M, Oh SJ, DiMauro S. Arch Neurol. 2004;61:1777–9.
107. Van Goethem G, Dermaut B, Lofgren A, Martin JJ, Van Broeckhoven C. Nat Genet. 2001;28:211–2.
108. Hakonen AH, Heiskanen S, Juvonen V, Lappalainen I, Luoma PT, Rantamaki M, Goethem GV, Lofgren A, Hackman P, Paetau A, Kaakkola S, Majamaa K, Varilo T, Udd B, Kaariainen H, Bindoff LA, Suomalainen A. Am J Hum Genet. 2005;77:430–41.
109. Van Goethem G, Luoma P, Rantamaki M, Al Memar A, Kaakkola S, Hackman P, Krahe R, Lofgren A, Martin JJ, De Jonghe P, Suomalainen A, Udd B, Van Broeckhoven C. Neurology. 2004;63:1251–7.
110. Longley MJ, Clark S, Yu Wai Man C, Hudson G, Durham SE, Taylor RW, Nightingale S, Turnbull DM, Copeland WC, Chinnery PF. Am J Hum Genet. 2006;78:1026–34.
111. Sarzi E, Goffart S, Serre V, Chretien D, Slama A, Munnich A, Spelbrink JN, Rotig A. Ann Neurol. 2007;62:579–87.
112. Spelbrink JN, Li FY, Tiranti V, Nikali K, Yuan QP, Tariq M, Wanrooij S, Garrido N, Comi G, Morandi L, Santoro L, Toscano A, Fabrizi GM, Somer H, Croxen R, Beeson D, Poulton J, Suomalainen A, Jacobs HT, Zeviani M, Larsson C. Nat Genet. 2001;28:223–31.
113. Salviati L, Sacconi S, Mancuso M, Otaegui D, Camano P, Marina A, Rabinowitz S, Shiffman R, Thompson K, Wilson CM, Feigenbaum A, Naini AB, Hirano M, Bonilla E, DiMauro S, Vu TH. Ann Neurol. 2002;52:311–7.
114. Mancuso M, Salviati L, Sacconi S, Otaegui D, Camano P, Marina A, Bacman S, Moraes CT, Carlo JR, Garcia M, Garcia-Alvarez M, Monzon L, Naini AB, Hirano M, Bonilla E, Taratuto AL, DiMauro S, Vu TH. Neurology. 2002;59:1197–202.
115. Nishino I, Spinazzola A, Papadimitriou A, Hammans S, Steiner I, Hahn CD, Connolly AM, Verloes A, Guimaraes J, Maillard I, Hamano H, Donati MA, Semrad CE, Russell JA, Andreu AL, Hadjigeorgiou GM, Vu TH, Tadesse S, Nygaard TG, Nonaka I, Hirano I, Bonilla E, Rowland LP, DiMauro S, Hirano M. Ann Neurol. 2000;47:792–800.
116. Bourdon A, Minai L, Serre V, Jais JP, Sarzi E, Aubert S, Chretien D, de Lonlay P, Paquis-Flucklinger V, Arakawa H, Nakamura Y, Munnich A, Rotig A. Nat Genet. 2007;39:776–80.
117. Kollberg G, Darin N, Benan K, Moslemi AR, Lindal S, Tulinius M, Oldfors A, Holme E. Neuromuscul Disord. 2009;19:147–50.
118. Fratter C, Raman P, Alston CL, Blakely EL, Craig K, Smith C, Evans J, Seller A, Czermin B, Hanna MG, Poulton J, Brierley C, Staunton TG, Turnpenny PD, Schaefer AM, Chinnery PF, Horvath R, Turnbull DM, Gorman GS, Taylor RW. Neurology. 2011;76:2032–4.
119. Takata A, Kato M, Nakamura M, Yoshikawa T, Kanba S, Sano A, Kato T. Genome Biol. 2011;12:R92.
120. Napoli L, Bordoni A, Zeviani M, Hadjigeorgiou GM, Sciacco M, Tiranti V, Terentiou A, Moggio M, Papadimitriou A, Scarlato G, Comi GP. Neurology. 2001;57:2295–8.
121. Palmieri L, Alberio S, Pisano I, Lodi T, Meznaric-Petrusa M, Zidar J, Santoro A, Scarcia P, Fontanesi F, Lamantea E, Ferrero I, Zeviani M. Hum Mol Genet. 2005;14:3079–88.
122. Ostergaard E, Christensen E, Kristensen E, Mogensen B, Duno M, Shoubridge EA, Wibrand F. Am J Hum Genet. 2007;81:383–7.
123. Ostergaard E, Schwartz M, Batbayli M, Christensen E, Hjalmarson O, Kollberg G, Holme E. Eur J Pediatr. 2010;169:201–5.
124. Carrozzo R, Dionisi-Vici C, Steuerwald U, Lucioli S, Deodato F, Di Giandomenico S, Bertini E, Franke B, Kluijtmans LA, Meschini MC, Rizzo C, Piemonte F, Rodenburg R, Santer R, Santorelli FM, van Rooij A, Vermunt-de Koning D, Morava E, Wevers RA. Brain. 2007;130:862–74.

125. Ostergaard E, Hansen FJ, Sorensen N, Duno M, Vissing J, Larsen PL, Faeroe O, Thorgrimsson S, Wibrand F, Christensen E, Schwartz M. Brain. 2007;130:853–61.
126. Cohn AC, Toomes C, Potter C, Towns KV, Hewitt AW, Inglehearn CF, Craig JE, Mackey DA. Am J Ophthalmol. 2007;143:656–62.
127. Stewart JD, Hudson G, Yu-Wai-Man P, Blakeley EL, He L, Horvath R, Maddison P, Wright A, Griffiths PG, Turnbull DM, Taylor RW, Chinnery PF. Neurology. 2008;71:1829–31.
128. Yu-Wai-Man P, Griffiths PG, Gorman GS, Lourenco CM, Wright AF, Auer-Grumbach M, Toscano A, Musumeci O, Valentino ML, Caporali L, Lamperti C, Tallaksen CM, Duffey P, Miller J, Whittaker RG, Baker MR, Jackson MJ, Clarke MP, Dhillon B, Czermin B, Stewart JD, Hudson G, Reynier P, Bonneau D, Marques Jr W, Lenaers G, McFarland R, Taylor RW, Turnbull DM, Votruba M, Zeviani M, Carelli V, Bindoff LA, Horvath R, Amati-Bonneau P, Chinnery PF. Brain. 2010;133:771–86.
129. Bykhovskaya Y, Casas K, Mengesha E, Inbal A, Fischel-Ghodsian N. Am J Hum Genet. 2004;74:1303–8.
130. Zeharia A, Shaag A, Pappo O, Mager-Heckel AM, Saada A, Beinat M, Karicheva O, Mandel H, Ofek N, Segel R, Marom D, Rotig A, Tarassov I, Elpeleg O. Am J Hum Genet. 2009;85:401–7.
131. Coenen MJ, Antonicka H, Ugalde C, Sasarman F, Rossi R, Heister JG, Newbold RF, Trijbels FJ, van den Heuvel LP, Shoubridge EA, Smeitink JA. N Engl J Med. 2004;351:2080–6.
132. Antonicka H, Sasarman F, Kennaway NG, Shoubridge EA. Hum Mol Genet. 2006;15:1835–46.
133. Valente L, Tiranti V, Marsano RM, Malfatti E, Fernandez-Vizarra E, Donnini C, Mereghetti P, De Gioia L, Burlina A, Castellan C, Comi GP, Savasta S, Ferrero I, Zeviani M. Am J Hum Genet. 2007;80:44–58.
134. Smeitink JA, Elpeleg O, Antonicka H, Diepstra H, Saada A, Smits P, Sasarman F, Vriend G, Jacob-Hirsch J, Shaag A, Rechavi G, Welling B, Horst J, Rodenburg RJ, van den Heuvel B, Shoubridge EA. Am J Hum Genet. 2006;79:869–77.
135. Galmiche L, Serre V, Beinat M, Assouline Z, Lebre AS, Chretien D, Nietschke P, Benes V, Boddaert N, Sidi D, Brunelle F, Rio M, Munnich A, Rotig A. Hum Mutat. 2011;32:1225–31.
136. Carroll CJ, Isohanni P, Poyhonen R, Euro L, Richter U, Brilhante V, Gotz A, Lahtinen T, Paetau A, Pihko H, Battersby BJ, Tyynismaa H, Suomalainen A. J Med Genet. 2013;50:151–9.
137. Miller C, Saada A, Shaul N, Shabtai N, Ben-Shalom E, Shaag A, Hershkovitz E, Elpeleg O. Ann Neurol. 2004;56:734–8.
138. Saada A, Shaag A, Arnon S, Dolfin T, Miller C, Fuchs-Telem D, Lombes A, Elpeleg O. J Med Genet. 2007;44:784–6.
139. Smits P, Saada A, Wortmann SB, Heister AJ, Brink M, Pfundt R, Miller C, Haas D, Hantschmann R, Rodenburg RJ, Smeitink JA, van den Heuvel LP. Eur J Hum Genet. 2011;19:394–9.
140. Gotz A, Tyynismaa H, Euro L, Ellonen P, Hyotylainen T, Ojala T, Hamalainen RH, Tommiska J, Raivio T, Oresic M, Karikoski R, Tammela O, Simola KO, Paetau A, Tyni T, Suomalainen A. Am J Hum Genet. 2011;88:635–42.
141. Scheper GC, van der Klok T, van Andel RJ, van Berkel CG, Sissler M, Smet J, Muravina TI, Serkov SV, Uziel G, Bugiani M, Schiffmann R, Krageloh-Mann I, Smeitink JA, Florentz C, Van Coster R, Pronk JC, van der Knaap MS. Nat Genet. 2007;39:534–9.
142. Talim B, Pyle A, Griffin H, Topaloglu H, Tokatli A, Keogh MJ, Santibanez-Koref M, Chinnery PF, Horvath R. Brain. 2013;136, e228.
143. Elo JM, Yadavalli SS, Euro L, Isohanni P, Gotz A, Carroll CJ, Valanne L, Alkuraya FS, Uusimaa J, Paetau A, Caruso EM, Pihko H, Ibba M, Tyynismaa H, Suomalainen A. Hum Mol Genet. 2012;21:4521–9.
144. Pierce SB, Chisholm KM, Lynch ED, Lee MK, Walsh T, Opitz JM, Li W, Klevit RE, King MC. Proc Natl Acad Sci U S A. 2011;108:6543–8.
145. Pierce SB, Gersak K, Michaelson-Cohen R, Walsh T, Lee MK, Malach D, Klevit RE, King MC, Levy-Lahad E. Am J Hum Genet. 2013;92:614–20.
146. Bayat V, Thiffault I, Jaiswal M, Tetreault M, Donti T, Sasarman F, Bernard G, Demers-Lamarche J, Dicaire MJ, Mathieu J, Vanasse M, Bouchard JP, Rioux MF, Lourenco CM, Li Z, Haueter C, Shoubridge EA, Graham BH, Brais B, Bellen HJ. PLoS Biol. 2012;10, e1001288.
147. Rankin J, Brown R, Dobyns WB, Harington J, Patel J, Quinn M, Brown G. Am J Med Genet A. 2010;152A:2079–84.
148. Belostotsky R, Ben-Shalom E, Rinat C, Becker-Cohen R, Feinstein S, Zeligson S, Segel R, Elpeleg O, Nassar S, Frishberg Y. Am J Hum Genet. 2011;88:193–200.
149. Riley LG, Cooper S, Hickey P, Rudinger-Thirion J, McKenzie M, Compton A, Lim SC, Thorburn D, Ryan MT, Giege R, Bahlo M, Christodoulou J. Am J Hum Genet. 2010;87:52–9.
150. Antonicka H, Ostergaard E, Sasarman F, Weraarpachai W, Wibrand F, Pedersen AM, Rodenburg RJ, van der Knaap MS, Smeitink JA, Chrzanowska-Lightowlers ZM, Shoubridge EA. Am J Hum Genet. 2010;87:115–22.
151. Haack TB, Kopajtich R, Freisinger P, Wieland T, Rorbach J, Nicholls TJ, Baruffini E, Walther A, Danhauser K, Zimmermann FA, Husain RA, Schum J, Mundy H, Ferrero I, Strom TM, Meitinger T, Taylor RW, Minczuk M, Mayr JA, Prokisch H. Am J Hum Genet. 2013;93:211–23.
152. Neeve VC, Pyle A, Boczonadi V, Gomez-Duran A, Griffin H, Santibanez-Koref M, Gaiser U, Bauer P, Tzschach A, Chinnery PF, Horvath R. Mitochondrion. 2013;13:743–8.
153. Baruffini E, Dallabona C, Invernizzi F, Yarham JW, Melchionda L, Blakely EL, Lamantea E, Donnini C, Santra S, Vijayaraghavan S, Roper HP, Burlina A, Kopajtich R, Walther A, Strom TM, Haack TB, Prokisch H, Taylor RW, Ferrero I, Zeviani M, Ghezzi D. Hum Mutat. 2013;34:1501–9.
154. McKenzie M, Lazarou M, Thorburn DR, Ryan MT. J Mol Biol. 2006;361:462–9.
155. Cotan D, Cordero MD, Garrido-Maraver J, Oropesa-Avila M, Rodriguez-Hernandez A, Gomez Izquierdo L, De la Mata M, De Miguel M, Lorite JB, Infante ER, Jackson S, Navas P, Sanchez-Alcazar JA. FASEB J. 2011;25:2669–87.
156. Mollet J, Delahodde A, Serre V, Chretien D, Schlemmer D, Lombes A, Boddaert N, Desguerre I, de Lonlay P, de Baulny HO, Munnich A, Rotig A. Am J Hum Genet. 2008;82:623–30.
157. Le Ber I, Dubourg O, Benoist JF, Jardel C, Mochel F, Koenig M, Brice A, Lombes A, Durr A. Neurology. 2007;68:295–7.
158. Quinzii CM, Kattah AG, Naini A, Akman HO, Mootha VK, DiMauro S, Hirano M. Neurology. 2005;64:539–41.
159. Quinzii C, Naini A, Salviati L, Trevisson E, Navas P, Dimauro S, Hirano M. Am J Hum Genet. 2006;78:345–9.
160. Salviati L, Sacconi S, Murer L, Zacchello G, Franceschini L, Laverda AM, Basso G, Quinzii C, Angelini C, Hirano M, Naini AB, Navas P, DiMauro S, Montini G. Neurology. 2005;65:606–8.
161. Heeringa SF, Chernin G, Chaki M, Zhou W, Sloan AJ, Ji Z, Xie LX, Salviati L, Hurd TW, Vega-Warner V, Killen PD, Raphael Y, Ashraf S, Ovunc B, Schoeb DS, McLaughlin HM, Airik R, Vlangos CN, Gbadegesin R, Hinkes B, Saisawat P, Trevisson E, Doimo M, Casarin A, Pertegato V, Giorgi G, Prokisch H, Rotig A, Nurnberg G, Becker C, Wang S, Ozaltin F, Topaloglu R, Bakkaloglu A, Bakkaloglu SA, Muller D, Beissert A, Mir S, Berdeli A, Varpizen S, Zenker M, Matejas V, Santos-Ocana C, Navas P, Kusakabe T, Kispert A, Akman S, Soliman NA, Krick S, Mundel P, Reiser J, Nurnberg P, Clarke CF, Wiggins RC, Faul C, Hildebrandt F. J Clin Invest. 2011;121:2013–24.
162. Mollet J, Giurgea I, Schlemmer D, Dallner G, Chretien D, Delahodde A, Bacq D, de Lonlay P, Munnich A, Rotig A. J Clin Invest. 2007;117:765–72.

163. Lopez LC, Schuelke M, Quinzii CM, Kanki T, Rodenburg RJ, Naini A, Dimauro S, Hirano M. Am J Hum Genet. 2006;79:1125–9.
164. Duncan AJ, Bitner-Glindzicz M, Meunier B, Costello H, Hargreaves IP, Lopez LC, Hirano M, Quinzii CM, Sadowski MI, Hardy J, Singleton A, Clayton PT, Rahman S. Am J Hum Genet. 2009;84:558–66.
165. Gempel K, Topaloglu H, Talim B, Schneiderat P, Schoser BG, Hans VH, Palmafy B, Kale G, Tokatli A, Quinzii C, Hirano M, Naini A, DiMauro S, Prokisch H, Lochmuller H, Horvath R. Brain. 2007;130:2037–44.
166. Vedrenne V, Gowher A, De Lonlay P, Nitschke P, Serre V, Boddaert N, Altuzarra C, Mager-Heckel AM, Chretien F, Entelis N, Munnich A, Tarassov I, Rotig A. Am J Hum Genet. 2012;91:912–8.
167. Di Fonzo A, Ronchi D, Lodi T, Fassone E, Tigano M, Lamperti C, Corti S, Bordoni A, Fortunato F, Nizzardo M, Napoli L, Donadoni C, Salani S, Saladino F, Moggio M, Bresolin N, Ferrero I, Comi GP. Am J Hum Genet. 2009;84:594–604.
168. Sanaker PS, Toompuu M, Hogan VE, He L, Tzoulis C, Chrzanowska-Lightowlers ZM, Taylor RW, Bindoff LA. Biochim Biophys Acta. 2010;1802:539–44.
169. Cameron JM, Janer A, Levandovskiy V, Mackay N, Rouault TA, Tong WH, Ogilvie I, Shoubridge EA, Robinson BH. Am J Hum Genet. 2011;89:486–95.
170. Janer A, Antonicka H, Lalonde E, Nishimura T, Sasarman F, Brown GK, Brown RM, Majewski J, Shoubridge EA. Am J Hum Genet. 2012;91:737–43.
171. Shadel GS, Clayton DA. Annu Rev Biochem. 1997;66:409–35.
172. Chinnery PF, Zeviani M. Neuromuscul Disord. 2008;18:259–67.
173. Tang S, Wang J, Lee NC, Milone M, Halberg MC, Schmitt ES, Craigen WJ, Zhang W, Wong LJ. J Med Genet. 2011;48:669–81.
174. Walter MC, Czermin B, Muller-Ziermann S, Bulst S, Stewart JD, Hudson G, Schneiderat P, Abicht A, Holinski-Feder E, Lochmuller H, Chinnery PF, Klopstock T, Horvath R. J Neurol. 2010;257:1517–23.
175. Spinazzola A, Invernizzi F, Carrara F, Lamantea E, Donati A, Dirocco M, Giordano I, Meznaric-Petrusa M, Baruffini E, Ferrero I, Zeviani M. J Inherit Metab Dis. 2009;32:143–58.
176. Kemp JP, Smith PM, Pyle A, Neeve VC, Tuppen HA, Schara U, Talim B, Topaloglu H, Holinski-Feder E, Abicht A, Czermin B, Lochmuller H, McFarland R, Chinnery PF, Chrzanowska-Lightowlers ZM, Lightowlers RN, Taylor RW, Horvath R. Brain. 2011;134:183–95.
177. Bonnefond L, Fender A, Rudinger-Thirion J, Giege R, Florentz C, Sissler M. Biochemistry. 2005;44:4805–16.
178. Smits P, Smeitink JA, van den Heuvel LP, Huynen MA, Ettema TJ. Nucleic Acids Res. 2007;35:4686–703.
179. Westermann B. Nat Rev Mol Cell Biol. 2010;11:872–84.
180. Detmer SA, Chan DC. Nat Rev Mol Cell Biol. 2007;8:870–9.
181. Santel A, Fuller MT. J Cell Sci. 2001;114:867–74.
182. Smirnova E, Griparic L, Shurland DL, van der Bliek AM. Mol Biol Cell. 2001;12:2245–56.
183. Alexander C, Votruba M, Pesch UE, Thiselton DL, Mayer S, Moore A, Rodriguez M, Kellner U, Leo-Kottler B, Auburger G, Bhattacharya SS, Wissinger B. Nat Genet. 2000;26:211–5.
184. Delettre C, Lenaers G, Griffoin JM, Gigarel N, Lorenzo C, Belenguer P, Pelloquin L, Grosgeorge J, Turc-Carel C, Perret E, Astarie-Dequeker C, Lasquellec L, Arnaud B, Ducommun B, Kaplan J, Hamel CP. Nat Genet. 2000;26:207–10.
185. Zuchner S, Mersiyanova IV, Muglia M, Bissar-Tadmouri N, Rochelle J, Dadali EL, Zappia M, Nelis E, Patitucci A, Senderek J, Parman Y, Evgrafov O, Jonghe PD, Takahashi Y, Tsuji S, Pericak-Vance MA, Quattrone A, Battaloglu E, Polyakov AV, Timmerman V, Schroder JM, Vance JM. Nat Genet. 2004;36:449–51.
186. Waterham HR, Koster J, van Roermund CW, Mooyer PA, Wanders RJ, Leonard JV. N Engl J Med. 2007;356:1736–41.
187. Quinzii CM, Hirano M. Dev Disabil Res Rev. 2010;16:183–8.
188. Quinzii CM, DiMauro S, Hirano M. Neurochem Res. 2007;32:723–7.
189. Jin H, May M, Tranebjaerg L, Kendall E, Fontan G, Jackson J, Subramony SH, Arena F, Lubs H, Smith S, Stevenson R, Schwartz C, Vetrie D. Nat Genet. 1996;14:177–80.
190. Tong WH, Rouault T. EMBO J. 2000;19:5692–700.
191. Koppen M, Metodiev MD, Casari G, Rugarli EI, Langer T. Mol Cell Biol. 2007;27:758–67.
192. Arnoldi A, Tonelli A, Crippa F, Villani G, Pacelli C, Sironi M, Pozzoli U, D'Angelo MG, Meola G, Martinuzzi A, Crimella C, Redaelli F, Panzeri C, Renieri A, Comi GP, Turconi AC, Bresolin N, Bassi MT. Hum Mutat. 2008;29:522–31.
193. Warnecke T, Duning T, Schwan A, Lohmann H, Epplen JT, Young P. Neurology. 2007;69:368–75.
194. Casari G, De Fusco M, Ciarmatori S, Zeviani M, Mora M, Fernandez P, De Michele G, Filla A, Cocozza S, Marconi R, Durr A, Fontaine B, Ballabio A. Cell. 1998;93:973–83.
195. Seyda A, Newbold RF, Hudson TJ, Verner A, MacKay N, Winter S, Feigenbaum A, Malaney S, Gonzalez-Halphen D, Cuthbert AP, Robinson BH. Am J Hum Genet. 2001;68:386–96.
196. Nishino I, Spinazzola A, Hirano M. Science. 1999;283:689–92.
197. Van Goethem G, Schwartz M, Lofgren A, Dermaut B, Van Broeckhoven C, Vissing J. Eur J Hum Genet. 2003;11:547–9.
198. Ferre M, Bonneau D, Milea D, Chevrollier A, Verny C, Dollfus H, Ayuso C, Defoort S, Vignal C, Zanlonghi X, Charlin JF, Kaplan J, Odent S, Hamel CP, Procaccio V, Reynier P, Amati-Bonneau P. Hum Mutat. 2009;30:E692–705.
199. Fuhrmann N, Alavi MV, Bitoun P, Woernle S, Auburger G, Leo-Kottler B, Yu-Wai-Man P, Chinnery P, Wissinger B. J Med Genet. 2009;46:136–44.
200. Honzik T, Tesarova M, Magner M, Mayr J, Jesina P, Vesela K, Wenchich L, Szentivanyi K, Hansikova H, Sperl W, Zeman J. J Inherit Metab Dis. 2012;35(5):749–59.
201. Koenig MK. Pediatr Neurol. 2008;38:305–13.
202. Scaglia F, Towbin JA, Craigen WJ, Belmont JW, Smith EO, Neish SR, Ware SM, Hunter JV, Fernbach SD, Vladutiu GD, Wong LJ, Vogel H. Pediatrics. 2004;114:925–31.
203. Haas RH, Parikh S, Falk MJ, Saneto RP, Wolf NI, Darin N, Cohen BH. Pediatrics. 2007;120:1326–33.
204. Gellerich FN, Mayr JA, Reuter S, Sperl W, Zierz S. Mitochondrion. 2004;4:427–39.
205. Wong LJ. Ann N Y Acad Sci. 2004;1011:246–58.
206. Wong LJ, Cobb BR, Chen TJ. Methods Mol Biol. 2006;336:135–43.
207. White HE, Durston VJ, Seller A, Fratter C, Harvey JF, Cross NC. Genet Test. 2005;9:190–9.
208. Bai RK, Wong LJ. Clin Chem. 2004;50:996–1001.
209. Chinault AC, Shaw CA, Brundage EK, Tang LY, Wong LJ. Genet Med. 2009;11:518–26.
210. Zeviani M, Bonilla E, DeVivo DC, DiMauro S. Neurol Clin. 1989;7:123–56.
211. Bai RK, Wong LJ. J Mol Diagn. 2005;7:613–22.
212. Whittaker RG, Blackwood JK, Alston CL, Blakely EL, Elson JL, McFarland R, Chinnery PF, Turnbull DM, Taylor RW. Neurology. 2009;72:568–9.
213. Mamanova L, Coffey AJ, Scott CE, Kozarewa I, Turner EH, Kumar A, Howard E, Shendure J, Turner DJ. Nat Methods. 2010;7:111–8.

Metabolic Disorders

11

Lisa Edelmann, Yaping Yang, Amy C. Yang, and Ruth Kornreich

Abstract

Inborn errors of metabolism represent a highly diverse group of genetic disorders. Although individually the disorders are rare, collectively they are estimated to affect as many as 1 in 600 individuals. This chapter discusses the molecular mechanisms of disease and the available genetic testing for selected metabolic disorders. Mutations in many of the metabolic diseases are genetically heterogeneous and diagnoses are still widely dependent on biochemical testing. DNA testing is critical for confirmatory studies, genetic counseling, carrier and prenatal testing, and genotype-phenotype correlation, and is widely used for carrier screening for metabolic disorders in certain populations that have a high frequency of specific mutations due to founder effects. With increasing use of next-generation sequencing technologies in the clinical laboratory, DNA testing for confirmatory studies of all newborn screening positive results likely will be available in the near future.

Keywords

Inborn errors of metabolism • Molecular testing • Newborn screening • Phenylketonuria • Medium-chain acyl CoA dehydrogenase deficiency • Maple syrup urine disease • Ornithine transcarbamylase deficiency • Lysosomal storage disorders • Tay-Sachs disease • Gaucher disease • Galactosemia • Hereditary fructose intolerance • Glycogen storage diseases • von Gierke disease • Pompe disease • Cori disease • Andersen disease • Very-long-chain acyl-CoA dehydrogenase deficiency • X-linked adrenoleukodystrophy • Canavan disease

Introduction

Inborn errors of metabolism represent a highly diverse group of genetic disorders. Individually the disorders are rare. The most prevalent disorder, phenylketonuria (PKU), affects approximately 1 in 10,000 individuals. However, because numerous metabolic disorders exist, collectively they are estimated to affect as many as 1 in 600 individuals. The clinical consequences of such disorders are broad and can be severe, with progressive neurological impairment, intellectual disability (ID), organomegaly, and high morbidity. The mode of inheritance is usually autosomal recessive but also can be X-linked. Metabolic disorders result from defects in the individual enzymes of pathways that govern many different aspects of metabolism in distinct compartments within the cell.

L. Edelmann, Ph.D.
Department of Genetics and Genomic Sciences, Icahn School of Medicine, Mount Sinai Medical Center, New York, NY, USA

Y. Yang, Ph.D.
Department of Molecular and Human Genetics, Medical Genetics Laboratory and Whole Genome Laboratory, Baylor College of Medicine, Houston, TX, USA

A.C. Yang, M.D.
Department of Genetics and Genomic Sciences, Division of Medical Genetics, Mount Sinai School of Medicine, New York, NY, USA

R. Kornreich, Ph.D. (✉)
Department of Genetics and Genomic Sciences, Mount Sinai School of Medicine, One Gustave L. Levy Place, Box 1497, New York, NY 10029, USA
e-mail: ruth.kornreich@mssm.edu

D.G.B. Leonard (ed.), *Molecular Pathology in Clinical Practice*, DOI 10.1007/978-3-319-19674-9_11

The onset of disease is most often after birth with the appearance of an apparently normal infant, but in some classes of metabolic disorders, multiple congenital anomalies also exist. For most metabolic disorders, disease symptoms begin in early infancy or childhood, but in less severe cases, adolescent or adult onset may occur. Therefore, early recognition with prompt therapeutic intervention when possible is critical for reducing damage due to the metabolic defect. For those diseases that are prevalent and for which early detection and intervention would have a beneficial outcome, neonatal screening is performed in the USA and in several countries around the world. In the USA, each state and the District of Columbia determine the diseases for which newborns are screened and the methods used for screening. With respect to metabolic disorders, all states now screen for PKU, congenital hypothyroidism, galactosemia, maple syrup urine disease, (MSUD), homocystinuria, biotinidase deficiency, congenital adrenal hyperplasia, and tyrosinemia. Since the American College of Medical Genetics and Genomics (ACMG) Newborn Screening Expert Group's recommendation in 2006, tandem mass spectrometry has been added to newborn screening programs in all states and can detect more than 20 metabolic disorders, including medium-chain acyl CoA dehydrogenase (MCAD) deficiency. DNA testing is currently used as a follow-up to an initial positive screen for certain disorders, such as MCAD deficiency and PKU.

This chapter discusses the molecular mechanisms of disease and the available genetic testing for selected metabolic disorders. The choice of disorders reflects population prevalence and current availability of molecular testing, as the mutations in many of the metabolic diseases are genetically heterogeneous and diagnoses are still widely dependent on biochemical testing. DNA testing often is critical for confirmatory studies, genetic counseling, carrier and prenatal testing, and genotype-phenotype correlation, and is widely used for carrier screening for metabolic disorders in certain populations that have a high frequency of specific mutations due to founder effects. With increasing use of next-generation sequencing technologies in the clinical laboratory, DNA testing for confirmatory studies of all newborn screening positive results likely will be available in the near future.

Amino Acidopathies

Amino acids derived from protein sources within the diet are metabolized via specific pathways. Enzyme deficiencies within these pathways lead to distinct clinical manifestations of amino acidopathies, such as PKU and MSUD.

Phenylketonuria

Molecular Basis of the Disease

PKU is an autosomal recessive disorder caused by the inability of the body to convert phenylalanine to tyrosine. PKU is the most common metabolic disease in Caucasians, with an incidence of 1 in 10,000 individuals. About 98 % of PKU cases are caused by defects in the phenylalanine hydroxylase (*PAH*) gene, which encodes the rate-limiting enzyme of the pathway. The other 2 % are caused by defects in the biosynthesis or regeneration of the cofactor of PAH, 6(R)-L-ERYTHRO-TETRAHYDROBIOPTERIN (BH4). Accumulation of phenylalanine can damage the development of the central nervous system and result in ID. PKU has a spectrum of phenotypes ranging from classic PKU, which is the most severe type with the least tolerance to dietary phenylalanine, to moderate PKU, mild PKU, and mild hyperphenylalaninemia (MHP). Patients with MHP have no clinical symptoms and do not require dietary treatment.

PKU is included in newborn screening programs in all 50 states and is a classic example of a genetic disease that meets the criteria for newborn screening: relatively high occurrence, availability of fast and economical screening methods, and therapeutic options. With early diagnosis and intervention, including a low-phenylalanine diet, the major disease phenotypes of ID and growth retardation can be prevented.

The *PAH* gene is located on 12q23.2 and spans a genomic region of 90 kilobases (kb). The coding region is about 4 kb with 13 exons. More than 600 mutations in *PAH* have been reported to date, of which approximately 81 % are point mutations, 14 % are small deletions or insertions and the remaining 5 % are gross deletions or duplications affecting one or multiple exons or even the entire gene (HGMD® Professional 2011.4) [1]. While the majority of the mutations are private mutations, seven of the most prevalent European mutations, p.R408W (31 %), c.1315+1G→A (11 %), c.1066-11G→A (6 %), p.I65T (5 %), p.Y414C (5 %), p.R261Q (4 %), and p.F39L (2 %), account for approximately two-thirds of all mutations [2].

Clinical Utility of Testing

Molecular testing for PKU serves several purposes, including assisting prognosis, confirmation of clinical and newborn screening results, carrier testing, prenatal diagnosis, and information for genetic counseling.

Available Assays

Several methods are currently used for the molecular detection of mutations in *PAH* associated with PKU. These methods include the following:

- Testing of a panel of common mutations detects up to 50 % of mutations, depending on the number of mutations included as well as the ethnic backgrounds of the patients.

- Denaturing high-performance liquid chromatography (DHPLC) detects approximately 96 % of mutations with scanning of the entire coding region of *PAH* [3]. However, the claimed detection rate is based on limited numbers of variants and does not necessarily reflect the real detection rate for each exonic position in the gene.
- Sanger sequencing, which is considered the gold standard for detecting small nucleotide changes, is utilized much more widely than DHPLC in clinical testing of the *PAH* gene. With high sensitivity and lower cost, Sanger sequencing should be the method of choice for mutation screening of the entire code region of the gene.
- Gross deletions and duplications, which usually cannot be detected by Sanger sequencing, have been reported in the *PAH* gene (HGMD® Professional 2011.4) [1]. The most commonly used methods to detect these types of mutations are array-based comparative genomic hybridization (aCGH), multiplex ligation-dependent probe amplification (MLPA), and quantitative PCR (qPCR). Finally, when molecular analysis fails to detect one or both mutant alleles, linkage studies using polymorphic markers within or very closely linked to the *PAH* gene may be considered.

Interpretation of Test Results

The variant interpretation guidelines from ACMG [4] should be followed, and include assessment of the evidence from in vitro studies, familial segregation data, or population data before a missense variant is classified as deleterious. Genotype may not be a good predictor of phenotype since environmental factors and/or modifier genes also can play a role in the clinical manifestations of the disease. For patients with mild mutations in the BH4 cofactor-binding region (p.V190A, p.R241C, p.A300S, p.A313T, p.E390G, p.A403V, and p.P407S), overloading with BH4 may increase PAH activity and may be used as an alternative to dietary restriction [5].

Maple Syrup Urine Disease

Molecular Basis of the Disease

MSUD is an autosomal recessive disorder characterized by a maple syrup odor in the urine and cerumen, and elevated branched-chain amino acids (leucine, valine, isoleucine, allo-isoleucine) in the blood. MSUD is caused by a deficiency of the branched-chain alpha-ketoacid dehydrogenase (BCKAD) complex. While it is relatively rare in the general population with an incidence of about 1 in 185,000 live births, due to founder effects, select populations such as the Ashkenazi Jewish and the Amish-Mennonites have a much higher incidence (1 in 26,000 and 1 in 380, respectively).

The BCKAD complex is comprised of four subunits; E1a, E1b, E2, and E3. Mutations in E1a (*BCKDHA*), E1b (*BKDHB*), or E2 (*DBT*) that give rise to MSUD are biochemically identical. Because the subunit E3 (*DLD*) also is shared with the pyruvate dehydrogenase and alpha-ketoglutarate complexes, a pathological defect in E3 also will cause lactic and/or metabolic acidosis, abnormal urine organic acids, and Leigh syndrome-like neuropathology, which are features not typically seen in MSUD. E3 deficiency also is called lipoamide dehydrogenase (LAD) deficiency and occurs at a higher frequency in the Ashkenazi Jewish population with two founder mutations.

Based on residual enzyme activity, an affected individual can be phenotypically classified as having classic, intermediate, or intermittent MSUD. Classic MSUD usually presents neonatally with poor feeding, lethargy, dystonia, and seizures. Intermediate types usually present with milder symptoms and later onset with developmental delays or ID. Intermittent types can have normal early development with acute, episodic mental status changes and/or psychosis during times of illness or stress. The treatment goal of protein and branched-chain restrictive diets is to maintain leucine, valine, and isoleucine at a therapeutic level and thus prevent neurotoxic effects from elevated metabolites. Liver transplantation is now a curative treatment for MSUD, with effective normalization of the branched-chain amino acid levels without dietary therapy. MSUD is included in newborn screening programs in all 50 states.

Table 11.1 shows the four genes implicated in MSUD, the protein involved, and notable pathological alleles. The p.T438N mutation on E1a has a carrier frequency of about 1 in 10 in the Amish-Mennonite population. The three common mutations on E1b found in the Ashkenazi Jewish population (p.R183P, p.G278S, and p.Q372X) have a combined carrier frequency of approximately 1 in 80 [6]. A pathological allele for LAD deficiency (p.G229C) has a carrier frequency of 1 in 94 in Ashkenazi Jews [7]. Excluding those with LAD deficiency, 45 % of patients have mutations in the *BCKDHA* gene, 35 % in the *BCKDHB* gene, and 20 % in the *DBT* gene [8].

Clinical Utility of Testing

Molecular testing for MSUD confirms clinical and newborn screening results. Carrier screening for the Mennonite and Ashkenazi Jewish populations is available and allows for preconceptual and prenatal genetic counseling and for immediate treatment of an affected infant after birth.

Available Assays

Targeted mutation analysis of the common alleles via multiplex PCR is a cost-effective and quick method for the Mennonite and Ashkenazi Jewish populations, with a mutation detection rate of over 98 % for *BCKDHA* and

Table 11.1 Genes, protein subunit, and founder alleles associated with MSUD

Gene	MSUD type	Locus	Size	Protein subunit	Exons	Founder mutations
BCKDHA	Ia	19q13	28 kb	E1a	9	p.T438N
BCKDHB	Ib	6q14	240 kb	E1b	11	p.R183P, p.G278S, p.Q372X
DBT	II	1p31	56 kb	E2	11	
DLD	III (aka. LAD deficiency)	7q31	30 kb	E3	14	p.G229C

BCKDHB, respectively [8]. For the general population, exon sequencing and deletion analysis of *BCKDHA*, *BCKDHB*, and *DBT*, and *DLD* are available.

Interpretation of Test Results

Mutations in *BCKDHA*, *BCKDHB*, and *DBT* do not have clear phenotype correlations, and treatment modality is essentially the same, regardless of the degree of biochemical phenotype. In a small study of 13 Ashkenazi Jewish families affected with LAD deficiency, homozygosity for the p. G229C allele appeared to be associated with a milder and later-onset disease, with no neurological manifestations [7].

Urea Cycle Disorders (Ornithine Transcarbamylase Deficiency)

Molecular Basis of the Disease

Defects in the urea cycle constitute a rare group of disorders resulting in the accumulation of urea precursors, mainly ammonium and glutamine. Ornithine transcarbamylase (OTC) deficiency, the most common inborn error of ureagenesis, is an X-linked disorder. Affected hemizygous males typically present in the neonatal period or later in childhood, with symptoms that include vomiting, lethargy, hypothermia, and apnea due to hyperammonemia, leading to coma or death. Recurrent episodes of metabolic crisis can result in ID. The only available treatment after an acute metabolic episode is liver transplantation, which should be performed as early as possible to prevent brain damage. In 15–20 % of carrier females, symptoms are evident. Symptomatic carrier females typically have a later onset but the disease can be fatal, presumably due to an unfavorable pattern of X-inactivation in the liver [9].

OTC is a homotrimeric mitochondrial matrix enzyme that catalyzes the synthesis of citrulline from ornithine and carbamyl phosphate, and is found almost exclusively in the liver and intestinal mucosa. Loss of OTC activity results in high plasma glutamine and ammonium, low plasma citrulline, and an excess of orotic acid in the urine, a combined metabolic profile that is diagnostic for OTC deficiency. However, a direct assay of OTC activity performed on tissue isolated from a liver biopsy specimen may be necessary to obtain unequivocal biochemical results.

The *OTC* gene is located on Xp21 and spans a region of 73 kb that contains ten exons and encodes a protein of 354 amino acids. The overall prevalence of the disease is estimated at 1 in 50,000 in the USA, with similar statistics reported in Japan. Mutations have been identified in all ten exons; however, disease-causing mutations are less frequent in exons 1 and 7, the least conserved exons, most likely reflecting their lesser relevance to the function of the enzyme [10].

Clinical Utility of Testing

Diagnosis of OTC deficiency by molecular testing is preferable to the more invasive liver biopsy that is necessary for the enzymatic test. Molecular screening for *OTC* mutations identifies approximately 80 % of mutations, while the remaining undetected mutations are expected to affect promoter function or splicing [11]. The *OTC* gene has an approximately 50:1 sperm-to-egg mutation rate ratio [9]. From 66–93 % of male probands inherit the mutation from their mothers, while only 20 % of manifesting females inherit the mutation, taking into account differences in new mutation rates between sperm and eggs, and lyonization effects for a female to manifest symptoms. Thus, a woman who has a son with OTC deficiency has a much higher chance of harboring the mutation than a woman who has an affected daughter. Due to the inheritability and the severity of the disease with the limited treatment available, molecular screening of at-risk couples for the purpose of prenatal testing may be beneficial. Additionally, mutation identification may be of prognostic value in OTC deficiency (see "Interpretation of Test Results" below).

Available Assays

Molecular testing using bidirectional sequencing of the entire coding region and intron-exon boundaries of the *OTC* gene is available in a number of clinical molecular laboratories. In addition, MLPA is used to detect large *OTC* coding region deletions/duplications. High-resolution aCGH can be used to detect exonic deletions/duplications or larger rearrangements that include the *OTC* gene as part of a contiguous gene deletion syndrome [12]. Approximately 300 mutations have been reported (http://www.cnmcresearch.org/OTC/). Most mutations (86 %) in the *OTC* gene are point mutations, with G to A transitions accounting for 34 % and C to T transitions accounting for 21 % of the total. Approximately one-third of all point mutations are at CpG dinucleotides, and 15 % are at splice junctions. Although the CpG sites are recurrent mutation sites, none accounts for more than 4 % of the total single-base substitutions.

Interpretation of Test Results

In general, the genotypic spectrum correlates with the severity of the phenotype, and mutations that result in complete loss of function or amino acid changes near the active site of the protein result in neonatal onset of disease. In contrast, amino acid changes that are not close to the active site and result in protein with residual enzymatic activity are associated with later onset and a milder disease course [12].

Lysosomal Storage Disorders

Lysosomal storage disorders are a group of diverse inherited metabolic diseases that result from the disruption of the lysosomal system and catabolism of macromolecules (for review, see Ref. 13). Mutations in genes encoding hydrolyzing enzymes, activator proteins, lysosomal membrane proteins, or proteins involved in the posttranslational modification or transport of lysosomal proteins can cause such storage disorders. More than 40 lysosomal storage disorders are known, and they have a collective incidence of approximately 1 in 5,000–8,000 live births in the USA. Most of the genes responsible for lysosomal storage disorders have been cloned, permitting molecular testing once a diagnosis is established by biochemical analyses. This information is valuable for genotype-phenotype correlation, selection of therapy, and genetic counseling. In this section, two lysosomal storage disorders are discussed: Tay-Sachs disease (TSD), which serves as a model for population screening, and Gaucher disease (GD), for which much effort has been concentrated on genotype-phenotype correlations.

Tay-Sachs Disease

Molecular Basis of the Disease

TSD is a neurodegenerative disorder resulting from deficiency of the lysosomal enzyme hexosaminidase A (HEX A), resulting in accumulation of the cell membrane glycolipid G_{M2} ganglioside within lysosomes (for review, see Refs. 14, 15). The clinical course of TSD is characterized by normal development for the first few months of life followed by progressive loss of motor skills, macrocephaly, seizures, blindness, and death usually before 4 years of age. Infantile TSD always is fatal and there is no effective treatment. Later-onset forms of TSD have slower disease progression. TSD is an autosomal recessive disease and has a carrier frequency of approximately 1 in 30 among Ashkenazi Jewish individuals and 1 in 250–300 in most other populations. Genetically isolated populations such as the French Canadians of Quebec, Cajuns from Louisiana, and the Amish in Pennsylvania also have carrier frequencies similar to the Ashkenazi Jews. The first carrier screening programs began in 1970 and used the measurement of HEX A activity in serum, leukocytes, or tears. When the *HEXA* gene encoding HEX A was cloned in 1987, disease-associated mutations were identified. Current testing for TSD utilizes both biochemical and molecular testing by various methods.

Clinical Utility of Testing

Carrier screening for TSD, which began in the 1970s and was later endorsed by the American College of Obstetricians and Gynecologists (ACOG) and the ACMG, has been a model for population screening programs. As a result, there has been a 90 % reduction in the incidence of TSD in the North American Ashkenazi Jewish population, such that the incidence of TSD is now three- to fourfold higher in non-Jews by comparison.

Available Assays

Clinical laboratories use several strategies to incorporate mutation testing into their screening programs. Some laboratories initially screen by enzyme analysis followed by molecular testing for individuals with a result in the carrier or inconclusive ranges. Other laboratories use molecular testing alone for selected populations. Molecular tests are performed using a variety of methods, including PCR amplification followed by allele-specific primer extension analysis, allele-specific oligonucleotide (ASO) hybridization or restriction enzyme digestion, allele-specific amplification, TaqMan probe technologies, or ligation chain reaction amplification. In Ashkenazi Jewish individuals, two common mutations in *HEXA* are associated with infantile TSD and one associated with an adult-onset form of the disease. A four-base pair insertion (c.1274_1277dupTATC) in exon 11 accounts for approximately 80 % of mutant alleles in the Ashkenazi Jewish population, and a splice defect in intron 12 (c.1421+1G>A; IVS12) accounts for another 15 %. A missense mutation, p.G269S, leads to an adult-onset form of TSD and accounts for approximately 2 % of carriers.

Interpretation of Test Results

A pseudodeficiency allele, p.R247W, is present in approximately 2 % of Ashkenazi Jewish individuals who are carriers by the enzymatic assay. The p.R247W variant decreases the activity of HEX A for the artificial substrate used in the laboratory but does not cause TSD since it does not affect HEX A activity for its natural substrate, GM2 ganglioside. About 36 % of non-Jewish individuals who are carriers by enzyme analysis have a pseudodeficiency allele (32 % p.R247W and 4 % p.R249W). In addition, screening for the three common Ashkenazi Jewish mutations and an additional mutation (c.1073+1G>A; IVS9) will identify approximately 95 % of Ashkenazi Jewish carriers, but only 40–50 % of disease-causing alleles in the non-Ashkenazi Jewish populations. Other populations who are at high risk, such as the French Canadians, Cajuns, and Pennsylvania Dutch, have their own common alleles. Therefore, the mutations included for population screening must target the specific mutations of the ethnic background of the individuals being tested.

Gaucher Disease

Molecular Basis of the Disease

GD is another prevalent autosomal recessive lysosomal storage disorder that is found with higher incidence in the Ashkenazi Jewish population. The carrier frequency is 1 in 15 in the Ashkenazi Jewish population and 1 in 100 in other populations [16] (for comprehensive review on GD, see Ref. 17). A defect in the enzyme glucocerebrosidase leads to the accumulation of glucocerebrosides in lysosomal compartments in macrophage/monocyte-derived cells, particularly in the liver, bone marrow, spleen, and lung. Several forms of GD exist. Type 1 GD has a wide range of clinical presentations, from asymptomatic to symptoms including bone disease, hepatosplenomegaly, anemia, and thrombocytopenia, but without primary central nervous system involvement. Types 2 and 3 have primary central nervous system involvement that varies by age of onset and rate of disease progression. Type 2 GD patients usually have an earlier age of onset than type 3 patients, with acute disease progression and death by approximately 2 years of age. Type 3 patients have onset in early childhood to adolescence and survive into their first to fourth decade of life. A perinatal-lethal form of GD also can occur, as well as a cardiovascular form characterized by aortic and mitral valve calcification, ophthalmologic abnormalities, and hydrocephalus.

The glucocerebrosidase gene (*GBA*) and its transcribed pseudogene (ψ*GBA*) are located on chromosome 1q21. Approximately 200 mutations causing GD have been identified. Many of the mutations are most likely due to gene conversion events with the pseudogene.

Clinical Utility of Testing

The demonstration of deficient glucocerebrosidase activity in leukocytes establishes a diagnosis of GD but is unreliable for carrier detection. Therefore, molecular testing is useful for carrier identification, prenatal testing, and genetic counseling.

Available Assays

Four mutations (p.N409S, c.115+1G>A, c.84dupG, p.L483P) are responsible for approximately 95 % of disease-causing alleles in Ashkenazi Jewish individuals and 50 % of disease-causing alleles in non-Ashkenazi Jewish individuals [16]. Most clinical molecular laboratories performing GD molecular testing assess at least these four mutations. Several factors must be considered when designing molecular testing for GD. Primers must be selected that avoid amplification of the pseudogene which is located 16 kb downstream and is approximately 96 % identical to the functional gene. Recombinant alleles, which are thought to result from unequal crossovers between exons 9 and 10 of the functional gene and pseudogene, contain two or more point mutations, including p.L483P. If p.L483P alone is tested, misdesignation of the genotype may occur. This may be important, as the recombinant allele is typically associated with a more severe genotype. Mistyping also is possible when a 55 base pair (bp) deletion in exon 9 (c.1263_1317del), is present in combination with the common p.N409S allele. Homozygosity of p.N409S would be observed even though the true genotype is p.N409S/55 bp deletion. Therefore, the 55 bp deletion should be analyzed in patients who are found to be homozygous for p.N409S.

Interpretation of Test Results

Genotype-phenotype correlations have been widely investigated in GD [18]. While overlaps occur, some generalizations can be made. The presence of a p.N409S allele is predictive of type 1 disease. Individuals with p.L483P in the presence of a null allele will usually have type 2 GD, while homozygosity for p.L483P typically results in type 3 GD. Homozygosity for the p.D448H allele has been associated with the rarer cardiovascular form of GD.

Disorders of Carbohydrate Metabolism

Galactosemia, fructosemia, and the glycogen storage diseases are discussed in this section, which addresses disorders of carbohydrate metabolism.

Galactosemia

Molecular Basis of the Disease

Galactosemia is an autosomal recessive disorder caused by deficient or absent activity of one of three enzymes involved in the metabolic pathway to convert galactose to glucose: galactokinase (GALK), galactose-1-phosphate uridyl transferase (GALT), and UDP-galactose 4′-epimerase (GALE). Classic galactosemia is due to a severe reduction or absence of the GALT enzyme, and has an incidence of 1 in 40,000–60,000 in European newborns (for review, see Ref. 19).

The symptoms of classic galactosemia in neonates include poor feeding, vomiting, failure to thrive, lethargy, jaundice, occasionally diarrhea, and *E. coli* sepsis. The symptoms in an affected newborn can be obviated if a lactose-free diet is initiated within the first 2 weeks of life. Newborn screening for galactosemia is included in all 50 states. Newborns with a positive screen are followed up with immediate dietary treatment and confirmatory biochemical analysis.

The *GALT* gene is located at 9q13, is about 4 kb in length, and consists of 11 exons. More than 150 mutations in the *GALT* gene have been reported, most of which are private mutations [20]. The p.Q188R mutation is the most frequent mutation associated with classic galactosemia in many populations, and accounts for 64 % of disease alleles in Europeans, 60–70 % in Americans, and 50–58 % in Mexican Hispanics [20, 21]. Ethnic-specific mutations include p.K285N, p.S135L, c.253-2A>G, and a 5 kb deletion in Caucasian, African-American, Hispanic, and Jewish patients, respectively.

Clinical Utility of Testing

Molecular testing is used for confirmation of diagnosis, carrier detection, prenatal diagnosis, prognosis, and genetic counseling. Because the detection rate of molecular testing is less than 100 % and biochemical testing is highly accurate, mutation detection is carried out in parallel with biochemical analysis.

Prenatal diagnosis for galactosemia can provide the opportunity for immediate dietary restriction of the newborn. Although galactosemia is considered "treatable," symptoms such as ID, growth delays, speech dyspraxia, abnormal motor function, and premature ovarian failure in women may still occur even with early intervention and lifetime dietary restrictions. These long-term phenotypes often are associated with specific mutations; for example, p.Q188R can cause premature ovarian failure and speech dyspraxia. Genetic counseling is very important for parents of affected fetuses before a choice regarding pregnancy outcome is made.

Available Assays

Initial molecular testing for the diagnosis of galactosemia focuses on the most prevalent mutations or the p.N314D mutation associated with Duarte galactosemia (Duarte-2) by quick and cost-effective methods, such as multiplex PCR followed by restriction enzyme digestion [22]. If only one mutation or no mutations are found, screening of all 11 exons and exon-intron boundaries by DNA sequencing can be performed [22]. A detection rate of 96 % can be achieved by a combination of testing for prevalent mutations and DNA sequencing [23]. Gross deletions and duplications are detected by aCGH or MLPA.

Interpretation of Test Results

Genotype-phenotype associations have been established for some mutations [20]. For example, p.Q188R, p.K285N, and p.L196P alleles have undetectable GALT activity and are associated with severe phenotypes, whereas p.S135L and p.T138M are less severe and are usually associated with a good prognosis. In addition to the classic form of galactosemia, which has less than 5 % of the normal GALT activity, the Duarte-2 variant associated with the p.N314D variant has 50 % of the normal GALT activity. The p.N314D allele is in linkage disequilibrium with four polymorphisms, c.329-27G>C, c.378-24G>A, c.507+62G>A, and c.-119_-116delGTCA. The symptoms of Duarte-2 patients are mild compared to the classic type, but Duarte-2 still results in long-term phenotypes such as ID and growth delays, speech dyspraxia, abnormal motor function, and premature ovarian failure in women.

Hereditary Fructose Intolerance

Molecular Basis of the Disease

Hereditary fructose intolerance (HFI) is an autosomal recessive disorder caused by deficient or absent activity of aldolase B. The aldolases are a group of tetrameric enzymes that are highly conserved and involved in the cleavage of fructose-1,6-biphosphate. Aldolase B also cleaves fructose-1-phosphate, and thus is a key player in fructose metabolism, as well as in gluconeogenesis and glycogenolysis. Aldolase A is found predominantly in muscles, whereas aldolase B is found predominantly in the liver, kidney, and intestine, and aldolase C is predominantly in the brain. Severe reduction or absence of only the aldolase B enzyme causes HFI, and has an incidence of 1 in 20,000–30,000 in European newborns (for review, see Ref. 24).

Typically in HFI, symptoms do not arise until an infant is exposed to fructose, sucrose, or sorbitol-containing foods, usually at the weaning of breast milk and introduction of table foods. Acute ingestion of the offending sugar can result in a variable presentation of abdominal pain, vomiting, progressive liver dysfunction, hypoglycemia, uric and lactic acidosis, and renal tubulopathy, depending on the dose of the sugar ingested, and timing and length of exposure. Chronic, low-dose ingestion of fructose-containing foods can cause a subacute picture of hepatomegaly and failure to thrive. Affected individuals typically have an aversion to sweets. The acute and chronic symptoms are, for the most part, reversible, if a fructose-free diet is initiated. Once on treatment, the prognosis is good with a normal life expectancy.

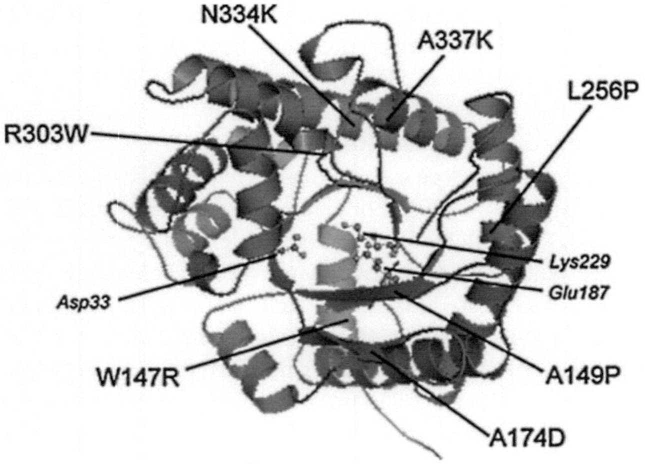

Figure 11.1 Location of some naturally occurring aldolase B mutations, shown on the crystal structure of human aldolase B (based on Protein Data Bank [PDB] structure file 1QO5, chain A) [26]. Only one monomer is shown for clarity. Active site residues are shown in a *ball and stick* representation and labeled in *italics*. Reprinted from Bouteldja N, Timson DJ. The biochemical basis of hereditary fructose intolerance. J Inherit Metab Dis 2010;33(2):105–12 [24], by permission of Springer

The *ALDOB* gene is located at 9q22.3, is about 14 kb in length, and consists of nine exons, eight of which are translated. More than 40 mutations have been identified (http://www.bu.edu/aldolase/HFI/hfidb/hfidb.html). The most common allele, p.A149P, accounts for 50–65 % of all mutations in the European population, and together with two other common mutations, p.A174D and p.N334K, account for more than 80 % of mutant alleles in the European population [25]. Most of the missense mutations are located in exons 5 and 9. Studies show that the p.A149P decreases the thermal stability of the enzyme. Figure 11.1 illustrates the locations of the most common variants in the aldolase B protein structure.

Clinical Utility of Testing

Molecular testing is used for confirmation of diagnosis, carrier detection, prenatal diagnosis, and genetic counseling. Enzymatic testing of aldolase B activity can only be performed from liver, kidney, or intestinal tissue. Thus, molecular testing is now the preferred method. Prenatal diagnosis for HFI can provide the opportunity for early dietary restriction and prevention of acute symptoms and liver disease.

Available Assays

Targeted mutation analysis of the common alleles using multiplex PCR is a cost effective and rapid method for the European population [27]. If only one mutation or no mutations are found, DNA sequencing of the entire coding region and exon-intron boundaries should be performed. For those not of European descent, DNA sequencing should be performed as a first-line method.

Interpretation of Test Results

Genotype-phenotype correlations are not clear. HPI patients with the same genotype have varied presentations and reactions to ingestion of fructose.

Glycogen Storage Diseases

Molecular Basis of the Disease

Glycogen storage diseases (GSD) are a group of heterogeneous genetic disorders characterized by the accumulation of glycogen in tissues and have an overall incidence of 1 in 20,000–25,000 live births [28]. Fourteen types of GSD that vary significantly in clinical phenotypes, age of onset, and affected organs have been identified (www.omim.org). They are caused by defects in one of 18 genes in glycogen metabolism. A summary of the 14 GSD types is presented in Table 11.2. The most common and severe types, GSD I, II, III, and IV, are discussed below.

GSD I (von Gierke disease) is characterized by hepatomegaly, kidney enlargement, growth retardation, hypoglycemia, hyperuricemia, and hyperlipidemia. GSD I has two major subgroups, GSD1a and GSD1b. The subgroup GSD1a has a deficiency of glucose-6-phosphatase (G6Pase), which converts glucose-6-phosphate to glucose and phosphate, the last step in glycogenolysis. The *G6PC* gene encoding G6Pase is located on 17q21. The subgroup GSD1b has a deficiency in glucose-6-phosphate translocase, encoded by *SLC37A4* gene located on 11q23. Common mutations vary in different ethnic groups [20]. The prevalent mutations for GSD1a in different ethnic groups are: p.R83C and p.Q347X in Caucasians; p.R83C in Ashkenazi Jews; c.459insTA and p.R83C in Hispanics; p.V166G in Muslim Arabs; p.R83H and p.G727T in Chinese; and p.G727T in Japanese. For GSD1b, two common mutations, p.G339C and c.1211delCT, are present in whites, while p.W118R is prevalent in Japanese.

GSD II, also known as Pompe disease, is a lysosomal storage disease caused by the inability to degrade glycogen due to defects in acid α-1,4-glucosidase. The phenotypes range from the most severe infantile disorder to juvenile- and late-onset adult myopathy. Patients with the infantile form usually die from cardiomyopathy before 2 years of age. Acid α-1,4-glucosidase is encoded by the gene *GAA* located at 17q25, and different forms of the protein are obtained by different proteolytic processing. Common mutations have been identified in different ethnic groups.

Patients affected with GSD III, also known as Cori disease, have symptoms similar to but milder than those associated with GSD I. GSD III is caused by mutations in the

Table 11.2 Glycogen storage disease types and subgroups

Disorder(s)	Defective enzymes	Gene symbol	Gene location	Inheritance pattern
GSD I (von Gierke disease)	GSD1a: Glucose-6-phosphatase, catalytic	*G6PC*	17q21.31	AR
	GSD1b: Solute carrier family 37 (glycerol-6-phosphate transporter), member 4	*SLC37A4*	11q23.3	AR
GSD II (Pompe disease)	Glucosidase, alpha acid	*GAA*	17q25.3	AR
GSD III (Cori disease)	Amylo-1,6-glucosidase, 4-alpha-glucanotransferase	*AGL*	1p21.2	AR
GSD IV (Andersen disease)	Glucan (1,4-alpha-) branching enzyme	*GBE1*	3p12.2	AR
GSD V (McArdle disease)	Phosphorylase, glycogen (muscle)	*PYGM*	11q13.1	AR
GSD VI (Hers disease)	Phosphorylase, glycogen (liver)	*PYGL*	14q22.1	AR
GSD VII	Phosphofructokinase, muscle	*PFKM*	12q13.11	AR
GSD IX (GSD VIII)	Phosphorylase kinase alpha 1 (muscle)	*PHKA1*	Xq13	XR
	Phosphorylase kinase alpha 2 (liver)	*PHKA2*	Xp22.13	XR
	Phosphorylase kinase, beta subunit	*PHKB*	16q12.1	AR
	Phosphorylase kinase, testis/liver, gamma 2	*PHKG2*	16p11.2	AR
GSD X	Phosphoglycerate mutase 2, muscle	*PGAM2*	7p13	AR
GSD XI	Lactate dehydrogenase A	*LDHA*	11p15.1	AR
GSD XII	Aldolase A	*ALDOA*	16P11.2	AR
GSD XIII	Enolase 3 (beta, muscle)	*ENO3*	17p13.2	AR
GSD XIV	Phosphoglucomutase 1	*PGM1*	1p31.3	AR

amylo-1-6-glucosidase (*AGL*) gene. GSD IV, also known as Andersen disease, is caused by deficiencies of the glycogen-branching enzyme encoded by the *GBE1* gene, resulting in abnormal and insoluble glycogen. Intracellular glycogen accumulations occur in the liver, brain, heart, skeletal muscles, and skin fibroblasts. Neonates with GSD IV appear normal at birth but develop hepatomegaly and failure to thrive in the first year of life. Patients develop progressive cirrhosis and usually die of liver failure by 2–5 years of age.

Clinical Utility of Testing

Due to the complex nature of molecular testing for GSD (large genes with numerous mutations), enzyme assays are usually used for the diagnosis of GSD. However, for prenatal diagnosis of GSD I, gene-based mutation testing or linkage analysis is the preferred method, since the enzymes are not present in amniocytes or chorionic villi, requiring a liver biopsy to obtain tissue containing the relevant enzyme. For prenatal diagnosis of other types of GSD, DNA testing can be used to complement and confirm biochemical results. Therapy for GSD I, II, III, and IV includes dietary management, and for GSD II, enzyme replacement is available (for complete review on treatment for GSD, see Refs. 28, 29).

Available Assays

Sanger sequencing tests are available clinically for all the GSD genes.

Fatty Acid Oxidation Disorders

During periods of fasting or prolonged aerobic exercise when glycogen stores are depleted, fatty acids become a main energy source by β-oxidation in the liver, and skeletal and cardiac muscles, via synthesis of acetyl-CoA and ketone bodies. The pathway for fatty acid oxidation occurs in the mitochondria and is complex, involving many steps. A number of disorders involving different enzymes in the pathway have been identified. Although the symptoms of the disorders have phenotypic overlap, several biochemical measurements can aid in the diagnosis of these disorders, including plasma carnitine levels which are usually low, plasma acylcarnitines, and urine acylglycines (for review, see Ref. 30). The most common of these disorders is medium-chain acyl-CoA dehydrogenase (MCAD) deficiency. Since the addition of the acylcarnitine profile to newborn screening, the prevalence for very-long-chain acyl-CoA dehydrogenase (VLCAD) deficiency is thought to be more common, and a new role for clinical molecular testing for VLCAD is emerging. At present, all 50 states within the USA employ tandem mass spectrometry in their newborn screening program, which allows detection of the abnormal plasma acylcarnitine profile characteristic of MCAD and VLCAD deficiencies.

Medium-Chain Acyl-CoA Dehydrogenase Deficiency

Molecular Basis of the Disease

MCAD is an intramitochondrial enzyme that is encoded by a nuclear gene. The normal function of MCAD is the initial dehydrogenation of acyl-CoAs with chain lengths of 4–12 carbons. Defective function leads to the accumulation of metabolites of the medium-chain fatty acids, mainly the dicarboxylic acids, acylglycine in urine, and acylcarnitine in plasma. These metabolites are at their highest concentration in the blood in the first few days of life, making the newborn period the ideal time for detection. Accordingly, the specificity of the newborn screening test is 100 %, as no false negatives have been reported. MCAD enzymatic activity also can be assayed in several different tissue types.

Because fatty acid oxidation fuels hepatic ketogenesis, the symptoms of MCAD deficiency appear after periods of prolonged fasting or intercurrent infections and include hypoketotic hypoglycemia, lethargy, seizures, coma, and, without treatment, death. Complications of the disease can include hepatomegaly, acute liver disease, and brain damage. The disease typically presents before 2 years of age but after the newborn period. However, individuals have been described who present with symptoms within the first few days of life as well as those who present as adults.

MCAD deficiency is an autosomal recessive disorder that is prevalent in individuals of northwestern European ancestry, with the highest overall frequency of 1 in 4,900 in northern Germany. The incidence in the USA is somewhat lower and is estimated to be 1 in 15,700. The MCAD gene, *ACADM,* spans a 44 kb region on chromosome 1p31 and contains 12 exons encoding a protein of 421 amino acids. A single founder mutation in exon 11, 985A>G, which results in the substitution of the acidic amino acid, glutamate, for the basic amino acid, lysine (p.K304E), represents 90 % of all alleles in the northern European population. However, recent studies of the US population, attributable to the expansion of newborn screening for MCAD deficiency, indicate that this mutation accounts for 79 % of the total mutant alleles in the US population (Table 11.3) [31]. The discrepancy between the two results is presumably due to the greater ethnic diversity of the US population.

Table 11.3 Genotypes of 57 MCAD-deficient newborns detected

Using MS/MS to screen more than 1.1 million newborns (Neo Gen Screening, Pittsburgh, PA, USA)	
Mutation position and type	**Number of patients identified**
c. 985 A→G/985 A→G	35
c. 985 A→G/199T→C (exon 3)	8
c. 985 A→G/deletion 343–348	2
c. 985 A→G/other[a]	5
c. 985 A→G/unidentified	5
c. 799 G→A/254 G→A	1
Unidentified/unidentified	1
Other mutations: seen with c. 985A→G	
c. 244 insertion T (exon 4)	
c. 362 C→T (exon 5)	
c. 489T→G (exon 7)	
IVS 5+1G→A	
IVS 8+6G→T	

Clinical Utility of Testing

Molecular testing for *ACADM* mutations usually is offered as confirmatory testing after the initial diagnosis of MCAD deficiency by biochemical testing. In addition, carrier testing for MCAD deficiency cannot be performed using biochemical metabolite profiles and must be done by molecular testing or by direct assay of MCAD activity in cultured fibroblasts.

MCAD deficiency is a disease that can be treated if promptly diagnosed in the early postnatal period. Precautions, such as avoidance of fasting and saturated fats and ingestion of carbohydrates prior to bedtime, can eliminate the symptoms and related complications of the disease. Although prenatal diagnosis on chorionic villus sampling or cultured amniocytes using biochemical or molecular testing, or both, is possible, with the inherent risks of the procedures, prenatal testing may offer no advantage to postnatal testing of acylcarnitines and other metabolites characteristic of the disease. Therefore, genetic counseling and discussion of the issues related to this disease are warranted when prenatal testing is being considered.

Available Assays

Initial molecular testing usually focuses on the high-prevalence p.K304E allele and is performed by PCR amplification followed by restriction enzyme digestion or other methods that can discriminate between single nucleotide changes, such as ASO hybridization or ligation chain reaction amplification. Clinical testing for this mutation is widely available. When an affected individual is found to be heterozygous for the p.K304E mutation or in the rare instance when an affected individual is negative for the mutation, all 12 exons of the *ACADM* gene are sequenced; however, relatively few laboratories offer *ACADM* gene sequencing. Additional mutations

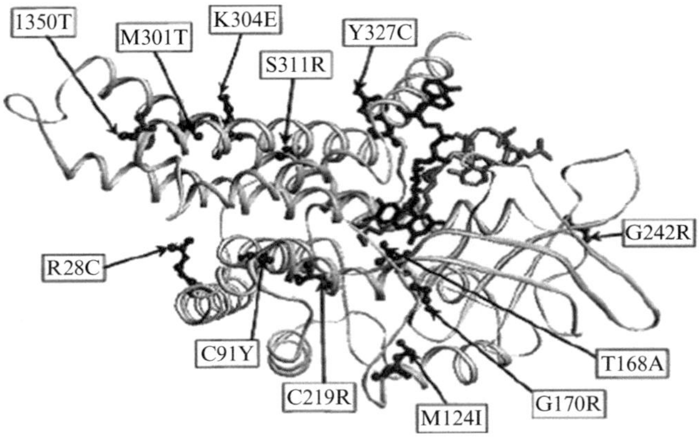

Figure 11.2 Schematic representation of a human MCAD monomer based on the crystal structure with cofactor flavin adenine dinucleotide (FAD) (*black*) and bound C8-CoA substrate (*darker gray*). The side chains for residues in which missense mutations have been published are shown in ball-and-stick representation. Only one of these mutations (T168A) is located in close proximity to the active site, forming a hydrogen bond to the flavin N(5) of FAD. Reprinted from Gregersen N, Andresen BS, Corydon MJ, et al. Mutation analysis in mitochondrial fatty acid oxidation defects: exemplified by acyl-CoA dehydrogenase deficiencies, with special focus on genotype-phenotype relationship. Hum Mutat 18(3):169–89 [32], by permission of Wiley-Liss, Inc., a subsidiary of John Wiley & Sons, Inc., ©2001

have been identified throughout the gene with no obvious mutation hotspot.

Interpretation of Test Results

The majority of mutations identified in *ACADM* are missense mutations located away from the active center of the enzyme, and are thought to affect the overall stability of the protein by affecting proper protein folding (Fig. 11.2) [32]. Most patients exhibit the classic MCAD phenotype; however, a small subset of patients has been identified that is compound heterozygous for the p.A304E mutation or for two other mutations, where at least one mutation is present that does not eliminate MCAD activity. These patients are much less likely to experience metabolic decompensation; however, even mildly symptomatic patients should avoid circumstances that could precipitate a metabolic crisis, since there is variability in age of onset even with classic MCAD deficiency.

Very-Long-Chain Acyl-CoA Dehydrogenase Deficiency

Molecular Basis of the Disease

VLCAD is an inner mitochondrial membrane enzyme encoded by the nuclear gene, *ACADVL*. VLCAD initiates the first reaction in β-oxidation of long, straight-chained acyl-CoAs of 14–20 carbons in length. Since the majority of dietary and endogenous fats are long chains, VLCAD function is an early crucial step for energy and ketone production from fat metabolism. Like MCAD deficiency, defective VLCAD activity leads to the accumulation of abnormal metabolites, mainly long-chain fatty acids and their conjugated moieties in the urine and plasma. Again, these metabolites are at their highest concentration in the first few days of life, due to the stressful and catabolic early neonatal period.

Because long-chained fats are the primary source of energy for the heart and during sustained skeletal muscle activity, the primary features of VLCAD deficiency, besides fasting hypoketotic hypoglycemia, are cardiomyopathy and skeletal myopathy with three main phenotypes. The severe, infantile-onset form presents with cardiomyopathy and arrhythmias which can lead to sudden death, hypotonia, and hepatomegaly. The childhood-onset form presents primarily with fasting hypoglycemia and liver disease, and rarely with cardiomyopathy. The late-onset form is mostly myopathic in presentation, with exercise intolerance, muscle cramping, and intermittent rhabdomyolysis during physical stress or times of illness. Patients are treated with a low-fat diet with supplemental medium-chain triglycerides, avoidance of fasting, intravenous glucose during hypoglycemic episodes, and intravenous fluids for rhabdomyolysis.

VLCAD deficiency is an autosomal recessive disorder with a prevalence of approximately 1 in 30,000. The VLCAD gene, *ACADVL*, is located on chromosome 17p13, is 5.4 kb in length, and contains 20 exons, encoding a protein of 701 amino acids. Unlike MCAD deficiency, there does not appear to be a prevalent mutant allele among a specific population. Mutations in all 20 exons have been reported.

Clinical Utility of Testing

An elevated C14:1-carnitine on the newborn screen taken at 48–72 h of life is highly indicative of VLCAD deficiency. However, borderline high levels can be equivocal in determining affected individuals from healthy carriers and normal neonates [33]. In addition, C14:1-carnitine levels can normalize with time, and attempts to confirm an abnormal acylcarnitine profile after 5 days can lead to a false-negative diagnosis [34]. Thus, molecular testing for *ACADVL* mutations is now offered as confirmatory testing of positive newborn screening results. VLCAD enzyme activity in lymphocytes or fibroblasts also is available. If two pathological *ACADVL* mutations are found, the diagnosis of VLCAD deficiency is confirmed. If only one mutation is found, an enzyme test using lymphocytes or fibroblasts is recommended.

Once diagnosis is confirmed, VLCAD deficiency is a disease that can be treated promptly in the early postnatal period to avoid cardiomyopathy, liver disease, and sudden hypoglycemic coma. With an identified *ACADVL* mutation, genetic counseling and carrier and prenatal testing can be made available to the patient and family, and genotype-phenotype correlations can be deduced (see below).

Available Assays

Because mutations causing VLCAD deficiency are heterogeneous, molecular testing is done through sequencing and deletion/duplication analysis. Sequencing of all 20 exons has a mutation detection rate of 85–93 % for individuals with clinical disease [35].

Interpretation of Test Results

Deleterious mutations identified in *ACADVL* include missense mutations, deletions, insertions, and splice-site changes. Mutations that lead to a null mutation, as in a truncation of protein or a premature stop codon, result in elimination of enzyme activity, while missense or single-amino acid deletions can still confer residual enzyme activity. The presence of two null mutations correlates with the severe infant-childhood phenotype. Conversely, patients with a milder disease phenotype more frequently have missense or single-amino acid deletions [36].

Peroxisomal Disorders (X-Linked Adrenoleukodystrophy)

Genetic disorders of peroxisomal biogenesis and function have severe phenotypic consequences that often result in death in early childhood. A number of important metabolic processes, including β-oxidation of long- and very-long-chain fatty acids and the degradation of peroxide (H_2O_2), take place in the unique microenvironment of the single-membrane-bound matrix of the peroxisome. Whereas the symptoms of most metabolic diseases manifest after birth, disorders of peroxisome biogenesis, such as Zellweger syndrome, are associated with multiple congenital anomalies (for review, see Ref. 37). In this section, X-linked adrenoleukodystrophy (X-ALD) is highlighted, as it is the most common disorder.

Molecular Basis of the Disease

X-ALD is a severe, often fatal, disease that manifests in a progressive demyelination of the central nervous system, dysfunction of the adrenal cortex, and testicular dysfunction in hemizygous males. The most common form has an early onset that typically appears at 4–8 years of age and results in a progressive irreversible dementia and often death. Less severe presentations of the disorder include adrenomyeloneuropathy (AMN), which has a later age of onset, neurological complications that are limited to the spinal cord and peripheral nerves, and frequently includes adrenal insufficiency [38]. Although the disease is inherited in an X-linked recessive manner, up to 20 % of carrier females manifest late onset neurological symptoms similar to AMN. More than 93 % of X-ALD patients inherit mutations from their mothers, while the remaining 5–7 % carry de novo mutations; mosaicism has been reported in less than 1 % of patients [39]. The primary biochemical defect is impaired peroxisomal β-oxidation of fatty acids with the subsequent accumulation of very-long-chain fatty acids (VLCFAs), most notably C26, in the plasma and tissues. Therefore, X-ALD is not a disorder of peroxisomal biogenesis, but rather a specific defect of peroxisomal function. The accumulation of VLCFAs and the accompanying inflammatory response are thought to mediate the severity of the disease phenotype. In the great majority of hemizygous males (99 %) and approximately 85 % of carrier females, the plasma concentration of VLCFAs is elevated, a measurement that can be used as a diagnostic marker for the disease [40].

Defects in the peroxisomal membrane protein, ALDP, a member of the ATP-binding cassette family of molecular transporters, cause the severe juvenile form of X-ALD and its milder associated forms. The X-ALD gene, *ABCD1*, is located on Xq28, spans 19 kb, contains ten exons, and encodes a protein of 745 amino acids. The overall incidence of X-ALD and all variant forms is 1 in 15,000, making X-ALD the most common genetic determinant of peroxisomal disease. More than 1,000 different mutations have been found in the *ABCD1* gene, with the vast majority being point mutations, although deletions and duplications also have been identified (http://www.x-ald.nl/). In addition, mutations in all ten exons have been reported. No genotype-phenotype correlations are apparent, and wide phenotypic variation has been reported within families.

Clinical Utility of Testing

Molecular testing is most useful for determining the carrier status of at-risk women and for prenatal diagnosis, since 15 % of carrier females will not have elevated VLCFA levels and therefore will have a false-negative result by biochemical methods.

Available Assays

Molecular testing of the *ABCD1* gene is clinically available with many of the mutations identified as private mutations specific to a particular family. PCR amplification and SSCP or direct sequencing of all ten exons successfully identifies mutations in the majority of cases [41], whereas Southern blotting and MLPA can be used to assess deletion and duplication status. Complications can arise during PCR amplification due to the presence of paralogous gene segments of *ABCD1* spanning exons 7–10 on chromosomes 2p11, 10p11,

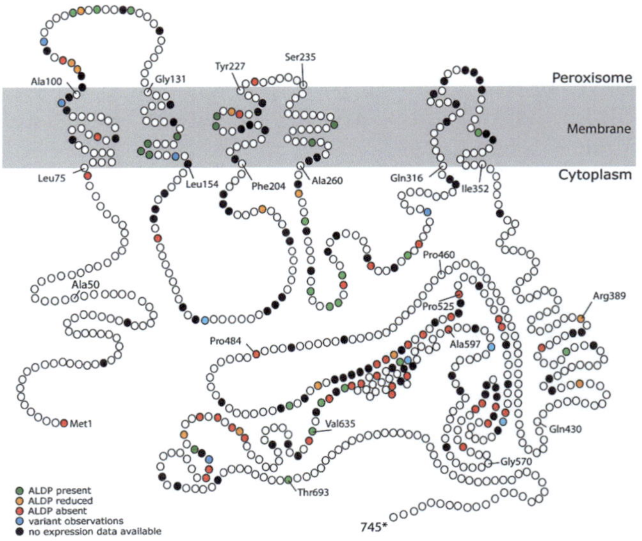

Figure 11.3 A hypothetical model of ALDP is shown. Individual amino acids are represented by *circles*. Missense mutations may affect the stability of ALDP. The effect of a missense mutation on ALDP stability by means of immunofluorescence (IF) in primary fibroblasts was investigated for >200 independent (non-recurrent) missense mutations. The results are presented in this figure. *Green circles* indicate missense mutations that do not affect protein stability; *red circles* those that result in no detectable ALDP (see remark below); *orange circles* represent mutations that result in reduced ALDP expression; *blue circles* indicate amino acid residues at which multiple missense mutations have been reported that result in different outcomes. The *black circles* indicate amino acids at which a missense mutation was identified, but for which no expression data are available. Overall, 69 % of all missense mutations result in reduced levels or absence of detectable ALDP [42]. All other mutations, including in-frame amino acid deletions and truncations near the carboxy terminus, result in the absence of detectable levels of ALDP. Reproduced from the Web site http://www.x-ald.nl/, with permission ©J. Berger and S. Kemp

16p11, and 22q11, but can be overcome by primer design that avoids amplification from the other chromosomes [41]. Although mutations have been identified throughout the entire *ABCD1* gene, a 2 bp AG deletion in exon 5 was found in 10.3 % of families with X-ALD and is therefore the most common mutation identified in the *ABCD1* gene [42]. Interestingly, this mutation, which is associated with all X-ALD phenotypes, does not represent a founder allele and is therefore a mutation hotspot within the *ABCD1* gene.

Interpretation of Test Results

The majority of mutations in *ABCD1* are missense mutations (61 %), with frameshifts and nonsense mutations accounting for 20 % and 10 % of mutation alleles, respectively, and amino acid insertions and deletions and whole exon deletions accounting for 4.6 % and 4 %, respectively. A recent study of the effects of missense mutations on ALDP stability demonstrated that approximately 70 % resulted in absent or reduced ALDP, indicating that most mutations in *ABCD1* result in complete loss of protein function (Fig. 11.3) [42]. These findings are consistent with the observed lack of genotype-phenotype correlation and lend support to the existence of additional genetic and environmental factors that modify the X-ALD phenotype.

Leukodystrophies (Canavan Disease)

The leukodystrophies are a group of degenerative metabolic diseases that involve the white matter of the brain, resulting predominately from disruption in the synthesis, transport, or catabolism of myelin. Examples include Krabbe disease and metachromatic leukodystrophy which affect lysosomal function and degradation of myelin, and Pelizaeus-Merzbacher disease, which is due to the abnormal synthesis of proteolipid protein. Another example, discussed in detail below, is Canavan disease, characterized by loss of axonal myelin sheaths and spongiform degeneration of the brain. Neurological deterioration in most leukodystrophies occurs after a period of normal development, and therapy is usually limited to the alleviation of symptoms.

Molecular Basis of the Disease

Canavan disease (CD) is an autosomal recessive disorder found mainly in Ashkenazi Jewish families and is caused by deficiency in the activity of the enzyme aspartoacylase (for review, see Ref. 43). The pathophysiologic relationship between the loss of this enzymatic activity and the development of CD remains to be elucidated. Diagnosis usually is established by the demonstration of increased levels of the substrate N-acetylaspartic acid in urine because enzymatic studies have been shown to be quite variable. Clinical symptoms associated with CD include macrocephaly, hypotonia, severe developmental delay, optic atrophy, poor head control, and death in childhood.

The gene encoding aspartoacylase (*ASPA*), located on the short arm of chromosome 17, is relatively small, with six exons spanning 30 kb of genomic sequence. Two point mutations, p.E285A and p.Y231X, are responsible for more than 97 % of mutant alleles in Ashkenazi Jews. Mutations in non-Jewish individuals are more heterogeneous; however, a panethnic mutation, p.A305E, accounts for 40–48 % of non-Jewish European alleles [44].

Clinical Utility of Testing

The genes responsible for many of the leukodystrophies have been cloned and characterized. Because the mutations in most of these genes are diverse, biochemical testing is still widely used for diagnosis, although molecular testing may be performed for carrier and subsequent prenatal testing. CD, however, occurs at increased frequency in the Ashkenazi Jewish population and screening for a limited number of specific mutations is feasible.

CD population screening of Ashkenazi Jewish individuals has demonstrated a carrier frequency of 1 in 40–59 (Refs. 45, 46 and our unpublished data). The carrier frequency for non-Jewish individuals has not been determined adequately, but it is far lower than that seen in the Ashkenazi Jewish population. As the carrier frequency is so high in the Ashkenazi Jewish population and the sensitivity of the assay is well above 90 %, ACOG and the ACMG recommended in 1998 that carrier screening for CD be performed preconceptually on couples with Ashkenazi Jewish ancestry.

Available Assays

A number of laboratories test for the two common Ashkenazi Jewish mutations, while some also test for p.A305E. A few laboratories also test for the less frequent non-Jewish mutation, c.433-2A>G. Testing methods commonly used for the detection of these mutations include PCR followed by ASO hybridization or restriction enzyme digestion, or allele-specific amplification. Miami Children's Hospital Research Institute holds a patent on the *ASPA* gene and CD testing, and requires laboratories to obtain a license, with a royalty fee for each test performed.

Interpretation of Test Results

If carrier screening indicates that both partners are carriers, prenatal testing should be offered. The preferred method of testing is DNA analysis of known mutations. For couples in which one partner is shown to be a carrier and the other partner is negative by targeted molecular testing, particularly if they are not Jewish, biochemical testing by measurement of the substrate in amniotic fluid is possible when the fetus has been shown to carry the one identified parental mutation.

Laboratory Issues

As discussed in this chapter, molecular genetic testing for metabolic disorders is used primarily as a follow-up to biochemical analyses for confirmation of findings, prognosis, carrier screening, or prenatal testing. Readers interested in learning which clinical laboratories perform individual tests should refer to the Genetic Test Registry (http://www.ncbi.nlm.nih.gov/gtr/). As testing for many of these disorders is performed in only a few laboratories, commercial test kits and proficiency testing is limited. Proficiency testing for TSD is available through the California Tay-Sachs Disease Prevention Program. For other disorders, interlaboratory exchange of samples is common practice. Several companies have developed assays for a panel of Ashkenazi Jewish disorders that include TSD, CD, and GD, among others. Although a large number of clinical laboratories offer Sanger sequencing and additional dosage sensitive methods for metabolic disorders, next-generation sequencing will allow assessment of large panels of genes related to metabolic disorders, though improved genotype-phenotype correlation will be needed before sequencing will replace biochemical testing as a first-line test.

References

1. Stenson PD, Mort M, Ball EV, Howells K, Phillips AD, Thomas NST, Cooper DN. The human gene mutation database: 2008 update. Genome Med. 2009;1(1):13.
2. Nowacki PM, Byck S, Prevost L, Scriver CR. PAH mutation analysis consortium database: 1997. Prototype for relational locus-specific mutation databases. Nucleic Acids Res. 1998;26:220–5.
3. Xiao W, Oefner PJ. Denaturing high-performance liquid chromatography: a review. Hum Mutat. 2001;17:439–74.
4. Richards CS, Bale S, Bellissimo DB, Das S, Grody WW, Hegde MR, Lyon E, Ward BE. Molecular Subcommittee of the ACMG Laboratory Quality Assurance Committee. ACMG recommendations for standards for interpretation and reporting of sequence variations: revisions 2007. Genet Med. 2008;10:294–300.
5. Erlandsen H, Stevens RC. The structural basis of phenylketonuria. Mol Genet Metab. 1999;68:103–25.
6. Edelmann L, Wasserstein MP, Kornreich R, et al. Maple syrup urine disease: identification and carrier-frequency determination of a novel founder mutation in the Ashkenazi Jewish population. Am J Hum Genet. 2001;69(4):863–8.
7. Shaag A, Saada A, Berger I, et al. Molecular basis of lipoamide dehydrogenase deficiency in Ashkenazi Jews. Am J Med Genet. 1999;82(2):177–82.
8. Strauss KA, Puffenberger EG, Morton DH. Maple syrup urine disease (updated [Dec 15, 2009]). In: GeneReviews at Genetests: medical genetics information resource (database online). Copyright, University of Washington, Seattle, 1997–2011. Available at http://www.genetests.org.
9. Brusilow SW, Horwich AL. Urea cycle enzymes. In: Scriver R, Beaudet al, Sly WS, Valle D, editors. The metabolic and molecular bases of inherited disease. 8th ed. New York: McGraw-Hill; 2001. p. 1909–63.
10. Tuchman M, Jaleel N, Morizono H, Sheehy L, Lynch MG. Mutations and polymorphisms in the human ornithine transcarbamylase gene. Hum Mutat. 2002;19:93–107.
11. Tuchman M, McCullough BA, Yudkoff M. The molecular basis of ornithine transcarbamylase deficiency. Eur J Pediatr. 2000;159 Suppl 3:S196–8.
12. McCullough BA, Yudkoff M, Batshaw ML, Wilson JM, Raper SE, Tuchman M. Genotype spectrum of ornithine transcarbamylase deficiency: correlation with the clinical and biochemical phenotype. Am J Med Genet. 2000;93:313–9.
13. Wenger DA, Coppola S, Liu SL. Lysosomal storage disorders: diagnostic dilemmas and prospects for therapy. Genet Med. 2002;4:412–9.
14. Gravel RA, Kaback MM, Proia RL, Sandhoff K, Suzuki K, Suzuki Y. The GM2 gangliosidoses. In: Scriver CR, Beaudet al, Sly WS, Valle D, editors. The metabolic and molecular bases of inherited disease. 8th ed. New York: McGraw-Hill; 2001. p. 3827–77.
15. Sutton VR. Tay-Sachs disease screening and counseling families at risk for metabolic disease. Obstet Gynecol Clin North Am. 2002; 29:287–96.
16. Grabowski GA. Gaucher disease: gene frequencies and genotype/phenotype correlations. Genet Test. 1997;1:5–12.
17. Beutler E, Grabowski GA. Gaucher disease. In: Scriver R, Beaudet al, Sly WS, Valle D, editors. The metabolic and molecular

bases of inherited disease. 8th ed. New York: McGraw-Hill; 2001. p. 3635–68.
18. Koprivica V, Stone DL, Park JK, et al. Analysis and classification of 304 mutant alleles in patients with type 1 and type 3 Gaucher disease. Am J Hum Genet. 2000;66:1777–86.
19. Holton JB, Walter JH, Tyfield LA. Galactosemia. In: Scriver CR, Beaudet al, Sly WS, Valle D, editors. The metabolic and molecular bases of inherited disease. 8th ed. New York: McGraw-Hill; 2001. p. 1553–87.
20. Tyfield L, Reichardt J, Fridovich-Keil J, et al. Classical galactosemia and mutations at the galactose-1-phosphate uridyl transferase (GALT) gene. Hum Mutat. 1999;13:417–30.
21. Elsas LJ, Langley S, Steele E, et al. Galactosemia: a strategy to identify new biochemical phenotypes and molecular genotypes. Am J Hum Genet. 1995;56:630–9.
22. Elsas LJ, Lai K. The molecular biology of galactosemia. Genet Med. 1998;1:40–8.
23. Yang Y-P, Corley N, Garcia-Heras J. Molecular analysis in newborns from Texas affected with galactosemia. Hum Mutat. 2002;19:82–3.
24. Bouteldja N, Timson DJ. The biochemical basis of hereditary fructose intolerance. J Inherit Metab Dis. 2010;33(2):105–12.
25. Tolan DR. Molecular basis of hereditary fructose intolerance: mutations and polymorphisms in the human aldolase B gene. Hum Mutat. 1995;6(3):210–8.
26. Dalby AR, Tolan DR, Littlechild JA. The structure of human liver fructose-1,6-bisphosphate aldolase. Acta Crystallogr D Biol Crystallogr. 2001;57(Pt 11):1526–33.
27. Costa C, Costa JM, Deleuze JF, et al. Simple, rapid nonradioactive method to detect the three most prevalent hereditary fructose intolerance mutations. Clin Chem. 1998;44(5):1041–3.
28. Chen Y-T. Glycogen storage diseases. In: Scriver CR, Beaudet al, Sly WS, Valle D, editors. The metabolic and molecular bases of inherited disease. 8th ed. New York: McGraw-Hill; 2001. p. 1521–51.
29. Hirschhorn R, Reuser AJJ. Glycogen storage disease type II: acid aglucosidase (acid maltase) deficiency. In: Scriver CR, Beaudet al, Sly WS, Valle D, editors. The metabolic and molecular bases of inherited disease. 8th ed. New York: McGraw-Hill; 2001. p. 3389–420.
30. Roe CR, Ding J. Mitochondrial fatty acid oxidation disorders. In: Scriver CR, Beaudet al, Sly WS, Valle D, editors. The metabolic and molecular bases of inherited disease. 8th ed. New York: McGraw-Hill; 2001. p. 2297–326.
31. Chace DH, Kalas TA, Naylor EW. The application of tandem mass spectrometry to neonatal screening for inherited disorders of intermediary metabolism. Annu Rev Genomics Hum Genet. 2002;3:17–45.
32. Gregersen N, Andresen BS, Corydon MJ, et al. Mutation analysis in mitochondrial fatty acid oxidation defects: exemplified by acyl-CoA dehydrogenase deficiencies, with special focus on genotype–phenotype relationship. Hum Mutat. 2001;18:169–89.
33. Liebig M, Schymik I, Mueller M, et al. Neonatal screening for very long-chain acyl-coA dehydrogenase deficiency: enzymatic and molecular evaluation of neonates with elevated C14:1-carnitine levels. Pediatrics. 2006;118(3):1065–9.
34. Boneh A, Andresen BS, Gregersen N, et al. VLCAD deficiency: pitfalls in newborn screening and confirmation of diagnosis by mutation analysis. Mol Genet Metab. 2006;88(2):166–70.
35. Leslie ND, Tinkle BT, Strauss AW, Shooner K, Zhang K. Very long-chain acyl-coenzyme A dehydrogenase deficiency (updated [Sept 22, 2011]). In: GeneReviews at Genetests: medical genetics information resource (database online). Copyright, University of Washington, Seattle, 1997–2012. Available at http://www.genetests.org.
36. Andresen BS, Olpin S, Poorthuis BJ, et al. Clear correlation of genotype with disease phenotype in very-long-chain acyl-CoA dehydrogenase deficiency. Am J Hum Genet. 1999;64(2):479–94.
37. Sacksteder KA, Gould SJ. The genetics of peroxisome biogenesis. Annu Rev Genet. 2000;34:623–52.
38. Moser HW, Smith KD, Watkins PA, Powers J, Moser AB. X-linked adrenoleukodystrophy. In: Scriver CR, Beaudet al, Sly WS, Valle D, editors. The metabolic and molecular bases of inherited disease. 8th ed. New York: McGraw-Hill; 2001. p. 3257–302.
39. Wang Y, Busin R, Reeves C. X-linked adrenoleukodystrophy: ABCD1 de novo mutations and mosaicism. Mol Genet Metab. 2011;104:160–6.
40. Moser HW, Loes DJ, Melhem ER, et al. X-Linked adrenoleukodystrophy: overview and prognosis as a function of age and brain magnetic resonance imaging abnormality: a study involving 372 patients. Neuropediatrics. 2000;31:227–39.
41. Boehm CD, Cutting GR, Lachtermacher MB, Moser HW, Chong SS. Accurate DNA-based diagnostic and carrier testing for X-linked adrenoleukodystrophy. Mol Genet Metab. 1999;66:128–36.
42. Kemp S, Pujol A, Waterham HR, et al. ABCD1 mutations and the X-linked adrenoleukodystrophy mutation database: role in diagnosis and clinical correlations. Hum Mutat. 2001;18:499–515.
43. Matalon R, Michals-Matalon K. Recent advances in Canavan disease. Adv Pediatr. 1999;46:493–506.
44. Kaul R, Gao GP, Matalon R, et al. Identification and expression of eight novel mutations among non-Jewish patients with Canavan disease. Am J Hum Genet. 1996;59:95–102.
45. Kronn D, Oddoux C, Phillips J, Ostrer H. Prevalence of Canavan disease heterozygotes in the New York metropolitan Ashkenazi Jewish population. Am J Hum Genet. 1995;57:1250–2.
46. Sugarman EA, Allitto BA. Carrier testing for seven diseases common in the Ashkenazi Jewish population: implications for counseling and testing. Obstet Gynecol. 2001;97:S38–9.

Fibroblast Growth Factor Receptor and Related Skeletal Disorders

12

Steven Sperber and Elaine Spector

Abstract

Osteochondrodysplasias are a heterogeneous group of disorders. To date, more than 450 skeletal conditions have been characterized. Many of the skeletal dysplasias arise during the prenatal period and are able to be diagnosed by ultrasonography. Fibroblast growth factor (FGF) signaling, including the ligands and their receptors, plays an important role in the function of chondrocytes and osteocytes that contribute to bone patterning. Two of the most common types of skeletal dysplasias are achondroplasia and thanatophoric dysplasia, emphasizing the importance of FGF signaling in skeletal development. This chapter focuses on the many distinct skeletal disorders arising from mutations in the FGF receptor (FGFR) family of genes that are responsible for forms of syndromic and non-syndromic craniosynostosis and chondrodysplasias.

Keywords

Osteochondrodysplasias • Skeletal dysplasia • Fibroblast growth factor • FGF • Fibroblast growth factor receptor • FGFR • Achondroplasia • Thanatophoric dysplasia • Craniosynostosis • Chondrodysplasias

Introduction

Osteochondrodysplasias are a heterogeneous group of disorders. To date, greater than 450 skeletal conditions have been characterized [1–3]. Many of the skeletal dysplasias arise during the prenatal period and can be clinically diagnosed by ultrasonography. The perinatal prevalence of skeletal dysplasias is conservatively suggested to be 2.3 in 10,000 with estimates as high as 1 in 4,000–5,000 births [4, 5]. Fibroblast growth factor (FGF) signaling, including the ligands and their receptors, play an important role in the function of chondrocytes and osteocytes that contribute to bone patterning. Two of the most common types of skeletal dysplasias are achondroplasia and thanatophoric dysplasia, emphasizing the importance of FGF signaling in skeletal development [6]. Since mutations found in the FGF receptor (FGFR) genes result in some of the most common types of skeletal dysplasias, genetic testing is an effective diagnostic tool for determination of the type of skeletal dysplasia and establishing recurrence risks. This chapter focuses on the many distinct skeletal disorders arising from mutations in the FGFR family of genes that are responsible for forms of syndromic and non-syndromic craniosynostosis and chondrodysplasias.

S. Sperber, M.S., Ph.D., F.A.C.M.G. (✉)
Department of Genetic and Genomic Sciences, Mount Sinai Genetic Testing Laboratory, Icahn School of Medicine at Mount Sinai, One Gustave L. Levy Place, Box 1497, New York, NY 10029, USA
e-mail: Steven.Sperber@mssm.edu

E. Spector, Ph.D., F.A.C.M.G.
Department of Pediatrics, Denver Genetic Laboratories, Children's Hospital Colorado, Aurora, CO, USA
e-mail: elaine.spector@childrenscolorado.org

Fibroblast Growth Factor Signaling

The FGF signaling pathway plays a prominent role in the growth and shaping of the skeletal system through regulation

D.G.B. Leonard (ed.), *Molecular Pathology in Clinical Practice*, DOI 10.1007/978-3-319-19674-9_12

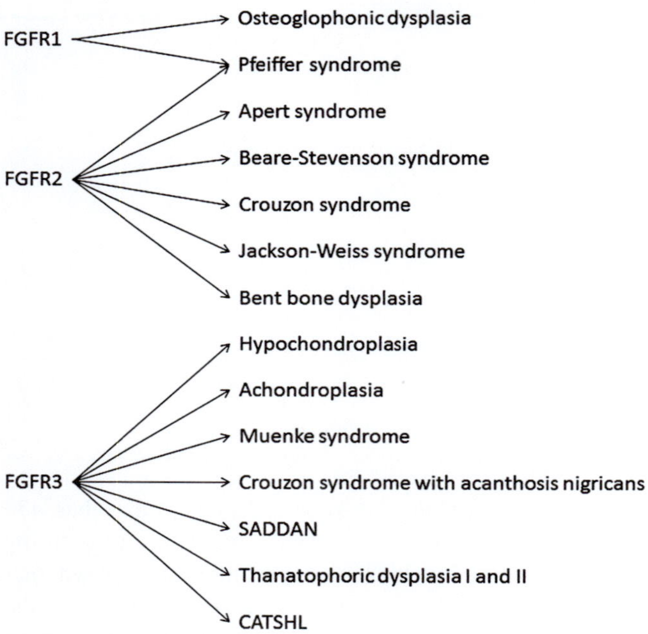

Figure 12.1 FGFR-associated syndromic conditions

Table 12.1 *FGFR1*, *-2*, and *-3* genes

Gene	OMIM	Chromosomal location	Gene organization
FGFR1	*136350	8p11.23-p11.22	18 exons, 17 coding
FGFR2	*176943	10q26.13	18 exons, 17 coding
FGFR3	*134934	4p16.3	18 exons, 17 coding

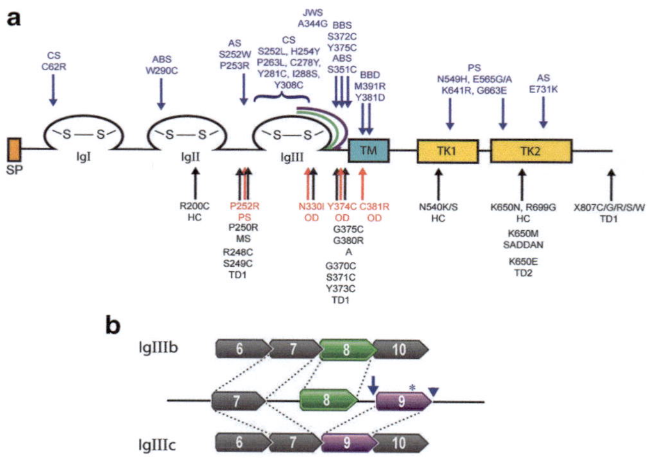

Figure 12.2 FGFR protein structure. (**a**) Common FGFR protein structure showing the signal peptide domain (SP, *orange*), the three immunoglobulin loops (IgI, IgII, and IgIII) with cysteine–cysteine disulfide bonds (S–S), the transmembrane domain (TM, *blue*), and the bifurcated tyrosine kinase domain (TK1 and TK2, *yellow*). The alternatively spliced carboxy-region of IgIII is illustrated as *green* and *purple lines*. Locations of selected mutations in *FGFR1* (*red*), *FGFR2* (*blue*), and *FGFR3* (*black*) are indicated by *arrows*, with the associated disease above or below the mutation. *A* achondrodysplasia, *ABS* Antley-Bixler syndrome, *AS* Apert syndrome, *BBD* bent bone dysplasia, *BSS* Beare-Stevenson syndrome, *CS* Crouzon syndrome, *HC* hypochondrodysplasia, *JWS* Jackson-Weiss syndrome, *MS* Muenke syndrome, *OD* osteoglophonic dysplasia, *PS* Pfeiffer syndrome, *TD1* and *TD2* thanatophoric dysplasia type 1 and 2, respectively. (**b**) Alternative splicing of exons 8 and 9 that code for the IgIII carboxy-terminal region. Isoform FGFR-IIIb (*top*) includes exon 8 (*green*). Isoform FGFR-IIIc (*bottom*) includes exon 9 (*purple*). Examples of *FGFR2* splicing mutations are shown: c.940-2A>G (*arrow*), c.1032G>A (A344A) (*asterisk*); and c.1084+3A>G (*arrowhead*)

of chondro- and osteoblastogenesis [7]. Twenty-three known FGF family members act as ligands to the FGFRs to influence cellular proliferation and differentiation. The FGF ligands interact with four high-affinity receptors (*FGFR1* through -4). Signaling is initiated by a FGFR monomer that binds to a FGF ligand, which requires heparin sulfate proteoglycan to facilitate the interaction [9]. FGF ligands bind to the FGFRs with different affinities and specificities [8]. Ligand binding induces homodimerization of the receptors and autophosphorylation of the tyrosine residues located in the cytoplasmic domain to propagate the intracellular signal [10, 11].

FGF Receptors

FGFRs are membrane-bound receptor tyrosine kinases. Of the four receptors, only mutations in *FGFR1*, *-2*, and *-3* (OMIM *136350, *176943, *134934) result in skeletal disorders (Fig. 12.1). The structures of the FGFR paralogs are very similar (Table 12.1). The FGFR paralogs share the same organization consisting of three immunoglobulin-like extracellular domains denoted as IgI, IgII, and IgIII, a membrane traversing hydrophobic region, and a bifurcated intracellular tyrosine kinase domain that propagates the signal to downstream pathways (Fig. 12.2a). The three immunoglobulin-like regions are stabilized by cysteine-cysteine disulfide bonds. The *FGFR1-3* genes produce alternative splicing of the IgIII domain, which generates two isoforms that exhibit tissue-specific expression. The amino aspect of the IgIII region is referred to as IgIIIa. The carboxy half of the IgIII loop contains one of two alternate exons (Fig. 12.2b) denoted as IgIIIb and IgIIIc that code for the C-terminal region of the IgIII domain [12, 13]. The two isoforms preferentially bind to particular FGF ligands and are differentially expressed in epithelial and mesenchymal tissues during development [14]. Studies indicate that it is the FGFR2c and FGFR3c isoforms, expressed in the mesenchyme, that are particularly involved in proper bone patterning [15].

Molecular Basis of Disease

Mutations in the *FGFR1*, *-2*, and *-3* genes account for approximately 15–20 % of all craniosynostosis and chondrodysplasias. FGFR-related skeletal anomalies are a result of gain-of-function variants that constitutively activate the receptor function [16–18]. Activated FGFRs receptors cause increased cellular proliferation and premature osteoblast differentiation [19–21]. The FGFR constitutive activation is by either a FGF ligand-dependent or -independent mechanism. Ligand-dependent mechanisms arise due to mutations that improve binding of FGF ligands and dimerization of the receptors prolonging signaling activity [22]. Alternatively, ligand-independent mechanisms include the following: (1) enhancement of receptor dimerization due to an immunoglobulin domain structural change such as a gain or loss of a cysteine residue within the loops; (2) augmentation of dimerization due to intramembrane domain changes in amino acid charge that increases hydrogen bonding; and (3) alterations in the kinase domain causing constitutively active phosphorylation [23–25].

Mutations causing FGFR-related craniosynostosis and/or chondrodysplasia tend to cluster in specific domains of the receptors (Fig. 12.2a). These clusters illustrate the importance of the domains in receptor function. Analogous mutations found in each of the different FGFRs tend to mirror phenotypic effects between the receptors. However, distinctions between analogous mutations in the different receptors and their phenotypes reveal their independent roles during normal skeletogenesis.

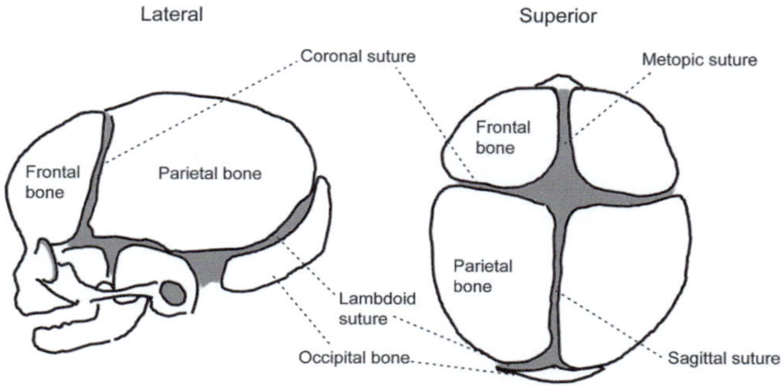

Figure 12.3 Skull sutures of a newborn. (*left*) Lateral view. (*right*) Superior view

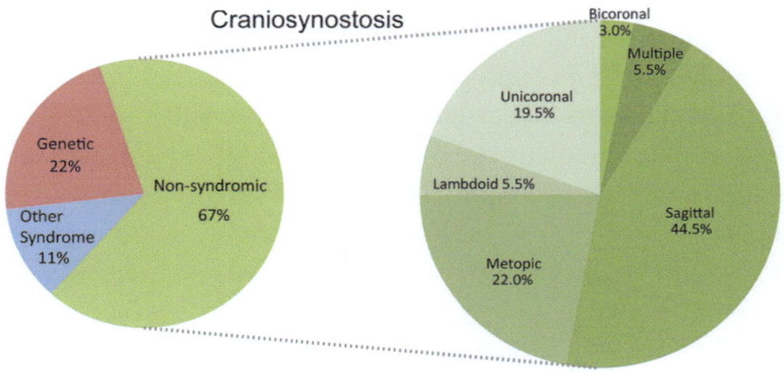

Figure 12.4 The prevalence of different forms of craniosynostosis derived from analysis of a 215-patient cohort affected with syndromic and nonsyndromic forms of craniosynostosis (*left*). Phenotypic categorization of nonsyndromic cases based upon affected sutures (*right*) (adapted with permission from Wilkie et al. 2010 [32])

Craniosynostosis and Chondrodysplasia

Craniosynostosis

Craniosynostosis arises from the premature fusion of one or more of the cranial sutures resulting in a dysmorphic skull. Distortions of the skull arise from uneven growth patterns between the sutures and depend on the location and timing of the fusion events [26]. The cranial sutures are the leading edges of the growing intramembranous bones that comprise the skull vault or calvaria. The calvaria consists of the left and right frontal, squamous occipital, squamous temporal, and the left and right parietal bones that will form the neurocranium (Fig. 12.3). At birth, the frontal bones are separated by the metopic suture. The coronal suture separates the frontal bones from the left and right parietal bones. The lambdoid suture separates the parietals from the occipital bone. The suture leading edges function as ossification centers. The calvaria of the neurocranium that forms the desmocranium ossifies as intramembranous bone forming the vault of the neurocranium. Normally, the metopic suture begins to close after the first year and closure is completed by the seventh year, generating the frontal bone [27]. The sagittal, coronal, and lambdoidal sutures generally complete fusion between 20 and 40 years of age. *De novo* or autosomal dominantly inherited mutations in the *FGFR1–3* genes that enhance signaling result in the inhibition of the osteogenic proliferation program, thereby causing premature fusion of cranial sutures [28]. Mutations associated with isolated nonsyndromic forms of craniosynostosis have been found in each of the *FGFR1–3* genes [29–31].

Nonsyndromic or isolated single-suture forms of craniosynostosis are more common than syndromic and number 1 in 2,100–3,000 live births [17]. Sagittal synostosis is the most common, followed by coronal, metopic, and then lambdoid suture synostosis (Fig. 12.4) [32, 33]. Nonsyndromic craniosynostosis is heterogeneous and many of the causes remain unknown. Often full sequencing of the *FGFR* genes may be requested to rule out the receptors and potentially detect *de novo* mutations.

Chondrodysplasias

In addition to influencing the growth of the neurocranium, FGF signaling also participates in the development of the skeletal system exemplified by its role in the growth of the long bones of the appendicular skeleton. Dominantly inherited and *de novo* gain-of-function mutations result in varying degrees of dwarfism as illustrated by particular *FGFR3* mutations that cause hypochondroplasia and achondroplasia. Observed in both craniosynostosis and chondrodysplasia cases, germline mutations due to advanced paternal age are a significant contributor to these disorders [34, 35].

Clinical Utility of Testing

Syndromic forms of *FGFR*-related craniosynostosis and chondrodysplasia are diagnosed clinically, based on their well-described phenotypes. Three-dimensional ultrasonography is able to detect early skeletal anomalies, including short bones, premature skull fusion, and other characteristic syndromic features [6, 36]. Molecular testing is performed to confirm the diagnosis and provide recurrence risks in pregnancies with either suspected germline mosaic transmission in families with a history of a previously affected fetus, or in families with an affected parent and a 50 % probability of passing on the deleterious allele. In such cases of inheritance, examination of the contributing parent may reveal a mild phenotype. For severe cases, *de novo* mutations occurring in the male germline may be responsible. Advanced paternal age is known to increase the risk of having affected offspring. Generally, targeted mutation analysis is sufficient to confirm a well-characterized phenotype and is the first tier of testing. Sequencing of all the exons may be performed if no mutation is found initially.

Available Assays

Different methods have been developed to identify mutations within the *FGFR* genes. The vast majority of mutations are missense and nonsense, with splicing and in-frame small insertions and deletions being much rarer. Detection methods include targeted mutation analysis, scanning of specific exons, and sequencing of all the coding regions as well as their intron/exon boundaries. Targeted analysis is based on testing the patient's DNA for previously described mutations. Using restriction fragment length polymorphism (RFLP) methods, regions of interest within the coding sequences can be amplified by polymerase chain reaction (PCR) and digested with restriction endonucleases that would characteristically identify specific mutations based on altered banding patterns observed by gel electrophoresis and staining (Fig. 12.5). Incomplete digestion of a restriction site may lead to aberrant results and an incorrect heterozygosity interpretation; therefore, both positive and negative digestion controls are essential for RFLP analysis. Alternatively, allele-specific oligonucleotide PCR with primers targeted to wild-type alleles and previously characterized mutations may be performed, resulting in identifiable amplicon patterns. The drawback to targeted analysis is that mutations outside the scope of the assay will be missed.

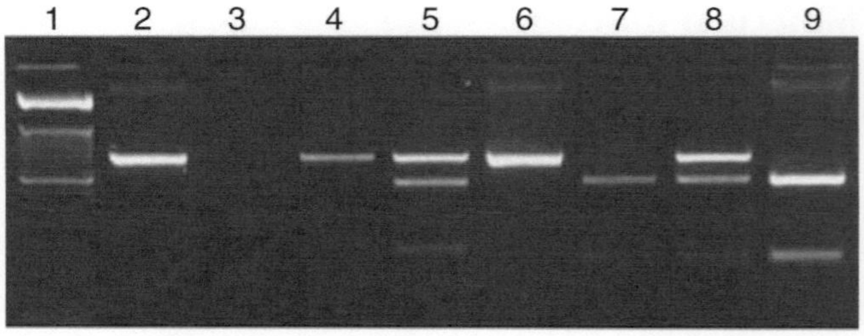

Figure 12.5 Thanatophoric dysplasia type 2 restriction fragment length polymorphism (RFLP) assay. Amplification of the *FGFR3* exon 15 and digestion of patient and control DNA give characteristic banding patterns diagnostic for the p.Lys650Glu mutation. *Lane 1*, 50 base pair (bp) size marker; *lane 2*, undigested 450 bp amplicon; *lane 3*, no DNA template PCR control; *lanes 4–6*, restriction digest with *Bsm*AI; *lanes 7–9*, digest with *Bbs*I. *Lanes 4, 6, 7,* and *9*, control DNA. *Lanes 5* and *8*, patient DNA. *Lanes 4–6* show a gain of a *Bsm*AI restriction site in the patient DNA (*lane 5*). *Lanes 7–9* demonstrate loss of a *Bbs*I digest site in the patient's DNA (*lane 8*)

Mutation scanning by denaturing high-performance liquid chromatography (DHPLC) has been employed to screen the exons of the FGFR genes whereby patient's profiles suggest potential mutations in comparison to unaffected and affected controls. Issues arise in scanning techniques such as DHPLC as well as high-temperature melting profiles and single-stranded conformational polymorphism in their inability to identify specific mutations or distinguish between known mutations and rare polymorphisms. Unique profiles identifying potential mutations must then be directly sequenced. Sequence analysis of the coding exons is the most comprehensive of the methods ensuring that any point mutation and small deletions and duplications will be identified within the amplified regions. Massively parallel sequencing, using next-generation sequencing platforms, also offers the option to perform sequence analysis on many samples concurrently through barcoding of individual patient's DNA and using bioinformatics to separate the reads by patient and analyze the sequence data.

Deletion/duplication analysis may be performed by multiplex ligation-dependent probe amplification or exon level array-based comparative genomic hybridization and then confirmed by quantitative PCR. These methods measure the relative amounts of each exonic region where probes are placed, comparing the quantitative results to internal controls, usually housekeeping gene(s) found on other chromosomes.

Interpretation of Test Results

The majority of *FGFR* mutations causing skeletal dysplasia are point mutations. Interpretation of novel missense variants is becoming easier as the knowledge base grows. To date, there are approximately 155 known mutations within the *FGFR1-2-3* that cause skeletal dysplasias. Current lists of mutations are available in the Human Gene Mutation Database (www.biobase-international.com/product/hgmd). Databases that include polymorphisms, such as dbSNP (www.ncbi.nlm.nih.gov/projects/SNP/), the 1000 Genomes Project (www.1000genomes.org/), and exome sequencing projects (Exome Aggregation Consortium [ExAC], exac.broadinstitute.org; Exome Variant Server, http://evs.gs.washington.edu/EVS/), provide information on the genetic variants and their frequencies in the general population [37, 38]. Variants of unknown significance can be evaluated using predictive algorithms that may provide insight into whether they are benign or pathogenic. These predictions take into consideration the biochemical properties of the amino acid change, including size, charge, polarity, steric constraints, and evolutionary conservation of the residue within the protein domain. Internet-based predictive tools, including PolyPhen2, SIFT, and Mutation Taster, provide analysis of the probable functional consequences of missense variants [39–41]. The results of these prediction tools have to be considered as one piece of evidence.

Rare splicing mutations causing skeletal dysplasia have been documented. Mutations, such as the synonymous change p.Ala344Ala (c.1032G>A) in the immunoglobulin IIIc (IgIIIc) domain of *FGFR2*, activate a cryptic splice donor site (Fig. 12.2b) [42]. Conversely, weakening the endogenous donor site (c.1084+3A>G and c.1084+1G>A) induces exon skipping and preferential splicing of the IgIIIb isoform [43–45]. Similarly, *FGFR2* mutations causing Pfeiffer syndrome affect the IgIIIc acceptor site (c.940-2A>G or A>T) [46]. Unknown variants found in the intronic regions of the gene can be analyzed through splicing algorithms, such as the Human Splice Finder (www.umd.be/HSF/) [47] and Netgene2 (www.cbs.dtu.dk/services/NetGene2/) [48], to predict their influence on the precursor mRNA.

Laboratory Issues

Commercial test kits for analyzing the *FGFR* genes are not available, so testing is performed using laboratory developed tests. Test development and validation may be achieved using cell lines obtained from the Coriell Cell Repository (http://ccr.coriell.org). Proficiency testing is available through the College of American Pathologists Molecular Genetics Laboratory sequencing surveys. Additionally, interlaboratory sample exchanges and internal repeat testing of blinded samples can be used to meet the proficiency testing requirements.

FGFR-Related Skeletal Syndromes

Apert Syndrome

Apert syndrome (OMIM#101200), also known as acrocephalosyndactyly, is characterized by craniosynostosis, facial hypoplasia, broad thumbs and great toes, and digit fusion of the hands and feet (syndactyly) described as a "mitten-hand" malformation. As the most common of the craniosynostosis syndromes, Apert syndrome accounts for approximately 4.5 % of all cases with an occurrence estimated as 1 in 65,000 to 80,000 [49, 50]. The majority of cases result from *de novo* mutations attributed to increasing paternal age [51].

The majority of cases (99 %) are caused by one of two point mutations in the *FGFR2* gene [52]. The common mutations are p.Ser252Trp, which accounts for approximately two-thirds of the cases, and p.Pro253Arg accounting for one third of cases. These mutations, located at the IgII-IgIII linker region, enhance ligand binding affinity [9]. Rarer mutations have been observed surrounding these two mutations in the linker region. Diagnostic testing can be performed by targeted Sanger sequencing.

Apert syndrome is clinically diagnosed. Identification of the specific mutation helps in determining the potential risk for further affected pregnancies due to germline mosaicism. With an affected parent, there is a 50 % probability that a pregnancy will result in an affected child.

Pfeiffer Syndrome

Patients presenting with Pfeiffer Syndrome (OMIM#101600) exhibit brachycephaly, hypertelorism, ocular proptosis, a flat midface, broad thumbs, and medially deviated great toes, and occasionally with hearing loss and variable cutaneous syndactyly [17]. Pfeiffer syndrome is a genetically heterogeneous disorder. Mutations have been found in both *FGFR1* and *FGFR2*. *FGFR2* mutations account for 95 % of patients' mutations. One activating mutation, p.Pro252Arg in the *FGFR1* gene, accounts for approximately 5 % of the diagnosed patients. Mutations in *FGFR2* are found in the IgIIIa and IgIIIc regions as well as the tyrosine kinase domain, and tend to be phenotypically more severe than the *FGFR1*-derived phenotype.

Crouzon Syndrome With or Without Acanthosis Nigricans

Crouzon syndrome (OMIM#123500) patients have multiple suture fusions or coronal fusions causing brachycephaly, trigonocephaly, and rare reports of cloverleaf skull malformation also known as kleeblattschädel [53, 54]. Attributes typically include hypertelorism, a small midface, beaked nose and protrusion of the eyes. Hands and feet are generally normal. Heterozygous mutations in the *FGFR2* gene show high penetrance and variability of the phenotype within families. Approximately half of the cases are inherited and the other half arise from *de novo* mutations. Increasing paternal age is a contributing factor for *de novo* mutations [35]. The prevalence is estimated as 1 in 65,000 live births [55].

Patients with Crouzon syndrome with acanthosis nigricans (OMIM#612247) are typically female, display hyperpigmentation of the skin, hyperkeratosis, and other skin findings. A specific *FGFR3* heterozygous mutation, p.Ala391Glu, has been identified and is located in the transmembrane domain [56].

Muenke Syndrome

Muenke syndrome (OMIM#602849) displays incomplete penetrance and a variable phenotype even within families [57]. Prevalence in the population is estimated to be 1 in 30,000 live births. Sporadic and familial cases have been reported. Characteristics include bi- or unicoronal synostosis, midfacial hypoplasia, ptosis, and downslanting palpebral fissures. Some affected individuals have additional features that may include sensorineural hearing loss, developmental delay, brachydactyly, and coned epiphyses in the hands and feet. Muenke craniosynostosis is a result of a specific heterozygous mutation, p.Pro250Arg, found in the linker region between domains IgII and IgIII of *FGFR3* [58–61]. Targeted testing may be performed by sequencing the seventh exon of *FGFR3* or by RFLP analysis using the *Msp*I endonuclease.

Beare-Stevenson Syndrome

Beare-Stevenson (OMIM#123790), also known as cutis gyrate syndrome of Beare and Stevenson, is a rare and severe disorder. Patients characteristically have body-wide skin furrows (cutis gyrate), acanthosis nigricans, skin tags, bifid scrotum, and anogenital anomalies. The craniosynostosis may be severe and present as a cloverleaf skull with hypertelorism, a broad nasal bridge, cleft palate, and hypodontia. Two heterozygous point mutations in the *FGFR2* gene, p.Ser372Cys and p.Tyr375Cys, account for 50–60 % of cases, suggesting locus heterogeneity. The resulting cysteine residues are thought to increase ligand-independent dimerization. These *de novo* mutations are analogous to the mutations in *FGFR3* causing thanatophoric dysplasia. An intragenic deletion, c.1506del63, has recently been described and is proposed to alter gene splicing in favor of the IgIIIb isoform of *FGFR2*. Loss of the 21 amino acids encoded by exons 8 and 9 is suggested to cause aberrant expression of *FGFR2b* [62].

Jackson-Weiss Syndrome

Jackson-Weiss Syndrome (OMIM#123150), inherited in an autosomal dominant manner, has been most prominently described in an extended Amish family with a p.Ala344Gly mutation in the IgIIIc domain of *FGFR2* [63–66]. Fully penetrant with variable severity, the characteristics of the syndrome include craniosynostosis with facial anomalies, broad great toes, and webbing of the second and third toes [67]. A few reports suggest mutations in *FGFR2* and *FGFR1* exhibit phenotypic traits similar to Jackson-Weiss syndrome indicating that Crouzon, Jackson-Weiss, and Pfeiffer syndromes may represent a spectrum of craniosynostotic and digit malformations [68, 69].

Antley-Bixler Syndrome Type 2

Antley-Bixler syndrome (ABS; trapezoidocephaly-synostosis syndrome) is a rare and severe heterogeneous disorder with mutations found in both the *FGFR2* gene (autosomal dominant; type 2; OMIM#207410) and the cytochrome P450 oxidoreductase (*POR*) gene (autosomal recessive; type 1; OMIM#201750). ABS type 2 is characterized by craniosynostosis of the coronal and lambdoid sutures, midfacial hypoplasia, radiohumeral and digit fusions, exophthalmos, and arachnodactyly [70, 71]. The mutations associated with ABS include p.Trp290Cys and p.Ser351Cys, both found in the IgIII domain of the *FGFR2* gene [72]. Mutations at these positions also have been associated with the milder phenotype of Crouzon syndrome [73].

Osteoglophonic Dysplasia

Osteoglophonic dysplasia (Fairbank-Keats syndrome; OMIM#166250), a very rare disorder, is typified by variable craniosynostosis and rhizomelic dwarfism with a "hollowed-out" appearance of the tubular bones on radiographs, depression of the nasal bridge, unerupted teeth, frontal bossing, and prognathism similar to achondroplasia. Mutations in *FGFR1* are found in the conserved amino acids clustered in the C-terminal region of the IgIII immunoglobulin domain, the linker region, and the transmembrane domain. The *FGFR1* p.Tyr372Cys mutation is analogous to both the *FGFR2* p.Tyr375Cys mutation that causes Beare-Stevenson syndrome and the p.Tyr373Cys *FGFR3* mutation that causes thanatophoric dwarfism type 1, indicating the importance of that amino acid position in the functional role of the receptors [74].

Achondroplasia

Achondroplasia (OMIM#100800) arises from mutations in the *FGFR3* gene that inhibit chondrocyte proliferation within the endochondral growth plate resulting in the shortening of long bones. Achondroplasia is the most common form of FGFR-related short-limbed dwarfism [75, 76], with an occurrence of 1 in 10,000 to 30,000 live births [4, 5]. Two common variants, c.1138G>A (~98 %) and c.1138G>C (1–2 %), result in a p.Gly380Arg mutation in the transmembrane domain of *FGFR3* [77]. The achondroplasia mutation is the most common *de novo* disease-causing mutation known. There is a strong paternal origin for the mutation, mostly in fathers over the age of 35 years [34]. A second mutation, described in several published accounts, suggests that p.Gly375Cys also causes achondroplasia [78–80].

Testing for the c.1138G>A mutation may be performed by RFLP digestion of exon 10 with the *Sfc*I restriction enzyme. It has been noted, however, that complete digestion is not consistently observed for the assay and other molecular methods may be required to differentiate between the G>A and the G>C mutations, the heterozygous form, and the lethal homozygous form [81–83].

Severe Achondroplasia, Developmental Delay, and Acanthosis Nigricans (SADDAN)

Severe achondroplasia, developmental delay and acanthosis nigricans (SADDAN; OMIM#187600), is caused by a c.1949A>T mutation (p.Lys650Met) in *FGFR3*. The substitution of a methionine residue at position 650 differentiates SADDAN from type 2 thanatophoric dysplasia, which arises from a glutamic acid substitution at the same position (c.1948A>G; Lys650Glu). The SADDAN amino acid change induces constitutive kinase activity that is threefold greater than normal [84].

Hypochondroplasia

Hypochondroplasia (OMIM#146000) is clinically diagnosed as a mild form of skeletal dysplasia. Clinical diagnosis is usually by short limbs detected on ultrasonography, which prompts diagnostic testing. The *FGFR3* c.1138G>A mutation that causes achondroplasia has been found in about 5 % of hypochondroplasia cases. *FGFR3* mutations account for only 50–70 % of cases, suggesting genetic heterogeneity. Of those mutations in *FGFR3*, 70 % are a recurrent p.Asn540Lys amino acid change located in the tyrosine kinase 1 domain (TK1), while others are rarer. Testing may be performed by RFLP analysis of an exon 13 PCR product, which will detect the two c.1659C>A/G, p.N540K mutations. A *Bsp*MI restriction site is abolished by the c.1620C>A mutation, and the c.1620C>G mutation creates a novel *Alu*I restriction site [85]. The other known mutations may be detected by sequencing exons 10, 13, and 15 of *FGFR3*.

Thanatophoric Dysplasia

Thanatophoric dysplasia (TD) is the most common lethal condition of short-limbed skeletal dysplasia with a distorted head and has an estimated incidence of 1 in 20,000 to 50,000 live births. Two types of TD are clinically diagnosed based on ultrasound and radiographic findings [86–88]. Type 1 (OMIM#187600) patients have prominently curved femurs, while type 2 (OMIM#187601) patients typically have a severe form of craniosynostosis often referred to as a cloverleaf skull and a small chest [89].

Several different gain-of-function mutations in *FGFR3* cause TD type 1. Mutations p.Arg248Cys, p.Ser249Cys, p.Ser371Cys, and p.Tyr373Cys create novel cysteine residues in the extracellular and intramembranous domains, while other mutations causing TD type 1, such as p. Ter807Arg, p.Ter807Cys, p.Ter807Gly, p.Ter807Ser, and p.Ter807Trp, obliterate the stop codon resulting in extension of the intracellular domain by an additional 141 amino acids [90, 91].

TD type 2 is caused by the *FGFR3* transition mutation c.1948A>G, coding for p.Lys650Glu [92, 93]. The mutation causes multiple cranial sutures to fuse prematurely resulting in a cloverleaf skull malformation. The importance of the lysine 650 codon, situated in the tyrosine kinase-domain activation loop of FGFR3, is emphasized by the wide range of clinical phenotypes observed based, on the different amino acid substitutions and their ability to influence kinase activity. Similar to the previously mentioned SADDAN p. Lys650Met mutation, substitution of the lysine 650 for a glutamine or asparagine residue is associated with a milder hypochondrodysplasia phenotype [94].

Bent Bone Dysplasia: FGFR2 Type

Bent bone dysplasia-FGFR2 type (OMIM#614592) has recently been attributed to two heterozygous mutations in the FGFR2 transmembrane domain, c.1172T>G (p.Met391Arg) and c.1141T>G (p.Tyr381Asp) that reduce its localization to the plasma membrane [95]. A phenotype of perinatal lethality with hypertelorism, midface hypoplasia, micrognathia, prematurely erupted prenatal teeth, low-set posteriorly rotated ears, and clitoromegaly in females. Distinct radiological findings include coronal craniosynostosis with poorly mineralized calvaria, curved appendicular skeletal defects, and clavicle hypoplasia. The nuances of the genotype-phenotype correlations are observed in the mutation of the tyrosine 381 residue to asparagine (p.Tyr381Asn, c.1141T>A) that causes Crouzon syndrome [96]. These studies suggest a spectrum of severity for altered FGFR2 activity.

Other *FGFR*-Associated Disorders

In addition to the activating mutations resulting in craniosynostosis and chondrodysplasia, loss-of-function mutations in the *FGFR* genes cause a variety of different syndromes.

CATSHL Syndrome

Dominantly inherited, camptodactyly, tall stature, scoliosis, and hearing loss (CATSHL; OMIM#610474) is caused by a *FGFR3* p.Arg621His heterozygous missense mutation residing within the tyrosine kinase domain generating a loss-of-function that promotes endochondral bone growth [97]. Recently, a novel homozygous *FGFR3* c.1167C>A p.Thr546Lys, mutation has been described as also causing skeletal overgrowth [98].

Kallmann Syndrome

Hypogonadotropic hypogonadism, also known as Kallmann syndrome (OMIM#308700), is a heterogenic disorder with mutations found most commonly in the *KAL* gene (KAL1, X-linked; OMIM *300836) as well as *FGFR1* (KAL2, OMIM#147950). Other genes that account for 5 % or less of cases include *PROKR2*, *PROK2*, *CHD7*, and *FGF8*, while an additional five genes are known to account for the autosomal recessive form. Sensitivity of testing for clinically diagnosed Kallmann syndrome is approximately 30 % for the aforementioned genes [99]. Loss-of-function mutations in *FGFR1* account for approximately 10 % of cases of type 2 Kallmann Syndrome with deletions being rare contributors to the disorder. Kallmann syndrome exhibits a 5:1 male to female ratio with an incidence of approximately 1 in 8,000 to 10,000 in males and 1 in 40,000 to 50,000 in females [100, 101]. Patients characteristically have olfactory bulb dysgenesis (anosmia) and hypogonadotropic hypogonadism, with boys also having micropenis and cryptorchidism. Mutations in the *FGFR1* gene also may result in cleft lip and/or palate, agenesis of the teeth, and digital malformations [102].

LADD Syndrome

Lacrimo-auriculo-dento-digital (LADD) syndrome (OMIM#149730; Levy-Hollister syndrome) is a dominant, heterogeneous disorder with mutations found in the *FGF10* gene as well as the tyrosine kinase domains of *FGFR2* (p.Ala648Thr, p.Ala628Thr) and *FGFR3* (p.Asp513Asn) [103–105]. Variants in the receptor kinase domain associated with LADD syndrome reduce phosphorylation activity [106]. Affected individuals typically exhibit hypoplasia/aplasia of the tear and salivary ducts, malformed ears and deafness, hypodontia, and digital anomalies mostly affecting the thumbs [107–109].

References

1. Superti-Furga A, Steinmann B, Gitzelmann R, Eich G, Giedion A, Bucher HU, Wisser J. A glycine 375-to-cysteine substitution in the transmembrane domain of the fibroblast growth factor receptor-3 in a newborn with achondroplasia. Eur J Pediatr. 1995; 154(3):215–9.
2. Warman ML, Cormier-Daire V, Hall C, Krakow D, Lachman R, LeMerrer M, Mortier G, Mundlos S, Nishimura G, Rimoin DL, Robertson S, Savarirayan R, Sillence D, Spranger J, Unger S, Zabel B, Superti-Furga A. Nosology and classification of genetic skeletal disorders: 2010 revision. Am J Med Genet A. 2011;155(5):943–68.
3. Krakow D. Skeletal Dysplasias. Clin Perinatol. 2015;42:301–19.
4. Orioli IM, Castilla EE, Barbosa-Neto JG. The birth prevalence rates for the skeletal dysplasias. J Med Genet. 1986;23(4):328–32.
5. Stoll C, Dott B, Roth M-P, Alembik Y. Birth prevalence rates of skeletal dysplasias. Clin Genet. 1989;35(2):88–92.
6. Krakow D, Alanay Y, Rimoin LP, Lin V, Wilcox WR, Lachman RS, Rimoin DL. Evaluation of prenatal-onset osteochondrodysplasias by ultrasonography: A retrospective and prospective analysis. Am J Med Genet A. 2008;146A(15):1917–24.
7. Ornitz DM, Itoh N. The Fibroblast Growth Factor signaling pathway. Wiley Interdiscip Rev Dev Biol. 2015;4(3):215–66.
8. Spivak-Kroizman T, Lemmon MA, Dikic I, Ladbury JE, Pinchasi D, Huang J, Jaye M, Crumley G, Schlessinger J, Lax I. Heparin-induced oligomerization of FGF molecules is responsible for FGF receptor dimerization, activation, and cell proliferation. Cell. 1994;79(6):1015–24.
9. Mohammadi M, Olsen SK, Ibrahimi OA. Structural basis for fibroblast growth factor receptor activation. Cytokine Growth Factor Rev. 2005;16(2):107–37.
10. Plotnikov AN, Schlessinger J, Hubbard SR, Mohammadi M. Structural basis for FGF receptor dimerization and activation. Cell. 1999;98(5):641–50.
11. Pellegrini L, Burke DF, von Delft F, Mulloy B, Blundell TL. Crystal structure of fibroblast growth factor receptor ectodomain bound to ligand and heparin. Nature. 2000;407(6807): 1029–34.
12. Givol D, Yayon A. Complexity of FGF receptors: genetic basis for structural diversity and functional specificity. FASEB J. 1992;6(15):3362–9.
13. Orr-Urtreger A, Bedford MT, Burakova T, Arman E, Zimmer Y, Yayon A, Givol D, Lonai P. Developmental localization of the splicing alternatives of fibroblast growth factor receptor-2 (FGFR2). Dev Biol. 1993;158(2):475–86.
14. Delezoide AL, Benoist-Lasselin C, Legeai-Mallet L, Le Merrer M, Munnich A, Vekemans M, Bonaventure J. Spatio-temporal expression of FGFR 1, 2 and 3 genes during human embryo-fetal ossification. Mech Dev. 1998;77(1):19–30.
15. Eswarakumar VP, Lax I, Schlessinger J. Cellular signaling by fibroblast growth factor receptors. Cytokine Growth Factor Rev. 2005;16(2):139–49.
16. Webster MK, Donoghue DJ. Constitutive activation of fibroblast growth factor receptor 3 by the transmembrane domain point mutation found in achondroplasia. EMBO J. 1996;15(3):520–7.

17. Muenke M, Gripp K, McDonald-McGinn D, Gaudenz K, Whitaker L, Bartlett S, Markowitz R, Robin N, Nwokoro N, Mulvihill J, Losken H, Mulliken J, Guttmacher A, Wilroy L, Clarke R, Hollway G, Adès L, Haan E, Mulley J, Cohen M, Bellus G, Francomano C, Moloney D, Wall S, Wilkie A, Zackai E. A unique point mutation in the fibroblast growth factor receptor 3 gene (FGFR3) defines a new craniosynostosis syndrome. Am J Hum Genet. 1997;60(3):555–64.
18. Cohen MM. Some chondrodysplasias with short limbs: molecular perspectives. Am J Med Genet. 2002;112(3):304–13.
19. Legeai-Mallet L, Benoist-Lasselin C, Delezoide A-L, Munnich A, Bonaventure J. Fibroblast growth factor receptor 3 mutations promote apoptosis but do not alter chondrocyte proliferation in thanatophoric dysplasia. J Biol Chem. 1998;273(21):13007–14.
20. Legeai-Mallet L, Benoist-Lasselin C, Munnich A, Bonaventure J. Overexpression of FGFR3, Stat1, Stat5 and p21Cip1 correlates with phenotypic severity and defective chondrocyte differentiation in FGFR3-related chondrodysplasias. Bone. 2004;34:26–36.
21. Holmes G, Rothschild G, Roy UB, Deng C-X, Mansukhani A, Basilico C. Early onset of craniosynostosis in an apert mouse model reveals critical features of this pathology. Dev Biol. 2009;328:273–84.
22. Monsonego-oran E, Adar R, Feferman T, Segev O, Yayon A. The transmembrane mutation G380R in fibroblast growth factor receptor 3 uncouples ligand-mediated receptor activation from down-regulation. Mol Cell Biol. 2000;20(2):516–22.
23. Sorokin A, Lemmon MA, Ullrich A, Schlessinger J. Stabilization of an active dimeric form of the epidermal growth factor receptor by introduction of an inter-receptor disulfide bond. J Biol Chem. 1994;269(13):9752–9.
24. Hart KC, Robertson SC, Donoghue DJ. Identification of tyrosine residues in constitutively activated fibroblast growth factor receptor 3 involved in mitogenesis, Stat activation, and phosphatidylinositol 3-kinase activation. Mol Biol Cell. 2001;12:931–42.
25. Ratisoontorn C, Fan GF, McEntee K, Nah DD. Activating (P253R, C278F) and dominant negative mutations of FGFR2: differential effects on calvarial bone cell proliferation, differentiation, and mineralization. Connect Tissue Res. 2003;44 Suppl 1:292–7.
26. Cohen MM. No man's craniosynostosis: the arcana of sutural knowledge. J Craniofac Surg. 2012;23(1):338–42. 310.1097/SCS.1090b1013e318241dbc318244.
27. Sperber G, Sperber S, Guttmann G. Craniofacial embryogenetics and development. Shelton, CT: People's Medical Publishing House; 2010.
28. Ornitz DM. Regulation of chondrocyte growth and differentiation by fibroblast growth factor receptor 3. Novartis Found Symp. 2001;232:63–80, 272–282.
29. Johnson D, Wall SA, Mann S, Wilkie AOM. A novel mutation, Ala315Ser, in FGFR2: a gene-environment interaction leading to craniosynostosis? Eur J Hum Genet. 2000;8(8):571–7.
30. Kress W, Petersen B, Collmann H, Grimm T. An unusual FGFR1 mutation (fibroblast growth factor receptor 1 mutation) in a girl with non-syndromic trigonocephaly. Cytogenet Cell Genet. 2000;91(1-4):138–40.
31. Barroso E, Pérez-Carrizosa V, García-Recuero I, Glucksman MJ, Wilkie AO, García-Minaur S, Heath KE. Mild isolated craniosynostosis due to a novel FGFR3 mutation, p.Ala334Thr. Am J Med Genet. A. 2011;155(12):3050–3.
32. Wilkie AOM, Byren JC, Hurst JA, Jayamohan J, Johnson D, Knight SJL, Lester T, Richards PG, Twigg SRF, Wall SA. Prevalence and complications of single-gene and chromosomal disorders in craniosynostosis. Pediatrics. 2010;126(2):e391–400.
33. Levi B, Wan DC, Wong VW, Nelson E, Hyun J, Longaker MT. Cranial suture biology: from pathways to patient care. J Craniofac Surg. 2012;23(1):13–9. doi:10.1097/SCS.1090b1013e318240c318246c318240.
34. Wilkin DJ, Szabo JK, Cameron R, Henderson S, Bellus GA, Mack ML, Kaitila I, Loughlin J, Munnich A, Sykes B, Bonaventure J, Francomano CA. Mutations in fibroblast growth-factor receptor 3 in sporadic cases of achondroplasia occur exclusively on the paternally derived chromosome. Am J Hum Genet. 1998;63(3):711–6.
35. Glaser RL, Jiang W, Boyadjiev SA, Tran AK, Zachary AA, Van Maldergem L, Johnson D, Walsh S, Oldridge M, Wall SA, Wilkie AOM, Jabs EW. Paternal origin of FGFR2 mutations in sporadic cases of Crouzon syndrome and Pfeiffer syndrome. Am J Hum Genet. 2000;66(3):768–77.
36. Krakow D, Williams J, Poehl M, Rimoin DL, Platt LD. Use of three-dimensional ultrasound imaging in the diagnosis of prenatal-onset skeletal dysplasias. Ultrasound Obstet Gynecol. 2003;21(5):467–72.
37. 1000 Genomes Consortium. A map of human genome variation from population scale sequencing. Nature. 2010;467(7319):1061–73.
38. Shendure J. Next-generation human genetics. Genome Biol. 2011;12(9):408.
39. Kumar P, Henikoff S, Ng PC. Predicting the effects of coding non-synonymous variants on protein function using the SIFT algorithm. Nat Protoc. 2009;4(8):1073–81.
40. Adzhubei IA, Schmidt S, Peshkin L, Ramensky VE, Gerasimova A, Bork P, Kondrashov AS, Sunyaev SR. A method and server for predicting damaging missense mutations. Nat Methods. 2010;7(4):248–9.
41. Schwarz JM, Rodelsperger C, Schuelke M, Seelow D. MutationTaster evaluates disease-causing potential of sequence alterations. Nat Methods. 2010;7(8):575–6.
42. Li X, Park WJ, Pyeritz RE, Jabs EW. Effect on splicing of a silent FGFR2 mutation in Crouzon syndrome. Nat Genet. 1995;9:232–3.
43. Cornejo-Roldan LR, Roessler E, Muenke M. Analysis of the mutational spectrum of the FGFR2 gene in Pfeiffer syndrome. Hum Genet. 1999;104(5):425–31.
44. Kan R, Twigg SRF, Berg J, Wang L, Jin F, Wilkie AOM. Expression analysis of an FGFR2 IIIc 5′ splice site mutation (1084+3A→G). J Med Genet. 2004;41(8):e108.
45. Traynis I, Bernstein JA, Gardner P, Schrijver I. Analysis of the alternative splicing of an FGFR2 transcript due to a novel 5′ splice site mutation (1084+1G>A): case report. Cleft Palate Craniofac J. 2011;49(1):104–8.
46. Lajeunie E, Ma HW, Bonaventure J, Munnich A, Le Merrer M, Renier D. FGFR2 mutations in Pfeiffer syndrome. Nat Genet. 1995;9:108.
47. Desmet F-O, Hamroun D, Lalande M, Collod-Béroud G, Claustres M, Béroud C. Human splicing finder: an online bioinformatics tool to predict splicing signals. Nucl Acids Res. 2009;37(9):e67.
48. Brunak S, Engelbrecht J, Knudsen S. Prediction of human mRNA donor and acceptor sites from the DNA sequence. J Mol Biol. 1991;220(1):49–65.
49. Cohen MM. Birth prevalence study of the Apert syndrome. Am J Med Genet. 1992;42:655–9.
50. Tolarova MM, Harris JA, Ordway DE, Vargervik K. Birth prevalence, mutation rate, sex ratio, parents' age, and ethnicity in Apert syndrome. Am J Med Genet. 1997;72(4):394–8.
51. Moloney DM, Slaney SR, Oldridge M, Wall SA, Sahlin P, Stenman G, Wilkie AOM. Exclusive paternal origin of new mutations in Apert syndrome. Nat Genet. 1996;13(1):48–53.
52. Wilkie AOM, Slaney SF, Oldridge M, Poole MD, Ashworth GJ, Hockley AD, Hayward RD, David DJ, Pulleyn LJ, Rutland P, Malcolm S, Winter RM, Reardon W. Apert syndrome results from localized mutations of FGFR2 and is allelic with Crouzon syndrome. Nat Genet. 1995;9(2):165–72.
53. Rohatgi M. Cloverleaf skull — a severe form of Crouzon's syndrome: a new concept in aetiology. Acta Neurochir. 1991;108(1):45–52.
54. Murdoch-Kinch CA, Bixler D, Ward RE. Cephalometric analysis of families with dominantly inherited Crouzon syndrome: an aid

to diagnosis in family studies. Am J Med Genet. 1998;77(5):405–11.
55. Cohen MM, Kreiborg S. Birth prevalence studies of the Crouzon syndrome: comparison of direct and indirect methods. Clin Genet. 1992;41(1):12–5.
56. Arnaud-López L, Fragoso R, Mantilla-Capacho J, Barros-Núñez P. Crouzon with acanthosis nigricans. Further delineation of the syndrome. Clin Genet. 2007;72(5):405–10.
57. Escobar LF, Hiett AK, Marnocha A. Significant phenotypic variability of Muenke syndrome in identical twins. Am J Med Genet A. 2009;149A(6):1273–6.
58. Bellus GA, Gaudenz K, Zackai EH, Clarke LA, Szabo J, Francomano CA, Muenke M. Identical mutations in three different fibroblast growth factor receptor genes in autosomal dominant craniosynostosis syndromes. Nat Genet. 1996;14(2):174–6.
59. Muenke M, Wilkie AOM. Craniosynostosis syndromes. In: Scriver C, Beaudet A, Sly W, et al., editors. The metabolic and molecular basis of inherited disease. New York, NY: McGraw-Hill; 2001.
60. Graham JM, Braddock SR, Mortier GR, Lachman R, Van Dop C, Jabs EW. Syndrome of coronal craniosynostosis with brachydactyly and carpal/tarsal coalition due to Pro250Arg mutation in FGFR3 gene. Am J Med Genet. 1998;77(4):322–9.
61. Lowry RB, Wang Jabs E, Graham GE, Gerritsen J, Fleming J. Syndrome of coronal craniosynostosis, Klippel-Feil anomaly, and sprengel shoulder with and without Pro250Arg mutation in the FGFR3 gene. Am J Med Genet. 2001;104(2):112–9.
62. Slavotinek A, Crawford H, Golabi M, Tao C, Perry H, Oberoi S, Vargervik K, Friez M. Novel FGFR2 deletion in a patient with Beare–Stevenson-like syndrome. Am J Med Genet A. 2009;149A(8):1814–7.
63. Cross HE, Opitz JM. Craniosynostosis in the Amish. J Pediatr. 1969;75:1037–44.
64. Jackson CE, Weiss L, Reynolds WA, Forman TF, Peterson JA. Craniosynostosis, midfacial hypoplasia and foot abnormalities: an autosomal dominant phenotype in a large Amish kindred. J Pediatr. 1976;88(6):963–8.
65. Jabs EW, Li X, Scott AF, Meyers G, Chen W, Eccles M, Mao J, Charnas LR, Jackson CE, Jaye M. Jackson-Weiss and Crouzon syndromes are allelic with mutations in fibroblast growth factor receptor 2. Nat Genet. 1994;8:275–9.
66. Heike C, Seto M, Hing A, Palidin A, Hu FZ, Preston RA, Ehrlich GD, Cunningham M. Century of Jackson-Weiss syndrome: further definition of clinical and radiographic findings in "lost" descendants of the original kindred*. Am J Med Genet. 2001;100(4):315–24.
67. Cohen MM. Jackson-Weiss syndrome. Am J Med Genet. 2001;100(4):325–9.
68. Meyers GA, Day D, Goldberg R, Daentl DL, Przylepa KA, Abrams LJ, Graham JM, Feingold M, Moeschler JB, Rawnsley E, Scott AF, Jabs EW. FGFR2 exon IIIa and IIIc mutations in Crouzon, Jackson-Weiss, and Pfeiffer syndromes: evidence for missense changes, insertions, and a deletion due to alternative RNA splicing. Am J Hum Genet. 1996;58(3):491–8.
69. Roscioli T, Flanagan S, Kumar P, Masel J, Gattas M, Hyland VJ, Glass IA. Clinical findings in a patient with FGFR1 P252R mutation and comparison with the literature. Am J Med Genet. 2000;93(1):22–8.
70. Antley R, Bixler D. Trapezoidocephaly, midfacial hypoplasia and cartilage abnormalities with multiple synostoses and skeletal fractures. Birth Defects Orig Artic Ser. 1975;11(2):397–401.
71. McGlaughlin KL, Witherow H, Dunaway DJ, David DJ, Anderson PJ. Spectrum of Antley-Bixler syndrome. J Craniofac Surg. 2010;21(5):1560–4.
72. Chun K, Siegel-Bartelt J, Chitayat D, Phillips J, Ray PN. FGFR2 mutation associated with clinical manifestations consistent with Antley-Bixler syndrome. Am J Med Genet. 1998;77(3):219–24.
73. Schaefer F, Anderson C, Can B, Say B. Novel mutation in the FGFR2 gene at the same codon as the Crouzon syndrome mutations in a severe Pfeiffer syndrome type 2 case. Am J Med Genet. 1998;75(3):252–5.
74. White KE, Cabral JM, Davis SI, Fishburn T, Evans WE, Ichikawa S, Fields J, Yu X, Shaw NJ, McLellan NJ, McKeown C, FitzPatrick D, Yu K, Ornitz DM, Econs MJ. Mutations that cause osteoglophonic dysplasia define novel roles for FGFR1 in bone elongation. Am J Hum Genet. 2005;76(2):361–7.
75. Shiang R, Thompson LM, Zhu Y-Z, Church DM, Fielder TJ, Bocian M, Winokur ST, Wasmuth JJ. Mutations in the transmembrane domain of FGFR3 cause the most common genetic form of dwarfism, achondroplasia. Cell. 1994;78(2):335–42.
76. Vajo Z, Francomano CA, Wilkin DJ. The molecular and genetic basis of fibroblast growth factor receptor 3 disorders: the achondroplasia family of skeletal dysplasias, Muenke craniosynostosis, and Crouzon syndrome with acanthosis nigricans. Endocr Rev. 2000;21(1):23–39.
77. Bellus GA, McIntosh I, Smith EA, Aylsworth AS, Kaitila I, Horton WA, Greenhaw GA, Hecht JT, Francomano CA. A recurrent mutation in the tyrosine kinase domain of fibroblast growth factor receptor 3 causes hypochondroplasia. Nat Genet. 1995;10(3):357–9.
78. Nishimura G, Fukushima Y, Ohashi H, Ikegawa S. Atypical radiological findings in achondroplasia with uncommon mutation of the fibroblast growth factor receptor-3 (fgfr-3) gene (gly to cys transition at codon 375). Am J Med Genet. 1995;59(3):393–5.
79. Superti-Furga A, Unger S. Nosology and classification of genetic skeletal disorders: 2006 revision. Am J Med Genet A. 2007;143A(1):1–18.
80. Foldynova-Trantirkova S, Wilcox WR, Krejci P. Sixteen years and counting: the current understanding of fibroblast growth factor receptor 3 (FGFR3) signaling in skeletal dysplasias. Hum Mutat. 2012;33(1):29–41.
81. Lanning RW, Brown CA. An improved methodology for the detection of the common mutation in the FGFR3 gene responsible for achondroplasia. Hum Mutat. 1997;10(6):496–9.
82. Etlik O, Koksal V, Tugba Arican-Baris S, Baris I. An improved tetra-primer PCR approach for the detection of the FGFR3 G380R mutation responsible for achondroplasia. Mol Cell Probes. 2008;22(2):71–5.
83. He X, Xie F, Ren Z-R (2012) Rapid detection of G1138A and G1138C mutations of FGFR3 gene in patients with achondroplasia using high-resolution melting analysis. Genet Test Mol Biomarkers (in press).
84. Tavormina PL, Bellus GA, Webster MK, Bamshad MJ, Fraley AE, McIntosh I, Szabo J, Jiang W, Jabs EW, Wilcox WR, Wasmuth JJ, Donoghue DJ, Thompson LM, Francomano CA. A novel skeletal dysplasia with developmental delay and acanthosis nigricans is caused by a Lys650Met mutation in the fibroblast growth factor receptor 3 gene. Am J Hum Genet. 1999;64(3):722–31.
85. Prinster C, Carrera P, Maschio MD, Weber G, Maghnie M, Vigone MC, Mora S, Tonini G, Rigon F, Beluffi G, Severi F, Chiumello G, Ferrari M. Comparison of clinical-radiological and molecular findings in hypochondroplasia. Am J Med Genet. 1998;75(1):109–12.
86. Langer LO, Yang SS, Hall JG, Sommer A, Kottamasu SR, Golabi M, Krassikoff N, Opitz JM, Bernstein J. Thanatophoric dysplasia and cloverleaf skull. Am J Med Genet. 1987;28(S3):167–79.
87. Chen C-P, Chern S-R, Shih J-C, Wang W, Yeh L-F, Chang T-Y, Tzen C-Y. Prenatal diagnosis and genetic analysis of type I and type II thanatophoric dysplasia. Prenat Diag. 2001;21(2):89–95.
88. Tonni G, Azzoni D, Ventura A, Ferrari B, Felice CD, Baldi M. Thanatophoric dysplasia type I associated with increased nuchal translucency in the first trimester: early prenatal diagnosis

using combined ultrasonography and molecular biology. Fetal Pediatr Pathol. 2010;29(5):314–22.
89. Naveen NS, Murlimanju BV, Kumar V, Pulakunta T, Jeeyar H. Thanatophoric dysplasia: a rare entity. Oman Med J. 2011;26(3):196–7.
90. Rousseau F, Saugier P, Merrer ML, Munnich A, Delezoide A-L, Maroteaux P, Bonaventure J, Narcy F, Sanak M. Stop codon FGFR3 mutations in thanatophoric dwarfism type 1. Nat Genet. 1995;10(1):11–2.
91. Rousseau F, El Ghouzzi V, Delezoide AL, Legeai-Mallet L, Le Merrer M, Munnich A, Bonaventure J. Missense FGFR3 mutations create cysteine residues in thanatophoric dwarfism type I (TD1). Hum Mol Genet. 1996;5(4):509–12.
92. Tavormina PL, Shiang R, Thompson LM, Zhu Y-Z, Wilkin DJ, Lachman RS, Wilcox WR, Rimoin DL, Cohn DH, Wasmuth JJ. Thanatophoric dysplasia (types I and II) caused by distinct mutations in fibroblast growth factor receptor 3. Nat Genet. 1995;9(3):321–8.
93. Martínez-Frías ML, Egüés X, Puras A, Hualde J, de Frutos CA, Bermejo E, Nieto MA, Martínez S. Thanatophoric dysplasia type II with encephalocele and semilobar holoprosencephaly: insights into its pathogenesis. Am J Med Genet A. 2011;155(1):197–202.
94. Bellus GA, Spector EB, Speiser PW, Weaver CA, Garber AT, Bryke CR, Israel J, Rosengren SS, Webster MK, Donoghue DJ, Francomano CA. Distinct missense mutations of the FGFR3 Lys650 codon modulate receptor kinase activation and the severity of the skeletal dysplasia phenotype. Am J Hum Genet. 2000;67(6):1411–21.
95. Merrill AE, Sarukhanov A, Krejci P, Idoni B, Camacho N, Estrada KD, Lyons KM, Deixler H, Robinson H, Chitayat D, Curry CJ, Lachman RS, Wilcox WR, Krakow D. Bent bone dysplaisa-FGFR2 type, a distinct skeletal disorder, has deficient canonical FGF signaling. Am J Hum Genet. 2012;90:550–7.
96. Collet C, Alessandri JL, Arnaud E, Balu M, Daire V, Di Rocco F. Crouzon syndrome and bent bone dysplasia associated with mutatins at the same Tyr-381 residue in FGFR2 gene. Clin Genet. 2013. doi:10.1111/cge.12213. Epub ahead of print.
97. Toydemir RM, Brassington AE, Bayrak-Toydemir P, Krakowiak PA, Jorde LB, Whitby FG, Longo N, Viskochil DH, Carey JC, Bamshad MJ. A novel mutation in FGFR3 causes camptodactyly, tall stature, and hearing loss (CATSHL) syndrome. Am J Hum Genet. 2006;79(5):935–41.
98. Makrythanasis P, Temtamy S, Aglan MS, Otaify GA, Hamamy H, Antonarakis SE. A Novel Homozygous Mutation in FGFR3 Causes Tall Stature, Severe Lateral Tibial Deviation, Scoliosis, Hearing Impairment, Camptodactyly, and Arachnodactyly. Hum Mutat. 2014;35(8):959–63.
99. Kaplan JD, Bernstein JA, Kwan A, Hudgins L. Clues to an early diagnosis of Kallmann syndrome. Am J Med Genet A. 2010;152A(11):2796–801.
100. Cadman SM, Kim SH, Hu Y, González-Martínez D, Bouloux PM. Molecular pathogenesis of Kallmann's syndrome. Horm Res. 2007;67(5):231–42.
101. Kulkarni M, Balaji M, Kulkarni A, Sushanth S, Kulkarni B. Kallmann's syndrome. Indian J Pediatr. 2007;74(12):1113–5.
102. Dode C, Levilliers J, Dupont J-M, De Paepe A, Le Du N, Soussi-Yanicostas N, Coimbra RS, Delmaghani S, Compain-Nouaille S, Baverel F, Pecheux C, Le Tessier D, Cruaud C, Delpech M, Speleman F, Vermeulen S, Amalfitano A, Bachelot Y, Bouchard P, Cabrol S, Carel J-C, Delemarre-van de Waal H, Goulet-Salmon B, Kottler M-L, Richard O, Sanchez- Franco F, Saura R, Young J, Petit C, Hardelin J-P. Loss-of-function mutations in FGFR1 cause autosomal dominant Kallmann syndrome. Nat Genet. 2003;33(4):463–5.
103. Milunsky JM, Zhao G, Maher TA, Colby R, Everman DB. LADD syndrome is caused by FGF10 mutations. Clin Genet. 2006;69(4):349–54.
104. Rohmann E, Brunner HG, Kayserili H, Uyguner O, Nurnberg G, Lew ED, Dobbie A, Eswarakumar VP, Uzumcu A, Ulubil-Emeroglu M, Leroy JG, Li Y, Becker C, Lehnerdt K, Cremers CWRJ, Yuksel-Apak M, Nurnberg P, Kubisch C, Schlessinger J, van Bokhoven H, Wollnik B. Mutations in different components of FGF signaling in LADD syndrome. Nat Genet. 2006;38(4):414–7.
105. Shams I, Rohmann E, Eswarakumar VP, Lew ED, Yuzawa S, Wollnik B, Schlessinger J, Lax I. Lacrimo-auriculo-dento-digital syndrome is caused by reduced activity of the fibroblast growth factor 10 (FGF10)-FGF receptor 2 signaling pathway. Mol Cell Biol. 2007;27(19):6903–12.
106. Lew ED, Bae JH, Rohmann E, Wollnik B, Schlessinger J. Structural basis for reduced FGFR2 activity in LADD syndrome: Implications for FGFR autoinhibition and activation. PNAS. 2007;104(50):19802–7.
107. Hollister DW, Klein SH, De Jager HJ, Lachman RS, Rimoin DL. The lacrimo-auriculo-dento-digital syndrome. J Pediatr. 1973;83(3):438–44.
108. Shiang EL, Holmes LB. The lacrimo-auriculo-dento-digital syndrome. Pediatrics. 1977;59(6):927–30.
109. Mathrawala N, Hegde R. Lacrimo-auriculo-dento-digital syndrome. J Indian Soc Pedod Prev Dent. 2011;29(2):168–70.

Cystic Fibrosis

13

Lora J.H. Bean and V.M. Pratt

Abstract

Cystic fibrosis (CF) is one of the most common lethal autosomal recessive diseases in whites, with an estimated incidence of 1 in 2,500–3,300 live births. CF, caused by mutations in the *CFTR* gene, is a complex multisystem disease, affecting the respiratory tract, pancreas, intestine, male genital tract, hepatobiliary system, and exocrine system. Recurrent infections that lead to respiratory failure are the major cause of morbidity. Due to the high frequency of CF, *CFTR* mutation analysis is useful for a variety of clinical indications, including newborn screening, diagnostic testing, carrier screening, and fetal diagnosis for at-risk pregnancies. A relatively small number of mutations account for the majority of CF alleles. The American College of Medical Genetics and the American Congress of Obstetricians and Gynecologists recommend first-tier *CFTR* mutation analysis using a panethnic panel of 23 mutations that occur at a frequency of >0.1 % in any of the major US ethnic groups. Commercial test kits are available to perform this testing. Reporting of CF results is complex because the detection in a targeted mutation assay is less than 100 %. The interpretation and subsequent recommendations are dependent on the indication for the test and the ethnicity and family history of the individual being tested, and may require consultation with a medical geneticist or genetic counselor.

Keywords

Cystic fibrosis • *CFTR* • Diagnostic testing • Carrier screening • Prenatal testing • Molecular testing

Introduction

Cystic fibrosis (CF) is one of the most common lethal autosomal recessive diseases in whites, with an estimated incidence of 1 in 2,500 to 1 in 3,300 live births. CF, caused by mutations in the *CFTR* gene, is a complex multisystem disease, affecting the respiratory tract, pancreas, intestine, male genital tract, hepatobiliary system, and exocrine system. Recurrent infections that lead to respiratory failure are the major cause of morbidity. Due to the high frequency of CF, *CFTR* mutation analysis is useful for a variety of clinical indications, including newborn screening (NBS), diagnostic testing, carrier screening, and fetal diagnosis for at-risk pregnancies. A relatively small number of mutations account for the majority of CF alleles. The American College of Medical Genetics (ACMG) and the American Congress of Obstetricians and Gynecologists (ACOG) recommend a panethnic panel of 23 mutations that occur at a frequency of >0.1 % in any of the major US ethnic groups be used for first-tier *CFTR* mutation analysis. Commercial kits are available to perform this testing. Reporting of CF results is complex because the detection in a targeted mutation assay is

L.J.H. Bean, Ph.D., F.A.C.M.G. (✉)
Department of Human Genetics, Emory Genetics Laboratory, Emory University, 615 Michael St., Suite 301, Atlanta, GA 30322, USA
e-mail: ljbean@emory.edu

V.M. Pratt, Ph.D., F.A.C.M.G.
Pharmacogenomics Laboratory, Department of Medical and Molecular Genetics, Indiana University School of Medicine, 975 W. Walnut St., IB-130, Indianapolis, IN 46202, USA
e-mail: vpratt@iu.edu

D.G.B. Leonard (ed.), *Molecular Pathology in Clinical Practice*, DOI 10.1007/978-3-319-19674-9_13

less than 100 %. The interpretation and subsequent recommendations are dependent on the indication for the test and the ethnicity and family history of the individual and may require consultation with a geneticist or genetic counselor.

Molecular Basis of Disease

CF is one of the most common lethal autosomal recessive diseases in Caucasians, with an estimated incidence of 1 in 2,500 to 3,300 live births. Approximately 30,000 children and adults in the USA are affected and approximately 1,000 individuals are newly diagnosed annually, the majority less than 1 year old. For a current, comprehensive review of clinical CF and molecular diagnostics for this disorder, see ref. 1.

The gene mutated in CF, the cystic fibrosis transmembrane conductance regulator (*CFTR*), spans approximately 230 kilobases (kb) on chromosome 7q31.2, contains 27 coding exons, produces a 6.5 kb mRNA product, and encodes a CFTR protein of 1,480 amino acids with a mass of approximately 170,000 Da. The CFTR protein is in the ATP-binding cassette family of transporter proteins, containing five domains: two membrane-spanning domains, a regulatory domain, and two nucleotide-binding domains that interact with adenosine triphosphate. Mutations that lead to an abnormal CFTR protein cause defective electrolyte transport in the apical membrane of epithelial cells resulting in complex multisystem disease affecting the respiratory tract, pancreas, intestine, male genital tract, hepatobiliary system, and exocrine system.

CF is characterized by viscous mucus secondary to faulty transport of sodium and chloride, which leads to salt loss, and affects water content of the extracellular space. CF has a highly variable presentation and clinical course. The clinical features of "classic" CF are dominated by pulmonary disease. The median age of diagnosis is 6–8 months, and nearly two-thirds of affected individuals are diagnosed by the age of 1 year; however, the advent of NBS for CF is enabling earlier diagnosis of presymptomatic individuals. Respiratory failure, often with recurrent respiratory infections, is the major cause of morbidity and mortality. Approximately 90 % of CF patients die from pulmonary complications with an overall median survival into the late 30s. Approximately 85 % of CF patients have pancreatic insufficiency as a result of obstruction of the pancreatic ducts and subsequent scarring and destruction of exocrine functions. Neonatal meconium ileus, which can present prenatally as echogenic bowel (EB), occurs in approximately 15 % of newborns with CF. Other manifestations include chronic sinusitis, nasal polyps, liver disease, pancreatitis, and, in males, congenital bilateral absence of the vas deferens (CBAVD) resulting in azoospermia.

Treatment for individuals with CF is palliative and includes chest percussion and use of inhaled medications or hypotonic saline to clear lung secretions, control of infections by antibiotic therapy, and improvement of nutritional status through dietary managements and pancreatic enzyme replacement. The goals of therapy are maintenance of adequate nutritional status, prevention of pulmonary and other complications, encouragement of physical activity, and provision of adequate psychosocial support. Although the development of new therapies for CF based on correction of electrolyte transport is a major research focus, there is currently no cure for CF. While lung transplantation can be used in selected CF patients with severe respiratory compromise, the success is not sustained and lung transplant does not address the other end-organ disease of CF [2].

A diagnosis of CF in a symptomatic or at-risk individual is suggested by clinical presentation and confirmed by a sweat test. In the presence of clinical symptoms (e.g., recurrent respiratory infections), a sweat chloride level above 60 mmol/L is diagnostic for CF. Although the results of this test are valid in a newborn as young as 24 h, collecting a sufficient sweat sample from a baby younger than 3 or 4 weeks old is difficult and must be performed by an experienced, Cystic Fibrosis Foundation-accredited sweat testing center. The sweat test also confirms the diagnosis in older children and adults but is not useful for carrier detection.

Since the identification of the *CFTR* gene, more than 1,800 mutations have been identified; a complete list can be found at www.cftr2.org/. A relatively small number of mutations account for the majority of CF alleles. The most frequent mutation is c.1521_1523delCTT (p.Phe508del), commonly known as deltaF508. This mutation is a 3-base pair deletion that accounts for approximately 70 % of CF chromosomes worldwide; thus, approximately half of CF patients are homozygous for deltaF508. The mutations and their frequency vary by ethnic group.

CFTR gene mutations and variants that reduce but do not destroy CFTR protein function are associated with "non-classic CF," the clinical spectrum of which includes chronic respiratory problems such as rhinosinusitis, chronic pancreatitis, and isolated CBAVD. The presence of a variant with less impact on CFTR protein function on one chromosome, in combination with a classic CF mutation on the opposite chromosome (in *trans*), may lead to non-classic clinical features of CF (Fig. 13.1). Males with CBAVD have an increased frequency of mutations in one or both *CFTR* alleles or an incompletely penetrant mutation (the intron 8-variant c.1210-12T[5T], commonly known as the 5T allele) in a noncoding region of *CFTR*. These men usually have no pancreatic disease and may have normal, borderline, or elevated sweat electrolytes. Small subsets of individuals with non-classic CF have chronic *Pseudomonas* bronchitis, normal pancreatic function, and normal or

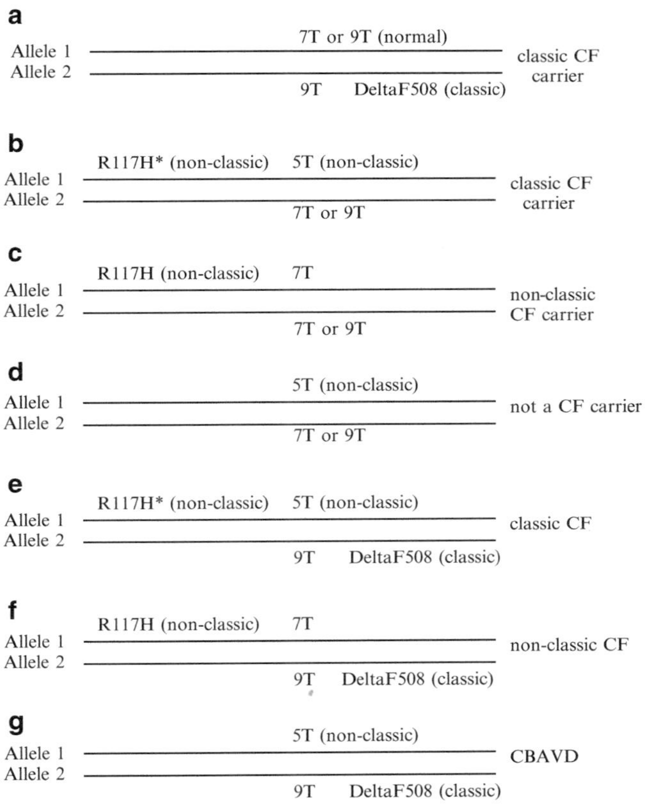

Figure 13.1 Examples of allelic configurations and their interpretations in carrier testing (**a–d**) and diagnostic testing (**e–g**) when classic or non-classic mutations are detected. *c.350G>A (p.R117H) and c.1210-12T (intron 8 5T/7T/9T) are the most frequently occurring non-classic *CFTR* gene variants. Other non-classic variants detectable by sequence analysis have been described

intermediate sweat electrolytes. Asymptomatic infants identified by NBS with an elevated immunoreactive trypsinogen (IRT), one classic *CFTR* gene mutation, and a borderline sweat test are given the diagnosis *CFTR*-related metabolic syndrome (CRMS) until it is known whether they will manifest clinical features of CF.

Clinical Utility of Testing

Due to the high frequency of CF, *CFTR* mutation analysis is useful for a variety of clinical indications, including NBS, diagnostic testing, carrier screening, and prenatal diagnosis for at-risk pregnancies. Biochemical testing is used to augment molecular methods for NBS and diagnostic testing. Carrier and prenatal testing relies solely on molecular testing.

Newborns with CF tend to have elevated levels of blood IRT. Although these levels fall within a few weeks after birth, elevated IRT is a reliable biochemical marker to identify newborns at increased risk for CF. NBS is performed in all states and many foreign countries using IRT alone or in combination with molecular testing. If IRT alone is used, a second sample is typically collected and those newborns with two elevated IRT results are called screen positive and are referred for further testing (IRT-IRT model). In a model where *CFTR* mutation analysis is performed on the original sample for those with an elevated IRT (IRT-DNA model), infants with one or two *CFTR* mutations identified are called screen positive, and those with two mutations have a presumptive diagnosis (for review, please see the CLSI Approved Guidelines for Newborn Screening for Cystic Fibrosis [3]). Diagnosis of infants with presymptomatic CF leads to better management and long-term outcomes, a fact underscored by a recommendation from the ACMG to include CF as one of their 29 recommended "core conditions" for uniform NBS in the USA [4].

In a symptomatic individual, the identification of two classic *CFTR* mutations is sufficient to establish a diagnosis for CF; however, sweat testing remains the diagnostic gold standard as recommended by the CF Foundation [5]. In the majority of classic CF cases, both mutations can be identified by a panel of common mutations. For symptomatic individuals in whom two of the common mutations are not identified, full *CFTR* gene sequencing and, if necessary, *CFTR* gene deletion/duplication analysis are useful to determine the likelihood that the individual's clinical features are part of a *CFTR*-related disorder. The availability of both biochemical and molecular diagnostic tests is particularly useful for individuals with non-classic clinical presentations and normal or borderline sweat tests, at-risk newborns from whom it is difficult to collect sufficient quantities of sweat, and individuals in whom one classic *CFTR* mutation and one *CFTR* variant of uncertain or unknown clinical significance have been identified. Identification of familial mutations is useful for testing at-risk relatives.

In 1997, a National Institutes of Health Consensus Development Conference recommended CF carrier testing for all couples planning a pregnancy, regardless of family history. However, at that time, there was no standardization of CF testing among laboratories and no commercially available reagents or kits. The largest challenges to standardize mutation panels were the ethnic diversity and admixture of the US population, which complicated the selection of mutations for a standardized screening panel. The ACMG and the ACOG recommended a panethnic panel of 23 mutations (which was revised from an original 25 mutations) that occur at a frequency of >0.1 % in any of the major US ethnic groups, plus reflex testing for four additional sequence variants under specified conditions (Table 13.1) ([6–8], revised 2011). These organizations developed and distributed an educational document entitled "Preconceptual and Prenatal Carrier Screening for Cystic Fibrosis" to the members of ACMG and ACOG, and established CF carrier screening as a standard of care in the USA.

Table 13.1 Recommended core mutation panel for general-population CF carrier-screening/legacy (common) nomenclature

c.254G>A/G85E	c.1624G>T/G542X	c.3846G>A/W1282X	c.1521_1523delCTT/ deltaF508	c.2657+5G>A/2789+5G>A
c.350G>A/R117H	c.1652G>A/G551D	c.3909C>G/N1303K	c.1585-1G>A/1717-1G>A	c.2988+1G>A/3120+1G>A
c.1000C>T/R334W	c.1657C>T/R553X	c.489+1G>T/621+1G>T	c.1766+1G>A/1898+1G>A	c.3527delC/3659delC
c.1040G>C/R347P	c.1679G>C/R560T	c.579+1G>T/711+1G>T	c.2052delA/2184delA	c.3718-2477C>T/3849+10kbC>T
c.1364C>A/A455E	c.3484C>T/R1162X	c.1519_1521delATC/deltaI507		
Reflex tests				
c.1210-12T/intron 8 5T/7T/9T; c.1516A>G/I506V, c.1519A>G/I507V, c.1523T>G/F508C				

Table 13.2 Commercially available molecular kits for targeted *CFTR* mutation analysis

Vendor	Abbott/Celera	Autogenomics	Elucigene/ GenProbe	Luminex	Hologic	Innogenetics	GenMarkDx	Illumina, Inc. (San Diego, CA)
Platform	PCR target amplification, OLA, and capillary electrophoresis	PCR target amplification, and hybridization to BioFilmChip microarray	ARMS target amplification, ARMS, and capillary electrophoresis	PCR target amplification, allele-specific primer extension, hybridization to universal tags, and sorting on Luminex 100 analyzer	PCR and signal amplification and FRET detection	PCR target amplification and reverse ASO	PCR target amplification, chip hybridization, and detection on an electronic microarray	Sequencing by synthesis
Product or platform name	Oligonucleotide Ligation Assay 16-capillary CEGA	INFINITI™ CFTR31	Elucigene CF-EU	TAG-IT CF39, TAG-IT CF60, TAG-IT CF71	InPlex	Inno-LiPA CFTR	eSensor® Cystic Fibrosis Genotyping Test	MiSeqDx Cystic Fibrosis 139-Variant Assay, MiSeqDx Cystic Fibrosis Clinical Sequencing Assay
Regulatory status	US FDA cleared	Research use only/CE marked	CE marked (not available in the USA)	US FDA cleared	US FDA cleared	Research use only	US FDA cleared	FDA-cleared

ARMS amplification refractory mutation system, *ASO* allele-specific oligonucleotide, *CEGA* capillary electrophoresis genetic analyzer, *FRET* fluorescence resonance energy transfer, *OLA* oligonucleotide ligation assay, *PCR* polymerase chain reaction

Prior to the cloning of the *CFTR* gene, couples learned that both parents were CF carriers upon the birth of an affected child. No robust assays were available to assess a subsequent pregnancy with a 1 in 4 risk of CF. Now, the most common indication for mutation analysis is direct heterozygote detection for carrier risk revision for a couple either for pregnancy planning or screening.

The ACMG/ACOG panel is not designed for diagnostic testing for individuals with clinical features of classic or non-classic CF or men with CBAVD, although the panel is often used as an initial screen in these clinical settings. A larger mutation panel provides increased detection for symptomatic individuals.

Analysis is used for fetal testing of pregnancies with a 1 in 4 risk for which both mutations have been identified in the two carrier parents. Fetal or prenatal testing often is offered in lower risk pregnancies presenting in the second trimester on ultrasound with fetal EB. EB is associated with an increased risk for CF (2–20 %) in the absence of a positive family history. Mutation analysis of the parents of a fetus with EB may reveal that both are carriers, but often neither or only one parent carries a common *CFTR* mutation. Fetal diagnosis can determine that a heterozygous parent has transmitted an identified mutation, but there is no additional testing offered to further clarify the fetal CF status. In such cases of EB, Bayesian analysis is used to modify the risk.

Furthermore, some clinicians submit a fetal sample without testing the parents, and formal genetic counseling may not be offered to the couple until the laboratory testing has been completed.

Available Assays

Currently, there are several available testing platforms. Technical standards and guidelines for CF mutation testing have been published by the ACMG ([6], revised 2011) and are available at www.acmg.net. These guidelines address the technology platforms used with commercial kits and reagents for laboratory-developed tests (LDTs) for CF mutations. Currently available commercial kits and reagents for LDTs are summarized in Table 13.2. All are robust and include at least the ACMG/ACOG minimum core mutation panel, but vary considerably with respect to criteria that laboratories consider for platform adoption: reagent/royalty costs, footprint of instrumentation, throughput, flexibility, and data analysis.

Reflex testing for the c.1210-12T (intron 8 5T/7T/9T) sequence variation is specifically recommended by ACOG/ACMG for individuals with an identified c.350G>A (R117H) mutation, since 5T vs 7T or 9T *in cis* increases CF severity in a compound heterozygote with a second CF mutation. Note that some assay platforms may only reveal the c.1210-12T (intron 8 5T/7T/9T) results if a c.350G>A (R117H) mutation is identified. Since some methodologies do not distinguish between c.1521_1523delCTT (deltaF508) and other alterations in close proximity, a second reflex to three exon 10 sequence variants [c.1516A>G (I506V), c.1519A>G (I507V), c.1523T>G (F508C)] is recommended when an unexpected homozygous c.1521_1523delCTT (deltaF508) or c.1519A>G (I507V) mutation is detected to avoid reporting of false-positive results due to interference by these surrounding polymorphisms. Most available kits or reagents include these nonpathogenic exon 10 reflex sequence variants.

The Abbott/Celera platform offers both semiautomated and automated detection and data analysis and requires capital purchase of an instrument with a relatively large footprint. The automated assay format is useful for high-volume testing.

The Innogenetics assay is a reverse allele-specific oligonucleotide test that can be semiautomated using a customized instrument. The assay is amenable to low and high test volumes. Manual analysis of the strip data is required.

The Elucigene assay features capillary electrophoresis detection of sequence-specific primer amplicons and provides an expanded mutation panel specific to European populations. This platform is not available in the USA.

The Luminex assays incorporate multiplex PCR and multiplex allele-specific primer extension with a proprietary universal tag sorting system (xTAG® Technology) on the Luminex 100/200 Analyzer. This is a high-throughput assay that incorporates automated software analysis for genotype calls.

The Autogenomics and GenMarkDx systems are microarray assays that are partially amenable to automation. With lower throughput than some other assays, these assays may be optimal for laboratories with small test volumes. Both platforms also have flexibility to use other non-CF reagents on the same system.

The Hologic assay only requires manual pipetting steps which can be automated using a liquid handler. Thus, this assay is potentially of low cost, requiring only a fluorescent plate reader. The assay is unique among CF assays by combining limited cycles of PCR with signal amplification using the Invader® FRET technology. Because this assay format cannot be multiplexed, the detection steps are performed on a custom "InPlex" card, in which reaction products are distributed to wells of dried-down reagents, each specific for the detection of a single-mutant allele.

DNA sequencing and deletion/duplication analyses are laboratory-developed tests validated and performed in high-complexity laboratories in the USA. *CFTR* gene sequencing refers to DNA sequencing of the *CFTR* exons and intronic borders. Newer sequencing technologies' cost is decreasing to perform the assay. In an affected individual, if two mutations are not identified by targeted mutation analysis and gene sequencing, or if unexpected homozygosity for a rare mutation is identified, deletion/duplication testing may be warranted. Commercial reagents are available (MRC-Holland, Amsterdam, the Netherlands) for laboratory-developed deletion/duplication testing.

Interpretation of Test Results

The majority of *CFTR* gene mutations can be detected by targeted mutation analyses, which have only three possible results: detection of no, one, or two mutations. However, reporting of CF results is complex because the mutation detection rate in a targeted mutation assay is less than 100 %. The interpretation and subsequent recommendations are dependent on the indication for the test and the ethnicity and family history of the individual. In cases where *CFTR* gene sequencing or deletion/duplication analysis is warranted, interpretation of test results is more complex and should be performed in a laboratory with experience in interpretation of these test results in collaboration with a medical geneticist or genetic counselor.

In the majority of CF NBS programs, infants with an elevated IRT NBS test result are tested for a panel of classic

CFTR mutations. An infant with two classic *CFTR* mutations is presumed to have a diagnosis of CF; however, confirmatory studies such as a sweat testing and molecular testing on a new blood sample are standard practice to assure proper identification of the infant specimen. Infants with one mutation identified are at an elevated risk for CF (approximately 1 in 10). In infants with an elevated IRT and one *CFTR* mutation, a normal sweat test confirms carrier status and an abnormal sweat test confirms a diagnosis of CF; however, a borderline sweat test may indicate non-classic CF. If the sweat test results indicate classic or non-classic CF, *CFTR* gene sequencing is indicated to identify rare or private *CFTR* gene mutations and variants. Infants with an elevated IRT and no classic *CFTR* mutation are presumed to be NBS false positives, but should be referred for further evaluation if symptoms of CF develop. It is important to note that infants with meconium ileus tend to have normal IRT levels and therefore a normal CF NBS.

For individuals with symptoms of CF, finding of two *CFTR* mutations confirms a diagnosis of CF. However, genotype-phenotype relationships are not adequately established to make prognostic interpretations for the many possible homozygous and compound heterozygous genotypes. The interpretation of one or no detected mutations for a symptomatic individual must include a statement of limitations of the targeted assay, a recommendation for *CFTR* gene sequencing and/or deletion/duplication analyses, and consultation with a CF specialist. Referrals for CF diagnostic testing may include older children and adults with features of non-classic CF, for example chronic respiratory problems, isolated pancreatitis, or male infertility. In such cases a *CFTR* classic mutation panel is unlikely to fully explain the clinical symptoms (Fig. 13.1), but identification of a single mutation would be a strong indicator that full gene sequencing and/or deletion/duplication analysis are warranted.

Since the publication of the ACMG/ACOG recommendations, more than 95 % of all DNA testing for CF is for carrier screening in a prenatal or pregnancy setting. Although the finding of one mutation in a couple is straightforward, the majority of these pregnancy planning carrier-screening tests are negative, with no mutations detected. In the setting of a negative test result, the physician must be informed that the revised carrier risk, while reduced from the prior risk, is not eliminated because the mutation detection is incomplete. As shown in Table 13.3, both the prior and revised carrier risks are dependent on individual ethnicity and family history. Prior carrier risks are based on pedigree analysis. For example, risks for a non-Hispanic Caucasian individual vary from a high of 2 in 3 for an individual with an affected sibling to approximately 1 in 25 for an individual with no family history.

Prior carrier risks for individuals without a family history of CF are calculated from the ethnic frequency of CF, which is highest among non-Hispanic Caucasians (1 in 25), lower in Hispanics (1 in 46) and non-Hispanics of African descent (1 in 62), and lowest among Asians (1 in 90). Revised risks also are based on the frequency of the tested mutations in the individual's ethnic group. The frequency of mutation detection using the ACMG/ACOG panel ranges from 97 % for individuals of Ashkenazi Jewish descent to 57 % for Hispanics, and 49 % for Asians. Risk revision is even more complicated for individuals of mixed heritage.

Table 13.3 Prior and residual CF risks for individuals with a negative carrier test for Caucasian, European: 90 % detection

Affected relative	Prior risk	Revised risk
No affected relative	1 in 25	1 in 241
Sibling	2 in 3	1 in 6
Niece/nephew/half-sibling	1 in 2	1 in 11
Aunt/uncle	1 in 3	1 in 21
First cousin	1 in 4	1 in 31

Responsible reporting for *CFTR* mutation test interpretation should include a clear statement of test limitations. Often, samples are referred for testing without individual ethnicity information provided to the testing laboratory for calculation of risk; therefore, a table of residual risks for Ashkenazi Jewish, Caucasian, Hispanic, African American, and Asian individuals for the test performed should be provided. Such a table is also useful for individuals of mixed ancestry since their residual risk would be intermediate between two or more groups. For individuals with a family history of CF a recommendation for a medical genetics consultation or genetic counseling is appropriate since a more precise risk assessment can be made if the familial mutations are known.

The published ACMG/ACOG recommendations include model laboratory reports for detection of no or one mutation in a carrier-screening context for individuals with a negative personal and family history [7]. These model reports also are included in the educational materials that have been distributed to the members of ACOG and ACMG. They contain a field for patient ethnicity, but the interpretation is not patient specific. In the model mutation-negative report, the prior and revised carrier risks for all ethnicities are presented in the interpretation field in a tabular format.

Laboratories can anticipate the most common reporting formats and prepare standard template reports. This approach accommodates high test volumes while maintaining reporting standards. Each report should contain a statement that the carrier risk of the consultant is reduced but that the risk for having a child affected by CF is also a function of the partner's carrier status. In this way, the non-zero value of the revised risk for a negative test is emphasized as well as the interplay of the genotypes of both parents.

Although the ACMG/ACOG mutation panel is designed for carrier screening of individuals without a family history of CF, individuals with an affected relative often are referred for carrier risk testing, and the same screening mutation panel is used. Often the affected family member has not been tested and the familial mutations are not known, or the mutation has been identified but the information is not available to the at-risk relative. Reports should clearly state that the intended use of the mutation panel is for individuals without a family history of CF to alert the physician that residual carrier risk after a negative test is modified by this history. Table 13.3 illustrates the benefit of identifying familial mutations, thereby allowing a yes or no answer to carrier status, vs not identifying the familial mutation and relying on risk reduction alone even when the affected individual is more distantly related. The report also may include a recommendation that the physician refer individuals with a positive family history for genetic counseling and Bayesian calculation of revised carrier risk (see Chap. 5). If a laboratory has the expertise and sufficiently reliable clinical information, individual-specific revised risks may be reported. All such reports should include an individual-specific revised risk calculation, a recommendation for genetic counseling and a statement that the residual risk would be significantly modified if the familial mutations are known.

Reporting for most of the possible positive results in a carrier test is straightforward and, as recommended by ACMG/ACOG, should always contain a recommendation for genetic counseling and a comment that at-risk relatives also may benefit from genetic counseling and mutation analysis for carrier risk revision. As recommended by ACMG/ACOG, interpretation of positive results for the c.350G>A (R117H) mutation should always be made in the context of the individual's genotype for the c.1210-12T (intron 8 5T/7T/9T) sequence, since expression of the c.350G>A (R117H) mutation in a compound heterozygous child is variable, depending on the specific genotypic combination (Fig. 13.1). The c.350G>A (R117H) mutation is most severe when on the same allele as the 5T variant. The reflex of an unexpected c.1521_1523delCTT (deltaF508) homozygous result in a healthy adult to testing for other exon 10 sequence variations [c.1516A>G (I506V), c.1519A>G (I507V), c.1523T>G (F508C)] is necessary to prevent false-positive results, since some detection platforms (e.g., probe hybridization) do not discriminate the c.1521_1523delCTT (deltaF508) mutation from these polymorphisms.

For fetal testing, laboratories may request or require CF carrier screening results of both partners. Parental results influence the interpretation of fetal results particularly when one or both are found to be carriers. Partners often have different last names, they may be tested at different times or in different laboratories, or the laboratory volume can be high enough that partners are not recognized during CF testing. The nongeneticist physician usually can communicate a 1 in 4 risk to couples who are both carriers, but may not have the experience to provide a fetal risk assessment when only one partner is a CF carrier and the other does not carry a common mutation. Effective ways to communicate the results and interpretations of a complex genetic test to a nongeneticist physician, enabling him or her to make appropriate management decisions, is an area of ongoing research [9, 10]. Successful carrier testing for CF depends on many factors, the most important of which is physician education to react appropriately to the complex scenarios that occur in patients and couples.

Laboratory Issues

Targeted mutation panels are designed to test for the most common variants, but rare variants can interfere with the assay and cause false results, for example due to allele drop-out. In some cases, the variants may occur under primers and probes and present as homozygosity for rare mutations or amplicons may fail to amplify. Laboratories often provide disclaimers on reports indicating the possibility of such rare events. In cases of homozygosity for rare mutations, follow-up by DNA sequencing and/or duplication/deletion analysis or family studies to establish biparental inheritance may be warranted. Additional family members also can be tested, if available, and may provide useful information for interpretation of results in the proband.

Predicting a genotype-based phenotype is imprecise and is not recommended as there are often additional variants or modifiers of mutations present. For example, two (or more) variants may be present on the same chromosome (in cis) and are often referred to as "complex alleles." Parental studies may be needed to confirm if complex alleles are present. A relatively common example is c.1210-12T (intron 8 5T/7T/9T) and c.350G>A (p.R117H).

Reference materials and controls are important for assay validation and quality control. Although kits and reagents for targeted CF mutation testing are commercially available, most do not include positive controls for all of the mutations. Commercially available controls can be obtained from several sources (www.cdc.gov/dls/genetics/rmmaterials). One source is Maine Molecular Quality Controls, Inc. (Scarborough, ME) that offers a variety of synthetic *CFTR* mutation panel control reagents, one of which includes the 23 ACMG/ACOG recommended mutations. In addition, the Coriell Cell Repository (Camden, NJ) offers a set of DNAs that contains a complete set of verified mutations in the ACMG/ACOG panel. The Coriell Cell Repository also has verified reference materials for several other CF mutations. The Centers for Disease Control and Prevention Newborn Screening Quality Assurance Program (NSQAP) provides reference materials for IRT-level testing and consultation and training for laboratories offering NBS for CF (www.cdc.gov/labstandards/nsqap).

Proficiency testing or external quality assessment programs for CF testing ensure the quality of the testing laboratory. For molecular testing, the College of American Pathologists (CAP), jointly administered by the ACMG and CAP, and European CF-EQA provide such programs. For NBS, NSQAP oversees proficiency testing for IRT and DNA tests.

References

1. Moskowitz SM, Chmiel JF, Sternen DL, Cheng E, Cutting GR (2008) CFTR-related disorders. Gene Rev [Internet]. www.ncbi.nlm.nih.gov/sites/GeneTests/. Accessed 1 Feb 2012.
2. Braun AT, Merlo CA. Cystic fibrosis lung transplantation. Curr Opin Pulm Med. 2011;17:467–72.
3. CLSI. Newborn screening for cystic fibrosis: approved guideline. Wayne, PA: Clinical Laboratory Standards Institute; 2011. CLSI document I/LA35-A.
4. Watson MS, Mann MY, Lloyd-Puryear MA, Rinaldo P, Howell RR. Newborn screening: toward a uniform screening panel and system. Genet Med. 2006;8(5):1s–250.
5. Farrell PM, Rosenstein BJ, White TB, Accurso FJ, Castellani C, Cutting GR, Durie PR, Legrys VA, Massie J, Parad RB, Rock MJ, Campbell 3rd P. Cystic Fibrosis Foundation Guidelines for diagnosis of cystic fibrosis in newborns through older adults: Cystic Fibrosis Foundation consensus report. J Pediatr. 2008;153(2):S4–14. doi:10.1016/j.jpeds.2008.05.005.
6. Amos J, Feldman G, Grody WW, Monaghan K, Palomaki G, Prior TW, Richards CS, Watson MS (2008, Revised 2011) American College of Medical Genetics Standards and Guidelines for Clinical Genetics Laboratories. ACMG. www.acmg.net. Accessed 1 Feb 2012.
7. Grody WW, Cutting GR, Klinger KW, Richards CS, Watson MS, Desnick RJ. Laboratory standards and guidelines for population-based cystic fibrosis carrier screening. Genet Med. 2001;3(2):149–54.
8. Watson MS, Cutting GR, Desnick RJ, Driscoll DA, Klinger K, Mennuti M, Palomaki GE, Popovich BW, Pratt VM, Rohlfs EM, Strom CM, Richards CS, Witt DR, Grody WW. Cystic fibrosis population carrier screening: 2004 revision of American College of Medical Genetics mutation panel. Genet Med. 2004;6(5):387–91.
9. Lubin IM, Caggana M, Constantin C, Gross SJ, Lyon E, Pagon RA, Trotter TL, Wilson JA, McGovern MM. Ordering molecular genetic tests and reporting results: practices in laboratory and clinical settings. J Mol Diagn. 2008;10(5):459–68. doi:10.2353/jmoldx.2008.080050.
10. Lubin IM, McGovern MM, Gibson Z, Gross SJ, Lyon E, Pagon RA, Pratt VM, Rashid J, Shaw C, Stoddard L, Trotter TL, Williams MS, Amos Wilson J, Pass K. Clinician perspectives about molecular genetic testing for heritable conditions and development of a clinician-friendly laboratory report. J Mol Diagn. 2009;11(2):162–71. doi:10.2353/jmoldx.2009.080130.

Deafness

14

A. Eliot Shearer, Robert W. Eppsteiner,
and Richard J.H. Smith

Abstract

Deafness is the most common sensory deficit in humans. Genetic diagnosis has traditionally been difficult due to extreme genetic heterogeneity and a lack of phenotypic variability. For these reasons multi-gene screening panels have been adopted. While these methods make comprehensive genetic testing possible, interpretation of the many variants is difficult, specifically, differentiating novel benign variants from novel deafness-causing variants. This chapter describes methods for the genetic diagnosis of deafness with particular attention to multi-gene screening panels.

Keywords

Hearing loss • Deafness • Genetic testing • Massively parallel sequencing • GJB2

Introduction

Deafness is the most common sensory deficit in humans, affecting 1 of 500 newborns [1]. The relative contributions of syndromic and non-syndromic deafness to the total deafness genetic load vary with age of ascertainment. About 70 % of congenital hereditary deafness is non-syndromic (non-syndromic hearing loss, NSHL) with the remaining 30 % accounted for by a large number of different syndromes (SHL). In developed countries, most NSHL (80 %) is due to a genetic cause. Because syndromes are generally straightforward to recognize, most are identified at birth with the notable exceptions of Usher syndrome and Pendred syndrome. With both of these common recessively inherited types of SHL, deafness is the only immediately apparent phenotype.

Comprehensive genetic testing for deafness has been difficult because of significant genetic heterogeneity: 57 NSHL genes have been identified since the first gene was cloned in 1995 (http://www.hereditaryhearingloss.org) and more than 1,100 causative allelic variants have been reported in these genes (http://www.deafnessvariationdatabase.org). Traditionally, hereditary deafness is distinguished from non-genetic causes of deafness (often referred to as acquired deafness) by medical and family history, physical examination, and audiologic testing, in some cases aided by ancillary tests such as temporal bone imaging, urinalysis, thyroid function studies, and electrocardiography. However, even using this test battery, an unequivocal distinction between heritable and environmental causes of deafness can be difficult. If comorbid conditions are identified, deafness may fall into one of more than 400 recognized types of SHL, but if hearing is the only abnormality, the basis for the diagnosis of hereditary deafness is often exclusionary in the absence of some type of genetic testing.

This paradigm is shifting rapidly with the use of massively parallel sequencing methods, which provide the ability to screen thousands or millions of DNA base pairs simultaneously. Genetic testing for NSHL is uniquely suited to take advantage of these technologies due to its genetic heterogeneity, which makes multi-gene screening panels the logical default option. Today, genetic testing for apparent NSHL is the first test that should be ordered after history,

A.E. Shearer, B.Sc. • R.W. Eppsteiner, M.D.
R.J.H. Smith, M.D. (✉)
Department of Otolaryngology – Head & Neck Surgery, University of Iowa Hospitals and Clinics,
200 Hawkins Drive, 21151-PFP, Iowa City, IA 52242, USA
e-mail: aiden-shearer@uiowa.edu; robert-eppsteiner@uiowa.edu; richard-smith@uiowa.edu

D.G.B. Leonard (ed.), *Molecular Pathology in Clinical Practice*, DOI 10.1007/978-3-319-19674-9_14

physical examination, and audiometry. This comprehensive genetic testing can unequivocally diagnose hereditary hearing loss, provide prognostic information, and help dictate further patient management.

While these technologies hold the promise of personalized genomic medicine, they are accompanied by specific challenges with respect to assay design and implementation, the interpretation of results, and the ethical issues that may arise. Particularly challenging is differentiating variants of unknown significance (VUS) or novel variants predicted to be pathogenic but without an established record of pathogenesis from true disease-causing mutations. With these technologies, the testing focus is heavily shifted towards data interpretation rather than data generation. At present, screening of a single gene, *GJB2*, using Sanger sequencing remains a cost-effective option and is prudent in patients with apparent congenital autosomal recessive NSHL (ARNSHL) prior to embarking on a multi-gene screen. For this reason, testing of this single gene is discussed separately from multi-gene screening strategies.

Molecular Basis of Disease

In 1994, Guilford et al. mapped the first locus for ARNSHL to chromosome 13q12-13 and named it DFNB1, nonsyndromic hearing loss and deafness (Online Mendelian Inheritance in Man [OMIM; database online] #220290) [2]. Three years later, the deafness-causing gene at this locus was identified as *GJB2* [3]. Of relevance to genetic testing, mutations in *GJB2* are causative in up to 50 % of individuals with severe-to-profound congenital ARNSHL in several worldwide populations. No other gene makes up such a significant proportion of genetic deafness [4].

Since the discovery of *GJB2*-related deafness, our understanding of the biology of hearing and deafness has advanced tremendously through the identification of genetic pathologies that lead to deafness in animal models and humans. Mutations have been identified that affect almost every part of the organ of Corti: the cellular cytoskeleton, including actins (*ACTG1*) and actin-associated genes (*TRIOBP* and *RDX*); myosins (*MYO7A*, *MYO15A*, *MYO6*, *MYO1A*, *MYH9*, *MYH14*); cell-cell junctions (*OTOA*, *CLDN14*); cell-cell attachments (*CDH23*, *PCDH15*); gap-junctions (*GJB2*, *GJB6*); transporters (*SLC26A4*); and ion channels (*KCNQ4*).

Clinical Utility of Testing

The primary goals in obtaining a molecular diagnosis of apparent NSHL are (1) to preclude unnecessary diagnostic testing (for example, CT scanning of the temporal bones) and define possible medical comorbidities (for example, visual problems that will develop in Usher syndrome); (2) to provide families with genetic counseling and allay parental/family concerns; and (3) in the future to guide treatment options to remediate the hearing loss [5–7].

Available Assays

GJB2 Single-Gene Screening

Historically, a number of mutation detection strategies have been used to screen *GJB2* for nucleotide changes, including restriction enzyme digestion, allele-specific polymerase chain reaction, single-strand conformation polymorphism (SSCP), heteroduplex analysis (HA), denaturing high-performance liquid chromatography, and Sanger sequencing. Of these methods, SSCP and HA were among the first and most commonly used methods because of their simplicity and cost-effectiveness. However, the gold standard is bidirectional Sanger sequencing.

Although *GJB2* is a small gene with only a single coding exon, more than 100 different allele variants are associated with both ARNSHL and autosomal dominant NSHL (ADNSHL). These variants, scattered throughout the gene, make mutation screening of the entire coding sequence essential. Phenotypic-genotypic studies of *GJB2*-associated deafness have provided important insights that are invaluable for genetic counselors. For example, cross-sectional analyses of *GJB2* genotypes against audiometric data from 1,531 persons with ARNSHL ranging from mild-to-profound identified a total of 177 different genotypes. The degree of hearing loss associated with biallelic truncating mutations was significantly more severe than the hearing loss associated with biallelic non-truncating mutations. Several common mutations (M34T, V37I, L90P) were associated with mild-to-moderate hearing loss (median 25–40 decibels [dB]), and two genotypes [35delG/R143W (median = 105 dB) and 35delG/del(GJB6-D13S1830) (median = 108 dB)] had significantly more severe hearing loss than 35delG homozygotes [8].

The identification of a single deafness-causing allele variant in *GJB2* is not uncommon and implies the presence of a "missed" variant in a noncoding region or coincidental carrier status in a person with deafness of another etiology. These types of challenges are multiplied when more comprehensive multi-gene panels are used for diagnosis and stress the need for phenomic approaches to the interpretation of genomic data.

Multi-Gene Panels

Massively parallel sequencing (MPS, also called next-generation sequencing or NGS) identifies many genetic variants and the interpretation of these variants is key to rendering a genetic diagnosis. As a bridge between Sanger sequencing of a single gene and exome or genome sequencing, targeted genomic enrichment (TGE) isolates a subset of genes from genomic DNA for more targeted sequencing. TGE is especially well suited to multi-gene screening panels and has been quickly adopted for several diseases, including deafness, because of a relatively low-cost but high-yield result. During library preparation, molecular barcodes can be added to an individual's DNA sample to ensure that data are correctly matched with a specific patient. Barcoding also allows multiple samples to be pooled in a single sequencing run, which improves the cost-effectiveness of the testing.

An alternative technology that has been used for genetic testing for deafness is resequencing arrays. While these arrays are cost effective, they are limited by the number of base pairs that can be sequenced on a single array. For deafness testing, no arrays are available that interrogate every base pair of every gene implicated in NSHL. In contrast, TGE followed by MPS provides a comprehensive genetic assessment for deafness.

MPS is extremely reliant on bioinformatic analysis of the sequencing data. Following TGE and sequencing, a typical workflow involves de-multiplexing sequencing reads, mapping reads to the human reference genome, and then identifying and annotating variants. Variants are then prioritized to determine the variant(s) most likely to cause deafness. Use of both publicly available databases (i.e., 1000 Genomes, dbSNP) and laboratory-developed databases is essential for variant filtering. A freely available central repository of variants specific to deafness is available at http://www.deafnessvariationdatabase.org.

Interpretation of Results

GJB2 Single-Gene Screening

Several databases of *GJB2* deafness-causing variants exist and should be consulted for interpretation of results (Connexin-deafness homepage http://davinci.crg.es/deafness/; http://www.deafnessvariationdatabase.org). The carrier rate for pathogenic *GJB2* variants is high enough that a single mutation is not diagnostic of *GJB2*-related deafness. If the full sequencing of *GJB2* (exon 1, coding regions, splice sites, and upstream deletions) does not identify two disease-causing variants, then testing with a multi-gene panel is recommended. Multi-gene panel testing also should be considered in instances of obvious *GJB2* genotype-phenotype discordance.

Table 14.1 Evaluation of targeted genomic enrichment assays: a sample summary of variants

Sample evaluation—targeted genomic enrichment	
Sample ID	112111-3
Phenotype	High-frequency SNHL
Exons targeted	1,357
Bases targeted	351,522 base pairs
Metric	**Result (reference range)**
Total reads	28.2 million (14–32 million)
% Reads mapped	97.2 % (94.3–98.7 %)
% Reads overlapping target	61.0 % (58.1–63.9 %)
Targets covered at 1×	98.8 % (98.6–98.9 %)
Targets covered at 10×	98.2 % (97.5–98.2 %)
Total variants identified	335 (300–400)
Rare variants (≤1 %)	87 (60–100)
Exonic or splice site variants	19 (10–30)
Non-synonymous/indel/splice site variants	7
Variants of unknown significance	4
Known disease-causing mutations	0
Candidate mutations for deafness	2

Multi-Gene Panels

Evaluation of the quality of the targeted enrichment and the sequence reads is essential. Typical metrics to consider are overall sequence data generation, read quality, percent of reads that map to the human genome, percent of reads that overlap the targeted genes, and the depth of coverage of the targeted regions (Table 14.1).

Variants are typically annotated with the following: gene, location (exonic/intronic/splice site/intergenic/noncoding RNA), nucleotide change, amino acid change, presence in publicly available databases (1000 Genomes, dbSNP), and scores in pathogenicity prediction algorithms (Polyphen, PhyloP, SIFT). Variants are then prioritized to identify those most likely to be disease causing; variants previously reported as disease-causing mutations (DCMs) are most likely to be causative. In general, if no DCMs are identified, the prioritization strategy adheres to two generally accepted tenants of human disease genetics: (1) DCMs will be rare; and (2) DCMs will have a significant functional impact on the protein. An algorithm for variant prioritization is included in Fig. 14.1.

Determining the population frequency of a variant is greatly facilitated by dbSNP and the 1000 Genomes Project, where millions of genomic variants from large sequencing projects are publicly available. Of particular importance are well-curated, locus-specific databases and laboratory-developed variant databases, which can provide significant

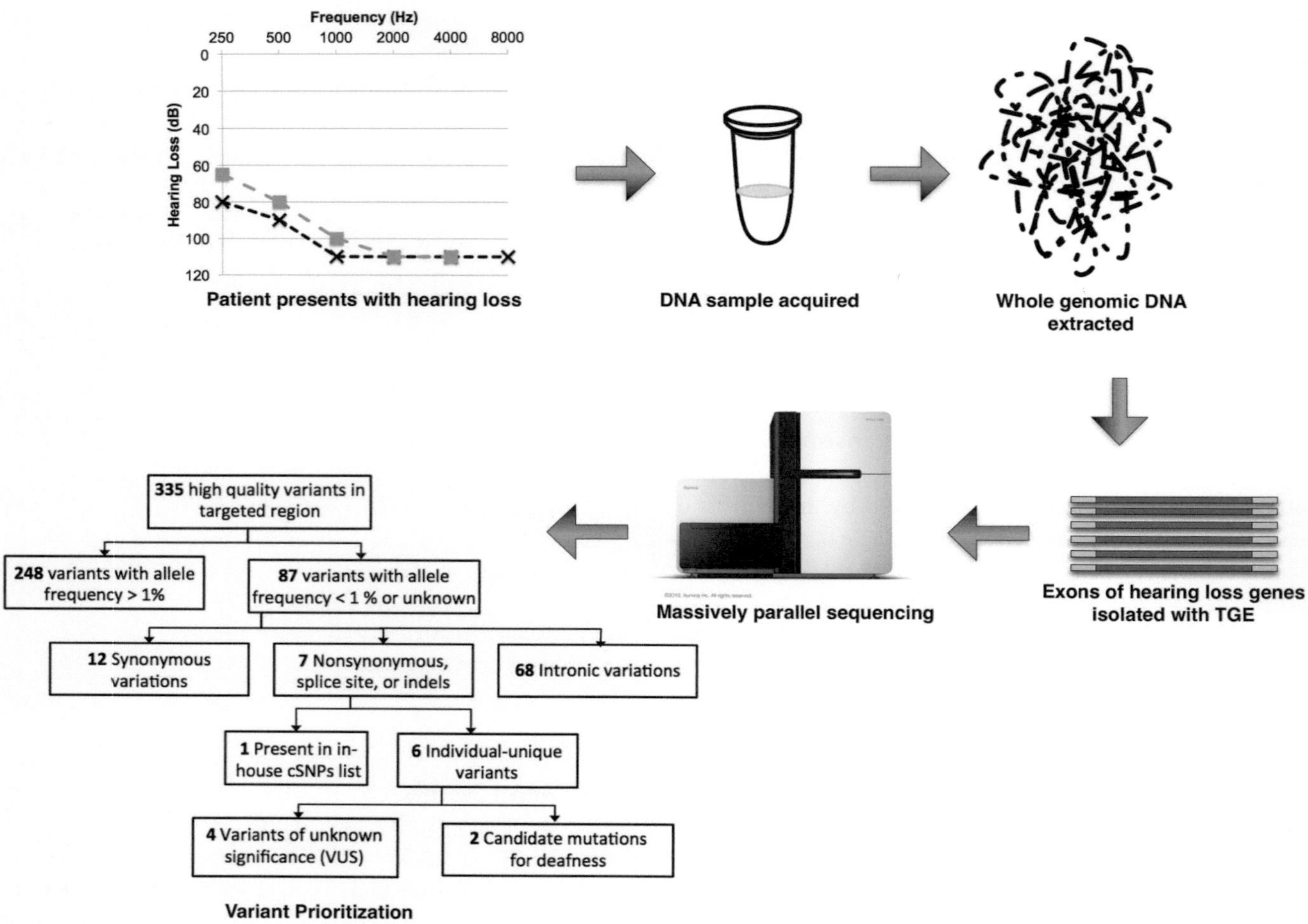

Figure 14.1 Overview of multi-gene screening panel for deafness using targeted genomic enrichment (TGE). After DNA is isolated, exons of interest (every exon of every known hearing loss gene) are isolated via TGE. Massively parallel sequencing yields millions of sequencing reads that are assessed for quality and aligned to the reference human genome. Variants are compared to the reference genome for annotation and prioritization to identify those changes that are most likely to be deafness causing, as described in detail in the text

data on variant frequency for TGE assays. The functional effect of a genetic variant is most easily interpretable when it is non-synonymous, affects a splice site, or is an insertion/deletion that causes a frameshift. Variants located outside the coding sequence are more difficult to interpret.

Frequently, several rare variants cannot be further prioritized based on database comparison and gene effect assessment. In silico pathogenicity algorithms can be used to predict the significance of these variants. For example, evolutionary conservation of the variant location (BLOSUM), comparison of the physical characteristics of the most common and the variant amino acids (Align-GVGD), and protein-specific annotation and functional consequence of changes (SIFT and PolyPhen) can provide insight into the possible pathogenicity of VUS. These in silico methods do not replace in vitro or in vivo experimentation, but provide the only mechanism to assess the large numbers of variants expeditiously. When these four specific methods are concurrent on pathogenicity, the positive predictive value is >94 % [9]. The alternative, to invest significant time and effort completing functional assays, would reduce the clinical usefulness of genetic testing in many instances.

A complementary technique for filtering is based on the patient's phenotype. In the case of NSHL, particularly ADNSHL, audiograms can be used to filter variants. For example, DCMs in *WFS1* are associated with an audio profile characterized by low-frequency NSHL; DCMs in *KCNQ4*, in contrast, cause high-frequency NSHL. Prioritizing the significance of identified variants based on a patient's clinical characteristics will play an increasingly large role as more genotype-phenotype correlation data are available.

Laboratory Issues

GJB2 Single-Gene Screening

Determination of *GJB2*-related deafness is dependent on the identification of mutations in the DNA of affected individuals. Sequencing of only exon 2 of *GJB2* by any technique is incomplete because there are several common noncoding, noncomplementary DFNB1-causing mutations that must be considered in persons heterozygous for a known *GJB2* deafness-causing variant. These mutations include those found in intron 1 and a few large deletions involving *GJB6* [DFNB1B (MIM 612645)] or both *GJB2* and *GJB6* that are easily detectable by sequencing across the breakpoint fragments or by MPS of a multi-gene panel for deafness. Based on the relative frequency of *GJB2* allele variants in the general population, the frequency of noncoding *GJB2* variants associated with deafness, and phenotype-genotype correlations, ongoing studies of *GJB2*-related deafness have confirmed the existence of at least one additional variation associated with the DFNB1 phenotype that lies outside the coding region of *GJB2* [10].

Multi-Gene Panels

Due to the capacity of next-generation sequencers, bar-coded genomic libraries from several individual patients frequently are pooled prior to sequencing. Due to the large output associated with these assays, data storage and the documentation and maintenance of the bioinformatics infrastructure are issues that must be addressed in any clinical laboratory using this testing method. Due to the speed at which genomics is advancing, annotation and prioritization methods must be updated frequently to ensure that variants are reported correctly. Laboratories must consider whether to implement processes to modify earlier reports as new data are generated that potentially change the interpretation of the previous report. Examples include the addition of new genes to these platforms and the inclusion of intronic and promoter regions to allow the identification of noncoding deafness-causing variants. One important advance already realized has been the ability to complete comprehensive copy-number variant analysis of the genes included on the multi-gene panels currently in use. This type of analysis can detect *GJB2* and *GJB6* deletions and has implicated deletions of *STRC* as a very frequent cause of mild-to-moderate ARNSHL.

Laboratories must determine through their validation process whether DCMs will be validated by an alternative method such as Sanger sequencing to confirm the MPS results that are predicted to be clinically significant. If possible, limited segregation analysis should be completed. Laboratories also must have procedures that define which data will be stored and for what length of time. Screening controls to determine the population carrier frequency of identified variants is no longer necessary due to the prevalence of publicly available data. Processes for reporting of VUS results to healthcare providers, patients, and families also should be defined by the laboratory in collaboration with the healthcare providers.

Conclusions and Future Directions

Inherited deafness is uniquely suited to TGE and MPS because of its extreme genetic heterogeneity. Over the last 5 years, these technologies have transformed genetic testing for deafness from a gene-by-gene approach to a comprehensive and all-inclusive test. For the short term, initial screening of persons with severe-to-profound presumed ARNSHL for variants in *GJB2* is an acceptable option, with a negative result triggering a multi-gene screen. However, the capacity of MPS is rapidly expanding and costs are decreasing, making single-gene methods of very limited use. The currently used TGE platform for deafness is sufficiently flexible that more genes can be easily added with follow-up validation, ensuring a continually up-to-date platform. As clinicians become more comfortable with genomic medicine, comprehensive genetic testing for hearing loss will be an integral part of the clinical evaluation of patients and become the test of choice for a diagnosis of NSHL.

Acknowledgements This work was supported in part by NIDCD RO1s DC003544, DC002842, and DC012049 to R.J.H.S. and NIDCD 1F30DC011674-01A1 to A.E.S.

References

1. Morton CC, Nance WE. Newborn hearing screening – a silent revolution. N Engl J Med. 2006;354:2151–64.
2. Guilford P, Ben Arab S, Blanchard S, et al. A non-syndrome form of neurosensory, recessive deafness maps to the pericentromeric region of chromosome 13q. Nat Genet. 1994;6:24–8.
3. Kelsell DP, Dunlop J, Stevens HP, et al. Connexin 26 mutations in hereditary non-syndromic sensorineural deafness. Nature. 1997;387:80–3.
4. Hilgert N, Smith RJ, Van Camp G. Forty-six genes causing nonsyndromic hearing impairment: which ones should be analyzed in DNA diagnostics? Mutat Res. 2009;681:189–96.
5. Cohn ES, Kelley PM, Fowler TW, et al. Clinical studies of families with hearing loss attributable to mutations in the connexin 26 gene (GJB2/DFNB1). Pediatrics. 1999;103:546–50.
6. Denoyelle F, Marlin S, Weil D, et al. Clinical features of the prevalent form of childhood deafness, DFNB1, due to a connexin-26 gene defect: implications for genetic counselling. Lancet. 1999;353:1298–303.
7. Green G, Mueller R, Cohn E, et al. Audiological manifestations and features of connexin 26 deafness. Audiol Med. 2003;1:5–11.
8. Snoeckx RL, Huygen PL, Feldmann D, et al. GJB2 mutations and degree of hearing loss: a multicenter study. Am J Hum Genet. 2005;77:945–57.
9. Ng SB, Turner EH, Robertson PD, et al. Targeted capture and massively parallel sequencing of 12 human exomes. Nature. 2009;461:272–6.
10. Azaiez H, Chamberlin GP, Fischer SM, et al. GJB2: the spectrum of deafness-causing allele variants and their phenotype. Hum Mutat. 2004;24:305–11.

Coagulation Disorders

15

Rajiv K. Pruthi, Michelle L. Kluge, and Aneel A. Ashrani

Abstract

The vascular system is a series of interconnected biologic conduits filled with fluid moving under pressure. This system is subject to injury, with exsanguination avoided by the functions of the hemostatic system. Normal hemostasis is a reparative process and consists of three major mechanisms: (1) vasospasm, (2) platelet plug formation, and (3) the procoagulant system. While inherited or acquired disorders of all three mechanisms can cause clinically abnormal bleeding, this chapter reviews the molecular basis of the more commonly inherited disorders of the procoagulant system (e.g., hemophilia A and B, and von Willebrand disease) associated with abnormal bleeding.

Keywords

Bleeding disorder • Coagulation • Hemophilia A • Factor VIII deficiency • F8 gene • Hemophilia B • Factor IX deficiency • F9 gene • von Willebrand disease • VWF gene • Thrombophilia • Factor V Leiden • F5 gene • Prothrombin • F2 gene • Venous thrombosis • Purpura fulminans neonatalis • Hyperhomocysteinemia • Homocystinuria • Molecular testing • Diagnostic testing

Introduction

Reduced to its simplest form, the vascular system is a series of interconnected biologic conduits filled with fluid moving under pressure. This system is subject to injury, with repair required to avoid exsanguination. This latter function is provided by the hemostatic system. Thus, normal hemostasis is a reparative process and consists of three major mechanisms: (1) vasospasm, which is the main mechanism for controlling bleeding after transection/avulsion injuries of large arteries, arterioles, and veins; (2) platelet plug formation; and (3) the procoagulant

R.K. Pruthi, M.B.B.S. (✉)
Division of Hematology, Department of Internal Medicine, Mayo Clinic College of Medicine, Rochester, MN USA
e-mail: pruthi.rajiv@mayo.edu

M.L. Kluge, M.S., C.G.C.
Department of Laboratory Medicine and Pathology, Division of Hematopathology and Laboratory Genetics, Mayo Clinic College of Medicine, Rochester, 200 First Street, SW, Rochester, MN 55905, USA

Mayo Comprehensive Hemophilia Center, Mayo Clinic Rochester, 200 First Street, SW, Rochester, MN 55905, USA

A.A. Ashrani, M.D., M.S.
Division of Hematology, Department of Internal Medicine, Mayo Clinic College of Medicine, Rochester, MN, USA

Special Coagulation Laboratory, Mayo Comprehensive Hemophilia Center, Rochester, MN, USA

Department of Laboratory Medicine and Pathology, Division of Hematopathology and Laboratory Genetics, Mayo Clinic Rochester, 200 First Street, SW, Rochester, MN 55905, USA

D.G.B. Leonard (ed.), *Molecular Pathology in Clinical Practice*, DOI 10.1007/978-3-319-19674-9_15

system. The procoagulant system consists of mechanisms by which fluid blood is converted into an insoluble hemostatic thrombus. While inherited or acquired disorders of all three mechanisms can cause clinically abnormal bleeding, this chapter reviews the molecular basis of the more commonly inherited disorders of the procoagulant system (e.g., hemophilia A (HA), hemophilia B (HB), and von Willebrand disease (VWD) associated with abnormal bleeding. Inherited vascular and platelet disorders associated with abnormal bleeding are not discussed.

Consider also that, once activated, the reparative (e.g., hemostatic) response to injury must be constrained such that the thrombus is limited to the site of injury, and is down-regulated such that the conversion of fluid blood to solid thrombus does not propagate throughout the lumen of the vessel. This latter function is provided by the anticoagulant and fibrinolytic systems. Inherited disorders (deficiencies) of the anticoagulant system (e.g., familial thrombophilia) are associated with venous thromboembolism (VTE) and complications of pregnancy. In addition, inherited abnormalities of selected procoagulant proteins are associated with VTE. Although biologically plausible, the association between familial thrombophilia and arterial thrombosis is unproven and will not be reviewed.

Inherited Bleeding Disorders

The initial hemostatic response to endothelial injury is platelet adhesion to exposed subendothelial matrix. Platelets circulate preferentially along the vessel luminal surface, as opposed to circulating evenly distributed throughout the blood. Thus, platelets can be viewed as a "surveillance" blood cell that is "searching" for sites of endothelial injury. Platelet adhesion at an injury site is mediated by the ligand, von Willebrand factor (VWF). VWF tethers platelets to the site of injury by binding to collagen within the subendothelial matrix exposed by the injury, and to the constitutively active platelet receptor, glycoprotein (GP)-Ib-IX-V complex. Firm platelet adhesion at the injury site is mediated by subsequent binding of the platelet GP-$\alpha_2\beta_1$ collagen receptor to subendothelial matrix collagen. VWF binding to platelet GP-Ib-IX-V generates transmembrane signals that activate platelets, converting the constitutively inactive platelet fibrinogen receptor, GP-$\alpha_{IIb}\beta_3$ (GP IIb/IIIa), to the fibrinogen-binding conformation. Subsequent platelet-to-platelet cohesion is mediated by fibrinogen or VWF binding to platelet GP-$\alpha_{IIb}\beta_3$. In addition, a scramblase protein within the platelet membrane phospholipid bilayer flips negatively charged phospholipids from the inside to the outside membrane bilayer leaflet. The newly exposed negatively charged phospholipids support assembly of the plasma procoagulant factors on the platelet membrane. Finally, platelets release contents of the dense granules (adenosine diphosphate [ADP], serotonin, etc.) and α-granules (fibrinogen, VWF, factors V and XI, etc.), which feed back to stimulate further platelet activation and support the plasma procoagulant system.

The plasma procoagulant system has been characterized as a "cascade" of amplifying enzymatic reactions leading to the activation of the final serine protease enzyme, thrombin from prothrombin. This cascade is initiated by exposure of the coagulation activator, tissue factor, to circulating blood. Tissue factor, located within the vascular walls and normally sequestered from the circulation, is exposed to blood after blood vessel injury. Exposed (or expressed) tissue factor binds to circulating factor VII_a ($FVII_a$) to form a "Factor X-ase" activation complex which either cleaves ("activates") FX to FX_a directly or activates FIX to FIX_a (Fig. 15.1). Factor IX_a binds $FVIII_a$ to form a second Factor X-ase activation complex. Factor X_a binds FV_a to form the "prothrombinase complex" that activates prothrombin (FII) to thrombin (FII_a). The X-ase and the prothrombinase complexes assemble on negatively charged phospholipids within the outer membrane of activated platelets. Thrombin produces a hemostatic thrombus by cleaving fibrinogen (factor I) to form fibrin monomers, by activating platelets, and by activating FXIII to $FXIII_a$ which cross-links strands of fibrin monomers to form an insoluble hemostatic thrombus. In a feedback amplification loop, thrombin also increases its own production by activating FV, FVIII, and FXI.

Hemophilia A

Overview

HA is an X-linked recessive bleeding disorder due to a deficiency in coagulation factor VIII (FVIII). HA affects approximately 1 in 10,000 live male births, among all ethnic populations. Approximately 30 % of cases result from new mutations occurring in families in whom there is no apparent family history of HA. The diagnosis of HA is established based on reduced or absent FVIII activity (FVIII:C) and is classified into severe (<1 %), moderate (1–5 %), or mild (>5–40 %) disease, with estimated prevalence of 43 %, 26 %, and 31 %, respectively [1].

Molecular Basis of Disease

The factor VIII gene (*F8*) is located on the long arm of the X chromosome (Xq28) (Fig. 15.2). *F8* is 186 kilobase pairs (kbp) with 26 relatively short exons, ranging from 69 to 262 base pairs (bp), and two long exons, exon 14 (3,106 bp) and exon 26 (958 bp). The resulting messenger RNA (mRNA) is approximately 9 kb, of which the coding sequence is 7,053 nucleotides. The intron/exon boundaries roughly correlate with the FVIII domains (Fig. 15.3). The introns are large (14–23 kb) with intron 22 being the largest (32 kb). A CpG island in intron 22 acts as a bi-directional promoter for two additional genes (Fig. 15.2). The first, termed *F8*-associated gene

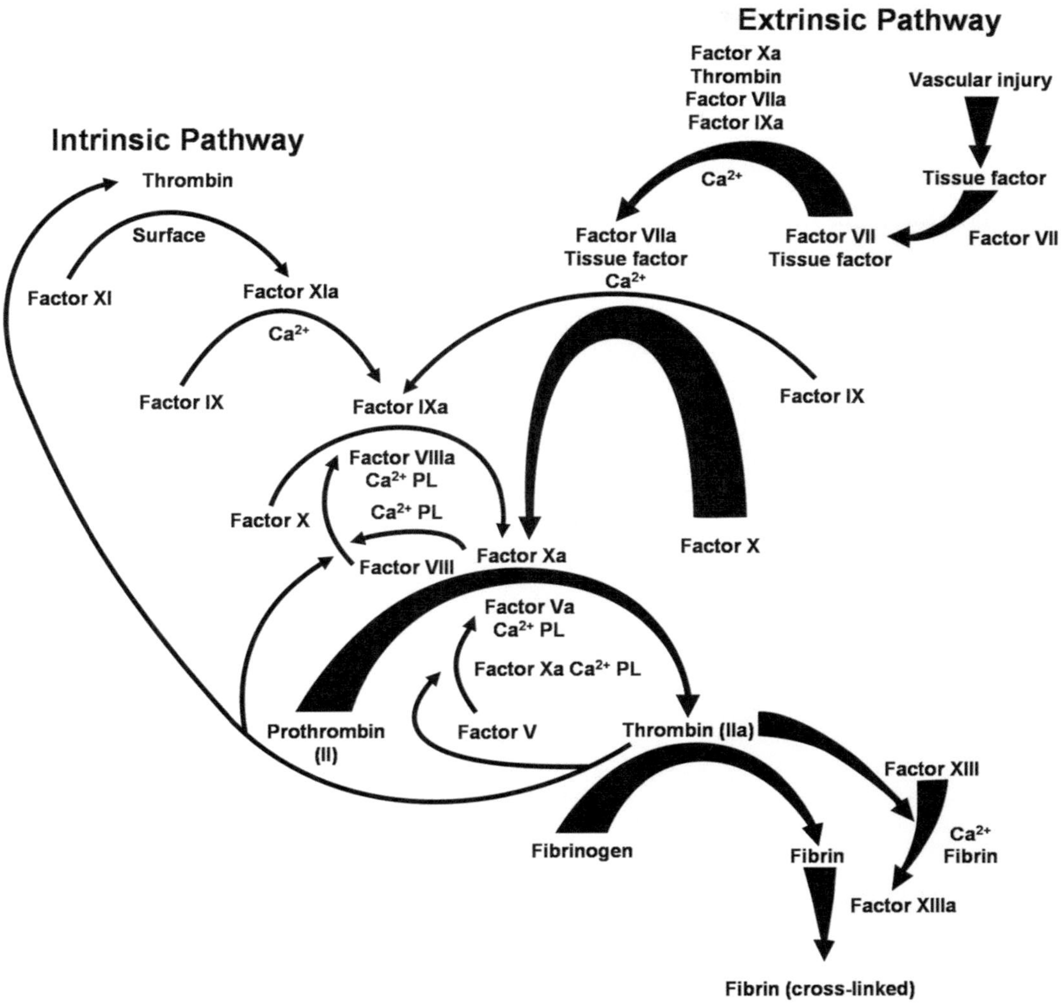

Figure 15.1 The Coagulation Cascade: *a* activated factor; *Ca2+* calcium; *PL* phospholipid. Reprinted with permission from Davie EW, Fujikawa K, Kisiel W. The coagulation cascade: initiation, maintenance and regulation. Biochemistry. 1991;30:10363. Copyright 1991 American Chemical Society

A (*F8A* or *Int22h-1*), is an intronless gene approximately 2 kb long and is transcribed in the opposite direction to *F8*. The second *F8*-associated gene B (*F8B*) is 2.5 kb long and transcribed in the same direction as *F8*. The *F8A* and *F8B* transcripts originate within 122 bases of each other and the functions of their potential protein products are unknown. The *F8A* sequence is replicated at least twice, approximately 500 kb telomeric to the *F8* gene and close to the tip of the X chromosome termed Int22h-2 (proximal) and Int22h-3 (distal). Int 22h-2 and -3 are about 100 kb apart and transcribed in the same direction as the *F8* gene. These three homologous repeats are involved in the intron 22 inversion mutation which is a frequent rearrangement of the *F8* gene, resulting in severe HA (Fig. 15.4). The putative promoter region is located 300 nucleotides 5′ to the gene and although a TATA box is not essential for transcription, liver-enriched transcription factors (e.g., HNF1, NFkB, C/EBPa, and C/EBPb) interact with the *F8* promoter region. The *F8* gene encodes a precursor protein of 2,351 amino acid residues consisting of a 19 amino acid leader peptide followed by 2,332 amino acids in the mature protein. The mature protein can be divided into several homologous domains termed A1-A2-B-A3-C1-C2 and is predominantly expressed in the liver.

Factor VIII is activated to FVIIIa via proteolytic cleavage, by either thrombin (FIIa) or factor Xa in the presence of phospholipid surfaces (Fig. 15.3). Although cleavages at amino acid positions 740 or 1,721 have no effect on coagulant activity, the cleavages at amino acid position 372 or 1,689 are important for FVIII procoagulant activity. Cleavage at 1,689 releases FVIII from VWF, permitting FVIII interaction with phospholipids and platelets. Missense mutations affecting these cleavage sites have been found in patients with HA and result in a form of hemophilia called "cross-reacting material positive (CRM+)-HA" with normal levels of FVIII antigen but low activity (1–7 %). Although missense mutations have been found in the A2 domain in HA and its value to FVIII coagulant activity has been confirmed by in vitro studies, the exact role of the A2 subunit remains unknown.

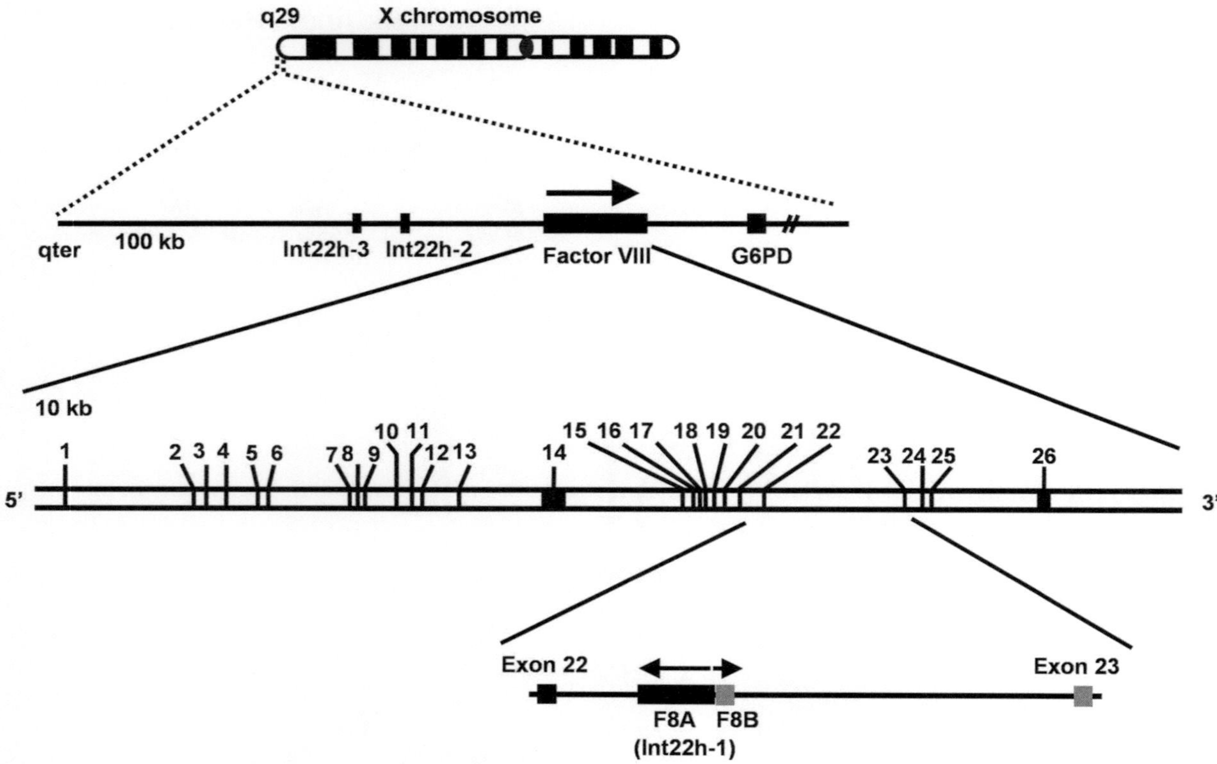

Figure 15.2 The location and structure of the *F8* gene: *G6PD* glucose 6 phosphate dehydrogenase, *kb* kilobases. Reprinted with permission from Kazazian HH, Tuddenham EGD, Stylianos EA. Hemophilia A: deficiency of coagulation factor VIII. In Scriver CR, Beaudet al, Valle D, et al., eds. The Metabolic and Molecular Basis of Inherited Disease. Copyright 2001 McGraw-Hill

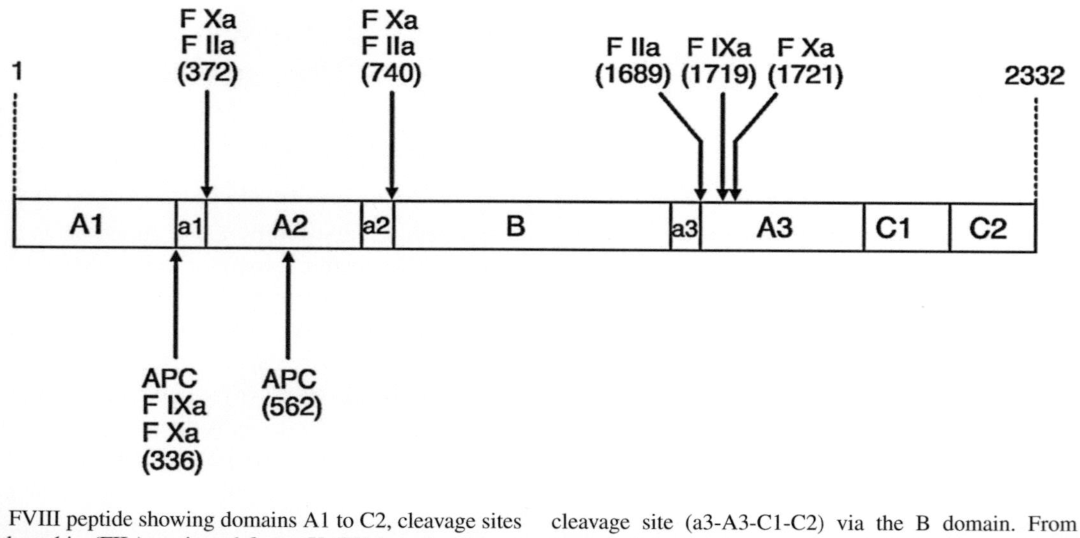

Figure 15.3 FVIII peptide showing domains A1 to C2, cleavage sites (*arrows*) for thrombin (FIIa), activated factor X (FXa), and activated protein C (APC): Amino acids are numbered in parentheses. The heavy-chain cleavage site (A1-a1-A2-a2) is linked to the light-chain cleavage site (a3-A3-C1-C2) via the B domain. From Pruthi RK, Nichols WL. Autoimmune factor VIII inhibitors. Curr Opin Hematol 6;314. Copyright 1999 Lippincott Williams and Wilkins. Reprinted with permission from Wolters Kluwer Health

The B domain is cleaved during proteolytic activation and is not directly required for procoagulant activity of FVIII. However, it may have a role in intracellular processing and/or secretion of FVIII as B-domain-deleted FVIII molecules are expressed at five- to ten-fold higher levels than non B-domain-deleted FVIII. Mutations in this region have been reported in HA.

VWF-bound FVIII is protected from inactivation by activated protein C (APC). The putative VWF-binding region on FVIII is felt to be at the N-terminus of the light chain of

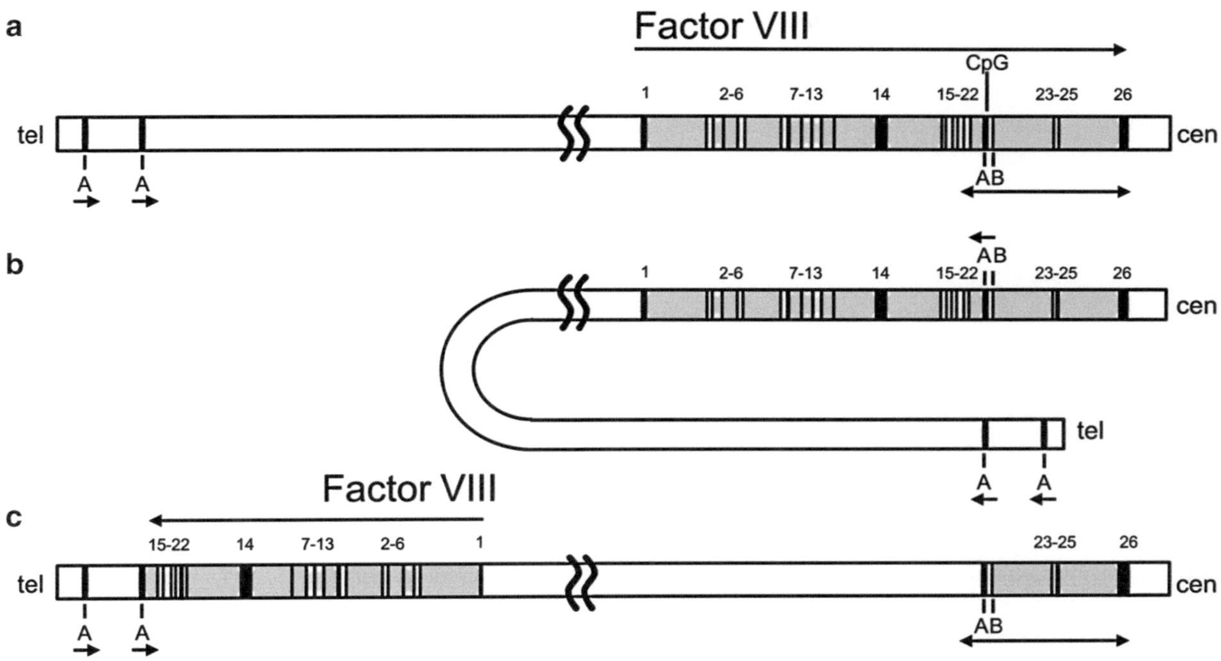

Figure 15.4 Intron 22 inversion mutation of the *F8* gene: (**a**) Orientation of the *F8* gene showing three copies of the *F8A* gene (A) and location of the *F8B* gene (B) transcript in intron 22. *Arrows* indicate the direction of transcription of the *F8* and internal *F8A* (A) and *F8B* (B) genes. (**b**) Proposed mechanism of homologous recombination between intron 22 gene *F8A* (A) and one of the two telomeric copies of gene *F8A* (A). (**c**) Results of proposed crossover. *cen* centromere, *tel* telomere. Reprinted with permission from Kazazian HH, Tuddenham EGD, Stylianos EA. Hemophilia A: deficiency of coagulation factor VIII. In Scriver CR, Beaudet al, Valle D, et al., eds. The metabolic and molecular basis of inherited disease. Copyright 2001 McGraw-Hill

FVIII and in the C2 domain. The binding site for FIXa has been localized to the A2 domain and regions of the light chain. In addition, the binding site to FX is localized to the C-terminus of the A1 domain. Binding to phospholipids, which is important for FX activation by FIXa and FVIIIa, occurs in the C1 and C2 domains of the light-chain FVIII. No deleterious mutations in HA patients have been identified in the inactivation cleavage sites of FVIII.

Deleterious Mutations in *F8* Gene

Deleterious mutations and polymorphisms are cataloged in an international database available on the Internet and updated periodically: http://hadb.org.uk. References for the amino acid numbering system used below can be accessed at this website.

Mutations have been found in the promoter and all coding regions of the *F8* gene. Of the approximately 1,492 unique reported mutations, missense mutations account for approximately 46 %, small deletions (<50 bp) 18 %, large deletions (>50 bp) 11 %, nonsense mutations 10 %, and splice-site mutations and insertions 7 % each. However, approximately 40 % of severe HA patients have an inversion mutation at the tip of the X chromosome that disrupts the *F8* gene [2]. Homologous recombination can occur when the *F8A* gene (Inth22-1) in intron 22 of *F8* pairs with one of the two homologous regions (Int22h-2 or Int22h-3) that are telomeric to the *F8* gene probably as a result of folding over of the tip of the X chromosome (Fig. 15.4). Upon unfolding, exons 1–22 are inverted and placed approximately 500 kb upstream of exons 23–26 and oriented in the opposite direction. Depending on which repeat the *F8A* pairs with, the inversion may be termed type I (distal) or type II (proximal). Rarely type III inversion mutations occur in patients with a third extragenic copy of *F8A*. Given that the majority of inversions originate in male meiosis, almost all mothers of patients with the inversion mutation are carriers. An additional inversion of exon 1 of the *F8* gene affecting up to 5 % of patients with severe HA has also been described [3].

Genotype-Phenotype Correlations

The types of *F8* mutations correlate with the severity of hemophilia and the risk of developing FVIII inhibitors. In addition to the inversion mutations, certain missense, insertion, and deletion mutations result in severe disease (<1 % FVIII activity). However, specific deletions of 156 bp of exon 22 or the 294 bp of exons 23 and 24 are associated with moderate disease, likely due to in-frame splicing of exon 21 to exon 23, or exon 22 to exon 25. Patients with large deletions are susceptible to formation of FVIII inhibitors (antibodies) in response to therapy with FVIII concentrates. In an analysis of the HA database, up to 40 % of patients with deletions develop FVIII inhibitors, whereas up to 60 % of patients with single-base pair changes resulting in nonsense mutations and 15 % of patients with single-base pair changes resulting in missense mutations developed inhibitors [4]. More recently, a meta-analysis of 30 studies involving over 5,000 patients concluded that the pooled odds ratios (OR) of inhibitor development in large deletions and nonsense mutations were 3.6 (95 % CI 2.3–5.7) and 1.4 (95 % CI 1.1–1.8), respectively, compared to intron 22 inversion mutations, with the remaining mutations (e.g., intron 1 inversions and splice-site mutations) posing an equivalent risk as an intron 22 inversion [5].

Single-base pair changes that result in missense mutations are spread throughout the *F8* gene. Although the structure-function relationships of some of the missense mutations are known or can be deduced (e.g., alteration of VWF-binding site, thrombin cleavage site), the structural consequences of most such mutations remain undefined.

Although HA predominantly affects males, some female carriers have reduced FVIII:C and may have clinically significant bleeding. The molecular basis of symptomatic females includes lyonization of the normal X chromosome and Turner syndrome (XO karyotype) where the dominant mutant *F8* gene is responsible for production of the abnormal FVIII. Rarely, a female known to be a carrier may have children with a known hemophilia patient; in this circumstance, each child regardless of gender has a 50 % chance of being affected.

Polymorphisms in the *F8* Gene

Polymorphisms present within the *F8* gene (intragenic) or outside the *F8* gene (extragenic) have been used to assign haplotypes (combination of polymorphisms) for linkage analysis. The putative defective *F8* gene can be tracked with polymorphisms that are closely linked to the gene. The carrier frequency of such polymorphisms varies with the ethnicity of the study population and needs to be considered when studying patients of diverse ethnic origin. A complete listing of polymorphisms is available in the *F8* mutation database at http://hadb.org.uk.

Clinical Utility of Testing

In a male patient suspected of being affected, the diagnosis of HA is established by assaying plasma FVIII:C. Given that FVIII relies on binding to VWF for its normal survival, all patients with a low FVIII:C should have VWB excluded. In addition, FVIII is a labile factor resulting in a potential artifactual loss of up to 15 % of FVIII:C with delayed processing of plasma specimens. Thus, mild reductions in FVIII:C should prompt repeat testing with careful attention to timely specimen processing.

In at-risk females, while reduced FVIII:C typically confirms carrier status, a normal FVIII:C does not exclude the possibility of carrier status. Given that FVIII:C may be normal in carriers and the fact that FVIII is an acute-phase reactant, it can be elevated with acute or chronic inflammation, liver disease, vasculitis, estrogen therapy, or pregnancy. Thus, molecular genetic testing would be the only option for diagnosis.

Knowledge of the causative *F8* mutation in the proband does not alter clinical management but may be useful in predicting the risk of developing FVIII inhibitors [4]. The causative mutation can be useful for carrier testing of family members. Asymptomatic females with no access to their familial *F8* genotype information will need their entire *F8* gene analyzed for carrier testing. This is not an uncommon situation for adopted females. For carriers, prenatal diagnosis during pregnancy provides useful information for management of labor and delivery and, occasionally, pregnancy termination. Advances in reproductive technology may permit preimplantation genetic diagnosis and circumvent the need for prenatal testing [6].

Available Assays

Several laboratories offer genetic testing for HA. A complete listing of clinical laboratories performing HA testing that have registered with GeneTests can be found on their website (www.genetests.org). An alternative source is the NCBI Genetic Testing Registry (http://www.ncbi.nim.nih.gov/gtr). In general, testing can be divided into direct mutation analysis and indirect testing based on haplotype, and selected laboratories offer prenatal testing.

Direct DNA Analysis

Direct DNA analysis for the intron 22 and 1 inversion mutations is typically performed by restriction digestion and Southern blot method. This detects the more common types: I and II inversions and the rare type III inversion. Polymerase chain reaction (PCR)-based assays also can be used [3, 7, 8]. Detection of hemizygous gene or exonic deletions in the *F8* gene in at-risk carriers by PCR amplification of individual exons may not be diagnostic given that the normal copy of the gene may be amplified. For this situation, linkage analysis may be required; however, the role of multiplex ligation-dependent probe amplification (MLPA) is evolving [9]. Different laboratories utilize varied approaches, including initial screening or direct sequencing of all the relevant regions of the *F8* gene [10]. The large size of the *F8* gene with 26 exons makes this a labor-intensive test. Thus alternate strategies have been utilized on a research basis which involves analysis of *F8* mRNA by RT-PCR [11] or other SSCP-based screening techniques [12].

Indirect DNA Analysis (Linkage Analysis)

The principle underlying genetic linkage analysis is the tendency for alleles close together on the same chromosome to be transmitted together as an intact unit through meiosis.

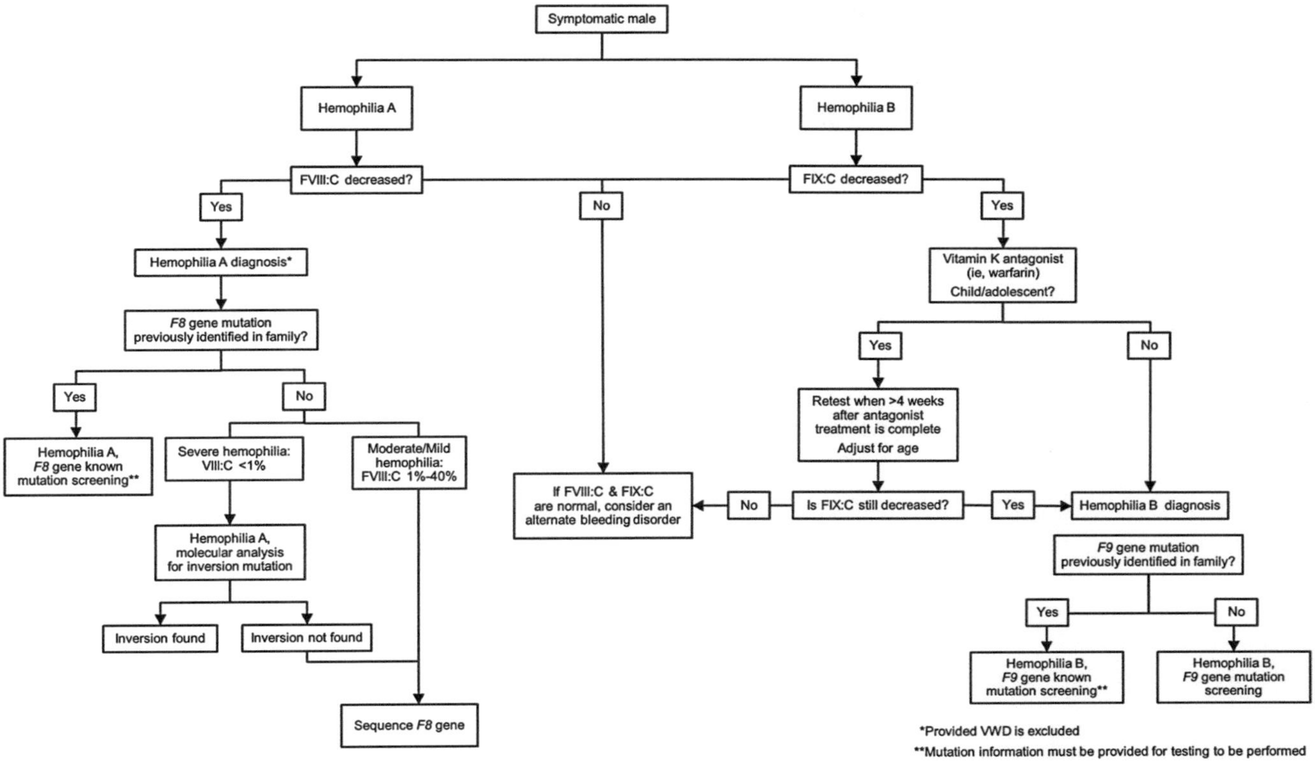

Figure 15.5 Hemophilia testing algorithm: symptomatic male. FVIII:C, FVIII activity; FIX:C, FIX activity; *F8*, FVIII gene; *F9*, factor IX gene. By permission of Mayo Foundation for Medical Education and Research. All rights reserved

Polymorphisms, within the *F8* gene (intragenic) or outside the *F8* gene (extragenic), are typically single-base pair changes or simple sequence repeats (CA^n repeats). Disadvantages of linkage analysis include the need for DNA samples from the proband and both parents, and the requirement that the proband's mother be heterozygous and thus "informative" for the polymorphism. A polymorphism is informative if the DNA sequence at a locus differs on the maternally inherited and paternally inherited chromosomes. Most families (up to 90 %) are informative with one or more DNA polymorphisms if both intragenic and extragenic polymorphisms are analyzed. The distance between the disease-causing mutation and the polymorphism increases the risk of recombination, which may lead to false-positive or false-negative results. This risk is lowest if intragenic markers are used. Rarely, families will only be informative for extragenic polymorphisms: misdiagnosis can occur in up to 6 % of carriers as a result of linkage disequilibrium. When an intragenic polymorphism is used for the diagnosis of carrier or affected status, the chance of an error is less than 1 %. A major drawback with linkage analysis is the possibility of identifying nonpaternity in the tested family. A complete listing and frequency of polymorphisms is available in the *F8* mutation database.

HA Testing Algorithms

HA genetic testing should be accompanied by pretest and posttest counseling, which is described below. For questions regarding any laboratory's sample requirement, testing, and reporting process, direct communication with the laboratory is critical. Most laboratories have a genetic counselor available for testing guidance. In general, genetic testing for hemophilia is ordered by healthcare providers familiar with the diseases, inheritance patterns, and testing options, but also is ordered by primary care providers who may not be familiar with testing options and counseling. Algorithms for testing symptomatic males and at-risk females are illustrated in Figs. 15.5 and 15.6 and described below.

For a symptomatic male, the diagnosis of HA is established based on plasma FVIII:C, which also classifies the disease as severe (<1 %), moderate (1–5 %), or mild (>5–40 %) (Fig. 15.5). In patients with a history of a bleeding disorder but who have normal FVIII:C, alternative bleeding disorders should be considered, e.g., HB (X-linked recessive) or VWD (autosomal dominant or recessive). If the specific *F8* mutation has been identified in an affected family member, the documentation of the specific familial mutation should be provided to the laboratory and testing should concentrate on identifying the presence or absence of the familial

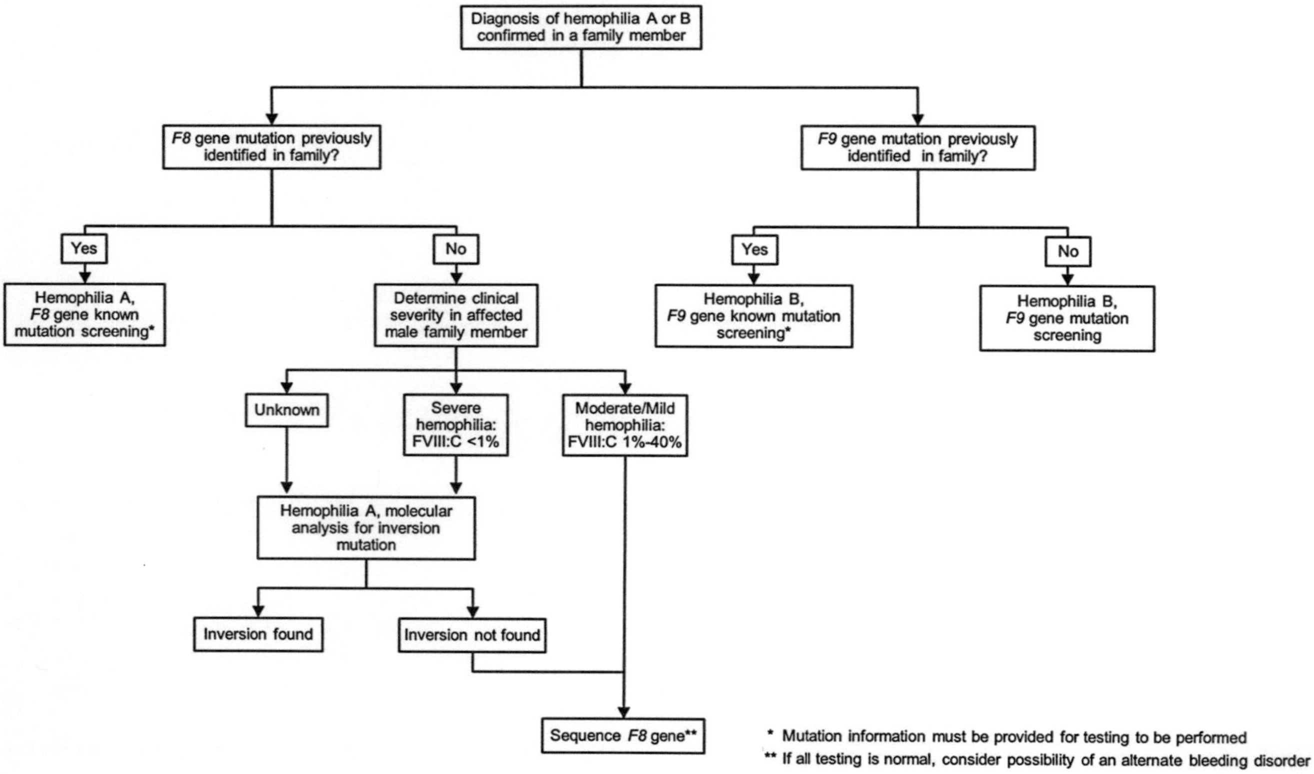

Figure 15.6 Hemophilia carrier testing algorithm: FVIII:C, FVIII activity; FIX:C, FIX activity; *F8*, FVIII gene; *F9*, factor IX gene. By permission of Mayo Foundation for Medical Education and Research. All rights reserved

mutation; typically, testing laboratories offer focused testing generically termed "known mutation analysis." If the familial mutation has not been identified, for symptomatic males with severe HA, initial testing is focused on the *F8* intron 22 inversion mutation and, if negative, the intron 1 inversion. For those with no detectable inversion mutation and for probands with moderate or mild HA, full gene analysis is required.

For at-risk females, a reduced FVIII:C confirms carrier status; however, a normal FVIII does not exclude HA carrier status, for which molecular testing is required. As with testing male patients, if the familial mutation is known, this information should be provided to the laboratory and testing should focus on the familial mutation (Fig. 15.6). For at-risk females without a known familial mutation, determining the clinical severity of hemophilia in an affected male family member will aid in a rational testing approach. Information on severity of the hemophilia may not be known to the at-risk female (especially if the proband was a distant relative). Communication with the local comprehensive hemophilia center that provided hemophilia care to the proband may be useful. For families with severe HA, initial testing is focused on the *F8* intron 22 inversion, and if negative, the intron 1 inversion. For those with no detectable inversion mutation and for families with moderate or mild HA, full *F8* gene analysis is required.

Identification of a causative mutation confirms the disease in symptomatic males, and carrier status in at-risk females. This carrier status confers a 50 % risk of each male child being affected with and a 50 % risk of each female child being a carrier for HA. All biological daughters of an affected male are obligate carriers. Lack of a detectable mutation in an at-risk female excludes carrier status if the familial mutation is known, but not if the familial mutation is unknown. Posttest counseling for a discussion on the aforementioned issues is vital in ensuring that the patient understands his or her own risk and the risk for offspring to be carriers of or affected with HA.

Interpretation of Test Results

Reduced FVIII:C is virtually diagnostic of HA, provided VWD and specimen artifact (see above) have been excluded. Rare instances of other genetic disorders that can have low FVIII activity include VWD type 2N (see section on VWD) and rare combined deficiencies of FV and FVIII. The latter occurs as a result of mutations in ERGIC-53, which is a protein necessary for efficient transport of FV and FVIII from the endoplasmic reticulum to the Golgi. FV and FVIII levels are typically in the 10–15 % range [13].

Detection of the presence of a deleterious mutation in a symptomatic male establishes the familial mutation and

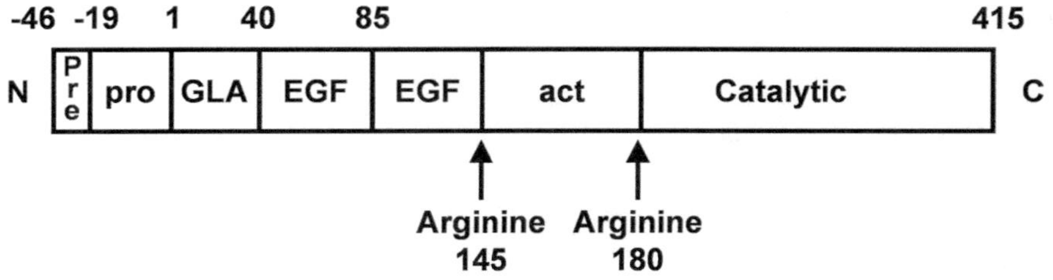

Figure 15.7 Factor IX peptide showing domains: *N* N-terminus, *C* C-terminus, *Pre* pre-propeptide, *pro* propeptide, *GLA* glutamic acid-rich domain, *EGF* epidermal growth factor domain, *act*, activation peptide

confirms carrier status in the at-risk female. Certain well-defined mutations (e.g., inversion, deletions, insertions, splice junction mutations, and nonsense mutations) have obviously deleterious effects. Determining the deleterious nature of previously uncharacterized missense mutations poses a challenge. However, identification of a variant of uncertain significance in hemizygous genes (*F8* and *F9*) in males without additional mutations provides reasonable evidence of its deleterious nature. Other criteria typically considered include genotype-phenotype correlation in the family if other family members are affected and tested, analysis of the degree of conservation of the respective residue among other species, and presence of a similar mutation in other patients. The best evidence of deleterious nature of a missense mutation is in vitro confirmation of its effect on protein function.

Laboratory Issues

As with any genetic test performed on peripheral blood leukocyte genomic DNA, high-quality DNA extracted from whole blood is essential. The specimen needs to be clearly identified and, given that testing is performed on peripheral blood leukocyte genomic DNA, history of allogeneic bone marrow or peripheral blood stem cell transplant needs to be provided. For testing performed on cord blood samples, a maternal peripheral blood sample should also be submitted for exclusion of maternal cell contamination of the cord blood which can cause incorrect test results.

Hemophilia B

Overview

HB is an X-linked recessive bleeding disorder due to a deficiency of FIX and is clinically indistinguishable from HA. HB affects 1 in 30,000 live male births across all ethnic groups. As with HA, up to 30 % of HB cases occur in families with no prior family history of HB. The diagnosis is established based on plasma FIX activity (FIX:C), which permits classification of HB disease severity as severe (<1 %), moderate (1–5 %), or mild (>5–40 %).

Molecular Basis of Disease

The factor IX gene (*F9*) is located on the long arm of the X chromosome (Xq27.1) and is 38 kb long with eight exons of varying lengths (25–1,935 bp). The *F9* mRNA is approximately 3 kb in length with a coding sequence of 1,390 nucleotides. The intron/exon boundaries roughly correlate with the FIX domains and bear a high degree of homology to members of the vitamin K-dependent protein family (FVII, FX, and protein C) (Fig. 15.7). The *F9* gene encodes a precursor protein of approximately 454 amino acids consisting of a propeptide followed by a glutamic acid-rich (Gla) domain, two epidermal growth factor domains, an activation peptide, and a catalytic domain.

Activation of FIX to FIXa occurs by cleavage by factor VIIa (FVIIa)-tissue factor (TF) and activated factor XI (FXIa). Cleavage releases the activation peptide, resulting in circulating light and heavy chains connected by a disulfide bond. Numerous posttranslational modifications are necessary for the normal function of FIXa, including tyrosine sulfation, serine phosphorylation, and *O*- and *N*-linked glycosylation. The relatively small size of the *F9* gene allows complete molecular testing, and mutations are catalogued in a database accessed at http://www.factorix.org.

Mutations in the *F9* Gene

The majority of *F9* mutations are single-base pair changes that result in missense, frameshift, or nonsense mutations. Short deletions (<30 nucleotides) account for approximately 7 %, larger deletions approximately 3 %, and insertions approximately 2 % of mutations. Many of the single-base pair changes occur at CpG doublets that are "hotspots" for mutation. However, a subset of recurrent mutations is due to a founder effect, which typically results in mild disease. Mutations have been detected in all regions of the *F9* gene, including the poly(A) signal.

Genotype-Phenotype Correlation

The numbering system for FIX peptide has evolved. The former numbering system was based on the Yoshitake numbering system [14] which is termed the legacy system in the FIX mutation database. An alternate and increasingly used system is the Human Genome Variation Society numbering system. The numbering system utilized in this chapter is the legacy system.

Missense mutations account for the majority of mutations that typically result in mild disease unless the mutations occur in residues critical for normal FIX function. Selected mutations in the promoter region of the *F9* gene result in a unique phenotype termed hemophilia B Leyden. This phenotype is characterized by severe disease at birth with progressive amelioration of severity through adolescence and puberty. However, some promoter mutations (e.g., Brandenburg mutation at −26) in the *F9* promoter result in lifelong severe disease. Nonsense mutations in the signal peptide and propeptide regions lead to severe HB. Selected missense changes, that lead to retention of FIX within hepatic cells (e.g., p.Ile-30 and p.Ile-19) or prevent cleavage of the propeptide, result in a dysfunctional FIX molecule (e.g., p.Arg-4) and result in hemophilia of varying severity (mild, moderate, or severe) depending on the amino acid substitution.

Mutations in the Gla domain disrupt γ-carboxylation (posttranslational modification) that is important for normal FIXa binding to collagen, activated platelets, and endothelial cells. Mutations in the EGF domains result in disruption of FIX binding to calcium that is essential for procoagulant activity, as well as impaired binding to its cofactor FVIII. Mutations in the catalytic domain typically disrupt the catalytic triad (p.His221, p.Asp269, and p.Ser365) essential for FIXa protease function.

An unusual FIX variant, due to mutation at p.Ala10, is characterized by normal baseline FIX:C. However, warfarin therapy results in a severe and disproportionate reduction in FIX:C (typically <1 %) and causes bleeding in patients being treated with warfarin who have an apparently therapeutic International Normalized Ratio. An indication of such a situation is a disproportionate prolongation of the activated partial thromboplastin time which should prompt testing for FIX:C levels. A second unusual variant, p.Arg338Leu (termed FIX Padua), results in a marked increase in FIX:C of up to 700 % of normal. In one case report, this mutation resulted in early-onset and recurrent VTE [15].

Polymorphisms in the *F9* Gene

Eight common polymorphisms that do not cause HB have been described in different ethnic populations of European and African descent. These polymorphisms, however, are much less common in Asian and other populations. The most informative polymorphism documented in the Asian population is what is termed the *Hha* I polymorphism (rs3117459 allele frequency = 0.17) located approximately 8 kb 3′ to *F9*. Recent reports [16] have described additional polymorphic loci in these populations, facilitating molecular diagnosis of non-Caucasian carriers and patients with HB. A polymorphism within the FIX-coding region, p.Ala148Thr, occurs within the activation peptide. This does not correlate with FIX activity or antigenic levels. The Thr allele occurs with a frequency of 0.3 in the Caucasian population; however, it is much less frequent in the African-American (0.053–0.15) and Asian (<0.01) populations.

Clinical Utility of Testing

The diagnosis of HB in a symptomatic patient is established by FIX:C testing, rather than by genetic testing. Given that FIX is a vitamin K-dependent protein, all patients with mild-to-moderate reductions in FIX activity should have vitamin K deficiency excluded. In addition, healthy normal children have a lower FIX activity that reaches adult reference ranges at puberty.

For the symptomatic male, knowledge of *F9* genotype does not alter clinical management of HB patients; however, the specific genotype may predict the risk of developing FIX inhibitors and anaphylaxis in response to FIX concentrate therapy [17]. Although knowledge of the proband's genotype information is important for carrier testing of at-risk female family members, the smaller size of the *F9* gene allows routine use of sequence analysis to identify the specific *F9* mutation causing HB. A reduced FIX:C in at-risk females typically confirms HB carrier status, provided that vitamin K deficiency has been excluded. However, normal FIX:C does not exclude the patient being a carrier. In this circumstance, molecular genetic testing would be the only option for diagnosis. See Fig. 15.5 for a recommended diagnostic testing algorithm for HB patients and Fig. 15.6 for recommended testing algorithm for HB carriers.

Available Assays

A listing of laboratories offering HB genetic testing that have registered with GeneTests can be found on their website (www.genetests.org). An alternative source is the NCBI Genetic Testing Registry (http://www.ncbi.nlm.nih.gov/gtr/). In general, testing can be divided into direct and indirect testing and selected laboratories offer prenatal testing.

Direct DNA Analysis

Generally, most patients with HB have mild disease. Since approximately 25 % of mild HB Caucasian patients have one of the three founder mutations (p.Gly60Ser, p.Ile397Thr, and p.Thr296Met) [18], a logical first step is to perform limited testing for these founder mutations. For symptomatic patients without one of the founder mutations, for severely affected patients, and for individuals at risk of being an HB carrier, the logical next step is *F9* gene mutation screening or sequencing regions of functional significance in the *F9* gene. Although the majority of HB patients have one deleterious mutation, approximately 1 % of HB patients have two mutations. Additional limitations of molecular testing as described in the section above on HA also apply for HB.

Indirect DNA Analysis (Linkage Analysis)

As discussed above for HA, indirect DNA analysis of an HB proband does not identify the familial mutation. Linkage analysis does assign a haplotype which identifies the abnormal *F9* gene and is useful for carrier testing of family members. Given the small size of the *F9* gene, direct sequencing is also feasible for carrier testing when the HB mutation is not a large *F9* gene deletion. As discussed in the section on HA, such mutations may be detected by MLPA.

Testing Algorithm

Pre- and posttest genetic counseling is critical for overall patient management. See section on HA above. A reduced, age-appropriate, FIX:C confirms the diagnosis of HB, provided that vitamin K deficiency or use of vitamin K antagonists (e.g., warfarin) can be excluded. The FIX:C level allows classification of the severity of disease as severe (<1 %), moderate (1–5 %), or mild (>5–40 %). If FIX:C is not reduced, consider testing for an alternate bleeding disorder, such as HA or VWD.

The preanalytical issues regarding knowledge of the familial mutation, as discussed in the section on HA above, also apply to HB. Thus, for probands or at-risk carriers with an identified familial mutation, focused testing is reasonable. If the familial mutation is not known or not available, *F9* gene sequencing is the most appropriate approach.

Interpretation of Test Results

See section on HA above.

Laboratory Issues

See section on HA above.

von Willebrand Disease

Overview

VWD is an autosomal dominant or recessive disorder characterized by a deficiency of VWF. VWD is the most commonly recognized congenital bleeding disorder, with a prevalence of 0.82–2 % [19]. Diagnosis is established based on a personal and family history of abnormal clinical bleeding and reduced plasma VWF antigen levels and/or functional activity (ristocetin cofactor activity), and analysis of the size distribution of the VWF multimers.

Molecular Basis of Disease

The *VWF* gene is located near the end of the short arm of human chromosome 12, spans 180 kb, and consists of 52 exons. The intron-exon boundaries roughly correlate with the VWF domains. The presence of an unprocessed partial pseudogene located on chromosome 22q11.2 corresponds to exons 23–34 of the *VWF* gene. VWF is synthesized in endothelial cells and megakaryocytes and is secreted from its storage sites (platelet alpha granule and endothelial cell Weibel-Palade bodies) into plasma. VWF is a 2,813-amino acid peptide consisting of a 22-amino acid signal peptide, a 741-amino acid propeptide, and a mature 2,050-amino acid VWF protein (Fig. 15.8). After removal of the signal peptide, the pro-VWF dimerizes by disulfide bonds at the C-terminal

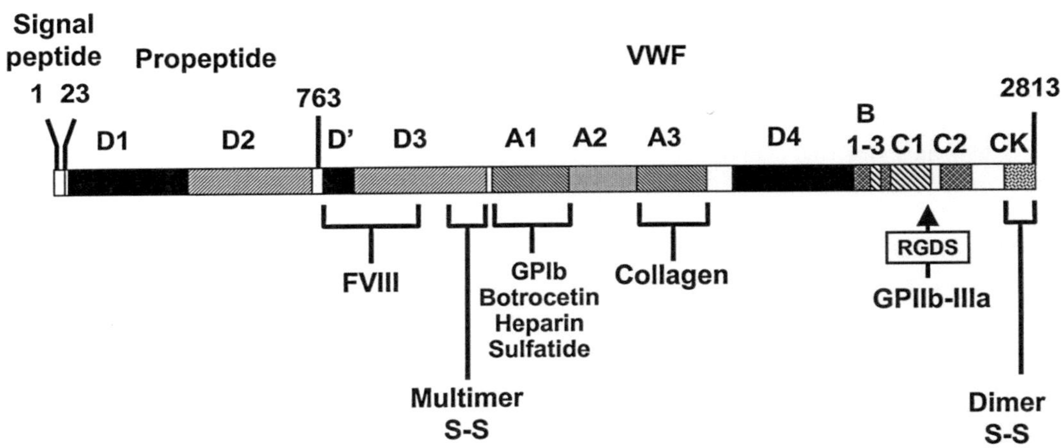

Figure 15.8 von Willebrand peptide domains: *FVIII* factor VIII, *S-S* disulphide bridge, *GPIb* glycoprotein Ib, *VWF* von Willebrand factor, *GPIIb–IIIa* glycoprotein IIb–IIIa, *RGDS* arginine (R), glycine (G), aspartic acid (D), serine (S)-binding sequence. Reprinted with permission from Sadler AJE. Von Willebrand disease. In Scriver, CR, Beaudet al, Valle D, et al., eds. The metabolic and molecular basis of inherited disease. Copyright 2001 McGraw-Hill

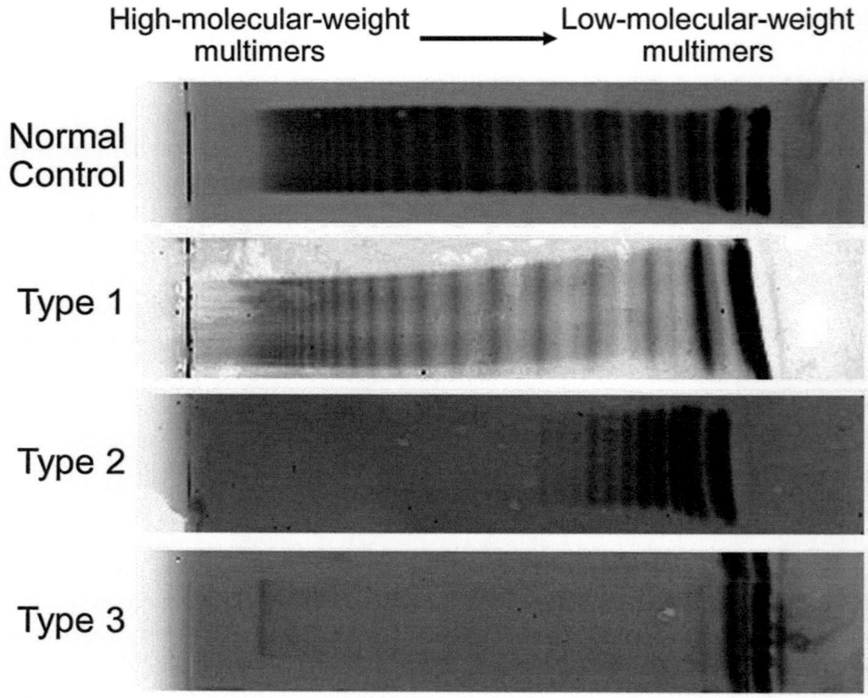

Figure 15.9 VWF multimer distribution: The protein gel demonstrates the size distribution of VWF multimers in a normal control and the three types of VWD. Type 1 has reduced multimers of normal size distribution, type 2 has reduced highest and intermediate molecular weight multimers, and type 3 lacks all multimers

ends and further polymerizes between the N-terminal ends resulting in multimers ranging in size from 500 kDa to over 10 million daltons. Binding sites for various ligands have been localized to different domains of the VWF subunit.

VWD can be divided into two broad categories based on quantitative (types 1 and 3) or qualitative (type 2) abnormalities of plasma VWF. Quantitative abnormalities include a mild reduction of qualitatively normal VWF (type 1) or absent VWF (type 3). Type 2 VWD is characterized by plasma VWF with defective structure and function, and typically results in the absence or reduction of the larger VWF multimers (Fig. 15.9).

Previously identified mutations and polymorphisms in the *VWF* gene are available in an international database at http://www.sheffield.ac.uk/VWF/.

Type 1 von Willebrand Disease

Type 1 VWD, which accounts for approximately 85 % of VWD cases in the USA, is typically autosomal dominant. Diagnosis is established by assays of VWF demonstrating proportionate reduction in plasma VWF antigen (VWF:Ag), ristocetin cofactor activity (VWF:RCo), and factor VIII activity (FVIII:C) with a normal distribution of VWF multimers. Although the most commonly diagnosed variant of VWD, the molecular pathogenesis of type 1 continues to be elucidated. Currently, apart from a few sporadic reports, few clearly deleterious *VWF* mutations have been identified in type 1 VWD. Although type 1 VWD appears to be linked to the *VWF* locus, animal data suggests locus heterogeneity as an explanation for the mild quantitative deficiency of VWF associated with type 1 VWD, e.g., defects in glycosylation of the VWF protein [20]. Selected patients with type 1 VWD are a result of heterozygous inheritance of a VWD type 3 defect which includes nonsense, frameshift, or deletion mutations; however, emerging information demonstrates a completely different mutation spectrum from VWD type 3, discussed below. A unique variant, type 1 Vicenza, is characterized by the presence of ultralarge VWF multimers with increased clearance from the circulation, and is due to a unique mutation p.Arg1205His in the D3 domain.

Type 1 VWD has heterogeneous clinical manifestations with variable penetrance that may be due to concordant or discordant reductions in platelet VWF. Some pedigrees are characterized by significant reductions in VWF levels which may be due to defects in multimer synthesis or secretion.

Type 3 von Willebrand Disease

Type 3 VWD, which accounts for approximately 5 % of VWD cases in the USA, is autosomal recessive and characterized by a severe reduction in VWF:Ag, VWF:RCo, and a concordant reduction in FVIII:C resulting in a more severe bleeding phenotype. Deleterious mutations include frameshifts, deletions, and nonsense mutations. Although most patients are typically compound heterozygous for such VWF mutations, homozygosity has been demonstrated in a few consanguineous families. Although most patients with type 3 VWD have two defective *VWF* alleles, many have clinically unaffected parents. Assays of VWF may be normal or exhibit only mild abnormalities. Full gene analysis would be required to document heterozygous carrier state. This poses a challenge in providing genetic counseling, due to the possibility of new mutations.

The prevalence of type 3 VWD is 0.5–3 per million and based on the Hardy-Weinberg equilibrium, heterozygotes should occur at an expected frequency of at least 1,400–3,500 per million population. However, the currently estimated prevalence of symptomatic type 1 VWD is at least tenfold lower. This discrepancy may be due to a distinct molecular pathogenesis of type 1 VWD compared to type 3 VWD (outlined above) or variable phenotypic expression of type 1 VWD. Although VWF levels may be lower in parents of patients with type 3 VWD, there is a variable expression with most parents being asymptomatic.

Type 2 von Willebrand Disease

Type 2 variants of VWD, which account for approximately 10 % of VWD cases in the USA, are characterized by qualitatively abnormal VWF with defective stability, function, or multimer distribution and include types 2A, B, N, and M. In general, mutations are well characterized and may disrupt dimerization, multimerization, impaired secretion, or increased susceptibility to proteolysis.

Type 2A von Willebrand Disease

Type 2A VWD is autosomal dominant and accounts for approximately 75 % of all type 2 VWD. There is a variable reduction in VWF antigen, with a discordant reduction in VWF:RCo, indicative of a qualitative VWF abnormality. The higher and intermediate plasma VWF multimers are reduced or absent, and the lower molecular weight multimers are relatively increased or have an abnormal infrastructure. Plasma and platelet multimer abnormalities may be concordant or discordant depending on the underlying molecular defect.

Missense mutations resulting in type 2A VWD occur predominantly in the A2 domain of VWF and result in abnormal VWF patterns by two distinct mechanisms. The first mechanism includes impairing the assembly and secretion of normal VWF multimers, resulting in decreased higher molecular weight VWF multimers in both plasma and platelets. The second mechanism includes normal assembly and secretion of VWF; however, the mutant VWF has an increased sensitivity to proteolytic degradation in plasma resulting in decreased plasma high-molecular-weight multimers but a normal platelet VWF multimer pattern.

Type 2B von Willebrand Disease

Type 2B VWD is autosomal dominant and accounts for approximately 20 % of all type 2 VWD. Type 2B is characterized by a variable reduction in the VWF:Ag, a discordant reduction in VWF:RCo with a loss of the higher and intermediate plasma VWF multimers, but normal distribution of platelet VWF multimers. Type 2B is distinguished from type 2A VWD by the presence of mild-to-moderate thrombocytopenia. This occurs as a result of an increased affinity of VWF for platelet GPIb, resulting in spontaneous binding of VWF to platelets and rapid clearance of the platelet-bound larger multimers from plasma. In addition, platelet aggregation in response to ristocetin demonstrates an exaggerated response. The few cases described of normal multimer distribution with hyperresponsiveness to ristocetin appear to represent a mild form of the type 2B defect. Causative missense mutations are found in the A domain of VWF and result in a dominant gain-of-function phenotype. Mutations in this region likely disrupt a regulatory site that normally inhibits the binding of the A1 domain to platelet GPIb.

Type 2B VWD must be distinguished from a pseudo-VWD or platelet-type VWD, which is similar in presentation. The latter group of patients has a primary platelet defect resulting from mutations in the platelet GPIb/IX receptor.

Type 2M von Willebrand Disease

In type 2M VWD, although the VWF:Ag and the distribution of VWF multimers are normal, the VWF:RCo is reduced, reflecting a functional defect of the VWF multimers. Mutations in the A1 domain of VWF can result in decreased binding affinity for platelet GPIb and thus a reduced VWF:RCo. However, not all reduced VWF:RCo represents VWD. A recent description of a polymorphism in the A1 domain, p.Asp1472His, found in 63 % of the African-American normal control population and 17 % of the Caucasian normal control population, results in a lower VWF:RCo in carriers of the mutation compared to noncarriers. Carriers of this mutation did not have bleeding symptoms [21].

Type 2N (Normandy) von Willebrand Disease

Mutations in the FVIII-binding domain of VWF result in suboptimal binding of FVIII to VWF. This binding defect results in a shorter half-life of plasma FVIII and thus plasma FVIII:C is reduced. Levels of VWF:Ag and VWF:RCo are normal as is the plasma VWF multimer distribution. This subtype mimics mild HA; however it is distinguished by an autosomal recessive pattern of inheritance rather than the X-linked recessive pattern of HA. In a recent international survey, type 2N VWD was detected in 4.8 % (58/1,198) of patients previously diagnosed as having mild HA. Three *VWF* gene mutations (p.Thr791Met, p.Arg816Trp, and p.Arg854Gln) accounted for 96 % of type 2N patients [22]. Type 2N VWD should be considered in patients with a diagnosis of "mild HA" with a non-X-linked inheritance pattern. Typically, heterozygotes have normal FVIII:C and homozygotes have reduced FVIII:C. However, apparent heterozygotes with low FVIII:C typically have inherited a second allele resulting in type 1 VWD (compound heterozygotes).

Clinical Utility of Testing

Currently, the most significant impact on clinical management and genetic counseling is the differentiation of type 2N VWD and mild HA. Both have a mild-to-moderate reduction in FVIII with normal levels of VWF:Ag and VWF:RCo. The autosomal inheritance pattern and the need for use of VWF concentrates in patients with VWD2N, rather than pure FVIII concentrates, make this an important distinction.

Differentiation of type 2A from 2B VWD alters clinical management, since therapeutic use of vasopressin (DDAVP) is contraindicated in patients with type 2B VWD given the potential for worsening the thrombocytopenia. Patients with type 2B VWD can have variable degrees of thrombocytopenia, such that a clear distinction between types 2A and 2B is not always possible based on platelet levels alone.

Currently, genetic testing is not useful for type 1 VWD, given its mild phenotype, the lack of well-characterized mutations, and the implication of locus heterogeneity. In contrast, type 3 VWD has well-characterized mutations and a severe phenotype. Although genotyping the index patient of a family would likely not affect their clinical management, the genotype would be useful for genetic counseling and prenatal diagnosis of the parents in anticipation of future pregnancies.

Available Assays

Functional assays that measure FVIII binding to VWF are available in selected laboratories and are considered the initial test of choice. Molecular testing confirms the genotype, but mutations are not consistently found in all patients with binding defects. Tests available include assays for determining the molecular basis of type 2N, and types 2A and 2B. Methods include restriction fragment length polymorphism analysis or direct sequencing. Indirect testing is available for VWD; however it is rarely indicated except for severe type 3 VWD. The laboratories offering such testing are listed with GeneTests and can be found on their website (genetests.org). An alternative source is the Genetic Testing Registry at http://www.ncbi.nim.nih.gov/gtr.

Interpretation of Test Results

Detection of mutation(s) in the FVIII-binding domains of *VWF* in a homozygous state is good evidence of the deleterious effect on protein function and presence of type 2N VWD. However, not all mutations have been characterized at a structural level and thus need to be viewed with caution. The presence of a heterozygous mutation in the setting of a low FVIII:C could reflect the presence of a second mutation in *VWF* (compound heterozygote). Although most known mutations in type 2A and 2B VWD are clustered within exon 28 of the *VWF* gene, type 2 variants with mutations outside this domain have been described.

Laboratory Issues

The large size of the *VWF* gene precludes efficient, cost-effective screening or sequencing on a clinical basis. In addition, (co)amplification of the unprocessed pseudogene, homologous to exons 23–34 of *VWF* gene, complicates mutational analysis of PCR products amplified from genomic DNA. However, use of primers designed specifically to amplify the *VWF* gene and not the pseudogene reduces this risk. Mutation analysis of mRNA on a research basis has been performed, but likely is not practical for clinical testing given the instability of mRNA in transported specimens; however current availability of stabilizing agents may make this a viable option. At the present time, mRNA-based sequencing is not available for clinical testing.

Inherited Thrombophilias

The term "thrombophilia" refers to hereditary or acquired disorders or clinical circumstances that are risk factors for venous or arterial thrombosis. Broadly speaking, within the coagulation system, predisposition to thrombosis can be caused by deficiencies of the anticoagulant and fibrinolytic components or unbridled activity of the procoagulant system. The known hereditary thrombophilia disorders are well-established risk factors for venous thrombosis and its complication, pulmonary embolism, which together are called VTE; however, although biologically plausible, the association of the hereditary thrombophilia disorders with arterial thrombosis is less well established.

The recognized plasma components of the anticoagulant system include antithrombin (AT), protein C (PC), and protein S (PS); the fibrinolytic system includes plasminogen and its activating proteins, plasminogen activator inhibitors 1 and 2 (PAI-1 and -2), as well as alpha-2 antiplasmin. The procoagulant system consists of members of the coagulation cascade (Fig. 15.1). Two key hemostasis regulatory proteins, factors V (FV) and VIII (FVIII), once activated to FV_a and $FVIII_a$, function as cofactors that markedly accelerate the rate of thrombin generation and fibrin thrombus formation. Thus, inactivation of these cofactors markedly downregulates thrombin generation (Fig. 15.10).

PC, a vitamin K-dependent zymogen, circulates in an inactive form and, for its anticoagulant activity, requires activation to activated protein C (APC). This activation occurs by the thrombin-thrombomodulin complex. Thrombomodulin is an integral membrane protein on the luminal surface of endothelial cells that binds circulating thrombin and changes its substrate specificity such that thrombin no longer cleaves fibrinogen nor activates platelets. Instead, thrombomodulin-bound thrombin activates PC to APC, which in turn exerts its

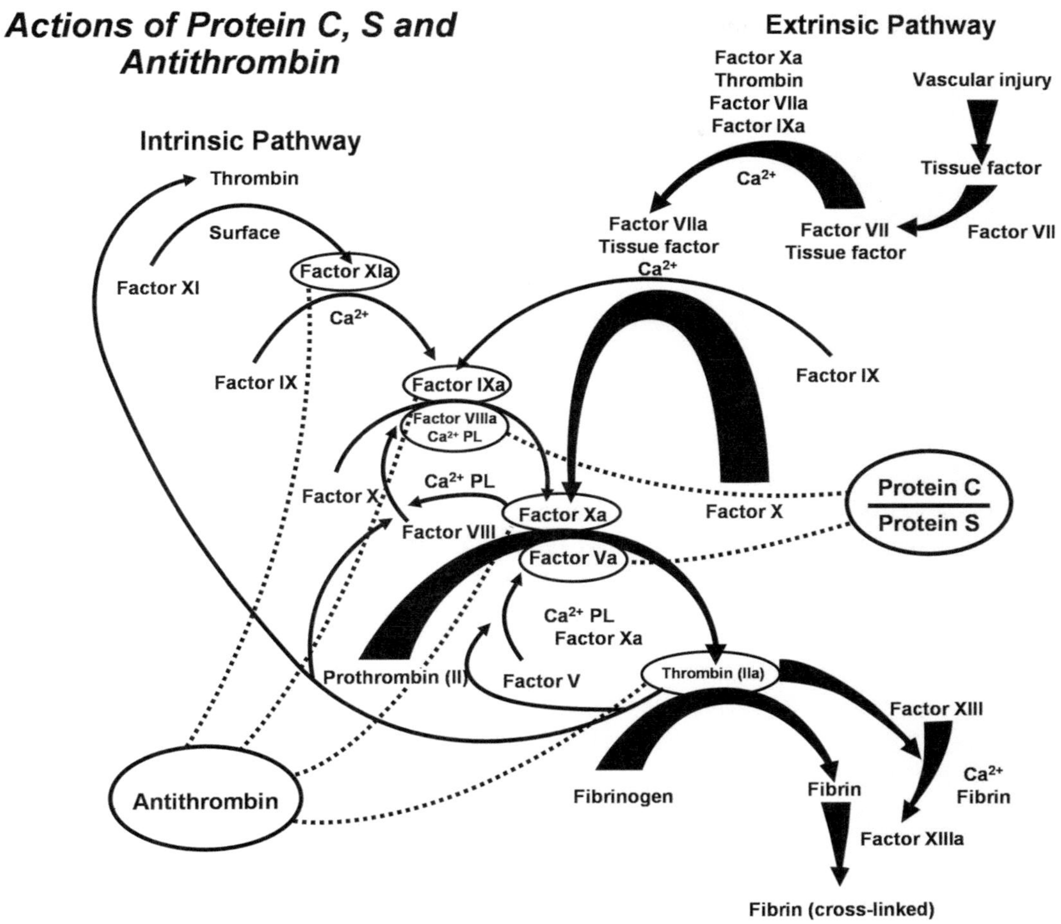

Figure 15.10 Sites of action of protein C, protein S, and antithrombin within the coagulation cascade: *a* activated factor; *Ca2+* calcium; *PL* phospholipid. Reprinted with permission from Davie EW, Fujikawa K, Kisiel W. The coagulation cascade: initiation, maintenance and regulation. Biochemistry. 1991;30:10363. Copyright 1991 American Chemical Society

anticoagulant activity by inactivating (via enzymatic cleavage) FV_a and $FVIII_a$ in the presence of PS.

AT is a serine protease inhibitor (SERPIN) and acts as a pseudo-substrate to irreversibly inhibit thrombin and procoagulant factors IX_a, X_a, XI_a, and XII_a by covalently binding the enzymatic active sites. AT anticoagulant activity is markedly enhanced by glycosaminoglycans (e.g., heparin).

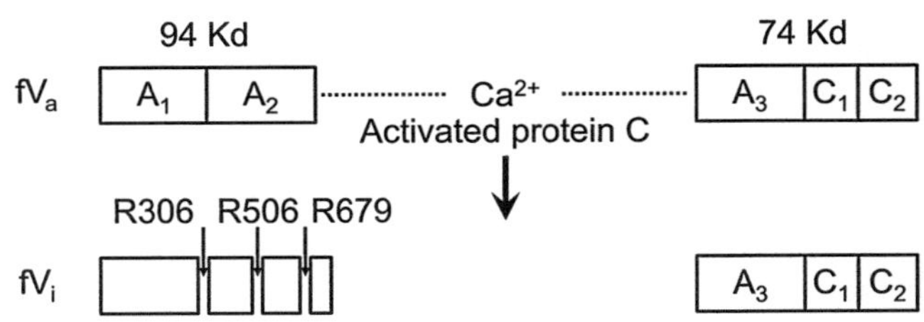

Figure 15.11 Cleavage sites for inactivation of activated factor V. *Ca2+* calcium, *FVa* activated factor V, *FVi* inactivated factor V, *Kd* kilodalton, *R* arginine, *thin arrows* cleavage sites. Reprinted with permission from Mayo Clinic

Activated Protein C Resistance Due to Factor V Leiden Mutation

Molecular Basis of Disease

APC inactivates FV_a by cleavage at two sites on FV. Described using legacy nomenclature (amino acid numbering starts 28 amino acids after standard HGVS nomenclature), an initial cleavage at arginine (R) 506 of FV_a facilitates subsequent cleavage at positions R306 and R679 (in the presence of phospholipid and PS) resulting in inactivation of FV_a (Fig. 15.11). Hereditary resistance to inactivation of FV_a by APC, termed activated protein C resistance (APCR), is an autosomal dominant condition and occurs as a result of a single-point mutation, guanine (G) to adenine (A) at the 1,691 nucleotide (G1691A) within exon 10 of the *F5* gene [called factor V Leiden (FVL), *F5* rs6025] on chromosome 1 (1q21-25) [23]. HGVS nomenclature describes the factor V Leiden mutation as *F5*:c1601G>A, p.Arg534Gln (p.R534Q).

This mutation encodes for substitution of a glutamine (Gln, Q) for arginine (Arg, R) at amino acid position 506 within the heavy chain of FV, one of the three APC-cleavage sites (R306, R506, R679). FVL promotes thrombosis by impaired downregulation of thrombin generation and by inhibition of fibrinolysis.

FVL is a founder mutation, arising between 21,000 and 34,000 years ago and after the evolutionary divergence of Africans from non-Africans and of Caucasoid from Mongoloid subpopulations. Worldwide, the FVL carrier frequency ranges from 2 % in Southern Europe to 15 % in Southern Sweden, and generally declines in native populations as one moves from west to east toward Asia, Africa, and Australasia. In the USA, about 3–7 % of asymptomatic white populations of northern European or Scandinavian ancestry are heterozygous carriers. FVL is much less common in other US populations, with a carrier frequency of 1.2 % in African Americans, 2.2 % in Hispanics, 1.2 % in Native Americans, and 0.45 % in Asian Americans.

Clinical Utiltity of Factor V Leiden Testing

Most patients with FVL go through their lives with no clinical events. For those developing clinical sequelae, VTE is the most common clinical presentation. The initial observations of an association with pregnancy-related complications, such as recurrent fetal loss, preeclampsia, and abruption, are currently being questioned [24].

Guidelines on FVL testing continue to evolve [25–27]. Currently, FVL testing is not recommended as a newborn or general population screen, nor is it indicated in asymptomatic prepubescent children, in patients with arterial thrombotic events, or as a risk stratification tool for deciding on type and duration of thromboprophylaxis. Routine testing prior to pregnancy or oral contraceptive use was not found to be cost effective [27]; however, in contrast to no testing, testing was felt to be cost effective prior to hormonal replacement therapy in postmenopausal women, but impact on overall patient management needs to be considered [27].

Testing for FVL may impact clinical management in patients with a history of recurrent VTE; a first VTE before 50 years of age; a first unprovoked VTE at any age; a first VTE at an unusual anatomic site such as the cerebral, mesenteric, portal, or hepatic veins; and a first VTE at any age in a subject with a first-degree family member with a VTE before age 50 years. However, a careful analysis of the impact on patient management should be considered.

Testing for FVL is controversial in young (age <50 years) women smokers with a myocardial infarction; older patients (age >50 years) with a first provoked VTE in the absence of cancer or an intravascular device; or a first VTE related to selective estrogen receptor modulators (SERMs).

After appropriate counseling, testing for FVL may also be indicated in asymptomatic adult family members of probands with known FVL, especially those with a strong family history of thrombosis at a young age (<50 years) and asymptomatic female family members that are pregnant or are considering oral contraceptives or pregnancy.

Available Assays

In most circumstances, a functional assay of plasma APCR is the preferred initial test. In the most commonly used assay, the patient's plasma is first mixed with FV-deficient plasma that contains a heparin neutralizer. The addition of the FV-deficient plasma corrects for deficiencies of other coagulation proteins and may dilute the effect of some lupus-like anticoagulants. The assay is essentially 100 % sensitive and specific for FVL and accurately distinguishes heterozygotes from homozygotes. This assay is unaffected by heparin or warfarin anticoagulation; however, it may still not be diagnostic if the baseline aPTT (after mixing with FV-deficient plasma) still is prolonged due to a lupus anticoagulant or a specific factor inhibitor. Moreover, the assay will miss patients with acquired APCR. Each laboratory must establish the normal range for this assay based on their patient population.

Direct DNA-based testing for FVL is widely available for diagnosis. Commonly used molecular methods involve PCR amplification of the region surrounding the mutation, followed by RFLP analysis, allele-specific PCR amplification, or allele-specific hybridization. Semiautomated assay methods include fluorescence detection of PCR products with allele-specific hybridization probes, and non-PCR signal amplification methods based on either enzymatic hybridization mismatch recognition using fluorescent allele-specific probes or linked fluorescent allele-specific pyrophosphorolysis-kinase reactions [26]. Each laboratory must insure that its method can distinguish FVL from an uncommon polymorphism A1696G.

Counseling Issues and Management

Pre- and post-test counseling should take into account the indications for testing and the potential impact on patient management. VTE is the most common known clinical consequence of APCR due to FVL. Given that VTE is a multifactorial disease, specific issues to review in women are the interaction of the FVL with oral contraceptives, pregnancy, hormonal replacement therapy, and use of SERM therapy (e.g., tamoxifen, raloxifene). Other environmental risk factors that interact with FVL include hospitalization (with or without surgery), nursing home care, trauma, malignant neoplasms (with or without chemotherapy), central venous catheterization, or a transvenous pacemaker, and serious neurologic disease with extremity paresis or paralysis [28].

Incidence of Venous Thromboembolism

The annual incidence of VTE in the general population (noncarriers of FVL) is approximately 1 per 1,000 person-years (0.1 % per year) and increases with age [28]. FVL prevalence among incident VTE cases varies from 12 to 50 %. In addition, individuals who are heterozygous for FVL have an eight-fold relative increased risk of VTE, while individuals with homozygous FVL have an 80- to 100-fold increased risk. In absolute terms, the data can be summarized as follows: individuals who are FVL heterozygous have a lifetime probability of developing VTE by age 65 years from 2.4 % [29] to 6 % [30] and the annual VTE incidence is 0.45 % [25].

VTE Risk with Oral Contraceptive Use

Depending on the study design, the relative increased risk of VTE is reported to vary from approximately 5- to 30-fold among women who are FVL heterozygous and taking oral contraceptives [27]. In absolute terms, the incidence of VTE among women of childbearing age who are not carriers of FVL and are not on oral contraceptives is approximately 1 per 10,000 woman-years [31], and that risk is increased about three-fold (to an incidence of 3 per 10,000 woman-years) among women taking oral contraceptives. Among women of childbearing age who are FVL heterozygous, the incidence of VTE is about 6 per 100,000 woman-years, and increased to approximately 30 per 100,000 woman-years when also taking oral contraceptives. While this represents a 30-fold relative risk, the incidence is still only 0.3 % per year (i.e., 99.7 % of carriers on oral contraceptives will not develop VTE during that year). In more recent studies, the annual absolute risk of VTE has been approximated to 0.35 per 100 person-years [32]. The acceptability of this mild increase in risk compared to the benefits of oral contraceptive use will vary with each patient.

VTE Risk During Pregnancy and Postpartum Period

The OR for VTE during pregnancy and the postpartum period is approximately 8-fold for women who are FVL heterozygous and 34-fold for women who are FVL homozygous [27]. This translates to an absolute annual incidence of 1.97 per 100 pregnancy-years for women who are heterozygous for FVL, compared to an annual incidence of 0.73 per 100 pregnancy-years for women without FVL [32].

Interaction with Postmenopausal Hormone Replacement Use

Postmenopausal women heterozygous for FVL had an OR for VTE of up to 15-fold higher when receiving estrogen replacement therapy. Given the baseline increased risk of VTE with age, this translated into an annual incidence of >1 % in this population of patients.

Interaction with Age

The incidence of VTE among individuals with FVL also varies by age, ranging from 2–3 per 1,000 person-years for ages 15–30 years to 7–11 per 1,000 person-years for age 60 years and older.

Impact on Patient Management

Empiric anticoagulation therapy is not recommended for asymptomatic FVL carriers; however, appropriate prophylaxis should be prescribed for medical and surgical hospitalizations [33–35]. The indication and type of VTE prophylaxis should not be based on results of thrombophilia testing. FVL carriers with acute VTE should receive standard anticoagulation therapy [36]. Given that VTE recurs frequently, with an estimated cumulative recurrence of 30 % by 10 years [28], research efforts are focused on determining predictive recurrence risk factors. Independent predictors of recurrence include older age, obesity, malignant neoplasm, and extremity paresis or paralysis. The recurrence risk in the presence of hereditary thrombophilia varies by study and thrombophilia type.

Although studies are conflicting, individuals who are FVL heterozygous are not felt to be at increased risk of recurrent VTE compared to non-carriers; however, this risk is significantly increased for individuals who are both heterozygous FVL and heterozygous prothrombin G20210A, and in individuals who are homozygous FVL. Recommendations on short- and long-term management of VTE have recently been reviewed [36].

Pre- and posttest counseling and the decision to perform thrombophilia testing in eligible women prior to prescribing oral contraception or hormone replacement therapy require a detailed discussion with the patients regarding their comfort level with the risk of VTE which needs to be balanced against the benefits of the prescribed hormones. Currently, FVL testing is not advised for pregnancy-associated complications other than VTE [24]. Prophylactic anticoagulation in pregnant, asymptomatic FVL carriers with no prior history of VTE is not routinely recommended. Decisions about providing prophylaxis should be individualized based on the FVL genotype (heterozygous vs homozygous) and coexisting risk factors. Asymptomatic women who do not receive anticoagulation should be followed closely throughout pregnancy and given prophylaxis during the postpartum period.

Prothrombin G20210GA Mutation

Molecular Basis of Disease

The prothrombin G20210A (*F2* G20210A, HGVS: c.*97G>A) mutation is a relatively common mutation that affects the 3′ terminal nucleotide of the 3′ untranslated region of *F2* [37]. The *F2* G20210A mutation causes a gain of function due to increased recognition of the polyadenylation cleavage signal, increased 3′ end RNA processing, mRNA accumulation, and increased protein synthesis [38]. A family-based study has shown close linkage between a quantitative trait locus determining plasma prothrombin activity and the *F2* G20210A mutation [39]. Plasma prothrombin concentration is a major determinant of plasma thrombin generation potential; thus, thrombin generation is increased in the plasma of individuals either heterozygous or homozygous for the *F2* G20210A mutation. High plasma prothrombin levels also inhibit APC-mediated inactivation of procoagulant factor V_a, further augmenting thrombin production. Although carriers of the *F2* G20210A mutation have higher median plasma prothrombin levels compared to non-carriers, there is considerable overlap of the range of prothrombin levels; thus, molecular testing is the only option for diagnosis of this thrombophilia disorder.

Based on haplotype analyses, the *F2* G20210A mutation also appears to be a founder mutation, arising 20,000–30,000 years ago and after the divergence of Africans from non-Africans and of Caucasoid from Mongoloid subpopulations. In Europe, the overall carrier frequency is 2 %, ranging from 1.7 % in northern Europe to 3 % in southern Europe. In the USA, the estimated overall carrier frequency is 1–2 %. The mutation is uncommon among African Americans and rarely seen among Asian Americans and Native Americans [40].

Clinical Utility of F2 G20210A Testing

As with FVL, the majority of patients with *F2* G20210A will go through their lives with no clinical events. For those developing clinical sequelae, the most common clinical presentation is VTE. Although initial studies suggested an association with pregnancy-related complications, e.g., recurrent fetal loss, preeclampsia, and abruption, currently this association is being questioned and testing is not recommended [24]. Recommendations for *F2* G20210A mutation testing and patient management are essentially the same as for FVL.

Available Assays

Although *F2* G20210A carriers have statistically higher plasma prothrombin activity, the normal range for plasma prothrombin activity is quite broad. Thus, plasma prothrombin activity cannot accurately distinguish *F2* G20210A carriers from non-carriers. Direct DNA-based testing for the specific mutation is required for diagnosis. Molecular testing methods available for the *F2* G20210A mutation are essentially the same as for FVL. Each laboratory must ensure that its method can distinguish the *F2* G20210A from an uncommon polymorphism at nucleotide *F2* C20209T, which is prevalent among the African-American population but is not associated with VTE.

Counseling Issues and Management

Issues pertaining to *F2* G20210A mutation and interactions with environmental risk factors for VTE are similar to those with FVL (see above). The *F2* G20210A mutation is a weaker risk factor for VTE, so the risk estimates and incidence of VTE are lower. Selected unique features of *F2* G20210A are as follows. Female *F2* G20210A carriers receiving oral contraception have an approximate 6-fold increased risk for deep vein thrombosis or VTE [27], and a 150-fold increased risk of cerebral vein thrombosis. The available data suggests that the absolute risk of VTE with oral contraceptive use or pregnancy is similar to that with FVL. No detailed studies are available on the risk of VTE in association with hormone replacement therapy; however the risks are likely similar to those for FVL.

Impact on Patient Management

Issues pertaining to patient management in carriers of *F2* G20210A are similar to those for FVL (see above).

Deficiencies of Anticoagulant Proteins

Molecular Basis of Disease

Genetic deficiencies of plasma AT, PC, or PS activity to approximately half of normal plasma activity are strongly associated with VTE. Altogether, deficiency of AT, PC, or PS is found in less than 10 % of patients with VTE. Comparing family members with inherited AT, PC, or PS deficiency to family members with no defect, the lifetime relative VTE risk is increased about seven- to eight-fold. Individuals who are homozygous or compound heterozygous for PC or PS mutations may develop severe full-thickness dermal and limb thrombotic infarction as neonatalis (called purpura fulminans neonatalis). Homozygous AT deficiency appears to be incompatible with life except for mutations that impair heparin binding to AT.

The AT gene, *SERPINCI*, is located at chromosome 1q23-q25, and mutations lead to type I (reduced antigen and activity) or type II (reduced activity and normal antigen) AT deficiency. Type II can be subdivided into reactive site (RS) mutations, heparin-binding site (HBS) mutations, and pleiotropic effect (PE) mutations. Reported mutations are catalogued in the AT mutation database at http://www.hgmd.cf.ac.uk/ac/index.php.

Mutations in the PC gene, *PROC*, located on chromosome 2q13-q21, lead to type I and II defects, as with AT deficiency. Reported *PROC* mutations are catalogued in the PC mutation database at http://www.hgmd.cf.ac.uk/ac/index.php.

The gene encoding PS, *PROS1*, is located on chromosome 3p11.1-q11.2. A homologous pseudogene, (*PROSP*) is approximately 95 % homologous to the *PROS1* gene. PS deficiency is classified into type 1 (reduced free and total PS antigen and activity), type II (normal total and free PS antigen and reduced PS activity), and type III (normal total reduced free PS antigen).

Clinical Utility of Testing

Although rare, patients with deficiency of PC, PS, or AT are at high lifetime risk of VTE with approximately 50 % of patients developing VTE by 50 years of age. Once symptomatic VTE has occurred, such patients are at a high lifetime risk of recurrent VTE (approximately 10 % per year) in the absence of anticoagulation. Testing patients who are young, have a strong family history of VTE, or experience a recurrent VTE is useful.

Avazilable Assays

Mutations causing impaired expression or function of AT, PC, or PS are rare and spread throughout their respective genes. Moreover, there are few data correlating specific mutations with a unique clinical thrombosis phenotype. Thus, for diagnosis, functional testing of plasma activities of AT, PC, or PS is preferred over genetic testing. Selected laboratories may offer gene sequencing on a research basis.

Recommendations for Testing

Given that knowledge of genotype-to-phenotype correlation is still developing, at the present time, genetic testing for PC, PS, and AT deficiency is not routinely recommended. Functional and antigenic assays for the proteins (AT, PC, and PS) should be the initial tests. It is important to remember that these proteins are produced in the liver; thus, patients with advanced liver diseases will have reduced levels. In addition, reference ranges for neonatalis are lower than those for adults. Finally, given that PC and PS are vitamin K-dependent proteins, levels are typically reduced in patients with vitamin K deficiency and those on vitamin K antagonists (warfarin).

Counseling Issues and Management

Asymptomatic family members who are tested as part of family screening have an annual risk of incident VTE that ranges from 0.7 to 1.7 per 100 person-years, a risk that is higher than with FVL or the *F2* gene mutation [32]. In addition, these patients have an annual risk of recurrent VTE that approaches approximately 10 % [41]. The annual risk of VTE in users of oral contraceptives approaches 4.6 per 100 person-years; thus oral contraceptive use is generally discouraged in patients with PC, PS, or AT deficiency.

Hyperhomocysteinemia

Molecular Basis of Disease

Homocysteine is an intermediary amino acid formed during metabolism of methionine to cysteine (Fig. 15.12) which is formed by intracellular demethylation of dietary methionine. Homocysteine is then converted to cysteine in a two-step transsulfuration pathway that requires initial condensation of homocysteine with serine to form cystathionine. The latter reaction is catalyzed by cystathionine-β-synthase (CBS) and requires the essential cofactor, pyridoxal 5-phosphate (vitamin B_6). In the second step, catalyzed by cystathionine γ-lyase, cystathionine is hydrolyzed to α-ketobutyrate and cysteine. Homocysteine can be remethylated to methionine via two pathways. In the first, a methyl

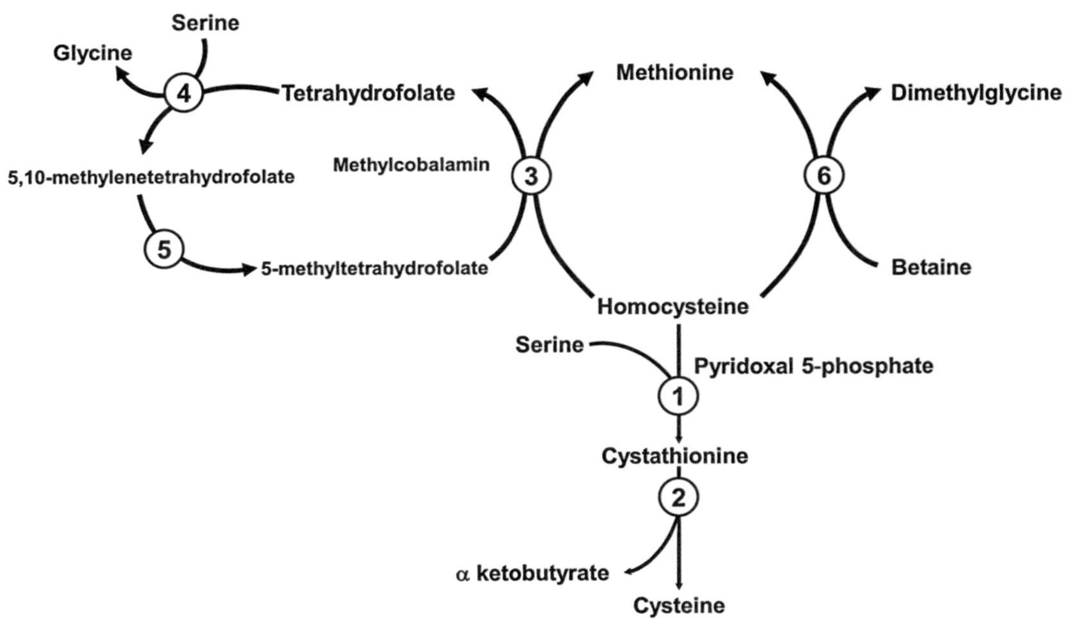

Figure 15.12 Homocysteine metabolism pathway. (*1*) Cystathionine βsynthetase (CBS); (*2*) cystathionine γ ligase; (*3*) methyltetrahydrofolate-homocysteine methyltransferase; (*4*) serine-glycine hydroxymethyltransferase; (*5*) 5,10-methylenetetrahydrofolate reductase (MTHFR); (*6*) betaine-homocysteine methyltransferase

group is donated by 5-methyltetrahydrofolate in a reaction catalyzed by methyltetrahydrofolate-homocysteine methyltransferase and requiring methyl-cobalamin (vitamin B_{12}). Tetrahydrofolate (folic acid) is remethylated to 5-methyltetrahydrofolate in a reaction that includes the intermediary 5,10-methylenetetrahydrofolate and requires the enzymes serine-glycine hydroxymethyl transferase and 5,10-methylenetetrahydrofolate reductase (MTHFR). In the second pathway, betaine (trimethyl-glycine) donates a methyl group to remethylate homocysteine to methionine in a reaction requiring betaine-homocysteine methyltransferase. Remethylation is primarily responsible for regulation of fasting homocysteine levels, while transsulfuration mainly regulates higher homocysteine levels as occur in the postprandial state or after methionine loading [42].

Homocystinuria is a rare inherited disorder affecting 3–5 per million of the general population, and usually is caused by severe deficiency of cystathionine β synthase (CBS). Most patients are homozygous or compound heterozygous for one or more of the three mutations (c.833T>C, c.919G>A, c.1224-2A>C) within the *CBS* gene located in the subtelomeric region of 21q22. CBS mutation heterozygotes often have normal basal plasma homocysteine levels, but develop hyperhomocysteinemia after a methionine load [42].

While rare, severe MTHFR deficiency due to mutations in the *MTHFR* gene also cause homocystinuria. Individuals who are homozygous for the common *MTHFR* C677T mutation (HGVS: c.665C>T) and become folate deficient may develop mild hyperhomocysteinemia. This mutation encodes p.Ala223Val. Approximately 1.5 % and 30 % of the US population are homozygous and heterozygous for the *MTHFR* C677T mutation, respectively. The role of a second commonly tested *MTHFR* variant, A1298C (HGVS: c.1286A>C), in the diagnosis and management of VTE is still being defined.

Clinical Utility of Testing

Testing for the *MTHFR* C677T and A1298C variants, in the presence of a normal plasma homocysteine level, provides little clinical utility. Patients with homocystinuria are at markedly increased risk for both atherosclerotic arterial occlusive disease and VTE. About 25 % of patients with homocystinuria develop a thrombotic vascular occlusive event by age 16 years, and about 50 % develop such an event by age 29 years [43]. Of these, about half are arterial occlusive events (e.g., stroke, myocardial infarction, or peripheral artery thrombosis), and the remainder are venous thromboembolic events. The event rate is significantly reduced by vitamin therapy in B_6-responsive patients [42].

Homocystinuric patients generally have plasma homocysteine levels of 100–300 μmol/L. Multiple case-control studies have found that milder hyperhomocysteinemia (e.g., 15–100 μmol/L) is a risk factor for both arterial occlusive disease and VTE, with OR of about 2.2–3.0 [42]. However, there is concern that these studies may have been confounded because plasma homocysteine levels may be elevated after thrombotic vascular events. Indeed, although fewer in number, prospective studies have provided conflicting results. Thus, hyperhomocysteinemia appears to be a weak risk factor for thrombotic arterial occlusive disease, while the risk for VTE remains uncertain. Individuals heterozygous for the *MTHFR* C677T mutation are not at risk for hyperhomocysteinemia, thrombotic arterial occlusive disease, or VTE. While individuals homozygous for the *MTHFR* C677T mutation are at increased risk for hyperhomocysteinemia, homozygosity for the *MTHFR* C677T mutation in the absence of hyperhomocysteinemia is not an independent risk factor for either arterial or venous thrombosis. There are no studies showing that reduction in plasma homocysteine levels by therapy with vitamins B_6, B_{12}, or folic acid reduces the risk for arterial or venous thrombosis. Testing for hyperhomocysteinemia is recommended for patients with documented atherosclerotic arterial occlusive disease (e.g., coronary artery, cerebrovascular, or peripheral vascular), while testing patients with VTE remains controversial. Genotyping for the *MTHFR* C677T mutation may provide insight into the etiology of hyperhomocysteinemia, but does not influence therapy or warrant family testing. Recently the American College of Medical Genetics released practice guidelines recommending that providers not order *MTHFR* polymorphism genotyping for a thrombophilia or recurrent pregnancy loss clinical evaluation. In addition, genotyping should not be conducted for at-risk family members [44].

Available Assays

Clinical assays for plasma homocysteine include HPLC and immunoassay [42]. Each laboratory should determine local gender and population-specific reference ranges. The basal plasma homocysteine level should be determined first, and, if elevated, further investigation regarding the potential cause as well as therapeutic intervention should be considered. The need for an overnight fast prior to testing plasma homocysteine levels is unclear. Because plasma homocysteine levels can be elevated for several months after myocardial infarction or stroke, testing should be postponed accordingly. In addition to vitamin deficiency, impaired renal function and hypothyroidism are other common causes of hyperhomocysteinemia. It is particularly important to exclude vitamin B_{12} deficiency prior to beginning therapy with high-dose folic acid which can precipitate acute B_{12} neuropathy. If the basal homocysteine level is normal, methionine loading (0.1 g/kg body weight or 3.8 g/m^2 body surface area with measurement of plasma homocysteine 4–6 h after the load) should be considered since 25–40 % of symptomatic patients develop hyperhomocysteinemia only after methionine loading. Therapy includes folic acid (0.5–1.0 mg/day), vitamin B_{12} (400–1,000 μg/day), and/or vitamin B_6 (20–50 mg/day) [42].

References

1. Soucie JM, et al. Occurrence of hemophilia in the United States. The Hemophilia Surveillance System Project Investigators. Am J Hematol. 1998;59:288–94.
2. Antonarakis SE, et al. Factor VIII gene inversions in severe hemophilia A: results of an international consortium study. Blood. 1995;86:2206–12.
3. Bagnall RD, et al. Recurrent inversion breaking intron 1 of the factor VIII gene is a frequent cause of severe hemophilia A. Blood. 2002;99:168–74.
4. Gilles JGG, et al. Factor VIII inhibitors. Thromb Haemost. 1997;78:641.
5. Gouw SC, et al. F8 gene mutation type and inhibitor development in patients with severe hemophilia A: systematic review and meta-analysis. Blood. 2012;119:2922–34.
6. ESHRE. ESHRE Preimplantation Genetic Diagnosis Consortium: data collection III (May 2001). Hum Reprod. 2002;17:233–46.
7. Liu Q, et al. Single-tube polymerase chain reaction for rapid diagnosis of the inversion hotspot of mutation in hemophilia A. Blood. 1998;92:1458–9.
8. Rossetti LC, et al. Developing a new generation of tests for genotyping hemophilia-causative rearrangements involving int22h and int1h hotspots in the factor VIII gene. J Thromb Haemost. 2008;6:830–6.
9. Payne AB, et al. Utility of multiplex ligation-dependent probe amplification (MLPA) for hemophilia mutation screening. J Thromb Haemost. 2012;10:1951–4.
10. Higuchi M, et al. Molecular characterization of severe hemophilia A suggests that about half the mutations are not within the coding regions and splice junctions of the factor VIII gene. Proc Natl Acad Sci U S A. 1991;88:7405–9.
11. Naylor JA, et al. Detection of three novel mutations in two haemophilia A patients by rapid screening of whole essential region of factor VIII gene. Lancet. 1991;337:635–9.
12. Buzin CH, et al. Scanning by DOVAM-S detects all unique sequence changes in blinded analyses: evidence that the scanning conditions are generic. Biotechniques. 2000;28:746–50. 752–3.
13. Nichols WC, et al. Mutations in the ER-Golgi intermediate compartment protein ERGIC-53 cause combined deficiency of coagulation factors V and VIII. Cell. 1998;93:61–70.
14. Yoshitake S, et al. Nucleotide sequence of the gene for human factor IX (antihemophilic factor B). Biochemistry. 1985;24:3736–50.
15. Simioni P, et al. X-linked thrombophilia with a mutant factor IX (factor IX Padua). N Engl J Med. 2009;361:1671–5.
16. de la Salle C, et al. Common intragenic and extragenic polymorphisms of blood coagulation factors VIII and IX are different in Chinese and Caucasian populations. Clin Genet. 1990;38:434–40.
17. Warrier I, et al. Factor IX inhibitors and anaphylaxis in hemophilia B. J Pediatr Hematol Oncol. 1997;19:23–7.
18. Ketterling RP, et al. Evidence that descendants of three founders constitute about 25% of hemophilia B in the United States. Genomics. 1991;10:1093–6.
19. Sadler JE. Von Willebrand disease. In: Scriver CR, Beaudet al, Valle D, et al., editors. The metabolic and molecular bases of inherited disease. 8th ed. New York: McGraw-Hill; 2001.
20. Mohlke KL, et al. Mvwf, a dominant modifier of murine von Willebrand factor, results from altered lineage-specific expression of a glycosyltransferase. Cell. 1999;96:111–20.
21. Bellissimo DB, et al. VWF mutations and new sequence variations identified in healthy controls are more frequent in the African-American population. Blood. 2012;119:2135–40.
22. Mazurier C, Meyer D. Factor VIII binding assay of von Willebrand factor and the diagnosis of type 2N von Willebrand disease—results of an international survey. On behalf of the Subcommittee on von Willebrand Factor of the Scientific and Standardization Committee of the ISTH. Thromb Haemost. 1996;76:270–4.
23. Bertina RM, et al. Mutation in blood coagulation factor V associated with resistance to activated protein C. Nature. 1994;369:64–7.
24. Lockwood C, Wendel G. Practice bulletin no. 124: inherited thrombophilias in pregnancy. Obstet Gynecol. 2011;118:730–40.
25. Middeldorp S, et al. The incidence of venous thromboembolism in family members of patients with factor V Leiden mutation and venous thrombosis. Ann Intern Med. 1998;128:15–20.
26. Press RD, et al. Clinical utility of factor V Leiden (R506Q) testing for the diagnosis and management of thromboembolic disorders. Arch Pathol Lab Med. 2002;126:1304–18.
27. Wu O, et al. Screening for thrombophilia in high-risk situations: systematic review and cost-effectiveness analysis. The Thrombosis: Risk and Economic Assessment of Thrombophilia Screening (TREATS) study. Health Technol Assess. 2006;10:1–110.
28. Heit JA, et al. The epidemiology of venous thromboembolism in the community. Thromb Haemost. 2001;86:452–63.
29. Rodeghiero F, Tosetto A. Activated protein C resistance and factor V Leiden mutation are independent risk factors for venous thromboembolism. Ann Intern Med. 1999;130:643–50.
30. Heit JA, et al. The incidence of venous thromboembolism among Factor V Leiden carriers: a community-based cohort study. J Thromb Haemost. 2005;3:305–11.
31. Vandenbroucke JP, et al. Increased risk of venous thrombosis in oral-contraceptive users who are carriers of factor V Leiden mutation. Lancet. 1994;344:1453–7.
32. van Vlijmen EF, et al. Thrombotic risk during oral contraceptive use and pregnancy in women with factor V Leiden or prothrombin mutation: a rational approach to contraception. Blood. 2011;118:2055–61. quiz 2375.
33. Falck-Ytter Y, et al. Prevention of VTE in orthopedic surgery patients: Antithrombotic Therapy and Prevention of Thrombosis, 9th ed: American College of Chest Physicians Evidence-Based Clinical Practice Guidelines. Chest. 2012;141:e278S–325.
34. Gould MK, et al. Prevention of VTE in nonorthopedic surgical patients: Antithrombotic Therapy and Prevention of Thrombosis, 9th ed: American College of Chest Physicians Evidence-Based Clinical Practice Guidelines. Chest. 2012;141:e227S–77.
35. Kahn SR, et al. Prevention of VTE in nonsurgical patients: Antithrombotic Therapy and Prevention of Thrombosis, 9th ed: American College of Chest Physicians Evidence-Based Clinical Practice Guidelines. Chest. 2012;141:e195S–226.
36. Kearon C, et al. Antithrombotic therapy for VTE disease: Antithrombotic Therapy and Prevention of Thrombosis, 9th ed: American College of Chest Physicians Evidence-Based Clinical Practice Guidelines. Chest. 2012;141:e419S–94.
37. Poort SR, et al. A common genetic variation in the 3′-untranslated region of the prothrombin gene is associated with elevated plasma prothrombin levels and an increase in venous thrombosis. Blood. 1996;88:3698–703.
38. Gehring NH, et al. Increased efficiency of mRNA 3′ end formation: a new genetic mechanism contributing to hereditary thrombophilia. Nat Genet. 2001;28:389–92.
39. Soria JM, et al. Linkage analysis demonstrates that the prothrombin G20210A mutation jointly influences plasma prothrombin levels and risk of thrombosis. Blood. 2000;95:2780–5.
40. McGlennen RC, Key NS. Clinical and laboratory management of the prothrombin G20210A mutation. Arch Pathol Lab Med. 2002;126:1319–25.
41. Brouwer JL, et al. High long-term absolute risk of recurrent venous thromboembolism in patients with hereditary deficiencies of protein S, protein C or antithrombin. Thromb Haemost. 2009;101:93–9.
42. Key NS, McGlennen RC. Hyperhomocyst(e)inemia and thrombophilia. Arch Pathol Lab Med. 2002;126:1367–75.
43. Mudd SH, Skoyby F, Levy HL, et al. The natural history of homocystinuria due to cystathionine beta-synthase deficiency. Am J Hum Genet. 1985;37:1–31.
44. Hickey SE, et al. ACMG Practice Guideline: lack of evidence for MTHFR polymorphism testing. Genet Med. 2013;15:153–6.

Hematologic Disorders: Hemochromatosis, Hemoglobinopathies, and Rh Incompatibility

16

Daniel B. Bellissimo and Archana Agarwal

Abstract

Hereditary hemochromatosis (HHC) is a disorder of iron metabolism and has been classified into six types having similar phenotypes but caused by mutations in different genes involved in the regulation of iron stores. Two allelic variants of the *HFE* gene, p.C282Y (c.845G>A) and p.H63D (c.187C>G), are significantly correlated with HHC, and most clinical studies have focused on these variants. Diagnosis of HHC is based on clinical, biochemical, histological, and molecular studies, specifically tests such as transferrin saturation, ferritin concentration, evaluation of iron stores by liver biopsy, and genotyping for p.C282Y and p.H63D mutations in *HFE*. Hemoglobinopathies are the most common single-gene diseases in the world. Approximately 5–7 % of the world's population is a carrier for one of the hemoglobin disorders. Two copies of the alpha (α) globin genes are present (α1 and α2) on each chromosome 16. The beta and beta-like chains (ε, Gγ, Aγ, and δ) are clustered on chromosome 11. The hemoglobinopathies are commonly divided into two broad categories: structural variants, and thalassemias that are characterized by reduced rates of production of α or β chains. Sickle hemoglobin results from a single nucleotide substitution (GAG→GTG) that changes codon 6 of the β-globin gene from a glutamic acid to a valine (Glu6Val). Homozygosity for this mutation causes sickle cell disease (SD), an autosomal recessive disorder. SD is a major cause of morbidity and mortality in Africa and in populations with individuals of African descent. The α-thalassemias are most commonly caused by deletions while the β-thalassemias are most likely due to single nucleotide substitutions or frameshift mutations. Single nucleotide changes causing either structural variants or thalassemias can be easily diagnosed by targeted mutation analysis or by sequencing. Gap-PCR or multiplex ligation dependent probe amplification assays are the common methods to detect deletions. The Rh antigen system is clinically important because antibodies to Rh antigens are involved in hemolytic transfusion reactions, autoimmune hemolytic anemia, and hemolytic disease of the fetus and newborn. The Rh antigens are expressed on proteins encoded by two distinct but highly homologous genes, *RHD* and *RHCE*, on chromosome 1p34.3-36.1. The D antigen is expressed from *RHD* and the C/c and E/e antigens are expressed from *RHCE*. Rh incompatibility cases require both phenotypic and genotypic testing of parental samples.

D.B. Bellissimo, Ph.D. (✉)
Obstetrics, Gynecology and Reproductive Sciences, University of Pittsburgh School of Medicine, Pittsburgh, PA, USA

Magee-Womens Hospital, 300 Italket St., Rm 1240, Pittsburgh, PA 15213, USA
e-mail: dbbellissimo@sbcglobal.net

A. Agarwal, M.D.
Department of Pathology, University of Utah, Salt Lake City, UT, USA

D.G.B. Leonard (ed.), *Molecular Pathology in Clinical Practice*, DOI 10.1007/978-3-319-19674-9_16

Keywords
Hereditary hemochromatosis • *HFE* gene • Hemoglobinopathies • Sickle cell disease • Thalassemia • Rh incompatibility • Blood group antigens • Hemolytic transfusion reactions • Autoimmune hemolytic anemia • Hemolytic disease of the fetus and newborn • Molecular testing • Diagnostic testing

Introduction

Hemochromatosis

Hereditary hemochromatosis (HHC) is a disorder of iron metabolism resulting from excess iron storage in the liver, skin, pancreas, heart, joints, testes, and pituitary gland. It is a disorder of iron metabolism and has been classified into six types having similar phenotypes but caused by mutations in different genes involved in the regulation of iron stores. Two allelic variants of the *HFE* gene, p.C282Y (c.845G>A) and p.H63D (c.187C>G), are significantly correlated with HHC, and most clinical studies have focused on these variants. These mutations are most common in populations of European descent. Diagnosis of HHC is based on clinical, biochemical, histological, and molecular studies, specifically tests such as transferrin saturation, ferritin concentration, evaluation of iron stores by liver biopsy, and genotyping for p.C282Y and p.H63D mutations in *HFE*, when necessary. These mutations can be accurately detected by polymerase chain reaction-restriction fragment length polymorphism (PCR-RFLP), allele-specific PCR (AS-PCR), allele-specific oligonucleotide (ASO) hybridization, single-nucleotide primer extension, and real-time PCR methods.

Hemoglobinopathies

Hemoglobinopathies are the most common single-gene diseases in the world; approximately 5–7 % of the world's population is a carrier for one of the hemoglobin disorders. There are two copies of the alpha (α) globin genes (α1 and α2) on each chromosome 16. The beta (β) and β-like chains (ε, Gγ, Aγ, and δ) are clustered on chromosome 11. The hemoglobinopathies are commonly divided into two broad categories: structural variants, and thalassemias that are characterized by reduced rates of production of α or β chains. Sickle hemoglobin results from a single nucleotide substitution (GAG→GTG) that changes codon 6 of the β-globin gene from a glutamic acid to a valine (Glu6Val). Homozygosity for this mutation causes sickle cell disease (SD), an autosomal recessive disorder. SD is a major cause of morbidity and mortality in Africa and in populations with individuals of African descent. The α-thalassemias are most commonly caused by deletions while the β-thalassemias are most likely due to single nucleotide substitutions or frameshift mutations. Single nucleotide changes causing either structural variants or thalassemias can be easily diagnosed by targeted mutation analysis or by sequencing the gene. Gap-PCR or multiplex ligation dependent probe amplification (MLPA) assays are the common methods to detect deletions.

Rh Incompatibility

The Rh antigen system is clinically important because antibodies to Rh antigens are involved in hemolytic transfusion reactions, autoimmune hemolytic anemia, and hemolytic disease of the fetus and newborn (HDFN). HDFN results from the alloimmunization of a mother to a paternally inherited fetal alloantigen. The most common cause for alloimmunization is fetomaternal hemorrhage. The severity of HDFN is variable; mild cases require either no treatment or phototherapy, while more severe cases require exchange transfusion at birth, or possibly intrauterine transfusion, and may result in fetal hydrops. The Rh antigens are expressed on proteins encoded by two distinct but highly homologous genes, *RHD* and *RHCE*, on chromosome 1p34.3-36.1. The most common RHD-negative allele results from the total deletion of *RHD*; however, there are a number of *RHD*-negative haplotypes that are positive for at least portions of the *RHD* gene. The c.307T>C, p.Ser103Pro, variation is responsible for the C and c antigens expressed from the *RHCE* gene. The assay formats are predominantly AS-PCR and real-time PCR with hydrolysis probes.

Hemochromatosis

Molecular Basis of Disease

HHC is a disorder of iron metabolism resulting from excess iron storage in the liver, skin, pancreas, heart, joints, testes, and pituitary gland. If left untreated, life-threatening complications such as cirrhosis, diabetes, liver cancer, and cardiomyopathy may result. Iron overload and the resulting clinical complications can be avoided by early diagnosis and periodic phlebotomy to reduce the body's iron stores. Extensive reviews on the *HFE* gene and HHC are available [1–4].

Table 16.1 Hereditary hemochromatosis classification

Type	OMIM#	Gene	Chr.	Protein	Inheritance	Age of onset
1	235200	*HFE*	6p22.2	Hereditary Hemochromatosis Protein	Autosomal recessive	Adult
2A	602390	*HJV*	1q21.1	Hemojuvelin	Autosomal recessive	Child to young adult
2B	602390	*HAMP*	19q13.12	Hepcidin	Autosomal recessive	Child to young adult
3	604250	*TFR2*	7q22.1	Transferrin Receptor Protein 2	Autosomal recessive	Young adult to adult
4A	606069	*SLC40A1*	2q32.2	Solute carrier family 40 member 1 (Ferroportin)	Autosomal dominant (LOF)	Adult
4B	606069	*SLC40A1*	2q32.2		Autosomal dominant (GOF)	Adult

GOF gain of function, *LOF* loss of function

Table 16.2 *HFE* genotype frequencies and their contribution to hereditary hemochromatosis

Genotype	Population frequency (%)	Pooled odds ratio	95 % CI	% HHC cases
p.C282Y/p.C282Y	0.4	4,383	1,374–>10,000	77.5
p.C282Y/p.H63D	2.0	32	18.5–55.4	5.3
p.H63D/p.H63D	2.0	5.7	3.2–10.1	1.5
p.C282Y/+	9.2	4.1	2.9–5.8	3
p.H63D/+	23	1.9	1.5–2.5	3

Source: Data are from Refs. 2, 7

HHC has been classified into six types that have similar phenotypes but are caused by mutations in different genes involved in the regulation of iron stores (Table 16.1). Types 1–3 are autosomal recessive disorders with mutations in genes that result in defective expression of the hepcidin (*HAMP*) gene. Hepcidin regulates iron homeostasis by binding SLC40A1, also known as ferroportin, causing degradation of this iron-transporting protein resulting in reduced iron export from enterocytes. Type 4 is an autosomal dominant disorder with mutations in the *SLC40A1* gene. The gain-of-function mutations in type 4B cause defective down regulation in response to hepcidin. The loss-of-function mutations in type 4A result in iron retention in monocytes and macrophages and cause a distinctly different phenotype than the other types of HHC. HHC typically has an age of onset in adults; however, types 2A and 2B are juvenile forms of HHC. Except for *HFE*-related HHC (type 1) which is the most common form of HHC, the other types of HHC are rare.

The HFE protein, a 343 amino acid transmembrane protein, is homologous to major histocompatibility class I molecules and associates with β_2-microglobulin. The HFE protein is found predominantly in hepatocytes. At the cell surface, HFE complexes with the transferrin receptor protein 1 (TfR1) and competes for binding of iron-loaded transferrin. Under conditions of high iron, HFE is displaced from TfR1 and binds to transferrin receptor protein 2 (TfR2). Although the mechanism is not understood, the HFE-TfR2 complex is believed to create an intercellular signal to increase hepcidin expression. The role of *HFE* in HHC and iron homeostasis is supported by the fact that an *HFE* knockout mouse develops iron overload similar to that seen in human HHC [5].

Two allelic variants of the *HFE* gene, p.C282Y (c.845G>A) and p.H63D (c.187C>G), are significantly correlated with HHC, and most of the clinical studies have focused on these variants [6]. These two variants are usually not found on the same chromosome. The p.C282Y mutation abolishes a conserved disulfide bond which disrupts secondary structure required for HFE-binding to β_2-microglobulin and subsequent transport to the cell surface. The p.C282Y HFE protein remains in the Golgi rather than being transported to the cell surface. The p.H63D protein product is expressed on the cell surface, but likely has an altered interaction with the transferrin receptor. Several other *HFE* allelic variants have been described, but little is known regarding their phenotypic effects. The p.S65C mutation has been implicated in HHC but its clinical significance is still unclear [2].

The frequency of the p.C282Y and p.H63D mutations in different ethnic groups has been reviewed [2]. These mutations are most common in populations of European descent. A pooled analysis of several Caucasian population studies found that the frequency of p.C282Y homozygosity was 0.4 % and heterozygosity was 9.2 % (Table 16.2). The frequency of p.H63D homozygosity was 2 % and heterozygosity was 23 %. Compound heterozygosity (p.C282Y/p.H63D) was 2 %. The frequency of *HFE* genotypes in HHC cases was 77.5 % for p.C282Y/p.C282Y, 5.3 % for p.C282Y/p.H63D, and 1.5 % for p.H63D/p.H63D. The pooled odds ratio (OR) for each *HFE* genotype indicated that individuals with the p.C282Y/p.C282Y and p.C282Y/p.H63D genotypes have the highest risk for iron overload with an OR of 4,383 and 32, respectively [7]. Individuals with the p.H63D/p.H63D and p.C282Y heterozygote (p.C282Y/+) genotypes are not considered to be at elevated risk for developing iron overload. The high frequency of HHC patients with the p.C282Y/p.C282Y genotype suggested that the penetrance for this genotype was very high. However, additional studies designed to estimate the penetrance suggested that the majority of p.C282Y homozygotes would not develop clinical disease resulting from iron overload. In a large prospective study, the proportion of p.C282Y homozygotes with documented iron-overload was 28.4 % for men and 1.2 % for women [8]. Currently, the estimates of the penetrance range from 1 % to 50 %. The penetrance of the p.C282Y/p.H63D genotype is much lower, ranging from 0.3 % to 1.4 %.

Clinical Utility of Testing

Diagnosis of HHC is based on clinical, biochemical, histological, and molecular studies, specifically tests such as transferrin saturation, ferritin concentration, evaluation of iron stores by liver biopsy, and genotyping for p.C282Y and p.H63D mutations in the *HFE* gene. Due to the reduced penetrance of p.C282Y/p.C282Y, the even lower penetrance of p.C282Y/p.H63D, and the presence of other mutations within *HFE* or in other genes related to HHC, the diagnosis or rule out of HHC cannot be made with a molecular test alone. However, in patients with clinical and biochemical symptoms of iron overload, molecular testing can be useful in confirming the diagnosis of HHC and may eliminate the need for liver biopsy. Typically, molecular testing is warranted in patients with transferrin saturation of >45 %. A genotyping result of p.C282Y/p.C282Y or p.C282Y/p.H63D is considered to confirm a diagnosis of HHC. A small number of cases (<5 %) will be identified as p.C282Y heterozygotes. It is possible these patients have other mutations in *HFE* or mutations in other genes involved in iron overload (Table 16.1).

Molecular testing also is used for carrier analysis and to identify relatives at risk for HHC. After the diagnosis of HHC is made in the proband, testing may be appropriate for other family members who may be at higher risk than the general population for developing iron overload. The iron status of these individuals can be monitored as appropriate. The *HFE* genotyping test can be used to identify individuals with the same genotype as the proband; these individuals would be at higher risk for developing iron overload than family members who did not inherit the mutations present in the proband. Requests for prenatal testing for HHC are highly unusual since HHC is a treatable adult onset disorder with low penetrance.

Soon after the identifications of the role of *HFE* mutations in iron overload, population screening for p.C282Y and p. H63D was considered. Since simple phlebotomy can prevent iron overload and its severe clinical complications, early identification of individuals at risk would be beneficial. However, given the low penetrance of the *HFE* genotypes, the majority of individuals identified with *HFE* mutations would be unlikely to develop clinical symptoms associated with HHC and yet might be subject to stigmatization and/or genetic discrimination as a result of the testing. At this time, population screening for HHC is not recommended due to these limitations.

Available Assays

As the p.C282Y and p.H63D mutations are single nucleotide polymorphisms (SNPs), they can be accurately detected using a variety of methods. As with all SNP assays, careful consideration must be given to the known sequence variants that may affect the assay method. The first method described for these mutations was an oligonucleotide ligation assay [6]. The primers described by this group to amplify the regions of the *HFE* gene have been used in a variety of assays. However, polymorphisms in one primer binding site sequence has been described and has the potential to result in a diagnostic error [9, 10]. Using primers that do not include the polymorphisms eliminates this potential error. The possible interference of the p.S65C mutation with the detection of p.H63D also should be considered in assay design. A number of additional assay methods for these mutations have been described, including PCR-RFLP, AS-PCR, ASO hybridization, single-nucleotide primer extension, and real-time PCR methods [11].

A simple method for detection of p.C282Y and p.H63D is PCR-RFLP. p.C282Y is detected by digestion of the PCR product with *Rsa*I, and H63D is detected by using *Bcl*I or *Mbo*I. The digested PCR products are analyzed by gel electrophoresis. The advantage of this method is that optimization is relatively straightforward and expensive equipment is not required. The disadvantage is a longer turnaround time for testing. AS-PCR assays distinguish the normal and mutant alleles directly with only gel electrophoresis of the PCR products, so the post-PCR processing is reduced. The AS-PCR reactions require careful optimization, and multiple reactions are required to determine the genotype.

Real-time PCR methods that couple PCR with detection of hybridization probes are commonly used to detect single nucleotide polymorphisms. These techniques are rapid, sensitive, have a wide dynamic range, and require no additional processing after PCR. A variety of chemistries are available such as FRET hybridization probes with melt curve analysis, hydrolysis probes, and molecular beacons. For each method, the appropriate negative and positive controls are required to demonstrate the specificity of the assay. A melting curve of the hybridization probe fluorescence is used to detect changes in thermal stability and therefore discriminate single base mutations in a single reaction (Fig. 16.1). An additional advantage of real-time PCR is that new sequence variations in the probe regions are detected. For example, the probe for

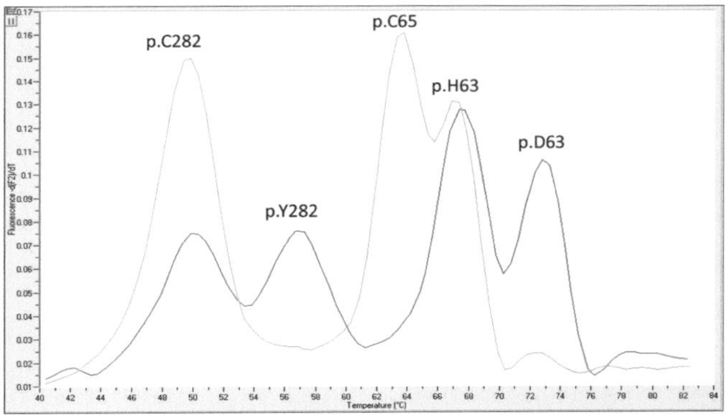

Figure 16.1 PCR-FRET hybridization probe with melt curve analysis for p.Cys282Tyr (p.C282Y) and p.His63Asp (p.H63D) alleles of the *HFE* gene. One set of probes distinguishes the p.C282Y alleles and the other set p.H63D alleles. The probes for p.H63D also overlap the p. S65C allele so it can also be identified. Each allele has a specific melting temperature. Since the melting temperatures of the probes do not overlap, this assay can be performed using a single fluorophore. An example of a p.C282Y/p.H63D compound heterozygous sample (*blue trace*) and a sample negative for p.C282Y and p.H63D and positive for p.S65C (*green trace*) are shown

p.H63D also detects the p.S65C mutation [12]. In cases where testing is indicated for additional *HFE* mutations or HHC types 2–4, *HFE*, *HJV*, *HAMP*, *TFR2*, and *SLC40A1* are analyzed by DNA sequencing.

Interpretation of Test Results

The analytic sensitivity for detecting these mutations should be >99 %. False positives and false negatives are rare. However, sequence variations in primers, probes, and restriction sites have the potential to lead to a diagnostic error. A polymorphism reported at the 3′ end of one of the primers described in the original publication [6] was later reported to prevent the amplification of wild-type p.C282Y alleles with some assay methods [9].

Interpretations should be made in the context of all clinical information and account for the reduced penetrance and variable expression observed with HHC. In individuals with biochemical evidence of iron overload, a genotype of p. C282Y/p.C282Y or p.C282Y/p.H63D confirms a diagnosis of *HFE*-related HHC. Up to 5 % of these individuals will be heterozygous for p.C282Y. Testing for other *HFE* mutations or mutations in other iron-related genes may be indicated. Individuals who test negative for p.C282Y are a heterogeneous group with other genetic causes of HHC or iron overload caused by liver disease or a metabolic disorder. Unaffected individuals with the p.C282Y/p.C282Y genotype have an increased risk of HHC with a penetrance of 1–50 %. p.C282Y heterozygotes may have elevated iron levels but rarely develop complications of iron overload.

Genetic counseling should be recommended when p.C282Y and p.H63D are identified in a family. Molecular testing will be useful in identifying carriers, homozygous individuals, and those who did not inherit the at-risk genotype. Most parents of the proband will be p.C282Y heterozygotes so the risk to siblings of a proband is 25 % but could be as high as 50 % if one of the parents is homozygous. The risk assessment should include the most current estimates of the disease penetrance.

Laboratory Issues

Proficiency testing for p.C282Y and p.H63D mutations in the *HFE* gene is available through the College of American Pathologists (CAP) Molecular Genetics Laboratory (MGL) survey. Cell-line controls can be purchased from Coriell Cell Repositories (http:/ccr.coriell.org/).

Hemoglobinopathies

Molecular Basis of Disease

Hemoglobinopathies are the most common single-gene diseases in the world; approximately 5–7 % of the world's population is a carrier for one of the hemoglobin disorders. The extensive study of these disorders has led to much of our knowledge regarding protein structure and function, mutational mechanisms, gene expression during development, and evolution. Extensive reviews of these disorders are available [13, 14]. A list of the numerous characterized mutant alleles is available at the Globin Gene Server (http://globin.cse.psu.edu) and the Human Gene Mutation Database (http://www.hgmd.cf.ac.uk/ac/index.php).

Hemoglobin (Hb) functions as an oxygen carrier in vertebrate red cells. The protein is a tetramer consisting of two α and two β chains. Each subunit contains a heme prosthetic group that is responsible for the oxygen-binding capacity of the protein. These chains are highly homologous to one another at the primary sequence level as well as in three-dimensional structure. Six different globin chains (α, β, γ, δ, ε, ζ) are found in normal human hemoglobins at various times during development [13–15]. The α and β chains are encoded by separate genetic loci (Fig. 16.2). The α and α-like chains (ζ, Ψζ, Ψα) are clustered on chromosome 16. In addition, two copies of the α-globin genes, α_1 and α_2, are located on each chromosome 16. The β and β-like chains (ε, Gγ, Aγ, Ψβ, δ) are clustered on chromosome 11.

The developmental regulation of these genes is important to the understanding of many of the hemoglobin disorders. The gene order in each cluster is identical to the order of expression during development. In each developmental stage, there is an equimolar production of α and β chains. Hb Gower 1 ($\zeta_2\varepsilon_2$), Hb Gower 2 ($\alpha_2\varepsilon_2$), and Hb Portland

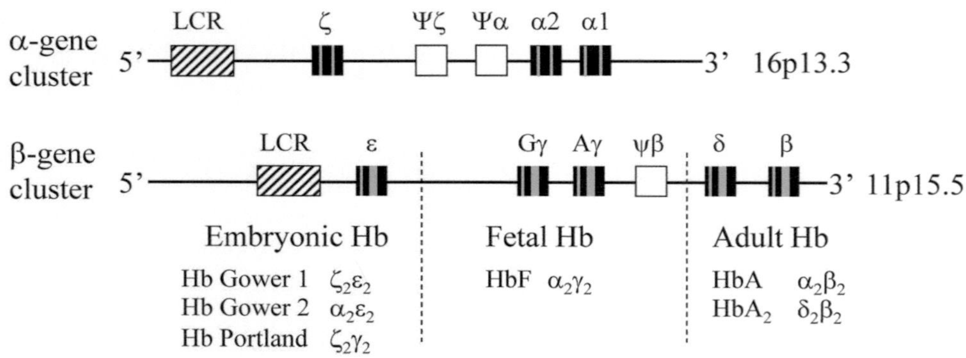

Figure 16.2 Genomic organization and developmental expression of the α- and β-globin gene clusters. The *boxes* identify the locus control region (LCR; *diagonal*), pseudogenes (*white*), exons (*black*), and introns (*gray*). The developmental time periods for the expression of the β-globin genes are indicated by the *dashed lines*. (Adapted from Stamatoyannopoulos G, Nienhuis AW. Hemoglobin switching. In: Stamatoyannopoulos G, Nienhuis AW, Majerus PW, Varmus H, eds. *The molecular basis of blood diseases*. Philadelphia: W.B. Saunders, 1994:107–55)

($\zeta_2\gamma_2$) are expressed in embryos. In the fetal stage, the Hb is predominantly $\alpha_2\gamma_2$ (HbF). In normal adults, the Hb is comprised of approximately 96 % $\alpha_2\beta_2$ (HbA), 2.5 % $\delta_2\beta_2$ (HbA2), and approximately 1 % $\alpha_2\gamma_2$ (HbF). In addition to promoters and enhancer elements, the locus control region (LCR) is responsible for developmental expression of these genes. The LCR for the β locus is approximately 20 kb upstream of the ε-globin gene and the LCR for the α locus is approximately 40 kb upstream from the ζ-globin gene. The LCR is required for expression of all the globin genes at the locus [13].

The difference in gene dosage and expression patterns between α and β genes is significant. Each diploid genome encodes four copies of the α gene and two copies of the β gene. Since γ globin is expressed during fetal life and shortly after birth, β globin mutations do not exert their deleterious effects during the prenatal period. In contrast, since α chains are expressed during fetal and postnatal life, mutations in the α chain can cause severe disease during both developmental stages.

The hemoglobinopathies are commonly divided into two broad categories: structural variants, and thalassemias that are characterized by reduced rates of production of α or β chains [13]. These categories are not exclusive, as structural variants, which result in unstable hemoglobins, can be associated with both α- and β-thalassemia phenotypes. Although an extensive number of abnormal hemoglobins have been described, this chapter focuses on two of the most common structural variants, sickle hemoglobin (HbS) and HbC, and the more common forms of α- and β-thalassemia.

Sickle hemoglobin results from a single nucleotide substitution (GAG→GTG) that changes codon 6 of the β-globin gene from a glutamic acid to a valine (p.Glu6Val). Using standard nomenclature this variant should be reported as p. Glu7Val; however, the extensive literature uses the numbering of the mature protein in which the first methionine is cleaved. Homozygosity for this mutation causes SD, an autosomal recessive disorder. SD is a major cause of morbidity and mortality in Africa and in populations with individuals of African descent such as the Mediterranean area, the Middle East, and India [13]. Under the condition of low oxygen tension in the microvasculature, HbS polymerizes into fibers that cause the erythrocytes to sickle. The poor deformability of the sickle red cells and their defective passage in the micro-circulation causes the vasoocclusive events that are the hallmark of SD. The shortened survival of these red cells leads to a chronic hemolytic anemia. The frequency of SD is 1 in 600 in African Americans; the heterozygote frequency in African Americans is approximately 8 %, but the frequency in Africa can be much higher [13]. The frequency of the HbS allele, as well as alleles causing thalassemia, is maintained by their protective effect against malaria. The heterozygous state, sickle cell trait, is clinically normal but may be at risk for vasoocclusive events when exposed to low oxygen tension such as flying at high altitude in an airplane with reduced cabin pressure.

The sickling disorders also include compound heterozygous states with the HbS mutation in association with another β-globin variant such as HbC, or β-thalassemia. Similar to HbS, HbC also has an amino acid substitution at position 6 of the β-globin gene (Glu6Lys). HbC is less soluble than HbA and leads to reduced deformability of the red cells and a mild hemolytic anemia. The allele is frequent in persons of African descent; approximately 3 % of African Americans are carriers [13]. Individuals with $\beta^S\beta^C$ have sickle cell hemoglobin (SC) disease. SC disease is a milder hemolytic disorder than SD and therefore may go unrecognized until a serious complication occurs.

The thalassemias result from the reduced synthesis or stability of either the α- or β-globin chain. The chains in excess due to the α:β imbalance precipitate within the red blood cells, leading to membrane damage and red cell destruction. The defect produces a hypochromic, microcytic anemia. The population distribution of thalassemia includes the Mediterranean, Middle East, portions of Africa, India, and Southeast Asia; however, the migration of these populations has resulted in the worldwide occurrence of these diseases [13].

The most common forms of α-thalassemia are caused by deletions. The genetics of α-thalassemia are complicated by the fact that each normal chromosome has two α genes and that there are haplotypes with either the loss of one (-α) (α+ thalassemia) or both (--) (α^o thalassemia) copies of the α gene. In addition to the normal genotype, four additional genotypes are possible: silent carrier (αα/-α), α-thalassemia trait (-α/-α or --/αα), HbH (β_4) disease (-α/--), and hydrops fetalis, Hb Barts: γ_4 (--/--). Individuals with HbH disease have a moderately severe hemolytic anemia, while the inheritance of no copies of the α gene (Hb Barts) is incompatible with life. Carriers of α-thalassemia trait have only a mild hypochromic microcytic anemia, but couples with these genotypes are at risk for having a fetus with hydrops fetalis or a child with HbH disease. The (--) genotype, and therefore the risk of hydrops fetalis, is largely restricted to Southeast Asia, while in other groups the (-α) genotype is more common [13, 14]. Distinguishing these two carrier states is important for accurate genetic counseling. The most widely occurring single α-globin gene deletions are $-\alpha^{3.7}$ and $-\alpha^{4.2}$. The double α-globin gene deletions $\alpha\text{-}^{SEA}$, $\alpha\text{-}^{FIL}$, and $\alpha\text{-}^{THAI}$ are common in Southeast Asia while $\alpha\text{-}^{MED}$ and $-(\alpha)^{20}$ are more common in the Mediterranean area. Nondeletion α-thalassemia alleles are rare, but the $\alpha^{Constant\ Spring}$, a mutation in the termination codon of the α_2 gene, is frequently present in Southeast Asia.

The β-thalassemias are mainly inherited in an autosomal recessive manner, although there are some dominant forms. Heterozygotes are asymptomatic but with recognizable hematologic parameters including an elevated HbA_2. Homozygotes and compound heterozygotes of HbE develop a severe anemia within the first year of life as the switch from γ to β chains occurs. In contrast to α-thalassemia, β-thalassemias are heterogeneous at the molecular level. The molecular mechanism of the mutations is equally varied. Most mutations are single-nucleotide substitutions or frameshift mutations. More than 200 disease-causing mutations have been identified in the β-globin gene; however, within each at-risk population there is a set of 4–10 mutations that account for the majority of disease-causing alleles (Table 16.3) [15]. HbE is a β-globin variant (Glu26Lys) that can cause a mild thalassemia phenotype. It is one of the most common Hb variants, and the frequency is high in Southeast Asia. Although HbE homozygotes are asymptomatic, compound heterozygotes with another β-thalassemia allele will have an abnormal phenotype [13]. Although deletions are rare, a 619 base pair (bp) deletion involving the 3′ end of the β-globin gene is common in India and Pakistan, accounting for approximately 30 % of the β-thalassemia alleles [13]. β-Thalassemia also may result from deletion of part of the globin gene cluster (e.g., 5P-thalassemia) or from deletions that start 50–100 kilobases (kb) upstream from the globin gene cluster and extend 3′ into the cluster (εγδβ-thalassemia). Some of these deletions lead to hereditary persistence of fetal hemoglobin. In addition, there are fusion chain variants such as Hb Lepore, a $\delta\beta^+$ thalassemia. Mutations either completely (β°-thalassemia) or partially (β^+-thalassemia) abolish β-chain production. Milder phenotypes have been recognized that can be explained at the molecular level by homozygosity or compound heterozygosity for mild or silent mutations, coinheritance of α-thalassemia, or coinheritance of a genetic determinant that increases the production of the γ chain.

Clinical Utility of Testing

Sickle cell disease and α- and β-thalassemias and their carrier states can be diagnosed using standard red-cell indices such as Hb, red blood cell number, mean corpuscular volume, and red cell distribution, along with Hb electrophoresis, high-performance liquid chromatography (HPLC) and isoelectric focusing (IEF). The main application of molecular testing is for prenatal diagnosis and genetic counseling. When a carrier is identified by abnormal hematologic analysis, the carrier's partner can be screened for carrier status. Molecular testing can be used to identify the disease-causing mutations. Prenatal molecular testing can be offered to couples whose gene mutations have been identified. Testing also can be used to identify mutations in partners with borderline or normal hematologic values when one partner is clearly a carrier, since these couples are at risk for having a fetus with thalassemia. This testing model has been successfully used in population screening to reduce the incidence of thalassemia.

In states where testings for hemoglobinopathies are included in the newborn screen, HbH disease or hydrops fetalis can be diagnosed by the presence of Hb Barts on HPLC, or IEF analysis. However, molecular confirmation might be necessary in these conditions to make a definitve diagnosis and also to know about the specific deletions for genetic counseling purposes. For α-thalassemia, prenatal diagnosis predominantly is used in situations where both members of the couple are carriers of the double α-gene deletion or one member has one α gene deletion and the other has double α gene deletions, as only these couples are at risk for having a fetus with hydrops fetalis and HbH disease, respectively. Although the α^o-gene is found almost exclusively in the Southeast Asian population, molecular testing can be used to identify and distinguish the two distinct types of α-thalassemia carrier states (-α/-α vs --/αα) because HPLC analysis is not helpful in these conditions. As these carrier states can present with microcytic anemia, the diagnosis is important in differentiating them from iron deficiency states to avoid unnecessary iron intake.

Table 16.3 Population-specific mutations in β-thalassemia

Population	Detection frequency (%)	[a]Nonstandard variant names	[b]Standard nomenclature
Mediterranean	91–95	-87 C→G IVS1-1G→A IVS1-6T→C IVS1-110 G→A cd 39C→T IVS2-745C→G	c.-136C>G c.92+1G>A c.92+6T>C c.93-21G>A c.118C>T c.316-106C>G
Middle East	91–95	cd8–AA cd 8/9+G IVS1-5G→C cd 39C→T cd 44-C IVS2-1G→A	c.25_26delAA c.27_28insG c.92+5G>C c.118C>T c.135delC c.315+1G>A
Indian	91–95	cd 8/9 +G IVS1-1G→T IVS1-5G→C cd41/42 –TTCT	c.27_28insG c.92+1G>T c.92+5G>C c.124_127delTTCT
Thai	91–95	-28 A→G 17 A→T 19 A→G IVS1-5 G→C 41/42-TTCT IVS2-654 C→T	c.-78A>G c.52A>T c.59A>G c.92+5G>C c.124_127delTTCT c.316-197C>T
Chinese	91–95	-28A→G 17A→T 41/42-TTCT IVS2-654 C→T	c.-78A>G c.52A>T c.124_127delTTCT c.316-197C>T
African/African American	75–80	-88C→T -29 A→G cd24T→A IVS2-849A→G, A→C	c.-138C>T c.-79A>G c.75T>A c.316-2A>G, A>C

Source: Reprinted with permission from Cao A, Galanello R. Beta-thalassemia. GeneReviews [database online]. ©University of Washington, Seattle, WA. Updated June 7, 2010
[a]Nonstandard variant designations in common use
[b]DNA nucleotide change designations follow current nomenclature guidelines

In addition to prenatal testing for β-thalassemia, molecular testing can be used to predict the clinical phenotype by identifying mild and silent alleles and for presymptomatic diagnosis of at-risk family members. HbE disorders are now becoming increasingly recognized in the US population due to migration. A β-thalassemia major phenotype also could be due to compound heterozygosity for a beta zero mutation and HbE disease. Molecular testing is the only way to make a definitive diagnosis in these cases. Molecular testing also may be useful in recognition of complex heterozygotes in populations where multiple hemoglobinopathies are common.

Available Assays

HbS and HbC are caused by single-base substitutions, so a number of methods are suitable as long as the mutations can be distinguished from one another. One of the most common methods is PCR-RFLP [16]. Modified primers are used to introduce restriction sites so the β^A, β^S, and β^C alleles can be identified using *Ava*I and *Sty*I restriction enzymes. A real-time PCR method using hybridization probes also has been described that can readily identify the β^E allele in addition to the β^A, β^S, and β^C alleles [17].

The conventional method for detecting α-gene deletions has been Southern blot using probes to the ζ- and α-globin genes. The ζ-globin probe is useful for detecting deletion breakpoint fragments because the α-globin probe will fail to hybridize to the α fragment in an α^o-thalassemia fetus [16]. A number of PCR-based methods including a gap PCR method which is widely used, have been described that detect the seven most common α^o and α+ deletions [18]. Since these deletions either partially or completely remove the α2 globin gene, its detection by PCR indicates heterozygosity when a deletion allele is present. The PCR assays are faster, less expensive, and easier to interpret than Southern blot, although the PCR has to be carefully optimized to faithfully amplify the GC-rich sequences at this locus. The remaining deletions not detected by this common deletion testing by PCR can be detected by MLPA [19]. If all these tests are negative, non-deletion mutations can be identified by α globin sequencing.

Since the mutations causing β-thalassemia are mainly single-nucleotide substitutions, assays using ASO hybridization, AS-PCR, PCR-RFLP [19], and real-time PCR with hybridization probes have been described [20]. These assays target population-specific mutations. If mutations are not identified by these methods, then direct sequencing of the β-globin gene including known 5′ promoter and 3′ polyadenylation site mutations can be performed. The size of the β-globin gene, about 1.6 kb containing three exons, is amenable to DNA sequencing. The advantage of DNA sequencing is that virtually all β-globin mutations can be detected. Deletions of the β-globin gene cluster can be detected by MLPA or gap PCR.

Interpretation of Test Results

Hematologic screens are more than 95 % accurate, with occasional problems detecting carriers with mild phenotypes. The analytic sensitivity for detecting gene mutations should be greater than 99 %. False positives and false negatives are rare. However, sequence variations in primers, probes, and restriction sites have the potential to lead to a diagnostic error. The mutation resulting in HbC occurs at 1 bp from the HbS mutation. There is the potential for a diagnostic error with a test that does not clearly distinguish these two mutations.

The mutation detection rate for α- and β-thalassemia will depend on the mutations in the panel and the patient's ethnicity. For α-thalassemia, greater than 95 % of the mutations are deletions; the majority of these deletions can be detected in the current assays. For β-thalassemia, if a mutation is not detected in a patient with symptoms, then DNA sequencing should be considered to identify the mutation. The detection rate using DNA sequencing for β-thalassemia is approximately 99 % depending on the actual coverage of the gene sequence. Deletions larger than the PCR product size or ones that abolish the PCR primer sites will not be detected by DNA sequencing. When interpreting the molecular analysis in relation to the clinical phenotype, the possible coinheritance of genetic determinants that could influence the phenotype must be considered. For example, inheritance of an α-thalassemia allele, silent or mild β-thalassemia allele, HPFH allele, or HbS allele would modify the phenotype. Family studies are useful in sorting out complex genotypes.

The possibility of maternal contamination should be considered in interpreting the molecular test result done for prenatal diagnosis. The contamination with maternal cells of both direct and cultured amniotic fluid and chorionic villus sampling (CVS) is well documented and therefore represents a potential source of error in prenatal diagnosis. Prenatal samples should be tested in parallel with a maternal sample, or both samples should be used to perform a separate analysis for maternal contamination using microsatellite markers, to rule out error due to maternal cell contamination. Laboratories should understand how their testing methods are affected by the presence and the amount of maternal cell contamination. The mutation status of one or both parents, as appropriate, should be tested prior to testing of fetal specimens, preferably within the same laboratory.

Laboratory Issues

Proficiency testing is available for HbS and HbC through the CAP MGL survey. Proficiency testing for α- and β-thalassemia usually can be accomplished through a sample exchange with another laboratory that performs the testing. DNA and cell-line controls for many of the hemoglobinopathies can be purchased from Coriell Cell Repositories (http://ccr.coriell.org/). Commercial kits for the HbS, HbC, and the common α- and β-thalassemia mutations are available from Bio-Rad Laboratories (Hercules, CA).

Rh Incompatibility

Molecular Basis of Disease

The Rh antigen system is clinically important because antibodies to Rh antigens are involved in hemolytic transfusion reactions, autoimmune hemolytic anemia, and HDFN. HDFN results from the alloimmunization of a mother to a paternally inherited fetal alloantigen. For example, an RhD-negative mother may make antibodies to the D antigen if the fetus inherits the *RHD* gene from the father. The most common cause for alloimmunization is fetomaternal hemorrhage. Other causes include unrecognized miscarriage, amniocentesis, CVS, cordocentesis, and transfusion. In subsequent pregnancies, these antibodies cross the placenta and may destroy the red blood cells of an antigen-positive fetus leading to hemolytic disease. The severity of HDFN is variable; mild cases require either no treatment or phototherapy, while more severe cases require exchange transfusion at birth, or possibly intrauterine transfusion, and may result in fetal hydrops. HDFN can occur when fetomaternal incompatibilities exist in several red cell antigen systems, including the RHD, C/c, E/e, Kell, Kidd, Duffy, and M. Anti-D accounts for the majority of HDFN cases followed by anti-K, anti-c, and anti-E [21]. The frequency of Rh-negative individuals, those at risk for making anti-D, is 15 % in Caucasians, 5 % in African Americans, 8 % in Hispanics, and low in Inuit, Native Americans, Japanese, and Asians.

The Rh antigens are expressed on proteins encoded by two distinct but highly homologous genes, *RHD* and *RHCE*, on chromosome 1p34.3-36.1 [22]. The *RHD* and *RHCE* genes are arranged in tandem and likely arose through duplication of a single ancestral gene (Fig. 16.3a) [23]. The D

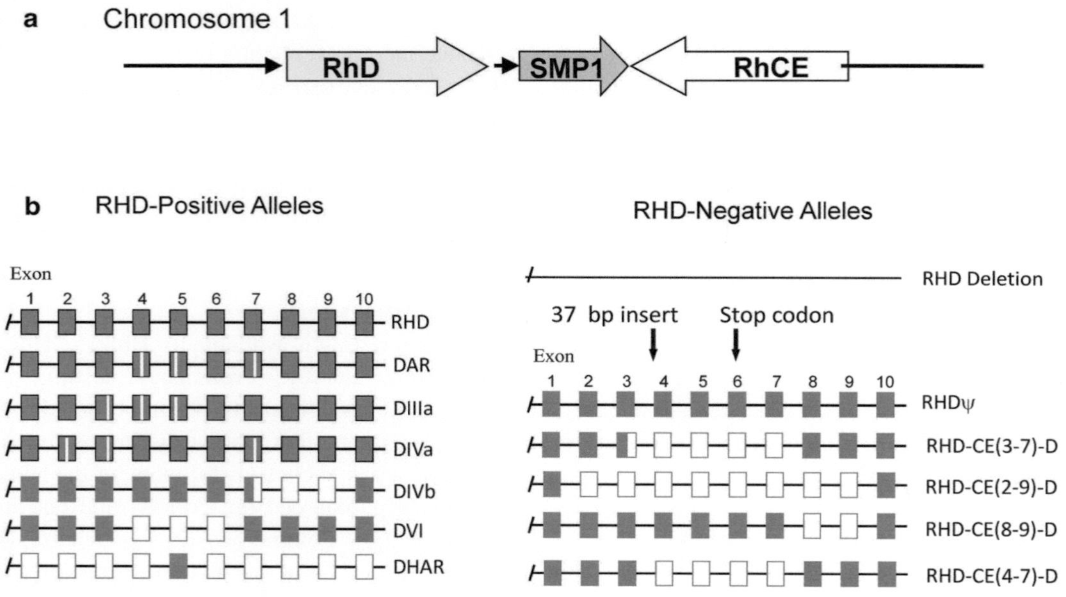

Figure 16.3 (**a**) Genomic organization of the RHD and RHCE genes on the short arm of chromosome 1. The RHD gene is flanked by two highly homologous Rhesus boxes (*black arrowheads*). (**b**) The listing of the most common *RHD* variant alleles illustrates why *RHD* genotyping assays require multiple targets within the *RHD* gene. Most variants are *RHD–RHCE* hybrid genes. *RHD* exons are indicated by the *square boxes*. *Grey boxes* indicate *RHD*-specific sequences and white indicates *RHCE*-specific sequences. The *RHDΨ* and *RHD-CE*(3-7)-*D* are frequently seen in the African-American population and may lead to false-positive results if not specifically targeted and detected. ((**b**) Used with kind permission of Springer Science+Business Media from Diagnostic molecular pathology in practice: a case based approach, 2011, Chap. 9, Rh Incompatibility by DB Bellissimo)

antigen is expressed from *RHD* and the C/c and E/e antigens are expressed from *RHCE*. The alleles from the *RHD* and *RHCE* are inherited as a haplotype. The eight possible haplotypes in order of frequency in the Caucasian population are DCe, dce, DcE, Dce, dCe, dcE, DCE, and dCE where d is the designation for the RHD-negative allele. The *RH* genes are more than 95 % homologous at the nucleotide sequence level and both genes consist of ten exons spanning over 75 kb. A number of sequence variations can be used to distinguish these two highly similar genes. However, it is important to be aware of a number of variant alleles that exist in this genetic system as the result of gene conversion events between the *RHD* and *RHCE* genes and from point mutations (Fig. 16.3b). Databases of these variants are available: Blood Group Antigen Gene Mutation Database (http://www.ncbi.nlm.nih.gov/projects/rbc) and the Rhesus Site (http://www.uni-ulm.de/~wflegel/RH/).

These hybrid *RHD-CE-D* alleles may result in either *RHD*-positive or *RHD*-negative haplotypes. Most variant *RHD*-positive alleles encode proteins that do not express all the RHD epitopes. Although an RHD-negative mother can be alloimmunized by a partial D antigen, hemolytic disease in these cases is rare. However, a mother with a partial D antigen can still be alloimmunized by the normal D antigen. The frequency of these variant alleles is low in the Caucasian population, but in some ethnic groups these alleles can be common [24]. The DAR allele is found in 17 % of South-African blacks, and DIIIa has been found in 18 % of blacks in New York and 28 % of blacks from Brazil.

The most common *RHD*-negative allele results from the total deletion of *RHD*; however, there are a number of *RHD-negative* haplotypes that are positive for at least portions of the *RHD* gene (Fig. 16.3b). In the African population, there are two *RHD*-positive, antigen D-negative alleles that are common and must be considered in any genotyping strategy. *RHDΨ* is present in 66 % of RHD-negative Africans and 24 % of African Americans and contains a 37 bp insertion at the junction of intron 3 and exon 4 that disrupts the reading frame and leads to a stop codon [25]. There are additional sequence variations in exon 4, 5, and 6 that distinguish *RHDΨ* from *RHD*. The Cde^s allele (RHD-CE(3-7)-D) is a hybrid allele containing exons 1 and 2, part of exon 3 from *RHD*, exons 3–7 from *RHCE* and exons 8–10, including intron 7, from *RHD*. Cde^s is found in 15 % of RHD-negative Africans. In addition, a significant percentage of RHD-negative Asians (27 %) are positive for the *RHD* gene.

The c.307T>C, p.Ser103Pro, sequence variation is responsible for the C and c antigens expressed from the *RHCE* gene. Genotyping for the *RHc* allele is straightforward, but the identification of the *RHC* allele is complicated by the fact that exon 2 of the *RHC* allele is identical to exon 2 of *RHD*. A 109 bp insertion found in intron 2 of the *RHC* allele can be used for genotyping [26]. The *Cdes* allele discussed above does express a C antigen but this allele will give a false-negative result with this intron 2 assay since the intron 2 is of *RHD* origin. The identification of *RHD* and *RHCE* sequences in exon 3 will indicate the possible presence of this variant allele. The c.676C>G, p. Pro226Ala, sequence variation is responsible for the RhE and Rhe antigens of the *RHCE* gene. Rare allelic variants involving exon 5 have been described that would lead to erroneous typing of the E/e polymorphism.

Clinical Utility of Testing

Algorithms for managing a first sensitized pregnancy and patients with a previously affected fetus or newborn have been described [27]. Maternal antibody titers, ultrasound, middle cerebral artery (MCA) Doppler, cordocentesis, and molecular testing are used to monitor these pregnancies. MCA Doppler has a sensitivity of 88 % and specificity of 82 % for the detection of severe hemolytic disease [28]. MCA Doppler has largely replaced the use of amniotic fluid ΔOD_{450} which requires serial amniocentesis and puts these patients at risk for additional alloimmunization. Molecular testing plays an important role in the proposed algorithms for the management of HDFN. The algorithms seek to identify fetuses at risk for HDFN and monitor the severity of the disease while minimizing invasive procedures that may increase maternal exposure to fetal red cells and worsen the sensitization. The main utility of molecular testing is to determine paternal zygosity and fetal genotype, and to characterize variant alleles.

Paternal zygosity is used to predict the risk of HDFN in each pregnancy. If the paternal sample is homozygous for the alloallele then the fetus is predicted to be positive for the alloallele and the fetus can be appropriately monitored and invasive procedures may be avoided. Prenatal testing of the fetus may still be indicated if non-paternity is a possibility. If the paternal sample is heterozygous, fetal DNA testing through amniocentesis, CVS, or the testing of free fetal DNA in maternal plasma can be used to determine whether the fetus is positive or negative for the alloallele. Zygosity determination is straightforward by serological or molecular methods in most biallelic antigen systems except for *RHD*. *RHD* zygosity can be predicted by the Rh phenotype and haplotype frequencies. However, the predictions are not reliable in some ethnic groups, especially African Americans. *RHD* zygosity is most accurately determined using molecular methods.

Genotyping assays for *RH* also can help identify variant alleles that may or may not be identified in the immunohematology laboratory or blood bank by their usual phenotypic characteristics. Some individuals will be typed as RhD-negative by serology, yet may have a weak or partial D that is not detected by the antibody reagent being used. Molecular testing is useful in detecting these variants and may help identify patients that require Rh immune globulin treatment.

There are a number of examples in the literature describing the loss or weakening of RhD expression, particularly in cancer patients [22]. In some instances this has been caused by deletion of the *RHD* gene or loss or abnormalities involving chromosome 1. Molecular assays can confirm the loss of genetic material encoding the *RHD* gene. In addition, molecular assays are useful in predicting blood group phenotype in the transfused patient [29].

Available Assays

The assay formats are predominantly AS-PCR and real-time PCR with hydrolysis probes. Both methods are well suited for detecting single base pair polymorphisms; however, the sensitivity of real-time assays is beneficial when the amount of DNA from a prenatal sample is limiting. Testing for two or more regions of the *RHD* gene is required for identification of allelic variants. Assays must distinguish the *RHD* gene from *RHCE*. A number of assays have been described using the various sequence differences between the genes in exons 3–7 and 9, introns 4 and 7, and the 3′ untranslated region of exon 10 [26, 30, 31]. Detection of the *RHDΨ* also should be included in all genotyping assays [25]. Targets for *RHDΨ* include a 37 bp insertion in exon 4 as well as single nucleotide variants in exons 5 and 6. Although exon 10 is a very sensitive marker for the *RHD* gene due to the unique sequence in this exon, it is important to be aware of possible false positives and false negatives caused by variant alleles. However, exon 10 is useful in recognizing the Cde^s haplotypes in RhD-negative individuals.

Molecular assays for *RHE/e* take advantage of polymorphisms within exon 5 that are specific to the *RHCE* gene [26]. *RHc* is detected directly using the C307 polymorphism, while the 109 bp intron 2 insertion is used to detect the *RHC* allele. Multiplex genotyping assays for *RHD* and *RHCc* also have been described [25]. The sensitivity for detecting the RHC allele can be improved by using an assay that detects the *RHC* allele associated Cde^s haplotype [26]. Although laboratory-developed tests are most commonly used, CE-marked kits for *RHCE* and *RHD* including partial and variant alleles are available from Bag Healthcare (Lich, Germany). A number of assays are being developed for genotyping patients and blood donors for red cell antigens [32]. Their use of these assays for prenatal testing has not been assessed.

The precise site of the *RHD* deletion has been defined, making detection of the deletion possible with a PCR-based assay [24]. Although the deletion is the most common *RHD-negative* allele in whites and African Americans, this assay will not correctly determine zygosity in RhD-negative alleles that contain RHD gene sequences such as Cde^s and *RHDΨ*. Real-time PCR assays or fragment analysis of fluorescently labeled PCR products potentially can be used for determining zygosity, as long as more than one region of the *RHD* gene is detected and the assay design takes into account possible genetic variants. A quantitative fluorescent PCR technique has been described that detects *RHD* exons 5 and 7 using *RHCE* exon 7 as an internal two copy control [33]. The presence of common Rh variants in Caucasians and African Americans is recognized when the *RHD* exon 5 copy number is discordant with exon 7. The exon 5 primers are specific for the *RHD* gene, such that *RHDΨ* is not detected. The exon 7 primers detect both the *RHD* and *RHDΨ* genes.

These methods are suitable for testing fetal DNA as well as genomic DNA from blood. Fetal DNA sources are typically amniotic fluid or chorionic villi, using either direct or cultured samples. Since fetal DNA preparations can be potentially contaminated with maternal DNA, laboratories must understand how maternal contamination will affect the assay results and have methods to determine the extent of contamination. Testing of variable number of tandem repeats (VNTR) or microsatellite loci in fetal and maternal DNA samples can be used to determine whether maternal cells contaminate the fetal sample.

Another potential source of fetal DNA is maternal plasma. Fetal DNA accounts for approximately 3 % of the total cell-free DNA in maternal plasma during the second trimester and increases throughout pregnancy. Since this method avoids invasive techniques that cause risk to the fetus, and prevents further sensitization of the mother, the method is of significant interest. Laboratories outside the USA have successfully performed these tests for almost 10 years. However, due to intellectual property issues, the maternal plasma assays have only recently become available in the USA. Several studies have demonstrated that fetal DNA in maternal plasma can be used to determine a fetal genotype using real-time PCR or mass spectrometry [31, 34, 35].

Interpretation of Test Results

Using a multiplex strategy, the sensitivity for detecting the *RHD* gene should be >99 % and the false-positive rate <1 %. However, the performance characteristics may vary with different testing strategies in different ethnic groups. The rate of false-positive results and positive predictive values for different PCR strategies in the European population has been described [30]. One rare *RHD* allele, DHar, would be missed by many genotyping assays as it contains only exon 5 of the *RHD* gene (*RHCE-D(5)-CE*). The frequency of variant *RHD* alleles is much greater in other ethnic groups, especially Africans (Fig. 16.3b). The most common RhD-negative variants are *Cdes* and *RHDΨ*. In most assay designs, the presence of a variant allele is identified by a missing or altered PCR product.

In a typical HDFN case, an Rh-D negative mother has developed an anti-D titer. *RHD* zygosity testing on a paternal sample determines whether the fetus is at 50 % or 100 % risk of inheriting an *RHD* allele. An example *RHD* genotyping assay that targets exon 7 and intron 4 in one reaction and exon 4 and intron 7 in a second reaction is shown (Fig. 16.4a). The size of the exon 4 band indicates whether RHDΨ is present. The maternal sample has only the control bands as expected for a *RHD*-negative sample. The exon 4 products in the paternal sample indicate the presence of the *RHD* gene and *RHDΨ*. The results indicate the fetus is RHD-positive and is at risk for HDFN. Figure 16.4b illustrates two more complex HDFN cases. In the first case, fetus F1 is positive for *RHD* but the maternal sample (M1) is also *RHD*-positive despite a D-negative phenotype. Unless the maternal variant can be identified, it cannot be determined whether the fetus has inherited the maternal or paternal *RHD* allele or both. Zygosity testing on the fetal sample can be used to determine whether the fetus has inherited one or two copies of *RHD*. If the fetus is homozygous, then the fetus inherited the paternal *RHD* and is at risk for HDFN. If the fetus is heterozygous, the test is inconclusive. The fetus should be consider at risk for HDFN with a 50 % chance of being RhD-negative. The second case involves an RhD-positive mother that has developed anti-D. Genotyping of the maternal sample (M2) indicates the absence of exon 7 most likely due to a *DAR* or *DIVa* allele (Fig. 16.3b). The fetus F2 genotypes as *RHD*-positive. The presence of the exon 7 band indicates the fetus inherited the paternal *RHD* gene and is at risk for HDFN.

These examples illustrate the importance of testing maternal and paternal samples. The detection of variant alleles by discrepancies between parental serotypes and genotypes will reduce the risk of false-negative and false-positive results. Variants easily will be identified in RhD-negative mothers that test positive for the *RHD* gene. As discussed above, if the mother is positive for only parts of the *RHD* gene, it still may be possible to tell if her fetus inherited a paternal *RHD* gene. Allelic variants can go undetected by serology and genotyping in paternal samples by the presence of a "normal" *RHD* allele. If the masked allele with an altered pattern of *RHD* products is detected, the genotype may not allow certain prediction whether the fetus will have an RhD-positive phenotype. In these cases, the fetus should be considered at risk for HDFN.

As discussed earlier, allelic variants of the *RHC* are common in individuals of African ancestry. In RHD-negative Africans, the *Cdes* allele will result in a 15–20 % false-negative result since intron 2 is of *RHD* origin. Clearly, in this ethnic group, testing a paternal sample for the presence of the *RHC* allele is important, especially in a C-negative fetus. The *DHar* allele (*RHCE-D5RHCE*) may cause a false negative for Rhe since exon 5, the location of the *RHE/e* polymorphism, is of *RHD* origin. Other rare alleles in the *RH* system may be misidentified in DNA typing assays. When maternal and paternal samples are not available, interpretation should include the possibility of a false-positive or false-negative result as relevant to the population being tested.

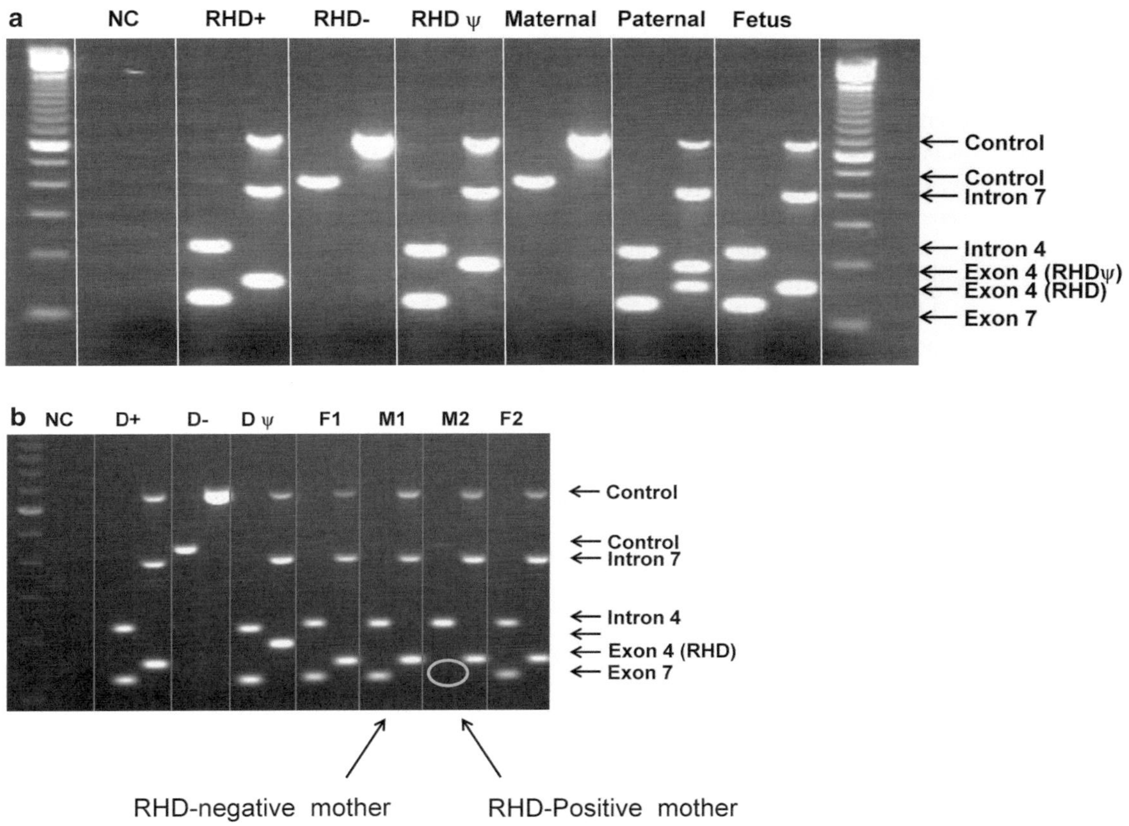

Figure 16.4 (**a**) *RHD* multiplex genotyping assay. There are two reactions per sample. The first reaction detects exon 7 and intron 4. The second reaction detects exon 4 and intron 7. If the *RHDΨ* is present, the size of the exon 4 PCR product is increased by 37 bp. Each PCR reaction also contains primers to a control gene. The control products for reactions 1 and 2 are of different sizes. The PCR products are identified by the *arrows*. (**b**) Complex HDFN cases with variant *RHD* alleles. Fetus (F1) is positive for *RHD* but the maternal sample (M1) is also *RHD*-positive despite a D-negative phenotype. M2 is RhD-positive with anti-D; exon 7 is absent (*circle*) most likely due to a DAR or DIVa allele (Fig. 16.3b). The fetus (F2) genotypes as *RHD*-positive. The presence of the exon 7 band indicates the fetus inherited the paternal *RHD* gene and is at risk for HDFN. ((**a**) Used with kind permission of Springer Science + Business Media from Diagnostic molecular pathology in practice: a case based approach, 2011, Chap. 9, Rh Incompatibility by DB Bellissimo)

Laboratory Issues

Many Rh incompatibility cases will require both phenotypic and genotypic testing of parental samples. Laboratories need to work in conjunction with an immunohematology laboratory, which is able to provide phenotypic data and assist in the analysis of variant alleles. Only simple *RHD* controls are available from Coriell Cell Repositories (http://ccr.coriell.org/). The immunohematology laboratory or blood bank are the best source of ethnic-specific assay controls. These tests are typically developed and validated by the laboratory. Proficiency testing for *RHD* is available in the CAP MGL survey but this survey does not challenge the laboratory's ability to identify variant *RHD* alleles. Proficiency testing can be accomplished through a sample exchange with another laboratory that performs the testing.

The key laboratory issue is understanding the sensitivity and specificity of the test and how this will be affected by ethnic group and if one or both of the parental samples are not available for testing. This is especially true for maternal plasma testing. Despite the high sensitivity and specificity of these assays, there is still a significant level of false-positive, false-negative, and inconclusive results compared to conventional testing [34]. The fetal DNA represents a minority of the total DNA in maternal plasma and the fetal copy number is variable. Internal controls are important to demonstrate that fetal DNA is present in sufficient quantity. This is especially true when the test result is *RHD*-negative. Y chromosome-specific sequences can be used when the fetus is male but other paternal-specific polymorphisms, dose, or fetal-specific markers may be required to provide the necessary internal control [36]. Finally, the laboratory needs to be aware whether the test on the fetus is being requested to determine if they are at risk for HDFN or soley predict the fetal blood type. Typically, Rh-negative blood is used when a fetus requires an intrauterine transfusion for HDFN. However, if multiple red cell antigen antibodies are present, the antigen-negative blood needed may be quite rare. Finding blood will be easier if the fetus is known to be RhD-positive and can be transfused with Rh-positive blood. A false-positive result in these instances has quite different medical management implications. In the fetus at risk for HDFN related to anti-D, a false-positive result will lead to increased monitoring of the fetus, whereas a false-positive result for transfusion could lead to an RhD-negative fetus being transfused with RhD-positive blood. When predicting red cell antigen phenotypes by genotyping, it is important to work with experts in transfusion medicine.

References

1. Imperatore G, Pinsky LE, Motulsky A, Reyes M, Bradley LA, Burke W. Hereditary hemochromatosis: perspectives of public health, medical genetics, and primary care. Genet Med. 2003;5:1–8.
2. Hanson EH, Imperatore G, Burke W. HFE gene and hereditary hemochromatosis: a HuGE review. Human Genome Epidemiology. Am J Epidemiol. 2001;154:193–206.
3. Weiss G. Genetic mechanisms and modifying factors in hereditary hemochromatosis. Nat Rev Gastroenterol Hepatol. 2010;7:50–8.
4. Kowdley KV, Bennet RL, Motulsky A. HFE-associated hereditary hemochromatosis. GeneReviews [serial online] 2012. Accessed 19 Apr, 12 A.D.
5. Zhou XY, Tomatsu S, Fleming RE, et al. HFE gene knockout produces mouse model of hereditary hemochromatosis. Proc Natl Acad Sci U S A. 1998;95:2492–7.
6. Feder JN, Gnirke A, Thomas W, et al. A novel MHC class I-like gene is mutated in patients with hereditary haemochromatosis. Nat Genet. 1996;13:399–408.
7. Burke W, Imperatore G, McDonnell SM, Baron RC, Khoury MJ. Contribution of different HFE genotypes to iron overload disease: a pooled analysis. Genet Med. 2000;2:271–7.
8. Allen KJ, Gurrin LC, Constantine CC, et al. Iron-overload-related disease in HFE hereditary hemochromatosis. N Engl J Med. 2008;358:221–30.
9. Somerville MJ, Sprysak KA, Hicks M, Elyas BG, Vicen-Wyhony L. An HFE intronic variant promotes misdiagnosis of hereditary hemochromatosis. Am J Hum Genet. 1999;65:924–6.
10. Beutler E, Gelbart T. A common intron 3 mutation (IVS3-48c→g) leads to misdiagnosis of the c.845G→A (C282Y) HFE gene mutation. Blood Cells Mol Dis. 2000;26:229–33.
11. Pointon JJ, Merryweather-Clarke AT, Carella M, Robson KJ. Detection of C282Y and H63D in the HFE gene. Genet Test. 2000;4:115–20.
12. Lyon E, Frank EL. Hereditary hemochromatosis since discovery of the HFE gene. Clin Chem. 2001;47:1147–56.
13. Weatherall DJ. The thalassemias: disorders of globin synthesis. In: Kaushansky K, Lichtman MA, Beutler E, Kipps TJ, Seligsohn U, Prchal JT, editors. Williams hematology. 8th ed. New York: McGraw-Hill; 2010. p. 675–707.
14. Higgs DR. Alpha thalassemia. In: Steinberg MH, Forget BG, Higgs DR, Weatherall DJ, editors. Disorders of hemoglobin: genetics, pathophysiology, and clinical management. 2nd ed. New York: Cambridge University Press; 2009. p. 241–323.
15. Cao A, Galanello R. Beta-thalassemia. GeneReviews [serial online] 2010.
16. Hatcher SL, Trang QT, Robb KM, Teplitz RL, Carlson JR. Prenatal diagnosis by enzymatic amplification and restriction endonuclease digestion for detection of haemoglobins A, S and C. Mol Cell Probes. 1992;6:343–8.
17. Hermann MG. Genotyping b-globin mutations (HbS, HbC, HbE) by muliplexing probe color and melting temperature. In: Meuer S, Wittwer CT, Nakagawara K, editors. Rapid cycle real-time PCR: methods and applications. Heidelberg: Springer; 2001. p. 119–25.
18. Tan AS, Quah TC, Low PS, Chong SS. A rapid and reliable 7-deletion multiplex polymerase chain reaction assay for alpha-thalassemia. Blood. 2001;98:250–1.
19. Tuzmen S, Schechter AN. Genetic diseases of hemoglobin: diagnostic methods for elucidating beta-thalassemia mutations. Blood Rev. 2001;15:19–29.
20. Moreno I, Bolufer P, Perez ML, Barragan E, Sanz MA. Rapid detection of the major Mediterranean beta-thalassaemia mutations by real-time polymerase chain reaction using fluorophore-labelled hybridization probes. Br J Haematol. 2002;119:554–7.
21. Bowman JM. Immune hemolytic disease. In: Nathan DG, Oski FA, editors. Hematology of infancy and childhood. 5th ed. Philadelphia: W.B. Saunders; 1998. p. 53–78.
22. Avent ND, Reid ME. The Rh blood group system: a review. Blood. 2000;95:375–87.
23. Wagner FF, Flegel WA. RHCE represents the ancestral RH position, while RHD is the duplicated gene. Blood. 2002;99:2272–3.
24. Reid ME, Lomas-Francis C. The blood group antigen facts book. 2nd ed. London: Academic; 2004.
25. Singleton BK, Green CA, Avent ND, et al. The presence of an RHD pseudogene containing a 37 base pair duplication and a nonsense mutation in Africans with the Rh D-negative blood group phenotype. Blood. 2000;95:12–8.
26. van der Schoot CE, Tax GH, Rijnders RJ, De Haas M, Christiaens GC. Prenatal typing of Rh and Kell blood group system antigens: the edge of a watershed. Transfus Med Rev. 2003;17:31–44.
27. Moise Jr KJ. Management of rhesus alloimmunization in pregnancy. Obstet Gynecol. 2008;112:164–76.
28. Oepkes D, Seaward PG, Vandenbussche FP, et al. Doppler ultrasonography versus amniocentesis to predict fetal anemia. N Engl J Med. 2006;355:156–64.
29. Reid ME, Rios M, Powell VI, Charles-Pierre D, Malavade V. DNA from blood samples can be used to genotype patients who have recently received a transfusion. Transfusion. 2000;40:48–53.
30. Wagner FF, Frohmajer A, Flegel WA. RHD positive haplotypes in D negative Europeans. BMC Genet. 2001;2:10.
31. Finning KM, Martin PG, Soothill PW, Avent ND. Prediction of fetal D status from maternal plasma: introduction of a new noninvasive fetal RHD genotyping service. Transfusion. 2002;42:1079–85.
32. Denomme GA, Johnson ST, Pietz BC. Mass-scale red cell genotyping of blood donors. Transfus Apher Sci. 2011;44:93–9.
33. Pirelli KJ, Pietz BC, Johnson ST, Pinder HL, Bellissimo DB. Molecular determination of RHD zygosity: predicting risk of hemolytic disease of the fetus and newborn related to anti-D. Prenat Diagn. 2010;30:1207–12.
34. Bombard AT, Akolekar R, Farkas DH, et al. Fetal RHD genotype detection from circulating cell-free fetal DNA in maternal plasma in non-sensitized RhD negative women. Prenat Diagn. 2011;31:802–8.
35. Tynan JA, Angkachatchai V, Ehrich M, Paladino T, van den Boom D, Oeth P. Multiplexed analysis of circulating cell-free fetal nucleic acids for noninvasive prenatal diagnostic RHD testing. Am J Obstet Gynecol. 2011;204:251–6.
36. Nygren AO, Dean J, Jensen TJ, et al. Quantification of fetal DNA by use of methylation-based DNA discrimination. Clin Chem. 2010;56:1627–35.

Cardiovascular Disease

17

Samantha M. Baxter and Birgit H. Funke

Abstract

During the last decade, techniques and advances in molecular genetics and genomics have yielded profound insights into the fundamental mechanisms and genetic underpinnings for many heritable cardiovascular diseases. The availability of clinical genetic testing has resulted in dramatic changes in our ability to: (1) identify preclinical/presymptomatic individuals by molecular testing, (2) characterize/clarify clinical diagnoses with phenotypic and genotypic overlap, and (3) in some cases, provide gene-specific or gene-targeted therapy including primary prevention in genotype-positive/phenotype-negative individuals. Sudden cardiac death (SCD) consumes more lives than any other medical condition in developed countries, with 1,000 SCDs occurring each day in the USA. Coronary artery disease (CAD) is the major cause of SCD, while other heritable diseases including cardiomyopathies and channelopathies also predispose to fatal ventricular arrhythmias. Characteristic hallmarks of most inherited cardiovascular diseases discussed in this chapter include a high degree of locus heterogeneity (many genes) as well as allelic heterogeneity (many different mutations within a gene). Multiple modes of inheritance usually exist and reduced penetrance and variable expressivity are common. All these factors can complicate the interpretation of genetic test results and highlight the critical importance of interpreting identified mutations in the context of an individual's clinical features as well as family history.

Keywords

Cardiovascular disease • Sudden cardiac death • Coronary artery disease • Cardiomyopathy • Channelopathy • Arrhythmia • Congenital heart disease • Long QT syndrome • Brugada syndrome • Idiopathic ventricular fibrillation • Catecholaminergic polymorphic ventricular tachycardia • Molecular genetic testing

Introduction

During the last decade, techniques and advances in molecular genetics and genomics have yielded profound insights into the fundamental mechanisms and genetic underpinnings for many heritable cardiovascular diseases. The availability of clinical genetic testing has resulted in dramatic changes in our ability to: (1) identify preclinical/presymptomatic individuals by molecular testing, (2) characterize/clarify clinical diagnoses with phenotypic and genotypic overlap, and (3) in some cases,

S.M. Baxter, M.S., C.G.C.
Laboratory for Molecular Medicine, Partners HealthCare, Cambridge, MA, USA

B.H. Funke, Ph.D., F.A.C.M.G. (✉)
Department of Pathology, Harvard Medical School, 65 Landsdowne St., Cambridge, MA, USA
e-mail: bfunke@partners.org

D.G.B. Leonard (ed.), *Molecular Pathology in Clinical Practice*, DOI 10.1007/978-3-319-19674-9_17

provide gene-specific or gene-targeted therapy including primary prevention in genotype-positive/phenotype-negative individuals. Cardiology has embraced new genetic discoveries. Sudden cardiac death (SCD) consumes more lives than any other medical condition in developed countries, with 1,000 SCDs occurring each day in the USA. Coronary artery disease (CAD) is the major cause of SCD, while other heritable diseases including cardiomyopathies and channelopathies also predispose to fatal ventricular arrhythmias. For example, over 4,000 deaths per year are attributed to long QT syndrome (LQTS) and in 10 to 15 % of those cases sudden death is the first symptom a patient experiences [1]. In this chapter, we review the current understanding of heritable cardiovascular diseases with a focus on the molecular pathogenic mechanisms and status of molecular testing for cardiomyopathies, channelopathies/arrhythmias, CAD, and congenital heart disease or defects (CHD), most of which of which render an individual susceptible to SCD.

Cardiomyopathies have a combined estimated prevalence of 1 in 390 individuals [2]. Many causal genes have been identified and extensively studied in individuals with hypertrophic cardiomyopathy (HCM), dilated cardiomyopathy (DCM), arrhythmogenic right ventricular cardiomyopathy (ARVC), restrictive cardiomyopathy (RCM), and isolated left ventricular non-compaction (LVNC) [3]. Cardiac channelopathies may account for a significant proportion of SCD and are characterized by a structurally normal heart, defined as no abnormalities seen at autopsy [4]. The main channelopathies/arrhythmias include congenital LQTS, Brugada syndrome (BrS), idiopathic ventricular fibrillation, and catecholaminergic polymorphic ventricular tachycardia (CPVT) [3]. CAD is a common disease with a complex interaction of many genetic susceptibility loci and environmental factors. Much progress has been made towards understanding genetic risk factors for CAD; however, clinical genetic testing is not yet within reach. Several rare monogenic diseases such as familial hypercholesterolemia predispose to CAD and provide a stepping stone to understand the common, complex form [5]. Finally, isolated CHDS are the most common birth defect with an estimated incidence of approximately 6 in 1,000 live births. While much of the genetic etiology of various types of CHD (such as Tetralogy of Fallot or various septal defects) is thought to be complex, monogenic forms exist and disease genes lending themselves to genetic testing have been identified [6].

Many genetic syndromes, such as Noonan syndrome and Marfan syndrome, have cardiovascular involvement. As with many of the diseases mentioned in this chapter, use of molecular testing has increasingly informed the clinical diagnosis of these syndromes, and helped characterize their phenotypic spectrum [7, 8]. Syndromes with cardiac involvement are discussed further in other chapters.

Characteristic hallmarks of most inherited cardiovascular diseases discussed in this chapter include a high degree of locus heterogeneity (many genes) as well as allelic heterogeneity (many different mutations within a gene). Multiple modes of inheritance usually exist and reduced penetrance (not everyone with a pathogenic mutation will present with disease in their lifetime) and variable expressivity (those with the mutation can present at various stages of life and with different symptoms) also are common. All of these factors can complicate the interpretation of genetic test results and highlight the critical importance of interpreting identified mutations in the context of an individual's clinical features as well as family history.

Expert Opinions and Guidelines on Genetic Testing for Inherited Cardiac Disease

Several expert opinions and practice guidelines on clinical management as well as genetic testing for inherited cardiomyopathies and channelopathies have been published over the last few years [3, 9–11]. General recommendations include obtaining a detailed family history of at least three generations, clinically screening at risk relatives, counseling for a possible heritable basis and considering genetic testing of the most clearly affected person in a family. It is recognized that the evidence implicating cardiomyopathy and channelopathy genes varies tremendously and that the level of evidence for a given gene correlates directly with a test's clinical validity (its ability to correctly detect the condition). Recent guidelines from the Heart Rhythm Society (HRS) and European Heart Rhythm Association (EHRA) based recommendations on the diagnostic, prognostic, and therapeutic impact of genetic testing [3]. Despite the availability of gene panels of rapidly increasing size, comprehensive testing is currently recommended only for a relatively small number of genes, which have high detection rates and/or strong genotype–phenotype correlations. One of the main benefits of genetic testing is the ability to test at-risk family members, when a pathogenic mutation is identified. The presence of a clearly pathogenic mutation in a presymptomatic relative enables implementation of lifestyle changes to avoid sudden death, while disease risk in mutation negative relatives is reduced to the general population risk. However, because genetic testing for inherited cardiovascular disease is still a relatively young discipline, the risk for identifying uninterpretable mutations, often referred to as variants of unknown significance (VUS), is still relatively high compared to other disease areas, reducing the clinical utility of currently available tests [3].

Genetic Testing for Inherited Cardiac Disease in the Era of Genomic Medicine

Until recently, the high cost of Sanger sequencing made comprehensive genetic testing challenging for genetically heterogeneous diseases. Gene panels were of limited size and usually did not include genes with low detection rates. With the advent of next-generation sequencing (NGS) technologies this limitation has been removed. A prime example is the titin (*TTN*) gene, which encodes the largest human protein. Due to its enormous size (383 exons), only with the clinical use of NGS testing is this gene now being sequenced in patients, which has led to the discovery that *TTN* is one of the most frequently mutated genes in DCM [12]. Gene panels covering tens to hundreds of genes are beginning to be broadly available in molecular testing laboratories. These comprehensive tests greatly facilitate the genetic testing process as they eliminate the costly and lengthy testing odysseys of one gene at a time that has dominated genetic testing for inherited cardiovascular disease for a decade. Although still costly and therefore not yet broadly available, exome or genome sequencing (ES/GS) is beginning to enter clinical practice though still mostly in the setting of clinically complex cases [13–15]. An important advantage of these large scale sequencing tests is that while the assay assesses all genes, the interpretation can focus on a clinically relevant subset of genes relevant to the patient's disease or symptoms. Despite obvious advantages, testing large gene sets has some important limitations. In the past, the limited size of gene panels provided a natural selection for well-established disease genes. With the ability to sequence virtually every gene it is critical to carefully review the evidence available for a published disease-gene association. It is not uncommon that a gene (particularly if disease-causing mutations are rare) is supported by a single or very small number of studies providing limited evidence. The inclusion of genes that have not yet been firmly associated with disease can lead to an inflation of VUS, which limit the clinical utility of large gene panels if no clear pathogenic mutation is detected.

Inherited Cardiomyopathies

Cardiomyopathies are diseases of the heart muscle that have traditionally been defined based solely on clinical features including ventricular morphology and function. While HCM, DCM, ARVC, and LVNC are generally recognized as distinct clinical entities, phenotypic overlap is increasingly recognized. For example, end stage HCM can resemble DCM [16]. Similarly, there is phenotypic overlap between DCM and ARVC, which can manifest with ventricular dilation [17]. Finally, features of LVNC can overlap with HCM, DCM, and RCM [18, 19]. With the characterization of the underlying genetic etiologies came the recognition of substantial and increasing genetic overlap (Table 17.1, reviewed in Refs. 3 and 20). Genes encoding proteins of the sarcomere, the contractile unit of myocytes, were first identified in patients with HCM but more recently also in patients with DCM, LVNC, and RCM [21–23]. Similarly, Z-disk genes have been implicated in DCM as well as HCM [24]. A growing number of genes have been associated with both DCM and ARVC. Genes encoding desmosomal proteins were initially only implicated in ARVC, but recent evidence suggests that mutations in these genes also cause DCM [25, 26]. The phenotypic spectrum of mutations in the desmin gene includes DCM, RCM, and recently also ARVC [27–29]. Finally, mutations in the *TTN* gene recently were shown to be a frequent cause of DCM [12] and emerging evidence also implicates the *TTN* gene in ARVC [30].

The amount of phenotypic overlap combined with genetic overlap has challenged the traditional paradigm of configuring test content strictly by clinical diagnosis. The large number of genes that can now be screened simultaneously has enabled test configurations that remove the need for sequential testing for those patients where the phenotype is not clearly defined.

Hypertrophic Cardiomyopathy

HCM is the most common inherited cardiomyopathy and affects approximately 1 in 500 individuals [3]. Asymmetric left ventricular hypertrophy (LVH) occurs in the absence of identifiable causes (e.g., uncontrolled hypertension), with myocyte hypertrophy, disarray, and interstitial fibrosis as the hallmark histological features of this disease [31, 32]. HCM typically follows an autosomal dominant mode of inheritance, although autosomal recessive forms have been identified (Table 17.1). Clinical manifestations are variable, ranging from an asymptomatic or mildly symptomatic course to severe heart failure and SCD [33]. HCM commonly manifests between the second and fourth decades of life but can manifest at the extremes of age [34, 35]. SCD can be the tragic sentinel event in children, adolescents, and young adults. Storage diseases such as Fabry disease and Danon disease also can present with apparently isolated LVH [36, 37]; however, these typically present with concentric LVH and, in males, are accompanied by other symptoms such as reduced sweating (Fabry disease) or cognitive impairment (Danon disease). In severe cases, HCM can progress, causing cell remodeling and an end stage phenotype that can resemble DCM [38, 39].

Table 17.1 Genes implicated in the etiology of inherited cardiomyopathies

Gene	Spectrum of clinical features						MOI	Location/function
	HCM	DCM	ARVC	RCM	LVNC	Other		
ABCC9		X					AD	Potassium channel
ACTC1	X	X		X	X		AD	Sarcomere
ACTN2	X	X					AD	Z-disk
ANKRD1	X	X					?	Z-disk
BAG3	X	X		X		Myofibrillar myopathy	AD	Z-disk
CASQ2					X	CPVT	AR	Sarcoplasmatic reticulum
CAV3	X	X				Myopathies, LongQT, HyerpCKaemia	AD, ?AR	Plasma membrane
CRYAB		X				Myofibrillar myopathy	AD, ?AR	Chaperone
CSRP3	X	X				Myopathy	AD	Z-disk
CTF1		X					?	cytokine
DES		X	X	X		Myopathy	AD	Intermediate filament
DMD		X				Muscular dystrophy	XL	Dystrophin-associated protein complex
DSC2		X	2–7 %				AD	Desmosome
DSG2		X	5–10 %				AD	Desmosome
DSP		X	2–12 %			Carvajal disease	AD, AR	Desmosome
DTNA					X		AD	Dystrophin-associated protein complex
EMD		X				Myopathy	XL	Nuclear membrane
FHL2		X						Z-disk
GLA	X					Fabry disease	XL	Lysosome
JUP			X			Naxos disease	AD, AR	Desmosome
LAMA4		X						Basement membrane
LAMP2	X	X				Danon disease	XL	Lysosome
LDB3	X	X			~5 %	Myofibrillar myopathy	AD	Z-disk
LMNA		5.3 %			X	Myopathy	AD	Nuclear membrane
Mt-DNA	X	X				Mitochondrial disease	M	Mitochondrium
MYBPC3	20–45 %	X		X	X		AD	Sarcomere
MYH6	X	X				CHD	AD	Sarcomere
MYH7	15–20 %	6.4 %		~5 %	X	Myopathy	AD	Sarcomere
MYL2	X						AD	Sarcomere
MYL3	X						AD	Sarcomere
MYLK2	X						?	Kinase
MYOZ2	X						AD	Z-disk
NEBL		X					?	Z-disk
NEXN	X	X					AD	Z-disk
PKP2		X	25–40 %				AD	Desmosome
PLN	X	X					AD	Sarcoplasmatic reticulum
PRKAG2	X					WPW	AD	Kinase
RBM20		X					AD	RNA-binding motif protein
SCN5A		2.6 %				Brugada, LQTS	AD	Sodium channel
SGCD		X				LGMD2F	AR; ?AD	Dystrophin-associated Protein complex
TAZ		X			X	Barth syndrome	XL	Mitochondrium
TCAP		X				LGMD2G	AR, AD	Z-disk
TMEM43			X				AD	Transmembrane protein
TNNC1	X	X					AD	Sarcomere
TNNI3	1–7 %	X		~5 %			AD, AR	Sarcomere

(continued)

Table 17.1 (continued)

Gene	Spectrum of clinical features						MOI	Location/function
	HCM	DCM	ARVC	RCM	LVNC	Other		
TNNT2	1–7 %	3.7 %		X	X		AD	Sarcomere
TPM1	X	X					AD	Sarcomere
TTN		18–25 %	X			Myopathy	AD	Sarcomere
TTR	X						AD	Transport protein
VCL		X			X		AD	Z-disk

All genes are reviewed in Ackerman_2011_21810866 and/or Teekakirikul_2013
? emerging but not yet well associated with the disease, *AD* autosomal dominant, *AR* autosomal recessive, *ARVC* arrhythmogenic right ventricular cardiomyopathy, *CHD* congenital heart defects, *CPVT* catecholaminergic polymorphic ventricular tachycardia, *DCM* dilated cardiomyopathy, *HCM* hypertrophic cardiomyopathy, *LGMDZF* limb-girdle muscular dystrophy type 2F, *LGMD2G* limb-girdle muscular dystrophy type 2G, *LVNC* left venricular non-compaction cardiomyopathy, *LQTS* long QT syndrome, *M* mitochondrial, *MOI* mode of inheritance, *RCM* restrictive cardiomyopathy, *WPW* Wolff-Parkinson-White syndrome, *XL* X-linked inheritance, *Unk* unknown, *X* disease causing mutations have been reported. Detection rates of >5 % in at least one study are detailed and highlighted

Molecular Basis of Disease

HCM is considered to be primarily a disease of the sarcomere, the contractile unit of myocytes. Disease-causing mutations have been identified in most sarcomere genes, with two genes (*MYH7* and *MYBPC3*) contributing almost 80 % of disease causing mutations [40]. Genes encoding Z-disk proteins, mitochondrial genes, and metabolic genes also have been implicated, though these are less frequently mutated. The majority of mutations are private (only seen in one family), and there is a high prevalence of missense mutations acting in a dominant negative fashion. Mutations leading to loss of function are less frequent but are prevalent in the *MYBPC3* gene. The known HCM-causing genes are listed in Table 17.1. Interestingly, very few genotype–phenotype correlations have been identified. Some general associations have emerged through analysis of case studies, though these are broad, usually are defined at the gene level, and may not be applicable to everyone with mutations in those genes. For example, HCM caused by mutations in *TNNT2* has been associated with a wide variety of clinical presentations and is usually associated with a reduced disease penetrance, a mild degree of hypertrophy, but a high incidence of SCD and more extensive myocyte disarray, although some mutations are associated with hypertrophy without risk of arrhythmias [41–43]. *MYBPC3*-related HCM has been associated with a reduced penetrance, relatively mild hypertrophy, a low incidence of SCD, late onset of clinical manifestations, and good prognosis before the age of 40 [44–46]. *PRKAG2* related HCM is associated with concentric hypertrophy and Wolff–Parkinson–White syndrome [47, 48]. Finally, *MYH7* mutations appear to be associated with severe LVH and an increased risk of heart failure and SCD [10].

Recent studies have shown that approximately 5 % of individuals with HCM have two pathogenic mutations, typically one inherited from each parent [49, 50]. Multiple mutations typically lead to a more severe presentation and an earlier age of onset than those seen with only one mutation [50].

Clinical Utility of Testing

One of the most important uses of genetic testing for HCM is the ability to identify asymptomatic family members who may be at risk to develop HCM. Multiple modes of inheritance have been described in HCM and knowing the genetic cause of an individual's disease allows for more accurate genetic counseling of family members. Since genotype–phenotype correlations for HCM are minimal, prognostic use of genetic testing is limited. Distinguishing the different genetic causes of heart muscle thickening is extremely important, as the treatment for HCM differs markedly from the treatment of other conditions. Fabry disease can present as isolated LVH in men and women and recent studies have suggested that approximately 6 % of males with late onset HCM had low α-Gal A enzyme activity [51, 52]. Identifying a pathogenic mutation in the *GLA* gene can provide a definitive diagnosis and enable lifesaving enzyme replacement therapy. Additionally, studies are emerging regarding therapeutic guidance for patients with sarcomeric HCM. Experimental studies and clinical trials of interventions (including diltiazem and angiotensin receptor/aldosterone blockade) show promise in delaying disease onset [53–55].

Available Assays

Clinical molecular testing for the HCM genes listed in Table 17.1 is currently available through several laboratories (www.genetests.org). The majority of testing for HCM is done by NGS using a targeted gene panel.

Interpretation of Test Results

Over 50 % of individuals with a clinical diagnosis of idiopathic HCM and up to 70 % of familial HCM will have a mutation in one of the genes listed in Table 17.1 [3, 20]. Therefore, a negative test result reduces but does not eliminate the likelihood that the individual carries a causative mutation. Copy number variants (CNVs), such as large deletions leading to loss of function, are generally suspected to exist in genes with a high prevalence of other loss-of-function variants (e.g., nonsense and frameshift variants). HCM genes that fit this description include *MYBPC3* and *LAMP2*. Deletion mutations have been described [56] but are thought to be rare. However, Sanger sequencing does not detect large deletions and thus, their prevalence will only emerge as technologies which can detect large deletions are more widely used for clinical testing. Methods of NGS data analysis are being developed to simultaneously detect small mutations as well as CNVs, which will provide a more accurate estimate of the prevalence of CNVs related to HCM and other inherited disorders.

Genetic studies have revealed that approximately 25 % of tested patients have a mutant allele but do not manifest a HCM phenotype (genotype-positive/phenotype-negative HCM) [57]. The variability in phenotypic expression of the mutations could be due to environmental influences (differences in lifestyle, risk factors, and exercise) or genetic modifiers. VUS are common and difficult to interpret and should not be used for predictive testing for at-risk family members. Genetic testing laboratories typically offer targeted testing of family members to establish whether a variant identified in the index family member segregates with the disease. These concordance studies can be helpful in clarifying the clinical significance of VUS. Functional tests, such as the investigation of a possible splice mutation, exist but are currently difficult to incorporate into routine clinical testing so are largely confined to research laboratories.

Laboratory Issues

The majority of molecular genetic testing for inherited cardiac diseases is done by sequencing the exons and splice sites of one or several disease genes because allelic heterogeneity is the norm for all diseases covered in this chapter. Similarly, the assays that are commonly used to detect small deletions or duplications (e.g., multiplex ligation-dependent probe amplification [MLPA] or array-based comparative genomic hybridization) are not unique to any given gene or disease; hence, the laboratory issues common to all genetic CVD testing are reviewed at the end of this chapter.

Dilated Cardiomyopathy

DCM is characterized by ventricular dilation and impaired systolic function affecting approximately 1 in 2,500 individuals ([58]; www.genereviews.org). The spectrum of clinical manifestations includes dyspnea, orthopnea, fatigue, edema, and ultimately heart failure. DCM is most commonly an end stage manifestation of acquired causes, such as ischemic injury from myocardial infarction, viral myocarditis, or thyroid disease, that damage the myocardium. DCM also is caused by environmental insults including drug related side effects or alcohol abuse.

Idiopathic DCM (IDC) is diagnosed when all other known causes have been ruled out. A molecular basis for IDC was first postulated after clinical studies demonstrated familial inheritance in 20–35 % of cases when first-degree relatives are screened carefully [59, 60]. Today, over 40 genes have been implicated in the genetic etiology of DCM (Table 17.1). The onset of clinical manifestations is age related, with only 20 % of gene mutation carriers under the age of 20 years of age manifesting the disease phenotype. Nearly two thirds of familial DCM has an autosomal dominant inheritance pattern with an isolated cardiac phenotype [61]. However, other modes of inheritance are known and include autosomal recessive, mitochondrial (maternal), and X-linked inheritance.

DCM also presents with arrhythmias and/or muscular involvement and can be the initial and/or predominant feature of Emery–Dreifuss muscular dystrophy, Barth syndrome, myofibrillar myopathy, and Duchenne muscular dystrophy [62, 63]. Recently, familial co-occurrence of peripartum cardiomyopathy (PPCM) and DCM have been observed, which led to the suggestion that PPCM is part of the phenotypic spectrum of familial DCM [64, 65].

Phenotypic overlap exists between DCM and end stage HCM as well as ARVC, which was initially believed to be restricted to a right ventricular defect but is now increasingly recognized to have a left ventricular contribution.

Molecular Basis of Disease

DCM is, by far, the most heterogeneous of the diseases discussed in this chapter. Mutations in *MYH7*, *LMNA*, *SCN5A*, *TNNI3*, and *TNNT2* make up roughly 20 % of familial DCM cases [3, 23]. Additional genes (Table 17.1) typically contribute a small fraction of the remaining DCM-causing mutations. The recent discovery that loss of function mutations in the *TTN* gene are responsible for as much as 25 % of genetic DCM is a notable exception and a radical improvement for genetic testing for DCM [12]. Missense mutations in the *LMNA* and *SCN5A* genes are responsible for inherited DCM with conduction system disease [66–68]. Autosomal recessive DCM is less frequent and is characterized by a significantly younger age of onset and a worse prognosis compared to the dominant form. This form is typically associated with skeletal myopathy and caused by mutations in the *SGCD* and *TCAP* genes. Additionally, autosomal dominant forms of DCM can present with skeletal myopathy and include mutations in the

CSRP3, *DES*, *DMD*, *EMD*, *LMNA*, *MYH7*, and *TTN* genes [3, 20] (Table 17.1). The *TAZ* gene is associated with Barth syndrome but DCM can be the first presenting feature [69–72]. In addition, recent studies have provided evidence that mutations in the *LAMP2* gene, which typically cause Danon disease in young boys, can cause DCM in the fourth decade of life in women [37]. Finally, there is emerging evidence of genetic overlap with ARVC as mutations in traditional ARVC genes have been detected in individuals with DCM [25, 26].

Clinical Utility of Testing

Molecular testing for DCM is most useful when there is a confirmed family history and/or conduction system disease in the proband or other affected family members. The profound genetic heterogeneity has long precluded a prominent role for molecular testing in isolated DCM, though this is rapidly changing. Multiple modes of inheritance have been described in DCM, and knowing the cause of an individual's disease allows for more accurate genetic counseling regarding the risk to other family members. Distinguishing the different genetic causes of heart muscle weakness is extremely important, as the clinical management for primary DCM can differ from DCM associated with other conditions. The prognostic utility of genetic testing is limited to a higher risk for SCD in *SCN5A* and *LMNA* mutation carriers, and screening for mitochondrial disease and skeletal myopathy in the genes associated with those features. For those individuals who are at risk for SCD due to arrhythmias caused by *SCN5A* and *LMNA* mutations, an implantable cardioverter defibrillator (ICD) can be implanted as a preventative measure.

Available Assays

Molecular testing for the DCM genes listed in Table 17.1 is currently available through clinical laboratories (www.genetests.org). Both Sanger sequencing and NGS methods are used.

Interpretation of Test Results

The detection rate of mutations in individuals with DCM is rapidly evolving. Until 2012, approximately 20 % of individuals with idiopathic DCM and more than 30 % of those with familial DCM were expected to have a mutation in one of the genes listed in Table 17.1 [3, 73]. With the discovery that *TTN* mutations may account for another 25 %, the detection rate for DCM is now approaching that of HCM. A negative test result reduces but does not eliminate the likelihood that an individual carries a causative mutation. The variability in phenotypic expression of mutations could be due to environmental influences or acquired traits (differences in lifestyle, risk factors, and exercise). Variants of unknown significance are difficult to interpret and should not be used for predictive testing for at-risk family members.

Arrhythmogenic Right Ventricular Cardiomyopathy

Initially termed arrhythmogenic right ventricular dysplasia (ARVD), this disease is now more commonly referred to as arrhythmogenic right ventricular cardiomyopathy (ARVC). ARVC is characterized by progressive degeneration and fibro-fatty replacement of the right ventricular myocardium, arrhythmias with a left bundle branch block profile, and increased risk of SCD in juveniles [74–76]. Although initially thought to affect predominantly the right ventricle, left ventricular involvement is now increasingly recognized, generating phenotypic overlap with other inherited cardiac disease of left ventricular origin [17]. Recent studies have revealed that the cellular defect underlying fibroadiposis is impaired WNT signaling, which leads to a redirection of myocyte fate to adipocyte fate [77, 78].

Molecular Basis of Disease

Two modes of inheritance, autosomal dominant and autosomal recessive, are observed with ARVC. This disease is often described as a disease of the desmosome because mutations are predominantly found in genes encoding this multiprotein complex. Desmosomes form cell–cell junctions and are prevalent in tissues that are subjected to mechanical stress (such as the heart and skin). To date, six genes (*PKP2*, *DSP*, *DSC2*, *DSG2*, *JUP*, and *TMEM43*) have been implicated in autosomal dominant ARVC and two of these genes (*DSP* and *JUP*) have been associated with rare autosomal recessive forms that have cutaneous involvement (wooly/kinky hair and palmoplantar hyperkeratosis) [79–82]. These variants are referred to as Naxos syndrome (OMIM: #601214) and Carvajal syndrome (OMIM: #605676). Autosomal dominant ARVC has incomplete penetrance and variable phenotypic expression [83]. Catecholaminergic polymorphic ventricular tachycardia (CPVT) is characterized by SCD during physical or emotional stress [84, 85]. Although considered clinically distinct, CPVT shares some features with ARVC and given that ARVC can be difficult to diagnose clinically, genetic testing sometimes includes the *RYR2* gene, which is the main gene associated with CPVT. A recent study provided convincing evidence for a role of the *TTN* gene, which is strongly associated with DCM, in ARVC [30].

Clinical Utility of Testing

The variability of phenotype, disease progression, and underlying genetic cause contribute to the difficulties of diagnosis and risk stratification in ARVC. Given these complexities, genetic testing can be helpful in providing a definitive diagnosis when a pathogenic mutation is found. Although a few patterns have emerged in relation to genotype–phenotype correlations, the evidence is limited and the prognostic and therapeutic implications of genetic testing are still being debated. Because the age of onset, symptoms, and penetrance vary so widely in ARVC, genetic testing may be more accurate at identifying at-risk relatives than clinical screening alone.

Available Assays

Molecular testing for the ARVC genes listed in Table 17.1 is currently available through clinical laboratories (www.genetests.org). Both Sanger sequencing and NGS methods are used.

Interpretation of Test Results

Approximately 50 % of individuals who meet task force criteria for ARVC have a pathogenic mutation in one of the six genes listed in Table 17.1 [86, 87]. *PKP2* mutations make up the majority of cases. Therefore, a negative test result reduces but does not eliminate the likelihood that the individual carries a causative mutation. The variability in phenotypic expression of the mutations could be due to environmental influences or acquired traits (differences in lifestyle, risk factors, and exercise). VUS are difficult to interpret and should not be used for predictive testing for at risk family members.

Restrictive Cardiomyopathy

RCM is a rare myocardial disorder characterized by increased stiffness, impaired diastolic filling of the left ventricle, and reduced diastolic volume in the presence of normal systolic function and normal myocardial thickness [33]. Although most frequently caused by diseases causing infiltration or fibrosis of the myocardium, RCM may be found in the absence of a precipitating condition in many patients and is then referred to as idiopathic RCM [88].

Molecular Basis of Disease

Idiopathic RCM is most commonly sporadic, but familial disease has been reported with autosomal dominant inheritance [89, 90]. Missense mutations in the *DES* (desmin) gene have been found in several families with desmin-related myopathy with and without RCM [91, 92]. Additionally, mutations in *ACTC*, *MYH7*, *TNNI3*, and *TNNT2* have been associated with RCM, confirming that RCM is part of the spectrum of hereditary sarcomeric contractile protein disease (reviewed in refs. 3, 20).

Clinical Utility of Testing

Given the low detection rate for RCM genetic testing, the diagnostic utility of genetic testing is limited to predictive testing for family members. No genotype–phenotype correlations have been established and genetic testing has limited prognostic value.

Available Assays

Tests for most genes which have been associated with RCM are available as single gene tests using Sanger sequencing. Most clinical laboratories do not offer panels of genes specifically tailored to RCM but all genes associated with RCM to date are part of panels offered for HCM testing.

Interpretation of Test Results

The clinical detection rate of the genes listed in Table 17.1 is estimated to be roughly 10–15 %; however, due to the unclear etiology of the disease and limited numbers, a true detection rate is unknown [3]. Therefore, a negative test result reduces but does not eliminate the likelihood that the individual carries a causative mutation. VUS are difficult to interpret and should not be used for predictive testing for at-risk family members.

Isolated Left Ventricular Noncompaction

Isolated LVNC is characterized by a hypertrophic left ventricle with deep trabeculations and poor systolic function with or without associated left ventricular dilation. LVNC is thought to be due to an arrest of myocardial morphogenesis during embryonic development leading to a failure to complete the normal compaction process [93, 94]. Others have proposed that LVNC may be an acquired process based on some individuals who developed LVNC after initially negative echocardiographic findings [95]. There is ongoing controversy whether LVNC is a distinct clinical entity. The World Health Organization as well as a position statement of the European Society of Cardiology lists LVNC as an unclassified cardiomyopathy (reviewed in ref. 95). In contrast, the American Heart Association classified LVNC as a primary genetic cardiomyopathy in 2006 [96].

Molecular Basis of Disease

Familial recurrence in LVNC is high and found in approximately 40 % of patients [94]. Gene mutations have been detected in sarcomere/Z-disk genes including *MYH7*, *MYBPC3*, *TNNT2*, *ACTC1*, and *LDB3* [97]. In addition, LVNC can be the presenting feature of Barth syndrome caused by mutations in the *TAZ* gene [98, 99].

Clinical Utility of Testing

The ability to identify asymptomatic family members who may be at risk of developing LVNC is the main utility of genetic testing for this disease. As multiple modes of inheritance (autosomal dominant and X-linked) have been described in LVNC families, knowing the cause of an individual's disease allows for more accurate genetic counseling regarding the risk to other family members. No genotype–phenotype correlations have been established and as such genetic testing has limited prognostic value.

Available Assays

Molecular testing for the LVNC genes listed in Table 17.1 is currently available through clinical laboratories (www.genetests.org). Both Sanger sequencing and NGS methods are used.

Interpretation of Test Results

Between 17 and 41 % of individuals who meet criteria for LVNC will have a pathogenic mutation in one of the genes listed in Table 17.1 [20, 100]. Therefore, a negative test results reduces but does not eliminate the likelihood that an individual carries a causative mutation. The variability in phenotypic expression of the mutations could be due to environmental influences or acquired traits (differences in lifestyle, risk factors, and exercise). VUS are difficult to interpret and should not be used for predictive testing for at-risk family members.

Cardiac Channelopathies and Primary Arrhythmia Syndromes

The molecular understanding of cardiac channelopathies and primary arrhythmias has exploded over the last decade. At the turn of the century genetic testing was only available through research laboratories. As of 2013 there are over 30 channelopathy and arrhythmia genes for which genetic testing is available through clinical laboratories (Genetic Testing Registry; http://www.ncbi.nlm.nih.gov/gtr/).

Congenital Long QT Syndrome

Molecular Basis of Disease

Congenital LQTS is an inherited cardiac channelopathy characterized by prolongation of the QT interval of the cardiac cycle and increased susceptibility for syncope, seizures, and sudden cardiac death secondary to polymorphic ventricular tachyarrhythmias (torsades de pointes). Congenital LQTS occurs in two main heritable forms: autosomal dominant LQTS, originally described as Romano–Ward syndrome, and autosomal recessive LQTS, originally described as the Jervell and Lange-Nielsen syndrome. LQTS is the first type of arrhythmia to be understood at the molecular level as a primary cardiac channelopathy [101–103].

Over thirteen LQTS genes have been identified. Mutations in *KCNQ1* (*KVLQT1*, LQT1) [104], and *KCNH2* (*HERG*, LQT2) [105] cause the majority (about half) of LQTS. In approximately 25 % of families with LQTS, a genetic defect cannot be identified in the currently known LQTS-causing genes (www.genereviews.com). *KCNQ1*, the gene responsible for LQTS type 1 (LQTS1), encodes the α-subunit of the slowly activating delayed rectifier potassium ion channel (I_{Ks}). LQTS mutations in this gene cause a loss-of-function; the loss of I_{Ks} channel function decreases the I_{Ks} current, resulting in prolongation of the action potential duration and ventricular repolarization. LQTS type 2 (LQTS2) is due to mutations in *KCNH2*, which codes for the α-subunit of the rapidly activating delayed rectifier potassium ion channel (I_{Kr}). Mutations in *KCNH2* reduce the I_{Kr} current, resulting in prolongation of the action potential duration and repolarization. LQTS type 3 (LQTS3) results from mutations in *SCN5A*, which encodes the α-subunit of the cardiac sodium channel [106]. In contrast to the other forms of LQTS, in which a reduction of repolarization causes the prolongation of the action potential, *SCN5A* mutations that cause LQTS3 cause a "gain-of-function" in the cardiac sodium channel with an increase in late sodium current [107]. Ankyrin-B (*ANK2*) is a member of a family of versatile membrane adapters [108]. This gene was the first non-cardiac channel gene implicated in LQTS. Since this discovery, other non-cardiac cannel genes (*CAV3*, *AKAP9*, and *SNT1*) have been associated with LQTS [109–111]. The remaining LQTS-causing genes and their associated mutations are shown in Table 17.2.

Interestingly, correlations have been identified between the type of mutation and phenotypic outcome. For example, loss-of-function and dominant negative mutations in *KCNJ2* are thought to cause 50 % of Andersen syndrome (AS), while gain-of-function mutations in the same gene are associated with short QT syndrome (SQTS). AS is a rare inherited disorder (approximately 200 cases reported) characterized by periodic paralysis, prolongation of the QT interval with ventricular arrhythmias, and characteristic dysmorphic features including low-set ears, micrognathia, short stature, scoliosis, hypertelorism, broad forehead, and clinodactyly [112, 113]. AS is inherited in an autosomal dominant manner [114], although many cases are sporadic. Gain-of-function mutations in *KCNH2*, *KCNQ1*, and *KCNJ2* result in short QT syndrome (SQTS), a cardiac arrhythmia characterized by shortening of the QT interval on electrocardiogram and

Table 17.2 Genes implicated in the etiology of channelopathies

Gene	ALIAS	MOI	Protein function	Detection rate	Other associated diseases	Key references (Author_year_PMID)
Romano–Ward Syndrome (autosomal dominant LQTS)						
KCNQ1	LQT1	AD	Potassium channel	30–35 %	Jervell and Lange-Nielsen syndrome, Short QT syndrome, AF	Ackerman_2011_21810866
KCNH2	LQT2	AD	Potassium channel	25–30 %	Short QT syndrome	Ackerman_2011_21810866
SCN5A	LQT3	AD	Sodium channel	5–10 %	Brugada, DCM, sick sinus syndrome, VF, heart block, AF	Ackerman_2011_21810866
ANK2	LQT4	AD	Na/Ca exchange	Unknown	Cardiac arrhythmia	Moss_2008_18835466
KCNE1	LQT5	AD	Potassium channel	~1 %	Jervell and Lange-Nielsen syndrome	Moss_2008_18835466
KCNE2	LQT6	AD	Potassium channel	<1 %	AF	Moss_2008_18835466
KCNJ2	LQT7	AD	Potassium channel	<1 %	Short QT syndrome, CPVT, AF	Moss_2008_18835466
CACNA1C	LQT8	AD	Calcium channel	Unknown	Brugada syndrome	Moss_2008_18835466
CAV3	LQT9	AD	Cell–cell communication	~1 %	HCM, skeletal muscle disease, muscular dystrophy, elevated serum creatine	Vatta_2006_17060380 Moss_2008_18835466
SCN4B	LQT10	AD	Sodium channel	Unknown	–	Moss_2008_18835466
AKAP9	LQT11	AD	Regulate channel activity	~1 %	–	Chen_2007_18093912
SNTA1	LQT12	AD	Synaptogenesis	~1 %	–	Ueda_2008_18591664
KCNJ5	LQT13	AD	Potassium channel	Unknown	Familial hyperaldosteronism	Yang_2010_20560207
Jervell and Lange-Nielsen Syndrome (autosomal recessive LQTS)						
KCNQ1	LQT1	AR	Potassium channel	85 %	Long QT syndrome (AD), Short QT syndrome, AF	Schwartz_2006_16461811
KCNE1	LQT5	AR	Potassium channel	9 %	Jervell and Lange-Nielsen syndrome	Schwartz_2006_16461811
Anderson Syndrome						
KCNJ2		AD	Potassium channel	50 %	Andersen syndrome, Short QT syndrome, CPVT, AF	Donaldson_2003_12796536
Brugada Syndrome						
SCN5A		AD	Sodium channel	20–30 %	Long QT syndrome (AD), DCM, sick sinus syndrome, VF heart block, AF	Ackerman_2011_21810866
GPD1L		AD	Sodium current	<1 %	–	Perrin_2012_23062665
CACNA1C		AD	Calcium channel	<5 %	Timothy syndrome	Perrin_2012_23062665
CACNB2		AD	Calcium channel	<5 %	–	Perrin_2012_23062665
SCN1B		AD	Sodium channel	<5 %	Febrile seizures, cardiac conduction defect	Perrin_2012_23062665
KCNE3		AD	Potassium channel	<5 %	–	Perrin_2012_23062665
SCN3B		AD	Sodium channel	<5 %	–	Perrin_2012_23062665
HCN4		AD	Hyperpolarization-activated cation currents	<5 %	Sick sinus syndrome	Ueda_2008_19165230
KCNJ8		AD	Potassium channel	<1 %	–	Perrin_2012_23062665

(continued)

Table 17.2 (continued)

Gene	ALIAS	MOI	Protein function	Detection rate	Other associated diseases	Key references (Author_year_PMID)
Catecholaminergic Polymorphic Ventricular Tachycardia (CPVT)						
RYR2		AD	Calcium-release channel	50–55 %	ARVC2	Ackerman_2011_21810866
CASQ2		AR	Calcium ion reservoir	1–2 %	LVNC	di Barletta_2006_15671604
KCNJ2		AD	Potassium channel	Unknown	Long QT syndrome, Short QT syndrome, Anderson syndrome, AF	Tester_2006_16818210

AD autosomal dominant, *AF* atrial fibrillation, *AR* autosomal recessive, *ARVC* 2 arrhythmogenic right ventricular cardiomyopath 2y, *CPVT* catecholaminergic polymorphic ventricular tachycardiaa, *DCM* dilated cardiomyopathy, *HCM* hypertrophic cardiomyopathy, *LQT* long QT, *LVNC* left venricular non-compaction cardiomyopathy, *M* mitochondrial, *MOI* mode of inheritance, *VF* ventricular fibrillation, *XL* X-linked inheritance

paroxysmal atrial and ventricular tachyarrhythmias (episodes of rapid heartbeats originating from the heart chambers). SQTS is associated with an increased risk of atrial fibrillation and sudden cardiac death, resulting from an accelerated cardiac atrial and ventricular repolarization [115–117]. Fewer than 30 cases of SQTS have been published since the condition was first described in 2000 [118]. Autosomal recessive LQTS (Jervell and Lange-Nielsen syndrome) is secondary to homozygous or compound heterozygous mutations in either *KCNQ1* (~90 %) or *KCNE1* [119]. By definition, both parents are heterozygous for a pathogenic mutation; however, they are typically asymptomatic with negligible QT interval prolongation [120]. In contrast, their affected offspring not only have a severe cardiac phenotype but also are deaf. The I_{Ks} channel plays a critical role in potassium homeostasis in the endolymph of the inner ear [121, 122].

Clinical Utility of Testing

In addition to the utility of known mutation testing in family members, knowing the molecular cause of an individual's LQTS also has prognostic implications. First, cardiac events occur more frequently at rest or during sleep in LQTS3, whereas cardiac events are typically related to emotion or exercise (particularly swimming) in LQTS1 [123, 124] and auditory stimuli in LQTS2 [124]. Second, the recurrence rate of cardiac events while on β-blocker therapy was significantly lower in patients with LQTS1 (19 %) compared to LQTS2 (41 %) and LQTS3 (50 %) [125]. These insights further justify the utility of molecular testing for patients with LQTS. Given the high risk of sudden death in individuals with LQTS, an ICD can be placed in individuals who are confirmed to have a pathogenic mutation. However, these associations are limited and clinical care should not be driven by genotype alone.

Available Assays

Molecular testing for the LQTS genes listed in Table 17.2 is currently available through clinical molecular laboratories (www.genetests.org). Mutational analyses of the known LQTS genes are performed by Sanger sequencing and NGS, as well as MLPA for deletions or duplications, which are known to be a considerable part of the mutation spectrum for LQTS.

Interpretation of Test Results

Molecular genetic testing for LQTS plays a critical complementary role in the diagnostic evaluation and risk stratification for LQTS. However, the present sensitivity of genetic testing is approximately 75 % [3]. As such, a negative LQTS gene screen will not provide sufficient objective evidence to exclude the diagnosis of LQTS. The variability in phenotypic expression of the mutations could be due to environmental influences or acquired traits (differences in lifestyle, risk factors, and exercise). VUS are difficult to interpret and should not be used for predictive testing for at-risk family members.

Brugada Syndrome

BrS is characterized clinically by syncope and increased risk of SCD, particularly in young men at night, electrocardiographically by a right bundle branch block pattern and ST segment elevation in the precordial leads V1–V3, and echocardiographically by a structurally normal heart [126, 127]. BrS has been considered a distinct subgroup of idiopathic ventricular fibrillation (IVF) and may account for at least 20 % of all patients with IVF [128]. IVF is classified as ventricular fibrillation without demonstrable cardiac or noncardiac causes [129] and accounts for approximately 5–12 % of all sudden deaths. IVF is associated with a high mortality rate and high recurrence rates of up to 30 % during the 5 years after an initial episode of survived cardiac arrest. For both BrS and IVF, the treatment of choice is principally ICD placement.

Molecular Basis of Disease

In 1998, Chen and colleagues reported the first gene linked to BrS [130]. Mutations in the cardiac sodium channel encoded by *SCN5A* were subsequently identified in three families. BrS-causing *SCN5A* mutations result in a loss-of-function and have been identified in approximately 20 % of patients with familial BrS [131, 132]. Mutations in *SCN5A* also have been associated with progressive conduction system disease (PCCD) as well as LQT3. In contrast to BrS and PCCD, mutations causing LQT3 result in a gain-of-function. Mutations in seven additional genes have now been identified, including *GPDL*, *CACNA1C*, *CACNB2*, *SCN1B*, *KCNE3*, *SCN3B*, and *HCN4*, each one contributing a small fraction of mutations found in patients with BrS [133].

Clinical Utility of Testing

In 2010 the HRS and EHRA released guidelines stating that comprehensive or *SCN5A* targeted BrS genetic testing can be useful for any patient with suspected BrS based on examination of the patient's clinical history, family history, and expressed electrocardiographic phenotype [3]. If a pathogenic mutation is identified, an ICD can be placed to prevent sudden cardiac death. Additionally, known mutation testing can be performed on asymptomatic family members to determine their risk for developing BrS.

Available Assays

Clinical testing for the eight genes associated with BrS is available from clinical molecular laboratories. Various sequencing technologies as well as deletion/duplication analysis (MLPA) are used to detect mutations that cause BrS.

Interpretation of Test Results

The clinical sensitivity of current BrS molecular genetic testing is approximately 25–40 %. As such, a negative Brugada gene screen cannot exclude the presence of BrS. VUS are difficult to interpret and should not be used for predictive testing for at-risk family members.

Catecholaminergic Polymorphic Ventricular Tachycardia

CPVT is a distinct arrhythmogenic entity in children and adolescents with structurally normal hearts characterized by episodes of ventricular arrhythmias (predominantly bidirectional ventricular tachycardias) resulting in syncope, seizures, or sudden death in response to physical activity or emotional stress [134].

Molecular Basis of Disease

CPVT can be transmitted in either an autosomal dominant or an autosomal recessive inheritance pattern [84, 135]. Ryanodine receptor (*RYR2*) gene mutations are the primary cause of autosomal dominant CPVT, though recent studies have suggested that *KCNJ2* could play a role as well [136]. Autosomal recessive CPVT is caused by missense mutations in the calsequestrin 2 (*CASQ2*) gene [137, 138]. It is currently estimated that approximately 50 % of autosomal dominant cases occur de novo, which is a direct consequence of the high mortality rate associated with CPVT. The identification of a variant that occurred de novo in an individual without a family history of the tested disease is commonly regarded as strong support for a pathogenic role.

Clinical Utility of Testing

Although only 55 % of CPVT has been elucidated genetically, some important genotype–phenotype relationships have emerged that support a role for molecular genetic testing in addition to the preclinical identification of asymptomatic carriers. Families with mutations in *RYR2* are more prone to stress-induced ventricular tachycardia at an earlier age than genotype-negative CPVT. In addition, males with *RYR2* mutations may be at greater risk for syncope than males lacking *RYR2* mutations [85]. However, there are no prognostic or therapeutic changes which would be made based on these results and the clinical utility is limited.

Available Assays

Sequence analysis of the *RYR2*, *CASQ2*, and *KCNJ2* genes is available clinically by Sanger sequencing and NGS methods (www.genetests.org).

Interpretation of Test Results

The sensitivity of molecular testing for the three CPVT-causing genes is greater than 55 %. A negative CPVT gene screen cannot rule out a diagnosis of CPVT. VUS are difficult to interpret and should not be used for predictive testing for at-risk family members.

Coronary Artery Disease

Atherosclerosis, or CAD, is the leading cause of death worldwide. It is a prime example of a common, complex disease caused by the interaction of many genetic, lifestyle, and environmental factors. A genetic component is evident by familial clustering and the heritability (the fraction of phenotypic variability that can be attributed to genetic variation) is estimated to be 63 % for premature myocardial infarction (reviewed in ref. 139). Affected physiologic processes include lipoprotein metabolism, coagulation, and inflammation. Among those, LDL cholesterol and blood pressure have an established strong association with and elevated risk for CAD (reviewed in ref. 5). As is typical for complex diseases, rarer Mendelian forms such as familial hypercholesterolemia (FH) have led to the identification of candidate genes for the more common forms. Today, many genome-wide association studies (GWAS) have successfully mapped a number of common susceptibility variants for CAD [140]. However, each one of those loci contributes only a small fraction of the overall genetic risk and translating these population risks to a personal risk for an individual carrying several of these risk alleles has proven challenging. Clinical testing for risk prediction is therefore not yet within reach. The following section discusses rare, Mendelian diseases predisposing to CAD.

Hyperlipidemias (Lipoprotein Metabolism)

Molecular Basis of Disease

Goldstein and Brown first reported one of the most important molecular mechanisms leading to atherosclerosis: defects of the low-density lipoprotein (LDL) receptor [141, 142].

Autosomal dominant FH is one of the most frequent hereditary disorders of lipid metabolism with a prevalence of approximately 1 in 500 in the general population (reviewed in ref. 5). FH is characterized by an isolated elevation of LDL particles leading to premature death from atherosclerosis. FH is caused mainly by defects in the genes encoding the LDL receptor (*LDLR*) [143, 144], apolipoprotein B (*APOB*) [145, 146], proprotein convertase subtilisin/kexin type 9 (*PCSK9*) [147–149], and other unidentified gene(s) at chromosome 16q22.1 [150]. More than 1,000 different *LDLR* mutations have been identified to date [151, 152] (HGMD.org).

Autosomal recessive hypercholesterolemia (ARH) is a very rare recessive disorder caused by mutations in a putative adaptor protein called ARH, and is characterized by severe hypercholesterolemia (elevation of LDL level), xanthomatosis, and premature CAD [153]. Additional genes shown in Table 17.3 have been associated with other rare CAD diseases. Examples are the *ABCG5* and *ABCG8* genes where mutations have been associated with sitosterolemia [154, 155].

Several CAD modifying genes have been identified. Apolipoprotein E (APOE) is a constituent of several plasma lipoproteins including chylomicrons (VLDL, IDL, and HDL-E), and may be a risk-stratifying biomarker for CAD. The *APOE* alleles (ε2, ε3, and ε4) have a strong and consistent influence on plasma lipids and CAD. Both, ε2 and ε4 are associated with higher plasma triglyceride concentrations and more than 90 % of patients with hyperlipoproteinemia type III (HLPIII) are homozygous for the ε2 allele. However, homozygosity for ε2 occurs with a frequency of 0.5–1 in 100 Caucasian individuals and only a fraction of those develop overt HLPIII. Therefore, ε2 is believed to contribute to but not be the sole cause of this disease [156]. Interleukin-6 (IL6) is an inflammatory cytokine associated with the development and severity of CAD [157]. The -174C allele of the *IL6* gene is associated with risk of CAD and high systolic blood pressure in men [158]. Endothelial nitric oxide synthase (NOS) is an enzyme catalyzing the synthesis of nitric oxide (NO) in vascular endothelium and effects vascular relaxation. Alterations in the NOS pathway leading to decreased generation or action of NO are potential mechanisms in the development of premature atherosclerosis [159].

Clinical Utility of Testing

Clinical genetic testing for FH has been implemented in several countries. For example, the National Institute for Health and Clinical Excellence in the UK recommends that all patients are offered a referral for DNA testing to enable identification of affected (presymptomatic) relatives [160].

Available Assays

Gene sequencing tests (*LDLR APOB*, *PCSK9*) as well as deletion/duplication analysis (*LDLR*) are available clinically. The three common *APOE* alleles (ε2, ε3, and ε4) can be assessed using various genotyping methods (www.genetests.org).

Interpretation of Test Results

Multi-mutation test panels covering between 20 and 200 mutations have been used and identify mutations in 50–70 % of patients with FH [5]. Gene sequencing can be performed when targeted mutation panels are negative. In the future, testing is expected to be carried out by NGS of gene panels or ultimately by ES/GS. For patients with a lipid profile characteristic of hyperlipoproteinemia type III, APOE analysis will detect the homozygous ε2 allele.

Isolated Congenital Heart Defects

Molecular Basis of Disease

Congenital heart defects (CHD) are the most common type of birth defects and can be caused by chromosome abnormalities, single gene mutations, teratogenic exposures, and other unknown etiological mechanisms. While some CHD occur as part of Mendelian syndromes or with other birth defects, the majority occur in isolation. The estimated incidence of moderate and severe CHD is approximately

Table 17.3 Primary hyperlipoproteinemias caused by known single-gene mutations

Disease	Clinical findings	Elevated lipoprotein	Gene	OMIM#	MOI	Estimated prevalence	Key reference (Author_year_PMID)
Autosomal dominant familial hypercholesterolemia	Tendon xanthomas, CAD	LDL	*LDLR*	606945	AD	1/500	Varret_2007_18028451
	Tendon xanthomas, CAD	LDL	*APOB*	107730	AD	1/1,000	Varret_2007_18028451
Familial dysbetalipoproteinemia	Palmar and tuberoeruptive xanthomas, CAD, PVD	Chylomicrons and VLDL remnants	*APOE*	107741	AD	1/10,000	Bersot_1983_6309903
Autosomal recessive hypercholesterolemia	Tendon xanthomas, CAD	LDL	*ARH*	605747	AR	<1/1,000,000	Soutar_2004_15630633
Sitosterolemia	Tendon xanthomas, CAD	LDL	*ABCG5* or *ABCG8*	605459 or 605460	AR	<1/1,000,000	Berge_2000_11099417
Lipoprotein lipase deficiency	Eruptive xanthomas, hepatosplenomegaly and pancreatitis	Chylomicrons	*LPL*	609708	AR	1/1,000,000	Devlin_1990_2294743
Familial apolipoprotein C-II deficiency	Eruptive xanthomas, hepatosplenomegaly and pancreatitis	Chylomicrons	*APOC2*	608083	AR	<1/1,000,000	Wilson_2003_12783430
Familial hepatic lipase deficiency	Premature atherosclerosis	VLDL remnants	*LIPC*	151670	AR	<1/1,000,000	Hegele_1991_1671786

AD autosomal dominant, *AR* autosomal recessive, *CAD* coronary artery disease, *LDL* low-density lipoprotein, *M* mitochondrial, *MOI* mode of inheritance, *PVD* peripheral vascular disease, *VLDL* very low-density lipoprotein, *XL* X-linked inheritance

6 per 1,000 live births, approximately half of which are cardiac septal defects (CSD) [161, 162]. Although much of CHD is thought to have a complex genetic and/or environmental etiology, an increasing number of families with monogenic CHD have been reported and disease genes are being identified [6].

CSD include atrial septal defects (ASD), ventricular septal defects (VSD), and atrioventricular septal defects (AVSD). CSD are characterized by openings in the septal wall between the left and right sides of the heart that allow oxygen-rich (red) blood to recirculate through the lungs instead of traveling to the rest of the body, resulting in increased pressure and stress in the lungs. Several genes have been identified as having a causative role, including *GATA4* and *NKX2-5*. A range of *GATA4* and *NKX2-5* mutations have been observed in both familial and isolated cases of CSD, and can be associated with additional CHD including tricuspid valve abnormalities (including Ebstein's anomaly), conotruncal anomalies (tetralogy of Fallot, double outlet right ventricle, interrupted aortic arch, and transposition of the great arteries), left sided lesions (hypoplastic left heart syndrome, coarctation, left ventricular hypertrophy), and pulmonary valve stenosis [163–169].

Cyanotic heart disease is a defect causing mixing of pure oxygen-rich blood with venous blood, resulting in a low blood oxygen concentration. The most common form is tetralogy of Fallot (TOF), which is characterized by a combination of four abnormalities: (1) VSD, (2) pulmonary stenosis (PS) or atresia (PA), (3) overriding aorta (the aorta lies directly over the VSD), and (4) right ventricular hypertrophy (RVH). TOF accounts for 6.8 % of all CHD [170], of which approximately 70 % occurs sporadically without another anomaly [171]. Mutations in *NKX2-5* are thought to account for up to 4–5 % of individuals with TOF [167, 168, 170]. Mutations in the Jagged 1 (*JAG1*) gene are the main cause of Alagille syndrome (AGS) but can also present as isolated CHD. The most common malformation in carriers of *JAG1* mutations is peripheral pulmonic stenosis (PPS), but other malformations such as isolated TOF, PS, or VSD with aortic dextroposition have been observed [172–174]. Of the cases of AGS caused by mutations in *JAG1*, the vast majority (88 %) are small sequence variants [174].

Clinical Utility of Testing

Genetic testing of clinically affected individuals with CHD and their relatives can help to confirm a clinical diagnosis and identify the cause of CHD in a particular family. Genetic testing also is useful to rule out a syndromic cause of CHD and to identify at-risk family members.

Available Assays

Sequencing assays for several CHD genes are offered clinically (genetests.org). A recent meta-analysis of published literature on CNVs in children with structural birth defects including CHD revealed that pathogenic CNVs appear to occur at increased frequency in this patient population [175]. Microarray based testing is widely available and can detect gross CNVs.

Interpretation of Test Results

Sensitivity and specificity are not known for most of the tests.

Laboratory Issues

The majority of molecular genetic testing for inherited cardiac diseases is done by sequencing one or several disease genes, usually the entire coding sequence, because allelic heterogeneity is the norm for all diseases covered in this chapter. Similarly, the assays that are commonly used to detect small deletions or duplications (e.g., MLPA or aCGH) are not unique to any given gene or disease. Hence, laboratory issues the physician (and patient) should be aware of do not differ by disease and are reviewed here instead of in the individual disease sections.

The majority of currently available tests are laboratory developed tests (LDTs), which (at the time of writing this chapter) are not subject to US FDA clearance, but are developed in laboratories accredited under the Clinical Laboratory Improvement Amendments (CLIA) regulations by the Centers for Medicare and Medicaid Services (CMS). Analytical performance (such as false-positive and false-negative rates) is established by the testing laboratory. The analytical sensitivity (the ability of the test to identify a mutation that is known to be present) is often not 100 % though typically very close [176]. Technical performance parameters have to be disclosed in the methods section of clinical reports issued by clinical molecular laboratories.

In addition to technical limitations that can lead to false negatives, the design of gene sequencing tests can impact mutation detection. For example, testing is typically limited to coding sequence (exons) as well as the splice consensus sequence. Therefore, mutations in noncoding regions that can affect gene regulation (e.g., promoter, enhancer, and the 3′ untranslated region) will not be detected. In addition, Sanger sequencing does not detect large copy number changes (such as partial or whole gene deletions/duplications) or structural mutations such as translocations. NGS technologies have the ability to detect these types of mutations but detection of these types of variants depends on the bioinformatics tools used by the laboratory for analysis of the sequencing data [177]. At the time of writing this chapter, gross structural changes are typically not part of the analysis offered by clinical molecular laboratories using NGS test methods, though this is expected to change rapidly.

Genetic testing laboratories commonly confirm any mutation that is detected using a second testing method. This is done because most technologies used are not immune to technical artifacts (false-positive mutations). A second use of confirmatory testing is to rule out a sample switch although this does not include a switch prior to the sample's arrival at the testing laboratory. It is therefore essential to reconcile the result with the phenotype of the tested individual and to contact the laboratory when a discrepancy (such as the absence of a familial pathogenic mutation in an affected family member) exists. While there are alternate explanations such as environmental phenocopies of a disease or the presence of more than one disease causing mutation in a family, genotype–phenotype discrepancies should trigger a thorough investigation of possible sample switch.

Conclusions

Since the completion of the Human Genome Project in 2003, the number of identified disease genes has increased dramatically. Testing for genetically heterogeneous cardiac disorders, which has long been challenging due to high test cost, is now increasingly used in clinical practice and medical management of patients. Recent technological breakthroughs have increased the size of genetic test panels by an order of magnitude and the $1,000 genome, which was unthinkable just 10 years ago is now within reach and is anticipated to radically change the landscape of genetic testing as we know it today. It is likely that with rapidly dropping test cost and increasing accuracy and coverage, genome sequencing will soon replace most if not all genetic tests we know today. It is possible (even likely) that clinical genome sequencing will be performed at birth. Once obtained, an individual's genome can be used in a predictive fashion. Alternatively, data can be stored and subsets can be analyzed as needed, for example initiated by the presence of a specific family history or the onset of a disease that is known to have a genetic etiology. These indications can trigger the analysis of disease specific gene sets or, if the diagnosis is not clear, the exome or genome.

Current challenges include the timely and accurate interpretation of the approximately three million variants that are present per genome. We are only beginning to be able to understand the complete spectrum of benign variation, which is critical to narrow the number of variants detected. Although tools and processes to analyze human genomes are still in their infancy, success stories where ES/GS successfully identified the cause of diagnostically challenging cases are inspiring and give an outlook to what will be common in the relatively near future. As we are beginning to sequence many genomes, we will undoubtedly identify so far elusive genetic etiologies for inherited cardiovascular disorders such that the clinical utility of genetic testing will dramatically improve.

References

1. Zareba W, Moss AJ, Schwartz PJ, Vincent GM, Robinson JL, Priori SG, Benhorin J, Locati EH, Towbin JA, Keating MT, et al. Influence of genotype on the clinical course of the long-QT syndrome. International Long-QT Syndrome Registry Research Group. N Engl J Med. 1998;339:960–5.
2. Raju H, Alberg C, Sagoo GS, Burton H, Behr ER. Inherited cardiomyopathies. BMJ. 2011;343:d6966.
3. Ackerman MJ, Priori SG, Willems S, Berul C, Brugada R, Calkins H, Camm AJ, Ellinor PT, Gollob M, Hamilton R, et al. HRS/EHRA expert consensus statement on the state of genetic testing for the channelopathies and cardiomyopathies this document was developed as a partnership between the Heart Rhythm Society (HRS) and the European Heart Rhythm Association (EHRA). Heart Rhythm. 2011;8:1308–39.
4. Prutkin JM, Sotoodehnia N. Genetics of sudden cardiac arrest. Prog Cardiovasc Dis. 2008;50:390–403.
5. Holmes MV, Harrison S, Talmud PJ, Hingorani AD, Humphries SE. Utility of genetic determinants of lipids and cardiovascular events in assessing risk. Nat Rev Cardiol. 2011;8:207–21.
6. Wessels MW, Willems PJ. Genetic factors in non-syndromic congenital heart malformations. Clin Genet. 2010;78:103–23.
7. Loeys BL, Dietz HC, Braverman AC, Callewaert BL, De Backer J, Devereux RB, Hilhorst-Hofstee Y, Jondeau G, Faivre L, Milewicz DM, et al. The revised Ghent nosology for the Marfan syndrome. J Med Genet. 2010;47:476–85.
8. Noonan JA. Noonan syndrome and related disorders: alterations in growth and puberty. Rev Endocr Metab Disord. 2006;7:251–5.
9. Hershberger RE, Cowan J, Morales A, Siegfried JD. Progress with genetic cardiomyopathies: screening, counseling, and testing in dilated, hypertrophic, and arrhythmogenic right ventricular dysplasia/cardiomyopathy. Circ Heart Fail. 2009;2:253–61.
10. Hershberger RE, Lindenfeld J, Mestroni L, Seidman CE, Taylor MR, Towbin JA. Genetic evaluation of cardiomyopathy–a Heart Failure Society of America practice guideline. J Card Fail. 2009;15:83–97.
11. Ingles J, McGaughran J, Scuffham PA, Atherton J, Semsarian C. A cost-effectiveness model of genetic testing for the evaluation of families with hypertrophic cardiomyopathy. Heart. 2011;98(8):625–30.
12. Herman DS, Lam L, Taylor MR, Wang L, Teekakirikul P, Christodoulou D, Conner L, DePalma SR, McDonough B, Sparks E, et al. Truncations of titin causing dilated cardiomyopathy. N Engl J Med. 2012;366:619–28.
13. Bamshad MJ, Ng SB, Bigham AW, Tabor HK, Emond MJ, Nickerson DA, Shendure J. Exome sequencing as a tool for Mendelian disease gene discovery. Nat Rev Genet. 2011;12:745–55.
14. Goh V, Helbling D, Biank V, Jarzembowski J, Dimmock D. Next-generation sequencing facilitates the diagnosis in a child with twinkle mutations causing cholestatic liver failure. J Pediatr Gastroenterol Nutr. 2012;54:291–4.
15. Worthey EA, Mayer AN, Syverson GD, Helbling D, Bonacci BB, Decker B, Serpe JM, Dasu T, Tschannen MR, Veith RL, et al. Making a definitive diagnosis: successful clinical application of whole exome sequencing in a child with intractable inflammatory bowel disease. Genet Med. 2011;13:255–62.
16. Biagini E, Coccolo F, Ferlito M, Perugini E, Rocchi G, Bacchi-Reggiani L, Lofiego C, Boriani G, Prandstraller D, Picchio FM, et al. Dilated-hypokinetic evolution of hypertrophic cardiomyopathy: prevalence, incidence, risk factors, and prognostic implications in pediatric and adult patients. J Am Coll Cardiol. 2005;46:1543–50.

17. Sen-Chowdhry S, Syrris P, Prasad SK, Hughes SE, Merrifield R, Ward D, Pennell DJ, McKenna WJ. Left-dominant arrhythmogenic cardiomyopathy: an under-recognized clinical entity. J Am Coll Cardiol. 2008;52:2175–87.
18. Biagini E, Ragni L, Ferlito M, Pasquale F, Lofiego C, Leone O, Rocchi G, Perugini E, Zagnoni S, Branzi A, et al. Different types of cardiomyopathy associated with isolated ventricular noncompaction. Am J Cardiol. 2006;98:821–4.
19. Kelley-Hedgepeth A, Towbin JA, Maron MS. Images in cardiovascular medicine. Overlapping phenotypes: left ventricular noncompaction and hypertrophic cardiomyopathy. Circulation. 2009;119:e588–9.
20. Teekakirikul P, et al. Inherited Cardiomyopathies: Molecular Genetics and Clinical Genetic Testing in the Post Genomic Era. J Mol Diagn. 2013;15(2):158–70.
21. Kaski JP, Syrris P, Burch M, Tome-Esteban MT, Fenton M, Christiansen M, Andersen PS, Sebire N, Ashworth M, Deanfield JE, et al. Idiopathic restrictive cardiomyopathy in children is caused by mutations in cardiac sarcomere protein genes. Heart. 2008;94:1478–84.
22. Klaassen S, Probst S, Oechslin E, Gerull B, Krings G, Schuler P, Greutmann M, Hurlimann D, Yegitbasi M, Pons L, et al. Mutations in sarcomere protein genes in left ventricular noncompaction. Circulation. 2008;117:2893–901.
23. Lakdawala NK, Funke BH, Baxter S, Cirino AL, Roberts AE, Judge DP, Johnson N, Mendelsohn NJ, Morel C, Care M, et al. Genetic testing for dilated cardiomyopathy in clinical practice. J Card Fail. 2012;18:296–303.
24. Bos JM, Poley RN, Ny M, Tester DJ, Xu X, Vatta M, Towbin JA, Gersh BJ, Ommen SR, Ackerman MJ. Genotype-phenotype relationships involving hypertrophic cardiomyopathy-associated mutations in titin, muscle LIM protein, and telethonin. Mol Genet Metab. 2006;88:78–85.
25. Elliott P, O'Mahony C, Syrris P, Evans A, Rivera Sorensen C, Sheppard MN, Carr-White G, Pantazis A, McKenna WJ. Prevalence of desmosomal protein gene mutations in patients with dilated cardiomyopathy. Circ Cardiovasc Genet. 2010;3:314–22.
26. Posch MG, Posch MJ, Geier C, Erdmann B, Mueller W, Richter A, Ruppert V, Pankuweit S, Maisch B, Perrot A, et al. A missense variant in desmoglein-2 predisposes to dilated cardiomyopathy. Mol Genet Metab. 2008;95:74–80.
27. Klauke B, Kossmann S, Gaertner A, Brand K, Stork I, Brodehl A, Dieding M, Walhorn V, Anselmetti D, Gerdes D, et al. De novo desmin-mutation N116S is associated with arrhythmogenic right ventricular cardiomyopathy. Hum Mol Genet. 2010;19:4595–607.
28. Otten E, Asimaki A, Maass A, van Langen IM, van der Wal A, de Jonge N, van den Berg MP, Saffitz JE, Wilde AA, Jongbloed JD, et al. Desmin mutations as a cause of right ventricular heart failure affect the intercalated disks. Heart Rhythm. 2010;7:1058–64.
29. van Tintelen JP, Hauer RN. Cardiomyopathies: New test for arrhythmogenic right ventricular cardiomyopathy. Nat Rev Cardiol. 2009;6:450–1.
30. Taylor M, Graw S, Sinagra G, Barnes C, Slavov D, Brun F, Pinamonti B, Salcedo EE, Sauer W, Pyxaras S, et al. Genetic variation in titin in arrhythmogenic right ventricular cardiomyopathy-overlap syndromes. Circulation. 2011;124:876–85.
31. Maron BJ. Hypertrophic cardiomyopathy. Lancet. 1997;350:127–33.
32. Maron BJ, Anan TJ, Roberts WC. Quantitative analysis of the distribution of cardiac muscle cell disorganization in the left ventricular wall of patients with hypertrophic cardiomyopathy. Circulation. 1981;63:882–94.
33. Richardson P, McKenna W, Bristow M, Maisch B, Mautner B, O'Connell J, Olsen E, Thiene G, Goodwin J, Gyarfas I, et al. Report of the 1995 World Health Organization/International Society and Federation of Cardiology Task Force on the Definition and Classification of cardiomyopathies. Circulation. 1996;93:841–2.
34. Maron BJ. Hypertrophic cardiomyopathy: a systematic review. JAMA. 2002;287:1308–20.
35. Popjes ED, St John Sutton M. Hypertrophic cardiomyopathy. Pathophysiology, diagnosis, and treatment. Geriatrics. 2003;58:41–6. quiz 47.
36. Havndrup O, Christiansen M, Stoevring B, Jensen M, Hoffman-Bang J, Andersen PS, Hasholt L, Norremolle A, Feldt-Rasmussen U, Kober L, et al. Fabry disease mimicking hypertrophic cardiomyopathy: genetic screening needed for establishing the diagnosis in women. Eur J Heart Fail. 2010;12:535–40.
37. Toib A, Grange DK, Kozel BA, Ewald GA, White FV, Canter CE. Distinct clinical and histopathological presentations of Danon cardiomyopathy in young women. J Am Coll Cardiol. 2010;55:408–10.
38. Elliott P, McKenna WJ. Hypertrophic cardiomyopathy. Lancet. 2004;363:1881–91.
39. Garcia-Pavia P, Vazquez ME, Segovia J, Salas C, Avellana P, Gomez-Bueno M, Vilches C, Gallardo ME, Garesse R, Molano J, et al. Genetic basis of end-stage hypertrophic cardiomyopathy. Eur J Heart Fail. 2011;13:1193–201.
40. Seidman CE, Seidman JG. Identifying sarcomere gene mutations in hypertrophic cardiomyopathy: a personal history. Circ Res. 2011;108:743–50.
41. Forissier JF, Carrier L, Farza H, Bonne G, Bercovici J, Richard P, Hainque B, Townsend PJ, Yacoub MH, Faure S, et al. Codon 102 of the cardiac troponin T gene is a putative hot spot for mutations in familial hypertrophic cardiomyopathy. Circulation. 1996;94:3069–73.
42. Moolman JC, Corfield VA, Posen B, Ngumbela K, Seidman C, Brink PA, Watkins H. Sudden death due to troponin T mutations. J Am Coll Cardiol. 1997;29:549–55.
43. Watkins H, McKenna WJ, Thierfelder L, Suk HJ, Anan R, O'Donoghue A, Spirito P, Matsumori A, Moravec CS, Seidman JG, et al. Mutations in the genes for cardiac troponin T and alpha-tropomyosin in hypertrophic cardiomyopathy. N Engl J Med. 1995;332:1058–64.
44. Charron P, Dubourg O, Desnos M, Bennaceur M, Carrier L, Camproux AC, Isnard R, Hagege A, Langlard JM, Bonne G, et al. Clinical features and prognostic implications of familial hypertrophic cardiomyopathy related to the cardiac myosin-binding protein C gene. Circulation. 1998;97:2230–6.
45. Muchir A, Medioni J, Laluc M, Massart C, Arimura T, van der Kooi AJ, Desguerre I, Mayer M, Ferrer X, Briault S, et al. Nuclear envelope alterations in fibroblasts from patients with muscular dystrophy, cardiomyopathy, and partial lipodystrophy carrying lamin A/C gene mutations. Muscle Nerve. 2004;30:444–50.
46. Niimura H, Bachinski LL, Sangwatanaroj S, Watkins H, Chudley AE, McKenna W, Kristinsson A, Roberts R, Sole M, Maron BJ, et al. Mutations in the gene for cardiac myosin-binding protein C and late-onset familial hypertrophic cardiomyopathy. N Engl J Med. 1998;338:1248–57.
47. Arad M, Benson DW, Perez-Atayde AR, McKenna WJ, Sparks EA, Kanter RJ, McGarry K, Seidman JG, Seidman CE. Constitutively active AMP kinase mutations cause glycogen storage disease mimicking hypertrophic cardiomyopathy. J Clin Invest. 2002;109:357–62.
48. Arad M, Maron BJ, Gorham JM, Johnson Jr WH, Saul JP, Perez-Atayde AR, Spirito P, Wright GB, Kanter RJ, Seidman CE, et al. Glycogen storage diseases presenting as hypertrophic cardiomyopathy. N Engl J Med. 2005;352:362–72.
49. Girolami F, Ho CY, Semsarian C, Baldi M, Will ML, Baldini K, Torricelli F, Yeates L, Cecchi F, Ackerman MJ, et al. Clinical

features and outcome of hypertrophic cardiomyopathy associated with triple sarcomere protein gene mutations. J Am Coll Cardiol. 2010;55:1444–53.
50. Maron BJ, Maron MS, Semsarian C. Double or compound sarcomere mutations in hypertrophic cardiomyopathy: a potential link to sudden death in the absence of conventional risk factors. Heart Rhythm. 2012;9:57–63.
51. Colucci WS, Lorell BH, Schoen FJ, Warhol MJ, Grossman W. Hypertrophic obstructive cardiomyopathy due to Fabry's disease. N Engl J Med. 1982;307:926–8.
52. Sachdev B, Takenaka T, Teraguchi H, Tei C, Lee P, McKenna WJ, Elliott PM. Prevalence of Anderson-Fabry disease in male patients with late onset hypertrophic cardiomyopathy. Circulation. 2002;105:1407–11.
53. Abozguia K, Elliott P, McKenna W, Phan TT, Nallur-Shivu G, Ahmed I, Maher AR, Kaur K, Taylor J, Henning A, et al. Metabolic modulator perhexiline corrects energy deficiency and improves exercise capacity in symptomatic hypertrophic cardiomyopathy. Circulation. 2010;122:1562–9.
54. Penicka M, Gregor P, Kerekes R, Marek D, Curila K, Krupicka J. The effects of candesartan on left ventricular hypertrophy and function in nonobstructive hypertrophic cardiomyopathy: a pilot, randomized study. J Mol Diagn. 2009;11:35–41.
55. Teekakirikul P, Eminaga S, Toka O, Alcalai R, Wang L, Wakimoto H, Nayor M, Konno T, Gorham JM, Wolf CM, et al. Cardiac fibrosis in mice with hypertrophic cardiomyopathy is mediated by non-myocyte proliferation and requires Tgf-beta. J Clin Invest. 2010;120:3520–9.
56. Yang Z, Funke BH, Cripe LH, Vick 3rd GW, Mancini-Dinardo D, Pena LS, Kanter RJ, Wong B, Westerfield BH, Varela JJ, et al. LAMP2 microdeletions in patients with Danon disease. Circ Cardiovasc Genet. 2010;3:129–37.
57. Maron BJ, Niimura H, Casey SA, Soper MK, Wright GB, Seidman JG, Seidman CE. Development of left ventricular hypertrophy in adults in hypertrophic cardiomyopathy caused by cardiac myosin-binding protein C gene mutations. J Am Coll Cardiol. 2001;38:315–21.
58. Codd MB, Sugrue DD, Gersh BJ, Melton 3rd LJ. Epidemiology of idiopathic dilated and hypertrophic cardiomyopathy. A population-based study in Olmsted County, Minnesota, 1975-1984. Circulation. 1989;80:564–72.
59. Grunig E, Tasman JA, Kucherer H, Franz W, Kubler W, Katus HA. Frequency and phenotypes of familial dilated cardiomyopathy. J Am Coll Cardiol. 1998;31:186–94.
60. Keeling PJ, Gang Y, Smith G, Seo H, Bent SE, Murday V, Caforio AL, McKenna WJ. Familial dilated cardiomyopathy in the United Kingdom. Br Heart J. 1995;73:417–21.
61. Mestroni L, Rocco C, Gregori D, Sinagra G, Di Lenarda A, Miocic S, Vatta M, Pinamonti B, Muntoni F, Caforio AL, et al. Familial dilated cardiomyopathy: evidence for genetic and phenotypic heterogeneity. Heart Muscle Disease Study Group. J Am Coll Cardiol. 1999;34:181–90.
62. Bonne G, Di Barletta MR, Varnous S, Becane HM, Hammouda EH, Merlini L, Muntoni F, Greenberg CR, Gary F, Urtizberea JA, et al. Mutations in the gene encoding lamin A/C cause autosomal dominant Emery-Dreifuss muscular dystrophy. Nat Genet. 1999;21:285–8.
63. Muntoni F, Lichtarowicz-Krynska EJ, Sewry CA, Manilal S, Recan D, Llense S, Taylor J, Morris GE, Dubowitz V. Early presentation of X-linked Emery-Dreifuss muscular dystrophy resembling limb-girdle muscular dystrophy. Neuromuscul Disord. 1998;8:72–6.
64. Morales A, Painter T, Li R, Siegfried JD, Li D, Norton N, Hershberger RE. Rare variant mutations in pregnancy-associated or peripartum cardiomyopathy. Circulation. 2010;121:2176–82.
65. van Spaendonck-Zwarts KY, van Tintelen JP, van Veldhuisen DJ, van der Werf R, Jongbloed JD, Paulus WJ, Dooijes D, van den Berg MP. Peripartum cardiomyopathy as a part of familial dilated cardiomyopathy. Circulation. 2010;121:2169–75.
66. Arbustini E, Pilotto A, Repetto A, Grasso M, Negri A, Diegoli M, Campana C, Scelsi L, Baldini E, Gavazzi A, et al. Autosomal dominant dilated cardiomyopathy with atrioventricular block: a lamin A/C defect-related disease. J Am Coll Cardiol. 2002;39:981–90.
67. Fatkin D, MacRae C, Sasaki T, Wolff MR, Porcu M, Frenneaux M, Atherton J, Vidaillet Jr HJ, Spudich S, De Girolami U, et al. Missense mutations in the rod domain of the lamin A/C gene as causes of dilated cardiomyopathy and conduction-system disease. N Engl J Med. 1999;341:1715–24.
68. Hershberger RE, Parks SB, Kushner JD, Li D, Ludwigsen S, Jakobs P, Nauman D, Burgess D, Partain J, Litt M. Coding sequence mutations identified in MYH7, TNNT2, SCN5A, CSRP3, LBD3, and TCAP from 313 patients with familial or idiopathic dilated cardiomyopathy. Clin Transl Sci. 2008;1:21–6.
69. Barth PG, Wanders RJ, Vreken P, Janssen EA, Lam J, Baas F. X-linked cardioskeletal myopathy and neutropenia (Barth syndrome) (MIM 302060). J Inherit Metab Dis. 1999;22: 555–67.
70. Bione S, D'Adamo P, Maestrini E, Gedeon AK, Bolhuis PA, Toniolo D. A novel X-linked gene, G4.5. is responsible for Barth syndrome. Nat Genet. 1996;12:385–9.
71. Cantlay AM, Shokrollahi K, Allen JT, Lunt PW, Newbury-Ecob RA, Steward CG. Genetic analysis of the G4.5 gene in families with suspected Barth syndrome. J Pediatr. 1999;135:311–5.
72. Ichida F, Tsubata S, Bowles KR, Haneda N, Uese K, Miyawaki T, Dreyer WJ, Messina J, Li H, Bowles NE, et al. Novel gene mutations in patients with left ventricular noncompaction or Barth syndrome. Circulation. 2001;103:1256–63.
73. Zimmerman RS, Cox S, Lakdawala NK, Cirino A, Mancini-DiNardo D, Clark E, Leon A, Duffy E, White E, Baxter S, et al. A novel custom resequencing array for dilated cardiomyopathy. Genet Med. 2010;12:268–78.
74. Basso C, Thiene G, Corrado D, Angelini A, Nava A, Valente M. Arrhythmogenic right ventricular cardiomyopathy. Dysplasia, dystrophy, or myocarditis? Circulation. 1996;94:983–91.
75. Corrado D, Thiene G, Nava A, Rossi L, Pennelli N. Sudden death in young competitive athletes: clinicopathologic correlations in 22 cases. Am J Med. 1990;89:588–96.
76. Nava A, Bauce B, Basso C, Muriago M, Rampazzo A, Villanova C, Daliento L, Buja G, Corrado D, Danieli GA, et al. Clinical profile and long-term follow-up of 37 families with arrhythmogenic right ventricular cardiomyopathy. J Am Coll Cardiol. 2000;36:2226–33.
77. Lombardi R, Marian AJ. Molecular genetics and pathogenesis of arrhythmogenic right ventricular cardiomyopathy: a disease of cardiac stem cells. Pediatr Cardiol. 2011;32:360–5.
78. Saffitz JE, Asimaki A, Huang H. Arrhythmogenic right ventricular cardiomyopathy: new insights into mechanisms of disease. Cardiovasc Pathol. 2010;19:166–70.
79. Alcalai R, Metzger S, Rosenheck S, Meiner V, Chajek-Shaul T. A recessive mutation in desmoplakin causes arrhythmogenic right ventricular dysplasia, skin disorder, and woolly hair. J Am Coll Cardiol. 2003;42:319–27.
80. McKoy G, Protonotarios N, Crosby A, Tsatsopoulou A, Anastasakis A, Coonar A, Norman M, Baboonian C, Jeffery S, McKenna WJ. Identification of a deletion in plakoglobin in arrhythmogenic right ventricular cardiomyopathy with palmoplantar keratoderma and woolly hair (Naxos disease). Lancet. 2000;355:2119–24.
81. Norgett EE, Hatsell SJ, Carvajal-Huerta L, Cabezas JC, Common J, Purkis PE, Whittock N, Leigh IM, Stevens HP, Kelsell DP. Recessive mutation in desmoplakin disrupts desmoplakin-intermediate filament interactions and causes dilated

cardiomyopathy, woolly hair and keratoderma. Hum Mol Genet. 2000;9:2761–6.
82. Protonotarios N, Tsatsopoulou A. Naxos disease and Carvajal syndrome: cardiocutaneous disorders that highlight the pathogenesis and broaden the spectrum of arrhythmogenic right ventricular cardiomyopathy. Cardiovasc Pathol. 2004;13:185–94.
83. Nava A, Thiene G, Canciani B, Scognamiglio R, Daliento L, Buja G, Martini B, Stritoni P, Fasoli G. Familial occurrence of right ventricular dysplasia: a study involving nine families. J Am Coll Cardiol. 1988;12:1222–8.
84. Laitinen PJ, Brown KM, Piippo K, Swan H, Devaney JM, Brahmbhatt B, Donarum EA, Marino M, Tiso N, Viitasalo M, et al. Mutations of the cardiac ryanodine receptor (RyR2) gene in familial polymorphic ventricular tachycardia. Circulation. 2001;103:485–90.
85. Priori SG, Napolitano C, Memmi M, Colombi B, Drago F, Gasparini M, DeSimone L, Coltorti F, Bloise R, Keegan R, et al. Clinical and molecular characterization of patients with catecholaminergic polymorphic ventricular tachycardia. Circulation. 2002;106:69–74.
86. den Haan AD, Tan BY, Zikusoka MN, Llado LI, Jain R, Daly A, Tichnell C, James C, Amat-Alarcon N, Abraham T, et al. Comprehensive desmosome mutation analysis in north americans with arrhythmogenic right ventricular dysplasia/cardiomyopathy. Circ Cardiovasc Genet. 2009;2:428–35.
87. Marcus FI, McKenna WJ, Sherrill D, Basso C, Bauce B, Bluemke DA, Calkins H, Corrado D, Cox MG, Daubert JP, et al. Diagnosis of arrhythmogenic right ventricular cardiomyopathy/dysplasia: proposed modification of the task force criteria. Circulation. 2010;121:1533–41.
88. Kushwaha SS, Fallon JT, Fuster V. Restrictive cardiomyopathy. N Engl J Med. 1997;336:267–76.
89. Aroney C, Bett N, Radford D. Familial restrictive cardiomyopathy. Aust N Z J Med. 1988;18:877–8.
90. Zachara E, Bertini E, Lioy E, Boldrini R, Prati PL, Bosman C. Restrictive cardiomyopathy due to desmin accumulation in a family with evidence of autosomal dominant inheritance. G Ital Cardiol. 1997;27:436–42.
91. Dalakas MC, Park KY, Semino-Mora C, Lee HS, Sivakumar K, Goldfarb LG. Desmin myopathy, a skeletal myopathy with cardiomyopathy caused by mutations in the desmin gene. N Engl J Med. 2000;342:770–80.
92. Goldfarb LG, Park KY, Cervenakova L, Gorokhova S, Lee HS, Vasconcelos O, Nagle JW, Semino-Mora C, Sivakumar K, Dalakas MC. Missense mutations in desmin associated with familial cardiac and skeletal myopathy. Nat Genet. 1998;19:402–3.
93. Chin TK, Perloff JK, Williams RG, Jue K, Mohrmann R. Isolated noncompaction of left ventricular myocardium. A study of eight cases. Circulation. 1990;82:507–13.
94. Ichida F, Hamamichi Y, Miyawaki T, Ono Y, Kamiya T, Akagi T, Hamada H, Hirose O, Isobe T, Yamada K, et al. Clinical features of isolated noncompaction of the ventricular myocardium: long-term clinical course, hemodynamic properties, and genetic background. J Am Coll Cardiol. 1999;34:233–40.
95. Oechslin E, Jenni R. Left ventricular non-compaction revisited: a distinct phenotype with genetic heterogeneity? Eur Heart J. 2011;32:1446–56.
96. Maron BJ, Towbin JA, Thiene G, Antzelevitch C, Corrado D, Arnett D, Moss AJ, Seidman CE, Young JB. Contemporary definitions and classification of the cardiomyopathies: an American Heart Association Scientific Statement from the Council on Clinical Cardiology, Heart Failure and Transplantation Committee; Quality of Care and Outcomes Research and Functional Genomics and Translational Biology Interdisciplinary Working Groups; and Council on Epidemiology and Prevention. Circulation. 2006;113:1807–16.
97. Finsterer J. Cardiogenetics, neurogenetics, and pathogenetics of left ventricular hypertrabeculation/noncompaction. Pediatr Cardiol. 2009;30:659–81.
98. Bleyl SB, Mumford BR, Brown-Harrison MC, Pagotto LT, Carey JC, Pysher TJ, Ward K, Chin TK. Xq28-linked noncompaction of the left ventricular myocardium: prenatal diagnosis and pathologic analysis of affected individuals. Am J Med Genet. 1997;72:257–65.
99. Bleyl SB, Mumford BR, Thompson V, Carey JC, Pysher TJ, Chin TK, Ward K. Neonatal, lethal noncompaction of the left ventricular myocardium is allelic with Barth syndrome. Am J Hum Genet. 1997;61:868–72.
100. Ackerman MJ, Siu BL, Sturner WQ, Tester DJ, Valdivia CR, Makielski JC, Towbin JA. Postmortem molecular analysis of SCN5A defects in sudden infant death syndrome. JAMA. 2001;286:2264–9.
101. Ackerman MJ. The long QT syndrome: ion channel diseases of the heart. Mayo Clin Proc. 1998;73:250–69.
102. Ackerman MJ, Clapham DE. Ion channels–basic science and clinical disease. N Engl J Med. 1997;336:1575–86.
103. Keating MT, Sanguinetti MC. Molecular and cellular mechanisms of cardiac arrhythmias. Cell. 2001;104:569–80.
104. Wang Q, Curran ME, Splawski I, Burn TC, Millholland JM, VanRaay TJ, Shen J, Timothy KW, Vincent GM, de Jager T, et al. Positional cloning of a novel potassium channel gene: KVLQT1 mutations cause cardiac arrhythmias. Nat Genet. 1996;12:17–23.
105. Curran ME, Splawski I, Timothy KW, Vincent GM, Green ED, Keating MT. A molecular basis for cardiac arrhythmia: HERG mutations cause long QT syndrome. Cell. 1995;80:795–803.
106. Wang Q, Shen J, Splawski I, Atkinson D, Li Z, Robinson JL, Moss AJ, Towbin JA, Keating MT. SCN5A mutations associated with an inherited cardiac arrhythmia, long QT syndrome. Cell. 1995;80:805–11.
107. Wang Q, Shen J, Li Z, Timothy K, Vincent GM, Priori SG, Schwartz PJ, Keating MT. Cardiac sodium channel mutations in patients with long QT syndrome, an inherited cardiac arrhythmia. Hum Mol Genet. 1995;4:1603–7.
108. Mohler PJ, Gramolini AO, Bennett V. Ankyrins. J Cell Sci. 2002;115:1565–6.
109. Chen L, Marquardt ML, Tester DJ, Sampson KJ, Ackerman MJ, Kass RS. Mutation of an A-kinase-anchoring protein causes long-QT syndrome. Proc Natl Acad Sci U S A. 2007;104:20990–5.
110. Ueda K, Valdivia C, Medeiros-Domingo A, Tester DJ, Vatta M, Farrugia G, Ackerman MJ, Makielski JC. Syntrophin mutation associated with long QT syndrome through activation of the nNOS-SCN5A macromolecular complex. Proc Natl Acad Sci U S A. 2008;105:9355–60.
111. Vatta M, Ackerman MJ, Ye B, Makielski JC, Ughanze EE, Taylor EW, Tester DJ, Balijepalli RC, Foell JD, Li Z, et al. Mutant caveolin-3 induces persistent late sodium current and is associated with long-QT syndrome. Circulation. 2006;114:2104–12.
112. Andersen ED, Krasilnikoff PA, Overvad H. Intermittent muscular weakness, extrasystoles, and multiple developmental anomalies. A new syndrome? Acta Paediatr Scand. 1971;60:559–64.
113. Sansone V, Griggs RC, Meola G, Ptacek LJ, Barohn R, Iannaccone S, Bryan W, Baker N, Janas SJ, Scott W, et al. Andersen's syndrome: a distinct periodic paralysis. Ann Neurol. 1997;42:305–12.
114. Canun S, Perez N, Beirana LG. Andersen syndrome autosomal dominant in three generations. Am J Med Genet. 1999;85:147–56.
115. Gaita F, Giustetto C, Bianchi F, Wolpert C, Schimpf R, Riccardi R, Grossi S, Richiardi E, Borggrefe M. Short QT Syndrome: a familial cause of sudden death. Circulation. 2003;108:965–70.
116. Gussak I, Brugada P, Brugada J, Wright RS, Kopecky SL, Chaitman BR, Bjerregaard P. Idiopathic short QT interval: a new clinical syndrome? Cardiology. 2000;94:99–102.

117. Schimpf R, Borggrefe M, Wolpert C. Clinical and molecular genetics of the short QT syndrome. Curr Opin Cardiol. 2008;23:192–8.
118. Crotti L, Taravelli E, Girardengo G, Schwartz PJ. Congenital short QT syndrome. Indian Pacing Electrophysiol J. 2010;10:86–95.
119. Schwartz PJ, Spazzolini C, Crotti L, Bathen J, Amlie JP, Timothy K, Shkolnikova M, Berul CI, Bitner-Glindzicz M, Toivonen L, et al. The Jervell and Lange-Nielsen syndrome: natural history, molecular basis, and clinical outcome. Circulation. 2006;113:783–90.
120. Schulze-Bahr E, Wedekind H, Haverkamp W, Borggrefe M, Assmann G, Breithardt G, Funke H. The LQT syndromes–current status of molecular mechanisms. Z Kardiol. 1999;88:245–54.
121. Drici MD, Arrighi I, Chouabe C, Mann JR, Lazdunski M, Romey G, Barhanin J. Involvement of IsK-associated K+ channel in heart rate control of repolarization in a murine engineered model of Jervell and Lange-Nielsen syndrome. Circ Res. 1998;83:95–102.
122. Romey G, Attali B, Chouabe C, Abitbol I, Guillemare E, Barhanin J, Lazdunski M. Molecular mechanism and functional significance of the MinK control of the KvLQT1 channel activity. J Biol Chem. 1997;272:16713–6.
123. Ackerman MJ, Tester DJ, Porter CJ. Swimming, a gene-specific arrhythmogenic trigger for inherited long QT syndrome. Mayo Clin Proc. 1999;74:1088–94.
124. Schwartz PJ, Priori SG, Spazzolini C, Moss AJ, Vincent GM, Napolitano C, Denjoy I, Guicheney P, Breithardt G, Keating MT, et al. Genotype-phenotype correlation in the long-QT syndrome: gene-specific triggers for life-threatening arrhythmias. Circulation. 2001;103:89–95.
125. Moss AJ, Zareba W, Hall WJ, Schwartz PJ, Crampton RS, Benhorin J, Vincent GM, Locati EH, Priori SG, Napolitano C, et al. Effectiveness and limitations of beta-blocker therapy in congenital long-QT syndrome. Circulation. 2000;101:616–23.
126. Brugada P, Brugada J. Right bundle branch block, persistent ST segment elevation and sudden cardiac death: a distinct clinical and electrocardiographic syndrome. A multicenter report. J Am Coll Cardiol. 1992;20:1391–6.
127. Martini B, Nava A, Thiene G, Buja GF, Canciani B, Scognamiglio R, Daliento L, Dalla Volta S. Ventricular fibrillation without apparent heart disease: description of six cases. Am Heart J. 1989;118:1203–9.
128. Remme CA, Wever EF, Wilde AA, Derksen R, Hauer RN. Diagnosis and long-term follow-up of the Brugada syndrome in patients with idiopathic ventricular fibrillation. Eur Heart J. 2001;22:400–9.
129. Viskin S, Belhassen B. Idiopathic ventricular fibrillation. Am Heart J. 1990;120:661–71.
130. Chen Q, Kirsch GE, Zhang D, Brugada R, Brugada J, Brugada P, Potenza D, Moya A, Borggrefe M, Breithardt G, et al. Genetic basis and molecular mechanism for idiopathic ventricular fibrillation. Nature. 1998;392:293–6.
131. Priori SG, Napolitano C, Gasparini M, Pappone C, Della Bella P, Brignole M, Giordano U, Giovannini T, Menozzi C, Bloise R, et al. Clinical and genetic heterogeneity of right bundle branch block and ST-segment elevation syndrome: A prospective evaluation of 52 families. Circulation. 2000;102:2509–15.
132. Priori SG, Napolitano C, Gasparini M, Pappone C, Della Bella P, Giordano U, Bloise R, Giustetto C, De Nardis R, Grillo M, et al. Natural history of Brugada syndrome: insights for risk stratification and management. Circulation. 2002;105:1342–7.
133. Lippi G, Montagnana M, Meschi T, Comelli I, Cervellin G. Genetic and clinical aspects of Brugada syndrome: an update. Adv Clin Chem. 2009;56:197–208.
134. Leenhardt A, Lucet V, Denjoy I, Grau F, Ngoc DD, Coumel P. Catecholaminergic polymorphic ventricular tachycardia in children. A 7-year follow-up of 21 patients. Circulation. 1995;91:1512–9.
135. Lahat H, Eldar M, Levy-Nissenbaum E, Bahan T, Friedman E, Khoury A, Lorber A, Kastner DL, Goldman B, Pras E. Autosomal recessive catecholamine- or exercise-induced polymorphic ventricular tachycardia: clinical features and assignment of the disease gene to chromosome 1p13-21. Circulation. 2001;103:2822–7.
136. Postma AV, Bhuiyan ZA, Bikker H. Molecular diagnostics of catecholaminergic polymorphic ventricular tachycardia using denaturing high-performance liquid chromatography and sequencing. Methods Mol Med. 2006;126:171–83.
137. Eldar M, Pras E, Lahat H. A missense mutation in the CASQ2 gene is associated with autosomal-recessive catecholamine-induced polymorphic ventricular tachycardia. Trends Cardiovasc Med. 2003;13:148–51.
138. Lahat H, Pras E, Olender T, Avidan N, Ben-Asher E, Man O, Levy-Nissenbaum E, Khoury A, Lorber A, Goldman B, et al. A missense mutation in a highly conserved region of CASQ2 is associated with autosomal recessive catecholamine-induced polymorphic ventricular tachycardia in Bedouin families from Israel. Am J Hum Genet. 2001;69:1378–84.
139. Patel RS, Ye S. Genetic determinants of coronary heart disease: new discoveries and insights from genome-wide association studies. Heart. 2011;97:1463–73.
140. Schunkert H, Konig IR, Kathiresan S, Reilly MP, Assimes TL, Holm H, Preuss M, Stewart AF, Barbalic M, Gieger C, et al. Large-scale association analysis identifies 13 new susceptibility loci for coronary artery disease. Nat Genet. 2011;43:333–8.
141. Brown MS, Goldstein JL. A receptor-mediated pathway for cholesterol homeostasis. Science. 1986;232:34–47.
142. Goldstein JL, Brown MS. Binding and degradation of low density lipoproteins by cultured human fibroblasts. Comparison of cells from a normal subject and from a patient with homozygous familial hypercholesterolemia. J Biol Chem. 1974;249:5153–62.
143. Lindgren V, Luskey KL, Russell DW, Francke U. Human genes involved in cholesterol metabolism: chromosomal mapping of the loci for the low density lipoprotein receptor and 3-hydroxy-3-methylglutaryl-coenzyme A reductase with cDNA probes. Proc Natl Acad Sci U S A. 1985;82:8567–71.
144. Yamamoto T, Davis CG, Brown MS, Schneider WJ, Casey ML, Goldstein JL, Russell DW. The human LDL receptor: a cysteine-rich protein with multiple Alu sequences in its mRNA. Cell. 1984;39:27–38.
145. Innerarity TL, Weisgraber KH, Arnold KS, Mahley RW, Krauss RM, Vega GL, Grundy SM. Familial defective apolipoprotein B-100: low density lipoproteins with abnormal receptor binding. Proc Natl Acad Sci U S A. 1987;84:6919–23.
146. Law SW, Lackner KJ, Hospattankar AV, Anchors JM, Sakaguchi AY, Naylor SL, Brewer Jr HB. Human apolipoprotein B-100: cloning, analysis of liver mRNA, and assignment of the gene to chromosome 2. Proc Natl Acad Sci U S A. 1985;82:8340–4.
147. Abifadel M, Varret M, Rabes JP, Allard D, Ouguerram K, Devillers M, Cruaud C, Benjannet S, Wickham L, Erlich D, et al. Mutations in PCSK9 cause autosomal dominant hypercholesterolemia. Nat Genet. 2003;34:154–6.
148. Allard D, Amsellem S, Abifadel M, Trillard M, Devillers M, Luc G, Krempf M, Reznik Y, Girardet JP, Fredenrich A, et al. Novel mutations of the PCSK9 gene cause variable phenotype of autosomal dominant hypercholesterolemia. Hum Mutat. 2005;26:497.
149. Soutar AK, Naoumova RP. Mechanisms of disease: genetic causes of familial hypercholesterolemia. Nat Clin Pract Cardiovasc Med. 2007;4:214–25.
150. Marques-Pinheiro A, Marduel M, Rabes JP, Devillers M, Villeger L, Allard D, Weissenbach J, Guerin M, Zair Y, Erlich D, et al. A fourth locus for autosomal dominant hypercholesterolemia maps at 16q22.1. Eur J Hum Genet. 2010;18:1236–42.

151. Heath KE, Gahan M, Whittall RA, Humphries SE. Low-density lipoprotein receptor gene (LDLR) world-wide website in familial hypercholesterolaemia: update, new features and mutation analysis. Atherosclerosis. 2001;154:243–6.
152. Wilson DJ, Gahan M, Haddad L, Heath K, Whittall RA, Williams RR, Humphries SE, Day IN. A World Wide Web site for low-density lipoprotein receptor gene mutations in familial hypercholesterolemia: sequence-based, tabular, and direct submission data handling. Am J Cardiol. 1998;81:1509–11.
153. Soutar AK, Naoumova RP. Autosomal recessive hypercholesterolemia. Semin Vasc Med. 2004;4:241–8.
154. Lee MH, Lu K, Hazard S, Yu H, Shulenin S, Hidaka H, Kojima H, Allikmets R, Sakuma N, Pegoraro R, et al. Identification of a gene, ABCG5, important in the regulation of dietary cholesterol absorption. Nat Genet. 2001;27:79–83.
155. Lu K, Lee MH, Hazard S, Brooks-Wilson A, Hidaka H, Kojima H, Ose L, Stalenhoef AF, Mietinnen T, Bjorkhem I, et al. Two genes that map to the STSL locus cause sitosterolemia: genomic structure and spectrum of mutations involving sterolin-1 and sterolin-2, encoded by ABCG5 and ABCG8, respectively. Am J Hum Genet. 2001;69:278–90.
156. Eichner JE, Dunn ST, Perveen G, Thompson DM, Stewart KE, Stroehla BC. Apolipoprotein E polymorphism and cardiovascular disease: a HuGE review. Am J Epidemiol. 2002;155:487–95.
157. Ridker PM, Rifai N, Stampfer MJ, Hennekens CH. Plasma concentration of interleukin-6 and the risk of future myocardial infarction among apparently healthy men. Circulation. 2000;101:1767–72.
158. Humphries SE, Luong LA, Ogg MS, Hawe E, Miller GJ. The interleukin-6 -174 G/C promoter polymorphism is associated with risk of coronary heart disease and systolic blood pressure in healthy men. Eur Heart J. 2001;22:2243–52.
159. Soufi M, Sattler AM, Maisch B, Schaefer JR. Molecular mechanisms involved in atherosclerosis. Herz. 2002;27:637–48.
160. Wierzbicki AS, Humphries SE, Minhas R. Familial hypercholesterolaemia: summary of NICE guidance. BMJ. 2008;337:a1095.
161. Hoffman JI. Incidence of congenital heart disease: II. Prenatal incidence. Pediatr Cardiol. 1995;16:155–65.
162. Hoffman JI, Kaplan S. The incidence of congenital heart disease. J Am Coll Cardiol. 2002;39:1890–900.
163. Benson DW, Silberbach GM, Kavanaugh-McHugh A, Cottrill C, Zhang Y, Riggs S, Smalls O, Johnson MC, Watson MS, Seidman JG, et al. Mutations in the cardiac transcription factor NKX2.5 affect diverse cardiac developmental pathways. J Clin Invest. 1999;104:1567–73.
164. Gioli-Pereira L, Pereira AC, Mesquita SM, Xavier-Neto J, Lopes AA, Krieger JE. NKX2.5 mutations in patients with non-syndromic congenital heart disease. Int J Cardiol. 2008;138:261–5.
165. Hamanoue H, Rahayuningsih SE, Hirahara Y, Itoh J, Yokoyama U, Mizuguchi T, Saitsu H, Miyake N, Hirahara F, Matsumoto N. Genetic screening of 104 patients with congenitally malformed hearts revealed a fresh mutation of GATA4 in those with atrial septal defects. Cardiol Young. 2009;19:482–5.
166. Ikeda Y, Hiroi Y, Hosoda T, Utsunomiya T, Matsuo S, Ito T, Inoue J, Sumiyoshi T, Takano H, Nagai R, et al. Novel point mutation in the cardiac transcription factor CSX/NKX2.5 associated with congenital heart disease. Circ J. 2002;66:561–3.
167. McElhinney DB, Geiger E, Blinder J, Benson DW, Goldmuntz E. NKX2.5 mutations in patients with congenital heart disease. J Am Coll Cardiol. 2003;42:1650–5.
168. Sarkozy A, Conti E, Neri C, D'Agostino R, Digilio MC, Esposito G, Toscano A, Marino B, Pizzuti A, Dallapiccola B. Spectrum of atrial septal defects associated with mutations of NKX2.5 and GATA4 transcription factors. J Med Genet. 2005;42:e16.
169. Tomita-Mitchell A, Maslen CL, Morris CD, Garg V, Goldmuntz E. GATA4 sequence variants in patients with congenital heart disease. J Med Genet. 2007;44:779–83.
170. Metcalfe K, Rucka AK, Smoot L, Hofstadler G, Tuzler G, McKeown P, Siu V, Rauch A, Dean J, Dennis N, et al. Elastin: mutational spectrum in supravalvular aortic stenosis. Eur J Hum Genet. 2000;8:955–63.
171. Greenway SC, Pereira AC, Lin JC, DePalma SR, Israel SJ, Mesquita SM, Ergul E, Conta JH, Korn JM, McCarroll SA, et al. De novo copy number variants identify new genes and loci in isolated sporadic tetralogy of Fallot. Nat Genet. 2009;41:931–5.
172. Eldadah ZA, Hamosh A, Biery NJ, Montgomery RA, Duke M, Elkins R, Dietz HC. Familial Tetralogy of Fallot caused by mutation in the jagged1 gene. Hum Mol Genet. 2001;10:163–9.
173. Krantz ID, Smith R, Colliton RP, Tinkel H, Zackai EH, Piccoli DA, Goldmuntz E, Spinner NB. Jagged1 mutations in patients ascertained with isolated congenital heart defects. Am J Med Genet. 1999;84:56–60.
174. Spinner NB, Hutchinson AL, Krantz ID, Kamath BM. Alagille Syndrome. (1993).
175. Southard AE, Edelmann LJ, Gelb BD. Role of copy number variants in structural birth defects. Pediatrics. 2012;129:755–63.
176. Mattocks CJ, Morris MA, Matthijs G, Swinnen E, Corveleyn A, Dequeker E, Muller CR, Pratt V, Wallace A. A standardized framework for the validation and verification of clinical molecular genetic tests. Eur J Hum Genet. 2010;18:1276–88.
177. Desai AN, Jere A. Next generation sequencing: ready for the clinics? Clin Genet. 2012;81(6):503–10.

Neurodegenerative Disorders

18

Maria Martinez-Lage

Abstract

Neurodegenerative disorders are characterized by progressive neuronal deterioration resulting in cognitive or mental degeneration, dementias, muscle weakness, and/or movement disorders. Some disorders, such as Alzheimer disease or Parkinson disease exhibit sporadic as well as familial forms, with familial forms generally developing at an earlier age. Others, such as Huntington disease, are always inherited. Molecular genetics has elucidated the basis for a number of neurodegenerative disorders, and molecular testing may identify familial mutations, allowing presymptomatic or prenatal testing for family members.

Keywords

Alzheimer's disease • Parkinson's disease • Frontotemporal degeneration • Amyotrophic lateral sclerosis • Hereditary dystonia • Spinocerebellar ataxia • Autosomal dominant cerebellar ataxias • Friedrich ataxia • Huntington disease

Introduction

Neurodegenerative disorders are characterized by progressive neuronal deterioration resulting in cognitive or mental degeneration, dementias, muscle weakness, and/or movement disorders. Some disorders, such as Alzheimer disease or Parkinson disease, exhibit sporadic as well as familial forms, with familial forms generally developing at an earlier age. Others, such as Huntington disease, are always inherited. Molecular genetics has elucidated the basis for a number of neurodegenerative disorders, and molecular testing may identify familial mutations, allowing presymptomatic or prenatal testing for family members.

M. Martinez-Lage, M.D. (✉)
Pathology and Laboratory Medicine, Neuropathology, Perelman School of Medicine at the University of Pennsylvania, 3400 Spruce St., 6 Founders, Philadelphia, PA 19104, USA
e-mail: maria.martinez-lage@uphs.upenn.edu

Alzheimer Disease

Molecular Basis of Disease

Alzheimer disease (AD) is an adult-onset, slowly progressive, and complex neurodegenerative disease that initially affects memory and later involves other cognitive and basic neurologic functions. AD is the most common form of dementia, particularly in the elderly. An estimated 5.2 million Americans had Alzheimer's disease in 2014, including approximately 200,000 individuals younger than age 65 [1]. The pathological hallmarks of AD are extracellular amyloid plaques composed of beta-amyloid (Aβ), and intracellular neurofibrillary tangles composed of phosphorylated tau protein, which can also be seen in the form of neuropil threads. AD can be clinically categorized as either late onset, presenting after 65 years of age, (LOAD) or early-onset disease (EOAD), which accounts for 1–5 % of all cases. Approximately 25 % of all AD is familial (i.e., ≥2 persons in a family have AD) of which approximately 95 % is LOAD [2].

Pathologic mutations in at least three genes have been associated with the development of early-onset familial Alzheimer disease (EOFAD) (Table 18.1). Approximately 10–15 % of EOFAD is associated with mutations in the

D.G.B. Leonard (ed.), *Molecular Pathology in Clinical Practice*, DOI 10.1007/978-3-319-19674-9_18

Table 18.1 Molecular genetic classification of Alzheimer disease (AD)

Gene symbol	Gene product	Chromosomal location	Key information
Definitive disease-causing genes (causative mutations of early onset Alzheimer disease)			
APP (AD1)	Amyloid precursor protein	21q21.3	Autosomal dominant, 25 pathogenic mutations, 16 % of early onset AD
PSEN1 (AD3)	Presenilin-1	14q24	Autosomal dominant, 185 pathogenic mutations, 66 % of early onset AD
PSEN2 (AD4)	Presenilin-2	1q31	Autosomal dominant, 12 pathogenic mutations
Genes with increased susceptibility (risk variants for late-onset Alzheimer disease)			
APOE (AD2)	Apolipoprotein E	19q13.32	
SORL1	Sortilin-related receptor	11q24.1	
ABCA7	ATP-binding cassette, subfamily A, member 7	19p13.3	
BIN1	Bridging integrator 1	2q14.3	
CD33 (*SIGLEC6*)	CD33 antigen/Sialic-acid binding immunoglobulin-like lectin 6	19q13.41	
CD2AP	CD2-associated protein	6p12.3	
CLU	Clusterin	8p21.1	
CR1	Complement component receptor 1	1q32.2	
EPHA1	Ephrin receptor EphA1	7q34-q35	
MS4A4E/*MS4A6A*	Membrane-spanning 4-domains, ubfamily A, members 6E, 4A	11q12.2	
PICALM	Phosphatidylinositol-binding clathrin assembly protein	11q14.2	

Source: OMIM (http://omim.org/entry/104300), Schellenberg GD, Montine TJ. The genetics and neuropathology of Alzheimer disease. Acta Neuropathol. 2012;124(3):305–23

gene encoding the amyloid precursor protein (APP), a 110–130 kDa ubiquitously expressed protein [2]. A small proteolytic fragment of APP, $A\beta_{1-42}$, is found as a major component of amyloid plaques, one of the neuropathological hallmarks of AD. Up to 25 pathogenic mutations have been identified to date, all of which are clustered in a 54 amino acid segment of APP that lies within or adjacent to the sequence encoding Aβ peptides [3]. The London mutation (V717I) is the most common APP mutation and results in increased levels of $A\beta_{1-42}$. The Swedish mutation involves two different codons (K670M and N671K) and increases total levels of Aβ production. The excess of Aβ is considered sufficient to cause AD, and this has been largely supported by the observation of a high prevalence of AD neuropathological changes and increased incidence of dementia in patients with trisomy 21 (Down syndrome), who carry an extra copy of the *APP* gene [2].

Mutations in presenilin-1 (*PSEN1*), located at chromosomal position 14q24.3, are responsible for the highest percentage of autosomal dominant EOFAD. Approximately 185 pathogenic mutations have been identified to date [3], all with complete penetrance by age 60–65 years. Presenilin-1 is the catalytic component of γ-secretase, a protein complex responsible for the cleavage of membrane proteins, including APP. Normal γ-secretase activity yields mainly $A\beta_{1-40}$ with smaller amounts of $A\beta_{1-42}$. *PSEN1* mutations alter the secretase activity [4], which likely increases the ratio of $A\beta_{1-42}$ to $A\beta_{1-40}$, facilitating the deposition of amyloidogenic species. Presenilin-2 (*PSEN2*), located at chromosomal position 1q31-q42, is highly homologous to *PSEN1* and participates in the γ-secretase complex as the catalytic domain in the absence of Presenilin-1. *PSEN2* mutations are less common than *PSEN1* variants, with only 13 pathogenic mutations identified to date [3]. Compared to *PSEN1*, patients with *PSEN2* mutations tend to have an older age of onset (accounting for the very small number of LOAD caused by an inherited mutation), longer course of disease, and more variable penetrance.

The association of the apolipoprotein E (*APOE*) ε4 allele with LOAD in non-Hispanic whites of European ancestry has been well known for more than a decade. ApoE is a plasma protein involved in the transport of cholesterol that exists as three isoforms determined by three alleles (ε2, ε3, and ε4). The ApoE ε2 and ε3 alleles are the most common in the general population. A single ApoE ε4 allele conveys a two-fold to three-fold increased risk of developing AD, whereas having two copies is associated with a five-fold increased risk, demonstrating an additive risk association. The ε2 allele is considered protective, also in an additive manner, so that a homozygous ε2/ε2 genotype confers a lower risk than just one ε2 allele. The ε4 allele s associated with not only a higher risk of developing the disease, but also an earlier age of onset; however, the presence of ε4 is neither sufficient nor necessary to develop AD, since approximately 45 % of AD patients do not have an ε4 allele [1]. Other susceptibility genes associated with increased risk for AD are shown in Table 18.1.

Clinical Utility of Testing

The use of *APOE* genotyping in the clinical setting remains controversial. As a diagnostic adjunct in the clinical evaluation of a patient with late-onset dementia, the test may have some clinical utility; however, there is general agreement that this test should not be used for predictive purposes and should never be considered for prenatal testing. In contrast, within the context of a high degree of clinical suspicion and the documentation of a family history of AD, clinical molecular testing for *APP*, *PSEN1*, and *PSEN2* has demonstrable utility. Confirmation of a pathologic mutation in a proband will establish a diagnosis and clarify the EOFAD subtype such that both presymptomatic testing for appropriate family members and prenatal testing for at-risk pregnancies could be offered to family members.

Available Assays

APOE genotyping can be performed by traditional polymerase chain reaction-restriction fragment length polymorphism (PCR-RFLP) analysis, Sanger sequencing, or TaqMan® SNP assay (Life Technologies, Grand Island, NY). Detection of pathologic mutations in *APP*, *PSEN1*, and *PSEN2* requires DNA sequencing, either Sanger sequencing or next-generation sequencing.

Interpretation of Test Results

Interpretation of an *APOE* genotype requires the concurrent evaluation of clinical information available at the time of testing and should never be interpreted in the absence of this information. As such, testing is limited to situations where the index of clinical suspicion for AD is quite high. In contrast, the identification of a pathologic *PSEN1* or *PSEN2* mutation in a symptomatic individual is diagnostic. While both presymptomatic as well as prenatal testing are theoretically possible in mutation-positive kindred, the possible existence of incomplete or reduced penetrance must be discussed during genetic counseling.

Laboratory Issues

APOE genotyping is commercially available in several reference laboratories. The College of American Pathologists (CAP) offers *APOE* genotyping proficiency testing challenges twice a year as part of the CAP/ACMG Biochemical and Molecular Genetics Survey. Methods-based sequencing challenges (Sanger or next-generation sequencing) are also available through CAP.

Parkinson Disease

Molecular Basis of Disease

Parkinson disease (PD) is a chronic, progressive, idiopathic neurodegenerative disorder of late onset, clinically characterized by the development of parkinsonism, which consists of rigidity, bradykinesia, resting tremor, and postural instability. Additional frequent non-motor symptoms include insomnia, depression, anxiety, rapid eye movement, behavior disorder, fatigue, constipation, dysautonomia, and anosmia. With progression of the disease, 15 % of affected individuals develop psychosis (visual hallucinations and delusions) and dementia. PD is the second most common neurodegenerative disorder, after AD [5]. The neuropathologic hallmark is the presence of α-synuclein positive intracytoplasmic inclusions called Lewy bodies, with selective degeneration of dopaminergic neurons in the pars compacta of the substantia nigra in the midbrain. Although most patients present with a late-onset sporadic form of the disease, the identification of familial forms of PD has clearly established the role of genetic factors in disease etiology and pathogenesis. Of note, the neuropathology of some forms of genetically based parkinsonism may differ significantly from the classic findings documented in classical PD, including nigral pathology in the absence of Lewy bodies [6].

Genes for ten familial forms of PD (PARK1, PARK2, PARK4, PARK6, PARK7, PARK8, PARK9, PARK12, PARK15, and PARK17) have been identified (Table 18.2). The inheritance patterns for PD include autosomal dominant (PARK1, PARK4, PARK8, and PARK17), autosomal recessive (PARK2, PARK6, PARK7, PARK9, and PARK15), and X-linked (PARK12). Three different but interconnected cellular processes appear to be involved in these forms: synaptic transmission, mitochondrial quality control, and lysosome-mediated autophagy [7].

PARK1 is associated with early-onset autosomal dominant PD. Despite an earlier age of onset, PARK1 patients have typical dopa-responsive parkinsonism symptoms with classic neuropathologic findings at autopsy. Three pathogenic missense mutations in the α-synuclein (*SNCA*) gene at 4q21 have been identified. The first, A53T, was found in 13 families of Italian–Greek descent [8] and the second, A30P, identified in a single German kindred [9]. A third point mutation, E46K, was described in a Spanish kindred with clinical manifestations of both parkinsonism and dementia, clinically similar to Lewy body dementia [10]. All three point mutations appear to be highly penetrant. Other pathogenic variants include gene duplications and triplications [3], some of which are responsible for the PARK4 phenotype with late-onset parkinsonism and extensive cortical Lewy bodies. α-Synuclein is a 140 amino acid protein predominantly expressed in neuronal tissues. Although the function of α-synuclein is not well characterized, this protein is one of the major protein

Table 18.2 Molecular genetic classification of Parkinson disease (PD)

Locus name	Gene	Gene product	Chromosomal location	Inheritance pattern
PARK1, PARK4	*SNCA*	Alpha-synuclein	4q21	Autosomal dominant
PARK2	*PARK2*	Parkin	6q25	Autosomal recessive
PARK6	*PINK1*	Serine/threonine protein kinase PINK1	1p35	Autosomal recessive
PARK7	*PARK7*	Protein DJ-1	1p36	Autosomal recessive
PARK8	*LRRK2*	Leucine-rich repeat serine/threonine protein kinase 2	12p11	Autosomal dominant
PARK9	*ATP13A2*	Probable cation-transporting ATPase 13A2	1p36	Autosomal recessive
PARK12	*TAF1*	Transcription initiation factor TFIID subunit 1	Xq21-q25	X-linked
PARK15	*FBX07*	F-box only protein 7	22q12.3	Autosomal recessive
PARK17	*VPS35*	Vacuolar protein sorting-associated protein 35	16q11.2	Autosomal dominant

Source: http://www.ncbi.nlm.nih.gov/books/NBK1223/

constituents of the Lewy body. One attractive hypothesis proposes that the mutant forms of the protein have a propensity to oligomerize and form toxic neuronal aggregates that contribute to the formation of insoluble fibrils through the disruption of the cellular ubiquitin–proteasome pathway and ultimately neuronal cell death via an apoptotic mechanism.

PARK2, or juvenile-onset autosomal recessive PD, is associated with mutations in the *PARK2* gene that maps to chromosome 6q25. The gene consists of 12 exons and encodes a 465 amino acid protein, parkin. Functionally, parkin contains an ubiquitin-like domain in the N-terminus and two RING finger domains in the C-terminus. Similar to other proteins containing RING finger domains, parkin has been shown to have an E3 ubiquitin ligase activity. The association of parkin mutations with an autosomal recessive form of PD suggests that it is the loss of E3 ubiquitin ligase activity that directly contributes to the pattern of neurodegeneration seen in PD. Like PARK1, this mechanism is thought to involve disruption of the ubiquitin–proteasome system, resulting in the abnormal accumulation of substrate proteins. To date, more than 127 pathologic loss-of-function *PARK2* mutations have been identified [7]. Mutations are generally exon rearrangements leading to deletions, duplications, triplications, or point mutations.

PARK6 is associated with mutations in the serine/threonine protein kinase gene (*PINK1*), with an autosomal recessive pattern of inheritance [5]. PARK7, another autosomal recessive form of PD, is caused by mutations (deletion and point mutations) in the *PARK7* gene. PARK9 defines a particular autosomal recessive phenotype with parkinsonism and iron accumulation in basal ganglia and is due to mutations in the cation-transporting ATPase 13A2 protein encoded by *ATP13A2*. PARK15, also known as pallido-pyramidal syndrome, is characterized by the presence of pyramidal tract signs in addition to parkinsonism, and is associated with mutations in *FBX07* [11].

PARK8 is a dominantly inherited late-onset form of PD associated with mutations in the leucine rich repeat kinase 2 gene (*LRRK2*). Nearly a dozen different pathogenic variants have been reported in LRRK2; the most common, p.Gly2019Ser, has been found in approximately 5–7 % of autosomal dominant PD. Of note, the frequency of this variant is substantially higher among individuals of Ashkenazi Jewish ancestry or Northern African ancestry [5].

Mutations of *TAF1* are the only known cause of PD with X-linked inheritance (PARK12), a rare event only found among individuals of Panayan (Philippines) origin [5].

Clinical Utility of Testing

Testing for *SNCA*, *PARK2*, *PINK1*, *PARK7*, and *LRRK2* mutations is available clinically. With a high degree of clinical suspicion and the documentation of a family history of PD, molecular testing has demonstrable utility. Confirmation of a pathologic mutation in a proband will establish a diagnosis and clarify the mode of inheritance such that both presymptomatic testing for appropriate family members and prenatal testing for at-risk pregnancies could be offered.

Available Assays

Testing for most of the PD genes can be performed by conventional Sanger sequencing of the mutation-containing exons. Testing for *PARK2* mutations generally necessitates the use of a semiquantitative PCR methodology to detect heterozygous exonic rearrangements (deletions, duplications, and triplications), which would not be detected by conventional non-quantitative PCR or Sanger sequencing [12]. Next-generation sequencing panels of multiple Parkinson-associated genes are available in international laboratories.

Interpretation of Results

The identification of a pathologic mutation in a symptomatic proband is diagnostic.

Laboratory Issues

No commercial in vitro diagnostic test kits or formal proficiency testing are currently available.

Amyotrophic Lateral Sclerosis and Frontotemporal Degeneration

Molecular Basis of Disease

Amyotrophic lateral sclerosis (ALS) is a progressive neurodegenerative condition affecting upper and lower motor neurons characterized by rapidly progressive weakness, hyperreflexia, spasticity, muscle wasting, and fasciculations, usually leading to death in a few years. The peak incidence of ALS is in the sixth decade for sporadic cases (SALS, 90 %), and 10 years earlier for the 5–10 % of familial cases (FALS) [13].

Frontotemporal degeneration (FTD) is a neurodegenerative disorder characterized clinically by progressive changes in social, behavioral, and/or language function and pathologically by degeneration of the frontal and/or anterior temporal lobes. Clinical and pathologic phenotypes of FTD are heterogeneous, with several subtypes recognized depending on the most prominent clinical manifestation. In contrast to AD, memory is relatively preserved in FTD until late stages of disease. FTD accounts for 5–15 % of all dementia and is the second most common cause in the presenile age group. A subset of patients with FTD have associated motor neuron disease or parkinsonism. Onset is usually between 35–75 years of age and a family history of a similar disease is present in approximately 40 % of patients.

About 5 % of patients with ALS also have clinically documented FTD, and up to 30–50 % have milder evidence of executive dysfunction, supporting the hypothesis that at least in a majority of cases, FTD and ALS are part of a disease continuum. The presence of pathological deposits of TDP-43 in most cases of ALS, in most cases with overlap between FTD and ALS (FTD-ALS), and in most cases of FTD provides a potential unifying mechanistic link [14]. Mutations in the gene coding for TDP-43 (*TARDBP*) cause FALS in a 1–4 % of families.

The first gene to be identified in ALS is associated with the ALS1 locus. The *SOD1* gene encodes copper-zinc superoxide dismutase, a metalloenzyme consisting of 153 amino acids with both copper and zinc binding sites. SOD1 catalyzes the conversion of superoxide anions to hydrogen peroxide and molecular oxygen and, as such, is thought to have a protective function in the cell by preventing oxidative damage caused by the accumulation of free radicals. More than 100 mutations have been reported in the *SOD1* gene, with one, A5V (previously known as A4V), accounting for approximately 50 % of all mutations found in North American families. Approximately 20 % of patients with FALS and 3 % of patients with SALS have *SOD1* mutations [13]. Incomplete penetrance has been documented in some families. Table 18.3 includes the gene products, chromosomal location, and clinical features of other ALS-related genes.

Several different genes and chromosomal loci have been associated with FTD, primarily with an autosomal dominant inheritance. Mutations in the microtubule (MT)-associated protein tau (*MAPT*) are responsible for 10–20 % of familial cases, and all these have tau-based neuropathology. The main function of these proteins is to stabilize the MTs and to promote MT assembly by binding to tubulin. More than 40 mutations in *MAPT* have been associated with FTD [3]. These cause disease by either altering the MT-binding properties of tau or by altering the splicing of exon 10 of *MAPT*, which alters the ratio of isoforms with 3 or 4 microtubule binding repeats.

A number of other FTD families with linkage to the same region on chromosome 17 as *MAPT* (17q21) but with no identifiable *MAPT* mutation and no significant tau pathology demonstrate mutations in the progranulin (*GRN*) gene, including frameshift, nonsense, and splice-site mutations. Progranulin (PGRN) is a 593 amino acid-secreted growth factor known to play a role in central nervous system development. The underlying disease mechanism is likely due to loss-of-function leading to protein haploinsufficiency, and the end point is TDP-43 neuropathology. *GRN* mutations account for approximately 20 % of familial FTD.

In 2011, GGGGCC hexanucleotide repeat expansions in the first intron of the *C9orf72* gene were identified as the most common genetic cause of both FTD and ALS [15, 16]. Normal individuals have between 2 and 32 GGGGCC repeats, whereas affected individuals with expansions usually have more than several hundred repeats [17]. The average mutation frequencies in North Americans and Europeans are 37 % for FALS, 6–7 % for SALS, 21–25 % for familial FTD, and 6 % for sporadic FTD (http://www.omim.org/entry/614260). Penetrance of the mutation is high, with 90 % of people with an expansion having onset of symptoms by age 70 years. No clear relationship between phenotype and expansion size has been determined. ALS patients with a *C9orf72* expansion have earlier age of onset and reduced survival compared to ALS patients without an expansion.

Clinical Utility of Testing

Within the context of a high degree of clinical suspicion and the documentation of a positive family history, clinical molecular testing for most of the above ALS and FTD related genes has demonstrable utility. Confirmation of a pathologic mutation in a proband will establish a diagnosis and clarify the

Table 18.3 Molecular genetic classification of amyotrophic lateral sclerosis (ALS) and frontotemporal lobar degeneration (FTD)

Locus name	Gene	Gene product	Chromosomal location	Inheritance pattern	Clinical presentation
ALS1	*SOD1*	Superoxide dismutase (Cu-Zn)	21q22.1	Autosomal dominant	20 % of FALS
ALS2	*ALS2*	Alsin	2q33	Autosomal recessive	
ALS3	*ALS3*	Unknown	18q21	Autosomal dominant	FALS
ALS4	*SETX*	Senataxin	9q34	Autosomal dominant	Juvenile motor neuropathy with pyramidal features
ALS5	*ALS5*	Unknown	15q15	Autosomal recessive	Juvenile ALS
ALS6	*FUS/TLS*	RNA-binding protein FUS	16p11.2	Autosomal recessive	ALS with or without FTD
ALS7	*ALS7*	Unknown	20p13	Autosomal dominant	Incomplete penetrance
ALS8	*VAPB*	Vesicle-associated membrane protein-associated protein B/C	20q13.32	Autosomal dominant	Finkel type SMA
ALS9	*ANG*	Angiogenin	14q11.2	Autosomal dominant	FALS
ALS10	*TARDBP*	TDP-43	1p36.22	Autosomal dominant	1–4 % of FALS; ALS with or without FTD, FTD
ALS 11	*FIG4*	Sac domain containing inositol phosphatase 3	6q21	Autosomal dominant	ALS, Yunis–Varon syndrome, CMT 4J
ALS12	*OPTN*	Optineurin	10p13	Autosomal recessive	FALS
ALS13	*ATXN2*	Ataxin-2	12q24.12	Autosomal dominant	SCA2
ALS14	*VCP*	Valosin-containing protein	9p13.3	Autosomal dominant	ALS with or without FTD, IBMPFD
ALS15	*UBQLN2*	Ubiquilin-2	Xp11.21	X-linked	ALS with or without FTD
ALS17	*CHMP2B*	Chromatin-modifying protein 2B	3p11.2	Autosomal dominant	FALS/familial FTD
ALS18	*PFN1*	Profilin-1	17p13.2	Autosomal dominant	FALS
C9FTD/ALS	*C9orf72*	Uncharacterized protein C9orf72	9p21.2	Autosomal dominant	Noncoding GGGGCC hexanucleotide repeat, 23–30 % of FTD/ALS
CHCHD10-ALS/FTD	*CHCHD10*	Coiled-coil-helix-coiled-coil-helix domain-containing protein 10, mitochondrial	22q11.23	Autosomal dominant	ALS, mitochondrial myopathy, SMA Jokela type
FTD-MAPT	*MAPT*	Tau protein	17q21	Autosomal dominant	FTD
FTD-GRN	*GRN*	Progranulin	17q21	Autosomal dominant	FTD

Sources: http://www.ncbi.nlm.nih.gov/books/NBK1450/, http://omim.org/entry/600274 *AD* Autosomal dominant, *AR* Autosomal recessive, *ALS* amyotrophic lateral sclerosis, *CMT* Charcot-Marie-Tooth syndrome, *FALS* familial amyotrophic lateral sclerosis, *FTD* frontotemporal dementia, *IBMPFD* inclusion body myopathy with early onset Paget disease and frontotemporal dementia, *SCA2* spinocerebellar ataxia type 2, *SMA* spinal muscular atrophy

mode of inheritance such that both presymptomatic testing for appropriate family members and prenatal testing for at-risk pregnancies could be offered. Clinical testing for a *C9orf72* hexanucleotide repeat expansion can help to confirm the diagnosis of ALS or FTD and be used for screening and genetic counseling of patients and family members after an affected family member has been found to carry an expansion.

Available Assays

Direct DNA sequencing analysis is most commonly used for ALS related genes (*SOD1*, *ALS2*, etc.), as well as for *GRN* and *MAPT*. When the mutation is known in the proband, directed sequencing is preferred in the screening of family members. Next-generation sequencing as well as Sanger sequencing panels that include many of these genes are currently available. The hexanucleotide expansion in *C9orf72* uses a combination of PCR-based amplification for normal alleles with expansion analysis, usually by Southern blot analysis, for homozygous PCR results, and is available at most reference laboratories.

Interpretation of Test Results

The identification of a pathogenic mutation in any of the above genes in a symptomatic proband is considered diagnostic. However, negative results must be interpreted with caution, because not all genetic causes of ALS and FTD have been identified. Once a mutation has been identified in the proband, directed gene mutation testing can be performed in affected family members as well as in unaffected adult family members who wish to know their mutation status, after presymptomatic genetic counseling with a certified genetic counselor. Prenatal testing may be considered; however, it is important to note that onset of disease is in the adult years and is variable. In addition, penetrance may not be 100 % with all mutations.

Normal, nonpathogenic alleles of *C9orf72* contain between 2 and 32 hexanucleotide repeats at this locus, while pathogenic expansions contain from 32 to >1,000 repeats. The clinical significance of alleles with 20–32 repeats is currently unclear and should be interpreted with caution.

Laboratory Issues

Formal proficiency testing is not available for any of these ALS/FTD associated genes.

Huntington Disease

Molecular Basis of Disease

Huntington disease (HD) is an autosomal dominant neurodegenerative disorder clinically characterized by the presence of choreiform movements, psychiatric symptoms, and cognitive decline. While >90 % of HD patients become symptomatic in adulthood, 5–10 % present before the age of 20 years (juvenile-onset) which is frequently associated with inheritance of the mutant allele from a symptomatic father. Unlike the adult-onset form, juvenile-onset HD is generally characterized by the presence of rapidly progressive rigidity, seizures, ataxia, dystonia, and intellectual decline [18].

The Huntington gene (*HTT*, formerly *IT15*) is at chromosomal location 4p16.3. The gene spans more than 200 kilobases (kb) and contains 67 exons. *HTT* encodes a 3,142 amino acid protein with an approximate molecular weight of 350 kilodaltons (kDa) that shares no known homologies with other characterized proteins. HD is caused by a toxic gain-of-function mechanism associated with the expansion of a polyglutamine tract within the protein that is translated from a CAG repeat region within exon 1 of the gene. The CAG repeat length is highly polymorphic in the general population, with the largest normal allele currently defined as carrying ≤26 CAG repeats. Alleles carrying ≥40 CAG repeats are considered diagnostic, since they have never been identified in the absence of HD pathology. Alleles with 27–35 CAG repeats are defined as "mutable normal or intermediate alleles." While alleles in this size range have yet to be convincingly associated with an HD phenotype, they can be meiotically unstable in sperm and result in the expansion of paternally derived alleles. Alleles of 36–39 CAG repeats are defined as "HD alleles with reduced penetrance," as they have been found in both clinically as well as neuropathologically confirmed HD patients and in elderly asymptomatic individuals [19].

Clinical Utility of Testing

As HD is largely a genetically homogeneous disease, molecular testing has been routinely utilized for confirmatory, predictive, and prenatal purposes. Professional standards strongly encourage that predictive test should be offered only to individuals 18 years of age or older. The recommended multidisciplinary presymptomatic protocol includes pretest counseling and evaluation by a clinical geneticist, genetic counselor, psychologist or psychiatrist, and neurologist over several visits, with the option to not receive test results even after testing has been completed. With few exceptions, interpretation of laboratory results is unambiguous and the resulting genetic counseling consultations follow those for other autosomal dominant adult-onset disorders. Prenatal testing can be performed using amniotic fluid cells or chorionic villus samples after a molecular diagnosis of HD in the family. Maternal cell contamination studies should be performed on every prenatal sample to confirm the fetal origin of the tested sample [19].

Available Assays

The presence of CAG repeat expansions can be determined by both PCR and Southern blot methods. For PCR, several sets of primers, assay conditions, amplicon separation, and detection techniques have been published. Regardless of the particular PCR test method employed, optimization of the assay conditions and post-PCR analyses is essential to ensure accurate and unambiguous quantitation of the HD CAG repeat length (Fig. 18.1), given that sizing anomalies have been observed in analyses utilizing agarose, capillary, and denaturing polyacrylamide gel electrophoretic (PAGE) methods [19]. As such, accurate quantitation of patient amplicon sizes should be empirically determined by comparison to appropriate external or internal standards [19].

As the length of the polymorphic CAG repeat alone is associated with HD, testing must be designed to amplify only the CAG repeat and not an adjacent CCG repeat [19]. The CCG repeat, which lies 12 base pairs (bp) 3′ of the HD

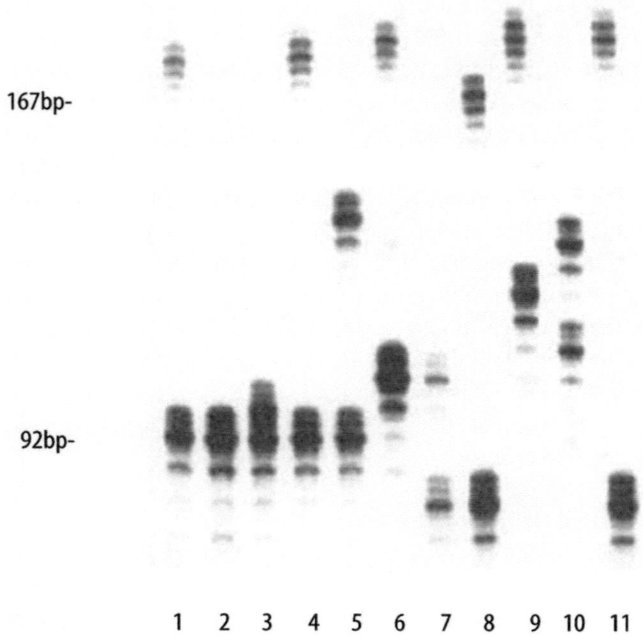

Figure 18.1 PCR genotyping of the Huntington disease polymorphic CAG repeat utilizing ^{32}P-dCTP incorporation and the Al/C2 primer pair [20, 21]. Separation and sizing of alleles was performed on a 35 cm × 43 cm 6 % denaturing polyacrylamide gel followed by autoradiography. The numbers of CAG repeats in each of the two alleles for patients in *lanes 1–11* are 17 and 44, 17 and 17, 17 and 18, 17 and 44, 17 and 25, 19 and 45, 15 and 19, 15 and 40, 22 and 45, 20 and 24, and 15 and 45, respectively

CAG repeat, is also polymorphic and as a result may lead to diagnostic inaccuracies for both normal and HD allele sizing. Furthermore, polymorphisms surrounding or within the CAG tract have been identified with a collective frequency of approximately 1 %. These nucleotide substitutions can be categorized into two groups: (1) those that modify primer-annealing sites and (2) those that result in the loss of sequence interruption between the CAG and CCG repeat tracts. With the first category, nucleotide changes may result in the misinterpretation of genotyping data due to an allele-specific amplification failure associated with improper primer annealing. In the second category, rare A to G substitutions within the intervening 12 bp segment between the CAG and CCG tracts can result in increased meiotic instability of the tract as well as miscalculation of uninterrupted CAG repeat length based on conventional calculation formulas [19].

Triplet-repeat primed PCR (TP PCR) allows for the rapid identification of large pathogenic repeats refractory to conventional PCR amplification by using a chimeric PCR approach that generates different sized amplicons due to multiple annealing sites on the template [22]. The forward primer is fluorescently labeled and the design of the chimeric reverse primer introduces nonspecific DNA amplification by hybridization to multiple sites within the expanded region originating PCR products of varying sizes. Capillary electrophoresis is used to separate the products and the true alleles are easily distinguished as the highest peaks, with a stutter peak of decreasing amplitude seen when an expanded allele is too large to be amplified by the assay (usually >101 repeats).

Southern blot methods, although not generally used for routine diagnostic testing, often are essential for the identification or confirmation of very large expansions typically associated with juvenile-onset HD. Furthermore, Southern blot or TP PCR may be used for confirmation testing of patients (generally children) who appear to be homozygous for two normal-sized alleles [19].

Interpretation of Test Results

PCR testing for the HD CAG repeat has a reported sensitivity of 99 % [23]. The remaining 1 % of patients represent HD phenocopies, and to date at least two distinct genetic loci, *HDL1* which corresponds to the prion protein gene *PRNP* (http://www.omim.org/entry/176640#0001) and *HDL2* which is discussed below in the section on dystonia, have been identified. Testing specificity is nearly 100 % [24]. In summary, the interpretative challenges in HD testing are primarily related to the need to recognize that CAG ranges and descriptors may be modified over time. For reporting of HD results, the American College of Medical Genetics and Genomics (ACMG) has recently established updated guidelines regarding the definitions of CAG repeat range descriptors and interpretative guidelines for test reporting and genetic counseling purposes [19].

Laboratory Issues

CAP offers HD proficiency challenges twice per year as part of the CAP/ACMG Molecular Genetics Laboratory (MGL2) Survey. Genotyped HD patient DNA for use as controls can be obtained from the Coriell Cell Repositories (Camden, NJ; http://ccr.coriell.org/).

Autosomal Dominant Cerebellar Ataxias and Friedreich Ataxia

Molecular Basis of Disease

The autosomal dominant cerebellar ataxias (ADCAs) or spinocerebellar ataxias (SCAs) represent a clinically and genetically heterogeneous group of neurological disorders with an autosomal dominant mode of inheritance. To date, at least 35 distinct loci have been identified, and clinical testing is presently available for most in which a causative gene has been identified. Because the collective incidence of these disorders is high in both unselected and selected ataxia cohorts [25, 26] and the degree of clinical overlap among the various ADCAs is extensive, molecular genetic testing is a valuable diagnostic tool. Most of the molecularly characterized ADCAs (dentatorubro pallidoluysian atrophy or DRPLA and SCA1, 2, 3, 6, 7, 8, 10, 12, 17, 31, and 36) are associated with reiterated repeat expansion mutations and neuropathologically share the presence of inclusions or aggregates. DRPLA and SCA1, 2, 3, 6, 7, 12, and 17 are associated with CAG trinucleotide repeat expansion, and SCA8 with a CTG trinucleotide repeat expansion. SCA10 is associated with an ATTCT pentanucleotide repeat expansion, SCA31 with a TGGAA pentanucleotide repeat expansion, and SCA36 with a GGCCTG hexanucleotide repeat expansion (Table 18.4). In general, larger repeat expansions correlate with earlier onset of disease and greater severity of disease symptoms. Also, expanded repeats are less stable and can change, and usually to a larger size of the repeat, when passed on to the next generation. This repeat expansion with passage to the next generation results in the clinical phenomenon of anticipation, which is the observation of an earlier age of onset and more severe disease when an expansion is passed on to the next generation.

In the majority of the ADCAs, the location of the repeat region is exonic (DRPLA and SCA1, 2, 3, 6, 7, and 17), and the mechanism of disease pathogenesis (with the exception of SCA6) is thought to involve a toxic gain of function in the protein. Genes associated with polyglutamine expansion ADCAs are involved in RNA metabolism, chromatin structure, transcription regulation, glutamate transmission, mitochondrial function, and their dysfunction can lead to the toxic accumulation of aggregates and intranuclear inclusions. The non-polyglutamine expansion ADCAs (SCA8, 10, 12, and 31) demonstrate expansions in noncoding regions which also can trigger a gain of function mechanism. These genes are associated with chromatin structure, RNA metabolism, mitochondrial function, and toxic accumulation of protein and RNA aggregates. The rest of the ADCAs, not associated with repeat expansion, are linked to conventional mutations, such as missense point mutations, insertions, and deletions. The genes involved in the ADCAs without repeat expansions are responsible for calcium homeostasis, glutamate transmission, mitochondrial function, axonal transport, tau metabolism, and potassium transmission [27].

Friedreich ataxia (FRDA) is the most common form of hereditary ataxia, with a prevalence of approximately 2–4 per 100,000 and a carrier frequency of approximately 1 in 90. The disease has an autosomal recessive mode of inheritance. FRDA is clinically characterized by the onset of gait and limb ataxia before the age of 25 years, decreased deep tendon reflexes, dysarthria, pyramidal signs, Babinski responses, and decreased position or vibration sense (or both) in the lower limbs. Approximately 65 % of patients also develop a cardiomyopathy, while approximately 10 % of patients develop diabetes. Atypical clinical presentations have been reported in approximately 25 % of patients and generally have included later ages of onset (after 25 years of age), retained reflexes, and slower disease progression. In addition, genetically confirmed patients with more complex phenotypes have recently been reported and include individuals with idiopathic spastic paraparesis, motor and sensory neuropathy, limb and axial dystonia, and chorea with myoclonus [28]. FRDA is caused by mutations in the *FXN* gene that encodes the 210 amino acid protein frataxin that localizes to the mitochondrial inner membrane, where it is required for mitochondrial iron homeostasis. Approximately 90–94 % of patients are homozygous for GAA expansion mutations within intron 1 of *FXN*, whereas 6–10 % of patients are compound heterozygotes for a GAA expansion on one allele and an inactivating point mutation or deletion on the other. As opposed to what occurs in most ADCA with trinucleotide repeat expansion, FRDA is not associated with the phenomenon of genetic anticipation [29].

Ataxia-telangiectasia (AT) is an autosomal recessive, early onset, progressive cerebellar ataxia with characteristic oculomotor apraxia, choreoathetosis, conjunctival telangiectasias, immunodeficiency, and increased risk for leukemia, lymphoma, and other malignancies. AT is caused by homozygous or compound heterozygous mutations in the *ATM* gene, encoding the ATM serine/threonine kinase protein. Mutations include missense, nonsense, and splice site mutations, small intragenic deletions/insertions, and, in 1–2 % of cases, large genomic deletions. Of note, in AT, DNA sequence analysis of *ATM* in search of mutations may have lower sensitivity than immunoblotting for intracellular ATM protein depletion [30].

Clinical Utility of Testing

The utility of offering testing for the molecularly characterized hereditary ataxias is very high. For the ADCAs with well-characterized genetic loci, diagnostic, predictive, as well as prenatal testing is available. Although allelic heterogeneity has been reported in FRDA (i.e., point mutations in compound heterozygotes), the vast majority of FRDA patients have homozygous expansions of the GAA repeat; hence, diagnostic, predictive, and prenatal testing also is available. As is the case with HD, predictive testing for the ADCAs should be offered only to individuals who have reached the statutory age of majority (generally 18 years). Before testing is performed for an asymptomatic family member at risk, a formal multidisciplinary predictive testing protocol, similar to the one utilized for HD predictive testing, should be offered to those desiring determination of their carrier status. Again, with few exceptions, interpretation of the laboratory result is unambiguous, and the resulting genetic counseling consultations follow those for other autosomal dominant adult-onset disorders. For FRDA and AT families, appropriate counseling consistent with an autosomal recessive pattern of inheritance is required. AT patients

Table 18.4 Molecular genetic classification of the autosomal dominant cerebellar ataxias (ADCA) and selected autosomal recessive ataxias

Locus name	Gene	Gene product	Chromosomal location	Key information
SCA1	*ATXN1*	Ataxin-1	6p22.3	Peripheral neuropathy, (CAG)*n* trinucleotide repeat
SCA2	*ATXN2*	Ataxin-2	12q24.12	Peripheral neuropathy, dementia, (CAG)*n* trinucleotide repeat
SCA3	*ATXN3*	Ataxin-3	14q32.12	Machado–Joseph disease, most common ADCA worldwide, (CAG)*n* trinucleotide repeat
SCA4	–	Unknown	16q22.1	SCA with sensory axonal neuropathy; same region but not allelic with SCA31
SCA5	*SPTBN2*	Spectrin, beta, non-erythrocytic 2	11q13.2	Early onset and slow progression, point mutations and deletions
SCA6	*CACNA1A*	P/Q-type voltage-gated calcium channel, transmembrane pore-forming alpha 1A subunit	19p13.2	Very slow progression, sometimes episodic ataxia, (CAG)*n* trinucleotide repeat
SCA7	*ATXN7*	Ataxin-7	3p14.1	SCA with pigmentary macular dystrophy, (CAG)*n* trinucleotide repeat
SCA8	*ATXN8, ATXN8OS*	Ataxin-8, Ataxin-8 opposite strand	13q21	'CTG*CAG' complementary repeat expansion of both genes
SCA10	*ATXN-10*	Ataxin-10	22q13.31	(ATTCT)*n* repeat
SCA11	*TTBK2*	Tau tubulin kinase-2	15q15.2	Relatively pure SCA, insertions/deletions
SCA12	*PPP2R2B*	Protein phosphatase PP2A, regulatory subunit beta	5q32	SCA with early tremor, (CAG)*n* trinucleotide repeat
SCA13	*KCNC3*	Potassium channel, voltage-gated, Shaw-related member 3	19q13.33	Point mutations
SCA14	*PRKCG*	Protein kinase C, gamma	19q13.42	Missense mutations, deletions
SCA15	*ITPR1*	Inositol 1,4,5-triphosphate (IP3) receptor type 1	3p26.1	Very slow progression, point mutations, and deletions
SCA17	*TBP*	TATA box-binding protein	6q27	SCA with seizures, psychiatric and cognitive symptoms; trinucleotide repeat encoding glutamine (CAG or CAA)
SCA18	*SCA18*	Unknown	7q22-q32	SCA with early sensory/motor neuropathy
SCA19/22	*KCND3*	Potassium channel, voltage-gated, Shal-related member 3	1p13.2	Point mutations, deletions
SCA20	–	–	11q12	SCA with early dysarthria and dysphonia, 260 kb contiguous gene duplication
SCA21	*TMEM240*	Transmembrane protein 240	1p36.33	SCA with cognitive impairment, point mutations
SCA23	*PDYN*	Prodynorphin	20p13	Point mutations
SCA25	*SCA25*	Unknown	2p21-p13	
SCA27	*FGF14*	Fibroblast growth factor-14	13q33.1	Point mutations, deletion
SCA28	*AFG3L2*	ATPase family gene 3-like 2	18p11.21	Point mutations, autosomal dominant; allelic with AR spastic ataxia 5
SCA29	*ITPR1*	Inositol 1,4,5-triphosphate (IP3) receptor type 1	3p26.1	Congenital nonprogressive cerebellar ataxia, missense mutations

(continued)

Table 18.4 (continued)

Locus name	Gene	Gene product	Chromosomal location	Key information
SCA31	*BEAN1*	Brain-expressed associated with NEDD4	16q21	Common in Japan, (TGGAA)*n* pentanucleotide repeats, same region but not allelic with SCA4
SCA35	*TGM6*	Transglutaminase-6	20p13	Point mutations
SCA36	*NOP56*	Homolog of S. Cerevisiae NOP56	20p13	SCA and fasciculations, (GGCCTG)*n* hexanucleotide repeat
DRPLA	*ATN1*	Atrophin-1	12p13.31	Dentatorubral-pallidoluysian atrophy, ataxia, dementia, myoclonic epilepsy, and choreoathetosis), (CAG)*n* trinucleotide repeat
ATM	*ATM*	ATM serine/threonine kinase (Ataxia-telangiectasia mutated gene)	11q22.3	Ataxia telangiectasia, AR, cerebellar ataxia, telangiectasias, immune defects, and cancer predisposition
FRDA	*FXN*	Frataxin	9q21.11	Friedreich ataxia, AR, slowly progressive ataxia with limb weakness, areflexia, sensory loss, and cardiomyopathy, biallelic (GAA)*n* trinucleotide repeat

Sources: http://www.ncbi.nlm.nih.gov/books/NBK1138/; http://omim.org/phenotypicSeries/PS164400
AR autosomal recessive, *SCA* spinocerebellar ataxia

and their families require genetic counseling and additional screening due to the increased risk of developing cancer, which also is a risk for unaffected carriers.

Available Assays

Detection and quantitation of the repeat expansions associated with the ADCAs can be determined by both PCR and Southern blot methods, and the choice of methodology is dependent on the characteristic size range for the disease-specific expansion mutation. For example, very large expansions, such as those routinely seen in SCA10, require Southern blot analysis, whereas those seen in other ADCAs (SCA6, for example) are amenable to detection by routine PCR analysis. Some notable exceptions, however, are described below. As noted above for HD, regardless of the particular PCR method used, assay conditions and post-PCR analyses should be optimized to ensure accurate and unambiguous quantitation of repeat length. Furthermore, CAG sizing anomalies for ADCA testing also have been observed in comparative studies of capillary and denaturing PAGE methods. As such, accurate quantitation of patient amplicon sizes should be empirically determined by comparison to appropriate external or internal standards.

One of the important methodological considerations for quantitation of expansion mutations in general is the recognition of the existence of "extreme expansions" associated with several of the SCAs. For example, both the infantile and juvenile-onset forms of SCA2 and SCA7 have been associated with large, or "extreme," expansions generally greater than 200 CAG repeats [31]. In a situation that is analogous to the large expansions of juvenile-onset HD, these alleles can be refractory to PCR amplification or difficult to separate using conventional PAGE. Test results that are apparently "homozygous normal" genotypes in infants or children with a high index of clinical suspicion of SCA2 or SCA7 should be confirmed using a Southern blot test that can detect large expansions (Fig. 18.2) [32]. As discussed above in reference to HD, TP-PCR is a novel, rapid and robust technique that can be used to detect large trinucleotide repeats in FRDA and ADCAs (SCA1, 2, 3, 6, 7, 8, and 17).

Analysis of the FRDA GAA expansion mutation is generally performed by long-template PCR (Fig. 18.3) or by Southern blot analysis. Although the fidelity of this assay is high, PCR artifacts resembling expansions can be seen, particularly in samples with two normal-sized alleles (Fig. 18.3a, lane 4). The expansion artifacts are thought to be heteroduplexes, as they do not appear when amplicons are analyzed under denaturing conditions. These artifacts should not result in significant diagnostic errors for patients who are clearly heterozygous for two normal-sized alleles, as the intensity of the true alleles is usually much greater than that of the heteroduplexes. Ambiguities may remain,

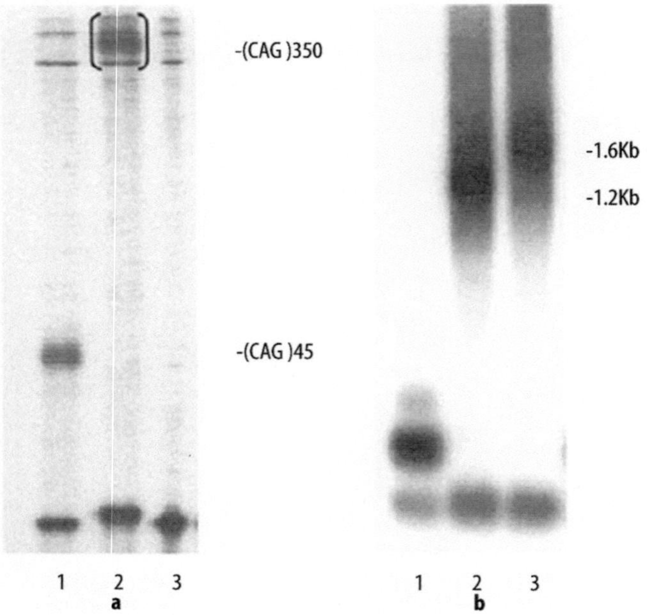

Figure 18.2 Molecular testing for the SCA2 CAG repeat. (**a**) PCR genotyping of the SCA2 polymorphic CAG repeat utilizing the UH13/UH10 primer pair [33] is shown for two related patients (*lane 1*: mother; *lane 2*: son) with adult-onset and juvenile-onset SCA2, respectively [31]. Separation and sizing of alleles was performed on a 35 cm × 43 cm 6 % denaturing polyacrylamide gel followed by autoradiography. The numbers of CAG repeats in each of the two alleles are 22 and 45 for the affected mother (*lane 1*), 23 and approximately 350 for the affected son (*lane 2*), and 22 and 22 for a normal unaffected control (*lane 3*). (**b**) PCR-Southern blot analysis [32] of the same mother-son samples shown in (**a**), confirming the presence of the extreme expansion in the affected son. Allele sizes are 22 and 45 for the affected mother (*lane 1*), 23 and approximately 350 for the affected son (*lane 2*), and 23 and approximately 400 for a positive extreme expansion control (*lane 3*). ((**b**) Courtesy of Dr. Karen Snow-Bailey, Auckland District Health Board, Auckland, New Zealand)

however, because the resolution of 1 % agarose gels for amplicons in the 500 bp range is limited. These can be clarified, if necessary, by either Southern blot or denaturing PAGE.

For screening purposes in a proband with no documented mutation, given the significant overlap between phenotypes in ADCAs, next-generation sequencing panels that include multiple genes in a single test have demonstrated significant value [35] allowing for a final diagnosis in patients that had been negative for multiple single gene tests over time. The caveat with this approach however is the possibility of novel variants that may need to be proven as pathogenic before clinical testing is offered to other family members.

Interpretation of Test Results

PCR tests for the ADCAs have a sensitivity of >99 %, and complete testing including Southern blot or TP PCR has a sensitivity of close to 100 %. For the reporting of results, interpretation of the findings requires the integration of available clinical information, repeat size, and its clinical descriptor (i.e., normal, intermediate, or abnormal). PCR tests for FRDA have a sensitivity of approximately 96 %, but the presence of a *FXN* point mutation must be considered in patients with a high degree of clinical suspicion and only one expanded GAA allele (Fig. 18.3b, lane 3; Fig. 18.4). In such situations, referral to a laboratory that offers point mutation analysis is strongly recommended.

Laboratory Issues

No commercial test kits are available for the ADCAs, FRDA, or AT. The CAP offers proficiency testing twice a year as part of the CAP/ACMG MGL Survey (MGL2) that includes challenges for several SCAs (1, 2, 3, 6, and 7) as well as FRDA.

Dystonia

Molecular Basis of Disease

While the dystonias are not strictly considered a neurodegenerative disease but rather a movement disorder, clinical and molecular descriptions of the dystonias have historically been found in texts describing neurodegenerative disorders. Neuropathological descriptions have traditionally been scant due to the scarcity of postmortem material, so the underlying histopathology of dystonia is still poorly understood [37]. The dystonias represent a clinically heterogeneous group of disorders characterized by sustained involuntary muscle contractions leading to repetitive twisting movements and abnormal postures. Many forms of dystonia (Table 18.5) can be distinguished on a genetic basis and several causative genes have been identified [38].

Dystonias are classified clinically into isolated and combined dystonias, where the latter demonstrate additional clinical features other than pure dystonia. The presence of other neurological symptoms such as parkinsonism, myoclonus, and dyskinesia define some of these combined dystonias. In addition, dystonia can be a prominent characteristic in other complex neurodegenerative disorders that can present both in childhood and in the adult, some of which are documented in Table 18.5 [38]. The isolated dystonias encompass three forms: DYT1, DYT6, and DYT25, all of which have an autosomal dominant pattern of inheritance. DYT1, also known as early-onset primary dystonia, is usually associated with reduced penetrance, since only 30 % of heterozygotes for a pathogenic variant of the gene will develop the disease. Essentially all patients with DYT1 (>99.9 %) have a 3 bp deletion (GAG) in the *TOR1A* gene, at chromosomal location 9q34 and encoding a 332 amino acid protein called torsin-1A. Torsin-1A is a member of the AAA super-family of ATPases prominently expressed in the

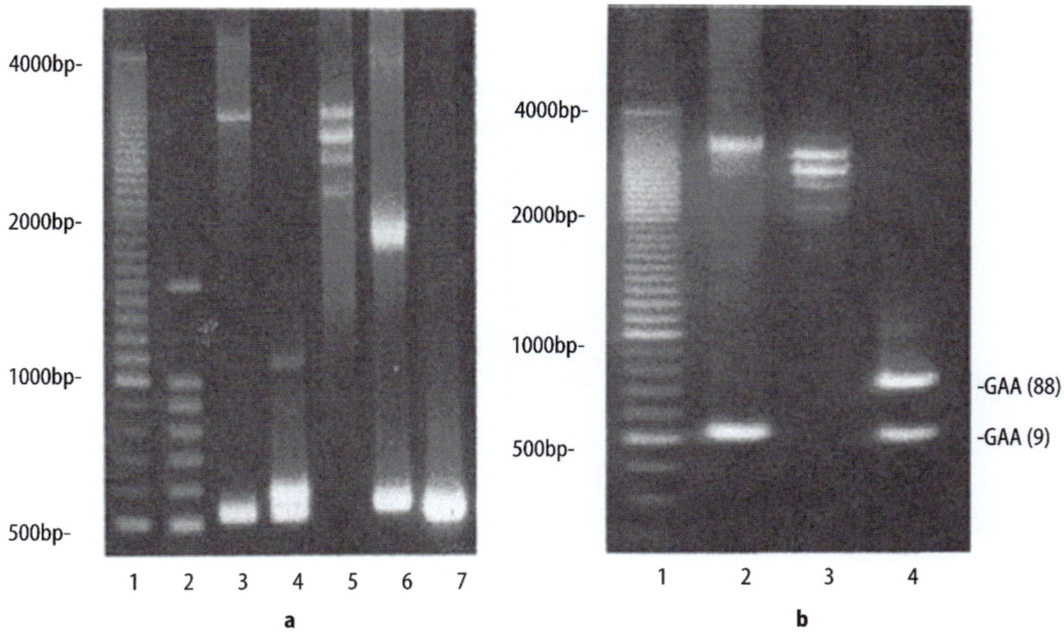

Figure 18.3 PCR analysis of the Friedreich ataxia (FRDA) polymorphic 4,000 bp GAA expansion mutation utilizing the 104F/629R primer pair [34] and the Expand Long Template PCR System (Roche Diagnostics, Mannheim, Germany). (**a**) *Lane 1*: 100 bp step ladder G6951 (Promega, Madison, WI); *lane 2*: 100 bp ladder G2101 (Promega); *lane 3*: 2,000 bp FRDA carrier with approximately 850 GAA repeats; *lane 4*: normal individual with allele sizes of 9 and 26 GAA repeats; *lane 5*: FRDA patient with allele sizes of approximately 800 and 900 GAA repeats; *lane 6*: FRDA carrier with approximately 450 GAA repeats; *lane 7*: normal control. (**b**) *Lane 1*: 100 bp step ladder G6951 (Promega); *lane 2*: FRDA compound heterozygote (see Fig. 18.4) with approximately 1,000 GAA repeats; *lane 3*: FRDA patient with allele sizes of approximately 800 and 900 GAA repeats; *lane 4*: FRDA carrier with allele sizes of 9 and 88 GAA repeats (confirmed by DNA sequencing). PCR products were separated through 1 % agarose on a 10.5 cm × 14 cm horizontal gel and the alleles visualized after ethidium bromide staining

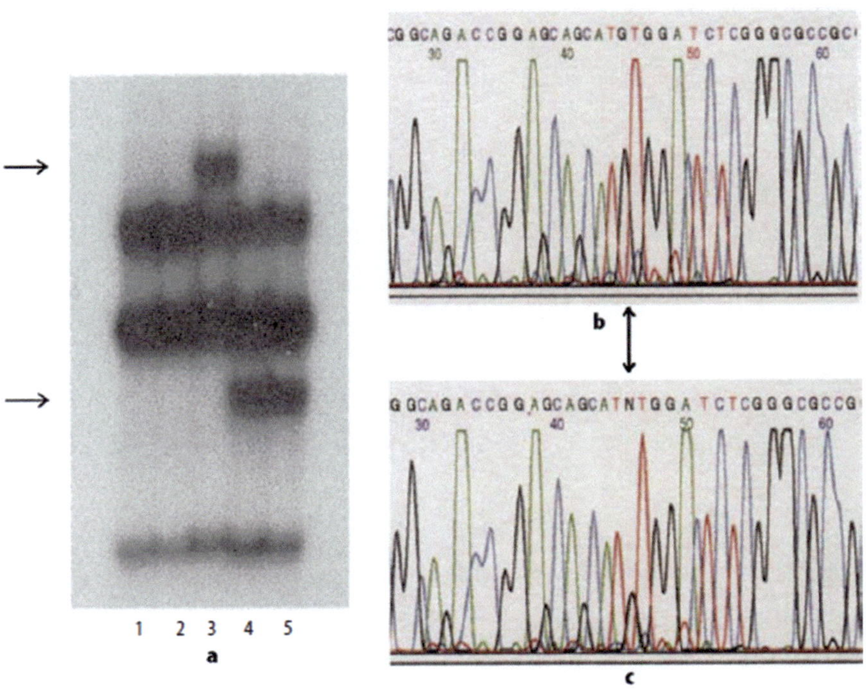

Figure 18.4 Example test results for Friedreich ataxia (FRDA). (**a**) SSCP analysis of the *FXN* gene exon 1 amplicon revealing the presence of abnormal conformers in two FRDA compound heterozygotes. *Lanes 1* and *2*, exon 1 amplicon from a normal control; *lane 3*, FRDA compound heterozygote carrying a G→A transition at nucleotide 3 of the *FXN* gene [36]; *lanes 4* and *5* (duplicate), FRDA compound heterozygote carrying an A→C transversion at nucleotide 1 of the *FRDA* gene. (**b**, **c**) Representative exon 1 electropherograms from a normal individual (**b**) and the 3G→A/GAA_{1000} FRDA compound heterozygote (**c**) shown in (**a**), *lane 3*, confirming the presence of the mutation in the heterozygous state (↕)

Table 18.5 Molecular genetic classification of the inherited (monogenic) dystonias

Locus name	Gene	Gene product	Chromosomal location	Inheritance pattern	Key information
Isolated dystonias					
DYT1	*TOR1A*	Torsin-1A (part of the AAA family of ATPases)	9q34.11	Autosomal dominant	Primary torsion dystonia with early-onset generalized dystonia, 3 bp deletion, GAG (delE302/303) most common change
DYT6	*THAP1*	THAP domain containing protein 1	8p11.21	Autosomal dominant	Adolescent-onset dystonia
DYT25	*GNAL*	Guanine nucleotide-binding protein, alpha-activating activity polypeptide, olfactory type	18q11.21	Autosomal dominant	Adult onset cranial-cervical dystonia
Dystonia plus parkinsonism					
DYT3	*TAF1*	TATA-binding protein (TBP)-associated factor-1 gene	Xq13.1	X-linked	Filippino founder effect, caused by a retrotransposon insertion
DYT5a/14	*GCH1*	GTP cyclohydrolase-1	14q22.1-q22.2	Autosomal dominant	Childhood-onset dopa-responsive dystonia
DYT5b	*TH*	Tyrosine hydroxylase	11p15.5	Autosomal recessive	Infantile-onset dopa-responsive dystonia (Segawa syndrome)
Not assigned	*SPR*	Sepiapterin reductase	2p13.2	Autosomal recessive	Infantile-onset dopa-responsive dystonia
DYT12	*ATP1A3*	Na+/K+ ATPase transporting alpha-3 polypeptide	19q13.2	Autosomal dominant	Rapid-onset dystonia-parkinsonism
Dystonia plus myoclonus					
DYT11	*SGCE*	Sarcoglycan, epsilon	7q21.3	Autosomal dominant	Myoclonic dystonia
Paroxysmal dystonia plus other dyskinesia					
DYT8	*PKND*	Probable hydrolase PNKD (formerly MR-1, myofibrillogenesis regulator-1)	2q35	Autosomal dominant	Paroxysmal nonkinesigenic dyskinesia
DYT10	*PRRT2*	Proline-rich transmembrane protein 2	16p11.2	Autosomal dominant	Paroxysmal kinesigenic dyskinesia
DYT9/18	*SLC2A1*	Solute carrier family 2 (facilitated glucose transporter) member 1 (formerly GLUT1)	1p34.2	Autosomal dominant	Paroxysmal exertion-induced dyskinesia
Complex dystonias: inherited neurodegenerative/metabolic disorders (selected)					
PKAN	*PANK2*	Pantothenate kinase 2	20p13	Autosomal recessive	Neurodegeneration with brain iron accumulation 1 or pantothenate kinase-associated neurodegeneration
WD	*ATP7B*	ATPase, Cu2+-transporting, beta polypeptide	13q14.3	Autosomal recessive	Wilson disease, accumulation of intracellular hepatic copper with hepatic dysfunction and neurologic symptoms
HDL2	*JPH3*	Junctophilin-3	16q24.3	Autosomal dominant	Huntington disease-like 2, juvenile onset, CTG repeat expansion

Sources: http://www.ncbi.nlm.nih.gov/books/NBK1155/; http://omim.org/phenotypicSeries/PS128100

substantia nigra pars compacta, and is present in cytoplasmic inclusion bodies in the brainstem of patients with confirmed DYT1 [39].

DYT5, or dopamine-responsive dystonia (DRD), is clinically characterized by dystonia plus parkinsonism with a dramatic response to treatment with levodopa, and is associated with mutations in three different genes. Homozygous as well as compound heterozygous mutations in the tyrosine hydroxylase (TH) gene at 11p15.5 are associated with the rare autosomal recessive form of DRD known as Segawa syndrome. A second form of autosomal recessive DRD is not assigned a DYT number, and is associated with mutations in the *SPR* gene, located at 2p13.2 and encoding the sepiapterin reductase protein. The more common autosomal dominant form of DRD is associated with mutations in the GTP cyclohydrolase I (*GCH1*) gene, at chromosomal location 14q22.1. DYT3 (X-linked dystonia-parkinsonism, also known as "lubag" from the Filipino word for "twisted") is associated with mutations in *TAF1* and is endemic to the Philippines. DYT11, or myoclonus-dystonia, is associated with loss-of-function mutations in the ε-sarcoglycan (*SGCE*) gene at 7q21 in a large number of families and represents a major locus for myoclonus-dystonia.

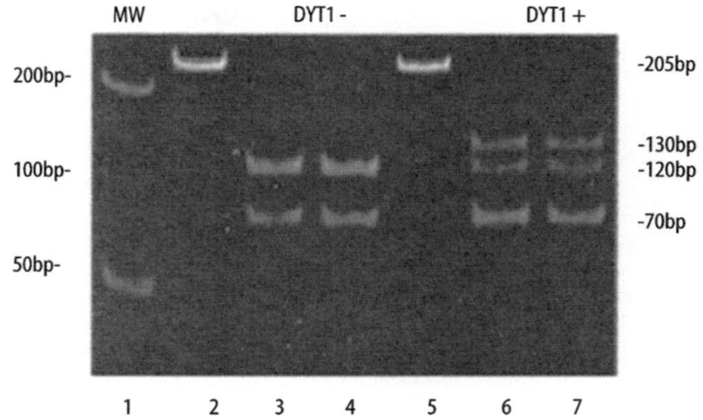

Figure 18.5 PCR-RFLP analysis of the *TOR1A* GAG deletion mutation associated with dominant early-onset torsion dystonia (DYT1). DNA was amplified with the 6419/H48 primer pair [36] and the resulting 25 bp amplicons digested with *Bse* RI. The presence of the GAG deletion mutations results in the loss of a *Bse* RI site on the mutant allele and the generation of a novel 130 bp DNA fragment in addition to the 120 bp and 70 bp DNA fragments generated from the normal allele. *Lane 1*: 100 bp ladder G2101 (Promega, Madison, WI); *lane 2*: undigested amplicons; *lanes 3* and *4*: *Bse* RI digests from two patients without DYT1; *lane 5*: undigested amplicons; *lanes 6* and *7*: *Bse* RI digests from two patients with DYT1 (note the presence of the novel 130 bp DNA fragment)

Clinical Utility of Testing

Clinical molecular testing is presently available for several of the dystonia genes (see http://www.ncbi.nlm.nih.gov/gtr/).

Available Assays

Molecular testing can be performed by PCR-RFLP analysis of the GAG-containing *DYT1* exon (Fig. 18.5). Determination of pathologic mutations in *GCH1* requires direct DNA sequencing of the gene.

Interpretation of Test Results

Essentially all patients with typical DYT1 carry the GAG deletion on one allele, and thus, the test sensitivity approaches 100 %. In contrast, the specificity of the assay is 60–70 %, because DYT1 is inherited as an autosomal dominant trait with reduced penetrance (30–40 %). Counseling of the parents of the proband should include an evaluation of their clinical status and consideration of molecular testing to determine parental origin of the mutation. The risk of inheriting a *TOR1A* mutation allele from a proband is 50 %; however, the probability that the mutation carrier will become symptomatic is estimated to be 30–40 %. Prenatal testing is clinically available for fetuses at 50 % risk of inheriting a *TOR1A* mutation allele, once the presence of the mutation has been confirmed in the family. New mutations, although rare, have been reported, but the de novo mutation rate is unknown.

Unlike in DYT1, other dystonia genes show a high frequency of diverse mutations, so clinical testing requires complete gene sequencing and is usually limited to diagnostic testing in a proband with the knowledge that testing sensitivity may reach only 60 %. If a mutation is detected, carrier testing or prenatal testing or both can be considered for family members.

Laboratory Issues

No commercial test kits are available for dystonia testing. Control DNA can be obtained from the Coriell Cell Repositories (Camden, NJ; http://ccr.coriell.org/). No formal proficiency testing is available.

Acknowledgement The author would like to acknowledge the previous author of this chapter, Nicholas T. Potter, Ph.D., F.A.C.M.G., for his generous donation of material and figures to be included in the current edition.

References

1. Alzheimer's Association. 2014 Alzheimer's disease facts and figures. Alzheimers Dement. 2014;10(2):e47–92.
2. Schellenberg GD, Montine TJ. The genetics and neuropathology of Alzheimer's disease. Acta Neuropathol. 2012;124(3):305–23.
3. Cruts M, Theuns J, Van Broeckhoven C. Locus-specific mutation databases for neurodegenerative brain diseases. Hum Mutat. 2012;33(9):1340–4.
4. Chau D-M, Crump CJ, Villa JC, Scheinberg DA, Li Y-M. Familial Alzheimer disease presenilin-1 mutations alter the active site conformation of γ-secretase. J Biol Chem. 2012;287(21):17288–96.
5. Farlow J, Pankratz ND, Wojcieszek J, Foroud T. Parkinson disease overview. In: Pagon RA, Adam MP, Ardinger HH, Bird TD,

Dolan CR, Fong C-T, et al., editors. GeneReviews(®) [Internet]. Seattle, WA: University of Washington, Seattle; 1993. Available from: http://www.ncbi.nlm.nih.gov/books/NBK1223/. Cited 16 Feb 2015.
6. Poulopoulos M, Levy OA, Alcalay RN. The neuropathology of genetic Parkinson's disease. Mov Disord. 2012;27(7):831–42.
7. Trinh J, Farrer M. Advances in the genetics of Parkinson disease. Nat Rev Neurol. 2013;9(8):445–54.
8. Polymeropoulos MH, Lavedan C, Leroy E, Ide SE, Dehejia A, Dutra A, et al. Mutation in the alpha-synuclein gene identified in families with Parkinson's disease. Science. 1997;276(5321):2045–7.
9. Krüger R, Kuhn W, Müller T, Woitalla D, Graeber M, Kösel S, et al. Ala30Pro mutation in the gene encoding alpha-synuclein in Parkinson's disease. Nat Genet. 1998;18(2):106–8.
10. Zarranz JJ, Alegre J, Gómez-Esteban JC, Lezcano E, Ros R, Ampuero I, et al. The new mutation, E46K, of alpha-synuclein causes Parkinson and Lewy body dementia. Ann Neurol. 2004;55(2):164–73.
11. Di Fonzo A, Dekker MCJ, Montagna P, Baruzzi A, Yonova EH, Correia Guedes L, et al. FBXO7 mutations cause autosomal recessive, early-onset parkinsonian-pyramidal syndrome. Neurology. 2009;72(3):240–5.
12. Lucking CB, Brice A. Semiquantitative PCR for the detection of exon rearrangements in the Parkin gene. In: Potter NT, editor. Neurogenetics: methods and protocols, vol. 217. Totowa, NJ: Humana Press; 2002. p. 13–26.
13. Kinsley L, Siddique T. Amyotrophic lateral sclerosis overview. In: Pagon RA, Adam MP, Ardinger HH, Bird TD, Dolan CR, Fong C-T, et al., editors. GeneReviews(®) [Internet]. Seattle, WA: University of Washington, Seattle; 1993. Available from: http://www.ncbi.nlm.nih.gov/books/NBK1450/. Cited 16 Feb 2015.
14. Neumann M, Sampathu DM, Kwong LK, Truax AC, Micsenyi MC, Chou TT, et al. Ubiquitinated TDP-43 in frontotemporal lobar degeneration and amyotrophic lateral sclerosis. Science. 2006;314(5796):130–3.
15. DeJesus-Hernandez M, Mackenzie IR, Boeve BF, Boxer AL, Baker M, Rutherford NJ, et al. Expanded GGGGCC hexanucleotide repeat in noncoding region of C9ORF72 causes chromosome 9p-linked FTD and ALS. Neuron. 2011;72(2):245–56.
16. Renton AE, Majounie E, Waite A, Simón-Sánchez J, Rollinson S, Gibbs JR, et al. A hexanucleotide repeat expansion in C9ORF72 is the cause of chromosome 9p21-linked ALS-FTD. Neuron. 2011;72(2):257–68.
17. Beck J, Poulter M, Hensman D, Rohrer JD, Mahoney CJ, Adamson G, et al. Large C9orf72 hexanucleotide repeat expansions are seen in multiple neurodegenerative syndromes and are more frequent than expected in the UK population. Am J Hum Genet. 2013;92(3):345–53.
18. Warby SC, Graham RK, Hayden MR. Huntington disease. In: Pagon RA, Adam MP, Ardinger HH, Bird TD, Dolan CR, Fong C-T, et al., editors. GeneReviews(®) [Internet]. Seattle, WA: University of Washington, Seattle; 1993. Available from: http://www.ncbi.nlm.nih.gov/books/NBK1305/. Cited 16 Feb 2015.
19. Bean L, Bayrak-Toydemir P. Committee on behalf of the ALQA. American College of Medical Genetics and Genomics Standards and Guidelines for Clinical Genetics Laboratories, 2014 edition: technical standards and guidelines for Huntington disease. Genet Med. 2014;16(12), e2.
20. Andrew SE, Goldberg YP, Theilman J, et al. A CCG repeat polymorphism adjacent to the CAG repeat in the Huntington disease gene: implications for diagnostic accuracy and predictive testing. Hum Mol Genet. 1994;3:65–7.
21. Margolis RL, Stine OC, Callahan C, et al. Two novel single-base-pair-substitutions adjacent to the CAG repeat in the Huntington disease gene (IT15): implications for diagnostic testing. Am J Hum Genet. 1999;64:323–6.
22. Jama M, Millson A, Miller CE, Lyon E. Triplet repeat primed PCR simplifies testing for Huntington disease. J Mol Diagn. 2013;15(2):255–62.
23. Palomaki GE, Richards CS. Assessing the analytic validity of molecular testing for Huntington disease using data from an external proficiency testing survey. Genet Med. 2012;14(1):69–75.
24. Saft C, Leavitt BR, Epplen JT. Clinical utility gene card for: Huntington's disease. Eur J Hum Genet [Internet]. 2014;22(5). Available from: http://www.nature.com/ejhg/journal/v22/n5/full/ejhg2013206a.html. Cited 22 Feb 2015.
25. Bird TD. Hereditary ataxia overview. In: Pagon RA, Adam MP, Ardinger HH, Bird TD, Dolan CR, Fong C-T, et al., editors. GeneReviews(®) [Internet]. Seattle, WA: University of Washington, Seattle; 1993. Available from: http://www.ncbi.nlm.nih.gov/books/NBK1138/. Cited 16 Feb 2015.
26. Potter NT, Nance MA. Ataxia Molecular Diagnostic Testing Group. Genetic testing for ataxia in North America. Mol Diagn. 2000;5(2):91–9.
27. Durr A. Autosomal dominant cerebellar ataxias: polyglutamine expansions and beyond. Lancet Neurol. 2010;9(9):885–94.
28. Bidichandani SI, Delatycki MB. Friedreich ataxia. In: Pagon RA, Adam MP, Ardinger HH, Bird TD, Dolan CR, Fong C-T, et al., editors. GeneReviews(®) [Internet]. Seattle, WA: University of Washington, Seattle; 1993. Available from: http://www.ncbi.nlm.nih.gov/books/NBK1281/. Cited 16 Feb 2015.
29. Bird TD. Alzheimer disease overview. In: Pagon RA, Adam MP, Ardinger HH, Bird TD, Dolan CR, Fong C-T, et al., editors. GeneReviews(®) [Internet]. Seattle, WA: University of Washington, Seattle; 1993. Available from: http://www.ncbi.nlm.nih.gov/books/NBK1161/. Cited 16 Feb 2015.
30. Gatti R. Ataxia-Telangiectasia. In: Pagon RA, Adam MP, Ardinger HH, Bird TD, Dolan CR, Fong C-T, et al., editors. GeneReviews(®) [Internet]. Seattle, WA: University of Washington, Seattle; 1993. Available from: http://www.ncbi.nlm.nih.gov/books/NBK26468/. Cited 23 Feb 2015.
31. Mao R, Aylsworth AS, Potter N, Wilson WG, Breningstall G, Wick MJ, et al. Childhood-onset ataxia: testing for large CAG-repeats in SCA2 and SCA7. Am J Med Genet. 2002;110(4):338–45.
32. Snow K, Mao R. Extreme expansion detection in spinocerebellar ataxia type 2 and type 7. In: Potter NT, editor. Neurogenetics: methods and protocols, vol. 217. Totowa, NJ: Humana Press; 2002. p. 41–50.
33. Imbert G, Saudou F, Yvert G, et al. Cloning of the gene for spinocerebellar ataxia 2 reveals a locus with high sensitivity to expanded CAG/glutamine repeats. Nat Genet. 1996;14:285–91.
34. Filla A, De Michelle G, Cavalcanti F, et al. The relationship between trinucleotide (GAA) repeat length and clinical features in Friedreich ataxia. Am J Hum Genet. 1996;59:554–60.
35. Németh AH, Kwasniewska AC, Lise S, Parolin Schnekenberg R, Becker EBE, Bera KD, et al. Next generation sequencing for molecular diagnosis of neurological disorders using ataxias as a model. Brain. 2013;136(Pt 10):3106–18.
36. Potter NT, Miller CA, Anderson IJ. Mutation detection in an equivocal case of Friedreich ataxia. Pediatr Neurol. 2000;22:413–5.
37. Paudel R, Hardy J, Revesz T, Holton JL, Houlden H. Review: genetics and neuropathology of primary pure dystonia. Neuropathol Appl Neurobiol. 2012;38(6):520–34.
38. Klein C, Marras C, Münchau A. Dystonia overview. In: Pagon RA, Adam MP, Ardinger HH, Bird TD, Dolan CR, Fong C-T, et al., editors. GeneReviews(®) [Internet]. Seattle, WA: University of Washington, Seattle; 1993. Available from: http://www.ncbi.nlm.nih.gov/books/NBK1155/. Cited 16 Feb 2015.
39. McNaught KSP, Kapustin A, Jackson T, Jengelley T-A, JnoBaptiste R, Shashidharan P, et al. Brainstem pathology in DYT1 primary torsion dystonia. Ann Neurol. 2004;56(4):540–7.

Polycystic Kidney Disease

19

Adrian Y. Tan, Jon Blumenfeld, and Hanna Rennert

Abstract

Polycystic kidney disease (PKD) is a group of monogenic disorders that result in renal cyst development, progressive chronic kidney disease, and are associated with extrarenal manifestations. The most common form, autosomal dominant PKD (ADPKD), is a multisystem disease most often diagnosed in adults and caused by mutations in *PKD1* and *PKD2*. The *PKD1* gene product, polycystin-1 (PC1), is a large receptor like protein. The *PKD2* gene product, polycystin-2 (PC2)' is a member of the transient receptor potential family (i.e., TRPP2) and is a nonselective cation channel that is permeable to calcium. Both PC1 and PC2 are located on non-motile cilia located on virtually all epithelia and other cell types.

Autosomal recessive PKD (ARPKD) usually presents during infancy with enlarged kidneys and hepatic fibrosis, but patients are increasingly being identified during childhood and early adulthood. ARPKD is caused by mutations in *PKHD1*. The protein encoded by this gene, polyductin, is localized to the basal body of non-motile cilia and can form a complex with PC2.

Molecular genetic testing plays an increasingly important role in the management of PKD. In ADPKD, testing enables early diagnosis of patients with inconclusive results by kidney imaging; this can clarify the disease status of a prospective related kidney donor. In both ADPKD and ARPKD, testing can inform pre-implantation genetic diagnosis (PGD). The purpose of this chapter is to review the clinical and laboratory characteristics of these disorders and to describe the application of emerging molecular technologies.

Keywords

ADPKD • Polycystic kidney disease • PKD genes • Gene variation • Mutation • Variants of uncertain significance

A.Y. Tan, Ph.D.
Department of Pathology, Weill Cornell Medical College, New York, NY, USA

J. Blumenfeld, M.D.
The Susan R. Knafel Polycystic Kidney Disease Center, The Rogosin Institute, New York, NY, USA

Clinical Medicine, Nephrology and Hypertension, Weill Cornell Medical College, New York, NY, USA

H. Rennert, Ph.D., F.A.C.M.G. (✉)
Department of Pathology and Laboratory Medicine, Weill Cornell Medical College, New York Presbyterian Hospital, 525 East 68th St., Room F544B, New York, NY 10021, USA
e-mail: Har2006@med.cornell.e.du

D.G.B. Leonard (ed.), *Molecular Pathology in Clinical Practice*, DOI 10.1007/978-3-319-19674-9_19

Introduction

Polycystic kidney disease (PKD) is a group of monogenic disorders that result in renal cyst development. Autosomal dominant PKD (ADPKD) (OMIM#173900; 173910) is the most common inherited renal disease and the fourth most common cause of end stage renal disease (ESRD) in adults. The prevalence of ADPKD is approximately 1 in 400-1,000 live births in all races [1], and affects approximately 12.5 million individuals worldwide, with 5,000–6,000 new cases diagnosed in the USA each year. The age of presentation of ADPKD varies largely, ranging from onset in utero with enlarged, cystic kidneys to incidental diagnosis in the elderly with adequate renal function [2]. The principal renal manifestation of ADPKD is the formation of cysts as a result of abnormal proliferation of renal tubular epithelial cells. Cysts increase gradually in both size and number, resulting in marked kidney enlargement and a progressive decline in renal function (Fig. 19.1).

Other common renal manifestations include hypertension, kidney stones, urinary tract infections, and hematuria. Extrarenal manifestations are highly prevalent, including cysts in the liver, pancreas, seminal vesicles, and arachnoid membranes, cardiac valve abnormalities, and aneurysms. These renal and extrarenal abnormalities are a significant cause of morbidity and mortality. The mean age of onset of hypertension is 20–30 years, usually occurring while renal function is still within the normal range; this is approximately one decade earlier than in the general population with essential hypertension [3]. The prevalence of intracranial aneurysm is about five times higher than in the general population [4]. Approximately 50 % of the ADPKD patients progress to ESRD by the seventh decade [5], and account for approximately 5 % of all patients requiring hemodialysis or kidney transplant [6].

Autosomal recessive PKD (ARPKD) (OMIM#263200) is characterized by non-obstructive dilation of the cortical collecting tubule in utero or during the neonatal period, resulting in massive renal enlargement. However, a subset is increasingly being identified in childhood, adolescence, or even adulthood. These cases with later onset diagnosis usually have milder kidney disease, but more significant complications of liver disease [7]. This is accompanied by a ductal plate malformation of the liver, resulting in congenital hepatic fibrosis. Approximately 2–5 % of ADPKD patients also present during the neonatal period with significant morbidity and mortality [8], and may only be differentiated from ARPKD at that time by histological or genetic analysis.

Many other pediatric disorders are associated with renal cysts or cystic dysplasia as a component of their phenotypes. However, they generally can be distinguished from ARPKD and ADPKD by a detailed physical examination, basic laboratory and imaging studies, and by their extrarenal clinical characteristics [9]. The prevalence of ARPKD has been estimated to be 1 in 20,000-40,000 live births, with a carrier frequency of 1 in 70 [7].

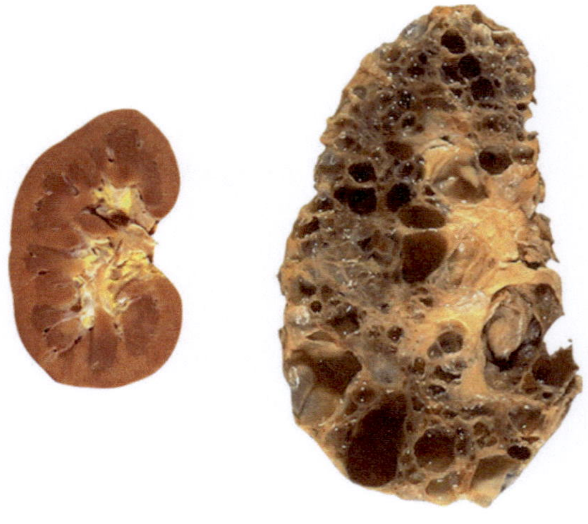

Figure 19.1 Normal and polycystic kidneys. A normal kidney is shown on the *left* and a kidney with a high number of variable-sized cysts that characterize polycystic kidney disease is shown on the *right*

Autosomal Dominant Polycystic Kidney Disease

Molecular Basis of Disease

ADPKD is genetically heterogeneous, caused mainly by mutations in two genes: *PKD1* and *PKD2*, located on chromosome 16p13.3 [10] and 4q21 [11], respectively.

PKD1 is a large gene, with 46 exons, occupying 50 kb of genomic sequence on chromosome 16, and encoding a large transcript with an open reading frame of 12,909 bp. The first 33 exons of *PKD1* are located in a region that is duplicated six times on chromosome 16 [12]. These homologous genes, also termed pseudogenes, have 97–99 % homology to *PKD1*, which complicates genetic testing [13]. *PKD2* consists of 15 exons, spanning 68 kb of genomic sequence, and encoding a transcript 2,904 bp [11]. De novo *PKD1* and *PKD2* mutations are reported to occur in approximately 10 % of affected individuals [14]. The reported prevalence of *PKD2* mutations among ADPKD patients is variable. In community-based studies, *PKD2* mutations accounted for approximately 29–36 % of cases [15], while in hospital-based studies, *PKD2* mutations comprised only 15 % of cases; the remainder had *PKD1* mutations. This discrepancy is likely due to a detection bias toward cases with more severe manifestation that characterize patients with *PKD1* gene mutations [15].

The *PKD1* gene encodes a large integral membrane protein, polycystin-1 (PC1), which has 11 transmembrane domains and an extracellular segment consisting of a variety of domains that occupy approximately 75 % of the entire protein. Overall, PC1 has the structure that is suggestive of a receptor or adhesion molecule and is thought to be a mechanical sensor of fluid flow [16]. The *PKD2* gene product, polycystin-2 (PC2), is a member of the transient receptor potential family (i.e., TRPP2) that functions as a nonselective cation channel that transports calcium [17]. PC1 and PC2 localize to the immotile cilia on renal tubule epithelium [18], where PC1 and PC2 interact with each other [19]. A current hypothesis is that the polycystin complex functions as a mechanoreceptor that senses fluid flow in the tubular lumen, triggering Ca^{2+} influx through TRPP2, consequently affecting the intracellular calcium and cyclic AMP (cAMP) levels [20]. Mutations in either *PKD1* or *PKD2* result in malfunction of the polycystin complex, leading to abnormal cross talk between the adenylate cyclase and receptor tyrosine kinase pathways. These abnormalities, together with reduced intracellular calcium concentration, promote renal tubular epithelial cell proliferation and fluid secretion, which are key phenotypic features of ADPKD [21].

The renal cysts of ADPKD have two distinctive characteristics: significant size variation and focal development. These features can be explained by a two hit model in which two separate inactivation events in either one of the PKD genes is required for cyst formation [22]. The first hit is a germline mutation, usually inherited from the affected parent, which is necessary but not sufficient for cyst formation. The second hit, a somatic mutation only occurring in an individual renal tubular cell, inactivates either the normal *PKD1* or *PKD2* allele, thus initiating abnormal, monoclonal proliferation of tubular epithelial cells and cyst formation [23, 24]. The somatic mutation can occur at any given point during the patient's lifetime, resulting in formation of cysts of different size. The size of the cyst typically correlates with the time the second mutation occurred. Although ADPKD is a dominant disease, the requirement of both a germline and a somatic mutation for cyst formation supports a recessive disease model at the cellular level. In a small number of families, germline mutations can be found in trans in *PKD1* and *PKD2*. This bilineal inheritance demonstrates that co-inheritance of a mutation in both genes is not necessarily lethal during embryogenesis, but is associated with a more severe disease phenotype [25]. Interestingly, somatic *PKD2* mutations can be detected in cysts of patients with *PKD1* germline mutations and vice versa, further supporting the two-hit model and the dosage effect hypothesis for cyst formation [26, 27].

Various cellular mechanisms have been implicated in the pathogenesis of ADPKD as a consequence of impaired interactions of PC1 and PC2. These can be summarized as negative growth regulation, G protein activation, and Wnt pathway modulation [28]. Increased proliferation of renal tubular epithelial cells has been attributed to loss of inhibition by the mammalian target of rapamycin complex (mTOR) and cyclin-dependent kinases, among others. These pathways have been the targets of treatment strategies [29].

At the population level, ADPKD presents great phenotypic variability, including interfamilial and intrafamilial variability. This phenomenon is best explained by three genetic levels of attributions: genic (gene), allelic, and gene modifier effects. Interfamilial heterogeneity is mainly explained by genic effects; *PKD1* gene mutations are associated with more severe disease and earlier age of ESRD onset [30]. The mean age of onset of ESRD is approximately 20 years earlier in patients with *PKD1* mutations compared to patients with *PKD2* mutations (54.3 years vs 74.0 years) [30]. The more severe phenotype, accounting for the younger age of diagnosis of ADPKD and earlier age of onset of ESRD in the *PKD1* population, is likely due to the development of renal cysts at an earlier age, rather than a faster rate of cyst growth [31]. *PKD1* patients also have a higher incidence of hypertension and hematuria.

Allelic effects in ADPKD are relatively small compared with genic effects. Patients with mutations in the 5′ region of *PKD1* have been reported to reach ESRD slightly earlier than patients with mutations in the 3′ region (53 years vs 56 years) [32]. They also have a higher prevalence of intracranial aneurysms as well as aneurysm rupture [33]. However, in a more recent study, the phenotype was found to be affected by the type of *PKD1* mutation, but not the position of the mutation in the gene [34]. No clear correlation has been reported between severity of disease phenotype and the position of the mutation in *PKD2*. Recently, hypomorphic alleles have been reported in both *PKD1* and *PKD2*, which usually are missense mutations and reduce the levels of gene activity, but do not totally inactivate gene function [35]. Patients with one hypomorphic allele have mild cystic disease, while patients who are homozygous or compound heterozygous for two hypomorphic alleles present with moderate to severe disease, with cyst formation similar to that observed in patients with pathogenic PKD mutations. A hypomorphic allele coexisting with a pathogenic mutation can cause early onset disease [35].

The significant intrafamilial phenotypic variability, both in the rate of progression of chronic kidney disease and in the array of extrarenal manifestations, has been attributed, at least in part, to gene modifier effects [36]. Analysis of the phenotypic variability in renal function between monozygotic twins and siblings supports the involvement of genetic modifiers [37, 38]. Heritable modifying factors were estimated to account for 18–50 % of the variability in disease severity [39]. Recently, a candidate gene approach has identified Dickkopf 3 (*DKK3*) as marginally associated with ADPKD disease severity; however, replication studies are needed to verify the association reported [40, 41]. The development of high-resolution single nucleotide polymorphism (SNP) arrays enables properly powered genome-wide association studies (GWAS) for mapping modifier genes in an unbiased way; however, the success of such studies is strongly dependent on the availability of clinically well-characterized, large ADPKD cohorts.

Clinical Utility of Testing

Genetic testing for ADPKD has two main clinical applications: (1) clarifying whether ADPKD is present in a young family member without kidney cysts who is considering kidney donation, and (2) identifying the PKD gene mutation in an affected individual for reproductive decision-making (e.g., preimplantation genetic diagnosis). The gold standard method for diagnosis of ADPKD is an age-specific renal phenotype, based on the number of cysts identified by renal ultrasonogram in an individual with a 50 % risk of inheritance, determined by a positive history of ADPKD in a first-degree relative [42]. However, these criteria were suboptimal for patients with *PKD2* mutations. A recent revision of the Ravine criteria has improved diagnostic performance for renal ultrasonography in patients with either PKD1 or PKD2 mutations [43]. Accordingly, in families of unknown genotype with an affected first-degree relative, the presence of three or more (unilateral or bilateral) renal cysts is sufficient for establishing the diagnosis of ADPKD in individuals aged 15–39 years; two or more cysts in each kidney is sufficient for individuals aged 40–59 years; and four or more cysts in each kidney is required for individuals 60 years of age or older. Conversely, fewer than two renal cysts in at-risk individuals aged 40 years or older is sufficient to exclude the disease [43]. Diagnostic imaging is sufficient for most patients; however, it is often ambiguous in young patients whose renal sonogram may not be conclusive or when the family history is unknown. A recent, single-center study found that magnetic resonance imaging has high sensitivity and specificity in patients at risk for ADPKD. Specifically, among subjects aged 16–40 years old, the presence of a total of more than 10 renal cysts was found to be sufficient for diagnosis [44].

Recently, Huang et al. proposed an algorithm that incorporates the use of DNA testing and imaging for donors with a family history of ADPKD [45]. They concluded that genetic testing, especially DNA sequencing, is cost effective because it shortens the waiting time for a living related transplant if at least one living donor per year results from every ten linkage or every five DNA sequencing tests performed, given that many individuals are on a transplant list for many years. Although genetic testing of *PKD1* and *PKD2* can be useful for clarifying the disease status in these individuals, the low sensitivity by the reference commercial laboratory (40–60 %) and high cost (approximately $6,000 per test) limits the use of widespread genotyping at this time [46].

Available Assays

Two methods are available for genetic testing of ADPKD: gene-based mutation screening and DNA linkage analysis. Molecular testing by gene-based mutation screening currently is the predominant method of ADPKD genetic testing. However, the marked allelic heterogeneity of the disease-associated mutations, the vast majority of which are private, and the duplicated structure of *PKD1* together with its large size, makes mutation screening a significant technical challenge. Although mutation analysis of the *PKD2* gene and the *PKD1* single copy region (exons 34–46) is straightforward, analysis of the duplicated 5′ region of *PKD1* is more complex because of its 98 % identity to the six *PKD1* pseudogenes on chromosome 16.

Several strategies are available for ADPKD genetic testing (Fig. 19.2). Prior to 2001, genetic analysis of ADPKD could be only performed for *PKD2* and the 3′ single copy region of *PKD1*. The first assay for analyzing the entire *PKD1*, developed in 2001, uses long-range PCR (LR-PCR) to specifically amplify the duplicated exon 1 to exon 33 regions, followed by nested PCR of the individual exons [47]. This method was later commercialized by Athena Diagnostics, Inc., which until recently had the exclusive license for analyzing *PKD1* and *PKD2* and was the sole provider of clinical ADPKD genotyping in the USA. Garcia-Gonzalez et al. evaluated the clinical utility of this commercially available test by analyzing a cohort of 82 ADPKD patients [48]. Definite pathogenic mutations were detected in 42 % of the patients and the maximal mutation detection rate was 78 %, after including missense, in-frame insertion/deletion, and atypical splice mutations that were likely to be pathogenic [48].

Although complete gene sequencing remains the gold standard for ADPKD genetic testing, it is expensive and time-consuming. Thus, several screening-based methods were developed to lower testing costs and minimize turnaround time. Denaturing gradient gel electrophoresis, a traditional

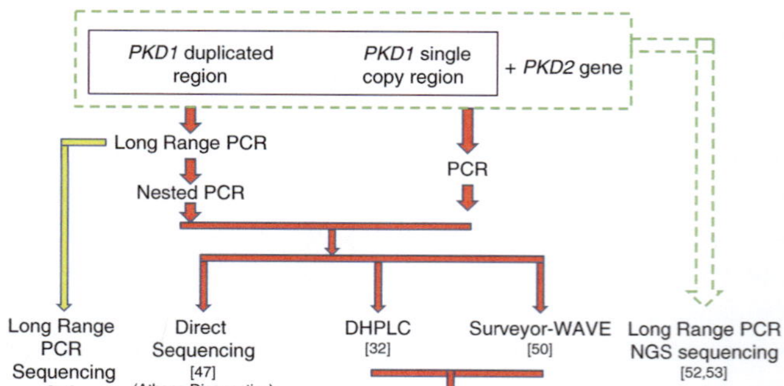

Figure 19.2 Strategies for ADPKD genotyping. *NGS* next-generation sequencing

gel-based heteroduplex analysis method, as well as single strand conformation polymorphism (SSCP) have been successfully used to screen both the single copy and the duplicated regions of the *PKD1* gene [49]. However, these methods suffer from a low mutation detection rate (30–40 %). Rossetti et al. [32] developed a denaturing high-performance liquid chromatography (DHPLC) screening method that was more sensitive than previous assays, with a detection rate of 64 % for definite pathogenic mutations. Further improvement in the utility of DHPLC for PKD genetic testing is the use of *CelI* endonuclease (SURVEYOR® nuclease, Transgenomic Inc.) and the Transgenomic WAVE® Nucleic Acid High Sensitivity Fragment Analysis System [50]. This method is 100 % sensitive when compared to the complete DNA sequencing method of the entire genes used by a commercial reference laboratory, with a detection rate of 64 % for definite pathogenic mutations, comparable to the rate reported in the literature [32].

An improved method for genetic analysis of ADPKD was developed by Tan et al. [51] using direct sequencing of the *PKD1* LR-PCR products. In this strategy, the entire *PKD1* coding region is amplified in nine LR-PCR reactions, generating products ranging in length from 2 to 6 kb, followed by column purification and direct sequencing with several pairs of walking primers. When compared with the direct sequencing result of the reference laboratory, this method was highly sensitive (100 %) and specific (98.5 %), circumventing the need for nested PCR of the *PKD1* duplicated region, and reducing the risk of PCR amplification carryover contamination that can lead to false-positive results. In addition, this method has decreased the number of required PCR reactions by 80 %, substantially lowering test cost by approximately 20 % and improving turn-around time compared with both the direct sequencing and the SURVEYOR-WAVE screening methods. Another advantage of the LR-PCR sequencing method is that it covers intronic regions extending 200–300 bp beyond the exon-intron junctions, enabling better detection of deep intronic mutations.

Next-generation sequencing (NGS) technology is revolutionizing the field of human genetics and has been recently applied to PKD genetic testing. Rossetti et al. [52] reported a mutation screening strategy for analyzing *PKD1* and *PKD2* genes using NGS by pooling LR-PCR amplicons and multiplexing barcoded libraries. To increase the throughput, amplicons from four patients and libraries of up to 12 patients were pooled together and analyzed in a single reaction using indexed DNA barcodes. Using this strategy, these authors detected definite and likely pathogenic variants in 115 (63 %) of 183 patients with typical ADPKD. When compared with Sanger sequencing, this approach had a sensitivity of 78 % and a specificity of 100 % for mutation detection. This method also enabled the identification of atypical mutations, including a gene conversion event, and the characterization of deep intronic variations.

A second NGS approach amplifies *PKD1* and *PKD2* genes in a total of ten LR-PCR reactions, using locus-specific primers [51]. Indexed libraries from up to 25 patients are pooled together and analyzed in a single flow-cell using the MiSeq system (Illumina Inc., San Diego, CA). Sequencing results are sorted according to the barcodes with the FASTX toolkit and aligned against the reference sequence using the BWA program (http://bio-bwa.sourceforge.net/). Sequence variants are called using the GATK software package (The Genome Analysis Toolkit, The Broad Institute), carefully following The Best Practice Guidelines recommended by GATK (Fig. 19.3). With addition of an improved bioinformatics analysis pipeline, this approach has a sensitivity of 100 % in mutation detection when compared with Sanger sequencing, while retaining high specificity [51]. Several typical genetic variations detected by this approach are shown in Fig. 19.4. NGS approaches have the potential to dramatically improve genetic testing for ADPKD by allowing simultaneous detection of point mutations and copy number variations in a single test. Accordingly, these methods can increase the mutation detection rate, particularly of deep intronic mutations, and significantly reduce testing costs and turnaround time.

Large DNA rearrangements also play a role in ADPKD causation, but their detection is complicated by the presence of the *PKD1* pseudogenes [53]. Field inversion gel electrophoresis followed by Southern blot analysis traditionally has been used to identify large deletions in *PKD1*. Recently, a multiplex ligation dependent probe assay (MLPA) was developed for detecting large genomic rearrangements in the PKD genes [54]. In this assay, a set of probes were designed to target *PKD1*, *PKD2*, and *PKD1–TSC2*, covering a total of 320 kb genomic region including flanking regions. The amplified products are analyzed using the Luminex FlexMAP technology in a single assay. Using this method, Consugar et al. identified large deletions in 31 % of the previously mutation-negative cases, accounting for approximately 4 % of all patients in a prospectively studied cohort of patients with ADPKD [54]. This method has been recently commercialized by MRC-Holland (MRC-Holland, Amsterdam, The Netherlands) and is available as a clinical test. An example of MLPA analysis results is shown in Fig. 19.5.

Family linkage analysis provides another approach to genetic testing for ADPKD. This strategy employs highly informative microsatellite markers flanking *PKD1* and *PKD2*. Once linkage analysis has been performed, haplotype reconstruction can be used to predict the disease status of other family members. However, this method is suitable in fewer than 50 % of families because of constraints such as an insufficient number of affected family members [55]. Although it is now seldom used for genetic testing in ADPKD, linkage analysis may be considered in situations

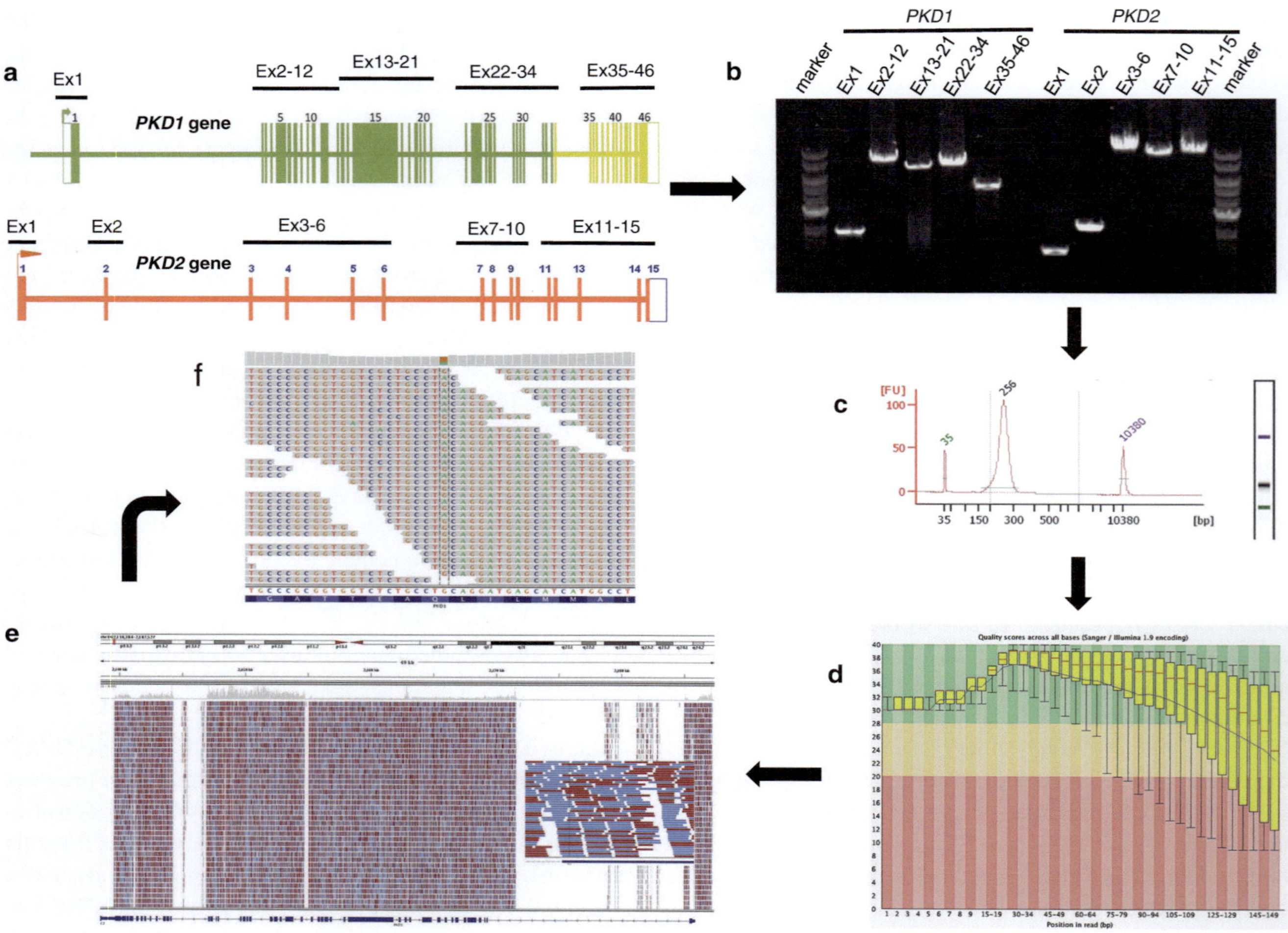

Figure 19.3 Schematic visualization of the NGS testing workflow for ADPKD. The workflow indicated by the *arrows* is as follows: (**a**) *PKD1* and *PKD2* sequences are individually amplified as ten locus-specific long-range PCR products (1.4–10.9 kb in size), covering all coding regions and most intronic regions for a total of ~80 kb. (**b**) Amplification quality verified using agarose gel electrophoresis with ethidium-bromide staining. (**c**) Amplicons from each individual sample are batched in equimolar ratios, fragmented, and subjected to library preparation using sample-specific barcodes. The indexed libraries are pooled and analyzed for quality using an Agilent Bioanalyzer. (**d**) Samples are sequenced on an Illumina MiSeq instrument, and the reads exported as FASTQ files, deconvoluted by bar code, and subjected to quality control analysis before proceeding with the mutation analysis bioinformatics pipeline. The quality score (Phred-like score) is shown at each specific bp location in *PKD1*. The *red line* in each box-and-whiskers plot shows the median value of the quality score at each bp position. The *yellow box* represents the inter-quartile range (25–75 %) of the quality score at each base. The *upper* and *lower* whiskers represent the 10 %th and 90 %th percentiles points, respectively. The *blue line* represents the mean quality score. Very good quality calls (Phred-like score within the green region at >28; chance of error 1:10,000), reasonable quality (Phred-like score within the orange region; chance of error 1:1,000), and calls of poor quality (Phred-like score within the red region; chance of error 1:100). (**e**) Reads were then mapped back to the genome with the BWA program. In this example, *PKD1* sequencing coverage and read depth for a single patient are shown. The *x*-axis represents *PKD1* genomic interval and the *y*-axis represents the number of reads. *Red lines*, reads from the plus DNA strands; *blue lines*, reads from the minus strands. The overall mean coverage of *PKD1* sequences was 668-fold. (**f**) Variant calls made by the GATK software

such as preimplantation genetic diagnosis (PGD), where low amounts of genomic DNA limit the utility of other genotyping approaches. Typing of several markers also is recommended to ensure against confounders such as allele dropout (see below), which can occur when amplifying very low amounts of DNA and/or when evaluating highly polymorphic genes such as *PKD1* [56].

Interpretation of Results

Mutations in *PKD1* and *PKD2* are usually private, highly variable and are distributed throughout the entire gene, with no mutation hot spot. This high level of allelic heterogeneity makes the interpretation of genotyping results challenging. The ADPKD Mutation Database at Mayo Clinic (http://pkdb.mayo.edu/) [57] is the most complete mutation data-

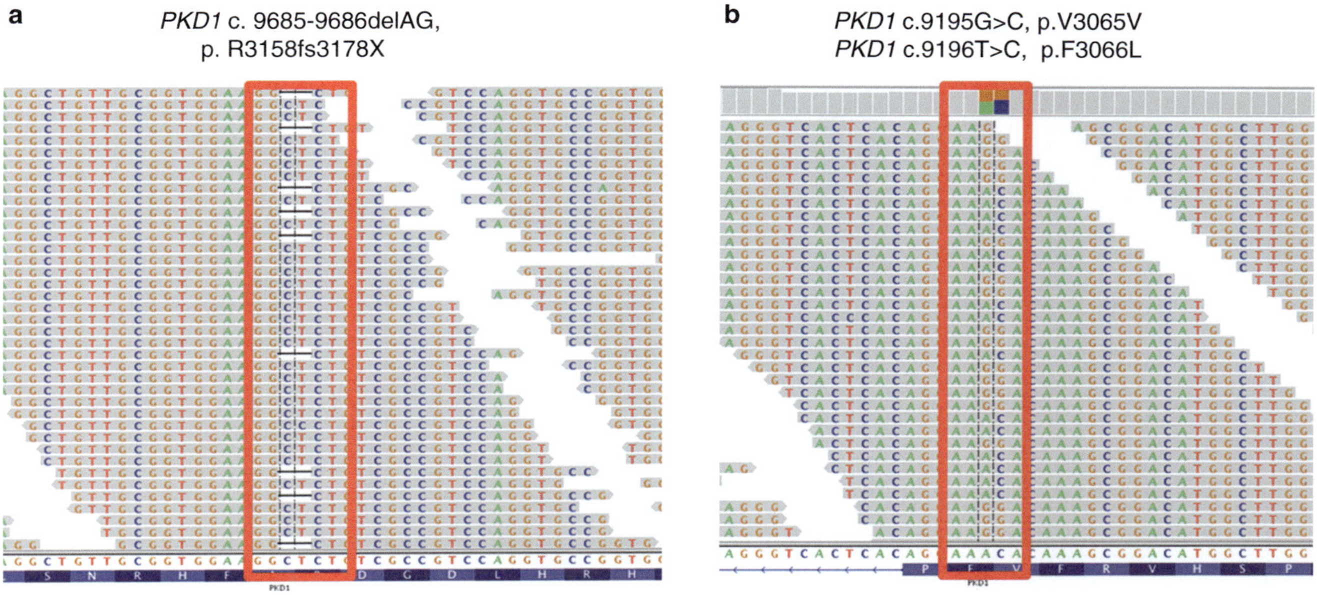

Figure 19.4 Typical alignment of *PKD1* NGS data and gene variation calls. (**a**) A two-base deletion (c.9685-9686delAG) resulting in a downstream truncation in the protein. (**b**) A synonymous (c.9195G>C; p. V3065V) variant. Minus strand is called. *Colored boxes* above each variant indicate the ratios of the two bases at the variant position. Sequence shown in Integrative Genomics Viewer (IGV), Broad Institute, Cambridge, MA

base for ADPKD. Mutation information has been reported for a total of 1,794 families: 1,420 (79 %) have *PKD1* mutations and the remaining 21 % have mutations in *PKD2* (as of November, 2013).

Genetic variations in the ADPKD Mutation Database are classified into 12 categories according to their characteristics at the DNA or protein level, including frameshift mutations, nonsense mutations, splice-site substitutions, intervening sequence (IVS), variations, silent changes, silent 5′ and 3′ untranslated region changes, synonymous changes, and rearrangements (deletions and duplications). Based on their predicted pathogenicity, those variations have been further classified into six categories: definitely pathogenic, highly likely pathogenic, likely pathogenic, hypomorphic, indeterminate, and likely neutral. A total of 1,923 changes for *PKD1* are reported in the ADPKD Mutation Database (Table 19.1), including 48.3 % pathogenic (with 32.2 % definitely pathogenic, 7.5 % highly likely pathogenic, and 8.6 % likely pathogenic), 0.5 % hypomorphic, 9.0 % indeterminate, and 42.2 % neutral. Large rearrangements account for 3 % of the pathogenic mutations reported for *PKD1*. A total of 241 *PKD2* changes are documented in the same database, consisting of 69.2 % pathogenic (with 53.5 % definitely pathogenic, 6.6 % highly likely pathogenic, and 9.1 % likely pathogenic), 0.4 % likely hypomorphic, 6.6 % indeterminate, and 23.7 % neutral (Table 19.1). Figure 19.6 shows the distributions of all known genomic changes in the *PKD1* (Fig. 19.6a) and *PKD2* (Fig. 19.6b) genes.

Determining the pathogenicity of gene variants that truncate the protein, such as frame-shift, nonsense, atypical splicing, or large rearrangements, can often be accomplished with a high level of certainty. However, interpretation of missense changes and other genetic variations that are not predicted to truncate the protein can be challenging. These groups of genetic changes, which are usually referred to as variants of uncertain significance (VUS), include synonymous and non-synonymous variants and small exonic in-frame deletions. Due to the high level of genetic variation found in *PKD1*, with an average of 10.1 variants per patient, ranging from 0 to 55 total variants, analyzing the pathogenic potential of VUS plays an important role in molecular testing for ADPKD [50].

Computational analysis of VUS includes evaluation of interspecies conservation and chemical differences of resulting amino acid substitutions. Rossetti et al. developed a method based on the Grantham Matrix Score (GMS) to predict the pathogenic effect of non-synonymous changes for ADPKD [58]. The GMS can be calculated online using Align-GVGD (http://agvgd.iarc.fr/) [59]. In addition to Align-GVGD, two other analysis programs can be used to predict pathogenicity of variants: SIFT (http://sift.jcvi.org/) [60] and PolyPhen (http://genetics.bwh.harvard.edu/pph/) [61]. SIFT and PolyPhen are based on principles similar to those used for GMS, but employ different analysis criteria. Both applications can search online databases and generate multiple sequence alignments [49].

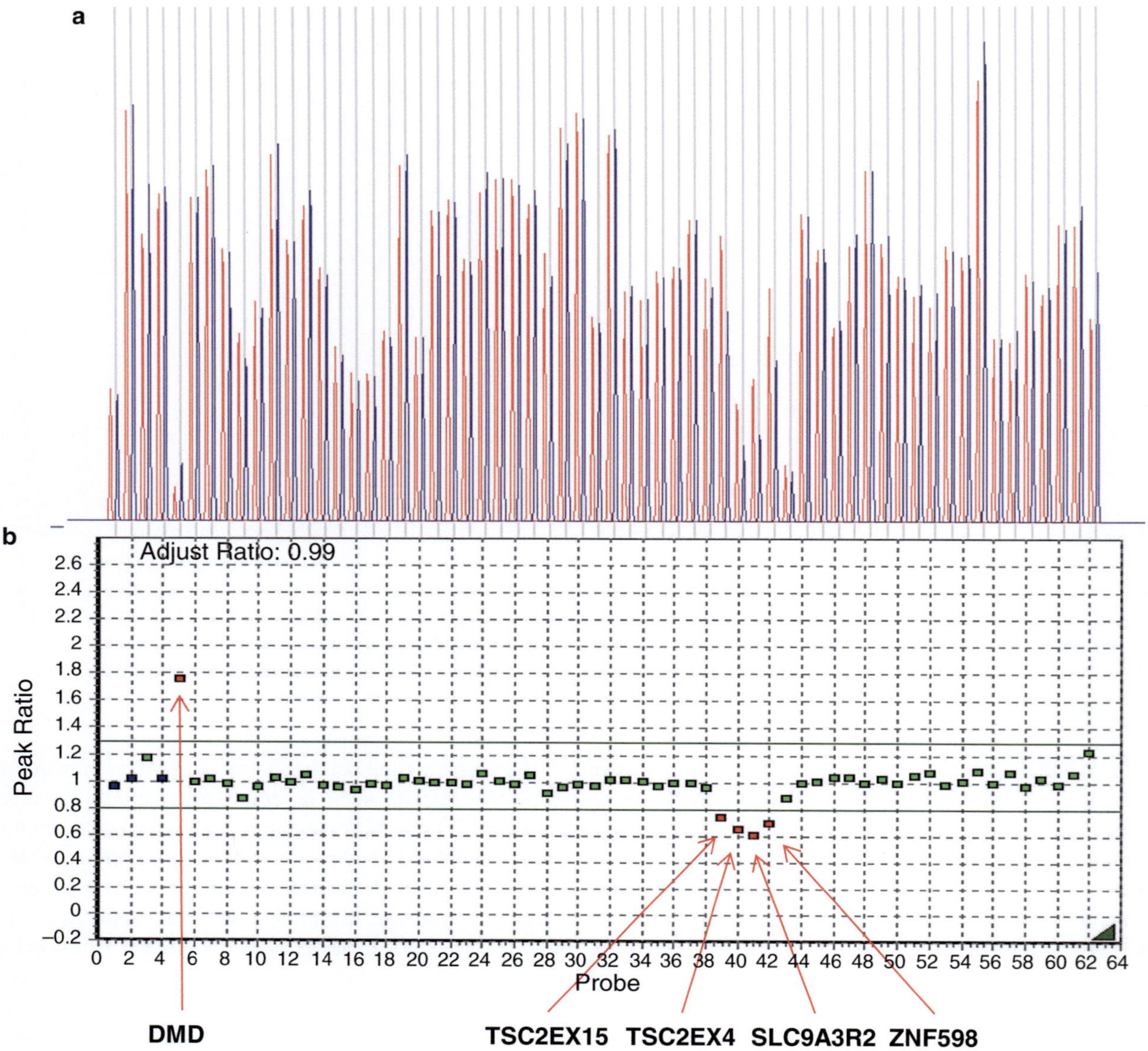

Figure 19.5 Multiplex ligation-dependent probe amplification (MLPA) analysis of a positive control DNA sample (Coriell, Camden, NJ), using probes covering the *PKD2* gene on chromosome 4 as well as numerous continuous genes (*PKD1*, *TSC2*, *SLC9A3*, *ZNF598*, and *TBL3*) on chromosome 16. Data were deconvoluted according to relative copy number compared to both the internal control genes as well as a normal control male sample using the GeneMarker software (Softgenetics, LLC; State College, PA, USA). (**a**) The *Dosage Histogram* displays the ratio of normalized peak intensities between the reference and the sample trace. Sample probes are represented by *blue bars* and control probes by *red bars*. (**b**) The *Ratio Plot* displays, in graphical form, the ratio of normalized peak intensities between the reference and the sample trace. Each *square* represents a specific probe. Analysis results show the expected deletions corresponding to one copy of *TSC2EX15*, *TSC2EX4*, *SLC9A3R2*, and *ZNF598* genes (*red squares* and *arrows*), and two copies of all *PKD1* and *PKD2* gene probes (*green squares*) and the two-copy internal controls (*blue squares*). The X-linked *DMD* control (*upper left side*) is indicated in *red*, demonstrating a patient-control peak ratio of approximately 1.8, consistent with a two-copy female DNA and a single-copy male reference control

In order to predict the potential splicing site mutation, several other programs based on different prediction principles have been developed to predict the impact of splice site variants. These include Splice Site Prediction by Neural Network (http://www.fruitfly.org/seq_tools/splice.html) [62], ESEfinder (http://rulai.cshl.edu/cgi-bin/tools/ESE3/esefinder.cgi) [63], and Human Splicing Finder (http://www.umd.be/HSF/) [64]. The prediction results of atypical splicing could be further confirmed by reverse transcription (RT)-PCR analysis, if the patient's RNA is available.

Assessing the functional impact of missense mutations is more difficult, especially for *PKD1*, particularly because of the large size and uncertain functions of the polycystins. For the CRISP cohort, 38 of 99 (38 %) missense changes were

Table 19.1 Distribution of *PKD1* and *PKD2* gene variants by type and pathogenicity (*N*=1,794 ADPKD families)

Gene	Mutation type	Definitely pathogenic	Highly likely pathogenic	Likely pathogenic	Likely hypomorphic	Indeterminate	Likely neutral	Total
PKD1 (*N*=1,420)	Nonsense	203	0	0	0	0	0	203
	Frameshift	310	0	0	0	0	0	310
	Splice	62	10	19	0	0	0	91
	Insertion	9	2	6	0	0	1	18
	Deletion	19	20	21	0	2	1	63
	Large deletion	15	0	0	0	0	0	15
	Large duplication	1	0	0	0	0	0	1
	Substitution	0	112	120	9	155	285	681
	IVS silent	0	0	0	0	1	188	189
	IVS unknown	0	0	0	0	15	0	15
	UTR silent	0	0	0	0	0	12	12
	Synonymous	0	0	0	0	0	325	325
	Sub Total	619	144	166	9	173	812	1,923
PKD2 (*N*=374)	Nonsense	40	0	0	0	0	0	40
	Frameshift	61	0	0	0	0	0	61
	Splice	23	2	6	0	0	0	31
	Insertion	1	0	0	0	2	0	3
	Deletion	0	1	3	0	0	0	4
	Large deletion	3	0	0	0	0	0	3
	Large duplication	1	0	0	0	0	0	1
	Substitution	0	13	13	1	13	25	65
	IVS silent	0	0	0	0	0	13	13
	IVS unknown	0	0	0	0	1	0	1
	Synonymous	0	0	0	0	0	6	19
	Sub Total	129	16	22	1	16	57	241
All		748	160	188	10	189	869	2,164

IVS intervening sequence; *UTR* untranslated region
Definitely pathogenic including nonsense, frameshift, typical splicing, and in-fame changes of five or more amino acids. The pathogenicity of other changes were assessed by a scoring system integrating Grantham Matrix Score, the likelihood for aberrant splicing, segregation analysis results (if available), and contextual information. A score ≥11 were classed as highly likely pathogenic; a score 5–10 as likely pathogenic; –4 to 4 as indeterminate; and ≤–5 as likely neutral [57]. Hypomorphic mean incompletely penetrant
Data derived from the ADPKD Mutation Database (http://pkdb.mayo.edu/), November 2013

predicted to be pathogenic, with 35 in *PKD1* and 3 in *PKD2* [58]. By including the probably pathogenic mutations, the mutation detection rate can be increased to over 85 % [50, 58]. In 10–15 % of individuals with clinical ADPKD, no mutation in either *PKD1* or *PKD2* could be detected. This could be due to other atypical genetic events such as deep intronic changes that affect splicing, gene conversion events not readily detected by current exon-based screening methods, or mutations in other yet undiscovered cyst related genes [65, 66]. Low-level mosaicism caused by de novo mutations can also account for these apparent mutation-negative cases [67].

Laboratory Issues

Most of the currently used genotyping methods for ADPKD employ nested PCR to amplify each individual exon of the duplicated sequences of *PKD1*. This approach requires ultra-high (10^5-fold) dilutions of the primary *PKD1* LR-PCR products, which then serve as template for the second round of nested PCR. This process is especially vulnerable to carryover of PCR amplification products, potentially leading to PCR contamination and false-positive results. Consequently, special precautions, such a second PCR set-up chamber, are needed.

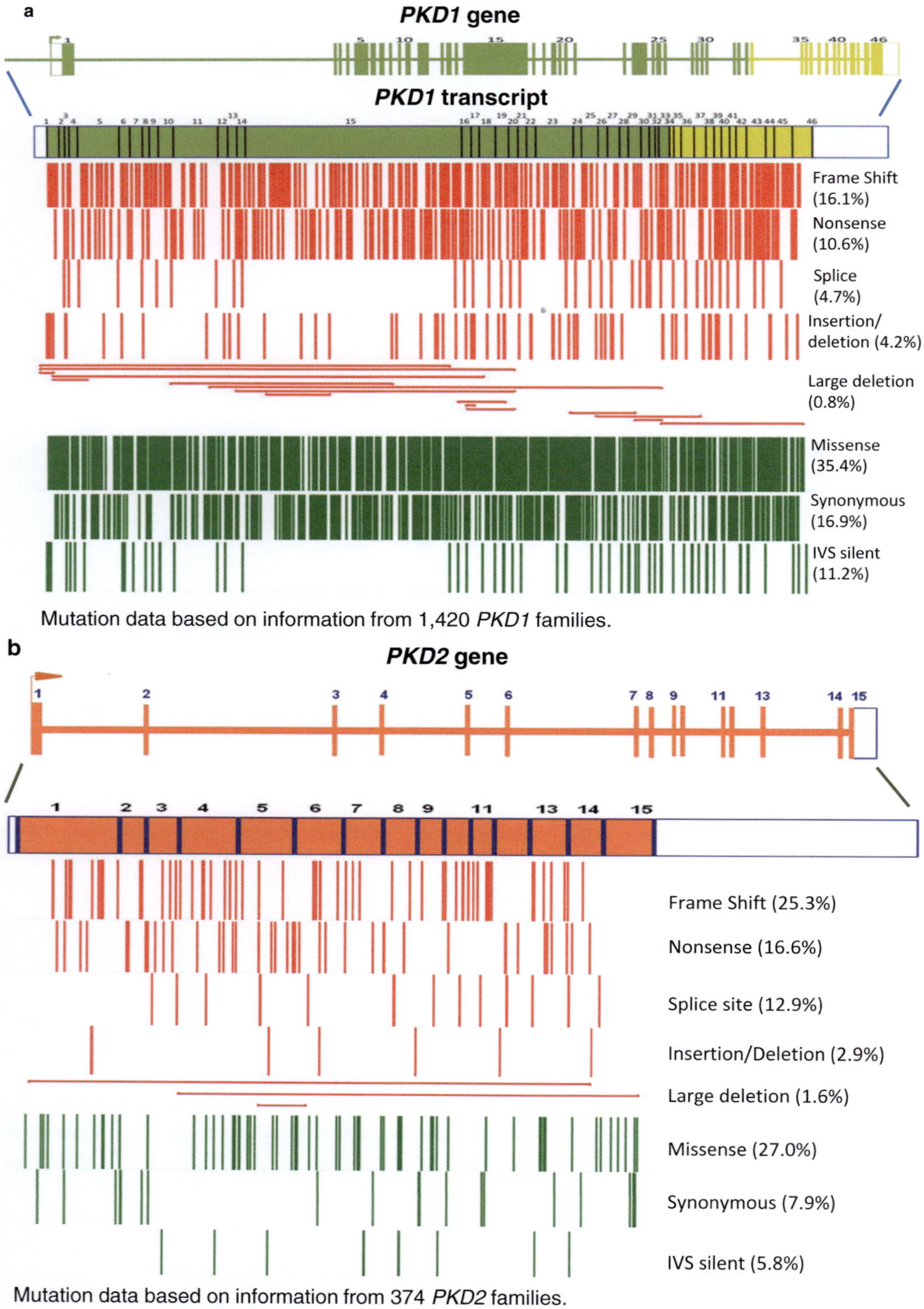

Figure 19.6 *PKD1* and *PKD2* gene structures and distribution of genetic variants. *Upper panels* show the gene and mRNA structure of *PKD1* (**a**) and *PKD2* (**b**), respectively. *Lower panels* show the spectrum and distribution of genetic variants for *PKD1* (**a**) and *PKD2* (**b**), grouped by mutation type, according to their relative position on the mRNA. Definite pathogenic mutations are colored *red*; other changes are colored *green*

PKD1 is highly polymorphic, increasing the chance that a SNP is located in the primer-binding region of an allele, resulting in lower or complete lack of amplification of one of the two alleles during the PCR reaction. This phenomenon, termed allele dropout or pseudo-homozygosity, has been well documented in ADPKD testing [50]. A homozygous mutation result in either *PKD1* or *PKD2* is most likely due to allele dropout, since homozygous mutations are thought to be embryonically lethal [68]. Therefore, the finding of a homozygous PKD gene mutation would warrant confirmation before reporting.

Another issue is the existence of the six highly identical *PKD1* pseudogenes. The primers used for amplifying these regions must complement the rare mismatch sites that distinguish the genuine *PKD1* gene from the pseudogenes to avoid amplification of the pseudogenes. Fortunately, it is relatively easy to distinguish whether these *PKD1* pseudogenes are co-amplified because they are enriched in polymorphisms and pathogenic variations that are not present in *PKD1*.

Autosomal Recessive Polycystic Kidney Disease

Molecular Basis of Disease

Despite the highly variable phenotype, genetic linkage studies indicate that mutations at a single locus are responsible for all ARPKD phenotypes [69]. The ARPKD gene, polycystic kidney and hepatic disease 1 (*PKHD1*), maps to locus 6p21 and is a large gene with 67 exons and a 470 kb genomic sequence [70]. *PKHD1* has a variety of alternatively spliced transcripts, and the longest open reading frame has 12,222 bp with 66 exons. *PKHD1* encodes a protein called polyductin or fibrocystin, which is a multidomain integral membrane protein with 4,074 amino acids [6]. The function of polyductin has not been defined. Based on the predicted structure with a highly glycosylated N-terminal extracellular domain, a single transmembrane domain, and a short cytoplasmic C-terminal tail, polyductin is thought to be an integral membrane receptor. Furthermore, polyductin complexes with PC2, and together with other proteins, localizes to primary cilia, thus it may execute its function through PC2 [71].

PKDH1 exhibits a high level of allelic heterogeneity, with 303 different mutations described in approximately 650 alleles; 40 % are truncation mutations and the remaining are in-frame changes, mainly missense mutations. About one-third of these mutations are unique private mutations with some mutations enriched in specific geographic areas. One missense mutation T36M, likely of European origin, accounts for approximately 17 % of all mutant alleles [72].

Clinical Utility

Similar to ADPKD, the diagnosis of ARPKD usually relies on imaging studies by renal ultrasonography. Clinical molecular testing can establish a diagnosis in 85 % of patients, but is not recommended for those in whom a diagnosis can be obtained by imaging techniques because of the high cost of genotyping. The clinical utility of molecular diagnosis in ARPKD is to confirm the diagnosis, especially in cases with a less severe phenotype, or when imaging results are not diagnostic. Due to the significant morbidity and mortality associated with ARPKD, many families with ARPKD seek prenatal and PGD testing. A robust molecular testing approach is critical for these indications.

Available Assays

DNA-based diagnostic testing for ARPKD is complicated by the large size of the *PKDH1* gene, its complex pattern of RNA splicing, and the unknown function of the encoded protein. There are two major approaches used for clinical molecular testing for ARPKD: sequencing-based mutation screening and family linkage analysis. Sequencing-based mutation screening can be achieved by directly sequencing all the exons of *PKDH1*, or by a mutation screening step before sequencing to lower the cost. Over the years, two approaches have been established for mutation screening of *PKHD1*: SSCP and DHPLC. SSCP has a mutation detection rate of 61 % while DHPLC achieves a detection rate of 85 %, for detection of both causative mutations in a family [73]. Direct sequencing was reported to have a slightly higher detection rate of 87 % [74], with at least one mutation detected in more than 95 % of ARPKD families [73]. Because of the existence of mutation hot spots, mutation screening approaches can be further simplified by analyzing only a subset of exons, accelerating the testing process [75].

If mutations are identified, prenatal and PGD testing for at-risk pregnancies can be performed by Sanger sequencing of the corresponding exons. Without prior knowledge of the causative mutation, PGD can only be performed by linkage analysis, requiring at least one affected individual in the family. A novel protocol method for PGD testing for ARPKD is genome amplification of single blastomeres and haplotype analysis with 20 novel STR loci. This approach can significantly reduce allele dropout. Large genomic rearrangements seen in ARPKD can be analyzed using MLPA, with *PKHD1-specific* probes.

Interpretation of Results

A locus-specific ARPKD mutation database is available at http://www.humgen.rwth-aachen.de/. All reported cases with two truncating mutations have the most severe disease, dying with respiratory distress by the end of the neonatal period. Patients surviving the neonatal period have at least one missense mutation, indicating that many missense variations have incomplete penetrance and some residual protein function. Missense mutations are significantly more prevalent than truncating mutations among patients with less severe disease manifestations, although some missense mutations are as deleterious as truncating mutation. No significant phenotype differences could be found between cases with two missense mutations and cases with a truncating and a missense mutation in trans [76].

Despite the fact that 60 % of mutations found in ARPKD are missense, an approach that can definitively assess the potential pathogenicity of these changes is still lacking. As discussed for ADPKD, computational algorithms can be used to predict the likelihood of whether or not a missense change is pathogenic, or an intronic change can affect splicing, and are crucial in characterization of newly identified VUS.

Laboratory Issues

The same issues discussed for ADPKD molecular diagnosis also apply for ARPKD, including PCR contamination and allele dropout that require special attention, especially when considering prenatal and PGD testing, where extremely low amounts of genomic DNA are available.

Conclusions and Future Directions

This chapter reviews the molecular mechanisms underlying PKD and the strategies used for clinical molecular testing for both ADPKD and ARPKD. Completion of the Human Genome Project, the rapid development of new molecular testing tools, improved bioinformatics applications, and the establishment of strong PKD mutation databases have greatly aided with mutation identification and characterization. Genetic testing for ADPKD and ARPKD is now available, in some instances becoming the method of choice for diagnosis. Better understanding of genotype–phenotype correlation will further enhance the development of novel diagnostic and prognostic biomarkers, as well as facilitate personalized patient management. This process will likely accelerate as more effective and personalized therapies for PKD become available. Among the biggest challenges in this field include the evaluation of new testing technologies for diagnosis of PKD, incorporation of new approaches for data analysis and management, and changing regulatory standards for clinical laboratories.

References

1. Peters DJ, Sandkuijl LA. Genetic heterogeneity of polycystic kidney disease in Europe. Contrib Nephrol. 1992;97:128–39.
2. Rossetti S, Burton S, Strmecki L, et al. The position of the polycystic kidney disease 1 (PKD1) gene mutation correlates with the severity of renal disease. J Am Soc Nephrol. 2002;13(5):1230–7.
3. Kelleher CL, McFann KK, Johnson AM, et al. Characteristics of hypertension in young adults with autosomal dominant polycystic kidney disease compared with the general U.S. population. Am J Hypertens. 2004;17(11, Pt 1):1029–34.
4. Torres VE, Harris PC, Pirson Y. Autosomal dominant polycystic kidney disease. Lancet. 2007;369(9569):1287–301.
5. Braun WE. Autosomal dominant polycystic kidney disease: emerging concepts of pathogenesis and new treatments. Cleve Clin J Med. 2009;76(2):97–104.
6. Harris PC. 2008 Homer W. Smith Award: insights into the pathogenesis of polycystic kidney disease from gene discovery. J Am Soc Nephrol. 2009;20(6):1188–98.
7. Fliegauf M, Benzing T, Omran H. When cilia go bad: cilia defects and ciliopathies. Nat Rev Mol Cell Biol. 2007;8(11):880–93.
8. Sedman A, Bell P, Manco-Johnson M, et al. Autosomal dominant polycystic kidney disease in childhood: a longitudinal study. Kidney Int. 1987;31(4):1000–5.
9. Sweeney Jr WE, Avner ED. Diagnosis and management of childhood polycystic kidney disease. Pediatr Nephrol. 2011;26(5):675–92.
10. Hughes J, Ward CJ, Peral B, et al. The polycystic kidney disease 1 (PKD1) gene encodes a novel protein with multiple cell recognition domains. Nat Genet. 1995;10(2):151–60.
11. Mochizuki T, Wu G, Hayashi T, et al. PKD2, a gene for polycystic kidney disease that encodes an integral membrane protein. Science. 1996;272(5266):1339–42.
12. Harris PC, Rossetti S. Molecular diagnostics for autosomal dominant polycystic kidney disease. Nat Rev Nephrol. 2010;6(4):197–206.
13. Consortium TIPKD. Polycystic kidney disease: the complete structure of the PKD1 gene and its protein. The International Polycystic Kidney Disease Consortium. Cell. 1995;81(2):289–98.
14. Reed B, McFann K, Kimberling WJ, et al. Presence of de novo mutations in autosomal dominant polycystic kidney disease patients without family history. Am J Kidney Dis. 2008;52(6):1042–50.
15. Torres VE, Harris PC. Autosomal dominant polycystic kidney disease: the last 3 years. Kidney Int. 2009;76(2):149–68.
16. Sandford R, Sgotto B, Aparicio S, et al. Comparative analysis of the polycystic kidney disease 1 (PKD1) gene reveals an integral membrane glycoprotein with multiple evolutionary conserved domains. Hum Mol Genet. 1997;6(9):1483–9.
17. Hanaoka K, Qian F, Boletta A, et al. Co-assembly of polycystin-1 and -2 produces unique cation-permeable currents. Nature. 2000;408(6815):990–4.
18. Yoder BK, Tousson A, Millican L, et al. Polaris, a protein disrupted in orpk mutant mice, is required for assembly of renal cilium. Am J Physiol Renal Physiol. 2002;282(3):F541–52.
19. Qian F, Germino FJ, Cai Y, et al. PKD1 interacts with PKD2 through a probable coiled-coil domain. Nat Genet. 1997;16(2):179–83.
20. Nauli SM, Alenghat FJ, Luo Y, et al. Polycystins 1 and 2 mediate mechanosensation in the primary cilium of kidney cells. Nat Genet. 2003;33(2):129–37.
21. Yamaguchi T, Wallace DP, Magenheimer BS, et al. Calcium restriction allows cAMP activation of the B-Raf/ERK pathway, switching cells to a cAMP-dependent growth-stimulated phenotype. J Biol Chem. 2004;279(39):40419–30.
22. Wu G, Tian X, Nishimura S, et al. Trans-heterozygous Pkd1 and Pkd2 mutations modify expression of polycystic kidney disease. Hum Mol Genet. 2002;11(16):1845–54.
23. Arnaout MA. Molecular genetics and pathogenesis of autosomal dominant polycystic kidney disease. Annu Rev Med. 2001;52:93–123.
24. Pei Y. A "two-hit" model of cystogenesis in autosomal dominant polycystic kidney disease? Trends Mol Med. 2001;7(4):151–6.
25. Pei Y, Paterson AD, Wang KR, et al. Bilineal disease and trans-heterozygotes in autosomal dominant polycystic kidney disease. Am J Hum Genet. 2001;68(2):355–63.

26. Hopp K, Ward CJ, Hommerding CJ, et al. Functional polycystin-1 dosage governs autosomal dominant polycystic kidney disease severity. J Clin Invest. 2012;122(11):4257–73.
27. Koptides M, Mean R, Demetriou K, et al. Genetic evidence for a trans-heterozygous model for cystogenesis in autosomal dominant polycystic kidney disease. Hum Mol Genet. 2000;9(3):447–52.
28. Chapin HC, Caplan MJ. The cell biology of polycystic kidney disease. J Cell Biol. 2010;191(4):701–10.
29. Torres VE, Harris PC. Polycystic kidney disease in 2011: connecting the dots toward a polycystic kidney disease therapy. Nat Rev Nephrol. 2011;8(2):66–8.
30. Hateboer N, v Dijk MA, Bogdanova N, et al. Comparison of phenotypes of polycystic kidney disease types 1 and 2. European PKD1-PKD2 Study Group. Lancet. 1999;353(9147):103–7.
31. Harris PC, Bae KT, Rossetti S, et al. Cyst number but not the rate of cystic growth is associated with the mutated gene in autosomal dominant polycystic kidney disease. J Am Soc Nephrol. 2006;17(11):3013–9.
32. Rossetti S, Chauveau D, Walker D, et al. A complete mutation screen of the ADPKD genes by DHPLC. Kidney Int. 2002;61(5):1588–99.
33. Rossetti S, Chauveau D, Kubly V, et al. Association of mutation position in polycystic kidney disease 1 (PKD1) gene and development of a vascular phenotype. Lancet. 2003;361(9376):2196–201.
34. Cornec-Le Gall E, Audrezet MP, Chen JM, et al. Type of PKD1 mutation influences renal outcome in ADPKD. J Am Soc Nephrol. 2013;24(6):1006–13.
35. Rossetti S, Kubly VJ, Consugar MB, et al. Incompletely penetrant PKD1 alleles suggest a role for gene dosage in cyst initiation in polycystic kidney disease. Kidney Int. 2009;75(8):848–55.
36. Geberth S, Ritz E, Zeier M, et al. Anticipation of age at renal death in autosomal dominant polycystic kidney disease (ADPKD)? Nephrol Dial Transplant. 1995;10(9):1603–6.
37. Peral B, Gamble V, San Millan JL, et al. Splicing mutations of the polycystic kidney disease 1 (PKD1) gene induced by intronic deletion. Hum Mol Genet. 1995;4(4):569–74.
38. Persu A, Duyme M, Pirson Y, et al. Comparison between siblings and twins supports a role for modifier genes in ADPKD. Kidney Int. 2004;66(6):2132–6.
39. Fain PR, McFann KK, Taylor MR, et al. Modifier genes play a significant role in the phenotypic expression of PKD1. Kidney Int. 2005;67(4):1256–67.
40. Liu M, Shi S, Senthilnathan S, et al. Genetic variation of DKK3 may modify renal disease severity in ADPKD. J Am Soc Nephrol. 2010;21(9):1510–20.
41. Rossetti S, Harris PC. Genotype-phenotype correlations in autosomal dominant and autosomal recessive polycystic kidney disease. J Am Soc Nephrol. 2007;18(5):1374–80.
42. Ravine D, Gibson RN, Walker RG, et al. Evaluation of ultrasonographic diagnostic criteria for autosomal dominant polycystic kidney disease 1. Lancet. 1994;343(8901):824–7.
43. Pei Y, Obaji J, Dupuis A, et al. Unified criteria for ultrasonographic diagnosis of ADPKD. J Am Soc Nephrol. 2009;20(1):205–12.
44. Pei Y, Hwang YH, Conklin J, et al. Imaging-based diagnosis of autosomal dominant polycystic kidney disease. J Am Soc Nephrol. 2015;26(3):746–53.
45. Huang E, Samaniego-Picota M, McCune T, et al. DNA testing for live kidney donors at risk for autosomal dominant polycystic kidney disease. Transplantation. 2009;87(1):133–7.
46. Blumenfeld JD. Pretransplant genetic testing of live kidney donors at risk for autosomal dominant polycystic kidney disease. Transplantation. 2009;87(1):6–7.
47. Rossetti S, Strmecki L, Gamble V, et al. Mutation analysis of the entire PKD1 gene: genetic and diagnostic implications. Am J Hum Genet. 2001;68(1):46–63.
48. Garcia-Gonzalez MA, Jones JG, Allen SK, et al. Evaluating the clinical utility of a molecular genetic test for polycystic kidney disease. Mol Genet Metab. 2007;92(1–2):160–7.
49. Perrichot R, Mercier B, Quere I, et al. Novel mutations in the duplicated region of PKD1 gene. Eur J Hum Genet. 2000;8(5):353–9.
50. Tan YC, Blumenfeld JD, Anghel R, et al. Novel method for genomic analysis of PKD1 and PKD2 mutations in auto somal dominant polycystic kidney disease. Hum Mutat. 2009;30(2):264–73.
51. Tan YC, Blumenfeld J, Michaeel A, et al. Development of a novel, and rapid genetic test for autosomal dominant polycystic kidney disease (ADPKD) genes, *PKD1* and *PKD2* using long-range PCR. J Mol Diagn. 2012;14:305–13.
52. Rossetti S, Hopp K, Sikkink RA, et al. Identification of gene mutations in autosomal dominant polycystic kidney disease through targeted resequencing. J Am Soc Nephrol. 2012;23(5):915–33.
53. Tan YC, Michaeel A, Liu G, et al. Molecular diagnosis of autosomal dominant polycystic kidney disease using next generation sequencing. J Mol Diagn. 2014;16(2):216–28.
54. Consugar MB, Wong WC, Lundquist PA, et al. Characterization of large rearrangements in autosomal dominant polycystic kidney disease and the PKD1/TSC2 contiguous gene syndrome. Kidney Int. 2008;74(11):1468–79.
55. Pei Y. Diagnostic approach in autosomal dominant polycystic kidney disease. Clin J Am Soc Nephrol. 2006;1(5):1108–14.
56. De Rycke M, Georgiou I, Sermon K, et al. PGD for autosomal dominant polycystic kidney disease type 1. Mol Hum Reprod. 2005;11(1):65–71.
57. Gout AM, Martin NC, Brown AF, et al. PKDB: Polycystic Kidney Disease Mutation Database—a gene variant database for autosomal dominant polycystic kidney disease. Hum Mutat. 2007;28(7):654–9.
58. Rossetti S, Consugar MB, Chapman AB, et al. Comprehensive molecular diagnostics in autosomal dominant polycystic kidney disease. J Am Soc Nephrol. 2007;18(7):2143–60.
59. Tavtigian SV, Deffenbaugh AM, Yin L, et al. Comprehensive statistical study of 452 BRCA1 missense substitutions with classification of eight recurrent substitutions as neutral. J Med Genet. 2006;43(4):295–305.
60. Ng PC, Henikoff S. Predicting deleterious amino acid substitutions. Genome Res. 2001;11(5):863–74.
61. Sunyaev S, Ramensky V, Koch I, et al. Prediction of deleterious human alleles. Hum Mol Genet. 2001;10(6):591–7.
62. Reese MG, Eeckman FH, Kulp D, et al. Improved splice site detection in Genie. J Comput Biol. 1997;4(3):311–23.
63. Cartegni L, Wang J, Zhu Z, et al. ESEfinder: a web resource to identify exonic splicing enhancers. Nucleic Acids Res. 2003;31(13):3568–71.
64. Desmet FO, Hamroun D, Lalande M, et al. Human Splicing Finder: an online bioinformatics tool to predict splicing signals. Nucleic Acids Res. 2009;37(9), e67.
65. King K, Flinter FA, Nihalani V, et al. Unusual deep intronic mutations in the COL4A5 gene cause X linked Alport syndrome. Hum Genet. 2002;111(6):548–54.
66. Paul BM, Consugar MB, Ryan-Lee M, et al. Evidence of a third ADPKD locus is not supported by reanalysis of designated PKD3 families. Kidney Int. 2014;85(2):383–92.
67. Tan YC, Blumenfeld J, Donahue S, et al. Autosomal dominant polycystic kidney disease due to somatic and germline mosaicism. Clin Genet. 2014: April 26. doi:10.1111/cge.12383 [Epub ahead of print].
68. Lu W, Peissel B, Babakhanlou H, et al. Perinatal lethality with kidney and pancreas defects in mice with a targeted Pkd1 mutation. Nat Genet. 1997;17(2):179–81.
69. Guay-Woodford LM, Muecher G, Hopkins SD, et al. The severe perinatal form of autosomal recessive polycystic kidney disease

maps to chromosome 6p21.1-p12: implications for genetic counseling. Am J Hum Genet. 1995;56(5):1101–7.

70. Ward CJ, Hogan MC, Rossetti S, et al. The gene mutated in autosomal recessive polycystic kidney disease encodes a large, receptor-like protein. Nat Genet. 2002;30(3):259–69.
71. Wang S, Zhang J, Nauli SM, et al. Fibrocystin/polyductin, found in the same protein complex with polycystin-2, regulates calcium responses in kidney epithelia. Mol Cell Biol. 2007;27(8):3241–52.
72. Bergmann C, Senderek J, Sedlacek B, et al. Spectrum of mutations in the gene for autosomal recessive polycystic kidney disease (ARPKD/PKHD1). J Am Soc Nephrol. 2003; 14(1):76–89.
73. Bergmann C, Senderek J, Schneider F, et al. PKHD1 mutations in families requesting prenatal diagnosis for autosomal recessive polycystic kidney disease (ARPKD). Hum Mutat. 2004;23(5): 487–95.
74. Losekoot M, Haarloo C, Ruivenkamp C, et al. Analysis of missense variants in the PKHD1-gene in patients with autosomal recessive polycystic kidney disease (ARPKD). Hum Genet. 2005;118(2): 185–206.
75. Bergmann C, Kupper F, Dornia C, et al. Algorithm for efficient PKHD1 mutation screening in autosomal recessive polycystic kidney disease (ARPKD). Hum Mutat. 2005;25(3): 225–31.
76. Bergmann C, Senderek J, Windelen E, et al. Clinical consequences of PKHD1 mutations in 164 patients with autosomal-recessive polycystic kidney disease (ARPKD). Kidney Int. 2005;67(3): 829–48.

Host Factor Pharmacogenetics for Treatment of Infectious Diseases

20

Patricia R. Slev and David R. Hillyard

Abstract

Progress in therapeutics and testing for infectious diseases over the past 100 years has resulted in dramatic reductions in morbidity and mortality. However, with developments of effective drugs has come the recognition that not all individuals respond the same to a given therapy, and this marked the beginning of initiatives to study human genetic variations as a factor in response to drug therapy. The pharmacogenetics of infectious diseases is in its infancy; however, the goal of maximizing drug efficacy while minimizing toxicity has important implications for clinical care and better understanding of the biology of the host-pathogen interface. This chapter provides an overview of the progress that has been made in pharmacogenetics and summarizes the challenges that remain for bridging the gap between research and clinical use. The few illustrative examples of genetic testing currently utilized as tools for patient management are discussed.

Keywords

Genetic factors for drug response • Pharmacogenetics • Genetic testing • Infectious diseases • Drug toxicity • Host-pathogen interactions

Introduction

Progress in therapeutics and testing for infectious diseases over the past 100 years has resulted in dramatic reductions in morbidity and mortality. However, with developments of effective drugs has come the recognition that not all individuals respond the same to a given therapy, marking the beginning of initiatives to study human genetic variations as a factor in response to drug therapy. The pharmacogenetics of infectious diseases is in its infancy; however, the goal of maximizing drug efficacy while minimizing toxicity has important implications for clinical care and better understanding of the biology of the host-pathogen interface.

Type A adverse drug reactions (ADRs) are dose dependent and therefore a large component of pharmacogenetics is genotyping for functionally important polymorphisms in genes that affect pharmacokinetics. These include genes that code for drug-metabolizing enzymes and transporter proteins, for example, phase I oxidative isozymes of the cytochrome P450 (CYP) superfamily, phase II conjugative

P.R. Slev, Ph.D., D.(A.B.C.C.) (✉)
Department of Pathology, School of Medicine, University of Utah, Salt Lake City, UT, USA

Serologic Hepatitis & Retrovirus Laboratory, ARUP Laboratories, MS 115 - Medical Directors, 500 Chipeta Way, Salt Lake City, UT 84108, USA

Immunology Core Laboratory, ARUP Laboratories, MS 115 - Medical Directors, 500 Chipeta Way, Salt Lake City, UT 84108, USA
e-mail: patricia.slev@aruplab.com

D.R. Hillyard, M.D.
Department of Pathology, School of Medicine, University of Utah, Salt Lake City, UT, USA

Molecular Infectious Disease Testing and Infectious Disease Sequencing Core, ARUP Laboratories, Salt Lake City, UT, USA
e-mail: hillyadr@aruplab.com

D.G.B. Leonard (ed.), *Molecular Pathology in Clinical Practice*, DOI 10.1007/978-3-319-19674-9_20

enzymes such as uridine diphosphate glucuronosyltransferase 1 (UGT1A1) and *N*-acetyltransferase 2 (NAT 2), P-glycoprotein (P-gp), and multidrug resistance proteins. CYP2C9, CYP2D6, and CYP2B19 as a group metabolize approximately 40 % of drugs currently on the market, including drugs used to treat various microbial infections. Many CYP, NAT, MDR, and other gene polymorphisms that affect pharmacokinetics of drugs used to treat infectious diseases have been identified, but there is little consensus regarding utilization of these associations for prospective screening.

There are several reasons that may explain why clinical use of pharmacogenetic variants affecting antimicrobial therapy is limited. First, pharmacogenetic testing is best suited for drugs that have a narrow therapeutic index. Second, genotype-phenotype correlation often is difficult, especially if multiple genes are involved in the metabolism of a single drug, or when drug-drug interactions and other non-genetic factors influence the phenotype. Third, there must be a clear relationship between drug concentration and effective drug response. Today, the most notable examples of applied pharmacogenetics as related to Type A ADRs are in the areas of oncology, psychiatry, and cardiology.

Type B ADRs are not dose dependent and are largely caused by immunoallergic reactions. As such, these ADRs are a consequence of pharmacodynamics, rather than pharmacokinetics resulting in drug toxicity. Growing evidence suggests that a significant proportion of these immunoallergic reactions have a strong HLA association [1]. HLA associations with hypersensitivity reactions to drugs, due to inappropriate HLA presentation and ensuing immune response, have become the more common reason for clinical determination of HLA genotype (excluding transplantation). HLA pharmacogenetic testing for prevention of this type of ADR is one of the most rapidly evolving fields with direct clinical application.

Until recently, the candidate gene approach based on known metabolic pathways or suspected etiology was the only option available for detecting relevant gene polymorphisms. With the advent of high-throughput platforms that can genotype thousands of single-nucleotide polymorphisms (SNPs) simultaneously, interrogation of the entire human genome is possible and can detect polymorphisms associated with a disease, treatment response, or an ADR. This strategy holds the promise of identifying functionally important polymorphisms in genes that have an unexpected role in drug metabolism or drug toxicity. Studies conducted utilizing this methodology known as genome-wide association studies (GWAS) have had little clinical impact as far as providing novel targets that would predict disease, treatment outcome, or toxicity. Although many variants associated with complex diseases have been identified, the variants themselves explain only a small fraction of the heritable contribution to disease risk or response to treatment [2, 3]. Advances in technology have increased discovery of host genetic markers that have provided critical insight into disease pathogenesis, pharmacokinetics, pharmacodynamics, and drug toxicity, but these have not altered clinical practice significantly.

An enormous amount of work has been dedicated to identifying functionally important human polymorphisms with the ultimate goal of improving patient care. Significant progress has been made in detecting such polymorphisms in drug-metabolizing genes, HLA and non-HLA immunity genes, and other host genetic markers that impact either susceptibility to infectious disease, therapy selection, or therapy response. One of the primary barriers to translating most of these genetic associations into the clinical setting is the weakness of the predictive value of any given association with an unfavorable outcome, be it disease risk, poor treatment response, or ADRs. Even in the rare cases where positive and negative predictive values approach 100 %, suggesting clinical utility, the lack of prospective studies addressing cost-effectiveness and demonstrating clear benefits with broad applicability across different ethnic populations precludes testing as part of routine medical practice. This chapter provides an overview of the progress that has been made in host pharmacogenetics and summarizes the challenges that remain for bridging the gap between research and clinical use. The few illustrative examples of genetic testing currently utilized as tools for patient management are discussed in detail.

HLA-B*5701 and Abacavir

HLA-B*5701 screening prior to administering abacavir to treat human immunodeficiency virus (HIV) infection is the best described and extensively studied example of a pharmacogenetic marker for infectious diseases. It also represents one of the few and arguably the most successful example of a pharmacogenetic marker that has been adopted into medical practice. Abacavir is a nucleoside reverse transcriptase inhibitor antiretroviral drug used to treat HIV infection. Abacavir hypersensitivity reaction syndrome (ABC-HSR) is a multi-organ reaction characterized by rash, fever, fatigue, and respiratory and gastrointestinal symptoms. These nonspecific symptoms can be easily confused with other etiologies such as unrelated viral disease or adverse reactions to concomitant medications. Distinguishing between ABC-HSR and other causes of the symptoms is important because continuing therapy with abacavir in those who develop this hypersensitivity reaction can result in serious illness and even death. ABC-HSR usually develops within the first six weeks of treatment and has been estimated to affect 5–8 % of patients treated with abacavir [4]. Although discontinuation of therapy reverses the symptoms, re-initiation of therapy can be life threatening [5].

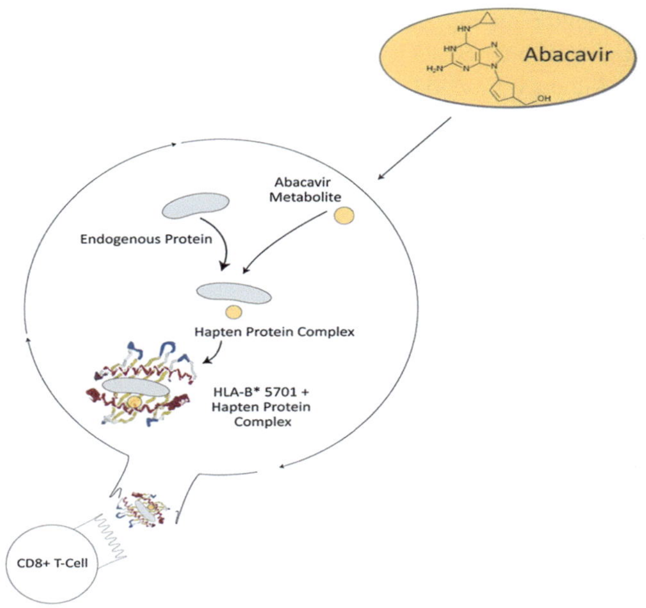

Figure 20.1 Proposed mechanism for HLA-B*5701 abacavir hypersensitivity

In 2002, initial reports of abacavir hypersensitivity reactions occurring in one family suggested a genetic component [6]. Further investigation demonstrated that prevalence of ABC-HSR varied among different ethnic populations, which reinforced the hypothesis of a genetic etiology [7]. Today, the genetics are no longer disputed as it is clear that ABC-HSR is indeed restricted to HLA-B*5701 carriers [4, 8]. Early clues that suggested an immunogenetic mechanism included the symptoms of abacavir hypersensitivity syndrome that had the hallmark features of a cellular delayed-type hypersensitivity reaction. Subsequent observational and experimental data confirmed this suspicion and provided insight into the immunopathogenesis of ABC-HSR [9, 10].

HLA-B*5701 is a class I HLA allele at the B locus, and successful binding of a pathogen-derived peptide by HLA-B*5701 results in presentation to CD8+ T cells and initiation of the adaptive cellular immune response. In this case, a hapten-carrier complex, composed of an abacavir metabolite and an endogenous protein, bind the HLA-B*5701 molecule possibly in the presence of HSP70, resulting in presentation to and activation of CD8+ T cells (Fig. 20.1) [11]. Each HLA-encoded molecule has exquisite specificity and as few as one or two amino acid differences in the peptide-binding cleft of an HLA molecule can change the subset of pathogen-derived peptides each HLA molecule can bind and present. Abacavir presentation is clearly HLA-B*5701 restricted which explains why ABC-HSR is not observed in those who carry closely related alleles such as HLA-B*5702 and HLA-B*5703 that only differ by a few amino acids in the HLA-binding groove.

Australia was one of the earliest countries to introduce routine HLA-B*5701 screening and results from the prospective study that was conducted between 2002 and 2005 demonstrated a significant reduction of ABC-HSR from 8 to 2 % [11, 12]. Additional studies with similar results prompted one of the largest pharmacogenetics clinical trials ever conducted, the Prospective Randomized Evaluation of DNA Screening in a Clinical Trial (PREDICT-1) [13]. This double-blind, randomized trial was also the first study to address the clinical utility of a pharmacogenetic marker to reduce toxicity of a drug. PREDICT-1 enrolled 1,956 patients, who were predominantly Caucasian, from 19 different countries. Patients were randomized into two groups. The control group received standard of care, meaning no screening and administration of abacavir without restriction. The second group received prospective HLA typing and abacavir was withheld from patients who tested positive for HLA-B*5701. One aspect that made this study unique was that all suspected cases of clinical ABC-HSR were confirmed by patch testing. The results obtained were important because prescreening eliminated all cases of patch-confirmed, immunologically mediated, HLA-related abacavir hypersensitivity and yielded 100 % negative predictive value.

Prior to PREDICT-1, reliance on clinical diagnosis had led to inaccurate estimates of the negative predictive value of HLA-B*5701 testing, casting doubts on the utility of prospective screening. This study provided robust evidence for preventive screening in Caucasians, but the lack of ethnic diversity in study participants limited generalization to other ethnic populations. The frequency of the HLA-B*5701 allele varies globally, with a high frequency of 8 % in Caucasians and only 2.5 % in African Americans [14]. The Study for Hypersensitivity to Abacavir and Pharmacogenetic Evaluation (SHAPE) confirmed the reduced prevalence of ABC-HSR in African Americans, but presented clear evidence that screening had applicability across races [15].

Further studies evaluated the cost-effectiveness of pretreatment screening and considered variables such as the frequency of HLA-B*5701 carriers, and the sensitivity and specificity of assays for detection of the HLA-B*5701 allele, as well as the cost of preventive screening, alternative therapies, and treatment of ABC-HSR. The conclusion was that pretreatment screening was a cost-effective approach and the evidence supported adoption of widespread implementation of prescreen testing [16, 17].

Clinical Utility

Clinical utility of prospective screening for HLA-B*5701 to prevent abacavir hypersensitivity reaction is well established. Genetic screening has now been widely adopted in most Western countries, particularly Australia, Ireland, the United Kingdom, and the USA. In 2007, guidelines from the US Department of Health and Human Services that address antiretroviral treatment recommended screening for HLA-B*5701 prior to initiation of abacavir therapy [18]. In 2008, the US Food and Drug Administration also revised the product label and added a black box warning for all abacavir-containing formulations to reflect the new guidelines for HLA-B*5701 screening.

Available Assays

One hurdle for widespread implementation of screening was the availability of a simple, reliable, and inexpensive assay to detect HLA-B*5701 carriers. Because of the level of resolution needed to discriminate between the many closely related alleles present at each locus, sequencing is the gold standard for HLA haplotyping. Generally, HLA-B*5701 haplotyping by sequencing is available only in highly specialized laboratories that perform tissue matching in the setting of organ transplantation. The expense, labor, and expertise required for the sequencing method are barriers to widespread availability of testing. In an effort to overcome these challenges, simplified molecular assays have been developed and some groups have even explored alternative, surrogate markers for HLA-B*5701. Rs2395029(G) allele in the HCP5 region of the HLA complex is in linkage disequilibrium with HLA-B*5701 and has been proposed as a substitute for HLA-B*5701 testing [19, 20]. Genotyping for the rs2395029 T/G SNP is technically less challenging than genotyping for HLA-B*5701, as this necessitates reliable discrimination between closely related alleles, and it is less expensive than sequencing methods; however, as discussed below, this marker does not always correlate with the presence of an HLA-B*5701 allele.

For direct detection of HLA-B*5701, allele-specific PCR methods with gel electrophoresis or melting curve analysis are available commercially [21, 22]. Flow cytometry-based typing is cost effective and also utilized by diagnostic laboratories. A Taqman allelic discrimination assay for the HCP5 rs2395029 T/G SNP has also been described [19]. Sequencing for HLA-B*5701 remains an alternative.

Interpretation of Results

The presence of one HLA-B*5701 allele is sufficient to predispose to ABC-HSR, because HLA expression is codominant. As reviewed above, HLA is extremely polymorphic; therefore, most individuals will be heterozygous at this locus and carry only one copy of the HLA-B*5701 allele. Laboratories may offer HLA-B*5701 allele detection but not all assays directly detect HLA-B*5701. Assays that rely on the detection of the HCP5 rs2395029(G) allele that is in linkage disequilibrium with HLA-B*5701 and is an indirect test for HLA-B*5701 are available in the USA. In the initial study using this approach, 100 % sensitivity and 99.4 % specificity were observed [19]. However, there are now multiple reports that HLA-B*5701 and the HCP5 rs2395029(G) allele are not in complete linkage disequilibrium and patients can be positive for HLA-B*5701 but negative for HCP5 rs2395029 [23, 24].

Although HLA-B*5701 allotype has a negative predictive value approaching 100 %, a negative HLA-B*5701 result does not absolutely preclude the development of ABC-HSR. Therefore, careful clinical observation for signs and symptoms associated with a hypersensitivity reaction remain a vital component of patient care. Abacavir therapy should be withdrawn in individuals with symptoms of a hypersensitivity reaction regardless of the HLA-B*5701 genotype result. Skin patch testing can be used to immunologically confirm ABC-HSR, but has no usefulness in prospective screening. As is typical for most HLA associations with disease or ADRs, the positive predictive value is often low and has been estimated to be only 47 % in this case [13]. In other words, only about half of patients that carry an HLA-B*5701 allele would be expected to develop ABC-HSR when placed on abacavir therapy. Clearly, other genetic or environmental factors contribute to the risk of developing ABC-HSR in patients who are HLA-B*5701 positive.

Hepatitis C and *IL28B* Genotyping

Chronic hepatitis C (HCV) infection affects millions of individuals worldwide with a substantial risk for liver cirrhosis and hepatocellular carcinoma decades after infection. Although the incidence of HCV infection has decreased, the number of patients that will be diagnosed and must be treated is expected to increase for years to come. Current therapeutic regimens can produce a sustained viral response (SVR) and slow or prevent these long-term complications [25]. Current therapy is based on the combined use of interferon and ribavirin (RBV) for infections with HCV genotypes 2 through 6, and beginning in 2011, the combined use of interferon, RBV, and a protease inhibitor for HCV genotype 1 infections [26].

The first important biomarker for guidance of therapy was pre-therapeutic viral genotyping. Genotype 1 infections require longer treatment and have substantially lower rates of SVR. Identification of HCV genotypes 2 or 3 infection allows for a reduction in the length of interferon RBV treatment to 24 weeks compared to 48 weeks for other genotypes. More recently, measurement of the kinetics of viral clearance during therapy has been implemented as standard of care to predict the likelihood of SVR for all HCV genotypes. A rapid viral response (RVR) defined as a fall in HCV viral load to undetectable levels after 4 weeks of therapy strongly predicts SVR. Although RVR is less likely to be achieved with an HCV genotype 1 infection, achieving an RVR is the best predictor of SVR compared to HCV genotype or host physiologic markers. This observation suggests the existence of host factors which affect the likelihood of achieving an

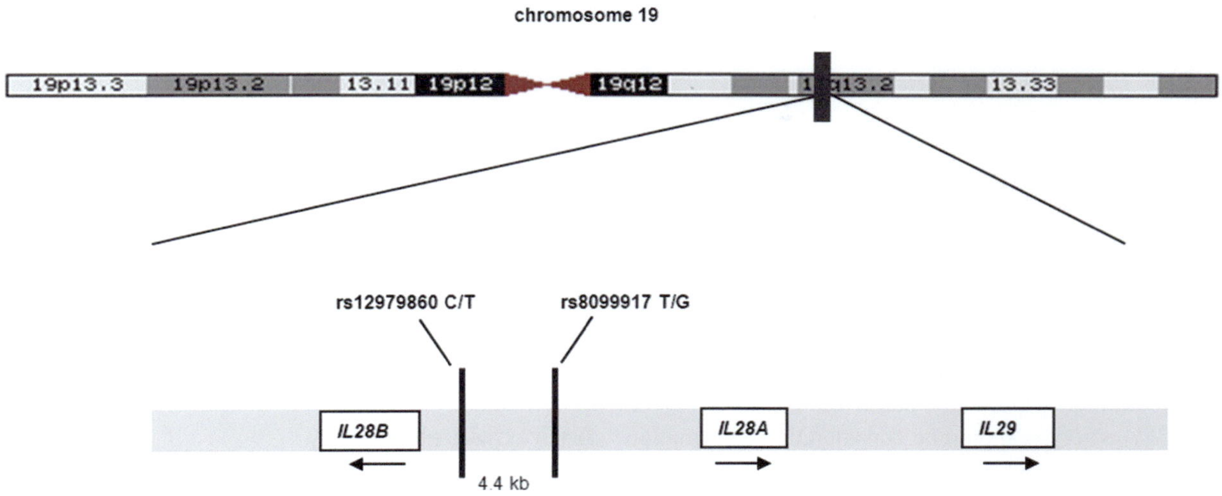

Figure 20.2 Location of SNPs in the *IL28* region

SVR. Until recently, no host genetic markers have been available to predict the likelihood of response or drug toxicity prior to therapy.

In late 2009, a series of papers was published by several groups that performed GWAS seeking biomarkers associated with HCV treatment outcome. Several SNPs were identified on chromosome 19 near the *IL28B* gene that were associated with both spontaneous and treatment-induced HCV clearance (Fig. 20.2) [27–31]. Two SNPs, rs12979860 and rs8099917, have been identified by multiple investigators as having the strongest predictive values for achieving an SVR in patient cohorts of varied ethnic background and have emerged as candidates for *IL28B*-associated genotyping assays. For the rs12979860 C/T SNP those with the CC genotype are two-fold more likely to achieve an SVR and 2.5 times more likely to clear HCV spontaneously, compared to CT heterozygotes or TT homozygotes [28, 29]. For rs8099917, the TT genotype predicts likelihood of an SVR, while TG heterozygotes and GG homozygotes have an increased risk of treatment failure [27].

These associations more powerfully predict spontaneous clearance and therapeutically driven SRV than all previously described host markers including gender, age, liver steatosis, and insulin resistance [32, 33]. In addition, they account for a significant component of the long-appreciated poor treatment outcomes for individuals of African descent. African-American populations have a much higher prevalence of the rs12979860 TT genotype compared to Caucasian or Hispanic populations. African Americans who carry the CC genotype fare better than those carrying CT or TT genotypes but still worse than Caucasian or Hispanic population with the same genotype, suggesting that IL28 explains much but not all of the long-observed differences in HCV spontaneous clearance and treatment response [29].

The mechanism by which *IL28B* genotype exerts its effects remains elusive. The two SNPs, rs 12979860 and rs 8099917, are in linkage disequilibrium, approximately 4 kb apart, and both are located upstream of *IL28B*. The *IL28* gene encodes a type III lambda interferon. Lambda interferons, like alpha interferons, stimulate antiviral effects through the JAK-STAT signaling pathway, but use a different cell surface receptor that is preferentially expressed in hepatocytes. Lambda interferons can inhibit HCV growth in vitro, but the precise mechanism for clearance of HCV in vivo remains uncertain [34, 35]. Further complicating interpretation is that both SNPs associated with HCV response are located upstream of the *IL28B* gene and not in the gene itself. This finding suggests that these SNPs affect transcription of the gene. However, initial messenger RNA expression studies have yielded conflicting results. Although the underlying mechanism has not been clarified, the predictive power of these *IL28B*-associated SNPs for HCV clearance has been unequivocally substantiated.

Clinical Utility

The significance of the *IL28B* genotype was originally discovered in patients infected with HCV genotype 1 who were undergoing standard-of-care (SOC) treatment with interferon and RBV. Subsequent studies have investigated *IL28B* genotype in patients infected with HCV genotypes 1, 2, and 4. Although the results from these investigations support the overall conclusion that favorable *IL28B* genotype is predictive of likelihood of response to treatment, *IL28B* genotype has lower predictive value in patients infected with HCV genotypes other than 1. Clinical trials and one study have investigated the utility of *IL28B* genotyping in the era of direct-acting antiviral therapies. Data demonstrate that those with a favorable *IL28B* genotype are more likely to have abbreviated therapy under this new treatment regimen [36–38]. Individuals with the favorable *IL28B* genotype have higher SVR rates with triple therapy as compared to SOC; therefore, no recommendation can be made for one therapy over another based on *IL28B* genotype.

In summary, *IL28B* genotyping is a strong pretreatment predictor of treatment response to interferon and RBV therapy, as well as protease inhibitor triple therapy, in patients infected with HCV genotype 1. Predictive value is lower in patients infected with HCV genotypes 2 and 3 [26, 33]. Currently, insufficient evidence exists to recommend one therapy over another for HCV genotype 1 or to recommend a specific duration of therapy based on *IL28B* genotype alone. *IL28B* genotype should be considered, if information regarding the likelihood of response and probable duration of response is needed [26].

Available Assays

Both TaqMan allelic discrimination and dual-color fluorescence resonance energy (FRET) probe assays for *IL28B* genotyping have been published and are commercially available [39].

Interpretation of Results

Caution must be taken in interpreting *IL28B* genotype results. First, *IL28B* genotype is primarily a predictive marker for likelihood of response and duration of treatment, but cannot be used to recommend a particular therapy and does not directly dictate duration of treatment. Second, not all individuals with a favorable genotype will achieve a positive treatment outcome, and conversely not all individuals with a risk genotype are destined to fail therapy. Third, *IL28B* genotype assays are now commercially available that genotype for the rs12979860 or the rs8099917 SNP or both, and it is clinically important to know which SNP is the target. These two SNPs are in linkage disequilibrium with *IL28B*, but the degree (strength) of linkage disequilibrium between these two SNPs varies with ethnic background [29, 31, 39, 40]. The two SNPs provide interchangeable information in Caucasians, but not in African Americans. Because both SNPs are tag SNPs and neither is the causal variant, it is not well established which of the two SNPs is more reflective of observed response in patients who are discordant for these two SNPs.

Future Directions

HCV and *ITPA*

GWAS for HCV infection and therapy markers discovered that polymorphisms in the inosine triphosphatase (*ITPA*) gene were associated with hemoglobin concentrations in patients treated with RBV. Follow-up studies identified two variants, rs1127354 and rs7270101, that cause inosine triphosphatase (ITPAse) deficiency and protect patients from RBV-induced hemolytic anemia [41–45]. The rs1127354 C-to-A polymorphism is a missense mutation and the rs7270101 is an A-to-C splice mutation, both of which are significantly and independently associated with enzyme deficiency and protective effects. The biological mechanism is not well defined, but the protective effects have been confirmed. Genotyping assays for *ITPA* polymorphisms are available clinically on a limited basis.

Antiretroviral Therapy

One of the most promising areas of pharmacogenetics is antiretroviral therapy. The introduction of highly active antiretroviral therapy (HAART) in the mid-1990s for treatment of HIV infection has proven to be extremely effective and has virtually transformed HIV infection into a manageable, chronic disease. Because HIV is never cleared, long-term antiretroviral therapy (ART) is necessary for suppressing viral replication and is often complicated not only by emergence of viral resistance, but also by the development of severe toxic syndromes and unexpected health consequences. For example, extended use of ART correlates with an increased risk of developing accelerated atherogenesis and cardiovascular complications (events). Consequently, the link between genetic variations in lipid metabolism or transport genes and dyslipidemia has been examined by many investigators. Polymorphisms in *APOC3*, *APOE*, and *APOA5* genes are believed to significantly contribute to increased triglyceride concentrations in patients on long-term ART, particularly those treated with ritonavir [46–49].

Other host-treatment associations of note include (1) HLA-DRB*0101 class II allele and nevirapine-associated hypersensitivity; (2) atazanavir- and indinavir-induced hyperbilirubinemia associated with *UGT1A1* primarily but also P-gp (formerly *MDR1*) SNPs; (3) tenofovir renal proximal tubulopathy associated with multidrug-resistance protein (MRP2) transporter variation; and (4) efavirenz-associated neurotoxicity attributed to *CYP2B6* differences [46, 47]. Genetic screening has been proposed for both *UGT1A1* and *CYP2B6* prior to atazanavir and efavirenz treatment, respectively. However, even for these well-established associations clinical utility of genetic testing remains controversial, because it is becoming increasingly clear that variation in more than one drug-metabolizing gene and multiple mechanisms may affect the pharmacokinetics of any one drug. The relative contribution of variation in all genes that impact metabolism of a drug has to be determined before utility of genotyping for one or multiple markers can be demonstrated. Currently, the majority of these associations are of research interest only due to the many limitations of pharmacogenetics, as discussed above. Perhaps the foremost limitations are the lack of widespread applicability and well-designed cost-effectiveness studies. Nevertheless, HLA-B*5701 is a great example that genetic associations can be successfully translated into clinical practice if the appropriate studies are conducted. There is considerable anticipation that personalized HAART pharmacogenetics will be possible in the near future.

Tuberculosis

Tuberculosis (TB) is an infectious disease with a long history. There is resurgence in the global morbidity and mortality caused by TB, primarily due to the emergence of antibiotic-resistant Mycobacterium strains and HIV coinfection. Globally, the prevalence of TB has been estimated at 30 %, with the highest burden in developing nations. SOC treatment for TB is a combination of multiple drugs: rifampicin, streptomycin/ethambutol, and pyrazinamide combined with isoniazid. Serious dose-dependent side effects associated with isoniazid therapy, mainly hepatotoxicity, were apparent as early as the 1970s. It is now well accepted that polymorphisms in *NAT2* are responsible for the differential extent of N-acetylation of isoniazid and observed phenotypes. Genetic testing for this marker could reduce dose-dependent ADRs in slow metabolizers while increasing efficacy in fast metabolizers or acetylators. Appropriate patient dosing based on genetic testing likely would increase patient compliance with the added benefit of minimizing drug resistance. Drug resistance is a growing problem and has led to combination therapy as the mainstay for TB treatment. Although *NAT2* testing is not recommended prior to prescribing isoniazid, pharmacogenetic information regarding the role of NAT2 in isoniazid metabolism is included in US drug labels. *NAT2* genotyping or phenotyping is not widely available.

Malaria

Malaria is one of the deadliest infectious diseases known to man, with an enormous human and financial toll. Ironically, one of the earliest examples of an ADR associated with host genetics was the recognition that those who have glucose-6-phosphate dehydrogenase (G6PD) deficiency develop severe hemolytic anemia when administered primaquine, an antimalarial drug introduced in 1950 [50]. Importantly, G6PD deficiency is still relevant to developing efficacious antimalarial drugs, and as recently as 2008, complications due to G6PD deficiency caused withdrawal of chlorproguanil/dapsone therapy [51–53]. Antimalarial drugs have been available for decades and were initially effective and relatively inexpensive. However, monotherapy approaches to treatment led to widespread resistance. Hope was restored around 2000 with the development of artemisinin combination therapies (ACT). ACT is predicated on different classes of drugs with different modes of action for parasite elimination, impeding the emergence of drug-resistant parasites. At the moment, the three ACT options widely utilized for TB management are amodiaquine and artesunate, artemether-lumefantrine, and artesunate-mefloquine [54].

The availability of ample data for both components of the amodiaquine-artesunate ACT therapy provides a good illustration of the potential for pharmacogenetic testing in the setting of malaria. Amodiaquine has a well-established association with severe toxicity. Concerns over high rates of lethal agranulocytosis and hepatoxicity observed in Caucasians prompted removal of this drug from the WHO Essential Medicines List, but it had to be reintroduced due to growing resistance to remaining therapeutic options [55–57]. The adverse reaction has been attributed to the *CYP2C8*2* polymorphism. Impaired amodiaquine metabolism by *CYP2C8*2* results in accumulation of a toxic metabolite and the severe adverse reactions. Despite the fact that other *CYP2C8* low activity-alleles, such as *3 and *4, have been identified in Zanzibar, the first line of therapy in this country is amodiaquine-artesunate, placing this population at increased risk of adverse events [58]. Overall, the percentage of individuals at risk for developing an ADR is small, but this translates into large absolute numbers due to the vast number of people who need to be treated. In contrast, therapy regimens including amodiaquine would be well suited to West Africa, where low-activity alleles are rarely found [51, 54].

Conversion of artesunate to the active metabolite dihydroartemisinin (DHA) is dependent on CYP2A6 [59]. *CYP2A6* is highly polymorphic with approximately 40 gene variants [60]. Many of these have decreased metabolizing function and some alleles have no activity in vivo. Clearly, prescribing therapy containing artesunate to individuals that do not have the ability to convert the drug to an active metabolite is futile. Furthermore, for those who have reduced metabolizing capacity, the concentration of active metabolite formed is insufficient, severely impairing parasite elimination and increasing the potential for development of drug resistance. Reports suggest that resistance to artesunate-based therapy is already as high as 10 % in some parts of the globe, such as Thailand [61]. Interestingly, Thailand has a high prevalence of low-activity alleles [62] and this may have contributed to the emergence of drug-resistant strains in this location [51].

For malaria and to some extent TB, it is not likely that personalized medicine would be possible, given the cost of genetic testing compared to treatment and the great number of patients that would require testing. For both, however, population-level application of pharmacogenetics could have important implications for global disease control. Simply knowing the frequencies of relevant genetic polymorphisms at the population level may shape a global strategy and drug policy for the developing world that would increase therapeutic efficacy, minimize adverse reactions, and diminish the potential for drug resistance. Drug resistance is an increasingly difficult problem that is even more acute in the context of a pathogen that infects 100 million people annually and for which only a limited number of effective drugs exist.

Summary

In summary, advances in technology coupled with intensive studies have improved our understanding of the underlying basis of the genetics associated with disease and drug response. Despite significant progress made from the biological perspective, translation to routine medical practice for most discoveries is lagging. Demonstration of the clinical utility of genetic association using large, well-designed prospective clinical trials is just the first step in translating a pharmacogenetic test into routine healthcare. Test endorsements in consensus statements and practice guidelines are pivotal for acceptance. Furthermore, the speed of adoption is often influenced by logistical considerations such as widespread access to a reliable and cost-effective test and reasonable reimbursement for the test. Nevertheless, good examples now exist of successful implementation of pharmacogenetic testing in medical practice and there is ample hope that future applications of pharmacogenomics are likely to become important in infectious disease treatment.

References

1. Becquemont L. HLA: a pharmacogenomics success story. Pharmacogenomics. 2010;11(3):277–81. doi:10.2217/pgs.10.38.
2. Goldstein DB. Common genetic variation and human traits. N Engl J Med. 2009;360(17):1696–8. doi:10.1056/NEJMp0806284.
3. Hirschhorn JN. Genome-wide association studies–illuminating biologic pathways. N Engl J Med. 2009;360(17):1699–701. doi:10.1056/NEJMp0808934.
4. Hetherington S, Hughes AR, Mosteller M, Shortino D, Baker KL, Spreen W, et al. Genetic variations in HLA-B region and hypersensitivity reactions to abacavir. Lancet. 2002;359(9312):1121–2.
5. Shapiro M, Ward KM, Stern JJ. A near-fatal hypersensitivity reaction to abacavir: case report and literature review. AIDS Read. 2001;11(4):222–6.
6. Peyriere H, Nicholas J, Siffert M, Demoly P, Hillaire-Buys D, Reynes J. Hypersensitivity related to abacavir in two members of a family. Ann Pharmacother. 2001;35(10):1291–2.
7. Hughes AR, Mosteller M, Bansal AT, Davies K, Hameline SA, Lai EH, et al. Association of genetic variations in HLA-B region with hypersensitivity to abacavir in some, but not all populations. Pharmaocogenomics. 2004;5(2):203–11.
8. Mallal S, Nolan D, Witt C, Masel G, Martin AM, Moore C, et al. Association between presence of HLA-B*5701, HLA-DR7 and HLA-DQ3 and hypersensitivity to HIV-1 reverse transcriptase inhibitor abacavir. Lancet. 2002;359(9308):727–32.
9. Chessman D, Kostenko L, Lethborg T, Purcell AW, Williamson NA, Zea C. Human leukocyte antigen class I-restricted activation of CD8+ T cells provides the immunogenetic basis of a systemic drug hypersensitivity. Immunity. 2008;29(1):165.
10. Phillips EJ, Wong GA, Kaul R, Shahabi K, Nolan DA, Knowles SR, et al. Clinical and immunogenetic correlates of abacavir hypersensitivity. AIDS. 2005;19(9):979–81.
11. Martin AM, Nolan D, Gaudieri S, Almeida CA, Nolan R, James I, et al. Predisposition to abacavir hypersensitivity conferred by HLA-B*5701 and a haplotypic Hsp70-Hom variant. Proc Natl Acad Sci U S A. 2004;10(12):4180–5.
12. Rauch A, Nolan D, Martin A, McKinnon E, Almeida C, Mallal S. Prospective genetic screening decreases the incidence of abacavir hypersensitivity reactions in the Western Australian HIV cohort study. Clin Infect Dis. 2006;43(1):99–102.
13. Mallal SA, Phillips E, Carosi G, Molina JM, Workman C, Jea T. HLA-B*5701 screening for hypersensitivity to abacavir. N Engl J Med. 2008;358(6):568–79.
14. Nolan D, Gaudieri S, Mallal S. Pharmacogenetics: a practical role in predicting antiretroviral drug toxicity? J HIV Ther. 2003;8(2):36–41.
15. Saag MS, Balu R, Phillips E, Brachman P, Martorell C, Burman W, et al. High sensitivity of human leukocyte antigen-B*5701 as a marker for immunologically confirmed abacavir hypersensitivity in white and black patients. Clin Infect Dis. 2008;46(7):1111–8.
16. Schackman BR, Scott CA, Walensky RP, Losina E, Freedberg KA, Sax PE. The cost-effectiveness of HLA-B*5701 genetic screening to guide initial antiretroviral therapy for HIV. AIDS. 2008;22(15):2025–33. doi:10.1097/QAD.0b013e3283103ce6.
17. Hughes DA, Vilar FJ, Ward CC, Alfirevic A, Park BK, Pirmohamed M. Cost-effectiveness analysis of HLA B*5701 genotyping in preventing abacavir hypersensitivity. Pharmacogenetics. 2004;14(6):335–42.
18. Department of Health and Human Services PoAGfAaA (2008) Guidelines for the Use of antiretroviral agents in HIV-1-infected adults and adolescents.
19. Colombo S, Rauch A, Rotger M. The HCP5 single-nucleotide polymorphism: a simple screening tool for prediction of hypersensitivity reaction to abacavir. J Infect Dis. 2008;198(9):1415.
20. Sanchez-Giron F, Villegas-Torres B, Jaramillo-Villafuerte K, Silva-Zolezzi I, Fernandez-Lopez JC, Jimenez-Sanchez G, Carnevale A. Association of the genetic marker for abacavir hypersensitivity HLA-B*5701 with HCP5 rs2395029 in Mexican Mestizos. Pharmacogenomics. 2011;12(6):809–14. doi:10.2217/pgs.11.31.
21. Martin AM, Nolan D, Mallal S. HLA-B*5701 typing by sequence-specific amplification: validation and comparison with sequence-based typing. Tissue Antigens. 2005;65(6):571–4. doi:10.1111/j.1399-0039.2005.00401.x.
22. Hammond E, Mamotte C, Nolan D, Mallal S. HLA-B*5701 typing: evaluation of an allele-specific polymerase chain reaction melting assay. Tissue Antigens. 2007;70(1):58–61. doi:10.1111/j.1399-0039.2007.00840.x.
23. Badulli C, Sestini R, Sbarsi I, Baroncelli M, Pizzochero C, Martinetti M, Porfirio B. Tag SNPs of the ancestral haplotype 57.1 do not substitute HLA-B*57:01 typing for eligibility to abacavir treatment in the Italian population. Pharmacogenomics. 2012;13(3):247–9. doi:10.2217/pgs.11.168.
24. Phillips E, Nolan D, Thornborn D, Schaefer M, Laird R, Rauch A, et al. Genetic factors predicting abacavir hypersensitivity and tolerance in HLA-B*5701 positive individuals. Eur J Dermatol. 2008;18(2):247.

25. Morgan T, Ghany M, Kim H, Snow K, Shiffman ML, De Santo J, Lee W, Di Bisceglie A, Bonkovsky H, Dienstag J, Morishima C, Lindsay K, Lok AS. Outcome of sustained virological responders with histologically advanced chronic hepatitis C. Hepatology. 2010;52:833–44.
26. Ghany MG, Nelson DR, Strader DB, Thomas DL, Seeff LB, American Association for Study of Liver D. An update on treatment of genotype 1 chronic hepatitis C virus infection: 2011 practice guideline by the American Association for the Study of Liver Diseases. Hepatology. 2011;54(4):1433–44. doi:10.1002/hep.24641.
27. Tanaka Y, Nishida N, Sugiyama M, Kurosaki M, Matsuura K, Sakamoto N, Nakagawa M, Korenaga M, Hino K, Hige S, Ito Y, Mita E, Tanaka E, Mochida S, Murawaki Y, Honda M, Sakai A, Hiasa Y, Nishiguchi S, Koike A, Sakaida I, Imamura M, Ito K, Yano K, Masaki N, Sugauchi F, Izumi N, Tokunaga K, Mizokami M. Genome-wide association of IL28B with response to pegylated interferon-alpha and ribavirin therapy for chronic hepatitis C. Nat Genet. 2009;41(10):1105–9. doi:10.1038/ng.449. ng.449 [pii].
28. Thomas DL, Thio CL, Martin MP, Qi Y, Ge D, O'Huigin C, Kidd J, Kidd K, Khakoo SI, Alexander G, Goedert JJ, Kirk GD, Donfield SM, Rosen HR, Tobler LH, Busch MP, McHutchison JG, Goldstein DB, Carrington M. Genetic variation in IL28B and spontaneous clearance of hepatitis C virus. Nature. 2009;461(7265):798–801. doi:10.1038/nature08463.
29. Ge D, Fellay J, Thompson AJ, Simon JS, Shianna KV, Urban TJ, Heinzen EL, Qiu P, Bertelsen AH, Muir AJ, Sulkowski M, McHutchison JG, Goldstein DB. Genetic variation in IL28B predicts hepatitis C treatment-induced viral clearance. Nature. 2009;461(7262):399–401. doi:10.1038/nature08309.
30. Suppiah V, Moldovan M, Ahlenstiel G, Berg T, Weltman M, Abate ML, Bassendine M, Spengler U, Dore GJ, Powell E, Riordan S, Sheridan D, Smedile A, Fragomeli V, Muller T, Bahlo M, Stewart GJ, Booth DR, George J. IL28B is associated with response to chronic hepatitis C interferon-alpha and ribavirin therapy. Nat Genet. 2009;41(10):1100–4. doi:10.1038/ng.447. ng.447 [pii].
31. Rauch A, Kutalik Z, Descombes P, Cai T, Di Iulio J, Mueller T, Bochud M, Battegay M, Bernasconi E, Borovicka J, Colombo S, Cerny A, Dufour JF, Furrer H, Gunthard HF, Heim M, Hirschel B, Malinverni R, Moradpour D, Mullhaupt B, Witteck A, Beckmann JS, Berg T, Bergmann S, Negro F, Telenti A, Bochud PY, Swiss Hepatitis CCS, Swiss HIVCS. Genetic variation in IL28B is associated with chronic hepatitis C and treatment failure: a genome-wide association study. Gastroenterology. 2010;138(4):1338–45. doi:10.1053/j.gastro.2009.12.056. 1345.e1331-1337.
32. Thompson AJ, Muir AJ, Sulkowski MS, Ge D, Fellay J, Shianna KV, Urban T, Afdhal NH, Jacobson IM, Esteban R, Poordad F, Lawitz EJ, McCone J, Shiffman ML, Galler GW, Lee WM, Reindollar R, King JW, Kwo PY, Ghalib RH, Freilich B, Nyberg LM, Zeuzem S, Poynard T, Vock DM, Pieper KS, Patel K, Tillmann HL, Noviello S, Koury K, Pedicone LD, Brass CA, Albrecht JK, Goldstein DB, McHutchison JG. Interleukin-28B polymorphism improves viral kinetics and is the strongest pretreatment predictor of sustained virologic response in genotype 1 hepatitis C virus. Gastroenterology. 2010;139(1):120–129.e118. doi:10.1053/j.gastro.2010.04.013.
33. Mangia A, Thompson AJ, Santoro R, Piazzolla V, Tillmann HL, Patel K, Shianna KV, Mottola L, Petruzzellis D, Bacca D, Carretta V, Minerva N, Goldstein DB, McHutchison JG. An IL28B polymorphism determines treatment response of hepatitis C virus genotype 2 or 3 patients who do not achieve a rapid virologic response. Gastroenterology. 2010;139(3):821–7. doi:10.1053/j.gastro.2010.05.079. 827.e821.
34. Robek MD, Boyd BS, Chisari FV. Lambda interferon inhibits hepatitis B and C virus replication. J Virol. 2005;79(6):3851–4. doi:10.1128/JVI.79.6.3851-3854.2005.
35. Thio CL, Thomas DL. Interleukin-28b: a key piece of the hepatitis C virus recovery puzzle. Gastroenterology. 2010;138(4):1240–3. doi:10.1053/j.gastro.2010.02.033.
36. Akuta N, Suzuki F, Hirakawa M, Kawamura Y, Yatsuji H, Sezaki H, Suzuki Y, Hosaka T, Kobayashi M, Kobayashi M, Saitoh S, Arase Y, Ikeda K, Chayama K, Nakamura Y, Kumada H. Amino acid substitution in hepatitis C virus core region and genetic variation near the interleukin 28B gene predict viral response to telaprevir with peginterferon and ribavirin. Hepatology. 2010;52(2):421–9. doi:10.1002/hep.23690.
37. Poordad F, Bronowicki JP, Gordon S, Zeuzem S, Jacobson IM, Sulkowski M, et al. IL28B polymorphism predicts virological response in patients with chronic hepatitis C genotype 1 treated with boceprevir (BOC) combination therapy. J Hepatol. 2011;54 suppl 1:S6.
38. Jacobson IM, Catlett I, Marcellin P, et al. Telaprevir substantially improves SVR rates across all IL28b genotypes in the advanced trial. J Hepatol. 2011;54(S1):S1369.
39. Melis R, Fauron C, McMillin G, Lyon E, Shirts B, Hubley LM, Slev PR. Simultaneous genotyping of rs12979860 and rs8099917 variants near the IL28B locus associated with HCV clearance and treatment response. J Mol Diagn. 2011;13(4):446–51. doi:10.1016/j.jmoldx.2011.03.008.
40. Tanaka Y, Nishida N, Sugiyama M, Tokunaga K, Mizokami M. lambda-Interferons and the single nucleotide polymorphisms: a milestone to tailor-made therapy for chronic hepatitis C. Hepatol Res. 2010;40(5):449–60. HEP671 [pii].
41. Tanaka Y, Kurosaki M, Nishida N, Sugiyama M, Matsuura K, Sakamoto N, Enomoto N, Yatsuhashi H, Nishiguchi S, Hino K, Hige S, Itoh Y, Tanaka E, Mochida S, Honda M, Hiasa Y, Koike A, Sugauchi F, Kaneko S, Izumi N, Tokunaga K, Mizokami M. Genome-wide association study identified ITPA/DDRGK1 variants reflecting thrombocytopenia in pegylated interferon and ribavirin therapy for chronic hepatitis C. Hum Mol Genet. 2011;20(17):3507–16. doi:10.1093/hmg/ddr249.
42. Sakamoto N, Tanaka Y, Nakagawa M, Yatsuhashi H, Nishiguchi S, Enomoto N, Azuma S, Nishimura-Sakurai Y, Kakinuma S, Nishida N, Tokunaga K, Honda M, Ito K, Mizokami M, Watanabe M. ITPA gene variant protects against anemia induced by pegylated interferon-alpha and ribavirin therapy for Japanese patients with chronic hepatitis C. Hepatol Res. 2010;40(11):1063–71. doi:10.1111/j.1872-034X.2010.00741.x.
43. Azakami T, Hayes CN, Sezaki H, Kobayashi M, Akuta N, Suzuki F, Kumada H, Abe H, Miki D, Tsuge M, Imamura M, Kawakami Y, Takahashi S, Ochi H, Nakamura Y, Kamatani N, Chayama K. Common genetic polymorphism of ITPA gene affects ribavirin-induced anemia and effect of peg-interferon plus ribavirin therapy. J Med Virol. 2011;83(6):1048–57. doi:10.1002/jmv.22069.
44. Fellay J, Thompson AJ, Ge D, Gumbs CE, Urban TJ, Shianna KV, Little LD, Qiu P, Bertelsen AH, Watson M, Warner A, Muir AJ, Brass C, Albrecht J, Sulkowski M, McHutchison JG, Goldstein DB. ITPA gene variants protect against anaemia in patients treated for chronic hepatitis C. Nature. 2010;464(7287):405–8. doi:10.1038/nature08825.
45. Thompson AJ, Santoro R, Piazzolla V, Clark PJ, Naggie S, Tillmann HL, Patel K, Muir AJ, Shianna KV, Mottola L, Petruzzellis D, Romano M, Sogari F, Facciorusso D, Goldstein DB, McHutchison JG, Mangia A. Inosine triphosphatase genetic variants are protective against anemia during antiviral therapy for HCV2/3 but do not decrease dose reductions of RBV or increase SVR. Hepatology. 2011;53:389. doi:10.1002/hep.24068.
46. Tozzi V. Pharmacogenetics of antiretrovirals. Antiviral Res. 2010;85(1):190–200. doi:10.1016/j.antiviral.2009.09.001.
47. Phillips EJ, Mallal SA. Pharmacogenetics and the potential for the individualization of antiretroviral therapy. Curr Opin Infect Dis. 2008;21(1):16–24. doi:10.1097/QCO.0b013e3282f42224.

48. Foulkes AS, Wohl DA, Frank I, Puleo E, Restine S, Wolfe ML, Dube MP, Tebas P, Reilly MP. Associations among race/ethnicity, ApoC-III genotypes, and lipids in HIV-1-infected individuals on antiretroviral therapy. PLoS Med. 2006;3(3):e52. doi:10.1371/journal.pmed.0030052.
49. Arnedo M, Taffe P, Sahli R, Furrer H, Hirschel B, Elzi L, Weber R, Vernazza P, Bernasconi E, Darioli R, Bergmann S, Beckmann JS, Telenti A, Tarr PE, Swiss HIVCS. Contribution of 20 single nucleotide polymorphisms of 13 genes to dyslipidemia associated with antiretroviral therapy. Pharmacogenet Genomics. 2007;17(9):755–64. doi:10.1097/FPC.0b013e32814db8b7.
50. Alving AS, Carson PE, Flanagan CL, Ickes CE. Enzymatic deficiency in primaquine-sensitive erythrocytes. Science. 1956;124(3220):484–5.
51. Roederer MW, McLeod H, Juliano JJ. Can pharmacogenomics improve malaria drug policy? Bull World Health Organ. 2011; 89(11):838–45.
52. Phillips-Howard PA, West LJ. Serious adverse drug reactions to pyrimethamine-sulphadoxine, pyrimethamine-dapsone and to amodiaquine in Britain. J R Soc Med. 1990;83(2):82–5.
53. GlaxoSmithKline. Update on GSK's malaria treatments: Dacart and Lapdap, 2008.
54. Piedade R, Gil JP. The pharmacogenetics of antimalaria artemisinin combination therapy. Expert Opin Drug Metab Toxicol. 2011;7(10):1185–200. doi:10.1517/17425255.2011.608660.
55. Raymond JM, Dumas F, Baldit C, Couzigou P, Beraud C, Amouretti M. Fatal acute hepatitis due to amodiaquine. J Clin Gastroenterol. 1989;11(5):602–3.
56. Olliaro P, Nevill C, LeBras J, Ringwald P, Mussano P, Garner P, Brasseur P. Systematic review of amodiaquine treatment in uncomplicated malaria. Lancet. 1996;348(9036):1196–201. doi:10.1016/S0140-6736(96)06217-4.
57. Ferreira PE, Cavaco I, Gil JP. Pharmacogenetic tools for malaria and TB in the Developing World. Fut Med. 2008;5(6):627–39.
58. Cavaco I, Stromberg-Norklit J, Kaneko A, Msellem MI, Dahoma M, Ribeiro VL, Bjorkman A, Gil JP. CYP2C8 polymorphism frequencies among malaria patients in Zanzibar. Eur J Clin Pharmacol. 2005;61(1):15–8. doi:10.1007/s00228-004-0871-8.
59. Ilett KF, Ethell BT, Maggs JL, Davis TM, Batty KT, Burchell B, Binh TQ, le Thu TA, Hung NC, Pirmohamed M, Park BK, Edwards G. Glucuronidation of dihydroartemisinin in vivo and by human liver microsomes and expressed UDP-glucuronosyltransferases. Drug Metab Dispos. 2002;30(9):1005–12.
60. Di YM, Chow VD, Yang LP, Zhou SF. Structure, function, regulation and polymorphism of human cytochrome P450 2A6. Curr Drug Metab. 2009;10(7):754–80.
61. White NJ. Qinghaosu (artemisinin): the price of success. Science. 2008;320(5874):330–4. doi:10.1126/science.1155165.
62. Noedl H, Socheat D, Satimai W. Artemisinin-resistant malaria in Asia. N Engl J Med. 2009;361(5):540–1. doi:10.1056/NEJMc0900231.

21 Pharmacogenetics

Stuart A. Scott and Elaine Lyon

Abstract

Pharmacogenetics is the study of the genetic determinants of drug response variability. Some pharmacogenetic tests can be used to explain or predict adverse events and/or non-responsiveness to therapy. The goal and promise of clinical pharmacogenetic testing is to deliver the right drug to the right person at the right dose. As such, when a genetic variant directly involved in drug response variability is identified in a patient prior to initiating therapy, adverse reactions, excessive use of ineffective drugs, or ineffective dosing can hopefully be prevented. Despite challenges to demonstrate clinical utility, clinical tests are currently available for selected genes where clinical validity has largely been established. This chapter describes pharmacogenetic applications for which clinical tests are currently available, including *CYP2D6*, *CYP2C19*, *CYP2C9* and *VKORC1*, *TPMT*, and *UGT1A1*.

Keywords

Pharmacogenetics • Drug metabolism • Cytochrome P450 • Thiopurine *S*-methyltransferase • Toxicity • Warfarin • Irinotecan

Introduction

Pharmacogenetics is the study of the genetic determinants of drug response variability. Accordingly, pharmacogenetic variant alleles often occur in genes that encode drug metabolism enzymes and alter their enzymatic activity. These enzymes can activate a prodrug to its active form or catalyze the inactivation and elimination of a drug or metabolite. Prominent among these enzymes are the cytochrome P450 (CYP450) superfamily, which directly influence the pharmacokinetics of many drugs. In addition, genetic variants in cell receptors can influence drug transport, which often plays a role in pharmacodynamics. Consequently, pharmacogenetic tests are now available that can be used to explain or predict adverse events or non-responsiveness to therapy. The goal and promise of clinical pharmacogenetic testing is to deliver the right drug to the right person at the right dose. As such, when a genetic variant directly involved in drug response variability is identified in a patient prior to initiating therapy, adverse reactions, excessive use of ineffective drugs, or ineffective dosing can potentially be prevented.

Despite many robust associations between specific variant alleles and drug response variability, the clinical utility of pharmacogenetic genotyping has been difficult to establish for some clinical applications. Important pharmacogenetic variants are often rare in the general population, which makes identifying enough individuals with a particular genotype in the research setting challenging. To achieve an adequate sample size, some studies group heterozygotes (one variant) and homozygotes or compound heterozygotes (two

S.A. Scott, Ph.D.
Department of Genetics and Genomic Sciences, Icahn School of Medicine at Mount Sinai, New York, NY, USA

Mount Sinai Genetic Testing Laboratory, New York, NY, USA

E. Lyon, Ph.D. (✉)
Department of Pathology, University of Utah School of Medicine, 500 Chipeta Way, MS-115, Salt Lake City, UT 84108, USA

Molecular Genetics and Genomics, ARUP Laboratories, 500 Chipeta Way, MS-115, Salt Lake City, UT 84108, USA
e-mail: lyone@aruplab.com

D.G.B. Leonard (ed.), *Molecular Pathology in Clinical Practice*, DOI 10.1007/978-3-319-19674-9_21

variants) together, yet many enzymes exhibit an autosomal recessive inheritance. By combining the two genotypes, the effect of two variants, and therefore the true "poor metabolizers," may not be evident.

Since genotyping may not detect all variants that affect drug metabolism, it does not necessarily replace the need for drug monitoring when indicated. Other factors such as concomitant medications, comorbidities, and diet often affect drug metabolism and drug levels. Despite these challenges, clinical genetic tests are currently available for selected genes where clinical validity has largely been established. This chapter describes clinical pharmacogenetic applications for which tests currently are available, including genotyping tests for variants in *CYP2D6*, *CYP2C19*, *CYP2C9* and *VKORC1*, *TPMT*, and *UGT1A1*.

CYP2D6

Cytochrome P450-2D6 (CYP2D6) is an important isoenzyme of the P450 superfamily that is involved in the metabolism of approximately 25 % of commonly prescribed drugs, including tamoxifen [1], alpha-blockers, analgesics [2], antidepressants [3], antihypertensives [4], antipsychotics [5], β-receptor blockers [6], norepinephrine reuptake inhibitors [7], and others. More than 100 *CYP2D6* alleles have been described (http://www.cypalleles.ki.se/cyp2d6.htm); however, many are rare in the general population. Although the effect of all of these variant alleles on enzyme activity has not been established, many of the commonly interrogated *CYP2D6* variants include nonfunctional, reduced-, and increased-function alleles. The combination of these alleles in a given genotype results in four predicted phenotype categories: ultrafast (ultrarapid), extensive (normal), intermediate, and poor metabolizers [8]. Depending on the drug, CYP2D6 may be involved in the activation of a prodrug or inactivation of an active drug. Consequently, reduced CYP2D6 activity due to loss-of-function alleles can result in ineffective treatment when activating a prodrug or adverse reactions by allowing toxic compounds to accumulate due to impaired drug inactivation.

Clinical Utility

Although the clinical utility of testing for *CYP2D6* variants has been difficult to establish for many medications, it has been shown for a few drugs. Tamoxifen is metabolized by CYP2D6 to its active metabolite endoxifen [9], although other cytochrome P450 enzymes also are involved (e.g., CYP2C19, CYP2C9, CYP3A4/5). As such, *CYP2D6* genotyping can be used to identify individuals in which tamoxifen is potentially less effective. Identification of a poor metabolizer may help in drug or dose adjustment. Less is understood for intermediate metabolizers, although a potential dose modification may be considered. However, routine testing for women being placed on tamoxifen is not currently recommended due to conflicting data in the literature [10].

The Clinical Pharmacogenetics Implementation Consortium (CPIC) has published practice guidelines for the use of *CYP2D6* genotyping to guide codeine therapy [11, 12] (Table 21.1). Evidence also exists for a role of *CYP2D6* genotyping for individualized treatment with tricyclic antidepressants, which also has prompted a recent CPIC guideline [13]. For example, CYP2D6 poor metabolizers treated with amitriptyline and nortriptyline have impaired drug metabolism and increased risks of side effects, whereas ultrafast metabolizers have elevated risks of reduced drug efficacy due to rapid drug elimination (Table 21.2). Evidence supporting a role for *CYP2D6* in selective serotonin reuptake inhibitor response variability also exists and a CPIC guideline is currently in development (http://www.pharmgkb.org/page/cpic).

Table 21.1 CPIC recommendations for *CYP2D6*-directed dosing of codeine[a]

Predicted CYP2D6 metabolism phenotype	Implications for codeine metabolism	Therapeutic recommendations
Ultrarapid metabolizer (UM)	Increased formation of morphine following codeine administration, leading to higher risk of toxicity	Avoid codeine use due to potential for toxicity
Extensive metabolizer (EM)	Normal morphine formation	Use label-recommended age- or weight-specific dosing
Intermediate metabolizer (IM)	Reduced morphine formation	Use label-recommended age- or weight-specific dosing. If no response, consider alternative analgesics such as morphine or a non-opioid
Poor metabolizer (PM)	Greatly reduced morphine formation following codeine administration, leading to insufficient pain relief	Avoid codeine use due to lack of efficacy

CPIC Clinical Pharmacogenetics Implementation Consortium
[a]Adapted from Crews et al. [12]

Table 21.2 CPIC recommendations for *CYP2D6*-directed dosing of tricyclic antidepressants[a,b]

Predicted CYP2D6 metabolism phenotype	Implications for tricyclic antidepressant metabolism	Therapeutic recommendations
Ultrarapid metabolizer (UM)	Increased metabolism of tricyclics to less active compounds when compared to extensive metabolizers. Lower plasma concentrations will increase the probability of pharmacotherapy failure	Avoid tricyclic use due to potential lack of efficacy. Consider alternative drug not metabolized by CYP2D6 If a tricyclic is warranted, consider increasing the starting dose. Utilize therapeutic drug monitoring to guide dose adjustments
Extensive metabolizer (EM)	Normal metabolism of tricyclics	Initiate therapy with recommended starting dose
Intermediate metabolizer (IM)	Reduced metabolism of tricyclics to less active compounds when compared to extensive metabolizers. Higher plasma concentrations will increase the probability of side effects	Consider 25 % reduction of recommended starting dose. Utilize therapeutic drug monitoring to guide dose adjustments
Poor metabolizer (PM)	Greatly reduced metabolism of tricyclics to less active compounds when compared to extensive metabolizers. Higher plasma concentrations will increase the probability of side effects	Avoid tricyclic use due to potential for side effects. Consider alternative drug not metabolized by CYP2D6 If a tricyclic is warranted, consider 50 % reduction of recommended starting dose. Utilize therapeutic drug monitoring to guide dose adjustments

CPIC Clinical Pharmacogenetics Implementation Consortium
[a]Adapted from Hicks et al. [13]
[b]Note that dosing guidelines for tricyclic antidepressants and *CYP2C19* genotype-directed therapy were also reported [13]. Optional dosing recommendations based on both *CYP2D6* and *CYP2C19* can be found in the supplemental material of Hicks et al. [13].

Available Assays

CYP2D6 genotyping typically is performed by platforms that simultaneously detect multiple variants across the gene (Fig. 21.1). Several commercial assays are currently available, including the AmpliChip® (Affymetrix/Roche [14]), Luminex [15], and AutoGenomics [16] assays, as well as other laboratory-developed tests (e.g., single-nucleotide extension assay) [17]. The AmpliChip® CYP450 Test (Roche Diagnostics, Indianapolis, IN) is an oligonucleotide microarray hybridization method that tests variants in both *CYP2D6* and *CYP2C19*. The Tag-It™ Luminex (Luminex Molecular Diagnostics, Toronto, Canada) platform is a bead array with oligonucleotides bound to microspheres and genotyping by allele-specific primer extension. The AutoGenomics (Carlsbad, CA) platform is a film-based microarray tested on the INFINITI® PLUS Analyzer. These assays typically interrogate 15–20 important *CYP2D6* variants including the deletion and duplication alleles.

Interpretation

CYP2D6 alleles are designated by the common star (*) allele nomenclature system, which often include multiple variants on the same haplotype. The *CYP2D6*1* allele is the wild-type haplotype encoding normal enzyme activity; however, this is typically assigned in the absence of other detected variants. Consequently, when **1* is reported by targeted genotyping, a rare *CYP2D6* star (*) allele not included in the genotyping panel would not be detected, which can only be identified by gene sequencing. Commonly interrogated *CYP2D6* alleles are summarized in Table 21.3.

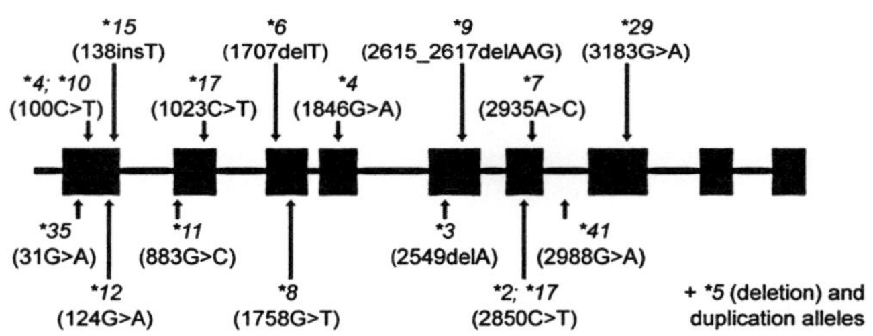

Figure 21.1 Gene diagram of *CYP2D6* (and chromosome location) indicating common alleles and their molecular alteration (in *parentheses*), including the deletion (*5) and duplication alleles. Note that variants are referred to by their common names (GenBank Accession Number M33388)

Two functional *CYP2D6* alleles or one functional and one reduced-function *CYP2D6* allele predict normal or extensive metabolizers. Two reduced-function alleles or one reduced-function and one nonfunctional allele predict intermediate metabolizers. Two nonfunctional alleles predict a poor metabolizer phenotype. Duplicated functional *CYP2D6* alleles predict an ultrarapid metabolizer phenotype [8]. In addition to duplicated functional alleles, duplicated non-functional or reduced-function alleles also have been described. As such, determining which *CYP2D6* allele is duplicated is important for proper interpretation when a

Table 21.3 Examples of commonly tested pharmacogenetic alleles and their effect on enzyme activity

Gene	Loss-of-function alleles	Reduced-function alleles	Increased-function alleles
CYP2D6	**3, *4, *5, *6, *7, *8, *12, *14*	**9, *10, *17, *29, *41*	Functional allele duplication
CYP2C19	**2, *3, *4, *5, *6, *7, *8*	**9, *10*	**17*
CYP2C9	**3, *6*	**2, *5, *8, *11*	–
TPMT	**2, *3A, *3B, *3C, *4*	–	–

gene duplication is identified in addition to a heterozygous genotype [18].

CYP2D6 genotyping is complicated by the fact that several variants occur on a number of important star (*) alleles and commercial assays cannot determine the phase of identified genotypes [19]. For example, the nonfunctional **4* allele is defined by several variants, including 100C>T and 1846G>A. The 1846G>A variant is the defining functional mutation for **4*, which disrupts exon splicing and results in a frameshift and loss of enzyme activity. However, the **10* reduced-function allele also has the 100C>T variant but without 1846G>A. Of note, 1846G>A can also exist on a haplotype without 100C>T (**4M*), and this allele is very rare. When one copy of each variant is detected, the most probable genotype is heterozygous **4* (one copy of a nonfunctional allele), since 100C>T and 1846G>A are presumed to be on the same haplotype. As genotyping platforms generally do not predict *CYP2D6* haplotypes, individual laboratories are responsible for interpreting results and reporting *CYP2D6* genotypes. Without haplotyping by more involved molecular assays, it is possible that one copy of both 100C>T and 1846G>A could be misinterpreted as a **4M/*10* compound heterozygote (one nonfunctional allele and one decreased-function allele). Although this scenario would be rare in the general population, the **4/*10* genotype is more appropriately defined by two copies of 100C>T and one copy of 1846G>A.

Further interpretation challenges exist when a duplication is detected with a reduced-function or nonfunctional allele, as most platforms are not capable of identifying which allele is duplicated. Furthermore, the number of duplicated *CYP2D6* copies on an allele is not typically determined. When in combination with a reduced-function allele, the number of copies may become clinically relevant in predicting the phenotype. Family studies (such as parental testing) may help determine the phase of identified variants in these scenarios, if warranted.

Laboratory Issues

The *CYP2D6* gene is highly homologous to a related pseudogene (*CYP2D7P1*), which complicates the design of PCR primers used for genotyping. As such, primers are designed to avoid co-amplification of pseudogenes by employing a specific long-range PCR of the entire *CYP2D6* gene. Given the technical challenges with long-range PCR, suboptimal or degraded DNA may not perform well for many commercial *CYP2D6* assays.

When a *CYP2D6* platform is unable to identify if a duplication is a functional or nonfunctional allele in a heterozygous sample, laboratories may report an "indeterminant" result. As noted above, family studies can facilitate identifying which allele is duplicated in these cases. Although laboratory guidelines for *CYP2D6* genotyping in relation to tamoxifen therapy have recently been reported [19], no current professional guidelines detail which alleles should be included in clinical *CYP2D6* assays. Therefore, different laboratories may include different *CYP2D6* alleles in their testing panels, which can result in conflicting *CYP2D6* genotypes and predicted phenotypes between laboratories.

CYP2C19

Cytochrome P450-2C19 (CYP2C19) is another important member of the cytochrome P450 superfamily that metabolizes commonly prescribed medications including anticonvulsants, antidepressants, antifungals, proton-pump inhibitors, antithrombotics, and chemotherapy, antimalarial, and antiulcer drugs [20]. Another drug metabolized by CYP2C19 is the antiplatelet agent clopidogrel, commonly prescribed for patients with acute coronary syndromes and those undergoing percutaneous coronary intervention (PCI). CYP2C19 converts clopidogrel in a two-step enzymatic reaction to an active metabolite, which binds irreversibly to platelet receptors and inhibits aggregation for the duration of the platelet life span. About 25 % of ACS/PCI patients have reduced platelet inhibition due in part to *CYP2C19* loss-of-function alleles [21], which reduces the effectiveness of clopidogrel treatment.

Although over 30 *CYP2C19* variant alleles have been identified, the effect of some rare alleles on enzyme function has not been established. Notable among the *CYP2C19* alleles are **2* to **8*, which impart loss of function, and **17*, which has been reported as an increased-function allele (http://www.cypalleles.ki.se/cyp2c19.htm). In contrast to the role of the *CYP2C19*2* to **8* alleles in reduced clopidogrel effectiveness, **17* may be associated with an enhanced response to clopidogrel and some antidepressants [22]. Variant *CYP2C19* allele frequencies vary between racial and ethnic groups, with **2* being present in approximately 30 %

Table 21.4 CPIC recommendations for *CYP2C19*-directed dosing of tricyclic antidepressants[a,b]

Predicted *CYP2C19* metabolism phenotype	Implications for tricyclic antidepressant metabolism	Therapeutic recommendations
Ultrarapid metabolizer (UM)	Increased metabolism of amitriptyline when compared to extensive metabolizers	Consider alternative drug not metabolized by *CYP2C19*. If a tricyclic is warranted, utilize therapeutic drug monitoring to guide dose adjustments
Extensive metabolizer (EM)	Normal metabolism of amitriptyline	Initiate therapy with recommended starting dose
Intermediate metabolizer (IM)	Reduced metabolism of amitriptyline when compared to extensive metabolizers	Initiate therapy with recommended starting dose
Poor metabolizer (PM)	Greatly reduced metabolism of amitriptyline when compared to extensive metabolizers. Higher plasma concentrations of amitriptyline will increase the probability of side effects	Consider 50 % reduction of recommended starting dose. Utilize therapeutic drug monitoring to guide dose adjustments

CPIC Clinical Pharmacogenetics Implementation Consortium
[a]Adapted from Hicks et al. [13]
[b]Note that dosing guidelines for tricyclic antidepressants and *CYP2D6* genotype-directed therapy were also reported [13]. Optional dosing recommendations based on both *CYP2D6* and *CYP2C19* can be found in the supplemental material of Hicks et al. [13]

Table 21.5 CPIC recommendations for *CYP2C19*-directed antiplatelet therapy when considering clopidogrel for ACS patients undergoing PCI[a]

Predicted *CYP2D6* metabolism phenotype	Implications for clopidogrel	Therapeutic recommendations
Ultrarapid metabolizer (UM)	Increased platelet inhibition; decreased residual platelet aggregation[b]	Clopidogrel label-recommended dosage and administration
Extensive metabolizer (EM)	Normal platelet inhibition; normal residual platelet aggregation	Clopidogrel label-recommended dosage and administration
Intermediate metabolizer (IM)	Reduced platelet inhibition; increased residual platelet aggregation; increased risk for adverse cardiovascular events	Alternative antiplatelet therapy (if no contraindication); e.g., prasugrel, ticagrelor
Poor metabolizer (PM)	Significantly reduced platelet inhibition; increased residual platelet aggregation; increased risk for adverse cardiovascular events	Alternative antiplatelet therapy (if no contraindication); e.g., prasugrel, ticagrelor

ACS acute coronary syndrome; *CPIC* Clinical Pharmacogenetics Implementation Consortium; *PCI* percutaneous coronary intervention
[a]Adapted from Scott et al. [23]
[b]The *CYP2C19*17* allele may be associated with increased bleeding risks [27]

of Asians and 15 % of Caucasians and African Americans, while *3 has a frequency of approximately 8 % in the Asian population, but is rare in other populations.

Clinical Utility

CYP2C19 genotyping can identify individuals who should avoid medications or may require modified doses of medications metabolized by CYP2C19. For ACS/PCI patients being treated with clopidogrel, *CYP2C19*2* and **3* carriers have reduced platelet inhibition compared to extensive metabolizers due to reduced metabolic activation of the prodrug. Consequently, an alternative antiplatelet agent has been recommended for ACS/PCI patients who are *CYP2C19* intermediate and poor metabolizers [23]. For tamoxifen, *CYP2C19*17* carriers have been shown to produce higher concentrations of the active endoxifen metabolite and may have a more favorable outcome than **1*, **2*, and **3* carriers [24]. CPIC guidelines are available for the use of *CYP2C19* genotyping results for patients treated with tricyclic antidepressants [13, 25] (Table 21.4) and clopidogrel [23, 25] (Table 21.5).

Available Assays

A number of multiplexed molecular assays are available to identify selected variant *CYP2C19* alleles. For example, *CYP2C19* is combined with *CYP2D6* in the AmpliChip® assay (Roche) described above. Additional *CYP2C19* assays are commercially available from Luminex Molecular Diagnostics (xTAG® CYP2C19 Kit), AutoGenomics (Infiniti® CYP2C19 Assay), Nanosphere (Verigene® CYP2C19 Test), GenMark Diagnostics (eSensor® 2C19 Test), Sequenom (iPLEX® ADME CYP2C19 Panel), and Spartan Bioscience (Spartan RX CYP2C19 Test). All these assays include the common nonfunctional alleles (**2* and **3*, with or without **4* to **8*), and some also include **17* and other variants (Fig. 21.2; Table 21.3).

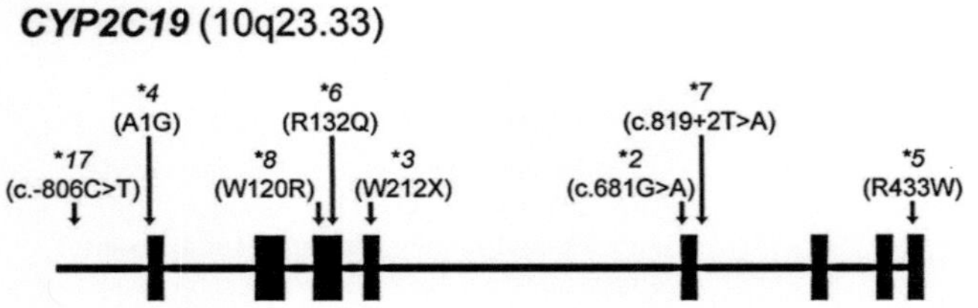

Figure 21.2 Gene diagram of *CYP2C19* (and chromosome location) indicating common alleles and their molecular alteration (in *parentheses*)

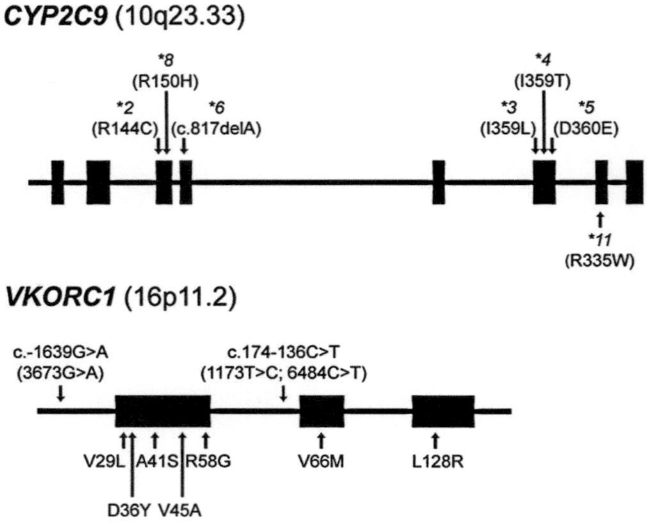

Figure 21.3 Gene diagrams of *CYP2C9* and *VKORC1* (and chromosome locations) indicating common alleles and their molecular alteration (in *parentheses*). Note the rare "warfarin-resistant" *VKORC1* mutations listed below the *VKORC1* gene, which are not commonly included in clinical *CYP2C9* and *VKORC1* genetic tests

Interpretation

Based on identified *CYP2C19* genotype, individuals typically are categorized as extensive (**1/*1*), intermediate (e.g., **1/*2*, **1/*3*), or poor (e.g., **2/*2*, **2/*3*) metabolizers [20]. The frequencies of *CYP2C19* poor metabolizers are 2–5 % of Caucasians and African Americans and approximately 15 % of Asians [23, 26]. Additionally, individuals who have at least one copy of the *CYP2C19*17* allele often are categorized as ultrarapid metabolizers (e.g., **17/*17*). However, given that **17* is unable to completely compensate for the **2* loss-of-function allele [27], **2/*17* compound heterozygotes can be classified as intermediate metabolizers, although some laboratories may report the predicted phenotype for this genotype as "unknown" or "indeterminate."

Laboratory Issues

Although most commercial assays include the common *CYP2C19*2* and **3* loss-of-function alleles, some assays also include the **4* to **8* alleles. Moreover, some assays include the **17* increased-function allele. Like other *CYP450* genotyping assays, the wild-type **1* allele is assigned in the absence of other detected alleles. Consequently, different laboratories may test different allele panels which can result in conflicting *CYP2C19* genotypes and predicted phenotypes depending on which alleles were interrogated.

CYP2C9 and VKORC1 (Warfarin Sensitivity)

Warfarin is a commonly prescribed vitamin K antagonist for the prevention of thromboembolism among patients with atrial fibrillation, deep vein thrombosis, and other indications. However, the drug has a very narrow therapeutic index and a large interindividual variability in response, in part due to inherited genetic variability within genes involved in warfarin pharmacokinetics and pharmacodynamics. For example, cytochrome P450-2C9 (CYP2C9) is the principal enzyme involved in S-warfarin inactivation and elimination. Like other cytochrome P450 genes, *CYP2C9* is highly polymorphic with several known variant alleles encoding reduced enzyme activity (http://www.cypalleles.ki.se/cyp2c9.htm). Importantly, in vitro studies have shown that the common **2* and **3* alleles are functionally defective, exhibiting only approximately 70 % and 5 % of wild-type activity toward S-warfarin, respectively [28]. Consequently, these *CYP2C9* alleles result in reduced warfarin inactivation, higher warfarin blood levels with standard warfarin doses, and increased bleeding risks [29, 30]. The frequencies of **2* and **3* are approximately 15 % and 6 %, respectively, among Caucasians and 2–4 % among Asians and African Americans [31]. Of note, other variant alleles are more prevalent in individuals of African descent (e.g., **5*, **6*, and **8*) [31], which may provide additional utility for genetically guided warfarin dosing in these populations.

Warfarin acts as a vitamin K antagonist by inhibiting the regeneration of reduced vitamin K, an essential cofactor for the clotting cascade. The target enzyme for warfarin is VKORC1, which catalyzes the rate-limiting step in the vitamin K cycle [32]. Importantly, common *VKORC1* haplotypes that result in reduced gene expression have been reproducibly implicated as the major genetic determinant of warfarin dose variability [33–38]. The most commonly interrogated *VKORC1* allele associated with warfarin sensitivity is the c.-1639G>A promoter polymorphism (Fig. 21.3) [38]. Like *CYP2C9*, the frequencies of *VKORC1* alleles vary between racial and ethnic groups, with c.-1639G>A allele frequencies of approximately 10 %, 45 %, and 70–90 %, among African-American, Caucasian, and Asian individuals, respectively [31]. Of note, rare *VKORC1* coding region mutations also have been identified that are strongly correlated with warfarin resistance.

Taken together, common *CYP2C9* and *VKORC1* variant alleles account for approximately 35 % of interindividual dose variability [36, 37], which can be used in conjunction with known clinical variables (e.g., age, race, body weight, gender) to predict individual therapeutic warfarin doses. These data prompted the US Food and Drug Administration (FDA) to modify the warfarin label noting the importance of pharmacogenetic testing with dosing recommendations based on *CYP2C9* and *VKORC1* genotypes (Table 21.6).

Clinical Utility

Using genotype information to guide initial warfarin dose has the potential to improve initial dosing accuracy, reduce the time to attain a stable dose, and lead to improved outcomes in warfarin-treated patients, such as decreased hemorrhagic or thrombotic events associated with supra- or subtherapeutic anticoagulation, respectively. Several dosing algorithms have been developed that incorporate demographic, clinical, and genetic variables (including variant *CYP2C9* and *VKORC1* alleles) [39], and some are freely available online (http://www.warfarindosing.org/) [36, 37]. As noted above, to facilitate physician interpretation of clinical *CYP2C9* and *VKORC1* genotyping, the FDA updated the "Dosage and Administration" section of the warfarin label in 2010 to include a table containing stable maintenance doses (Table 21.6). Although these label dosing recommendations are likely to be more accurate than empiric dosing (i.e., 5 mg/day), a retrospective study has shown that pharmacogenetic-guided dose prediction is more accurate than both empiric dosing and the dosing guideline table listed on the warfarin label [40]. However, recently reported randomized clinical trials indicate that although pharmacogenetic-guided dosing is more accurate than routine fixed dosing [41], a dosing algorithm with only three *CYP2C9* and *VKORC1* variants common among Caucasians is not superior to a clinical variable dosing algorithm, particularly among individuals of African ancestry [42]. As such, a major issue behind pharmacogenetic-guided warfarin dosing continues to be the appropriate selection of *CYP2C9* and *VKORC1* variants for a given ethnicity and the ongoing debate over clinical utility [43, 44].

Available Assays

Most commercial assays for warfarin genotyping include the *CYP2C9*2* and **3* alleles and *VKORC1* c.-1639G>A (or the linked c.174-136C>T [1173C>T] allele) together in a multiplexed assay. FDA-approved or FDA-cleared *CYP2C9*–*VKORC1* genotyping platforms include the INFINITI® Warfarin Assay (AutoGenomics, Inc., Vista, CA), eSensor® Warfarin Sensitivity Test (GenMark Diagnostics, Inc., Carlsbad, CA), Verigene® Warfarin Metabolism Nucleic Acid Test (Nanosphere, Northbrook, IL), and the eQ-PCR™ LC Warfarin Genotyping Kit (TrimGen, Sparks, MD). Other assays, many with additional variant alleles, not currently FDA-approved, are available from AutoGenomics, Inc., GenMark Diagnostics, Inc., and Luminex Molecular Diagnostics. Importantly, analytical performance for these platforms is very good, with high concordance being reported for the AutoGenomics, Luminex, Invader, and pyrosequencing assays [45].

Interpretation

The American College of Medical Genetics and Genomics has published guidelines on *CYP2C9* and *VKORC1* genotyping for warfarin sensitivity [46]. *CYP2C9* results are reported with a predicted metabolizer status (e.g., extensive, intermediate, poor) and *VKORC1* c.-1639G>A results with a predicted degree of sensitivity (e.g., G/G, low; G/A, intermediate; A/A, high). Since most currently available *CYP2C9* and *VKORC1* genotyping tests do not include the rare *VKORC1* coding region mutations, they will not be able to assess warfarin resistance.

Laboratory Issues

Some assays will interrogate the *VKORC1* c.1173C>T allele that is in linkage disequilibrium (LD) with c.-1639G>A [46]. Although this allele will provide results consistent with c.-1639G>A for most populations, the LD is reduced in individuals of African descent [38], which may result in c.1173C>T being less predictive for warfarin dosing. As mentioned above, other variables influence warfarin dose variability such as gender, body mass, other medications, and age. If laboratories do not provide a predicted therapeutic dose in their reports, they should include where physicians can incorporate genotype results with other clinical variables into pharmacogenetic dosing algorithms. Two commonly used algorithms are available online (http://www.warfarindosing.org/ and http://www.pharmgkb.org/guideline/PA166104949) and are recommended by CPIC practice guidelines when genotype results are available [47].

Table 21.6 Range of expected therapeutic warfarin doses based on *CYP2C9* and *VKORC1* genotypes[a]

	CYP2C9					
***VKORC1* (c.-1639G>A)**	***1/*1**	***1/*2**	***1/*3**	***2/*2**	***2/*3**	***3/*3**
G/G	5–7 mg	5–7 mg	3–4 mg	3–4 mg	3–4 mg	0.5–2 mg
G/A	5–7 mg	3–4 mg	3–4 mg	3–4 mg	0.5–2 mg	0.5–2 mg
A/A	3–4 mg	3–4 mg	0.5–2 mg	0.5–2 mg	0.5–2 mg	0.5–2 mg

[a]Adapted from the warfarin product insert: http://www.accessdata.fda.gov/drugsatfda_docs/label/2010/009218s108lbl.pdf

TPMT

Thiopurine *S*-methyltransferase (TPMT) inactivates azathioprine, 6-mercaptopurine (6-MP), and 6-thioguanine. These drugs are used to treat acute lymphoblastic leukemia [48], autoimmune diseases [49, 50], and inflammatory bowel disease [51, 52], as well as to prevent rejection of solid organ transplants [53]. They are metabolized to 6-thioguanine nucleotides (6-TGN) by hypoxanthine-guanine phosphoribosyltransferase (HGPRT). The TGNs are incorporated into the DNA of dividing cells and inhibit several metabolic pathways; the exact mechanism of action is not known but likely is a combination of inducing apoptosis and inhibiting cell metabolism.

About 10 % of the population have intermediate levels of TPMT activity and 0.3 % have low or undetectable enzyme activity and are considered TPMT deficient. Individuals with low TPMT activity are at risk for 6-thioguanine-mediated toxicity, but may be treated successfully with decreased doses. When TPMT enzyme activity is reduced, proportionately more 6-MP may be converted into the active and cytotoxic TGNs. Since TPMT catalyzes the metabolism of TGNs, low TPMT activity results in the accumulation of the active/cytotoxic metabolites. Excess 6-thioguanine in the bone marrow inhibits purine synthesis, thus inhibiting cell proliferation, and contributes to excess myelosuppression. Accordingly, individuals at risk for 6-thioguanine-mediated toxicity can be treated with decreased doses of thiopurine drugs. Identifying at-risk individuals prior to treatment can be accomplished by genotyping the most common *TPMT* variant alleles (Fig. 21.4; Table 21.3); however, genotyping alone does not replace the need for clinical monitoring of patients treated with thiopurine drugs.

Clinical Utility

TPMT genotyping is used to identify patients prior to initiating therapy who may be at risk for severe myelosuppression with standard dosing. One copy of a nonfunctional *TPMT* allele is associated with intermediate enzyme activity and an increased risk for bone marrow toxicity. Two copies of nonfunctional alleles result in lack of TPMT activity and a high risk for severe myelosuppression. Carriers of one copy may need a dose reduction, while individuals who have two nonfunctional alleles require significant dose reduction. A CPIC guideline with dosing recommendations for azathioprine, mercaptopurine, and thioguanine based on *TPMT* genotype is available [54] (Table 21.7).

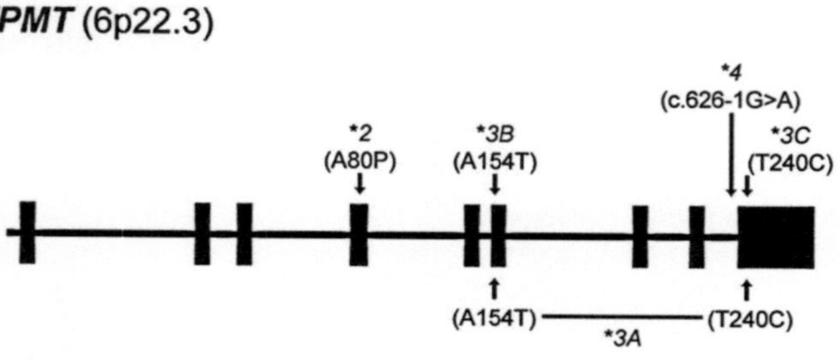

Figure 21.4 Gene diagram of *TPMT* (and chromosome location) indicating common alleles and their molecular alteration (in *parentheses*)

Available Assays

Among the over 20 variants described in *TPMT*, three common alleles (**2*, **3A*, and **3C*) are often included in testing panels [55, 56]; however, panels with additional variants also are available [57]. PCR-based assays that interrogate the three common variants detect 80–95 % of low and intermediate enzyme activity individuals in the Caucasian, African-American, and Asian populations [58]. The analytical performance of *TPMT* genotyping is generally high for most testing platforms. Of note, *TPMT* genotyping tests have high specificity and positive predictive values, but lower sensitivity and negative predictive values [59].

Interpretation

Patients with reduced-function or nonfunctional alleles are at high risk of bone marrow toxicity and require significant dose reduction (ten-fold lower than the standard dose) [54]. One copy of a nonfunctional or reduced-function allele may be associated with an increased risk of toxicity, with possible dose reductions of 30–50 % [54]. Therapeutic drug monitoring may help optimize dosing for individuals with one or two *TPMT* mutations; however, myelosuppression may be due to other factors, such as drug-drug interactions. When none of the targeted *TPMT* mutations are detected, patients are presumed to have normal TPMT activity, be at low risk of bone marrow toxicity, and treated with the standard dose. However, unless the gene is sequenced, the patient still may have an undetected and/or rare *TPMT* variant that affects enzyme activity.

Laboratory Issues

In addition to genotyping assays, TPMT phenotyping for enzyme activity and metabolite tests also are available. However, enzyme phenotype testing should be done prior to treatment because the drug or metabolites may directly interfere with assay performance. Given that other polymorphic enzymes are involved in mercaptopurine metabolism (e.g., inosine triphosphatase [ITPA]) and that not all *TPMT* variants are detected by genotyping, *TPMT* genotype results may not always correlate with phenotype test results. For example, selected studies on azathioprine-treated rheumatic patients suggest that *TPMT* genotyping alone may not be sufficient to personalize azathioprine dosage and that TPMT enzyme and azathioprine metabolite

Table 21.7 CPIC recommendations for *TPMT*-directed dosing of azathioprine[a]

Predicted TPMT phenotype	Implications for azathioprine metabolism	Therapeutic recommendations
Homozygous wild-type or normal, high activity (two functional **1* alleles)	Lower concentrations of TGN metabolites, higher methyl-TIMP; normal	Start with normal starting dose (e.g., 2–3 mg/kg/day) and adjust doses of azathioprine based on disease-specific guidelines. Allow 2 weeks to reach steady state after each dose adjustment
Heterozygote or intermediate activity (one functional allele—**1*, plus one nonfunctional allele—**2*, **3A*, **3B*, **3C*, or **4*)	Moderate to high concentrations of TGN metabolites; low concentrations of methyl-TIMP	If disease treatment normally starts at the "full dose," consider starting at 30–70 % of target dose (e.g., 1–1.5 mg/kg/day) and titrate based on tolerance. Allow 2–4 weeks to reach steady state after each dose adjustment
Homozygous variant, mutant, low, or deficient activity (two nonfunctional alleles—**2*, **3A*, **3B*, **3C*, or **4*)	Extremely high concentrations of TGN metabolites; fatal toxicity possible without dose decrease; no methyl-TIMP metabolites	Consider alternative agents. If using azathioprine start with drastically reduced doses (reduce daily dose by ten-fold and dose thrice weekly instead of daily) and adjust doses of azathioprine based on the degree of myelosuppression and disease-specific guidelines. Allow 4–6 weeks to reach steady state after each dose adjustment. Azathioprine is the likely cause of myelosuppression

CPIC Clinical Pharmacogenetics Implementation Consortium; *TGN* 6-thioguanine nucleotide; *TIMP* 6-thioinosine monophosphate; *TPMT* thiopurine S-methyltransferase

[a]Adapted from Relling et al. [54]. Note that this CPIC guideline also has *TPMT*-directed guidelines for mercaptopurine and thioguanine

assays may be warranted in this context [49]. However, given the reliability of *TPMT* genotyping and that performing both genotyping and phenotyping is not typically feasible, genotyping may be considered the primary choice for pretreatment evaluation of TPMT function before initiation of thiopurine therapy [60].

UGT1A1

The UDP-glucuronosyltransferases (UGT) are a superfamily of enzymes that aid in drug excretion by conjugating glucuronic acid, which renders drugs and endogenous compounds more hydrophilic and amenable to biliary or renal elimination. A number of UGT family members have been identified and one of the most commonly studied is encoded by the *UGT1A1* gene [61]. The most important variant *UGT1A1* alleles is **28*, which is a promoter polymorphism comprised of seven thymine-adenine (TA) dinucleotide repeats $[(TA)_7TAA]$ [62], compared to the normal *UGT1A1*1* allele with six TA repeats $[(TA)_6TAA]$ (Fig. 21.5). Importantly, the length of the TA repeat sequence is inversely correlated with UGT1A1 activity [63]. Consequently, *UGT1A1*28* heterozygotes and homozygotes have an approximately 25 % and 70 % reduction in enzyme activity, respectively [63]. Five $[(TA)_5TAA]$ and eight $[(TA)_8TAA]$ repeats also have been reported, but due to their rarity, they are not well studied. In addition, **28* has been associated with Gilbert's syndrome, an inherited unconjugated hyperbilirubinemia that does not indicate liver damage but affects the metabolism of several substances [64].

UGT1A1 **(2q37.1)**

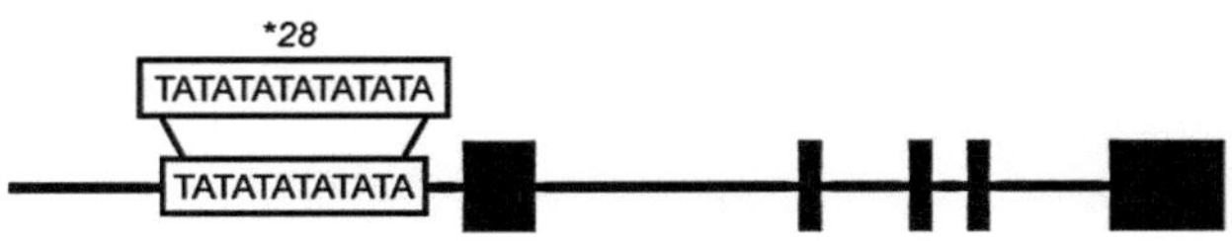

Figure 21.5 Gene diagram of *UGT1A1* (and chromosome location) indicating the **28* allele associated with irinotecan sensitivity

Irinotecan commonly is used to treat advanced stage colorectal cancer and may be used for the treatment of lung, brain, and breast cancers. Irinotecan is a prodrug that is activated to SN-38, which is then conjugated by UGT1A1 to excretory glucuronides (SN-38G). Patients with the *UGT1A1*28* allele are at higher risk for irinotecan toxicity (e.g., neutropenia), particularly when administered at higher doses, since they express lower levels of UGT1A1-mediated glucuronidation activity [65–67]. These data prompted the FDA, in 2005, to modify the irinotecan drug label with information on toxicity risk due to *UGT1A1*28* and the availability of clinical genetic testing. Like other variant pharmacogenetic alleles, the frequencies of *UGT1A1*28* vary between populations with the **28/*28* genotype ranging from 1 to 2 % in Asians to approximately 10 % and 20 % in Caucasians and individuals of African descent, respectively [61].

Clinical Utility

The most commonly tested *UGT1A1* alleles are the promoter TA dinucleotide repeats that influence gene transcription and UGT1A1 activity. The wild-type **1* allele (six TA repeats) is associated with normal enzyme activity and the **28* allele (seven TA repeats) is associated with reduced activity. This test can be used prior to irinotecan administration to predict toxicity or after exposure to explain adverse effects such as severe diarrhea and neutropenia. However, no study has prospectively documented the potential benefits (reduced adverse drug events) or harms (reduced proportion of responsive tumors) from changes in irinotecan dosing based on *UGT1A1*28* genotyping.

Available Assays

Several assays are available that detect the *UGT1A1* TA repeat polymorphism. The most straightforward assay is a laboratory-developed test involving fluorescent PCR amplification and size separation by capillary electrophoresis. This assay also detects the less common five and eight TA repeat alleles. One *UGT1A1*28* genotyping test has been FDA-approved, the Invader® UGT1A1 Molecular Assay from Hologic, Inc. (Madison, WI). The analytic validity of current *UGT1A1* genetic testing methods is adequate, and available data indicate that both analytic sensitivity and specificity for the **1* and **28* alleles are high [68].

Interpretation

One or two copies of the *UGT1A1*28* allele predict irinotecan sensitivity. The rare five repeat allele is assumed to maintain efficient transcription, while the rare eight repeat allele indicates irinotecan sensitivity similar to the seven repeat allele (**28*). Although the Evaluation of Genomic Applications in Practice and Prevention (EGAPP) Working Group found that the evidence was insufficient to recommend for or against the routine use of *UGT1A1* genotyping in patients with metastatic colorectal cancer who are treated with irinotecan [68], the Royal Dutch Pharmacists Association – Pharmacogenetics Working Group has evaluated therapeutic dose recommendations for irinotecan based on *UGT1A1* genotype and recommended dose reduction for **28* homozygous patients receiving more than 250 mg/m^2 [25].

Laboratory Issues

Genotyping assays that interrogate *UGT1A1* need to be robust, since often the patient is being treated with chemotherapy and may have low white cell counts, yielding minimal DNA from a peripheral blood specimen. Some research gaps reported by the EGAPP include the need for prospective studies of *UGT1A1* genotyping and clinical decision-making with clinical outcomes, which are needed to answer the overarching question of clinical utility.

Future Perspectives

The continued progression of translational genomics research will undoubtedly identify more DNA variants associated with drug response variability. In addition, future studies are warranted to assess the clinical utility of pharmacogenetic-guided therapy, including cost-effectiveness studies. Although the FDA continues to modify labels by adding pharmacogenetic information and genetic testing recommendations, a number of obstacles remain for effective clinical use of pharmacogenetic test results, including physician education, regulatory issues, rapid turnaround time testing [69], and reimbursement [70]. To address some of these issues, some large academic medical centers are deploying progressive preemptive pharmacogenetic testing for specific patient populations [71–74]. In addition, ongoing whole-exome and genome sequencing programs will undoubtedly change the future landscape of clinical pharmacogenomics by enabling the rapid identification of additional genetic variants implicated in drug response. Of great importance is the continued study of the clinical utility of pharmacogenetics and the incorporation of both genetic and nongenetic variables for the most effective use of personalized medicine.

References

1. Higgins MJ, Stearns V. CYP2D6 polymorphisms and tamoxifen metabolism: clinical relevance. Curr Oncol Rep. 2010;12(1):7–15.
2. Samer CF, Daali Y, Wagner M, Hopfgartner G, Eap CB, Rebsamen MC, et al. Genetic polymorphisms and drug interactions modulating CYP2D6 and CYP3A activities have a major effect on oxycodone analgesic efficacy and safety. Br J Pharmacol. 2010;160(4):919–30.
3. D'Empaire I, Guico-Pabia CJ, Preskorn SH. Antidepressant treatment and altered CYP2D6 activity: are pharmacokinetic variations clinically relevant? J Psychiatr Pract. 2011;17(5):330–9.
4. Rau T, Wuttke H, Michels LM, Werner U, Bergmann K, Kreft M, et al. Impact of the CYP2D6 genotype on the clinical effects of metoprolol: a prospective longitudinal study. Clin Pharmacol Ther. 2009;85(3):269–72.
5. Cacabelos R, Hashimoto R, Takeda M. Pharmacogenomics of antipsychotics efficacy for schizophrenia. Psychiatry Clin Neurosci. 2011;65(1):3–19.
6. Ong FS, Deignan JL, Kuo JZ, Bernstein KE, Rotter JI, Grody WW, et al. Clinical utility of pharmacogenetic biomarkers in cardiovascular therapeutics: a challenge for clinical implementation. Pharmacogenomics. 2012;13(4):465–75.
7. Michelson D, Read HA, Ruff DD, Witcher J, Zhang S, McCracken J. CYP2D6 and clinical response to atomoxetine in children and adolescents with ADHD. J Am Acad Child Adolesc Psychiatry. 2007;46(2):242–51.
8. Owen RP, Sangkuhl K, Klein TE, Altman RB. Cytochrome P450 2D6. Pharmacogenet Genomics. 2009;19(7):559–62.
9. Brauch H, Murdter TE, Eichelbaum M, Schwab M. Pharmacogenomics of tamoxifen therapy. Clin Chem. 2009;55(10):1770–82.
10. Hertz DL, McLeod HL, Irvin Jr WJ. Tamoxifen and CYP2D6: a contradiction of data. Oncologist. 2012;17(5):620–30.
11. Crews KR, Gaedigk A, Dunnenberger HM, Klein TE, Shen DD, Callaghan JT, et al. Clinical Pharmacogenetics Implementation

Consortium (CPIC) guidelines for codeine therapy in the context of cytochrome P450 2D6 (CYP2D6) genotype. Clin Pharmacol Ther. 2012;91(2):321–6.
12. Crews KR, Gaedigk A, Dunnenberger HM, Leeder JS, Klein TE, Caudle KE, et al. Clinical Pharmacogenetics Implementation Consortium guidelines for cytochrome P450 2D6 genotype and codeine therapy: 2014 update. Clin Pharmacol Ther. 2014;95(4):376–82.
13. Hicks JK, Swen JJ, Thorn CF, Sangkuhl K, Kharasch ED, Ellingrod VL, et al. Clinical Pharmacogenetics Implementation Consortium guideline for CYP2D6 and CYP2C19 genotypes and dosing of tricyclic antidepressants. Clin Pharmacol Ther. 2013;93(5):402–8.
14. de Leon J. AmpliChip CYP450 test: personalized medicine has arrived in psychiatry. Expert Rev Mol Diagn. 2006;6(3):277–86.
15. Melis R, Lyon E, McMillin GA. Determination of CYP2D6, CYP2C9 and CYP2C19 genotypes with Tag-It mutation detection assays. Expert Rev Mol Diagn. 2006;6(6):811–20.
16. Savino M, Seripa D, Gallo AP, Garrubba M, D'Onofrio G, Bizzarro A, et al. Effectiveness of a high-throughput genetic analysis in the identification of responders/non-responders to CYP2D6-metabolized drugs. Clin Lab. 2011;57(11–12):887–93.
17. Sistonen J, Fuselli S, Levo A, Sajantila A. CYP2D6 genotyping by a multiplex primer extension reaction. Clin Chem. 2005;51(7):1291–5.
18. Ramamoorthy A, Skaar TC. Gene copy number variations: it is important to determine which allele is affected. Pharmacogenomics. 2011;12(3):299–301.
19. Lyon E, Gastier Foster J, Palomaki GE, Pratt VM, Reynolds K, Sabato MF, et al. Laboratory testing of CYP2D6 alleles in relation to tamoxifen therapy. Genet Med. 2012;14(12):990–1000.
20. Scott SA, Sangkuhl K, Shuldiner AR, Hulot JS, Thorn CF, Altman RB, et al. PharmGKB summary: very important pharmacogene information for cytochrome P450, family 2, subfamily C, polypeptide 19. Pharmacogenet Genomics. 2012;22(2):159–65.
21. Shuldiner AR, O'Connell JR, Bliden KP, Gandhi A, Ryan K, Horenstein RB, et al. Association of cytochrome P450 2C19 genotype with the antiplatelet effect and clinical efficacy of clopidogrel therapy. JAMA. 2009;302(8):849–57.
22. Sim SC, Risinger C, Dahl ML, Aklillu E, Christensen M, Bertilsson L, et al. A common novel CYP2C19 gene variant causes ultrarapid drug metabolism relevant for the drug response to proton pump inhibitors and antidepressants. Clin Pharmacol Ther. 2006;79(1):103–13.
23. Scott SA, Sangkuhl K, Stein CM, Hulot JS, Mega JL, Roden DM, et al. Clinical pharmacogenetics implementation consortium guidelines for CYP2C19 genotype and clopidogrel therapy: 2013 update. Clin Pharmacol Ther. 2013;94(3):317–23.
24. Schroth W, Antoniadou L, Fritz P, Schwab M, Muerdter T, Zanger UM, et al. Breast cancer treatment outcome with adjuvant tamoxifen relative to patient CYP2D6 and CYP2C19 genotypes. J Clin Oncol. 2007;25(33):5187–93.
25. Swen JJ, Nijenhuis M, de Boer A, Grandia L, Maitland-van der Zee AH, Mulder H, et al. Pharmacogenetics: from bench to byte—an update of guidelines. Clin Pharmacol Ther. 2011;89(5):662–73.
26. Martis S, Peter I, Hulot JS, Kornreich R, Desnick RJ, Scott SA. Multi-ethnic distribution of clinically relevant CYP2C genotypes and haplotypes. Pharmacogenomics J. 2013;13(4):369–77.
27. Sibbing D, Gebhard D, Koch W, Braun S, Stegherr J, Morath T, et al. Isolated and interactive impact of common CYP2C19 genetic variants on the antiplatelet effect of chronic clopidogrel therapy. J Thromb Haemost. 2010;8(8):1685–93.
28. Lee CR, Goldstein JA, Pieper JA. Cytochrome P450 2C9 polymorphisms: a comprehensive review of the in-vitro and human data. Pharmacogenetics. 2002;12(3):251–63.
29. Aithal GP, Day CP, Kesteven PJ, Daly AK. Association of polymorphisms in the cytochrome P450 CYP2C9 with warfarin dose requirement and risk of bleeding complications. Lancet. 1999;353(9154):717–9.
30. Higashi MK, Veenstra DL, Kondo LM, Wittkowsky AK, Srinouanprachanh SL, Farin FM, et al. Association between CYP2C9 genetic variants and anticoagulation-related outcomes during warfarin therapy. JAMA. 2002;287(13):1690–8.
31. Scott SA, Khasawneh R, Peter I, Kornreich R, Desnick RJ. Combined CYP2C9, VKORC1 and CYP4F2 frequencies among racial and ethnic groups. Pharmacogenomics. 2010;11(6):781–91.
32. Owen RP, Gong L, Sagreiya H, Klein TE, Altman RB. VKORC1 pharmacogenomics summary. Pharmacogenet Genomics. 2010;20(10):642–4.
33. Rieder MJ, Reiner AP, Gage BF, Nickerson DA, Eby CS, McLeod HL, et al. Effect of VKORC1 haplotypes on transcriptional regulation and warfarin dose. N Engl J Med. 2005;352(22):2285–93.
34. Sconce EA, Khan TI, Wynne HA, Avery P, Monkhouse L, King BP, et al. The impact of CYP2C9 and VKORC1 genetic polymorphism and patient characteristics upon warfarin dose requirements: proposal for a new dosing regimen. Blood. 2005;106(7):2329–33.
35. Wadelius M, Chen LY, Downes K, Ghori J, Hunt S, Eriksson N, et al. Common VKORC1 and GGCX polymorphisms associated with warfarin dose. Pharmacogenomics J. 2005;5(4):262–70.
36. Gage BF, Eby C, Johnson JA, Deych E, Rieder MJ, Ridker PM, et al. Use of pharmacogenetic and clinical factors to predict the therapeutic dose of warfarin. Clin Pharmacol Ther. 2008;84(3):326–31.
37. International Warfarin Pharmacogenetics Consortium, Klein TE, Altman RB, Eriksson N, Gage BF, Kimmel SE, et al. Estimation of the warfarin dose with clinical and pharmacogenetic data. N Engl J Med. 2009;360(8):753–64.
38. Limdi NA, Wadelius M, Cavallari L, Eriksson N, Crawford DC, Lee MT, et al. Warfarin pharmacogenetics: a single VKORC1 polymorphism is predictive of dose across 3 racial groups. Blood. 2010;115(18):3827–34.
39. Lubitz SA, Scott SA, Rothlauf EB, Agarwal A, Peter I, Doheny D, et al. Comparative performance of gene-based warfarin dosing algorithms in a multiethnic population. J Thromb Haemost. 2010;8(5):1018–26.
40. Finkelman BS, Gage BF, Johnson JA, Brensinger CM, Kimmel SE. Genetic warfarin dosing: tables versus algorithms. J Am Coll Cardiol. 2011;57(5):612–8.
41. Pirmohamed M, Burnside G, Eriksson N, Jorgensen AL, Toh CH, Nicholson T, et al. A randomized trial of genotype-guided dosing of warfarin. N Engl J Med. 2013;369(24):2294–303.
42. Kimmel SE, French B, Kasner SE, Johnson JA, Anderson JL, Gage BF, et al. A pharmacogenetic versus a clinical algorithm for warfarin dosing. N Engl J Med. 2013;369(24):2283–93.
43. Zineh I, Pacanowski M, Woodcock J. Pharmacogenetics and coumarin dosing—recalibrating expectations. N Engl J Med. 2013;369(24):2273–5.
44. Scott SA, Lubitz SA. Warfarin pharmacogenetic trials: is there a future for pharmacogenetic-guided dosing? Pharmacogenomics. 2014;15(6):719–22.
45. King CR, Porche-Sorbet RM, Gage BF, Ridker PM, Renaud Y, Phillips MS, et al. Performance of commercial platforms for rapid genotyping of polymorphisms affecting warfarin dose. Am J Clin Pathol. 2008;129(6):876–83.
46. Flockhart DA, O'Kane D, Williams MS, Watson MS, Gage B, Gandolfi R, et al. Pharmacogenetic testing of CYP2C9 and VKORC1 alleles for warfarin. Genet Med. 2008;10(2):139–50.
47. Johnson JA, Gong L, Whirl-Carrillo M, Gage BF, Scott SA, Stein CM, et al. Clinical Pharmacogenetics Implementation Consortium Guidelines for CYP2C9 and VKORC1 genotypes and warfarin dosing. Clin Pharmacol Ther. 2011;90(4):625–9.
48. Meeker ND, Yang JJ, Schiffman JD. Pharmacogenomics of pediatric acute lymphoblastic leukemia. Expert Opin Pharmacother. 2010;11(10):1621–32.

49. Tani C, Mosca M, Colucci R, Gori G, d'Ascanio A, Ghisu N, et al. Genetic polymorphisms of thiopurine S-methyltransferase in a cohort of patients with systemic autoimmune diseases. Clin Exp Rheumatol. 2009;27(2):321–4.
50. Nguyen TM, Daubard M, Le Gall C, Larger M, Lachaux A, Boulieu R. Monitoring of azathioprine metabolites in pediatric patients with autoimmune hepatitis. Ther Drug Monit. 2010;32(4): 433–7.
51. Smith MA, Marinaki AM, Sanderson JD. Pharmacogenomics in the treatment of inflammatory bowel disease. Pharmacogenomics. 2010;11(3):421–37.
52. Teml A, Schaeffeler E, Herrlinger KR, Klotz U, Schwab M. Thiopurine treatment in inflammatory bowel disease: clinical pharmacology and implication of pharmacogenetically guided dosing. Clin Pharmacokinet. 2007;46(3):187–208.
53. Anglicheau D, Legendre C, Thervet E. Pharmacogenetics in solid organ transplantation: present knowledge and future perspectives. Transplantation. 2004;78(3):311–5.
54. Relling MV, Gardner EE, Sandborn WJ, Schmiegelow K, Pui CH, Yee SW, et al. Clinical Pharmacogenetics Implementation Consortium guidelines for thiopurine methyltransferase genotype and thiopurine dosing. Clin Pharmacol Ther. 2011;89(3): 387–91.
55. Yates CR, Krynetski EY, Loennechen T, Fessing MY, Tai HL, Pui CH, et al. Molecular diagnosis of thiopurine S-methyltransferase deficiency: genetic basis for azathioprine and mercaptopurine intolerance. Ann Intern Med. 1997;126(8):608–14.
56. Evans WE, Hon YY, Bomgaars L, Coutre S, Holdsworth M, Janco R, et al. Preponderance of thiopurine S-methyltransferase deficiency and heterozygosity among patients intolerant to mercaptopurine or azathioprine. J Clin Oncol. 2001;19(8):2293–301.
57. Okada Y, Nakamura K, Wada M, Nakamura T, Tsukamoto N, Nojima Y, et al. Genotyping of thiopurine methyltransferase using pyrosequencing. Biol Pharm Bull. 2005;28(4):677–81.
58. Zhou S. Clinical pharmacogenomics of thiopurine S-methyltransferase. Curr Clin Pharmacol. 2006;1(1):119–28.
59. Donnan JR, Ungar WJ, Mathews M, Rahman P. Systematic review of thiopurine methyltransferase genotype and enzymatic testing strategies. Ther Drug Monit. 2011;33(2):192–9.
60. Hindorf U, Appell ML. Genotyping should be considered the primary choice for pre-treatment evaluation of thiopurine methyltransferase function. J Crohns Colitis. 2012;6(6):655–9.
61. Marques SC, Ikediobi ON. The clinical application of UGT1A1 pharmacogenetic testing: gene-environment interactions. Hum Genomics. 2010;4(4):238–49.
62. Perera MA, Innocenti F, Ratain MJ. Pharmacogenetic testing for uridine diphosphate glucuronosyltransferase 1A1 polymorphisms: are we there yet? Pharmacotherapy. 2008;28(6):755–68.
63. Zhang D, Zhang D, Cui D, Gambardella J, Ma L, Barros A, et al. Characterization of the UDP glucuronosyltransferase activity of human liver microsomes genotyped for the UGT1A1*28 polymorphism. Drug Metab Dispos. 2007;35(12):2270–80.
64. Strassburg CP. Pharmacogenetics of Gilbert's syndrome. Pharmacogenomics. 2008;9(6):703–15.
65. Innocenti F, Iyer L, Ratain MJ. Pharmacogenetics of anticancer agents: lessons from amonafide and irinotecan. Drug Metab Dispos. 2001;29(4 Pt 2):596–600.
66. Innocenti F, Undevia SD, Iyer L, Chen PX, Das S, Kocherginsky M, et al. Genetic variants in the UDP-glucuronosyltransferase 1A1 gene predict the risk of severe neutropenia of irinotecan. J Clin Oncol. 2004;22(8):1382–8.
67. Hoskins JM, Goldberg RM, Qu P, Ibrahim JG, McLeod HL. UGT1A1*28 genotype and irinotecan-induced neutropenia: dose matters. J Natl Cancer Inst. 2007;99(17):1290–5.
68. Evaluation of Genomic Applications in Practice and Prevention (EGAPP) Working Group. Recommendations from the EGAPP Working Group: can UGT1A1 genotyping reduce morbidity and mortality in patients with metastatic colorectal cancer treated with irinotecan? Genet Med. 2009;11(1):15–20.
69. Scott SA. Clinical pharmacogenomics: opportunities and challenges at point of care. Clin Pharmacol Ther. 2013;93(1):33–5.
70. Scott SA. Personalizing medicine with clinical pharmacogenetics. Genet Med. 2011;13(12):987–95.
71. Pulley JM, Denny JC, Peterson JF, Bernard GR, Vnencak-Jones CL, Ramirez AH, et al. Operational implementation of prospective genotyping for personalized medicine: the design of the Vanderbilt PREDICT project. Clin Pharmacol Ther. 2012;92(1):87–95.
72. O'Donnell PH, Bush A, Spitz J, Danahey K, Saner D, Das S, et al. The 1200 patients project: creating a new medical model system for clinical implementation of pharmacogenomics. Clin Pharmacol Ther. 2012;92(4):446–9.
73. Gottesman O, Scott SA, Ellis SB, Overby CL, Ludtke A, Hulot JS, et al. The CLIPMERGE PGx Program: clinical implementation of personalized medicine through electronic health records and genomics-pharmacogenomics. Clin Pharmacol Ther. 2013;94(2):214–7.
74. Rasmussen-Torvik LJ, Stallings SC, Gordon AS, Almoguera B, Basford MA, Bielinski SJ, et al. Design and anticipated outcomes of the eMERGE-PGx project: a multicenter pilot for preemptive pharmacogenomics in electronic health record systems. Clin Pharmacol Ther. 2014;96(4):482–9.

Section II

Inherited Cancers

Section Editor: Hanna Rennert

Inherited Breast Cancer

22

Rachel Michaelson-Cohen, Rachel Beeri, Eliahu Golomb, and Ephrat Levy-Lahad

Abstract

Inherited mutations in high-risk breast cancer-predisposing genes explain approximately 10 % of all breast cancer cases. Most of these mutations are in the *BRCA1* and *BRCA2* genes, as part of hereditary breast and ovarian cancer (HBOC). Others are in genes associated with syndromes which include a wider spectrum of malignancies and/or distinct clinical features. Molecular analysis, guided by clinical criteria and application of risk assessment models, currently reveal the underlying cause in roughly half of hereditary breast cancer families. Women who have inherited mutations in the *HBOC* genes have a high lifetime risk for both breast cancer and ovarian cancer. In *BRCA1* and *BRCA2* carriers, effective surveillance and prevention measures (such as risk-reduction salpingo-oophorectomy) reduce morbidity and mortality, and mutation status can enable targeted therapy (such as PARP inhibitors).

Clinical genetic analysis for suspected inherited predisposition to breast cancer, previously mostly limited to Sanger sequencing of *BRCA1* and *BRCA2*, has been transformed by next-generation sequencing (NGS) technology, which enables rapid and simultaneous analysis of multiple genes. The ability of NGS assays to accurately and cost-effectively detect all classes of mutations, including large rearrangements, offers an important advantage over previous testing strategies. However, clinical interpretation of variants remains a significant challenge even in the well-studied *BRCA1* and *BRCA2* genes, let alone other breast cancer-associated genes. Testing numerous individuals is revealing an ever greater number of rare variations, whose effect on gene and protein function remains unclear. Reporting such variants of unknown significance is not driven by their clinical utility, and there is an urgent need for improved strategies to assess their functional and clinical effects. Testing genes beyond *BRCA1* and *BRCA2* is further complicated by the current lack of evidence-based guidelines for surveillance and prevention measures, even for carriers of mutations in genes considered to be clear moderate-risk predisposition genes.

R. Michaelson-Cohen, M.D. • E. Levy-Lahad, M.D. (✉)
Hebrew University Medical School, Jerusalem, Israel

Medical Genetics Institute, Shaare Zedek Medical Center, Jerusalem, Israel
e-mail: lahad@szmc.org.il

R. Beeri, Ph.D.
Medical Genetics Institute, Shaare Zedek Medical Center, Jerusalem, Israel

E. Golomb, M.D., Ph.D.
Department of Pathology, Shaare Zedek Medical Center, Medical Genetics Institute, Jerusalem, Israel

D.G.B. Leonard (ed.), *Molecular Pathology in Clinical Practice*, DOI 10.1007/978-3-319-19674-9_22

Nevertheless, identifying cancer-predisposing mutations is increasingly feasible, will lead to optimized, personalized care for mutation carriers, and is likely to provide insights of broader relevance to cancer.

Keywords
Breast cancer • *BRCA1* • *BRCA2* • HBOC (hereditary breast and ovarian cancer) • Risk assessment • NGS (next-generation sequencing) • PARP inhibitors • RR-BSO (risk-reducing salpingo-oophorectomy) • Multiple gene testing panels

Introduction

Breast cancer is the most common invasive cancer in women and in Western countries is the leading cause of cancer deaths in women after lung cancer. Breast cancer risk is affected by both environmental/behavioral and genetic factors, reflecting complex disease etiology. Established risk factors include age, family history of breast cancer, reproductive behavior, hormonal exposures, lifestyle habits, and personal breast-specific history (e.g., mammographic density, previous breast cancer, breast biopsy features of benign lesions) [1]. Family history of breast cancer is the most significant risk factor after female gender and older age. In the Swedish Family-Cancer Database, the attributable risk of a positive family history was estimated at about 11 % [2]. The risk to relatives of a person with breast cancer increases with closer degree of relationship and with younger age at cancer diagnosis [3]. Presence of an affected first-degree relative confers a relative risk of 1.76–2.96, depending on the age at diagnosis and the tumor's receptor status [4]. Male breast cancer is rare in general and has a higher genetic component than female breast cancer [5].

The Molecular Basis of Inherited Breast Cancer

Inherited mutations in high-risk breast cancer-predisposing genes explain 8–10 % of all breast cancer cases [6]. Most of these mutations are in the *BRCA1* and *BRCA2* genes, which were identified in 1994 and 1995, respectively, as the bases of hereditary breast-ovarian cancer syndrome (HBOC). More rarely, breast cancer predisposition is caused by mutations in genes associated with other syndromes which include a wider spectrum of malignancies and/or distinct clinical features. Examples include *TP53* (Li-Fraumeni syndrome), *PTEN* (Cowden syndrome), and *STK11* (Peutz-Jeghers syndrome). Molecular analysis guided by clinical criteria [7, 8] and application of risk assessment models (see below) currently reveal the underlying cause in roughly half of hereditary breast cancer families [9].

The remaining cases have been the subject of intense investigation in the past 15 years, but this has not led to the discovery of additional major breast cancer genes. Although some familial aggregates may be explained by mutations conferring moderate (two- to three-fold) risks, e.g., *CHEK2* or *ATM* mutations, or by combinations of low-risk alleles [10], a plausible explanation is that non-*BRCA1–BRCA2* hereditary breast cancer is caused by high-risk mutations in a large number of genes, with each gene mutated in only a small proportion of families [11]. This hypothesis is being tested, with the advent of genome sequencing in clinical practice. Indeed, *RAD51C* [12] and *RAD51D* [13] mutations have been identified as rare causes of HBOC (approximately 1 % of non-*BRCA1–BRCA2* families), and a significant number of new genes can be expected to be identified in the near future.

BRCA1 and *BRCA2* Structure and Function

BRCA1 (NG_005905.2) and *BRCA2* (NG_012772.1) were identified as genes mutated in HBOC, by genetic analysis in families with multiple cases of these malignancies [14, 15]. The *BRCA1* gene on chromosome 17 encodes a 7.8 kb transcript composed of 24 coding exons that is translated to a 1,863 amino acid (220 kD) protein [16]. BRCA1 is a chromatin-interacting protein with an amino-terminal RING domain that has E3 ubiquitin ligase activity, a nuclear localization signal, and the BRCA1 C-terminal (BRCT) phosphopeptide-binding domain, which is conserved in multiple proteins involved in the DNA damage response (DDR). The *BRCA2* gene on chromosome 13 encodes a 10.4 kb transcript composed of 27 exons that is translated to a 3,418 amino acid (380 kD) protein. BRCA2 contains a DNA-binding domain (DBD) that binds both single-stranded DNA (ssDNA) and double-stranded DNA (dsDNA), eight BRC repeats that bind RAD51, a key protein in homologous recombination (HR), and a C-terminal NLS [17].

Both BRCA1 and BRCA2 play important roles in the DDR, the cellular defense mechanism against genotoxic stress. The DDR is a multistage process that includes sensing ssDNA and dsDNA breaks (DSBs), mediating between sensors and repair effectors, and repairing DNA damage. Impairment of the DDR can lead to genomic/chromosomal instability, a hallmark of many malignancies, and indeed, cells lacking either BRCA1 or BRCA2 have multiple chromosomal aberrations, suggesting that both proteins function as "caretakers" of genomic integrity (reviewed in Ref. 17). Additional BRCA1 roles include estrogen receptor (ER) signaling [18], TP53 stabilization, and transcription modulation including heterochromatin-mediated silencing [19]. BRCA2 has more limited functions and, by recruiting RAD51, is primarily a co-effector of DNA repair by HR, in which the undamaged sister chromatid is used as an accurate template for DSB repair. The BRCA1-PALB2 complex is required for BRCA2 recruitment [17], and RAD51 binding to the BRCA2-BRC repeats facilitates recruitment of RAD51 to DSBs [20].

BRCA1 and *BRCA2* Mutations

Mutational analysis is complicated by the large size of the *BRCA1* and *BRCA2* genes and the wide variety and distribution of mutations. Interpretation of test results is complicated by occurrence of variants of unknown significance (VUS, see below). Both public and commercial databases curate *BRCA1* and *BRCA2* mutations. The National Human Genome Research Institute hosts the Breast Cancer Information Core (BIC) (see URL list), which at the time of this writing includes 15,311 entries for *BRCA1*, with 1,787 distinct mutations, polymorphisms, and variants, 981 of which had been reported only once. For *BRCA2*, BIC contains 14,914 entries, including 2,000 distinct mutations, polymorphisms, and variants, 1,065 of which have been reported only once. Additional online databases include the Human Gene Mutation Database (HGMD, see URL list), the Leiden Open Variation Database (LOVD), and ClinVar (see URL list).

Founder Mutations

The frequency and spectrum of *BRCA1* and *BRCA2* mutations are highly dependent on ethnicity [21, 22]. While the majority of mutations are rare, "private" mutations observed in single cases or families, some mutations recur in particular ethnic groups and are called founder mutations. These founder mutations are thought to have occurred once in the history of an ethnic group and predominate because of population isolation and expansion. *BRCA1* and *BRCA2* testing is obviously simplified when founder mutations account for a high proportion of mutations in a specific ethnic group.

Founder *BRCA1* and *BRCA2* mutations have been described worldwide including in Norway [23], Sweden [24], Poland [25], and numerous other countries, as well as in many ethnic groups [21], including people of African ancestry [26]. Perhaps the most prominent examples are the founder mutations in Ashkenazi Jews (Jews of European origin) and in Iceland. Among Ashkenazi Jews, two *BRCA1* mutations (185delAG and 5382insC) and one *BRCA2* mutation (6174delT) are found in approximately 2.5 % of healthy individuals and account for approximately 10 % of all breast cancer cases, approximately one quarter of breast cancers diagnosed before age 40, and approximately 40 % of ovarian cancer at any age [27, 28]. Other *BRCA1* and *BRCA2* mutations are rare [29].

In Iceland, the frequency of the common *BRCA2* mutation (999del5) is 0.4 % and accounts for 8.5 % and 7.9 % of breast cancer and ovarian cancer patients, respectively [30]. In addition, a rare *BRCA1* founder mutation (G5193A) is present in 1 % of cases of breast cancer and ovarian cancer [21]. In males, these Icelandic founder mutations are responsible for about half of male breast cancer cases and a large percentage of prostate cancer in breast cancer families. Founder mutations also include deletions and duplications. The 6 kbp *BRCA1* exon 13 duplication is an ancestral British mutation found in 10 of 1,831 (0.5 %) of affected families [31]. Three *BRCA1* genomic deletions in exons 22, 13, and 13–16 account for as much as 36 % of *BRCA1* mutations in families of Dutch ancestry [32].

Clinical Utility of *BRCA1* and *BRCA2* Testing

Cancer Risks in *BRCA1* and *BRCA2* Mutation Carriers

Women who have inherited mutations in the *BRCA1* and *BRCA2* genes have a high lifetime risk of breast cancer (56–84 %) [27, 33–35], an increased risk of contralateral breast cancer [27, 36–39], and a substantial lifetime risk of ovarian cancer (11–62 %, depending on the gene involved and the population studied) [27, 36, 37, 40, 41]. The average age at diagnosis of both breast and ovarian cancer is generally younger for *BRCA1* carriers than for *BRCA2* carriers, but each can manifest as breast cancer in the 20s. In addition to breast and ovarian cancer, an excess of male breast cancer occurs in *BRCA2* families and to a lesser extent in *BRCA1* families [29]. Lifetime risk of breast cancer is about 6 % for male *BRCA2* carriers and is probably lower for male *BRCA1* carriers. *BRCA2* mutations also are associated with an excess risk for prostate cancer in males and for pancreatic cancer and melanoma in both sexes.

In fact, *BRCA2* has been considered an important pancreatic cancer predisposition gene for many years [42], and more recent reports have estimated that it accounts for 6–12 % of pancreatic cancer families [43, 44]. *BRCA1* and *BRCA2* mutation carriers have a 2.5-fold and 3.5- to 10-fold increased risk of pancreatic cancer, respectively [45, 46], although absolute risks are low (<2 %) [47].

Risk Management in *BRCA1* and *BRCA2* Mutation Carriers

Effective cancer risk management strategies are available for *BRCA1* and *BRCA2* carriers as well as for families with a high clinical suspicion of genetic predisposition. HBOC management includes both surveillance and preventive measures, e.g., early breast cancer surveillance (from age 25 to 30 years) by annual mammography and breast MRI, chemoprevention for breast (e.g., tamoxifen) and ovarian (e.g., oral contraceptives) cancers, and risk-reducing (RR) surgery by mastectomy (RRM) and salpingo-oophorectomy (RRSO). Two large prospective studies [48, 49] showed that in *BRCA1* and *BRCA2* carriers, RRSO reduces overall mortality by 60–77 %. Breast cancer-specific mortality was reduced by 56 % and ovarian cancer-specific mortality by 79 % [48].

Testing Family Members

In the setting of a known familial mutation, identifying a relative as a noncarrier obviates the need for aggressive surveillance and prevention measures and provides reassurance to the individuals tested as well as to their offspring. Identifying that a person is a *BRCA1* or *BRCA2* carrier provides an opportunity for effective interventions.

Therapeutic Implications

Testing may have clinical implications for individuals newly or previously diagnosed with breast or ovarian cancer. Some evidence indicates that tumors in *BRCA1* and *BRCA2* mutation carriers are particularly sensitive to platinum-based chemotherapy (reviewed in Ref. 50), and a new class of compounds, poly-ADP-ribose-polymerase (PARP) inhibitors, were designed specifically to target BRCA-associated tumors. PARP inhibitors target the ssDNA repair pathway. Unrepaired ssDNA breaks convert to DSBs, which cannot be repaired by BRCA-deficient cells, resulting in selective synthetic lethality of these tumor cells [51]. A PARP inhibitor has already been approved by the FDA for advanced ovarian cancer in *BRCA* mutation carriers [52, 53], heralding the therapeutic utility of *BRCA1* and *BRCA2* testing in treatment selection. Responses have also been observed in BRCA carriers with pancreatic cancer, and clinical trials are underway with various PARP inhibitors in a variety of BRCA and BRCA-pathway-associated tumors [52, 54, 55].

BRCA1 and *BRCA2* Testing

Breast Cancer Pathology in *BRCA1* and *BRCA2* Mutation Carriers

Gene expression analysis studies indicate five major breast cancer types: luminal A, luminal B, "normal breast-like," HER2 amplified, and basal [56, 57]. Luminal A tumors tend to be of lower grade, showing tubule formation, lower proliferative activity, cellular pleomorphism, and estrogen (ER) and progesterone receptors (PR) expression, and lack of HER2 amplification. Luminal B tumors tend to be high grade (show high proliferative activity and pleomorphism, with little or no tubule formation), express ER and PR, and show variable HER2 expression and amplification. Basal-type carcinomas tend to be high grade, not to express ER, PR, or HER2 (i.e., are triple negative), and express the high molecular weight cytokeratins: 5/6 and 14 and/or EGFR1. This basal group includes medullary and atypical medullary breast carcinomas. The *HER2* oncogene amplification subtype tends to be high grade and not to express ER or PR.

BRCA1-associated breast cancers tend to be basal-type, high grade, and show a syncytial growth pattern with metaplastic features more than sporadic and other familial breast cancers. Basal-type carcinomas are 27 times more likely to be associated with a *BRCA1* mutation compared to other breast cancer subtypes [58]. In contrast, *BRCA2*-associated breast cancers have less distinct morphological characteristics. *BRCA2*-associated breast cancers tend to have luminal B-type features, i.e., tubule formation, "pushing" borders, high mitotic counts and proliferative activity (by Ki-67 immunostaining), and ER and PR expression. A differentiating point between *BRCA2*-associated tumors and characteristic sporadic tumors may lie in the discrepancy between their high proliferative activity relative to the "quiescent" features of hormone receptor expression and tubule formation [58] and in the tendency to have "pushing" borders [59]. However, pathological and expression profile differences are neither sufficiently sensitive nor specific to preclude *BRCA1* or *BRCA2* testing in cases lacking these features.

Immunohistochemistry for BRCA1 and BRCA2

Lack of BRCA1 or BRCA2 protein expression occurs in BRCA1- and BRCA2-associated tumors of almost all carriers (except those with missense mutations). This is a result of loss of the normal (nonmutant) allele. In affected persons, tumor BRCA1 and BRCA2 immunohistochemistry (IHC) is a plausible screening test to identify potential carriers, similar to IHC for mismatch repair protein expression to screen for hereditary nonpolyposis colon cancer (HNPCC). IHC for

BRCA1 was originally confounded by conflicting evidence regarding its subcellular localization and lack of robust antibodies, and evidence suggested that it did not reliably identify *BRCA1* carriers [60]. More recent studies demonstrated a 52 % positive predictive value (PPV) in ovarian cancer cases (86 % sensitivity and 78 % specificity for germline mutations) [61] and 80 % sensitivity and 100 % specificity in breast cancers [62]. These studies all used a nuclear staining monoclonal antibody (Ab-1/MS110) against the N-terminus. A reliable BRCA1 C-terminal antibody is not commercially available, precluding distinction between wild-type and truncated BRCA1 proteins. For BRCA2, IHC combining both N-terminal and C-terminal antibodies has been shown to be highly sensitive (95 %) and specific (98 %) in identifying potential carriers of *BRCA2* truncating mutations [63]. However, BRCA1 and BRCA2 IHC is not widely used, probably due to lack of robust BRCA1 IHC, the lack of identification of missense mutations in either gene, and the existence of other mechanisms, e.g., promoter methylation, leading to loss of BRCA1 protein (Meisel et al. 2014).

Refining the morphological and IHC characteristics of carcinomas associated with specific mutations, and quantitative assessment of these associations, may still play a role in prioritizing genetic analysis. Even if new sequencing methods render prioritization superfluous, these correlates remain important for assessment of VUS, both in *BRCA1* and *BRCA2*, and in other susceptibility genes.

BRCA1 and *BRCA2* Genetic Testing Methods

Clinical and Pathological Correlates of *BRCA1* and *BRCA2* Mutations

The complexity of full molecular analysis of *BRCA1* and *BRCA2* has led to attempts to identify clinical, pathological, and gene expression correlates of mutations in these genes, to aid in selecting cases to test and prioritize the genes to be analyzed. Despite the excess of male breast and other cancers in *BRCA2* vs *BRCA1* families, breast and ovarian cancer are the predominant malignancies in both cases, so generally the types of cancers in a family cannot reliably distinguish *BRCA1* from *BRCA2*. More importantly, approximately half of the affected female carriers do not have a significant family history that would have led to testing before their cancer diagnosis [27, 64].

Probability Models

Probability models were developed to estimate the likelihood that an individual or family has a *BRCA1* or *BRCA2* mutation. Testing costs were a major impetus for developing these models, and testing is commonly considered as indicated if the probability of mutation detection is at least 10 % (common in the USA and for privately funded testing) or 20 % (for public health services, e.g., the UK NHS NICE guidelines; see URL list). Although decreasing testing costs and increasing therapeutic implications lessen the relevance of such thresholds, estimating the likelihood of a HBOC mutation remains important because of the complexity of interpreting test results. In particular, the significance of a VUS is in part determined by the PPV calculated a priori by a prediction model.

Two broadly used models are BRCAPRO and Myriad II. BRCAPRO ([65], also see Cancer Pro in URL list) is a computer-based Bayesian probability model that uses breast and/or ovarian cancer family history to determine the probability that a *BRCA1* or *BRCA2* mutation accounts for cancer in the index case. The main parameters integrated in the risk assessment are the population prevalence of mutations, age-specific risks for carriers, and Ashkenazi Jewish heritage. The model is frequently updated, and the recent addition of breast tumor markers (hormone receptor and HER2 status) has improved prediction accuracy [66]). Myriad II (see URL list) is an online set of frequently updated prevalence tables categorized by ethnic ancestry (Ashkenazi Jewish or other), age of breast cancer diagnosis (<50 years or >50 years), and personal or family history of ovarian cancer. Myriad II is based on test results from the Myriad Genetic Laboratories commercial testing service [29]. Both models predict mutation presence more accurately than family cancer history alone and are part of the publicly available, convenient CancerGene software package (Cancer Pro, see URL list), which simultaneously calculates results for both models. In a direct comparison, BRCAPRO had higher sensitivity and similar specificity to Myriad II [67].

Other probability models include the Breast and Ovarian Analysis of Disease Incidence and Carrier Estimation Algorithm (BOADICEA) [68, 69], which performs as well as BRCAPRO [70], Tyrer-Cuzick [34, 71], and the Manchester Scoring System [72]. Notably, most prediction models were developed using data from non-Hispanic Caucasian women and may be less accurate in other populations. Both BOADICEA and BRCAPRO have poorer performance in African Americans and Hispanics [73], and BRCAPRO and Myriad II underpredicted Asian carriers [74].

Standard Genetic Testing Methods

Targeted Mutation Analysis

In relevant populations, targeted founder mutation testing remains the first step in *BRCA1* and *BRCA2* analysis. Because targeted analysis is simple, inexpensive, and detects only clearly pathological mutations, it can be offered to all women affected with breast/ovarian cancer in populations with founder mutations, even without prior risk assessment as detailed above [64]. Targeted mutation analysis techniques include PCR-RFLP which requires postamplification restriction enzyme digestion and TaqMan real-time allelic discrimination which is more rapid and scalable to high-throughput genotyping. If no founder mutation is detected, full analysis is considered based on the residual likelihood that a *BRCA1* or *BRCA2* germline mutation is present in the particular individual.

Mutation Scanning and Sanger Sequencing

Because Sanger sequencing large genes is both time- and cost-intensive, historically, various scanning techniques were used to detect *BRCA1* and *BRCA2* mutations, e.g., single-strand conformation polymorphism (SSCP) and high-performance liquid chromatography (HPLC). However, sensitivity of scanning is low, with nearly one-third of *BRCA1* and *BRCA2* mutations detectable by sequencing are missed by scanning methods [75]. Therefore, despite higher costs, Sanger sequencing of *BRCA1* and *BRCA2* coding exons and flanking intronic sequences has been the gold standard for non-rearrangement mutation analysis. An important concern with any sequencing technique is identification of VUS which are found in 5–10 % of all fully sequenced individuals ([76] and discussed below).

BRCA1 and *BRCA2* Genomic Rearrangement Testing

Large deletions or insertions are estimated to account for 12–18 % of *BRCA1* mutations but are less frequent in *BRCA2* and in Ashkenazi Jews [77–79]. Such rearrangements are not detectable by Sanger sequencing. In the USA, until many claims of the Myriad patent for *BRCA1* and *BRCA2* testing was invalidated by the US Supreme Court, standard testing included both Sanger sequencing and screening for four large deletions and duplications in *BRCA1*, specifically large deletions in exons 13, 14–20, and 22, and duplication of exon 13. In a study of 20,000 patients, 66 of 2,634 (2.5 %) deleterious mutations were rearrangements [80]. The exon 13 duplication represented 80 % of rearrangement mutations and 2 % of total mutations, making this the most prevalent non-Ashkenazi mutation [80]. Outside the USA, testing for large rearrangements has been comprehensive, revealing that approximately 10 % of *BRCA1* and *BRCA2* mutations are genomic rearrangements ([79], [81]). Genomic rearrangement testing has usually been performed using PCR-based quantitative methods such as multiplex ligation-dependent probe amplification (MLPA) [82]. Even with the advent of next-generation sequencing (NGS) technologies, detection of large genomic rearrangements remains challenging, requiring very high coverage, so complementing NGS with specific rearrangement testing has been advocated [83, 84].

Next-Generation Sequencing of *BRCA1* and *BRCA2*

BRCA1 and *BRCA2* testing has become integral to the clinical management of women with a personal or family history of breast or ovarian cancer [77] and has significantly increased the number of tests performed. In parallel, NGS testing methods allow higher throughput and lower cost per sequenced base. NGS can generate gigabases of nucleotides of sequence data in a single instrument run [85, 86], enabling sequencing of human exomes and genomes (NGS as a method is described in Chap. 59). NGS testing for *BRCA1* and *BRCA2* analysis [83, 87–91] has become routine in many clinical laboratories in the last five years.

NGS for point/small mutation analysis was originally reported using the GAIIx-Illumina MPS platform on templates produced by long-range PCR of the *BRCA1*, *BRCA2*, and *TP53* genes [87] or by in-solution capture using custom-designed complementary RNA oligonucleotide baits for 21 breast/ovarian cancer predisposition genes including *BRCA1* and *BRCA2* [82]. A multiplex bar-coded amplicon pyrosequencing method for *BRCA1* and *BRCA2* analysis was also reported (Roche/GS-FLX) [88, 89], with 98 % sensitivity. Only 3 of 133 (2 %) variants were not detected, which were all deletions or duplications in homopolymers of ≥7 nucleotides, a known limitation of pyrosequencing [88, 89]. All other studies ([82, 87], Hernan et al. 2012, [91]) reported 100 % sensitivity for point mutations and small insertions/deletions (indels). Specificity ranged from 84 % [87] to 100 % [82, 88, 89]. Bar coding strategies that enable pooling samples in one run are available and further reduce sequencing costs without compromising accuracy.

Next-Generation Sequencing for *BRCA1* and *BRCA2* Genomic Rearrangements

Detecting genomic rearrangements is possible with some but not all NGS strategies. De Leeneer et al. reported a lack of detection of large rearrangements, which is typical of NGS using short reads from short-fragment libraries [88, 89]. In contrast, Walsh identified all six large rearrangements tested (160 bp to 101 kbp in size) by comparing the number of reads at each base pair in each sample to the number of reads at the same base pair for all other samples [82]. This read depth analysis was possible because of significantly higher read depth (>1,200 vs 38 in Ref. 88, 89) and use of a mate-paired library template. In mate-paired libraries, template DNA fragments of known size (typically 2–5 kbp) are circularized and re-sheared, so that both ends of the original fragment are adjacent to each other ("mates") in a new fragment which is sequenced. The original distance between the sequenced "mates" is known and can be compared to the expected distance in the reference sequence. This approach is now commonly used in genome-wide detection of structural rearrangements [92, 93].

The ability of NGS assays to accurately and cost-effectively detect all classes of mutations, including large rearrangements, offers an important advantage compared to previous testing strategies, which required multiple techniques to achieve comprehensive *BRCA1* and *BRCA2* analysis.

NGS Testing for Breast Cancer Predisposition Genes Beyond *BRCA1* and *BRCA2*: Advantages and Challenges

In recent years, testing has expanded to cancer predisposition genes other than *BRCA1* and *BRCA2*. These genes can be defined as genes in which rare mutations confer a greater than two-fold relative breast cancer risk [94]. Advances in technology have allowed development of multiplex gene panels in which many genes can be assessed simultaneously by NGS. NGS has made large-scale, high-throughput testing available and affordable. The advantage of this approach is an efficient evaluation that may be only slightly more expensive than standard-of-care genetic testing (or in the case of serial testing even less expensive) [95]. For familial cancer conditions, exome sequencing is gradually becoming more successful and is identifying new breast cancer risk genes [96, 97]. Identification of non-syndromic genes will remain challenging until it is possible to interpret data from testing of thousands of individuals. Analytical prioritization strategies will thus have high utility over the next few years [98].

Identifying a cancer-predisposing mutation will lead to optimized, personalized care for mutation carriers and will probably provide insights of broader relevance to cancer.

Currently, over 20 breast cancer predisposition genes are associated with at least a moderately increased risk for breast cancer, including *BRCA1, BRCA2, TP53, PTEN, STK11, CHEK2, ATM, BRIP1, PALB2, CDH1, RAD51C, RAD51D*, and more genes are likely to be identified in the future [99]. Although approximately 5 % of high-risk patients with negative *BRCA* results can be expected to carry a mutation in *CHEK2* or *TP53* [77], these and other genes were often tested only selectively [100] because of the low expected yield per gene, compounded by high sequencing costs. NGS testing has revolutionized the possibility of multiple gene testing. NGS testing of over 20 genes has been reported at less than half the cost of commercial testing of only *BRCA1* and *BRCA2* [82], and NGS-based panels of multiple cancer-related genes are available in clinical laboratories. Multiple gene testing is also being performed for other familial cancers, such as in Lynch (HNPCC) syndrome and pancreatic cancer [101]. In 278 young onset (<40 years) breast cancer patients in which previous *BRCA1* and *BRCA2* testing was negative, a 20-gene NGS panel revealed a deleterious or likely deleterious mutation in 11 % [102]. A similar yield of 11.4 %, after excluding *BRCA1* and *BRCA2* mutations, was observed in a study of 198 persons including a mix of affected and unaffected high-risk individuals [103].

NGS panels also present a number of challenges. Multiple genes present in current clinical testing panels were chosen based on their participation in cancer pathways (particularly the Fanconi anemia pathway) or on other hypothetical grounds, without previous epidemiological or clinical evidence that they are indeed hereditary cancer predisposition genes [94]. Overestimation of a likely causal link between the presence of a gene variant and cancer in an individual is not rare, since rare coding variations, including putative deleterious mutations, are collectively common [98, 104]. For example, heterozygosity for *MUTYH* mutations was found in 2.2 % of young-onset breast cancer cases, yet *MUTYH* has not been previously shown to be a breast cancer predisposition gene [102]. Furthermore, VUS are more commonly observed as new genes are added to panels, particularly genes for which the full extent of benign variation is not yet described. Currently, the VUS rate is approximately 20 % for a 22-gene panel, with VUS being more common in non-Whites [102]. The extent of VUS will reflect a balance between increasing knowledge of existing variation and the number of genes added to panels. Finally, with respect to clinical utility, it must be recognized that even for genes considered to be clear moderate-risk predisposition genes, evidence-based guidelines for surveillance or prevention measures in mutation carriers are not available [95, 102].

Interpretation of *BRCA1* and *BRCA2* Test Results

Sequencing of *BRCA1* and *BRCA2* generates 36,000 nucleotides of sequence per person, posing problems of data management and leading to detection of multiple variants, often novel. Nonsense mutations, frameshift mutations, and large rearrangements are clearly deleterious, i.e., associated with loss of gene function and highly increased cancer risks. However, in the absence of simple assays for either BRCA1 or BRCA2 function in the presence of identified variants, the clinical significance of missense variants, leading to amino acid substitutions, is more difficult to determine. This is also true of splice site mutations with no clear biological implications, intronic variants, small in-frame indels (inserting or deleting only a single or few amino acids), and silent mutations (nucleotide substitutions that do not change the amino acid). Although over time a large number of such variants have been classified as either pathogenic or benign, many remain unclassified, and full *BRCA1* and *BRCA2* sequencing detects VUS in 5–10 % of individuals tested [76, 105]. VUS pose difficult challenges in genetic counseling and clinical management and are currently assessed using a number of tools, described below.

Literature and Database Searches and Analysis of Control Noncancer Groups

Online databases, e.g., the Breast Cancer Information Core (BIC) database, the BReast CAncer genes IARC database, and ClinVar (see URL list) include information on the possible clinical significance of reported variants. Comparing the frequency of a variant between cancer cases and controls also can indicate if a VUS is pathogenic, if found in the cases with a significantly higher frequency than the controls.

In Silico Assessment of Missense Mutations

Missense variants can be assessed for location within a functional domain of the protein (e.g., the BRCA1-RING finger), evolutionary conservation, and severity of modification of the biophysical characteristics due to the amino acid change. Examples of public, in silico tools for all proteins include SIFT (Sorting Intolerant From Tolerant) and PolyPhen (Polymorphism Phenotyping, see URL list) which predict the possible impact of an amino acid substitution on the structure and function of a specific protein based on sequence homology and comparative physical methods [106, 107]. An in silico analysis using a combination of evolutionary conservation and the Grantham score (a measure of the chemical difference between the normal and mutant amino acids) enabled tentative classification of 50 % of missense VUS observed during clinical testing of *BRCA1* with 50 of 314 missense variants and 2 of 8 in-frame deletions classified as probably deleterious and 92 of 314 missense variants as probably neutral [108, 109].

Assessment of Effects on Splicing

Variants can affect splicing, even if they are located outside exon-intron junctions, e.g., by affecting exonic splicing elements. Therefore, VUS should be analyzed in silico using splicing prediction models and experimentally using RNA-based assays. The BReast CAncer genes IARC database (see URL list) has a *BRCA1*- and *BRCA2*-specific tool which assesses effect of variants on splicing. In a study of VUS using five splicing prediction programs and experimental assays, 10 of 53 VUS were predicted to affect splicing by two or more programs, and four of these predictions were confirmed by splicing assays. Experimental assays showed that another five intra-exonal VUS, though not predicted to alter splicing in silico, caused variable levels of exon skipping [110].

Co-segregation with Cancer in the Family

In families with multiple cases of cancer, a pathogenic mutation is expected to segregate with the disease, i.e., be present in affected relatives and absent in healthy older relatives. Lack of segregation decreases the likelihood that a VUS is pathogenic. However, segregation studies are often not possible, because of small family size, or limited availability of family data and DNA samples, especially for deceased relatives.

Co-occurrence with a Pathologic Mutation

Based on the lethality of both *BRCA1* and *BRCA2* knockout mice, biallelic deleterious mutations in *BRCA1* or *BRCA2* are expected to be lethal or associated with a severe developmental phenotype. Indeed, biallelic *BRCA2* mutations cause Fanconi anemia-type D1 which can include various congenital anomalies [111], and rare biallelic *BRCA1* mutations are associated with severe developmental abnormalities [112, 113]. Therefore, determining that a VUS is in trans with a known deleterious mutation supports its classification as neutral. In general, proving that variants are in trans is complicated by the need to test additional family members to determine the phasing of the mutations based on inheritance patterns in the family [109].

Loss of Heterozygosity in the Tumor

Based on Knudson's two-hit hypothesis, *BRCA*-associated tumors are expected to show loss of heterozygosity (LOH) at the *BRCA* locus more frequently than sporadic tumors [114], mainly through loss of the normal allele. If a VUS is identified in an affected person whose tumor is available, LOH information can be incorporated into integrated models to assess the pathogenicity of the VUS [76].

Tumor Pathological Characteristics

As detailed above, *BRCA1*-associated tumors have characteristic features, which can be helpful in determining VUS pathogenicity [115]. In particular, *BRCA1*-associated breast cancer is more often "triple negative" (lack of ER, PR, and HER2 expression) with a basal-like expression profile and medullary morphology.

Functional Assays

A few studies have utilized functional assay results to refine the likelihood of pathogenicity of missense changes in *BRCA1* or *BRCA2* [116, 117]. A functional assay measuring the effect of missense mutations on BRCA2 activity in HR DNA repair and centriole amplification demonstrated a strong correlation between the functional assay and the likelihood model [116]. Functional assays also have been developed for BRCA1 (reviewed in Ref. 118) and BRCA2 [119].

Classification and Reclassification of *BRCA1* and *BRCA2* Variants

BRCA1 and *BRCA2* are among the largest genes frequently sequenced in the clinical setting, which led to early realization of the issue of VUS, which has become a general issue since NGS testing has moved into clinical care. The *BRCA*-testing community established a research-based consortium, ENIGMA (evidence-based network for the interpretation of germline mutant alleles; see URL list), which aims to facilitate classification of variants through collaborative large-scale projects by sharing data and improving classification methods [120]. This consortium also intends to analyze variants in other cancer predisposition genes and develop generally applicable strategies.

Clinically, *BRCA1* and *BRCA2* VUS pose a significant dilemma for carriers, who must make difficult decisions regarding risk-reduction surgeries based on inconclusive test results. Although a VUS may be reclassified to natural or pathologic over time, clinical decisions must be made in the present, leading some patients to undergo irreversible procedures before VUS reclassification is achieved. Of 107 women who received a *BRCA* VUS result between 1998 and 2009, 11 (10.3 %) pursued RRM and 22 (20.6 %) pursued RRSO [105]. These uptake rates overlap rates for women both with and without clearly pathogenic mutations. Reclassification of VUS occurred up to 9 years after testing, but five of 22 (22.7 %) women, followed up for 8 years or longer, continued to have a VUS result.

Laboratory Issues

Implementing a molecular genetic test for clinical use is a complex process involving many levels of assessment and validation. This is particularly true for implementation of a completely novel technology and is the major laboratory issue confronting cancer predisposition testing. Principles of validation and verification in the area of human molecular genetic testing have been delineated by the EuroGentest Validation Group [121] and by the College of American Pathologists' Molecular Pathology Resource Committee [122]. Use of NGS has only recently transitioned from the research to the clinical setting, and criteria for clinical NGS testing, as well as better delineation of the types of NGS errors, are still evolving [88, 89, 123]. NGS involves multiple steps, including sample preparation, enrichment and capture strategies, library preparation, sequence generation, and sequence analysis including result interpretation and reporting. Furthermore, the volume of data generated by NGS requires new protocols for data transfer, storage, secondary processing, and security [124].

Quality management practices are obviously essential at all stages of the testing process to ensure accuracy and utility. Although proficiency testing/external quality assessment (PT/EQA) schemes for Sanger sequencing of *BRCA1* and *BRCA2* exist, the list of genes for which PT is not available is rapidly growing and potentially encompasses all human genes [125]. Furthermore, a single gene/mutation PT/EQA process is inadequate to assess multigene NGS tests [126]. One alternative is methods-based proficiency testing (MBPT), an EQA scheme that is based on method rather than on each individual gene or specific mutation analyzed. MBPT approaches, such as PT for NGS, would allow assessment of many tests for which formal PT is not available and are likely to be the most efficient, practical, and cost-effective method to measure laboratory proficiency in genome-based sequencing analyses [126]. *BRCA* mutation analysis tests are complex processes, and validation and quality control will be necessary both for sequencing and data-analysis platforms and for the specific tests performed.

Conclusions

Assessment of genetic risk for individuals and families with suspected hereditary predisposition to breast cancer has important clinical implications. Such risk assessment should be performed in the context of genetic counseling and culminate in genetic analysis of relevant genes. Currently, the genetic basis for cancer predisposition can be determined in approximately half of high-risk families, and mutation testing can distinguish between carriers who are at risk and noncarriers who are at background risk. The most commonly mutated genes in HBOC are *BRCA1* and *BRCA2*, and effective surveillance and prevention measures, in addition to targeted therapy, reduce morbidity and mortality in *BRCA1* and *BRCA2* carriers.

Mutation detection and interpretation for the *BRCA1* and *BRCA2* genes is still technically challenging. The large variety and extensive distribution of mutation types mandates the use of multiple mutation detection methods to achieve complete sensitivity, and clinical interpretation is beleaguered by the high prevalence of VUS. Although Sanger sequencing has been the gold standard for clinical *BRCA1* and *BRCA2* testing, new sequencing technologies are producing a sea change in this field, leading to identification of novel breast cancer predisposition genes and enabling large-scale, multiple gene testing.

Web Site URLs

BRCAPro: http://www4.utsouthwestern.edu/breasthealth/cagene/CGdownload.asp

CancerGene Software Package (Cancer Pro, The University of Texas Southwestern Medical Center at Dallas): http://www4.utsouthwestern.edu/breasthealth/cagene/

ClinVar (public archive of reports of the relationships among human variations and phenotypes): http://www.ncbi.nlm.nih.gov/clinvar/

Corresponding consensus coding sequence IDs (CCDS): http://www.ncbi.nlm.nih.gov/CCDS/CcdsBrowse.cgi

ENIGMA (Evidence-Based Network for the Interpretation of Germline Mutant Alleles): http://www.enigmaconsortium.org

Myriad II: http://www.myriad-tests.com/provider/brca-mutation-prevalence.htm

PolyPhen (Polymorphism Phenotyping): http://genetics.bwh.harvard.edu/pph2/

SIFT (Sorting Intolerant From Tolerant): http://sift.jcvi.org

The BReast CAncer genes IARC database: http://brca.iarc.fr/index.php/

The Cancer Genome Atlas: http://cancergenome.nih.gov/

The Human Gene Mutation Database (HGMD): http://www.hgmd.cf.ac.uk/ac/all.php

The Leiden Open Variation Database (LOVD): http://chromium.liacs.nl/LOVD2/cancer/home.php?select_db=BRCA1

The National Human Genome Research Institute hosts the Breast Cancer Information Core (BIC): http://research.nhgri.nih.gov/bic/

The National Institutes of Health genetic sequence database genomic reference sequence records (RefSeq): http://www.ncbi.nlm.nih.gov/refseq/rsg/

The UK NHS NICE (National Institute for Health and Clinical Excellence) guidelines: http://guidance.nice.org.uk/CG164/NICEGuidance/pdf/English

http://pathways.nice.org.uk/pathways/familial-breast-cancer

References

1. Parkin DM, Boyd L, Walker LC. The fraction of cancer attributable to lifestyle and environmental factors in the UK in 2010. Br J Cancer. 2011;105 Suppl 2:S77–81.
2. Hemminki K, Granstrom C, Czene K. Attributable risks for familial breast cancer by proband status and morphology: a nationwide epidemiologic study from Sweden. Int J Cancer. 2002;100:214–9.
3. Pharoah PD, Day NE, Duffy S, et al. Family history and the risk of breast cancer: a systematic review and metaanalysis. Int J Cancer. 1997;71:800–9.
4. Mavaddat N, Pharoah P, Blows F, et al. Familial relative risks for breast cancer by pathological subtype: a population-based cohort study. Breast Cancer Res. 2010;12(1):R10.
5. Bevier M, Sundquist K, Hemminki K. Risk of breast cancer in families of multiple affected women and men. Breast Cancer Res Treat. 2012;132(2):723–8.
6. Anglian Breast Cancer Study Group. Prevalence and penetrance of BRCA1 and BRCA2 mutations in a population-based series of breast cancer cases. Br J Cancer. 2000;83:1301–8.
7. Offit K. Risk Counseling and Management Clinical Cancer Genetics. New York: Wiley-Liss; 1998.
8. Daly MB, Axilbund JE, Buys S, et al. Genetic/familial high-risk assessment: breast and ovarian. National Comprehensive Cancer Network. J Natl Compr Canc Netw. 2010;8(5):562–94.
9. de Jong MM, Nolte IM, Meerman GJ, et al. Genes other than BRCA1 and BRCA2 involved in breast cancer susceptibility. J Med Genet. 2002;39:225–42.
10. Meijers-Heijboer H, van den Ouweland A, Klijn J, et al. Low-penetrance susceptibility to breast cancer due to CHEK2(*)1100delC in noncarriers of BRCA1 or BRCA2 mutations. Nat Genet. 2002;31:55–9.
11. McClellan J, King MC. Genetic heterogeneity in human disease. Cell. 2010;141(2):210–7.
12. Meindl A, Hellebrand H, Wiek C, et al. Germline mutations in breast and ovarian cancer pedigrees establish RAD51C as a human cancer susceptibility gene. Nat Genet. 2010;42(5):410–4.
13. Loveday C, Turnbull C, Ramsay E, Breast Cancer Susceptibility Collaboration (UK), et al. Germline mutations in RAD51D confer susceptibility to ovarian cancer. Nat Genet. 2011;43(9):879–82.
14. Miki Y, Swensen J, Shattuck-Eidens D, et al. A strong candidate for the breast and ovarian cancer susceptibility gene BRCA1. Science. 1994;266:66–71.
15. Wooster R, Bignell G, Lancaster J, et al. Identification of the breast cancer susceptibility gene BRCA2. Nature. 1995;378:789–92.
16. Chen Y, Farmer AA, Chen CF, et al. BRCA1 is a 220-kDa nuclear phosphoprotein that is expressed and phosphorylated in a cell cycle-dependent manner. Cancer Res. 1996;56:3168–72.
17. Roy R, Chun J, Powell SN. BRCA1 and BRCA2: different roles in a common pathway of genome protection. Nat Rev Cancer. 2011;12(1):68–78.
18. Fan S, Wang J, Yuan R, et al. BRCA1 inhibition of estrogen receptor signaling in transfected cells. Science. 1999;284:1354–6.
19. Zhu Q, Pao GM, Huynh AM, et al. BRCA1 tumour suppression occurs via heterochromatin-mediated silencing. Nature. 2011;477:179–84.
20. Venkitaraman AR. Cancer susceptibility and the functions of BRCA1 and BRCA2. Cell. 2002;108:171–82.
21. Ferla R, CaloV, Cascio S et al. (2007). Founder mutations in BRCA1 and BRCA2 genes. Ann. Oncol. 18 Suppl 6, vi93-vi98.
22. Szabo CI, King MC. Population genetics of BRCA1 and BRCA2. Am J Hum Genet. 1997;60:1013–20.
23. Moller P, Heimdal K, Apold J, et al. Genetic epidemiology of BRCA1 mutations in Norway. Eur J Cancer. 2001;37:2428–34.
24. Einbeigi Z, Bergman A, Kindblom LG, et al. A founder mutation of the BRCA1 gene in Western Sweden associated with a high incidence of breast and ovarian cancer. Eur J Cancer. 2001;37:1904–9.
25. Menkiszak J, Gronwald J, Gorski B, et al. Hereditary ovarian cancer in Poland. Int J Cancer. 2003;106:942–5.
26. Olopade OI, Fackenthal JD, Dunston G, et al. Breast cancer genetics in African Americans. Cancer. 2003;97(suppl):236–45.
27. King MC, Marks JH, Mandell JB. Breast and ovarian cancer risks due to inherited mutations in BRCA1 and BRCA2. Science. 2003;302(5645):643–6.
28. Moslehi R, Chu W, Karlan B, et al. BRCA1 and BRCA2 mutation analysis of 208 Ashkenazi Jewish women with ovarian cancer. Am J Hum Genet. 2000;66(4):1259–72.
29. Frank TS, Deffenbaugh AM, Reid JE, et al. Clinical characteristics of individuals with germline mutations in BRCA1 and BRCA2: analysis of 10,000 individuals. J Clin Oncol. 2002;20:1480–90.
30. Thorlacius S, Sigurdsson S, Bjarnadottir H, et al. Study of a single BRCA2 mutation with high carrier frequency in a small population. Am J Hum Genet. 1997;60:1079–84.

31. The BRCA1 Exon 13 Duplication Screening Group. The exon 13 duplication in the BRCA1 gene is a founder mutation present in geographically diverse populations. Am J Hum Genet. 2000;67(1):207–12.
32. Petrij-Bosch A, Peelen T, van Vliet M, et al. BRCA1 genomic deletions are major founder mutations in Dutch breast cancer patients. Nat Genet. 1997;17:341–5.
33. Ford D, Easton DF, Stratton M, et al. Genetic heterogeneity and penetrance analysis of the BRCA1 and BRCA2 genes in breast cancer families. The Breast Cancer Linkage Consortium. Am J Hum Genet. 1998;62(3):676–89.
34. Antoniou AC, Pharoah PD, Easton DF, et al. BRCA1 and BRCA2 cancer risks. J Clin Oncol. 2006;24(20):3312–4.
35. Struewing JP, Hartge P, Wacholder S, et al. The risk of cancer associated with specific mutations of BRCA1 and BRCA2 among Ashkenazi Jews. N Engl J Med. 1997;336(20):1401–8.
36. Antoniou AC, Pharoah PD, Narod S, et al. Average risks of breast and ovarian cancer associated with BRCA1 or BRCA2 mutations detected in case Series unselected for family history: a combined analysis of 22 studies. Am J Hum Genet. 2003;72:1117–30.
37. Ford D, Easton DF, Bishop DT, et al. Risks of cancer in BRCA1 mutation carriers. Lancet. 1994;343:692–5.
38. Lizarraga I, Sugg S, Weigel R, et al. Review of risk factors for the development of contralateral breast cancer. Am J Surgery. 2013;206:704–8.
39. Metcalfe K, Gershman S, Lynch HT, et al. Predictors of contralateral breast cancer in BRCA1 and BRCA2 mutation carriers. Br J Cancer. 2011;104:1384–92.
40. Finch A, Beiner M, Lubinski J, et al. Salpingo-oophorectomy and the risk of ovarian, fallopian tube, and peritoneal cancers in women with a BRCA1 or BRCA2 Mutation. JAMA. 2006;296:185–92.
41. Risch HA, McLaughlin JR, Cole DC, et al. Prevalence and penetrance of germline BRCA1 and BRCA2 mutations in a population of 649 women with ovarian cancer. Am J Hum Genet. 2001;68:700–10.
42. Murphy KM, Brune KA, Griffin C, et al. Evaluation of candidate genes MAP2K4, MADH4, ACVR1B, and BRCA2 in familial pancreatic cancer: deleterious BRCA2 mutations in 17%. Cancer Res. 2002;62:3789–93.
43. Canto MI, Harinck F, Hruban RH, et al. International Cancer of the Pancreas Screening (CAPS) Consortium summit on the management of patients with increased risk for familial pancreatic cancer. Gut. 2013;62:339–47.
44. Slater EP, Langer P, Fendrich V, et al. Prevalence of BRCA2 and CDKN2a mutations in German familial pancreatic cancer families. Fam Cancer. 2010;9:335–43.
45. Thompson D, Easton DF. Cancer Incidence in BRCA1 mutation carriers. J Natl Cancer Inst. 2002;94:1358–65.
46. Van Asperen CJ, Brohet RM, Meijers-Heijboer EJ, et al. Cancer risks in BRCA2 families: estimates for sites other than breast and ovary. J Med Genet. 2005;42:711–9.
47. Iqbal J, Ragone A, Lubinski J, et al. The incidence of pancreatic cancer in BRCA1and BRCA2 mutation carriers. Br J Cancer. 2012;107(12):2005–9.
48. Domchek SM, Friebel TM, Singer CF, et al. Association of risk-reducing surgery in BRCA1 or BRCA2 mutation carriers with cancer risk and mortality. JAMA. 2010;304(9):967–75.
49. Finch AP, Lubinski J, Møller P, et al. Impact of oophorectomy on cancer incidence and mortality in women with a BRCA1 or BRCA2 mutation. J Clin Oncol. 2014;32(15):1547–53.
50. Bayraktar S, Glück S. Systemic therapy options in BRCA mutation-associated breast cancer. Breast Cancer Res Treat. 2012;135(2):355–66.
51. Fong PC, Boss DS, Yap TA, et al. Inhibition of poly(ADP-ribose) polymerase in tumors from BRCA mutation carriers. N Engl J Med. 2009;361(2):123–34.
52. Kaufman B, Shapira-Frommer R, Schmutzler RK, et al. Olaparib monotherapy in patients with advanced cancer and a germline BRCA1/2 mutation. J Clin Oncol. 2015;33(3):244–50.
53. American Association for Cancer Research (2015). Olaparib Approved for Advanced Ovarian Cancer. Cancer Discov. (ahead of print).
54. Bhalla A, Saif MW. PARP-inhibitors in BRCA-associated pancreatic cancer. JOP. 2014;15(4):340–3.
55. Brough R, Frankum JR, Costa-Cabral S, et al. Searching for synthetic lethality in cancer. Curr Opin Genet Dev. 2011;21:34–41.
56. Carey LA, Perou CM, Livasy CA, et al. Race, Breast Cancer Subtypes, and Survival in the Carolina Breast Cancer Study. JAMA. 2006;295:2492–502.
57. Turner NC, Reis-Filho JS. Basal-like breast cancer and the BRCA1 phenotype. Oncogene. 2006;25:5846–53.
58. Bane AL, Beck JC, Bleiweiss I, et al. BRCA2 mutation-associated breast cancers exhibit a distinguishing phenotype based on morphology and molecular profiles from tissue microarrays. Am J Surg Pathol. 2007;31:121–8.
59. Lakhani SR, Gusterson BA, Jacquemier J, et al. The pathology of familial breast cancer: histological features of cancers in families not attributable to mutations in BRCA1 or BRCA2. Clin Cancer Res. 2000;6:782–9.
60. Perez-Valles A, Martorell-Cebolla M, Nogueira-Vazquez, et al. The usefulness of antibodies to the BRCA1 protein in detecting the mutated BRCA1 gene. An immunohistochemical study. J Clin Pathol. 2001;54(6):476–80.
61. Meisel JL, Hyman DM, Garg K, et al. The performance of BRCA1 immunohistochemistry for detecting germline, somatic, and epigenetic BRCA1 loss in high-grade serous ovarian cancer. Ann Oncol. 2014; 25(12):2372–8.
62. Vaz FH, Machado PM, Brandao RD, et al. Familial breast/ovarian cancer and BRCA1/2 genetic screening: The role of immunohistochemistry as an additional method in the selection of patients. J Histochem Cytochem. 2007;55:1105–13.
63. Watson P, Lieberman R, Snyder C, et al. Detecting BRCA2 protein truncation in tissue biopsies to identify breast cancers that arise in BRCA2 gene mutation carriers. J Clin Oncol. 2009;27(24):3894–900.
64. Gabai-Kapara E, Lahad A, Kaufman B, et al. Population-based screening for breast and ovarian cancer risk due to BRCA1 and BRCA2. Proc Natl Acad Sci U S A. 2014;111(39):14205–10.
65. Parmigiani G, Berry D, Aguilar O. Determining carrier probabilities for breast cancer-susceptibility genes BRCA1 and BRCA2. Am J Hum Genet. 1998;62(1):145–58.
66. Biswas S, Tankhiwale N, Blackford A, et al. Assessing the added value of breast tumor markers in genetic risk prediction model BRCAPRO. Breast Cancer Res Treat. 2012;133(1):347–55.
67. van Harssel JJ, van Roozendaal CE, Detisch Y, et al. Efficiency of BRCAPRO and Myriad II mutation probability thresholds versus cancer history criteria alone for BRCA1/2 mutation detection. Fam Cancer. 2010;9(2):193–201.
68. Antoniou AC, Cunningham AP, Peto J, et al. The BOADICEA model of genetic susceptibility to breast and ovarian cancers: updates and extensions. Br J Cancer. 2008;98:1457–66.
69. Antoniou AC, Hardy R, Walker L, et al. Predicting the likelihood of carrying a BRCA1 or BRCA2 mutation: validation of BOADICEA, BRCAPRO, IBIS, Myriad and the Manchester scoring system using data from UK genetics clinics. J Med Genet. 2008;45(7):425–31.
70. Schneegans SM, Rosenberger A, Engel U, et al. Validation of three BRCA1/2 mutation-carrier probability models Myriad, BRCAPRO and BOADICEA in a population-based series of 183 German families. Fam Cancer. 2011;11(2):181–8.
71. Tyrer JP, Duffy SW, Cuzick J. A breast cancer prediction model incorporating familial and personal risk factors. Stat Med. 2004;23(7):1111–30.

72. Evans GR, Lalloo F. Development of a scoring system to screen for BRCA1/2 mutations. Methods Mol Biol. 2010;653:237–47.
73. Kurian AW, Gong GD, John EM, et al. Performance of prediction models for BRCA mutation carriage in three racial/ethnic groups: findings from the Northern California Breast Cancer Family Registry. Cancer Epidemiol Biomarkers Prev Biomarkers Prev. 2009;18(4):1084–91.
74. Kurian AW, Gong GD, Chun NM, et al. Performance of BRCA1/2 mutation prediction models in Asian Americans. J Clin Oncol. 2008;26(29):4752–8.
75. Gerhardus A, Schleberger H, Schleberger B, et al. Diagnostic accuracy of methods for the detection of BRCA1 and BRCA2 mutations: a systematic review. Eur J Hum Genet. 2007;6:619–27.
76. Spearman AD, Sweet K, Zhou XP, et al. Clinically applicable models to characterize BRCA1 and BRCA2 variants of uncertain significance. J Clin Oncol. 2008;26(33):5393–400.
77. Walsh T, Casadei S, Coats KH, et al. Spectrum of mutations in BRCA1, BRCA2, CHEK2, and TP53 in families at high risk of breast cancer. JAMA. 2006;295(12):1379–88.
78. Palma MD, Domchek SM, Stopfer J, et al. The relative contribution of point mutations and genomic rearrangements in BRCA1 and BRCA2 high risk breast cancer families. Cancer Res. 2008;68(17):7006–14.
79. Sluiter MD, van Rensburg EJ. Large genomic rearrangements of the BRCA1 and BRCA2 genes: review of the literature and report of a novel BRCA1 mutation. Breast Cancer Res Treat. 2011;125(2):325–49.
80. Hendrickson B, Judkins T, Ward BD, et al. Prevalence results for five previously reported and recurrent BRCA1 genetic rearrangement mutations in 20,000 patients from hereditary breast/ovarian cancer families. Genes Chromosomes Cancer. 2005;43:309–13.
81. Judkins T, Rosenthal E, Arnell C, et al. Clinical significance of large rearrangements in BRCA1 and BRCA2. Cancer. 2012;118(21): 5210–6.
82. Schouten JP, McElgunn CJ, Waaijer R et al. (2002). Relative quantification of 40 nucleic acid sequences by multiplex ligation-dependent probe amplification. Nuc. Acid Res. 30(12):e57.
83. Walsh T, Lee MK, Casadei S, et al. Detection of inherited mutations for breast and ovarian cancer using genomic capture and massively parallel sequencing. Proc Natl Acad Sci U S A. 2010;107(28):12629–33.
84. Cheeseman K, Rouleau E, Vannier A, et al. A diagnostic genetic test for the physical mapping of germline rearrangements in the susceptibility breast cancer genes BRCA1 and BRCA2. Hum Mutat. 2012;33(6):998–1009.
85. Berglund EC, Kiialainen A, Syvänen AC, et al. Next-generation sequencing technologies and applications for human genetic history and forensics. Investigative Genet. 2011;2:23.
86. Metzker ML. Sequencing technologies—the next generation. Nat Rev. 2010;11:31–46.
87. Morgan JE, Carr IM, Sheridan E, et al. Genetic diagnosis of familial Breast Cancer using clonal sequencing. Hum Mutat. 2010;4:484–91.
88. De Leeneer K, De Schrijver J, Clement L, et al. Practical tools to implement massive parallel pyrosequencing of PCR products in next generation molecular diagnostics. PLoS One. 2011;6(9), e25531.
89. De Leeneer K, Hellemans J, De Schrijver J, et al. Massive parallel amplicon sequencing of the breast cancer genes BRCA1 and BRCA2: opportunities, challenges, and limitations. Hum Mutat. 2011;32(3):335–44.
90. Herman I, Borrás E, de Sousa DM, et al. Detection of genomic variations in BRCA1 and BRCA2 genes by long-range PCR and next-generation sequencing. J Mol Diagn. 2012;14(3):286–93.
91. Ozcelik H, Shi X, Chang MC, et al. Long-Range PCR and Next-Generation Sequencing of BRCA1 and BRCA2 in Breast Cancer. J Mol Diagn. 2012;14(5):467–75.
92. Korbel JO, Urban AE, Affourtit JP, et al. Paired-end mapping reveals extensive structural variation in the human genome. Science. 2007;318:420–6.
93. Campbell PJ, Stephens PJ, Pleasance ED, et al. Identification of somatically acquired rearrangements in cancer using genome-wide massively parallel paired-end sequencing. Nat Genet. 2008;40:722–9.
94. Rahman N. Realizing the promise of cancer predisposition genes. Nature. 2014;505(7483):302–8.
95. Domchek SM, Nathanson KL. Panel testing for inherited susceptibility to breast, ovarian, and colorectal cancer. Genet Med. 2014;16(11):827–9.
96. Comino-Mendez I, Gracia-Aznárez FJ, Schiavi F, et al. Exome sequencing identifies MAX mutations as a cause of hereditary pheochromocytoma. Nat Genet. 2011;43:663–7.
97. Smith MJ, O'Sullivan J, Bhaskar SS, et al. Loss-of-function mutations in SMARCE1 cause an inherited disorder of multiple spinal meningiomas. Nat Genet. 2013;45(3):295–8.
98. Snape K, Ruark E, Tarpey P, et al. Predisposition gene identification in common cancers by exome sequencing: insights from familial breast cancer. Breast Cancer Res Treat. 2012;134(1):429–33.
99. Turnbull C, Rahman N. Genetic predisposition to breast cancer: past, present, and future. Ann Rev Genomics Hum Genet. 2008;9:321–45.
100. Berry DA, Iversen ES, Gudbjartsson DF, et al. BRCAPRO validation, sensitivity of genetic testing of BRCA1/BRCA2, and prevalence of other breast cancer susceptibility genes. J Clin Oncol. 2002;20(11):2701–12.
101. Ghiorzo P. Genetic predisposition to pancreatic cancer. World J Gastroenterol. 2014;20(31):10778–89.
102. Maxwell KN, Wubbenhorst B, D'Andrea K (2014). Prevalence of mutations in a panel of breast cancer susceptibility genes in BRCA1/2-negative patients with early-onset breast cancer. Genet Med. doi: 10.1038/gim.2014.176. [Epub ahead of print]
103. Kurian AW, Hare EE, Mills MA. Clinical evaluation of a multiple-gene sequencing panel for hereditary cancer risk assessment. J Clin Oncol. 2014;32(19):2001–9.
104. Abecasis GR, et al. An integrated map of genetic variation from 1,092 human genomes. Nature. 2012;491:56–65.
105. Murray ML, Cerrato F, Bennett RL, et al. Follow-up of carriers of BRCA1 and BRCA2 variants of unknown significance: Variant reclassification and surgical decisions. Genet Med. 2011;13(12):998–1005.
106. Ng PC, Henikoff S. Accounting for human polymorphisms predicted to affect protein function. Genome Res. 2002;12(3): 436–46.
107. Ramensky V, Bork P, Sunyaev S, et al. Human non-synonymous SNPs: server and survey. Nucleic Acids Res. 2002;30(17): 3894–900.
108. Abkevich V, Zharkikh A, Deffenbaugh A, et al. Analysis of missense variation in human BRCA1 in the context of interspecific sequence variation. J Med Genet. 2004;41(7):492–507.
109. Tavtigian SV, Samollow PB, de Silva D, et al. An analysis of unclassified missense substitutions in human BRCA1. Fam Cancer. 2006;5(1):77–88.
110. Théry JC, Krieger S, Gaildrat P, et al. Contribution of bioinformatics predictions and functional splicing assays to the interpretation of unclassified variants of the BRCA genes. Eur J Hum Genet. 2001;10:1052–8.
111. Alter BP, Rosenberg PS, Brody LC. Clinical and molecular features associated with biallelic mutations in FANCD1/BRCA2. J Med Genet. 2007;44:1–9.

112. Domchek SM, Tang J, Stopfer J, et al. Biallelic deleterious BRCA1 mutations in a woman with early-onset ovarian cancer. Cancer Discov. 2013;3(4):399–405.
113. Sawyer SL, Tian L, Kähkönen M, et al. Biallelic mutations in BRCA1 cause a new Fanconi anemia subtype. Cancer Discov. 2015;5(2):135–42.
114. Collins N, McManus R, Wooster R, et al. Consistent loss of the wild type allele in breast cancers from a family linked to the BRCA2 gene on chromosome 13q12-13. Oncogene. 1995;10(8):1673–5.
115. Hofstra RM, Spurdle AB, Eccles D, Unclassified Genetic Variants Working Group IARC, et al. Tumor characteristics as an analytic tool for classifying genetic variants of uncertain clinical significance. Hum Mutat. 2008;29:1292–303.
116. Farrugia DJ, Agarwal MK, Pankratz VS, et al. Functional assays for classification of BRCA2 variants of uncertain significance. Cancer Res. 2008;68(9):3523–31.
117. Iversen ES, Couch FJ, Goldgar DE, et al. A computational method to classify variants of uncertain significance using functional assay data with application to BRCA1. Cancer Epidemiol Biomarkers Prev. 2011;20(6):1078–88.
118. Millot GA, Carvalho MA, Caputo SM, on behalf of the ENIGMA (Evidence-based Network for the Interpretation of Germline Mutant Alleles) Consortium Functional Assay Working Group, et al. A guide for functional analysis of BRCA1 variants of uncertain significance. Hum Mutat. 2012;33(11):1526–37.
119. Hendriks G, Morolli B, Calléja FM, et al. An efficient pipeline for the generation and functional analysis of human BRCA2 variants of uncertain significance. Hum Mutat. 2014;11:1382–91.
120. Spurdle AB, Healey S, Devereau A, et al. ENIGMA-evidence-based network for the interpretation of germline mutant alleles: an international initiative to evaluate risk and clinical significance associated with sequence variation in the BRCA1 and BRCA2 genes. Hum Mutat. 2012;33(1):2–7.
121. Mattocks CJ, Morris MA, Matthijs G, Group EGV, et al. A standardized framework for the validation and verification of clinical molecular genetic tests. Eur J Hum Genet. 2010;18(12):1276–88.
122. Jennings L, Van Deerlin VM, Gulley ML. Recommended Principles and Practices for Validating Clinical Molecular Pathology Tests. Arch Pathol Lab Med. 2009;133:743–55.
123. Haas J, Katus HA, Meder B. Next-generation sequencing entering the clinical arena. Mol Cell Probes. 2011;25(5-6):206–11.
124. Gullapalli RR, Lyons-Weiler M, Petrosko P, et al. Clinical integration of next-generation sequencing technology. Clin Lab Med. 2012;32(4):585–99.
125. Kalman LV, Lubin IM, Barker S, et al. Current landscape and new paradigms of proficiency testing and external quality assessment for molecular genetics. Arch Pathol Lab Med. 2013;137(7):983–8.
126. Schrijver I, Aziz N, Jennings LJ, et al. Methods-based proficiency testing in molecular genetic pathology. J Mol Diagn. 2014;16:283–7.

Familial Adenomatous Polyposis and Turcot and Peutz–Jeghers Syndromes

23

Kandelaria M. Rumilla

Abstract

To date the majority of colorectal cancers are thought to be sporadic. However, familial predisposition has been well recognized for years. Familial adenomatous polyposis coli, Turcot syndrome, Gardner syndrome, and Peutz–Jeghers syndrome are examples of hereditary syndromes that predispose individuals to colorectal adenocarcinoma as well as a host of other malignant, hamartomatous, and benign growths. While not comprehensive of all familial colorectal predisposition syndromes, a summary of these syndromes is provided in this chapter.

Keywords

Familial adenomatous polyposis coli • FAP • *APC* • Turcot syndrome • Gardner syndrome • Attenuated polyposis • Desmoid tumors • Epidermoid cyst • Duodenal adenocarcinoma • Papillary thyroid carcinoma • CNS tumors • Hepatoblastoma • CHRPE • Peutz-Jeghers syndrome • *STK11* • Juvenile polyposis • Intussusception • Peutz-Jeghers polyps • Mucocutaneous pigmentation

To date the majority of colorectal cancer are thought to be sporadic. However, familial predisposition has been well recognized for years. Familial adenomatous polyposis coli, Turcot syndrome, Gardner syndrome, and Peutz–Jeghers syndrome are examples of hereditary syndromes that predispose individuals to colorectal adenocarcinoma as well as a host of other malignant, hamartomatous, and benign growths. While not comprehensive of all familial colorectal predisposition syndromes, a summary of these syndromes is provided in this chapter.

K.M. Rumilla, M.D. (✉)
Department of Laboratory Medicine and Pathology, Laboratory Genetics, Mayo Clinic, 200 First Street SW, Rochester, MN 55905, USA
e-mail: rumilla.kandelaria@mayo.edu

Familial Adenomatous Polyposis Coli

Familial adenomatous polyposis coli (FAP) is estimated to account for approximately 1 % of colorectal adenocarcinoma in the general population. The reported incidence ranges from 1 in 7,500 [1] to 1 in 30,000 [2] and the penetrance is approximately 100 % by age 40 [3]. Early references to this autosomal dominant disorder date back to the 1880s. By 1960, the association with epidermoid cysts, osteomas [4], and central nervous system tumors had been described [5]. The disease is caused by constitutional mutations in the adenomatous polyposis coli (*APC*) gene identified in 1991 [6]. Variants of FAP also are described and include attenuated FAP (AFAP), Gardner syndrome, and Turcot syndrome.

D.G.B. Leonard (ed.), *Molecular Pathology in Clinical Practice*, DOI 10.1007/978-3-319-19674-9_23

Clinical Features

Familial Adenomatous Polyposis Coli

While the diagnostic criteria for FAP rests primarily in the number of adenomatous polyps that are identified in the distal colorectum at an early age (>100 colorectal adenomatous polyps), the true impact of this syndrome is seen in the risk for colorectal cancer and other neoplasms. If untreated, virtually 100 % of affected individuals will develop colorectal adenocarcinoma. The average age of diagnosis is 39 years in the classic presentation. The risk for malignant neoplasm is not limited to the colorectum. Individuals with this syndrome are also at increased risk of other malignancies compared to the general population. Adenocarcinomas from other gastrointestinal primary sites (small intestine, including duodenum and periampullary) occur in 4–12 % of patients, while pancreatic adenocarcinoma and papillary thyroid carcinoma (PTC) occur in approximately 2 % of FAP patients. Although this is a small percent of FAP patients, both pancreatic adenocarcinoma and PTC are much less common in the general population; there is 0.2 % incidence of PTC in the general population [7]. FAP is associated with a specific histologic subtype of PTC, the cribriform-morular variant [8], but is not pathognomonic [9]. Gastric adenocarcinoma and medulloblastoma [10] occur in less than 1 % of FAP patients, while hepatoblastoma occurs in approximately 1 of 150 FAP patients under the age of 5. Other malignant tumors arising from the bile duct or adrenal gland are associated with FAP, but are infrequent.

The clinical diagnosis rests on the identification of numerous pre-cancerous adenomatous polyps. Colonic adenomatous polyps can be identified in affected patients at young ages; polyps are present in 50 % of affected individuals by age 16 years, and in 95 % by age 35. Adenomatous polyps can be seen in the stomach of approximately 10 % of patients. Adenomatous polyps of the duodenum and ampulla of Vater can present as intussusception and obstructive pancreatitis, respectively.

Desmoid tumors (proliferation of myofibroblasts) occur in 3.5–32 % of FAP patients. Although most common after surgery, desmoid tumors may occur in the absence of prior surgery and are the presenting symptom in approximately 16 % of FAP patients. Characteristic features, such as abdominal location, may help distinguish FAP-associated and non-FAP-associated desmoid tumors. Gender does not correlate between FAP and non-FAP cases as women have more desmoids than men in both the FAP and non-FAP groups [11].

Hamartomatous and benign lesions seen in FAP include gastric fundic gland polyps (50 % of FAP cases), lipomas, fibromas, sebaceous, and epidermoid cysts [12], osteomas usually affecting the long bones, mandible, or skull, nasal angiofibromas, dental abnormalities ranging from unerupted teeth to absent or supernumerary teeth (17 % of FAP cases). Congenital hypertrophy of the retinal pigment epithelium (CHRPE) is a benign finding which does not affect visual acuity but can be the presenting finding.

Attenuated Familial Adenomatous Polyposis Coli

AFAP is an important clinical phenotypic variant of FAP. AFAP has fewer polyps (from 30 to 100 polyps) which are located more proximal in the colon, and has a later age of onset [13]. The AFAP phenotype can overlap with other syndromes, including MYH-associated polyposis and Lynch syndrome (Hereditary Non-polyposis Colon Cancer, HNPCC). Several criteria have been proposed for clinical diagnosis of AFAP, with most including a lower number of polyps present at slightly older ages with family history, polyposis, or cancer. One example is less than 100 polys by 25 years and an autosomal dominant family history [14]. Most of these proposals do not include mutation status of the *APC* gene, exclusion of other predisposing syndromes, or consideration of other noncolonic manifestations, which likely limits the sensitivity of such diagnostic criteria in clinical practice.

Gardner Syndrome

Gardner syndrome is a clinical diagnosis that includes colorectal adenocarcinoma and colorectal polyposis as seen with FAP plus osteomas, fibromas, or epidermoid cysts within the individual or family.

Turcot Syndrome

Widely recognized as a subset of FAP and Lynch syndrome, Turcot syndrome is defined by the combination of primary colonic neoplasms with synchronous or metachronous malignant central nervous system tumors. As originally described, Turcot syndrome overlaps both FAP and DNA mismatch repair (MMR) defective tumor syndromes with *APC* gene mutations identified in approximately two-thirds of affected individuals. The type of cancer to which patients are predisposed depends in part on the affected gene. For example, the risk of medulloblastoma with an *APC* gene mutation is 92 times greater than for the general population, but the lifetime risk remains low (less than 1 %). *APC* mutations also are associated with astrocytomas and ependymomas. Individuals with mutations in a MMR gene (e.g., *MLH1*, *MSH2*, *PMS2*) are predisposed to glioblastoma.

Prevention and Surveillance

Familial Adenomatous Polyposis Coli

Prevention and surveillance target the detection of malignant and premalignant lesions characteristic of FAP. Evaluation of patients 18 years or younger identified that 68 % were already symptomatic, which led to the recommendation that colonoscopy screening begin at age 10 years [15]. Controversy remains regarding the use and frequency of some screening tests, such as for hepatoblastoma (alpha-fetoprotein and hepatic ultrasound). The mainstay of screening remains colonoscopy every 1–2 years prior to colectomy. Screening methods also continue to evolve; for example, more recent work done in screening for PTC suggests that ultrasound is more effective than palpation [7]. Other gastrointestinal manifestations also require screening, including esophagogastroduodenoscopy (EGD) for small bowel disease starting at about age 25 years, although the age to start and frequency of screening is not clear. Flexible sigmoidoscopy may be sufficient for initial diagnosis, but insufficient for surveillance in carriers who have not undergone colectomy. For prophylactic colectomy, the extent of resection also is debated [16]. For those who have not had molecular testing or do not have an identified mutation such that the diagnosis is based on clinical diagnosis alone, and first-degree relatives, the recommendation is to have regular colon/sigmoidoscopy from 10 years of age until multiple polyps are found or the patient reaches age 50 years, and then to follow routine population-based colon cancer screening recommendations [17].

As surveillance and prophylactic methods result in longer survival for affected individuals, such that other lesions (including nonmalignant lesions) are becoming more significant as their impact on morbidity and mortality grows. Most notably, 5–20 % of FAP patients who develop desmoid tumors, which can cause compression or obstruction, have significant morbidity or mortality [18]. Fortunately, nonsurgical options are available for treating desmoid tumors, including hormonal therapy, embolization, and chemotherapy, since surgery can trigger the growth of desmoids [19].

Attenuated Familial Adenomatous Polyposis Coli

Surveillance recommendations are similar to FAP with modifications for the lesser severity and later onset of the disease. AFAP surveillance includes colonoscopy every 2–3 years starting at age 18–20 years of age, and EGD by 25 years of age and every 1–3 years depending on extent of small bowel disease observed.

Gardner Syndrome

Appropriate surveillance is similar to FAP for gastrointestinal disease. Recommendations to address other manifestations of Gardner syndrome are less specific, but include physical examinations. Some patients come to clinical attention for cosmetic reasons related to superficial fibromas, or epidermoid cysts.

Turcot Syndrome

Appropriate surveillance is similar to FAP or HNPCC with additional screening and awareness of the increased risk for CNS tumors.

Genetics

Familial Adenomatous Polyposis Coli

Mutations located in the *APC* gene located at 5q21 cause FAP [6]. *APC* encodes a 2,843-amino acid protein, 75 % of which is encoded by the last exon historically numbered exon 15. Approximately 20 % of families with a clinical diagnosis do not have an identifiable mutation using current testing methods. Several possible explanations for this include mutations in regions of the gene not typically tested (introns for example); mutation in a different gene; and de novo mutations that are not represented in the bone marrow. One-third of affected individuals are thought to have a de novo mutation, and may have a more variable phenotype, lack a significant family history, and testing from peripheral blood may be negative or mosaic depending on the sensitivity of the method used for analysis. Genetic counseling is important due to the limitations of testing, and the medical implications of genetic testing. In general, genetic testing is considered standard of care [20]. Additionally, the fact that FAP includes childhood onset of tumors with recommendations for surveillance procedures to begin at 10–12 years of age, genetic screening prior to the age of 18 is medically and ethically supported.

Attenuated Familial Adenomatous Polyposis Coli

Less than 30 % of individuals with AFAP have a germline mutation identified in *APC* [21]. One likely reason for this lower detection rate is the greater degree of overlap in the phenotypic spectrum with other predisposing syndromes, including *MUTYH*-associated adenomatous polyposis syndrome.

Gardner Syndrome

Gardner syndrome is caused by mutations in the *APC* gene, as described above for FAP.

Turcot Syndrome

Turcot syndrome can be caused by *APC* mutations, but also may be caused by mutations in MMR genes. In addition, several different inheritance patterns have been reported, including autosomal dominant, autosomal recessive, and compound heterozygous changes involving *APC* and the MMR genes. Of Turcot syndrome families, 66–80 % have an identifiable mutation in *APC* and 20–33 % have a mutation in one of the MMR genes.

Molecular Mechanism

Familial Adenomatous Polyposis Coli/Attenuated Familial Adenomatous Polyposis Coli

APC functions as a classic tumor suppressor with a role in signal transduction and modulation of transcription factors, which in turn regulate a number of cellular processes including cell division and cell adhesion. The normal APC protein product interacts with a number of components of the Wnt signaling pathway. APC regulates cytoplasmic beta-catenin levels by ubiquitination and degradation, thereby reducing the beta-catenin available to localize to the nucleus and resulting in reduced activation of genes involved in promoting cell proliferation, including *MYC* and cyclin D1 (*CCND1*). Therefore, loss of APC function results in increased levels of beta-catenin by reducing its degradation rate and increased cell proliferation. The increased beta-catenin expression can be seen in the cytoplasm and nucleus by immunohistochemistry. This APC loss of function mechanism for FAP is consistent with the finding that the majority of germline mutations are truncating mutations or result in decreased expression of APC [24].

Genotype–Phenotype Correlation

Familial Adenomatous Polyposis Coli

Although genotype–phenotype correlations involving the locations of mutations in *APC* can be made, variation of the phenotype can be seen between and within families. While some correlations are useful clinically to focus screening procedures, the associations are not definitive. In classic FAP cases, the FAP phenotype is usually clear, but by young adulthood a spectrum that ranges from florid polyposis to a few adenomatous polyps can be seen [22, 23].

Nomenclature of the *APC* gene located on 5q21 can be confusing as there are multiple transcripts with varying numbers of exons. The more common transcript has 15 translated exons that produce a 2,843 amino acid protein [22]. The protein has a number of functional domains including binding sites for beta-catenin, DNA, axin, and microtubules, as well as a nuclear export motif. Two "hot spot" germline mutations occur at codons 1061 and 1309 which together represent approximately 28 % of FAP [17, 24]. Two other important variants in the *APC* gene are p. I1307K and p.E1317Q. Testing for p.I1307K in the Ashkenazi Jewish population has been controversial. The *APC* p.I1307K mutation increases the lifetime risk of colorectal carcinoma to 10–20 %, with an odds ratio of 1.85. The p.I1307K mutation is found in approximately 6 % of the Ashkenazi Jewish population but has been reported in up to 28 % of patients with a family history of colorectal cancer. It is important to note that this mutation is not sufficient to cause a polyposis phenotype and does not alter clinical management of carriers, as many carriers would already be undergoing increased screening due to their family history. Since p.I1307K does not result in a nonfunctional protein, the theorized mechanism by which this mutation results in increased cancer risk is different than typical FAP. The p. I1307K change is thought to create a hypermutable site in *APC* which leads to loss of protein function mutations [25]. Whether or not the p.E1317Q variant confers an increased risk of colorectal carcinoma is not as well established, and the clinical significance remains debatable.

The classic FAP phenotype is associated with mutations involving codons 168–1600, while severe expression of the disease based on number of polyps is associated with mutations in codons 1350–1464. Other associated lesions have also been correlated with the location of the mutation in the *APC* gene, including extra colonic manifestations such as CHRPE which has been associated with mutations in codons 1403–1578 and codons 463 and 1387. Osteomas and desmoids appear to have the highest association with mutations in codons 1395 and 1560. In general, mutations at either end of the *APC* gene, before codon 400 and after codon 1500, and whole gene deletions, have been associated with the attenuated phenotype and have more variable expressivity [24, 26]. Somatic mutations also are common in *APC* but the location of these mutations is more restricted, with about 80 % occurring between codons 1284 and 1580, a region designated as the mutation cluster region [24].

Attenuated Familial Adenomatous Polyposis Coli

AFAP is associated with mutations in different regions of the gene, including: (1) 5′ to codon 157 in exon 4; (2) alternative splice in exon 9; (3) 3′ to codon 1595 in exon 15; and (4) some in-frame deletions [27].

Gardner Syndrome

Desmoid tumors are more strongly associated with *APC* mutations between codons 1444 and 1580 than with mutations either 5′ or 3′ of this region [28].

Turcot Syndrome

Although *APC* mutations between codons 457–1309 have been associated with brain tumors [23], specific genotype–phenotype correlations within the *APC* gene are not widely used. Importantly, medulloblastomas are associated with *APC* mutations and glioblastomas are associated with MMR gene mutations (Lynch syndrome).

Clinical Testing and Laboratory Issues

The methods used for clinical testing of the *APC* gene have changed over the years with direct germline sequencing of the entire coding region becoming more common than targeted testing for specific mutations. Unlike screening assays, sequencing can detect changes in the coding region, flanking sequences and intron/exon boundaries, and can identify novel mutations. Depending on the sequencing method and platform used, there are various pitfalls including inability to detect large deletions and duplications and the interpretation of novel nontruncating alterations that are likely to be classified as variants of unknown significance (VUS). While Sanger sequencing is still commonly used for testing this is being quickly replaced by next-generation sequencing (NGS) and will likely continue to gain momentum as bioinformatics improves and larger insertions/deletions (indels) and copy number variants can be detected by NGS. Large deletion/duplication analysis is routinely performed using multiplex ligation dependent probe amplification assays (MLPA) or array comparative genomic hybridization (aCGH) technologies.

The protein truncation test (PTT) is a screening method that is still used in some clinical laboratories for several reasons. PTT allows for higher throughput mutation screening for the large last exon of *APC* where many mutations are located. Since PTT detects truncated protein products, the underlying mutations are almost certainly deleterious. PTT does have drawbacks, however. For example, missense alterations that have an effect on protein function will likely not be detected, and several gene regions will not be well covered in terms of mutation detection, including alterations outside of the coding regions and mutations that are located at the 5′ or 3′ ends of the segments. Additionally, follow-up sequencing is required to identify the exact sequence change detected by PTT.

Although once common, linkage analysis is rarely performed, but may be useful in cases where sequencing or MLPA fail to detect a specific mutation. This process requires informative markers and participation of affected and unaffected family members, although not all families are large enough or have informative markers to allow for successful linkage analysis. Since a third of cases are de novo, linkage analysis will not be useful for these families.

Other largely historical screening methods include denaturing high-performance liquid chromatography, single strand conformation polymorphism, and denaturing gradient gel electrophoresis. Much like PTT, these methods also require follow-up sequencing for positive results. Other methods, such as allele-specific oligonucleotide hybridization, are useful in specific populations with founder or limited numbers of common mutations (such as p.I1307K), but will not detect other changes.

Testing for AFAP, Gardner syndrome, and Turcot syndrome is similar to testing for FAP. Given the lower detection rate, additional genes should also be considered and can be tested in tandem or parallel to *APC*. Due to the overlap with Lynch syndrome, testing of both *APC* and MMR genes should be considered for patients with a diagnosis of Turcot syndrome.

In general genetic counseling is recommended for a patient undergoing germline testing for a tumor predisposition syndrome. As one of the syndromes in which children can be affected, testing individuals under the age of 18 is acceptable and recommended when the familial mutation is known or the child has symptoms.

Other laboratory issues, such as proficiency testing (PT), have evolved in recent years. Where once a laboratory would have been running PT for each gene/assay, the Collage of American Pathologists (CAP) and the International Program RIQAS are moving towards more platform-based PT, in particular for well-established technologies such as Sanger sequencing. Interlaboratory exchanges also are used to meet PT requirements. Similarly the number and kind of controls that are run with clinical patients has also evolved. As it is impossible to have controls for all possible alterations, representative alterations are often chosen for each platform being used.

Genetic Testing Interpretation and Utility

The clinical sensitivity of *APC* sequencing is approximately 70 % in cases with a clinical diagnosis and family history. Copy number assays for large deletions and insertions add about 5–10 % to the detection rate. Linkage analysis can accurately detect 95–99 % of carriers. In families in which a mutation is identified, genetic testing for the identified mutation in at-risk family members can be useful for determining recommendation and need for surveillance for individuals. Testing and early screening improves the life expectancy of individuals with FAP. There are limitations to testing, as discussed above since mutations are not detected in 20 % of clinically diagnosed cases. There are several possible explanations for this, including that the disease tracking in the family may be a phenocopy of FAP or the mutation in the *APC* gene may be located in an untested region.

Peutz-Jeghers Syndrome

Patients with Peutz-Jeghers syndrome (PJS) have characteristic polyps of the gastrointestinal tract which have low malignant potential, hyperpigmented mucocutaneous lesions, and a family history. PJS occurs in approximately 1 in 8,300–200,000 live births and has an autosomal dominant inheritance pattern. PJS was first reported in 1921 by Johannes Laurentius Augustinus Peutz, with a follow up study of the same family by Westerman [29], and by Harold Joseph Jeghers in 1949 [30].

Depending on the criteria used to classify individuals, up to 25 % are defined as sporadic cases. The clinical diagnostic criteria as established by the World Health Organization are as follows: a positive family history plus either histology-confirmed PJS type hamartomatous polyps or characteristic hyperpigmented mucocutaneous lesions. In the absence of a family history, the clinical criteria for diagnosis of PJS is three Peutz-Jeghers-type polyps or any number of other types of polyps, plus the characteristic pigmentation pattern [31].

Clinical Features

The age of clinical presentation due to symptoms varies widely, with an average age of presentation of 29 years. Variation may be partly due to ascertainment and severity bias, and the availability of genetic testing for clinically asymptomatic individuals. Despite this variation between individuals, the most common presentation due to the gastrointestinal lesions is small bowel intussusception. Other presentations include colon obstruction, GI bleeding, intermittent abdominal pain, and/or rectal prolapse.

Individuals with PJS are predisposed to a number of neoplasms: colon (39 %); small intestine (13 %); stomach (29 %); pancreas (7–36 %); lung (15 %); breast (54 %); benign ovarian sex-cord stromal tumors with annular tubules (21 %); uterus (9 %); adenoma malignum of the cervix (10 %); and estrogen producing sertoli-cell tumors that can lead to precocious puberty and gynecomastia in the testis (9 %) [32–34]. The sites of the pre-cancerous lesions in individuals with PJS reflect the organs that are commonly associated with related malignant neoplasms. One of the two most characteristically associated lesions is the PJS polyp with its pathognomonic smooth muscle extending to the lamina propria with a branching tree-trunk like pattern [35]. Approximately 90 % of these polyps occur in the small intestine and colorectum, and although once thought to be hamartomatous, 33 % can be mixed with an adenomatous component. The other characteristic feature is the hyperpigmented mucocutaneous lesions that often develop prior to the age of 5 years. This feature is not pathognomonic as these lesions are present in approximately 15 % of the general population, as well as with other syndromes/complexes such as Carney's complex [36]. Typically, these dark blue to brown pigmented macules are clustered at mucocutaneous junctions such as the buccal mucosa, perioral areas, nostrils, eyes, and perianal areas, as well as the axillae, hands, and feet. This feature is not consistent within families or within individuals as they tend to fade with increasing age.

In a recent Dutch cohort, the median age of death was 45 years and the median age of living patients was 34 years. The most common cause of death was cancer (67 %), giving a lifetime cumulative cancer risk of 76 %. Overall, this is ten times the risk of the general Dutch population. The authors note that the second-most-common cause of death was intussusception and that deaths from this cause had occurred prior to 1970 and that the ages of these individuals ranged from 3 to 20 years [37].

Prevention and Surveillance

Clinical management of individuals with PJS has primarily centered on surveillance programs that allow for early detection of cancer and management of the cancers that do occur. The debate regarding which organs to monitor, when to start screening, at what time intervals, and by which modalities continues. Several recommendations have recently been proposed. Colonoscopy starting at age 8–10 years with the frequency dependent on the colonoscopy findings, similar time frame for video capsule endoscopy or magnetic resonance enterography and barium follow-through for the small bowel. For women, monthly breast self-examinations beginning at age 18 years, annual breast MRI starting at age 25 years, and standard cervical screening protocols are recommended. For men, the recommendations include yearly testicular exams with ultrasound if abnormalities are detected [33, 38]. Management for these individuals is also likely to undergo changes in the coming years based on the development of new therapeutic options. Potential inhibitor therapy is being assessed in clinical trials using mTOR inhibition with rapamycin or everolimus [39], and inhibitors targeting PI3CA, AKT, and PDK1 are on the horizon.

Genetics

STK11 (previously called *LKB1*) located on chromosome 19p13.3, has been identified as the causative gene for PJS [40, 41]. Over time, the percent of individuals who meet clinical criteria in whom mutations are found has varied widely, ranging from 10–96 % [37, 42, 43]. While it has been suggested that locus heterogeneity may be present [44], a second locus has yet to be positively identified.

Molecular Mechanism

The *STK11* gene, a tumor suppressor, encodes a 433-amino acid protein that is expressed in both the cytoplasm and nucleus. The STK11 kinase domain (codons 50–337) shares homology with other serine-threonine and tyrosine kinase family members. STK11 is involved in a number of cellular functions, including regulation of cell cycle arrest via CDKN1A (also known as WAF1 and p21) signaling [45]; TP53 mediated apoptosis [46]; cell polarity [47]; metabolism and energy homeostasis [48]; regulation of the WNT signaling pathway [49]; the TSC pathway; and the MTOR pathway [38, 50]. Multiple types of mutations have been identified, including truncating mutations, missense mutations, and deletions.

Genotype–Phenotype Correlation

Mutations have been identified throughout the *STK11* gene and genotype–phenotype correlations have yet to be definitively identified [34, 51].

Clinical Testing and Laboratory Issues

Clinical testing is available and methods most commonly include Sanger sequencing and MLPA, but NGS is rapidly replacing these methods, allowing for larger gene panel testing. Estimated detection rates are associated with the presence or absence of family history, approaching 100 % with a positive family history. Reasons for decreased detection rates in sporadic cases and cases with atypical phenotypes include the disease tracking in the family may be a phenocopy of PJS or the mutation in *STK11* may be located in an untested region, as was discussed above for FAP.

In general, genetic counseling is recommended for a patient undergoing germline testing for a tumor predisposition syndrome. As one of the syndromes in which children can be affected, testing individuals under the age of 18 is acceptable and recommended when the familial mutation is known or the child has symptoms.

Other laboratory issues, such as PT, have evolved in recent years. Where once a laboratory would have been running PT for each gene/assay, the CAP and EQA have been moving towards more platform-based PT, in particular for well-established technologies such as Sanger sequencing. Interlaboratory exchanges also are used to meet PT requirements. Similarly the number and kind of controls that are run with clinical patients has also evolved. As it is impossible to have controls for all possible alterations, representative alterations are often chosen for each platform being used.

Genetic Testing Interpretation and Utility

Regardless of methodology used, careful consideration must be given to the clinical significance and pathogenicity of identified variants. Identification of the germline mutation in individuals with PJS not only can confirm the diagnosis (particularly in individuals who do not have a family history), but once identified can be used to screen at-risk family members who would then be offered appropriate cancer screening. Genetic counseling is an integral part of the process for both the proband and family members at risk. While a number of pathogenic mutations have been identified and are well established, novel alterations continue to be identified and interpretation of the pathogenicity of these alterations may not be clear. The distinction between mutation, VUS, and polymorphism is crucial for the appropriate diagnosis of the affected individual and screening of asymptomatic at risk family members.

References

1. Bulow S, Faurschou Nielsen T, Bulow C, Bisgaard ML, Karlsen L, Moesgaard F. The incidence rate of familial adenomatous polyposis. Results from the Danish Polyposis Register. Int J Colorectal Dis. 1996;11:88–91.
2. Jarvinen HJ. Epidemiology of familial adenomatous polyposis in Finland: impact of family screening on colorectal cancer rate and survival. Gut. 1992;1992(33):357–60.
3. American Gastroenterology Association. AGA technical review on hereditary colorectal cacner and genetic testing. Gastroenterology. 2001;121:198–213.
4. Gardner EJ. A genetic and clinical study of intestinal polyposis, a predisposing factor for carcinoma of the colon and rectum. Am J Hum Genet. 1951;3:167–76.
5. Turcot J, Despres JP, St Pierre F. Malignant tumors of the central nervous system associated with familial polyposis of the colon: report of two cases. Dis Colon Rectum. 1959;2:465–8.
6. Kinzler KW, Nilbert MC, Su LK, Vogelstein B, Bryan TM, Levy DB, et al. Identification of FAP locus genes from chromosome 5q21. Science. 1991;253:661–5.
7. Jarrar AM, Milas M, Mitchell J, Laguardia L, O'Malley M, Berber E, et al. Screening for thyroid cancer in patients with familial adenomatous polyposis. Ann Surg. 2011;253:515–21. doi:10.1097/SLA.0b013e3181fcba8a.
8. Harach HR, Williams GT, Williams ED. Familial adenomatous polyposis associated thyroid carcinoma: a distinct type of follicular cell neoplasm. Histopathology. 1994;25:549–61.
9. Nose V. Thyroid cancer of follicular cell origin in inherited tumor syndromes. Adv Anat Pathol. 2010;17:428–36. doi:10.1097/PAP.0b013e3181f8b028.

10. Hamilton SR, Liu B, Parsons RE, Papadopoulos N, Jen J, Powell SM, et al. The molecular basis of Turcot's syndrome. N Engl J Med. 1995;332:839–47. doi:10.1056/NEJM199503303321302.
11. Fallen T, Wilson M, Morlan B, Lindor NM. Desmoid tumors—a characterization of patients seen at Mayo Clinic 1976–1999. Fam Cancer. 2006;5:191–4. doi:10.1007/s10689-005-5959-5.
12. Gardner EJ, Richards RC. Multiple cutaneous and subcutaneous lesions occurring simultaneously with hereditary polyposis and osteomatosis. Am J Hum Genet. 1953;5:139–47.
13. Spirio L, Olschwang S, Groden J, Robertson M, Samowitz W, Joslyn G, et al. Alleles of the APC gene: an attenuated form of familial polyposis. Cell. 1993;75:951–7.
14. Knudsen AL, Bisgaard ML, Bulow S. Attenuated familial adenomatous polyposis (AFAP). A review of the literature. Fam Cancer. 2003;2:43–55.
15. Alkhouri N, Franciosi JP, Mamula P. Familial adenomatous polyposis in children and adolescents. J Pediatr Gastroenterol Nutr. 2010;51:727–32. doi:10.1097/MPG.0b013e3181e1a224.
16. Parc Y, Piquard A, Dozois RR, Parc R, Tiret E. Long-term outcome of familial adenomatous polyposis patients after restorative coloproctectomy. Ann Surg. 2004;239:378–82.
17. Al-Sukhni W, Aronson M, Gallinger S. Hereditary colorectal cancer syndromes: familial adenomatous polyposis and lynch syndrome. Surg Clin North Am. 2008;88(4):819–844 vii. doi:10.1016/j.suc.2008.04.012.
18. Latchford A, Volikos E, Johnson V, Rogers P, Suraweera N, Tomlinson I, et al. APC mutations in FAP-associated desmoid tumours are non-random but not 'just right'. Hum Mol Genet. 2007;16:78–82. doi:10.1093/hmg/ddl442.
19. Nieuwenhuis MH, Mathus-Vliegen EM, Baeten CG, Nagengast FM, van der Bijl J, van Dalsen AD, et al. Evaluation of management of desmoid tumours associated with familial adenomatous polyposis in Dutch patients. Br J Cancer. 2011;104:37–42. doi:10.1038/sj.bjc.6605997.
20. Robson ME, Storm CD, Weitzel J, Wollins DS, Offit K. American Society of Clinical Oncology policy statement update: genetic and genomic testing for cancer susceptibility. J Clin Oncol. 2010;28:893–901. doi:10.1200/JCO.2009.27.0660.
21. Lefevre JH, Rodrigue CM, Mourra N, Bennis M, Flejou JF, Parc R, et al. Implication of MYH in colorectal polyposis. Ann Surg. 2006;244:874–9. doi:10.1097/01.sla.0000246937.54435.50. discussion 879-880.
22. Soravia C, Berk T, Madlensky L, Mitri A, Cheng H, Gallinger S, et al. Genotype-phenotype correlations in attenuated adenomatous polyposis coli. Am J Hum Genet. 1998;62:1290–301. doi:10.1086/301883.
23. Wallis YL, Morton DG, McKeown CM, Macdonald F. Molecular analysis of the APC gene in 205 families: extended genotype-phenotype correlations in FAP and evidence for the role of APC amino acid changes in colorectal cancer predisposition. J Med Genet. 1999;36:14–20.
24. Sieber OM, Tomlinson IP, Lamlum H. The adenomatous polyposis coli (APC) tumor suppressor -genetics, function and disease. Mol Med Today. 2000;6:462–9.
25. Laken SJ, Petersen GM, Gruber SB, Oddoux C, Ostrer H, Giardiello FM, et al. Familial colorectal cancer in Ashkenazim due to a hypermutable tract in APC. Nat Genet. 1997;17:79–83. doi:10.1038/ng0997-79.
26. Kerr SE, Thomas CB, Thibodeau SN, Ferber MJ, Halling KC. APC germline mutations in individuals being evaluated for familial adenomatous polyposis: a review of the Mayo Clinic experience with 1591 consecutive tests. J Mol Diagn. 2013;15:31–43.
27. Nielsen M, Bik E, Hes FJ, Breuning MH, Vasen HF, Bakker E, et al. Genotype-phenotype correlations in 19 Dutch cases with APC gene deletions and a literature review. Eur J Hum Genet. 2007;15:1034–42. doi:10.1038/sj.ejhg.5201871.
28. Friedl W, Caspari R, Sengteller M, Uhlhaas S, Lamberti C, Jungck M, et al. Can APC mutation analysis contribute to therapeutic decisions in familial adenomatous polyposis? Experience from 680 FAP families. Gut. 2001;48:515–21.
29. Westerman AM, Entius MM, de Baar E, Boor PP, Koole R, van Velthuysen ML, et al. Peutz-Jeghers syndrome: 78-year follow-up of the original family. Lancet. 1999;353:1211–5.
30. Jeghers H, Mc KV, Katz KH. Generalized intestinal polyposis and melanin spots of the oral mucosa, lips and digits; a syndrome of diagnostic significance. N Engl J Med. 1949;241:1031–6. doi:10.1056/NEJM194912292412601.
31. Hamilton SR, Aaltonen LA. Pathology and genetics of tumours of the digestive system. In: Kleihues P, Sobin LH, editors. World Health Organization classification of tumours. Lyon, France: IARC Press; 2000. p. 251.
32. Giardiello FM, Brensinger JD, Tersmette AC, Goodman SN, Petersen GM, Booker SV, et al. Very high risk of cancer in familial Peutz-Jeghers syndrome. Gastroenterology. 2000;119:1447–53.
33. van Lier MG, Wagner A, Mathus-Vliegen EM, Kuipers EJ, Steyerberg EW, van Leerdam ME. High cancer risk in Peutz-Jeghers syndrome: a systematic review and surveillance recommendations. Am J Gastroenterol. 2010;105:1258–64. doi:10.1038/ajg.2009.725. author reply 1265.
34. Hearle N, Schumacher V, Menko FH, Olschwang S, Boardman LA, Gille JJ, et al. Frequency and spectrum of cancers in the Peutz-Jeghers syndrome. Clin Cancer Res. 2006;12:3209–15. doi:10.1158/1078-0432.CCR-06-0083.
35. Jass JR, Williams CB, Bussey HJ, Morson BC. Juvenile polyposis–a precancerous condition. Histopathology. 1988;13:619–30.
36. McCarthy PM, Piehler JM, Schaff HV, Pluth JR, Orszulak TA, Vidaillet Jr HJ, et al. The significance of multiple, recurrent, and "complex" cardiac myxomas. J Thorac Cardiovasc Surg. 1986;91:389–96.
37. van Lier MG, Westerman AM, Wagner A, Looman CW, Wilson JH, de Rooij FW, et al. High cancer risk and increased mortality in patients with Peutz-Jeghers syndrome. Gut. 2011;60:141–7. doi:10.1136/gut.2010.223750.
38. Beggs AD, Latchford AR, Vasen HF, Moslein G, Alonso A, Aretz S, et al. Peutz-Jeghers syndrome: a systematic review and recommendations for management. Gut. 2010;59:975–86. doi:10.1136/gut.2009.198499.
39. Wei C, Amos CI, Zhang N, Wang X, Rashid A, Walker CL, et al. Suppression of Peutz-Jeghers polyposis by targeting mammalian target of rapamycin signaling. Clin Cancer Res. 2008;14:1167–71. doi:10.1158/1078-0432.CCR-07-4007.
40. Hemminki A, Markie D, Tomlinson I, Avizienyte E, Roth S, Loukola A, et al. A serine/threonine kinase gene defective in Peutz-Jeghers syndrome. Nature. 1998;391:184–7. doi:10.1038/34432.
41. Jenne DE, Reimann H, Nezu J, Friedel W, Loff S, Jeschke R, et al. Peutz-Jeghers syndrome is caused by mutations in a novel serine threonine kinase. Nat Genet. 1998;18:38–43. doi:10.1038/ng0198-38.
42. Volikos E, Robinson J, Aittomaki K, Mecklin JP, Jarvinen H, Westerman AM, et al. LKB1 exonic and whole gene deletions are a common cause of Peutz-Jeghers syndrome. J Med Genet. 2006;43, e18. doi:10.1136/jmg.2005.039875.
43. Aretz S, Stienen D, Uhlhaas S, Loff S, Back W, Pagenstecher C, et al. High proportion of large genomic STK11 deletions in Peutz-Jeghers syndrome. Hum Mutat. 2005;26:513–9. doi:10.1002/humu.20253.
44. Mehenni H, Gehrig C, Nezu J, Oku A, Shimane M, Rossier C, et al. Loss of LKB1 kinase activity in Peutz-Jeghers syndrome, and evidence for allelic and locus heterogeneity. Am J Hum Genet. 1998;63:1641–50.

45. Tiainen M, Vaahtomeri K, Ylikorkala A, Makela TP. Growth arrest by the LKB1 tumor suppressor: induction of p21(WAF1/CIP1). Hum Mol Genet. 2002;11:1497–504.
46. Karuman P, Gozani O, Odze RD, Zhou XC, Zhu H, Shaw R, et al. The Peutz-Jegher gene product LKB1 is a mediator of p53-de pendent cell death. Mol Cell. 2001;7:1307–19.
47. Morton DG, Roos JM, Kemphues KJ. par-4, a gene required for cytoplasmic localization and determination of specific cell types in Caenorhabditis elegans embryogenesis. Genetics. 1992;130:771–90.
48. Alessi DR, Sakamoto K, Bayascas JR. LKB1-dependent signaling pathways. Annu Rev Biochem. 2006;75:137–63. doi:10.1146/annurev.biochem.75.103004.142702.
49. Lin-Marq N, Borel C, Antonarakis SE. Peutz-Jeghers LKB1 mutants fail to activate GSK-3beta, preventing it from inhibiting Wnt signaling. Mol Genet Genomics. 2005;273:184–96. doi:10.1007/s00438-005-1124-y.
50. Corradetti MN, Inoki K, Bardeesy N, DePinho RA, Guan KL. Regulation of the TSC pathway by LKB1: evidence of a molecular link between tuberous sclerosis complex and Peutz-Jeghers syndrome. Genes Dev. 2004;18:1533–8. doi:10.1101/gad.1199104.
51. Mehenni H, Resta N, Guanti G, Mota-Vieira L, Lerner A, Peyman M, et al. Molecular and clinical characteristics in 46 families affected with Peutz-Jeghers syndrome. Dig Dis Sci. 2007;52:1924–33. doi:10.1007/s10620-006-9435-3.

Hereditary Nonpolyposis Colorectal Cancer and Lynch Syndrome

24

James P. Grenert

Abstract

Hereditary nonpolyposis colorectal cancer (HNPCC) is an autosomal dominant cancer disorder associated with a greatly increased risk of colorectal, uterine, and other cancers. Most cases of HNPCC are due to inherited mutations in DNA mismatch repair (MMR) genes and their encoded proteins which correct errors made during DNA replication. HNPCC associated with inherited MMR defects is also called Lynch syndrome. Additionally, sporadic cancers occurring in individuals without HNPCC may have diminished expression of MMR protein(s) due to epigenetic silencing. Defective MMR function leads to reduced fidelity of DNA synthesis and microsatellite instability (MSI), the accumulation of mutations in repetitive sequences of DNA called microsatellites. Testing for defective MMR can be done directly by immunohistochemical staining for MMR proteins or indirectly by PCR fragment analysis of microsatellites.

Keywords

Lynch syndrome • Hereditary nonpolyposis colorectal cancer • HNPCC • Microsatellite instability • MSI • Mismatch repair • BRAF V600E • MLH1 methylation • MSH2 • MSH6 • PMS2

Hereditary nonpolyposis colorectal cancer (HNPCC) is an autosomal dominant cancer disorder. Initially defined clinically, a distinct subset of HNPCC can be identified through molecular testing and is responsible for approximately 3 % of all colorectal carcinomas.

Clinical Characteristics

The use of the term HNPCC has a long and problematic history. It was first coined by Dr. Harry T. Lynch and colleagues in 1984 to differentiate what were known as the cancer family syndrome (CFS), characterized by early-onset, predominantly proximal colorectal cancer as well as other cancers, and hereditary site-specific colon cancer (HSSCC), which differed from CFS in that non-colorectal cancers were not increased, from familial adenomatous polyposis (FAP) [1]. HNPCC has significant descriptive shortcomings. While these families do not exhibit the numerous colonic polyps characteristic of FAP, their colorectal cancers (CRC) nevertheless arise from adenomatous polyps. Additionally, despite its name, HNPCC is associated with not only a greatly increased risk of CRC but also of several other cancers, most commonly endometrial cancer of the uterus. These limitations led many researchers to adopt the alternative designation of Lynch syndrome, in place of HNPCC, and in both the literature and common usage, the terms are often used interchangeably.

Since the discovery of the underlying molecular basis for most cases of HNPCC, specifically, a heritable defect in DNA mismatch repair (MMR, discussed below), some authors have advocated for the use of Lynch syndrome to specifically refer to those that fit the clinical picture of HNPCC and

J.P. Grenert, M.D., Ph.D. (✉)
University of California, San Francisco, 1001 Potrero Avenue, Building 3, room 102, San Francisco, CA 94110, USA
e-mail: James.grenert@ucsf.edu

D.G.B. Leonard (ed.), *Molecular Pathology in Clinical Practice*, DOI 10.1007/978-3-319-19674-9_24

Table 24.1 Clinical criteria for identification of Lynch syndrome carriers

Amsterdam Criteria II
There should be at least three relatives with an HNPCC-associated cancer (CRC, cancer of the endometrium, small bowel, ureter, or renal pelvis)
One should be a first-degree relative of the other two
At least two successive generations should be affected
At least one should be diagnosed before age 50 years
Familial adenomatous polyposis should be excluded in the CRC case(s), if any
Tumors should be verified by pathological examination
Revised Bethesda Guidelines
CRC in a patient who is less than 50 years of age
Presence of synchronous, metachronous colorectal, or other HNPCC-associated tumors,[a] regardless of age
CRC with the MSI-H histology[b] diagnosed in a patient who is less than 60 years of age
CRC diagnosed in one or more first-degree relatives with an HNPCC-related tumor, with one of the cancers being diagnosed under age 50 years
CRC diagnosed in two or more first- or second-degree relatives with HNPCC-related tumors, regardless of age

[a]Hereditary nonpolyposis colorectal cancer (HNPCC)-related tumors include colorectal, endometrial, stomach, ovarian, pancreas, ureter and renal pelvis, biliary tract, and brain (usually glioblastoma as seen in Turcot syndrome) tumors, sebaceous gland adenomas and keratoacanthomas in Muir–Torre syndrome, and carcinoma of the small bowel
[b]Presence of tumor infiltrating lymphocytes, Crohn's-like lymphocytic reaction, mucinous/signet ring differentiation, or medullary growth pattern
CRC colorectal cancer, *HNPCC* hereditary nonpolyposis coli, *MSI-H* microsatellite instability-high

demonstrate MMR deficiency, while reserving HNPCC for cases where no MMR abnormality is identified [2–4]. HNPCC, then, encompasses two groups: Lynch syndrome and a second, possibly heterogeneous group that has been called "familial colorectal cancer type X." A number of explanations have been proposed to account for type X, including familial environmental causes, undiscovered genetic syndromes, and even aggregation of cancers occurring by chance [5, 6]. In the absence of a well-defined, testable etiology for type X, the focus of this chapter will be HNPCC-associated cancers that fit the current definition of Lynch syndrome and other tumors caused by defective MMR.

HNPCC is characterized by a greatly increased risk of malignancies, particularly CRC and endometrial carcinomas, which occur at a younger age than is typical for these tumors. These often striking clinical features have led to the development of clinical criteria for the diagnosis of HNPCC. The earliest system in widespread use was that created by the International Collaborative Group on Hereditary Non-Polyposis Colorectal Cancer (ICG-HNPCC) at a 1990 meeting in Amsterdam, subsequently referred to as the "Amsterdam Criteria." These criteria emphasized multigenerational disease, early age of onset (<50 years), and the lack of a polyposis syndrome [7]. Recognizing some deficiencies in the system, most notably the lack of extracolonic cancers in the criteria, the ICG-HNPCC updated these criteria in 1998 (Amsterdam Criteria II) [8]. A second group at an HNPCC workshop at the National Cancer Institute in Bethesda, MD, which included some of the members of the ICG-HNPCC, developed guidelines for identification of tumors that should undergo microsatellite instability (MSI) testing for evidence of defective MMR and published their conclusions in 1997 (the "Bethesda Guidelines"). These guidelines focused on not only the clinical features and family history of the patient but also on pathological features of the tumor including site and histologic appearance/subtype [9]. The Bethesda Guidelines were revised in 2004 to include less-restrictive age criteria and eliminate testing of adenomas in young people [10]. The updated Amsterdam and Bethesda systems are shown in Table 24.1. The reported clinical performance of these criteria varies widely. While some authors report nearly 100 % sensitivity and specificity for the Bethesda Guidelines, it is unlikely that such performance can be achieved in all settings [11, 12]. A large study of 500 patients from the Ohio State University found only 39 and 72 % sensitivity for the Amsterdam and Bethesda criteria, respectively [13]. In particular, the age limits have the potential to exclude Lynch carriers who present at more advanced age.

CRC arising in the setting of defective MMR has a tendency toward a number of pathologic features, including location in the proximal colon, mucinous or signet ring differentiation, poor differentiation, and prominent lymphocytic inflammation in and around the tumor. Examples of histologic features of MMR-deficient tumors are shown in Fig. 24.1. Recognition of histologic patterns has been shown to be highly sensitive for tumors with defective MMR, with reported sensitivity in some studies greater than 90 %. The specificity of histology, however, is only 55–67 %, making additional testing a necessary component of tumor evaluation [14–16].

Lynch syndrome is associated with several other cancers (listed among the Bethesda Guidelines). The association of some of these cancers with CRC has been noted by medical researchers over the years, and these have been given eponymous syndromes such as Turcot (glioblastoma) and Muir–Torre (keratoacanthoma and sebaceous tumors) syndromes. The importance of gynecologic cancers in the disease burden

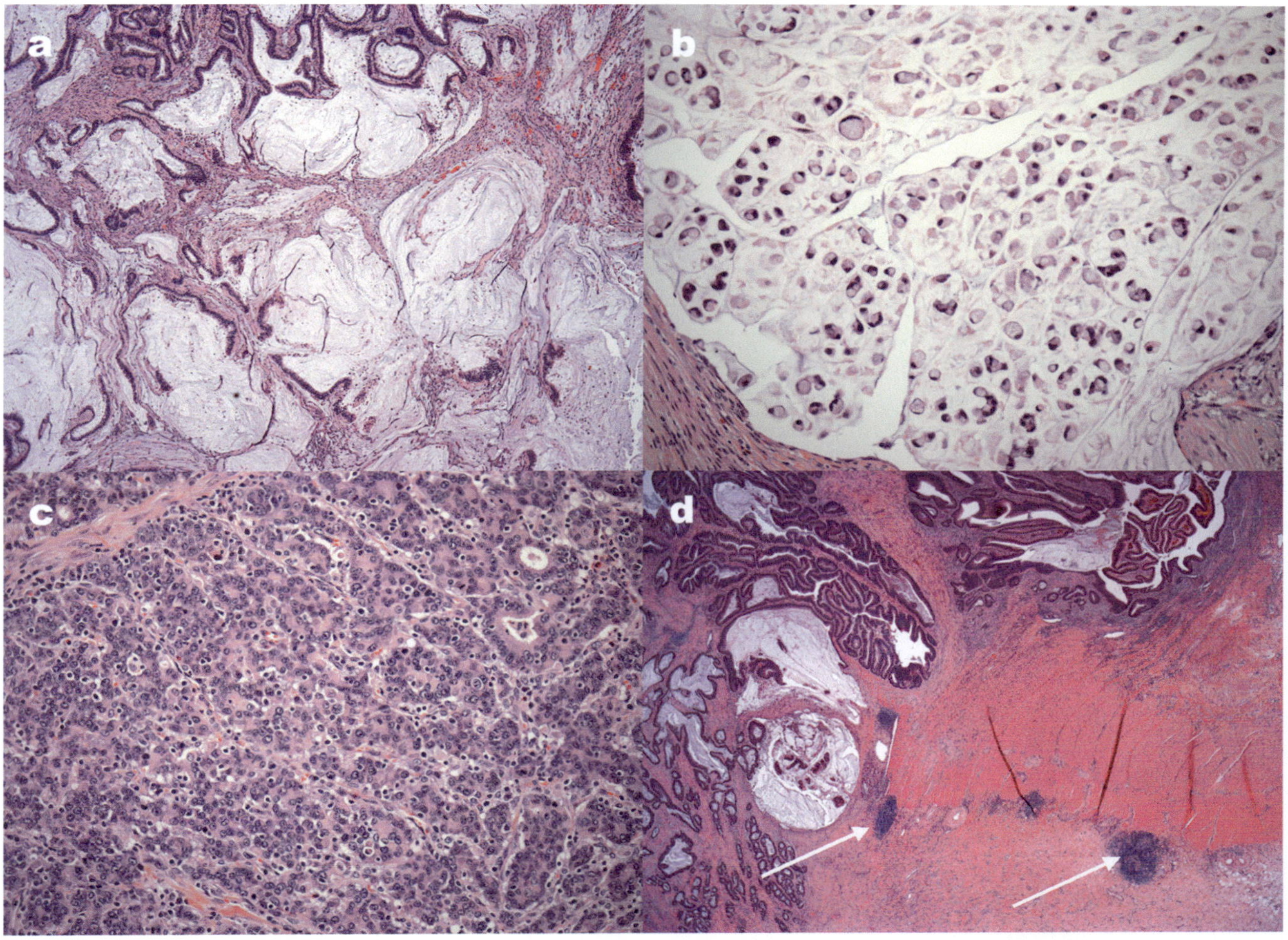

Figure 24.1 Examples of histological features of colorectal carcinomas with defective DNA mismatch repair. (**a**) Extracellular mucin pools in a mucinous adenocarcinoma. (**b**) Signet ring cell adenocarcinoma with tumor cells containing a single, large mucin vacuole. (**c**) Tumor-infiltrating lymphocytes are seen as small, round cells, often with a surrounding clear "halo," infiltrating among tumor cell glands or aggregates. (**d**) Crohn's-like lymphocytic response is illustrated by discrete lymphocytic aggregates (*arrows*) away from the tumor, resembling the transmural inflammation of Crohn's disease

cannot be stressed enough, with uterine and ovarian cancer comprising half of the presenting cancers in women with Lynch syndrome [17]. The overall risk of CRC by age 70 in Lynch carriers has been reported as high as 82 %, although some studies have shown a lower risk of 30–74 %, with men at significantly higher risk than women [18–20]. The risk of uterine cancer in women with Lynch syndrome is 34–60 % [18, 20, 21]. For some less common tumors such as gastric, small bowel, and urinary tract cancers, the lifetime risk of cancer is approximately 5–15 % [22].

Molecular Basis of Disease

In 1993, through the work of multiple groups working independently, the molecular basis for Lynch syndrome began to be uncovered. This was first recognized in HNPCC tumors as changes in the size of microsatellites, tandem repetitive sequences of DNA which make up about 3 % of the human genome. The repeating sequence in these microsatellites ranges in size from 1 to 13 bases, although microsatellites longer than 5 bases are not typically used in testing. In HNPCC tumors, the number of repeats in microsatellites expanded or contracted, resulting in a shift in the size of the microsatellites. These changes were called replication errors or microsatellite instability (originally abbreviated MIN but now usually shown as MSI). MSI was found to be much more common in tumors of families with HNPCC than in sporadic CRC [23–25].

Soon after the discovery of MSI in HNPCC, the phenomenon was linked to defective function of proteins involved in the repair of errors introduced during DNA replication. These proteins have homologs, MutS and MutL, originally described in *E. coli*, whose function is to recognize and correct DNA heteroduplexes of mismatched base pairs [26]. Microsatellites, due to the repetitive nature of their sequences, appear to represent a "slippery" template along which DNA polymerase is prone to skip forward or backward during replication, creating small loops of unpaired bases in the process [27]. Depending on the direction of the slippage, the newly synthesized strand will contain a greater or lesser number of repeats than the template. Single base–base mismatches can occur when an incorrect nucleotide is incorporated into the new strand. An intact MMR system recognizes these alterations and directs a multistep process of strand breakage, excision of the error, and resynthesis of the strand, thereby resulting in a corrected sequence. The connection between the MSI and the MMR system was first shown by the identification of germline mutations in *MSH2*, the human homolog of *mutS*, in families with Lynch syndrome, and later in the MutL homolog *MLH1* [28, 29]. Most of these mutations result in a premature stop codon and a truncated protein. Less commonly, missense mutations affect protein-protein interactions that are essential for MMR function.

CRC arising in Lynch syndrome are believed to follow a typical adenoma–carcinoma sequence in common with non-Lynch tumors. This has been shown through the presence of adenomas adjacent to early carcinomas identified in prophylactic colectomies performed in Lynch syndrome carriers [30]. Furthermore, adenomas arising in Lynch syndrome, particularly those that show high histologic grade, often have evidence of MSI prior to the development of invasive carcinoma [31]. While there have been reports of MSI in histologically normal cells and tissues of patients with Lynch syndrome, in most cases, testing of normal tissue in Lynch syndrome carriers does not demonstrate MSI, and the presence of MMR proteins can be demonstrated with immunohistochemical staining [32–35]. Thus, despite the loss of one functional copy of a MMR gene, DNA MMR largely remains intact until a second genetic hit results in deletion or mutation of the functioning allele.

At least seven MMR proteins involved in DNA repair during mitosis have been identified in humans [36]. Four of these, MLH1, PMS2, MSH2, and MSH6, appear to be largely responsible for Lynch syndrome, with mutations in MLH1 and MSH2 causing approximately 90 % of cases [37]. The MMR proteins function as heterodimers, and MLH1 and MSH2 serve as the obligate components of dimers homologous to the bacterial *mutL* and *mutS*, respectively. MLH1 primarily pairs with PMS2 but can also be paired with PMS1 or MSH3. MSH2 pairs primarily with MSH6, and MSH3 is a secondary partner [36]. The specific combinations formed determine the types of DNA mismatches that are corrected. For example, MSH2 and MSH6 can repair single base pair mismatches as well as longer insertions and deletions, while MSH2 and MSH3 mainly correct larger mismatches [26]. The different pairings and their functions seem to have clinical relevance, as shown by the fact that different Lynch mutations do not appear to be equal with respect to the clinical manifestations of the syndrome and the associated cancer risk. Carriers with mutations in the obligate components MLH1 and MSH2, without which MMR dimers cannot function, have an approximately four-fold higher risk of CRC than do those with an MSH6 mutation [21]. This may be explained by substitution of MSH6 by MSH3 in the MutS-type dimer, partially compensating for MSH6 loss. The effect of this substitution is restoration of repair of longer mutations, while single base errors may go uncorrected [38].

In addition to HNPCC-associated cancers, sporadic CRC (i.e., those not associated with a strong family history of CRC) also can have MSI [39]. These microsatellite-unstable tumors make up approximately 15–25 % of sporadic CRC, a much greater number of tumors than those attributable to Lynch syndrome [40]. Like Lynch-associated CRC, sporadic tumors with MSI have a tendency toward a right-sided proximal location in the colon, but the age of onset of these tumors does not differ significantly from MMR-proficient tumors [41, 42]. The precursor lesion of these cancers, sessile serrated adenoma, lacks the cellular atypia of tubular adenomas that precede Lynch-associated tumors and has the saw-toothed microscopic appearance of a common hyperplastic polyp. However, the sessile serrated adenoma differs from hyperplastic polyps by increased architectural complexity, which is due to altered distribution of proliferating cells in colonic glands [43]. Analysis of MMR genes showed that most of the sporadic tumors lack either germline or somatic mutations in MMR genes, yet immunohistochemical staining for MMR proteins shows that these tumors commonly lack expression of MLH1 [44]. This apparent discrepancy was explained by the recognition that the *MLH1* promoter was epigenetically silenced via hypermethylation in sporadic CRC with MSI [45]. Further, *MLH1* hypermethylation is closely linked to the activating V600E mutation in the BRAF kinase, with *BRAF* mutation seen in 31–87 % of CRC with silenced MLH1. Significantly for diagnostic purposes, BRAF mutation is virtually never seen in Lynch syndrome-associated CRC [46–48]. A causal relationship between *BRAF* mutation and *MLH1* silencing has yet to be discovered. *MLH1* hypermethylation also has been demonstrated in sporadic endometrial cancers with MSI. However, in stark contrast with what is seen in the colon, these tumors consistently lack *BRAF* mutation, suggesting that *MLH1* hypermethylation can occur independently of *BRAF* mutation [49]. Thus, *BRAF* mutation may indicate an *MLH1*-methylated CRC but may not be the underlying etiology. Rarely, constitutional MLH1 methylation may be inherited, resulting in Lynch syndrome without protein-coding mutations in MMR genes. While this constitutes <1% of all Lynch syndrome patients, it is an important Lynch etiology in individuals who are MLH1-deficient but negative for MLH1 mutation [50].

While DNA replication errors in microsatellites can be used as an indicator of defective mismatch repair function, it is not clear what role MSI may play in vivo in cancer pathogenesis. The Human Genome Project has revealed that many microsatellites are located in the coding regions of hundreds of genes. These include genes encoding proteins with important roles in signal transduction (TGFBII and IGFIIR, receptors for TGFB and insulin-like growth factor, respectively), tumor suppression (PTEN), and apoptosis (BAX). Ironically, the genes for two of the MMR proteins, MSH3 and MSH6, also contain microsatellites. Supporting the idea that instability in these and other microsatellite-containing genes can affect colon carcinogenesis is the observation that frameshift mutations in these genes have been identified in tumors from HNPCC families, and this instability can occur as early as the adenoma stage [51, 52].

Clinical Utility of Testing

The primary goal of most testing for defective mismatch repair is to screen for Lynch syndrome carriers. The high risk of malignancy in this population makes their identification, increased surveillance, and consideration of medical and surgical prophylaxis of critical importance in preventing morbidity and mortality. Carriers of MMR protein mutations do not have an increased rate of development of precancerous adenomas, but progression from adenoma to carcinoma appears to be accelerated [53]. For this reason, the recommended interval for colonoscopy in this population is every 1–2 years, shorter than the 5-year interval for non-carriers. Increased frequency of colonoscopy in surveillance appears to result in fewer invasive cancers due to removal at the adenoma stage [54, 55].

In addition to increased surveillance, another strategy under investigation to protect against cancer is chemoprevention. Aspirin has been used in a long-term trial (CAPP2) with Lynch carriers to see if it lowers the incidence of CRC. After nearly 5-year average follow-up, participants taking aspirin had a nearly 40 % reduction in CRC risk compared to those taking placebo [56]. The most definitive preventive measure is surgical resection of organs at high risk of malignancy, including subtotal or greater colectomy for Lynch carriers undergoing CRC resection. This is a complex issue that is beyond the scope of this chapter, but it has been addressed by a number of authors and been shown to be both medically effective and cost effective [55, 57, 58].

Once one Lynch carrier has been identified, the specific germline MMR gene mutation detected can be assayed in the patient's blood relatives, greatly expanding the importance of the initial detection. The first-degree relatives of a Lynch carrier each have a 50 % risk of being a carrier. Given the potential interventions for Lynch syndrome carriers, some have advocated for universal screening of all CRC for evidence of defective MMR [59, 60]. While the specific recommendations for screening method differ, universal screening may be cost effective [13, 61, 62].

Determination of MMR status has prognostic and predictive significance. Clinical studies of patients with MMR-deficient CRC have shown that these tumors present with more advanced local disease (have deeper invasion into the colonic wall), yet paradoxically, patients with these tumors have a longer survival than those with MMR-proficient cancer [63–65]. A very thorough review of survival studies by Popat et al. estimated the survival advantage of patients with MMR-deficient CRC to be 15 % or more [66]. Although both sporadic and Lynch-associated MMR-deficient tumors have a better prognosis, this effect is most pronounced in patients with Lynch syndrome [63]. It is unlikely that the younger age of presentation of patients with Lynch syndrome completely explains the improved survival. When early-onset CRC patients were compared with respect to MMR function, there remained a trend toward improved survival in those with defective MMR [67]. For reasons that are not clear, MMR-deficient tumors show less aggressive behavior in terms of lymphatic and distant metastasis and prolonged time to recurrence [63, 68, 69].

The improved survival in patients with MMR-deficient tumors means there is less opportunity for benefit from chemotherapy. Patients and their physicians may feel that the adverse effects of chemotherapy outweigh the modest improvement in survival (5 % at 5 years in stage II patients) that has been associated with adjuvant treatment [70]. Additionally, in patients with stage II and III disease, studies have shown that while fluorouracil treatment of tumors with intact MMR improves survival, patients with MMR-deficient tumors may not benefit [71, 72].

Available Assays

The majority of testing is directed toward identifying tumors with defective MMR, both as a means of screening for potential Lynch carriers and for its prognostic and therapeutic implications. Once potential carriers have been identified, additional testing can identify the presence of a germline mutation in an MMR protein to confirm a Lynch syndrome diagnosis and to allow counseling and targeted testing of family members for carrier status. However, since most MMR-deficient tumors arise sporadically, the number of patients who require germline mutation testing is relatively small, and the focus of this section is on screening assays. Protocols for germline testing have been published and involve both direct sequencing for small mutations and denaturing high-pressure liquid chromatography for large rearrangements [73]. Hundreds of Lynch syndrome mutations have been identified and are catalogued online by the

International Society for Gastrointestinal Hereditary Tumours (InSiGHT; http://www.insight-group.org) [74]. Different Lynch syndrome mutations have different cancer risks, with *MLH1* and *MSH2* mutations associated with approximately four-fold greater risk of cancer than *MSH6* mutation [21]. Thus, identification of the specific mutation can provide useful information for counseling carriers and their family members.

Immunohistochemistry

The most readily available assay for detecting MMR deficiency is immunohistochemical (IHC) staining of tissue sections for MMR proteins. This can be performed by most histology laboratories using standard protocols with commercial antibodies against MLH1, PMS2, MSH2, and MSH6. This technique directly detects the presence or absence of these MMR proteins in the tumor but does not assay for the activity of the MMR proteins. MMR mutations result in a truncated or otherwise nonfunctional protein that is then degraded by the cell [75, 76]. IHC, then, identifies the loss of one or more mismatch repair proteins in a tumor.

Related to their function to ensure the fidelity of DNA replication, MMR proteins are normally found in the nucleus. In a tumor with a functioning MMR system, staining for each MMR protein will reveal positive staining in the nuclei of tumor cells. This system is also at work in non-tumor cells, which also should have positive nuclear staining. Evaluation of non-tumor cells can serve as an internal positive control for each stain [77]. Although every cell in a MMR-proficient tumor is expected to be positive if the MMR proteins are intact, in practice, this is usually not the case. As is seen with many IHC stains, staining often is variable throughout the tumor. Indeed, non-tumor cells may show the same inconsistency in staining [78]. It is unclear if this represents variable fixation/antigen retrieval issues which abound with IHC, biologic variability at the cell level, or a combination of these factors. In general, MMR proteins that are nonfunctional will fail to dimerize and will be degraded. Using IHC, this typically corresponds to widespread loss of nuclear staining in the tumor cells [77]. Similarly, epigenetic silencing of MLH1 expression also results in a loss of staining [44]. An example of loss of MMR staining by IHC is shown in Fig. 24.2.

MMR protein heterodimer composition allows prediction of the underlying molecular defect based on the pattern of protein loss. Usually, when the obligatory partner of a MMR component is lost, that protein will be lost as well. On the other hand, MMR proteins that may dimerize with multiple partners can still be present if one of the partners is deficient. For example, PMS2 can only pair with MLH1, and therefore, loss of MLH1 most often results in lack of staining for both MLH1 and PMS2. MLH1, on the other hand, can pair with proteins other than PMS2, and loss of PMS2 may occur without MLH1 loss. Table 24.2 demonstrates the common protein loss patterns and the causative genetic defects. Although definitive diagnosis of Lynch syndrome requires identification of a germline mutation in one of the MMR genes, this information from IHC testing can direct the germline testing to a specific MMR gene.

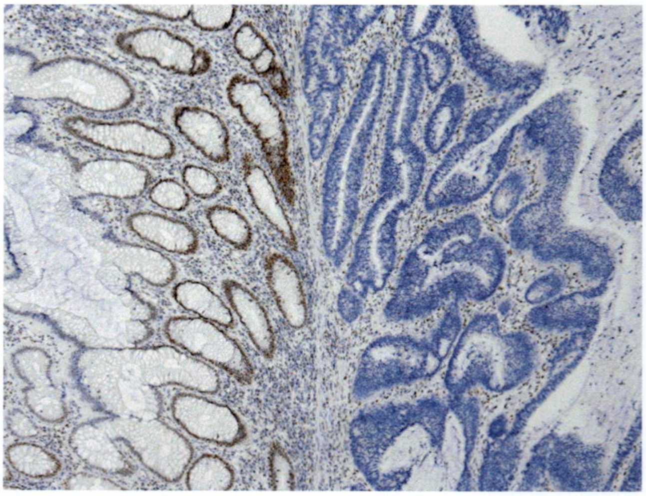

Figure 24.2 Example of loss of immunohistochemical staining for the mismatch repair protein PMS2 in a colon carcinoma. The normal glands on the *left* show positive, brown staining for PMS2 in cell nuclei, while the cancerous glands on the *right* lack the brown staining. The blue staining present in the nucleus is a counterstain to show the tissues. Note that even in the normal tissue on the left, not every cell will stain positively

Table 24.2 Interpretation of protein loss patterns in MMR immunohistochemistry

Protein(s) lost	Possible gene defect[a]
MLH1 and PMS2	The most common pattern of loss. Both sporadic and hereditary tumors may show this pattern, but most are sporadic. *MLH1* hypermethylation in sporadic tumors. *MLH1* mutation in hereditary tumors.
MSH2 and MSH6	The most common exclusively hereditary pattern. *MSH2* mutation.
MSH6 only	Uncommon. *MSH6* mutation.
PMS2 only	Rare. *PMS2* mutation or, less likely, *MLH1* mutation.

[a]MMR immunohistochemistry is not diagnostic for Lynch syndrome, and suspected gene mutation must be confirmed.
MMR mismatch repair

Although IHC should ideally clearly show that a MMR protein is either present or absent in a tumor, IHC results can be ambiguous. Tumor cells often show variable staining, making interpretation difficult, and even tumors that harbor MMR gene mutations may still demonstrate detectable protein staining [78–80]. One MLH1 truncation mutation has been reported to avoid degradation and stains positively by IHC, while its partner PMS2 is destabilized and shows protein loss, a pattern which would normally indicate PMS2 mutation [81]. It has been suggested that IHC staining for only two MMR proteins, MSH6 and PMS2, may be as effective as staining for all four MMR proteins as a screening test, since one of these should be lost in any of the most common Lynch syndrome scenarios [82]. This has a cost advantage, but many laboratories may choose to use all four stains to help clarify difficult cases and to provide immediate guidance for gene testing.

Sometimes, a tumor that is otherwise completely negative for a protein may show scattered positive nuclei. These may actually represent staining of benign lymphocytes admixed with tumor, the intratumoral lymphocytes (ITL) that are one of the histologic features of MMR-deficient tumors. One feature that can distinguish this artifact from true tumor staining is if the staining is limited to uniform, small, round nuclei characteristic of lymphocytes. Occasionally, apoptotic cells may aberrantly stain for a MMR protein that is absent in the tumor. It is often helpful to review the histologic appearance of the tumor for the presence of ITL and apoptotic cells. Another potential source of misinterpretation is diminished MSH6 staining in rectal carcinomas that have been treated with chemoradiation. Although the staining may be completely absent in these tumors, some may not have an MSH6 mutation or evidence of MSI. If a pretreatment specimen is available, staining is likely to be more representative of the true MSH6 status [83]. Finally, the interpretation of IHC testing should be reported as having MMR proteins "present" or "absent," rather than positive or negative, to avoid possible misinterpretation by the recipient of the test results; "positive" may be incorrectly read as "positive for MMR deficiency."

Microsatellite Instability PCR

PCR testing of DNA microsatellites represents an indirect functional assay for MMR proteins. After DNA is extracted from tumor tissue and from a non-tumor control tissue from the same patient, a panel of microsatellites is amplified by PCR using primers adjacent to but not including the repetitive sequence. The size of the PCR products is then analyzed by capillary electrophoresis, or less commonly by gel electrophoresis. Because defective MMR causes frameshift mutations in microsatellites, instability is shown by a change in the size of the PCR products from the microsatellite. Commonly used panels of microsatellites for MSI testing in the USA are the NCI panel (three dinucleotide [*D2S123*, *D5S346*, and *D17S250*] and two mononucleotide [Big Adenine Tract, *BAT-25*and *BAT-26*] microsatellites) and the panel supplied in a commercial kit available from Promega (Madison, WI) with five mononucleotide repeats (*BAT-25*, *BAT-26*, *NR-21*, *NR-24*, and *MONO-27*) [84]. Different microsatellites vary in their ability to identify tumors with defective MMR, with mononucleotide repeat loci generally superior to dinucleotide loci in both sensitivity and specificity [85]. This may be particularly true with MSH6 deficiency, which preferentially causes errors in mononucleotide repeats, as described earlier. The Promega panel includes two additional pentanucleotide repeats which are not evaluated to identify MSI but are used to ensure correct pairing of a patient's tumor and normal DNA. These repeats are highly polymorphic in the population, and different patterns seen between a patient's samples raise the possibility of specimen contamination or a labeling error.

As established by criteria from the National Cancer Institute, tumors exhibiting stability in all of the microsatellites tested are called microsatellite stable (MSS). Those with instability in ≥30–40 % of tested microsatellites are designated microsatellite instability-high (MSI-H). The third category, microsatellite instability-low (MSI-L), encompasses tumors that have at least one unstable microsatellite, but not enough to meet MSI-H criteria [86]. In common practice with the 5-microsatellite Promega or NCI panels, MSS, MSI-L, and MSI-H correspond to zero, one, or two or more unstable microsatellites, respectively. MSS tumors usually have intact MMR function, while MSI-H tumors correlate with MMR deficiency. MSI-L tumors have not been shown to be associated with defective MMR and are usually regarded as equivalent to MSS in the absence of solid evidence for Lynch syndrome. Instability is defined by a change in the length of a microsatellite in tumor DNA when compared to non-tumor ("normal") DNA from the same patient. When compared with the normal control, an unstable allele will appear as a novel allele or a shift in the length of the allele.

The types of patterns seen in MSI testing depend upon whether dinucleotide or mononucleotide repeats are being evaluated. Dinucleotide repeats are polymorphic in the population, and a patient will often have alleles of different sizes on the maternal and paternal chromosomes. Thus, the normal sample will show two peaks, each representing one allele. One or both of these may change in length in the tumor as a result of defective MMR. The presence of two peaks in the normal DNA may mask a shift if the novel allele is obscured by an overlapping normal allele. Mononucleotide repeats, on the other hand, are generally very homogeneous ("quasi-monomorphic"), with same-sized alleles inherited from each parent. Thus, the normal sample will typically

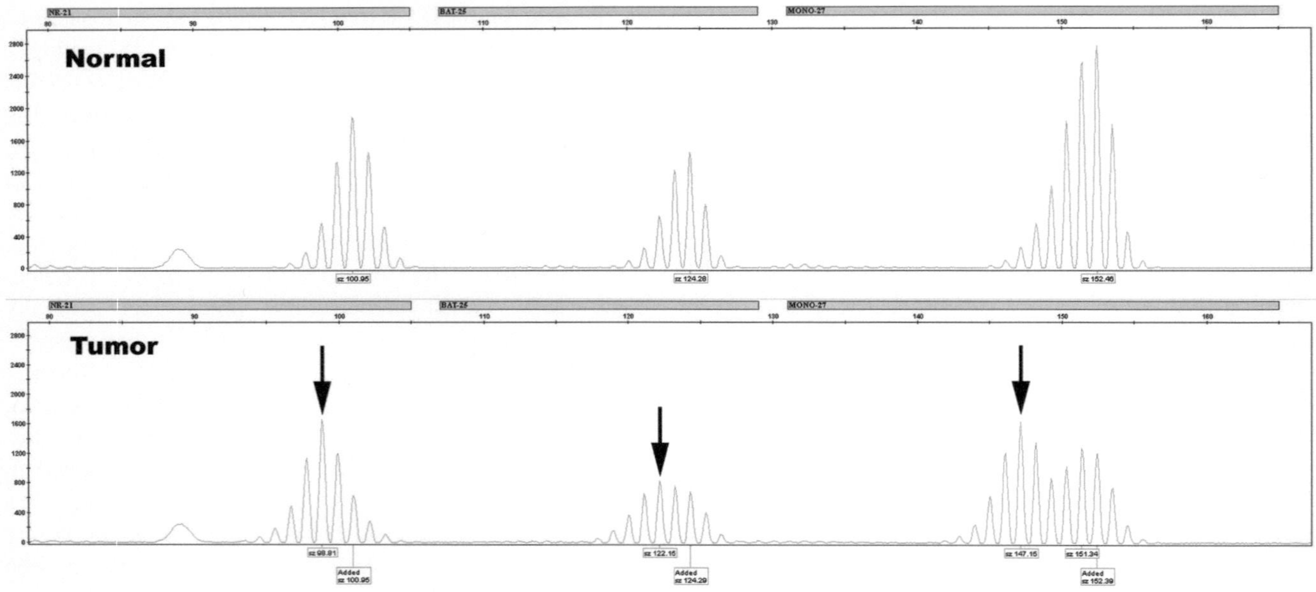

Figure 24.3 Three microsatellites with instability. Capillary electrophoresis data for three microsatellites, *NR-21*, *BAT-26*, and *MONO-27*, is shown for a patient's normal (*above*) and tumor (*below*) DNA. *Arrows* point to changes in the size of microsatellites in the tumor, indicative of stability. Note that the subtle 2-bp size change in *NR-21* and *BAT-26* may be difficult to appreciate unless a comparison with the normal sample is made

show only a single peak for each microsatellite. Tumor instability will be demonstrated as a shift in length for that peak or the presence of a second peak that was not seen in the normal tissue. Examples of unstable mononucleotide microsatellite alleles are shown in Fig. 24.3.

The effectiveness of MSI testing is closely related to the panel of microsatellites used in the assay. Poor performance of some markers may result in MSI-L designation, and when many microsatellites are tested, the percentage of MSI-L tumors increases [87]. The percentage of MSI-L tumors in older reports, before the use of only mononucleotide panels, is as high as 35 % [88]. In contrast, when mononucleotide repeats are used exclusively, MSI-L tumors become very uncommon [89]. The significance of MSI-L when testing with a mononucleotide panel is unclear, and these patients should be offered genetic counseling. Fortunately, the percentage of unstable microsatellites in MSI-H tumors is usually 80–100 % when mononucleotide repeats are used [90]. Note that the pentanucleotide repeats in the Promega panel may show instability themselves in MSI-H tumors, and this can cause confusion if used to match a patient's tumor and normal samples [89].

Recognition of some general patterns of instability in mononucleotide microsatellites can be helpful in MSI interpretation. First, mononucleotide markers nearly always shift to a smaller size when unstable. While larger sizes can be seen, their presence may indicate another genetic event such as an insertion, rather than instability. Second, the magnitude of a shift is usually no greater than approximately 10–12 bases, and large shifts often have some intermediate-sized alleles present as well. These intervening peaks are due to heterogeneous instability in the tumor. Shifts greater than approximately 12 bases may be the result of a deletion, and a deletion would not be expected to show the intermediate-sized alleles. A third pattern to be aware of is heterozygosity for a mononucleotide microsatellite. While most individuals have inherited alleles of the same size for a mononucleotide microsatellite, occasionally, patients have two different-sized alleles. This will be evident in both tumor and normal samples. Because heterozygosity is uncommon (only occurring in up to 5 % of cases), it is unlikely to be present in more than one or two microsatellites, and cases with more than this should be carefully evaluated for the possibility of specimen mislabeling or contamination of the normal DNA sample with tumor DNA. Finally, the minimum size of a shift is one base, the length of the repeating unit. Since identification of such a small shift is difficult, some clinical laboratories require a minimum of a two-base shift to score a microsatellite unstable. Fortunately, if a mononucleotide panel is being used, most MSI-H tumors will show 3–5 clearly unstable microsatellites.

Some authors have suggested that the nearly monomorphic character of certain mononucleotide repeats (i.e., nearly all alleles in the population are approximately the same length) precludes the need for a non-tumor sample for testing. Because the expected allele size is very limited, any deviation indicates instability [90]. Although rational, some circumstances can only be resolved if a non-tumor sample is tested in parallel with the tumor sample. Every tumor sample, unless obtained with laser capture microdissection, contains non-tumor cells such as fibroblasts, blood vessels, and inflammatory cells. These cells will dilute the tumor DNA and make shifted alleles more difficult to detect. Adding further difficulty is the presence of "stutter" peaks, a distribution of secondary peaks around the true size of the microsatellite. Stutter peaks occur because *Taq* polymerase used in the PCR reaction also slips on the microsatellite template, and in the absence of an in vitro MMR system, the errors are retained. When the change in microsatellite size is small, only a subtle shift may be evident on the electropherogram, largely masked by normal DNA and stutter peaks. Without a normal sample for comparison, such a shift may not be evident.

BRAF V600E and *MLH1* Methylation

Testing for the BRAF V600E mutation and hypermethylation of the *MLH1* promoter are important adjuncts to IHC and MSI testing. Because *BRAF* mutation in an MSI-H colorectal tumor is a very strong indication of a sporadic tumor, it can help rule out Lynch syndrome. The specific mutation seen in these tumors is a T-to-A transversion at position 1799, which produces an amino acid change from valine to glutamate at codon 600 (V600E). The uniformity of this mutation allows for many methods of detection, including Sanger sequencing, pyrosequencing, allele-specific PCR, and hybridization probe melting analysis. The high degree of specificity with which the BRAF V600E mutation can identify a sporadic MSI-H tumor has led the Association for Molecular Pathology to recommend testing for this mutation in all CRC [91].

Detection of *MLH1* hypermethylation, the underlying defect causing sporadic loss of MLH1, nearly always points to a sporadic tumor. Nevertheless, it is important to correlate MLH1 results with clinical and family history, since rare cases of MLH1 methylation may represent an inherited epimutation that is the underlying cause in up to 13% of MLH1-deficient but mutation-negative Lynch families [92]. Sequencing, restriction digestion, or methylation-specific PCR following bisulfite treatment of tumor DNA can be used to identify this epigenetic modification of the promoter region of the *MLH1* gene. However, this assay is more difficult to perform and interpret compared to *BRAF* testing, so is less commonly available in clinical laboratories. *MLH1* hypermethylation testing has one advantage over *BRAF* testing in that it is suitable for use in testing MSI-H endometrial tumors of the uterus, which have not been shown to have *BRAF* mutations [93–95].

Laboratory Issues

Biopsies from the colon, endometrium, or elsewhere are typically small, perhaps no more than a few millimeters in size. While in theory these small tumors may be suitable for IHC and MSI testing, this specimen type has limitations. For IHC testing, irregular staining in a tumor may result in the appearance of MMR loss in a small specimen, especially when the amount of tumor is scant. Testing of a larger resection specimen is more likely to include areas where the protein can be demonstrated with IHC. MSI testing requires a relatively pure sample of tumor for testing (usually >20 % tumor cells) and a normal sample not contaminated by tumor cells. Biopsies often have intimately intermixed tumor and non-tumor tissue in a very small physical space. Unless laser capture microdissection is used, separation of tumor and normal cells for DNA extraction may not be possible. If the tumor tissue is adequate, the limitation on the normal tissue may be overcome with the use of the patient's peripheral blood or a previous non-tumor specimen. Biopsies of precancerous colorectal adenomas often do not demonstrate MSI or MMR protein loss unless they are advanced stage (high-grade dysplasia/intramucosal carcinoma), so while adenomas of Lynch carriers may test positive, a negative result does not rule out Lynch syndrome [31, 35]. Testing of unselected young patients with adenoma does not appear to be an effective means of screening for Lynch syndrome [96].

An important decision for the clinical laboratory is the selection of testing method(s) to screen for defective MMR, as well as which cases to screen. This is likely to be driven in no small part by the technology available locally. While most pathology practices have ready access to IHC, molecular testing may be difficult to obtain. Other nonanalytical considerations include cost and turnaround time. When test performance is compared, both IHC and PCR are highly effective. MMR IHC is estimated to be 76–88 % sensitive in detection of an inherited mutation in a MMR protein, while MSI PCR is 76–90 % sensitive. The best performance is with MMR gene sequencing, which is over 99 % sensitive and specific; it is the primary test used to confirm a diagnosis of Lynch syndrome [91]. Arguments in favor of IHC and PCR have been put forth [97, 98]. Analytically, an advantage of IHC is the ability to detect MSH6 mutations that could be missed by MSI, while a disadvantage is variable/patchy staining, especially for MSH6, which may also have decreased staining following chemoradiation [83, 97, 99]. In favor of MSI is "indifference" to the underlying defect, which includes MMR proteins that cannot be tested by IHC, and a high rate of interlaboratory concordance (98 %) [98]. Decreased sensitivity of MSI to MSH6 defects has already been discussed, but this disadvantage may be of lesser importance with the current use of mononucleotide repeat panels.

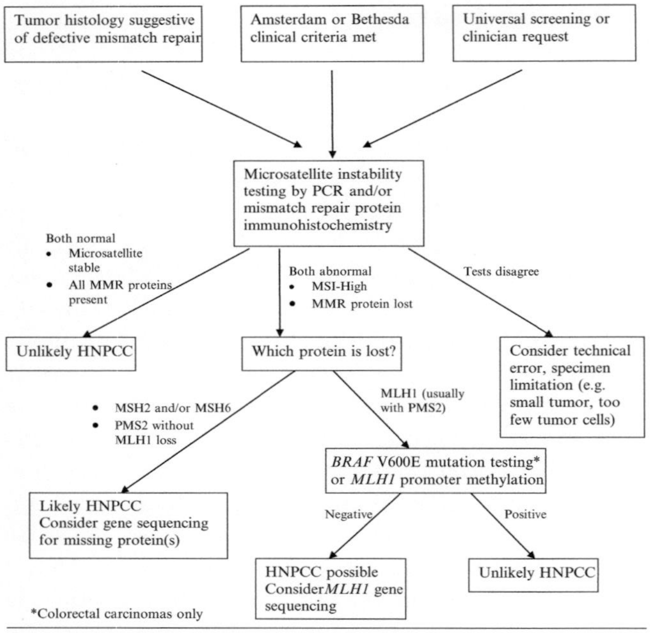

Figure 24.4 HNPCC testing algorithm

While IHC and PCR results have greater than 90 % concordance, neither test is superior in all cases [100].

Independent of analytical performance, each assay has distinct advantages. IHC results can guide MMR gene mutation testing; MSI testing can immediately be followed with *BRAF* or *MLH1* methylation testing on the same sample (if the tumor is MSI-H). The combination of IHC and PCR was shown to have 100 % sensitivity in a review of four large case series [91]. Thus, many laboratories elect to use both tests in some or all cases. A suggested testing protocol is shown in Fig. 24.4. Recent guidelines from the Association for Molecular Pathology have recommended simultaneous testing with MMR IHC, MSI PCR, and *BRAF* mutation testing [91]. Tumors which are MSS and stain positively for all four MMR proteins, which will make up the great majority of cases (approximately 75–85 %), are unlikely to represent Lynch syndrome and do not require MMR gene sequencing. MSI-H and MLH1-deficient tumors occurring in conjunction with the BRAF V600E mutation also do not require gene sequencing, unless there is other clinical, family, or historical information raising concern for Lynch syndrome. Thus, only those MSI-H tumors lacking *BRAF* mutation, or those tumors with loss of only MSH2, MSH6, or PMS2, should be considered for MMR gene sequencing, with a referral of the patient for genetic counseling prior to sequencing.

Finally, development of systems for Lynch syndrome testing requires a team approach, including pathologists, oncologists, surgeons, medical geneticists, genetic counselors, and other healthcare providers. This begins with selection of which tumors to screen. Some institutions or regulatory bodies may conclude that testing for defective MMR is similar enough to genetic testing that patient consent is required, while others may decide that only gene mutation testing requires consent. If all tumors are not screened, who should initiate testing? Pathologists may want to test tumors that show histology suggestive of MMR deficiency, and a decision should be made whether this can be ordered by the pathologist or requires discussion with the healthcare provider for the patient. Adequate genetic counseling resources are required for follow-up on patient results. Some testing algorithms may recommend genetic counseling for all patients with abnormal test results (i.e., MSI-H, MSI-L, or MMR loss). If all CRC are screened, up to 20–25 % of patients with these tumors will require the opportunity for a genetic consultation. Once these plans are in place, a reliable reporting system must be established to ensure that all testing results will be communicated to clinicians and/or genetic counselors to arrange proper patient follow-up.

References

1. Lynch HT, et al. Hereditary nonpolyposis colorectal cancer (Lynch syndromes I and II). I Clinical description of resource. Cancer. 1985;56(4):934–8.
2. Bellizzi AM, Frankel WL. Colorectal cancer due to deficiency in DNA mismatch repair function: a review. Adv Anat Pathol. 2009;16(6):405–17.
3. Boland CR. Evolution of the nomenclature for the hereditary colorectal cancer syndromes. Fam Cancer. 2005;4(3):211–8.
4. Jass JR. Hereditary non-polyposis colorectal cancer: the rise and fall of a confusing term. World J Gastroenterol. 2006;12(31):4943–50.
5. Lindor NM. Familial colorectal cancer type X: the other half of hereditary nonpolyposis colon cancer syndrome. Surg Oncol Clin N Am. 2009;18(4):637–45.
6. Lindor NM, et al. Lower cancer incidence in Amsterdam-I criteria families without mismatch repair deficiency: familial colorectal cancer type X. JAMA. 2005;293(16):1979–85.
7. Vasen HF, et al. The International Collaborative Group on HNPCC. Anticancer Res. 1994;14(4B):1661–4.
8. Vasen HF, et al. New clinical criteria for hereditary nonpolyposis colorectal cancer (HNPCC, Lynch syndrome) proposed by the International Collaborative group on HNPCC. Gastroenterology. 1999;116(6):1453–6.
9. Rodriguez-Bigas MA, et al. A National Cancer Institute workshop on hereditary nonpolyposis colorectal cancer syndrome: meeting highlights and Bethesda guidelines. J Natl Cancer Inst. 1997;89(23):1758–62.
10. Umar A, et al. Revised Bethesda Guidelines for hereditary nonpolyposis colorectal cancer (Lynch syndrome) and microsatellite instability. J Natl Cancer Inst. 2004;96(4):261–8.
11. Rodriguez-Moranta F, et al. Clinical performance of original and revised Bethesda guidelines for the identification of MSH2/MLH1 gene carriers in patients with newly diagnosed colorectal cancer: proposal of a new and simpler set of recommendations. Am J Gastroenterol. 2006;101(5):1104–11.
12. Wolf B, et al. Efficiency of the revised Bethesda guidelines (2003) for the detection of mutations in mismatch repair genes in Austrian HNPCC patients. Int J Cancer. 2006;118(6):1465–70.

13. Hampel H, et al. Feasibility of screening for Lynch syndrome among patients with colorectal cancer. J Clin Oncol. 2008; 26(35):5783–8.
14. Truta B, et al. Tumor histology helps to identify Lynch syndrome among colorectal cancer patients. Fam Cancer. 2008;7(3):267–74.
15. Jenkins MA, et al. Pathology features in Bethesda guidelines predict colorectal cancer microsatellite instability: a population-based study. Gastroenterology. 2007;133(1):48–56.
16. Alexander J, et al. Histopathological identification of colon cancer with microsatellite instability. Am J Pathol. 2001;158(2):527–35.
17. Lu KH, et al. Gynecologic cancer as a "sentinel cancer" for women with hereditary nonpolyposis colorectal cancer syndrome. Obstet Gynecol. 2005;105(3):569–74.
18. Dunlop MG, et al. Cancer risk associated with germline DNA mismatch repair gene mutations. Hum Mol Genet. 1997;6(1):105–10.
19. Jenkins MA, et al. Cancer risks for mismatch repair gene mutation carriers: a population-based early onset case-family study. Clin Gastroenterol Hepatol. 2006;4(4):489–98.
20. Aarnio M, et al. Cancer risk in mutation carriers of DNA-mismatch-repair genes. Int J Cancer. 1999;81(2):214–8.
21. Bonadona V, et al. Cancer risks associated with germline mutations in MLH1, MSH2, and MSH6 genes in Lynch syndrome. JAMA. 2011;305(22):2304–10.
22. Engel C, et al. Risks of less common cancers in proven mutation carriers with lynch syndrome. J Clin Oncol. 2012;30(35):4409–15.
23. Aaltonen LA, et al. Clues to the pathogenesis of familial colorectal cancer. Science. 1993;260(5109):812–6.
24. Ionov Y, et al. Ubiquitous somatic mutations in simple repeated sequences reveal a new mechanism for colonic carcinogenesis. Nature. 1993;363(6429):558–61.
25. Thibodeau SN, Bren G, Schaid D. Microsatellite instability in cancer of the proximal colon. Science. 1993;260(5109):816–9.
26. Kunkel TA, Erie DA. DNA mismatch repair. Annu Rev Biochem. 2005;74:681–710.
27. Strand M, et al. Destabilization of tracts of simple repetitive DNA in yeast by mutations affecting DNA mismatch repair. Nature. 1993;365(6443):274–6.
28. Fishel R, et al. The human mutator gene homolog MSH2 and its association with hereditary nonpolyposis colon cancer. Cell. 1993;75(5):1027–38.
29. Bronner CE, et al. Mutation in the DNA mismatch repair gene homologue hMLH1 is associated with hereditary non-polyposis colon cancer. Nature. 1994;368(6468):258–61.
30. Jass JR. Colorectal adenomas in surgical specimens from subjects with hereditary non-polyposis colorectal cancer. Histopathology. 1995;27(3):263–7.
31. Iino H, et al. DNA microsatellite instability and mismatch repair protein loss in adenomas presenting in hereditary non-polyposis colorectal cancer. Gut. 2000;47(1):37–42.
32. Parsons R, et al. Mismatch repair deficiency in phenotypically normal human cells. Science. 1995;268(5211):738–40.
33. Vilkki S, et al. Extensive somatic microsatellite mutations in normal human tissue. Cancer Res. 2001;61(11):4541–4.
34. Ichikawa Y, et al. Microsatellite instability and immunohistochemical analysis of MLH1 and MSH2 in normal endometrium, endometrial hyperplasia and endometrial cancer from a hereditary nonpolyposis colorectal cancer patient. Jpn J Clin Oncol. 2002;32(3):110–2.
35. Pino MS, et al. Deficient DNA mismatch repair is common in Lynch syndrome-associated colorectal adenomas. J Mol Diagn. 2009;11(3):238–47.
36. Li GM. Mechanisms and functions of DNA mismatch repair. Cell Res. 2008;18(1):85–98.
37. de la Chapelle A. Genetic predisposition to colorectal cancer. Nat Rev Cancer. 2004;4(10):769–80.
38. Verma L, et al. Mononucleotide microsatellite instability and germline MSH6 mutation analysis in early onset colorectal cancer. J Med Genet. 1999;36(9):678–82.
39. Liu B, et al. Mismatch repair gene defects in sporadic colorectal cancers with microsatellite instability. Nat Genet. 1995;9(1):48–55.
40. Peltomaki P. Role of DNA mismatch repair defects in the pathogenesis of human cancer. J Clin Oncol. 2003;21(6):1174–9.
41. Kim H, et al. Clinical and pathological characteristics of sporadic colorectal carcinomas with DNA replication errors in microsatellite sequences. Am J Pathol. 1994;145(1):148–56.
42. Young J, et al. Features of colorectal cancers with high-level microsatellite instability occurring in familial and sporadic settings: parallel pathways of tumorigenesis. Am J Pathol. 2001;159(6):2107–16.
43. Snover DC, et al. Serrated polyps of the large intestine: a morphologic and molecular review of an evolving concept. Am J Clin Pathol. 2005;124(3):380–91.
44. Thibodeau SN, et al. Altered expression of hMSH2 and hMLH1 in tumors with microsatellite instability and genetic alterations in mismatch repair genes. Cancer Res. 1996;56(21):4836–40.
45. Kane MF, et al. Methylation of the hMLH1 promoter correlates with lack of expression of hMLH1 in sporadic colon tumors and mismatch repair-defective human tumor cell lines. Cancer Res. 1997;57(5):808–11.
46. Deng G, et al. BRAF mutation is frequently present in sporadic colorectal cancer with methylated hMLH1, but not in hereditary nonpolyposis colorectal cancer. Clin Cancer Res. 2004;10(1 Pt 1): 191–5.
47. Domingo E, et al. BRAF screening as a low-cost effective strategy for simplifying HNPCC genetic testing. J Med Genet. 2004;41(9): 664–8.
48. Rajagopalan H, et al. Tumorigenesis: RAF/RAS oncogenes and mismatch-repair status. Nature. 2002;418(6901):934.
49. Mutch DG, et al. RAS/RAF mutation and defective DNA mismatch repair in endometrial cancers. Am J Obstet Gynecol. 2004;190(4):935–42.
50. Crepin M, et al. Evidence of constitutional MLH1 epimutation associated to transgenerational inheritance of cancer susceptibility. Hum Mutat. 2012;33(1):180–8.
51. Planck M, et al. Somatic frameshift alterations in mononucleotide repeat-containing genes in different tumor types from an HNPCC family with germline MSH2 mutation. Genes Chromosomes Cancer. 2000;29(1):33–9.
52. Woerner SM, et al. Microsatellite instability of selective target genes in HNPCC-associated colon adenomas. Oncogene. 2005;24(15):2525–35.
53. Dove-Edwin I, et al. Prospective results of surveillance colonoscopy in dominant familial colorectal cancer with and without Lynch syndrome. Gastroenterology. 2006;130(7):1995–2000.
54. Vasen HF, et al. One to 2-year surveillance intervals reduce risk of colorectal cancer in families with Lynch syndrome. Gastroenterology. 2010;138(7):2300–6.
55. Lindor NM, et al. Recommendations for the care of individuals with an inherited predisposition to Lynch syndrome: a systematic review. JAMA. 2006;296(12):1507–17.
56. Burn J, et al. Long-term effect of aspirin on cancer risk in carriers of hereditary colorectal cancer: an analysis from the CAPP2 randomised controlled trial. Lancet. 2011;378(9809):2081–7.
57. Yang KY, et al. A cost-effectiveness analysis of prophylactic surgery versus gynecologic surveillance for women from hereditary non-polyposis colorectal cancer (HNPCC) Families. Fam Cancer. 2011;10(3):535–43.
58. Parry S, et al. Metachronous colorectal cancer risk for mismatch repair gene mutation carriers: the advantage of more extensive colon surgery. Gut. 2011;60(7):950–7.
59. Terdiman JP. It is time to get serious about diagnosing Lynch syndrome (hereditary nonpolyposis colorectal cancer with defective

DNA mismatch repair) in the general population. Gastroenterology. 2005;129(2):741–4.
60. Hampel H. Point: justification for Lynch syndrome screening among all patients with newly diagnosed colorectal cancer. J Natl Compr Canc Netw. 2010;8(5):597–601.
61. Mvundura M, et al. The cost-effectiveness of genetic testing strategies for Lynch syndrome among newly diagnosed patients with colorectal cancer. Genet Med. 2010;12(2):93–104.
62. Ladabaum U, et al. Strategies to identify the Lynch syndrome among patients with colorectal cancer: a cost-effectiveness analysis. Ann Intern Med. 2011;155(2):69–79.
63. Benatti P, et al. Microsatellite instability and colorectal cancer prognosis. Clin Cancer Res. 2005;11(23):8332–40.
64. Lothe RA, et al. Genomic instability in colorectal cancer: relationship to clinicopathological variables and family history. Cancer Res. 1993;53(24):5849–52.
65. Barnetson RA, et al. Identification and survival of carriers of mutations in DNA mismatch-repair genes in colon cancer. N Engl J Med. 2006;354(26):2751–63.
66. Popat S, Hubner R, Houlston RS. Systematic review of microsatellite instability and colorectal cancer prognosis. J Clin Oncol. 2005;23(3):609–18.
67. Perea J, et al. Approach to early-onset colorectal cancer: clinicopathological, familial, molecular and immunohistochemical characteristics. World J Gastroenterol. 2010;16(29):3697–703.
68. Halling KC, et al. Microsatellite instability and 8p allelic imbalance in stage B2 and C colorectal cancers. J Natl Cancer Inst. 1999;91(15):1295–303.
69. Hutchins G, et al. Value of mismatch repair, KRAS, and BRAF mutations in predicting recurrence and benefits from chemotherapy in colorectal cancer. J Clin Oncol. 2011;29(10):1261–70.
70. Gray R, et al. Adjuvant chemotherapy versus observation in patients with colorectal cancer: a randomised study. Lancet. 2007;370(9604):2020–9.
71. Ribic CM, et al. Tumor microsatellite-instability status as a predictor of benefit from fluorouracil-based adjuvant chemotherapy for colon cancer. N Engl J Med. 2003;349(3):247–57.
72. Sargent DJ, et al. Defective mismatch repair as a predictive marker for lack of efficacy of fluorouracil-based adjuvant therapy in colon cancer. J Clin Oncol. 2010;28(20):3219–26.
73. Hegde MR, Roa BB. Genetic testing for hereditary nonpolyposis colorectal cancer (HNPCC). Curr Protoc Hum Genet. 2009;Chapter 10:Unit 10 12.
74. Ou J, et al. A database to support the interpretation of human mismatch repair gene variants. Hum Mutat. 2008;29(11):1337–41.
75. Peltomaki P, Vasen HF. Mutations predisposing to hereditary nonpolyposis colorectal cancer: database and results of a collaborative study. The International Collaborative Group on Hereditary Nonpolyposis Colorectal Cancer. Gastroenterology. 1997;113(4):1146–58.
76. Boland CR, et al. The biochemical basis of microsatellite instability and abnormal immunohistochemistry and clinical behavior in Lynch syndrome: from bench to bedside. Fam Cancer. 2008;7(1):41–52.
77. Mangold E, et al. Tumours from MSH2 mutation carriers show loss of MSH2 expression but many tumours from MLH1 mutation carriers exhibit weak positive MLH1 staining. J Pathol. 2005; 207(4):385–95.
78. Overbeek LI, et al. Interpretation of immunohistochemistry for mismatch repair proteins is only reliable in a specialized setting. Am J Surg Pathol. 2008;32(8):1246–51.
79. Muller A, et al. Challenges and pitfalls in HNPCC screening by microsatellite analysis and immunohistochemistry. J Mol Diagn. 2004;6(4):308–15.
80. Wahlberg SS, et al. Evaluation of microsatellite instability and immunohistochemistry for the prediction of germ-line MSH2 and MLH1 mutations in hereditary nonpolyposis colon cancer families. Cancer Res. 2002;62(12):3485–92.
81. Zighelboim I, et al. Epitope-positive truncating MLH1 mutation and loss of PMS2: implications for IHC-directed genetic testing for Lynch syndrome. Fam Cancer. 2009;8(4):501–4.
82. Shia J, et al. Immunohistochemistry as first-line screening for detecting colorectal cancer patients at risk for hereditary nonpolyposis colorectal cancer syndrome: a 2-antibody panel may be as predictive as a 4-antibody panel. Am J Surg Pathol. 2009;33(11): 1639–45.
83. Bao F, et al. Neoadjuvant therapy induces loss of MSH6 expression in colorectal carcinoma. Am J Surg Pathol. 2010;34(12):1798–804.
84. College of American Pathologists 2012 MSI-A participant summary; 2012. College of American Pathologists.
85. Bacher JW, et al. Development of a fluorescent multiplex assay for detection of MSI-High tumors. Dis Markers. 2004;20(4-5): 237–50.
86. Boland CR, et al. A National Cancer Institute Workshop on Microsatellite Instability for cancer detection and familial predisposition: development of international criteria for the determination of microsatellite instability in colorectal cancer. Cancer Res. 1998;58(22):5248–57.
87. Laiho P, et al. Low-level microsatellite instability in most colorectal carcinomas. Cancer Res. 2002;62(4):1166–70.
88. Tomlinson I, et al. Does MSI-low exist? J Pathol. 2002;197(1):6–13.
89. Murphy KM, et al. Comparison of the microsatellite instability analysis system and the Bethesda panel for the determination of microsatellite instability in colorectal cancers. J Mol Diagn. 2006;8(3):305–11.
90. Suraweera N, et al. Evaluation of tumor microsatellite instability using five quasimonomorphic mononucleotide repeats and pentaplex PCR. Gastroenterology. 2002;123(6):1804–11.
91. Funkhouser Jr WK, et al. Relevance, pathogenesis, and testing algorithm for mismatch repair-defective colorectal carcinomas: a report of the association for molecular pathology. J Mol Diagn. 2012;14(2):91–103.
92. Peltomaki P. Epigenetic mechanisms in the pathogenesis of Lynch syndrome. Clin Genet. 2014;85(5):403–12.
93. Esteller M, et al. MLH1 promoter hypermethylation is associated with the microsatellite instability phenotype in sporadic endometrial carcinomas. Oncogene. 1998;17(18):2413–7.
94. Feng YZ, et al. BRAF mutation in endometrial carcinoma and hyperplasia: correlation with KRAS and p53 mutations and mismatch repair protein expression. Clin Cancer Res. 2005; 11(17):6133–8.
95. Peterson LM, et al. Molecular characterization of endometrial cancer: a correlative study assessing microsatellite instability, MLH1 hypermethylation, DNA mismatch repair protein expression, and PTEN, PIK3CA, KRAS, and BRAF mutation analysis. Int J Gynecol Pathol. 2012;31(3):195–205.
96. Velayos FS, et al. Low rate of microsatellite instability in young patients with adenomas: reassessing the Bethesda guidelines. Am J Gastroenterol. 2005;100(5):1143–9.
97. Shia J. Immunohistochemistry versus microsatellite instability testing for screening colorectal cancer patients at risk for hereditary nonpolyposis colorectal cancer syndrome. Part I The utility of immunohistochemistry. J Mol Diagn. 2008;10(4):293–300.
98. Zhang L. Immunohistochemistry versus microsatellite instability testing for screening colorectal cancer patients at risk for hereditary nonpolyposis colorectal cancer syndrome. Part II The utility of microsatellite instability testing. J Mol Diagn. 2008;10(4):301–7.
99. Radu OM, et al. Challenging cases encountered in colorectal cancer screening for Lynch syndrome reveal novel findings: nucleolar MSH6 staining and impact of prior chemoradiation therapy. Hum Pathol. 2011;42(9):1247–58.
100. Grenert JP, et al. Concordance between Microsatellite Instability (MSI) testing and Mismatch Repair Protein Immunohistochemistry (MMR IHC) and analysis of discordant cases. Mod Pathol. 2011;24 Suppl 1:149A.

Multiple Endocrine Neoplasia Syndromes

25

Barbara A. Zehnbauer

Abstract

Multiple endocrine neoplasias (MEN) are familial cancer syndromes which feature autosomal dominant inheritance of genetic risks for a variety of endocrine gland tumors. Patients with multiple endocrine neoplasia type 1 (MEN1) have a high frequency of peptic ulcer disease and abnormalities involving the parathyroids, pancreatic islets, and anterior pituitary. Patients with MEN2 (MEN2A, MEN2B, or familial medullary thyroid carcinoma [FMTC]) exhibit a high frequency of medullary thyroid carcinoma, pheochromocytoma, parathyroid hyperplasia plus mucosal neuromas (lips and tongue), ganglioneuromas of the gastrointestinal tract, and marfanoid habitus (in MEN2B only). These tumors are typically diagnosed at an earlier age and with bilateral or multiple sites of tumor compared to the general population risk for the same tumors. Germline mutations in the *MEN1* gene and the *RET* gene are identified in nearly all families affected with these syndromes. Presymptomatic genetic testing provides early diagnosis of disease risk and facilitates clinical intervention at earlier stages of tumor development with increased likelihood of improved patient outcomes.

Keywords

Familial cancer syndrome • Autosomal dominant • MEN1 • Menin • Tumor suppressor • MEN2 • RET • Receptor tyrosine kinase • Genetic risk • Presymptomatic screening • Genotype–phenotype

Introduction

Multiple endocrine neoplasia (MEN) syndromes include several types of inherited autosomal dominant familial cancer syndromes, each characterized by a different pattern of endocrine gland tumors in affected individuals. The two major types are MEN type 1 or MEN1 (Wermer syndrome) and MEN type 2 or MEN2 (Sipple syndrome). MEN1 is characterized by a high frequency of peptic ulcer disease and primary endocrine abnormalities involving the parathyroids (90–97 % of patients), pancreatic islets (30–80 % of patients; including adenoma, prolactinoma, insulinoma, glucagonoma, gastrinoma, etc.), and anterior pituitary (15–50 % of patients) [1]. MEN2 includes subtypes MEN2A, MEN2B, and familial medullary thyroid carcinoma (FMTC, non-MEN), with the primary clinical features of medullary thyroid carcinoma (MTC; 95 % of patients), pheochromocytoma (50 % of patients with MEN2A and MEN2B but not in FMTC), parathyroid hyperplasia (15–30 % of patients with MEN2A and rarely MEN2B) plus mucosal neuromas of the lips and tongue, ganglioneuromas of the gastrointestinal tract, and marfanoid habitus (only in patients with MEN2B) [1]. The MEN2A diagnostic category characterizes approximately 60–90 % of patients with MEN2, FMTC accounts for 5–35 %, and MEN2B for about 5 % [2]. In MEN2, MTC usually presents as bilateral or multifocal neoplasia rather than the unilateral tumors in sporadic occurrences.

B.A. Zehnbauer, Ph.D., F.A.C.M.G., F.A.C.B. (✉)
Centers for Disease Control and Prevention,
1600 Clifton Road NE, MailStop G23, Atlanta, GA 30333, USA
e-mail: bzehnbauer@cdc.gov

D.G.B. Leonard (ed.), *Molecular Pathology in Clinical Practice*, DOI 10.1007/978-3-319-19674-9_25

An earlier age of onset of these tumors is also observed in these familial cancer syndromes with children as young as 5 years of age diagnosed with MTC in MEN2A rather than 50–60 years of age in the sporadic incidence of MTC. MEN2B is the most aggressive form with children less than 3 years of age diagnosed with MTC with metastases in cervical lymph nodes. FMTC is least aggressive with MTC presenting between 20 and 40 years of age.

Penetrance of both MEN1 and MEN2 is nearly complete by 60 years of age [1, 3]. While these syndromes are uncommon (1 in 10,000–100,000 for MEN1 and 1 in 25,000–30,000 for MEN2), diagnosis of these autosomal dominant disorders has important implications for other family members because first-degree relatives have a 50 % risk of inheriting the causative mutation and developing the disease. Early detection is critical for the most effective intervention with the goal of treatment prior to tumor metastasis. However, these two syndromes and their underlying molecular pathology present very different challenges for the clinical molecular laboratory as a study in contrast to allelic heterogeneity and detection sensitivity.

MEN1

Molecular Basis of Disease

The *MEN1* gene maps to human chromosome 11q13 and was cloned in 1997 [4]. *MEN1* is a tumor suppressor gene [5] that contains 10 exons (the first one is untranslated) and encodes a ubiquitously expressed 2.8 kilobase (kb) transcript. The predicted 610-amino-acid (67 kDa) protein product, termed menin, exhibits no apparent similarities to any previously known proteins or consensus protein motifs but acts as a tumor suppressor to prevent MEN1 neoplasias [6]. Menin is a nuclear protein that interacts with proteins involved in transcription and cell growth regulation, control of the cell cycle, and genomic stability. More than 1,000 different *MEN1* loss-of-function mutations (nonsense, frameshift, insertion, deletion, missense, and splicing defects) have been described and are distributed throughout the 9.8 kb of genomic DNA comprising the *MEN1* gene (Fig. 25.1) [3, 7]. At least 75 % of all reported *MEN1* mutations will produce an inactivating, truncated menin protein primarily by nonsense and frameshift mutations.

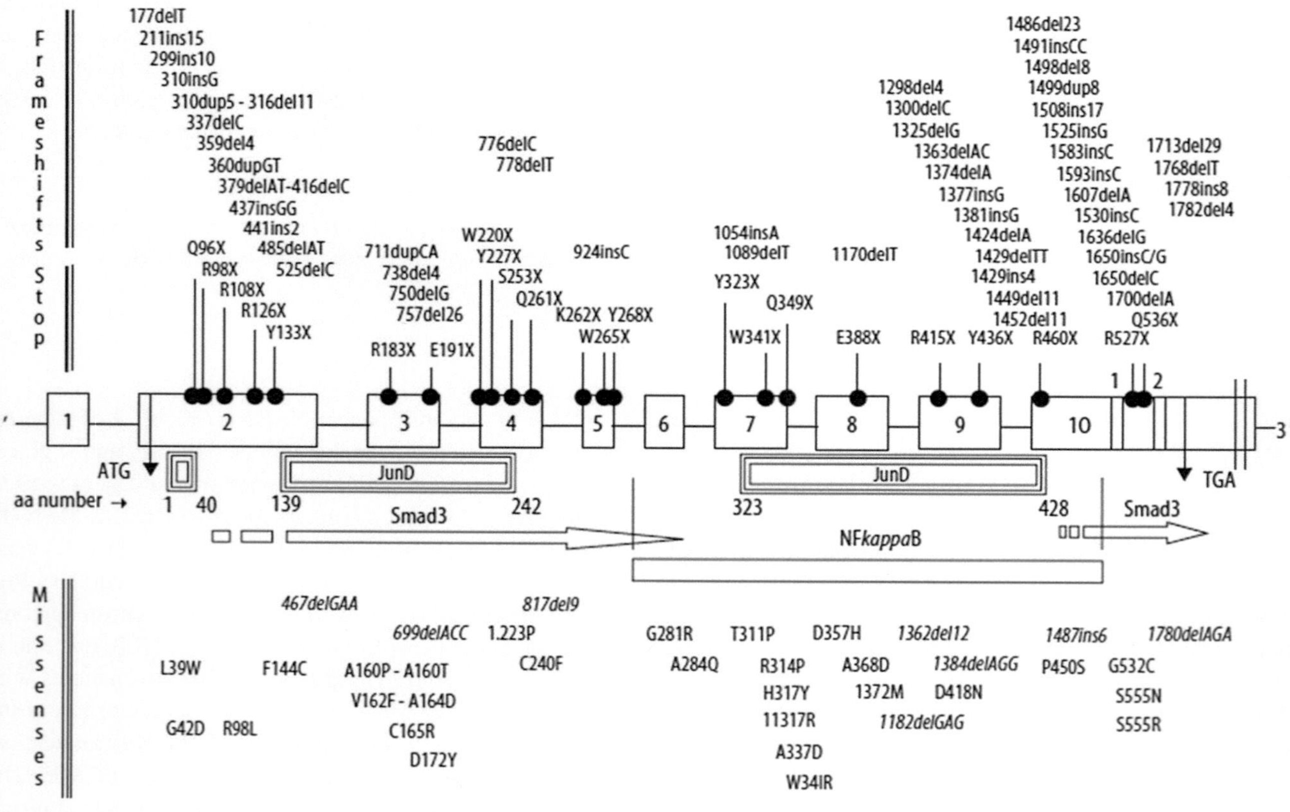

Figure 25.1 Schematic representation of the *MEN1* gene indicating the intron–exon organization, as well as the relative location, type, and distribution of germline mutations characterized in patients with MEN1. Functional domains of menin that interact with JUND, SMAD3, and NFKB are indicated below the gene map. Regions 1 and 2 within exon 10 note the locations of the nuclear localization signals 1 and 2 of the menin protein. From Wautot V, Vercherat C, Lespinasse J, et al. Germline mutation profile of MEN1 in multiple endocrine neoplasias type 1: search for correlations between phenotype and the functional domains of the MEN1 protein. Hum Mutat 2002;20:35–47, copyright © 2002 [3]. Reprinted with permission from John Wiley and Sons

Missense and in-frame genomic alterations have been described in the domains of menin that interact with *JUND*, *SMAD3*, and *NFKB1*, three major effectors in transcription and cell growth regulation pathways [8]. These and other alterations that predict a loss of menin function are consistent with a role of *MEN1* as a tumor suppressor gene [3]. In mouse models of MEN1, loss of both *MEN1* alleles in the mouse germline is lethal in the embryo but does not result in tumor formation [9]. Conditional gene knockouts targeted to pancreatic islet β-cells or parathyroid cells result in growth of insulinomas or parathyroid adenomas, respectively [10, 11]. No correlation has been observed between *MEN1* genotype and MEN1 phenotype [1, 3, 7, 12]. In approximately 20 % of MEN1 families, no mutation in the *MEN1* gene has been identified [13]. While this cancer syndrome displays an autosomal dominant pattern of inheritance of a single germline mutation, at the cellular level, *MEN1*-associated tumors are caused by inactivation of both copies of this tumor suppressor gene [13]. Extensive listing and descriptions of *MEN1* mutations are available online from the Human Gene Mutation Database Cardiff (http://www.hgmd.cf.ac.uk/ac/index.php, accessed 10/2/2014) and the Weizmann Institute of Science GeneCards (http://www.genecards.org/cgi-bin/carddisp.pl?%20gene=MEN1, accessed 10/2/2014).

Clinical Utility of Testing

Genetic testing for *MEN1* gene mutations is performed for three main reasons: (1) confirmation of a clinical diagnosis of MEN1, (2) identification of a presymptomatic at-risk relative, and (3) cessation of clinical screening in relatives who do not carry a mutation previously identified in affected family members. Approximately 50 % of patients with MEN1 will die as a result of their disease; thus, genetic screening to identify family members with germline *MEN1* mutations may lead to closer monitoring, earlier identification and treatment of tumors, improved outcomes, and longer survival. Confirmation of the diagnosis relies on identification of an *MEN1* germline mutation. Primary hyperparathyroidism is present in 100 % of patients with MEN1 by the age of 50 years [14], but parathyroid carcinomas are rarely seen. In addition, pancreatic islet cell adenomas may be observed in about 60 % of patients with MEN1 and are most commonly classified as gastrinomas or insulinomas. Pituitary adenomas also occur in approximately 30 % of MEN1 patients, but pituitary carcinomas are not usually detected. Variable expressivity and reduced penetrance also have been reported in many MEN1 families, making distinction of a familial condition difficult to discern from sporadic tumor occurrence. Absence of a detectable germline *MEN1* mutation does not exclude the diagnosis of MEN1. Genetic variability in other genes with which the menin protein interacts also may contribute to variable phenotypes of family members with the same *MEN1* allele.

Identification of carriers of *MEN1* gene mutations has not been very successful in either predicting or preventing the course of MEN1. The utility of *MEN1* mutation detection in directing individual patient care is limited by the absence of very sensitive imaging methods for early detection and treatment of MEN1-associated tumors, coupled with the lack of adequate treatment options for the types of tumors observed in MEN1 [12]. Knowledge of the carrier status is not an indicator for prophylactic surgery as in MEN2; thus, mutation screening in MEN1 patients does not avoid or cure the malignancy but may assist in clinical monitoring and lifestyle decisions. Predictive testing of at-risk relatives or prenatal screening requires that a disease-causing *MEN1* mutation has been previously detected in the family. When a family-specific mutation can be identified, the clinical significance of a subsequent negative genetic analysis in an at-risk relative can aid the genetic counselor in reassuring that family member and reducing screening to that of the general population. Targeting therapy to the menin protein has not been attempted because its function and the protein domains required for tumorigenesis have not been identified [13]. However, some small-molecule drug therapies are in development (see Conclusions and Future Directions below).

Available Assays

The mutations in the 9.8 kb genomic DNA of the *MEN1* gene that are associated with the MEN1 syndrome are diverse in both type and distribution. The initial molecular pathology screening of affected members of MEN1 families should include analysis of the entire gene. Up to 95 % of patients will have a *MEN1* mutation identified [15] when a combination of complete gene sequencing and deletion/duplication analyses is employed. Most approaches incorporate polymerase chain reaction (PCR) amplification of each exon with a survey for sequence variants by dideoxy fingerprinting [4], heteroduplex analysis (HA), single-strand conformation polymorphism (SSCP), or direct DNA sequencing [3, 12, 16]. PCR products from exons showing sequence variants by conformational changes usually are sequenced to identify the specific mutation. These strategies will identify mutations in 80–90 % of MEN1 families [17]. As in most PCR-based screening procedures, some types of mutations can be missed, including large deletions or insertions, point mutations in the 5′ regulatory or untranslated regions, nucleotide changes in the introns, or at the sites of PCR primer annealing, which may adversely affect PCR amplification efficiency. The majority of mutations are nonsense or frameshift mutations that predict expression of a truncated menin protein with loss of function [15]. Missense mutations in *MEN1* are primarily clustered in the domains that interact with the transcription factors, JUND (*MEN1* codons 1–40, 139–242, 323–428), SMAD3 (distal to *MEN1* codon 478), and NFKB (*MEN1* codons 276–479), of key cell growth pathways

(Fig. 25.1) [18]. Additional analysis using Southern hybridization [19, 20], long-range PCR, quantitative PCR, multiplex ligation-dependent probe amplification, or targeted genomic hybridization arrays will detect larger deletion and duplication mutations in MEN1 families following negative findings of direct DNA sequencing approaches. Clinical laboratories also may use next-generation sequencing methods to detect a broader range of mutations in a single test, including single-nucleotide variants, as well as small and large insertions and deletions. Thirty-seven Clinical Laboratory Improvement Amendments (CLIA)-certified clinical laboratories are listed in the Genetic Testing Registry database (www.ncbi.nlm.nih.gov/gtr/ accessed 6/25/15) as offering clinical testing for MEN1 [21]; while all of these laboratories indicate that DNA sequencing is performed, 25 also indicate that deletion and duplication analysis is included. Linkage analysis methods may be used to define familial haplotypes that confer genetic predisposition to MEN1.

Interpretation of Results

For any clinical molecular genetic test, the ability to identify a specific gene mutation to correlate with the disease status of an affected individual depends on the sensitivity of the assay. A well-defined clinical phenotype is essential for accurate interpretation and reporting of molecular test results to the healthcare professional. Genotype–phenotype correlations are either imperfect or nonexistent for MEN1.

Approximately 95 % of patients with MEN1 will have a germline mutation identified in the *MEN1* gene coding for the menin protein [15, 17]. *MEN1* germline mutations also have been identified in nearly two-thirds of patients with sporadic MEN1 [12]. There is presently no specific genotype–phenotype association of *MEN1* mutations to predict the clinical course or onset of this disease [15, 17]. More than 1,000 different mutations have been described [7], and some have been reported in multiple, independent kindreds. Characterization of these same genetic variations in newly diagnosed individuals supports the role of the mutant allele in the disease etiology and is very helpful for interpretation of the identified variant. As in many genetic syndromes, molecular identification of a pathogenic *MEN1* mutation in a family member with clinical features of MEN1 is most significant in the risk assessment of other first-degree relatives. Approximately 20 % of patients with familial isolated hyperparathyroidism, characterized by parathyroid adenoma or hyperplasia in the absence of other endocrine neoplasias, carry germline *MEN1* gene mutations [17, 22].

As reviewed by Guo and Sawicki [12], *MEN1* mutations are not limited to patients with MEN1. A significant number of sporadic endocrine tumors also may harbor *MEN1* mutations but not with the same prevalence as the same types of tumors in the syndromic cases. *MEN1* mutations do not provide clinically useful information for sporadic tumor staging [13]. While one third of MEN1 patients will develop pituitary tumors and have germline *MEN1* mutations, only about 1 % of sporadic pituitary tumors have *MEN1* mutations. The frequency of *MEN1* mutations also differs between different types of pancreatic endocrine tumors. In sporadic gastrinomas, the rate of *MEN1* mutations is 37 % in contrast to 15 % of sporadic nongastrinoma pancreatic tumors. Insulinomas, another pancreatic endocrine tumor of MEN1, develop in MEN1 knockout mice [23], but *MEN1* mutations have not been found in sporadic insulinomas [24]. Clearly the role of menin in familial and sporadic tumors is not the same. Sporadic parathyroid and pituitary adenomas with no detectable *MEN1* mutation may be characterized as phenocopies of MEN1, particularly when there is no family history of MEN1 [12].

Information about the penetrance and expressivity of the mutations in *MEN1* described to date suggests that carriers of a familial *MEN1* mutation have a 100 % risk of developing MEN1 by the age of 60 years [3]. Mutations leading to expression of a truncated menin protein create a loss of functional menin protein. Missense mutations may disrupt menin interaction with cell growth regulatory molecules or its cellular localization. These mutations also may decrease the stability of menin protein and lead to its degradation.

Laboratory Issues

Complete analysis of the *MEN1* gene sequence by PCR amplification of each exon and untranslated regions followed by direct DNA sequencing fails to identify mutations in 10–20 % of patients with MEN1. Some *MEN1* mutations have been identified repeatedly in apparently unrelated families, suggesting some tendency for mutational hot spots within *MEN1*, with mutation clusters at codons 83–84, 516, and 210–211 accounting for approximately 12 % of all mutations [7]. Caution must be used in the interpretation of the pathogenic functional consequences of DNA sequence variants. Predicting abnormal protein function from a DNA sequence change is imperfect. Approximately 24 polymorphisms of *MEN1* have been reported. For example, Arg171Gln and Ala541Thr produce amino acid substitutions featuring different polar side chains but are not associated with a disease phenotype [12]. Missense mutations in amino acids surrounding these same codons are consistent with MEN1 incidence in affected families [3]. Classification of polymorphisms as benign may change with long-term follow-up or ascertainment of additional MEN1 kindreds. Some frameshift or nonsense mutations do not completely abolish normal protein function. The existence of phenocopies (clinical presentations that may mimic familial disorders) also should be a consideration due to the relatively high frequency of sporadic parathyroid and pituitary adenomas [12], particularly in the absence of a family history of MEN1.

Genotype–phenotype prediction may be further complicated by variable expression among family members or different families with the same sequence change or by slow growth of an MEN1 tumor even after a gene mutation has been characterized. Once a sequence change has been documented as present in individuals with clinical features of MEN1 and absent in unaffected individuals, one can be reasonably certain of the significance of the finding as a true disease-associated mutation.

Approximately 70 % of reported mutations are nonsense, frameshift, or splice-site mutations that predict the expression of a truncated menin protein product. An in vitro protein truncation test (PTT) for diagnostic MEN1 screening proved to be too problematic for routine clinical laboratory implementation, given the problems inherent in (1) the instability of abnormal mRNA in peripheral blood lymphocytes of patients with MEN1 and (2) the scarcity of methionine residues for ^{35}S-methionine substitution in labeling the amino terminus polypeptides of the menin protein. Newer approaches with nonisotopic PTT [25, 26] may be more successful in applying this strategy to MEN1 mutation detection. Identification of large deletions by Southern blot or fluorescence in situ hybridization analysis may be useful for mutation screening because deletion of an entire exon or exons will result in amplification and sequencing of the remaining, normal allele and a false-negative test result, although next-generation sequencing can detect large deletions. Genetic variants in the regulatory regions of *MEN1*, including promoter mutations or methylation defects, may indicate abnormal gene expression but have not yet been documented.

For the MEN1 patients with no demonstration of germline MEN1 gene mutation, biochemical screening is an alternative course for monitoring disease. Careful biochemical screening may reveal evidence of neoplasia, including hyperparathyroidism, 10 years prior to the expression of overt clinical symptoms [20].

Formal proficiency testing programs are not available for MEN1 molecular testing. Clinical laboratories must meet the proficiency testing requirements by alternative proficiency assessment methods.

Conclusions and Future Directions

Currently, no preventive measures are available for prophylaxis or cure of MEN1-associated tumors. Radiologic imaging for identification of MEN1-associated tumors generally has low sensitivity in asymptomatic individuals. Biochemical screening for the tumor-secreted hormones may help detect early disease in asymptomatic mutation carriers [27]. Treatment usually involves surgery to remove the tumors, sparing unaffected tissue to preserve normal hormone production. Several clinical trials of drug therapies for patients with MEN1 have been launched. Various approaches focus on the modulation of the hypercalcemia and hypercalciuria of primary hyperparathyroidism by administration of the calcium-sensing receptor agonist, cinacalcet [28], or high-dose somatostatin with octreotide-LAR [29]. More extensive studies are needed to establish the efficacy of these molecules for clinical use.

MEN2

Molecular Basis of Disease

In 1993, the *RET* proto-oncogene ("*re*arranged during *t*ransfection"), located on chromosome 10q11, was cloned and characterized as encoding a transmembrane tyrosine kinase with a cysteine-rich extracellular receptor domain (Fig. 25.2) present on neuroendocrine cells of neural crest origin [30, 31]. *RET* spans 60 kb with 21 exons encoding a protein of approximately 1,100 amino acids [1]. Glial cell-derived neurotrophic factor and neurturin are two ligands for the *RET* receptor domain [32]. The ligands initiate homodimerization of *RET* protein molecules resulting in phosphorylation and activation of the tyrosine kinase domain, leading to downstream signal transduction [32]. *RET* is the only gene known to be associated with MEN2. Missense mutations in the *RET* gene were characterized in individuals with the MEN2 syndromes [30, 31, 33, 34] with a very restricted pattern of vari-

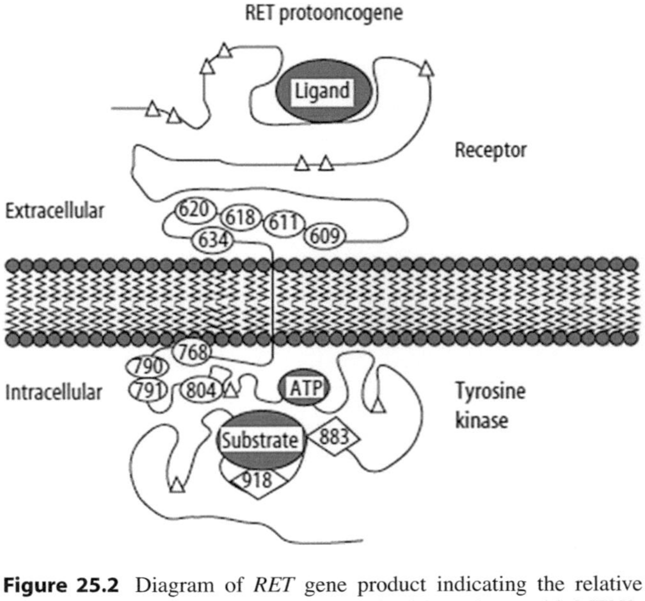

Figure 25.2 Diagram of *RET* gene product indicating the relative location of germline mutations characterized in patients with MEN2. *Ovals* are numbered to represent the codons that commonly contain germline missense mutations associated with MEN2A and FMTC. *Diamonds* are numbered to represent the codon location of germline mutations in MEN2B. *Triangles* indicate the positions of mutations in hereditary Hirschsprung disease. From Phay JE, Moley JF, Lairmore TC. Multiple endocrine neoplasias. Semin Surg Oncol 2000;18:324–32, copyright © 2000 [1]. Reprinted with permission from John Wiley and Sons

Table 25.1 Common *RET* gene mutations in MEN2 and associated clinical phenotypes

		MEN2 phenotype[b]			
***RET* location**	**Mutation[a]**	***FMTC***	***MEN2A***	***MEN2B***	**ATA risk[c]**
Exon 10	C609Y, F, G, R, or S	Y	Y	N	B
	C611Y, F, G, R, S, or W	Y	Y	N	B
	C618Y, F, G, R, or S	Y	Y	N	B
	C620Y, F, G, R, S, or W	Y	Y	N	B
Exon 11	C634R	N	Y	N	C
	C634Y, F, G, S, or W	Y	Y	N	C
Exon 13	E768D	Y	Y	N	A
Exon 14	V804M or V804L	Y	Y	N	A
	V804M+E805K	N	N	Y	D
	V804M+Y806C	N	N	Y	D
Exon 14/15	V804M+S904C	N	N	Y	D
Exon 15	A883F	N	N	Y	D
Exon 16	M918 ATG	N	N	Y	D

[a]Single letter amino acid abbreviations are indicated for each codon
[b]*Y* yes, *N* no, *FMTC* familial medullary thyroid carcinoma
[c]American Thyroid Association (ATA) medullary thyroid cancer guideline [39]

ations (Fig. 25.2). In patients with MEN2A or FMTC, nearly all the mutations in this gene are activating, gain-of-function missense mutations localized to exons 10, 11, and 13–15. Most commonly, heterozygous missense mutations are found in a cysteine-rich, extracellular domain adjacent to the transmembrane domain of the RET protein including six conserved cysteine residues in *RET* exon 10 (codons 609, 611, 618, and 620) and exon 11 (codons 630 and 634) (Table 25.1 and Fig. 25.2) [30, 31, 33]. Most of these mutations replace a cysteine with another amino acid that cannot form intramolecular disulfide bonds. The unpaired cysteine is then able to form a disulfide bond with another RET protein molecule producing constitutive dimerization and increased kinase activation of the aberrant RET protein [35, 36]. Missense mutations in codons 768 and 804, located in exons 13 and 14, respectively (Table 25.1), affect the intracellular portions of the RET protein next to the transmembrane domain (Fig. 25.2) [37, 38]. Nearly 95 % of all patients diagnosed with MEN2B have been characterized with a single missense mutation in codon 918 of *RET* exon 16, M918T, replacing a methionine residue with a threonine [33, 34]. Another 2–3 % of patients have an Ala833Phe mutation in exon 15. Both variants affect the intracellular tyrosine kinase catalytic domain (Fig. 25.2), altering substrate recognition, which leads to cellular transformation [35]. In each case, these common *RET* mutations produce a gain-of-function change for the aberrant RET protein. Online information about many other *RET* mutations is available from the Human Gene Mutation Database Cardiff (http://www.hgmd.cf.ac.uk/ac/index.php, accessed 10/2/2014), the Weizmann Institute of Science GeneCards (http://www.genecards.org/cgi-bin/carddisp.pl?gene=RET&search=RET, accessed 10/2/2014), and the ARUP Institute for Clinical and Experimental Pathology (http://www.arup.utah.edu/database/MEN2/MEN2_welcome.php, accessed 10/2/2014).

Hirschsprung disease (HSCR), an absence of enteric ganglia in the colon, also is associated with somatic or germline *RET* mutations, either in codons 609, 618, or 620, or distributed throughout other regions of the *RET* gene [40, 41]. Some families have been described in which HSCR cosegregates with either MEN2A or FMTC [42]. *RET* mutations in patients with HSCR may produce either loss or gain of RET protein function and include frameshift and nonsense mutations. Papillary thyroid carcinoma is associated with somatic gene rearrangements of the *RET* gene [43].

Clinical Utility of Testing

In an autosomal dominant inherited disorder, an individual with a single *RET* allele mutation has (1) a high likelihood of developing MTC (approximately 95 % of carriers) and (2) a 50 % risk of transmitting this risk allele and the high likelihood of developing MTC to each offspring. Genetic testing for *RET* mutations is the accepted best practice for confirmation of the diagnosis of MEN2, predictive risk-assessment testing for family members, and prenatal diagnosis of MEN2. Approximately 25 % of all MTC occurs as part of MEN2. Early detection of a pathogenic *RET* mutation improves the prognosis for presymptomatic individuals by offering an opportunity for therapeutic intervention prior to advanced disease, metastasis, or both [44–46]. Reduced morbidity and mortality is achieved by increased clinical monitoring, prophylactic thyroidectomy (followed by thyroid hormone replacement therapy plus autotransplantation of the parathyroids), or both [1, 47]. This can be a very effective treatment to prevent disease metastasis. Resected thyroid tissue from children and adults with positive genetic findings demonstrates C cell hyperplasia or microscopic foci of malignancy in the absence of biochemical screening abnormalities or clinical symptoms [46]. Thus, genetic testing for *RET* mutations is a more sensitive and specific screening tool than either physiological testing or histopathologic examination of the thyroid for assessing familial cancer risk for MEN2 in these families [44–46].

The clinical significance of identifying a *RET* mutation is considerable, given that there is virtually 100 % penetrance of these mutations for MTC. But genetic findings alone cannot predict the age of disease onset; thus, continued surveillance for residual or recurrent MTC plus adrenal tumors is included in the follow-up care of MEN2 patients and asymptomatic carriers. About 50 % of MEN2 patients (both subtypes A and B) will develop pheochromocytoma, while 20–30 % of MEN2A patients develop parathyroid hyperplasia [1]. Patients with FMTC typically develop only MTC and none of the other clinical manifestations of MEN2A or MEN2B. Each subtype appears to be consistent within a family. Any RET mutation in codon 634 in exon 11 results in a higher incidence of pheochromocytomas and hyperparathyroidism. In particular, the C634R (Cys to Arg) mutation has been associated with a higher incidence of metastases at diagnosis; the allele is virtually absent in patients with FMTC [48]. Families with both MEN2A or FMTC and HRSC most frequently have germline *RET* mutations in codons 609, 618, or 620 in exon 10 [49]. Individuals within the same family who carry the same RET mutation may still display a variable phenotype indicating that additional modifier gene functions or environmental or epigenetic factors affect the expression of altered RET protein function and tumorigenesis. Concomitant mutations in genes coding for RET ligands or coreceptors are the most likely modifier molecules.

Genetic screening and mutation identification are currently recommended by 5 years of age for children who are at risk in MEN2A families. Children should be screened at birth if MEN2B has been diagnosed in close relatives, due to the earlier age of onset and aggressive clinical course of the MEN2B type [44, 45]. Patients with MEN2B should be treated as soon as the diagnosis is made. Some of the other advantages of DNA testing in MEN2 are that the test is relatively noninvasive and low risk, it is usually better tolerated by the patient than biochemical screening by metabolic challenge [47], genotype results are not subject to physiologic status, and serial genotype testing is not necessary. Individuals in MEN2 families who are not carriers of the familial *RET* mutation have the lower, general population risk for sporadic incidence of these endocrine neoplasias and do not require the same frequent monitoring for abnormal thyroid or adrenal function in the absence of clinical symptoms.

Several tyrosine kinase inhibitors that inhibit the activated (mutant) RET are being tested in clinical trials for treatment of MEN2 neoplasms (see Conclusions and Future Directions).

Available Assays

Screening for *RET* proto-oncogene mutations to confirm MEN2 diagnosis or to determine predisposition for MEN2 in asymptomatic relatives may be accomplished with a focused survey of a few exons of the *RET* gene. The majority of pathogenic mutations have been characterized in exons 10, 11, 13, 14, 15, and 16, including codons 609, 611, 618, 620, 634, 768, 804, 883, and 918, with few exceptions [48, 49]. In addition, all mutations of these *RET* codons associated with MEN2 are missense substitutions [30, 31, 33, 34, 37, 38]. Direct DNA sequencing of these exons or the entire *RET* coding sequence is the most commonly used strategy for detecting mutations in patients with MTC with no prior family history of MEN2. A targeted sequencing approach limited to exon 16 or specific codons also is used to screen or confirm a diagnosis of MEN2B or 2A in an at-risk family member when a familial mutation has been previously identified in an affected family member. These methods usually confer a 95–98 % frequency of *RET* mutation detection in patients with MEN2. Currently, the Genetic Testing Registry database (www.ncbi.nlm.nih.gov/gtr/, accessed 6/25/2015) lists 76 CLIA-certified clinical laboratories which offer genetic testing for MEN2. Fifty-six of these laboratories indicate that sequencing of all *RET* coding regions is available, while 21 offer this assay for selected exons or targeted variants (some laboratories offer both types of testing).

The *RET* cysteine codons are not mutated with equal frequency, with the majority of patients with MEN2A having alterations of codon C634 (Fig. 25.3). Nearly every base position of these TGC cysteine codons has been a point of allelic variation, generating more than 20 distinct alleles; thus, mutation detection methods must be designed with the capability to interrogate each nucleotide position of the cysteine codons. In clinical molecular laboratory practice, the preferred approach is to first characterize the causative (pathogenic) mutation in an affected individual using a comprehensive PCR plus direct DNA sequencing or next-generation sequencing approach either of the commonly

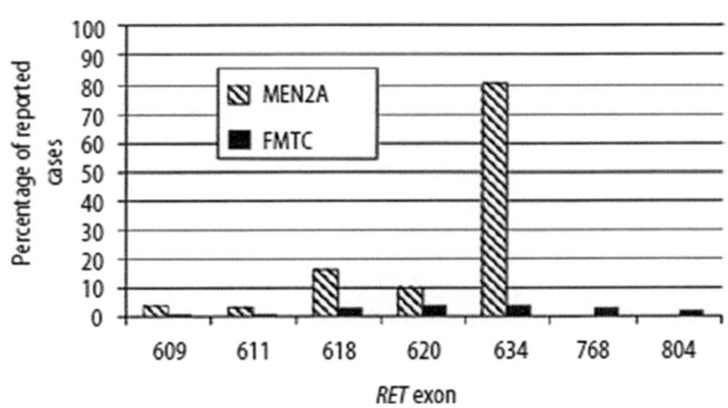

Figure 25.3 Distribution of *RET* mutations in MEN2A and FMTC. Summarized from the literature. Codon 634 in exon 11 represents a mutation hot spot for MEN2A

altered exons (Table 25.1) or of the entire *RET* gene. With decreasing costs and analytical improvements in DNA sequencing chemistry and data analysis, this has become the preferred method for comprehensive and direct *RET* mutation identification [50]. Nonsense and frameshift mutations in *RET* have not been observed in MEN2, and small, in-frame deletions or insertions are rarely identified [51].

Other physical detection methods for rapid discovery of DNA sequence variations such as denaturing gradient gel electrophoresis (DGGE) [52], SSCP [51, 53, 54], HA [55], and denaturing high-performance liquid chromatography (DHPLC) [55] have been used extensively in research studies but are less specific than direct DNA sequencing in the clinical laboratory. The utility of these indirect approaches for initial localization of a single-nucleotide sequence variation remains as a valuable diagnostic screening tool with some well-recognized analytical limitations. The high GC content of some *RET* sequences can confound physical detection methods by reducing the sensitivity of resolution between homoduplex and heteroduplex DNA molecules. Confirmation by direct DNA sequencing identifies both the exact position and nature of the base change localized by conformational screening methods. One major advantage of many of these conformational techniques is that they are frequently performed with automated instrumentation. Most of these methods identify a single-nucleotide sequence change by the altered mobility caused by the DNA conformational change using electrophoretic or melting profile shift analysis in comparison to the wild-type nucleotide sequence for the same DNA fragment. Sensitivity in the detection of the mobility shift is optimal in fragments of 200–400 base pairs (bp) for these approaches and may include 50–600 bp targets or up to 1.5 kb with DHPLC. Determination of the exact position of the base change within these fragments (e.g., TGC to TAC or TGC to GGC) can sometimes be deduced by comparison with an extensive panel of controls of defined mutant alleles previously confirmed by DNA sequencing [52, 55].

Increasingly, mutation scanning approaches have been replaced by high-resolution melting (HRM) analysis as a rapid, cost-effective method to analyze PCR amplicons and avoid contamination during post-amplification analyses [56]. In addition to PCR amplification primers, HRM requires oligonucleotide hybridization probes with sequences specific for each variant nucleotide. HRM analysis detects the mutant allele nucleotide substitution by using specific oligonucleotide probe sequences to distinguish normal and mutant sequences by virtue of their different melting temperatures conferred by the nucleotide substitution. The probes may be fluorescently labeled or unlabeled with fluorescent dye detection of the hybridization duplexes. *RET* missense mutations are more challenging to distinguish with these probes because several positions in the same codon may be variable and unique mutations may have similar or identical melting temperatures. Margraf and colleagues addressed this complexity by designing a two-stage *RET* genotyping assay in which mutation-specific probes for unambiguous genotyping of more than 50 *RET* sequence variations were simplified by the use of a masking technique [57].

Following the identification of the specific pathogenic mutation in an affected relative, other family members may be tested for just this allele with a more targeted, follow-up test of a single codon within one exon of *RET*. The molecular methodology may not be limited to direct DNA sequencing [47]. For example, many missense mutations identified in the comprehensive screening also may be directly detected by PCR–restriction fragment length polymorphism (RFLP) using a variety of enzymes [47], DGGE, DHPLC, SSCP, HA, or single-nucleotide polymorphism (SNP) testing methods [58]. Site-specific, single-base extension assays, such as those used for single-nucleotide polymorphism detection, have been described [58] for detection of many of the *RET* mutations. Linkage analysis is feasible [59] when direct mutation analysis fails to identify one of the common mutations in a family with a clear pattern of heritable disease.

Interpretation of Results

At least 95 % of patients with MEN2 will have one of a limited number of well-characterized mutations in the *RET* gene leading to a gain of function and activation of RET tyrosine kinase activity. Some genotype–phenotype specificity has been determined for the separate MEN2 subtypes, as summarized in Table 25.1 and Refs. 60 and 61. Significant overlap of clinical symptoms and missense variations occurs for any of six conserved cysteine codons (609, 611, 618, 620, 630, 634) which may be diagnostic for either MEN2A (95 %) or FMTC (80 %) (Fig. 25.3). Mutations at codon 634 account for about 85 % of kindreds with MEN2A and are the most common *RET* mutations associated with expression of hyperparathyroidism and pheochromocytomas. Mutations at codons 768, 804, and 891 in exons 13, 14, and 15, respectively, were initially described as consistent with the diagnosis of FMTC [37]; however, these variants also occur in rare families with MEN2A [60, 61]. In addition, some double heterozygous combinations of point mutations in addition to V804M are diagnostic for rare cases of MEN2B. The substitution of methionine at codon 918 with threonine, M918T, is diagnostic for MEN2B and is observed in 95–98 % of MEN2B patients. The substitution of alanine by phenylalanine at codon 883 of exon 15 (A883F) also is diagnostic for MEN2B. About half of the patients with MEN2B have de novo *RET* mutations and thus lack a family history for this syndrome. Somatic mutations at codon 918 have been frequently observed in patients who do not have a family history of MTC. The sensitivity of *RET* mutation screening requires concise clinical description of the patient's phenotype. The specificity of *RET* mutation detection for these disorders, MEN2A, FMTC, and MEN2B, is nearly 100 % [62].

The American Thyroid Association (ATA) Guidelines Task Force has completed evidence-based recommendations for clinical management of patients with MTC to establish current, rational, and optimal medical practice [39] (Table 25.1). Several of the recommendations specifically address the role of *RET* mutation testing in MEN2 syndromes. A key feature of the guidelines is the assignment of levels of risk (D through A) for development of aggressive MTC [39]. The highest risk, level D, is defined for *RET* mutations associated with MEN2B, i.e., M918T and A883F; a high risk, C, is assigned to C634R and other codon 634 missense mutations; a less high risk, B, applies to all exon 10 substitutions in the commonly mutated cysteine codons (609, 611, 618, 620); and the least high risk applies to all other point mutations and rare insertions and duplications in exons 5, 8, 10, 11, 13, 14, 15, and 16. Two variant alleles that had been thought to be pathogenic, S649L and Y791F, have now been reclassified as polymorphisms rather than disease-associated alleles. The ATA Guidelines further recommend that the ages for *RET* testing should be at diagnosis or <1 year of age for level D risk and <3–5 years of age for risk levels C through A. Patients as young as 5 years of age with M918T germline mutations have been diagnosed with MTC and distant metastases, conferring a greatly diminished likelihood of a surgical cure [63], and thus, the need for the earliest possible diagnosis with *RET* screening.

Interpretation should be conducted within the context of family history and the clinical presentation of the types of endocrine tumors in an affected family member, when available. Specific classification of a patient's MEN2 subtype is essential for the most accurate prognosis and effective clinical management. Distinguishing FMTC or MEN2A may be difficult in small kindreds, with limited or relatively young affected family members, or when scant family medical history is documented, because pheochromocytomas or parathyroid hyperplasia may primarily manifest in older relatives.

FMTC is considered as a reduced penetrance, phenotypic variant of MEN2A rather than a distinctly separate syndrome in the ATA recommendations [39]. Identical point mutations have been observed in families with only FMTC and in those with MEN2A as well as in kindreds that have MEN2A plus HSCR. Thus, the genotype–phenotype associations of MEN2 demonstrate variable expressivity and are not solely defined by *RET* mutations alone. Within particular kindreds, the clinical presentation is fairly consistent, considering the variable expression of tumor types in MEN2A. As a membrane tyrosine kinase molecule, the RET protein interacts with several coreceptor molecules and ligands including GDNF, neurturin, persephin, and artemin [64]. Base substitutions at the key conserved cysteine codons create amino acid substitutions which affect intermolecular associations, disrupt normal signaling, and change the activity or specificity of the kinase, or both [35]. It is hoped that clearer elucidation of concomitant variations in these other "modifier" genes will aid in the definition of more precise genotype–phenotype effects.

MEN2 syndromes account for approximately 25–30 % of MTC cases, based on epidemiological studies of new index cases. The remainder of MTC cases are sporadic, unilateral, or manifest in older adults with negative genetic findings of germline *RET* mutations. A significant proportion of the sporadic tumors (30–67 %) have somatic M918T mutations of *RET* in the absence of a constitutive germline mutation in leukocyte DNA of the same patient [65, 66]. Sporadic MTC also may feature a much more diverse type and distribution of *RET* mutations than MEN2A and FMTC. Disease-causing germline *RET* mutations also have been reported in 1–24 % of individuals with apparent sporadic MTC in the absence of previous family history of MEN2 but may be attributed to incomplete penetrance of some genetic variations [67]. Somatic *RET* mutations have not been detected in sporadic pheochromocytoma [66], but this tumor may also occur in von Hippel–Lindau (VHL) disease and neurofibromatosis type 1 (NF1). Neumann and colleagues showed the utility of additional mutation screening of the *VHL* gene associated with VHL disease in individuals with pheochromocytoma, but no other MEN2 symptoms and no identifiable *RET* gene mutation [68]. Screening for mutations in *VHL* and *NF1* genes should be considered in familial cases of pheochromocytoma with no detectable germline mutation in *RET*. HSCR is generally characterized by a broader spectrum of mutations distributed throughout the *RET* gene than those typical of MEN2, in both the familial and sporadic HSCR presentations [41, 42]. The rare occurrence of MEN2 family with no identifiable *RET* mutation may be tested by linkage analysis to identify the disease-associated haplotype if the disease is truly associated with an unidentified *RET* mutation, or perhaps a clinical misdiagnosis if the disease is caused by mutation of another gene. Many polymorphic markers are tightly linked to the *RET* gene, assuring high accuracy for linkage analysis.

Laboratory Issues

Overall, germline DNA sequencing for *RET* mutations is favored in clinical molecular laboratories because the mutations are localized, with limited regions to sequence and a low false-negative rate (approximately 5 %). Some of the limitations of *RET* genetic testing approaches can be attributed to the inherent technical aspects of PCR, DNA sequencing, restriction endonuclease digestion, fragment comigration, and nonpathogenic sequence changes. PCR primer and target fragment design are critical for sensitive detection of mutations by DNA conformation methods. DNA fragment size and base composition directly influence the melting profile of the PCR product and alter the optimal analytic conditions for heteroduplex and homoduplex separation (temperature, buffer concentrations, resolution). Conformational changes or mobility shifts in mutation screening methods should be confirmed with targeted direct DNA sequencing of the same fragment. DNA sequence polymorphisms within the PCR product at positions other than the ones being scored for pathogenic changes can alter the fragment mobility, prompting false-positive results. For example, a frequent silent polymorphism at *RET* codon 769 of exon 13 changes one leucine codon, CTT, to another leucine codon, CTG. This may produce altered mobility of the fragment, which could be attributed to a change at the adjacent codon 768, consistent with FMTC. Careful comparison with both wild-type and previously characterized mutant alleles as positive controls may assist with the appropriate interpretation of these variations, as it will direct DNA sequence confirmation of the same template.

When reviewing DNA sequence electropherograms from automated instruments, both the base sequence indicated by the software and the nucleotide-specific peaks or signals in the trace must be critically examined, because true heterozygous base positions, such as the common cysteine codon substitutions in exons 10 and 11 of *RET*, may be difficult to discern. The peaks should overlap with signals of nearly equal intensity, a condition that may be adversely affected by flanking sequence composition. For example, short repeats of G or C nucleotides may display decreasing peak heights for the more distal residues, thereby quenching adjacent signal intensity. Sequencing of both strands of the amplified DNA fragment should confirm the heterozygous base detection and is the standard approach in many clinical laboratories using sequencing technology for clinical molecular testing. The DNA oligonucleotide primers used for direct cycle sequencing reactions may be the same or nested within the PCR fragment but should be positioned 20–40 bases from the codons being scored in the mutation screening to optimize clear sequence interpretation. Some fluorescent dye chemistries used in automated DNA sequence techniques yield high background signals (particularly of thymidine nucleotides) resulting from incomplete removal of unincorporated dye terminator reagents prior to electrophoresis.

A few pitfalls specific to *RET* mutation screening have been encountered. We observed preferential (or biased) PCR amplification resulting from specific DNA sequence polymorphisms in primer binding regions. The polymorphisms caused poor primer annealing and failed amplification of the allele sequences adjacent to the polymorphism. We observed this variable performance with some *RET* PCR primer sequences for exon 11 in clinical genetic testing for direct detection of mutations in codon 634. Both affected and at-risk family members were screened by PCR–RFLP for the C634Y mutation (TGC>TAC) in codon 634 in *RET* exon 11 using the *Rsa*I enzyme. One individual had a DNA fragment pattern consistent with two copies of the mutant allele and no wild-type allele, which was unlikely in this autosomal dominant disorder. The patient's disease presentation and course were not dissimilar (neither more severe, nor more extensive, nor at an earlier age) from other affected relatives who were heterozygous for the same allele. Direct DNA sequencing of the PCR product did not resolve the problem. We next selected PCR primers that flanked the same region of exon 11 but did not overlap the original primer binding sites. These primers amplified both the mutant and wild-type alleles to demonstrate that the individual was heterozygous, and both PCR–RFLP and DNA sequencing detected both alleles with the new PCR primers. A downstream DNA polymorphism (codon 691) was identified in a cis configuration with the wild-type allele at codon 634. The original primer that overlapped this polymorphic region annealed poorly and did not amplify the adjacent wild-type C634 allele, resulting in efficient amplification of only the C634Y allele and a false homozygous mutant pattern (Fig. 25.4). Another solution to restore the amplification of both alleles was to lower the annealing temperature slightly for the first primer pair, thus allowing the mismatch and facilitating the efficient PCR amplification of both alleles. Consequently, our standard procedure for *RET*

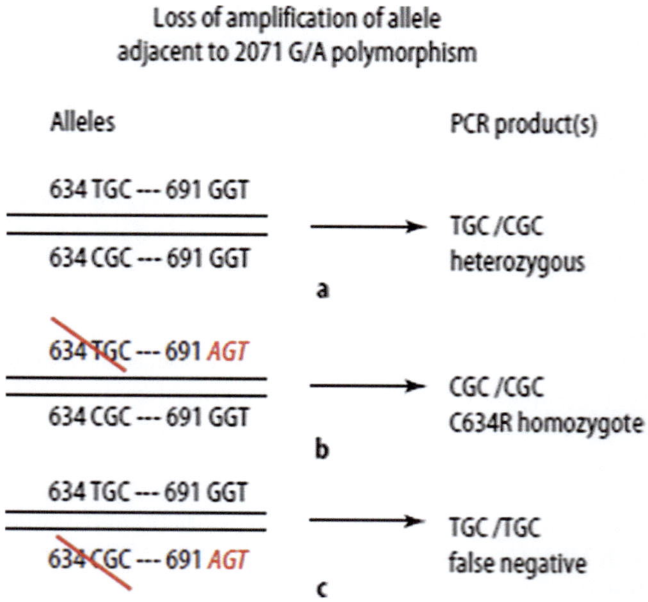

Figure 25.4 Schematic representation of the basis of unequal amplification of codon 634 in *RET*. When the GGT sequence is present at codon 691, complete homology with the PCR primer results in efficient amplification of the upstream, adjacent 634 codon on both alleles (**a**). When AGT is present at codon 691 on one *RET* allele, the match with the PCR primer is imperfect resulting in poor or absent amplification of the codon 634 region. The heterozygous condition, produces preferential amplification of only the 634 allele adjacent to the GGT 691 codon, producing either a false-positive (**b**; homozygous mutant, e.g., C634R) or a false-negative (**c**; wild type) genotype depending on whether the AGT variant is positioned in *trans* (**b**) or *cis* (**c**) configuration relative to the mutant C634 allele. Only the 634 alleles (mutant or wild type) linked to GGT at codon 691 are amplified efficiently

screening employs two independent sets of PCR primers to amplify each exon, followed by enzymatic digestion of each product or DNA sequencing of both strands of the PCR products. Findings from both PCR products must be concordant before a test interpretation is reported. In our standard quality control practice, positive (same mutant allele) and negative (no mutation) DNA controls are analyzed in parallel every time the assay is performed. A PCR with no added nucleic acid is also included in each test run and must be free of amplified DNA fragments, indicative of contamination, in all reported assays. In some reactions, small primer-dimer products (<30 bp) may appear, but are distinct from diagnostic DNA patterns.

The clustering of these common mutations in a limited region of the *RET* proto-oncogene allows the use of pyrosequencing technology as an alternative DNA-based diagnostic method of screening [69]. Reports of novel *RET* DNA alterations affecting noncysteine codons within exons 10 and 11 [50] require extended family studies to determine the clinical significance and the *RET* activation status of these variants.

Conclusions and Future Directions

Genetic testing for *RET* mutations can direct clinical care decisions to prevent and cure MEN2-associated cancers. Mortality from MTC and pheochromocytoma has been significantly reduced with earlier identification, prophylactic surgical thyroidectomy, or improved pharmacological therapy. Many clinical trials are currently testing small-molecule tyrosine kinase inhibitors (TKIs) for ability to target the RET protein or disrupt the RET signaling pathways as therapy for MTC, both sporadic cases and those associated with MEN2. The TKIs are not specific for RET, because most were developed to target other oncogenic proteins (such as EGFR, PDGFR, KIT, BRAF, and cMET), but several have activity against the RET kinase and tumor growth [36]. Trials of imatinib, vandetanib, motesanib, sorafenib, sunitinib, and XL-184 have overall produced modest or minimal partial responses (2–33 % of patients enrolled) for hereditary and sporadic MTC. Responses did not correlate with codon 618, 620, 634, or 918 mutations in *RET*. Somatic *RET* mutations were present in 70–80 % of the sporadic MTC tumors, primarily at codon 918 [36]. Comparisons across these trials are imperfect due to many differences in the activity of each TKI against RET, the extent of MTC tumor progression and aggressiveness, and the tolerated dose profiles for each TKI within various clinical disease groups. Development of RET-specific targeted therapies is an area for future work perhaps coupled with many approaches for the components of the RAS/RAF/MTE/MAPK or PI3K/AKT/mTOR intracellular pathways of signal transduction regulating proliferation and angiogenesis. Drug resistance to TKIs will probably challenge the efficacy of anti-RET therapies as has been observed with the treatment of other cancers with TKIs.

References

1. Phay JE, Moley JF, Lairmore TC. Multiple endocrine neoplasias. Semin Surg Oncol. 2000;18:324–32.
2. Eng C. Seminars in medicine of the Beth Israel Hospital, Boston. The RET proto-oncogene in multiple endocrine neoplasia type 2 and Hirschsprung's disease. N Engl J Med. 1996;335:943–51.
3. Wautot V, Vercherat C, Lespinasse J, et al. Germline mutation profile of MEN1 in multiple endocrine neoplasias type 1: search for correlations between phenotype and the functional domains of the MEN1 protein. Hum Mutat. 2002;20:35–47.
4. Chandrasekharappa SC, Guru SC, Manickam P, et al. Positional cloning of the gene for multiple endocrine neoplasia-type 1. Science. 1997;276:404–7.
5. Gagel RF, Marx SJ. Multiple endocrine neoplasias. In: Larsen PR, Kronenberg H, Melmed S, Polonsky K, editors. Williams textbook of endocrinology. 10th ed. Orlando, FL: WB Saunders; 2002. p. 17171762.
6. Thakker RV. Multiple endocrine neoplasia type 1(MEN1). Best Pract Res Clin Endocrinol Metab. 2010;24:355–70.
7. Lemos MC, Thakker RV. Multiple endocrine neoplasia type 1 (MEN1): analysis of 1336 mutations reported in the first decade following identification of the gene. Hum Mutat. 2008;29: 22–32.
8. Agarwal SK, Guru SC, Heppner C, et al. Menin interacts with the AP1 transcription factor JunD and represses JunD-activated transcription. Cell. 1999;96:143–52.
9. Bertolino P, Radovanovic I, Casse H, et al. Genetic ablation of the tumor suppressor menin causes lethality at mid-gestation with defects in multiple organs. Mech Dev. 2003;120:549–60.
10. Crabtree JS, Scacheri PC, Ward JM, et al. Of mice and MEN1: insulinomas in a conditional mouse knockout. Mol Cell Biol. 2003;23:6075–85.
11. Libutti SK, Crabtree JS, Lorang D, et al. Parathyroid gland-specific deletion of the mouse Men1 gene results in parathyroid neoplasia and hypercalcemic hyperparathyroidism. Cancer Res. 2003;63:8022–8.
12. Guo SS, Sawicki MP. Molecular and genetic mechanisms of tumorigenesis in multiple endocrine neoplasia type 1. Mol Endocrinol. 2001;15:1653–64.
13. Marx SJ. Molecular genetics of multiple endocrine neoplasia types 1 and 2. Nat Rev Cancer. 2005;5:367–75.
14. Agarwal SK, Lee Burns A, Sukhodets KE, Kennedy PA, et al. Molecular pathology of the MEN1 gene. Ann N Y Acad Sci. 2004;1014:189–98.
15. Chandrasekharappa SC, The BT. Functional studies of the MEN1 gene. J Intern Med. 2003;253:606–15.
16. Mutch MG, Dilley WG, Sanjurjo F, et al. Germline mutations in the multiple endocrine neoplasias type 1 gene: evidence for frequent splicing defects. Hum Mutat. 1999;13:175–85.
17. Fachetti A, Marini F, Brandi ML. Multiple endocrine neoplasia type 1. In: GeneReviews at GeneTests: Medical genetics information resource (database online). Copyright, University of Washington, Seattle. 1997–2011. Available at http://www.genetests.org. Accessed 12/2/2011.
18. Agarwal SK, Kester MB, Debelenko LV, et al. Germline mutations in the MEN1 gene in familial multiple endocrine neoplasias type 1 and related states. Hum Mol Genet. 1997;6:1169–75.
19. Kishi M, Tsukada T, Shimizu S, et al. A large germline deletion of the MEN1 gene in a family with multiple endocrine neoplasia type 1. Jpn J Cancer Res. 1998;89:1–5.
20. Lairmore TC, Piersall LD, DeBenedetti MK, et al. Clinical genetic testing and early surgical intervention in patients with multiple endocrine neoplasias type1 (MEN1). Ann Surg. 2004;239:637–47.
21. GeneTests: Medical Genetics Information Resource (database online). University of Washington, Seattle. 1993–2011. Available at http://www.genetests.org. Accessed 12/2/2011.

22. Hannan FM, Nesbit MA, Christie PT, Fratter C, Dudley NE, Sadler GP, Thakker RV. Familial isolated primary hyperparathyroidism caused by mutations of the MEN1 gene. Nat Clin Pract Endocrinol Metab. 2008;4:53–8.
23. Crabtree JS, Scacheri PC, Ward JM, et al. A mouse model of multiple endocrine neoplasia, type 1, develops multiple endocrine tumors. Proc Natl Acad Sci U S A. 2001;98:1118–23.
24. Cupisti K, Hoppner W, Dotzenrath C, et al. Lack of MEN1 gene mutations in 27 sporadic insulinomas. Eur J Clin Invest. 2000;30:325–9.
25. Gite S, Lim M, Carlson R, et al. A high-throughput non-isotopic protein truncation test. Nat Biotechnol. 2003;21:194–7.
26. Traverso G, Shuber A, Levin B, et al. Detection of APC mutations in fecal DNA from patients with colorectal tumors. N Engl J Med. 2002;346:311–20.
27. Marsh DJ, Gimm O. Multiple endocrine neoplasia: types 1 and 2. Adv Otorhinolaryngol. 2011;70:84–90.
28. Falchetti A, Cilotti A, Vaggelli L, Masi L, Amedei A, Cioppi F, Tonelli F, Brandi ML. A patient with MEN1-associated hyperparathyroidism, responsive to cinacalcet. Nat Clin Pract Endocrinol Metab. 2008;4:351–7.
29. Faggiano A, Tavares LB, Tauchmanova L, Milone F, Mansueto G, Ramundo V, DeCaro ML, Lombardi F, DeRosa G, Colao A. Effect of treatment with depot somatostatin analogue octreotide on primary hyperparathyroidism (PHP) in multiple endocrine neoplasia type 1 (MEN1) patients. Clin Endocrinol. 2008;69:756–62.
30. Mulligan LM, Kwok JB, Healey CS, et al. Germ-line mutations of the RET proto-oncogene in multiple endocrine neoplasias type 2A. Nature. 1993;363:458–60.
31. Donis-Keller H, Dou S, Chi D, et al. Mutations in the RET protooncogene are associated with MEN2A and FMTC. Hum Mol Genet. 1993;2:851–6.
32. Pichel JG, Shen L, Sheng HZ, et al. Defects in enteric innervation and kidney development in mice lacking GDNF. Nature. 1996;382:73–6.
33. Hofstra RM, Landsvater RM, Ceccherini I, et al. A mutation in the RET proto-oncogene associated with multiple endocrine neoplasias type 2B and sporadic medullary thyroid carcinoma. Nature. 1994;367:375–6.
34. Carlson KM, Dou S, Chi D, et al. Single missense mutation in the tyrosine kinase catalytic domain of the RET proto-oncogene associated with multiple endocrine neoplasia type 2B. Proc Natl Acad Sci U S A. 1994;91:1579–83.
35. Santoro M, Carlomagno F, Romano A, et al. Activation of RET as a dominantly transforming gene by germline mutations of MEN2A and MEN2B. Science. 1995;267:381–3.
36. Phay JE, Shah MH. Targeting RET receptor tyrosine kinase activation in cancer. Clin Cancer Res. 2010;16:5936–41.
37. Bolino A, Schuffenecker I, Luo Y, et al. RET mutations in exons 13 and 14 of FMTC patients. Oncogene. 1995;10:2415–9.
38. Eng C, Smith DP, Mulligan LM, et al. A novel point mutation in the tyrosine kinase domain of the RET proto-oncogene in sporadic medullary thyroid carcinoma. Oncogene. 1995;10:509–13.
39. American Thyroid Association Guidelines Task Force. Medullary thyroid cancer: management guidelines of the American Thyroid Association. Thyroid. 2009;19:565–612.
40. Edery P, Lyonnet S, Mulligan LM, et al. Mutations of the RET protooncogene in Hirschsprung's disease. Nature. 1994;367:378–80.
41. Romeo G, Ronchetto P, Luo Y, et al. Point mutations affecting the tyrosine kinase domain of the RET proto-oncogene in Hirschsprung's disease. Nature. 1994;367:377–8.
42. Borst MJ, VanCamp JM, Peacock ML, Decker RA. Mutational analysis of multiple endocrine neoplasias type 2A associated with Hirschsprung's disease. Surgery. 1995;117:386–91.
43. Grieco M, Santoro M, Berlingieri MT, et al. PTC is a novel rearranged form of the RET proto-oncogene and is frequently detected in vivo in human thyroid papillary carcinomas. Cell. 1990;60:557–63.
44. Ledger GA, Khosla S, Lindor NM, et al. Genetic testing in the diagnosis and management of multiple endocrine neoplasia type II. Ann Intern Med. 1995;122:118–24.
45. Gagel RF, Core GJ, Bugalho MJMG, et al. Clinical use of molecular information in the management of multiple endocrine neoplasia type 2A. J Intern Med. 1995;238:331–41.
46. Lips CJM, Landsvater RM, Hoppener JWM, et al. Clinical screening as compared with DNA analysis in families with multiple endocrine neoplasia type 2A. N Engl J Med. 1994;331:828–35.
47. Wells Jr SA, Chi DD, Toshima K, et al. Predictive DNA testing and prophylactic thyroidectomy in patients at risk for multiple endocrine neoplasia type 2A. Ann Surg. 1994;220:237–50.
48. Moline J, Eng C. (Updated 5/4/2010) Multiple Endocrine Neoplasia Type 2. In: GeneReviews at GeneTests: Medical Genetics Information Resource (database online). Copyright, University of Washington, Seattle. 1997–2011. Available at http://www.genetests.org. Accessed 12/2/2011.
49. Eng C. Common alleles of predisposition in endocrine neoplasia. Curr Opin Genet Dev. 2010;20:251–6.
50. Ahmed SA, Snow-Bailey K, Highsmith WE, Sun W, Fenwick RG, Mao R. Nine novel germline gene variants in the RET proto-oncogene identified in twelve unrelated cases. J Mol Diagn. 2005;7:283–8.
51. Musholt PB, Musholt TJ, Goodfellow PJ, et al. Cold single-stranded conformational variants for mutation analysis of the RET protooncogene. Surgery. 1997;122:363–70.
52. Peacock ML, Borst MJ, Sweet JD, Decker RA. Detection of RET mutations in multiple endocrine neoplasias type 2A and familial medullary thyroid carcinoma by denaturing gradient gel electrophoresis. Hum Mutat. 1996;7:100–4.
53. Ceccherini I, Hofstra RMW, Luo Y. DNA polymorphisms and conditions for SSCP analysis of the 20 exons of the RET protooncogene. Oncogene. 1994;9:3025–9.
54. Siegelman M, Mohabeer A, Fahey III TJ, et al. Rapid, nonradioactive screening for mutations in exons 10, 11, and 16 of the RET protooncogene associated with inherited medullary thyroid carcinoma. Clin Chem. 1997;43:453–7.
55. Liu W, Smith DI, Rechtzigel KJ, et al. Denaturing high performance liquid chromatography (DHPLC) used in the detection of germline and somatic mutations. Nucleic Acids Res. 1998;26:1396–400.
56. Margraf RL, Mao R, Highsmith WE, Holtegaard LM, Wittwer CT. RET proto-oncogene genotyping using unlabeled probes, the masking technique, and amplicon high-resolution melting analysis. J Mol Diagn. 2007;9:184–96.
57. Margraf RL, Mao R, Wittwer CT. Masking selected sequence variation by incorporating mismatches into melting analysis probes. Hum Mutat. 2006;27:269–78.
58. Chen X, Zehnbauer B, Gnirke A, et al. Fluorescence energy transfer detection as a homogeneous DNA diagnostic method. Proc Natl Acad Sci U S A. 1997;94:10756–61.
59. Howe JR, Lairmore TC, Mishra SK, et al. Improved predictive test for MEN2, using flanking dinucleotide repeats and RFLPs. Am J Hum Genet. 1992;51:1430–42.
60. Aiello A, Cioni K, Gobbo M, Collini P, et al. The familial medullary thyroid carcinoma-associated RET E768D mutation in a multiple endocrine neoplasia type 2A case. Surgery. 2005;137:574–6.
61. Jimenez C, Dang GT, Schultz PN, El-Naggar A, et al. A novel point mutation of the RET protooncogene involving the second intracellular tyrosine kinase domain in a family with medullary thyroid carcinoma. J Clin Endocrinol Metab. 2004;89:3521–6.
62. Noll WW. Utility of RET mutation analysis in multiple endocrine neoplasia type 2. Arch Pathol Lab Med. 1999;123:1047–9.
63. Machens A, Dralle H. Genotype-phenotype based surgical concept of hereditary medullary thyroid carcinoma. World J Surg. 2007;31:957–68.
64. Baloh RH, Tansey MG, Lampe PA, et al. Artemin, a novel member of the GDNF ligand family, supports peripheral and central neurons

and signals through the GFRa3-RET receptor complex. Neuron. 1998;21:1291–302.
65. Zedenius J, Larsson C, Bergholm U, et al. Mutations of codon 918 in the RET proto-oncogene correlate with poor prognosis in sporadic medullary thyroid carcinomas. J Clin Endocrinol Metab. 1995;80:3088–90.
66. Eng C, Mulligan LM. Mutations of the RET proto-oncogene in the multiple endocrine neoplasias type 2 syndromes, related sporadic tumors, and Hirschsprung disease. Hum Mutat. 1997;9:97–109.
67. Falchetti A, Marini F, Giusti F, Cavalli L, Cavalli T, Brandi ML. DNA-based test: when and why to apply it to primary hyperparathyroidism clinical phenotypes. J Intern Med. 2009;266:69–83.
68. Neumann HPH, Eng C, Mulligan LM, et al. Consequences of direct genetic testing for germline mutations in the clinical management of families with multiple endocrine neoplasia type II. JAMA. 1995;274:1149–51.
69. Kruckeberg KE, Thibodeau SN. Pyrosequencing technology as a method for the diagnosis of multiple endocrine neoplasia type 2. Clin Chem. 2004;50:522–9.

26 Von Hippel-Lindau Disease

Catherine A. Stolle

Abstract

Von Hippel-Lindau disease (VHLD) is an autosomal dominant cancer predisposition syndrome characterized by tumors of the brain and spine, retina, kidney, adrenal glands, and several other organs. Point mutations and deletions in the *VHL* tumor suppressor gene have been identified in virtually 100 % of patients who meet strict clinical criteria. Molecular diagnostic testing consists of DNA sequence analysis of the coding region (~72 % of mutations) as well as deletion analysis (~28 % of mutations). Most cases are inherited; however about 20 % of cases are the result of de novo mutations; individuals mosaic for a VHL gene mutation have been reported. Molecular testing may be used to confirm a clinical diagnosis in an affected patient or rule out the disease in individuals with a single typical tumor. In families with a known mutation, molecular testing may be used for predictive testing of at-risk members or for prenatal testing.

Keywords

Von Hippel-Lindau disease • *VHL* gene • Tumor suppressor • De novo mutations • Molecular testing • Diagnostic testing • Predictive testing • Prenatal testing

Introduction

Von Hippel-Lindau disease (VHLD; OMIM#19330) is an autosomal dominant cancer predisposition syndrome that gives rise to hemangioblastomas of the brain and spine, retinal angiomas, clear cell renal cell carcinoma, pheochromocytoma, endolymphatic sac tumors, tumors of the epididymis or broad ligament, and pancreatic tumors or cysts [1]. The incidence of VHLD is approximately 1 in 36,000 live births [2]. Onset is typically between the second and fourth decades of life, with penetrance for the disease nearly complete by the age of 65 years. In most cases, a family history of the disorder is apparent. In about 20 % of cases, however, the proband appears to have acquired a new mutation [3].

C.A. Stolle, Ph.D. (✉)
Department of Pathology and Laboratory Medicine, The Children's Hospital of Philadelphia, ARC 714G, 34th and Civic Center Boulevard, Philadelphia, PA 19104, USA
e-mail: stolle@email.chop.edu

Molecular Basis of Disease

The *VHL* tumor suppressor gene was isolated by positional cloning in 1993 [4]. The gene, which consists of three exons spanning about 10 kilobases (kb) of genomic DNA on the short arm of chromosome 3 (3p25.3), is highly conserved among worms, flies, frogs, fish, chickens, humans, and other mammals (reviewed in Refs. 5 and 6). Two transcripts, 6.0 and 6.5 kb in size, are almost ubiquitously expressed and encode proteins of 213 and 160 amino acid residues, respectively. The latter isoform is the major product in most tissues and results from initiation of translation from an internal methionine codon at position 54. Both protein isoforms appear to be functional.

The VHL protein has been implicated in a variety of functions including transcriptional regulation, posttranscriptional gene expression, apoptosis, extracellular matrix formation, and ubiquitylation (reviewed in Refs. 5 and 6). The role of VHL in the regulation of hypoxia-inducible genes through the targeted ubiquitylation and degradation of hypoxia-inducible factor 1 alpha subunit (HIF1A) has been elucidated, leading

D.G.B. Leonard (ed.), *Molecular Pathology in Clinical Practice*, DOI 10.1007/978-3-319-19674-9_26

to a model of how disruption of the *VHL* gene results in the production of highly vascularized tumors.

Normal VHL binds to the protein elongin C, which forms a complex with elongin B, cullin-2 (CUL2), and Rbx1. This complex resembles the SKP1-CUL1-F-box protein (SCF) ubiquitin ligase or E3 complex in yeast that catalyzes the polyubiquitylation of specific proteins and targets them for degradation by proteosomes. Under normoxic conditions, HIF1A is hydroxylated at a specific asparagine residue by a member of the egg-laying deficiency protein nine-like (EGLN) protein family of prolyl hydroxylase enzymes. VHL binds to hydroxylated HIF1A and targets it for degradation. Under hypoxic conditions, HIF1A is not hydroxylated, VHL does not bind, and HIF1A subunits accumulate. HIF1A forms heterodimers with HIF1B and activates transcription of a variety of hypoxia-inducible messenger RNAs (i.e., *VEGF*, *EPO*, *TGFA*, *PDGFB*). Likewise, when VHL is absent or mutated, HIF1A subunits accumulate, resulting in cell proliferation and the neovascularization of tumors characteristic of VHLD [5].

Predisposition to VHLD is inherited in an autosomal dominant manner. However, tumor formation requires inactivation of the second allele (i.e., through loss of heterozygosity, methylation, or point mutation), and so the disease is recessive at the level of the cell. Mutations known to result in predisposition to VHLD include partial or complete deletions of the gene and point mutations (missense, nonsense, frameshift, and splice site). Point mutations are predicted either to truncate the protein, alter protein folding, or interfere with the binding of VHL to elongin C, HIF1A, or other target proteins [5, 7]. Although a handful of mutations and one mutation "hotspot" in exon 3 are common, point mutations are distributed over all three exons of the gene from codon 54 (internal initiator methionine) to the stop codon.

Four VHLD phenotypes have been described based on the likelihood of pheochromocytoma or renal cell carcinoma [8]. Type 1 is characterized by a low risk for pheochromocytoma. Truncating mutations or missense mutations that are predicted to grossly disrupt the folding of the VHL protein [7] are associated with VHLD type 1. VHLD type 2 is characterized by a high risk for pheochromocytoma. Most patients with VHLD type 2 have missense mutations of *VHL*. VHLD type 2 is further subdivided into those with a low risk (type 2A) and those with a high risk (type 2B) of renal cell carcinoma, as well as individuals at risk for pheochromocytoma only (type 2C). Some missense mutations correlate with a specific type 2 VHLD phenotype [6, 8].

A novel genotype-phenotype correlation has been reported, but is not yet considered to be a separate VHL type [9]. Individuals with a complete deletion of the *VHL* gene are more likely to present with multiple hemangioblastomas of the brain or spine or both as the first or only symptom of disease. Pheochromocytoma and renal cell carcinoma are less likely or may present at a later stage in life. At present, it is not clear why a complete deletion of the *VHL* gene would result in a phenotype distinctly different from that caused by a partial deletion or truncating mutation (i.e., VHL type 1). However, deletion of a neighboring gene(s) at the same locus may contribute to this phenotype [6].

Clinical Utility

Clinical molecular testing for VHLD has proven to be virtually 100 % effective at detecting germline mutations in patients with pathology-proven disease [10]. For this reason, molecular testing may be used to confirm a clinical diagnosis in an affected patient, screen for a mutation in an unaffected individual with a family history of VHLD, or rule out the disease in individuals with one VHLD-like tumor but no family history. When the mutation in the family is known, molecular testing may be used for diagnostic or presymptomatic testing of at-risk family members or for prenatal testing.

A clinical diagnosis of VHLD may be made in an individual with at least two typical VHLD tumors with or without a family history of VHLD or in an individual with at least one typical tumor and a significant family history [1]. In such cases, a *VHL* gene mutation is almost invariably found. Identification of a *VHL* mutation confirms the clinical diagnosis, establishes the need for periodic clinical screening, and facilitates presymptomatic testing of at-risk relatives.

Presymptomatic testing of at-risk family members for a known *VHL* gene mutation permits identification of presymptomatic mutation carriers and leads to early detection of tumors, timely intervention, and improved outcome. Identification of mutation-negative individuals eliminates the need for costly annual clinical screening. Genetic testing for a known *VHL* gene mutation is definitive.

Since the detection rate for germline mutations is high, and since approximately 20 % of patients have VHLD due to a de novo mutation, testing is indicated in individuals with a single VHLD-type tumor and no family history of the disease. A negative-mutation screen greatly reduces the risk of VHLD in this circumstance. Since tumors have been reported in children as young as 4 years of age, and since the mutation status of at-risk individuals affects clinical care, presymptomatic testing of asymptomatic children is appropriate. Prenatal testing for a *VHL* gene mutation is possible when the disease-causing mutation in an affected parent is known. However, prior to testing, consultation with a genetic counselor knowledgeable about the natural history of the disease and available treatment options is strongly recommended.

Available Assays

A 100 % mutation detection rate has been reported in individuals with a germline mutation in the *VHL* gene using a combination of deletion analysis and DNA sequence analysis [10]. A variety of methods, including quantitative Southern blot analysis [10], fluorescence in situ hybridization [11], real-time quantitative PCR [12], multiplex ligation-dependent probe amplification (MLPA; [13]), and array comparative genomic hybridization [14], have been used for the analysis of deletions in the *VHL* gene. MLPA is commonly used in clinical molecular laboratories for deletion analysis of the *VHL* gene since it is a relatively simple and rapid technique. Partial and complete gene deletions account for approximately 28 % of all cases of VHLD, with complete deletions occurring in 3–5 % of patients. Duplications have not as yet been reported to cause VHL disease.

PCR amplification and DNA sequence analysis of exons 1–3 of the *VHL* gene (including the adjacent splice donor and acceptor sequences) will detect all disease-causing point mutations. The *VHL* gene has few benign polymorphisms. DNA sequence analysis is typically performed by Sanger sequencing using fluorescently labeled dideoxy terminator nucleotides. Analysis for known point mutations in the *VHL* gene using next-generation sequencing technologies is available from several clinical molecular laboratories as part of a panel of cancer-related genes.

Interpretation of Results

Using a combination of deletion analysis and DNA sequence analysis, germline mutations in the *VHL* gene have been identified in over 300 consecutive patients with well-documented (pathology-proven) VHL disease seen at the National Cancer Institute since 1995. The sensitivity and specificity of the assays used to detect *VHL* gene mutations, therefore, are very high.

If a disease-causing mutation is identified in an affected or at-risk individual, that individual will be predisposed to developing tumors characteristic of VHLD. Periodic screening of target organ systems is recommended for early detection and treatment of tumors. Molecular testing of offspring would be appropriate, as they are at 50 % risk of inheriting the disease-causing mutation. The parents of the proband should be offered molecular testing, as they may have unappreciated disease. The risk to siblings depends on the mutation status of the parents, since the mutations in approximately 20 % of patients are de novo.

The interpretation of a negative-mutation screen depends on the circumstances surrounding the testing and the strength of the clinical diagnosis in the affected family member. A negative test in an individual at risk for a known *VHL* gene mutation is definitive, and the individual is not at risk for developing VHLD and need not undergo clinical screening for VHLD-associated tumors.

In screening of an unaffected at-risk individual for an unknown mutation in the *VHL* gene (i.e., first-degree relative of a patient with a clinical diagnosis of VHLD but no identified *VHL* mutation), a negative-mutation screen indicates only that the individual does not have a germline *VHL* gene mutation. This may be because (1) the individual did not inherit the mutant allele in the affected relative (i.e., a parent), (2) the affected relative does not have VHLD (i.e., as a result of an incorrect or inconclusive diagnosis), or (3) if the unaffected individual is the parent, he or she may be mosaic for a mutation that was transmitted to the affected offspring. Whenever possible, careful clinical evaluation or molecular analysis of an affected family member is suggested to improve the accuracy of the test interpretation for at-risk family members.

For an individual with a clinical diagnosis of VHLD but no family history, a negative-mutation screen indicates that either the patient is a phenocopy (coincidental occurrence of tumors typical of VHLD but without a gene mutation) or a mosaic (with a mutation in some, but not all, cells of the body). Mosaicism has been documented in the affected but mutation-negative parents of patients with a germline *VHL* gene mutation [3]. The frequency of mosaicism is not known but is believed to be low (i.e., <5 %). If the diagnosis of VHLD is supported by pathologic findings, i.e., magnetic resonance imaging of brain or spine, eye examination, abdominal ultrasound or computed tomography scan, urinary catecholamines, etc., then the patient is more likely to be mosaic and should be periodically screened for additional tumors characteristic of VHLD. Offspring (if any) should be considered at risk and should be considered for periodic clinical screening for tumors or molecular testing. The degree of risk (0–50 %) depends on the extent of mosaicism and the potential for transmitting the mutant allele, neither of which can be determined by clinical molecular testing at this time.

For patients who do not fulfill the clinical criteria for VHLD diagnosis because they have a single type of tumor and no family history, a negative-mutation screen would indicate that they are very unlikely to have VHLD; however, mosaicism cannot be entirely ruled out. Although routine clinical surveillance for characteristic VHLD tumors would not appear warranted, regular follow-up visits to a physician regarding the initial tumor would be expected. Likewise, routine screening of offspring would not be indicated unless the proband develops additional tumors (especially of another typical organ system) or if the offspring begin to develop symptoms of VHLD.

Occasionally, a base change in the *VHL* gene will be detected that is neither a known disease-causing mutation nor a known polymorphism. These "variants of unknown significance" with regard to VHLD are generally missense mutations or mutations in introns outside the consensus splice sequences. Novel mutations may be evaluated as disease-causing mutations or polymorphisms using criteria described by Cotton and Scriver [15] and in silico programs such as SIFT and PolyPhen. In such cases, it is helpful to test other affected or unaffected family members or both to determine whether the mutation segregates with the disease in the family.

Laboratory Issues

Point mutation analysis of the *VHL* gene is performed as a laboratory-developed test. PCR primers and conditions have been published [10]. A kit for deletion analysis of the *VHL* gene by MLPA is available from MRC Holland (Amsterdam, the Netherlands). No organized proficiency testing program is available for VHLD; therefore, proficiency testing may be performed either by interlaboratory exchange or by repeat testing of previously analyzed samples.

Various sources of DNA are suitable for use in DNA sequencing and MLPA assays. Ethylenediaminetetraacetic acid anticoagulated peripheral blood is the most commonly submitted specimen; however, DNA, frozen tissue, cultured cells, saliva, paraffin-embedded tissue, cheek epithelial cells (buccal swab), unspun amniocytes, or direct chorionic villus sampling specimens may be used as well. Mutation screening by MLPA and DNA sequence analysis can be completed in approximately 1 week. Interpretation of the assays is fairly straightforward (described above). Point mutations may be compared to an online database of human gene mutations, either at the Human Gene Mutation Database at http://www.hgmd.org/hosted by the Institute of Medical Genetics in Cardiff or a list of *VHL* gene mutations in the Universal VHL-Mutation Database (http://www.umd.be/) [16].

The mutation detection rate quoted by laboratories in the USA varies from 95 % to greater than 99 %. Since all laboratories are using the same basic methodologies, this variability is likely due to uncertainty regarding the patient's diagnosis or inadequate clinical information rather than the inability to detect germline mutations in the *VHL* gene.

References

1. Glenn GM, Choyke PL, Zbar B, et al. von Hippel-Lindau disease: clinical review and molecular genetics. Probl Urol. 1990;4:312–30.
2. Maher ER, Iselius L, Yates JR, et al. Von Hippel-Lindau disease: a genetic study. J Med Genet. 1991;28:443–7.
3. Sgambati MT, Stolle C, Choyke PL, et al. Mosaicism in von Hippel-Lindau disease: lessons from kindreds with germline mutations identified in offspring with mosaic parents. Am J Hum Genet. 2000;66:84–91.
4. Latif F, Tory K, Gnarra J, et al. Identification of the von Hippel-Lindau disease tumor suppressor gene. Science. 1993;260:1317–20.
5. Kaelin Jr WG. Molecular basis of the VHL hereditary cancer syndrome. Nat Rev Cancer. 2002;2:673–82.
6. Nordstrom-O'Brien M, van der Luijt RB, van Rooijen E, et al. Genetic analysis of von Hippel-Lindau disease. Hum Mutat. 2010;31:521–37.
7. Stebbins CE, Kaelin Jr WG, Pavletich NP. Structure of the VHL-elongin C-elongin B complex: implications for VHL tumor suppressor function. Science. 1999;284:455–61.
8. Zbar B, Kishida T, Chen F, et al. Germline mutations in the von Hippel-Lindau disease (VHL) gene in families from North America, Europe and Japan. Hum Mutat. 1996;8:348–57.
9. Hes F, Zewald R, Peeters T, et al. Genotype-phenotype correlations in families with deletions in the von Hippel-Lindau (VHL) gene. Hum Genet. 2000;106:425–31.
10. Stolle C, Glenn G, Zbar B, et al. Improved detection of germline mutations in the von Hippel-Lindau disease tumor suppressor gene. Hum Mutat. 1998;12:417–23.
11. Pack SD, Zbar B, Pak E, et al. Constitutional von Hippel-Lindau (VHL) gene deletions detected in VHL families by fluorescence in situ hybridization. Cancer Res. 1999;59:5560–4.
12. Hoebeeck J, van der Luijt R, Poppe B, et al. Rapid detection of VHL exon deletions using real-time quantitative PCR. Lab Invest. 2005;85:24–33.
13. Banks RE, Tirukonda P, Taylor C, et al. Genetic and epigenetic analysis of von Hippel-Lindau (VHL) gene alterations and relationship with clinical variables in sporadic renal cancer. Cancer Res. 2006;66:2000–11.
14. Wallerstein RJ, Brooks SS, Streck DL, et al. Exclusion of APC and VHL gene deletions by array based comparative hybridization in two patients with microscopically visible chromosomal aberrations. Cancer Genet Cytogenet. 2007;178:151–4.
15. Cotton RGH, Scriver CR. Proof of "disease causing" mutation. Hum Mutat. 1998;12:1–3.
16. Beroud C, Joly D, Gallou C, et al. Software and database for the analysis of mutations in the VHL gene. Nucleic Acids Res. 1998;26:256–8.

Hereditary Skin Cancer

27

Dani Bercovich and Inbal Kedar

Abstract

Skin cancer can be divided into three categories: basal cell carcinoma, squamous cell carcinoma, and melanoma. Because of the heterogeneity of the skin cancer phenotypes as well as the unknown exact correlation to genotypes, genetic testing is not offered on routine bases for all types of skin cancers. Several approaches are being used by clinicians, to determine the possible genetic components, which may be involved after complete skin examination by a dermatologist as a screening tool for skin cancer and family history determination. Molecular genetics of melanoma can be both diagnostically and therapeutically useful. When candidate's genes are known, according to the skin cancer phenotypes or the syndrome, Sanger sequencing and gene copy number variations (MLPA or RT-PCR) are applied. More recently, the use of comparative genomic hybridization (CGH), analysis of copy number in known miRNA genes, and exome sequencing, followed by screening of targeted genes in melanoma, helps to elucidate the genetic background of several skin cancers and the appropriate therapeutic approach. Referral of individuals affected or at risk for skin cancers to a genetic counselor or hereditary cancer center that routinely tests skin cancers patients is recommended.

Keywords

Hereditary • Skin • Cancer • Melanoma • Clinical testing • NGS

Skin cancer can be divided into three categories: basal cell carcinoma, squamous cell carcinoma, and melanoma. Basal cell carcinoma (BCC) is the most common and the least aggressive, although it can be very destructive to local tissue. BCC can be treated with surgery or topical chemotherapy and has a hereditary factor. Squamous cell carcinoma (SCC) is the second most common type of skin cancer and accounts for approximately 20 % of cutaneous malignancies. Although most cancer registries do not include information on the incidence of nonmelanoma skin cancer, annual incidence estimates range from 1 million to 3.5 million cases in the USA [1]. Mortality is rare from SCC; however, the morbidity and costs associated with treatment of SCC are considerably high. Sun exposure is the major known environmental factor associated with the development of skin cancer of all types; however, different patterns of sun exposure are associated with each major type of skin cancer [2]. In addition to environmental radiation, exposure to therapeutic radiation is another risk factor for SCC. Individuals with skin disorders treated with psoralen plus ultraviolet-A radiation (PUVA) have a three-fold to six-fold increase in SCC [3]. Current or previous cigarette smoking has been associated with a 1.5- to 2-fold increase in SCC risk [4]. Available evidence suggests that the effect of smoking on cancer risk seems to be greater for SCC than for BCC. Malignant melanoma is a neoplasm of pigment-producing cells called melanocytes that occurs most often in the skin but may also occur in the eyes, ears, gastrointestinal tract, leptomeninges, and oral and genital mucous membranes [5].

D. Bercovich, Ph.D. (✉)
GGA—Galil Genetic Analysis; Biotechnology Program, Tel Hai College, P. O. Box 3664, Kazerin 12900, Israel
e-mail: danib@gga.org.il; dannyb@telhai.ac.il

Inbal Kedar, M.S.
Cancer Genetics, The Raphael Recanati Genetics Institute, Rabin Medical Center, Beilinson Hospital, Petah Tikva, Israel

D.G.B. Leonard (ed.), *Molecular Pathology in Clinical Practice*, DOI 10.1007/978-3-319-19674-9_27

Table 27.1 Skin cancers and associated syndromes

Skin cancer type	Associated syndromes
Cutaneous basal cell carcinoma	Basal cell nevus syndrome (BCNS)
	Bazex syndrome
	Rombo syndrome
	Brooke-Spiegler syndrome
	Muir-Torre syndrome
	Xeroderma pigmentosum
Squamous cell carcinoma	Xeroderma pigmentosum
	Ferguson-Smith syndrome
	Oculocutaneous albinism type 1
	Oculocutaneous albinism type 2
	Hermansky-Pudlak syndrome
	Chediak-Higashi syndrome
	Griscelli syndrome
	Dystrophic epidermolysis bullosa (DEB)
	Junctional epidermolysis bullosa (JEB)
	Fanconi anemia—FANCA
	Dyskeratosis congenital
	Rothmund-Thomson syndrome
	Bloom syndrome
	Werner syndrome
Cutaneous malignant melanoma (CMM)	–

Molecular Basis of Disease

Cutaneous BCC is the most common cancer among people of European ancestry [6]. The primary environmental risk factor for BCC is sun exposure, but genetic risk factors also have a substantial role. Susceptibility to BCC is a genetically heterogeneous trait. Some of the sequence variants that confer susceptibility seem to operate through their association with fair-pigmentation traits common among Europeans, resulting in reduced protection from the damaging effects of ultraviolet (UV) radiation. Genes which are known to be associated with fair skin or sensitivity to sun in BCC are *ASIP*, *TYR*, and *SHEP5* [7]. Other sequence variants have no obvious role in pigmentation or UV susceptibility but, instead, function in the contexts of growth and differentiation of the basal layers of the skin. BCC occurs as a feature of multiple syndromes, including basal cell nevus syndrome (BCNS), Bazex syndrome, Rombo syndrome, Brooke-Spiegler syndrome, Muir-Torre syndrome, and xeroderma pigmentosum (XP) (Table 27.1). Somatic mutations within the catalytic domain of the *RASA1* gene and four mutations within its C-terminal SH2 region occur in BCC syndromes. The region in which these mutations are clustered is A/T rich, raising the possibility that UV radiation is a contributing factor [8, 37]. For sporadic BCCs, mutations occur in the *PTCH1* and *PTCH2* genes [9, 10].

XP is a rare autosomal recessive hereditary disorder affecting approximately one in one million individuals in the USA and Europe but is more common in Japan, North Africa, and the Middle East. XP is caused by dysfunction of nucleotide excision repair that results in cutaneous malignancies in the first decade of life. Affected individuals have an increased sensitivity to sunlight, resulting in a markedly increased risk of SCC, BCC, and melanoma. One report found that non-melanoma skin cancer was increased 150-fold in individuals with XP; for those younger than 20 years, the prevalence was almost 5,000 times the general population incidence [11]. Seven complementation groups plus one variant form of XP are based on the underlying genetic cause of the disease. Complementation group A, due to mutations in *XPA*, accounts for approximately 10 % of cases [12]. Approximately 40 % of the XP cases in complementation group C are due to mutations in the *XPC* gene. *ERCC2* (*XPD*) mutations are present in about 20 % of the affected individuals and constitute complementation group D. Other mutated genes in this disorder include *ERCC3* (XP group B), *DDB2* (XP group E), *ERCC4* (XP group F), and *ERCC5* (XP group G). Carriers of a mutation in one XP gene are generally asymptomatic. Founder mutations in *XPA* (R228A) and *XPC* (V548A fs X572) have been identified in North African populations, and direct screening for these mutations has been proposed for this group of patients [13]. The variant form of XP, or type V XP, is caused by mutations in the *POLH* gene, which encodes a polymerase required in S-phase of the cell cycle.

Ferguson-Smith syndrome is an autosomal dominant disorder characterized by invasive skin tumors that are histologically identical to sporadic cutaneous SCC, which resolve spontaneously without intervention. Linkage analysis of affected families has shown loss of the long arm of chromosome 9, and haplotype analysis has localized this gene to 9q22.3 between D9S197 and D9S1809. *PTCH* (mutated in BCNS) and *XPA* are among the candidate genes located in this chromosomal region; however, neither one of these genes has been found to be mutated in the families affected with Ferguson-Smith syndrome. Two fructose bisphosphatase genes (*FBP1* and *FBP2*), a possible membrane alanine aminopeptidase (*C9orf3*), and three other genes of unknown function (*AL133071*, *FLJ14753*, and *CDC14B*) are additional candidates [14, 15].

Two types of oculocutaneous albinism are associated with increased risk of SCC of the skin. Oculocutaneous albinism type 1, or tyrosinase-related albinism, is caused by mutations in the tyrosinase gene, *TYR*, located on the long arm of chromosome 11. The *OCA2* gene, also known as the P gene, is mutated in oculocutaneous albinism type 2, or tyrosinase-positive albinism. Both disorders have an autosomal recessive inheritance pattern, with frequent compound heterozygosity [16]. Mutations in the genes *MATP* (*OCA4*) and *TYRP1* (tyrosinase-related protein) are associated with less common types of oculocutaneous albinism. Several other albinism syndromes such as Hermansky-Pudlak syndrome also are inherited in an autosomal recessive manner but may have a pseudodominant inheritance pattern in Puerto Rican families, due to its high prevalence in this population. The underlying cause is believed to be a defect in melanosome and lysosome transport in skin cells. A number of mutations at disparate loci have been associated with this syndrome, including *HPS1*, *HPS3*, *HPS4*, *HPS5*, *HPS6*, *HPS7* (*DTNBP1*), and *HPS8* (*BLOC1S3*) [17].

Two autosomal recessive syndromes, Chediak-Higashi syndrome and Griscelli syndrome, are caused by mutations in the *LYST* and *MYO5A* genes, respectively [18]. Approximately 95 % of individuals with the heritable disorder dystrophic epidermolysis bullosa have a detectable germline mutation in the gene *COL7A1*, located at 3p21.3, which is expressed in the basal keratinocytes of the epidermis and encodes for type VII collagen [19].

Junctional epidermolysis bullosa (JEB) is an autosomal recessive type of epidermolysis bullosa. JEB results in considerable mortality with approximately 50 % of cases dying within the first year of life. Mutations in any of the genes encoding the three basic subunits of laminin 332, previously known as laminin 5 or *COL17A1*, can result in this syndrome [19].

Fanconi anemia is a complex disorder that is characterized by increased incidence of hematologic and solid tumors, including SCC of the skin. Thirteen complementation groups defined by the underlying causative genetic factors have been identified for Fanconi anemia, of which Fanconi anemia complementation group A (FANCA) is the most common [20]. Individuals with dyskeratosis congenita have an incidence of SCC of approximately 1.5 %, and the median age at diagnosis is 21 years. These SCCs are generally managed as any other SCC of the skin. Several genes associated with telomere function (including *DKC1*, *TERC*, *TINF2*, *NHP2*, *NOP10*, and *TERT*) have been implicated in dyskeratosis congenita [21].

Rothmund-Thomson syndrome, also known as poikiloderma congenitale, is a heritable disorder characterized by chromosomal instability. The precise increased risk of skin cancer is not well characterized, but the point prevalence of nonmelanoma skin cancer, including both BCC and SCC, is 2–5 % in young individuals affected by this syndrome. A mutation in the *RECQL4* gene, located at 8q24.3, is present in 66 % of clinically affected individuals and has an autosomal recessive inheritance pattern. *RECQL4* encodes the ATP-dependent DNA helicase Q4, which promotes DNA unwinding to allow for cellular processes such as replication, transcription, and repair [22]. Loss of genomic stability is also the major cause of Bloom syndrome (*BLM* gene) and Werner syndrome (*WRN* gene). Approximately 20 % of the cancers reported in these syndromes are cutaneous, with melanoma and SCC of the skin accounting for 14 % and 5 %, respectively [23].

Susceptibility loci for several forms of familial cutaneous malignant melanoma (CMM) have been mapped, including *CMM1* on chromosome 1p36. Other familial CMM susceptibility loci include CMM2 which has been found to be affected by mutations in the *CDKN2A* gene on chromosome 9p21 and CMM3 by mutations in the *CDK4* gene on chromosome 12q14. *CMM4* has been mapped to chromosome 1p22. Susceptibility to melanoma has been associated with polymorphisms in the *MC1R* (*CMM5*) and *XRCC3* (*CMM6*) genes. The melanocortin 1 receptor (MC1R or alpha melanocyte-stimulating hormone receptor) is a key protein regulating skin and hair pigmentation. *CMM7* has been mapped to chromosome 20q11.22. The *CDKN2A* gene encodes proteins that regulate two critical cell cycle regulatory pathways, the TP53 pathway and the RB1 pathway. Through the use of shared coding regions and alternative reading frames, the *CDKN2A* gene produces two major proteins: p16 (INK4), which is a cyclin-dependent kinase inhibitor, and p14 (ARF), which binds the p53-stabilizing protein MDM2 [24]. Sporadic somatic mutations causing malignant melanoma have also been identified in several genes, including *BRAF*, *STK11*, *PTEN*, *TRRAP*, *DCC*, *GRIN2A*, *ZNF831*, and *BAP1*. A large percentage of melanomas (40–60 %) carry an activating somatic mutation in the *BRAF* gene, most often the missense mutation V600E [25] (Table 27.2).

Melanoma Risk Assessment

Family history of melanoma increases risk of melanoma by about two-fold. A family cancer registry study assessed over 20,000 individuals with melanoma and found a standardized incidence ratio of 2.62 for offspring of individuals with melanoma and 2.94 for siblings [38]. A study looking at the contribution of family history to melanoma risk showed a population-attributable fraction ranging from <1 % in northern Europe to 6.4 % in Australia [39], suggesting that only a small percentage of melanoma cases are caused by familial factors. Rarely in some families, many generations and multiple individuals develop melanoma and are at much higher risk. For individuals from these families, the incidence of melanoma is higher for sun-protected rather than sun-exposed skin [40]. The major hereditary melanoma susceptibility gene, *CDKN2A*, is mutated in approximately 35–40 % of families with three or more melanoma cases. To date, more than half of the families with multiple cases of melanoma have no identified mutation [41].

Patients with a personal history of melanoma or dysplastic nevi should be asked to provide information regarding a family history of melanoma and other cancers to detect the presence of familial melanoma. Age at diagnosis in family members and pathologic confirmation should also be sought. The presence of multiple primary melanomas in the same individual may also provide a clue to an underlying genetic

Table 27.2 Skin cancer types, known genes, and common mutations

Skin cancer type	Genes	Common mutations or variants
Cutaneous basal cell carcinoma	*TYR*	R402Q, rs1126809[A], rs1042602[C]
	SHEP5	
	RASA1	1 mutation within the catalytic domain and 4 mutations within the C-terminal SH2 region
	PTCH1	c.1291delC, c.2619C>A, c.2196_2197delCT, c.863G>A, c.3499G>A, c.3440 T>G, c.3244_3246dup, c.1347+6G>A, c.1504-1G>A, c.2251-3C>G, c.2560+1G>T
	PTCH2	1170delCT
	SMO	c.536C>T, c.IVS537+18C>T, c.582A>G
	ASIP	8818A>G, rs1015362[G], rs4911414[T]
	SLC24A4	rs12896399[T]
	KITLG	rs12821256[C]
	OCA2	rs1667394[A], rs7495174[A]
	TPCN2	rs35264875[T], rs3829241[A]
	TYRP1	rs1408799[T]
Squamous cell carcinoma	*XPA*	R228A
	XPC	V548A fs X572
	ERCC2 (*XPD*), *ERCC3* (*XPB*), *DDB2* (*XPE*), *ERCC4* (*XPF*), *ERCC5* (*XPG*)	K751Q (rs13181)
	PTCH	
	FBP1	
	FBP2	
	C9orf3	
	AL133071	
	FLJ14753	
	CDC14B	
	TYR	R402Q
	OCA2 (P gene)	
	MATP (*OCA4*)	
	TYRP1	
	HPS1, *HPS3*, *HPS4*, *HPS5*, *HPS6*, *HPS7* (*DTNBP1*), and *HPS8* (*BLOC1S3*)	
	LYST	
	MYO5A	
	COL7A1	
	Laminin genes	
	DKC1, *TERC*, *TINF2*, *NHP2*, *NOP10*, *TERT*	
	RECQL4	
	BLM	
	WRN	
Cutaneous malignant melanoma	*CMM1*, *CMM2* (*CDKN2A*), *CMM3* (*CDK4*), *CMM4*, *CMM5* (*XRCC3*), *CMM7*	
	MC1R, *CMM6*	R151C, R160W, D294H
	TP53	
	p16 (*INK4*)	G259S, R232T, 19-bp founder deletion in exon 2, 6-BP DEL, NT363, 3-BP DUP, R105INS, M53I, R24P, duplication of a 24-bp repeat present in the 5-prime region, -34G-T, A94E, V126D, IVS2, A-G, -105, G122R, V59G, L113L, P114S, S56I, G89D

(continued)

Table 27.2 (continued)

Skin cancer type	Genes	Common mutations or variants
Cutaneous malignant melanoma (continued)	p14 (*ARF*)	
	BRAF	V600E
	STK11	
	PTEN	
	TRRAP	
	DCC	
	GRIN2A	
	ZNF831	
	BAP1	
	KIT	

susceptibility. Approximately 30 % of affected individuals in hereditary melanoma kindreds have more than one primary melanoma, compared to 4 % of sporadic melanoma patients [42]. Family histories should be updated regularly.

For individuals without a personal history of melanoma, several models have been suggested for prediction of melanoma risk. Data including gender, age, family history of melanoma, number of severe sunburns, number of moles larger than 3 mm on the limbs, and hair color were used to create a model for prediction of melanoma risk [43].

Clinical Utility of Testing

Because of the heterogeneity of the skin cancer phenotypes as well as the unknown exact correlation to genotypes, genetic testing is not routinely offered for all types of skin cancers. Several approaches are used clinically for monitoring for the presence of skin cancer, including a complete skin examination by a dermatologist and a family history assessment. A physical examination in conjunction with ancillary diagnostic techniques such as epiluminescence microscopy, more commonly known as dermoscopy (dermatoscopy), may incline the physician to biopsy a suspicious skin lesion early in its evolution. An appropriate biopsy that is representative of the entire lesion is mandatory for an accurate histologic diagnosis of skin cancer; this is especially true for the diagnosis and staging of melanoma. Currently, the definitive diagnosis of melanoma and nonmelanoma skin cancers is by histopathologic evaluation of skin lesion resection specimens.

With a family history consistent of a hereditary form of skin cancer, appropriate genetic counseling and targeted genetic testing appropriate to the family history are used. Identification of the familial mutation can be used to screen of other family members to identify those with the mutation who will require close monitoring and avoidance of sun exposure and those without the mutation who are at the population risk for skin cancer. For severe forms of inherited skin cancer syndromes, prenatal testing or preimplantation genetic diagnosis may be offered to family members of childbearing age.

Molecular genetics of melanoma can be both diagnostically and therapeutically useful [26]. When candidates' genes are known, according to the skin cancer phenotypes or the syndrome, Sanger sequencing and gene copy number variation testing such as multiple ligation probe amplification (MLPA) or reverse-transcription PCR (RT-PCR) can be used. More recently, array-based comparative genomic hybridization (aCGH), analysis of copy number in known miRNA genes, and exome sequencing (by next-generation sequencing, NGS) followed by screening of targeted genes in melanoma are being used to elucidate the genetic background of several skin cancer syndromes and the appropriate therapeutic approach. Distinct patterns of genetic alterations, both chromosomal aberrations and the frequency of specific gene mutations, suggest that the subtypes of melanoma arise from separate mechanistic routes in response to different selective influences. For example, melanoma patients without chronic sun-induced damage have frequent losses of chromosome 10 and frequent mutations in the *BRAF* gene, while melanomas on skin with chronic sun-induced damage had frequent increases in the number of copies of the *CCND1* gene and infrequent mutations in *BRAF* [27]. The oncogene *KIT* has been identified as a potential therapeutic target in melanomas of mucosal membranes, acral skin, and skin with chronic sun-induced damage. This is of value, as this subset of melanomas infrequently has mutations in *BRAF*. The observation of such chromosomal aberrations in melanoma, and a virtual deficiency of abnormalities in benign nevi, leads to the possibility that chromosomal analysis could be used diagnostically in melanocytic lesions that are ambiguous based on our current methods of assessment [28]. Identifying such causative genetic alterations also offers targets for therapy. For example, a major response has been noted using imatinib mesylate in *KIT*-mutated melanoma and in a phase II trial of patients with metastatic melanoma having at least one protein tyrosine kinase mutation [29].

Available Assays

Both the general population and members of families with a history of skin cancer should have a complete skin examination by a dermatologist as a screening tool for skin cancer. The American Cancer Society recommends using the ABCDE mnemonic (asymmetry, border irregularity, color abnormalities, diameter greater than 5 mm, and evolving) to identify lesions that may require further evaluation by biopsy for histopathologic examination. The diagnostic utility of the dermatologist's visual examination technique has been confirmed and studies have shown that its sensitivity in the diagnosis of skin cancer ranges from 65 to 97 %, with a positive predictive value of 35–75 % [30]. Dermatoscopy is a noninvasive visualization technique that uses optical lenses and fluid immersion to closely examine suspicious cutaneous lesions, allowing the detailed inspection of skin pigment, vascular structures, and subtle skin color changes.

For molecular genetic testing, denaturing high-performance liquid chromatography, single-strand conformation polymorphism, and denaturing gradient gel electrophoresis are mutation screening methods that may be used in conjunction with Sanger or NGS sequencing for the analysis of the entire coding region or sequence analysis of select exons in the *CDKN2A* and *CDK4* genes. Deletions and duplications are most commonly detected by MLPA or quantitative real-time PCR (qPCR). For somatic mutation analysis of skin cancer specimens, Sanger or NGS sequencing of the full coding regions or selective single-nucleotide polymorphisms of candidates genes, such as *MC1R*, *BRAF*, *TP53*, *PTEN*, *KIT*, and *CCND1*, are available in some clinical molecular laboratories [44]. Melanomas can be characterized by somatic changes such as copy number variants and structural variants using aCGH [32].

Interpretation of Test Results

The sensitivity or accuracy of genetic tests varies by the method used and the phenotypic characterization (which depends on the examination by a dermatologist as a screening tool for skin cancer and/or genetic consultants). In the *CDKN2A* gene, germline mutations can be detected in 15–20 % of patients with melanoma [33, 34]. Mutations in the *CDKN2A* gene are melanoma predisposition alleles with high penetrance, although they have low population frequencies. In contrast, variants of *MC1R* confer much lower melanoma risk but are common in European populations. Three MC1R variants (R151C, R160W, and D294H) increase risk of melanoma with a hazard ratio of 3.72 and are associated with red hair, fair skin, and skin sensitivity to ultraviolet light [35]. *BRAF* somatic missense mutations are found in up to 66 % of malignant melanomas [36]. All mutations are within the BRAF kinase domain, with a single substitution, V600E, originally reported as V599E, accounting for 80 % of the mutations. Mutated BRAF proteins have elevated kinase activity and are transforming in NIH 3 T3 cells. BRAF is a serine/threonine kinase that is commonly activated by somatic point mutation in many human cancer types, which provides new therapeutic opportunities for treatment of melanoma.

Laboratory Issues

Genetic counseling is recommended before genetic testing is ordered. Referral of individuals affected or at risk for skin cancers to a genetic counselor or hereditary cancer center that routinely tests skin cancers patients is recommended.

Future Directions

MicroRNA (miRNA) expression signatures are not only found in cancer tissue but also in the blood of cancer patients. Specifically, miRNA detection in blood offers the prospect of a noninvasive analysis tool. Blood samples of melanoma patients and healthy individuals can be well differentiated from each other based on miRNA expression analysis [31]. In miRNA expression analysis using a subset of 16 significantly deregulated miRNAs, a pathogenicity classification accuracy of 97.4 % was achieved, with a specificity of 95 % and a sensitivity of 98.9 % by supervised analysis [31].

NGS technologies have enabled genome-wide identification of germline and somatic mutations in large-scale cancer sample sets [45]. Population screening of high-risk families will be the gold standard in the coming years to identify individuals who may be at high risk of skin cancer and should take proper preventive actions.

References

1. Rogers HW, Weinstock MA, Harris AR, et al. Incidence estimate of nonmelanoma skin cancer in the United States, 2006. Arch Dermatol. 2010;146(3):283–7.
2. Gallagher RP, Hill GB, Bajdik CD, et al. Sunlight exposure, pigmentation factors, and risk of nonmelanocytic skin cancer. II. Squamous cell carcinoma. Arch Dermatol. 1995;131(2):164–9.
3. Lindelöf B, Sigurgeirsson B, Tegner E, et al. PUVA and cancer risk: the Swedish follow-up study. Br J Dermatol. 1999;141(1):108–12.
4. Grodstein F, Speizer FE, Hunter DJ. A prospective study of incident squamous cell carcinoma of the skin in the nurses' health study. J Natl Cancer Inst. 1995;87(14):1061–6.
5. Habif, TP. Clinical dermatology. 5th edn. St. Louis: Mosby/Elsevier. 2009.

6. Stacey SN, Sulem P, Masson G, Gudjonsson SA, et al. New common variants affecting susceptibility to basal cell carcinoma. Nat Genet. 2009;41:909–14.
7. Rafnar T, Sulem P, Stacey SN, Geller F, et al. Sequence variants at the TERT-CLPTM1L locus associate with many cancer types. Nat Genet. 2009;41:221–7.
8. Friedman E, Gejman PV, Martin GA, McCormick F. Nonsense mutations in the C-terminal SH2 region of the GTPase activating protein (GAP) gene in human tumours. Nat Genet. 1993;5:242–7.
9. Ding L, Kim M, Kanchi KL, et al. Clonal architecures and driver mutations in metastatic melanomas.
10. Aszterbaum M, Rothman A, Johnson RL, Fisher M, et al. Identification of mutations in the human PATCHED gene in sporadic basal cell carcinomas and in patients with the basal cell nevus syndrome. J Invest Dermatol. 1998;110:885–8.
11. Smyth I, Narang MA, Evans T, Heimann C, et al. Isolation and characterization of human Patched 2 (PTCH2), a putative tumour suppressor gene in basal cell carcinoma and medulloblastoma on chromosome 1p32. Hum Mol Genet. 1999;8:291–7.
12. Kraemer KH, Lee MM, Andrews AD, et al. The role of sunlight and DNA repair in melanoma and nonmelanoma skin cancer. The xeroderma pigmentosum paradigm. Arch Dermatol. 1994;130(8):1018–21.
13. Moussaid L, Benchikhi H, Boukind EH, et al. Cutaneous tumors during xeroderma pigmentosum in Morocco: study of 120 patients. Ann Dermatol Venereol. 2004;131(1 Pt 1):29–33.
14. Messaoud O, Ben Rekaya M, Cherif W, et al. Genetic homogeneity of mutational spectrum of group-A xeroderma pigmentosum in Tunisian patients. Int J Dermatol. 2010;49(5):544–8.
15. Richards FM, Goudie DR, Cooper WN, et al. Mapping the multiple self-healing squamous epithelioma (MSSE) gene and investigation of xeroderma pigmentosum group A (XPA) and PATCHED (PTCH) as candidate genes. Hum Genet. 1997;101(3):317–22.
16. Bose S, Morgan LJ, Booth DR, et al. The elusive multiple self-healing squamous epithelioma (MSSE) gene: further mapping, analysis of candidates, and loss of heterozygosity. Oncogene. 2006;25(5):806–12.
17. Luande J, Henschke CI, Mohammed N. The Tanzanian human albino skin. Natural history. Cancer. 1985;55(8):1823–8.
18. Morgan NV, Pasha S, Johnson CA, et al. A germline mutation in BLOC1S3/reduced pigmentation causes a novel variant of Hermansky-Pudlak syndrome (HPS8). Am J Hum Genet. 2006;78(1):160–6.
19. Ménasché G, Ho CH, Sanal O, et al. Griscelli syndrome restricted to hypopigmentation results from a melanophilin defect (GS3) or a MYO5A F-exon deletion (GS1). J Clin Invest. 2003;112(3):450–6.
20. Bruckner-Tuderman L. Hereditary skin diseases of anchoring fibrils. J Dermatol Sci. 1999;20(2):122–33.
21. Rosenberg PS, Greene MH, Alter BP. Cancer incidence in persons with Fanconi anemia. Blood. 2003;101(3):822–6.
22. Mehenni Marrone A, Walne A, Tamary H, et al. Telomerase reverse-transcriptase homozygous mutations in autosomal recessive dyskeratosis congenita and Hoyeraal-Hreidarsson syndrome. Blood. 2007;110(13):4198–205.
23. Petkovic M, Dietschy T, Freire R, et al. The human Rothmund-Thomson syndrome gene product, RECQL4, localizes to distinct nuclear foci that coincide with proteins involved in the maintenance of genome stability. J Cell Sci. 2005;118(Pt 18):4261–9.
24. Tsuchiya H, Tomita K, Ohno M, et al. Werner's syndrome combined with quintuplicate malignant tumors: a case report and review of literature data. Jpn J Clin Oncol. 1991;21(2):135–42.
25. Robertson KD, Jones PA. Tissue-specific alternative splicing in the human INK4a/ARF cell cycle regulatory locus. Oncogene. 1999;18:3810–20.
26. Pollock PM, Harper UL, Hansen KS, Yudt LM, et al. High frequency of BRAF mutations in nevi. Nat Genet. 2003;33:19–20.
27. Bastian BC. Molecular genetics of melanocytic neoplasia: practical applications for diagnosis. Pathology. 2004;36(5):458–61.
28. Curtin JA, Busam K, Pinkel D, Bastian BC. Somatic activation of KIT in distinct subtypes of melanoma. J Clin Oncol. 2006;24(26):4340–6.
29. Bauer J, Bastian BC. Distinguishing melanocytic nevi from melanoma by DNA copy number changes: comparative genomic hybridization as a research and diagnostic tool. Dermatol Ther. 2006;19(1):40–9.
30. Kim KB, Eton O, Davis DW, et al. Phase II trial of imatinib mesylate in patients with metastatic melanoma. Br J Cancer. 2008;99(5):734–40.
31. Koh HK, Caruso A, Gage I, et al. Evaluation of melanoma/skin cancer screening in Massachusetts. Preliminary results. Cancer. 1990;65:375–9.
32. Leidinger P, Keller A, Borries A, Reichrath J, Rass K, Jager SU, et al. High-throughput miRNA profiling of human melanoma blood samples. BMC Cancer. 2010;10:262.
33. Jalas JR, Vemula S, Bezrookove V, Leboit PE, Simko JP, Bastian BC. Metastatic melanoma with striking adenocarcinomatous differentiation illustrating phenotypic plasticity in melanoma. Am J Surg Pathol. 2011;35(9):1413–8.
34. Monzon J, Liu L, Brill H, Goldstein AM, Tucker MA, From L, et al. CDKN2A mutations in multiple primary melanomas. N Engl J Med. 1998;338:879–87.
35. Molven A, Grimstvedt MB, Steine SJ, Harland M, Avril M-F, Hayward NK, et al. A large Norwegian family with inherited malignant melanoma, multiple atypical nevi, and CDK4 mutation. Genes Chromosomes Cancer. 2005;44:10–8.
36. Box NF, Duffy DL, Chen W, Stark M, Martin NG, Sturm RA, et al. MC1R genotype modifies risk of melanoma in families segregating CDKN2A mutations. Am J Hum Genet. 2001;69:765–73.
37. Davies H, Bignell GR, Cox C, Stephens P, et al. Mutations of the BRAF gene in human cancer. Nature. 2002;417:949–54.
38. Brandt A, Sundquist J, Hemminki K. Risk of incident and fatal melanoma in individuals with a family history of incident or fatal melanoma or any cancer. Br J Dermatol. 2011;165(2):342–8.
39. Olsen CM, Carroll HJ, Whiteman DC. Familial melanoma: a meta-analysis and estimates of attributable fraction. Cancer Epidemiol Biomarkers Prev. 2010;19(1):65–73.
40. Hemminki K, Zhang H, Czene K. Incidence trends and familial risks in invasive and in situ cutaneous melanoma by sun-exposed body sites. Int J Cancer. 2003;104(6):764–71.
41. Goldstein AM, Chan M, Harland M, et al. High-risk melanoma susceptibility genes and pancreatic cancer, neural system tumors, and uveal melanoma across GenoMEL. Cancer Res. 2006;66(20):9818–28.
42. Greene MH. The genetics of hereditary melanoma and nevi 1998 update. Cancer. 1999;86(11 Suppl):2464–77.
43. Cho E, Rosner BA, Feskanich D, et al. Risk factors and individual probabilities of melanoma for whites. J Clin Oncol. 2005;23(12):2669–75.
44. Woetmann A, Glue C, Røpke MA, Skov L, Odum N, Queille-Roussel C, et al. Diagnostic microRNA profiling in cutaneous T-cell lymphoma (CTCL). Blood. 2011;118(22):5891–900.
45. Jia P, Zhao Z. VarWalker: personalized mutation network analysis of putative cancer genes from next-generation sequencing data. PLoS Comput Biol. 2014;6:10(2).

28 Li-Fraumeni Syndrome

Arupa Ganguly and Zhao Chen

Abstract

Li-Fraumeni syndrome (LFS) is a rare familial cancer-predisposing syndrome, which is inherited in an autosomal dominant pattern. LFS patients often present with multiple primary tumors and an early age of onset. The lifetime risk of cancer is estimated to be 73 % for males and nearly 100 % for females. Germline mutations in the tumor suppressor gene, *TP53*, are associated with LFS and can be detected in more than 60 % of classic LFS families. Clinical genetic testing for *TP53* is available for individuals with a suspected or known clinical diagnosis of LFS or a molecular diagnosis based on a history of an identified *TP53* mutation in a family member. Although preventive and surveillance options for LFS are currently limited, presymptomatic genetic testing can provide early diagnosis of individuals at risk of cancer, closer surveillance, earlier detection, and treatment for cancers and an increased likelihood of improved outcomes.

Keywords

Li-Fraumeni syndrome • Familial cancer • Brain tumor • Osteosarcoma • Breast cancer • *TP53* gene • Genetic testing and counseling

Introduction

Li-Fraumeni syndrome (LFS) (OMIM #151623) is a rare familial cancer syndrome, which is inherited in an autosomal dominant pattern. Li and Fraumeni first reported this cancer predisposition syndrome in 1969 [1]. Individuals with LFS often present with a specific set of primary cancers in early childhood that include osteosarcoma, soft-tissue sarcoma, brain tumor, and adrenocortical carcinoma. Adult onset cancers in LFS include colorectal cancer, breast cancer, and other cancers (Fig. 28.1). Among the various cancers, osteosarcoma, breast cancer, soft-tissue sarcoma, colorectal cancer, brain tumor, and adrenocortical carcinomas are referred to as the "core" cancers of LFS and account for the majority of cancers observed. LFS is also referred to as *s*arcoma, *b*reast, *l*eukemia, and *a*drenal gland (SBLA) syndrome or sarcoma family syndrome of Li and Fraumeni. The lifetime risk of cancer in LFS is estimated to be 73 % for males and nearly 100 % for females, which is higher due to the increased risk for breast cancer [2].

LFS is an autosomal dominant disease. This means inheritance of a single copy of the mutated gene predisposes an individual to the disease. Based on clinical presentation, two forms of LFS are recognized: classic Li-Fraumeni syndrome (LFS) and Li-Fraumeni-like syndrome (LFL). Classic LFS is defined by the following criteria: a proband with a sarcoma diagnosed before 45 years of age, a first-degree relative with any cancer under 45 years of age, and a first- or second-degree relative with any cancer under 45 years of age or a sarcoma at any age [1]. LFL is characterized by a proband with any childhood cancer or sarcoma, brain tumor, or adrenal cortical tumor diagnosed before 45 years of age, a first- or

A. Ganguly, Ph.D. (✉) • Z. Chen, Ph.D.
Department of Genetics, Perelman School of Medicine, University of Pennsylvania, 415 Curie Boulevard, Room 500, Philadelphia, PA 19104, USA
e-mail: ganguly@mail.med.upenn.edu

D.G.B. Leonard (ed.), *Molecular Pathology in Clinical Practice*, DOI 10.1007/978-3-319-19674-9_28

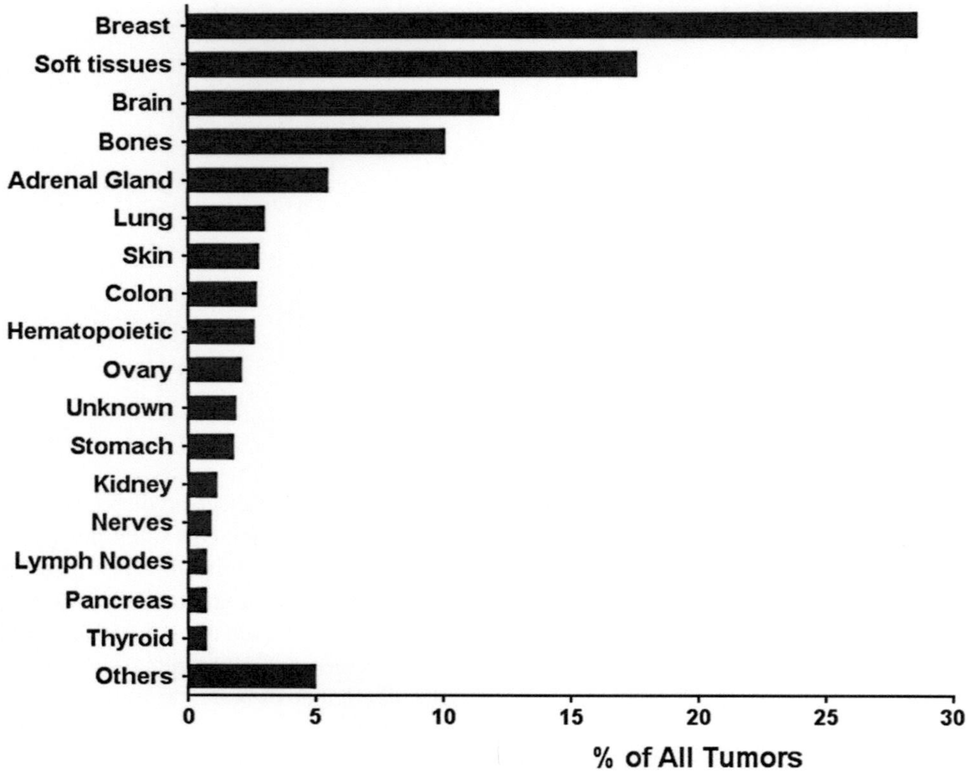

Figure 28.1 Tumor spectrum in individuals affected with LFS or LFL. The proportion of specific types of tumors among a total of 822 tumors reported in patients with LFS or LFL features is illustrated in the *bar graph*. Adapted from the International Association for Research on Cancer (IARC) database (R17, November 2013, http://p53.iarc.fr/)

second-degree relative with a typical LFS cancer (sarcoma, breast cancer, brain tumor, adrenal cortical tumor, or leukemia) at any age, and a first- or second-degree relative with any cancer under the age of 60 years [3]. A second definition of LFL is that the affected person can have two first- or second-degree relatives with LFS-related malignancies at any age [4]. The classic LFS criteria were refined and broadened to facilitate identification of individuals without immediate family history.

Breast cancer, brain tumor, and soft-tissue sarcoma account for more than 50 % of the tumors reported in patients with LFS or LFL features (Fig. 28.1) [5, 6]. Meanwhile, individuals with LFS are more likely to develop cancer at younger ages. Age-specific penetrance for cancer in LFS is about 50 % by age 30 years and 90 % by age 60 years. For individuals with LFS carrying germline mutations in the *TP53* gene, the median age of cancer onset can be even earlier [7–9]. In contrast, only 2 % of cancers occur under the age of 30 years in the general population [10]. Genetic testing is recommended for patients with multiple tumors, two of which represent characteristic LFS tumors diagnosed at age 36 or younger, or patients with adrenocortical carcinoma diagnosed at any age, regardless of family history [11].

Molecular Basis of Disease

Germline mutations in the tumor suppressor gene, *TP53*, are associated with LFS and LFL. The human *TP53* gene is located on chromosome 17p13.1. This gene spans approximately 20 kb on chromosome 17p13 with 11 exons of which exon 1 is not translated. The gene has multiple promoters and can give rise to multiple isoforms by alternate splicing. The *TP53* gene encodes the tumor protein p53 (TP53) that plays an important role in cell cycle control and apoptosis. As a DNA-binding protein, TP53 is composed of several functional domains: N-terminal transcription activation domains (TAD, consists of AD1 and AD2), the central DNA-binding domain (DBD), and the C-terminal tetramerization domain. Other important structural elements include the proline-rich domain, the C-terminal regulatory domain, and several nuclear localization or export signals. The central DNA-binding domain is crucial to the TP53 protein-DNA interaction and is the most frequent site for mutations, especially at codons 248, 273, and 213 (Fig. 28.2). Most of the posttranslational modification sites are localized in the C-terminal or N-terminal domains, which regulate the stability and activity of TP53 [12].

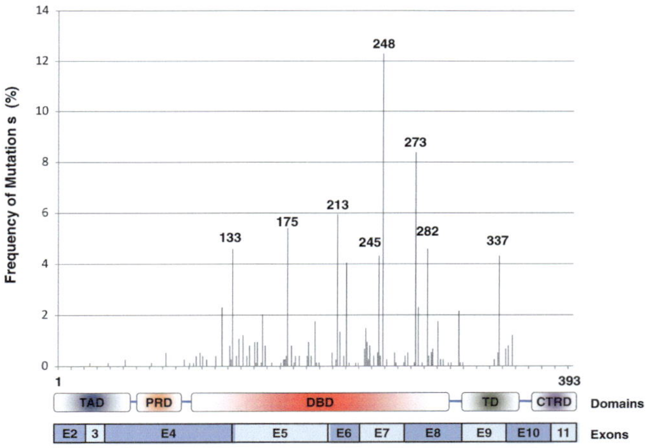

Figure 28.2 Structural organization of the coding exons of the *TP53* gene and functional domains of TP53 are illustrated at the *bottom* of the figure. Relative frequencies and codon positions of germline *TP53* mutations found in LFS and LFL families are *plotted*. Only single base substitutions and insertions/deletions in the codons are listed. Adapted from the International Association for Research on Cancer (IARC) database (R17, November 2013, http://p53.iarc.fr/)

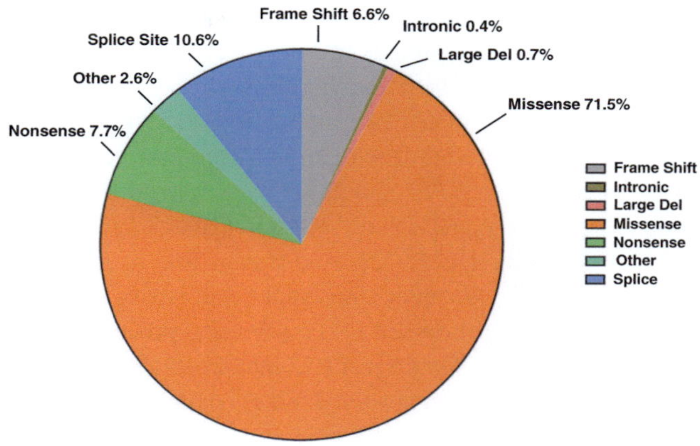

Figure 28.3 Types of germline mutations in the *TP53* gene found in LFS and LFL cases. *Pie chart* shows the percentage of the different types of observed mutations. Adapted from the International Association for Research on Cancer (IARC) database (R17, November 2013, http://p53.iarc.fr/)

The *TP53* gene is regarded as the guardian of the genome and is the most extensively studied tumor suppressor gene. In response to diverse cellular stresses, TP53 regulates a wide variety of genes involved in various cellular processes, including apoptosis, cell cycle, DNA damage repair, senescence, and cellular metabolism. In response to DNA damage caused by ionizing radiation or ultraviolet (UV) light, TP53 protein is stabilized by dissociation from its negative regulator, murine double minute 2 (MDM2). TP53 then translocates to the nucleus and activates the expression of relevant downstream genes, especially CDKN1A (*CIP1–WAF1*) [13]. CDKN1A protein can function as a cyclin-dependent kinase inhibitor and mediate the TP53-dependent G1-S cell cycle arrest through targeting cyclin-dependent kinases, such as CDK2 and CDK4. The activation of the cell cycle checkpoint facilitates the repair of damaged DNA [14].

Somatic *TP53* mutations occur in almost every type of cancer at varying frequencies, and they are more frequent in advanced stage or in more aggressive tumor types [15]. The International Agency for Research on Cancer (IARC) maintains a regularly updated database of all known *TP53* gene variations and mutations (germline and somatic) identified in human tumor samples (http://TP53.iarc.fr/). As of November 2013, the R17 release of IARC TP53 database contains 750 germline mutations, 28,000 somatic mutations, and TP53 mutation status of 2,700 cell lines. The database also includes functional data of 2,314 mutant TP53 proteins. The codon distribution and relative frequencies of germline mutations in *TP53* as observed in LFS or LFL families are summarized in Fig. 28.2. The spectrum of different types of *TP53* mutations observed in LFS and LFL is summarized in Fig. 28.3 (R17, November 2013) [5, 6, 16].

The majority of the germline mutations (83.7 %) reside within the central DBD, which can interfere with the ability of TP53 to bind to its target DNA sequences. Common mutations found in LFS and LFL families occur in codons 175, 213, 245, 248, 273, and 337 and account for 39 % of all the single base substitutions. Many tumor suppressor genes like *RB1* and *APC* are mainly altered by nonsense or truncating mutations. In contrast, the majority of germline *TP53* mutations found in LFS and LFL families are missense substitutions (71.5 %). Other alterations include splice site mutations (10.6 %), nonsense mutations (7.7 %), frameshift mutations (6.6 %), and other infrequent alterations such as large deletion (<1 %) and deep intronic mutations (<1 %) (Fig. 28.3) [5, 6]. Heterozygous deletion of the entire *TP53* gene has been observed in one of 79 LFS families without any coding sequence mutation in *TP53* [17]. Attwooll and colleagues detected a single nucleotide deletion within the *TP53* promoter region in two of 18 LFS/LFL families without an identifiable *TP53* coding sequence mutation. Later, their data indicated that this mutation does not have any functional consequence and is a rare polymorphism [18].

The results of sequence analysis of the entire coding region of *TP53* indicate that 60–80 % classic LFS families carry germline *TP53* mutations, while only 8–22 % of individuals with LFL have detectable mutations [19]. The frequency of de novo mutations in LFS is approximately 7–20 % [8, 9]. The reasons for a lower detection rate of *TP53* mutations in LFS families include undetected intronic or cytogenetic lesions of the *TP53* gene, other genes predisposing to LFS, or the presence of mutations in modifier genes.

The variability of the cancer spectrum and age of onset within LFS families suggests the presence of modifier genes. One of the plausible candidate genes is *MDM2*, which is a negative regulator of TP53 through its E3 ubiquitin ligase activity [20]. A single nucleotide polymorphism (SNP) within the promoter region of *MDM2*, SNP309 T>G (dbSNP ID, rs2279744), has been associated with earlier onset of tumors among germline *TP53* mutation carriers [21, 22]. It has also been suggested that there is a cumulative effect in cases where both *MDM2*-SNP309 polymorphism and *TP53* codon 72Arg variant (R72P, dbSNP ID, rs1042522) are present in LFS patients [21, 22]. A different line of evidence from Tabori and colleagues suggested the presence of accelerated telomere attrition in LFS families and postulated that the shorter telomere length in *TP53* mutant carriers can predict genetic anticipation observed in LFS patients and serves as a rational biological marker [23].

The relatively low frequency of detectable germline mutations in *TP53* in many LFS and LFL probands suggests the possible involvement of other genes, which may or may not directly involve in the TP53 pathway. The candidates include but are not limited to *p63*, *p73*, *BCL10*, *BAX*, *CDKN2A*, *PTEN*, *BRCA1*, *BRCA2*, *CHEK1*, and *CHEK2* genes. However, despite numerous efforts to screen these genes for mutations, studies have not detected any high-penetrance mutations [19, 24, 25]. For example, 1100delC and I157T mutations in the *CHEK2* gene have been recurrently found in LFS families and possibly represent low-penetrance mutations, which confer increased risk for breast, prostate, and thyroid cancer [19].

It has been generally accepted that mutation in all tumor suppressor genes will act in a recessive manner, which means both alleles should be inactivated to cause tumor initiation and progression [26]. Although the majority of *TP53* mutations are missense mutations that reside within the central DNA-binding domain, loss of heterozygosity is only identified in approximately 60 % of tumors [27, 28]. Approximately two-thirds of the tumors arising in LFS patients carry missense mutations on one allele of *TP53* while the other *TP53* allele remains as wild type. One explanation is that the mutant form of TP53 can exert a dominant negative effect and functionally inactivate the wild-type TP53. Various lines of evidence further indicate that certain *TP53* mutations may result in new TP53 functions that contribute to tumor initiation and progression and are referred to as gain-of-function mutations [29].

Clinical Utility of Testing

According to the practice guidelines in oncology (v.1.2010, of National Comprehensive Cancer Network (NCCN) http://www.nccn.org/professionals/physician_gls/f_guidelines.asp), *TP53* gene testing is considered necessary for individuals with a known family history of a *TP53* mutation, or with a suspected or known clinical diagnosis of LFS or LFL, or with a diagnosis of early-onset breast cancer before 30 years with a negative *BRCA1* and *BRCA2* test. Testing also is recommended if there is a family history of sarcoma, brain tumor, or adrenocortical carcinoma. Several general recommendations and guidelines are available regarding diagnostic testing for germline *TP53* mutations among cancer-prone individuals [30]. Individuals chosen for genetic testing on the basis of their family histories should be given current, relevant information on the test to make an informed voluntary decision.

Since cancers occur with high frequency among children in LFS families, testing these children (rather than delaying testing until young adulthood) is recommended. However, as children mature, obtaining of their assent or dissent to testing is appropriate, as well as the consent of their parents. Annual surveillance strategies are recommended for at-risk children and include complete physical examination, urinalysis, blood count, and abdominal ultrasound examination. Additional organ-targeted surveillance based on family history (e.g., imaging studies of the head if a relative had a childhood brain tumor) also is recommended.

For women with early-onset breast cancer with a negative *BRCA1* and *BRCA2* gene mutation, *TP53* gene testing is only meaningful in the context of a family history characteristic of classic LFS or LFL criteria. Several studies have shown that the likelihood of a germline *TP53* mutation in this population can range from 0–7 %, even if no family history of cancer is present [8, 9, 31, 32]. Females with a germline *TP53* mutation have the option of prophylactic mastectomy to reduce the risk of breast cancer [33]. Routine mammograms and clinical breast examinations are effective in women over age 40 years, but have not been proven to be beneficial for younger women with LFS or LFL. However, controversy exists regarding the use of routine mammograms in women with LFS, because of possible radiation sensitivity associated with *TP53* mutations [10, 34]. In addition, based on family history of specific cancers, colonoscopies or full-body MRI examination or PET scan has been suggested

Available Assays

Several approaches to clinical testing for *TP53* are used, but most use sequence analysis due to the distribution of mutations throughout the gene. A comprehensive list of available clinical tests is available through the Genetic Testing Registry database (http://www.ncbi.nlm.nih.gov/gtr/).

For sequence analysis, PCR amplification of the entire coding region of TP53 (exons 2–11) and the immediate flanking intronic sequences is performed on genomic DNA isolated from blood or saliva of the proband(s). Direct sequencing is performed using traditional automated fluorescent dideoxynucleotide sequencing. Approximately 75 % of disease-causing mutations can be identified in exons 5–8 of the *TP53* gene by sequence analysis [27]. Identified sequence variations can be classified as pathogenic mutations, benign variants, or variations of unknown clinical significance. Splice site mutations are common (12 %) in LFS and LFL probands [5, 6]. Further interpretation of the results of molecular analysis is usually based on the clinical presentation and family history of the patient.

Traditional direct sequencing strategies described above cannot identify mutations within the promoter region or deep intronic regions and will also miss genomic rearrangements involving partial or entire *TP53* gene. In cases where no coding sequence mutations are detected, deletion/duplication analysis should be used to determine the relative copy numbers of the coding exons of *TP53*. Several methods including quantitative PCR (copy number analysis), multiplex ligation-dependent probe amplification (MLPA), long-range PCR, or array-based comparative genomic hybridization (aCGH) are available. For detection of deep intronic splice site mutations, reverse-transcription polymerase chain reaction (RT-PCR) of RNA followed by sequencing can be used. IHC staining for TP53 is extensively utilized in clinical histopathology laboratories. The rationale of this method is based on the observation that mutant TP53 usually has a much longer half-life than wild-type protein and gives rise to a diffuse nuclear staining. However, the correlation between an abnormal TP53 staining pattern and the presence of sequence mutations can be imperfect [35].

Presymptomatic screening has been effective and beneficial to high-risk family members of some common hereditary cancer syndromes (Lynch syndrome, hereditary breast and ovarian cancers, etc.). But whether genetic screening for LFS can affect prognosis positively is still under debate because no preventive treatment options are currently available to high-risk individuals [19]. Also, presymptomatic testing raises concerns about the potential adverse psychological impact of positive results, risks to relationships with family members, and insurability or even employability [36].

Prenatal testing and preimplantation genetic diagnosis (PGD) are available for families with LFS in which the disease-causing mutation has been or can be identified. For prenatal diagnosis, fetal DNA can be obtained by chorionic villus sampling (CVS) which is performed at 10–12 weeks of gestation or by amniocentesis performed at 15–18 weeks of gestation. PGD has recently been offered for couples with an inherited predisposition for genetic diseases including LFS. Using a standard in vitro fertilization procedure, single cells from 8- to 16-cell-stage embryos are tested for different mutations predisposing to disease, and embryos without a mutation are selected and transferred back to the uterus of the mother for implantation. Despite existing controversy on the use of PGD, existing data demonstrate the usefulness of this approach as the only acceptable option for at-risk couples to avoid the birth of children with an inherited predisposition to cancer and to have a healthy child [37].

Interpretation of Results

Currently, the classification of LFS and LFL is based on clinical criteria, which means the family history or pedigree must meet the diagnostic guidelines of the diseases. In order to confirm the suspected diagnosis of LFS or LFL in a proband, or identify at-risk individuals among LFS/LFL families, sequencing of the *TP53* gene is recommended following the clinical diagnosis. Approximately 60–80 % of families with LFS have an identifiable germline *TP53* mutation, and the detection rate is even lower in LFL families [19, 38]. The percent of families with LFL syndrome who have an identifiable *TP53* mutation varies from 8 % using Eele's definition to 22 % using Birch's definition [10]. Classic LFS criteria have been estimated to have a high positive predictive value and a high specificity, but the sensitivity is reported to be relatively low (approximately 40 %). The sensitivity of the LFL criteria has been estimated to be higher, although the estimated specificity is relatively low [8, 9]. Special attention should be paid to the cases of de novo germline *TP53* mutations, because these families, which are infrequent, may not be classified as LFS or LFL by classic clinical criteria due to the absence of a family history [2].

Irrespective of the *TP53* mutation status, LFS is a highly penetrant cancer syndrome. Individuals with LFS are also at increased risk for developing multiple primary tumors. A retrospective study of 200 affected members of families with LFS found that 15 % had developed a second cancer, 4 % a third cancer, and 2 % a total of four cancers. In this cohort, survivors of childhood cancers were found to have the highest risks for developing additional malignancies [39].

Due to variable expression and differential penetrance of different *TP53* mutations, genotype-phenotype correlation for LFS is complicated. Even for the same codon, multiple mutations can occur at different frequencies and confer different phenotypes. For example, three different mutations have been documented at codon 337, which is located in the homo-oligomerization domain of TP53: R337H (CGC>CAC, 80 %), R337C (CGC>TGC, 13.9 %), and R337P (CGC>CAC, 6.1 %). The R337H mutation is presumed to be preferentially associated with cancer development in the adrenal cortex and may have a pH-dependent defect in oligomerization. Due to the fact that the R337H mutant may still largely maintain wild-type TP53 activity in vivo, it may be less penetrant with respect to tumor predisposition when compared to other variants, like R337S [40–42]. However, another study indicates that the spectrum of cancers seen in families with R337H mutation is similar to that of LFL families carrying other types of *TP53* mutations [5, 6].

The mean ages of tumor onset are reported to vary significantly between patients with missense mutations compared to other types of mutations (splicing, nonsense, and deletions) in *TP53*. Various lines of evidence further indicate that the *TP53* missense mutations are gain-of-function mutations that can contribute to tumor initiation and progression [29, 31]. At the same time, certain kinds of mutations in *TP53*, such as missense mutations that involve codons 152 and 158, are known to confer a lower cancer risk [43]. Large heterozygous deletions that encompass the entire *TP53* gene as well as up to 2 Mb of upstream and downstream sequences do not seem to confer increased cancer risk when the remaining allele is intact [44]. Therefore, not all *TP53* mutations are functionally equivalent, and different amino acid substitutions can lead to different consequences for TP53 structure and function that, in turn, may significantly influence clinical outcome.

Laboratory Issues

DNA sequencing is the most commonly used method for *TP53* genetic testing due to the wide distribution of mutations throughout the *TP53* gene. General practice guidelines for both the sequencing procedure and the interpretation of data all apply in the clinical testing for *TP53* mutation. First of all, the samples for genetic testing should be collected, identified, shipped, stored, and processed under quality-controlled conditions that maintain the DNA integrity and proper identification of the specimen. Genomic DNA from peripheral blood lymphocytes is typically used for testing. Alternative sources such as saliva, tumor tissue, formalin-fixed paraffin-embedded (FFPE) tissue, cultured amniocytes, or CVS can be used but require special quality control measures during sample processing, sequencing reactions, data analysis, and interpretation. For example, DNA from FFPE tissue generally yields poorer sequence reads because of degradation and/or chemical cross-linking. Special caution should be exercised to recover as much usable DNA as possible from FFPE tissue. Decreasing the amplicon size (<300 bp) also may improve the efficiency of PCR and sequencing.

The standard quality control measures for DNA sequencing, such as inclusion of both negative and positive controls, should be routinely performed. To eliminate the possibility of sample mix-up, all identified mutations in *TP53* can be confirmed by an independent sequencing assay on a DNA sample isolated at a different time from the first isolation. Bidirectional sequencing is also recommended for confirmation of heterozygous or homozygous mutations. The presence of a de novo or mosaic mutation requires careful analysis of bidirectional sequence reads.

False-negative results can occur for several reasons. Allele dropout due to presence of SNPs or indels (INsertion/DELetion) at the binding sites of sequencing primers can lead to allele dropout (amplification failure of one allele). Primers should be designed outside of the known polymorphic regions. Low-level tissue mosaicism, the preferential amplification of the smaller allele caused by a large indel, and exon or gene deletion also can produce false-negative results. Also of note, traditional sequencing panels that include only the coding exons and limited flanking intronic regions cannot detect deep intronic mutations, translocations, inversions, or copy number variations involving large chromosome regions. Other technologies, such as long-range PCR, MLPA, SNP array hybridization assays, aCGH, and next-generation sequencing technology, can address these issues.

Conclusions

LFS and LFL are autosomal dominantly inherited cancer predisposition syndromes. Mutations in the *TP53* gene are associated with 60–80 % of LFS and 8–22 % of LFL families. Irrespective of the *TP53* mutation status, the risk of specific LFS-associated cancers in first-degree relatives of a proband with LFS is significantly higher compared to the general population. Genetic testing for *TP53* mutations can identify presymptomatic individuals at risk of cancer and have important implications for clinical diagnosis, counseling, monitoring, and clinical management of LFS and LFL individuals. The benefits of surveillance and genetic testing in changing disease-related morbidity and mortality are still evolving.

References

1. Li FP, Fraumeni Jr JF. Soft-tissue sarcomas, breast cancer, and other neoplasms. A familial syndrome? Ann Intern Med. 1969;71(4):747–52.
2. Chompret A, Brugieres L, et al. P53 germline mutations in childhood cancers and cancer risk for carrier individuals. Br J Cancer. 2000;82(12):1932–7.
3. Birch JM, Hartley AL, et al. Prevalence and diversity of constitutional mutations in the p53 gene among 21 Li-Fraumeni families. Cancer Res. 1994;54(5):1298–304.
4. Eeles RA. Germline mutations in the TP53 gene. Cancer Surv. 1995;25:101–24.
5. Petitjean A, Achatz MI, et al. TP53 mutations in human cancers: functional selection and impact on cancer prognosis and outcomes. Oncogene. 2007;26(15):2157–65.
6. Petitjean A, Mathe E, et al. Impact of mutant p53 functional properties on TP53 mutation patterns and tumor phenotype: lessons from recent developments in the IARC TP53 database. Hum Mutat. 2007;28(6):622–9.

7. Lustbader ED, Williams WR, et al. Segregation analysis of cancer in families of childhood soft-tissue-sarcoma patients. Am J Hum Genet. 1992;51(2):344–56.
8. Gonzalez KD, Noltner KA, et al. Beyond Li Fraumeni Syndrome: clinical characteristics of families with p53 germline mutations. J Clin Oncol. 2009;27(8):1250–6.
9. Gonzalez KD, Buzin CH, et al. High frequency of de novo mutations in Li-Fraumeni syndrome. J Med Genet. 2009;46:689–93.
10. Varley JM, Evans DG, et al. Li-Fraumeni syndrome–a molecular and clinical review. Br J Cancer. 1997;76(1):1–14.
11. Chompret A et al. Sensitivity and predictive value of criteria for p53 germline mutation screening. J Med Genet. 2001;38:43–7.
12. Whibley C, Pharoah PD, et al. p53 polymorphisms: cancer implications. Nat Rev Cancer. 2009;9(2):95–107.
13. Lakin ND, Jackson SP. Regulation of p53 in response to DNA damage. Oncogene. 1999;18(53):7644–55.
14. Harper JW, Adami GR, et al. The p21 Cdk-interacting protein Cip1 is a potent inhibitor of G1 cyclin-dependent kinases. Cell. 1993;75(4):805–16.
15. Olivier M, Hollstein M, et al. TP53 mutations in human cancers: origins, consequences, and clinical use. Cold Spring Harb Perspect Biol. 2010;2(1):a001008.
16. Olivier M, Eeles R, et al. The IARC TP53 database: new online mutation analysis and recommendations to users. Hum Mutat. 2002;19(6):607–14.
17. Bougeard G, Brugieres L, et al. Screening for TP53 rearrangements in families with the Li-Fraumeni syndrome reveals a complete deletion of the TP53 gene. Oncogene. 2003;22(6):840–6.
18. Attwooll CL, McGown G, et al. Identification of a rare polymorphism in the human TP53 promoter. Cancer Genet Cytogenet. 2002;135(2):165–72.
19. Malkin D. Li-Fraumeni syndrome. Genes Cancer. 2011;2(4):475–84.
20. Takagi M, Absalon MJ, et al. Regulation of p53 translation and induction after DNA damage by ribosomal protein L26 and nucleolin. Cell. 2005;123(1):49–63.
21. Bond GL, Hirshfield KM, et al. MDM2 SNP309 accelerates tumor formation in a gender-specific and hormone-dependent manner. Cancer Res. 2006;66(10):5104–10.
22. Bougeard G, Baert-Desurmont S, et al. Impact of the MDM2 SNP309 and p53 Arg72Pro polymorphism on age of tumour onset in Li-Fraumeni syndrome. J Med Genet. 2006;43(6):531–3.
23. Tabori U, Nanda S, et al. Younger age of cancer initiation is associated with shorter telomere length in Li-Fraumeni syndrome. Cancer Res. 2007;67(4):1415–8.
24. Bougeard G, Limacher JM, et al. Detection of 11 germline inactivating TP53 mutations and absence of TP63 and HCHK2 mutations in 17 French families with Li-Fraumeni or Li-Fraumeni-like syndrome. J Med Genet. 2001;38(4):253–7.
25. Evans DG, Wu CL, et al. BRCA2: a cause of Li-Fraumeni-like syndrome. J Med Genet. 2008;45(1):62–3.
26. Knudson Jr AG. Mutation and cancer: statistical study of retinoblastoma. Proc Natl Acad Sci U S A. 1971;68(4):820–3.
27. Varley JM. Germline TP53 mutations and Li-Fraumeni syndrome. Hum Mutat. 2003;21(3):313–20.
28. Berger AH, Pandolfi PP. Haplo-insufficiency: a driving force in cancer. J Pathol. 2011;223(2):137–46.
29. Oren M, Rotter V. Mutant p53 gain-of-function in cancer. Cold Spring Harb Perspect Biol. 2010;2(2):a001107.
30. Li FP, Garber JE, et al. Recommendations on predictive testing for germ line p53 mutations among cancer-prone individuals. J Natl Cancer Inst. 1992;84(15):1156–60.
31. Bougeard G, Sesboue R, et al. Molecular basis of the Li-Fraumeni syndrome: an update from the French LFS families. J Med Genet. 2008;45(8):535–8.
32. Ginsburg OM, Akbari MR, et al. The prevalence of germ-line TP53 mutations in women diagnosed with breast cancer before age 30. Fam Cancer. 2009;8(4):563–7.
33. Thull DL, Vogel VG. Recognition and management of hereditary breast cancer syndromes. Oncologist. 2004;9(1):13–24.
34. Eng C, Hampel H, et al. Genetic testing for cancer predisposition. Annu Rev Med. 2001;52:371–400.
35. Kressner U, Inganas M, et al. Prognostic value of p53 genetic changes in colorectal cancer. J Clin Oncol. 1999;17(2):593–9.
36. Lammens CR, Aaronson NK, et al. Genetic testing in Li-Fraumeni syndrome: uptake and psychosocial consequences. J Clin Oncol. 2010;28(18):3008–14.
37. Simpson JL, Carson SA, et al. Preimplantation genetic diagnosis (PGD) for heritable neoplasia. J Natl Cancer Inst Monogr. 2005;34:87–90.
38. Nichols KE, Malkin D, et al. Germ-line p53 mutations predispose to a wide spectrum of early-onset cancers. Cancer Epidemiol Biomarkers Prev. 2001;10(2):83–7.
39. Hisada M, Garber JE, et al. Multiple primary cancers in families with Li-Fraumeni syndrome. J Natl Cancer Inst. 1998;90(8):606–11.
40. DiGiammarino EL, Lee AS, et al. A novel mechanism of tumorigenesis involving pH-dependent destabilization of a mutant p53 tetramer. Nat Struct Biol. 2002;9(1):12–6.
41. Ribeiro RC, Sandrini F, et al. An inherited p53 mutation that contributes in a tissue-specific manner to pediatric adrenal cortical carcinoma. Proc Natl Acad Sci U S A. 2001;98(16):9330–5.
42. Pinto EM, Ribeiro RC, et al. TP53-associated pediatric malignancies. Genes Cancer. 2011;2(4):485–90.
43. Varley JM, McGown G, et al. Are there low-penetrance TP53 Alleles? evidence from childhood adrenocortical tumors. Am J Hum Genet. 1999;65(4):995–1006.
44. Shlien A, Baskin B, et al. A common molecular mechanism underlies two phenotypically distinct 17p13.1 microdeletion syndromes. Am J Hum Genet. 2010;87(5):631–42.

29 Retinoblastoma

Arupa Ganguly and Zhao Chen

Abstract

Retinoblastoma (RB) is the most common primary intraocular malignancy of childhood associated with blindness and mortality. Mortality from RB has been significantly reduced with earlier diagnosis and improved methods of treatment. Biallelic inactivation of the tumor suppressor gene, *RB1*, is the cause of retinoblastoma. Multistep genetic analyses, including DNA sequencing, Southern blot, transcript promoter methylation analysis, and real-time PCR, have been used to characterize potential genetic abnormalities of *RB1*. Predisposing germline *RB1* mutations can be detected in 90–95 % of probands with heritable RB, while the detection rate is about 13 % for individuals with unilateral RB. Due to the presence of low-level mosaicism, chromosome rearrangements, or deep intronic splice site changes, detection of mutations can be challenging. The absence of detectable *RB1* mutations in a subset of unilateral RB tumors or in bilateral cases suggests the presence of alternate genetic mechanisms. A subset of unilateral RB tumors is associated with amplification of the *MYCN* oncogene.

Keywords

Retinoblastoma • Childhood onset cancer • Ocular malignancy • *RB1* gene • Genetic test • Genetic counseling

Introduction

Retinoblastoma (RB) is the most common intraocular cancer in children and occurs at a frequency of approximately 1 in 20,000 live births with about 300 new cases diagnosed each year in the USA and about 5,000 cases worldwide [1, 2]. Clinically, RB can present as bilateral (both eyes) or unilateral (one eye) disease, with or without a family history. The individuals with a family history of RB have the hereditary form. Individuals with hereditary RB most often present with bilateral disease at an early age of onset and infrequently as unilateral disease with multiple foci (Table 29.1) [3, 4]. From 5–15 % of patients with hereditary RB develop "trilateral" RB, defined as an additional pineoblastoma, a primitive neuroectodermal tumor located in the pineal region of the brain. The chance of pineoblastoma is only 0.5 % among unilateral cases [5]. Individuals with heritable RB also have higher risk for second primary tumors, such as osteosarcomas, soft tissue sarcomas, or melanomas. These non-ocular tumors usually occur in adolescence or adulthood. For patients who have been exposed to external beam radiation, the incidence of second non-ocular tumors can increase up to 50 % [6, 7]. Individuals with unilateral disease usually have the nonhereditary form of RB. In the past 25 years, the genetic basis of RB has been unraveled and new insights into the molecular pathogenesis of RB have evolved. This understanding has allowed for more effective approaches to clinical management and resulted in greater than 85–90 % cure rate for RB in developed countries. A subset of unilateral RB tumors without detectable mutation in the *RB1* gene is associated with amplification of the *MYCN* oncogene [8].

A. Ganguly, Ph.D. (✉) • Z. Chen, Ph.D.
Department of Genetics, Perelman School of Medicine, University of Pennsylvania, 415 Curie Boulevard, Room 500, Philadelphia, PA 19104, USA
e-mail: ganguly@mail.med.upenn.edu

D.G.B. Leonard (ed.), *Molecular Pathology in Clinical Practice*, DOI 10.1007/978-3-319-19674-9_29

Table 29.1 Features that distinguish heritable from nonheritable retinoblastoma

Tumor type	Heritable retinoblastoma	Nonheritable retinoblastoma
Eyes affected	Bilateral in 90–95 % of cases	Unilateral in 100 % of cases
	Unilateral in remaining cases	
Age of onset	Usually < 1 year	Variable — < 1–5 years
Presence of family history	10–20 % of newly diagnosed cases	Negative
Risk of second malignancy	5–15 %	0.5 %
Recurrence risk	50 % risk of passing on an *RB1* mutation to an offspring	Almost zero. Very low risk of passing on an *RB1* mutation due to presence of germline mosaicism

Molecular Basis of Disease

RB is caused by biallelic inactivation of the *RB1* gene. Friend and colleagues identified the *RB1* gene in 1986, the first tumor suppressor gene to be cloned [9]. The gene consists of 27 exons that span 183 kilobases of genomic DNA on chromosome 13q14 (Fig. 29.1). *RB1* encodes a 928 amino acid protein known as RB1, which is a nuclear phosphoprotein that plays a critical role in regulating cell cycle progression at the G1 to S phase transition. The regulatory activity of RB1 results from its ability to bind to and inhibit the function of the E2F families of transcription factors, which regulate multiple genes involved in S-phase entry. Unphosphorylated RB1 binds to the E2F/DP (dimerization partners of E2F) complex through a critical functional region containing RB1 A/B pocket domains. The pocket domains are encoded by exons 12 through 17 and 20 through 22 of the *RB1* gene and are hotspots for inactivating mutations in RB and other cancers. The C-terminal region of RB1 contains the nuclear localization signal and the interaction motif that is the target site of cyclin-CDK (cyclin-dependent kinase) complexes. The C-terminal region can also bind to the nuclear c-Abl tyrosine kinase and MDM2 (Mdm2, TP53 E3 ubiquitin protein ligase homolog [mouse]), which have oncogenic properties (Fig. 29.1). In the presence of mitogenic or oncogenic stimuli, RB1 is phosphorylated by CDKs (CDK4 and CDK6) and dissociates from E2F/DP complexes, which leads to the release of inhibition of E2F target genes and progression through the cell cycle (Fig. 29.2) [10, 11].

Inactivation of the RB1 pathway through direct perturbation of the *RB1* gene (deletion, mutation, or epigenetic mechanisms) leads to deregulated cell proliferation and ultimately tumorigenesis. Recent evidence suggests that *RB1* also plays important roles in multiple cellular processes beyond cell cycle regulation, such as mitochondria biogenesis, cell senescence, and others [12]. Inactivation of the RB1 pathway also can cause a mitotic defect, and genomic instability and aneuploidy [12, 13].

RB has served as the paradigm for the "two-hit" model of tumorigenesis [14]. The Knudson hypothesis is that inactivation of both alleles of *RB1* (two "hits") is necessary to develop RB. In children with hereditary RB, the first hit is the germline mutation on one allele of *RB1*. The second hit is a somatic inactivation event on the remaining allele which

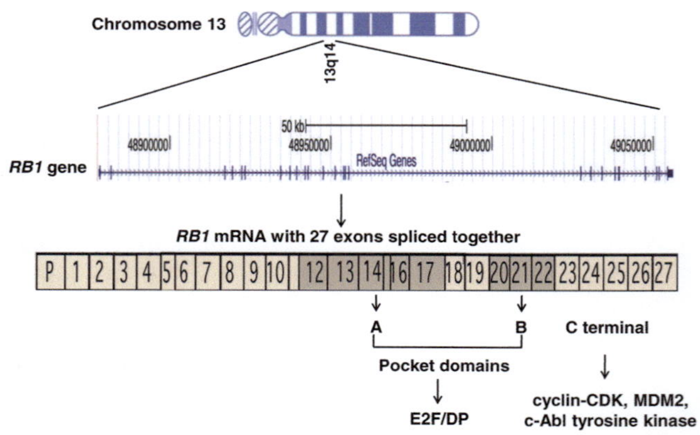

Figure 29.1 Genomic location and structure of the *RB1* gene on chromosome 13q14 and spanning 183,000 bases. The 27 exons encode the 928 amino acid RB1 protein. The *shaded exons* encode the pocket domains A and B of RB1, which mediate interactions with the E2F and DP families of transcription factors

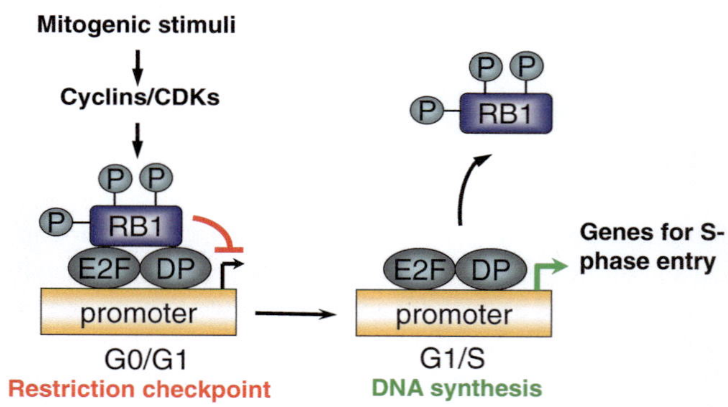

Figure 29.2 A simplified model for RB1 function. RB1 is hypophosphorylated during the G0/G1 phase of the cell cycle and interacts with E2F/DP family of transcription factors that inhibit transcription of downstream genes. In the presence of mitogenic stimuli, the cyclin-dependent kinase 4 (CDK4) protein phosphorylates RB1, which releases the E2F/DP factors and induces gene expression leading to the G1/S transition and progression through the cell cycle

includes point mutations, intragenic rearrangements, or hypermethylation of the promoter region and causes inactivation of RB1 protein and initiation of RB. In about 65 % of the RB cases, the second hit to the *RB1* gene is accomplished by the mechanism of loss of heterozygosity (LOH), which can result from deletions or chromosomal rearrangements affecting *RB1* [15]. In children with nonhereditary RB, the tumors develop as the result of two somatic *RB1* inactivation events in a retinal progenitor or precursor cell during embryonic development.

The presentation of RB can be classified in three categories: familial hereditary (5–10 %), de novo hereditary (20–30 %), or sporadic (60–70 %) [16]. Familial hereditary cases are characterized by a positive family history and germline mutations in *RB1* in individuals that present with bilateral disease in most cases and unilateral disease in 10–15 % of cases. However, only 20 % of bilateral cases and 15 % of unilateral cases have a positive family history and inherit the mutation from one of the parents. For individuals carrying a germline mutation in *RB1*, the risk of transmission of the mutation to an offspring is 50 %. In 80 % of newly diagnosed bilateral cases, the family history is negative and RB is caused by a de novo germline mutation on one of the parental germ cells. These represent the 20–30 % of sporadic hereditary cases with de novo mutations. In 90 % of these sporadic bilateral cases, the de novo mutation occurs on the paternal allele [17]. Approximately 60 % of RB cases are sporadic and nonheritable, with a unilateral presentation. Germline mutations are not present in the sporadic unilateral cases, and the risk of passing on the mutant allele to offspring is very low. There are reports of gonadal mosaicism in the parents of children with RB. In this setting, instead of being a single de novo event in one germ cell, a subset of the parental gametes carries the mutant *RB1* allele. The degree of mosaicism determines the risk of transmitting the mutant allele to future offspring. Thus, the risk of RB in the siblings of a sporadic heritable RB case should not be underestimated.

Almost all types of mutations have been identified in the *RB1* gene, including point mutations, deletions, translocations, insertions, and epigenetic changes. Conventional cytogenetic analysis of peripheral blood lymphocytes can identify deletions or rearrangements involving 13q14 in approximately 8 % of bilateral cases and 1–5 % of sporadic unilateral cases [15]. Smaller deletions in the *RB1* region are identified in approximately 10 % of bilateral RB cases by Southern blot analysis [15]. Approximately half of all defined *RB1* mutations are caused by single-base substitutions in coding exons, one third by small frameshift mutations, and another 10 % by rearrangements, such as intragenic or intergenic deletions or duplications involving chromosome 13q. These rearrangements may be limited to the *RB1* gene or include genes flanking the *RB1* locus [15, 18–21]. Nichols et al. carried out an investigation of a total of 180 RB cases, and the frequencies of germline mutations detected in bilateral, familial unilateral, and sporadic unilateral cases were 91 %, 70 %, and 7 %, respectively. Of the identified mutations, 76 % were coding sequence mutations, and 14 % were deletions of individual or multiple exons or the whole *RB1* gene [22].

The majority (70 %) of mutations identified in *RB1* are nonsense mutations or frameshift mutations, which lead to premature termination codons. Approximately 76 % of these nonsense mutations are recurrent CGA>TGA transitions affecting one of the 12 CGA codons within the open reading frame of *RB1*. Approximately 10 % of identified single-base substitutions are missense mutations, most of which localize to the pocket domains of RB1. Very few mutations have been identified in the promoter region of *RB1* or exons 25–27, although this region contains two CGA codons [15]. A recent study reported the presence of a germline frameshift mutation in exon 27 in an unaffected father of a child with unilateral RB. Interestingly, the mutant transcript showed reduced expression, which might explain the milder unilateral disease manifestation [23]. Thus, unlike similar mutations located elsewhere in the gene, truncating mutations in the last exon of *RB1* may be unique in their clinical presentations.

In addition to coding sequence variations, mutations affecting the conserved nucleotides in 5′ and 3′ splice sites within *RB1* introns are observed in approximately 18 % of RB cases [15]. *RB1* has 26 introns and the sizes of the introns range from small (intron 15 with 80 base pairs [bp]) to very large (intron 17 with 71,500 bp). While splice site mutations at the exon–intron junctions can be detected by routine sequence analysis, mutations located deep within the introns can be missed without analysis of the *RB1* mRNA. A few cases harboring deep intronic mutations have been documented by cDNA analysis. These deep intronic mutations usually generate cryptic splice sites and cause retention of intronic sequences, which lead to subsequent frameshift and premature termination of translation [22, 24, 25]. Furthermore, missense or nonsense mutations that flank the consensus sequences of splice sites also may give rise to aberrant splicing [22]. Hypermethylation of CpG dinucleotides within the promoter region of *RB1* can lead to gene silencing and is a somatic event in approximately 10 % of RB tumors and is almost never observed in constitutional cells [26, 27].

As described earlier, RB has a high rate of de novo mutations, which can originate at the preconception or postconception stage leading to germline or somatic mosaicism, respectively. Preconception mutation events occur mainly during spermatogenesis [17, 28]. Postzygotic events can occur at earlier stages of embryo development, and the mosaicism may extend to various organs and tissues, including retina or even gonads. Postzygotic germline mosaicism can occur on either paternal or maternal alleles, and the mosaic mutations can be detected in lymphocyte DNA in some cases [28, 29]. Mosaicism for *RB1* mutation should always be taken into account in genetic diagnosis, counseling, and disease management. In 1998, Sippel and colleagues reported that germline mosaicism occurs in up to 10 % of families with newly diagnosed RB using combined technologies of single-strand conformational polymorphism and pedigree analysis [30].

Approximately 10 % of RB cases are caused by heterozygous deletions of chromosome 13q that include the *RB1* gene. The sizes of the deletions vary from small (4,000 bases) to large (34 million bases) and the breakpoints are usually nonrecurrent [31]. Because larger deletions may involve many other genes besides *RB1*, individuals with deletions of 13q14 can exhibit other clinical manifestations in addition to RB. As might be expected, the length of the deletion seems to define the spectrum of clinical manifestations, with smaller deletions (those confined to 13q14) associated with macrocephaly, tall stature, obesity, and motor and/or speech delays, and larger deletions manifesting with characteristic craniofacial features, microcephaly, psychomotor delays, and other findings such as constipation and feeding problems [3, 31–33]. Interestingly, deletions larger than 1 Mb and encompassing the *MED4* gene, which encodes a mediator of RNA polymerase type II, are associated with a milder phenotype (i.e., unilateral eye involvement and less penetrant disease) [31]. The mechanism by which deletion of *MED4* lessens the severity of RB disease is unclear; however, reduced expression and nonpenetrance in carriers of large deletions might result from the loss of one or more genes contiguous with *RB1* that are important for basic cellular functions. In a susceptible retinal cell, loss of the second copy of these critical genes may lead to cell death as opposed to tumor formation.

Finally, interfamilial or intrafamilial variations of phenotypic expression of identical *RB1* mutations have been observed among RB families. This indicates that additional genetic factors modify genotype–phenotype correlations in RB [3, 34, 35]. For example, Klutz et al. reported the parent-of-origin effect in two unrelated families that segregate an identical base substitution within intron 6 of *RB1* gene. The substitution leads to exon skipping and a frameshift mutation that creates a premature termination codon. In addition to the fact that both families show incomplete penetrance, carriers who inherited the mutant allele from the maternal germline are unaffected, while carriers who inherited the mutant allele from the paternal germline are affected [3, 34, 35].

The identification and characterization of the *RB1* gene has provided critical insights into the biology of RB, and also many other tumor types, including lung, brain, breast, and bladder cancers. In the latter cases, somatic inactivation of the RB1 pathway is essential for tumorigenesis [36]. Since tumor development is associated with the sequential acquisition of multiple mutations that drive unregulated proliferation and/or reduced cell death [37, 38], it is apparent that alterations in other critical signaling pathways underlie RB tumorigenesis. For example, in addition to deletions flanking the *RB1* gene, karyotype analysis has identified various recurrent chromosome imbalances in RB, which include isochromosome 6p, trisomy 1q, monosomy 16, add(1p), double-minute chromosomes, and homogeneously staining regions involving the *MYCN* and *INT1* oncogenes [39].

The tumor suppressor protein, TP53, is a master regulator of cell cycle, apoptosis, and DNA damage and is the most frequently mutated gene in human cancer. But many studies have shown that the *TP53* gene is not mutated in RB [40, 41]. In 2006, Laurie and colleagues shed light on this issue by demonstrating that the TP53 pathway is also inactivated by the MDM (murine double minute) family of proteins following loss of *RB1* during retina development [42]. The MDM family of proteins, such as MDM2 and MDM4 (MDMX), are known inhibitors of TP53 and both are expressed in RB cells [43]. Additionally, a single-nucleotide polymorphism (SNP) located in the promoter region of *MDM2* (rs2279744, SNP309, 309 T>G) is correlated with enhanced MDM2 expression and attenuation of the TP53 pathway [44]. It has been postulated that the *MDM2* 309 T>G SNP behaves as a modifier gene in RB [45]. Another similar study pointed out that the *TP53* p.Arg72Pro SNP (rs1042522), which correlates with increased expression of *MDM2* and compromised TP53 pro-apoptotic activity, is significantly associated with onset of RB [46]. Collectively, these data strongly support that inactivation of the TP53 pathway is an important cooperating event in the development of RB.

In addition to TP53, genetic lesions in other signaling pathways might contribute to RB malignancy. A recent report implicated the involvement of oncogenic microRNA cluster miR-17~92 in RB tumorigenesis in a mouse model and possibly also in humans [47]. In another study, Zhang and his colleagues performed whole-genome sequencing of RB tumor samples and matched normal DNA utilizing next-generation sequencing technology. Surprisingly, they observed very few recurrent genetic lesions, except in *RB1* and *MYCN*. But gene expression and epigenetic analyses identified changes in other cancer-related genes, such as the protooncogene *SYK* [48].

Clinical Utility of Testing

The diagnosis of RB is essentially based on clinical examination of the fundus of the eye, which is confirmed by imaging technologies including B scan ultrasonography and computerized tomography or magnetic resonance imaging scans. Once diagnosis is established, *RB1* genetic testing is indicated. For individuals with bilateral or familial RB, the goal of genetic testing is to identify the predisposing germline *RB1* mutation, which can be detected in approximately 94 % of cases [22]. The identification of the germline *RB1* mutation enables appropriate primary tumor treatment and surveillance for additional ocular tumors and/or non-ocular malignancies. Furthermore, the identification of a germline mutation allows risk estimation for siblings and offspring. One of the main benefits of genetic testing is to rule out germline mutations in other young at-risk relatives of the proband to avoid unnecessary screening of children under anesthesia for early detection of RB. For individuals with sporadic unilateral RB, genetic testing focuses on identification of somatic mutations in the tumor (when available), followed by germline testing. Once mutations are identified in the tumor, peripheral blood DNA should be tested to determine whether one of the mutations is actually a predisposing germline mutation, which is estimated to exist in 13 % of sporadic unilateral cases [49].

Prenatal diagnosis and preimplantation genetic diagnosis (PGD) are available for at-risk pregnancies, which require the prior identification of predisposing germline mutations within the families. Prenatal genetic testing options include the molecular analysis of DNA isolated from the cells of the developing fetus through chorionic villus sampling or amniocentesis. More recently, PGD is available at a limited number of institutions [50–52]. PGD is performed in combination with in vitro fertilization and offers a way to test an individual's embryos for genetic disorders before transfer of unaffected embryos into the uterus. A recent report demonstrated the feasibility of PGD based on the inheritance of SNPs that are tightly associated with a wild-type or mutant *RB1* allele [52]. This approach is used when genetic screening for mutation detection is not readily available or the disease-causing mutation has not been identified. However, this approach can lead to erroneous conclusions in the presence of gonadal mosaicism and should be used with caution [53].

Available Assays

A broad spectrum of mutations ranging from point mutations, deletions/insertions, chromosomal rearrangements, and epigenetic silencing has been documented in the *RB1* gene. Accordingly, various types of molecular testing are used by clinical molecular laboratories for *RB1* mutation analysis. The genetic tests to identify mutations involve multiple testing approaches, which should be adjusted according to the diagnosis, family history, and availability of genetic materials.

For individuals with bilateral or multifocal unilateral RB, or unilateral tumor with a positive family history, clinical genetic testing for germline mutations starts with sequence analysis of the *RB1* coding exons, flanking introns, and the promoter region using DNA isolated from peripheral blood lymphocytes. Given the fact that larger deletions and insertion involving the whole *RB1* gene or certain exons are not readily detectable by sequence analysis, alternative methods can be applied, including fluorescence in situ hybridization (FISH), multiplex ligation-dependent probe amplification, quantitative real-time PCR, targeted array-based comparative genomic hybridization, and heterozygosity testing based on informative polymorphic markers. Cytogenetically visible deletions or rearrangements involving *RB1* can be detected by karyotype and FISH analyses, respectively, and are estimated to occur in 5 % of unilateral cases and 7.5 % of bilateral cases [49]. To detect deeper intronic mutations, reverse transcription-polymerase chain reaction methods can be used to test RNA isolated from RB tumor tissues or peripheral blood lymphocytes, followed by evaluation for abnormalities in the size and sequence of *RB1* transcripts [25]. Through the use of multiple sequential testing methods, the sensitivity of mutation detection has reached 90–95 % for probands with heritable RB [22, 49].

Mutation screening for nonhereditary unilateral RB cases is more complicated because only approximately 13 % of patients have germline mutations [49]; so genetic testing is more effective when tumor tissue is available. In the ideal scenario, if two inactivating *RB1* mutations are identified in the tumor, then it is straightforward to test lymphocyte DNA for the presence of the tumor-associated alterations.

In addition to the methods mentioned above, methylation analysis of the *RB1* promoter region or LOH analysis by comparing polymorphic markers flanking and inside the *RB1* gene between tumor and peripheral blood DNA can be performed. To evaluate hypermethylation of the *RB1* promoter, genomic DNA isolated from tumors is digested with two restriction endonucleases whose activities depend on the presence or absence of methylated cytosines in CpG dinucleotides [35]. The products of these digestions are quantified and compared, using sequence-specific primers and PCR. The results can demonstrate the degree of methylation in CpG dinucleotides within the promoter region of the *RB1* gene that can lead to gene silencing. Individuals with unilateral RB and no detectable germline mutation in *RB1* are generally classified as sporadic, nonheritable cases; however, there is a small possibility that the affected individuals carry low-level germline mosaic mutation which is beyond the detection limits of the testing method.

Currently, Sanger sequencing is the major method used to screen the *RB1* gene for mutations. However, the detection of mosaic mutations by Sanger sequencing is technically challenging and the threshold of detection of the mutant allele is only 10–20 %. Allele-specific PCR strategies can detect 11 recurrent nonsense mutations (CGA>TGA) within the *RB1* gene and can increase the sensitivity of the detection of mosaic mutations. Using this technology, the frequency of germline mosaicism is estimated to be 5.5 % in bilateral and 3.8 % in unilateral RB patients [54]. Next-generation sequencing has been used for genetic analysis for *RB1* mutations and has significantly increased sensitivity of detection of mosaic mutations [55].

A systematic approach to mutation detection that is designed to detect most *RB1* germline alterations facilitates the clinical management and genetic counseling of RB patients. The Genetic Diagnostic Laboratory at the University of Pennsylvania uses a sequence of test methods, beginning with PCR amplification and DNA sequencing of the 27 *RB1* coding exons and flanking intronic sequences, as well as 1,000 bp of the *RB1* promoter region. The DNA for this testing is isolated from peripheral blood lymphocytes, saliva, or frozen/formalin-fixed paraffin-embedded (FFPE) tumor sections following standard procedures. The results are compared with data reference *RB1* gene sequence to identify mutations, including nucleotide substitutions and small insertions or deletions. If no mutations are identified, samples are analyzed using quantitative dosage-sensitive PCR to identify rearrangements encompassing 1 or more of the 27 *RB1* coding exons. Whole-genome SNP arrays are used to identify the boundaries of larger genomic deletions or duplications when present. If no mutations are identified, testing for the methylation status of the *RB1* promoter or alterations in the *RB1* transcript by RNA analysis is performed.

Since 2001, the Genetic Diagnostic Laboratory has performed testing for a total of 545 individuals with bilateral RB, 37 cases with hereditary unilateral RB, and 561 probands with sporadic unilateral RB. For the bilateral and hereditary unilateral RB cases, the sensitivity of mutation detection approaches 96 % with a coding sequence mutation in approximately 80 % of patients and a partial- or whole-gene deletion/duplication involving the *RB1* locus in approximately 16 % of patients. Mosaic mutations account for at least an additional 4 % of these RB cases. For the 561 sporadic unilateral RB cases, germline *RB1* mutations were identified in about 13 %, among which 53 mutations (10 %) lead to silent, missense, nonsense, or frameshift changes, and 16 mutations (3 %) lead to intragenic deletions or duplications involving the *RB1* gene.

Interpretations of Results

The sensitivity of mutation detection using peripheral blood DNA is 90–95 % for probands with familial or bilateral RB and approximately 13 % for individuals with nonhereditary unilateral RB [49]. The reason the sensitivity of mutation detection is less than 100 % could be due to undetectable intronic mutations or intragenic rearrangements of *RB1* or very low-level mosaicism. It is also possible that additional genes are associated with RB.

For individuals with bilateral or familial RB, the chance of detecting a disease-causing *RB1* mutation in the DNA of the peripheral white blood cells is very high (more than 90 %). The identification of a mutation usually indicates the presence of a germline mutation. For unilateral cases without a family history, tumor tissue becomes the primary resource to detect the two somatic mutations. When the mutations detected in the tumor are not present in constitutional DNA, the probability of carrying a germline mutation is very low. Additionally, approximately 80 % of RB cases are due to a de novo mutation, which implies that the mutations identified in affected children are usually not present in the germline of the parents. It should be noted that germline mosaic mutations may not be uncommon in the unaffected parents and the risk of RB in their offspring should not be underestimated [30].

RB1 mutation carriers show variable phenotypic expression and penetrance, which is determined to a certain extent by the nature of the predisposing *RB1* mutations. Generally, carriers of an *RB1* mutant allele with nonsense or frameshift mutations have a very high risk of developing bilateral RB. But when these mutations exist in a mosaic form, the phenotypic expression can be milder [3]. Additionally, splice site mutations, small in-frame deletions, or missense mutations are usually associated with a milder phenotype, which exhibits incomplete penetrance and reduced expressivity. The effects of these mutations on RB1 protein function are considered to be less pronounced compared to nonsense mutations. For example, only a few missense mutations outside the RB1 pocket domains have been reported with putative oncogenic effect, and most of the cases show incomplete penetrance [20]. With splice site mutations, a fraction of the total transcripts usually are still processed as normal mRNA. In contrast, cryptic splice site mutations that result in change of the reading frame are usually associated with more severe phenotypes. Additionally, for mutations occurring in the promoter region of *RB1* gene, the expression of RB1 is less likely to be completely compromised and usually leads to milder phenotypes.

Laboratory Issues

DNA sequencing is the most commonly used method for *RB1* genetic testing. Adherence to best clinical laboratory practices for both the sequencing and data interpretation are important to ensure the quality of test performance. First, the samples for genetic testing should be collected, identified, shipped, stored, and processed under quality-controlled conditions. Genomic DNA from peripheral white blood cells is the typical starting material. Alternative sources such as saliva, tumor tissue, FFPE tissue, cultured amniocytes, or chorionic villi require special quality controls during sample processing, sequencing, and data interpretation. For example, DNA from FFPE tissue generally does not result in good sequence data and has a high failure rate because of degradation or chemical cross-linking. DNA isolation procedures should be optimized to recover as much usable DNA as possible. More importantly, to ensure the success of PCR and sequencing, special attention should be paid to the primer design, making sure all the amplicons are less than 300 bp in length when using FFPE tissue as a specimen type.

The standard quality control measures for DNA sequencing, such as inclusion of known negative control and positive controls should be routinely performed. Bi-directional sequencing is recommended for confirmatory mutation testing. Also, laboratories may confirm any mutation identified in an affected individual by repeat testing of an independent DNA sample to ensure no sample carry-over or specimen misidentification during testing.

False-negative results can occur for several reasons. Allele dropout can be caused by SNPs or insertion/deletions at the binding sites of PCR or sequencing primers. If allele dropout is suspected, alternate sequencing primers outside of the polymorphic regions can be used. Lower-level mosaicism, deep intronic cryptic splice mutations, preferential amplification of the smaller allele in a large insertion, or regional deletion/insertion can also introduce false-negative results. These limitations apply to most PCR-based sequencing methods currently used for any gene including *RB1* and are not limited to any specific gene test.

Accurate and unambiguous mutation nomenclature is important for the communication between clinical molecular laboratories, physicians, genetic consultants, and other healthcare providers. The mutation type, nucleotide base, or amino acid changes should be specified following the recommended nomenclature developed by Human Genome Variation Society (HGVS) [56]. *RB1* mutations are commonly annotated with reference to a specific genomic reference sequence (GenBank accession number L11910) [15]. Additionally, several databases are useful for interpretation of test results, including the RB1 Mutation Database (http://rb1-lovd.d-lohmann.de/home.php), the Human Gene Mutation Database (HGMD, http://www.hgmd.cf.ac.uk/ac/index.php), and dbSNP (http://www.ncbi.nlm.nih.gov/projects/SNP/).

Conclusions and Future Directions

Although RB remains the most common primary intraocular malignancy of infancy and childhood, mortality from RB has been significantly reduced with earlier diagnosis and improved methods of treatment. However, in cases with low-level mosaicism or deep intronic splice mutations, the mutations may not be easily detected. More exhaustive techniques such as next-generation sequencing technology may overcome these barriers. Also the absence of detectable *RB1* mutations in some patients suggests the presence of alternative underlying genetic mechanisms which requires better understanding of molecular pathology of RB.

Acknowledgements The authors are grateful to Dr. Carol Shields, Wills Eye Institute, Thomas Jefferson University, and Dr. Anna Meadows, Children's Hospital of Philadelphia, for their support and encouragement to pursue retinoblastoma research. This work was supported in part by grants from NIH/NCI (RO1CA118580).

References

1. Shields CL, Shields JA. Diagnosis and management of retinoblastoma. Cancer Control. 2004;11(5):317–27.
2. Broaddus E, Topham A, et al. Incidence of retinoblastoma in the USA: 1975-2004. Br J Ophthalmol. 2009;93(1):21–3.
3. Lohmann DR, Gallie BL. Retinoblastoma: revisiting the model prototype of inherited cancer. Am J Med Genet C: Semin Med Genet. 2004;129C(1):23–8.
4. Lohmann D. Retinoblastoma. Adv Exp Med Biol. 2010;685:220–7.
5. Kivela T. Trilateral retinoblastoma: a meta-analysis of hereditary retinoblastoma associated with primary ectopic intracranial retinoblastoma. J Clin Oncol. 1999;17(6):1829–37.
6. Kleinerman RA, Yu CL, et al. Variation of second cancer risk by family history of retinoblastoma among long-term survivors. J Clin Oncol. 2012;30(9):950–7.
7. Wong FL, Boice Jr JD, et al. Cancer incidence after retinoblastoma. Radiation dose and sarcoma risk. JAMA. 1997;278(15):1262–7.
8. Rushlow DE, Mol BM, et al. Characterisation of retinoblastomas without RB1 mutations: genomic, gene expression, and clinical studies. Lancet Oncol. 2013;14(4):327–34.
9. Friend SH, Bernards R, et al. A human DNA segment with properties of the gene that predisposes to retinoblastoma and osteosarcoma. Nature. 1986;323(6089):643–6.
10. Dick FA. Structure-function analysis of the retinoblastoma tumor suppressor protein – is the whole a sum of its parts? Cell Div. 2007;2:26.
11. Knudsen ES, Knudsen KE. Tailoring to RB: tumour suppressor status and therapeutic response. Nat Rev Cancer. 2008;8(9): 714–24.
12. Viatour P, Sage J. Newly identified aspects of tumor suppression by RB. Dis Model Mech. 2011;4(5):581–5.
13. Sage J, Straight AF. RB's original CIN? Genes Dev. 2010;24(13):1329–33.
14. Knudson AG. Mutation and cancer: statistical study of retinoblastoma. PNAS. 1971;68:820–3.
15. Lohmann DR. RB1 gene mutations in retinoblastoma. Hum Mutat. 1999;14(4):283–8.
16. Gallie BL. Predictive testing for retinoblastoma comes of age. Am J Hum Genet. 1997;61(2):279–81.
17. Dryja TP, Morrow JF, et al. Quantification of the paternal allele bias for new germline mutations in the retinoblastoma gene. Hum Genet. 1997;100(3-4):446–9.
18. Blanquet V, Turleau C, et al. Spectrum of germline mutations in the RB1 gene: a study of 232 patients with hereditary and non hereditary retinoblastoma. Hum Mol Genet. 1995;4(3):383–8.

19. Yilmaz S, Horsthemke B, et al. Twelve novel RB1 gene mutations in patients with hereditary retinoblastoma. Mutations in brief no. 206. Online. Hum Mutat. 1998;12(6):434.
20. Klutz M, Horsthemke B, et al. RB1 gene mutations in peripheral blood DNA of patients with isolated unilateral retinoblastoma. Am J Hum Genet. 1999;64(2):667–8.
21. Dundar M, Lanyon GW, et al. Detection of mutations in the RB1 gene by single strand conformation polymorphism (SSCP) analysis, amplification mismatch detection (AMD) analysis and polymerase chain reaction sequencing. Proc Natl Sci Counc Repub China B. 2001;25(3):166–73.
22. Nichols KE, Houseknecht MD, et al. Sensitive multistep clinical molecular screening of 180 unrelated individuals with retinoblastoma detects 36 novel mutations in the RB1 gene. Hum Mutat. 2005;25(6):566–74.
23. Mitter D, Rushlow D, et al. Identification of a mutation in exon 27 of the RB1 gene associated with incomplete penetrance retinoblastoma. Fam Cancer. 2009;8(1):55–8.
24. Dehainault C, Michaux D, et al. A deep intronic mutation in the RB1 gene leads to intronic sequence exonisation. Eur J Hum Genet. 2007;15(4):473–7.
25. Zhang K, Nowak I, et al. Patterns of missplicing caused by RB1 gene mutations in patients with retinoblastoma and association with phenotypic expression. Hum Mutat. 2008;29(4):475–84.
26. Sakai T, Toguchida J, et al. Allele-specific hypermethylation of the retinoblastoma tumor-suppressor gene. Am J Hum Genet. 1991;48(5):880–8.
27. Ohtani-Fujita N, Dryja TP, et al. Hypermethylation in the retinoblastoma gene is associated with unilateral, sporadic retinoblastoma. Cancer Genet Cytogenet. 1997;98(1):43–9.
28. Munier FL, Thonney F, et al. Evidence of somatic and germinal mosaicism in pseudo-low-penetrant hereditary retinoblastoma, by constitutional and single-sperm mutation analysis. Am J Hum Genet. 1998;63(6):1903–8.
29. Barbosa RH, Vargas FR, et al. Hereditary retinoblastoma transmitted by maternal germline mosaicism. Pediatr Blood Cancer. 2008;51(5):598–602.
30. Sippel KC, Fraioli RE, et al. Frequency of somatic and germ-line mosaicism in retinoblastoma: implications for genetic counseling. Am J Hum Genet. 1998;62(3):610–9.
31. Mitter D, Ullmann R, et al. Genotype-phenotype correlations in patients with retinoblastoma and interstitial 13q deletions. Eur J Hum Genet. 2011;19(9):947–58.
32. Lohmann D, Gallie B et al. Clinical utility gene card for: retinoblastoma. Eur J Hum Genet. 2010;19(3), doi:10.1038/ejhg.2010.200; published online 8 December 2010.
33. Albrecht P, Ansperger-Rescher B, et al. Spectrum of gross deletions and insertions in the RB1 gene in patients with retinoblastoma and association with phenotypic expression. Hum Mutat. 2005;26(5):437–45.
34. Klutz M, Brockmann D, et al. A parent-of-origin effect in two families with retinoblastoma is associated with a distinct splice mutation in the RB1 gene. Am J Hum Genet. 2002;71(1):174–9.
35. Taylor M, Dehainault C, et al. Genotype-phenotype correlations in hereditary familial retinoblastoma. Hum Mutat. 2007;28(3):284–93.
36. Burkhart DL, Sage J. Cellular mechanisms of tumour suppression by the retinoblastoma gene. Nat Rev Cancer. 2008;8(9):671–82.
37. Hanahan D, Weinberg RA. The hallmarks of cancer. Cell. 2000;100(1):57–70.
38. Hanahan D, Weinberg RA. Hallmarks of cancer: the next generation. Cell. 2011;144(5):646–74.
39. Mairal A, Pinglier E, et al. Detection of chromosome imbalances in retinoblastoma by parallel karyotype and CGH analyses. Genes Chromosomes Cancer. 2000;28(4):370–9.
40. Kato MV, Shimizu T, et al. Loss of heterozygosity on chromosome 17 and mutation of the p53 gene in retinoblastoma. Cancer Lett. 1996;106(1):75–82.
41. Nork TM, Poulsen GL, et al. p53 regulates apoptosis in human retinoblastoma. Arch Ophthalmol. 1997;115(2):213–9.
42. Laurie NA, Donovan SL, et al. Inactivation of the p53 pathway in retinoblastoma. Nature. 2006;444(7115):61–6.
43. Guo Y, Pajovic S, et al. Expression of p14ARF, MDM2, and MDM4 in human retinoblastoma. Biochem Biophys Res Commun. 2008;375(1):1–5.
44. Bond GL, Hu W, et al. A single nucleotide polymorphism in the MDM2 promoter attenuates the p53 tumor suppressor pathway and accelerates tumor formation in humans. Cell. 2004;119(5):591–602.
45. Castera L, Sabbagh A, et al. MDM2 as a modifier gene in retinoblastoma. J Natl Cancer Inst. 2010;102(23):1805–8.
46. Epistolato MC, Disciglio V, et al. p53 Arg72Pro and MDM2 309 SNPs in hereditary retinoblastoma. J Hum Genet. 2011;56(9):685–6.
47. Conkrite K, Sundby M, et al. miR-17~92 cooperates with RB pathway mutations to promote retinoblastoma. Genes Dev. 2011;25(16):1734–45.
48. Zhang J, Benavente CA, et al. A novel retinoblastoma therapy from genomic and epigenetic analyses. Nature. 2012;481(7381): 329–34.
49. Lohmann DR, Gallie BL (2010) Retinoblastoma. GeneReviews. http://www.ncbi.nlm.nih.gov/books/NBK1116/. Accessed May 2012.
50. Girardet A, Hamamah S, et al. First preimplantation genetic diagnosis of hereditary retinoblastoma using informative microsatellite markers. Mol Hum Reprod. 2003;9(2):111–6.
51. Xu K, Rosenwaks Z, et al. Preimplantation genetic diagnosis for retinoblastoma: the first reported liveborn. Am J Ophthalmol. 2004;137(1):18–23.
52. Dhanjal S, Kakourou G, et al. Preimplantation genetic diagnosis for retinoblastoma predisposition. Br J Ophthalmol. 2007;91(8):1090–1.
53. Castera L, Gauthier-Villars M, et al. Mosaicism in clinical practice exemplified by prenatal diagnosis in retinoblastoma. Prenat Diagn. 2011;31(11):1106–8.
54. Rushlow D, Piovesan B, et al. Detection of mosaic RB1 mutations in families with retinoblastoma. Hum Mutat. 2009;30(5):842–51.
55. Chen Z, Moran K, et al. Enhanced sensitivity for detection of low-level germline mosaic RB1 mutations in sporadic retinoblastoma cases using deep semiconductor sequencing. Hum Mutat. 2014;35(3):384–91.
56. Antonarakis SE. Recommendations for a nomenclature system for human gene mutations. Nomenclature Working Group. Hum Mutat. 1998;11(1):1–3.

30 Hereditary Paraganglioma and Pheochromocytoma

Fang-Yuan Li and Lee-Jun C. Wong

Abstract

Paragangliomas (PGLs) and pheochromocytomas (PCCs) are rare neuroendocrine tumors, which predominantly occur in the head and neck. They can be part of a syndrome, such as multiple endocrine neoplasia (MEN), neurofibromatosis (NF) type 1, and von Hippel-Lindau syndrome (VHL). Hereditary PGLs/PCCs are caused by molecular defects in the mitochondrial respiratory chain complex II, also known as the succinate dehydrogenase (SDH) complex, which contains protein subunits and assembly factors encoded by the nuclear genes, *SDHA*, *SDHB*, *SDHC*, *SDHD*, and *SDHAF2*. This chapter focuses on molecular mechanisms, available clinical molecular tests, interpretation of test results, and the clinical utility of molecular testing for hereditary PGL/PCC caused by mutations in the *SDH* genes. In general, diagnosis can be achieved by immunohistochemical studies of tumors, sequence analysis of *SDH* genes in germline cells and tumor tissues, and detection of large heterozygous deletions or duplications by microarray-based technology. Detailed clinical evaluation and family history are vital to appropriate prioritization of the diagnostic testing and for interpretation of test results.

Keywords

Paragangliomas • Pheochromocytomas • Hereditary paragangliomas • Mitochondrial respiratory chain complex II • Succinate dehydrogenase (SDH) • *SDHA* • *SDHB* • *SDHC* • *SDHD* • *SDHAF2*

Introduction

Paragangliomas (PGLs) and pheochromocytomas (PCCs) are rare neuroendocrine tumors, which predominantly occur in the head and neck. PGLs are vascularized neuroendocrine tumors that arise from paraganglia of neural crest origin. PGL can be categorized into two groups. The sympathetic PGLs are confined to the adrenal medulla, called pheochromocytoma (PCC), and usually secrete catecholamines. The nonsecretory extra-adrenal parasympathetic PGLs occur predominantly in the head and neck, for example, in the carotid body, the chemoreceptive organ responsible for sensing of and adaptation to hypoxia in the blood. PGLs/PCCs have a prevalence of one in 2,500–6,500 with an annual incidence of 500–1,600 in the USA [1].

Most PGLs/PCCs are benign and occur predominantly at age 40–60 years. Familial cases develop tumors earlier and are more likely to have bilateral tumors [2]. The predisposition for PGL/PCC tumors is inherited in an autosomal dominant mode, with loss of heterozygosity (LOH) in tumors. PGL/PCC can be part of a syndrome, such as multiple endocrine neoplasia syndrome types 2A and 2B (MEN types 2A and 2B), von Hippel-Lindau (VHL) disease, and neurofibromatosis (NF) type 1. Hereditary PGL/PCC syndrome may also result from defects in mitochondrial complex II function.

F.-Y. Li, M.D., Ph.D. • L.-J. C. Wong, Ph.D., F.A.C.M.G. (✉)
Department of Molecular and Human Genetics, Baylor Miraca Genetics Laboratory, Baylor College of Medicine, One Baylor Plaza, NAB 2015, Houston, TX, USA
e-mail: ljwong@bcm.edu

D.G.B. Leonard (ed.), *Molecular Pathology in Clinical Practice*, DOI 10.1007/978-3-319-19674-9_30

Table 30.1 Number of germline mutations identified in the *SDHB*, *SDHC*, and *SDHD* genes in PGL/PCC

Gene	Study 1 (%)	Study 2 (%)	Study 3[a] (%)
SDHB	16 (8.4)	24 (4.8)	38 (24.7)
SDHC	2 (1.1)	4 (0.8)	2 (1.3)
SDHD	3 (1.6)	47 (9.4)	31 (20.1)
Total cases	190 (11.1)	501 (15)	154 (46.1)

Study 1: [10]
Study 2: [14]
Study 3: Cases tested during July 2007 to January 2012 in the Medical Genetics Laboratories (MGL), Baylor College of Medicine (BCM)
[a]The higher mutation rate in Study 3 is likely due to the selection bias of specimens tested because samples were sent to MGL specifically for mutation analysis of *SDH* genes

Currently, ten genes are associated with PGL/PCC: *RET*, *VHL*, *NF1*, *MAX*, *TMEM127*, *SDHA*, *SDHB*, *SDHC*, *SDHD*, and *SDHAF2 (SDH5)*. This chapter will focus on PGL/PCC due to defects in the mitochondrial respiratory chain complex II also called the succinate dehydrogenase (SDH) complex. Five different PGL phenotypes have been identified, with each related to mutations in a different gene: *SDHA* (PGL5), *SDHB* (PGL4), *SDHC* (PGL3), *SDHD* (PGL1), and *SDHAF2* (PGL2).

The SDH complex is at the crossroad of the tricarboxylic acid cycle and the respiratory chain for adenosine triphosphate generation, which oxidizes succinate to fumarate and transfers electrons from $FADH_2$ to coenzyme Q (CoQ). Of the five mitochondrial respiratory chain complexes, SDH is the only one for which all of the subunits are encoded by the nuclear genome. The SDH complex has two functional domains: the catalytic domain consisting of SDHA and SDHB and the mitochondrial inner membrane anchor domain composed of SDHC and SDHD. Assembly of complex II requires at least two proteins, SDHAF1 [3] and SDHAF2 [4].

The association of PGL/PCC with mitochondrial complex II defects was first established by the identification of mutations in the *SDHD* gene [5]. Mutations in *SDHB*, *SDHC*, *SDHA*, and *SDHAF2* (*SDH5*) also cause PGL/PCC [4, 6–8]. Germline mutations in the *SDH* genes occur in 25–45 % of familial PGL/PCC cases, depending on clinical findings and classification, and in approximately 12 % of sporadic cases [9–11]. The mutation detection rate in patients with a family history is very high (>90 %). Large germline deletions also occur but are less frequent (<5 %) [12–14]. Mutations are identified more often in *SDHD* and *SDHB* than in *SDHC* [13] (Table 30.1). The only gene that is part of mitochondrial complex II subunits and assembly that has not been associated with PGL/PCC is *SDHAF1*. Autosomal recessive mutations in the *SDHAF1* gene, however, have been identified in patients with mitochondrial complex II deficiency [3].

Molecular Basis of Disease

The molecular mechanism underlying *SDH* mutations in PGL/PCC has yet to be identified. A proposed mechanism is that mutations in the *SDH* genes may cause a cascade of molecular events, leading to the abnormal stabilization of hypoxia-inducible factor (HIF) under normoxic conditions known as pseudo-hypoxia. The pseudo-hypoxia may lead to increased angiogenesis in the PGL/PCC tumor tissue [7]. Defects in the SDH complex cause an accumulation of succinate that inhibits prolyl-4-hydroxylases (PHDs) and subsequently impairs prolyl-hydroxylation of HIF [15, 16], leading to tumorigenesis, possibly via a glycolytic shift (Warburg effect). Glycolytic shift is observed in solid tumors, in which tumor cells generate energy from glycolysis followed by lactic acid fermentation [16–20]. Stabilized HIF activates transcription of genes downstream of the HIF pathway, resulting in cell proliferation and angiogenesis, and ultimately tumorigenesis [21].

The HIF pathway, which has been proposed to be defective in tumorigenesis caused by *SDH* mutations, normally functions to control cells' responses to low O_2 in vivo. Mammalian cells have complicated machineries to respond to O_2 deprivation. A key modulator is HIF. HIF is a heterodimer consisting of one O_2-labile α subunit and one O_2-stable β subunit. The α subunit has three forms: HIF1α, HIF2α (EPAS1), and HIF3α (IPAS). HIF1α exists ubiquitously. In the normoxic state, approximately 20 % of the HIFα subunits are hydroxylated at conserved proline residues and then degraded via the E3 ubiquitin pathway after forming a complex with the VHL protein [18, 22]. However, in hypoxic conditions, HIFα is stabilized and activates transcription of genes adaptive to hypoxic conditions. Accumulation of succinate due to mutations in *SDH* genes can inhibit the degradation of HIF1α protein, resulting in increased transcription of genes important for response to hypoxic conditions. In moderate hypoxic conditions (1.5 % O_2), mitochondria stimulate the production of cellular reactive oxygen species that may inhibit HIFα degradation. These oxygen radicals are specifically formed from complex III of the mitochondrial respiratory chain [23, 24].

The molecular mechanism underlining PGL/PCC caused by mutations in *SDH* genes may differ from those associated with mutations in *VHL*, *RET*, *NF1*, and *TMEM127*. A study of the expression profile of PGL/PCC tumors using microarray technology demonstrated a different expression pattern in tumors with mutations in the *SDH* genes compared to tumors with mutations in *VHL*, *RET*, *NF1*, or *TMEM172*. A somatic point mutation may function similarly to LOH in causing PGL/PCC tumors [10].

The study of *SDHD* knockout mice showed that $SDHD^{-/-}$ mice died in early embryonic stage (<7.5 days post conception)

and $SDHD^{+/-}$ mice had a deficiency of SDH activity. However, tumorigenesis in these $SDHD^{+/-}$ mice was not increased, indicating differences of the pathophysiology between human and mouse [25].

SDHA

The *SDHA* gene is located at human chromosome 5p15.33 [26] and codes for the largest subunit of the SDH complex. The gene consists of 15 exons and produces a 2,286 nucleotide transcript, which encodes a 644 amino acid polypeptide of 70 kDa. SDHA is a flavoprotein, which forms the SDH catalytic domain in complex with SDHB, an iron-sulfur protein. Disease-related mutations in the *SDHA* gene were first identified in Leigh syndrome patients with mitochondrial respiratory chain complex II deficiency [27], which is inherited in an autosomal recessive fashion. In 2010, the first case of an *SDHA* mutation associated PGL/PCC syndrome was reported in a patient with an extra-adrenal PGL [7], which is also categorized as paraganglioma syndrome type 5 (PGL5, OMIM #600857). The mutation was a germline heterozygous missense mutation, c.1765C>T (p.R589W), identified in the patient's blood sample. However, in the patient's tumor tissue, the mutant molecules were found to be predominant (much greater than 50 %), suggesting LOH, which was confirmed by array comparative genomic hybridization (aCGH) analysis. The predisposition to PGL/PCC tumors due to an *SDHA* germline mutation is inherited as an autosomal dominant trait at the pedigree level, but recessive at the cellular level, requiring a second mutation to lead to tumorigenesis.

Twenty-eight (28) point mutations in the *SDHA* gene have been reported in Human Genome Mutation Database (HGMD) (as of November 2014). Five mutations are associated with PGL/PCC. The remaining mutations are associated with Leigh syndrome, optic atrophy, ataxia, and myopathy [27–32]. The germline mutations were found in sporadic cases of PGL/PCC with negative SDHA immunostaining and LOH in their tumor tissues. The penetrance of *SDHA* mutations may be low. For example, the p.R31* and p.R585W mutations were found at a frequency of 0.3 % and 0.1 %, respectively, in the general population who are not affected with PGL/PCC, suggesting a low penetrance [33].

SDHB

The *SDHB* gene is located at chromosome 1p36.13 and consists of eight exons encoding a 30 kDa protein of 280 amino acids. The SDHB protein is an iron-sulfur protein forming part of the SDH complex catalytic domain with the SDHA subunit. *SDHB* is the most commonly mutated gene in PGL/PCC (PGL4, OMIM #185470). Currently, 195 *SDHB* mutations associated with PGL/PCC have been recorded in the HGMD, in contrast to the number of mutations in the other *SDH* genes (5 in *SDHA*, 44 in *SDHC*, 144 in *SDHD*, and 2 in *SDHAF2*) (Table 30.2). *SDHB* mutations are more frequently found in secreting PGL and malignant tumors [8, 34]. However, the penetrance of *SDHB* mutations is low (approximately 18 % at age 60) [35], which may explain why *SDHB* mutations are more common in sporadic PGLs/PCCs. Since the survival rate for patients with SDHB-immunonegative tumors is lower than for patients with SDHB-immunopositive tumors, *SDHB* germline mutation may serve as a prognostic marker for patients with PGL/PCC [36].

Table 30.2 Types of mutations in *SDH* genes associated with paragliomas and pheochromocytomas based on data from the Human Genome Mutation Database (HGMD; November 2014)

	Missense	Nonsense	Splicing	Small indels	Gross indels	Total
SDHA	4	1	0	0	0	5
SDHB	78	16	26	53	22	195
SDHC	19	7	6	5	7	44
SDHD	39	20	12	57	16	144
SDHAF2	1	0	0	1	0	2

SDHC

The *SDHC* gene is located at chromosome 1q23.3 and has at least four alternatively spliced isoforms, although the functional significance of the isoforms is not well understood. The longest isoform (NM_003001.3) consists of six exons. The SDHC protein is located in the mitochondrial inner membrane and together with SDHD forms an anchor domain for the mitochondria respiratory chain complex II. *SDHC* was the second SDH gene associated with PCC/PGL [8]. Mutations in *SDHC* have been found in paraganglioma syndrome type 3 (PGL3, OMIM #602413) but are much less frequent than those in *SDHB* or *SDHD* (Table 30.1). *SDHC* mutations are mostly found in head and neck PGL, although PGLs/PCCs in other loci caused by *SDHC* mutations have been reported [37, 38]. Germline deletion of exon 3 of the *SDHC* gene has been identified in a patient in a study of 190 patients affected with PGL/PCC. The patient had germline deletion of *SDHC* exon 3, but LOH was not found in the tumor. Instead, there was a gain of the entire 1q harboring the mutated *SDHC* gene with exon 3 deletion in the tumor tissue, suggesting that the mutant allele was duplicated [10].

SDHD

SDHD is the smallest subunit in the SDH complex and was the first protein subunit in the SDH complex identified to cause paraganglioma syndrome type 1 (PGL1, OMIM #168000) [5]. The *SDHD* gene is located at chromosome 11q23.1 and has four exons encoding a 159-amino-acid polypeptide. *SDHD* mutations are predominantly found in head and neck PGL [34, 39]. Although PGL/PCC with an *SDHD* mutation is transmitted in an autosomal dominant mode, inheritance is almost exclusively through paternal transmission, which suggests maternal imprinting (inactivation) even though the *SDHD* gene itself is not imprinted [5]. Hensen and colleagues studied 23 SDHD-linked tumors and found all had lost the entire maternal chromosome 11. Thus, they hypothesized that PGL/PCC caused by *SDHD* mutations might require three hits: an *SDHD* germline mutation, the loss of or a somatic mutation in the wild-type *SDHD* gene in the tumor, and defects in another paternally imprinted tumor suppressor gene on chromosome 11, most likely 11p15 where the only imprinted gene cluster on chromosome 11 is located [40]. However, one definitive adrenal PCC case had maternal transmission of the *SDHD* mutation. Molecular studies on tumor and blood demonstrated a germline mutation, a loss of the wild-type paternal *SDHD*, and a loss of the maternal 11p region. Although lacking the typical paternal transmission, this case also supports a 3-hit hypothesis [41].

SDHAF2 (SDH5)

SDHAF2 (SDH5) is the latest SDH complex gene found to be involved in the tumorigenesis of PGL/PCC. *SDHAF2 (SDH5)* is located at chromosome 11q12.2, about 50 Mb away from the *SDHD* gene, and consists of four exons encoding a 166-amino-acid polypeptide. SDHAF2 interacts with SDHA and is required for the flavination of SDHA. Thus, mutations in *SDHAF2* destroy SDH activity, reduce the stability of the SDH complex, and result in paraganglioma syndrome type 2 (PGL2, OMIM #601650) [4]. Inheritance of the risk for PGL/PCC due to an *SDHAF2* mutation is also via an autosomal dominant mechanism but shows parent-of-origin effects. Similar to *SDHD* mutations, *SDHAF2* mutations are paternally inherited for tumor susceptibility, and maternally transmitted mutations do not result in tumors [4]. By studying a large family with an *SDHAF2* mutation, Kunst et al. found that 12 of 16 carriers who inherited the mutation from their fathers were affected. Twenty-four tumors were found in 11 affected family members (one patient's clinical information was unavailable) and 10 of the 11 patients had at least two tumors. All tumors were found in the head and neck with the majority in the carotid body (17/24 or 71 %) [42]. Currently, two mutations have been reported. One mutation, c.232G>A (p.G78R), was identified in a large Dutch family and a Spanish family [4, 42, 43]. A study of 443 sporadic PGL/PCC patients who had no mutations identified in the *SDHB*, *SDHC*, or *SDHD* genes did not identify any germline mutations or gross deletions in the *SDHAF2* gene, suggesting a very low incidence [43]. The other mutation, c.358dupT, was reported in a sporadic patient with head and neck paraganglioma in the right carotid body [44].

Available Assays

In general, immunostaining of tumor tissues is a straightforward assay for the prediction of mutated genes and can be used as a first step in screening. SDHB immunostaining can be diagnostic based on a study of 200 PGL/PCC tumors in which all 102 PGLs/PCCs with an *SDHB*, *SDHC*, or *SDHD* mutation lacked SDHB protein staining, while all 65 PGLs/PCCs associated with MEN2, VHL, and NF1, and 47 of the 53 PGLs/PCCs without identifiable germline mutations had SDHB immunostaining [45]. This study supports that hypothesis that the major effect of an *SDH* mutation is to alter assembly or stability of the SDH complex, as opposed to disruption of catalytic dysfunction [45]. Later, SDHB-immunonegative staining was found in all eight PGLs/PCCs with a heterozygous *SDHA* germline mutation [7, 33]. Based on clinical findings such as family history, malignancy and location of tumors, and clinical symptoms, the appropriate candidate gene(s) may be sequenced. For example, a patient with a sporadic malignant, SDHB-immunonegative, extra-adrenal tumors is highly suggestive of an *SDHB* germline mutation. Lack of SDHA immunostaining may be quite specific for an *SDHA* germline mutation. Based on a study of 316 PGL/PCC tumors using SDHA immunostaining, six of seven SDHA-negative staining tumors were found to have a heterozygous *SDHA* germline mutation. The remaining one did not have enough DNA for *SDHA* sequence analysis [33].

Sequence analysis of the *SDH* genes is the gold standard for mutation detection of point mutations and small deletions and insertions. Currently, the most widely used method is Sanger sequencing. Each coding exon and approximately 50 base pairs of flanking intronic sequences are amplified using polymerase chain reaction (PCR), followed by sequencing of the PCR products using dideoxy chain termination Sanger sequencing, and analysis on an automated DNA sequencer. The sequencing results are compared to reference sequences to determine nucleotide changes. This testing approach is widely used in clinical molecular laboratories.

For detection of large deletions and duplications involving the *SDH* genes, aCGH technology can be performed. The aCGH technology compares the genomic DNA isolated from a patient and a control. The optimal microarray for *SDH* gene assessment contains oligonucleotide probes across the entire human genome with dense probes targeted to exons of genes involved in mitochondrial and metabolic disorders [46]. A custom-designed oligonucleotide microarray (MitoMet oligonucleotide microarray, developed by Medical Genetics Laboratories at the Baylor College of Medicine, http://www.bcm.edu/geneticlabs/) has been successfully used to detect a deletion involving exon 2 of the *SDHC* gene.

Interpretation of Results

Negative immunostaining of SDHB (i.e., lack of SDHB staining) is diagnostic of a germline mutation in one of the *SDH* genes [45]. Thus, sequence analysis of the *SDHB*, *SDHC*, and *SDHD* genes should be performed. SDHA-negative immunostaining of a tumor tissue is specific for an *SDHA* germline mutation. Thus, sequence analysis of the *SDHA* gene is highly recommended.

Sanger sequencing of the *SDH* genes has 98 % sensitivity; however, interpretation of the pathogenicity of an identified variant, especially a novel change, may be challenging. Information regarding clinical findings, detailed family history, testing of other affected and unaffected family members, molecular analyses of tumor tissues, the effect of the variant on protein structure, and the conservation of the base and/or codon across species may help with the correct interpretation of a novel variant. Databases such as Human Gene Mutation Database (HGMD; http://www.hgmd.org/) and dbSNP (http://www.ncbi.nlm.nih.gov/snp/) are excellent resources to help with the evaluation of a novel variant. Currently, approximately 390 *SDH* gene mutations have been reported in HGMD. It is worth noting that even though recessive mutations in the *SDHC* and *SDHD* genes have not been reported in the literature, the possibility that severe mitochondrial respiratory chain complex II deficiency caused by two recessive mutations in these genes cannot be ruled out.

The penetrance of mutations in the *SDH* genes is variable. The available data for penetrance studies focused on the two most commonly mutated *SDHB* and *SDHD* genes. The penetrance of *SDHB* mutations is 40–55 % at age 40 years and 70–95 % at age 60 years [34, 47, 48]. The differences among studies may be due to the limited number of family members studied, especially the members who do not have clinical presentations, the particular mutations involved in a family, and family-specific modifiers. Another study used a modified algorithm to recalculate the penetrance based on the same datasets and found that the penetrance is 8 % (4–11 %) at 40 years old and 18 % (10–26 %) at 60 years old [35]. The penetrance of an *SDHD* mutation is approximately 80 % at age of 50 years [34, 47].

Recessive *SDHA* mutations cause severe mitochondrial respiratory chain complex II deficiency and Leigh syndrome in early childhood [27, 29, 31]. However, a dominant *SDHA* germline mutation may result in PGL5 with LOH in the tumors, late-onset optic atrophy, ataxia, and myopathy, or gastrointestinal stromal tumors [7, 28, 30, 33]. As described by Korpershoek and colleagues, some *SDHA* mutations in PGL/PCC may occur in sporadic cases and may exhibit low penetrance. Therefore, an accurate clinical evaluation, family history, immunohistochemical and enzymatic analyses on tumor tissues, LOH study, and an estimated allelic frequency of a particular variant in the population must be considered for the proper interpretation of a variant.

An accurate detailed family history is especially important for the interpretation of mutations in the *SDHD* and *SDHAF2* genes due to their parent-of-origin effects. The tumors are exclusively from paternally inherited alleles [4, 5]. Thus, a paternal transmission pattern in a family pedigree is highly suggestive of an *SDHD* or *SDHAF2* germline mutation.

Clinical Utility of Testing

Although the majority of PGLs are benign, about 10 % may develop malignant features. Up to 65 % of PGLs in children/adolescents (<20 years old) are malignant [48]. Malignancy of PGL/PCC is defined by the presence of metastases, not by local invasion. Malignancy is not easy to determine by imaging or histochemistry. The prognosis for malignant PCC is about 50 % 5-year survival [1, 2]. Approximately 29 % of head and neck PGL produce significant amounts of catecholamines [50]. Excessive catecholamines may cause a variety of clinical symptoms including hypertension, palpitations, headache, sweating, and pallor.

Early detection of a PGL/PCC tumor with confirmed molecular testing is useful for disease prognosis and patient care. The primary goals for molecular testing of the *SDH* genes in patients affected with PGL/PCC are to confirm a clinical diagnosis, to improve medical management for the patients, and to facilitate carrier testing and genetic counseling for family members. Confirmation of the clinical diagnosis by the identification of a causative mutation may help clinicians to focus on the proper treatment and patient management rather than further expensive screening for differential diagnosis. Since *SDH* genes are tumor suppressor genes with an autosomal dominant mode of inheritance, identification of a mutation warrants testing of at-risk family members, including parents, children, and siblings of the proband. First-degree relatives have a 50 % carrier risk. If the mutation is not found in the parents, the mutation may be considered de novo, although gonadal mosaicism, which has not been documented, cannot be ruled out. Familial testing may find the mutation in young, presymptomatic relatives. Those presymptomatic mutation carriers could be closely monitored, for example, by regular computed tomography (CT) scanning or magnetic resonance imaging (MRI). Thus, a tumor may be identified at an early stage, which may allow early removal of the tumor to cure the disease. Surgery is still the primary treatment of PGL/PCC. Laparoscopic surgery is the first choice for resection of adrenal and extra-adrenal tumors. Other treatments include chemotherapy, radiotherapy, and/or [^{131}I] meta-iodobenzylguanidine [1]. Those relatives who have tested negative for the familial mutation may be spared the monitoring procedures.

Quality Control and Laboratory Issues

Although lack of SDHB immunostaining of tumor tissues is highly suggestive of a mutation in the *SDH* genes, the specific gene is not identified by this test. Other information including family history, location and malignancy of the tumor, and the number of tumors may help to prioritize candidate genes. Sequence analysis of *SDHB* should be the top priority if a sporadic patient is affected with malignant PGL/PCC. *SDHD* sequencing is highly recommended for a patient with a family history, especially if all the affected family members show inheritance from their fathers. While Sanger sequencing has high sensitivity for detection of point mutations in the coding regions, some mutations may be missed. For example, single nucleotide polymorphisms at PCR primer sites may result in allele dropout due to lack of or reduced PCR amplification of that allele and mutations in the promoter and deep intronic regions, and large heterozygous deletions/duplications may not be detected by sequencing. These drawbacks can be overcome by careful test design. For instance, two pairs of primers amplifying the same exon may be designed to avoid reduced amplification due to SNPs at the primer sites, and PCR primers may be used to amplify promoter and deep intronic regions for mutation testing. Large heterozygous germline deletion mutations have been reported [14]. If clinical findings strongly suggest an *SDH* mutation and sequence analysis is negative, aCGH testing or MLPA should be considered [46].

Special attention is required for the test design for *SDHA* sequence analysis due to the existence of a highly homologous pseudogene, which is located on chromosome 3q29. The homologous region involves exons 3–14. When clinical manifestation and other laboratory results strongly suggest an *SDHA* germline mutation but a mutation cannot be found by routine *SDHA* sequence analysis, the other factors mentioned above need to be considered. For example, long-range PCR (LR-PCR) may be used to avoid amplification of the pseudogene. Additional pairs of PCR primers may be used to avoid SNPs in PCR primer sites. In our laboratory (Medical Genetics Laboratories at the Baylor College of Medicine), we design LR-PCR primers that are located in nonhomologous regions to specifically amplify the *SDHA* gene and not the pseudogene. The LR-PCR products are then used as templates for PCR amplification of each exon that has homologous sequence in the genome. This strategy can avoid interference from homologous sequences. Even though the *SDHD* gene has a processed pseudogene on chromosome 1, sequence analysis may not be an issue because PCR primers are usually designed to include partial introns where sequences are locus specific. Due to existence of homologous sequences for the *SDHA* and *SDHD* genes, aCGH may not be useful to detect exonic deletions/duplications. In these cases, MLPA analysis is an option.

Proficiency testing programs are not available for the *SDH* genes, so laboratories must meet the proficiency testing requirements through interlaboratory sample exchange.

References

1. Chen H, Sippel RS, O'Dorisio MS, Vinik AI, Lloyd RV, Pacak K. The North American Neuroendocrine Tumor Society consensus guideline for the diagnosis and management of neuroendocrine tumors: pheochromocytoma, paraganglioma, and medullary thyroid cancer. Pancreas. 2010;39:775–83.
2. Lloyd RV. Adrenal cortical tumors, pheochromocytomas and paragangliomas. Mod Pathol. 2011;24:S58–65.
3. Ghezzi D, Goffrini P, Uziel G, Horvath R, Klopstock T, et al. SDHAF1, encoding a LYR complex-II specific assembly factor, is mutated in SDH-defective infantile leukoencephalopathy. Nat Genet. 2009;41:654–6.
4. Hao H-X, Khalimonchuk O, Schraders M, Dephoure N, Bayley J-P, et al. SDH5, a gene required for flavination of succinate dehydrogenase, is mutated in paraganglioma. Science. 2009;325:1139–42.
5. Baysal BE, Ferrell RE, Willett-Brozick JE, Lawrence EC, Myssiorek D, et al. Mutations in SDHD, a mitochondrial complex II gene, in hereditary paraganglioma. Science. 2000;287:848–51.
6. Astuti D, Latif F, Dallol A, Dahia PLM, Douglas F, et al. Gene mutations in the Succinate Dehydrogenase Subunit SDHB cause susceptibility to familial pheochromocytoma and to familial paraganglioma. Am J Hum Genet. 2001;69:49–54.
7. Burnichon N, Brière J-J, Libé R, Vescovo L, Rivière J, et al. SDHA is a tumor suppressor gene causing paraganglioma. Hum Mol Genet. 2010;19:3011–20.
8. Niemann S, Muller U. Mutations in SDHC cause autosomal dominant paraganglioma, type 3. Nat Genet. 2000;26:268–70.
9. Amar L, Bertherat J, Baudin E, Ajzenberg C, Bressac-de Paillerets B, et al. Genetic testing in pheochromocytoma or functional paraganglioma. J Clin Oncol. 2005;23:8812–8.
10. Burnichon N, Vescovo L, Amar L, Libé R, de Reynies A, et al. Integrative genomic analysis reveals somatic mutations in pheochromocytoma and paraganglioma. Hum Mol Genet. 2011;20:3974–85.
11. Gimenez-Roqueplo A-P, Burnichon N, Amar L, Favier J, Jeunemaitre X, Plouin P-F. Recent advances in the genetics of phaeochromocytoma and functional paraganglioma. Clin Exp Pharmacol Physiol. 2008;35:376–9.
12. Bayley JP, Grimbergen AE, van Bunderen PA, van der Wielen M, Kunst HP, et al. The first Dutch SDHB founder deletion in paraganglioma-pheochromocytoma patients. BMC Med Genet. 2009;10:34.
13. Burnichon N, Rohmer V, Amar L, Herman P, Leboulleux S, et al. The succinate dehydrogenase genetic testing in a large prospective

series of patients with paragangliomas. J Clin Endocrinol Metab. 2009;94:2817–27.
14. Mannelli M, Castellano M, Schiavi F, Filetti S, Giacchè M, et al. Clinically guided genetic screening in a large cohort of italian patients with pheochromocytomas and/or functional or nonfunctional paragangliomas. J Clin Endocrinol Metab. 2009;94:1541–7.
15. Briere JJ, Favier J, Benit P, El Ghouzzi V, Lorenzato A, et al. Mitochondrial succinate is instrumental for HIF1alpha nuclear translocation in SDHA-mutant fibroblasts under normoxic conditions. Hum Mol Genet. 2005;14:3263–9.
16. Selak MA, Armour SM, MacKenzie ED, Boulahbel H, Watson DG, et al. Succinate links TCA cycle dysfunction to oncogenesis by inhibiting HIF-alpha prolyl hydroxylase. Cancer Cell. 2005;7:77–85.
17. Dahia PL, Ross KN, Wright ME, Hayashida CY, Santagata S, et al. A HIF1alpha regulatory loop links hypoxia and mitochondrial signals in pheochromocytomas. PLoS Genet. 2005;1:72–80.
18. Majmundar AJ, Wong WJ, Simon MC. Hypoxia-inducible factors and the response to hypoxic stress. Mol Cell. 2010;40:294–309.
19. Raimundo N, Baysal BE, Shadel GS. Revisiting the TCA cycle: signaling to tumor formation. Trends Mol Med. 2011;17:641–9.
20. Selak MA, Duran RV, Gottlieb E. Redox stress is not essential for the pseudo-hypoxic phenotype of succinate dehydrogenase deficient cells. Biochim Biophys Acta. 2006;1757:567–72.
21. Gottlieb E, Tomlinson IP. Mitochondrial tumour suppressors: a genetic and biochemical update. Nat Rev Cancer. 2005;5:857–66.
22. Kaelin Jr WG, Ratcliffe PJ. Oxygen sensing by metazoans: the central role of the HIF hydroxylase pathway. Mol Cell. 2008;30:393–402.
23. Klimova T, Chandel NS. Mitochondrial complex III regulates hypoxic activation of HIF. Cell Death Differ. 2008;15:660–6.
24. Sudarshan S, Sourbier C, Kong HS, Block K, Valera Romero VA, et al. Fumarate hydratase deficiency in renal cancer induces glycolytic addiction and hypoxia-inducible transcription factor 1alpha stabilization by glucose-dependent generation of reactive oxygen species. Mol Cell Biol. 2009;29:4080–90.
25. Piruat JI, Pintado CO, Ortega-Sáenz P, Roche M, López-Barneo J. The mitochondrial SDHD gene is required for early embryogenesis, and its partial deficiency results in persistent carotid body glomus cell activation with full responsiveness to hypoxia. Mol Cell Biol. 2004;24:10933–40.
26. Morris AAM, Farnsworth L, Ackrell BAC, Turnbull DM, Birch-Machin MA. The cDNA sequence of the flavoprotein subunit of human heart succinate dehydrogenase. Biochim Biophys Acta. 1994;1185:125–8.
27. Bourgeron T, Rustin P, Chretien D, Birch-Machin M, Bourgeois M, et al. Mutation of a nuclear succinate dehydrogenase gene results in mitochondrial respiratory chain deficiency. Nat Genet. 1995;11:144–9.
28. Birch-Machin MA, Taylor RW, Cochran B, Ackrell BA, Turnbull DM. Late-onset optic atrophy, ataxia, and myopathy associated with a mutation of a complex II gene. Ann Neurol. 2000;48:330–5.
29. Horvath R, Abicht A, Holinski-Feder E, Laner A, Gempel K, et al. Leigh syndrome caused by mutations in the flavoprotein (Fp) subunit of succinate dehydrogenase (SDHA). J Neurol Neurosurg Psychiatry. 2006;77:74–6.
30. Pantaleo MA, Astolfi A, Indio V, Moore R, Thiessen N, et al. SDHA loss-of-function mutations in KIT-PDGFRA wild-type gastrointestinal stromal tumors identified by massively parallel sequencing. J Natl Cancer Inst. 2011;103:983–7.
31. Parfait B, Chretien D, Rotig A, Marsac C, Munnich A, Rustin P. Compound heterozygous mutations in the flavoprotein gene of the respiratory chain complex II in a patient with Leigh syndrome. Hum Genet. 2000;106:236–43.
32. Van Coster R, Seneca S, Smet J, Van Hecke R, Gerlo E, et al. Homozygous Gly555Glu mutation in the nuclear-encoded 70 kDa flavoprotein gene causes instability of the respiratory chain complex II. Am J Med Genet A. 2003;120A:13–8.
33. Korpershoek E, Favier J, Gaal J, Burnichon N, van Gessel B, et al. SDHA immunohistochemistry detects germline SDHA gene mutations in apparently sporadic paragangliomas and pheochromocytomas. J Clin Endocrinol Metab. 2011;96:E1472–6.
34. Neumann HP, Pawlu C, Peczkowska M, Bausch B, McWhinney SR, et al. Distinct clinical features of paraganglioma syndromes associated with SDHB and SDHD gene mutations. JAMA. 2004;292:943–51.
35. Schiavi F, Milne RL, Anda E, Blay P, Castellano M, et al. Are we overestimating the penetrance of mutations in SDHB? Hum Mutat. 2010;31:761–2.
36. Blank A, Schmitt AM, Korpershoek E, van Nederveen F, Rudolph T, et al. SDHB loss predicts malignancy in pheochromocytomas/sympathetic paragangliomas, but not through hypoxia signalling. Endocr Relat Cancer. 2010;17:919–28.
37. Mannelli M, Ercolino T, Giache V, Simi L, Cirami C, Parenti G. Genetic screening for pheochromocytoma: should SDHC gene analysis be included? J Med Genet. 2007;44:586–7.
38. Peczkowska M, Cascon A, Prejbisz A, Kubaszek A, Cwikla BJ, et al. Extra-adrenal and adrenal pheochromocytomas associated with a germline SDHC mutation. Nat Clin Pract Endocrinol Metab. 2008;4:111–5.
39. Erlic Z, Rybicki L, Peczkowska M, Golcher H, Kann PH, et al. Clinical predictors and algorithm for the genetic diagnosis of pheochromocytoma patients. Clin Cancer Res. 2009;15:6378–85.
40. Hensen EF, Jordanova ES, van Minderhout IJ, Hogendoorn PC, Taschner PE, et al. Somatic loss of maternal chromosome 11 causes parent-of-origin-dependent inheritance in SDHD-linked paraganglioma and phaeochromocytoma families. Oncogene. 2004;23:4076–83.
41. Yeap PM, Tobias ES, Mavraki E, Fletcher A, Bradshaw N, et al. Molecular analysis of pheochromocytoma after maternal transmission of SDHD mutation elucidates mechanism of parent-of-origin effect. J Clin Endocrinol Metab. 2011;96:E2009–13.
42. Kunst HPM, Rutten MH, de Mönnink J-P, Hoefsloot LH, Timmers HJLM, et al. SDHAF2 (PGL2-SDH5) and hereditary head and neck paraganglioma. Clin Cancer Res. 2011;17:247–54.
43. Bayley JP, Kunst HP, Cascon A, Sampietro ML, Gaal J, et al. SDHAF2 mutations in familial and sporadic paraganglioma and phaeochromocytoma. Lancet Oncol. 2010;11:366–72.
44. Piccini V, Rapizzi E, Bacca A, Di Trapani, Pulli R, et al. Head and neck paragangliomas: genetic spectrum and clinical variability in 79 consecutive patients. Endocr Relat Cancer. 2012;149–55.
45. van Nederveen FH, Gaal J, Favier J, Korpershoek E, Oldenburg RA, et al. An immunohistochemical procedure to detect patients with paraganglioma and phaeochromocytoma with germline SDHB, SDHC, or SDHD gene mutations: a retrospective and prospective analysis. Lancet Oncol. 2009;10:764–71.
46. Wong L-JC, Dimmock D, Geraghty MT, Quan R, Lichter-Konecki U, et al. Utility of oligonucleotide array–based comparative genomic hybridization for detection of target gene deletions. Clin Chem. 2008;54:1141–8.
47. Benn DE, Gimenez-Roqueplo A-P, Reilly JR, Bertherat J, Burgess J, et al. Clinical presentation and penetrance of pheochromocytoma/paraganglioma syndromes. J Clin Endocrinol Metab. 2006;91:827–36.
48. Ricketts C, Woodward ER, Killick P, Morris MR, Astuti D, et al. Germline SDHB mutations and familial renal cell carcinoma. J Natl Cancer Inst. 2008;100:1260–2.
49. King KS, Prodanov T, Kantorovich V, Fojo T, Hewitt JK, et al. Metastatic pheochromocytoma/paraganglioma related to primary tumor development in childhood or adolescence: significant link to SDHB mutations. J Clin Oncol. 2011;29:4137–42.
50. van Duinen N, Steenvoorden D, Kema IP, Jansen JC, Vriends AH, et al. Increased urinary excretion of 3-methoxytyramine in patients with head and neck paragangliomas. J Clin Endocrinol Metab. 2010;95:209–14.

Section III

Solid Tumors

Section Editor: Antonia R. Sepulveda

Colorectal Cancer

31

Antonia R. Sepulveda, Deqin Ma, Kathryn C. Behling, and Helen Fernandes

Abstract

Molecular testing of colorectal cancer (CRC) has become the standard practice in the management of patients who are candidates for chemotherapy and gene- or pathway-targeted therapies, providing critical information for precision therapy. Current and emerging testing approaches and guidelines used to select *EGFR* pathway-targeted therapies for CRC are reviewed, as well as the use of DNA mismatch repair deficiency testing in CRC for identification of patients who might not benefit from conventional therapies containing 5-fluorouracil (5FU). Recent recommendations for extended *RAS* mutation testing encompassing exons 2, 3, and 4 of *KRAS* and *NRAS* in CRC are highlighted. An overview of laboratory considerations includes the critical role of tumor tissue evaluation by pathologists, in order to select the best areas of tumor for testing. In addition to a number of conventional testing platforms, given the increasing number of gene mutations that may be critical to achieve targeted therapy efficacy in CRC, advances in the use of gene panels for mutation analysis with platforms that permit detection of hundreds of mutations in a single sample, such as next-generation sequencing (NGS) gene panels, are described.

Keywords

Mutation testing recommendations • Mutation detection assays • *RAS* mutation • *BRAF* mutation • Microsatellite instability • Colorectal cancer • Targeted therapy

Molecular Basis of Colorectal Cancer

Colorectal cancer (CRC) is the third most common cause of cancer in men and women in the USA with approximately 140,000 new cases annually [1, 2]. The majority of CRCs arise from precursor adenomas or from serrated polyps [3, 4]. The classifications of CRC based on molecular alterations have been centered on genomic and epigenomic alterations, leading to CRC molecular subtypes with chromosomal instability (CIN), CpG island methylator phenotype (CIMP), and microsatellite instability (MSI) [5–7]. Based on these genomic and epigenomic changes, five CRC types with prognostic significance have been defined: CIN only (58.2 %), MSI associated (12.6 %), CIMP only (5.3 %), CIMP+/CIN+ (13.4 %), and triple negative (10.6 %) [7].

A.R. Sepulveda, M.D., Ph.D. (✉)
Department of Pathology and Cell Biology, Columbia University Medical Center, New York, NY, USA
e-mail: as4400@columbia.edu

D. Ma, M.D., Ph.D.
Department of Pathology, University of Iowa Hospitals and Clinics, Iowa City, IA, USA

K.C. Behling, M.D., Ph.D.
Department of Biomedical Sciences, Cooper Medical School of Rowan University, Camden, NJ, USA

Department of Pathology, Cooper University Hospital, Camden, NJ, USA

H. Fernandes, Ph.D.
Department of Pathology and Laboratory Medicine, Weill Cornell Medical College, New York, NY, USA

D.G.B. Leonard (ed.), *Molecular Pathology in Clinical Practice*, DOI 10.1007/978-3-319-19674-9_31

The CIN pathway CRCs arise through the conventional adenoma-to-carcinoma progression and are characterized by widespread imbalances in chromosome numbers and alterations of multiple tumor suppressor genes and oncogenes, including adenomatous polyposis coli (*APC*), deleted in colorectal cancer (*DCC*), and deleted in pancreatic cancer 4 (*DPC4, SMAD4*), *TP53*, *KRAS*, and *CTNNB1* [3]. The CIMP pathway CRCs are characterized by methylation of CpG islands in genes associated with CRC carcinogenesis such as the *CDKN2A* tumor suppressor gene, *THBS1*, *MLH1*, and other cancer-related genes [8, 9].

MSI occurs in both sporadic and hereditary CRCs, however, by different mechanisms. The MSI pathway utilized by sporadic CRCs is characteristic of tumors with loss of expression of *MLH1* resulting from CIMP-associated CpG promoter methylation of the promoter region of this DNA mismatch repair (MMR) gene [9, 10]. In contrast, in hereditary nonpolyposis colorectal cancer (HNPCC), also known as Lynch syndrome, which represents 3–6 % of all CRC cases, MSI is due to germline mutations in one of the MMR genes. In both cases, deficient MMR function results in ineffective repair of DNA polymerase slippage errors in microsatellites and repetitive nucleotide sequences during DNA synthesis, resulting in changes in the number of nucleotides in these repeats, which is called MSI [11, 12]. Notably, CIMP is not a feature of HNPCC CRCs [13]. HNPCC patients inherit germline mutations of *MLH1*, *MSH2*, *MSH6*, or *PMS2*, in approximately 40 %, 40 %, 10 %, and 5 % of HNPCC cases, respectively [14].

Recently, The Cancer Genome Atlas (TCGA) project reported the results of a comprehensive analysis of 276 CRCs that included exome and DNA copy number analysis, CpG methylation assessment, and messenger RNA and microRNA expression [5]. The TCGA exome sequence analysis revealed two CRC groups: hypermutated and non-hypermutated tumors, consistent with previous studies [5]. Most hypermutated tumors (70 %) had high levels of MSI (MSI-H), with the majority showing *MLH1* promoter methylation, and most but not all cases showed overlapping CIMP. The remainder of the hypermutated tumors (30 %) lacked MSI-H, CIMP, or *MLH1* promoter methylation, but had somatic mutations in MMR genes or the *POLE* gene [5]. The most frequently mutated genes in the hypermutated tumors were *ACVR2A*, *APC*, *TGFBR2*, *MSH3*, *MSH6*, *SLC9A9*, *TCF7L2*, and *BRAF* (specifically the V600E mutation). The most frequent mutations in non-hypermutated tumors were detected in the following genes: *APC*, *TP53*, *KRAS*, *PIK3CA*, *FBXW7*, *SMAD4*, *TCF7L2*, and *NRAS* [5]. The TCGA report provided a detailed analysis of altered pathways in CRC, summarized below [5].

WNT Signaling Pathway

Alteration of the WNT signaling pathway occurs in 93 % of all CRCs, and inactivation of *APC* or activating mutations of *CTNNB1* occur in approximately 80 % of tumors. The WNT receptor frizzled (*FZD10*) was overexpressed in approximately 17 % of cases [5].

PI3K, RAS, and MAPK Signaling Pathways

Among non-hypermutated CRCs, 55 % have alterations in *KRAS*, *NRAS*, or *BRAF*, with significant mutual exclusivity. *IGF2* and *IRS2* overexpression was seen in some tumors. Mutually exclusive mutations in *PIK3R1* and *PIK3CA* and deletions in *PTEN* occur in 2 %, 15 %, and 4 % of non-hypermutated tumors, respectively. Co-occurrence of alterations involving the RAS and PI3K pathways occur in one-third of tumors, suggesting that simultaneous inhibition of the RAS and PI3K pathways may be required to achieve therapeutic benefit when treating these CRCs [5].

TGF-β Signaling Pathway

Genomic alterations in *TGFBR1*, *TGFBR2*, *ACVR2A*, *ACVR1B*, *SMAD2*, *SMAD3*, and *SMAD4* occur in 27 % of non-hypermutated and in 87 % of hypermutated CRCs [5].

TP53 Pathway

Alterations in *TP53* occur in 59 % of non-hypermutated CRCs. Alterations in ATM, a kinase that phosphorylates and activates TP53 after DNA damage, are seen in 7 % of non-hypermutated tumors. Alterations in these two genes trend toward mutual exclusivity [5].

Role of MYC in CRC

Integrated analysis of copy number, gene expression, methylation, and pathway data show that most CRCs have changes in the genes that are transcriptionally regulated by MYC. Activation of the WNT signaling pathway and inactivation of the TGF-β signaling pathway, resulting in increased activity of MYC, were nearly always present in CRC [5].

Molecular Testing of Colorectal Cancer for Targeted and Conventional Therapies

In clinical practice, molecular testing of CRCs is used to identify gene mutations that help oncologists select the therapeutic regimen for individual patients and to evaluate MMR deficiency to identify patients with HNPCC or sporadic MSI CRCs. Testing for DNA MMR in CRC is discussed in Chap. 24. This chapter reviews current and emerging testing approaches used to (1) select EGFR pathway-targeted therapies for CRC treatment and (2) identify patients who might not benefit from conventional therapies containing 5-fluorouracil (5-FU).

Table 31.1 Frequencies of mutations in EGFR pathway genes in colorectal cancer

Pathway	Genes	Frequency (%)
MAPK pathway	*KRAS*	40–45
	NRAS	2.5
	BRAF	5–10
PI3K pathway	*PIK3CA*	15
	PTEN	10–20
	AKT	5

Targeting EGFR Signaling Pathways in CRC

Aberrant activation of EGFR signaling pathways is frequent in CRC and is primarily associated with activating mutations of genes in the MAPK and PI3K pathways [1, 15]. In contrast to lung cancers, activating mutations in the *EGFR* gene itself have not been identified in CRC [1, 15]. The frequencies of mutations in EGFR pathway genes in CRC are shown in Table 31.1 [16]. Combined mutations of *KRAS* or *NRAS* and *PIK3CA* (5–10 %) also occur. Together, *BRAF* and *KRAS* are mutated in about half of all CRC cases, and *KRAS* and *BRAF* mutations are mutually exclusive [17, 18]). Activating mutations in the *KRAS* gene are associated with lack of responsiveness to monoclonal antibody-based therapy for CRC that targets EGFR. *KRAS* mutations occur mostly at exon 2 (codon 12 [70–80 %] or 13 [20–30 %]), followed by mutations in exon 3 at codon 61 and in exon 4 at codon 146 [19]. Mutations at codons 59 and 117 have also been recently reported (Table 31.2). A similar spectrum of *NRAS* mutations is seen in CRC (Table 31.2).

The most frequent *BRAF* mutations in CRC occur in exon 15 with a T-to-A transversion at nucleotide position 1,796, which leads to the substitution of valine for glutamate (V600E) [16]. The *BRAF* V600E mutation occurs in 4–12 % of MMR-proficient (microsatellite stable) CRCs and in 40–74 % of MLH1-deficient/MSI-H sporadic CRCs, but is not found in MLH1-deficient MSI-H CRC in HNPCC CRCs [17, 22, 23]. Therefore, determination of *BRAF* V600E mutation status may differentiate sporadic from hereditary MSI-H CRC, since hereditary CRC will not have a *BRAF* V600E mutation.

Mutations in the PI3K pathway have been reported in approximately 20 % of all CRCs [16, 17]. Interestingly, mutations involving genes in the two EGFR signaling pathways are not mutually exclusive, and about 5–10 % of CRCs carry mutations in genes from both the MAPK and PIK3 signaling pathways [16, 17].

Cetuximab and panitumumab are antibodies that bind to the extracellular domain of EGFR, block EGF and binding of other endogenous ligands to the EGFR, and thereby block EGFR signaling. Targeted EGFR therapies improve progression-free and overall survival in metastatic CRC [24].

Table 31.2 Overall *RAS* mutations in CRCs without mutations in *KRAS* codons 12 and 13

	OPUS trial (% of total CRCs)	CRYSTAL trial (% of total CRCs)
CRCs with other *RAS* mutations (WT *KRAS* C12 and C13)	27.9	17.0
Other *KRAS* mutations	15.2	8.9
Exon 3: C59 and C61	5.9	3.3
Exon 4: C117 and C146	9.3	5.6
***NRAS* mutations**	12.7	8.1
Exon 2: C12 and C13	6.8	3.5
Exon 3: C59 and C61	5.1	2.8
Exon 4: C117 and C146	0.8	0.9

The cutoff used for scoring mutation positivity was 5 % in both OPUS and CRYSTAL trials [20, 21]
C codon, *WT* wild type

For patients with metastatic CRC with wild-type *KRAS*, treatment with cetuximab significantly improved overall survival (median 9.5 vs 4.8 months) as compared to supportive care alone (Karapetis et al. [25]). In contrast, patients with mutated *KRAS* CRCs showed no significant difference between those who were treated with cetuximab and those who were not, leading to the conclusion that patients with CRC carrying a mutated *KRAS* do not benefit from cetuximab, whereas patients with wild-type *KRAS* CRC benefit from cetuximab therapy because the antibody effectively blocks the activating EGFR signaling at the cell surface [25]. The mutations tested for in the first trials were limited to *KRAS* exons 12 and 13 [24]. Further evidence from phase II and III clinical trials using monoclonal antibodies as monotherapy or in combination with chemotherapy for metastatic CRC (stage IV: any T, any N, M1) demonstrated that CRC with a *KRAS* mutation in codons 12, 13, or 61 did not benefit from treatment with cetuximab or panitumumab [26]. Based on the available clinical trial data in 2009, the American Society of Clinical Oncology recommended that patients with metastatic CRC who are candidates for anti-EGFR antibody therapy should have their tumor tested for *KRAS* mutations in a CLIA-accredited laboratory [26].

Up to 40 % of patients with a CRC without a *KRAS* mutation respond to anti-EGFR antibody therapy, while the remaining 60 % of patients with *KRAS* wild-type tumors did not respond [26]. The lack of response may be due to (1) mutations in genes downstream of KRAS, (2) the presence of *KRAS* mutations in exons not tested in the assay used for *KRAS* mutation testing, (3) mutations in *NRAS*, or (4) changes in other oncogenic pathways in individual cancers. For CRC with mutant *KRAS*, a number of drugs targeted to inhibit downstream signaling molecules, such as inhibitors of mTOR, RAF, and MEK, are under evaluation [27].

The role of *BRAF* mutation for prediction of response to anti-EGFR therapy in CRC is still pending results from larger studies [28, 29]. One study reported that colon cancer cells were unresponsive to the BRAF inhibitor vemurafenib due to rapid feedback activation of EGFR, blunting the benefit of vemurafenib [30]. However, the low proportion of CRC cases with *BRAF* mutations and the poor prognosis associated with *BRAF* mutations make determination of a definitive impact on outcomes difficult [28, 29].

Conflicting roles of *PIK3CA* mutations in tumor response to anti-EGFR antibody therapy have been reported in a number of small studies [31, 32]. However, a large study found that the presence of a *PIK3CA* mutation is associated with a poor response to cetuximab [17]. In this study, *BRAF*, *NRAS*, and *PIK3CA* exon 20 mutations were significantly associated with a poor response to cetuximab, and objective response rates were improved by stratifying patients by genotype of *BRAF*, *NRAS*, and *PIK3CA* exon 20 mutations in the *KRAS* wild-type population and excluding patients with any mutation from the treatment arm [17, 33]. However, guidelines for testing CRC of patients who are candidates for anti-EGFR antibody therapy for *BRAF* and *PIK3CA* mutations have not yet been reported.

Tissue Sample and Gene Testing Considerations for CRC-Targeted Therapies

The standard of practice for selection of patients with metastatic CRC who are candidates for targeted therapies with anti-EGFR antibodies has been primarily based on the mutation status of *KRAS* [26]. However, as discussed above, the mutation status of *BRAF*, *NRAS*, *PI3KCA*, and other genes downstream of EGFR may affect the tumor response to anti-EGFR therapy [33]. Therefore, testing for mutations in other genes may be indicated in candidate patients, particularly in the setting of clinical trials, at the present time. *EGFR* mutation testing is not indicated for CRC since activating *EGFR* mutations in CRC are rare and were not demonstrated to confer sensitivity to tyrosine kinase inhibitors or to cetuximab therapy [34].

In addition to *KRAS* mutations in codons 12 and 13 of exon 2, *KRAS* mutations in codons 59 and 61 of exon 3 and codons 117 and 146 of exon 4 and similar mutation hot spots in *NRAS* need to be considered when selecting true *RAS* wild-type patients who will benefit from cetuximab therapy for metastatic CRC (Tables 31.2 and 31.3) [20, 21, 35]. Further, the addition of cetuximab therapy for patients with any *RAS* mutation is of no benefit [20, 21, 35]. Therefore, patients with metastatic CRC should undergo expanded testing for all known activating *RAS* mutations, to avoid use of cetuximab in patients whose CRCs will not respond [20, 21, 35]. Interestingly, in contrast to other activating mutations in *KRAS*, use of cetuximab for patients with chemotherapy-refractory CRC with the *KRAS* G13D mutation may be associated with longer overall and progression-free survival than with other *KRAS* activating mutations [18], although this has not been supported by some studies.

Table 31.3 Effect of cetuximab in true *RAS* wild-type CRC: results from the CRYSTAL and OPUS clinical trials [20, 21]

Clinical trial	ORR (%)	PFS (months)	OS (months)
OPUS	57.9 % vs 28.6 %	12 vs 5.8	19.8 vs 17.8
	$p=0.008$	$p=0.062$	$p=$NS
CRYSTAL	66.3 % vs 38.6 %	11.4 vs 8.4	28.4 vs 20.2
	$p<0.0001$	$p=0.0002$	$p=0.0024$

ORR overall response rate, *OS* overall survival, *PFS* progression-free survival

Regarding the choice of tissue for DNA mutation analysis, since *KRAS* mutations occur early in colorectal carcinogenesis, most clinical trials have tested the primary tumor. Published studies show a good correlation between *KRAS* mutation status in primary and metastatic CRC lesions with an average concordance of 93 % (76–100 %) [36, 37]. Therefore, testing tumor tissue from either the primary site or from a metastatic lesion is appropriate, and a metastatic lesion when available is preferred. Pathologists should select a block of formalin-fixed, paraffin-embedded (FFPE) tissue with the highest proportion of viable tumor and highest percentage of tumor cells as possible, understanding that all cells present in the tissue contribute DNA, so this percentage is of all cells, namely, those that normally compose the colonic wall and variable amounts of inflammatory cells. For small samples, adequate DNA amount can be obtained by pooling macro- or microdissected tumor tissue from multiple tissue levels. This procedure may also provide a larger sampling of the tumor, including areas of mutational heterogeneity, thereby improving mutation detection. Importantly, a pretreatment biopsy sample may be preferable for testing rather than a resection specimen removed after neoadjuvant therapy, as is the case in rectal cancers, where minimal numbers of residual viable tumor cells may persist, making these tissues inadequate for molecular testing. Cytology specimens, particularly from metastatic lesions, also provide an adequate source of tumor for DNA extraction and mutation analysis.

In summary, *RAS* mutation analysis of CRC tumor tissues is recommended as the standard of care in patients who are candidates for anti-EGFR antibody therapy [20, 21, 35]. Additional mutation testing of other EGFR signaling pathway genes may be helpful to better select patients for targeted therapies with improved outcomes, but a general consensus about which genes should be tested is not yet established. In large practice centers, the trend is to test all CRCs for *RAS* and *BRAF* V600E mutations and for MMR deficiency (with the use of immunohistochemical and/or MSI testing), thus allowing for selection of patients for conventional therapy as well as targeted therapy [38]. The use of gene panels for mutation analysis with platforms that permit detection of hundreds of mutations in a single sample, such as next-generation sequencing (NGS) gene panels, may provide further insight into the issue of which genes should be tested. However, determination of which mutations should be considered for CRC treatment selection or exclusion still needs to be better defined based on data from clinical trials. The practice of Genomic Tumor Boards to address the use of gene mutation results and other molecular test results is evolving and is being used in some centers to evaluate treatment options other than established treatment protocols by providing clinical trial options for individual patients.

DNA Mismatch Repair Defects and Microsatellite Instability

Approximately 15 % of all CRCs have a deficient MMR system and are characterized by MSI. In 3–5 % of MMR-deficient/MSI-positive CRCs, patients have germline mutations in MMR genes diagnostic of HNPCC or Lynch syndrome, while the remaining are sporadic-type CRCs [39, 40]. In cells with deficient MMR, errors in DNA replication accumulate and are detectable in short tandem repeats of microsatellite regions but also in functional gene coding regions, which results in changes in the length of repeats at any one location (known as MSI) [41–43]. MSI, specifically when a tumor is identified to have a high level of MSI (MSI-H), is a genomic marker of deficient DNA MMR [43]. Six different genes (*MSH2*, *MLH1*, *PMS1*, *PMS2*, *MSH6*, and *MLH3*) encode the MMR system [44]. In HNPCC, as in other hereditary cancer syndromes, recessive mutation of one allele followed by somatic inactivation of the other is the main mechanism of gene silencing [45]. In contrast, in sporadic CRCs, the most frequent mechanism of DNA MMR gene downregulation is biallelic inactivation by CpG methylation and transcriptional silencing of the *MLH1* promoter region [46, 47].

MSI status of CRC can be tested by immunohistochemistry (IHC) of CRC tissue sections to assess expression of the MMR proteins or by PCR-based DNA testing for MSI to detect instability at microsatellite sequences [43, 48]. One advantage of IHC is that the protein identified as showing lost or reduced expression in tumor cell nuclei can be an indicator of which MMR gene has a mutation, which is particularly useful in the workup of HNPCC patients, helping to focus the germline mutation analysis on the most likely affected MMR gene. In addition, combining testing for the *BRAF* V600E activating mutation and CpG island methylation status of the promoter region of *MLH1* can be done to help determine whether a MSI-positive CRC with loss of *MLH1* expression is likely to be an inherited HNPCC CRC (*BRAF* mutation negative and *MLH1* promoter methylation negative) or sporadic-type CRC (*BRAF* mutation positive in up to 70 % of cases and *MLH1* promoter methylation positive) [49].

MSI positivity in CRCs is a prognostic marker for improved survival [42]. MSI was detected in 17 % of CRCs of patients < 50 years of age and was associated with (1) a lower likelihood of tumor metastasis to regional lymph nodes as well as distant organs, contributing to improved survival through tumor downstaging, and (2) an overall survival advantage independent of stage of disease [50]. In addition, no significant difference in survival was found between patients with MSI due to hereditary (HNPCC) CRC compared to sporadic CRC [50, 51]. A reported survival benefit for patients with HNPCC CRC is mainly determined by a diagnosis at younger age and less advanced tumor stage as compared with sporadic MSI-H CRC patients [51].

Deficient DNA MMR and MSI status are predictive of response to therapy in some subsets of deficient MMR CRCs [52]. Both the tumor stage and whether the CRC is sporadic or hereditary (HNPCC) are important factors for selection of adjuvant therapy for CRC patients. Patients with stage II CRCs with MMR-deficient/MSI-positive status receiving 5-FU have no improvement in disease-free survival, and treatment is associated with reduced overall survival [53]. The effect of deficient MMR/MSI in stage III CRC on response to therapy has been more difficult to establish, which may be related to heterogeneity of the studied populations in terms of the proportions of sporadic and HNPCC cases. Some studies showed improved outcomes with chemotherapy for advanced stage III CRCs that were MSI-H [54], but other studies did not [55]. In patients with stages II and III CRC, MMR-deficient CRC patients receiving 5-FU had no improvement in disease-free survival [53]. Sinicrope et al. reported that distant recurrences were reduced by 5-FU-based adjuvant treatment in MMR-deficient stage III CRCs, and a subset analysis suggested that any treatment benefit was restricted to suspected inherited CRCs as compared to sporadic tumors [56]. In summary, larger trials are needed to determine with certainty the utility of MMR and MSI status for treatment selection in routine patient care [56, 57]. Current data support the concept that MMR-deficient/MSI-H stage II and III CRC patients do not benefit from 5-FU-based adjuvant therapy, although one study of stage III MMR-deficient CRC patients showed a treatment benefit restricted to patients with suspected hereditary (HNPCC) CRC.

Assays for CRC Mutation Testing for Selection of Therapy

Many technical approaches and assays are used for mutation testing by clinical molecular laboratories. Laboratory-developed tests (LDTs) are frequently used and follow requirements for validation and interpretation as dictated by CLIA and state regulations, while some commercial in vitro diagnostic (IVD) test kits also are used. Assay methods for mutation detection include Sanger sequencing, pyrosequencing, multiplex PCR with primer extension, fluorescent bead detection assays, MassARRAY matrix-assisted laser desorption/ionization time-of-flight (MALDI-TOF) mass spectrometry, allele-specific PCR such as amplification refractory mutation system/scorpions (ARMS/S), melt curve analysis (as performed in Taq-Man assays using real-time quantitative PCR (qPCR)), and, most recently, NGS [58–62]. Table 31.4 compares three technologies commonly used for mutation detection in cancer-related genes in CRC. Until a few years ago, Sanger sequencing of PCR products was a commonly used method for mutation detection. Recent studies comparing Sanger sequencing with other approaches have highlighted its limited analytical sensitivity for clinical testing of DNA from solid tumor samples, requiring 20–50 % mutant alleles in the amplified products [62, 63].

A number of commercial IVD and LDT assays are available to detect the most common mutations in *KRAS* and *BRAF*. Many of the early assays only tested for a small number of mutations, limiting the correlation between mutation status and drug response in early clinical trials. Of note, early assays for *KRAS* mutation analysis performed both in clinical laboratories and as part of clinical trials were limited to codons 12 and 13 in exon 2, excluding other mutation hot spots. Clinical trials have demonstrated the importance of mutations in previously excluded codons of *KRAS*, in exons 2, 3, and 4, as well as the corresponding codons in *NRAS*. Additionally, mutations in other genes downstream of EGFR in the EGFR signaling pathway also are clinically significant for patient management decisions, as discussed above.

For mutation testing, genomic DNA can be extracted from fresh, frozen, or FFPE tissue using standard molecular laboratory methods. For solid tumor testing, histologic slides should be reviewed by an anatomic pathologist to assess the percent of tumor cells relative to total cells on the slide and to prioritize areas for macro- or microdissection, if necessary, to increase the percentage of tumor cells in the sample used for testing.

Pyrosequencing Assays

Pyrosequencing is a DNA sequencing technique based on the sequencing-by-synthesis principle [64], which is used for analysis of gene regions that are frequently mutated. A pyrosequencing result (pyrogram) for *BRAF* exon 15 is shown in Fig. 31.1. Non-mutated samples show the wild-type sequence

Table 31.4 Comparison of three technologies commonly used for mutation testing for colorectal cancer

Platform	Sanger sequencing	Pyrosequencing	Next-generation sequencing[a]
Principle of technology	Synthesis by addition of labeled nucleotide	Synthesis by nucleotide followed by release of pyrophosphate	Semiconductor: synthesis by nucleotide followed by release of proton
Detection method	Single sequence of varying length by high-resolution (capillary) electrophoresis	Single sequence of limited length using pyrosequencer	Multiple sequences of varying length using chip-based technology
Amplification	Incorporation of labeled nucleotides for strand elongation	Incorporation of unlabeled nucleotides followed by light emission	Incorporation of unlabeled nucleotides followed by pH change
Enzymes	DNA polymerase	DNA polymerase, ATP sulfurylase, luciferase, and apyrase	DNA polymerase
Advantages	Successfully call repeats. Good visual discrimination for interpretation	Fast. Accurate for short sequence reads. Good visual discrimination for easy interpretation	Emulsion PCR and indexing/bar coding allows for high-throughput multiplexing
Disadvantages	Low throughput	Relatively low throughput. Need to input sequence. Difficult to read repeats and homopolymers	Labor-intensive. Difficult to read repeats and homopolymers
Cost	+++ Reagents are expensive	++ Slightly less expensive than Sanger sequencing	+ Comparatively less expensive than both
Turnaround time	8 h/gene sequence	6 h for up to 4 gene sequences	24–36 h for up to 16 gene sequences
Technical issues	++	+	+++
Sensitivity	+	++	++

[a]Next-generation sequencing using the Ion Torrent PGM instrument (Life Technologies, Grand Island, NY)

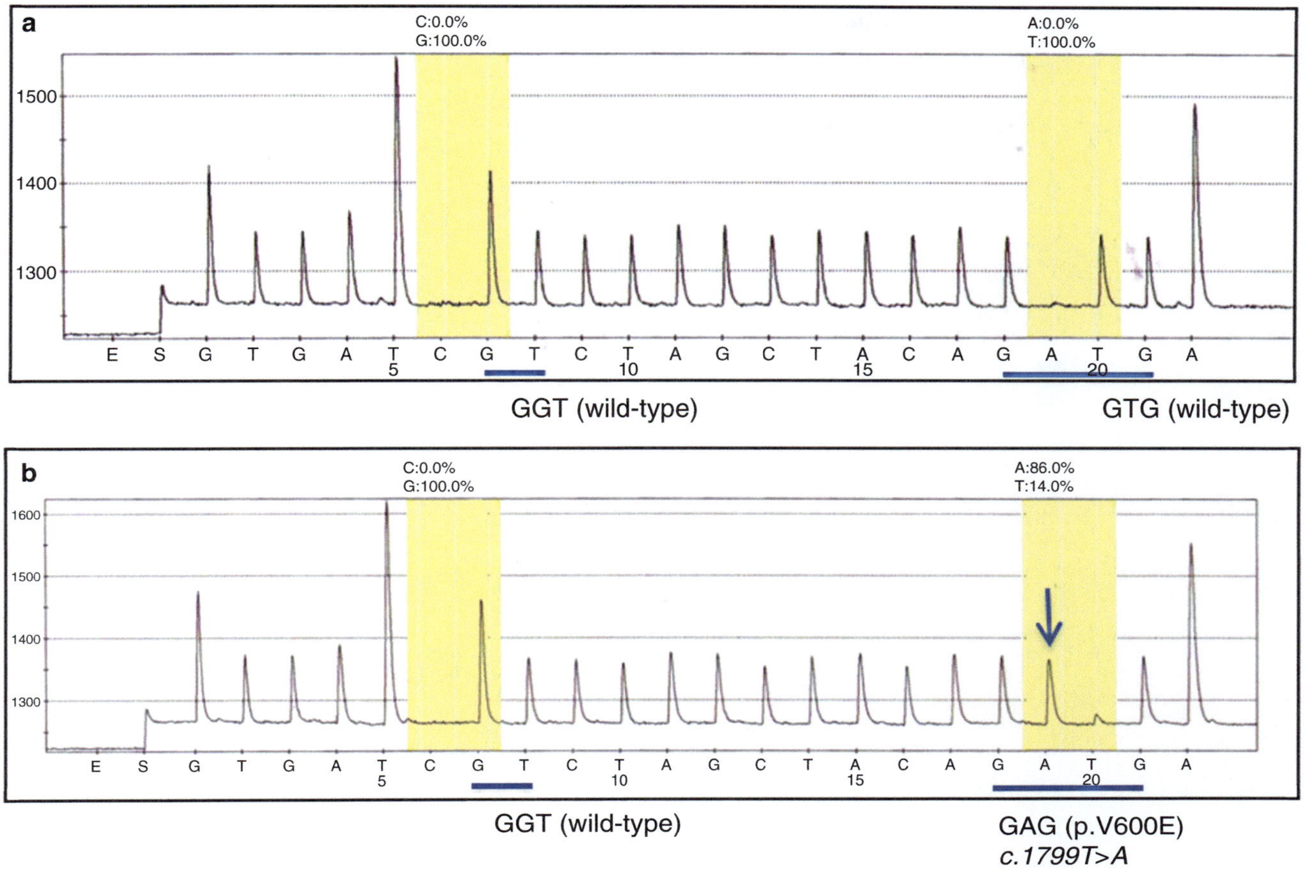

Figure 31.1 Pyrosequencing analysis of *BRAF* exon 15. (**a**) Wild-type *BRAF* sequence. (**b**) An "A" peak (*downward blue arrow*) is present instead of the "T" peak in the wild-type *BRAF* sequence, due to a T>A mutation (c.1799T>A), which results in an amino acid change from valine to glutamic acid in the BRAF protein (p.V600E)

with appropriate peaks and peak heights. Mutations are indicated as different peaks compared to the wild-type sequence or alterations in the height of wild-type peaks relative to a neighboring peak or compared to the reference peak. A reference peak is usually the first peak on each pyrogram. If the background is too high or the peaks are too low, pyrosequencing should be repeated. Indeterminate cases can be verified by Sanger sequencing or other available assays. Examples of *BRAF* mutation testing by pyrosequencing from CRCs of two different patients are shown in Fig. 31.2.

Compared to Sanger sequencing, which has an analytic sensitivity of 20 % mutant alleles, pyrosequencing has a higher sensitivity of approximately 5 % using FFPE tissue [65–69]. With its short read length (approximately 50 base pairs), pyrosequencing is optimal for scanning for mutations in hot spot gene regions and has been used to detect mutations in *KRAS* codons 12, 13, 61, and 146 and the *BRAF* V600E mutation [70–72]. Pyrosequencing is suitable for single-nucleotide polymorphism (SNP) genotyping [73] and DNA methylation analysis [74, 75], such as *MLH1* methylation in CRC [76, 77]. The assay can be performed in 96- or 384-well plates and scaled for sequencing hundreds of megabases of DNA using a large-scale parallel pyrosequencing system.

The limitations of pyrosequencing include the short read length of DNA sequences and sequencing errors in homopolymer regions, since the light intensity in such regions is not proportional to the number of nucleotides incorporated.

Multiplexed Primer Extension Assays

The primer extension method is a template-directed dye termination assay designed to detect the base immediately 3′ to the sequencing primer [78]. After the sequence of interest is amplified by PCR and the unincorporated nucleotides are removed, primer extension can be performed in a single reaction tube using, for example, the SNaPshot Multiplex kit (Applied Biosystems, Foster City, CA). The four major

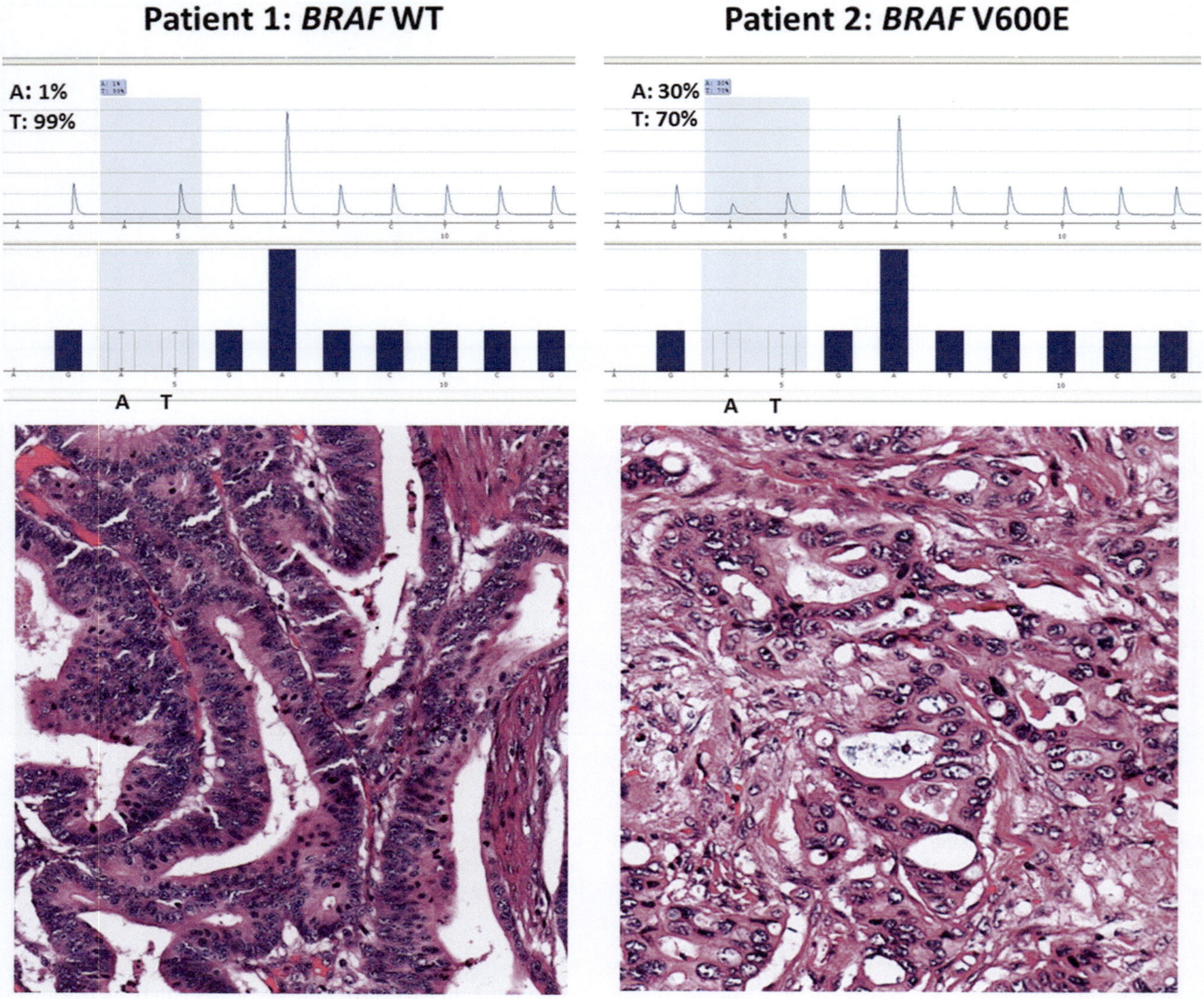

Figure 31.2 Colorectal cancers from two patients tested for *BRAF* V600E mutation by pyrosequencing. Patient 1 (*left*) has a wild-type (WT) gene (99 % T allele at position 1,799) and patient 2 (*right*) is positive for the *BRAF* V600E mutation (30 % A allele at position 1,799). Note that the "A" allele is only present at 30 % of total alleles due to DNA from non-tumor cells in the tissue section that have only the wild-type T allele

steps in a primer extension assay are (1) PCR amplification and column purification of the PCR product; (2) primer extension; (3) alkaline phosphatase digestion and heat inactivation; and (4) capillary electrophoresis of the fluorescently labeled products. Concurrent detection of mutations at multiple sites is possible by multiplexing at the PCR step [79]. When multiplex reactions are run, the primer extension probes are designed with varying lengths of deoxythymidine monophosphate homopolymers at their 5′ end to allow for discrimination of the probe for each site of interrogation by size.

An example of a multiplex primer extension assay for concurrent detection of *BRAF* V600 and K601 and *KRAS* exons 2 and 3 mutations in CRC is shown in Fig. 31.3. Genomic DNA from FFPE CRC tissue is isolated, and the coding sequences for *BRAF* exon 15 and *KRAS* codons 12, 13, and 61 are amplified using specific primers in a multiplex PCR reaction. The probes for primer extension are either in the sense or antisense direction and end one base 5′ of the following positions: nucleotides 1,799 and 1,801 of the *BRAF* gene and nucleotides 34, 35, 37, 38, 181, 182, and 183 of the *KRAS* gene. The probes allow for detection of common variants present in codons V600 and K601 of the *BRAF* gene and codons 12, 13, and 61 of the *KRAS* gene. After amplification, the PCR products are incubated with the unlabeled oligonucleotide primer extension probes, four dideoxynucleotide triphosphates (ddNTPs) labeled with different fluorescent colors, and DNA polymerase. During this primer

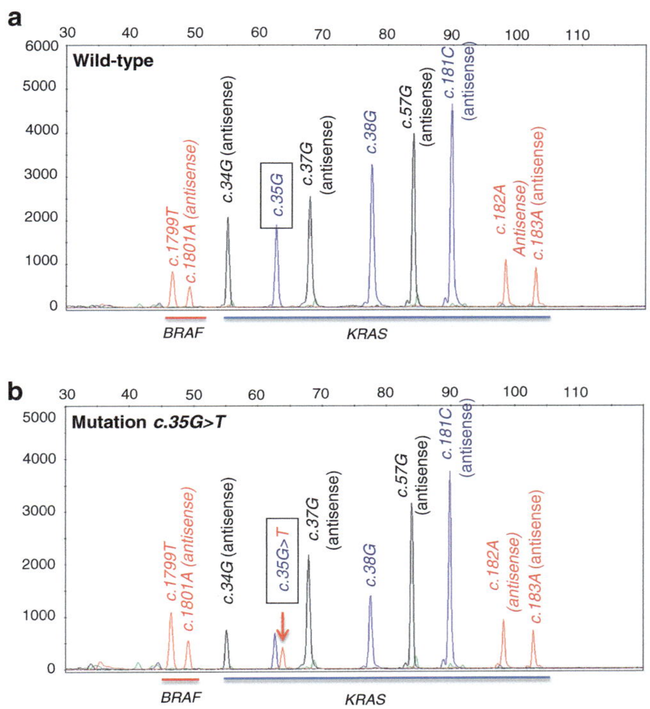

Figure 31.3 Multiplex primer extension assay for detection of *KRAS* codons 12, 13, and 61 mutations and *BRAF* V600E mutations. FFPE tissue section of CRC was manually macro-dissected and used for genomic DNA extraction. *KRAS* codons 12, 13, and 61 and *BRAF* codon 600 sequences were PCR amplified in a multiplex reaction and primer extension was performed. (**a**) No mutation is detected (wild type). (**b**) An extra peak is detected at nucleotide position 2 of the 3-nucleotide codon 12 of *KRAS*, which corresponds to a G>T mutation (c.35G>T) which results in an amino acid change of glycine to valine (p.G12V) in KRAS.

extension step, only the next complementary 5′ nucleotide is added to each probe. The primer extension products are analyzed by capillary electrophoresis. The base at the mutation site is determined by detection of the fluorescent color of the ddNTP that is incorporated.

Controls for primer extension assays included with each run are a wild-type or negative patient sample and a positive sensitivity control (cell line DNA or plasmid). The negative control should show amplification of the valid sizes and colors for all of the normal- or wild-type peaks for the primer extension products. Each patient's PCR and primer extension product serves as its own internal control for extraction and amplification. If no mutation is present, amplification of the valid size and color for the wild-type sequence is seen. If a mutation is present, the mutant peak(s) will be present admixed with the wild-type product. Failure to amplify a product may be due to poor quality or insufficient quantity of DNA or nucleotide polymorphism(s) or mutation(s) that prevents proper annealing of the primer to the DNA template. In the latter situation, an alternate method such as pyrosequencing or Sanger sequencing can be used to confirm the findings.

Primer extension assays combine the specificity of template-directed incorporation of nucleotide by DNA polymerase and the sensitivity of fluorescence polarization in SNP genotyping [79]. Since both wild-type and mutant DNAs are amplified, the limit of detection is determined to some extent by the degree of resolution of the ratio of wild-type to mutant signal. The analytical sensitivity is approximately 2–5 % [80, 81] and the reaction only requires 5–10 ng of genomic DNA [81].

MassARRAY technology (Sequenom, San Diego, CA) is another primer extension method which uses MALDI-TOF for analysis. After PCR amplification and primer extension reactions, nanoliter volumes of the primer extension products are spotted onto a matrix-array chip. The chip is analyzed using MALDI-TOF, and raw data is analyzed using manufacturer's analysis software [82, 83]. The number of assays that can be multiplexed into a single well for MALDI-TOF analysis is dependent on the mutation type and sequencing chemistry, with multiplexing limited to 40 assays for constitutional genetics and eight to ten assays for somatic mutations using iPLEX chemistry [84]. The analytical sensitivity for the MassARRAY platform is approximately 2.5–10 % for somatic mutations [83]. This platform has been used to develop assay panels that include mutations important for predictive and prognostic testing for CRC treatment, including mutations in *KRAS*, *BRAF*, *PI3KCA*, and *PTEN* [83].

Liquid Bead Array Assays

Liquid bead array assays are easy to perform and interpret using predetermined, laboratory-validated cutoffs for positive and negative results. Tumor DNA is used for PCR amplification of the multiple gene region(s) to be analyzed plus an additional conserved genetic sequence, which serves as an amplification control. Biotin-labeled primers are used and are incorporated into the PCR products. The labeled PCR products are hybridized to capture probes, which are covalently bound to fluorescently labeled beads with the color of each bead corresponding to a specific capture probe. The fluorescently labeled beads are incubated with streptavidin-phycoerythrin, a reporter for the presence of the biotin-labeled PCR product, and are analyzed by flow cytometry, to simultaneously detect the presence or absence of hybridized biotin-labeled PCR products and the fluorescent identity of the corresponding bead. Typically, a minimum of 50 beads are assessed for each analyte, and based on the collective fluorescence, the mean fluorescence intensity (MFI) is calculated. The MFI cutoffs for reporting of positive and negative results are validated by the clinical molecular laboratory. The assay result is considered positive when the MFI for an analyte exceeds the predetermined cutoff. When none of the analyte MFI

a

Patient	G12V	G12A	G13D	G12C	G12D	G12S	G12R	EC	Result
Patient 1	161	91	103	74	5120	150.5	120	6766	G12D Positive
Patient 1	150	119	87	42	5295	203	204	6832	G12D Positive
Patient 2	55	118	2604	54	32	206	170	6874	G13D Positive
Patient 2	109	50	2915	25	48	158	169	6933	G13D Positive
Patient 3	116.5	108	92	19	79	179	154	6687	Negative
Patient 3	120.5	100	31	16	59	178	197	6220	Negative
Control Negative	168	78	72.5	1	133	1654	159	8547	Negative
Control NTC	128	40	50.5	0	49.5	143	113	52	No Amp
Control Positive	112.5	74.5	2393	25	19	118	201.5	7671	G13D Positive

b

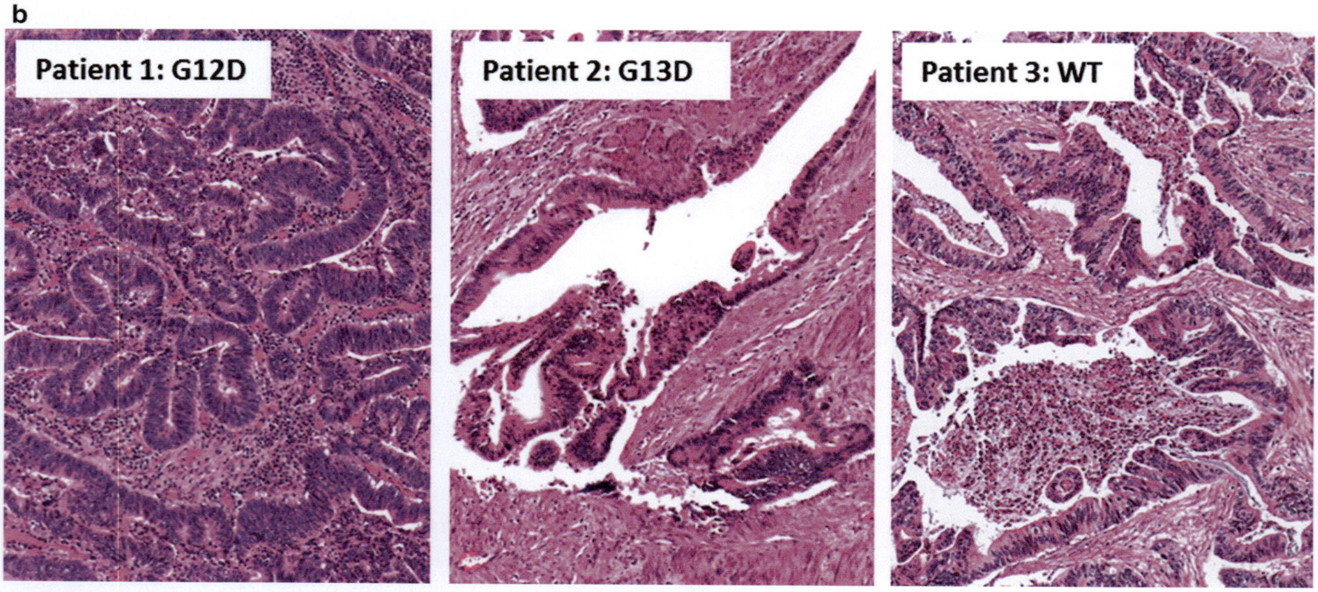

Figure 31.4 Results from a single run of *KRAS* mutation testing using a bead array assay. Results for three patients are shown, as well as results of the controls, including negative, positive, and no-template (NTC) controls. *EC* external positive control, *AMP* amplification

values exceed their cutoffs, but the amplification control is positive, the assay result is reported as negative. Specimen results are reported as inconclusive when MFI values for all analytes and the endogenous control fail to exceed their cutoff values [85].

A liquid bead array assay for the seven most common mutations in the *KRAS* gene is commercially available for the Luminex (Austin, TX) flow cytometer. The assay is relatively easy to perform with a total assay time of approximately 4 h, excluding DNA extraction. This assay has a clinical sensitivity of approximately 98 % and an analytical sensitivity of approximately 1 % mutant DNA in a background of wild-type DNA [86]. Pre-analytical variables, such as DNA amount and extraction method, can affect the analytical sensitivity of this assay, especially in samples with low tumor percentages [87]. Appropriate positive and negative controls are analyzed on all runs with clinical specimens. Cell line or plasmid DNA with one of the seven *KRAS* mutations detected by the assay can be used as a positive control while DNA from a cell line without a *KRAS* mutation can be used as a negative control. A water (no template) control is used as a control for reagent contamination with DNA or amplification products [85]. Figure 31.4 shows the results of *KRAS* mutation detection in three

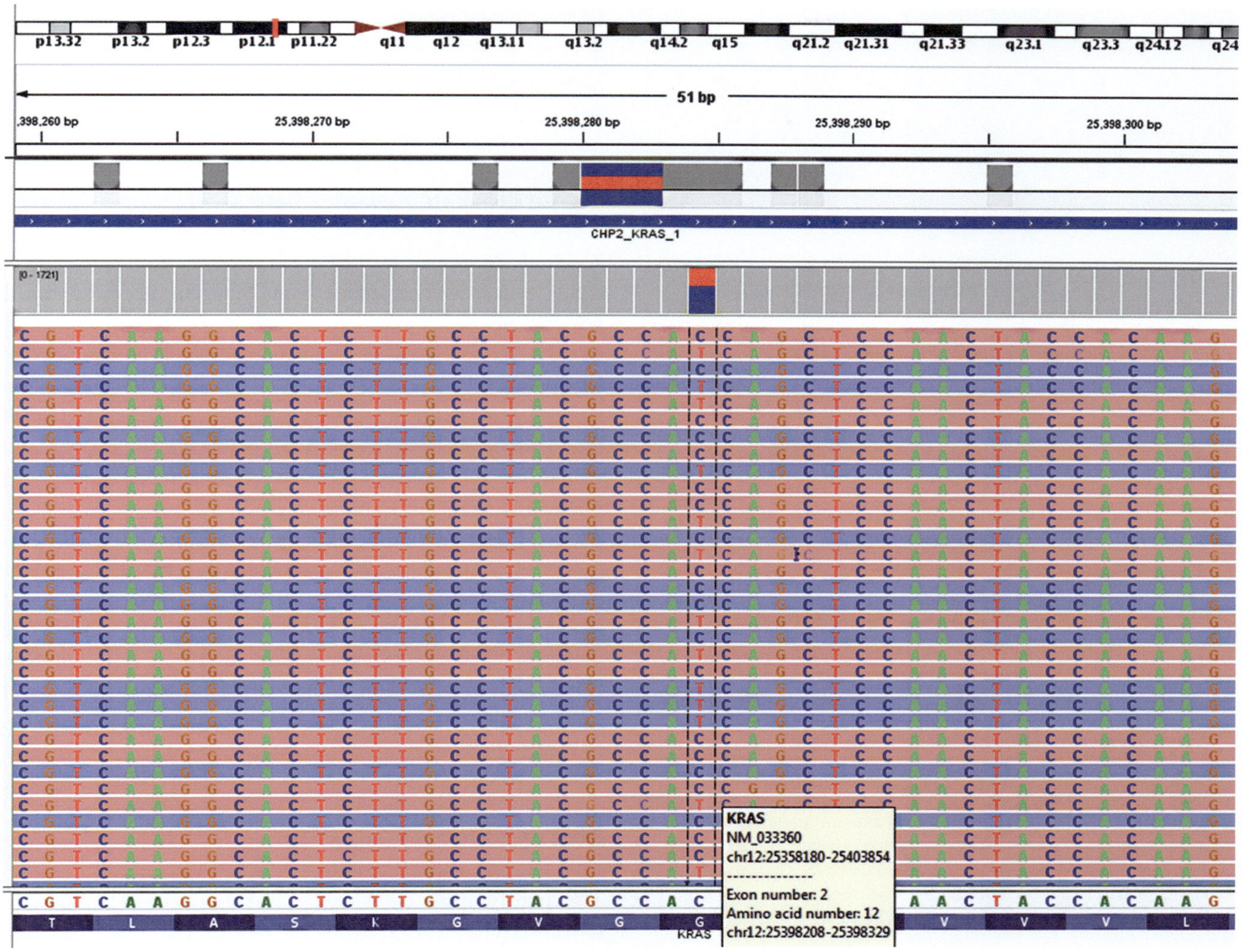

Figure 31.5 Next-generation sequencing results for a 41 bp region of *KRAS* showing a c.35G>A mutation at codon 12, resulting in a G12D mutation in the protein. The location of this region in the context of the human chromosome hg19 is shown above. The different colors of each row (*blue* or *red*) represent the sequences of the forward and the reverse strand, respectively. The heterozygous configuration of the variant is clearly identifiable in the demarcated column (*vertical dashed lines*) with both C and T nucleotides present

CRCs. Patient 1 CRC has a G12D mutation, patient 2 a G13D mutation, and patient 3 a wild-type sequence at codons 12 and 13 of *KRAS*.

Next-Generation Sequencing Assays

Assessment of multiple clinically actionable mutations using targeted NGS testing has greatly advanced cancer testing in the clinical molecular laboratory (see Chap. 59 for a description of the NGS method and Chap. 60 for cancer NGS). Information obtained from targeted NGS cancer panels is useful for concurrent assessment of a panel of hot spots directly related to cancer, for classification and diagnosis of tumor type, prognosis, and for the determination of response to EGFR-targeted therapy.

Sanger sequencing has been the gold standard for identification of mutations and variants in the clinical molecular laboratory. Modifications such as pyrosequencing were subsequently developed to enhance the sensitivity and detect 1–5 % mutant alleles in a background of wild-type DNA. NGS testing offers more information than other assays, combining sequence information and high analytical sensitivity for detection of actionable mutations in cancer tissues. NGS platforms work with minimal FFPE tissue and simultaneously detect many known and novel genetic variants in genes important for CRC. However, NGS testing validation, standardization, quality assurance, and quality control must be performed by the individual clinical molecular laboratory under CLIA and other regulatory standards, such as those of the College of American Pathologists and the New York State Department of Health. Figure 31.5 shows an example of a

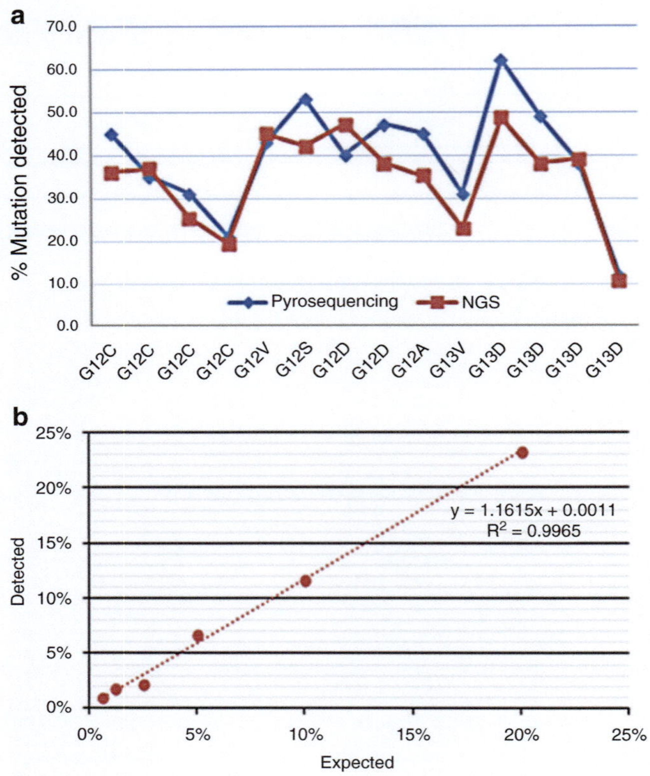

Figure 31.6 Comparison of pyrosequencing and next-generation sequencing (NGS) testing for detection of *KRAS* mutations commonly identified in CRC. (**a**) Quantifications of mutant allele percentages by both test methods show good concordance. Variant percentages from 10 % and above were accurately identified by NGS. (**b**) Analytical sensitivity of *KRAS* mutation detected by NGS showed linearity from 1 % to 20 % mutant allele in a wild-type background

KRAS C>T heterozygous mutation detected by NGS. In addition to *KRAS*, *BRAF*, and *EGFR*, CRCs have detectable mutations in additional genes, such as *PDGFRA*, *APC*, *FGFR3*, *MET*, and *TP53,* using an NGS gene panel test.

Comparison of Technologies

Table 31.4 provides an overview of the features of three technologies (Sanger sequencing, pyrosequencing, and NGS) commonly used to detect mutations in genes related to CRC. A comparison of pyrosequencing and NGS (Ion Torrent PGM, Life Technologies) assays for detection of representative CRC gene mutations is shown in Fig. 31.6a and shows excellent correlation of testing results by the two technologies. The graph (Fig. 31.6b) shows linearity from 1 % to 20 % for the NGS assay, indicating that the assay is able to detect 1 % of (homozygous) mutant DNA in a background of wild-type DNA.

Laboratory Issues

Molecular testing for gene mutations in CRCs requires attention to specific laboratory issues.

Tissue Block Review and Selection

A pathologist with expertise in anatomic or surgical pathology should select a tissue block containing non-necrotic, and if possible non-mucinous, regions of the CRC, with the most cancer cells. Necrotic and mucinous regions do not provide high-quality or significant amounts of DNA. Consideration must be given to the percentage of tumor cells compared to the total cells in the section, since all cells contribute DNA and will dilute the cancer DNA, including inflammatory cells, fibroblasts, noncancer epithelial cells, and other normal cells. Agreed criteria and training for the estimation of the percent of cancer cells relative to the total cells in a tissue section for molecular testing should be developed, for reproducible reporting of the percent of tumor cells. For most cancer gene mutation detection tests, a minimum of 10–25 % tumor cells is required. The pathologist may circle the highest density of cancer cells in a tissue section to allow for appropriate micro- or macro-dissection.

DNA Quality and Quantity

The quality of the DNA can be affected by necrosis or prolonged fixation times, as well as suboptimal storage conditions for FFPE tissue blocks. High-quality DNA is needed for most molecular testing. Accurate DNA quantification may not be significant for some molecular tests, but is essential for NGS testing. Quantification of DNA using qPCR or measurement of double-stranded DNA (dsDNA) using fluorometry provides accurate quantification of the amount of dsDNA prior to library amplification.

Conclusions and Future Directions

Currently, *RAS* mutation analysis of CRC tissues is recommended as the standard of care in patients who are candidates for targeted anti-EGFR antibody therapy. Additional mutation testing of other EGFR signaling pathway genes may be helpful to better select patients for targeted therapies with improved outcomes, but a general consensus regarding which genes should be tested is not yet established for CRC patient management. In academic medical centers, the trend is to test all CRCs for *RAS* and *BRAF* V600E mutations and for microsatellite instability, thus allowing for selection of patients for conventional therapy as well as targeted therapy [38]. The use of gene panels for mutation analysis, tested with platforms that permit detection of hundreds of mutations in a single sample, such as NGS gene panels, is a powerful and promising approach that provides the mutation status for multiple critical genes of cancer driver pathways. Genomic Tumor Boards which address the integrated use of gene mutation and other molecular test results for the clinical management of cancer patients are becoming more common to evaluate treatment options as well as enrollment in ongoing clinical trials of targeted therapies for individual patients.

References

1. Kozuch P, Malamud S, Wasserman C, Homel P, Mirzoyev T, Grossbard M. Phase II trial of erlotinib and capecitabine for patients with previously untreated metastatic colorectal cancer. Clin Colorectal Cancer. 2009;8(1):38–42.
2. Siegel R, Desantis C, Jemal A. Colorectal cancer statistics, 2014. CA Cancer J Clin. 2014;64(2):104–17.
3. Fearon ER, Vogelstein B. A genetic model for colorectal tumorigenesis. Cell. 1990;61(5):759–67.
4. Snover DC. Update on the serrated pathway to colorectal carcinoma. Hum Pathol. 2011;42(1):1–10.
5. Cancer Genome Atlas N. Comprehensive molecular characterization of human colon and rectal cancer. Nature. 2012;487(7407): 330–7.
6. Pancione M, Remo A, Colantuoni V. Genetic and epigenetic events generate multiple pathways in colorectal cancer progression. Patholog Res Int. 2012;2012:509348.
7. Simons CC, Hughes LA, Smits KM, Khalid-de Bakker CA, de Bruine AP, Carvalho B, Meijer GA, Schouten LJ, van den Brandt PA, Weijenberg MP, van Engeland M. A novel classification of colorectal tumors based on microsatellite instability, the CpG island methylator phenotype and chromosomal instability: implications for prognosis. Ann Oncol. 2013;24(8):2048–56.
8. Toyota M, Ohe-Toyota M, Ahuja N, Issa JP. Distinct genetic profiles in colorectal tumors with or without the CpG island methylator phenotype. Proc Natl Acad Sci U S A. 2000;97(2):710–5.
9. Weisenberger DJ, Siegmund KD, Campan M, Young J, Long TI, Faasse MA, Kang GH, Widschwendter M, Weener D, Buchanan D, Koh H, Simms L, Barker M, Leggett B, Levine J, Kim M, French AJ, Thibodeau SN, Jass J, Haile R, Laird PW. CpG island methylator phenotype underlies sporadic microsatellite instability and is tightly associated with BRAF mutation in colorectal cancer. Nat Genet. 2006;38(7):787–93.
10. Herman JG, Umar A, Polyak K, Graff JR, Ahuja N, Issa JP, Markowitz S, Willson JK, Hamilton SR, Kinzler KW, Kane MF, Kolodner RD, Vogelstein B, Kunkel TA, Baylin SB. Incidence and functional consequences of hMLH1 promoter hypermethylation in colorectal carcinoma. Proc Natl Acad Sci U S A. 1998;95(12): 6870–5.
11. Umar A. Lynch syndrome (HNPCC) and microsatellite instability. Dis Markers. 2004;20(4-5):179–80.
12. Lynch HT, Lynch PM, Lanspa SJ, Snyder CL, Lynch JF, Boland CR. Review of the Lynch syndrome: history, molecular genetics, screening, differential diagnosis, and medicolegal ramifications. Clin Genet. 2009;76(1):1–18.
13. Alemayehu A, Sebova K, Fridrichova I. Redundant DNA methylation in colorectal cancers of Lynch-syndrome patients. Genes Chromosomes Cancer. 2008;47(10):906–14.
14. Umar A, Boland CR, Terdiman JP, Syngal S, de la Chapelle A, Ruschoff J, Fishel R, Lindor NM, Burgart LJ, Hamelin R, Hamilton SR, Hiatt RA, Jass J, Lindblom A, Lynch HT, Peltomaki P, Ramsey SD, Rodriguez-Bigas MA, Vasen HF, Hawk ET, Barrett JC, Freedman AN, Srivastava S. Revised Bethesda Guidelines for hereditary nonpolyposis colorectal cancer (Lynch syndrome) and microsatellite instability. J Natl Cancer Inst. 2004;96(4):261–8.
15. Fisher GA, Kuo T, Ramsey M, Schwartz E, Rouse RV, Cho CD, Halsey J, Sikic BI. A phase II study of gefitinib, 5-fluorouracil, leucovorin, and oxaliplatin in previously untreated patients with metastatic colorectal cancer. Clin Cancer Res. 2008;14(21): 7074–9.
16. Bardelli A, Siena S. Molecular mechanisms of resistance to cetuximab and panitumumab in colorectal cancer. J Clin Oncol. 2010;28(7):1254–61.
17. De Roock W, Claes B, Bernasconi D, De Schutter J, Biesmans B, Fountzilas G, Kalogeras KT, Kotoula V, Papamichael D, Laurent-Puig P, Penault-Llorca F, Rougier P, Vincenzi B, Santini D, Tonini G, Cappuzzo F, Frattini M, Molinari F, Saletti P, De Dosso S, Martini M, Bardelli A, Siena S, Sartore-Bianchi A, Tabernero J, Macarulla T, Di Fiore F, Gangloff AO, Ciardiello F, Pfeiffer P, Qvortrup C, Hansen TP, Van Cutsem E, Piessevaux H, Lambrechts D, Delorenzi M, Tejpar S. Effects of KRAS, BRAF, NRAS, and PIK3CA mutations on the efficacy of cetuximab plus chemotherapy in chemotherapy-refractory metastatic colorectal cancer: a retrospective consortium analysis. Lancet Oncol. 2010;11(8):753–62.
18. De Roock W, Jonker DJ, Di Nicolantonio F, Sartore-Bianchi A, Tu D, Siena S, Lamba S, Arena S, Frattini M, Piessevaux H, Van Cutsem E, O'Callaghan CJ, Khambata-Ford S, Zalcberg JR, Simes J, Karapetis CS, Bardelli A, Tejpar S. Association of KRAS p. G13D mutation with outcome in patients with chemotherapy-refractory metastatic colorectal cancer treated with cetuximab. JAMA. 2010;304(16):1812–20.
19. Bos JL, Fearon ER, Hamilton SR, Verlaan-de Vries M, van Boom JH, van der Eb AJ, Vogelstein B. Prevalence of ras gene mutations in human colorectal cancers. Nature. 1987;327(6120):293–7.
20. Bokemeyer C, Kohne CH, Ciardiello F, Lenz HJ, Heinemann V, Klinkhardt U, Beier F, Duecker K, T. S. (2014). Treatment outcome according to tumor RAS mutation status in OPUS study patients with metastatic colorectal cancer (mCRC) randomized to FOLFOX4 with/without cetuximab. ASCO 2014 Annual Meeting, Chicago, Illinois, J Clin Oncol.
21. Ciardiello F, Lenz HJ, Kohne CH, Heinemann V, Tejpar S, Melezinek I, Beier F, Stroh C, CutsemE V. (2014). Treatment outcome according to tumor RAS mutation status in CRYSTAL study patients with metastatic colorectal cancer (mCRC) randomized to FOLFIRI with/without cetuximab. ASCO 2014 Annual Meeting, Chicago, Illinois, J Clin Oncol.
22. Deng G, Bell I, Crawley S, Gum J, Terdiman JP, Allen BA, Truta B, Sleisenger MH, Kim YS. BRAF mutation is frequently present in sporadic colorectal cancer with methylated hMLH1, but not in hereditary nonpolyposis colorectal cancer. Clin Cancer Res. 2004;10(1 Pt 1):191–5.
23. Palomaki GE, McClain MR, Melillo S, Hampel HL, Thibodeau SN. EGAPP supplementary evidence review: DNA testing strategies aimed at reducing morbidity and mortality from Lynch syndrome. Genet Med. 2009;11(1):42–65.
24. Grothey A. EGFR antibodies in colorectal cancer: where do they belong? J Clin Oncol. 2010;28(31):4668–70.
25. Karapetis CS, Khambata-Ford S, Jonker DJ, O'Callaghan CJ, Tu D, Tebbutt NC, Simes RJ, Chalchal H, Shapiro JD, Robitaille S, Price TJ, Shepherd L, Au HJ, Langer C, Moore MJ, Zalcberg JR. K-ras mutations and benefit from cetuximab in advanced colorectal cancer. N Engl J Med. 2008;359(17):1757–65.
26. Allegra CJ, Jessup JM, Somerfield MR, Hamilton SR, Hammond EH, Hayes DF, McAllister PK, Morton RF, Schilsky RL. American Society of Clinical Oncology provisional clinical opinion: testing

for KRAS gene mutations in patients with metastatic colorectal carcinoma to predict response to anti-epidermal growth factor receptor monoclonal antibody therapy. J Clin Oncol. 2009;27(12):2091–6.
27. Prenen H, Tejpar S, Van Cutsem E. New strategies for treatment of KRAS mutant metastatic colorectal cancer. Clin Cancer Res. 2010;16(11):2921–6.
28. Flaherty KT, Puzanov I, Kim KB, Ribas A, McArthur GA, Sosman JA, O'Dwyer PJ, Lee RJ, Grippo JF, Nolop K, Chapman PB. Inhibition of mutated, activated BRAF in metastatic melanoma. N Engl J Med. 2010;363(9):809–19.
29. Hutchins G, Southward K, Handley K, Magill L, Beaumont C, Stahlschmidt J, Richman S, Chambers P, Seymour M, Kerr D, Gray R, Quirke P. Value of mismatch repair, KRAS, and BRAF mutations in predicting recurrence and benefits from chemotherapy in colorectal cancer. J Clin Oncol. 2011;29(10):1261–70.
30. Prahallad A, Sun C, Huang S, Di Nicolantonio F, Salazar R, Zecchin D, Beijersbergen RL, Bardelli A, Bernards R. Unresponsiveness of colon cancer to BRAF(V600E) inhibition through feedback activation of EGFR. Nature. 2012;483(7387):100–3.
31. Prenen H, De Schutter J, Jacobs B, De Roock W, Biesmans B, Claes B, Lambrechts D, Van Cutsem E, Tejpar S. PIK3CA mutations are not a major determinant of resistance to the epidermal growth factor receptor inhibitor cetuximab in metastatic colorectal cancer. Clin Cancer Res. 2009;15(9):3184–8.
32. Sartore-Bianchi A, Martini M, Molinari F, Veronese S, Nichelatti M, Artale S, Di Nicolantonio F, Saletti P, De Dosso S, Mazzucchelli L, Frattini M, Siena S, Bardelli A. PIK3CA mutations in colorectal cancer are associated with clinical resistance to EGFR-targeted monoclonal antibodies. Cancer Res. 2009;69(5):1851–7.
33. De Roock W, De Vriendt V, Normanno N, Ciardiello F, Tejpar S. KRAS, BRAF, PIK3CA, and PTEN mutations: implications for targeted therapies in metastatic colorectal cancer. Lancet Oncol. 2011;12(6):594–603.
34. Ogino S, Meyerhardt JA, Cantor M, Brahmandam M, Clark JW, Namgyal C, Kawasaki T, Kinsella K, Michelini AL, Enzinger PC, Kulke MH, Ryan DP, Loda M, Fuchs CS. Molecular alterations in tumors and response to combination chemotherapy with gefitinib for advanced colorectal cancer. Clin Cancer Res. 2005;11(18): 6650–6.
35. Sorich MJ, Wiese MD, Rowland A, Kichenadasse G, McKinnon RA, Karapetis CS. Extended RAS mutations and anti-EGFR monoclonal antibody survival benefit in metastatic colorectal cancer: a meta-analysis of randomized, controlled trials. Ann Oncol. 2014;00:1–9.
36. Baas JM, Krens LL, Guchelaar HJ, Morreau H, Gelderblom H. Concordance of predictive markers for EGFR inhibitors in primary tumors and metastases in colorectal cancer: a review. Oncologist. 2011;16(9):1239–49.
37. Cejas P, Lopez-Gomez M, Aguayo C, Madero R, Moreno-Rubio J, Carpeno JD, Belda-Iniesta C, Barriuso J, Garcia VM, Diaz E, Burgos E, Gonzalez-Baron M, Feliu J. Analysis of the concordance in the EGFR pathway status between primary tumors and related metastases of colorectal cancer patients: Implications for cancer therapy. Curr Cancer Drug Targets. 2011;12(2): 124–31.
38. Funkhouser Jr WK, Lubin IM, Monzon FA, Zehnbauer BA, Evans JP, Ogino S, Nowak JA. Relevance, pathogenesis, and testing algorithm for mismatch repair-defective colorectal carcinomas: a report of the association for molecular pathology. J Mol Diagn. 2012;14(2):91–103.
39. Liu B, Farrington SM, Petersen GM, Hamilton SR, Parsons R, Papadopoulos N, Fujiwara T, Jen J, Kinzler KW, Wyllie AH, et al. Genetic instability occurs in the majority of young patients with colorectal cancer. Nat Med. 1995;1(4):348–52.
40. de la Chapelle A, Hampel H. Clinical relevance of microsatellite instability in colorectal cancer. J Clin Oncol. 2010;28(20): 3380–7.
41. Ionov Y, Peinado MA, Malkhosyan S, Shibata D, Perucho M. Ubiquitous somatic mutations in simple repeated sequences reveal a new mechanism for colonic carcinogenesis. Nature. 1993;363(6429):558–61.
42. Thibodeau SN, Bren G, Schaid D. Microsatellite instability in cancer of the proximal colon. Science. 1993;260(5109):816–9.
43. Hagemann IS, Sepulveda AR. Cancer Predisposition Syndromes of the Gastrointestinal Tract. Molecular Pathology of Neoplastic Gastrointestinal Diseases. A. R. Sepulveda and J. L. Lynch, Springer, LLC, New York, NY: 109-130, (2013).
44. Miyaki M, Konishi M, Tanaka K, Kikuchi-Yanoshita R, Muraoka M, Yasuno M, Igari T, Koike M, Chiba M, Mori T. Germline mutation of MSH6 as the cause of hereditary nonpolyposis colorectal cancer. Nat Genet. 1997;17(3):271–2.
45. Moslein G, Tester DJ, Lindor NM, Honchel R, Cunningham JM, French AJ, Halling KC, Schwab M, Goretzki P, Thibodeau SN. Microsatellite instability and mutation analysis of hMSH2 and hMLH1 in patients with sporadic, familial and hereditary colorectal cancer. Hum Mol Genet. 1996;5(9):1245–52.
46. Veigl ML, Kasturi L, Olechnowicz J, Ma AH, Lutterbaugh JD, Periyasamy S, Li GM, Drummond J, Modrich PL, Sedwick WD, Markowitz SD. Biallelic inactivation of hMLH1 by epigenetic gene silencing, a novel mechanism causing human MSI cancers. Proc Natl Acad Sci U S A. 1998;95(15):8698–702.
47. Toyota M, Ahuja N, Ohe-Toyota M, Herman JG, Baylin SB, Issa JP. CpG island methylator phenotype in colorectal cancer. Proc Natl Acad Sci U S A. 1999;96(15):8681–6.
48. Stone JG, Robertson D, Houlston RS. Immunohistochemistry for MSH2 and MHL1: a method for identifying mismatch repair deficient colorectal cancer. J Clin Pathol. 2001;54(6):484–7.
49. EGAPP. Recommendations from the EGAPP Working Group: routine testing for Factor V Leiden (R506Q) and prothrombin (20210G>A) mutations in adults with a history of idiopathic venous thromboembolism and their adult family members. Genet Med. 2011;13(1):67–76.
50. Gryfe R, Kim H, Hsieh ET, Aronson MD, Holowaty EJ, Bull SB, Redston M, Gallinger S. Tumor microsatellite instability and clinical outcome in young patients with colorectal cancer. N Engl J Med. 2000;342(2):69–77.
51. Benatti P, Gafa R, Barana D, Marino M, Scarselli A, Pedroni M, Maestri I, Guerzoni L, Roncucci L, Menigatti M, Roncari B, Maffei S, Rossi G, Ponti G, Santini A, Losi L, Di Gregorio C, Oliani C, Ponz de Leon M, Lanza G. Microsatellite instability and colorectal cancer prognosis. Clin Cancer Res. 2005;11(23):8332–40.
52. Ribic CM, Sargent DJ, Moore MJ, Thibodeau SN, French AJ, Goldberg RM, Hamilton SR, Laurent-Puig P, Gryfe R, Shepherd LE, Tu D, Redston M, Gallinger S. Tumor microsatellite-instability status as a predictor of benefit from fluorouracil-based adjuvant chemotherapy for colon cancer. N Engl J Med. 2003;349(3):247–57.
53. Sargent DJ, Marsoni S, Monges G, Thibodeau SN, Labianca R, Hamilton SR, French AJ, Kabat B, Foster NR, Torri V, Ribic C, Grothey A, Moore M, Zaniboni A, Seitz JF, Sinicrope F, Gallinger S. Defective mismatch repair as a predictive marker for lack of efficacy of fluorouracil-based adjuvant therapy in colon cancer. J Clin Oncol. 2010;28(20):3219–26.
54. Bertagnolli MM, Niedzwiecki D, Compton CC, Hahn HP, Hall M, Damas B, Jewell SD, Mayer RJ, Goldberg RM, Saltz LB, Warren RS, Redston M. Microsatellite instability predicts improved response to adjuvant therapy with irinotecan, fluorouracil, and leucovorin in stage III colon cancer: Cancer and Leukemia Group B Protocol 89803. J Clin Oncol. 2009;27(11):1814–21.

55. Kim GP, Colangelo LH, Wieand HS, Paik S, Kirsch IR, Wolmark N, Allegra CJ. Prognostic and predictive roles of high-degree microsatellite instability in colon cancer: a National Cancer Institute-National Surgical Adjuvant Breast and Bowel Project Collaborative Study. J Clin Oncol. 2007;25(7):767–72.
56. Sinicrope FA, Foster NR, Thibodeau SN, Marsoni S, Monges G, Labianca R, Kim GP, Yothers G, Allegra C, Moore MJ, Gallinger S, Sargent DJ. DNA mismatch repair status and colon cancer recurrence and survival in clinical trials of 5-fluorouracil-based adjuvant therapy. J Natl Cancer Inst. 2011;103(11):863–75.
57. Kerr DJ, Midgley R. Defective mismatch repair in colon cancer: a prognostic or predictive biomarker? J Clin Oncol. 2010;28(20):3210–2.
58. Newton CR, Graham A, Heptinstall LE, Powell SJ, Summers C, Kalsheker N, Smith JC, Markham AF. Analysis of any point mutation in DNA. The amplification refractory mutation system (ARMS). Nucleic Acids Res. 1989;17(7):2503–16.
59. Thelwell N, Millington S, Solinas A, Booth J, Brown T. Mode of action and application of Scorpion primers to mutation detection. Nucleic Acids Res. 2000;28(19):3752–61.
60. Ausch C, Buxhofer-Ausch V, Oberkanins C, Holzer B, Minai-Pour M, Jahn S, Dandachi N, Zeillinger R, Kriegshauser G. Sensitive detection of KRAS mutations in archived formalin-fixed paraffin-embedded tissue using mutant-enriched PCR and reverse-hybridization. J Mol Diagn. 2009;11(6):508–13.
61. Angulo B, Garcia-Garcia E, Martinez R, Suarez-Gauthier A, Conde E, Hidalgo M, Lopez-Rios F. A commercial real-time PCR kit provides greater sensitivity than direct sequencing to detect KRAS mutations: a morphology-based approach in colorectal carcinoma. J Mol Diagn. 2010;12(3):292–9.
62. Oliner K, Juan T, Suggs S, Wolf M, Sarosi I, Freeman DJ, Gyuris T, Baron W, Bakker A, Parker A, Patterson SD. A comparability study of 5 commercial KRAS tests. Diagn Pathol. 2010;5:23.
63. Gallegos Ruiz MI, Floor K, Rijmen F, Grunberg K, Rodriguez JA, Giaccone G. EGFR and K-ras mutation analysis in non-small cell lung cancer: comparison of paraffin embedded versus frozen specimens. Cell Oncol. 2007;29(3):257–64.
64. Ronaghi M, Uhlen M, Nyren P. A sequencing method based on real-time pyrophosphate. Science. 1998;281(5375):363, 365.
65. Ogino S, Kawasaki T, Brahmandam M, Yan L, Cantor M, Namgyal C, Mino-Kenudson M, Lauwers GY, Loda M, Fuchs CS. Sensitive sequencing method for KRAS mutation detection by Pyrosequencing. J Mol Diagn. 2005;7(3):413–21.
66. Tan YH, Liu Y, Eu KW, Ang PW, Li WQ, Salto-Tellez M, Iacopetta B, Soong R. Detection of BRAF V600E mutation by pyrosequencing. Pathology. 2008;40(3):295–8.
67. Setty P, Hammes J, Rothamel T, Vladimirova V, Kramm CM, Pietsch T, Waha A. A pyrosequencing-based assay for the rapid detection of IDH1 mutations in clinical samples. J Mol Diagn. 2010;12(6):750–6.
68. Sundstrom M, Edlund K, Lindell M, Glimelius B, Birgisson H, Micke P, Botling J. KRAS analysis in colorectal carcinoma: analytical aspects of Pyrosequencing and allele-specific PCR in clinical practice. BMC Cancer. 2010;10:660.
69. Curry JL, Torres-Cabala CA, Tetzlaff MT, Bowman C, Prieto VG. Molecular Platforms Utilized to Detect BRAF V600E Mutation in Melanoma. Semin Cutan Med Surg. 2012;31(4):267–73.
70. Bihl MP, Hoeller S, Andreozzi MC, Foerster A, Rufle A, Tornillo L, Terracciano L. KRAS mutation testing in colorectal cancer: comparison of the results obtained using 3 different methods for the analysis of codons G12 and G13. Diagn Mol Pathol. 2012;21(1):14–23.
71. Cykowski MD, Allen RA, Fung KM, Harmon MA, Dunn ST. Pyrosequencing of IDH1 and IDH2 Mutations in Brain Tumors and Non-neoplastic Conditions. Diagn Mol Pathol. 2012;21(4):214–20.
72. Lade-Keller J, Romer KM, Guldberg P, Riber-Hansen R, Hansen LL, Steiniche T, Hager H, Kristensen LS. Evaluation of BRAF mutation testing methodologies in formalin-fixed paraffin-embedded cutaneous melanomas. J Mol Diagn. 2012;15(1):70–80.
73. Alderborn A, Kristofferson A, Hammerling U. Determination of single-nucleotide polymorphisms by real-time pyrophosphate DNA sequencing. Genome Res. 2000;10(8):1249–58.
74. Tost J, Gut IG. DNA methylation analysis by pyrosequencing. Nat Protoc. 2007;2(9):2265–75.
75. Lof-Ohlin ZM, Nilsson TK. Pyrosequencing assays to study promoter CpG site methylation of the O6-MGMT, hMLH1, p14ARF, p16INK4a, RASSF1A, and APC1A genes. Oncol Rep. 2009;21(3):721–9.
76. Yu J, Freimuth RR, Culverhouse R, Marsh S, Watson MA, McLeod HL. DNA methylotype analysis in colorectal cancer. Oncol Rep. 2008;20(4):921–7.
77. Kwok CT, Ward RL, Hawkins NJ, Hitchins MP. Detection of allelic imbalance in MLH1 expression by pyrosequencing serves as a tool for the identification of germline defects in Lynch syndrome. Fam Cancer. 2010;9(3):345–56.
78. Chen X, Kwok PY. Template-directed dye-terminator incorporation (TDI) assay: a homogeneous DNA diagnostic method based on fluorescence resonance energy transfer. Nucleic Acids Res. 1997;25(2):347–53.
79. Kwok PY (2004). High-throughput genotyping with primer extension fluorescent polarization detection. Current protocols in human genetics/editorial board, Jonathan L. Haines … [et al.] **Chapter 2**: Unit 2 11.
80. Magnin S, Viel E, Baraquin A, Valmary-Degano S, Kantelip B, Pretet JL, Mougin C, Bigand M, Girardo B, Borg C, Ferrand C. A multiplex SNaPshot assay as a rapid method for detecting KRAS and BRAF mutations in advanced colorectal cancers. J Mol Diagn. 2011;13(5):485–92.
81. Lovly CM, Dahlman KB, Fohn LE, Su Z, Dias-Santagata D, Hicks DJ, Hucks D, Berry E, Terry C, Duke M, Su Y, Sobolik-Delmaire T, Richmond A, Kelley MC, Vnencak-Jones CL, Iafrate AJ, Sosman J, Pao W. Routine multiplex mutational profiling of melanomas enables enrollment in genotype-driven therapeutic trials. PLoS One. 2012;7(4), e35309.
82. Jurinke C, Oeth P, van den Boom D. MALDI-TOF mass spectrometry: a versatile tool for high-performance DNA analysis. Mol Biotechnol. 2004;26(2):147–64.
83. Arcila M, Lau C, Nafa K, Ladanyi M. Detection of KRAS and BRAF mutations in colorectal carcinoma roles for high-sensitivity locked nucleic acid-PCR sequencing and broad-spectrum mass spectrometry genotyping. J Mol Diagn. 2011;13(1):64–73.
84. Sequenom (2012). Sequenom MassARRAY®System for Somatic Mutation Screening. Doc. No. WKI 35-175, R1.0, CO No. 100004. 2012, from http://www.sequenom.com.
85. Laosinchai-Wolf W, Ye F, Tran V, Yang Z, White R, Bloom K, Choppa P, Labourier E. Sensitive multiplex detection of KRAS codons 12 and 13 mutations in paraffin-embedded tissue specimens. J Clin Pathol. 2011;64(1):30–6.
86. Wang HL, Lopategui J, Amin MB, Patterson SD. KRAS mutation testing in human cancers: the pathologist's role in the era of personalized medicine. Adv Anat Pathol. 2010;17(1):23–32.
87. Labourier E. Do pre-analytical parameters explain KRAS test sensitivity disparities? J Mol Diagn. 2012;14(6):631–3. author reply 632-633.

Lung Cancer

32

Dara L. Aisner, Robert C. Doebele,
Marileila Varella-Garcia, and Wilbur A. Franklin

Abstract

Molecular classification of lung cancer, specifically non-small cell lung cancer (NSCLC), is increasingly utilized to determine optimal treatment. Recent advances have demonstrated the utility of testing for specific alterations such as *EGFR* mutations and *ALK* rearrangements, as these determinations guide utilization of targeted therapies. Assays to detect mutations must balance comprehensiveness of detection of mutations and the need to achieve analytic sensitivity which can reliably detect mutations in mixed cell populations. Assays to detect rearrangements must balance comprehensiveness of identification of alterations and ease of use. As the number of targets for testing increases, greater emphasis will be placed on technologies which simultaneously detect multiple molecular variants from small tissue samplings.

Keywords

NSCLC • ALK • EGFR • KRAS • Fluorescence in situ hybridization (FISH) • Tyrosine kinase inhibitor (TKI) • Gene fusions • Sequencing

Introduction

Lung cancer is the leading cause of cancer-related mortality in males and the second most common cause of cancer-related death in females worldwide [1]. For much of the twentieth century, lung cancer was not only the leading cause of cancer-related death in the USA but also the fastest growing cause of cancer-related mortality. A sharp decline in this growth was noted beginning in the 1990s and has been attributed mostly to successful efforts to curb smoking [2].

The majority of lung cancer patients have advanced disease at the time of diagnosis which is unfortunately associated with a 5-year relative survival rate below 5 %. Even for those with early-stage disease, the 5-year relative survival is only approximately 50 %, which reflects the high lung cancer recurrence rate [2, 3].

Traditionally, the classification of lung cancer is based on a morphologic distinction between small-cell lung carcinoma (SCLC) and non-small cell lung carcinoma (NSCLC). With advances in molecular pathology, distinct entities with unique molecular underpinnings are increasingly recognized. Although many of the molecular alterations in SCLC are known, few have been translated into clinically actionable findings. In contrast, in NSCLC, the identification of molecular markers for targeted therapies has advanced rapidly in the last decade. Within NSCLC, the majority of findings that have become adopted in routine practice are most applicable to adenocarcinoma; thus, the focus of this chapter will be on molecular testing of NSCLC, with examples drawn from testing in pulmonary adenocarcinoma.

D.L. Aisner, M.D., Ph.D. (✉)
Department of Pathology, University of Colorado,
Mail Stop 8104, 12801 E. 17th Ave, Room 5102, Aurora, CO 80045, USA
e-mail: dara.aisner@ucdenver.edu

R.C. Doebele, M.D., Ph.D. • M. Varella-Garcia, Ph.D.
Division of Medical Oncology, University of Colorado Denver, Aurora, CO, USA

W.A. Franklin, M.D.
Department of Pathology, University of Colorado Denver, Aurora, CO, USA

D.G.B. Leonard (ed.), *Molecular Pathology in Clinical Practice*, DOI 10.1007/978-3-319-19674-9_32

Molecular Basis of Disease

The molecular profile of lung cancer is complex and vastly heterogeneous, which, until recently, has slowed the progress of clinical molecular applications. As specific molecular alterations have been identified, the focus has been on the evaluation of specific oncogenic pathways for targeted therapy development. Chief among these have been the epidermal growth factor receptor (EGFR) and other receptor tyrosine kinase (TK) signaling pathways.

The identification of *EGFR* mutation status as a predictor of response to tyrosine kinase inhibitors (TKIs) emerged from the convergence of clinical advances and laboratory science. Underpinning this work were the original isolation of EGF from mouse salivary gland in 1962 [4], demonstration of its binding to a cell membrane receptor [5], and sequencing of the receptor [6]. In the 1990s, EGFR was found to be highly expressed in squamous cell carcinoma. When monoclonal antibodies against EGFR that could be used to evaluate formalin-fixed, paraffin-embedded (FFPE) tissues became available, EGFR was found to be strongly expressed in lung adenocarcinomas [7]. EGFR overexpression in NSCLC is closely linked to *EGFR* gene amplification [8].

In 2004, two laboratories reported that mutation of the EGFR TK domain was largely responsible for the sensitivity of some pulmonary adenocarcinomas to TKIs [9, 10]. Mutations cluster in the ATP-binding pocket of the intracellular domain of *EGFR* and most commonly consist of either a single base substitution in exon 21 (c.2573G>C, p.L858R) or an in-frame deletion within exon 19 ranging from 9 to 18 base pairs. These and other less commonly identified mutations in *EGFR* have been associated with sensitivity to TKI therapy. Although the common mutations are understood to result in strong auto-activation of EGFR, the degree to which this is true for the less commonly identified mutations is not well understood.

Resistance to TKI therapy inevitably develops in treated patients. The two best studied mechanism of resistance to EGFR TKI therapy are *MET* amplification and a single point mutation in exon 20 of *EGFR* (c.2369C>T, p.T790M) [11–15]. In the latter, a bulky methionine side chain is thought to alter affinity of EGFR for the inhibitor [11, 16]. Tumor cells with the p.T790M mutation may exist in low numbers in untreated tumors and emerge through selective pressure exerted by targeted therapy [17]. The p.T790M mutation is found as a germline change in rare individuals [18]. In addition, some other mutations, such as insertions in exon 20 of *EGFR*, which can be found in untreated tumors, are predominantly associated with primary resistance to TKI therapy, although the mechanism of this resistance is unclear [19].

Mutations in *KRAS* are more common in lung cancer than *EGFR* mutations and, unlike *EGFR* mutations, occur predominantly in smokers [20, 21]. Coexistence of *KRAS* and *EGFR* mutation is uncommon but has been reported [22]. KRAS is a member of a superfamily of guanosine-5-triphosphatase (GTPase) proteins that also includes NRAS and HRAS [23]. The role of these proteins is to transduce stimuli from surface growth factor receptors along a pathway leading to transcriptional changes. As multiple simultaneous sources of signals from different receptors and ligands have been identified, the RAS proteins are increasingly recognized as integrators and processors of signals from the cell surface and not just transducers. RAS proteins activate an intracellular signaling cascade that involves numerous effector molecules including PI3K and MAPK. Because of its position "downstream" of EGFR signaling, the hypothesis that an activating mutation in *KRAS* would render a tumor unresponsive to TKI therapy has been extensively investigated with conflicting results [24].

Mutations are not the only molecular driver mechanisms in lung cancer. Overexpression of oncogenes also is driven by gene activation through chromosomal rearrangements. Rearrangements that fuse constitutively activated gene promoters to the TK domain of growth factors, growth factor receptors, or transcription factors can result in inappropriate signaling from the fusion product. Examples of activation by gene fusion in lung cancer involve *ALK*, *ROS1*, and *RET*. In 2007, Soda et al. discovered a transcript derived from a patient with NSCLC that could transform 3T3 cell line fibroblasts [25]. Further investigation demonstrated the transcript to be derived from the fusion of a gene called echinoderm microtubule-associated protein-like 4 (*EML4*) with the anaplastic lymphoma kinase (*ALK*) gene, which is also rearranged in large cell lymphomas. The rearrangement has been detected in 4–7 % of pulmonary adenocarcinomas, with increasing proportion seen when cohorts are selected based on clinicopathologic features such as never-smoker or light-smoker history, signet-ring subtype [26–30]. The driver of tumorigenesis with this rearrangement is thought to be inappropriately expressed ALK, which is not typically expressed in adult lung tissue. Fusions involving ALK lead to inappropriate constitutive activation of its kinase domain through dysregulation driven by a 5′ fusion partner, such as EML4, which is expressed in adult lung tissue [25, 31].

In less than 5 years from the initial discovery of the *EML4-ALK* rearrangement, over 10,000 lung cancers have been tested for the presence of this rearrangement, with more than 13 molecular variants of *EML4-ALK* fusion identified [27, 32], including two other gene partners for *ALK* [33, 34]. A novel targeted therapeutic agent, crizotinib, is effective against tumors driven by ALK overexpression [35] and received approval for treatment of NSCLC with *ALK*

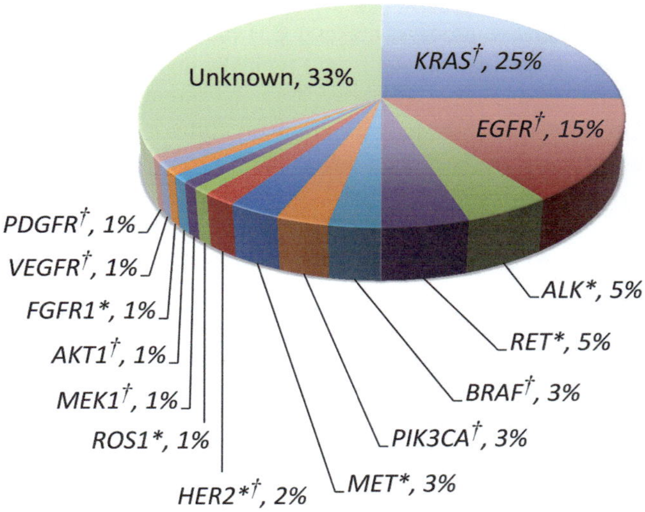

Figure 32.1 Approximate prevalence of identified "driver mutations" in unselected pulmonary adenocarcinoma. While many of these alterations are typically seen in isolation, others, such as *PIK3CA*, are often seen concurrently with other gene mutations. The spectrum of changes is different from that seen in squamous cell carcinoma of lung and varies by smoking status. *Asterisk* indicates a rearrangement or amplification; *dagger* indicates mutation [41] Ding L et al. 2008

rearrangement by the US Food and Drug Administration (FDA) [36].

These three examples, *EGFR* and *KRAS* mutations and *ALK* rearrangements, underscore the diversity of molecular alterations in NSCLC. "Driver mutations" are present in a significant proportion of lung cancers (Fig. 32.1). Efforts to exploit these alterations are underway with a wide array of targeted therapies.

Clinical Utility of Testing

Molecular testing significantly drives clinical therapeutic decision making for patients with NSCLC. Three commonly performed molecular tests, *EGFR* mutation testing, *KRAS* mutation testing, and *ALK* rearrangement testing usually by fluorescence in situ hybridization (FISH), illustrate three different scenarios for the clinical utility of molecular testing in NSCLC.

EGFR TKIs, including erlotinib and gefitinib, gained regulatory approval in unselected populations of NSCLC patients in the USA and Europe. The response rate in early studies of unselected lung cancer patients was only 10–15 % but was of marked degree in those patients who did respond. Later, activating *EGFR* mutations were identified to confer sensitivity to EGFR TKIs and accounted for the subset of tumors with response to therapy in early studies [9, 37] and that such therapy results in significantly higher overall response rates and progression free survival compared to standard chemotherapy. For patients without "sensitizing" *EGFR* mutations, chemotherapy without TKIs was clearly superior [37–39]. Thus, despite the broad indication for these drugs, the use of EGFR TKIs has dramatically shifted to their preferential early use in patients with proven "sensitizing" *EGFR* mutations. Patients without a "sensitizing" *EGFR* mutation also can benefit from the use of EGFR TKI in maintenance or later lines of therapy, but the benefit is modest [40, 41].

The oral kinase inhibitor, crizotinib, first entered clinical trials as a MET inhibitor for patients with *MET* gene amplification or activating mutations. After the discovery of *ALK* gene fusions in approximately 5 % of NSCLC patients, the trial was amended to include patients who demonstrated evidence of an *ALK* gene rearrangement by FISH. Following phase I and II data with overall response rates of 55–63 %, crizotinib gained provisional FDA approval for this highly selected group of patients [34, 42]. Unlike EGFR TKIs, which are approved for all patients with pulmonary adenocarcinoma, crizotinib is only approved for the treatment of patients with lung cancer carrying an *ALK* rearrangement, although its utility in other molecular subtypes, such as *ROS1* rearrangement-positive tumors, is under investigation [44, 45].

KRAS activating mutations occur in approximately 25 % of patients with NSCLC. Unfortunately, no KRAS-targeted therapies are currently FDA approved. The presence of a *KRAS* mutation, however, is still informative. The overlap of *KRAS* mutations with either sensitizing *EGFR* mutations, *ALK* gene rearrangements, or other oncogenic abnormalities is infrequent [46]. The presence of a *KRAS* mutation thus augments the negative predictive value of a negative *EGFR* mutation test or a negative *ALK* FISH test. Likewise, the presence of a *KRAS* mutation predicts a lack of tumor response from an EGFR TKI, although it does not necessarily predict a complete lack of benefit from an EGFR TKI [40, 41]. The detection of *KRAS* mutations can identify patients for participation in clinical trials. Currently, inhibition of MEK and PI3K pathways, both of which are downstream of KRAS, is under investigation in lung and other cancers. Thus, directing patients with a *KRAS* mutation-positive lung cancer to these clinical trials may enrich for patients who are likely to benefit from these strategies. Conversely, the presence of a *KRAS* mutation may provide a useful negative selection criterion for clinical trials that are targeting pathways upstream of KRAS [47].

In summary, molecular testing can provide guidance for prioritizing therapies to those patients most likely to receive the greatest benefit (*EGFR* mutations). Alternatively, molecular testing can identify patients with proven benefit from a targeted therapy (*ALK* gene rearrangements). Finally, molecular testing can provide clinicians with a rationale to guide certain patients toward clinical trials of targeted therapeutics

(*KRAS* mutations). These selected examples of targets are by no means the only ones of interest in NSCLC, in which a growing number of molecularly targeted agents are under investigation in association with specific molecular alterations. This includes mutations in *BRAF*, *HER2*, *PIK3CA*, and rearrangements in *RET*, among others [47].

Available Assays

Specimen Type, Quality, and Tumor Content

A discussion of the practical elements of molecular testing in NSCLC necessitates an understanding of the variability of specimen types likely to be encountered. As the majority of NSCLC patients present with advanced disease, they are not surgical candidates, and the diagnostic tumor sample is often the only tissue available for testing. This has driven the need to undertake evaluation of small specimens obtained from diagnostic biopsies, fine needle aspirations (FNA), and body cavity fluids. Cytopathology specimens are suitable for molecular testing, including cell block preparations as well as smeared and imprinted slides [49–55]. For small specimens, the quality of the specimen is often more important than the quantity [52, 56]. Individual laboratories are responsible for validation of the adequacy of all specimen types for each test.

Of paramount importance for any specimen type is the evaluation of the specimen by a pathologist with experience in the assessment of pathology specimens for molecular analysis. The tumor content of the specimen should be assessed for the presence of adequate non-necrotic tumor cells, as well as an estimation of the percent of tumor cells relative to all nucleated cells, which meets the criteria for acceptability for testing set by the clinical molecular laboratory [53]. Features suggesting that the specimen may not be of optimal quality include extensive necrosis, paucity of tumor cells, low abundance of tumor cells compared to other non-tumor cells in the specimen, and exposure to reagents which negatively impact molecular testing (e.g. decalcification) [52, 57, 58].

Some specimens are not sufficiently tumor rich to be utilized without tumor enrichment methods. Tumor enrichment methods include manual macrodissection, manual microdissection, and laser capture microdissection (LCM) [59]. Manual macrodissection is when a region of interest is scraped from a slide or carved from a paraffin block without microscope assistance. Manual microdissection is performed with a dissecting or light microscope, often using a scalpel, needle tip, or hollow bore pipette to preferentially isolate tumor cells and using a microscopically marked guide slide. LCM utilizes computer-aided imaging to select specific cells for capture from specially coated slides. However, the cost of equipment and specialized consumables, combined with a labor intensive process, makes LCM the costliest approach to tumor enrichment, and assays typically do not require this degree of precision. However, in some circumstances, the use of LCM may increase the ability to utilize low-sensitivity assays for some specimen types [60–62].

Common Driver Mutations Assays

Evaluation of mutation status in genes such as *EGFR* and *KRAS* can be accomplished using a variety of platforms. Historically, Sanger sequencing has been the "gold standard" for *EGFR* and *KRAS* mutation detection. Because of the comparatively low analytic sensitivity of Sanger sequencing, numerous other platforms have been developed with higher analytic sensitivity but typically assess only specific known mutations (Fig. 32.2) [56, 63]. The compromise for these mutational assays is the loss of detection of rare alterations. However, the clinical relevance of rare mutations is often not well established, and thus, many clinical laboratories find that the ease of use of a targeted assay, combined with improved analytic sensitivity (thus reducing the degree to which tumor enrichment must be achieved), is an acceptable trade-off. Owing to the rapid evolution of the recommendations for which specific genes and alleles should be tested, specific recommendations are not elaborated herein, and recent guidelines should be consulted [64]. The more common methods for cancer gene mutation testing are described here.

Sanger Sequencing

The primary advantage of Sanger sequencing for somatic mutation detection in NSCLC is the comprehensive assessment of the sequenced gene regions. The importance of comprehensive gene mutation assessment differs for different genes. Some of these assessments are influenced by the degree to which a specific target gene has been evaluated. For example, extensive evaluation of mutations in *EGFR* in NSCLC has demonstrated that a small number of mutations comprise the majority of changes. Thus, comprehensive assessment may only seldom identify a rare mutation not detected using targeted assays. In contrast, evaluation of mutations in *DDR2* in squamous cell carcinoma has been undertaken to a lesser degree in recent years, and the data to date suggest a wide distribution of mutations, indicating that the advantages of Sanger sequencing are indeed relevant.

Modifications to Sanger Sequencing

A number of modifications to Sanger sequencing, including *c*o-amplification at *l*ower *d*enaturation *t*emperature-PCR (COLD-PCR) [65, 66] and *i*mprove and *c*omplete *e*nrichment COLD-PCR (ICE-COLD-PCR) [67], leverage the advantages of Sanger sequencing, i.e., comprehensive

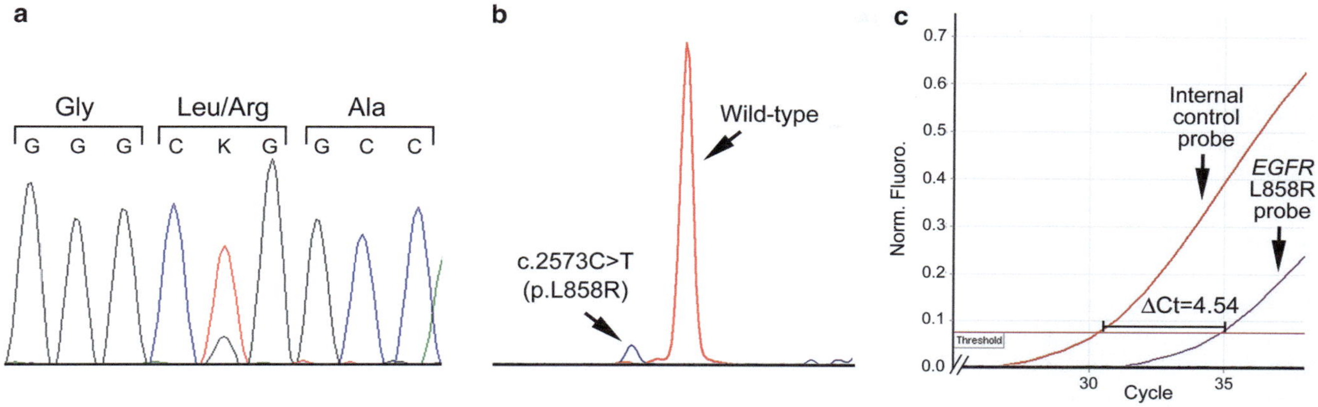

Figure 32.2 Different analytic sensitivities of mutation detection methods. (**a**) Sanger sequencing showing an *EGFR* c.2573T>G (p. L858R) mutation at 12.5 % allelic burden. (**b**) Single nucleotide base extension assay (SNaPshot®) showing the same mutation detectable at 6 % allelic burden. (**c**) Real-time PCR assay demonstrating the same mutation detectable at 1 % allelic burden

assessment, while achieving improved analytic sensitivity. These methods typically utilize alterations in cycling parameters to achieve imbalanced amplification favoring mutated alleles, thus increasing analytic sensitivity, followed by Sanger sequencing.

Restriction Fragment Length Polymorphism and PCR Fragment Sizing

A common method for *EGFR* mutation detection is combined PCR fragment sizing and restriction fragment length polymorphism (RFLP) for exon 19 deletions and L858R (c.2573C>T), respectively [68]. This approach is straightforward and has an analytic sensitivity of approximately 5 % mutant allele detection and excellent ease of use. The major disadvantage to this approach is the limitation in mutations detected, specifically that a number of mutations in *EGFR* which are not common, but similarly are not exceptionally rare, are not detected by this approach. Recent guidelines suggest that all mutations which are seen with a frequency of at least 1 % of *EGFR*-mutated lung adenocarcinomas, should be included in routine screening, which would not be accomplished by this approach [64].

Real-Time PCR

Multiple (non-FDA approved) commercial real-time PCR test kits are available for the detection of specific mutations in some genes, including *EGFR*, *KRAS*, and *BRAF*. Many of these kits indicate an analytic sensitivity of approximately 1 % mutant allele detection. A major advantage of real-time PCR is the high analytic sensitivity, which therefore reduces the likelihood of a false-negative result based on insufficient tumor content in the specimen [63]. In mid-2013, two real-time PCR-based assays (therascreen EGFR RGQ PCR Kit [Qiagen, Manchester, the United Kingdom] and cobas® EGFR Mutation Test [Roche, Pleasanton, CA]) were approved by the FDA for the evaluation of common *EGFR* mutations.

PCR Screening Methods

High-resolution melting curve analysis and denaturing high-performance liquid chromatography allow for rapid assessment of whether an alteration is present in a targeted region but do not identify the specific gene variation [69, 70]. The major advantage of mutation screening approaches is a rapid initial assessment of the status of a target region. However, precisely defining the alteration requires a follow-up test method to confirm and delineate the finding.

Pyrosequencing

Pyrosequencing has greater analytic sensitivity compared to Sanger sequencing and, rather than a purely targeted approach, does allow for the evaluation of short stretches of sequence. Pyrosequencing can be used for the detection of most single base substitutions and, although more challenging to interpret, can also be utilized for deletions and insertions (such as are commonly seen in *EGFR*) [71, 72]. The major advantages of pyrosequencing include better analytic sensitivity, ability to design custom nucleotide dispensations to query specific changes, and comprehensive evaluation over short stretches of sequence.

Ultrahigh Sensitivity Methods

Specific alterations may indicate the need for ultrasensitive methods for detection. One example of this is *EGFR* T790M (c.2369C>T), which is known to exist at varying percentages within the tumor cell population, due to both variable degrees of *EGFR* amplification and subclonality of the alteration. Multiple methods to achieve analytic sensitivities below 1 % allelic burden include locked nucleic acid assays and PCR assays utilizing restriction endonucleases to cleave wild-type sequences and beads, emulsion, amplification, and magnetics (BEAMing) [73–77]. The implementation of these approaches is dependent upon the clinical need for enhanced sensitivity in mutant allele detection, for example, in approaches which evaluate circulating tumor DNA, which are under evaluation [76].

Multiplex Methods

Increasingly, test methods which allow for the simultaneous detection of many mutations in a number of genes are used by clinical molecular laboratories. These include multiplexed single nucleotide base extension assays and mass spectrometry-based assays [78–80]. These assays rely on the development of multiplex PCR amplification followed by interrogation by multiple probes with spacer sequences and base extension reactions to allow for discrimination based on size or molecular weight. In addition, next generation sequencing (NGS) can query numerous entire genes, and the implementation of this approach into the clinical molecular laboratory is undergoing rapid adoption with the evaluation of appropriate metrics for quality assurance [81, 82]. Importantly, depending on methodology utilized for NGS, an assay may be able to identify selected gene rearrangements and copy number alterations.

Gene Rearrangements Assays

FISH Assays

The *EML4-ALK* fusion is generated by a paracentric chromosomal inversion in the short arm of chromosome 2, between bands p21 and p23.2. These two genes originally are separated by approximately 12.8 MB. The other described *ALK* fusions in lung cancer, *KIF5B-ALK* [34] and *TFG-ALK* [33], are caused by chromosomal translocations t(2;10)(p23.2;p11.22) and t(2;3)(p23.2;q12.1), respectively.

Numerous technical platforms are available for molecular diagnosis of *ALK* rearrangements in lung cancer, but the most commonly used for clinical testing is FISH. The standard FISH assay uses a dual-color break-apart probe set encompassing the 3′ and the 5′ sequences immediately adjacent to the breakpoint area in *ALK* (intron 19), labeled in orange and in green fluorophores, respectively (Fig. 32.3) [83].

The *ALK* BA FISH probe was used in the initial clinical trials for crizotinib [35, 84] and is approved by the FDA as a companion diagnostic test. The *ALK* BA FISH assay is DNA based and is thus robust and resistant to technical artifacts. Other advantages include being highly suitable for detection in FFPE tissue sections, detecting all variants of EML4-*ALK*, and detection of translocations with and of the reported or uncharacterized partner genes. On the other hand, the FISH platform requires specialized resources (fluorescence microscope, light-protected laboratory space) and highly trained personnel.

Two other receptor kinase genes were identified as activated in lung cancers by fusions, *ROS1* [33] and *RET* [85]. Integrated molecular and histopathologic screening systems have been successful in detecting a large number of fusion partners in lung cancer for these two genes, and preclinical studies have confirmed their tumorigenic potential [34]. Additionally, targeted therapy may have a role for these molecular subsets, which are predominantly identified using FISH assays [44, 45, 86].

Reverse-Transcription PCR

Reverse-transcription PCR (RT-PCR) can be used to detect and identify gene rearrangements. Messenger RNA (mRNA) is isolated from tumor tissue and reverse transcribed to complementary DNA (cDNA). Amplification with polymerase is performed using primers that bind sequences within the 5′ gene fusion partner (e.g., *EML4*) and the 3′ end of the fusion gene encoding the kinase domain of the oncogene (e.g., *ALK*). The presence of a gene fusion can thus be detected and identified by size discrimination assays and sequencing of the amplification product. To date, over ten *EML4-ALK* variants have been reported, involving eight different *EML4* exons and exon 20 of *ALK* [31]. Although methods exist to identify unknown gene fusion partners, such as inverse PCR and 5′ rapid amplification of cDNA ends (RACE), high-throughput targeted assays will typically only allow known fusion partners and variants to be detected [32]. Specific primers are designed for each *EML4* variant, which can be multiplexed for PCR amplification, as long as the amplicons are of different sizes and/or labeled with different fluorophores. Amplicon size must be kept relatively small (up to 150–200 base pairs) to allow the use of FFPE tissue, since frozen tissue is not routinely available. The implementation of these assays in the clinical molecular laboratory requires either follow up on testing for negative findings (i.e., extensive analysis of RNA quality), separate amplifications for each variant, or design of assays to minimize amplicon size [32].

Other Methods

Immunohistochemistry (IHC) using antibodies specific for the C-terminal region of the ALK protein is a surrogate method to detect the presence of an *ALK* gene rearrangement in NSCLC [87, 88]. The most commonly used antibodies are ALK1 (DAKO, Carpinteria, CA), 5A4 (Novocastra, Newcastle, the United Kingdom, and Abcam, Cambridge, MA), and D5F3 (Cell Signaling Technology, Danvers, MA). IHC is a favored test method due to rapid turnaround time and low cost. However, for ALK IHC, the methods are not standardized, and method variations include antibody dilu-

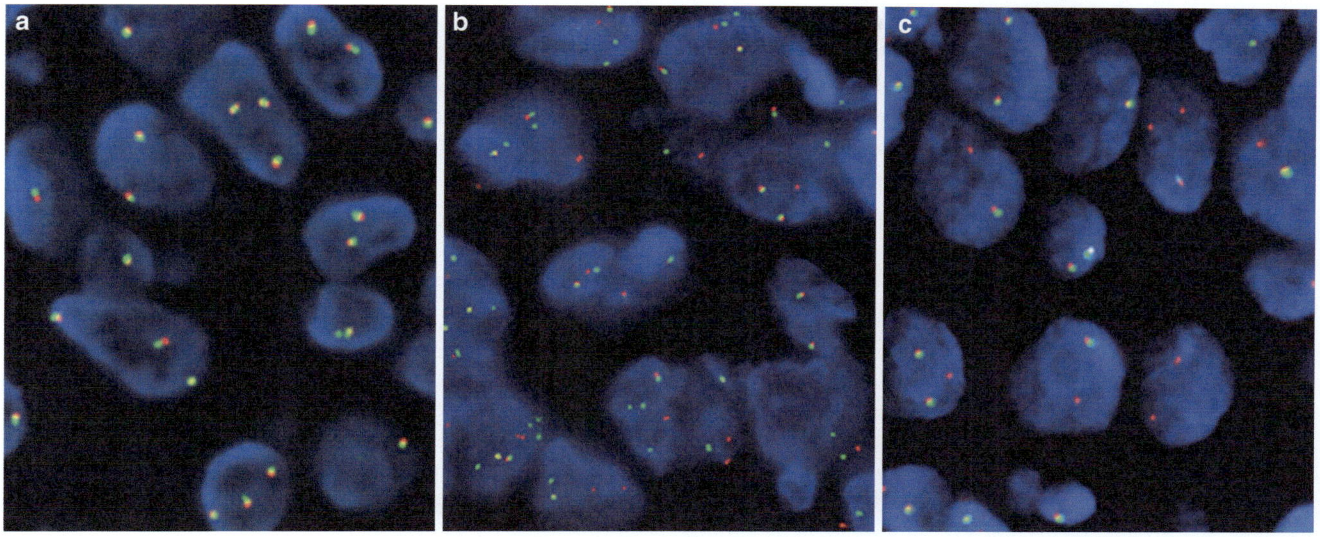

Figure 32.3 Lung adenocarcinoma specimens hybridized with the Vysis *ALK* Break Apart FISH Probe (Abbott Laboratories, Abbot Park, IL). (**a**) *ALK*-negative pattern (only native *orange/green* fused fluorescent signals), (**b**) *ALK*-positive pattern (split *orange-green* signals), and (**c**) *ALK*-positive pattern (single *orange* signals)

tions, detection systems with or without signal amplification, scoring criteria (qualitative, semiquantitative, and image-based), and cutoffs for classifying positive specimens, limiting the utility of IHC in the clinical molecular laboratory. However, extensive study is underway to define the concordance and reproducibility of this methodology with the expectation that following large-scale evaluations, IHC may become a dominant approach [89, 90, 91].

Quantitative real-time PCR (qPCR) techniques, using primers that amplify a portion of the 3′ end of the *ALK* gene (encoding the kinase domain), detect higher *ALK* mRNA expression in comparison with a housekeeping gene [92]. Both IHC and qPCR rely on the observation that ALK is not typically expressed in normal lung tissue or in NSCLC without an *ALK* gene rearrangement. Both techniques thus infer the presence of an *ALK* gene rearrangement but could also detect aberrant expression of native, full-length ALK.

Gene Amplification Assays

Oncogene activation is also achieved through amplification of gene copies. Mechanisms for gene amplification include the extrachromosomal double minutes and the intrachromosomal homogenously staining regions, both of which are easily detected by FISH assays.

In NSCLC, numerous genes can be amplified and typically confers a poor prognosis. Amplification of the *EGFR* gene is associated with response to EGFR inhibitors [93], although, at least in patients of Asian ethnicity, this association may largely reflect the amplification of activated mutant alleles [94] and the degree of this association is relatively weak compared to the evaluation of *EGFR* mutation status. Amplification of the *MET* gene has been associated with poor overall survival [95] and with acquired resistance to EGFR TK inhibitors [96], which is thought to arise from positive selection of low-level clones carrying the alteration [97]. *MET* amplification evaluation may also have relevance for the selection of targeted therapy as studies evaluating this analyte with respect to inhibitors of hepatocyte growth factor receptor (HGFR, the protein product of the *MET* gene) are ongoing [48]. A number of other genes encoding growth factors, growth factor receptors, and transcription factors can be amplified in lung cancer, such as *HER2*, *FGFR1–FGFR2*, *SOX2*, and *PIK3CA*. The availability of novel therapeutic agents that specifically inhibit these proteins has created an increased interest in testing for these molecular markers in order to select patients who are more likely to be sensitive (or resistant) to the targeted therapies [48].

Interpretation of Results

Driver Mutation Detection Assays

One of the key issues in the interpretation of somatic mutation testing is correlation between the preanalytic specimen features, preanalytic processing (especially tumor enrichment), testing method, and test results. This is especially relevant for negative results, which should be interpreted in the context of the above-listed features. Given that assessments of tumor cellularity are highly subjective and only a single specimen may be available for testing, a laboratory may elect to test a borderline specimen with a low percentage of tumor cells, because a positive result would be informative, even though a negative result may be inconclusive.

With gene sequencing assays, the interpretation of rare mutations can be challenging. For many gene targets, mutational hotspots have been identified, and a finding of a mutation outside of one of these known regions must be carefully interpreted for clinical significance. Since FFPE tissue is frequently used for somatic mutation testing, the possibility that a rare mutation represents a procedural artifact must be considered. Furthermore, as especially relevant to testing in NSCLC, using extremely limited tissue and DNA quantities, as may be seen with some small specimens, can also lead to sequencing artifacts [98]. Thus, rare mutations must be interpreted with these procedural artifacts in mind, especially for genes which have been extensively characterized. Rare mutation findings should be repeated from the earliest feasible stage of testing and potentially with an alternate testing method. If a rare mutation is confirmed, the report should reflect that the clinical implications are not well understood, unless the scientific medical literature supports an interpretation of clinical significance. Public databases for interpretation of cancer gene mutations include the Catalogue of Somatic Mutations in Cancer (COSMIC) [99] and dbSNP through NCBI. These resources are especially valuable in identifying literature relevant for the interpretation of a specific mutation.

For gene mutations which are previously reported with a known clinical significance, the molecular pathology report should include an interpretive statement as to the clinical relevance of the finding. The implications of a particular result with respect to prognosis or responsiveness to a targeted therapy can change rapidly with new clinical studies, and efforts should be undertaken to ensure the most up-to-date clinically validated implications are noted.

Gene Rearrangement Assays

FISH

Usually, interpretation of FISH results using the *ALK* BA probe is straightforward. However, the fact that the *EML4* and *ALK* genes are separated by a small distance (12.8 MB) makes the identification of split signals subtle and challenging in a fraction of tumor cells. In the native copy of *ALK*, the orange and green probes recognize homologous sequences that are physically close to each other and show up as a fused orange (red)/green fluorescent signal (Fig. 32.3a). Therefore, fusion fluorescent signals in this setting indicate a normal copy of the *ALK* gene. When the break occurs around the *ALK* intron 19, the orange (red) signals from the 3′ probe sequences separate from the green signals of the 5′ probe sequences (Fig. 32.3b). When *EML4-ALK* fusion occurs, the sequences recognized by the green probe are positioned approximately 12.8 MB more centromeric to their original locus. Because of the relatively small genomic distance between these signals, scoring criteria require that the split seen be at least two signal diameters wide. In approximately 30 % of the rearrangements involving *ALK*, chromosomal deletions also occur in association with the inversion causing loss of the genomic sequences recognized by the green-labeled 5′ end sequences (Fig. 32.3c). Thus, the split between orange (red) and green signals and the presence of single orange (red) signals are interpreted as a rearrangement of the *ALK* gene. A minimum of 50 cells should be counted for assay scoring, and when greater than 15 % of cells are scored as positive (either split pattern or single orange (red) pattern), the result is interpreted as positive for an *ALK* rearrangement. Additional scoring criteria for the FDA-approved companion diagnostic include an equivocal range of percent positive cells with requirement for a second reader in such cases, although a routine two-reader practice is recommended.

Reverse-Transcription PCR

Interpretation of RT-PCR assays for the detection of ALK rearrangements has particular benefits in that it provides the most direct evidence of a gene rearrangement. Furthermore, this technique can provide the details not only of the 5′ gene fusion partner identity in each case but also the specific exon fusion (Fig. 32.4). In *ALK* gene-rearranged NSCLC, there are at least three different 5′ gene fusion partners (*EML4*, *KIF5B*, and *TFG*) and multiple different fusion variants in which different exons of *EML4* (and occasionally *ALK*) have been detected for *EML4-ALK* gene fusions [32–34, 100, 101]. Distinction of which specific fusion partner is involved in the rearrangement can be accomplished through size analysis for some assays, wherein specific fusions produce products of predictable size or may require sequencing of the fusion gene product. For assays which identify fusion events based on the presence of an amplicon of specific size, sequencing should be routinely performed on the amplification product to ensure that the amplicon detected is actually a gene fusion transcript and not the results of false priming. If the assay is designed in a directed fashion (i.e., uses bidirectional primers for the detection of specific fusion variants), negative results must always be interpreted in the context of known fusion partners not detected by the assay and also consider false-negatives attributable to novel fusion partners not yet described. Additionally, as these assays are based on RNA which is typically derived from FFPE tissue, consideration of false negatives attributable to low RNA quality is imperative, and appropriate quality control metrics (such as independent measures of RNA quality) should be

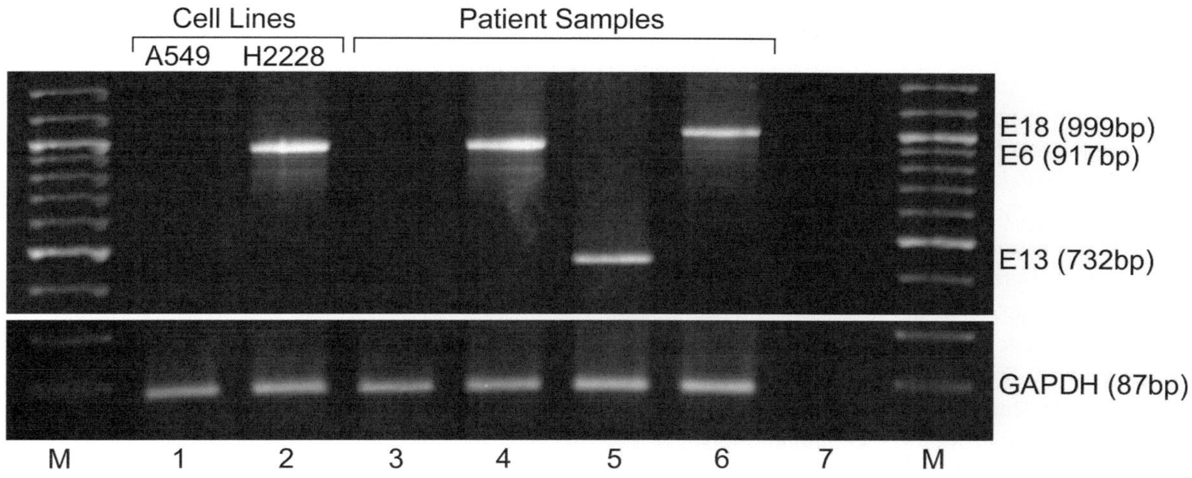

Figure 32.4 Reverse-transcription PCR (RT-PCR) for the detection of known *ALK* fusions from frozen non-small cell lung cancer (NSCLC) tissue. Multiplex RT-PCR including forward primers to exons 2 and 13 of *EML4* and one reverse primer to exon 20 of *ALK* are utilized in a single reaction. *Lanes 1* and *2* are results for negative (A549) and positive (H2228) cell lines, respectively. *Lane 3* is a patient sample negative for *ALK* rearrangement. *Lanes 4–6* are patient samples with *ALK* rearrangements with different *EML4* breakpoints. *Lane 7* is a no template control. *GAPDH* mRNA control reactions are shown in the *lower panel*. Negative results from an assay with amplicons >200–250 bp should be interpreted with caution, and multiplex primers can be designed with amplicon size aimed for detection in FFPE [31, 97]. *M* molecular weight markers

included and evaluated for assays of this nature. If such quality metrics are suboptimal, reporting should include caveats about potential false negatives. Finally, this technique has the potential to be extremely sensitive because of the combined effects of PCR amplification and the lack of background signal as only the fusion gene transcript is detected by this assay.

Gene Amplification Assays

Interpretation of results in FISH assays for copy number analysis is relatively simple. The number of copies per cell of a probe for the target gene sequence is compared with the number of copies of a reference probe, commonly represented by the centromere of the chromosome containing the target gene. Other gene sequences mapped in the same chromosome arm or in the opposite arm of the target gene are acceptable as reference sequences and sometimes even preferable, for instance, when complex rearrangements involve loss of centromeric sequences. Gene amplification is determined when the copy number ratio between the target and reference probe signals is greater than a prespecified value, commonly 2.0.

When a target gene is located close to the chromosomal centromere, both the target gene and the centromeric region may be amplified, making interpretation using a ratio greater than 2.0 inappropriate. *EGFR* maps at 7p12 near the centromere and is amplified in approximately 10 % of NSCLC [102]. With *EGFR* gene amplification, the chromosome 7 centromeric sequences also can be amplified, in which case the ratio between the mean *EGFR* probe signals per cell and the mean centromere 7 probe signals per cell will be approximately 1. Customized scoring systems have been developed to account for such phenomenon, when more than two probe signals for both the *EGFR* gene and the centromere 7 are identified [103].

Laboratory Issues

A question which often arises is which patients should be tested. Numerous approaches to this issue have been proposed, and while ultimately such decisions are made by the treating oncologist, some general principles have emerged. First and foremost, for patients with advanced stage disease, testing for *EGFR* mutations and *ALK* rearrangements is the standard of care, because the results impact first-line therapy selection. Regardless of the determinations of which patients to test, it is critical that results be available in a timeframe to allow therapeutic decisions to be based on the test results. This leads to the question of whether to test concurrently or in sequence. Despite the low prevalence of *ALK* rearrangement in NSCLC and the finding that co-occurrence of *EGFR* mutation and *ALK* rearrangement is uncommon, in order to meet the goal of returning results in a clinically actionable timeframe, concurrent testing may be preferable from a clinical perspective.

One significant challenge of clinical molecular testing for NSCLC is the need to perform testing on diagnostic small biopsy or FNA specimens. As the majority of NSCLC patients are not surgical candidates at the time of diagnosis, small samples are common for initial diagnosis. When considering the common need for IHC evaluation, which often requires multiple rounds of facing of a paraffin block, the residual material remaining after histopathologic diagnosis can be exceedingly limited. However, given appropriate methods, testing on such specimens can be accommodated. Implementation of appropriate tumor enrichment techniques is essential, as is evaluation of the specimen by a pathologist prior to testing, selection of an appropriate testing method, and reporting of results in an integrated format. Cytopathology specimens, including cell blocks and direct smears, are often adequate specimens for testing. Of paramount logistical relevance is the need to institute measures for maximal preservation of tissue from small diagnostic specimens to allow for molecular testing following histopathologic diagnosis. This includes efforts to limit the degree to which paraffin blocks are multiply faced and reduction in the use of IHC and duplicative controls. As the number of clinically validated molecular targets for testing grows, the need to preserve tissue will become ever more paramount. Part of the management of tissue for this purpose will be a growing recognition of the need to establish prioritization of clinical testing. While clinical parameters may be associated with some of the molecular subtypes of NSCLC, they are not sufficiently specific to dictate choice of testing. However, they may be useful in determining prioritization of testing for limited specimens.

Conclusions and Future Directions

As the number of defined targets for clinical molecular testing that drive therapy selection grows, the need to implement testing which evaluates as many of these oncogenic variants simultaneously is an inevitable necessity. The one-at-a-time model for testing for individual mutations has already been supplanted in some centers by multiplex testing for dozens of mutations simultaneously [104, 105]. As the clinical use of NGS advances, testing is likely to migrate to platforms which can accommodate the evaluation of dozens to hundreds of genes and variants concurrently.

Acknowledgments The authors thank Jerry Haney, Anh Le, and Lisa Litzenberger for assistance in making figures.

References

1. Jemal A, Bray F, Center MM, Ferlay J, Ward E, Forman D. Global cancer statistics. CA Cancer J Clin. 2011;61(2):69–90.
2. Jemal A, Siegel R, Xu J, Ward E. Cancer statistics, 2010. CA Cancer J Clin. 2010;60(5):277–300.
3. Chaft JE, Arcila ME, Paik PK, Lau C, Riely GJ, Pietanza MC, Zakowski MF, Rusch V, Sima CS, Ladanyi M, Kris MG. Coexistence of PIK3CA and other oncogene mutations in lung adenocarcinoma-rationale for comprehensive mutation profiling. Mol Cancer Ther. 2012;11(2):485–91.
4. Cohen S. Isolation of a mouse submaxillary gland protein accelerating incisor eruption and eyelid opening in the new-born animal. J Biol Chem. 1962;237:1555–62.
5. Carpenter G, Lembach KJ, Morrison MM, Cohen S. Characterization of the binding of 125-I-labeled epidermal growth factor to human fibroblasts. J Biol Chem. 1975;250(11):4297–304.
6. Ullrich A, Coussens L, Hayflick JS, Dull TJ, Gray A, Tam AW, Lee J, Yarden Y, Libermann TA, Schlessinger J, et al. Human epidermal growth factor receptor cDNA sequence and aberrant expression of the amplified gene in A431 epidermoid carcinoma cells. Nature. 1984;309(5967):418–25.
7. Franklin WA, Veve R, Hirsch FR, Helfrich BA, Bunn Jr PA. Epidermal growth factor receptor family in lung cancer and premalignancy. Semin Oncol. 2002;29(1 Suppl 4):3–14.
8. Hirsch FR, Varella-Garcia M, Bunn Jr PA, Di Maria MV, Veve R, Bremmes RM, Baron AE, Zeng C, Franklin WA. Epidermal growth factor receptor in non-small-cell lung carcinomas: correlation between gene copy number and protein expression and impact on prognosis. J Clin Oncol. 2003;21(20):3798–807.
9. Lynch TJ, Bell DW, Sordella R, Gurubhagavatula S, Okimoto RA, Brannigan BW, Harris PL, Haserlat SM, Supko JG, Haluska FG, Louis DN, Christiani DC, Settleman J, Haber DA. Activating mutations in the epidermal growth factor receptor underlying responsiveness of non-small-cell lung cancer to gefitinib. N Engl J Med. 2004;350(21):2129–39.
10. Paez JG, Janne PA, Lee JC, Tracy S, Greulich H, Gabriel S, Herman P, Kaye FJ, Lindeman N, Boggon TJ, Naoki K, Sasaki H, Fujii Y, Eck MJ, Sellers WR, Johnson BE, Meyerson M. EGFR mutations in lung cancer: correlation with clinical response to gefitinib therapy. Science. 2004;304(5676):1497–500.
11. Pao W, Miller VA, Politi KA, Riely GJ, Somwar R, Zakowski MF, Kris MG, Varmus H. Acquired resistance of lung adenocarcinomas to gefitinib or erlotinib is associated with a second mutation in the EGFR kinase domain. PLoS Med. 2005;2(3):e73.
12. Bean J, Brennan C, Shih JY, Riely G, Viale A, Wang L, Chitale D, Motoi N, Szoke J, Broderick S, Balak M, Chang WC, Yu CJ, Gazdar A, Pass H, Rusch V, Gerald W, Huang SF, Yang PC, Miller V, Ladanyi M, Yang CH, Pao W. MET amplification occurs with or without T790M mutations in EGFR mutant lung tumors with acquired resistance to gefitinib or erlotinib. Proc Natl Acad Sci U S A. 2007;104(52):20932–7.
13. Nguyen KS, Kobayashi S, Costa DB. Acquired resistance to epidermal growth factor receptor tyrosine kinase inhibitors in non-small-cell lung cancers dependent on the epidermal growth factor receptor pathway. Clin Lung Cancer. 2009;10(4):281–9.
14. Suda K, Murakami I, Katayama T, Tomizawa K, Osada H, Sekido Y, Maehara Y, Yatabe Y, Mitsudomi T. Reciprocal and complementary role of MET amplification and EGFR T790M mutation in acquired resistance to kinase inhibitors in lung cancer. Clin Cancer Res. 2010;16(22):5489–98.
15. Sequist LV, Waltman BA, Dias-Santagata D, Digumarthy S, Turke AB, Fidias P, Bergethon K, Shaw AT, Gettinger S, Cosper AK, Akhavanfard S, Heist RS, Temel J, Christensen JG, Wain JC, Lynch TJ, Vernovsky K, Mark EJ, Lanuti M, Iafrate AJ, Mino-Kenudson M, Engelman JA. Genotypic and histological evolution of lung cancers acquiring resistance to EGFR inhibitors. Sci Transl Med. 2011;3(75):75ra26.
16. Yun CH, Mengwasser KE, Toms AV, Woo MS, Greulich H, Wong KK, Meyerson M, Eck MJ. The T790M mutation in EGFR kinase

causes drug resistance by increasing the affinity for ATP. Proc Natl Acad Sci U S A. 2008;105(6):2070–5.
17. Inukai M, Toyooka S, Ito S, Asano H, Ichihara S, Soh J, Suehisa H, Ouchida M, Aoe K, Aoe M, Kiura K, Shimizu N, Date H. Presence of epidermal growth factor receptor gene T790M mutation as a minor clone in non-small cell lung cancer. Cancer Res. 2006;66(16):7854–8.
18. Girard N, Lou E, Azzoli CG, Reddy R, Robson M, Harlan M, Orlow I, Yatabe Y, Nafa K, Ladanyi M, Viale A, Kris MG, Riely G, Miller V, Klein RJ, Matsuo K, Pao W. Analysis of genetic variants in never-smokers with lung cancer facilitated by an Internet-based blood collection protocol: a preliminary report. Clin Cancer Res. 2010;16(2):755–63.
19. Yasuda H, Kobayashi S, Costa DB. EGFR exon 20 insertion mutations in non-small-cell lung cancer: preclinical data and clinical implications. Lancet Oncol. 2012;13(1):e23–31.
20. Ahrendt SA, Decker PA, Alawi EA, Zhu Yr YR, Sanchez-Cespedes M, Yang SC, Haasler GB, Kajdacsy-Balla A, Demeure MJ, Sidransky D. Cigarette smoking is strongly associated with mutation of the K-ras gene in patients with primary adenocarcinoma of the lung. Cancer. 2001;92(6):1525–30.
21. Riely GJ, Kris MG, Rosenbaum D, Marks J, Li A, Chitale DA, Nafa K, Riedel ER, Hsu M, Pao W, Miller VA, Ladanyi M. Frequency and distinctive spectrum of KRAS mutations in never smokers with lung adenocarcinoma. Clin Cancer Res. 2008;14(18):5731–4.
22. Benesova L, Minarik M, Jancarikova D, Belsanova B, Pesek M. Multiplicity of EGFR and KRAS mutations in non-small cell lung cancer (NSCLC) patients treated with tyrosine kinase inhibitors. Anticancer Res. 2010;30(5):1667–71.
23. Malumbres M, Barbacid M. RAS oncogenes: the first 30 years. Nat Rev Cancer. 2003;3(6):459–65.
24. Roberts PJ, Stinchcombe TE, Der CJ, Socinski MA. Personalized medicine in non-small-cell lung cancer: is KRAS a useful marker in selecting patients for epidermal growth factor receptor-targeted therapy? J Clin Oncol. 2010;28(31):4769–77.
25. Soda M, Choi YL, Enomoto M, Takada S, Yamashita Y, Ishikawa S, Fujiwara S, Watanabe H, Kurashina K, Hatanaka H, Bando M, Ohno S, Ishikawa Y, Aburatani H, Niki T, Sohara Y, Sugiyama Y, Mano H. Identification of the transforming EML4-ALK fusion gene in non-small-cell lung cancer. Nature. 2007;448(7153):561–6.
26. Rodig SJ, Mino-Kenudson M, Dacic S, Yeap BY, Shaw A, Barletta JA, Stubbs H, Law K, Lindeman N, Mark E, Janne PA, Lynch T, Johnson BE, Iafrate AJ, Chirieac LR. Unique clinicopathologic features characterize ALK-rearranged lung adenocarcinoma in the western population. Clin Cancer Res. 2009;15(16):5216–23.
27. Sasaki T, Rodig SJ, Chirieac LR, Janne PA. The biology and treatment of EML4-ALK non-small cell lung cancer. Eur J Cancer. 2010;46(10):1773–80.
28. Takahashi T, Sonobe M, Kobayashi M, Yoshizawa A, Menju T, Nakayama E, Mino N, Iwakiri S, Sato K, Miyahara R, Okubo K, Manabe T, Date H. Clinicopathologic features of non-small-cell lung cancer with EML4-ALK fusion gene. Ann Surg Oncol. 2010;17(3):889–97.
29. Pillai RN, Ramalingam SS. The biology and clinical features of non-small cell lung cancers with EML4-ALK translocation. Curr Oncol Rep. 2012;14(2):105–10.
30. Shaw AT, Yeap BY, Mino-Kenudson M, Digumarthy SR, Costa DB, Heist RS, Solomon B, Stubbs H, Admane S, McDermott U, Settleman J, Kobayashi S, Mark EJ, Rodig SJ, Chirieac LR, Kwak EL, Lynch TJ, Iafrate AJ. Clinical features and outcome of patients with non-small-cell lung cancer who harbor EML4-ALK. J Clin Oncol. 2009;27(26):4247–53.
31. Soda M, Takada S, Takeuchi K, Choi YL, Enomoto M, Ueno T, Haruta H, Hamada T, Yamashita Y, Ishikawa Y, Sugiyama Y, Mano H. A mouse model for EML4-ALK-positive lung cancer. Proc Natl Acad Sci U S A. 2008;105(50):19893–7.
32. Sanders HR, Li HR, Bruey JM, Scheerle JA, Meloni-Ehrig AM, Kelly JC, Novick C, Albitar M. Exon scanning by reverse transcriptase-polymerase chain reaction for detection of known and novel EML4-ALK fusion variants in non-small cell lung cancer. Cancer Genet. 2011;204(1):45–52.
33. Rikova K, Guo A, Zeng Q, Possemato A, Yu J, Haack H, Nardone J, Lee K, Reeves C, Li Y, Hu Y, Tan Z, Stokes M, Sullivan L, Mitchell J, Wetzel R, Macneill J, Ren JM, Yuan J, Bakalarski CE, Villen J, Kornhauser JM, Smith B, Li D, Zhou X, Gygi SP, Gu TL, Polakiewicz RD, Rush J, Comb MJ. Global survey of phosphotyrosine signaling identifies oncogenic kinases in lung cancer. Cell. 2007;131(6):1190–203.
34. Takeuchi K, Choi YL, Togashi Y, Soda M, Hatano S, Inamura K, Takada S, Ueno T, Yamashita Y, Satoh Y, Okumura S, Nakagawa K, Ishikawa Y, Mano H. KIF5B-ALK, a novel fusion oncokinase identified by an immunohistochemistry-based diagnostic system for ALK-positive lung cancer. Clin Cancer Res. 2009;15(9):3143–9.
35. Kwak EL, Bang YJ, Camidge DR, Shaw AT, Solomon B, Maki RG, Ou SH, Dezube BJ, Janne PA, Costa DB, Varella-Garcia M, Kim WH, Lynch TJ, Fidias P, Stubbs H, Engelman JA, Sequist LV, Tan W, Gandhi L, Mino-Kenudson M, Wei GC, Shreeve SM, Ratain MJ, Settleman J, Christensen JG, Haber DA, Wilner K, Salgia R, Shapiro GI, Clark JW, Iafrate AJ. Anaplastic lymphoma kinase inhibition in non-small-cell lung cancer. N Engl J Med. 2010;363(18):1693–703.
36. FDA Approval for Crizotinib. Retrieved 15 Feb 2012, from http://www.cancer.gov/cancertopics/druginfo/fda-crizotinib
37. Mok TS, Wu YL, Thongprasert S, Yang CH, Chu DT, Saijo N, Sunpaweravong P, Han B, Margono B, Ichinose Y, Nishiwaki Y, Ohe Y, Yang JJ, Chewaskulyong B, Jiang H, Duffield EL, Watkins CL, Armour AA, Fukuoka M. Gefitinib or carboplatin-paclitaxel in pulmonary adenocarcinoma. N Engl J Med. 2009;361(10):947–57.
38. Pao W, Chmielecki J. Rational, biologically based treatment of EGFR-mutant non-small-cell lung cancer. Nat Rev Cancer. 2010;10(11):760–74.
39. Mitsudomi T. Erlotinib, gefitinib, or chemotherapy for EGFR mutation-positive lung cancer? Lancet Oncol. 2011;12(8):710–1.
40. Cappuzzo F, Ciuleanu T, Stelmakh L, Cicenas S, Szczesna A, Juhasz E, Esteban E, Molinier O, Brugger W, Melezinek I, Klingelschmitt G, Klughammer B, Giaccone G. Erlotinib as maintenance treatment in advanced non-small-cell lung cancer: a multicentre, randomised, placebo-controlled phase 3 study. Lancet Oncol. 2010;11(6):521–9.
41. Douillard JY, Shepherd FA, Hirsh V, Mok T, Socinski MA, Gervais R, Liao ML, Bischoff H, Reck M, Sellers MV, Watkins CL, Speake G, Armour AA, Kim ES. Molecular predictors of outcome with gefitinib and docetaxel in previously treated non-small-cell lung cancer: data from the randomized phase III INTEREST trial. J Clin Oncol. 2010;28(5):744–52.
42. Ding L, Getz G, Wheeler DA, et al. Somatic mutations affect key pathways in lung adenocarcinoma. Nature. 2008;455(7216):1069–75.
43. Riely GJ, Kim D, Crino L, Janne PA, Blackhall FH, Camidge DR, Hirsch V, Mok TSK, Solomon B, Soria JC, Park K, Gadgeel SM, Martins RG, Han J, De Pas T, Bottomely A, Polli A, Petersen JA, Tassell VR, Shaw AT. Phase 2 data for crizotinib (PF-02341066) in ALK-positive advanced non-small cell lung cancer (NSCLC): PROFILE 1005. J Thoracic Oncol. Proceedings of the 14th World Conference on Lung Cancer. 2011;O31.05.
44. Bergethon K, Shaw AT, Ou SH, Katayama R, Lovly CM, McDonald NT, Massion PP, Siwak-Tapp C, Gonzalez A, Fang R, Mark EJ, Batten JM, Chen H, Wilner KD, Kwak EL, Clark JW,

Carbone DP, Ji H, Engelman JA, Mino-Kenudson M, Pao W, Iafrate AJ. ROS1 rearrangements define a unique molecular class of lung cancers. J Clin Oncol. 2012;30(8):863–70.

45. Davies KD, Le AT, Theodoro MF, Skokan MC, Aisner DL, Berge EM, Terracciano LM, Cappuzzo F, Incarbone M, Roncalli M, Alloisio M, Santoro A, Camidge DR, Varella-Garcia M, Doebele RC. Identifying and targeting ROS1 gene fusions in non-small cell lung cancer. Clin Cancer Res. 2012;18(17):4570–9.
46. Kris MG, Johnson BE, Kwiatkowski DJ, Iafrate AJ, Wistuba II, Aronson SL, Engelman JA, Shyr Y, Khuri FR, Rudin CM, Garon EB, Pao W, Schiller JH, Haura EB, Shirai K, Giaccone G, Berry LD, Kugler K, Minna JD, Bunn Jr PA. Identification of driver mutations in tumor specimens from 1,000 patients with lung adenocarcinoma: the NCI's Lung Cancer Mutation Consortium (LCMC). J Clin Oncol. 2011;29(Suppl):abstr CRA7506.
47. Karapetis CS, Khambata-Ford S, Jonker DJ, O'Callaghan CJ, Tu D, Tebbutt NC, Simes RJ, Chalchal H, Shapiro JD, Robitaille S, Price TJ, Shepherd L, Au HJ, Langer C, Moore MJ, Zalcberg JR. K-ras mutations and benefit from cetuximab in advanced colorectal cancer. N Engl J Med. 2008;359(17):1757–65.
48. Pao W, Girard N. New driver mutations in non-small-cell lung cancer. Lancet Oncol. 2011;12(2):175–80.
49. Boldrini L, Gisfredi S, Ursino S, Camacci T, Baldini E, Melfi F, Fontanini G. Mutational analysis in cytological specimens of advanced lung adenocarcinoma: a sensitive method for molecular diagnosis. J Thorac Oncol. 2007;2(12):1086–90.
50. Aisner DL, Deshpande C, Baloch Z, Watt CD, Litzky LA, Malhotra B, Sepulveda AR, Langer C, Evans T, Van Deerlin VM. Evaluation of EGFR mutation status in cytology specimens: an institutional experience. Diagn Cytopathol. 2011;41:316–23.
51. Betz BL, Roh MH, Weigelin HC, Placido JB, Schmidt LA, Farmen S, Arenberg DA, Kalemkerian GP, Knoepp SM. The application of molecular diagnostic studies interrogating EGFR and KRAS mutations to stained cytologic smears of lung carcinoma. Am J Clin Pathol. 2011;136(4):564–71.
52. da Cunha Santos G, Saieg MA, Geddie W, Leighl N. EGFR gene status in cytological samples of nonsmall cell lung carcinoma: controversies and opportunities. Cancer Cytopathol. 2011;119(2):80–91.
53. Malapelle U, Bellevicine C, Zeppa P, Palombini L, Troncone G. Cytology-based gene mutation tests to predict response to anti-epidermal growth factor receptor therapy: a review. Diagn Cytopathol. 2011;39(9):703–10.
54. Rekhtman N, Brandt SM, Sigel CS, Friedlander MA, Riely GJ, Travis WD, Zakowski MF, Moreira AL. Suitability of thoracic cytology for new therapeutic paradigms in non-small cell lung carcinoma: high accuracy of tumor subtyping and feasibility of EGFR and KRAS molecular testing. J Thorac Oncol. 2011;6(3):451–8.
55. Santis G, Angell R, Nickless G, Quinn A, Herbert A, Cane P, Spicer J, Breen R, McLean E, Tobal K. Screening for EGFR and KRAS mutations in endobronchial ultrasound derived transbronchial needle aspirates in non-small cell lung cancer using COLD-PCR. PLoS One. 2011;6(9):e25191.
56. Pirker R, Herth FJ, Kerr KM, Filipits M, Taron M, Gandara D, Hirsch FR, Grunenwald D, Popper H, Smit E, Dietel M, Marchetti A, Manegold C, Schirmacher P, Thomas M, Rosell R, Cappuzzo F, Stahel R. Consensus for EGFR mutation testing in non-small cell lung cancer: results from a European workshop. J Thorac Oncol. 2010;5(10):1706–13.
57. Greer CE, Peterson SL, Kiviat NB, Manos MM. PCR amplification from paraffin-embedded tissues. Effects of fixative and fixation time. Am J Clin Pathol. 1991;95(2):117–24.
58. Hunt JL. Molecular pathology in anatomic pathology practice: a review of basic principles. Arch Pathol Lab Med. 2008;132(2):248–60.
59. Hunt JL, Finkelstein SD. Microdissection techniques for molecular testing in surgical pathology. Arch Pathol Lab Med. 2004;128(12):1372–8.
60. Smouse JH, Cibas ES, Janne PA, Joshi VA, Zou KH, Lindeman NI. EGFR mutations are detected comparably in cytologic and surgical pathology specimens of nonsmall cell lung cancer. Cancer. 2009;117(1):67–72.
61. Chowdhuri SR, Xi L, Pham TH, Hanson J, Rodriguez-Canales J, Berman A, Rajan A, Giaccone G, Emmert-Buck M, Raffeld M, Filie AC. EGFR and KRAS mutation analysis in cytologic samples of lung adenocarcinoma enabled by laser capture microdissection. Mod Pathol. 2011;25:548–55.
62. Malapelle U, de Rosa N, Rocco D, Bellevicine C, Crispino C, Illiano A, Piantedosi FV, Nappi O, Troncone G. EGFR and KRAS mutations detection on lung cancer liquid-based cytology: a pilot study. J Clin Pathol. 2012;65(1):87–91.
63. Pao W, Ladanyi M. Epidermal growth factor receptor mutation testing in lung cancer: searching for the ideal method. Clin Cancer Res. 2007;13(17):4954–5.
64. Lindeman NI, Cagle PT, Beasley MB, Chitale DA, Dacic S, Giaccone G, Jenkins RB, Kwiatkowski DJ, Saldivar JS, Squire J, Thunnissen E, Ladanyi M. Molecular testing guideline for selection of lung cancer patients for EGFR and ALK tyrosine kinase inhibitors: guideline from the College of American Pathologists, International Association for the Study of Lung Cancer, and Association for Molecular Pathology. Arch Pathol Lab Med. 2013;137(6):828–60.
65. Li J, Makrigiorgos GM. COLD-PCR: a new platform for highly improved mutation detection in cancer and genetic testing. Biochem Soc Trans. 2009;37(Pt 2):427–32.
66. Milbury CA, Correll M, Quackenbush J, Rubio R, Makrigiorgos GM. COLD-PCR enrichment of rare cancer mutations prior to targeted amplicon resequencing. Clin Chem. 2012;58(3):580–9.
67. Milbury CA, Li J, Makrigiorgos GM. Ice-COLD-PCR enables rapid amplification and robust enrichment for low-abundance unknown DNA mutations. Nucleic Acids Res. 2011;39(1):e2.
68. Pan Q, Pao W, Ladanyi M. Rapid polymerase chain reaction-based detection of epidermal growth factor receptor gene mutations in lung adenocarcinomas. J Mol Diagn. 2005;7(3):396–403.
69. Cohen V, Agulnik JS, Jarry J, Batist G, Small D, Kreisman H, Tejada NA, Miller Jr WH, Chong G. Evaluation of denaturing high-performance liquid chromatography as a rapid detection method for identification of epidermal growth factor receptor mutations in nonsmall-cell lung cancer. Cancer. 2006;107(12):2858–65.
70. Do H, Krypuy M, Mitchell PL, Fox SB, Dobrovic A. High resolution melting analysis for rapid and sensitive EGFR and KRAS mutation detection in formalin fixed paraffin embedded biopsies. BMC Cancer. 2008;8:142.
71. Ogino S, Kawasaki T, Brahmandam M, Yan L, Cantor M, Namgyal C, Mino-Kenudson M, Lauwers GY, Loda M, Fuchs CS. Sensitive sequencing method for KRAS mutation detection by Pyrosequencing. J Mol Diagn. 2005;7(3):413–21.
72. Dufort S, Richard MJ, Lantuejoul S, de Fraipont F. Pyrosequencing, a method approved to detect the two major EGFR mutations for anti EGFR therapy in NSCLC. J Exp Clin Cancer Res. 2011;30:57.
73. Li J, Wang L, Janne PA, Makrigiorgos GM. Coamplification at lower denaturation temperature-PCR increases mutation-detection selectivity of TaqMan-based real-time PCR. Clin Chem. 2009;55(4):748–56.
74. Arcila ME, Oxnard GR, Nafa K, Riely GJ, Solomon SB, Zakowski MF, Kris MG, Pao W, Miller VA, Ladanyi M. Rebiopsy of lung cancer patients with acquired resistance to EGFR inhibitors and enhanced detection of the T790M mutation using a locked nucleic acid-based assay. Clin Cancer Res. 2011;17(5):1169–80.

75. Li J, Janne PA, Makrigiorgos GM. Biotinylated probe isolation of targeted gene region improves detection of T790M epidermal growth factor receptor mutation via peptide nucleic acid-enriched real-time PCR. Clin Chem. 2011;57(5):770–3.
76. Taniguchi K, Uchida J, Nishino K, Kumagai T, Okuyama T, Okami J, Higashiyama M, Kodama K, Imamura F, Kato K. Quantitative detection of EGFR mutations in circulating tumor DNA derived from lung adenocarcinomas. Clin Cancer Res. 2011;17(24):7808–15.
77. Zhao J, Huang J, Chen Y, Jiang J, Wu W, Wang P, Liu L, Li L, Wu L, Wang M, Chen W. A novel method for detection of mutation in epidermal growth factor receptor. Lung Cancer. 2011;74(2):226–32.
78. Dias-Santagata D, Akhavanfard S, David SS, Vernovsky K, Kuhlmann G, Boisvert SL, Stubbs H, McDermott U, Settleman J, Kwak EL, Clark JW, Isakoff SJ, Sequist LV, Engelman JA, Lynch TJ, Haber DA, Louis DN, Ellisen LW, Borger DR, Iafrate AJ. Rapid targeted mutational analysis of human tumours: a clinical platform to guide personalized cancer medicine. EMBO Mol Med. 2010;2(5):146–58.
79. Beadling C, Heinrich MC, Warrick A, Forbes EM, Nelson D, Justusson E, Levine J, Neff TL, Patterson J, Presnell A, McKinley A, Winter LJ, Dewey C, Harlow A, Barney O, Druker BJ, Schuff KG, Corless CL. Multiplex mutation screening by mass spectrometry evaluation of 820 cases from a personalized cancer medicine registry. J Mol Diagn. 2011;13(5):504–13.
80. Su Z, Dias-Santagata D, Duke M, Hutchinson K, Lin YL, Borger DR, Chung CH, Massion PP, Vnencak-Jones CL, Iafrate AJ, Pao W. A platform for rapid detection of multiple oncogenic mutations with relevance to targeted therapy in non-small-cell lung cancer. J Mol Diagn. 2011;13(1):74–84.
81. Voelkerding KV, Dames SA, Durtschi JD. Next-generation sequencing: from basic research to diagnostics. Clin Chem. 2009;55(4):641–58.
82. Gargis AS, Kalman L, Berry MW, Bick DP, Dimmock DP, Hambuch T, Lu F, Lyon E, Voelkerding KV, Zehnbauer BA, Agarwala R, Bennett SF, Chen B, Chin EL, Compton JG, Das S, Farkas DH, Ferber MJ, Funke BH, Furtado MR, Ganova-Raeva LM, Geigenmuller U, Gunselman SJ, Hegde MR, Johnson PL, Kasarskis A, Kulkarni S, Lenk T, Liu CS, Manion M, Manolio TA, Mardis ER, Merker JD, Rajeevan MS, Reese MG, Rehm HL, Simen BB, Yeakley JM, Zook JM, Lubin IM. Assuring the quality of next-generation sequencing in clinical laboratory practice. Nat Biotechnol. 2012;30(11):1033–6.
83. Camidge DR, Kono SA, Flacco A, Tan AC, Doebele RC, Zhou Q, Crino L, Franklin WA, Varella-Garcia M. Optimizing the detection of lung cancer patients harboring anaplastic lymphoma kinase (ALK) gene rearrangements potentially suitable for ALK inhibitor treatment. Clin Cancer Res. 2010;16(22):5581–90.
84. Shaw AT, Yeap BY, Solomon BJ, Riely GJ, Gainor J, Engelman JA, Shapiro GI, Costa DB, Ou SH, Butaney M, Salgia R, Maki RG, Varella-Garcia M, Doebele RC, Bang YJ, Kulig K, Selaru P, Tang Y, Wilner KD, Kwak EL, Clark JW, Iafrate AJ, Camidge DR. Effect of crizotinib on overall survival in patients with advanced non-small-cell lung cancer harbouring ALK gene rearrangement: a retrospective analysis. Lancet Oncol. 2011;12(11):1004–12.
85. Ju YS, Lee WC, Shin JY, Lee S, Bleazard T, Won JK, Kim YT, Kim JI, Kang JH, Seo JS. A transforming KIF5B and RET gene fusion in lung adenocarcinoma revealed from whole-genome and transcriptome sequencing. Genome Res. 2012;22:436–45.
86. Drilon A, Wang L, Hasanovic A, Suehara Y, Lipson D, Stephens P, Ross J, Miller V, Ginsberg M, Zakowski MF, Kris MG, Ladanyi M, Rizvi N. Response to Cabozantinib in patients with RET fusion-positive lung adenocarcinomas. Cancer Discov. 2013;3(6):630–5.
87. Mino-Kenudson M, Chirieac LR, Law K, Hornick JL, Lindeman N, Mark EJ, Cohen DW, Johnson BE, Janne PA, Iafrate AJ, Rodig SJ. A novel, highly sensitive antibody allows for the routine detection of ALK-rearranged lung adenocarcinomas by standard immunohistochemistry. Clin Cancer Res. 2010;16(5):1561–71.
88. Paik JH, Choe G, Kim H, Choe JY, Lee HJ, Lee CT, Lee JS, Jheon S, Chung JH. Screening of anaplastic lymphoma kinase rearrangement by immunohistochemistry in non-small cell lung cancer: correlation with fluorescence in situ hybridization. J Thorac Oncol. 2011;6(3):466–72.
89. Shaw AT, Solomon B, Kenudson MM. Crizotinib and testing for ALK. J Natl Compr Canc Netw. 2011;9(12):1335–41.
90. Weickhardt AJ, Aisner DL, Franklin WA, Varella-Garcia M, Doebele RC, Camidge DR. Diagnostic assays for identification of anaplastic lymphoma kinase-positive non-small cell lung cancer. Cancer. 2013;119(8):1467–77.
91. Kim H, Yoo SB, Choe JY, Paik JH, Xu X, Nitta H, Zhang W, Grogan TM, Lee CT, Jheon S, Chung JH. Detection of ALK gene rearrangement in non-small cell lung cancer: a comparison of fluorescence in situ hybridization and chromogenic in situ hybridization with correlation of ALK protein expression. J Thorac Oncol. 2011;6(8):1359–66.
92. Hout D, Xue L, Choppa P, Handshoe J, Bloom K, Ross D, Nickols J, Morris SW. Insight ALK ScreenTM, a highly sensitive and specific RT-qPCR first-line screening assay for comprehensive detection of all oncogenic anaplastic lymphoma kinase (ALK) fusions: clinical validation. Proceedings of the 102nd Annual Meeting of the American Association for Cancer Research. 2011;Abstract #2220.
93. Cappuzzo F, Camidge DR, Varella-Garcia M. Is FISH floating or still swimming in the lung cancer ocean? Ann Oncol. 2011;22(3):493–9.
94. Fukuoka M, Wu YL, Thongprasert S, Sunpaweravong P, Leong SS, Sriuranpong V, Chao TY, Nakagawa K, Chu DT, Saijo N, Duffield EL, Rukazenkov Y, Speake G, Jiang H, Armour AA, To KF, Yang JC, Mok TS. Biomarker analyses and final overall survival results from a phase III, randomized, open-label, first-line study of gefitinib versus carboplatin/paclitaxel in clinically selected patients with advanced non-small-cell lung cancer in Asia (IPASS). J Clin Oncol. 2011;29(21):2866–74.
95. Cappuzzo F, Marchetti A, Skokan M, Rossi E, Gajapathy S, Felicioni L, Del Grammastro M, Sciarrotta MG, Buttitta F, Incarbone M, Toschi L, Finocchiaro G, Destro A, Terracciano L, Roncalli M, Alloisio M, Santoro A, Varella-Garcia M. Increased MET gene copy number negatively affects survival of surgically resected non-small-cell lung cancer patients. J Clin Oncol. 2009;27(10):1667–74.
96. Engelman JA, Zejnullahu K, Mitsudomi T, Song Y, Hyland C, Park JO, Lindeman N, Gale CM, Zhao X, Christensen J, Kosaka T, Holmes AJ, Rogers AM, Cappuzzo F, Mok T, Lee C, Johnson BE, Cantley LC, Janne PA. MET amplification leads to gefitinib resistance in lung cancer by activating ERBB3 signaling. Science. 2007;316(5827):1039–43.
97. Turke AB, Zejnullahu K, Wu YL, Song Y, Dias-Santagata D, Lifshits E, Toschi L, Rogers A, Mok T, Sequist L, Lindeman NI, Murphy C, Akhavanfard S, Yeap BY, Xiao Y, Capelletti M, Iafrate AJ, Lee C, Christensen JG, Engelman JA, Janne PA. Preexistence and clonal selection of MET amplification in EGFR mutant NSCLC. Cancer Cell. 2010;17(1):77–88.
98. Akbari M, Hansen MD, Halgunset J, Skorpen F, Krokan HE. Low copy number DNA template can render polymerase chain reaction error prone in a sequence-dependent manner. J Mol Diagn. 2005;7(1):36–9.
99. COSMIC. Retrieved 1 Oct 2011, from http://www.sanger.ac.uk/genetics/CGP/cosmic/

100. Takeuchi K, Choi YL, Soda M, Inamura K, Togashi Y, Hatano S, Enomoto M, Takada S, Yamashita Y, Satoh Y, Okumura S, Nakagawa K, Ishikawa Y, Mano H. Multiplex reverse transcription-PCR screening for EML4-ALK fusion transcripts. Clin Cancer Res. 2008;14(20):6618–24.
101. Doebele RC, Pilling AB, Aisner D, Kutateladze TG, Le AT, Weickhardt AJ, Kondo KL, Linderman DJ, Heasley LE, Franklin WA, Varella-Garcia M, Camidge DR. Mechanisms of resistance to crizotinib in patients with ALK gene rearranged non-small cell lung cancer. Clin Cancer Res. 2012;18:1472–82.
102. Cappuzzo F, Hirsch FR, Rossi E, Bartolini S, Ceresoli GL, Bemis L, Haney J, Witta S, Danenberg K, Domenichini I, Ludovini V, Magrini E, Gregorc V, Doglioni C, Sidoni A, Tonato M, Franklin WA, Crino L, Bunn Jr PA, Varella-Garcia M. Epidermal growth factor receptor gene and protein and gefitinib sensitivity in non-small-cell lung cancer. J Natl Cancer Inst. 2005;97(9):643–55.
103. Solomon B, Varella-Garcia M, Camidge DR. ALK gene rearrangements: a new therapeutic target in a molecularly defined subset of non-small cell lung cancer. J Thorac Oncol. 2009;4(12):1450–4.
104. Sequist LV, Heist RS, Shaw AT, Fidias P, Rosovsky R, Temel JS, Lennes IT, Digumarthy S, Waltman BA, Bast E, Tammireddy S, Morrissey L, Muzikansky A, Goldberg SB, Gainor J, Channick CL, Wain JC, Gaissert H, Donahue DM, Muniappan A, Wright C, Willers H, Mathisen DJ, Choi NC, Baselga J, Lynch TJ, Ellisen LW, Mino-Kenudson M, Lanuti M, Borger DR, Iafrate AJ, Engelman JA, Dias-Santagata D. Implementing multiplexed genotyping of non-small-cell lung cancers into routine clinical practice. Ann Oncol. 2011;22(12):2616–24.
105. SEER Stat Fact Sheet: Lung & Bronchus. Retrieved 1 Oct 2011, from http://seer.cancer.gov/statfacts/html/lungb.html

Breast Cancer

33

Carolyn Mies

Abstract

Breast cancer treatment has evolved over the past 50 years, often as a direct consequence of molecular testing advances. In fact, molecular testing of predictive markers in breast cancer, including hormone receptors and HER2, is the model for personalized cancer treatment. Clinical practice guidelines specify that every primary invasive breast cancer and putative recurrence be tested for ER, PR, and HER2 expression to identify those cancers likely to respond to corresponding targeted treatments. The newest tests for breast cancer management are the tissue-based prognostic and/or predictive molecular assays, which identify patients with biologically indolent breast cancer who will not benefit from cytotoxic chemotherapy and those with intrinsically aggressive disease who may benefit. This chapter reviews clinically standard predictive marker and Oncotype DX® testing, as well as several emerging molecular testing systems.

Keywords

Breast cancer • Predictive markers • Estrogen receptor • HER2 • Immunohistochemistry In situ hybridization • Prognostic molecular assays • Intrinsic subtypes

Introduction

Breast carcinoma is the most common malignancy in women in the USA and occurs in two major forms: sporadic and hereditary. Sporadic breast cancer is the topic of this chapter; hereditary breast cancer, caused by mutations in *BRCA1* and *BRCA2* and other germline DNA mutation syndromes, is discussed in Chap. 22. Molecular assays for detecting circulating tumor cells are discussed in Chap. 39.

C. Mies, M.D. (✉)
Genomic Health Inc., 301 Penobscot Drive, Redwood City, CA 94063, USA
e-mail: cmies@genomichealth.com

Molecular Pathogenesis of Breast Cancer

The cause of common, sporadic breast cancer and the reasons for its progression are unknown. What is amply clear is that no simple, single alteration is responsible for sporadic breast cancer. Putative oncogenic processes include impaired cell-number regulation, mutated oncogenes and tumor suppressor genes, dysfunctional epigenetic controls, and deranged intercellular interaction [1]. In addition, emerging evidence supports a theory that transforming epithelia communicate aberrantly with their surrounding mammary stroma, such that the entire tissue region is likely involved in the oncogenic process. Collectively, these processes determine the behavior of a specific breast cancer.

Two dominant models of mammary carcinogenesis are (1) the stochastic clonal evolution model and (2) the cancer stem cell model (both reviewed in Ref. 2). The stochastic clonal evolution model proposes that random mutational events occur in any mammary cell; uncontrolled cell division results when a cell accumulates a sufficient number

D.G.B. Leonard (ed.), *Molecular Pathology in Clinical Practice*, DOI 10.1007/978-3-319-19674-9_33

and type of mutations to gain a selective growth advantage. In this model, the expanding aberrant clone acquires additional DNA alterations that enable it to invade adjacent stroma and spread to distant sites via lymphatics and blood vessels. The clone "evolves" to an invasive and metastatic phenotype.

The cancer stem cell hypothesis derives from the theoretical normal breast parenchymal development pathway. A breast stem cell divides asymmetrically to produce a daughter stem cell (self-renewal) and a common progenitor cell, which can divide and differentiate into either a myoepithelial cell or a luminal progenitor cell. The latter is the parent of two more-differentiated lineages: luminal and ductal epithelia [2]. The cancer stem cell hypothesis posits that the initiating carcinogenic event occurs in one of the small number of mammary stem cells or their uncommitted progenitors but never in differentiated luminal or myoepithelial cells. Following initiation, clonal evolution may progress to the fully malignant phenotype. An appealing variation of the cancer stem cell hypothesis has cancer initiation restricted to the second generation common progenitor cell, usually a common luminal progenitor. If correct, this would explain why global gene expression profiling parses human breast cancers into four to five major molecular classes (intrinsic subtypes), which include luminal A and B groups [3–5].

Anatomic Classification of Breast Cancer

The vast majority of breast cancers arise in the hormonally sensitive, physiologically active, terminal duct lobular units; only a small percentage arise in the larger ducts. The two morphologic subtypes of breast cancer, ductal and lobular, are named for the histologic structures from which they appear to arise, the terminal ducts and the lobules, respectively. Both ductal and lobular carcinomas occur in invasive and in situ forms; this chapter focuses on invasive carcinoma.

Invasive ductal carcinoma (IDC) is the most common form of invasive breast cancer, accounting for approximately 85 % of cases. Several lines of evidence indicate that IDC directly evolves from ductal carcinoma in situ (DCIS). Invasive lobular carcinoma (ILC) accounts for fewer cases of invasive breast cancer (approximately 15 %). Like IDC, ILC appears to evolve from a morphologic precursor lesion, lobular carcinoma in situ (LCIS). At the genomic level, IDC is far more heterogeneous than ILC. While the two subtypes share some recurrent molecular alterations, they differ at many more loci. Invasive ductal and lobular carcinomas are managed clinically in the same way.

Overview of the Clinical Management of Breast Cancer

Breast cancer treatment has evolved over the past 50 years, often as a direct consequence of molecular testing advances. Currently, potentially curable, early invasive breast cancer (Stages I, II, and III) is treated both as local-regional and systemic disease. The goal of local-regional treatment is to eradicate cancer from the breast and regional lymph nodes, whereas systemic treatment seeks to eliminate occult microscopic deposits of cancer at remote sites in the body.

Treatment selection rests on two sets of clinicopathologic factors: (1) anatomic staging [6] to estimate prognosis, which is the likelihood that a person will survive the disease independent of systemic treatment, and (2) results of predictive marker tests, which estimate the likelihood a breast cancer will respond to specific targeted treatments. Only two targeted treatments are in current common use for breast cancer: antiestrogens (e.g., tamoxifen, aromatase inhibitors) and trastuzumab (Herceptin™; Genentech, South San Francisco, CA), a monoclonal antibody targeting the human epidermal growth factor receptor-2 protein (simplified to HER2 in this chapter). Currently, tests for these predictive markers are used to determine the use of these targeted therapies for breast cancer: estrogen receptor (ER) levels and progesterone receptor (PR) levels for the antiestrogens and HER2 overexpression for trastuzumab.

Molecular testing of prognostic and predictive markers in breast cancer has a long, successful history and is a paradigm for personalized cancer treatment. Clinical practice guidelines specify that every primary invasive breast cancer and putative recurrence be tested for expression of ER, PR, and HER2 [7, 8]. These are called predictive markers because they predict the likelihood a cancer will respond to antiestrogen and anti-HER2 treatment. The next sections describe the standard and emerging molecular tests for newly diagnosed breast cancer, including ER and PR tests, HER2 tests, molecular profiling for intrinsic breast cancer subtypes, and the commercially marketed prognostic and/or predictive tests for breast cancer management.

Hormone Receptors in Breast Cancer

Molecular Basis for Targeting Hormone Receptor Expression in Breast Cancer

Like normal mammary glandular tissue, most invasive breast cancers (75–80 %) express ER and/or PR [9]. These receptors, which bind endogenous estrogen and progesterone, are ligand-inducible transcription factors that bind to regulatory DNA sequences associated with target genes, activating a variety of cellular events that give cancer cells a survival advantage [10, 11]. Aside from this direct DNA interface, ER also interacts with cytoplasmic proteins that have an indirect action on gene transcription [12]. Interfering with this key hormone-receptor interaction is a mainstay of ER-positive breast cancer treatment.

Estrogen receptor protein exists in two isoforms, ERα and ERβ, which are encoded by two highly homologous genes, *ESR1* and *ESR2*, respectively. ERα (*ESR1*) is the clinically important isoform of ER in breast cancer. Similarly, there are two PR isoforms (A and B), which are products of the same gene. PR isoform A is a truncated form of B [12]. Estrogen receptor-ligand complexes activate the transcription of PR; thus, nearly all ER-positive breast cancers also express PR. The ER test result dominates clinical decision-making. Antiestrogen treatment is recommended for all ER-positive (>1 % cells) cancers. The small fraction (approximately 3 %) of ER-negative, PR-positive cancers also are treated with antiestrogens because they are presumed to have partially intact ER transcriptional activity [13].

Three therapeutic approaches are used to nullify estrogen's ER-mediated effects on breast cancer: (1) remove the ovaries to reduce endogenous estrogen, (2) pharmacologically inactivate ER, and (3) medicate to prevent inactive forms of endogenous estrogen from converting to active molecules. Surgical oophorectomy, the oldest endocrine treatment for breast cancer, still has a role in some circumstances [14]. Inactivating ER directly is accomplished by treatment with tamoxifen (Nolvadex), one of the most commonly used targeted therapies. Tamoxifen is an oral medication that binds stably to the ER to form an unwieldy complex that is sterically incapable of binding to DNA to activate gene transcription. Lastly, aromatase inhibitors (AIs), such as anastrozole (Arimidex) and exemestane (aromasin), bind to the aromatase enzyme to prevent adrenal androgens, the main source of endogenous estrogen after menopause, from being converted to estrogen. AIs are most useful in postmenopausal patients, reducing circulating estradiol to near zero levels [13, 68].

Clinical Utility of ER/PR Expression Testing

ER/PR testing is critical because the ER content of a breast cancer is the strongest predictor of antiestrogen treatment efficacy, regardless of how the estrogen-reduced state is achieved (oophorectomy, tamoxifen, or AI). Breast cancers that entirely lack ER do not respond to antiestrogens and are omitted from the therapeutic plan [15]. All patients (women and men) with ER-positive invasive breast cancer based on ER/PR test results are offered antiestrogen treatment, unless contraindicated by specific comorbid conditions [9, 16]. The decision whether to use antiestrogen therapy is highly significant because adjuvant tamoxifen reduces mortality by at least 33 % at 15 years [15, 17].

Available Assays for Hormone Receptor Content Testing

Currently, immunohistochemistry (IHC) of formalin-fixed, paraffin-embedded (FFPE) tissue sections is the standard method for ER/PR testing. IHC testing for ER/PR expression has many advantages: ER/PR in invasive cancer cells can be assessed specifically and normal tissue expression ignored; results are not confounded by endogenous hormone levels; no requirement for fresh or frozen tissue, so that IHC can be applied retrospectively and to small (≤1.0 cm) invasive cancers, which are now commonplace; and lastly, IHC staining kits and instrumentation are widely available in nonacademic centers, where most breast cancers are diagnosed and treated. Any proposed new testing platform must retain or improve on these advantages to supplant IHC hormone receptor testing.

In late 2008, The American Societ of Clinical Oncology (ASCO) partnered with the College of American Pathologists (CAP) to convene a panel to determine best practices for ER/PR testing in breast cancer. The standardization effort was driven by academic oncologists who discovered significant discordances between local and central predictive marker testing results for patients entered in clinical trials. The panel analyzed numerous published studies and clinical trials' results correlating the ER/PR content to outcomes of antiestrogen treatment [8, 18]. The resulting 2010 ASCO/CAP Guideline Recommendations for IHC Testing of ER/PR in Breast Cancer were widely adopted and remain the standard practice [8].

The guideline recommends using IHC of FFPE tissue sections to test all primary invasive breast cancers and putative recurrences for ER/PR content, whenever tissue is available. The guideline defines how to control and document preanalytic, analytic, and postanalytic variables to ensure analytic and clinical validity and clinical utility [8].

Preanalytic Standardization

The 2010 ASCO/CAP Guideline Recommendations for IHC testing of ER/PR in Breast Cancer specify how to handle FFPE tissues that are likely to be tested (see summary below). The overall goal is to standardize three key preanalytic variables: tissue handling, fixation type, and fixation duration [8, 18]. Preanalytic factors are most easily controlled in the core biopsy setting which, therefore, is the preferred tissue for testing.

Documenting cold ischemia time requires cooperation between persons performing the breast cancer biopsies and resections with pathology personnel, which can be a challenge. Adding designated spaces for this biopsy or resection timing data to the surgical pathology requisition form or in the electronic ordering process can aid clinicians in providing the data. Reporting templates help the pathologist to document the preanalytic factors in the report.

Summary of ASCO/CAP Guideline Recommendations for Preanalytic Variables for Hormone Receptor and HER2 Immunohistochemistry:

- Minimize cold ischemia time (time from excision to initiation of fixation) to 1 h or less.
- Use 10 % neutral buffered formalin (NBF) as the standard fixative.
- If nonstandard fixatives or those containing decalcifying agents are used, add a disclaimer to the report.
- Do not use microwave-type processors for ER/PR staining, because results have not been clinically validated.
- Fix the cancer in NBF for at least 6 h, but no more than 72 h, before paraffin embedding.

Analytic Standardization

Antibodies and controls are the key analytic variables for ER/PR testing. The 2010 ASCO/CAP Guideline Recommendations for IHC Testing of ER/PR in Breast Cancer advise using specific ER antibody clones (1D5, 6F11, SP1, and 1D5+ER.2.123), which have slightly different staining profiles but have been sufficiently validated to provide comparable results. Test kits with validated scoring schemes that are approved or cleared by the US Food and Drug Administration (FDA) are considered optimal. Laboratory developed tests (LDTs) are acceptable, if stringently validated [8].

The interpreting pathologist must verify that the internal and external controls stain appropriately. Internal controls consist of immunoreactive benign mammary epithelia in the same section or in another equivalently processed section from the same specimen [8]. Where appropriate internal controls are lacking, an apparently negative ER or PR stain is considered uninterpretable. Breast biopsies are rarely problematic, but lung and bone, which are common sites of metastasis, may be more difficult to interpret. In this context, the pathologist should add a disclaimer that a negative staining result cannot be confirmed as accurate in tissues that do not normally express ER/PR (no internal control). Also, bone from pathologic fractures due to metastatic cancer typically must be decalcified. With decalcification, an apparently negative ER/PR stain must be interpreted cautiously and a disclaimer added to the report for a negative result, noting that decalcification can adversely affect antigen preservation in tissue and result in a false-negative stain. Finally, it is essential for a laboratory initiating IHC for ER/PR to validate the assays; the CAP provides guidelines for validation [19].

Postanalytic Standardization

The 2010 ASCO/CAP Guideline Recommendations for IHC Testing of ER/PR in Breast Cancer allow the pathologist to choose a scoring system (Allred system, *H*-score, etc.) but recommend that the report indicates both the percentage of stained invasive carcinoma cell nuclei and the stain intensity (see below). Some FDA-approved or FDA-cleared staining systems mandate the use of a specific scoring system to ensure clinical validity. For example, the FDA 510(k)-cleared DakoCytomation ER/PR pharmDx™ (Dako Corp, Carpinteria, CA) staining kit requires pathologists to report stain results using the Allred scoring scheme [20]. Semiquantitative visual estimates of nuclear staining are sufficient for guiding clinical decisions. Computer-assisted imaging is more expensive and does not add value to testing, given that antiestrogen treatment is considered for any level of staining ≥1 %.

Interpreting ER/PR stains (adapted from Ref. 8):

- ER- or PR-positive cancer is one in which ≥1 % of invasive carcinoma cell nuclei are immunoreactive.
- ER- or PR-negative cancer is one in which <1 % of invasive carcinoma cell nuclei are immunoreactive.
- ER and/or PR status is not interpretable when no invasive carcinoma cell nuclei are immunoreactive and appropriately stained controls are lacking.

Laboratory and Regulatory Issues

The Clinical Laboratory Improvement Amendments (CLIA) of 1988 and the derived CLIA regulations provide the analytic validity standards for predictive factor assays such as ER, PR, and HER2 tests. Laboratories performing these high complexity tests must be surveyed semiannually, with defined criteria and actions required when performance is deficient [21]. Semiannual proficiency testing for ER/PR analysis is now a mandatory part of the CAP Laboratory Accreditation Program (LAP) (http://www.cap.org/web/home/lab/accreditation/laboratory-accreditation-program. Accessed 3/10/2015). Competence is assessed by periodic review of test performance against peers and failure mandates remediation.

Future Directions

Transitioning routine ER/PR expression testing to a molecular platform, for example, a reverse transcription-polymerase chain reaction (RT-PCR) analysis using paraffin tissues, would not be straightforward. IHC has many advantages, including wide availability, and a strong evidence base that allows ER/PR results to be used to triage cancers for additional molecular testing, as discussed later.

The 2010 ASCO/CAP Guideline Recommendations for IHC Testing of ER/PR in Breast Cancer require new ER/PR tests be validated clinically and operationally [8]. Although

ER/PR expression profiling results are provided with the Oncotype DX® Recurrence Score (Genomic Health™, Redwood City, CA), these may serve to confirm IHC stain results but have not been validated for clinical decision-making [8, 21]. It is likely that paraffin-IHC will remain the platform of choice for some time.

HER2 in Breast Cancer

Molecular Basis for Targeting HER2 Expression in Breast Cancer

The other important predictive marker in breast cancer is HER2, a cell-surface membrane glycoprotein involved in cell proliferation control. *HER2* gene amplification, leading to protein overexpression, is found in 15–20 % of invasive breast cancers [21]. Early investigations used Southern blot analysis to identify *HER2* gene amplification in fresh or frozen samples of breast cancer and showed that patients with *HER2*-amplified breast cancers had higher recurrence and death rates than those with *HER2*-normal cancers [22, 23]. Defining *HER2* as a possible prognostic marker drove the first laboratory testing efforts using monoclonal antibodies for IHC staining [24]. Later, as HER2 became far more important as a drug target, the goals of testing shifted to predicting therapeutic response to drugs targeting the HER2 protein.

The first anti-HER2-targeted treatment, trastuzumab (Herceptin™; Genentech, South San Francisco, CA), was developed in the mid-1990s and is now the standard treatment for HER2-overexpressing breast cancers. Trastuzumab is a recombinant humanized monoclonal antibody that specifically binds to the extracellular juxtamembrane domain of HER2 and inactivates its intracellular tyrosine kinase function by several possible mechanisms, resulting in reduced growth and reduced survival of HER2-dependent cancers [25]. Trastuzumab is most effective when combined with chemotherapy agents active against breast cancer, such as taxanes, doxorubicin, and cyclophosphamide, with trastuzumab monotherapy not being the standard care at this time (http://www.nccn.org/professionals/physician_gls/pdf/breast.pdf. Accessed 03/19/2015).

Following the landmark Genentech-sponsored trials that demonstrated the efficacy of trastuzumab in HER2-overexpressing metastatic breast cancer, trastuzumab was marketed with a companion diagnostic IHC assay, HercepTest™ (Dako Corp, Carpinteria, CA). In 1998, the FDA approved the HercepTest™ designed to identify HER2 overexpression in invasive breast cancer to select patients for trastuzumab treatment [26]. The FDA advocates the importance of companion diagnostic testing for all emerging targeted cancer treatments.

Other anti-HER2 agents (pertuzumab, lapatinib, and ado-trastuzumab emtansine [T-DM1]) are in the clinical trial pipeline. Testing for HER2 overexpression/amplification is also used to select patients for these newer agents [21].

Clinical Utility of HER2 Expression Testing

Following trastuzumab's introduction, HER2 joined ER/PR expression as a standard predictive marker in breast cancer management. The ASCO Tumor Marker Guidelines Panel added routine HER2 expression testing of all invasive breast cancers to its 2001 recommendations [7]. Because DCIS is never treated with chemotherapy and trastuzumab, DCIS should not be tested for HER2 amplification.

The goal of HER2 expression testing is to identify patients who are likely to benefit from trastuzumab treatment, i.e., those with breast cancers that overexpress HER2 protein and/or have *HER2* gene amplification by in situ hybridization (ISH). Trastuzumab can be lifesaving for patients with HER2-overexpressing breast cancer but requires a costly (approximately $100,000), yearlong course of intravenous therapy that is not risk-free. As is true for ER/PR expression testing, accurate, reliable, and reproducible testing is essential to direct anti-HER2 treatment to those who can benefit and spare those who will not.

Whether trastuzumab benefits patients with HER2-negative or HER2-equivocal cancers has been controversial, although the weight of evidence from early exploratory trials suggested little, if any, effect [21, 25]. A prospective randomized clinical trial (NSABP B-47; NCT01275677) will answer this question definitively, but current clinical practice is to treat only HER2-positive invasive breast cancer with trastuzumab [21, 27].

Available Assays for HER2 Overexpression/ HER2 Amplification Testing

Clinical laboratories can use IHC to test for HER2 overexpression or ISH to detect *HER2* gene amplification. Gene amplification is the preponderant mechanism for HER2 overexpression in breast cancer. IHC and ISH share several advantages over Southern blot analysis: (1) the signals are interpreted in the context of the histopathology on tissue sections, permitting specific scoring in morphologically confirmed invasive cancer cells; (2) standard FFPE tissues are acceptable specimens, whereas Southern blot analysis requires fresh or frozen tissue to obtain intact DNA, not fragmented by the fixation and embedding processes; and (3) small cancer specimens, such as core needle biopsies, are acceptable for IHC and ISH, whereas larger specimens are needed for Southern blot analysis, which requires a large amount of DNA [21, 26]. ISH testing, especially fluorescence ISH (FISH), has the disadvantages of being more labor-intensive and costly than IHC;

because of expense, ISH is a second-line, confirmatory test in most clinical settings. Newer bright-field ISH platforms mitigate some of these disadvantages and may have a future in testing.

The optimal procedures for HER2 IHC testing, scoring, and reporting of results have been long debated. Some phase III clinical trials of trastuzumab found significant discordances between local and central laboratory results for HER2, highlighting the need to standardize HER2 testing [27]. Accurate testing for HER2 expression in the clinical trial context is critically important, because treating cancers with false-positive HER2 overexpression results can confound interpretation of treatment efficacy [21, 27]. Obviously, accurate testing in the patient care context is no less essential.

The ASCO and the CAP came together in 2006 to address HER2 testing inaccuracy (both false-positive and false-negative results) and develop guidelines for testing and interpretation. They convened an expert panel to (1) determine the optimal testing algorithm for HER2 testing, and (2) develop strategies to ensure optimal performance, interpretation, and reporting of results across US laboratories. The first ASCO/CAP HER2 Guideline Recommendations were published in 2007 [28]. An updated guideline in 2013 was informed by new clinical trial data and stakeholder suggestions and addresses newer testing platforms, such as FDA-cleared bright-field ISH assays ([21, 29]; http://www.asco.org/guidelines/her2; http://www.cap.org. Accessed 03/10/2015). Molecular pathologists can expect periodic guideline updates as investigators publish new clinical trial data for anti-HER2 agents.

Testing, Interpreting, and Reporting HER2 Test Results

The 2013 ASCO/CAP HER2 Guidelines recommend using IHC or ISH (FISH or bright-field ISH) on FFPE tissue sections to test all primary and recurrent invasive breast cancers for HER2 overexpression. Increasingly, oncologists biopsy suspected breast cancer recurrences to obtain tissue for accurate HER2 and ER/PR results to guide the treatment of metastatic disease.

The goal of the ASCO/CAP HER2 Guidelines is the same as for ER/PR testing: to standardize preanalytic, analytic, and postanalytic variables to ensure analytic and clinical validity and clinical utility [21, 28]. If available, a core biopsy sample of the primary cancer is used for the first HER2 test. If clearly positive, no further testing of the resected primary cancer is recommended. If the result is negative, no further testing is recommended, unless there are concerns about the core biopsy tissue handling, histopathologic discordance, or tumor heterogeneity, in which case testing can be repeated on the resection specimen [21].

Preanalytic Standardization

The 2013 ASCO/CAP HER2 Guidelines for tissue handling of primary invasive breast cancers and putative recurrences are identical to those for ER/PR expression testing [see section above and Refs. 8, 21].

Analytic Standardization

Antibodies and controls are the key analytic variables for IHC HER2 testing. ASCO/CAP, as well as the maker of trastuzumab and pertuzumab (Genentech, South San Francisco, CA), recommends using FDA-approved or FDA-cleared assays for HER2 testing. The FDA-approved HercepTest™ (Dako Corp, Carpinteria, CA) has validated scoring schemes and is considered optimal. As is true for ER/PR expression testing, LDTs are acceptable, if stringently validated [21].

Ideally, a new HER2 assay should be validated using well-annotated breast cancer specimens from prospective therapeutic trials of anti-HER2 therapy. This task is difficult to accomplish because such specimens are relatively rare and limited. As a substitute, ASCO/CAP will endorse HER2 assays that show high-level concordance with other established HER2 tests, as long as concordance studies use data sets with a representative distribution of HER2 overexpression/*HER2* amplification states.

The interpreting pathologist must verify that the controls stain appropriately. Benign mammary epithelia, which have normal *HER2* gene copy number and do not overexpress HER2 protein, function as negative controls. External controls are extremely important as positive controls and include known HER2-overexpressing and HER2-nonoverexpressing invasive breast carcinomas, which must be run concurrently. The HercepTest™ kit (Dako Corp, Carpinteria, CA) is an IHC test kit that includes three FFPE cell line controls with different HER2 copy numbers that stain negative (score 0), negative (score 1+), and positive (score 3+), respectively. Where appropriately stained controls are lacking, or nonstandard conditions have occurred, an apparently negative HER2 stain must be considered uninterpretable and be accompanied by a disclaimer noting the problem [21, 28]. HER2 staining results are interpreted as positive (3+), equivocal (2+), or negative (score 0 or 1+), as summarized below.

Interpreting IHC for HER2 overexpression status (adapted from Ref. 21):

1. IHC-positive (3+) carcinoma shows:
   - Circumferential complete, intense membrane staining in >10 % of contiguous and homogeneous cancer cells
2. IHC-equivocal (2+) carcinoma shows:
   - Complete, circumferential intense membrane staining in ≤10 % of cancer cells

- Circumferential membrane staining that is incomplete and/or weak/moderate intensity in >10 % of contiguous and homogeneous cancer cells

3. IHC-negative (1+) carcinoma shows:
   - Incomplete, faint/barely perceptible membrane staining in >10 % of cancer cells
4. IHC-negative (0) carcinoma shows:
   - No staining
   - Incomplete, faint/barely perceptible membrane staining in ≤10 % of cancer cells

The 2013 ASCO/CAP HER2 Guidelines indicate that ISH for *HER2* gene amplification may be single-probe (*HER2* alone) or dual-probe (*HER2* and chromosome 17 centromere, CEP17). The first FDA-approved, dual-probe FISH test for HER2 is the PathVysion *HER2* DNA Probe Kit (Abbott Molecular, Des Plaines, Illinois) and is used by most laboratories in the USA. Dual-probe FISH has been the standard method of detecting and semiquantitating *HER2* gene amplification in breast cancer since the late 1990s but has some disadvantages: suboptimal morphologic detail, which can make identification of carcinoma cells difficult; signals that fade quickly, not allowing for review; a 2–3-day turnaround time (TAT); and significant cost due to the need for a fluorescence imaging system and specially trained personnel. These drawbacks have stimulated development of more user-friendly bright-field approaches.

Bright-field ISH offers better microscopic detail, permanent signals that allow later review, less hands-on technician time, easier identification of tumor heterogeneity using low-power magnification, and lower cost (conventional light microscope) [30–32]. An important question has been whether bright-field ISH is as sensitive as FISH. While 15–20 % of invasive breast cancers have *HER2* amplification, among FISH-positive cases, nearly half (47 %) have only borderline or low levels of *HER2* amplification [33].

The most favored bright-field ISH platform is chromogenic ISH (CISH), which entails hybridizing DNA probe(s) to the target *HER2* DNA in tissue sections and then detecting the probe(s) using reagents similar to those used in IHC. Both single- and dual-probe approaches are feasible, and the signals appear as brown granules on tissue sections examined with a light microscope. Dual-probe approaches require two parallel cut sections, one for each probe; in this case, the two probes are to *HER2* and the chromosome 17 centromere.

Bhargava et al. [30] used tissue microarrays and a CISH *HER2* kit with a polymer detection system that enhances hybridization signals (Zymed Laboratories, South San Francisco, CA) to study 113 breast cancers selected from a much larger sample of tumors that had been tested previously for *HER2* amplification using FISH on tissue sections. The study set was designed to include ample proportions of negative and borderline-, low-, and high-amplified FISH-positive samples. Among 102 cases analyzed successfully for both probes ("dual-probe"), concordance between FISH and CISH was 100 % in categorizing a cancer as *HER2* amplified or not amplified. The use of a single *HER2* probe only resulted in discordant results (no amplification vs borderline or low-level *HER2* amplification) in three cases, 2.9 %, that were positive by FISH [30].

CISH has the same 2–3-day TAT as FISH but requires less hands-on technician time and the pathologist can interpret a CISH slide in approximately half the time, because it is easier to recognize carcinoma cells and count signals [30]. CISH may be especially useful in cases where morphologic detail is challenging: small invasive carcinomas; cases with an intimate admixture of in situ and invasive components; and cases where carcinoma insidiously invades benign parenchyma as single cells. Laboratories not currently set up for FISH but regularly performing IHC can consider CISH as a good alternative for HER2 expression testing [30].

Additional studies have shown good correlation between CISH and FISH for identifying *HER2* amplification [31]. Disadvantages are that not all signals appear crisply discrete and may be difficult to count against background. In addition, the CEP17 probe must be evaluated in a second reaction on a separate, parallel tissue section [30, 34].

Bright-field ISH should be interpreted on the basis of a comparison between normal breast and cancer cells. If the cancer cell pattern is neither normal nor clearly amplified, then expert opinion should be sought. Nonneoplastic cells in the same section serve as an internal control. A cancer should not be reported as "not amplified" unless one or two signals per nucleus are evident in benign cells. ISH criteria for *HER2* amplification status are summarized below.

ISH criteria for HER2 amplification status, based on counting at least 20 cells within the area (adapted from Ref. 21):

1. ISH-positive carcinoma fulfills one of the following criteria:
   - Dual-probe: HER2:CEP17 is >2.0, with average HER2 copy number >4 signals/cell.
   - Dual-probe: HER2:CEP17 is >2.0, with average HER2 copy number <4 signals/cell.
   - Dual-probe: HER2:CEP17 is <2.0, with average HER2 copy number >6 signals/cell.
   - Single-probe: Average HER2 gene copy number is >6 signals/nucleus.
2. ISH-equivocal carcinoma fulfills one of the following criteria:
   - Dual-probe: HER2:CEP17 is <2, with average HER2 gene copy number >4 but <6 signals/nucleus.
   - Single-probe: ISH average HER2 gene copy number is >4 and <6 signals/nucleus.

3. ISH-negative carcinoma fulfills one of the following criteria:
   - Dual-probe: HER2:CEP17 is <2, with average HER2 gene copy number <4 signals/nucleus.
   - Single-probe: Average HER2 gene copy number is <4 signals/nucleus.

Postanalytic Standardization

A HER2-positive (3+) breast cancer has evidence of protein overexpression by IHC or gene amplification by ISH. A HER2-negative (0, 1+) cancer lacks both. HER2-equivocal (2+) carcinoma has borderline features and requires confirmatory (reflex) testing by a second method. Most commonly, this refers to cases with equivocal IHC results, but some laboratories also do follow up testing of cancers that are IHC "triple-negative" (ER-, PR-, and HER2-negative) to ISH as further assurance that tissue quality has not led to spurious negative results. ISH-equivocal results should be confirmed by IHC, although many oncologists prefer to treat such patients regardless of the IHC staining results. Retesting using both approaches may be in order for results that seem discordant with clinical circumstances, e.g., HER2 overexpression in an ILC or a subcentimeter tubular ductal carcinoma, which usually do not overexpress HER2 [21].

Laboratory and Regulatory Issues

The CLIA requirements for laboratories performing HER2 expression testing are the same as for ER/PR expression testing. The 2013 ASCO/CAP HER2 Guidelines recommend that proficiency testing be through the CAP or another entity. Mandatory proficiency testing surveys for HER2 expression testing, identical to those for ER/PR evaluation, were added to the CAP LAP in 2007. The CAP has observed increased levels of proficiency testing and fewer deficiencies since the 2007 HER2 Guideline was published ([21], data supplement).

The 2013 ASCO/CAP HER2 Guideline recommendations allow the use of LDTs for HER2 expression testing, as long as the test has been prospectively validated clinically and operationally in the same clinical laboratory that will perform it, which entails demonstrating high concordance with a validated HER2 test on a sufficiently large and representative set of breast cancers [21]. This has been accomplished for bright-field ISH approaches such as CISH. Notably, HER2 expression profiling results provided with the Oncotype DX® Recurrence Score (Genomics Health™) may serve to confirm IHC stain results but have not been validated for clinical decision-making [8, 21].

Standard and Emerging Molecular Tests

Just as tamoxifen and trastuzumab and their corresponding predictive tests were "game changers" in breast cancer treatment, adjuvant systemic chemotherapy also has an important role in improving breast cancer survival. Berry et al. [35] note that breast cancer mortality declined 26 % between 1975 and 1990 and ascribe at least 50 % of the reduction to use of adjuvant systemic chemotherapy.

The persistent challenge has been to direct adjuvant systemic chemotherapy to those who can benefit most from the intervention and avoid treating those who will not. Overall, two groups of patients will *not* benefit from systemic chemotherapy: (1) those with biologically indolent cancer whose chances of survival are so good that the toxicities and risks of chemotherapy are greater than the benefits, and (2) patients with biologically aggressive cancers that will not respond to currently available chemotherapy agents. The new "game changers" in breast cancer management are the recently developed, tissue-based prognostic/predictive molecular assays, which aim to identify patients who do not need chemotherapy (prognostic) or who either will or will not respond to chemotherapy (predictive) [36].

Approximately 75–80 % of patients are diagnosed with ER-positive breast cancer. Without specific contraindications, these patients will be treated with antiestrogens and have an excellent outcome: 80 % of these patients will survive 10 years or more. Within this ER-positive group, however, 20 % recur within 10 years. The challenge has been to identify these patients at the time of diagnosis and add additional treatment to the antiestrogen treatment, in hopes of improving outcome. Thus, the second part of the challenge is to identify, within the ER-positive breast cancer patients, those who will benefit from added chemotherapy.

In this context of deciding whether chemotherapy will provide benefit for a patient, molecular tests have two actionable tasks:

1. Determine prognosis for the individual cancer patient with ER-positive cancer, which is either node negative (largest group) or node positive (second largest group), with the goal being to identify the low-residual risk group, in whom risks of adjuvant systemic chemotherapy outweigh predicted benefit
2. Among the patients with high residual risk, identify those who are likely to respond to systemic chemotherapy (and even better, a specific chemotherapy regimen).

The molecular profiling test endorsed by the major oncology and health-care organizations in the USA and abroad to date is the Oncotype DX® test (Genomic Health, Inc.). Several other tests are available, including MammaPrint®

(Agendia Inc., USA; Irvine, CA) and PAM50-based Prosigna Breast Cancer Prognostic Gene Signature Assay, simplified to Prosigna in this chapter (NanoString Technologies, Seattle, WA). All of these tests are LDTs that are validated and performed by a commercial reference laboratory.

Typically, oncologists and/or surgeons order one of the molecular profiling tests and pathologists select and ship FFPE tissue sections to the commercial laboratory, with estimated shipping/processing times of 7–10 days. The Prosigna test is the only one that has an option for local performance of the test through purchase of a testing system (http://prosigna.com/. Accessed 3/04/2015). All these tests presume that the test result will be used in the context of other clinicopathologic features (patient age, tumor size, lymph node status, standard predictive markers) and that women with ER-positive cancer will be treated with tamoxifen or aromatase inhibitors.

Oncotype DX®

The Oncotype DX® test provides a result as a 21-gene recurrence score (RS), which has been incorporated into ASCO, NCCN, St. Gallen, and NICE clinical practice guidelines ([37–39]; http://www.nccn.org/. Accessed 3/04/2015; https://www.nice.org.uk/. Accessed 3/04/2015). Oncotype DX® is a commercially available test that uses quantitative RT-PCR (qRT-PCR) to profile the expression of 21 genes (16 cancer-related; 5 reference) in FFPE breast cancer tissue.

The original clinical validation studies for Oncotype DX® examined archived tumors from patients enrolled in the National Surgical Adjuvant Breast and Bowel (NSABP) clinical trials B-14 and B-20, which compared different treatment outcomes in women with node-negative, ER-positive breast cancer [40, 41]. NSABP B-14 demonstrated the benefit of adjuvant tamoxifen compared to no adjuvant treatment, whereas the B-20 trial compared results of adjuvant tamoxifen plus chemotherapy to tamoxifen therapy alone. The investigators developed a high-throughput real-time RT-PCR method to quantitate gene expression levels in FFPE tissues and selected 250 candidate genes from prior publications, genomic databases, and intrinsic subtyping studies, discussed below [3]. Archived cancers were analyzed to assess the relationship between the expression of the candidate genes and breast cancer recurrence in patients with known outcome [40]. From these results, they further refined the candidate gene panel to 16 cancer-related genes and 5 reference genes, which were analyzed in prospective-retrospective studies of archived tumors from NSABP B-14 and B-20 trial patients. To quantitate the likelihood of distant recurrence in patients with node-negative, ER-positive breast cancer treated with adjuvant tamoxifen or not, they designed an algorithm based on the expression of the 21 genes. The test assigns a continuous RS between 1 and 100 and a risk category of low ($RS < 18$), intermediate ($18 \leq RS \leq 30$), or high ($RS \geq 31$) to each tumor [40]. The same strategy was applied to other clinical trial specimens from patients treated with either tamoxifen with systemic chemotherapy or tamoxifen only [41].

The RS quantitates the 10-year recurrence risk in tamoxifen-treated patients with node-negative, ER-positive breast cancer [40, 42]. In addition, the RS predicts the magnitude of chemotherapy benefit in this cohort: the higher the RS, the more likely that chemotherapy will be beneficial. Patients whose cancer has a low RS have minimal, if any, response to adjuvant systemic chemotherapy [41]. Further, the Oncotype DX® RS has clinical utility as a prognosticator for tamoxifen therapy for patients with ER-positive, node-positive ($N1 = 1–3$ nodes) breast cancer, as well as clinical utility for selecting patients likely to benefit from adjuvant systemic chemotherapy [43, 44].

Dowsett et al. [45] further validated the RS in the Arimidex, Tamoxifen Alone, or in Combination (ATAC) study, showing improved risk stratification in postmenopausal women treated with anastrozole or tamoxifen. A subsequent study showed that combining RS with clinicopathologic features could enhance the prognostic accuracy of the RS [43]. This group further showed that IHC4, an IHC panel consisting of ER, PR, HER2, and Ki67, a proliferation marker, provides risk information similar to that of the RS [46]. Further studies are needed to extend these early comparisons of the lower cost IHC4 method, which could be performed by many laboratories.

Two prospective, randomized clinical trials are in progress to assess the correlation between Oncotype DX and response to adjuvant systemic chemotherapy. The *T*rial *A*ssigning *I*ndividua*L*ized *O*ptions for Treatment (*Rx*) TAILORx trial is testing the value of adjuvant chemotherapy in tamoxifen-treated patients with ER-positive, node-negative breast cancer that yields an Oncotype DX® RS in the 11–25 range. The trial is now closed to accrual and is expected to yield the first mature data in 2015 (https://clinicaltrials.gov/ct2/show/NCT00310180?term=TailoRx&rank=2. Accessed 3/04/2015).

MammaPrint®

The MammaPrint® test began as a 70-gene prognostic signature developed by scientists at the Netherlands Cancer Institute [47, 48]. These investigators used gene expression microarrays to study archived snap-frozen breast cancers from a group of 117 patients with early breast cancer (tumors ≤5.0 cm size, node negative) who had not received adjuvant systemic chemotherapy. The expression of 231 genes was found to correlate with outcome at 5 years, identifying an early recurrence subgroup of patients who had developed metastatic disease within the first 5 years after treatment and a larger group who remained disease-free at this endpoint. This group of genes was then further refined to a 70-gene classifier that could optimally parse the two groups [47].

The 70-gene classifier was assessed with another cohort of 295 patients composed of early breast cancer patients with both node-negative and node-positive diseases. The 70-gene classifier parsed the cancers into those with a "poor prognosis" signature ($N=180$) and those with a "good prognosis" signature ($N=115$). At 10 years, the overall survival of those patients with "poor prognosis" cancers was 54.6 % compared to 94.5 % for the patients with "good prognosis" cancers. Patients with node-negative and node-positive breast cancer were evenly distributed in the two groups, indicating the signatures were independent of lymph node status. The prognostic signature was a strong independent factor in predicting disease outcome and added to risk assessment [48].

The 70-gene classifier was clinically validated for node-negative breast cancer by a retrospective multi-institutional European TRANSBIG consortium (http://www.breastinternationalgroup.org. Accessed 03/09/2015) that examined archived frozen cancers from 302 patients who had not been treated with adjuvant systemic chemotherapy or endocrine therapy [49]. Microarray analysis was performed at Agendia Laboratories (Irvine, CA), a spin-off company of the Netherlands Cancer Institute, which custom-designed an array chip given the name MammaPrint™, which was manufactured by Agilent Technologies using their oligonucleotide microarray platform [49]. The aim of the validation study was to examine whether the 70-gene signature had prognostic value independent of the best clinical risk classifications in a patient cohort in which adjuvant treatment could not confound the results. The TRANSBIG consortium used Adjuvant! Online (AOL) (http://www.adjuvantonline.com. Accessed 03/09/2015) to classify patient risk using conventional clinicopathologic attributes. Results showed MammaPrint™ was a strong prognostic marker for time to distant metastasis and overall survival for the node-negative breast cancer patients who had received no adjuvant systemic treatment and the prognostic value of the result was independent of the clinical risk stratification. Further, where there were discordances between clinical risk category (low vs high) generated by AOL and the MammaPrint™ result, the latter provided stronger prognostic information [49].

The ability of MammaPrint™ to effectively parse node-negative breast cancer patients into low- and high-risk categories was prospectively tested in the observational microarRAy-prognoSTics-in-breast-cancER (RASTER) study conducted at 16 community hospitals in the Netherlands using archived frozen cancers from 427 patients. MammaPrint™ performance was again compared to AOL clinical risk categories [50]. Adjuvant systemic chemotherapy decisions were based on the Dutch CBO 2004 guidelines, the MammaPrint™ result, and doctors' and patients' preferences. After a median follow-up of 5 years, MammaPrint™ outperformed AOL in prognostication, but the study had a number of limitations including the inhomogeneous approach to adjuvant systemic treatment. Despite the design drawbacks, omitting chemotherapy for patients with a low-risk gene signature did not appear to compromise outcome, an important aspect of clinical utility. Another prospective randomized clinical trial to demonstrate the clinical validity and utility of MammaPrint™ is underway in the MINDACT trial, which expects to report results after 2019 [51].

One of the disadvantages of using MammaPrint™ in routine clinical practice is that it requires snap-frozen tumor for testing, a distinct inconvenience in the clinical setting and one that may restrict use to larger tumors, where there is sufficient excess tumor tissue after standard pathologic staging and margin assessment in breast conserving procedures. Agendia Inc., USA (Irvine, CA), is in the process of validating MammaPrint™ for use with FFPE breast cancer tissues.

Intrinsic Subtype Profiling

Virtually all of the prognostic and predictive molecular tests are in some way informed by seminal gene profiling studies that are now more than 10 years old. Perou et al. [3] studied gene expression profiles of a small set of frozen invasive breast cancers ($N=38$), normal breast tissues ($N=3$), and 17 breast cancer cell lines, looking for evidence of molecularly defined breast cancer subtypes. Using an 8,100-gene complementary DNA (cDNA) microarray, these investigators honed this gene expression set to a smaller "intrinsic" gene expression list, whose transcripts showed significantly greater variation in expression between tumors from different patients than between paired samples from the same patient's tumor [3]. Using unsupervised cluster array analysis to organize the data, the samples were segregated based on the overall similarity in their gene expression patterns [3].

Four molecular signatures or subtypes emerged: ER+/luminal-like, basal-like, HER2-enriched, and normal breast-like, with expression of genes related to ER, PR, and HER2 largely driving placement into one of these groups. Later work using the same methods parsed the original ER+/luminal-like group into two subgroups, luminal A and luminal B, that differed primarily in the expression of proliferation related genes [4, 5]. Most importantly, intrinsic subtypes correlated with different patient outcomes. The "normal breast-like" cancers, accounting for 3–6 % of cancers in most studies, lack a distinct signature; there is evidence that they are a spurious category caused by artifactual contamination by excessive normal tissue RNA [52, 53].

Intrinsic subtypes are biologically plausible, conforming to tumor biology as it is understood on the basis of the standard predictive markers (ER/PR/HER2) and treatments, and the signatures have proven robust across multiple genomic profiling platforms [5, 54–57]. Breast cancers from different racial/ethnic groups partition into the same five groups, although the signatures can vary in distribution. For example, African Americans enrolled in two population-based breast cancer cohorts had a lower prevalence of luminal A cancers and a higher prevalence of basal-like cancers relative to non-Hispanic Whites [58]. Similarly, male breast cancers have intrinsic profiles that skew largely to the luminal A/B subtypes [59].

Research studies have used three different strategies for intrinsic subtyping: (1) microarray gene expression assays, (2) IHC stains, and (3) quantitative RT-PCR (qRT-PCR) [3, 58]. Microarray gene expression profiling is the gold standard approach but requires fresh or frozen tumor, which is impractical for routine clinical use. Standard IHC predictive marker stains (ER/PR/HER2) supplemented with a proliferation marker stain (e.g., Ki67) can parse FFPE breast cancers of any size into four clinicopathologic groups that are reasonable, but imperfect, surrogates for the intrinsic subtypes [60]. Lastly, qRT-PCR classifiers that can be applied to FFPE tissues are more practical clinically than microarray gene expression profiling and more quantitative than IHC stains. One qRT-PCR classifier is PAM50-based Prosigna™, which is described below.

PAM50-Based Prosigna™ Breast Cancer Prognostic Gene Signature Assay

Parker et al. [52] adapted microarray-based gene expression profiling to a clinically applicable test by developing a qRT-PCR assay using RNA extracted from FFPE tissues as a substrate. An expanded "intrinsic" gene set was derived from previous microarray studies and narrowed down to a 50-gene expression profiling set, with special weighting given to a set of proliferation-associated genes that could reproducibly predict the intrinsic subtypes. The final classifier was constructed using the Prediction Analysis for Microarrays (PAM) algorithm, hence the name "PAM50" ([3, 4, 5, 52, 61]). The PAM50 test was developed using FFPE tumors and the nCounter® platform (NanoString Technologies, Seattle, WA). The test is now marketed as the PAM50-based Prosigna™ Breast Cancer Prognostic Gene Signature Assay and nCounter® Dx Analysis System (NanoString Technologies, Seattle, WA), simplified to Prosigna™ in this discussion.

The clinical utility of Prosigna™ was assessed using a cohort of patients with node-negative breast cancer who had not received adjuvant systemic chemotherapy and found that the intrinsic subtypes showed prognostic significance that remained valid in multivariable analyses that incorporated standard clinicopathologic variables. The subtype plus tumor size performed best among several models as a risk of relapse (ROR) predictor and classified patients into low-, intermediate- or high-risk categories. Prosigna™ estimates prognosis for all types of breast cancer, irrespective of the status of ER and lymph node metastases [62]. The lowest ROR group contained only luminal A cancers; thus, like what Oncotype DX® does for node-negative, ER-positive patients, Prosigna™ identified an excellent prognosis group of patients who can reasonably forgo chemotherapy.

The clinical value of Prosigna™ has also been assessed using independent cohorts of ER-positive, tamoxifen-treated patients and shown to be superior to clinicopathologic features (e.g., using AOL) in estimating residual risk after antihormonal treatment and its similarity to Oncotype DX® in identifying a very low-risk cohort for whom antiestrogens alone are adequate treatment [53]. In node-positive patients, Prosigna™ is a better predictor than IHC profiling of standard markers, but late relapses and death occur in even the lowest risk category of patients; thus, an outcomes prediction test for a node-positive cohort that is adequately treated by antiestrogens alone is not yet available [53].

The ATAC study looked at outcome in women with ER-positive breast cancer who had received either tamoxifen or Arimidex (an aromatase inhibitor) [63] and compared, head-to-head, the ability of the Prosigna™ ROR score, the Oncotype DX® RS, Prosigna™ ROR, and IHC4 (an expanded stain panel: ER, PR, HER2, Ki67), to predict the 10-year risk of distant recurrence after endocrine therapy. The Prosigna™ analysis was done on the same RNA sample as the Oncotype DX® analysis. A significant difference is that the Oncotype DX® test was performed in one central laboratory (Genomic Health Inc., Redwood City, CA), whereas the Prosigna™ test was done with instruments distributed to multiple testing sites. Investigators compared the three molecular predictors to standard clinicopathologic features (stage, grade, age, and type of endocrine treatment). Distant recurrence (DR) risks predicted by the Prosigna™ ROR score were distinctly different in node-positive and node-negative patients: a 10-year DR of 10 % was predicted by a ROR score 42 in node-negative patients, whereas it was predicted by a ROR score of 25 in node-positive (N1, 1–3 nodes) patients [63]. Prosigna™ ROR was more accurately prognostic than Oncotype DX® RS with respect to scores and their corresponding 10-year DR rate. The number of patients characterized as low risk was similar between ROR and RS, but ROR categorized more patients as high risk and fewer as intermediate risk [63].

The difference in Prosigna™ and Oncotype DX® test performance characteristics, however, has little impact on clinical decision-making at this time, because of the way scores and categories are used to recommend treatment: without specific contraindication, all low-risk ER-positive breast cancer patients (Oncotype DX® or Prosigna™), by physician and patient preference, are treated with endocrine therapy alone following surgical resection. Most patients with intermediate-risk cancers and all with high-risk cancers, irrespective of specific score, are offered adjuvant systemic chemotherapy (ASCO treatment guidelines). The ATAC study showed the two tests performed similarly in this important regard [63]. Results from clinical trials to determine the benefit of adjuvant systemic chemotherapy for patients categorized as either intermediate or high risk by Oncotype DX® and/or Prosigna™ are eagerly awaited, since this prognostic/predictive classification has important impact on breast cancer patient management.

A second question is whether response to different types of chemotherapy will align with scores or with intrinsic subtype identified by Prosigna™. A phase III chemotherapy trial comparing response to three different chemotherapy regimens found that higher continuous ROR score was associated with worse outcome [64]. Although intrinsic subtypes did not predict treatment benefit, subgroup analysis suggested that subtype (nonluminal vs luminal) predicted taxane benefit [64]. Other clinical trials examining this question are in progress.

Prosigna™ was validated for analytical precision in a study testing five breast cancer RNA samples across three sites. Reproducibility was measured by testing replicate tissue sections from 43 FFPE tumor blocks across three sites [65]. Hospital laboratories have the option of sending tissue for the Prosigna™ test to a central commercial laboratory (Agendia Inc., USA; Irvine, CA) or purchasing an nCounter Dx Analysis System and performing and interpreting the assay.

Summary and Conclusions

The evolution of breast cancer testing and treatment has become the leading paradigm for personalized cancer treatment. In breast cancer, the first era began with the standardization of adjuvant tamoxifen treatment for ER-expressing breast cancers, which yielded dramatic improvements in survival. The next phase was dominated by the development and standardization of trastuzumab for HER2-overexpressing breast cancers. The third epoch, now 15 years old, began with global genome profiling and statistical algorithms for parsing molecular signatures into biologically distinct groups. Linking molecular profiles of archived FFPE cancers to outcomes from prospective-retrospective clinical trials translated gene profiling into clinically useful prognostic/predictive molecular tests that, combined with standard clinical and pathologic features, can better identify patients with biologically indolent cancer, who will not benefit from cytotoxic chemotherapy, and estimate the probability of chemotherapy response in patients with biologically aggressive cancer.

Molecular testing advances will continue to light the path leading to new and better breast cancer treatments. Research focus is now shifting to next-generation sequencing (NGS) and its ability to identify mutations that may be amenable to targeted treatments effective for similarly mutated non-breast cancer types. Moreover, genomic information derived from NGS also has the potential to drive new drug development and testing in breast cancer [66]. The translational task going forward is formidable because of the extreme genomic diversity of breast cancer and the daunting task of identifying and validating targets, as well as clinical response to treatments [67]. Because improvements in computational science have paralleled remarkable advances in the speed, precision, and affordability of genomic sequencing, many are optimistic that we are on the threshold of yet another new era of personalized breast cancer treatment.

Acknowledged Conflict of Interest Dr. Carolyn Mies is an employee of Genomic Health, Inc.

References

1. Hanahan D, Weinberg RA. Hallmarks of cancer: the next generation. Cell. 2011. doi:10.1016/j.cell.2011.02.013.
2. Bombonati A, Sgroi DC. The molecular pathology of breast cancer progression. J Pathol. 2011;223:307–17.
3. Perou CM, Sørlie T, Eisen MB, et al. Molecular portraits of human breast tumours. Nature. 2000;406:747–52.
4. Sørlie T, Perou CM, Tibshirani R, et al. Gene expression patterns of breast carcinomas distinguish tumor subclasses with clinical implications. Proc Natl Acad Sci. 2001;98:10869–74.
5. Sorlie T, Tibshirani R, Parker J, et al. Repeated observation of breast tumor subtypes in independent gene expression data sets. Proc Natl Acad Sci. 2003;100:8418–23.
6. American Joint Commission on Cancer. AJCC staging manual. 7th ed. New York: Springer; 2010.
7. Bast RC, Ravdin P, Hayes DF, et al. 2000 update of recommendations for the use of tumor markers in breast and colorectal cancer: clinical practice guidelines of the American Society of Clinical Oncology. J Clin Oncol. 2001;19:1865–78.
8. Hammond MEH, Hayes DF, Allred DC, et al. American Society of Clinical Oncology/College of American Pathologists guideline recommendations for immunohistochemical testing of estrogen and progesterone receptors in breast cancer (unabridged version). Arch Pathol Lab Med. 2010;134:e48–72.
9. Burstein HJ, Temin S, Anderson H, et al. Adjuvant endocrine therapy for women with hormone receptor-positive breast cancer: American Society of Clinical Oncology clinical practice guideline focused update. J Clin Oncol. 2014;32:2255–69.
10. Evans RM. The steroid and thyroid hormone receptor superfamily. Science. 1988;240:889–95.
11. Beato M. Gene regulation of steroid hormones. Cell. 1989;56:335–44.
12. Bjornstrom L, Sjoberg M. Mechanisms of estrogen receptor signaling: convergence of genomic and nongenomic actions on target genes. Mol Endocrinol. 2005;19:833–42.
13. Dowsett M, Cuzick J, Ingle J, et al. Meta-analysis of breast cancer outcomes in adjuvant trials of aromatase inhibitors versus tamoxifen. J Clin Oncol. 2010;28:509–18.
14. Beatson GT. On the treatment of inoperable cases of carcinoma of the mamma: suggestions for a new method of treatment with illustrative cases. Lancet. 1896;2:104–7.

15. Early Breast Cancer Trialists' Collaborative Group (EBCTCG), Davies C, Godwin J, et al. Relevance of breast cancer hormone receptors and other factors to the efficacy of adjuvant tamoxifen: patient-level meta-analysis of randomized trials. Lancet. 2011;378:771–84.
16. Tung N. What is the optimal endocrine therapy for postmenopausal women with hormone receptor-positive early breast cancer? J Clin Oncol. 2013;31:1391–7.
17. Burstein HJ, Griggs JJ. Deep time: the long and the short of adjuvant endocrine therapy for breast cancer. J Clin Oncol. 2012. doi:10.1200/JCO.2011.40.1455.
18. Yaziji H, Taylor CR, Goldstein NS, et al. Consensus recommendations on estrogen receptor testing in breast cancer by immunohistochemistry. Appl Immunohistochem Mol Morphol. 2008;16:513–20.
19. Fitzgibbons PL, Murphy DA, Hammond ME, et al. Recommendations for validating estrogen and progesterone receptor immunohistochemistry assays. Arch Pathol Lab Med. 2010;134:930–50.
20. Harvey JM, Clark GM, Osborne CK, et al. Estrogen receptor status by immunohistochemistry is superior to the ligand-binding assay for predicting response to adjuvant endocrine therapy in breast cancer. J Clin Oncol. 1990;17:1474–81.
21. Wolff AC, Hammond EH, Hicks DG et al. Recommendations for human epidermal growth factor receptor 2 testing in breast cancer: American Society of Clinical Oncology/College of American Pathologist Clinical Practice Guideline Update. J Clin Oncol 2013 [Published ahead of print on October 7, 2013 as 10.1200/JCO.2013.50.9984]
22. Slamon D, Clark GW, Wong SG, et al. Human breast cancer: correlation of relapse and survival with amplification of the HER-2/neu oncogene. Science. 1987;235:177–82.
23. Slamon D, Godolphin W, Jones L, et al. Studies of the HER-2/neu proto-oncogene in human breast and ovarian cancer. Science. 1989;244:707–12.
24. Press MF, Pike MC, Chazin VR, et al. Her-2/neu expression in node-negative breast cancer: direct tissue quantitation by computerized image analysis and associated of overexpression with increased risk of recurrent disease. Cancer Res. 1993;53:4960–70.
25. Hudis CA. Trastuzumab—mechanism of action and use in clinical practice. N Engl J Med. 2007;357:39–51.
26. Press MF, Slamon DJ, Flom KJ, et al. Evaluation of HER-2/neu gene amplification and overexpression: comparison of frequently used assay methods in a molecularly characterized cohort of breast cancer specimens. J Clin Oncol. 2002;20:3095–105.
27. Perez EA, Suman VJ, Davidson NE, et al. HER2 testing by local, central, and reference laboratories in specimens from the North Central Cancer Treatment Group N9831 Intergroup Adjuvant Trial. J Clin Oncol. 2006;24:3032–8.
28. Wolff AC, Hammond EH, Schwartz JN, et al. American Society of Clinical Oncology/College of American Pathologists guideline recommendations for human epidermal growth factor receptor 2 testing in breast cancer. Arch Pathol Lab Med. 2007;131:18–43.
29. Perez EA, Dueck AC, McCullough AE, Reinholz MM, Tenner KS, Davidson NE, Gralow J, Harris LN, Kutteh LA, Hillman DW, Jenkins RB, Chen B. Predictability of adjuvant trastuzumab benefit in N9831 patients using the ASCO/CAP HER2-positivity criteria. J Natl Cancer Inst. 2012;104:159–62.
30. Bhargava R, Lal P, Chen B. Chromogenic in situ hybridization for the detection of HER-2/neu amplification in breast cancer with an emphasis on tumors with borderline- and low-level amplification. Am J Clin Pathol. 2005;123:237–43.
31. Gruver AM, Peerwani Z, Tubbs RR. Out of the darkness and into the light: bright field in situ hybridisation for delineation of ERBB2 (HER2) status in breast carcinoma. J Clin Pathol. 2010;63:210–9.
32. Mansfield AS, Sukov WR, Eckel-Passow JE, et al. Comparison of fluorescence in situ hybridization (FISH) and dual-ISH (DISH) in the determination of HER2 status in breast cancer. Am J Clin Pathol. 2013;139:144–50.
33. Lal P, Salazar PA, Hudis CA, et al. HER-2 testing in breast cancer using immunohistochemical analysis and fluorescence in situ hybridization: a single-institution experience of 2,279 cases and comparison of dual-color and single-color scoring. Am J Clin Pathol. 2004;121:631–6.
34. Clark BZ, Bhargava R. Bright-field microscopy for HER2 gene assessment: not just DISH-ful thinking? Am J Clin Pathol. 2013;139:137–9.
35. Berry DA, Cronin KA, Plevritis SK, et al. Effect of screening and adjuvant therapy on mortality from breast cancer. N Engl J Med. 2005;353:1784–92.
36. Hayes DF. Targeting adjuvant chemotherapy: a good idea that needs to be proven! J Clin Oncol. 2012;30:1264–7.
37. Harris L, Fritsche H, Mennel R, et al. American Society of Clinical Oncology 2007 update of recommendations for the use of tumor markers in breast cancer. J Clin Oncol. 2007;25:5287–312.
38. Gnant M, Harbeck N, Thomssen C. St. Gallen 2011: summary of the consensus discussion. Breast Care (Basel). 2011;6:136–41.
39. Harbeck N, Thomssen C, Gnant M. St. Gallen 2013: brief preliminary summary of the consensus discussion. Breast Care (Basel). 2013;8:102–9.
40. Paik S, Shak S, Tang G, et al. A multigene assay to predict recurrence of tamoxifen-treated, node-negative breast cancer. N Engl J Med. 2004;351:2817–26.
41. Paik S, Tang G, Shak S, et al. Gene expression and benefit of chemotherapy in women with node-negative, estrogen receptor-positive breast cancer. J Clin Oncol. 2006;24:3726–34.
42. Habel LA, Shak S, Jacobs M, et al. A population-based study of tumor gene expression and risk of breast cancer death among lymph node-negative patients. Breast Cancer Res. 2006;2006:R25.
43. Tang G, Cuzick J, Costantino JP, et al. Risk of recurrence and chemotherapy benefit for patients with node-negative, estrogen receptor-positive breast cancer: recurrence score alone and integrated with pathologic and clinical factors. J Clin Oncol. 2011;33:4365–72.
44. Albain KS, Barlow WE, Shak S, et al. Prognostic and predictive value of the 21-gene recurrence score assay in postmenopausal women with node-positive, oestrogen-receptor-positive breast cancer on chemotherapy: a retrospective analysis of a randomised trial. Lancet Oncol. 2010;11:55–65.
45. Dowsett M, Cuzick J, Wale C, et al. Prediction of risk of distant recurrence using the 21-gene recurrence score in node-negative and node-positive postmenopausal patients with breast cancer treated with anastrozole or tamoxifen: a TransATAC study. J Clin Oncol. 2010;28:1829–34.
46. Cuzick J, Dowsett M, Pineda S, et al. Prognostic value of a combined estrogen receptor, progesterone receptor, Ki-67, and human epidermal growth factor receptor 2 immunohistochemical score and comparison with the genomic health recurrence score in early breast cancer. J Clin Oncol. 2011;32:4273–8.
47. van't Veer LJ, Dai J, van de Vijver MJ, et al. Gene expression profiling predicts clinical outcome of breast cancer. Nature. 2002;415:530–6.
48. van de Vijver MJ, He YD, van't Veer LJ, et al. A gene-expression signature as a predictor of survival in breast cancer. N Engl J Med. 2002;347:1999–2009.
49. Buyse M, Loi S, van't Veer L, et al. Validation and clinical utility of a 70-gene prognostic signature for women with node-negative breast cancer. J Natl Cancer Inst. 2006;98:1183–92.
50. Drukker CA, Bueno-de-Mesquita JM, van Harten WH, et al. A prospective evaluation of a breast cancer prognosis signature in the observational RASTER study. Int J Cancer. 2013;133:929–36.
51. Hornberger J, Alvarado MD, Chien R, et al. Clinical validity/utility, change in practice patterns, and economic implications of risk strat-

ifiers to predict outcomes for early-stage breast cancer: a systematic review. J Natl Cancer Inst. 2012;104:1068–79.
52. Parker JS, Mullins M, Cheang MCU, et al. Supervised risk predictor of breast cancer based on intrinsic subtypes. J Clin Oncol. 2009;27:1160–7.
53. Nielsen TO, Parker JS, Leung S. A comparison of PAM50 intrinsic subtyping with immunohistochemistry and clinical prognostic factors in tamoxifen-treated estrogen receptor-positive breast cancer. Clin Cancer Res. 2010;16:52222–5232.
54. Yu K, Lee CH, Tan PH, et al. Conservation of breast cancer molecular subtypes and transcriptional patterns of tumor progression across distinct ethnic populations. Clin Cancer Res. 2004;10:5508–17.
55. Hu Z, Fan C, Oh DS, et al. The molecular portraits of breast tumors are conserved across microarray platforms. BMC Genomics. 2006;7:96–107.
56. Cancer genome atlas network. Comprehensive molecular portraits of human breast tumors. Nature. 2012;490:61–70.
57. Chavez-Macgregor M, Liu S, De Melo-Gagliato D, et al. Differences in gene and protein expression and the effects of race/ethnicity on breast cancer subtypes. Cancer Epidemiol Biomarkers Prev. 2013. doi:10.1158/1055-9965.EPI-13-0929.
58. Sweeney C, Bernard PS, Factor RE, et al. Intrinsic subtypes from PAM50 gene expression assay in a population-based breast cancer cohort: differences by age, race, and tumor characteristics. Cancer Epidemiol Biomarkers Prev. 2014;23:714–24.
59. Kornegoor R, Verschuur-Maes AHJ, Buerger H, et al. Molecular subtyping of male breast cancer by immunohistochemistry. Mod Pathol. 2011;25:398–404.
60. Blows FM, Driver KE, Schmidt MK, et al. Subtyping of breast cancer by immunohistochemistry to investigate a relationship between subtype and short and long term survival: a collaborative analysis of data for 10,159 cases from 12 studies. PLoS Med. 2010;7(5):e1000279. doi:10.1371/journal.pmed.1000279.
61. Tibshirani R, Hastie T, Narasimhan B, et al. Diagnosis of multiple cancer types by shrunken centroids of gene expression. Proc Natl Acad Sci. 2002;99:6567–72.
62. Sorlie T. Introducing molecular subtyping of breast cancer into the clinic? J Clin Oncol. 2009;27:1153–4.
63. Dowsett M, Sestak I, Lopez-Knowles E, et al. Comparison of PAM50 risk of recurrence score with Oncotype DX and IHC4 for predicting risk of distant recurrence after endocrine therapy. J Clin Oncol. 2013;31:2783–90.
64. Liu S, Chapman J-AW, Burnell MJ, et al. Prognostic and predictive investigation of PAM50 intrinsic subtypes in the NCIC CTG MA.21 phase III chemotherapy trial. Breast Cancer Res Treat. 2015. doi:10.1007/s10549-014-3259-1.
65. Nielsen TO, Wallden B, Schaper C. Analytic validation of PAM50-based Prosigna breast cancer prognostic gene signature assay and nCounter analysis system using formalin-fixed paraffin-embedded breast tumor specimens. BMC Cancer. 2014;14:177.
66. Hansen AR, Bedard PL. Clinical application of high-throughput genomic technologies for treatment selection in breast cancer. Breast Cancer Res. 2013;15:R97.
67. Gray J, Druker B. The breast cancer landscape. Nature. 2012;486:328–9.
68. Bliss JM, Kilburn LS, Coleman RE, et al. Disease-related outcomes with long-term follow-up: an updated analysis of the intergroup exemestane study. J Clin Oncol. 2012;30:709–17.
69. Jensen EV, Jordan VC. The estrogen receptor: a model for molecular medicine. Clin Cancer Res. 2003;9:1980–9.
70. McShane LM, Hayes DF. Publication of tumor marker research results: the necessity for complete and transparent reporting. J Clin Oncol. 2012;30:4223–32.

Urothelial Carcinoma

34

Kevin C. Halling

Abstract

Our understanding of urothelial carcinoma (UC) has advanced significantly over the past three decades to provide a better understanding of the molecular basis of these tumors and the different clinical behaviors of low- and high-grade urothelial carcinoma. Fluorescence in situ hybridization is currently used to monitor UC patients for recurrent tumor and to detect new bladder tumors in patients with hematuria. The detection of cells with FGFR3 mutations in urine shows promise as a way to detect low-grade UC. Assessing upper urinary tract UC for defective mismatch repair with microsatellite instability testing or immunostains for MLH1, PMS2, MSH2, and MSH6 helps identify patients that may have Lynch syndrome. While targeted therapies are being investigated for use in advanced bladder cancer, progress has been slow and molecular profiling of urothelial carcinoma for guiding targeted therapy of UC is not currently clinically indicated.

Keywords

Bladder cancer • Urothelial carcinoma • UroVysion • Fluorescence in situ hybridization • FGFR3 • P16 • Microsatellite instability • Lynch syndrome

Introduction

The two main types of urothelial carcinoma (UC) are papillary UC (pTa) and "flat" UC (pTis), also known as carcinoma in situ (CIS). Approximately 80 % of UC are papillary and approximately 20 % are CIS. Most UC arise from the bladder, but UC also originate from the ureters and renal pelvis, and patients sometimes have tumor involving both the lower and upper urinary tract. Papillary tumors tend to recur but not progress to invasive cancer. CIS is aggressive and tends to progress to muscle-invasive cancer. UC tumorigenesis is a multistep process. Papillary UC may arise from areas of urothelial hyperplasia or from urothelial papillomas. Although most papillary tumors are low-grade and have little tendency to progress to invasive tumors, a small proportion are high grade and have significant potential to progress to invasive UC. Most invasive UC arise through the following sequence of events: normal urothelium to dysplasia to CIS to invasive cancer (Fig. 34.1). The schema used for staging UC of the bladder is shown in Table 34.1.

Molecular Basis of Disease

At the chromosomal level, the majority of low-grade papillary tumors are diploid or near-diploid, while the majority of high-grade papillary UC, CIS, and invasive UC (pTa tumors) are aneuploid. Based on array-based comparative genomic hybridization and fluorescence in situ hybridization (FISH) studies, noninvasive, low-grade pTa papillary UC have relatively few chromosomal abnormalities except for loss of all or part of chromosome 9, while CIS, high-grade pTa, and invasive UC (pT1 tumors) have a high number

K.C. Halling, M.D., Ph.D. (✉)
Department of Laboratory Medicine and Pathology, Division of Laboratory Genetics, Mayo Clinic, 200 1st Street SW, Hilton 920B, Rochester, MN 55905, USA
e-mail: halling.kevin@mayo.edu

D.G.B. Leonard (ed.), *Molecular Pathology in Clinical Practice*, DOI 10.1007/978-3-319-19674-9_34

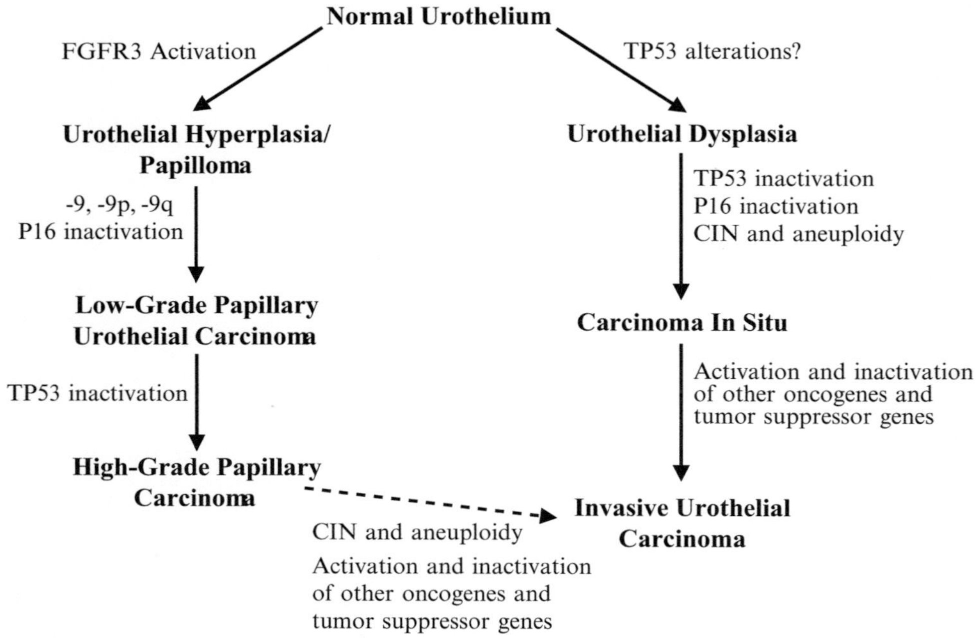

Figure 34.1 Genetic pathways for urothelial carcinoma tumorigenesis. Noninvasive papillary tumors are characterized by early activating mutations of the *FGFR3* gene, inactivating mutations or epigenetic alterations of the *P16* gene, and a diploid or near-diploid DNA content. Carcinoma in situ (CIS) and invasive tumors are characterized by early inactivating mutations within the *TP53* and *P16* genes, chromosomal instability (CIN), and an aneuploid DNA content. A small proportion of papillary tumors may acquire *TP53* alterations or alterations of other unknown genes that cause invasive potential of these tumors

Table 34.1 Pathologic staging of primary bladder urothelial carcinoma

Stage	Description
pTa	Noninvasive papillary
pTis	Carcinoma in situ
pT1	Invasion into lamina propria
pT2	Invasion into muscularis propria
pT3	Invasion through the muscularis propria and into bladder adventitia
pT4	Invasion into surrounding organs (e.g., colon)

of chromosomal gains and losses [1, 2]. The pT1 tumors also have loss of all or part of chromosome 9 but have numerous additional chromosomal abnormalities, which include whole or partial chromosomal losses and gains. Frequent sites of allelic imbalance (AI) in UC include 3p, 4p, 8p, 9p, 9q, 11p, 13q, 17p, and 18q based on microsatellite analysis (MA) [3–5]. Regions with high rates of AI are the sites of known or putative tumor suppressor genes. Many of the regions that show high rates of AI correspond to the areas of chromosomal gains and losses detected by aCGH.

Two important molecular genetic alterations that contribute to UC tumorigenesis are mutational and epigenetic alterations that inactivate the *P16* and *TP53* tumor suppressor genes. *P16* loss is one of the earliest events in the development of both papillary and flat/invasive UC [1, 5–7]. Mutations that inactivate *TP53* are found primarily in CIS and invasive UC and not low-grade papillary tumors and in part may be responsible for the aggressive behavior of these tumors [8, 9]. According to the Catalogue of Somatic Mutations in Cancer (COSMIC) database, other oncogenes and tumor suppressor genes mutated in decreasing order of frequency in UC include *FGFR3*, *PIK3CA*, *CDKN2A*, *HRAS*, *KRAS*, *PTEN*, *AKT1*, *APC*, *CTNB1*, and *NRAS* (http://www.sanger.ac.uk/genetics/CGP/cosmic/).

Defective DNA mismatch repair (MMR) is manifested as MSI at >30 % of microsatellite markers examined and in most cases is associated with a loss of expression of one of the DNA MMR proteins, hMSH2, hMLHl, hMSH6, or hPMS2. MMR is rarely observed in UC of the bladder but is found in approximately 20–30 % of upper urinary tract UC [10, 11]. The finding of defective MMR in an upper tract UC should prompt an investigation into the possibility that the patient may have hereditary nonpolyposis colorectal cancer (HNPCC) and a germline mutation of one of the DNA MMR genes.

Chromosomal instability (CIN) is present in invasive UC and CIS. It is likely that genes that maintain genomic stability are inactivated early during invasive UC tumorigenesis. CIN drives tumorigenesis and tumor progression by accelerating the mutation rate in tumor cells [12]. The genes responsible for CIN in invasive UC are not known, and the role of *TP53* inactivation in CIN has been a matter of debate. pTa tumors show little evidence of CIN but, as noted above, tend to be diploid or near-diploid tumors with relatively few chromosomal alterations. Chromosome 9 and *P16* alterations play a major role in the formation of low-grade pTa tumors.

In addition, most low-grade papillary UC and urothelial papillomas have missense mutations of the fibroblast growth factor 3 (*FGFR3*) gene, while mutations of this gene are less common in invasive UC and CIS [13].

Taken together, two genetic pathways lead to the development of UC [1, 7]. One pathway leads to the formation of noninvasive papillary UC and the other to the development of CIS/invasive UC (Fig. 34.1). The pathway for noninvasive papillary UC is characterized by the presence of *FGFR3* mutations and/or chromosome 9 alterations and *P16* inactivation. The pathway for invasive UC is characterized by early alterations in the *TP53* and *P16* genes, late alterations of other tumor suppressor genes and oncogenes, chromosomal instability, and aneuploidy. The genetic differences between noninvasive papillary and CIS/invasive tumors likely explain the markedly different behavior and prognosis of these tumors [14].

Clinical Utility of Testing

In general, clinical molecular tests for solid tumors can be categorized as being useful for predicting predisposition to developing tumor, aiding in a diagnosis of the tumor type, detecting the presence of tumor, predicting prognosis, or guiding therapy. Examples of assays that are currently being used or investigated for each of these indications for UC are presented below.

Available Assays

The most clinically useful clinical molecular tests, as described below, are the following:

- MSI analysis and DNA MMR protein immunohistochemistry (IHC) of upper urinary tract UC to assess for Lynch syndrome (LS)
- FISH for UC detection
- *FGFR3* mutation analysis for UC detection

Numerous assays with a variety of clinical purposes for UC have been investigated but have not yet transitioned into the clinical use. *TP53* mutations are common in UC, especially in high-grade UC [15]. Assays that assess for *TP53* status could potentially be used to assess prognosis and detect tumor recurrence. Some studies have shown that TP53 overexpression detected by IHC analysis of formalin-fixed, paraffin-embedded tumors is associated with worse prognosis and higher risk of muscle invasion [8, 16], while others have not [17]. IHC analysis of bladder tumors for TP53 expression has not been widely utilized by urologists or pathologists. A few studies have shown that the antiapoptotic protein survivin may be a sensitive and specific marker for the detection of recurrent UC [18], but blinded prospective studies are needed to further evaluate the clinical utility of this assay. Alterations in certain genes, such as glutathione S-transferase M1 and N-acetyltransferase that encode proteins that metabolize carcinogens, may increase an individual's risk of developing bladder cancer, especially among smokers, but assays for these alterations also have not been used clinically.

Interpretation of Results

MSI Analysis and DNA MMR Protein IHC of Upper Tract UC to Assess for LS

Defective DNA MMR is rarely observed in UC of the bladder but is found in approximately 20–30 % of upper tract UC [10, 11]. Patients with early onset upper tract UC or an upper tract UC and a family history of LS-related tumors should be evaluated for LS. This evaluation can consist of assessing the tumor for defective DNA MMR with MSI testing and/or DNA MMR IHC. Patients whose tumors exhibit high-level MSI (MSI-H phenotype) have defective DNA MMR and almost always show loss of expression of one or more of the DNA MMR proteins by IHC. Most histopathology laboratories perform immunostains for four DNA MMR proteins: MLH1, PMS2, MSH2, and MSH6. The most common pattern of protein expression loss in tumors that exhibit defective DNA MMR is loss of MLH1 and PMS2 with retention of staining for MSH2 and MSH6. This pattern of expression is most often due to epigenetic silencing of the *MLH1* gene through promoter hypermethylation. However, some patients with MLH1 and PMS2 loss have a germline mutation in the *MLH1* gene and consequently have HNPCC. Less common IHC staining patterns are loss of MSH2 and MSH6 with retention of MLH1 and PMS2, loss of MSH6 alone, or loss of PMS2 alone. These three patterns are strongly associated with the presence of a germline mutation in the *MSH2*, *MSH6*, and *PMS2* genes, respectively. Patients with genetically proven LS are at risk of developing various tumors such as colorectal cancer, endometrial cancer, upper tract UC, gastric cancer, and sebaceous skin tumors and should undergo regular surveillance for these tumors.

Fluorescence In Situ Hybridization for UC Detection

Urine cytology has been the primary laboratory method for diagnosing and monitoring UC for the past 50 years. Urine cytology has excellent specificity but poor sensitivity for the detection of UC [19]. The problem with false-negative urine cytology test results, if combined with a negative cystoscopy, is that clinical surveillance regimens recommend rescreening in 3 months, allowing an undetected tumor to progress to a higher, potentially incurable state before it is detected. This is of particular concern for grade 3 UC, which routinely progress if not removed or treated. The suboptimal sensitivity of urine cytology has prompted the development of new tests with improved sensitivity for UC detection.

Most UC are characterized by numerical and structural chromosomal abnormalities and a marked degree of CIN with variation in the chromosomal abnormalities found from cell to cell. The finding of aneusomy (i.e., abnormal chromosome copy number) and CIN in a population of cells by FISH is strongly correlated with the presence of malignancy. UroVysion (Abbott Molecular, Des Plaines, IL) is a FISH assay that has been developed for the detection of UC in urine. This assay utilizes four FISH probes, CEP3, CEP7, CEP17, and LSI 9p21, that are labeled with red, green, aqua, and yellow fluorophores, respectively [2, 19]. UroVysion received FDA approval in 2001 for monitoring UC patients for tumor recurrence and FDA approval in 2005 for assessing patients with hematuria (gross or microscopic) for bladder cancer. Representative examples of patients with FISH-positive and FISH-negative findings are shown in Fig. 34.2.

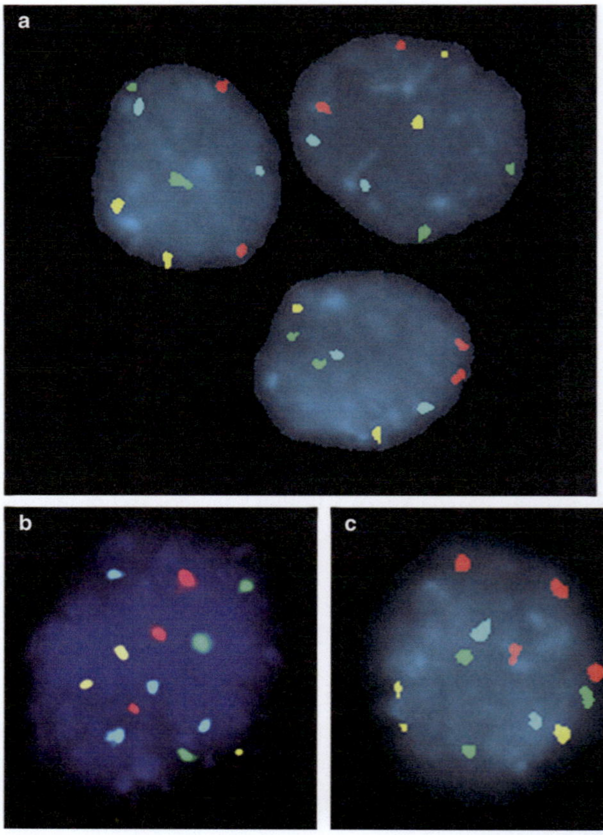

Figure 34.2 Representative examples of FISH results for nonneoplastic urothelial cells (*panel* **a**) and UC cells (*panels* **b** and **c**) using the UroVysion FISH assay (Abbott Molecular, Des Plaines, IL). Nonneoplastic cells generally have two signals for each of the four probes, though occasional nonneoplastic cells show only one signal for one or more of the probes due to random overlap of signals or imperfect hybridization efficiency. UC cells generally have gains for two or more of the probes (i.e., polysomy) of the UroVysion probe set. The finding of just a few cells with polysomy has high specificity for the presence of malignancy. *Panel* **b** shows UC cells with a gains of all four probe signals, CEP3(*red*), CEP7(*green*), CEP17 (*aqua*) and LSI 9p21 (*yellow*). *Panel* **c** shows UC cells with gain of CEP3 (*red*) and CEP7 (*green*) probe signals.

Meta-analysis of the sensitivity and specificity of UroVysion was 72 % (69–75 %) and 83 % (82–85 %), respectively [20]. The sensitivity of UroVysion for the detection of CIS, invasive UC, and high-grade papillary tumors is > 95 % [21]. The sensitivity of UroVysion is lower for low-grade papillary tumors than other UC, but is still significantly better than cytology for low-grade tumors. Though further studies are needed, it is possible that the low-grade tumors not detected by FISH have lower invasive potential and the intervals between cystoscopy could be extended. Studies suggest that UroVysion can detect recurrent UC before it is clinically evident by cystoscopy [21–24]. In the trial that led to FDA approval [23], Sarosdy et al. reported that 36 patients had a negative cystoscopic examination but a positive FISH result. With continued follow-up, 15 (41.7 %) of these cases were found to have biopsy-proven tumor recurrence with time-to-tumor diagnosis of 3–16 months (mean 6.0 months). Conversely, among 68 patients who had a negative cystoscopy and a negative FISH result, only 13 (19.1 %) had a biopsy-proven recurrence at 3–19 months (mean 11.2 months). The time to recurrence was significantly less ($p=0.014$) for the patients with a positive FISH result but a negative cystoscopy than for patients with a negative FISH result and a negative cystoscopy [23].

UroVysion FISH testing has several other clinical uses. The clinical management of patients with equivocal cytology results is challenging because fewer than half of these patients will have bladder cancer on clinical follow-up. Equivocal cytology results can lead to unnecessary and expensive clinical investigations. Patients with an equivocal cytology and positive FISH result are at higher risk for having bladder cancer and should be followed more aggressively [25, 26]. FISH is also useful for assessing noninvasive bladder cancer patients undergoing bacillus Calmette-Guerin (BCG) treatment for reduction of recurrence risk following therapy. A 2005 study by Kipp et al. found that patients with a positive FISH result following intravesical therapy were 4.6 times more likely to have recurrent bladder cancer and 9.4 times more likely to have follow-up muscle-invasive bladder cancer than patients with a negative FISH result [27]. Similar results were obtained by Mengual et al. [28] and Savic et al. [29], who found that patients with a positive post-BCG FISH result had 3.0 and 3.8 times higher risk of tumor recurrence, respectively.

Although other tumor markers are currently available for diagnosing bladder cancer (e.g. BTA stat [Polymedco, Inc., Cortlandt Manor, NY]; NMP22 [Alere, Orlando, FL]), the high sensitivity and specificity of the UroVysion FISH probe set makes this test one of the most commonly used molecular markers for detecting UC in urine cytology specimens. The primary disadvantage of the FISH assay is that it requires more effort than conventional cytology or point-of-care assays such as the BTA stat test. Typical turnaround time for the FISH assay is 1–2 days, though the test can be performed in a single day. Automated FISH enumeration instruments such as the Metasystems (Newton, MA), BioView (Billerica, MA), and Ikonisys (New Haven, CT) systems are used by some clinical laboratories. These systems may increase the ease of FISH test performance, reduce the cost of testing, and increase the throughput and sophistication of the data that can be obtained. Another shortcoming of the FISH test is its inability to detect some low-grade papillary tumors. An assay for UC cells that harbor *FGFR3* mutations (see *FGFR3* Mutation Analysis for UC Detection section below) may complement FISH and allow for the detection of virtually all UC.

FGFR3 Mutation Analysis for UC Detection

The detection of cells with *FGFR3* mutations in the urine is a promising way to detect the low-grade papillary tumors that are not detected by cystoscopy, cytology, or assays such as FISH [13, 30, 31]. FGFR3 is a tyrosine kinase receptor. Germline point mutations in various domains of *FGFR3* are associated with human skeletal disorders such as hypochondroplasia and achondroplasia, and somatic mutations of *FGFR3* have been identified in bladder cancer and myeloma. Interestingly, two groups have demonstrated a high frequency of somatic *FGFR3* point mutations in low-grade papillary UC and urothelial papilloma but not in high-grade papillary UC, CIS, or invasive UC [13, 30]. Billerey et al. found that the frequency of *FGFR3* mutations by stage was pTa 74 %, pTis 0 %, pT1 21 %, and pT2 to pT4 16 % [13]. UC of grade 1 showed 84 %, grade 2 showed 55 %, and grade 3 showed 7 %. The most common *FGFR3* mutation was an S249C mutation (33 of 48 tumors; 69 %), but R248C, G372C, Y375C, and K652E mutations also were identified. The difference in the frequency of *FGFR3* mutations between low-grade and high-grade tumors was highly significant ($p < 0.0001$) and is consistent with the current model of bladder tumor progression in which the most common precursor of invasive UC is CIS (Fig. 34.1). A commercial test kit for *FGFR3* mutation analysis is not available currently.

Laboratory Issues

Laboratory tests can be broadly divided into FDA-cleared/approved tests and laboratory-developed tests (LDT). Laboratories should verify that they can reproduce the performance characteristics that are published in the package inserts of FDA-approved tests. Laboratories that develop LDTs are responsible for establishing the performance characteristics of the LDT. Analytical validation of an LDT should include determining the accuracy, precision (reproducibility), reportable range, reference range, analytical sensitivity, and analytical specificity of the assay. In addition, the laboratory should conduct or be able to cite studies that demonstrate the clinical validity and utility of the LDT, including the positive and negative predictive values of the test. For a diagnostic assay, clinical validation would address the clinical sensitivity and specificity of the assay. For a prognostic assay, evidence of clinical validity would come from studies with Kaplan-Meier analyses and likelihood or hazard ratios.

As with all clinical tests, appropriate controls should be included with each run. For PCR-based tests, this would include positive, negative, and "no DNA" controls and analytical sensitivity and precision controls when a quantitative result is produced. Positive and negative controls for the UroVysion FISH test can be obtained from Abbott Molecular, Inc. These controls are non-hybridized slides prepared from cultured normal male lymphoblast cells and cultured bladder cancer cell lines. Each control slide consists of two separate target areas in which each of the different cell types has been applied. Clinical laboratories must enroll in proficiency testing when available and if not available establish internal methods to assess proficiency. Proficiency testing is available for UroVysion testing through the College of American Pathologists (CAP) Cytogenetics resource committee and for microsatellite instability (MSI) testing through the CAP Molecular Oncology resource committee.

Conclusions and Future Directions

Relatively few clinical molecular tests are used for the diagnosis and management of patients with UC. The main tests that are currently being used or developed are intended for bladder cancer detection in urine specimens. Messenger RNA expression profiling assays (e.g., Oncotype DX [Genomic Health, Redwood City, CA] and MammaPrint [Agendia, Inc., Irvine, CA]) have been used for prognosis and to guide therapy for patients for some tumor types such as breast cancer. Similar assays are not available for UC patients yet but could have clinical utility. Currently, no therapies are directed to specific molecular targets in UC. Therapies that target the FGFR3 tyrosine kinase receptor are being developed, and it is possible that the mutation status of the *FGFR3* gene may identify patients who are most likely to respond to these therapies [32]. In the near future it is likely that next-generation sequencing of UC will guide targeted therapy.

Conflict of Interest Dr. Halling receives industry funding from Abbott Laboratories and royalties from the sale of the UroVysion probe set.

References

1. Richter J, Jiang F, Gorog JP, et al. Marked genetic differences between stage pTa and stage pT1 papillary bladder cancer detected by comparative genomic hybridization. Cancer Res. 1997;57:2860.
2. Sokolova IA, Halling KC, Jenkins RB, et al. The development of a multitarget, multicolor fluorescence in situ hybridization assay for the detection of urothelial carcinoma in urine. J Mol Diagn. 2000;2:116.
3. Dalbagni G, Presti Jr JC, Reuter VE, et al. Molecular genetic alterations of chromosome 17 and p53 nuclear overexpression in human bladder cancer. Diagn Mol Pathol. 1993;2:4.
4. Knowles MA, Elder PA, Williamson M, et al. Allelotype of human bladder cancer. Cancer Res. 1994;54:531.
5. Rosin MP, Cairns P, Epstein JI, et al. Partial allelotype of carcinoma in situ of the human bladder. Cancer Res. 1995;55:5213.
6. Ruppert JM, Tokino K, Sidransky D. Evidence for two bladder cancer suppressor loci on human chromosome 9. Cancer Res. 1993;53:5093.
7. Cairns P, Shaw ME, Knowles MA. Initiation of bladder cancer may involve deletion of a tumour-suppressor gene on chromosome 9. Oncogene. 1993;8:1083.
8. Esrig D, Elmajian D, Groshen S, et al. Accumulation of nuclear p53 and tumor progression in bladder cancer. N Engl J Med. 1994;331: 1259.
9. Tsutsumi M, Sugano K, Yamaguchi K, et al. Correlation of allelic loss of the P53 gene and tumor grade, stage, and malignant progression in bladder cancer. Int J Urol. 1997;4:74.
10. Gonzalez-Zulueta M, Ruppert JM, Tokino K, et al. Microsatellite instability in bladder cancer. Cancer Res. 1993;53:5620.
11. Hartmann A, Zanardo L, Bocker-Edmonston T, et al. Frequent microsatellite instability in sporadic tumors of the upper urinary tract. Cancer Res. 2002;62:6796.
12. Jallepalli PV, Lengauer C. Chromosome segregation and cancer: cutting through the mystery. Nat Rev Cancer. 2001;1:109.
13. Billerey C, Chopin D, Aubriot-Lorton MH, et al. Frequent FGFR3 mutations in papillary non-invasive bladder (pTa) tumors. Am J Pathol. 2001;158:1955.
14. Sauter G, Mihatsch MJ. Pussycats and baby tigers: non-invasive (pTa) and minimally invasive (pT1) bladder carcinomas are not the same! J Pathol. 1998;185:339.
15. Uchida T, Wada C, Ishida H, et al. p53 mutations and prognosis in bladder tumors. J Urol. 1995;153:1097.
16. Sarkis AS, Dalbagni G, Cordon-Cardo C, et al. Nuclear overexpression of p53 protein in transitional cell bladder carcinoma: a marker for disease progression. J Natl Cancer Inst. 1993;85:53.
17. Shariat SF, Weizer AZ, Green A, et al. Prognostic value of P53 nuclear accumulation and histopathologic features in T1 transitional cell carcinoma of the urinary bladder. Urology. 2000;56:735.
18. Smith SD, Wheeler MA, Plescia J, et al. Urine detection of survivin and diagnosis of bladder cancer. J Am Med Assoc. 2001;285:324.
19. Halling KC, King W, Sokolova IA, et al. A comparison of cytology and fluorescence in situ hybridization for the detection of urothelial carcinoma. J Urol. 2000;164:1768.
20. Hajdinjak T. UroVysion FISH test for detecting urothelial cancers: meta-analysis of diagnostic accuracy and comparison with urinary cytology testing. Urol Oncol. 2008;26:646.
21. Halling KC, Kipp BR. Bladder cancer detection using FISH (UroVysion assay). Adv Anat Pathol. 2008;15:279.
22. Bubendorf L, Grilli B, Sauter G, et al. Multiprobe FISH for enhanced detection of bladder cancer in voided urine specimens and bladder washings. Am J Clin Pathol. 2001;116:79.
23. Sarosdy MF, Schellhammer P, Bokinsky G, et al. Clinical evaluation of a multi-target fluorescent in situ hybridization assay for detection of bladder cancer. J Urol. 2002;168:1950.
24. Skacel M, Fahmy M, Brainard JA, et al. Multitarget fluorescence in situ hybridization assay detects transitional cell carcinoma in the majority of patients with bladder cancer and atypical or negative urine cytology. J Urol. 2003;169:2101.
25. Lotan Y, Bensalah K, Ruddell T, et al. Prospective evaluation of the clinical usefulness of reflex fluorescence in situ hybridization assay in patients with atypical cytology for the detection of urothelial carcinoma of the bladder. J Urol. 2008;179:2164.
26. Kipp BR, Halling KC, Campion MB, et al. Assessing the value of reflex fluorescence in situ hybridization testing in the diagnosis of bladder cancer when routine urine cytological examination is equivocal. J Urol. 2008;179:1296.
27. Kipp BR, Karnes RJ, Brankley SM, et al. Monitoring intravesical therapy for superficial bladder cancer using fluorescence in situ hybridization. J Urol. 2005;173:401.
28. Mengual L, Marin-Aguilera M, Ribal MJ, et al. Clinical utility of fluorescent in situ hybridization for the surveillance of bladder cancer patients treated with bacillus Calmette-Guerin therapy. Eur Urol. 2007;52:752.
29. Savic S, Zlobec I, Thalmann GN, et al. The prognostic value of cytology and fluorescence in situ hybridization in the follow-up of nonmuscle-invasive bladder cancer after intravesical Bacillus Calmette-Guerin therapy. Int J Cancer. 2009;124:2899.
30. van Rhijn BW, Montironi R, Zwarthoff EC, et al. Frequent FGFR3 mutations in urothelial papilloma. J Pathol. 2002;198:245.
31. van Rhijn BW, Lurkin I, Chopin DK, et al. Combined microsatellite and FGFR3 mutation analysis enables a highly sensitive detection of urothelial cell carcinoma in voided urine. Clin Cancer Res. 2003;9:257.
32. Guagnano V, Furet P, Spanka C, et al. Discovery of 3-(2,6-dichloro-3,5-dimethoxy-phenyl)-1-{6-[4-(4-ethyl-piperazin-1-yl)-phenylamin o]-pyrimidin-4-yl}-1-methyl-urea (NVP-BGJ398), a potent and selective inhibitor of the fibroblast growth factor receptor family of receptor tyrosine kinase. J Med Chem. 2011;54:7066.

Prostate Cancer

35

Priti Lal

Abstract

The diagnosis and management of prostate cancer (PCa) was revolutionized by monitoring of prostate specific antigen (PSA), with a reduction in the mortality rate for men between the ages of 60 and 79 years, which correlates with a decrease in the incidence of metastatic disease. The monitoring of PSA levels also has led to overdiagnosis of clinically insignificant PCa, while highly aggressive PCa continues to be underrecognized. Over the last decade, advances in gene expression techniques and the introduction of sophisticated bioinformatics tools, have increased the momentum for discovery of more accurate clinicopathologic testing algorithms. Many potentially useful molecular biomarkers are using diverse specimen types, such as blood, urine, and tissue. This chapter describes the biomarkers used for diagnosis and prognosis for PCa.

Keywords

Prostate cancer • Prostate specific antigen, PSA • Androgen receptor gene, *AR* • *PTEN* • *MYC* • *AKT1* • Molecular testing • *TMPRSS2* • *SLC45A3* and *NDRG1* • ETS transcription factors • *ETV1* • *ERG*

Introduction

Prostate specific antigen (PSA), first isolated from prostatic tissue in 1970 [1], rapidly revolutionized the diagnosis and management of prostate cancer (PCa). According to the Surveillance, Epidemiology, and End Results Program of the National Institutes of Health, the mortality rate from PCa for men between 60–79 years of age has decreased to below that found before the introduction of serum PSA level testing. This decrease in mortality has been accompanied by a decrease in the incidence of metastatic disease [1, 2]. Multicenter trials have shown that patients with PSA values 3–10 ng/ml may have localized disease and may benefit from curative treatment [3]. However because of the low sensitivity of the PSA test, a negative biopsy rate of 70–80 % is noted in patients with PSA in the 3–10 ng/ml range. Several parameters, including prostate size, PSA density, PSA velocity, age-adjusted cutoff for PSA values, and free PSA have been added to improve the specificity of PSA. Despite these efforts, overdiagnosis of clinically insignificant PCa and underrecognition of a small proportion of highly aggressive PCa continue to be problems.

Despite its initial success as a screening tool, serum PSA is neither cancer-specific nor predictive of biological behavior. More specific tests that can enhance our ability to accurately predict disease progression, response to therapy, and survival are needed. Over the last decade, advances in gene expression techniques and the introduction of sophisticated bioinformatics tools have increased the momentum for discovery of more accurate clinicopathologic testing algorithms [2]. Many potentially useful molecular biomarkers using diverse specimen types, such as blood, urine, and tissue, are being evaluated.

P. Lal, M.D., F.A.C.P. (✉)
Pathology and Laboratory Medicine, Anatomic Pathology, University of Pennsylvania,
6 Founders Bldg., 3400 Spruce Street, Philadelphia, PA 19104, USA
e-mail: Priti.Lal@uphs.upenn.edu

D.G.B. Leonard (ed.), *Molecular Pathology in Clinical Practice*, DOI 10.1007/978-3-319-19674-9_35

Cancer biomarkers are either produced by the tumor or by the body in response to the tumor. Depending on their individual characteristics, biomarkers may be used as tools for early detection, specific diagnosis in difficult cases, prognosis, prediction of therapeutic response, and therapeutic targets, or as markers of surrogate end-points [3]. Biomarkers with proven clinical usefulness are designated by the College of American Pathologists (CAP) as Category I factors. In current clinical practice, PSA, TNM stage, Gleason grade, and surgical margins are defined as Category I factors. CAP Category II factors are those that have been studied extensively but await statistically robust trials and include tumor volume, histologic type, and DNA ploidy analysis. CAP Category III markers are those that need additional studies to ensure their clinical utility before undergoing further clinical trials. The majority of the currently emerging molecular markers fall into CAP Category III.

The advent of technologies such as next-generation sequencing [4–8] and proteomic platforms, together with advancements in computational and statistical tools, has led to an accelerated growth in our knowledge of the molecular changes in PCa. Significant progress made during the past few years has elucidated that the clinically heterogeneous entity of PCa is in fact a collection of homogeneous molecular subtypes. The ability to sequence many or all genes simultaneously has made comprehensive genomic classification of PCa possible. The completion of an accurate molecular classification is the first step towards development of biomarkers to distinguish aggressive from indolent disease and of targeted therapies. As high throughput technology has become more cost effective, gene panels for specific diagnoses, targeted treatment, and accurate prediction of prognosis are rapidly becoming mainstream, finally bringing the paradigm of comprehensive genomic medicine closer to routine practice of PCa management.

Multiple commercial molecular test kits are now available for PCa. Prostate cancer antigen 3 (PCA3) test (Progensa, Gen-Probe, San Diego, CA) and ConfirMDx (MDx Health, Irvine, CA) improve diagnostic specificity. Once PCa is detected, discrimination between clinically indolent and clinically significant disease is of paramount importance. Two multi-gene signature tests are used to stratify patients for definitive treatment and active surveillance: the cell cycle progression (CCP) score marketed as the Prolaris test (Myriad Genetics, Salt Lake City, UT), and the 17-gene RT-PCR panel algorithmically combined to calculate the Genomic Prostate Score (GPS) by Oncotype DX (Genomic Health, Redwood City, CA). Other tests differentiate patients who would benefit most from adjuvant treatment following prostatectomy. Decipher genomic classifier (Genome Dx Biosciences Vancouver, British Columbia, Canada) is designed to predict early metastasis and disease-specific mortality after radical prostatectomy using a 22-gene expression signature. The CCP (Prolaris) and GPS (Oncotype DX) scores show an association with adverse outcome following prostatectomy. In addition to RNA tests, a DNA test that uses copy number alterations (Genomic Evaluators of Metastatic Prostate Cancer) at 36 loci has been validated to predict biochemical failure in men at high risk of recurrence and is found to be better than clinical risk-stratification alone. This is the only test to be validated in a cohort of African-American patients with PCa treated by prostatectomy. This test was not commercially available at the time of writing this chapter.

Immense progress has been made in developing new prognostic and diagnostic tests for PCa. These tests need to be validated on a larger scale to truly empower patients and treating physicians to make well informed and scientifically sound decisions. Currently available models of risk-stratification at all stages of PCa management are limited in their ability to predict true aggressiveness. Ongoing evaluation of these tests and integration of genomic profiling into risk-assessment models will be critical to realizing the potential benefits for patients.

Molecular Basis of Prostatic Adenocarcinoma

PCa is driven by multiple genetic alterations. The majority of PCa harbor recurrent *ETS* gene fusions [2, 9–12]. Genomic and transcriptomic analyses of PCa have defined new PCa classifications based on gene-expression and somatic copy number aberration signatures [13–17]. Cardinal genetic alterations that activate oncogenes and inactivate tumor suppressor genes are now recognized as drivers of PCa (Table 35.1). Deletion of *NKX3.1* and the phosphatase and tensin homologue tumor suppressor gene (*PTEN*), and amplifications of the androgen receptor (*AR*) and *MYC* genes are some of the most common structural genomic alterations. Protein-altering mutations are rare in PCa. Genes with point mutations most commonly include *AR*, *PTEN,* and *AKT1* [18, 19], but mutations are rare and seen in approximately 1 % of primary PCa [14].

A significant percentage of PCa harbor gene-fusions involving androgen-regulated 5′ gene partners (*TMPRSS2*, *SLC45A3*, and *NDRG1*) and ETS transcription factors (e.g., *ETV1* and *ERG*) [5, 12].

While the implications of the ETS transcription factors as partners in gene fusion events in PCa are not currently understood, the fact that these gene partners are androgen-responsive may play a role in PCa development and progression. Numerous other genetic alterations, somatic mutations, and epigenetic changes occur during carcinogenesis and progression of PCa (see Table 35.1).

Table 35.1 Common genetic and epigenetic changes in prostate cancer

Change	Gene	Encodes	Location	Function
Tumor Suppressor Genes	*NKX3.1*	Prostate restricted homeobox protein	8p21.2	Suppresses cell proliferation
	PTEN	Phosphatase and tensin homolog	10q23.31	Suppresses cell proliferation and increases apoptosis
	CDKN1B	Cyclin-dependent kinase inhibitor p27	12p13.1-p12	Cell cycle inhibitor
	TP53	TP53	17p13.1	Many tumor suppressor functions: • Cell cycle arrest in response to DNA damage • Senescence in response to telomere dysfunction • Induction of apoptosis
Oncogenes	*MYC*	Transcription factor	8p24	Regulates cell proliferation, senescence, apoptosis and cell metabolism
	ERG	Proposed new oncogene in prostate cancer	21q22.3	Fusion transcript with androgen-regulated *TMPRSS* gene found in all stages of prostate cancer
	ETV1-ETV4	Proposed new oncogenes in prostate cancer	7p21.3; 19q13.12; 1q21-q23; 17q21.31	Fusion transcripts with androgen-regulated *TMPRSS* gene found in all stages of prostate cancer
	AR	Androgen receptor	Xq11-12	Protein over expressed in most prostate cancers
Other Changes	*GSTP1*	Glutathione S-transferase pi 1	11q13	Detoxifies carcinogens; inactivated in 90 % of cancers by hypermethylation
	Activation of telomerase			Activated via MYC leading to telomere shortening
	Telomere dysfunction			Shortening of telomere and chromosomal instability
	Multiple genes with hypermethylation of CpG islands			

Blood-Based Molecular Tests

Total PSA and PSA Isoforms

Total PSA

While Total PSA (t-PSA) has been used as a marker for PCa, the expression levels of t-PSA are highly variable across individuals and also in the same individual at different times. A single t-PSA result therefore has little clinical value [20]. Multiple factors account for the variations in t-PSA, including preanalytical specimen handling, different detection methods, biologic variations such as prostate size, and nonneoplastic processes such as hypertrophy and inflammation. In addition, no single t-PSA cutoff separates men at high risk for PCa from men at low risk.

The Prostate Cancer Prevention Trial demonstrated that as many as 15 % of men with a normal digital rectal examination (DRE) and a serum t-PSA of less than 4.0 ng/ml have PCa [21], and of these men, as many as 15 % may harbor a high Gleason grade disease. However, lowering the t-PSA threshold below 4 ng/ml did not improve early detection and long-term survival. Studies suggest that a rise in t-PSA level begins years or even decades before the diagnosis of PCa. Slowly rising t-PSA levels may reflect the long duration of PCa carcinogenesis.

Many efforts have focused on improving the performance of the t-PSA test over the years, including normalizing PSA to the size of the prostate gland, monitoring change in velocity (tPSAV) and PSA doubling time (tPSADT), and measurement of PSA isoforms (Pro-PSA) and alternate PSA forms. Given the limitations of t-PSA, targeting of the various molecular forms of PSA is being used to improve the predictive value of PSA testing and are discussed below.

Complex PSA vs Free PSA

Serum PSA exists in two forms, the bound form also known as complex PSA (c-PSA) and the unbound, enzymatically inactive form called free PSA (f-PSA). Serum c-PSA concentration correlates with the presence of PCa. Serum f-PSA levels are elevated in patients with benign prostatic hyperplasia (BPH) [22–25].

Large prospective studies have demonstrated that use of the percentage of f-PSA (%f-PSA) of total PSA improves the specificity of PSA screening for PCa in men with a normal DRE with serum PSA concentration in the "grey zone" of PSA (between 4 and 10 ng/ml) [26]. Based on these findings, the US Food and Drug Administration (FDA) approved the use of %f-PSA for PCa screening. In a recent meta-analysis of 66 studies, %f-PSA outperformed t-PSA and c-PSA as a predictor of biopsy outcomes [27]. This was more true in older men (≥50 years of age) than in younger men (44–50 years of age). Vickers et al. [28] found that the combined performance of %f-PSA, hK2 (human kallikrein-2), and t-PSA improved predictive ability when t-PSA was in the range of 1.2–2.0 ng/ml.

Subsequent studies noted a decrease in performance of %f-PSA. Explanation for these inconsistencies may lie in the limited stability of f-PSA in blood, particularly in stored sera [29, 30]. In addition performance of %f-PSA decreases with increased prostate size. In men with large prostates, %f-PSA increases even in the presence of cancer, thereby lowering the sensitivity of the test for PCa detection [31].

ProPSA and Prostate Health Index

ProPSA is a precursor form of PSA that contains a seven amino acid pro leader peptide that is cleaved by hk2 and trypsin to form active PSA. ProPSA is a component of free PSA (fPSA) and levels of proPSA are more closely associated with PCa. Truncated forms of proPSA in serum contain five, four, or two amino acids more than the total number of amino acids in PSA; the form with two additional amino acids is noted as proPSA (-2), [-2]proPSA, or p2PSA. FDA approved the Prostate Health Index (phi) developed by Beckman Coulter (Indianapolis, IN) in partnership with the NCI's Early Detection Research Network in 2012. Phi, a mathematical formula using three biomarkers ($[\text{p2PSA}/\text{f-PSA}] \times \sqrt{\text{PSA}}$), has been found to be useful in distinguishing men with PCa from those with benign prostatic conditions, when tPSA is in the grey zone (between 4 and 10 ng/ml) and the DRE is negative. Additionally, p2PSA levels and phi improve the detection of PCa with a Gleason score of 7 or higher; and in men with family history of PCa, phi score significantly outperforms tPSA and %fPSA for detection of aggressive PCa [32].

C-PSA remains to be evaluated as an alternative test. Currently the only c-PSA assay approved by the FDA is based on antibody-mediated elimination of all f-PSA followed by measurement of the remaining PSA (Bayer Immuno1 c-PSA Assay, Bayer Diagnostics, Tarrytown, NY).

Human Kallikrein-2

The human tissue kallikrein family of serine proteases consists of 15 members, known as kallikrein-related peptidases 1–15 (KLK 1–15) located together in a gene cluster at chromosomal region 19q13.3-13.4 [33–40]. The first identified kallikreins, the so-called classical kallikreins (KLK1, hK2, and PSA), contain a unique 11-amino acid-long kallikrein loop. Human Kallikrein-2 (hK2) shares 78 % homology with the amino acid sequence of PSA and has overlapping biological functions. Similar to PSA, hK2 occurs in two forms; one complexes with various plasma protease inhibitors, and the other occurs free in circulation. Unlike PSA, the majority of hK2 in serum is found in the free, unbound form. Total hK2 mRNA amounts to 10–50 % of t-PSA mRNA in the prostate tissue but in serum and seminal plasma, hK2 concentration is only 1–3 % of t-PSA. The highest concentrations of hK2 and PSA are found in seminal and prostatic fluid, but they are also present at lower concentrations in breast milk, breast cyst fluid, saliva, urine, and plasma [41–43]. Within the prostate, the expression of hK2 and PSA is regulated by androgens through the androgen receptor (AR) [44, 45]. Androgen response elements are located in the PSA promoter region [46–48].

Serum levels of hK2 and its ratio to f-PSA and %f-PSA have been reported to outperform t-PSA for PCa detection [49, 50] and could improve the discrimination of men with PCa from men without PCa [49, 51]. Two large studies tested the ability of serum hK2 to improve PCa screening in men with PSA levels below 10 ng/ml [52, 53]. Although the ratio of hK2 to f-PSA did not outperform %f-PSA, these studies showed that the hK2: f-PSA ratio is an independent predictive factor compared to %f-PSA.

Additionally, preoperative serum levels of hK2 appear to better predict biochemical failure (BCF), which is defined as post-treatment elevation of PSA level predictive of PCa recurrence. The predictive value of preoperative serum hK2 in patients undergoing prostatectomy for clinically localized disease was estimated at 0.721 (concordance index) vs 0.691 for tPSA. This difference in predictive accuracy was more pronounced in men with a tPSA <10 ng/ml (0.739 for hK2 vs 0.599 for tPSA, $p < 0.0005$), a category of men where a more accurate predictor is clinically useful.

Histological studies suggest that unlike t-PSA, hK2 expression increases with higher-stage and-grade tumors. It has also been suggested that hK2 could predict poor differentiation, extra-prostatic extension (EPE), and biochemical recurrence (BCR) in patients treated with radical prostatectomy [51, 54]. While intriguing, these findings need further validation [55].

In the grey zone of t-PSA levels, hK2 may add statistically and clinically important information for PCa detection and more importantly for prognostication. This is especially true in the USA where, due to aggressive PSA screening, most men diagnosed with PCa have a t-PSA less than 10 ng/ml, at which level the risk stratification using only t-PSA is not accurate.

Because of the extensive overlap in their amino acid sequence, clinical assays specific for hK2 without cross reactivity to PSA, yet sensitive enough to detect picogram/ml concentrations of hK2, have been difficult to develop. Currently these assays are only available in research laboratories.

A panel of four kallikreins, total PSA, f-PSA, intact PSA, and hK2, were combined to generate the 4K score [26, 28, 56, 57]. Studies suggest that the 4K score could be used to distinguish between pathologically insignificant and aggressive disease and reduce unnecessary biopsies [26]. The 4K score test is anticipated to be available through OURLab Urologic Reference Laboratory (OPKO Health, Inc., Miami, FL) in the future.

Other Blood-Based Molecular Markers

Between 15–40 % of patients treated for localized PCa will experience BCR as evidenced by rising PSA levels [58]. Androgen deprivation therapy is an accepted standard of care for patients who develop metastasis after definitive treatment [59, 60]. Despite adjuvant therapy, the mortality rate in these patients is high (also known as castrate resistant prostate cancer). Currently available tools for predicting disease-free survival are statistical models such as the Kattan nomogram that use PSA, Gleason Score, Clinical and Pathologic stage, and other clinical parameters to predict the probability of BCR-free survival at 5 years after radical prostatectomy [61]. Integration of blood-based predictive biomarkers to the currently available nomograms will increase their predictive power.

The uroKinase plasminagen activator (uPA) pathway or axis includes potential markers for PCa by being involved in various phases of tumor development and progression through degradation of extracellular matrix. Elevated levels of circulating uPA [62] and its receptor (uPAR) are linked to PCa stage and bone metastasis. Large multi-institutional studies are ongoing to further validate these findings [63–65].

TGF-β1 is a growth factor which regulates several cellular mechanisms such as proliferation, immune response, differentiation, and angiogenesis [66]. Increased levels of TGF-beta1 have been associated with cancer progression, occult and documented metastasis, and BCR [67–69]. Serum levels of IL6, a cytokine, and its receptor (IL6R) are elevated in patients with metastatic and treatment refractory disease. Elevated levels of IL6 may thus predict progression PCa [70, 71].

Endoglin is a transmembrane glycoprotein that is associated with angiogenesis. Elevation of preoperative plasma Endoglin may be associated with metastasis to regional lymph nodes [72]. Taking these into account, preoperative plasma levels of a combination of TGF-beta1, soluble IL6R, IL6, Endoglin, vascular endothelial growth factor, and vascular cell adhesion molecule were found to improve the predictive accuracy of the Kattan preoperative nomogram [73] by approximately 15 % (71.6–86.6 %) [2, 74, 75]. Additionally the inclusion of preoperative serum levels of these biomarkers to the traditional base model (tPSA, surgical margin status, extracapsular extension, seminal vesicles invasion, lymph node involvement, and pathologic Gleason sum) statistically significantly improved prediction of BCR.

Urine-Based Molecular Markers

PCA3/DD3: A Cancer-Specific Marker

PCA3, also known as *DD3*, is a noncoding RNA that was initially identified by Bussemakers et al. [76], and is currently the most specific clinically available marker for PCa. *PCA3* RNA is highly overexpressed in PCa compared to normal or benign prostate tissue. Hessels et al. [77] reported a median of 66-fold upregulation of *PCA3* in PCa tissue compared with normal prostate tissue. No other normal tissue or cancer expresses *PCA3*. In addition, *PCA3* is upregulated in prostate

Table 35.2 Performance of *PCA3* in urinary sediments after digital rectal examination

Authors	Sensitivity (%)	Specificity (%)	NPV (%)
Tinzl et al. [79]	82	76	87
Hessels et al. [77]	67	83	90

tissues with a low volume cancer load (less than 10 % PCa cells). Since PCa cells are shed into the urine, *PCA3* RNA can be measured not only in prostate tissue specimens but also in urine and in urine sediments after DRE. Given the specificity for PCa and the ease of analysis in urine sediments, *PCA3* is currently the most specific PCa marker. Several versions of *PCA3* urine tests are available [78].

In phase two of biomarker development for *PCA3*, a second generation reverse transcription-polymerase chain reaction (RT-PCR) assay was developed to detect *PCA3* transcripts in urinary sediments obtained after DRE from a cohort of men who were recommended for prostate needle biopsy based on a total serum PSA value above 3 ng/ml [77]. This study, and three subsequent independent studies [78–82], showed that *PCA3* had a high sensitivity and specificity using prostatic biopsies as the gold standard for the presence of a tumor (Table 35.2). DiagnoCure (Quebec, Canada) developed the first generation version of the *PCA3* RT-PCR test. Gen-Probe (San Diego, CA) acquired the exclusive worldwide diagnostic rights for the PCA3 test from DiagnoCure and developed a *PCA3* test using their APTIMA platform Progensa™ PCA3 test (Hologic, Inc., San Diego, CA).

Progensa™ PCA3 test (Hologic, Inc.) measures the concentration of *PCA3* RNA and *PSA* RNA molecules in serum and calculates the ratio of the two. The Progensa™ test was FDA-approved for use in men who have a suspicion of PCa based on elevated PSA level and/or an abnormal DRE and/or one or more negative biopsy results in the context of a clinical suspicion of PCa. A Progensa™ PCA3 score below 25 is interpreted as negative and is associated with a low likelihood of PCa [83–85]. Based on 11 clinical studies (including 6 multicenter studies and 5 from individual centers) that encompassed a total of 2,737 men, the Progensa™ PCA3 score had an area under the curve (AUC) ranging from 0.66 to 0.75. The average sensitivity and specificity for the Progensa™ PCA3 score quoted by various studies are 66 % and 76 %, respectively, compared to the sensitivity of 47 % for serum PSA alone [84, 86].

To increase the predictive accuracy of biopsy outcome and identify men at risk for PCa, novel biopsy nomograms that include *PCA3* levels have been created. Incorporation of *PCA3* test results improved the diagnostic accuracy of the Prostate Cancer Prevention Trial Risk Calculator [87, 88]. It is expected that inclusion of *PCA3* test results in future nomograms will be clinically useful for deciding whether to biopsy the prostate. Multiple studies [85, 89, 90] have suggested that PCA3 scores fulfill the criterion of being a valuable predictor of low-volume, insignificant cancer and could be of great help in selecting patients with PCa who are candidates for active surveillance.

PCA3 score predicts PCa risk independent from prostate volume, age, and the principal known non-neoplastic causes of increase in PSA, such as BPH and prostatitis. More than 90 % of high-grade prostate intraepithelial neoplasia (PIN) tissues express *PCA3* [91]. The PCA3 test score may therefore help monitor patients with high-grade PIN (HGPIN), such that increasing PCA3 scores may trigger a decision to biopsy the prostate.

TMPRSS-ERG Translocation: A Cancer-Specific Translocation

The combined use of a DNA microarray expression data and a novel bioinformatics algorithm called Cancer Outlier Profile Analysis (COPA) identified gene over-expression of two ETS family transcription factors, ERG and ETV1 in PCa [14, 15]. Further characterization of cases with ERG or ETV1 outlier expression subsequently lead to the identification of fusion of the 5′ untranslated region of the prostate specific androgen-induced trans-membrane protease serine 2 gene (*TMPRSS2*), to the 3′ end of an *ETS* family transcription factor gene [16]. *TMPRSS2* fusion with the *ETS* family member *ERG* is the predominant variant and is seen in 40–70 % (average 50 %) of patients with PCa, making the *TMPRSS2-ERG* gene fusion the most common genetic aberration described to date in human solid tumors [2]. *ERG* is regarded as a key PCa oncogene. Numerous other *ETS* member genes also can fuse to *TMPRSS2*, but are found at a much lower frequency in PCa. Similarly, variability in the 5′ gene fusion partner has been identified. Five major partners are known, and divided into classes based on their tissue-specificity and the sensitivity to androgens (Table 35.3) [9–12, 92, 93]. Class I is reserved for *TMPRSS2*; Class II includes other genes with prostate-specific, androgen-inducible 5′ UTR elements or endogenous retroviral elements; Class III includes the prostate-specific but androgen-repressed gene partners; Class IV includes the non-tissue-specific promoters that are ubiquitously expressed (housekeeping genes); and Class V consists of *ETV1*-specific rearrangements, including the localization of the entire *ETV1* locus to the prostate specific locus, 14q13.2-14q21.1. ETS fusion seems to be an early event in the development of PCa [4, 17]. To date none of the published literature has found this translocation to be present in benign prostate tissue, making it specific for PCa.

Use of ETS Fusion in the Diagnosis and Treatment of Prostate Cancer

The presence of the *TMPRSS2–ERG* translocation can be assessed by immunohistochemistry (IHC) and fluorescent in-situ hybridization (FISH). Mosquera et al. [94], using a

Table 35.3 Classification of 5′ partner of *ETV* associated translocations

5′ Partner	Class	3′ Partner	Initial reference
TMPRSS2	I	*ERG, ETV1, ETV4*	11, 12
TMPRSS2	I	*ETV5*	[144]
*HERV-K*_22q11.23		*ETV1*	[10]
SLC45A3	II		
KLK2 and *CANT1*	II	*ETV4*	[93]
ACSL3	II	*ETV1*	[91, 100]
SLC45A3	II	*ERG*	[145]
FLJ35294	II	*ETV1*	[145]
SLC45A3	II	*ETV5*	[144]
EST14, HERVK17, FOXP1	II	*ETV1*	[94]
SLC45A3	II	*ELK4*	[146]
NDRG1	II	*ERG*	[147]
C15orf21	III	*ETV1*	[10]
DDX5	IV	*ETV1*	[145]
HNRPA2B1	IV	*ETV1*	[10]
SLC45A3 and *ESRP1*	*ETS* neg	*BRAF*[a]	[148]

[a]3′ partners that are not members of the *ETS* family
Numerous alternative *ETS* members can fuse to *TMPRSS2*, but at a much lower frequency. Variability in 5′ partners are divided into five classes: Class I, Reserved for *TMPRSS2*; Class II, Prostate specific androgen inducible 5′ UTR or endogenous retroviral elements; Class III, Associated with prostate specific but androgen repressed partners; Class IV, Non-tissue-specific promoters that are ubiquitously expressed; Class V, *ETV1*-specific rearrangements, including the localization of the entire *ETV1* locus to prostate specific locus 14q13.2-14q21.1

FISH assay for *ERG* gene rearrangements in PIN, found a strong correlation with the presence of cancer. Based on these findings *TMPRSS2–ERG* FISH study on isolated PIN may identify men with a high likelihood of having unsampled PCa. In addition, *TMPRSS2–ERG* FISH may help identify patients undergoing transition to invasive carcinoma and for the work-up of atypical small acinar proliferations which are suspicious for, but quantitatively insufficient for, a definitive diagnosis of PCa on needle biopsy. Assessment for the presence of the *TMPRSS2-ERG* gene fusion therefore may not only be useful for early diagnosis [17, 18] but also may help stratify diagnostically difficult cases.

Knockdown of *TMPRSS-ERG* in fusion-positive cells inhibits tumor growth in xenograft assays [95, 96]. ETS fusions are therefore attractive therapeutic targets. Evaluation for targeting ETS fusion and its downstream targets is ongoing. Most 5′ *ETS* fusion partners including *TMPRSS2* are androgen-responsive and it is likely that current and future therapeutic strategies that target androgen signaling may function at least in part through inhibition of ETS fusions [97, 98]. Phase 1 and Phase 2 trials analyzing the response to abiraterone, a small molecule inhibitor of cytochrome P, found evidence of *ERG* translocation in circulating tumor cells of 41 % men with castrate-resistant PCa prior to treatment [99]. After treatment with abiraterone, 80 % of the patients with *ERG* rearrangements had more than 90 % decline of PSA levels. In patients showing less than 90 % decline in PSA, only 30 % had a translocation [99, 100]. In this cohort of patients, a decline in PSA was associated with a decline in circulating tumor cells and an increased survival rate. Phase 3 trials incorporating fusion status are ongoing. The usefulness of *ETS* gene fusion status as a prospective marker of androgen-dependence in castrate-resistant PCa remains to be seen. In addition to the therapeutic implications, these studies provide evidence that castrate-resistant PCa may remain dependent on androgen signaling [101]. *TMPRSS2–ERG* translocation may predict tumor sensitivity to poly (adenosine diphosphate-ribose) polymerase 1 (PARP1) inhibition and in conjunction with *PTEN* deletion may add prognostic information [91, 102, 103].

While TMPRSS2–ERG translocation is very specific for prostate cancer, it is only present in approximately 50 % of cancer, and hence has limited use as a diagnostic tool on its own. Its use as a diagnostic test therefore lies in multiplexed assays with other biomarkers such as *PCA3* [104, 105]. A study of more than 1,300 men demonstrated that combined measurement of *PCA3* mRNA levels and *TMPRSS2–ERG* gene-fusion in urine outperformed serum PSA for PCa diagnosis [105].

Immunohistochemical Assays of TMRPSS2-ETS Fusion Protein

Multiple anti-ERG monoclonal antibodies standardized for IHC on formalin-fixed paraffin-embedded (FFPE) tissue are commercially available. Expression of ERG on IHC (Fig. 35.1) is considered a marker for the translocation with a sensitivity and specificity of approximately 86 % [106–109]. IHC expression of ERG can therefore be utilized as a surrogate marker for the translocation.

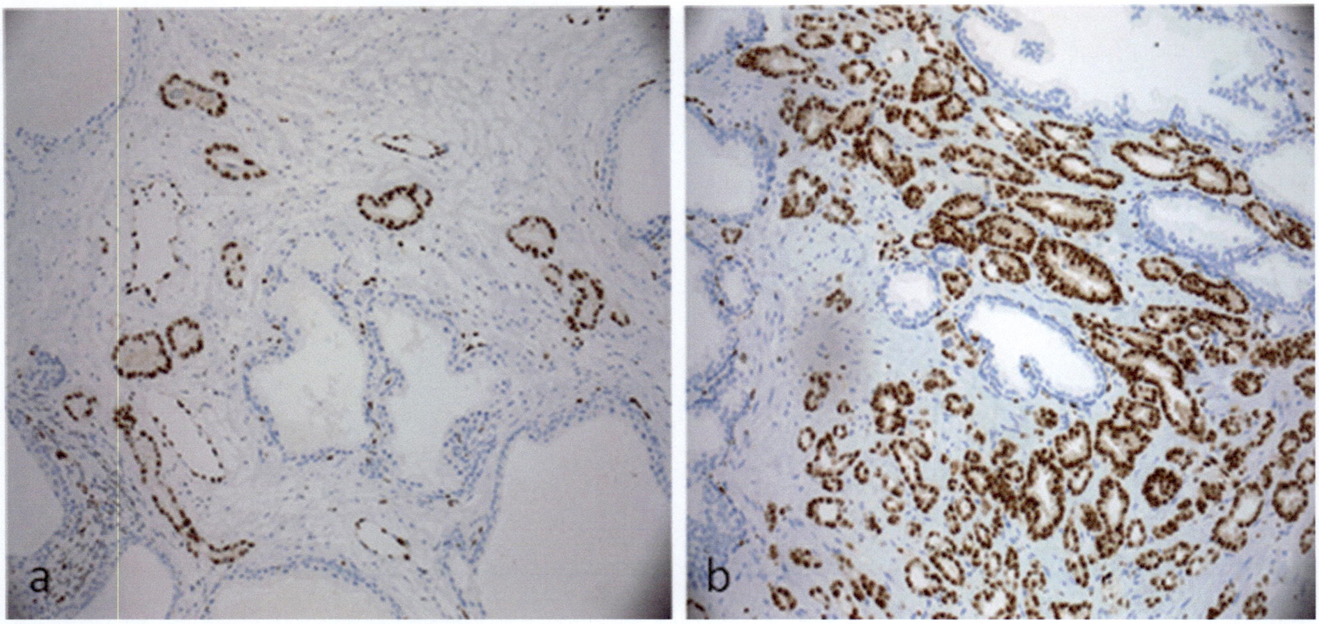

Figure 35.1 Immunohistochemical stain for ERG demonstrates negative staining of the stroma and normal glands. Normal endothelial cells are positive and act as internal controls. (**a**) Strong diffuse nuclear staining of a small cluster of atypical glands supports the diagnosis of prostatic adenocarcinoma. (**b**) Strong diffuse nuclear staining of ERG in prostatic adenocarcinoma. (Slides provided by Drs. Kyung Park and Mark A. Rubin, Department of Pathology and Laboratory Medicine, Weill Cornell Medical College, New York, NY)

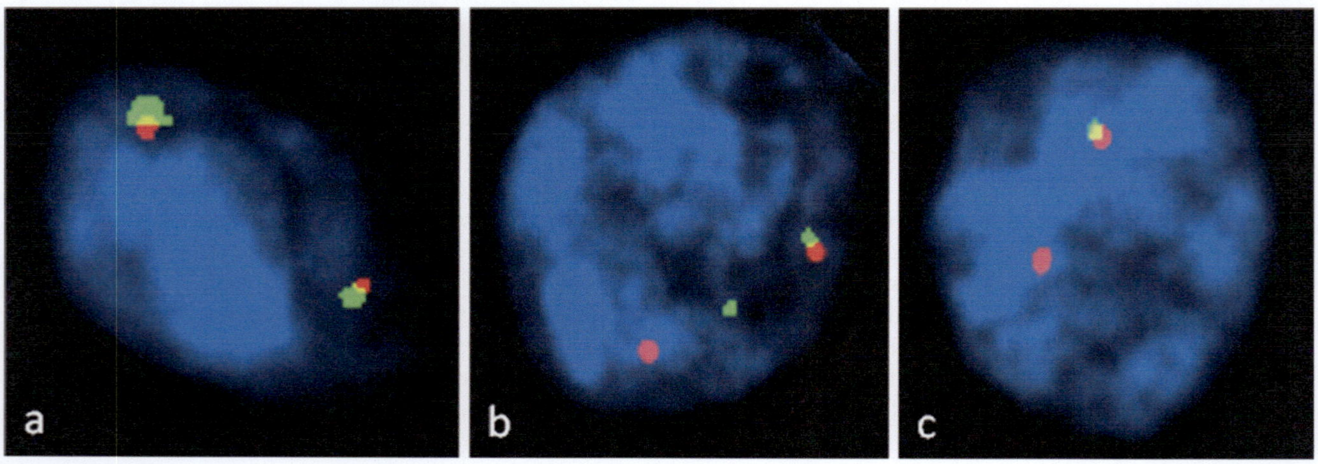

Figure 35.2 Dual Color *TMPRSS-ERG* FISH pattern in formalin-fixed, paraffin-embedded prostatic adenocarcinoma. A probe telomeric to the *ERG* gene is labeled green and a probe centromeric to *ERG* is labeled red. Overlapping green and red signals in normal cells produce a yellow color signal. (**a**) Normal cells without *TMPRSS-ERG* translocation with two overlapping red and green signals. (**b**) A cell positive for *TMPRSS-ERG* translocation with separation of one red and green signal. (**c**) Cell with *ERG* deletion resulting in loss of one green signal. (Slides provided by Drs. Kyung Park and Mark A. Rubin, Department of Pathology and Laboratory Medicine, Weill Cornell Medical College, New York, NY)

FISH Assays for Detection of *TMPRSS2–ETS* Gene Fusion

Traditionally, two strategies for FISH detection of *TMPRSS2–ERG* fusion included the two and three color break-apart assays. The two-color break-apart FISH assays (Fig. 35.2) are designed to identify rearrangements in specific *ETS* family gene partners [110, 111]. Probes were designed to label regions telomeric (green) and centromeric (red) of *ERG* locus on 21q22.3. This set of probes appears yellow due to the overlap of the red centromeric and green telomeric probe in the nontranslocated allele. If a break occurs between the two probes, each color can be separately detected indirectly supporting the *TMPRSS2–ERG* gene fusion [2]. By this method, confirmation of fusion between two genes and identification of the specific 5′ partner is not possible because the probes are not specific for any single gene.

The three-color break-apart assay developed by Yoshimoto et al. [112] utilizes three probes. Two probes flank the *ERG* gene at the 3′ (BAC clone RP11-476D17 RED) and 5′ (BAC clone RP11-95121 GREEN) regions, and the third probe is specific for the 5′ region of *TMPRSS2* (RP11-535H11 BLUE) or for the transcriptional regulatory sequences (telomeric) of *TMPRSS2* (RP11-35C4; RP11-891L10; RP11-260O11). The use of this probe configuration not only enables detection of *ERG* rearrangement but also allows the detection of the mechanism of the rearrangement as explained below. With three color FISH, rearrangement as a result of deletion (Edel) results in co-localization of the 3′ *ERG* and *TMPRSS2* signals and an absence of the 5′ *ERG* signal. Less frequently a genomic rearrangement leading to insertion of those sequences elsewhere in the genome to an unknown chromosome location can occur resulting in the separation of the 5′ *ERG* signals from the co-localization of the 3′ *ERG* and *TMPRSS2* signals, thus described as ERG split or Class Esplit. In either scenario the unaffected chromosome 21 will display a class N (or normal) signal configuration. The presence of more than one copy of the *TMPRSS2–ERG* gene fusion is identified as Class 2+Edel. In summary, in Class N, where no *ERG* rearrangement has occurred, the two *ERG* signals (3′ BAC clone RP11-476D17 in RED and 5′ BAC clone RP11-95121 GREEN) co-localize and are visualized as a yellow signal and the 5′ *TMPRSS2* signal is a separate blue probe signal. In Class Edel, the 3′ *ERG* probe (RED) co-localizes with the *TMPRSS2* probe signals (BLUE) with absence of the 5′ *ERG* signal, representing rearrangement with the loss of the intervening sequence; the unaffected chromosome 21 will display a Class N configuration. In Class Esplit, the 3′ *ERG* signal (RED) co-localizes with the *TMPRSS2* signal (BLUE) with retention of 5′ ERG signal (GREEN) elsewhere in the nucleus; the unaffected chromosome 21 displays Class N configuration.

RT-PCR for Determining Gene Fusion Status

The RT-PCR technique is dependent on detection of hybrid transcripts; however RT-PCR assays do not differentiate between the different genomic mechanisms such as Edel vs Esplit. To date, up to 17 different fusion transcripts and splice variations have been characterized. The most commonly found fusion transcript is composed of exon 1 of *TMPRSS2* fused to exon 4 of *ERG* [109, 113]. Of the transcripts described, one produces a genuine TMPRSS2-ERG fusion protein and eight contain premature stop codons and are unlikely to result in ERG over-expression [12, 113–116].

Wang et al. [113] characterized in detail the expression of *TMPRSS2-ERG* fusion mRNAs and correlated the isoforms and their respective expression levels with clinical outcome in cancers from men undergoing radical prostatectomy. Significant variation was identified in the alternatively spliced isoforms expressed in different cancers. Expression of an isoform, in which the native ATG in exon 2 of the *TMPRSS2* gene is in frame with exon 4 of the *ERG* gene, was associated with clinical and pathologic variables of aggressive disease. Expression of other isoforms, in which the native *ERG* ATG in exon 3 was the first in-frame ATG, was associated with seminal vesicle invasion, which is correlated with poor outcome following radical prostatectomy.

Clark et al. [115, 116] have described the great diversity that exists in the precise structure of *TMPRSS2-ERG* hybrid transcripts found in human PCa. Fourteen distinct hybrid transcripts were characterized, each containing different combinations of sequences from the *TMPRSS2* and *ERG* genes. Distinct patterns of hybrid transcripts were found in samples taken from separate regions of individual cancer-containing prostates, suggesting that *TMPRSS2-ERG* gene fusions may arise independently in different regions of a single prostate.

Indirect Methods for Detection of *ETS* Rearrangement Status

Analysis of array comparative genomic hybridization (aCGH) data, specifically the 21q22.2.3 region, may permit identification of Class Edel *TMPRSS2-ERG* gene fusions [117, 118]. Class Esplit retains the intervening sequence within the nucleus, in a copy-neutral manner and consequently aCGH cannot identify this arrangement. Gene expression microarray may indirectly indicate the presence of an ETS rearrangement by identifying overexpression of *ETS* gene family transcripts. A novel multiplexing technology developed to detect disease-specific biomarkers, including differentiation of various fusion transcripts, uses nano-structured microelectrodes that are integrated into a chip [119].

Tissue-Based Molecular Tests

Several commercial laboratories have developed LDT tests which combine multiple biomarkers for PCa into a single molecular test with a prognostic or predictive score as the result. These tests are not cleared or approved by FDA, but are offered nationally under each laboratory's CLIA permit which requires demonstration of analytical and clinical validity. A concern in using these tests is uncertainty of the validation studies and the lack of demonstration of clinical utility.

Oncotype DX

Oncotype DX (Genomic Health Inc., Redwood City, CA) was developed to test small 1 mm PCa using FFPE needle biopsies. The test assigns a GPS [57] by measuring 12 genes related to four molecular pathways. The genes are *AZGP1*, *KLK2*, *SRD5A2*, and *RAM13C* of the androgen pathway, *FLNC*, *GSN*, *TPM2*, and *GSTM2* of the cellular organization pathway, *TPX2* of the proliferation pathway, and *BGN*, *COL1A1*, and *SFRP4* genes of the stromal response pathway. In addition, five reference genes are used to normalize and control preanalytical and analytical variability. Together with the National Comprehensive Cancer Network risk criteria [120–122], the GPS [123] provides a risk stratification of PCa into very low, low, and modified intermediate risk to help clinicians select appropriate candidates for active surveillance.

Prolaris Score

The Polaris score (Myriad Genetics, Salt Lake City, UT) focuses on tumor cell growth characteristics to stratify risk of progression. The test uses either biopsy or prostatectomy FFPE tissue and includes 46 genes including 31 cell cycle genes and 15 housekeeping genes. A low expression of these genes is associated with low risk of progression whereas high expression is associated with high risk of progression [124, 125]. Patients with a high risk of progression may be offered closer clinical follow-up or additional therapy.

ConfirmHDx

This multiplex polymerase chain reaction (PCR) assay from MDx Health (Irvine, CA) measures DNA methylation of three genes *GSTP1*, *APC*, and *RASSF1*. Methylation of these genes is associated with PCa but can also be seen in histologically normal prostate tissue adjacent to PCa in a "halo" effect. The ConfirmHDx test guides urologists in distinguishing patients who have a true negative biopsy from those who may have an occult cancer (false-negative biopsy). A multiplexed testing approach is useful for smaller tissue volumes and works well on older tissues with small quantities of poor quality DNA [126]. Core-specific methylation pattern-identification has been validated by ConfirMDx with an 80–90 % negative predictive value on follow-up biopsy [127, 128].

Emerging Prognostic Factors Amenable to FFPE Tissue Evaluation

In addition to the commercially available tests mentioned above, a number of emerging prognostic factors are amenable to FFPE tissue evaluation, including oncogenes (*BCL2*, *MYC*, *EZH2*, and *HER2*), a proliferation index marker (Ki-67), tumor suppressor genes (*TP53*, *P21*, *P27*, *NKX3.1*, and *PTEN*), adhesion molecules (CD44 and E-cadherin), and AR. These biomarkers can be assessed using FISH (DNA or mRNA expression) or IHC (protein expression). Once validated for clinical use on FFPE tissue sections, the tests are easy to perform and have the added advantage of interpretation of many glands maintained within their histologic context. The information can be gathered as an adjunct to histological prognostic parameters (such as Gleason score) during routine histopathologic evaluation. IHC assays, such as those for TP53 and Ki67, are poised for transition to clinical use if clinically significant evidenced thresholds are established.

Deletion of *PTEN* at 10q23.3 occurs in approximately 40 % of PCa and can lead to genomic instability [129]. The genomic instability induced by the loss of *PTEN* leads to acquisition of other genomic rearrangements, and continuing instability generates genotypic heterogeneity. Loss of PTEN function leads to accumulation of PIP3 that activates the AKT/PKB signaling pathway with selective advantage for tumor progression. PTEN-null tumors are associated with an aggressive metastatic potential, poor prognosis, and androgen independence [130–134]. Hemizygous loss of *PTEN* carries an unfavorable prognosis in human disease. Homozygous deletion of *PTEN* is strongly associated with metastasis and hormone refractory PCa. Abnormalities of PTEN have been observed not only in prostate carcinoma but also in pre-neoplastic lesions of the prostate [135, 136]. Multiple inhibitors of the PI3K/AKT/mTOR pathway are in clinical trials, with much attention focused on mTOR inhibition. Interestingly, Yoshimoto et al. [103] and Reid et al. [134] observed that in PCa with a *TMPRSS2-ERG* translocation, a loss of *PTEN* was associated with less favorable outcomes. Patients lacking both *PTEN* deletion and *ERG–ETV1* gene rearrangements comprise a good prognosis population with favorable cancer-specific survival. The loss of *PTEN* in the absence of *ERG–ETV1* gene rearrangements is associated with a patient population (6 %) with poorer cancer-specific survival as compared to the good prognosis group. *ERG* rearrangements and *PTEN* deletion can be studied using FFPE tissue by FISH and IHC (Figs. 35.1, 35.2, 35.3, and 35.4).

Chinnaiyan et al. [137] tested seven putative PCa biomarkers using a multiplexed quantitative real-time PCR test

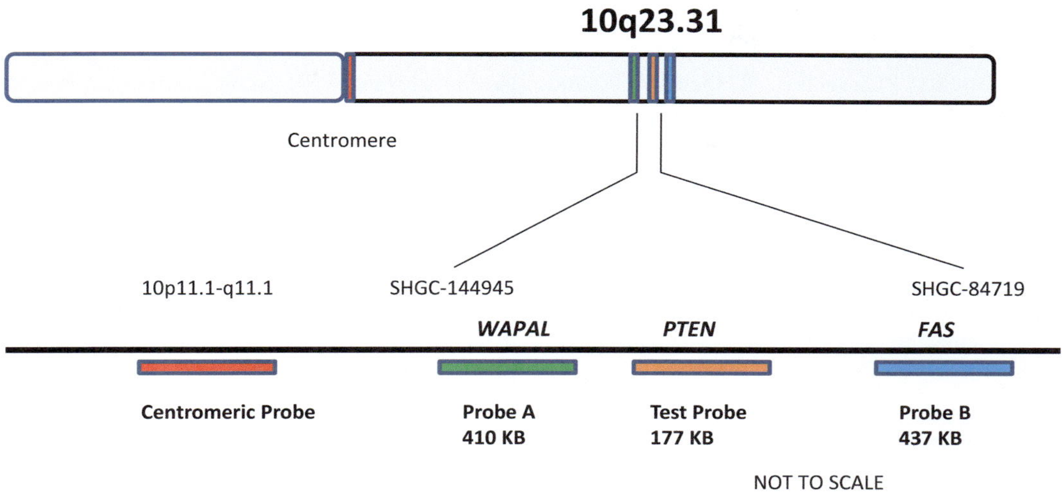

Figure 35.3 *PTEN* construct and ideogram. The localization of the four *PTEN* probes is shown above. The centromeric probe is labeled red and hybridizes to the centromere. The *PTEN* probe is labeled orange. A probe centromeric to *PTEN* is labeled green and hybridizes to *WAPAL*. A probe telomeric to *PTEN* is labeled aqua and hybridizes to the *FAS* gene. See Fig. 35.4 for examples of the signals with different *PTEN* mutations. (*PTEN* ideogram provided by Mohammed Harris, Director of Technical Service and Research, CymoGen Dx, New Windsor, NY)

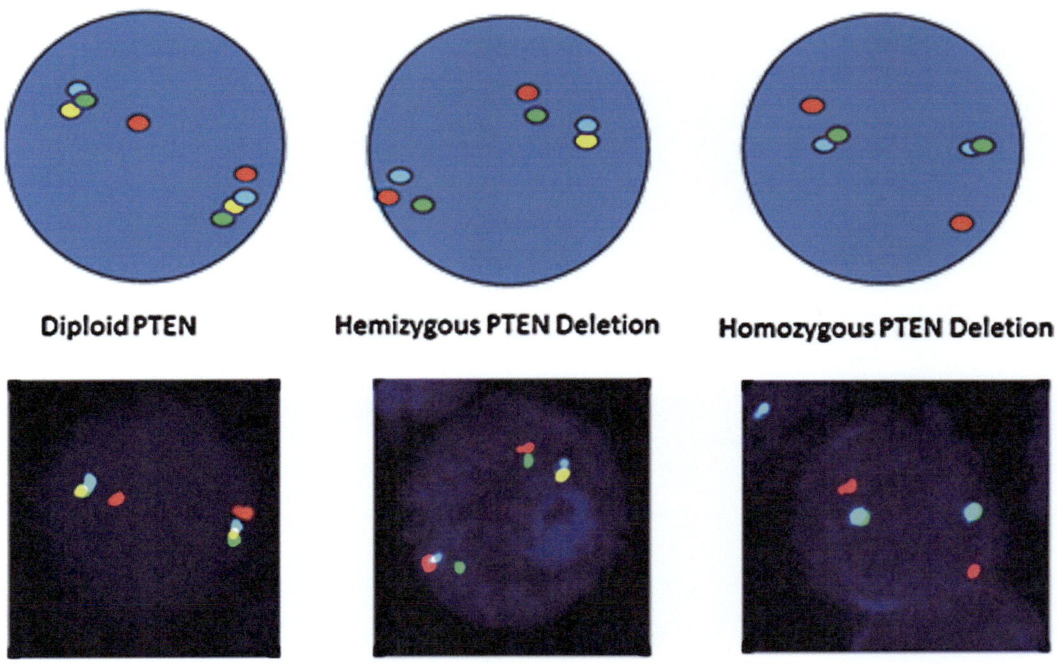

Figure 35.4 Four-Color *PTEN* FISH pattern in formalin-fixed, paraffin-embedded prostatic adenocarcinoma. *Left Panel*: Normal cell with preservation of all four signals, hence no evidence of TMPRSS2–ERG translocation. *Middle Panel*: Absence of gold/orange signal in one cluster and preservation in the other cluster, which indicates hemizygous deletion of *PTEN*. *Right Panel*: Absence of gold/orange signal in both clusters along with the absence of green, which is an example of homozygous deletion of *PTEN*. (*PTEN* FISH figures provided by Mohammed Harris, Director of Technical Service and Research, CymoGen Dx, New Windsor, NY)

in 138 patients with PCa and 96 patients with negative prostate needle biopsies. The biomarkers included those that are generally overexpressed in PCa such as *PCA3*, *AMACR*, and *GOLPH2*, as well as those that are overexpressed in subsets of PCa such as *ERG* and *SPINK1*. In the initial univariate analysis, *GOLPH2*, *PCA3*, *SPINK1*, and *TMPRSS2-ERG* showed significant discrimination between patients with and without PCa. Additionally, AUC analysis of these individual biomarkers for the ability to detect PCa showed that *GOLPH2*, *PCA3*, and *SPINK1* expression levels had better correlation with the presence of PCA than serum PSA.

Clinical Use of Prostate Cancer Tests for Patient Management

Compared to the other solid organ and hematologic malignancies, PCa diagnosis and management has been lagging far behind in utilization of molecular tools for diagnosis and personalized treatment. Only in the last 4–5 years have advances in our understanding of the genetic basis of PCa enabled scientists to design molecular panels for each step in the management of PCa. Integration of these novel molecular tools in routine clinical practice will help physicians better differentiate patients with PCa from those who have an elevated PSA secondary to other reasons. Currently available PCa molecular assays, including the PCA3 test, the phi, and *TMPRSS-ERG* translocation tests, are all standardized for use on urine samples. Integration of these cancer-specific tools as post-PSA screening tests can help identify patients at high risk of having PCa.

Despite their promise, the true ability of these newer tests to reduce the number of unnecessary biopsies has yet to be determined. A comparison of watchful waiting compared to treatment based on these test results would clarify their utility in routine clinical practice. Eventually the ability of these tests to reduce unnecessary biopsy procedures will depend on the tolerance of patients and physicians for the risk of occult cancer and also on the confidence index of the tests. Future tests may eventually include a panel of cancer-specific genes included in one test rather than individual biomarkers forming multiple individual tests.

Upon diagnosis of PCa on a needle biopsy, genomic tests such as Oncotype DX and Prolaris predict clinically indolent and clinically significant cancers. Integration of such tests into clinical algorithms will help confidently differentiate

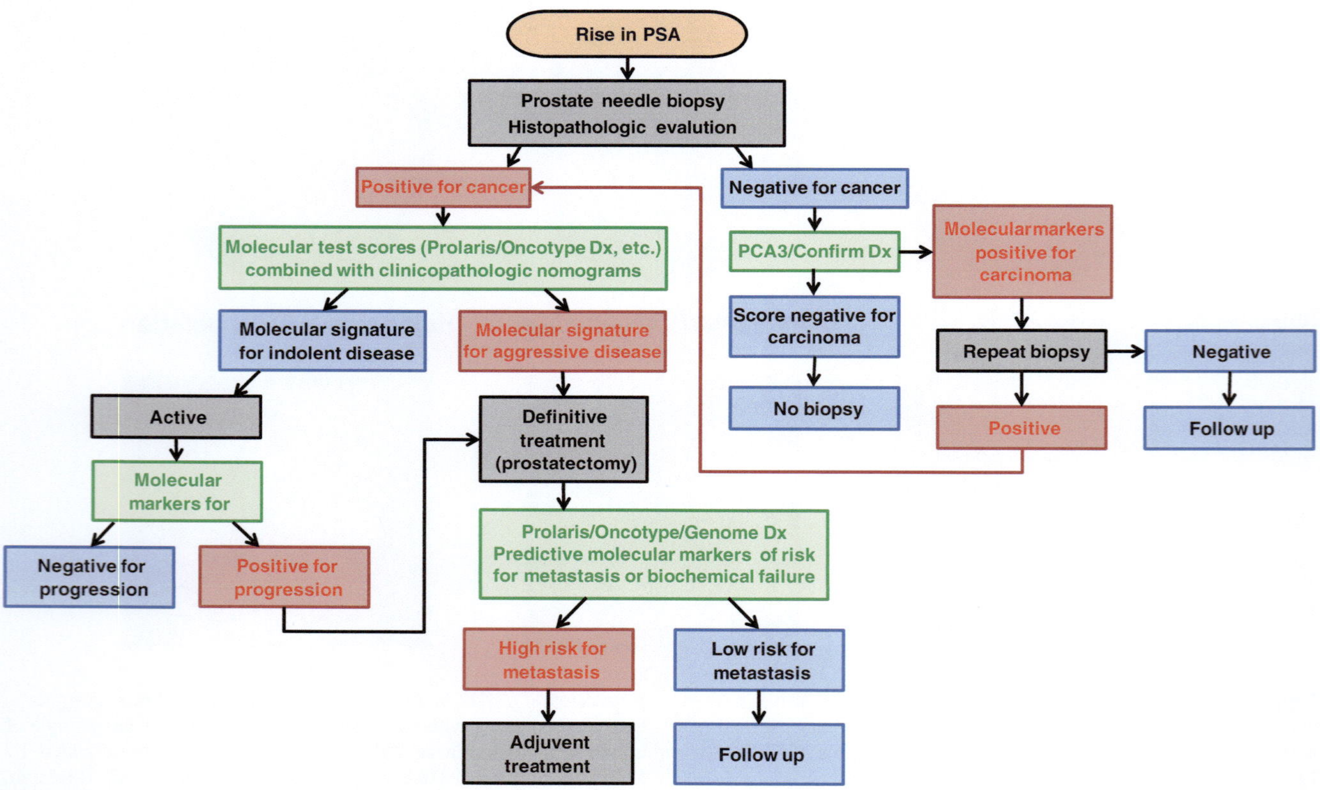

Figure 35.5 Potential algorithm for integration of molecular tests into clinical practice. Molecular tests can be integrated into each step of prostate cancer (PCa) diagnosis, treatment, and long-term management. Patients with an initial negative biopsy may be triaged further into those who have a high likelihood of cancer and hence in need of an early follow-up biopsy and those who are truly negative. Molecular tests can help stratify patients with a first time diagnosis of PCa into those who should get definitive treatment and those who should receive active surveillance. Patients who receive definitive treatment can then be further divided into those who are at low risk of metastasis and those who are at high risk of metastasis and hence need adjuvant therapy

patients who would benefit from active surveillance [138] from patients with more aggressive disease needing definitive treatment [139]. An algorithm for the use of molecular tests in clinical practice is shown in Fig. 35.5.

After radical prostatectomy, the currently available diagnostic models have predictive accuracies ranging from 78–89 % [140–143]. Use of recently discovered urine, blood, and tissue biomarkers may enhance the performance of currently available nomograms. The profiling of blood proteins, TGF-b1 and IL-6sR, in preoperative plasma improves the predictive accuracy of the Kattan [143] preoperative nomogram by a significant margin, but is not yet widely used in clinical practice.

Future Directions

From our current understanding of PCa, no single biomarker can provide high sensitivity and specificity to predict PCa behavior or aid in early diagnosis. Using single markers to predict the presence of PCa and outcomes does not take into account the genetic heterogeneity of PCa. The important issue in evaluating a new biomarker is not its independent predictive value, but its ability to improve the predictive accuracy for patients when combined with established biomarkers. An ideal test therefore will seek to identify the correct permutation and combination of the newly emerging biomarkers in association with established predictive factors. An extensive list of serum, urine, and tissue PCa biomarkers are currently in various phases of development. Multiplex assays that use a combination of biomarkers hold the most promise in the future. With advances in biotechnology, diverse techniques including a spectrum of "omics" are being explored. Future approaches may integrate proteomic, transcriptomic, and genomic approaches to identify the optimal combination of biomarkers for detection of PCa, differentiation of indolent from aggressive PCa, and for directing adjuvant treatment. The development of these future tests will require careful attention to the populations and clinical scenarios in which the tests are validated and used.

References

1. Flocks RH, Urich VC, Patel CA, Opitz JM. Studies on the antigenic properties of prostatic tissue. I. J Urol. 1960;84:134–43.
2. Perner S, Demichelis F, Beroukhim R, et al. TMPRSS2:ERG fusion-associated deletions provide insight into the heterogeneity of prostate cancer. Cancer Res. 2006;66:8337–41.
3. Shariat SF, Semjonow A, Lilja H, Savage C, Vickers AJ, Bjartell A. Tumor markers in prostate cancer I: blood-based markers. Acta Oncol. 2011;50 Suppl 1:61–75.
4. Bentley DR, Balasubramanian S, Swerdlow HP, et al. Accurate whole human genome sequencing using reversible terminator chemistry. Nature. 2008;456:53–9.
5. Kumar-Sinha C, Tomlins SA, Chinnaiyan AM. Recurrent gene fusions in prostate cancer. Nat Rev Cancer. 2008;8:497–511.
6. Margulies M, Egholm M, Altman WE, et al. Genome sequencing in microfabricated high-density picolitre reactors. Nature. 2005;437:376–80.
7. Shendure J, Porreca GJ, Reppas NB, et al. Accurate multiplex polony sequencing of an evolved bacterial genome. Science. 2005;309:1728–32.
8. Smith DR, Quinlan AR, Peckham HE, et al. Rapid whole-genome mutational profiling using next-generation sequencing technologies. Genome Res. 2008;18:1638–42.
9. Tomlins SA, Bjartell A, Chinnaiyan AM, et al. ETS gene fusions in prostate cancer: from discovery to daily clinical practice. Eur Urol. 2009;56:275–86.
10. Tomlins SA, Laxman B, Dhanasekaran SM, et al. Distinct classes of chromosomal rearrangements create oncogenic ETS gene fusions in prostate cancer. Nature. 2007;448:595–9.
11. Tomlins SA, Mehra R, Rhodes DR, et al. TMPRSS2:ETV4 gene fusions define a third molecular subtype of prostate cancer. Cancer Res. 2006;66:3396–400.
12. Tomlins SA, Rhodes DR, Perner S, et al. Recurrent fusion of TMPRSS2 and ETS transcription factor genes in prostate cancer. Science. 2005;310:644–8.
13. Demichelis F, Setlur SR, Beroukhim R, et al. Distinct genomic aberrations associated with ERG rearranged prostate cancer. Genes Chromosomes Cancer. 2009;48:366–80.
14. Taylor BS, Schultz N, Hieronymus H, et al. Integrative genomic profiling of human prostate cancer. Cancer Cell. 2010;18:11–22.
15. Setlur SR, Mertz KD, Hoshida Y, et al. Estrogen-dependent signaling in a molecularly distinct subclass of aggressive prostate cancer. J Natl Cancer Inst. 2008;100:815–25.
16. Lapointe J, Li C, Higgins JP, et al. Gene expression profiling identifies clinically relevant subtypes of prostate cancer. Proc Natl Acad Sci U S A. 2004;101:811–6.
17. Lapointe J, Li C, Giacomini CP, et al. Genomic profiling reveals alternative genetic pathways of prostate tumorigenesis. Cancer Res. 2007;67:8504–10.
18. Boormans JL, Korsten H, Ziel-van der Made AC, van Leenders GJ, Verhagen PC, Trapman J. E17K substitution in AKT1 in prostate cancer. Br J Cancer. 2010;102:1491–4.
19. Forbes SA, Tang G, Bindal N, et al. COSMIC (the Catalogue of Somatic Mutations in Cancer): a resource to investigate acquired mutations in human cancer. Nucleic Acids Res. 2010;38:D652–7.
20. Shariat SF, Park S, Trinh QD, Roehrborn CG, Slawin KM, Karakiewicz PI. Plasminogen activation inhibitor-1 improves the predictive accuracy of prostate cancer nomograms. J Urol. 2007;178:1229–36. discussion 36-7.
21. Thompson IM, Pauler DK, Goodman PJ, et al. Prevalence of prostate cancer among men with a prostate-specific antigen level < or =4.0 ng per milliliter. N Engl J Med. 2004;350:2239–46.
22. Stenman UH. Detection of complexes between prostate-specific antigen and protease inhibitors in plasma. Clin Chem. 2010;56:1895–6.
23. Stenman UH, Hakama M, Knekt P, Aromaa A, Teppo L, Leinonen J. Serum concentrations of prostate specific antigen and its complex with alpha 1-antichymotrypsin before diagnosis of prostate cancer. Lancet. 1994;344:1594–8.
24. Stenman UH, Leinonen J, Alfthan H, Rannikko S, Tuhkanen K, Alfthan O. A complex between prostate-specific antigen and alpha 1-antichymotrypsin is the major form of prostate-specific antigen in serum of patients with prostatic cancer: assay of the complex improves clinical sensitivity for cancer. Cancer Res. 1991;51:222–6.
25. Stenman UH, Leinonen J, Zhang WM. Standardization of PSA determinations. Scand J Clin Lab Invest Suppl. 1995;221:45–51.
26. Carlsson S, Maschino A, Schroder F, et al. Predictive value of four kallikrein markers for pathologically insignificant compared with

aggressive prostate cancer in radical prostatectomy specimens: results from the European Randomized Study of Screening for Prostate Cancer section Rotterdam. Eur Urol. 2013;64:693–9.
27. Roddam AW, Duffy MJ, Hamdy FC, et al. Use of prostate-specific antigen (PSA) isoforms for the detection of prostate cancer in men with a PSA level of 2-10 ng/ml: systematic review and meta-analysis. Eur Urol. 2005;48:386–99. discussion 98-9.
28. Voigt JD, Zappala SM, Vaughan ED, Wein AJ. The Kallikrein Panel for prostate cancer screening: its economic impact. Prostate. 2014;74:250–9.
29. Ulmert D, Becker C, Nilsson JA, et al. Reproducibility and accuracy of measurements of free and total prostate-specific antigen in serum vs plasma after long-term storage at -20 degrees C. Clin Chem. 2006;52:235–9.
30. Vickers AJ, Cronin AM, Aus G, et al. A panel of kallikrein markers can reduce unnecessary biopsy for prostate cancer: data from the European Randomized Study of Prostate Cancer Screening in Goteborg, Sweden. BMC Med. 2008;6:19.
31. Meyer A, Jung K, Lein M, Rudolph B, Schnorr D, Loening SA. Factors influencing the ratio of free to total prostate-specific antigen in serum. Int J Cancer. 1997;74:630–6.
32. Abrate A, Lazzeri M, Lughezzani G, et al. Clinical performance of Prostate Health Index (PHI) for prediction of prostate cancer in obese men: data from a multicenter European prospective study, PROMEtheuS project. BJU Int. 2015;115:537–45.
33. Harvey TJ, Hooper JD, Myers SA, Stephenson SA, Ashworth LK, Clements JA. Tissue-specific expression patterns and fine mapping of the human kallikrein (KLK) locus on proximal 19q13.4. J Biol Chem. 2000;275:37397–406.
34. Gan L, Lee I, Smith R, et al. Sequencing and expression analysis of the serine protease gene cluster located in chromosome 19q13 region. Gene. 2000;257:119–30.
35. Yousef GM, Chang A, Scorilas A, Diamandis EP. Genomic organization of the human kallikrein gene family on chromosome 19q13.3-q13.4. Biochem Biophys Res Commun. 2000;276:125–33.
36. Yousef GM, Diamandis EP. The expanded human kallikrein gene family: locus characterization and molecular cloning of a new member, KLK-L3 (KLK9). Genomics. 2000;65:184–94.
37. Yousef GM, Magklara A, Diamandis EP. KLK12 is a novel serine protease and a new member of the human kallikrein gene family-differential expression in breast cancer. Genomics. 2000;69:331–41.
38. Yousef GM, Scorilas A, Diamandis EP. Genomic organization, mapping, tissue expression, and hormonal regulation of trypsin-like serine protease (TLSP PRSS20), a new member of the human kallikrein gene family. Genomics. 2000;63:88–96.
39. Yousef GM, Scorilas A, Magklara A, Soosaipillai A, Diamandis EP. The KLK7 (PRSS6) gene, encoding for the stratum corneum chymotryptic enzyme is a new member of the human kallikrein gene family—genomic characterization, mapping, tissue expression and hormonal regulation. Gene. 2000;254:119–28.
40. Lundwall A, Clauss A, Olsson AY. Evolution of kallikrein-related peptidases in mammals and identification of a genetic locus encoding potential regulatory inhibitors. Biol Chem. 2006;387:243–9.
41. Shaw JL, Diamandis EP. Regulation of human tissue kallikrein-related peptidase expression by steroid hormones in 32 cell lines. Biol Chem. 2008;389:1409–19.
42. Denmeade SR, Lovgren J, Khan SR, Lilja H, Isaacs JT. Activation of latent protease function of pro-hK2, but not pro-PSA, involves autoprocessing. Prostate. 2001;48:122–6.
43. Denmeade SR, Sokoll LJ, Chan DW, Khan SR, Isaacs JT. Concentration of enzymatically active prostate-specific antigen (PSA) in the extracellular fluid of primary human prostate cancers and human prostate cancer xenograft models. Prostate. 2001;48:1–6.
44. Lawrence MG, Lai J, Clements JA. Kallikreins on steroids: structure, function, and hormonal regulation of prostate-specific antigen and the extended kallikrein locus. Endocr Rev. 2010;31:407–46.
45. Andriole GL, Catalona WJ. Prostate carcinoma. Annu Rev Med. 1994;45:351–9.
46. Riegman PH, Vlietstra RJ, van der Korput HA, Romijn JC, Trapman J. Identification and androgen-regulated expression of two major human glandular kallikrein-1 (hGK-1) mRNA species. Mol Cell Endocrinol. 1991;76:181–90.
47. Riegman PH, Vlietstra RJ, van der Korput JA, Brinkmann AO, Trapman J. The promoter of the prostate-specific antigen gene contains a functional androgen responsive element. Mol Endocrinol. 1991;5:1921–30.
48. Cleutjens KB, van der Korput HA, van Eekelen CC, van Rooij HC, Faber PW, Trapman J. An androgen response element in a far upstream enhancer region is essential for high, androgen-regulated activity of the prostate-specific antigen promoter. Mol Endocrinol. 1997;11:148–61.
49. Becker C, Piironen T, Pettersson K, et al. Discrimination of men with prostate cancer from those with benign disease by measurements of human glandular kallikrein 2 (HK2) in serum. J Urol. 2000;163:311–6.
50. Darson MF, Pacelli A, Roche P, et al. Human glandular kallikrein 2 expression in prostate adenocarcinoma and lymph node metastases. Urology. 1999;53:939–44.
51. Haese A, Graefen M, Steuber T, et al. Human glandular kallikrein 2 levels in serum for discrimination of pathologically organ-confined from locally-advanced prostate cancer in total PSA-levels below 10 ng/ml. Prostate. 2001;49:101–9.
52. Becker C, Piironen T, Pettersson K, Hugosson J, Lilja H. Clinical value of human glandular kallikrein 2 and free and total prostate-specific antigen in serum from a population of men with prostate-specific antigen levels 3.0 ng/mL or greater. Urology. 2000;55:694–9.
53. Partin AW, Catalona WJ, Finlay JA, et al. Use of human glandular kallikrein 2 for the detection of prostate cancer: preliminary analysis. Urology. 1999;54:839–45.
54. Haese A, Graefen M, Becker C, et al. The role of human glandular kallikrein 2 for prediction of pathologically organ confined prostate cancer. Prostate. 2003;54:181–6.
55. Kurek R, Nunez G, Tselis N, et al. Prognostic value of combined "triple"-reverse transcription-PCR analysis for prostate-specific antigen, human kallikrein 2, and prostate-specific membrane antigen mRNA in peripheral blood and lymph nodes of prostate cancer patients. Clin Cancer Res. 2004;10:5808–14.
56. Bjartell AS. Next-generation prostate-specific antigen test: ready to use? Eur Urol. 2013;64:700–2.
57. Sartori DA, Chan DW. Biomarkers in prostate cancer: what's new? Curr Opin Oncol. 2014;26:259–64.
58. Ward JF, Moul JW. Biochemical recurrence after definitive prostate cancer therapy. Part II: treatment strategies for biochemical recurrence of prostate cancer. Curr Opin Urol. 2005;15:187–95.
59. Bastian PJ, Boorjian SA, Bossi A, et al. High-risk prostate cancer: from definition to contemporary management. Eur Urol. 2012;61:1096–106.
60. Heidenreich A, Bastian PJ, Bellmunt J, et al. EAU guidelines on prostate cancer. Part II: treatment of advanced, relapsing, and castration-resistant prostate cancer. Eur Urol. 2014;65:467–79.
61. Kattan MW, Vickers AJ, Yu C, et al. Preoperative and postoperative nomograms incorporating surgeon experience for clinically localized prostate cancer. Cancer. 2009;115:1005–10.

62. Gupta A, Lotan Y, Ashfaq R, et al. Predictive value of the differential expression of the urokinase plasminogen activation axis in radical prostatectomy patients. Eur Urol. 2009;55:1124–33.
63. Shariat SF, Roehrborn CG, McConnell JD, et al. Association of the circulating levels of the urokinase system of plasminogen activation with the presence of prostate cancer and invasion, progression, and metastasis. J Clin Oncol. 2007;25:349–55.
64. Miyake H, Hara I, Yamanaka K, Gohji K, Arakawa S, Kamidono S. Elevation of serum levels of urokinase-type plasminogen activator and its receptor is associated with disease progression and prognosis in patients with prostate cancer. Prostate. 1999;39:123–9.
65. Hienert G, Kirchheimer JC, Pfluger H, Binder BR. Urokinase-type plasminogen activator as a marker for the formation of distant metastases in prostatic carcinomas. J Urol. 1988;140:1466–9.
66. Shariat SF, Shalev M, Menesses-Diaz A, et al. Preoperative plasma levels of transforming growth factor beta(1) (TGF-beta(1)) strongly predict progression in patients undergoing radical prostatectomy. J Clin Oncol. 2001;19:2856–64.
67. Shariat SF, Kattan MW, Traxel E, et al. Association of pre- and postoperative plasma levels of transforming growth factor beta(1) and interleukin 6 and its soluble receptor with prostate cancer progression. Clin Cancer Res. 2004;10:1992–9.
68. Shariat SF, Kim JH, Andrews B, et al. Preoperative plasma levels of transforming growth factor beta(1) strongly predict clinical outcome in patients with bladder carcinoma. Cancer. 2001;92:2985–92.
69. Ivanovic V, Melman A, Davis-Joseph B, Valcic M, Geliebter J. Elevated plasma levels of TGF-beta 1 in patients with invasive prostate cancer. Nat Med. 1995;1:282–4.
70. Michalaki V, Syrigos K, Charles P, Waxman J. Serum levels of IL-6 and TNF-alpha correlate with clinicopathological features and patient survival in patients with prostate cancer. Br J Cancer. 2004;90:2312–6.
71. Nakashima J, Tachibana M, Horiguchi Y, et al. Serum interleukin 6 as a prognostic factor in patients with prostate cancer. Clin Cancer Res. 2000;6:2702–6.
72. Karam JA, Svatek RS, Karakiewicz PI, et al. Use of preoperative plasma endoglin for prediction of lymph node metastasis in patients with clinically localized prostate cancer. Clin Cancer Res. 2008;14:1418–22.
73. Kattan MW, Shariat SF, Andrews B, et al. The addition of interleukin-6 soluble receptor and transforming growth factor beta1 improves a preoperative nomogram for predicting biochemical progression in patients with clinically localized prostate cancer. J Clin Oncol. 2003;21:3573–9.
74. Shariat SF, Karakiewicz PI, Ashfaq R, et al. Multiple biomarkers improve prediction of bladder cancer recurrence and mortality in patients undergoing cystectomy. Cancer. 2008;112:315–25.
75. Shariat SF, Karam JA, Walz J, et al. Improved prediction of disease relapse after radical prostatectomy through a panel of preoperative blood-based biomarkers. Clin Cancer Res. 2008;14:3785–91.
76. Bussemakers MJ, van Bokhoven A, Verhaegh GW, et al. DD3: a new prostate-specific gene, highly overexpressed in prostate cancer. Cancer Res. 1999;59:5975–9.
77. Hessels D, Klein Gunnewiek JM, van Oort I, et al. DD3(PCA3)-based molecular urine analysis for the diagnosis of prostate cancer. Eur Urol. 2003;44:8–15.
78. Hessels D, Schalken JA. The use of PCA3 in the diagnosis of prostate cancer. Nat Rev Urol. 2009;6:255–61.
79. Tinzl M, Marberger M, Horvath S, Chypre C. DD3PCA3 RNA analysis in urine–a new perspective for detecting prostate cancer. Eur Urol. 2004;46:182–6. discussion 7.
80. Hessels D, van Gils MP, van Hooij O, et al. Predictive value of PCA3 in urinary sediments in determining clinico-pathological characteristics of prostate cancer. Prostate. 2010;70:10–6.
81. Hessels D, Klein Gunnewiek JM, van Oort I, et al. DD3(PCA3)-based molecular urine analysis for the diagnosis of prostate cancer. Eur Urol. 2003;44:8–15. discussion -6.
82. de Kok JB, Verhaegh GW, Roelofs RW, et al. DD3(PCA3), a very sensitive and specific marker to detect prostate tumors. Cancer Res. 2002;62:2695–8.
83. Crawford ED, Rove KO, Trabulsi EJ, et al. Diagnostic performance of PCA3 to detect prostate cancer in men with increased prostate specific antigen: a prospective study of 1,962 cases. J Urol. 2012;188:1726–31.
84. Vlaeminck-Guillem V, Ruffion A, Andre J, Devonec M, Paparel P. Urinary prostate cancer 3 test: toward the age of reason? Urology. 2010;75:447–53.
85. Auprich M, Bjartell A, Chun FK, et al. Contemporary role of prostate cancer antigen 3 in the management of prostate cancer. Eur Urol. 2011;60:1045–54.
86. van Gils MP, Hessels D, van Hooij O, et al. The time-resolved fluorescence-based PCA3 test on urinary sediments after digital rectal examination; a Dutch multicenter validation of the diagnostic performance. Clin Cancer Res. 2007;13:939–43.
87. Ankerst DP, Groskopf J, Day JR, et al. Predicting prostate cancer risk through incorporation of prostate cancer gene 3. J Urol. 2008;180:1303–8. discussion 8.
88. Perdona S, Cavadas V, Di Lorenzo G, et al. Prostate cancer detection in the "grey area" of prostate-specific antigen below 10 ng/ml: head-to-head comparison of the updated PCPT calculator and Chun's nomogram, two risk estimators incorporating prostate cancer antigen 3. Eur Urol. 2011;59:81–7.
89. Nakanishi H, Groskopf J, Fritsche HA, et al. PCA3 molecular urine assay correlates with prostate cancer tumor volume: implication in selecting candidates for active surveillance. J Urol. 2008;179:1804–9. discussion 9-10.
90. Whitman EJ, Groskopf J, Ali A, et al. PCA3 score before radical prostatectomy predicts extracapsular extension and tumor volume. J Urol. 2008;180:1975–8. discussion 8-9.
91. Attard G, Clark J, Ambroisine L, et al. Duplication of the fusion of TMPRSS2 to ERG sequences identifies fatal human prostate cancer. Oncogene. 2008;27:253–63.
92. Hermans KG, van der Korput HA, van Marion R, et al. Truncated ETV1, fused to novel tissue-specific genes, and full-length ETV1 in prostate cancer. Cancer Res. 2008;68:7541–9.
93. Hermans KG, Bressers AA, van der Korput HA, Dits NF, Jenster G, Trapman J. Two unique novel prostate-specific and androgen-regulated fusion partners of ETV4 in prostate cancer. Cancer Res. 2008;68:3094–8.
94. Mosquera JM, Perner S, Genega EM, et al. Characterization of TMPRSS2-ERG fusion high-grade prostatic intraepithelial neoplasia and potential clinical implications. Clin Cancer Res. 2008;14:3380–5.
95. Wang J, Cai Y, Yu W, Ren C, Spencer DM, Ittmann M. Pleiotropic biological activities of alternatively spliced TMPRSS2/ERG fusion gene transcripts. Cancer Res. 2008;68:8516–24.
96. Sun C, Dobi A, Mohamed A, et al. TMPRSS2-ERG fusion, a common genomic alteration in prostate cancer activates C-MYC and abrogates prostate epithelial differentiation. Oncogene. 2008; 27:5348–53.
97. Attard G, Sarker D, Reid A, Molife R, Parker C, de Bono JS. Improving the outcome of patients with castration-resistant prostate cancer through rational drug development. Br J Cancer. 2006;95:767–74.
98. Marcucci G, Baldus CD, Ruppert AS, et al. Overexpression of the ETS-related gene, ERG, predicts a worse outcome in acute myeloid leukemia with normal karyotype: a Cancer and Leukemia Group B study. J Clin Oncol. 2005;23:9234–42.
99. Attard G, Swennenhuis JF, Olmos D, et al. Characterization of ERG, AR and PTEN gene status in circulating tumor cells from patients with castration-resistant prostate cancer. Cancer Res. 2009;69:2912–8.
100. Attard G, Reid AH, Yap TA, et al. Phase I clinical trial of a selective inhibitor of CYP17, abiraterone acetate, confirms that

castration-resistant prostate cancer commonly remains hormone driven. J Clin Oncol. 2008;26:4563–71.
101. Chen Y, Sawyers CL, Scher HI. Targeting the androgen receptor pathway in prostate cancer. Curr Opin Pharmacol. 2008;8:440–8.
102. Brenner JC, Ateeq B, Li Y, et al. Mechanistic rationale for inhibition of poly(ADP-ribose) polymerase in ETS gene fusion-positive prostate cancer. Cancer Cell. 2011;19:664–78.
103. Yoshimoto M, Joshua AM, Cunha IW, et al. Absence of TMPRSS2:ERG fusions and PTEN losses in prostate cancer is associated with a favorable outcome. Mod Pathol. 2008;21:1451–60.
104. Hessels D, Smit FP, Verhaegh GW, Witjes JA, Cornel EB, Schalken JA. Detection of TMPRSS2-ERG fusion transcripts and prostate cancer antigen 3 in urinary sediments may improve diagnosis of prostate cancer. Clin Cancer Res. 2007;13:5103–8.
105. Tomlins SA, Aubin SM, Siddiqui J, et al. Urine TMPRSS2:ERG fusion transcript stratifies prostate cancer risk in men with elevated serum PSA. Sci Transl Med. 2011;3:94ra72.
106. Chaux A, Albadine R, Toubaji A, et al. Immunohistochemistry for ERG expression as a surrogate for TMPRSS2-ERG fusion detection in prostatic adenocarcinomas. Am J Surg Pathol. 2011;35:1014–20.
107. Park K, Tomlins SA, Mudaliar KM, et al. Antibody-based detection of ERG rearrangement-positive prostate cancer. Neoplasia. 2010;12:590–8.
108. van Leenders GJ, Boormans JL, Vissers CJ, et al. Antibody EPR3864 is specific for ERG genomic fusions in prostate cancer: implications for pathological practice. Mod Pathol. 2011;24:1128–38.
109. Furusato B, Tan SH, Young D, et al. ERG oncoprotein expression in prostate cancer: clonal progression of ERG-positive tumor cells and potential for ERG-based stratification. Prostate Cancer Prostatic Dis. 2010;13:228–37.
110. Mehra R, Tomlins SA, Shen R, et al. Comprehensive assessment of TMPRSS2 and ETS family gene aberrations in clinically localized prostate cancer. Mod Pathol. 2007;20:538–44.
111. Zhang S, Pavlovitz B, Tull J, Wang Y, Deng FM, Fuller C. Detection of TMPRSS2 gene deletions and translocations in carcinoma, intraepithelial neoplasia, and normal epithelium of the prostate by direct fluorescence in situ hybridization. Diagn Mol Pathol. 2010;19:151–6.
112. Yoshimoto M, Joshua AM, Chilton-Macneill S, et al. Three-color FISH analysis of TMPRSS2/ERG fusions in prostate cancer indicates that genomic microdeletion of chromosome 21 is associated with rearrangement. Neoplasia. 2006;8:465–9.
113. Wang J, Cai Y, Ren C, Ittmann M. Expression of variant TMPRSS2/ERG fusion messenger RNAs is associated with aggressive prostate cancer. Cancer Res. 2006;66:8347–51.
114. Soller MJ, Isaksson M, Elfving P, Soller W, Lundgren R, Panagopoulos I. Confirmation of the high frequency of the TMPRSS2/ERG fusion gene in prostate cancer. Genes Chromosomes Cancer. 2006;45:717–9.
115. Clark J, Merson S, Jhavar S, et al. Diversity of TMPRSS2-ERG fusion transcripts in the human prostate. Oncogene. 2007;26:2667–73.
116. Clark J, Attard G, Jhavar S, et al. Complex patterns of ETS gene alteration arise during cancer development in the human prostate. Oncogene. 2008;27:1993–2003.
117. Watson RW, Schalken JA. Future opportunities for the diagnosis and treatment of prostate cancer. Prostate Cancer Prostatic Dis. 2004;7 Suppl 1:S8–13.
118. Ishkanian AS, Mallof CA, Ho J, et al. High-resolution array CGH identifies novel regions of genomic alteration in intermediate-risk prostate cancer. Prostate. 2009;69:1091–100.
119. Fang Z, Soleymani L, Pampalakis G, et al. Direct profiling of cancer biomarkers in tumor tissue using a multiplexed nanostructured microelectrode integrated circuit. ACS Nano. 2009;3:3207–13.
120. Kawachi MH, Bahnson RR, Barry M, et al. NCCN clinical practice guidelines in oncology: prostate cancer early detection. J Natl Compr Canc Netw. 2010;8:240–62.
121. Mohler J, Bahnson RR, Boston B, et al. NCCN clinical practice guidelines in oncology: prostate cancer. J Natl Compr Canc Netw. 2010;8:162–200.
122. Mohler JL. The 2010 NCCN clinical practice guidelines in oncology on prostate cancer. J Natl Compr Canc Netw. 2010; 8:145.
123. Knezevic D, Goddard AD, Natraj N, et al. Analytical validation of the Oncotype DX prostate cancer assay—a clinical RT-PCR assay optimized for prostate needle biopsies. BMC Genomics. 2013;14:690.
124. Bishoff JT, Freedland SJ, Gerber L, et al. Prognostic utility of the cell cycle progression score generated from biopsy in men treated with prostatectomy. J Urol. 2014;192:409–14.
125. Freedland SJ, Gerber L, Reid J, et al. Prognostic utility of cell cycle progression score in men with prostate cancer after primary external beam radiation therapy. Int J Radiat Oncol Biol Phys. 2013;86:848–53.
126. Van Neste L, Bigley J, Toll A, et al. A tissue biopsy-based epigenetic multiplex PCR assay for prostate cancer detection. BMC Urol. 2012;12:16.
127. Stewart GD, Van Neste L, Delvenne P, et al. Clinical utility of an epigenetic assay to detect occult prostate cancer in histopathologically negative biopsies: results of the MATLOC study. J Urol. 2013;189:1110–6.
128. Partin AW, Van Neste L, Klein EA, et al. Clinical validation of an epigenetic assay to predict negative histopathological results in repeat prostate biopsies. J Urol. 2014;192:1081–7.
129. Alimonti A, Carracedo A, Clohessy JG, et al. Subtle variations in Pten dose determine cancer susceptibility. Nat Genet. 2010;42:454–8.
130. Yoshimoto M, Cunha IW, Coudry RA, et al. FISH analysis of 107 prostate cancers shows that PTEN genomic deletion is associated with poor clinical outcome. Br J Cancer. 2007;97:678–85.
131. Sircar K, Yoshimoto M, Monzon FA, et al. PTEN genomic deletion is associated with p-Akt and AR signalling in poorer outcome, hormone refractory prostate cancer. J Pathol. 2009;218:505–13.
132. Koksal IT, Dirice E, Yasar D, et al. The assessment of PTEN tumor suppressor gene in combination with Gleason scoring and serum PSA to evaluate progression of prostate carcinoma. Urol Oncol. 2004;22:307–12.
133. Koksal IT, Yasar D, Dirice E, et al. Differential PTEN protein expression profiles in superficial versus invasive bladder cancers. Urol Int. 2005;75:102–6.
134. Reid AH, Attard G, Ambroisine L, et al. Molecular characterisation of ERG, ETV1 and PTEN gene loci identifies patients at low and high risk of death from prostate cancer. Br J Cancer. 2010;102:678–84.
135. Bismar TA, Yoshimoto M, Duan Q, Liu S, Sircar K, Squire JA. Interactions and relationships of PTEN, ERG, SPINK1 and AR in castration-resistant prostate cancer. Histopathology. 2012;60:645–52.
136. Bismar TA, Yoshimoto M, Vollmer RT, et al. PTEN genomic deletion is an early event associated with ERG gene rearrangements in prostate cancer. BJU Int. 2011;107:477–85.
137. Rhodes DR, Sanda MG, Otte AP, Chinnaiyan AM, Rubin MA. Multiplex biomarker approach for determining risk of prostate-specific antigen-defined recurrence of prostate cancer. J Natl Cancer Inst. 2003;95:661–8.
138. Cooperberg MR, Carroll PR, Klotz L. Active surveillance for prostate cancer: progress and promise. J Clin Oncol. 2011; 29:3669–76.

139. van den Bergh RC, Ahmed HU, Bangma CH, Cooperberg MR, Villers A, Parker CC. Novel tools to improve patient selection and monitoring on active surveillance for low-risk prostate cancer: a systematic review. Eur Urol. 2014;65:1023–31.
140. Stephenson AJ, Scardino PT, Eastham JA, et al. Postoperative nomogram predicting the 10-year probability of prostate cancer recurrence after radical prostatectomy. J Clin Oncol. 2005;23:7005–12.
141. Kattan MW, Eastham JA, Stapleton AM, Wheeler TM, Scardino PT. A preoperative nomogram for disease recurrence following radical prostatectomy for prostate cancer. J Natl Cancer Inst. 1998;90:766–71.
142. Kattan MW, Scardino PT. Prediction of progression: nomograms of clinical utility. Clin Prostate Cancer. 2002;1:90–6.
143. Kattan MW, Scardino PT. Prostate cancer: nomograms and risk assessment models. J Natl Compr Canc Netw. 2003;1 Suppl 3:S-49–54.
144. Helgeson BE, Tomlins SA, Shah N, et al. Characterization of TMPRSS2:ETV5 and SLC45A3:ETV5 gene fusions in prostate cancer. Cancer Res. 2008;68(1):73–80.
145. Han B, Mehra R, Dhanasekaran SM, Yu J, et al. A fluorescence in situ hybridization screen for E26 transformation-specific aberrations: identification of DDX5-ETV4 fusion protein in prostate cancer. Cancer Res. 2008;68(18):7629–37.
146. Rickman DS, Pflueger D, Moss B, et al. SLC45A3-ELK4 is a novel and frequent erythroblast transformation-specific fusion transcript in prostate cancer. Cancer Res. 2009;69(7):2734–8.
147. Pflueger D, Rickman DS, Sboner A, et al. N-myc downstream regulated gene 1 (NDRG1) is fused to ERG in prostate cancer. Neoplasia. 2009;11(8):804–11.
148. Palanisamy N, Ateeq B, Kalyana-Sundaram S, et al. Rearrangements of the RAF kinase pathway in prostate cancer, gastric cancer and melanoma. Nat Med. 2010;16(7):793–8.

Thyroid Cancer

36

Marina N. Nikiforova and Yuri E. Nikiforov

Abstract

Thyroid cancer is the most common type of endocrine malignancy. Initiation and progression of thyroid cancer involves multiple genetic and epigenetic alterations, of which mutations leading to the activation of the MAPK and PI3K/PTEN/AKT signaling pathways are crucial for tumor initiation and progression. Common mutations found in thyroid cancer are point mutations of the *BRAF* and *RAS* genes, as well as *RET/PTC* and *PAX8/PPARG* chromosomal rearrangements. More recently, a number of other mutations have been characterized, which occur in this cancer type with significantly lower frequency, but are associated with specific phenotypic and biological properties. These somatic mutations are useful diagnostic and prognostic markers for thyroid cancer and are being incorporated into clinical practice, offering a valuable tool for management of patients with thyroid nodules and cancer.

Keywords

Thyroid cancer • Thyroid nodules • FNA cytology • Molecular diagnostics • BRAF • RAS • RET/PTC • ALK

Introduction

Thyroid cancer is the most common endocrine malignancy, with a steadily growing incidence in the USA and other industrialized countries [1, 2]. The vast majority of thyroid tumors originate from follicular epithelial cells. The follicular cell-derived cancers are further subdivided into well-differentiated papillary carcinoma and follicular carcinoma, poorly differentiated carcinoma, and anaplastic (undifferentiated) carcinoma (Fig. 36.1) [3, 4]. Papillary carcinoma is the most common thyroid malignancy (80–85 %). In addition to classic-type papillary carcinoma, common histopathologic variants are microcarcinoma, follicular variant, and tall cell variant. Follicular carcinomas account for approximately 15 % of thyroid cancers and are subdivided into conventional type and oncocytic (Hürthle) type. Follicular adenoma is a benign tumor that is considered a precursor for follicular carcinomas (Fig. 36.1). Less differentiated thyroid cancers, i.e., poorly differentiated carcinoma and anaplastic carcinoma, can develop de novo, although many arise through the process of stepwise dedifferentiation of papillary and follicular carcinomas (Fig. 36.1). Medullary thyroid carcinoma originates from thyroid parafollicular or C cells, accounts for 3–5 % of thyroid cancers, can be a manifestation of an inherited genetic disease, and, therefore, is not discussed in this chapter.

Thyroid cancer occurs in thyroid nodules. Thyroid nodules are common in adults, particularly with increased age, and are typically detected by palpation or imaging [5–7]. However, most nodules are benign, and the rate of cancer in medically evaluated thyroid nodules ranges from 5–15 % [7–9]. A clinical challenge is to accurately diagnose cancer in these nodules and to avoid unnecessary thyroid surgery for benign disease. Sampling of thyroid nodules using fine needle aspiration (FNA) under ultrasound guidance followed by subsequent cytologic examination is the most accurate

M.N. Nikiforova, M.D. • Y.E. Nikiforov, M.D., Ph.D. (✉)
Department of Pathology and Laboratory Medicine, Division of Molecular and Genomic Pathology, University of Pittsburgh Medical Center, 3477 Euler Way, Pittsburgh, PA 15213, USA
e-mail: nikiforovye@upmc.edu

D.G.B. Leonard (ed.), *Molecular Pathology in Clinical Practice*, DOI 10.1007/978-3-319-19674-9_36

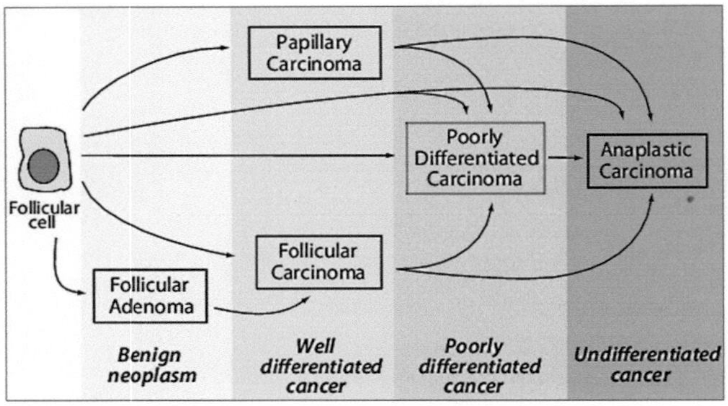

Figure 36.1 Pathways for thyroid cancer development from thyroid follicular cells

and widely used diagnostic tool at this time. FNA provides a definitive diagnosis of a malignant or benign nodule in the majority of cases. However, in about 25 % of nodules, FNA cytology cannot reliably exclude cancer, and such cases are placed in one of the indeterminate categories, hampering clinical management of these patients [6, 8, 10, 11]. By the current Bethesda System for Reporting Thyroid Cytopathology, the indeterminate categories include three specific cytologic diagnoses: atypia of undetermined significance/follicular lesion of undetermined significance (AUS/FLUS); follicular or oncocytic (Hürthle cell) neoplasm/suspicious for follicular or oncocytic (Hürthle cell) neoplasm (FN/SFN); and suspicious for malignant cells (SMC), with a predicted probability of cancer of 5–15 %, 15–30 %, and 60–75 %, respectively [12, 13]. Because FNA is unable to provide a definitive diagnosis for these indeterminate nodules, most patients with indeterminate cytology undergo diagnostic surgery to establish a histopathologic diagnosis. However, only 10–40 % of surgically resected indeterminate thyroid nodules are malignant [12]. The unneeded operations, with their attendant expenses and risks, may be avoided if the FNA procedure could reliably establish the presurgical diagnosis of a benign nodule. Additionally, since the standard of care is to offer a second surgery for total thyroidectomy if the diagnostic lobectomy confirms a cancer, a more optimal surgical management would be a single total thyroidectomy procedure that is planned when the diagnosis of cancer is established preoperatively.

Although well-differentiated thyroid cancer is a disease with an overall favorable outcome, some tumors entail a substantially worse prognosis and have to be treated more aggressively [14–16]. Multiple prognostic systems for differentiated thyroid cancer based on demographic and pathologic factors exist [17], but none of the systems accurately stratify thyroid tumors into appropriate risk categories. The rapidly expanding knowledge of the molecular genetics of thyroid cancer is being translated into clinical practice, offering significant improvement in the accuracy of the preoperative diagnosis of thyroid cancer and better tumor prognosis.

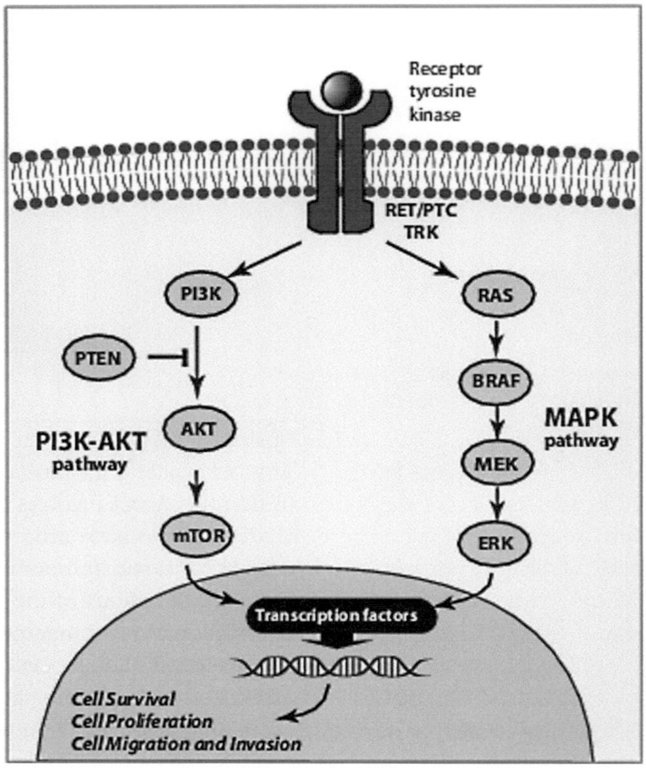

Figure 36.2 Thyroid cancer development and progression typically involves the activation of the mitogen-activated protein kinase (MAPK) and PI3K/PTEN/AKT signaling pathways. In thyroid cancer, the MAPK pathway is activated via point mutations of the *BRAF* or *RAS* gene, or chromosomal rearrangements involving the *RET* gene (known as RET/PTC rearrangement) or the *NTRK1* gene (TRK rearrangement). These non-overlapping genetic events are commonly found in well-differentiated papillary carcinomas and in some follicular carcinomas. Mutations in the genes coding for the effectors of the PI3K/PTEN/AKT pathway, such as *PIK3CA* (encoding a subunit of PI3K), *AKT1*, and *PTEN*, are found more frequently in follicular carcinomas and in more advanced and less-well-differentiated cancers

Molecular Basis of Disease

Thyroid cancer initiation and progression occurs through gradual accumulation of genetic and epigenetic alterations, including activating and inactivating somatic mutations, alteration in gene expression patterns, and miRNA dysregulation. Most mutations in thyroid cancer involve the effectors of the mitogen-activated protein kinase (MAPK) signaling pathway and the PI3K/PTEN/AKT signaling pathway (Fig. 36.2). Critical genes are frequently mutated in thyroid cancer via two distinct molecular mechanisms, point mutation or chromosomal rearrangement. MAPK activation frequently occurs via mutations in the cell membrane receptor tyrosine kinases RET and NTRK1, which are involved in chromosomal rearrangements, or through intracellular signal transducers BRAF and RAS, which are typically activated as a result of a point mutation. These mutually exclusive mutations occur in approximately 70 % of papillary thyroid carcinomas

(Table 36.1) [18–21]. In follicular carcinomas, mutations in the *RAS* genes are the most common, followed by *PAX8/PPARG* rearrangement. Thyroid cancer progression and dedifferentiation involves a number of additional mutations that affect the PI3K/PTEN/AKT signaling pathway and other cell signaling pathways (Table 36.1).

BRAF Mutations

BRAF is a serine-threonine kinase that is activated by RAS binding and protein recruitment to the cell membrane. BRAF phosphorylation leads to activation of MEK and other downstream targets along the MAPK signaling pathway (Fig. 36.2). In thyroid cancer, BRAF can be activated by point mutations, small in-frame deletions or insertions, or chromosomal rearrangement. The most common mechanism of activation is a point mutation of a thymine to adenine substitution at nucleotide 1799 (c.T1799A), resulting in a substitution of valine to glutamate at residue 600 (p.V600E) [19, 22]. The *BRAF* V600E mutation constitutes 95–99 % of all *BRAF* mutations found in thyroid cancer. Other alterations are *BRAF* p.K601E point mutation and small in-frame insertions or deletions surrounding codon 600 [23–26], as well as *AKAP9/BRAF* rearrangement [27]. The *BRAF* rearrangement seen in thyroid carcinomas is a paracentric inversion of chromosome 7q leading to the fusion of 3′ portion of the *BRAF* gene to the 5′ portion of the *AKAP9* gene and is more common in papillary carcinomas associated with radiation exposure [27]. More recently, several other fusion partners of *BRAF* have been identified in papillary carcinomas [28].

BRAF V600E is the most common genetic alteration in papillary thyroid carcinoma and is found in approximately 45 % of papillary thyroid tumors (Table 36.1) [29]. *BRAF* V600E also occurs in 10–20 % of poorly differentiated carcinomas and 30–40 % of anaplastic carcinomas arising from papillary carcinoma [30–33]. This mutation is typically found in papillary carcinomas with classic papillary histology and in the tall cell variant and is rare in the follicular variant of papillary carcinoma [18, 29]. In contrast, tumors with the *BRAF* K601E mutation are typically the follicular variant of papillary carcinoma [26]. *BRAF* V600E is not found in follicular carcinomas and benign thyroid nodules and therefore, among primary thyroid lesions, represents a specific marker of papillary carcinoma and related tumor types.

RAS Mutations

Point mutations of *RAS* are found in follicular carcinomas, papillary carcinomas, and follicular adenomas. Human *HRAS*, *KRAS*, and *NRAS* genes encode highly related G proteins that reside at the inner surface of the cell membrane and propagate signals arising from cell membrane receptors and G-protein-coupled receptors along the MAPK, PI3K/AKT, and other signaling pathways. Activating point mutations typically affect codons 12, 13, and 61 of the *RAS* genes. In thyroid cancer, *NRAS* codon 61 and *HRAS* codon 61 mutations are most common, followed by *KRAS* codon 12 and 13, although mutations have been found in different hot spots of all three genes. *RAS* mutations are present in 10–20 % of papillary carcinomas, 40–50 % of follicular carcinomas, and 20–40 % of poorly differentiated and anaplastic carcinomas [34–40]. Among papillary carcinomas, virtually all tumors with a *RAS* mutation belong to the follicular variant [18, 31]. *RAS* mutations also occur in 20–40 % of benign follicular adenomas [35, 36]. The finding of *RAS* mutations in benign adenomas as well as in follicular-patterned carcinomas suggests that *RAS* mutation positive follicular adenomas may serve as a precursor for *RAS* mutation positive follicular carcinoma and follicular variant of papillary carcinomas. Furthermore, *RAS* mutation may predispose well-differentiated cancers to dedifferentiation and anaplastic transformation [41–44]. Therefore, detection of this mutation at early stages may guide the therapy to prevent tumor progression.

RET/PTC Rearrangements

The *RET/PTC* chromosomal rearrangement is a characteristic of papillary thyroid cancer [45]. The rearrangement forms a fusion between the 3′ portion of the *RET* receptor tyrosine kinase gene and the 5′ portion of different partner genes. All chimeric genes contain the intact tyrosine kinase domain of *RET* fused to an active promoter of another gene that drives the expression and ligand-independent dimerization of the RET/PTC protein, leading to chronic stimulation of MAPK signaling (Fig. 36.2) [46–48]. The two most common fusions, *RET/PTC1* and *RET/PTC3*, are paracentric inversions since both *RET* and its respective fusion partners, *CCDC6* (*H4*) and *NCOA4* (*ELE1*), reside on the long arm of chromosome 10. In contrast, *RET/PTC2* and nine more recently discovered types of *RET/PTC* fusions are all interchromosomal rearrangements formed by *RET* fusion to genes located on different chromosomes (Table 36.2) [49].

RET/PTC is found in approximately 10–20 % of adult sporadic papillary carcinomas [18, 49] but occurs with higher incidence in patients with a history of radiation exposure (50–80 %) and in papillary carcinomas from children and young adults (40–70 %) [50–52]. The distribution of *RET/PTC* rearrangement within the tumor may be quite heterogeneous, varying from involving almost all neoplastic cells (clonal *RET/PTC*) to being detected only in a small fraction of tumor cells (non-clonal *RET/PTC*) [53, 54]. Although a low level of *RET/PTC* rearrangement has been

Table 36.1 Average prevalence of mutations in thyroid cancer

Tumor type	Genes	Prevalence of common mutations (%)
Papillary carcinoma		
	BRAF	40–45
	RET/PTC	10–20
	RAS	10–20
	NTRK1	<5
	NTRK3	<5
	ALK	<5
Follicular carcinoma		
	RAS	40–50
	PAX8-PPARG	30–35
	PIK3CA	<10
	PTEN	<10
Poorly differentiated carcinoma		
	RAS	20–40
	TP53	20–30
	CTNNB1	<10
	BRAF	10–20
	AKT1	5–10
	PIK3CA	5–10
Anaplastic (undifferentiated) carcinoma		
	TP53	50–80
	CTNNB1	50–60
	RAS	20–40
	BRAF	20–40
	PIK3CA	10–20
	PTEN	5–15
	AKT1	5–10

reported in adenomas and other benign thyroid lesions in studies that used ultrasensitive detection techniques, the clonal *RET/PTC* (i.e., rearrangement that is found in most cells within the tumor) is specific for papillary thyroid carcinoma [49, 53]. Proper techniques for the clinically relevant detection of *RET/PTC* are discussed later in the chapter. Among different rearrangement types, *RET/PTC1* is typically the most common, followed by *RET/PTC3*, whereas *RET/PTC2* and other novel rearrangement types are rare (Table 36.2) [49].

NTRK1 and *NTRK3* Rearrangements

Chromosomal rearrangements involving the *NTRK1* and *NTRK3* receptor tyrosine kinase genes also occur in papillary thyroid carcinomas, although with a significantly lower prevalence. The *NTRK1* gene resides on chromosome 1q22 and can be fused to at least three different partner genes located on the same or different chromosomes, leading to the *TRK* rearrangement (Table 36.2) [55–57]. *NTRK* rearrangements occur in less than 5 % of papillary thyroid carcinomas [28]. Fusions involving another *NTRK* family gene, *NTRK3*, also occur in papillary thyroid cancer. *ETV6-NTRK3* fusions occur in approximately 2 % of sporadic papillary thyroid cancers and with a significantly higher prevalence (approximately 15 %) in tumors associated with exposure to ionizing radiation [28, 58].

ALK Rearrangements

Recently, rearrangements involving the *ALK* gene were identified in thyroid cancer. The most common fusion partner of *ALK* is the striatin (*STRN*) gene [59]. *ALK* fusions are found in 1–2 % of papillary carcinomas and with higher frequency (5–10 %) in poorly differentiated and anaplastic thyroid cancers [28, 59].

PPARG Rearrangements

PAX8/PPARG rearrangement is a t(2;3)(q13;p25) translocation that leads to fusion between a portion of the *PAX8* gene, which encodes a paired domain transcription factor, and the peroxisome proliferator-activated receptor (*PPARG*) gene [60]. *PAX8/PPARG* rearrangement leads to strong overexpression of the PPARG protein, although the mechanisms of cell transformation induced by this genetic event are not understood. Several types of *PAX8/PPARG* rearrangement occur, formed by the fusion of four *PAX8* gene regions (exons 1–7, 1–8, 1–9, or 1–7 plus 9) to *PPARG* exons 1–6. These different *PAX8* gene region fusions are apparently a result of the alternate splicing involving exons 8 and 9 known to affect the wild-type *PAX8*. The most commonly expressed *PAX8/PPARG* transcripts in follicular thyroid carcinomas contain exons 1–9 and 1–7 plus 9 of *PAX8*. In addition to *PAX8/PPARG*, the *PPARG* gene can fuse with the *CREB3L2* gene; however, this type of fusion is rare (Table 36.2) [61].

PAX8/PPARG is characteristically found in 30–35 % of follicular thyroid carcinoma [62–64]. This rearrangement also occurs in a small proportion (1–5 %) of the follicular variant of papillary carcinomas and in some (2–13 %) follicular adenomas [62–66]. Follicular adenomas with a *PAX8/PPARG* rearrangement typically have a thick capsule and show the immunohistochemical profile characteristic of thyroid cancer, suggesting preinvasive (in situ) follicular carcinomas or malignant tumors where invasion was overlooked during histological examination [63]. *PAX8/PPARG* rearrangements and *RAS* point mutations rarely occur in the same tumor, suggesting that they represent distinct oncogenic pathways in the development of follicular thyroid carcinoma [63].

Table 36.2 Common chromosomal alterations in thyroid cancer

	Tumor type	Fusion name	Fusion genes	Chromosomal alterations	Prevalence of subtypes
RET Fusions	PTC	*RET/PTC1*	*RET/CCDC6(H4)*	inv(10)(q11.2;q21)	60–70 %
		RET/PTC2	*RET/RIα*	t(10;17)(q11.2;q23)	<5 %
		RET/PTC3	*RET/NCOA4(ELE1)*	inv(10)(q11.2)	20–30 %
		RET/PTC4	*RET/NCOA4 (ELE1)*	inv(10)(q11.2), v.2	<1 %
		RET/PTC5	*RET/GOLGA5*	t(10;14) (q11.2;q?)	<1 %
		RET/PTC6	*RET/HTIF1*	t(7;10)(q32;q11.2)	<1 %
		RET/PTC7	*RET/RFG7*	t(1;10)(p13;q11.2)	<1 %
			RET/ELKS	t(10;12)(q11.2;p13)	<1 %
			RET/KTN1	t(10;14)(q11.2;q22.1)	<1 %
			RET/RFG9	t(10;18)(q11.2;q21-22)	<1 %
			RET/PCM1	t(8;10)(p21-22;q11.2)	<1 %
			RET/RFP	t(6;10)(p21;q11.2)	<1 %
			RET/HOOK3	t(8;10)(p11.21;q11.2)	<1 %
NTRK Fusions	PTC		*NTRK1/TPM3*	inv(1)(q23.1;q21.3)	Equally prevalent
			NTRK1/TPR	inv(1)(q23.1;q25)	
			NTRK1/TFG	t(1;3)(q21;q11)	
			ETV6-NTRK3	t(12;15)(p13;q25)	
ALK Fusions	PTC		*STRN/ALK*	inv(2)(p22;p23)	70 %
			EML4/ALK	inv(2)(p21;p23)	30 %
PPARG Fusions	FTC, PTC, FV		*PAX8/PPARG*	t(2;3)(q13;p25.2)	98 %
			CREB3L2/PPARG	t(7;3)(q33;p25.2)	2 %

FTC follicular thyroid carcinoma, *FV* follicular variant, *PTC* papillary thyroid carcinoma

TERT Mutations

Mutations of the telomerase reverse transcriptase (*TERT*) gene promoter were first described in melanoma at two specific hot spots (chr5:1295228C→T, termed C228T, and chr5:1295250C→T, termed C250T) and lead to increased transcriptional activity and expression of the gene [67, 68]. The C228T and C250T *TERT* promoter mutations occur with variable prevalence in different types of thyroid cancer and have strong association with tumor recurrence, distant metastasis, and tumor-related mortality [69–72]. *TERT* mutations are not found in benign thyroid nodules and therefore are useful diagnostically; they can also play a role in prognostication of thyroid cancer.

Mutations Associated with Tumor Dedifferentiation

Thyroid cancer progression and dedifferentiation is more frequent in tumors with *BRAF* and *RAS* mutations and typically involves the accumulation of additional genetic alterations (Table 36.1). Point mutations affecting the *TP53* gene are very common in anaplastic carcinomas (50–80 % of cases) [73–76] but less frequent in poorly differentiated carcinomas and extremely rare in well-differentiated thyroid cancer. *TP53* mutations are most common in exons 5–8 and lead to loss of function of this important cell cycle regulator. The *CTNNB1* gene frequently mutates in anaplastic carcinoma and encodes β-catenin that is involved in cell adhesion and the wingless (Wnt) signaling. Point mutations in exon 3 of *CTNNB1* occur in up to 60 % of anaplastic carcinomas and with lower prevalence in poorly differentiated thyroid carcinomas [77, 78]. In addition, mutations in *PIK3CA*, *PTEN*, and *AKT1* genes are found in anaplastic and poorly differentiated carcinomas, but they are less common [33, 79–82].

Gene Expression and miRNA Expression

Thyroid papillary carcinomas and other types of thyroid cancer have distinct alterations in gene expression [21, 83–86]. Gene expression changes include downregulation of genes responsible for specialized thyroid function such as thyroid hormone synthesis, upregulation of many genes involved in cell adhesion, motility, cell-cell interaction, and different patterns of deregulation of genes coding for cytokines and other proteins involved in inflammation and immune response. Among papillary carcinomas, different mRNA expression profiles correlate with classic papillary histology, follicular variant, and tall cell variant [83, 87]. Moreover, presence of *BRAF*, *RAS, RET/PTC*, and *NTRK1* mutations correlates with different patterns of gene expression, providing a molecular basis for distinct phenotypic and biologic features associated with each mutation type [21, 83].

Many miRNAs are deregulated in thyroid cancer [88–91]. Generally, miRNA expression profiles are different between papillary carcinoma, follicular carcinoma, and other types of thyroid tumors [92]. Several specific miRNAs, such as miR-146b, miR-221, and miR-222, have increased expression in papillary carcinomas and may play a role in the development of these tumors [89, 91, 92]. Possible target genes for these miRNAs are the regulator of the cell cycle *p27(Kip1)* gene and the thyroid hormone receptor (*THRB*) gene [93, 94]. Several abnormally expressed miRNAs were found in follicular carcinomas (miR-197, miR-346, miR-155, miR-224) [90, 95] and anaplastic carcinomas (miR-30d, miR-125b, miR-26a, and miR-30a-5p) [96].

Clinical Utility of Testing

Preoperative Diagnosis of Thyroid Cancer

Molecular markers are helpful in improving the preoperative diagnosis of cancer in thyroid nodules. Despite the high diagnostic value of FNA cytology, it cannot reliably diagnose cancer in 20–30 % of nodules, and such cases are considered as indeterminate for malignancy. The inability to rule out cancer in these nodules leads to diagnostic lobectomy for most of these patients, although most surgically removed thyroid nodules are benign [12]. Additionally, those patients that are found to have cancer on surgery have to undergo a second surgery to complete thyroidectomy. Both the unnecessary surgeries and two-step surgical management can be avoided with more accurate preoperative diagnosis of cancer. The current American Thyroid Association's management guidelines recommend testing for mutational markers for nodules with indeterminate FNA cytology to help guide clinical management [97].

Mutational markers that have been most extensively validated and clinically used for preoperative diagnosis of thyroid cancer in FNA samples include *BRAF* and *RAS* point mutations and *RET/PTC*, *PAX8/PPARG*, and *NTRK1* rearrangements [98–101]. Finding of any of these mutations in thyroid FNA samples is a strong predictor of malignancy in thyroid nodules irrespective of the cytological diagnosis [98–100]. *BRAF* mutation has been studied most extensively, and in a meta-analysis of 22 studies of thyroid FNA samples, *BRAF* mutation correlated with malignant outcome in 99.3 % of cases [102]. The presence of a *RET/PTC* or *PAX8/PPARG* rearrangement also correlates with malignancy in close to 100 % of cases. Therefore, patients with these mutations would be candidates for total thyroidectomy irrespective of the cytologic diagnosis (Fig. 36.3). This would eliminate the need for intraoperative pathology consultation and subsequent second surgery for complete thyroidectomy, reducing costs and additional morbidity. Detection of a *RAS* mutation, which is the second most common mutation after *BRAF*, conferred a 74–87 % probability of malignancy [98, 99, 103]. Importantly, *RAS* mutations are found in tumors which are difficult to diagnose by cytology alone, i.e., follicular variant of papillary carcinoma and follicular carcinoma [104]. The remaining *RAS*-positive nodules are diagnosed as a benign follicular adenoma, which is most likely a precursor lesion for follicular carcinoma [63]. Therefore, surgical removal of follicular adenomas that carry this oncogenic mutation by lobectomy may be considered as justifiable to prevent tumor progression.

Testing for a seven-gene panel (*BRAF*, *NRAS*, *HRAS*, *KRAS*, *RET/PTC1*, *RET/PTC3*, and *PAX8/PPARG*) is particularly helpful in nodules with indeterminate cytology. In a prospective study of 1,056 consecutive thyroid FNA samples with indeterminate cytology, detection of any mutation in specific categories of indeterminate cytology, i.e., AUS/FLUS, FN/SFN, and SMC, conferred a risk of histologic malignancy in 88 %, 87 %, and 95 % of nodules, respectively [103]. The risk of cancer in mutation-negative nodules was 6 % in the AUS/FLUS group, 14 % in FN/SFN, and 28 % in SMC [103]. The clinical algorithm outlined in Fig. 36.3 recommends that any positive result in the mutational panel is an indication for total thyroidectomy in all categories of indeterminate cytology as the initial surgical approach [103]. This avoids a repeat of FNA and proceeds with optimal surgical management without delay. This clinical approach also eliminates the need for the current two-step surgery, i.e., diagnostic lobectomy followed by completion thyroidectomy for most patients with malignant nodules. In a series of 471 patients with thyroid nodules that had indeterminate cytology (AUS/FLUS or FN/SFN), patients with no access to mutation testing were 2.5-fold more likely to require a two-stage surgery [105]. A mutation-negative result of the seven-gene panel does not eliminate the risk of cancer, as expected based on its sensitivity of approximately 70 %. Therefore, diagnostic lobectomy is justified as the initial surgical intervention for mutation-negative nodules with FN/SFN and SMC cytology, whereas conservative management with ultrasound follow-up and repeat FNA can be considered for nodules with AUS/FLUS cytology (Fig. 36.3). Although larger gene panels are available, even the seven-gene panel, when applied routinely to thyroid FNA samples with indeterminate cytology, leads to an overall cost saving for patients with thyroid nodules due to the up-front offering of optimal surgical management [106].

The expansion of knowledge on driver mutations in thyroid cancer and the availability of new high-throughput tech-

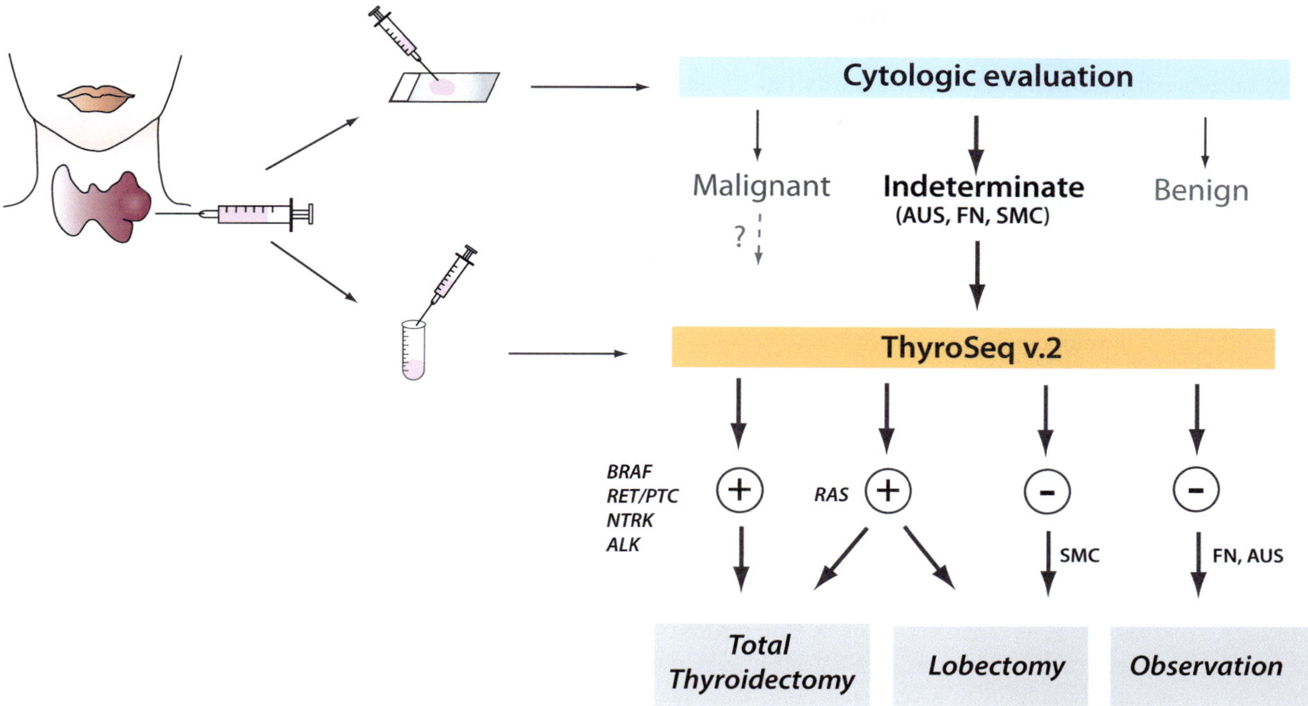

Figure 36.3 Clinical management of patients with thyroid nodules based on the combination of cytological examination and ThyroSeq v.2 mutational analysis of fine needle aspiration (FNA) samples. Molecular testing is particularly helpful for nodules with indeterminate cytology. Due to a high risk of cancer in nodules with *BRAF* mutations or *RET/PTC*, *PAX8/PPARG*, and *TRK* rearrangement, surgical treatment can proceed directly to total thyroidectomy. *RAS* mutations confer a 70–80 % risk of cancer, and these patients may benefit from either total thyroidectomy or lobectomy, depending on the additional clinical and imaging findings. Nodules without mutations found on ThyroSeq v.2 panel that have a cytologic diagnosis of follicular neoplasm/suspicious for follicular neoplasm (FN/SFN) or atypia of undetermined significance/follicular lesion of undetermined significance (AUS/FLUS) have a 4–5 % residual probability of cancer and may be followed conservatively. Nodules with suspicious for malignant cells (SMC) cytology and negative for mutations have approximately 20 % residual risk of cancer and should be managed by lobectomy.

nologies for simultaneous detection of multiple genetic mutations provided the basis for expanding gene panels for thyroid FNA samples. A 12-gene panel of selected gene regions from *AKT1*, *BRAF*, *CTNNB1*, *GNAS*, *PIK3CA*, *TP53*, *TSHR*, *PTEN*, *HRAS*, *KRAS*, *NRAS*, and *RET* (e.g., ThyroSeq [107]) utilizes next generation sequencing (NGS) to expand the original seven-gene panel and test for mutations in additional genes implicated in thyroid tumors. Detection of additional mutations together with higher sensitivity of detecting all mutations offered increased test performance. A study on 228 thyroid nodule samples including 51 FNA samples showed accurate detection of multiple mutations with a sensitivity of 3–5 % [107]. Common *BRAF* and *RAS* mutations were identified at low level in 27 tumors by NGS, which were not detected by the Sanger sequencing. This indicates that NGS-based panels not only can assess additional genes and hot spots mutations in a single test but also detect common driver mutations at a higher rate, thereby increasing the sensitivity and negative predictive value (NPV) of cancer detection in thyroid nodules [107]. Although most thyroid tumors had a single oncogenic mutation, this panel identified 2–3 mutations in each of the nine tumors, most of which presented at a higher stage, with dedifferentiation on histopathology [107]. As a result, identification of multiple mutations may be used to preoperatively identify those patients that need a significantly more aggressive treatment plan to maximize the chances for disease cure.

Commercially available NGS gene panels, such as AmpliSeq, contain many of the genes important to thyroid carcinogenesis. One study analyzed 34 indeterminate FNA samples using DNA obtained from cell blocks or from stained smears and tested them for mutations in 50 genes (AmpliSeq panel) [108]. Mutations in *BRAF*, *NRAS*, *KRAS*, and *PTEN* were detected in these samples, and the presence of a mutation in any of these genes was a strong indicator of cancer. In this study, the residual risk of cancer in nodules with indeterminate cytology and a negative molecular test result was 8 %.

Expansion of the gene panels to include additional and more recently discovered point mutations and gene fusions further increases the sensitivity and overall performance of gene tests for cancer diagnosis in thyroid nodules. An NGS gene panel that includes 56 genes and gene fusions (ThyroSeq®

v.2, UPMC/CBLPath, Rye Brook, NY) was validated with 143 thyroid nodules with FN/SFN cytology and known surgical outcome and showed both high sensitivity (90 %) and specificity (93 %) for cancer detection, with the NPV of 96 % [109]. Based on the high sensitivity and specificity, the NPV and positive predictive value (PPV) are expected to remain high in a broad range of cancer prevalence in the tested population.

Another approach to cancer detection in thyroid nodules is through the analysis of gene expression changes associated with cancer development. A commercial test, known as Afirma Thyroid FNA Analysis (Veracyte, South San Francisco, CA), utilizes the mRNA expression profiles of 142 genes to classify indeterminate thyroid nodules into a benign or suspicious category using a proprietary algorithm [110, 111]. This test was validated in a multi-institutional prospective double-blind study that included 265 nodules with indeterminate cytology [111]. The study showed high NPV in nodules with AUS/FLUS (95 %) and FN/SFN (94 %) cytology, whereas the PPV remained low (38 % for AUS/FLUS and 37 % for FN/SFN) [111]. High NPV suggests that this test is particularly helpful as a "rule-out" test, thereby helping to avoid unnecessary surgeries [112, 113].

Prognostic and Treatment Implications

Among prognostic markers, one of the best studied is the *BRAF* V600E mutation. *BRAF* V600E is associated with poor prognostic factors in papillary thyroid cancer such as extrathyroidal invasion, lymph node metastases, and tumor recurrence (reviewed in Ref. 114). In thyroid FNA specimens, preoperative testing that identifies a *BRAF* V600E mutation may be associated with disease persistence and recurrence [14], although some studies did not find such association [115–117]. A meta-analysis of multiple studies encompassing almost 2,500 patients demonstrated that a *BRAF* V600E mutation was significantly associated with tumor recurrence or persistent disease, which was found in 25 % of tumors with a *BRAF* V600E mutation compared to 13 % of *BRAF* mutation-negative tumors [118]. In addition, a large, multicenter study of 1,849 patients found the presence of the *BRAF* V600E mutation to be significantly associated with increased mortality from papillary thyroid cancer [119]. The overall mortality was 5 % in patients with a *BRAF* V600E mutation and 1 % in patients with a *BRAF* mutation-negative tumor. The results of these studies indicate that *BRAF* V600E is overall a sensitive but not specific marker of unfavorable outcome.

The presence of multiple driver mutations in thyroid cancer is associated with more aggressive tumor behavior. Coexisting mutations in the early driver genes, such as *BRAF* or *RAS*, with mutations in *PIK3CA*, *AKT1*, or *TP53* in the same tumor occur in poorly differentiated and anaplastic tumors [79, 81, 120]. More recently, an NGS-based mutation analysis demonstrated that approximately 4 % of well-differentiated papillary cancers have more than one mutation, and these tumors are aggressive and typically present with distant metastases [107].

TP53 mutation is a well-characterized genetic event governing thyroid tumor dedifferentiation and is found with high frequency in poorly differentiated and anaplastic thyroid cancer [73, 74]. However, *TP53* mutation also occurs in some well-differentiated cancers such as papillary thyroid carcinoma and oncocytic follicular carcinoma [107]. Well-differentiated cancers carrying a *TP53* mutation may have greater tumor dedifferentiation and a more aggressive clinical course.

Another prognostic molecular marker for thyroid cancer is a *TERT* mutation. The C228T and C250T mutations have a significantly higher prevalence in aggressive thyroid tumors including widely invasive oncocytic (Hürthle cell) carcinoma and anaplastic thyroid carcinoma [69–72]. In the largest study of thyroid cancer reported to date, *TERT* promoter mutations were an independent risk factor for persistent disease, distant metastases, and disease-specific mortality for well-differentiated thyroid cancer and separately for papillary carcinoma and follicular carcinoma [72]. Overall, testing for specific mutations and their combinations may provide important prognostic information and accurately identify patients who may benefit from more extensive initial thyroid surgery to prevent tumor recurrence and from more frequent monitoring of disease recurrence.

Patients with advanced thyroid cancer carrying activating mutations in the MAPK and PI3K pathways may benefit from treatment with tyrosine kinase inhibitors (sorafenib, vandetanib, axitinib, sunitinib) [121]. Also, selective inhibitors of the V600E mutant BRAF kinase (vemurafenib, PLX4032) showed promising early results in clinical trials, as well as inhibitors of ALK and NTRK kinases.

Available Assays

Testing for Mutations

For preoperative diagnosis of thyroid cancer, FNA samples can be tested for a shorter or broader panel of mutations. Those should contain most frequently occurring alterations including point mutations (*BRAF*, *HRAS*, *NRAS*, *KRAS*) and chromosomal rearrangements (*RET/PTC1*, *RET/PTC3*, *PAX8/PPARG*).

Detection of point mutations can be performed using many different methods, including Sanger sequencing, real-time PCR, pyrosequencing, allele-specific PCR, snapshot array, or restriction fragment polymorphism analysis

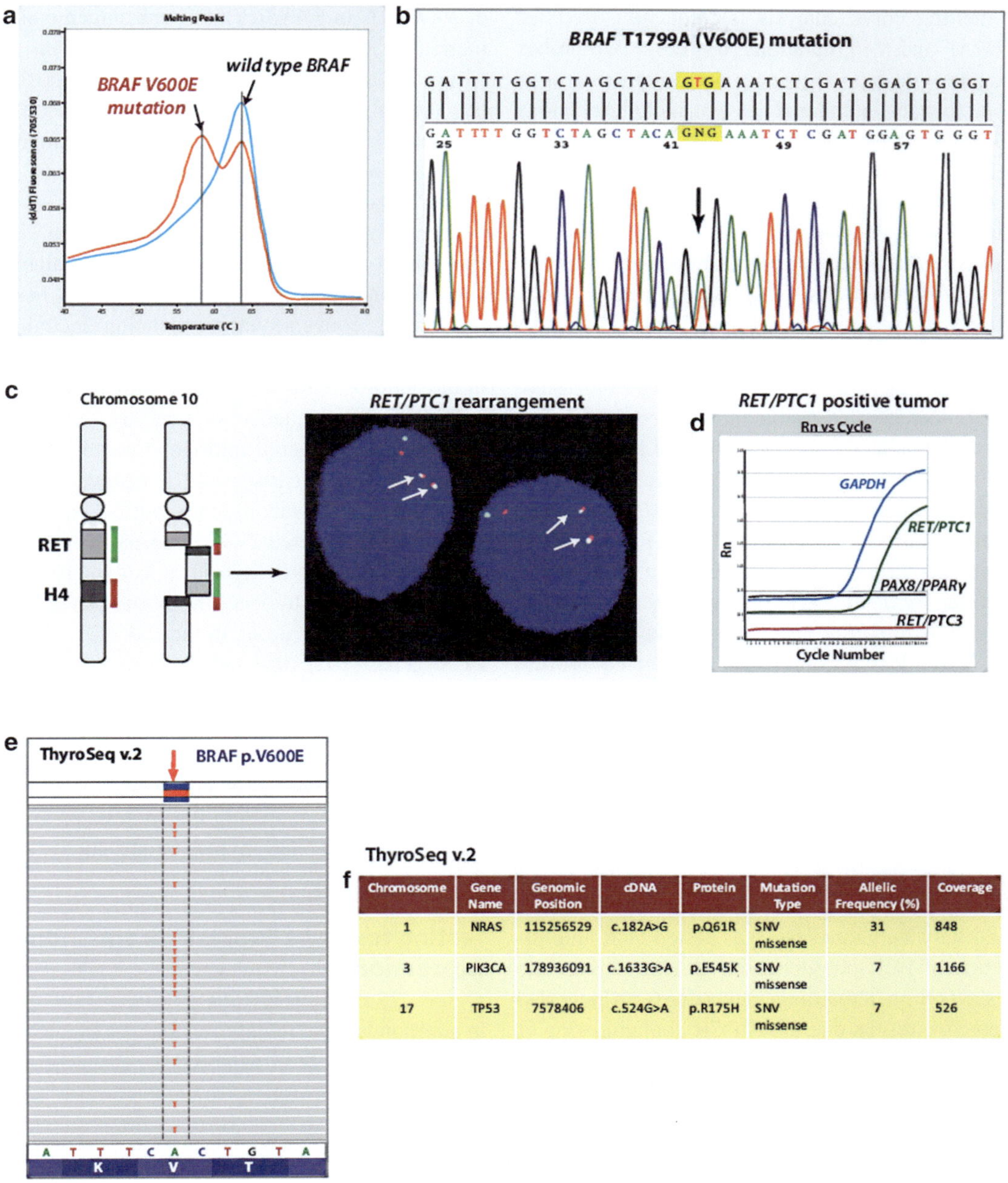

Chromosome	Gene Name	Genomic Position	cDNA	Protein	Mutation Type	Allelic Frequency (%)	Coverage
1	NRAS	115256529	c.182A>G	p.Q61R	SNV missense	31	848
3	PIK3CA	178936091	c.1633G>A	p.E545K	SNV missense	7	1166
17	TP53	7578406	c.524G>A	p.R175H	SNV missense	7	526

Figure 36.4 Laboratory techniques for detection of mutations in thyroid cancer. (**a**) Real-time PCR with post-PCR fluorescence melting curve analysis showing two melting peaks, one corresponding to a wild-type allele and the other to a mutant *BRAF* c.T1799A (p.V600E) allele. (**b**) Sanger sequencing detection of a *BRAF* c.T1799A (p.V600E) mutation, with vertical arrow indicating the heterozygous T and A nucleotides of the heterozygous wild-type and V600E alleles. (**c**) FISH detection of *RET/PTC1* rearrangement (arrows) using the fusion probe design. (**d**) Real-time RT-PCR analysis showing *RET/PTC1* rearrangement and no *RET/PTC3* and *PAX8/PPARG* rearrangements. (**e**) Detection of *BRAF* c.T1799A (p.V600E) mutation using targeted next generation sequencing gene panel. (**f**) Results of testing of a thyroid FNA sample using a 56-gene mutation panel showing the presence of three mutations involving the *NRAS*, *PIK3CA*, and *TP53* genes, which indicates a high risk of cancer in this nodule and suggests that the cancer may be prone to dedifferentiation and more aggressive biological behavior

(Fig. 36.4a, b) [19, 31, 122–126]. Other methods can be used for more sensitive detection of point mutations, e.g., coamplification at lower denaturation polymerase chain reaction (COLD-PCR), locked nucleic acids (LNA)-PCR, and others [103, 127]. In one study, detection of *BRAF* mutations was compared using probe-specific real-time PCR, real-time allele-specific PCR, direct sequencing, and a colorimetric assay and showed similar sensitivity in *BRAF* detection in archival FNA samples [125].

Real-time PCR methods are rapid, easy to perform, cost-efficient, and run in a closed PCR system that reduces the risk of PCR amplicon contamination. Real-time PCR followed by fluorescence melting curve analysis is frequently used for detection of *BRAF* and *RAS* mutations [63, 128]. Two probes complementary to wild-type sequences are designed to span the mutation site for each mutational hot spot, including codons 12, 13, and 61 of the *RAS* genes and codons 600 and 601 of the *BRAF* gene. If no mutation is present, probes will bind perfectly to the sample DNA and melt at a higher temperature, showing a single peak on post-PCR melting curve analysis (Fig. 36.4a). In contrast, if a heterozygous mutation is present, probes will bind to mutant DNA imperfectly, i.e., with one nucleotide mismatch, and will melt (dissociate) earlier, producing two melting peaks (Fig. 36.4a). Each nucleotide substitution produces a melting peak at a specific melting temperature (T_m). This method detects all possible mutation variants at the interrogated hot spot using a minimal amount of DNA.

The two most common approaches for detection of chromosomal rearrangements (*RET/PTC*, *PAX8/PPARG*, and *TRK*) are reverse transcription PCR (RT-PCR) and fluorescent in situ hybridization (FISH). RT-PCR is a reliable and sensitive technique for detection of fusion transcripts in fresh FNA samples and frozen tissue specimens. Assays frequently use real-time RT-PCR with fluorescently labeled probes, which increase the specificity of transcript detection and allow quantification of the amplified product (Fig. 36.4c) [98]. Amplification of a housekeeping gene in each RT-PCR reaction monitors RNA quality and quantity. When RT-PCR is used for detection of rearrangements from formalin-fixed paraffin-embedded (FFPE) tissue samples, amplification of short PCR products can overcome poor-quality RNA and avoid false-negative results.

Highly sensitivity techniques (such as nested PCR amplification or blotting of PCR products with specific probes) are not optimal for detection of rearrangements due to an increased risk of false-positive results due to RT-PCR contamination or amplification of nonspecific sequences and require rigorous use of negative controls. In addition, ultrasensitive techniques may result in the detection of rearrangements that are present in a small fraction of the tumor. This is particularly problematic for the detection of the *RET/PTC* rearrangement, which can vary from involving almost all neoplastic cells (clonal *RET/PTC*) to involving only a small fraction of tumor cells (non-clonal *RET/PTC*) [53, 54]. Since only clonal *RET/PTC* rearrangement is specific for papillary carcinoma [45, 53], the sensitivity of detection will not be greater than 1 % of tumor cells (i.e., detection of 1 % or more tumors cells in the background of normal cells) to avoid detecting non-clonal rearrangements, which have no clinical implications at this time.

For detection of gene rearrangements in FFPE samples, where RNA is degraded, FISH is a reliable method (Fig. 36.4d). FISH utilizes fluorescently labeled DNA probes for targeted detection of gene rearrangements in interphase or metaphase nuclei. The FISH probes are relatively large in size, ranging from 20 to 200 kb. Currently, probes for detection of *RET/PTC* or *PAX8/PPARG* rearrangements are not commercially available, but bacterial artificial chromosomes clones are available [53, 54, 60]. Several positive and negative controls are required to validate the scoring criteria for accurate FISH results. For *RET/PTC* rearrangement, the cutoff level for positive test results is 7–30 % positive cells, depending on the probe design [53, 129].

Introduction of NGS technology has enabled high-throughput detection of multiple genetic alterations in both constitutional and cancer genomes. NGS has clear advantages over conventional sequencing techniques, such as Sanger sequencing, by allowing sequencing of large regions of the genome at lower cost and with higher sensitivity. NGS can be used to sequence the genome, exome, transcriptome (mRNA), and targeted multigene panels. While genome or exome analyses are essential for discovery projects, targeted gene panels are advancing into routine clinical testing of thyroid cancer. Targeted NGS gene panels include testing for common mutations in thyroid cancer and for multiple genetic alterations known to occur in thyroid cancer with low prevalence, such as mutations in the *PIK3CA*, *AKT1*, *PTEN*, and *TP53* genes [102, 108] and chromosomal rearrangements of the *BRAF*, *ALK*, and *NTRK* genes. An NGS-based panel that includes 56 genes and gene fusions (ThyroSeq v.2) has been recently validated for preoperative diagnosis of thyroid nodules [109]. Commercially available targeted NGS gene panels that offer sequencing for mutations in cancer-related genes or custom NGS thyroid panels can be used.

Testing for Gene Expression and miRNA Expression

In addition to gene mutations, changes in mRNA and miRNA expression have been explored for diagnostic use in thyroid samples. Search for a limited number of differentially expressed genes that can be used diagnostically appears to be promising. Upregulation of the *HMGA2* gene in malignant thyroid tumors has been found in several studies and may be of diagnostic utility for thyroid nodule FNA samples [130, 131]. Aberrant expression of *MET*, *TPO*, *TIMP1*, *DPP*, and other genes was observed in several studies and explored for diagnostic use [83–85, 131, 132]. At least one company is exploring the use of gene expression profiling of thyroid FNA samples as a tool for determining the benign or malignant potential of thyroid nodules [110]. The possibility of applying a combination of cytological evaluation, mutational analysis, and gene expression markers to improve the FNA diagnosis of thyroid nodules may improve clinical care for these patients.

The diagnostic utility of miRNA expression in thyroid FNA samples has been also explored [88, 92, 133, 134]. In one study, preoperative assessment of several miRNAs (miR-221, miR-222, miR-146b, miR-224, miR-155, miR-197, miR-187) in thyroid nodule FNA samples demonstrated that upregulation of three or more of these miRNAs can predict papillary or follicular thyroid cancer with 98 % accuracy [92]. This demonstrates the feasibility of miRNA detection in thyroid FNA samples and provides initial evidence for its possible diagnostic use pending further validation.

Laboratory Issues

Collection of FNA Sample

Freshly collected and fixed FNA and resection specimens can be used for clinical molecular testing. Collection of fresh FNA samples during routine FNA procedures is simple, does not prolong the FNA procedure, and yields DNA and RNA of excellent quality. Typically, the FNA procedure is conducted under ultrasound guidance to ensure sampling of the nodule, with thyroid cells collected using a 23, 25, or 27 gauge needle and sent for cytological evaluation. In most cases, 3–4 FNA needle passes are performed. To collect a sample for molecular testing during an FNA procedure, either one entire pass is taken for molecular testing or most of the aspirated sample from the first two passes (the most representative sample) is used for direct cytology smears for cytological evaluation, with the residual material in the needle and the needle wash from both passes placed into a tube containing nucleic acid preservative solution, e.g., RNAlater (Qiagen) or Trizol (Invitrogen) (Fig. 36.3). The latter approach allows successful sampling of the nodule in 90–98 % of cases [98, 103]. After collection, the FNA specimen for molecular testing can be stored at −20 or −80 °C until molecular testing is performed. If collection of fresh FNA material is not possible, fixed cytology FNA material, i.e., stained cytology smear or cytology cell block, can be used for molecular testing. Use of a fixed specimen provides reliable detection of point mutations but is not ideal for detection of chromosomal rearrangements due to the suboptimal quality of the RNA.

Quality Assurance

The quantity and quality of nucleic acids isolated from FNA specimens can be assessed either by spectrophotometric measurements or by PCR amplification. Real-time PCR can be used to assess the quantity and quality of nucleic acids in a simple and cost-efficient way via evaluating PCR amplification of the *RAS* or *BRAF* genes for DNA and amplification of the *GAPDH* housekeeping gene for RNA.

Fresh FNA samples should be evaluated for sample adequacy prior to molecular testing to assess the proportion of thyroid epithelial cells and tumor cells within the sample. Thyroid FNA samples may contain a number of "contaminant" cells, i.e., lymphocytes, other white blood cells, and stromal cells. An abundance of these non-epithelial cells may decrease sensitivity of detection and lead to a false-negative result. Assessment of the proportion of thyroid epithelial cells within an FNA sample can be performed by comparing the expression of the universal housekeeping gene (i.e., *GAPDH*), which is uniformly expressed in all cell types, with the expression of a gene that is expressed only in thyroid cells or in several types of epithelial cells including thyroid cells, such as the thyroid peroxidase (*TPO*) gene, the thyroglobulin (*TG*) gene, and cytokeratin genes (*KRT7* and *KRT19*) [103, 135].

For assurance of quality of molecular testing, a set of positive and negative controls at different levels of allelic frequencies has to be used during each analytical run. Some controls are available through the commercial sources, e.g., Horizon Diagnostics (Cambridge, UK). In addition, the College of American Pathologists offers proficiency testing for several of the most commonly mutated genes in thyroid cancer, including *BRAF* and *KRAS*.

Conclusions

Our understanding of the molecular changes in thyroid cancers is improving the clinical management of patients with thyroid nodules. Molecular testing can enhance the accuracy of cancer diagnosis in thyroid nodules, cancer prognosis, and will likely be important for selection of targeted therapies for thyroid cancer. The most significant impact of molecular testing is the improved diagnosis of cancer in nodules with indeterminate cytology results. Research discoveries using NGS technologies will lead to identification of novel mutations and other genetic and epigenetic events in thyroid cancer with the potential for further improvement in the care of patients with thyroid cancer.

References

1. Davies L, Welch HG. Increasing incidence of thyroid cancer in the United States, 1973–2002. JAMA. 2006;295:2164–7.
2. Albores-Saavedra J, Henson DE, Glazer E, et al. Changing patterns in the incidence and survival of thyroid cancer with follicular phenotype–papillary, follicular, and anaplastic: a morphological and epidemiological study. Endocr Pathol. 2007;18:1–7.
3. DeLellis RA, Lloyd RV, Heitz PU, et al., editors. World Health Organization classification of tumours. Pathology and genetics of tumours of endocrine organs. Lyon: IARC Press; 2004.
4. Nikiforov YE. Thyroid tumors: Classification and general considerations. In: Nikiforov YE, Biddinger PW, Thompson LDR, editors. Diagnostic pathology and molecular genetics of the thyroid. Baltimore, MD: Lippincott Williams & Wilkins; 2009. p. 94–102.
5. Mazzaferri EL. Thyroid cancer in thyroid nodules: finding a needle in the haystack. Am J Med. 1992;93:359–62.

6. Gharib H. Changing trends in thyroid practice: understanding nodular thyroid disease. Endocr Pract. 2004;10:31–9.
7. Frates MC, Benson CB, Doubilet PM, et al. Prevalence and distribution of carcinoma in patients with solitary and multiple thyroid nodules on sonography. J Clin Endocrinol Metab. 2006;91: 3411–7.
8. Cooper DS, Doherty GM, Haugen BR, et al. Management guidelines for patients with thyroid nodules and differentiated thyroid cancer. Thyroid. 2006;16:109–42.
9. Papini E, Guglielmi R, Bianchini A, et al. Risk of malignancy in nonpalpable thyroid nodules: predictive value of ultrasound and color-Doppler features. J Clin Endocrinol Metab. 2002;87: 1941–6.
10. Sclabas GM, Staerkel GA, Shapiro SE, et al. Fine-needle aspiration of the thyroid and correlation with histopathology in a contemporary series of 240 patients. Am J Surg. 2003;186:702–9. discussion 709–10.
11. Yassa L, Cibas ES, Benson CB, et al. Long-term assessment of a multidisciplinary approach to thyroid nodule diagnostic evaluation. Cancer. 2007;111:508–16.
12. Baloch ZW, LiVolsi VA, Asa SL, et al. Diagnostic terminology and morphologic criteria for cytologic diagnosis of thyroid lesions: a synopsis of the National Cancer Institute Thyroid Fine-Needle Aspiration State of the Science Conference. Diagn Cytopathol. 2008;36:425–37.
13. Ali SZ, Cibas ES. The Bethesda system for reporting thyroid cytopathology. New York, NY: Springer; 2010.
14. Xing M, Clark D, Guan H, et al. BRAF mutation testing of thyroid fine-needle aspiration biopsy specimens for preoperative risk stratification in papillary thyroid cancer. J Clin Oncol. 2009;27:2977–82. doi:10.1200/JCO.2008.20.1426.
15. Elisei R, Ugolini C, Viola D, et al. BRAF(V600E) mutation and outcome of patients with papillary thyroid carcinoma: a 15-year median follow-up study. J Clin Endocrinol Metab. 2008;93:3943–9.
16. Yip L, Nikiforova MN, Carty SE, et al. Optimizing surgical treatment of papillary thyroid carcinoma associated with BRAF mutation. Surgery. 2009;146:1215–23.
17. Nikiforov YE. Thyroid tumors: classification, staging and general considerations. In: Nikiforov Y, Biddinger PW, THompson LDR, editors. Diagnostic pathology and molecular genetics of the thyroid. Baltimore, MD: Lippincott Williams & Wilkins; 2012. p. 108–18.
18. Adeniran AJ, Zhu Z, Gandhi M, et al. Correlation between genetic alterations and microscopic features, clinical manifestations, and prognostic characteristics of thyroid papillary carcinomas. Am J Surg Pathol. 2006;30:216–22.
19. Kimura ET, Nikiforova MN, Zhu Z, et al. High prevalence of BRAF mutations in thyroid cancer: genetic evidence for constitutive activation of the RET/PTC-RAS-BRAF signaling pathway in papillary thyroid carcinoma. Cancer Res. 2003;63:1454–7.
20. Soares P, Trovisco V, Rocha AS, et al. BRAF mutations and RET/PTC rearrangements are alternative events in the etiopathogenesis of PTC. Oncogene. 2003;22:4578–80.
21. Frattini M, Ferrario C, Bressan P, et al. Alternative mutations of BRAF, RET and NTRK1 are associated with similar but distinct gene expression patterns in papillary thyroid cancer. Oncogene. 2004;23:7436–40.
22. Cohen Y, Xing M, Mambo E, et al. BRAF mutation in papillary thyroid carcinoma. J Natl Cancer Inst. 2003;95:625–7.
23. Trovisco V, Vieira de Castro I, Soares P, et al. BRAF mutations are associated with some histological types of papillary thyroid carcinoma. J Pathol. 2004;202:247–51.
24. Hou P, Liu D, Shan Y, et al. Genetic alterations and their relationship in the phosphatidylinositol 3-kinase/Akt pathway in thyroid cancer. Clin Cancer Res. 2007;13:1161–70. doi:10.1158/1078-0432.CCR-06-1125.
25. Chiosea S, Nikiforova M, Zuo H, et al. A novel complex BRAF mutation detected in a solid variant of papillary thyroid carcinoma. Endocr Pathol. 2009;20:122–6.
26. Basolo F, Torregrossa L, Giannini R, et al. Correlation between the BRAF V600E mutation and tumor invasiveness in papillary thyroid carcinomas smaller than 20 millimeters: analysis of 1060 cases. J Clin Endocrinol Metab. 2010;95:4197–205.
27. Ciampi R, Knauf JA, Kerler R, et al. Oncogenic AKAP9-BRAF fusion is a novel mechanism of MAPK pathway activation in thyroid cancer. J Clin Invest. 2005;115:94–101.
28. Cancer Genome Atlas Research N. Integrated genomic characterization of papillary thyroid carcinoma. Cell. 2014;159:676–90. doi:10.1016/j.cell.2014.09.050.
29. Xing M. BRAF mutation in thyroid cancer. Endocr Relat Cancer. 2005;12:245–62. doi:10.1677/erc.1.0978.
30. Namba H, Nakashima M, Hayashi T, et al. Clinical implication of hot spot BRAF mutation, V599E, in papillary thyroid cancers. J Clin Endocrinol Metab. 2003;88:4393–7.
31. Nikiforova MN, Kimura ET, Gandhi M, et al. BRAF mutations in thyroid tumors are restricted to papillary carcinomas and anaplastic or poorly differentiated carcinomas arising from papillary carcinomas. J Clin Endocrinol Metab. 2003;88:5399–404.
32. Begum S, Rosenbaum E, Henrique R, et al. BRAF mutations in anaplastic thyroid carcinoma: implications for tumor origin, diagnosis and treatment. Mod Pathol. 2004;17:1359–63.
33. Ricarte-Filho JC, Ryder M, Chitale DA, et al. Mutational profile of advanced primary and metastatic radioactive iodine-refractory thyroid cancers reveals distinct pathogenetic roles for BRAF, PIK3CA, and AKT1. Cancer Res. 2009;69:4885–93.
34. Suarez HG, du Villard JA, Severino M, et al. Presence of mutations in all three ras genes in human thyroid tumors. Oncogene. 1990;5:565–70.
35. Esapa CT, Johnson SJ, Kendall-Taylor P, et al. Prevalence of Ras mutations in thyroid neoplasia. Clin Endocrinol (Oxf). 1999;50:529–35.
36. Motoi N, Sakamoto A, Yamochi T, et al. Role of ras mutation in the progression of thyroid carcinoma of follicular epithelial origin. Pathol Res Pract. 2000;196:1–7.
37. Manenti G, Pilotti S, Re FC, et al. Selective activation of ras oncogenes in follicular and undifferentiated thyroid carcinomas. Eur J Cancer. 1994;30A:987–93.
38. Namba H, Rubin SA, Fagin JA. Point mutations of ras oncogenes are an early event in thyroid tumorigenesis. Mol Endocrinol. 1990;4:1474–9.
39. Karga H, Lee JK, Vickery Jr AL, et al. Ras oncogene mutations in benign and malignant thyroid neoplasms. J Clin Endocrinol Metab. 1991;73:832–6.
40. Ezzat S, Zheng L, Kolenda J, et al. Prevalence of activating ras mutations in morphologically characterized thyroid nodules. Thyroid. 1996;6:409–16.
41. Fagin JA. Minireview: branded from the start-distinct oncogenic initiating events may determine tumor fate in the thyroid. Mol Endocrinol. 2002;16:903–11.
42. Saavedra HI, Knauf JA, Shirokawa JM, et al. The RAS oncogene induces genomic instability in thyroid PCCL3 cells via the MAPK pathway. Oncogene. 2000;19:3948–54.
43. Basolo F, Pisaturo F, Pollina LE, et al. N-ras mutation in poorly differentiated thyroid carcinomas: correlation with bone metastases and inverse correlation to thyroglobulin expression. Thyroid. 2000;10:19–23.
44. Garcia-Rostan G, Zhao H, Camp RL, et al. ras mutations are associated with aggressive tumor phenotypes and poor prognosis in thyroid cancer. J Clin Oncol. 2003;21:3226–35.
45. Santoro M, Carlomagno F, Hay ID, et al. Ret oncogene activation in human thyroid neoplasms is restricted to the papillary cancer subtype. J Clin Invest. 1992;89:1517–22.

46. Jhiang SM, Sagartz JE, Tong Q, et al. Targeted expression of the ret/PTC1 oncogene induces papillary thyroid carcinomas. Endocrinology. 1996;137:375–8.
47. Santoro M, Chiappetta G, Cerrato A, et al. Development of thyroid papillary carcinomas secondary to tissue-specific expression of the RET/PTC1 oncogene in transgenic mice. Oncogene. 1996;12:1821–6.
48. Powell Jr DJ, Russell J, Nibu K, et al. The RET/PTC3 oncogene: metastatic solid-type papillary carcinomas in murine thyroids. Cancer Res. 1998;58:5523–8.
49. Nikiforov YE. RET/PTC rearrangement in thyroid tumors. Endocr Pathol. 2002;13:3–16.
50. Nikiforov YE, Rowland JM, Bove KE, et al. Distinct pattern of ret oncogene rearrangements in morphological variants of radiation-induced and sporadic thyroid papillary carcinomas in children. Cancer Res. 1997;57:1690–4.
51. Rabes HM, Demidchik EP, Sidorow JD, et al. Pattern of radiation-induced RET and NTRK1 rearrangements in 191 post-chernobyl papillary thyroid carcinomas: biological, phenotypic, and clinical implications. Clin Cancer Res. 2000;6:1093–103.
52. Fenton CL, Lukes Y, Nicholson D, et al. The ret/PTC mutations are common in sporadic papillary thyroid carcinoma of children and young adults. J Clin Endocrinol Metab. 2000;85:1170–5.
53. Zhu Z, Ciampi R, Nikiforova MN, et al. Prevalence of RET/PTC rearrangements in thyroid papillary carcinomas: effects of the detection methods and genetic heterogeneity. J Clin Endocrinol Metab. 2006;91:3603–10.
54. Unger K, Zitzelsberger H, Salvatore G, et al. Heterogeneity in the distribution of RET/PTC rearrangements within individual post-Chernobyl papillary thyroid carcinomas. J Clin Endocrinol Metab. 2004;89:4272–9.
55. Radice P, Sozzi G, Miozzo M, et al. The human tropomyosin gene involved in the generation of the TRK oncogene maps to chromosome 1q31. Oncogene. 1991;6:2145–8.
56. Greco A, Pierotti MA, Bongarzone I, et al. TRK-T1 is a novel oncogene formed by the fusion of TPR and TRK genes in human papillary thyroid carcinomas. Oncogene. 1992;7:237–42.
57. Miranda C, Minoletti F, Greco A, et al. Refined localization of the human TPR gene to chromosome 1q25 by in situ hybridization. Genomics. 1994;23:714–5.
58. Leeman-Neill RJ, Kelly LM, Liu P, et al. ETV6-NTRK3 is a common chromosomal rearrangement in radiation-associated thyroid cancer. Cancer. 2014 Mar 15;120(6):799–807. doi:10.1002/cncr.28484.
59. Kelly LM, Barila G, Liu P, et al. Identification of the transforming STRN-ALK fusion as a potential therapeutic target in the aggressive forms of thyroid cancer. Proc Natl Acad Sci U S A. 2014;111(11):4233–8. doi:10.1073/pnas.1321937111.
60. Kroll TG, Sarraf P, Pecciarini L, et al. PAX8-PPARgamma1 fusion oncogene in human thyroid carcinoma [corrected]. Science. 2000;289:1357–60.
61. Lui WO, Kytola S, Anfalk L, et al. Balanced translocation (3;7) (p25;q34): another mechanism of tumorigenesis in follicular thyroid carcinoma? Cancer Genet Cytogenet. 2000;119:109–12.
62. French CA, Alexander EK, Cibas ES, et al. Genetic and biological subgroups of low-stage follicular thyroid cancer. Am J Pathol. 2003;162:1053–60. doi:10.1016/S0002-9440(10)63902-8.
63. Nikiforova MN, Lynch RA, Biddinger PW, et al. RAS point mutations and PAX8-PPAR gamma rearrangement in thyroid tumors: evidence for distinct molecular pathways in thyroid follicular carcinoma. J Clin Endocrinol Metab. 2003;88:2318–26.
64. Dwight T, Thoppe SR, Foukakis T, et al. Involvement of the PAX8/ peroxisome proliferator-activated receptor gamma rearrangement in follicular thyroid tumors. J Clin Endocrinol Metab. 2003;88:4440–5.
65. Nikiforova MN, Biddinger PW, Caudill CM, et al. PAX8-PPARgamma rearrangement in thyroid tumors: RT-PCR and immunohistochemical analyses. Am J Surg Pathol. 2002;26: 1016–23.
66. Marques AR, Espadinha C, Catarino AL, et al. Expression of PAX8-PPAR gamma 1 rearrangements in both follicular thyroid carcinomas and adenomas. J Clin Endocrinol Metab. 2002;87: 3947–52.
67. Horn S, Figl A, Rachakonda PS, et al. TERT promoter mutations in familial and sporadic melanoma. Science. 2013;339:959–61. doi:10.1126/science.1230062.
68. Huang FW, Hodis E, Xu MJ, et al. Highly recurrent TERT promoter mutations in human melanoma. Science. 2013;339:957–9. doi:10.1126/science.1229259.
69. Landa I, Ganly I, Chan TA, et al. Frequent somatic TERT promoter mutations in thyroid cancer: higher prevalence in advanced forms of the disease. J Clin Endocrinol Metab. 2013;98:E1562–6. doi:10.1210/jc.2013-2383.
70. Liu T, Wang N, Cao J, et al. The age- and shorter telomere-dependent TERT promoter mutation in follicular thyroid cell-derived carcinomas. Oncogene. 2013. doi:10.1038/onc.2013.446.
71. Liu X, Bishop J, Shan Y, et al. Highly prevalent TERT promoter mutations in aggressive thyroid cancers. Endocr Relat Cancer. 2013;20:603–10. doi:10.1530/ERC-13-0210.
72. Melo M, Rocha AG, Vinagre J, et al. TERT promoter mutations are a major indicator of poor outcome in differentiated thyroid carcinomas. J Clin Endocrinol Metab. 2014;99(5):754–65. doi:10.1210/jc.2013-3734.
73. Fagin JA, Matsuo K, Karmakar A, et al. High prevalence of mutations of the p53 gene in poorly differentiated human thyroid carcinomas. J Clin Invest. 1993;91:179–84.
74. Donghi R, Longoni A, Pilotti S, et al. Gene p53 mutations are restricted to poorly differentiated and undifferentiated carcinomas of the thyroid gland. J Clin Invest. 1993;91:1753–60.
75. Dobashi Y, Sugimura H, Sakamoto A, et al. Stepwise participation of p53 gene mutation during dedifferentiation of human thyroid carcinomas. Diagn Mol Pathol. 1994;3:9–14.
76. Ito T, Seyama T, Mizuno T, et al. Unique association of p53 mutations with undifferentiated but not with differentiated carcinomas of the thyroid gland. Cancer Res. 1992;52:1369–71.
77. Garcia-Rostan G, Camp RL, Herrero A, et al. Beta-catenin dysregulation in thyroid neoplasms: down-regulation, aberrant nuclear expression, and CTNNB1 exon 3 mutations are markers for aggressive tumor phenotypes and poor prognosis. Am J Pathol. 2001;158:987–96.
78. Garcia-Rostan G, Tallini G, Herrero A, et al. Frequent mutation and nuclear localization of beta-catenin in anaplastic thyroid carcinoma. Cancer Res. 1999;59:1811–5.
79. Garcia-Rostan G, Costa AM, Pereira-Castro I, et al. Mutation of the PIK3CA gene in anaplastic thyroid cancer. Cancer Res. 2005;65:10199–207.
80. Santarpia L, El-Naggar AK, Cote GJ, et al. Phosphatidylinositol 3-kinase/akt and ras/raf-mitogen-activated protein kinase pathway mutations in anaplastic thyroid cancer. J Clin Endocrinol Metab. 2008;93:278–84.
81. Hou P, Liu D, Xing M. Functional characterization of the T1799-1801del and A1799-1816ins BRAF mutations in papillary thyroid cancer. Cell Cycle. 2007;6:377–9.
82. Dahia PL, Marsh DJ, Zheng Z, et al. Somatic deletions and mutations in the Cowden disease gene, PTEN, in sporadic thyroid tumors. Cancer Res. 1997;57:4710–3.
83. Giordano TJ, Kuick R, Thomas DG, et al. Molecular classification of papillary thyroid carcinoma: distinct BRAF, RAS, and RET/PTC mutation-specific gene expression profiles discovered by DNA microarray analysis. Oncogene. 2005;24:6646–56.
84. Chevillard S, Ugolin N, Vielh P, et al. Gene expression profiling of differentiated thyroid neoplasms: diagnostic and clinical implications. Clin Cancer Res. 2004;10:6586–97.

85. Huang Y, Prasad M, Lemon WJ, et al. Gene expression in papillary thyroid carcinoma reveals highly consistent profiles. Proc Natl Acad Sci U S A. 2001;98:15044–9.
86. Mazzanti C, Zeiger MA, Costouros NG, et al. Using gene expression profiling to differentiate benign versus malignant thyroid tumors. Cancer Res. 2004;64:2898–903.
87. Finley DJ, Arora N, Zhu B, et al. Molecular profiling distinguishes papillary carcinoma from benign thyroid nodules. J Clin Endocrinol Metab. 2004;89:3214–23.
88. Chen YT, Kitabayashi N, Zhou XK, et al. MicroRNA analysis as a potential diagnostic tool for papillary thyroid carcinoma. Mod Pathol. 2008;21:1139–46.
89. He H, Jazdzewski K, Li W, et al. The role of microRNA genes in papillary thyroid carcinoma. Proc Natl Acad Sci U S A. 2005;102:19075–80.
90. Nikiforova MN, Chiosea SI, Nikiforov YE. MicroRNA expression profiles in thyroid tumors. Endocr Pathol. 2009;20:85–91.
91. Pallante P, Visone R, Ferracin M, et al. MicroRNA deregulation in human thyroid papillary carcinomas. Endocr Relat Cancer. 2006;13:497–508. doi:13/2/497 [pii] 10.1677/erc.1.01209.
92. Nikiforova MN, Tseng GC, Steward D, et al. MicroRNA expression profiling of thyroid tumors: biological significance and diagnostic utility. J Clin Endocrinol Metab. 2008;93(5):1600–8.
93. Visone R, Russo L, Pallante P, et al. MicroRNAs (miR)-221 and miR-222, both overexpressed in human thyroid papillary carcinomas, regulate p27Kip1 protein levels and cell cycle. Endocr Relat Cancer. 2007;14:791–8.
94. Jazdzewski K, Boguslawska J, Jendrzejewski J, et al. Thyroid hormone receptor beta (THRB) is a major target gene for microRNAs deregulated in papillary thyroid carcinoma (PTC). J Clin Endocrinol Metab. 2011;96:546–53.
95. Weber F, Teresi RE, Broelsch CE, et al. A limited set of human MicroRNA is deregulated in follicular thyroid carcinoma. J Clin Endocrinol Metab. 2006;91:3584–91.
96. Visone R, Pallante P, Vecchione A, et al. Specific microRNAs are downregulated in human thyroid anaplastic carcinomas. Oncogene. 2007;26:7590–5.
97. Cooper DS, Doherty GM, Haugen BR, et al. Revised American Thyroid Association management guidelines for patients with thyroid nodules and differentiated thyroid cancer. Thyroid. 2009;19:1167–214.
98. Nikiforov YE, Steward DL, Robinson-Smith TM, et al. Molecular testing for mutations in improving the fine-needle aspiration diagnosis of thyroid nodules. J Clin Endocrinol Metab. 2009;94:2092–8.
99. Cantara S, Capezzone M, Marchisotta S, et al. Impact of proto-oncogene mutation detection in cytological specimens from thyroid nodules improves the diagnostic accuracy of cytology. J Clin Endocrinol Metab. 2010;95:1365–9.
100. Ohori NP, Nikiforova MN, Schoedel KE, et al. Contribution of molecular testing to thyroid fine-needle aspiration cytology of "follicular lesion of undetermined significance/atypia of undetermined significance". Cancer Cytopathol. 2010;118:17–23.
101. Kim SK, Hwang TS, Yoo YB, et al. Surgical results of thyroid nodules according to a management guideline based on the BRAF(V600E) mutation status. J Clin Endocrinol Metab. 2011;96:658–64. doi:10.1210/jc.2010-1082.
102. Nikiforov YE, Nikiforova MN. Molecular genetics and diagnosis of thyroid cancer. Nat Rev Endocrinol. 2011;7(10):569–80. doi:10.1038/nrendo.2011.142 nrendo.2011.142 [pii].
103. Nikiforov Y. Impact of mutational testing on the diagnosis and management of patients with cytologically indeterminate thyroid nodules: a prospective analysis of 1056 FNA samples. J Clin Endocrinol Metab. 2011;96:3390–7.
104. Mehta RS, Carty SE, Ohori NP, et al. Nodule size is an independent predictor of malignancy in mutation-negative nodules with follicular lesion of undetermined significance cytology. Surgery. 2013;154:730–6. doi:10.1016/j.surg.2013.05.015. discussion 736–8.
105. Yip L, Wharry L, Armstrong M, et al. A clinical algorithm for fine-needle aspiration molecular testing effectively guides the appropriate extent of initial thyroidectomy. Ann Surg. 2014;260(1):163–8. doi:2010.1097/SLA.0000000000000215.
106. Yip L, Nikiforova M, Carty SE, et al. Cost impact of molecular testing for indeterminate thyroid nodule fine needle aspiration biopsies. J Clin Endocrinol Metab. 2012.
107. Nikiforova MN, Wald AI, Roy S, et al. Targeted next-generation sequencing panel (ThyroSeq) for detection of mutations in thyroid cancer. J Clin Endocrinol Metab. 2013;98:E1852–60. doi:10.1210/jc.2013-2292.
108. Le Mercier M, D'Haene N, De Neve N, et al. Next-generation sequencing improves the diagnosis of thyroid FNA specimens with indeterminate cytology. Histopathology. 2015;66(2):215–24. doi:10.1111/his.12461.
109. Nikiforov YE, Carty SE, Chiosea SI, et al. Highly accurate diagnosis of cancer in thyroid nodules with follicular neoplasm/suspicious for a follicular neoplasm cytology by ThyroSeq v2 next-generation sequencing assay. Cancer. 2014. 120(23):3627–34. doi:10.1002/cncr.29038.
110. Chudova D, Wilde JI, Wang ET, et al. Molecular classification of thyroid nodules using high-dimensionality genomic data. J Clin Endocrinol Metab. 2010;95(12):5296–304.
111. Alexander EK, Kennedy GC, Baloch ZW, et al. Preoperative diagnosis of benign thyroid nodules with indeterminate cytology. N Engl J Med. 2012;367:705–15. doi:10.1056/NEJMoa1203208.
112. Alexander EK, Schorr M, Klopper J, et al. Multicenter clinical experience with the Afirma gene expression classifier. J Clin Endocrinol Metab. 2014;99:119–25. doi:10.1210/jc.2013-2482.
113. Duick DS, Klopper JP, Diggans JC, et al. The impact of benign gene expression classifier test results on the endocrinologist-patient decision to operate on patients with thyroid nodules with indeterminate fine-needle aspiration cytopathology. Thyroid. 2012;22:996–1001. doi:10.1089/thy.2012.0180.
114. Xing M. BRAF mutation in papillary thyroid cancer: pathogenic role, molecular bases, and clinical implications. Endocr Rev. 2007;28:742–62. doi:10.1210/er.2007-0007.
115. Ito Y, Yoshida H, Maruo R, et al. BRAF mutation in papillary thyroid carcinoma in a Japanese population: its lack of correlation with high-risk clinicopathological features and disease-free survival of patients. Endocr J. 2009;56:89–97.
116. Kim TY, Kim WB, Song JY, et al. The BRAF mutation is not associated with poor prognostic factors in Korean patients with conventional papillary thyroid microcarcinoma. Clin Endocrinol (Oxf). 2005;63:588–93. doi:10.1111/j.1365-2265.2005.02389.x.
117. Liu RT, Chen YJ, Chou FF, et al. No correlation between BRAFV600E mutation and clinicopathological features of papillary thyroid carcinomas in Taiwan. Clin Endocrinol (Oxf). 2005;63:461–6. doi:10.1111/j.1365-2265.2005.02367.x.
118. Tufano RP, Teixeira GV, Bishop J, et al. BRAF mutation in papillary thyroid cancer and its value in tailoring initial treatment: a systematic review and meta-analysis. Medicine. 2012;91:274–86.
119. Xing M, Alzahrani AS, Carson KA, et al. Association between BRAF V600E mutation and mortality in patients with papillary thyroid cancer. JAMA. 2013;309:1493–501.
120. Liu Z, Hou P, Ji M, et al. Highly prevalent genetic alterations in receptor tyrosine kinases and phosphatidylinositol 3-kinase/akt and mitogen-activated protein kinase pathways in anaplastic and follicular thyroid cancers. J Clin Endocrinol Metab. 2008;93:3106–16. doi:10.1210/jc.2008-0273.
121. Schlumberger M, Sherman SI. Approach to the patient with advanced differentiated thyroid cancer. Eur J Endocrinol. 2012;166:5–11. doi:10.1530/EJE-11-0631.
122. Sapio MR, Posca D, Troncone G, et al. Detection of BRAF mutation in thyroid papillary carcinomas by mutant allele-specific PCR amplification (MASA). Eur J Endocrinol. 2006;154:341–8.
123. Rowe LR, Bentz BG, Bentz JS. Detection of BRAF V600E activating mutation in papillary thyroid carcinoma using PCR with

allele-specific fluorescent probe melting curve analysis. J Clin Pathol. 2007;60:1211–5.
124. Hayashida N, Namba H, Kumagai A, et al. A rapid and simple detection method for the BRAF(T1796A) mutation in fine-needle aspirated thyroid carcinoma cells. Thyroid. 2004;14:910–5.
125. Jin L, Sebo TJ, Nakamura N, et al. BRAF mutation analysis in fine needle aspiration (FNA) cytology of the thyroid. Diagn Mol Pathol. 2006;15:136–43.
126. Magnin S, Viel E, Baraquin A, et al. A multiplex SNaPshot assay as a rapid method for detecting KRAS and BRAF mutations in advanced colorectal cancers. J Mol Diagn. 2011;13:485–92. doi:10.1016/j.jmoldx.2011.05.010.
127. Arcila M, Lau C, Nafa K, et al. Detection of KRAS and BRAF mutations in colorectal carcinoma roles for high-sensitivity locked nucleic acid-PCR sequencing and broad-spectrum mass spectrometry genotyping. J Mol Diagn. 2011;13:64–73. doi:10.1016/j.jmoldx.2010.11.005.
128. Elenitoba-Johnson KS, Bohling SD, Wittwer CT, et al. Multiplex PCR by multicolor fluorometry and fluorescence melting curve analysis. Nat Med. 2001;7:249–53.
129. Unger K, Zurnadzhy L, Walch A, et al. RET rearrangements in post-Chernobyl papillary thyroid carcinomas with a short latency analysed by interphase FISH. Br J Cancer. 2006;94:1472–7. doi:10.1038/sj.bjc.6603109.
130. Lappinga PJ, Kip NS, Jin L, et al. HMGA2 gene expression analysis performed on cytologic smears to distinguish benign from malignant thyroid nodules. Cancer Cytopathol. 2010;118: 287–97.
131. Prasad NB, Somervell H, Tufano RP, et al. Identification of genes differentially expressed in benign versus malignant thyroid tumors. Clin Cancer Res. 2008;14:3327–37.
132. Lubitz CC, Fahey 3rd TJ. The differentiation of benign and malignant thyroid nodules. Adv Surg. 2005;39:355–77.
133. Vriens MR, Weng J, Suh I, et al. MicroRNA expression profiling is a potential diagnostic tool for thyroid cancer. Cancer. 2011. doi:10.1002/cncr.26587.
134. Mazeh H, Mizrahi I, Halle D, et al. Development of a microRNA-based molecular assay for the detection of papillary thyroid carcinoma in aspiration biopsy samples. Thyroid. 2011;21:111–8. doi:10.1089/thy.2010.0356.
135. Schreinemakers JM, Pieterman CR, Scholten A, et al. The optimal surgical treatment for primary hyperparathyroidism in MEN1 patients: a systematic review. World J Surg. 2011;35:1993–2005. doi:10.1007/s00268-011-1068-9.

Sarcomas and Related Mesenchymal Tumors

37

Giovanni Tallini, Dario de Biase, and Pei Hui

Abstract

Understanding the molecular pathology of sarcomas and related mesenchymal lesions is often essential for their diagnosis. Cytogenetics and molecular cytogenetics have contributed significantly to the identification of recurrent chromosomal changes, fostering a continual refinement in the classification of these tumors. The recognition of distinctive rearrangements in tumor subsets is providing powerful tools to a field in which pathological diagnosis and clinical management are often difficult, due to both the variety of tumor phenotypes and their relative rarity. Novel technical approaches, including next-generation sequencing, are increasing the speed and throughput of molecular analysis and the application of genomic knowledge into clinical practice may radically change the management of patients with sarcomas.

Keywords

Sarcoma • Soft tissue tumor • Mesenchymal lesion • Chromosomal translocation • Chromosomal amplification • Gene rearrangement • Fusion transcript • Gene mutation • Oncogene • Real-time PCR • Reverse transcription-PCR • Next-generation sequencing • FISH • Karyotyping

Introduction

Oncologic molecular pathology focuses on identifying and understanding molecular and genetic alterations underlying the development and progression of neoplastic processes. Sarcomas and related tumors may be classified into two main pathogenetic types: sarcomas with complex genetic alterations and sarcomas with specific recurrent chromosomal translocations. The type with complex genetic alterations includes the majority of high-grade, pleomorphic mesenchymal malignancies, for example, undifferentiated pleomorphic sarcoma (malignant fibrous histiocytoma), osteogenic sarcoma, and leiomyosarcoma. In the second type, that accounts for approximately 20 % of the cases, tumors are translocation specific, with a recurrent chromosomal translocation leading to an in-frame fusion of coding sequences from each of the two rearranged genes [1]. The translocation typically results in the production of a chimeric transcript encoding a fusion protein with oncogenic activity. Histologically, the translocation-specific sarcomas are generally a monomorphic proliferation of neoplastic cells. This two-category pathogenetic classification of sarcomas is biologically relevant and is best illustrated by the sarcoma types observed in Li–Fraumeni syndrome. Li–Fraumeni patients, with a *TP53* germline mutation, are prone to sarcomas with complex karyotypes, such as osteogenic sarcoma and undifferentiated pleomorphic sarcoma, which constitute major mesenchymal cancers. On the other hand, translocation-specific sarcomas virtually never occur in Li–Fraumeni patients [2]. Other mesenchymal tumors that do not fall into these main pathogenic groups are

G. Tallini, M.D. (✉) • D. de Biase
Anatomic Pathology, Bologna University School of Medicine, Ospedale Bellaria, Via Altura 3, Bologna 40139, Italy
e-mail: giovanni.tallini@unibo.it

P. Hui, M.D.
Department of Pathology, Yale University School of Medicine, New Haven, CT, USA

D.G.B. Leonard (ed.), *Molecular Pathology in Clinical Practice*, DOI 10.1007/978-3-319-19674-9_37

characterized by amplification of specific chromosomal regions or specific mutations.

Tremendous progress has been made in characterizing the molecular alterations of sarcomas. The identification of tumor-specific molecular changes has not only reshaped their classification, but in many instances is having an impact on patient therapy and prognosis. Chromosomal translocations and associated fusion genes can be so specific and occur in such a high prevalence in a given sarcoma type that they are essentially used to define the neoplasm at both the pathobiological and clinical diagnostic levels and are therefore the main focus of this chapter [3–7].

Molecular Basis of Disease

Chromosomal Translocations and Gene Rearrangements

Chromosomal rearrangements (translocations, inversions, deletions, and insertions) are associated with DNA recombination of the genes located at the DNA breakpoints. If the breakpoint occurs within the involved gene, an altered gene structure arises. If the breakpoint occurs outside the gene, it may involve control elements critical for gene expression. In either case, the result can be a dramatic change in the gene structure, expression levels, or both. Molecular analysis has identified two general mechanisms through which chromosomal translocations result in altered gene function (Fig. 37.1).

The first mechanism by which chromosomal translocations result in altered gene function is by gene fusion (Fig. 37.1), in which chimeric or fusion genes are the result of joining of two parent genes (one upstream, or 5′, and the other downstream, or 3′, to the breakpoint). Both genes are truncated by the translocation involving the coding portions of the parent genes. In general, translocation breakpoints are located in noncoding introns, and the normal splicing mechanism removes the chimeric intron sequence. The exons are spliced "in frame" for the translational reading frame and can be translated into a novel fusion protein. In rare instances, the breakpoints are located in the exons of the parent genes. This may result in a novel chimeric product if the translational reading frame is maintained, or it may produce a truncated protein (encoded by the 5′ gene sequence) if the reading frame is lost. Transcription of chimeric genes is usually under the control of the upstream parent gene promoter but may be influenced by DNA sequences in or close to the downstream gene.

The second mechanism through which chromosomal translocations result in altered gene function is promoter exchange, in which the breakpoint occurs at the 5′ end of the coding region of the involved gene (Fig. 37.1). This results in the replacement of the gene's promoter region with enhancer elements or with the promoter from the translocation partner. Promoter exchange leads to transcriptional activation with abnormal gene expression, but the protein is wild-type.

Numerous fusion genes have been identified in malignant tumors of the soft tissues and in mesenchymal tumors in general (Table 37.1). The majority of sarcoma translocations

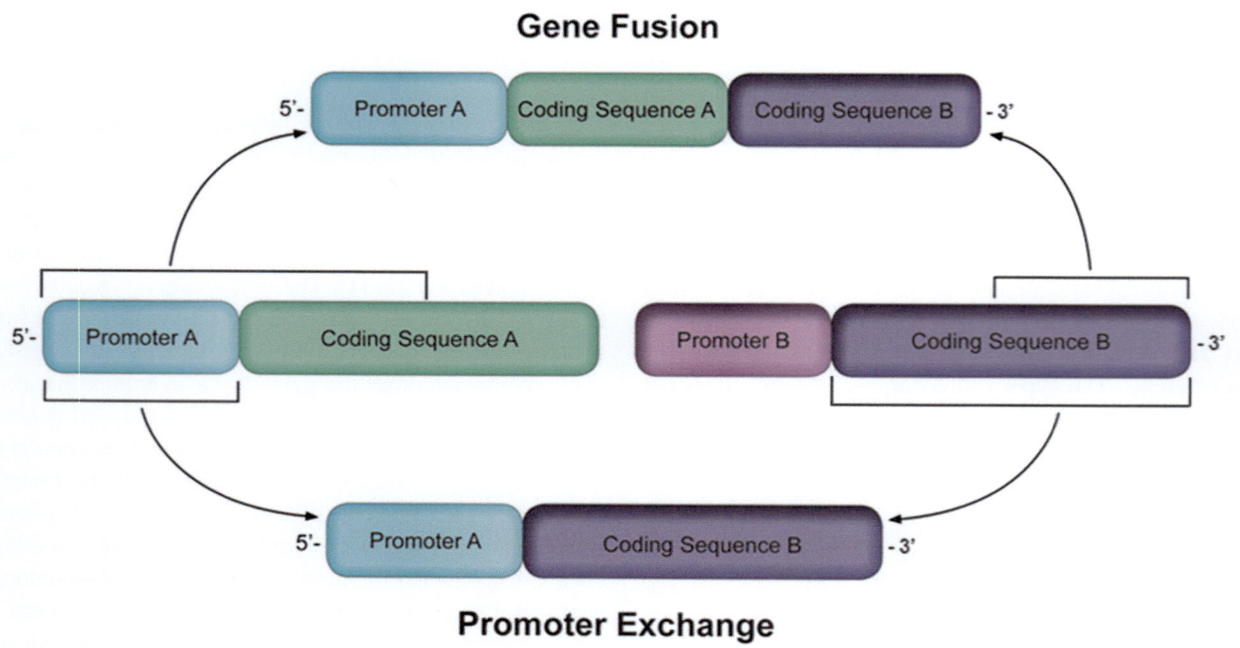

Figure 37.1 Mechanisms of chromosomal DNA rearrangement leading to altered gene expression by either gene fusion (*top pathway*) or promoter exchange (*bottom pathway*)

Table 37.1 Chromosomal alterations and aberrant gene products in sarcomas and related tumors

Tumor type	Chromosomal change	Fusion gene	Prevalence (%)	Number of fusion transcript variants	Function	Reference
Round cell tumors						
Desmoplastic small round cell tumor (DSRCT)	t(11;22)(p13;q12)	*EWSR1–WT1*	100	Small (3)	Transcription	Ladanyi. *Cancer Res* 1994;54:2837
Ewing's sarcoma (ES)/ Peripheral	t(11;22)(q24;q12)	*EWSR1–FLI1*	>90	Large (18)	Transcription	Delattre. *Nature* 1992;359:162
Neuroectodermal tumor (PNET)	t(21;22)(q22;q12)	*EWSR1–ERG*	5	Large (4)	Transcription	Sorensen. *Nat Genet* 1994;6:146 Zucman. *EMBO J* 1993;12:4481
	t(7;22)(p22;q12)	*EWSR1–ETV1*	<5	Uncertain	Transcription	Jeon. *Oncogene* 1995;10:1229
	t(17;22)(q12;q12)	*EWSR1–E1AF*	<5	Uncertain	Transcription	Urano. *Biochem Biophys Res Commun* 1996;219:608
	t(2;22)(q33;q12)	*EWSR1–FEV*	<5	Uncertain	Transcription	Peter. *Oncogene* 1997; 14:1159
	t(16;21)(p11;q22)	*FUS–ERG*	<5	Small (2)	Transcription	Shing. *Cancer Res* 2003;63:4568
Rhabdomyosarcoma, alveolar type (ARMS)	t(2;13)(q35;q14)	*PAX3–FOXO1*	60	None (1)	Transcription	Galili. *Nat Genet* 1993;5:230 Shapiro. *Cancer Res* 1993;53:5108
	t(1;13)(p36;q14)	*PAX7–FOXO1*	20	None (1)	Transcription	Davis. *Cancer Res* 1994;54:2869
	t(2;2)(p23;q35)	*PAX3–NCOA1*	<5	Small (2)	Transcription	Sumegi. *Genes Chromosomes Cancer* 2010;49:224
	t(2;8)(q35;q13)	*PAX3–NCOA2*	<5	None (1)	Transcription	Sumegi. *Genes Chromosomes Cancer* 2010;49:224
	t(X;2)(q13;q35)	*PAX3–FOXO4*	<5	None (1)	Transcription	Barr. *Cancer Res* 2002;62:4704
Spindle cell tumors						
Dermatofibrosarcoma protuberans/giant cell fibroblastoma	t(17;22)(q22;q13)	*COL1A1–PDGFB*	100	Large (>8)	Dysregulated cell growth (autocrine)	Simon. *Nat Genet* 1997;15:95
Fibrosarcoma, congenital type	t(12;15)(p13;q25)	*ETV6–NTRK3*	100	None (1)	Signaling (tyrosine kinase receptor)	Knezevich. *Nat Genet* 1998;18:184
Inflammatory myofibroblastic tumor[a]	t(1;2)(q25;p23)	*TPM3–ALK*	20	None (1)	Signaling (TKR)	Griffin. *Cancer Res* 1999;59:2776
	Inv(2)(p21;p23.2)	*EML4–ALK*	10	Large (>10)	Signaling (TKR)	Antonescu. *Am J Surg Pathol.* 2015
	t(2;19)(p23;p13)	*TPM4–ALK*	10	None (1)	Signaling (TKR)	Lawrence. *Am J Pathol* 2000;157:377
	6q22 alterations	*ROS1* rearrangements (*TFG* and other genes)	10	Uncertain	Signaling (TKR)	Antonescu. *Am J Surg Pathol.* 2015
	t(2;17)(p23;q23)	*CLTC–ALK*	Uncertain	None (1)	Signaling (TKR)	Bridge. *Am J Pathol* 2001;159:41
	t(2;11)(p23;p15)	*CARS–ALK*	Uncertain	None (1)	Signaling (TKR)	Cools. *Genes Chromosomes Cancer* 2002;34:354
	t(2;2)(p23;q13)	*RANBP2–ALK*	Uncertain	None (1)	Signaling (TKR)	Ma. *Genes Chromosomes*
	Various loci	Other *TK* (*PDGFRB, RET*)	<5	Uncertain	Signaling (TKR)	Antonescu. *Am J Surg Pathol* 2015 *Cancer* 2003;37:98

(continued)

Table 37.1 (continued)

Tumor type	Chromosomal change	Fusion gene	Prevalence (%)	Number of fusion transcript variants	Function	Reference
Low-grade fibromyxoid	t(7;16)(q33;p11)	*FUS–CREB3L2*	>75	Large (>4)	Transcription	Mertens. *Lab Invest* 2005;85:408
Sarcoma/hyalinizing spindle cell tumor with giant rosettes						Reid. *Am J Surg Pathol* 2003;27:1229 Guillou. *Am J Surg Pathol* 2007;31:1387
	t(11;16)(p11;p11)	*FUS–CREB3L1*	<10	Small (2)	Transcription	Mertens. *Lab Invest* 2005;85,408
Nodular fasciitis	t(17;22)(p13;q13)	*MYH9–USP6*	75	Uncertain	Signaling	Erickson-Johnson. *Lab Invest* 2011;91:1427
Spindle cell tumors with pericytic differentiation (pericytoma)	t(7;12) (p21-22;q13–15)	*ACTB–GLI*	Uncertain	Large (6)	Transcription	Dahlén. *Am J Pathol* 2004;164:1645
Synovial sarcoma	t(X;18)(p11;q11)	*SS18–SSX1*	65	None (1)	Transcription	Clark. *Nat Genet* 1994;7:502
	t(X;18)(p11;q11)	*SS18–SSX2*	30	None (1)	Transcription	Crew. *EMBO J* 1995;14:2333 De Leeuw. *Hum Mol Genet* 1995;4:1097
	t(X;18)(p11;q11)	*SS18–SSX4*	<5	None (1)	Transcription	Skytting. *J Natl Cancer Inst* 1999;91:974
	Marker chromosome with 20q13.3/Xp11 rearrangement	*SS18L1–SSX1*	<5	None (1)	Transcription	Skytting. *J Natl Cancer Inst* 1999;91:974
Lipomatous tumors						
Lipoblastoma	8q11–13	*HAS2–PLAG1*	>90	None (1)	Transcription	Hibbard. *Cancer Res* 2000;60:4869
	t(7;8)(q22;q12)	*COL1A2–PLAG1*	Uncertain	None (1)	Transcription	Hibbard. *Cancer Res* 2000;60:4869
Lipoma	t(3;12) (q27–28;q14–15)	*HMGA2–LPP*	50[b]	None (1)	Transcription	Ashar. *Cell* 1995;82:57
	Other t(12q15)	Other *HMGA2* rearrangements				Schoenmakers. *Nat Genet* 1995;10:436 Petit, *Genomics* 1996;36:118
	t(6p21)	*HMGA1* rearrangement	10[b]		Transcription	Tkachenko. *Cancer Res* 1997;57:2276
Liposarcoma, myxoid/round cell type	t(12;16)(q13;p11)	*FUS–DDIT3*	>90	Small (3)	Transcription	Crozat. *Nature* 1993;363:640 Rabbitts. *Nat Genet* 1993;4:175
	t(12;22)(q13;q12)	*EWSR1–DDIT3*	2–5	Uncertain	Transcription	Panagopoulos. *Oncogene* 1996;12:489
Liposarcoma, well-differentiated/atypical lipomatous tumor	12q13–15 amplification	*MDM2*, *CDK4*, other genes (*HMGA2*, *GLI*, *SAS*)	>70		Dysregulated cell growth	Pedeutour. *Genes Chromosomes Cancer* 1994;10:85 Fletcher. *Am J Pathol* 1996;148:623 Meza-Zepeda. *Cancer* 2001;31:264

Other soft tissue tumors						
Aggressive angiomyxoma	12q13–15	*HMGA2* rearrangement	Uncertain		Transcription	Nucci. *Genes Chromosomes Cancer* 2001;32:172
Alveolar soft part sarcoma	der(17)t(X;17)(p11;q25)	*ASPL–TFE3*	100	Small (2)	Transcription	Ladanyi. *Oncogene* 2001;20:48
Angiomatoid fibrous histiocytoma	t(2;22)(q33;q12)	*EWSR1–CREB1*	>50	None (1)	Transcription	Antonescu. *Genes Chromosomes Cancer* 2007;46:1051
	t(12;22)(q13;q12)	*EWSR1–ATF1*	30	None (1)	Transcription	Hallor. *Genes Chromosomes Cancer* 2005;44:97
	t(12;16)(q13;p11)	*FUS–ATF1*	10	Uncertain	Transcription	Waters. *Cancer Genet Cytogenet* 2000;121:109
Clear cell sarcoma (malignant melanoma of soft parts)	t(12;22)(q13;q12)	*EWSR1–ATF1*	>80	Large (4)	Transcription	Zucman. *Nat Genet* 1993;4:341 Wang. *Mod Pathol* 2009; 22:1201
	t(2;22)(q33;q12)	*EWSR1–CREB1*	<10	None (1)	Transcription	Antonescu. *Clin Cancer Res* 2006;12:5356
Endometrial stromal tumors	t(7;17)(p15;q21)	*JAZF1–JJAZ1*	40–100	None (1)	Transcription	Koontz. *Proc Natl Acad Sci USA* 2001;98:6348
	t(6;7)(p21;p15)	*JAZF1–PHF1*	<10	Small (2)	Transcription	Micci. *Cancer Res* 2006;66:107
	t(6;10;10)(p21;q22;p11)	*PHF1–EPC1*	<10	None (1)	Transcription	Micci. *Cancer Res* 2006;66:107
Epithelioid sarcoma	del(22q11.2) or 22q11.2 rearrangement	*INI1* inactivation[c]	<10–50[c]		Loss of tumor suppressor	Kohashi. *Hum Pathol* 2009;40:349 Modena. *Cancer Res* 2005;65:4012
Extraskeletal myxoid chondrosarcoma	t(9;22)(q22;q12)	*EWSR1–NR4A3*	70	Large (>4)	Transcription	Labelle. *Hum Mol Genet* 1995;4:2219 Clark. *Oncogene* 1996;12:229
	t(9;17)(q22;q11)	*TAF15–NR4A3*	25	None (1)	Transcription	Sjogren. *Cancer Res* 1999;59:5064 Panagopoulos. *Oncogene* 1999;18:7594 Attwooll. *Oncogene* 1999;18:7599
	t(9;15)(q22;q21)	*TCF12–NR4A3*	<5	None (1)	Transcription	Sjogren. *Cancer Res* 2000;60:6832
	t(3;9)(q11;q22)	*TGF–NR4A3*	<5	None (1)	Transcription	Hisaoka. *Genes Chromosomes Cancer* 2004;40:325
Fibrosarcoma, sclerosing epithelioid type	t(7;16)(q33;p11)	*FUS–CREB3L2*	10	Large (>4)	Signaling	Wang. *Mod Pathol* 2012;25:846
Hemangioendothelioma, epithelioid type	t(1;3)(p36;q25)	*WWTR1–CAMTA1*	>90	Small (2)	Transcription	Errani. *Genes Chromosomes Cancer* 2011;50:644
Hemangioendothelioma, pseudomyogenic	t(7;19)(q22;q13)	*SERPINE–FOSB*	15	Uncertain	Transcription	Walther. *J Pathol* 2014;232:534
Hemangioma, epithelioid with atypia	t(3;19)(q25.1;q13.32)	*WWTR1–FOSB*	<5	None (1)	Transcription	Antonescu. *Genes Chromosomes Cancer* 2014;53:951

(continued)

Table 37.1 (continued)

Tumor type	Chromosomal change	Fusion gene	Prevalence (%)	Number of fusion transcript variants	Function	Reference
Hemangioma, epithelioid with atypia	del19(q13.2–q13.32) or t(19;19)(q13.2;q13.32)	*ZFP36–FOSB*	15	Small (2)	Transcription	Antonescu. *Genes Chromosomes Cancer* 2014;53:951
Malignant rhabdoid tumor	del(22q11.2) or 22q11.2 rearrangement	*INI1* inactivation[c]	>90		Loss of tumor suppressor	Jackson. *Clin Cancer Res* 2009;15:1923
Myoepithelial tumors of soft tissue and bone[d]	t(6;22)(p21;q12)	*EWSR1–POU5F1*	10	Uncertain	Transcription	Antonescu. *Genes Chromosomes Cancer* 2010;49:1114
	t(1;22)(q23;q12)	*EWSR1–PBX1*	10	Uncertain	Transcription	Brandal. *Genes Chromosomes Cancer* 2008;47:558
	t(9;22)(q33;q12)	*EWSR1–PBX3*	10	None (1)	Transcription	Agaram. *Genes Chromosomes Cancer* 2015;54:63
	t(19;22)(q13;q12)	*EWSR1–ZNF444*	<5	Uncertain	Transcription	Brandal. *Genes Chromosomes Cancer* 2009;48:1051
Myxoinflammatory fibroblastic sarcoma/hemosiderotic fibrolipomatous tumor	t(1;10)(p22;q24)	*TGFBR3–MGEA5*	80	Uncertain	Transcription	Antonescu. *Genes Chromosomes Cancer* 2011;50:757
	3p11–12 amplification	*VGLL3, CHMP2B*	80		Transcription	Hallor. *J Pathol* 2009;217:716
Tenosynovial giant cell tumor	t(1;2)(p13;q37)	*CSF1–COL6A3*	Uncertain	Large (4)	Transcription	Möller. *Genes Chromosomes Cancer* 2008;47:21
Bone tumors						
Aneurysmal bone cyst	t(16;17)(q22;p13)	*USP6–CDH11*	20	None (1)	Signaling	Oliveira. *Am J Pathol* 2004;5:1773
	Other t(17p13)	Other *USP6* rearrangements (*TRAP150, ZNF9, OMD, COL1A1*, others)	40			Oliveira. *Am J Pathol* 2004;5:1773

Chondrosarcoma, mesenchymal type	t(8;8)(q13;q21)	*HEY1–NCOA2*	>90	Small (2)	Transcription	Wang. *Genes Chromosomes Cancer* 2012;51:127
Chondrosarcoma, secondary peripheral type (sporadic)	del(8q24)	*EXT1* (homozygous inactivation)	10[e]		Biosynthesis of heparan sulfate	de Andrea. *Oncogene* 2012; 31:1095
Osteochondroma (sporadic)	del(8q24)	*EXT1* (homozygous inactivation)	80[e]		Biosynthesis of heparan sulfate	Hameetman. *J Natl Cancer Inst* 2007;99:396
Osteosarcoma, low-grade (central and parosteal)	12q13–15 amplification	*MDM2*, *CDK4*, other genes (*HMGA2*, *GLI*, *SAS*)	>70		Dysregulated cell growth	Gisselsson. *Genes Chromosomes Cancer* 2002;33:133 Yoshida. *Modern Pathology* 2010;23:1279

TKR tyrosine kinase receptor

[a]The overall proportion of inflammatory myofibroblastic tumors with *ALK* gene rearrangement is 35 %

[b]Percentages indicate the proportion of tumors with abnormal karyotypes which have 12q13–15 or 6p21 chromosomal alterations. (*Sources*: Heim S & Mitelman F: Cancer Cytogenetics, 3rd Ed., Wiley-Blackwell, New York, 2009; Mitelman Database of Chromosome Aberrations and Gene Fusions in Cancer (2012). Mitelman F, Johansson B and Mertens F (Eds.), http://cgap.nci.nih.gov/Chromosomes/Mitelman; Fletcher CD,Akerman M, Dal Cin P, et al. Correlation between clinicopathological features and karyotype in lipomatous tumors. A report of 178 cases from the Chromosomes and Morphology (CHAMP) Collaborative Study Group. Am J Pathol. 1996;148:623–630)

[c]Loss of *INI1* expression by immunohistochemistry occurs in malignant rhabdoid tumors (renal, soft tissue, central nervous system-atypical teratoid/rhabdoid tumor of the CNS), epithelioid sarcoma, and in a variety of other tumors, often with "rhabdoid" features, including renal medullary carcinoma, myoepithelial carcinoma, extraskeletal myxoid chondrosarcoma, and epithelioid malignant peripheral nerve sheath tumors. The link between INI1 expression loss and genomic alterations is strong only in the case of malignant rhabdoid tumors; in the other tumors, the link is not clear, where epigenetic silencing or other mechanisms are a likely cause of *INI1* loss of expression

[d]*EWSR1* rearrangement without an identified fusion partner has been reported by FISH in a significant proportion of myoepithelial tumors of soft tissue and bone (approximately 30 % of cases)

[e]Exostosin 1 (*EXT1*, at 8q24) or exostosin 2 (*EXT2*, at 11p11–13) gene inactivation causes the multiple osteochondroma (MO) syndrome (previously known as hereditary multiple exostoses, inherited as an autosomal dominant trait) in 65 % and 35 % of cases, respectively. The percentage in the table refers to non-syndromic cases

result in in-frame fusion genes, resulting in abnormal chimeric transcription factors [4]. In a few cases, the gene fusion results in an aberrant tyrosine kinase or an autocrine growth factor [8–10]. The der(17) associated with the nonreciprocal t(X;17)(p11.2;q25) of human alveolar soft part sarcoma produces a chimeric transcript between the transcription factor gene *TFE3* and *ASPL*, a novel gene at 17q25 [11]. *ASPL* encodes a UBX-like domain at the C-terminus of the encoded protein. In alveolar soft part sarcoma, the 5′ end of *ASPL* is fused to exon 3 or 4 of *TFE3*, resulting in a fusion protein retaining the C-terminal TFE3 DNA-binding domain, a possible aberrant transcriptional regulator.

A recurrent t(7;17)(p15;q21) has been identified in endometrial stromal tumors [12]. Two new zinc finger genes are fused as a result of the translocation: *JAZF1* and *JJAZ1*. Protein products of the zinc finger genes usually function as transcriptional regulators via specific DNA binding through the zinc finger motif. The chimeric protein in endometrial stromal tumors has a tumor-specific mRNA transcript containing 5′ *JAZF1* and 3′ *JJAZ1* sequences including the zinc finger encoding regions from both parent genes. Since gene expression of wild-type *JAZF1* is present in normal endometrial stromal cells, the *JAZF1–JJAZ1* fusion gene present in endometrial stromal tumors likely results in aberrant transcriptional regulation in a lineage-specific manner.

Oncogenic Nature of Fusion Transcripts

Sarcomas theoretically develop from mesenchymal stem cells that are present in all compartments of the body. Unlike many epithelial neoplasms, where diverse genetic alterations usually underlie the stepwise progression of precursor lesions leading ultimately to the emergence of malignant clones, soft tissue malignancies have no identifiable precursor lesions and usually have a single genetic alteration typical of a particular type of sarcoma. In addition, chromosomal fusions in soft tissue sarcomas do not seem to represent a form of generalized genomic instability, as occurs with germline *TP53* mutations [6] or with microsatellite instability associated with colon carcinoma [13]. Benign tumor counterparts of soft tissue sarcomas usually carry quite different genetic or chromosomal abnormalities or both. For example, the specific sets of chromosomal alterations found in soft tissue lipomas are not among those consistently observed in liposarcoma [14, 15]. Similar to leukemogenesis and lymphomagenesis, the fusion gene in a given sarcoma is speculated to be oncogenic only in a specific cell type at a specific differentiation stage [16] and explains why in some instances the same fusion transcripts can be identified in unrelated tumors. For instance, *FUS–ERG* is present in both Ewing's sarcoma (ES)/peripheral neuroectodermal tumor (PNET) and acute myeloid leukemia, while *EWSR1–CREB1* is present in both angiomatoid fibrous histiocytoma and clear cell sarcoma, two soft tissue tumors that are clearly distinct both histologically and clinically [17]. In general, the genes involved in sarcoma translocations are transcription factors or cofactors. Many of the chimeric proteins include a strong transcriptional activator N-terminal domain encoded by one partner gene fused with a DNA-binding domain encoded by the other partner gene. In fact, fusion of domains capable of activating transcription with other domains featuring specific DNA-binding function appears to be a common theme shared among neoplasms of mesenchymal derivation, such as soft tissue tumors and leukemia. EWSR1 (and its homologous FUS) is a powerful transcription activator [18] and provides a paradigm for this type of oncogenic mechanism, as also indicated by its "promiscuity" as a fusion partner (Table 37.1).

Available data indicate that the fusion genes produced in translocation-specific sarcomas are the initiating oncogenic events, although additional alterations are important for the genesis of the malignant tumor. The fact that fusion genes are early events is supported by the observation that in biphasic tumors like synovial sarcoma, *SS18–SSX* is present in both spindle cell and epithelial components of the tumor. In vitro and in vivo experiments have shown evidence of tumorigenesis with the expression of these fusion genes. The most common chromosomal translocation in myxoid liposarcomas, t(12;16)(q13;p11), creates a *FUS–DDIT3* (*TLS–CHOP*) fusion gene. Transgenic mice expressing the altered form of FUS–DDIT3 created by an in-frame fusion of the FUS domain to the carboxy end of DDIT3 develop liposarcomas. No tumors of other tissues were found in these transgenic mice despite widespread activity of the transgene. The results provided evidence that the FUS domain of *FUS–DDIT3* plays a specific and critical role in the pathogenesis of liposarcoma [19]. Alveolar rhabdomyosarcoma (ARMS) is consistently associated with the characteristic translocations t(2;13)(q35;q14) or t(1;13)(p36;q14), which encode the PAX3–FOXO1 (PAX3–FKHR) or PAX7–FOXO1 (PAX7–FKHR) fusion oncoproteins, respectively. PAX3–FOXO1 fusion protein contributes to oncogenesis through abnormal control of growth, apoptosis, differentiation, or cell migration [20].

Specific Amplification of Chromosomal Regions

Amplification of specific chromosomal regions may lead to the occurrence of ring or giant marker chromosomes in the context of a simple karyotype. Chromosomal region amplifications occur in atypical lipomatous tumors/well-differentiated liposarcoma and in low-grade osteosarcoma, including both low-grade central osteosarcoma and parosteal osteosarcoma [21, 22]. In both instances the amplified chromosomal region

Table 37.2 Specific oncogenic mutations in sarcomas and related tumors

Tumor type	Chromosomal site	Gene	Mutation type	Function	Mutation prevalence (%)	Reference
Gastrointestinal stromal tumor (GIST)	4q11–q12	*KIT*	All mutations	Signaling (TKR)	80 (of all mutated GIST)	Corless. *Nat Rev Cancer* 2011;11:865. Hirota. Science 1998;279:577. Heinrich. *JCO* 2003;21:4342. Heinrich. *JCO* 2008;26:5360
			KIT exon 11 (deletions, insertions, single nucleotide changes)		65	
			KIT exon 9 (AY502-503 insertion)		10	
			Other *KIT* mutations		5	
	4q11–q12	*PDGFRA*	All mutations	Signaling (TKR)	5–10 (of all mutated GIST)	Heinrich. *Science* 2003;299:708. Corless. *JCO* 2005;23;5357
			PDGFRA exon 18 (D842V)		5	
			Other *PDGFRA* mutations		<5	
	7q34	*BRAF*		Signaling (MAPK)	<5 (~10 % of *KIT* and *PDGFRA* wild-type GIST)	Agaram. *Genes Chromosomes and Cancer* 2008;47:853
		Other genes (e.g., *RAS, SDH*) or unknown			5–10	Corless. *Nat Rev Cancer* 2011;11:865
Desmoid tumor (aggressive fibromatosis)	3p22–p21.3	*CTNNB1*		Signaling (Wnt)	85[a]	Lazar. *Am J Pathol* 2008;173:1518
Fibrous dysplasia of bone	20q13.3	*GNAS1*		Signaling (cAMP)	90[b]	Idowu. Histopathology 2007;50:691
Intramuscular myxoma	20q13.3	*GNAS1*		Signaling (cAMP)	60[b]	Delaney. Mod Pathol 2009;22:718

cAMP adenosine 3′5′ cyclic monophosphate, *MAPK* mitogen-activated protein kinase, *TKR* tyrosine kinase receptor, *Wnt* wingless-INT pathway

[a]The percentage refers to sporadic cases, not associated with the familial adenomatous polyposis (FAP) syndrome

[b]The percentage refers to sporadic cases, not associated with the McCune–Albright (MAS, polyostotic fibrous dysplasia, endocrine hyperfunction, café au lait spots) or Mazabraud (intramuscular myxoma and fibrous dysplasia) syndromes

is 12q13–15 where several genes with a role for tumor development are located, including *MDM2*, *CDK4*, *HMGA2*, *GLI*, and *SAS* [22–25]. *MDM2*, encoding a negative regulator of TP53, and *CDK4*, encoding a catalytic subunit of the protein kinase complex that promotes cell cycle progression, are the most consistently amplified genes [24, 25]. *HMGA2*, encoding a transcription cofactor, is often amplified and rearranged in atypical lipomatous tumors [25, 26].

Mutations

Specific and characteristic oncogenic mutations occur in mesenchymal tumors (Table 37.2). Gastrointestinal stromal tumors (GIST) are characterized by specific, mutually exclusive oncogenic mutations that affect primarily the receptor tyrosine kinase KIT or platelet-derived growth factor receptor-α (PDGFRA), in approximately 80 % and 5–10 %

of cases, respectively. In the remaining 10–15 % of GIST cases, mutations of other oncogenes, notably *BRAF*, have been identified [27]. The oncogenic role of *KIT* or *PDGFRA* mutations has been confirmed by numerous studies, and transgenic mice expressing mutated *KIT* develop stromal tumors with features of human GIST [28]. Mutations in GIST are in general heterozygous, but in 15 % of cases, the wild-type *KIT* allele is lost, an occurrence that has been associated with more aggressive behavior of the tumor [29]. GIST are mesenchymal neoplasms, thought to derive from the interstitial cells of Cajal, the pacemakers for peristaltic contractions in the gastrointestinal tract. Like their putative cell of origin, tumor cells express the KIT (CD117) protein that is detectable by immunohistochemistry in 95 % of cases, regardless of the presence of a mutation. Strictly speaking, GIST are gastrointestinal tumors, but because of their biologic and clinical features, they are included with other soft tissue sarcomas in the National Comprehensive Cancer Network guidelines [30]. GIST are relatively uncommon, but are very effectively treated with the tyrosine kinase inhibitor imatinib (STI571, Gleevec), developed to block the BCR-ABL tyrosine kinase of chronic myelogenous leukemia. Mutational analysis for *KIT* and *PDGFRA* genes is thus essential not only to define the diagnosis of GIST and to guide therapy [27, 31]; thus, mutation testing is included in the College of American Pathologists' protocol for GIST [32]. Correlation between genotype and phenotype is remarkable. *KIT* exon 11 mutations are associated with poor prognosis in untreated GIST [33]. Among exon 11 alterations, deletions, especially those involving codon 557 and/or codon 558, are a marker for poor outcome, when compared with other changes [34]. In contrast, GIST with mutations in *PDGFRA* generally have lower malignant potential, usually a gastric location, and variable, sometimes negative, immunohistochemical KIT expression [27]. Secondary resistance to imatinib treatment, which eventually develops in the large majority of patients, is usually caused by new mutations, which are almost always in the same gene and allele as the primary *KIT* or *PDGFRA* mutation. Unlike primary *KIT* mutations that predominate in exons 11 and 9, secondary mutations develop in specific regions of the KIT kinase domain that is the target of imatinib.

Mutations that prevent β-catenin degradation and activate Wnt signaling occur in a high proportion of desmoid tumors, including sporadic cases, not associated with the familial adenomatous polyposis syndrome [35]. Activating mutations of the *GNAS1* gene, encoding the stimulatory G protein α subunit (Gs-α) that couples receptor binding by several hormones to activation of the adenylate cyclase pathway, are present in most cases of fibrous dysplasia of bone and intramuscular myxoma [36, 37]. Inactivating *INI1* mutations are present in approximately 50 % of malignant rhabdoid tumors, a group of rare and highly aggressive cancers composed of large polygonal cells similar to rhabdomyoblasts. Like rhabdomyoblasts, rhabdoid tumor cells have vesicular nuclei with prominent nucleoli and aggregates of intermediate filaments resulting in intracytoplasmic eosinophilic inclusions. These tumors typically affect children and arise in the kidney, in soft tissue, or intracranially. Intracranial rhabdoid tumors are called atypical teratoid/rhabdoid tumor of the central nervous system. *INI1* encodes one subunit of an ATP-dependent chromatin remodeling complex that functions as a tumor suppressor, and biallelic inactivation through a combination of mutations, deletions, and loss of heterozygosity has been shown in more than 90 % of rhabdoid tumor cases [38].

Available Assays and Interpretation

A significant number of sarcomas have consistent abnormalities that are detectable by standard cytogenetics or molecular genetic approaches (Fig. 37.2) [4, 6, 7, 39]. Sarcomas in this group should be defined by their specific molecular and cytogenetic alterations, although determining the sensitivity and specificity of these translocations for specific sarcoma types and the relative roles of molecular and histological classification of each sarcoma will continue to be refined.

Karyotyping

Karyotyping is the classic cytogenetic approach for identifying chromosomal alterations including translocations in sarcomas [40]. Optimally, the procedure requires a substantial volume of viable, sterile tumor tissue, usually 1–2 cm^3. The specimen should be harvested, placed in culture medium as soon as possible, and transported to the laboratory. Specimens can be transported over a long distance at either room temperature or refrigerated for up to 48 h. Small samples (limited incisional or needle biopsies) can be successfully cultured and karyotyped, although they may require a longer incubation time (1–2 weeks) to obtain enough dividing tumor cells for analysis. Characteristic and diagnostic chromosomal alterations seen in human soft tissue tumors are listed in Table 37.1.

The major advantage of karyotyping over molecular genetic methods is the global assessment of the chromosome complement in a tumor cell in one assay, including both numerical and structural alterations. Moreover, primary and secondary chromosome alterations can be studied, and sarcoma translocations involving variant partner chromosome(s) can be easily identified. An obvious drawback of conventional cytogenetic analysis is the requirement of adequate tumor cell growth to obtain metaphase spreads. If tumor cells do not grow, a false-negative result of a normal karyotype

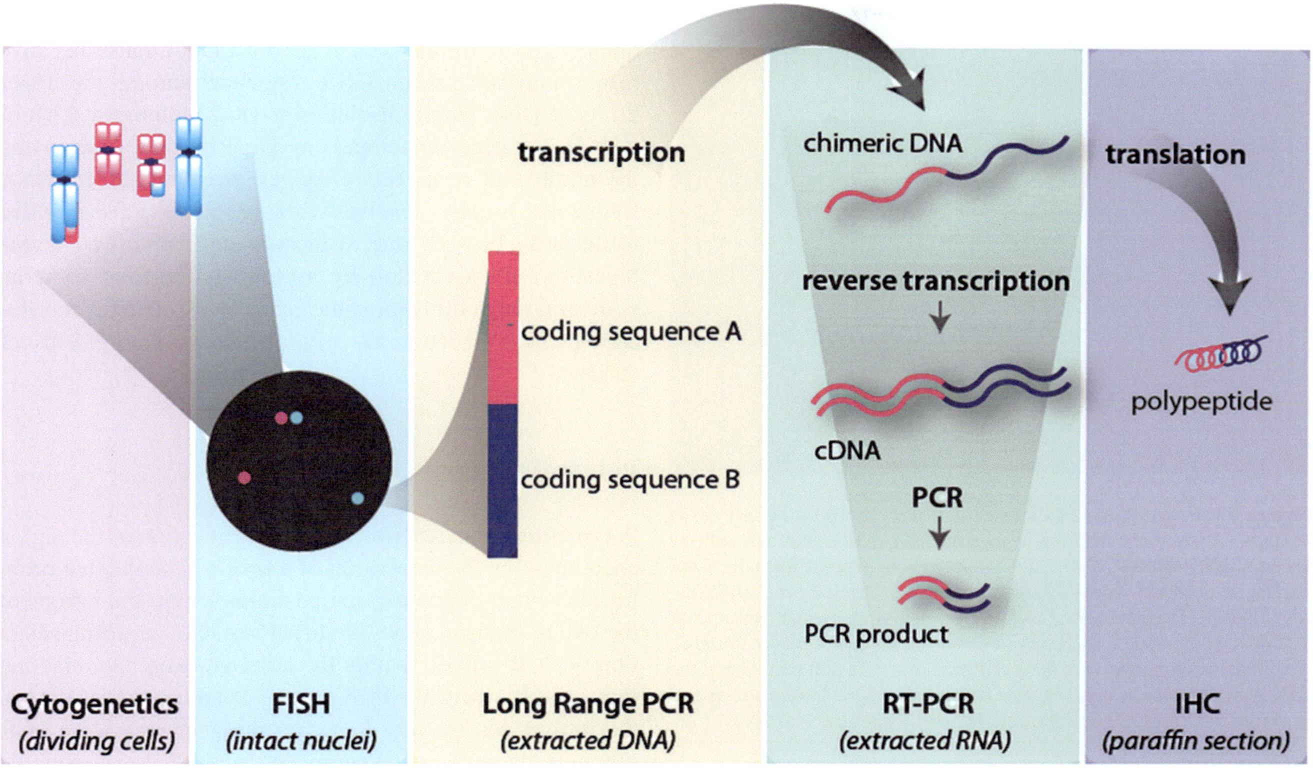

Figure 37.2 Methods to identify chromosomal translocation and fusion gene products (modified from Mertens et al. Semin Oncol 2009;36:312–323)

may occur due to the presence of normal fibroblasts in the specimen. Another pitfall of karyotyping is its limited resolution for identification of cryptic alterations, which may occur in sarcomas. Complex chromosomal changes also can make identification of sarcoma-specific translocations difficult. Furthermore, translocations involving specific chromosomal regions may not necessarily represent the characteristic gene fusion for a specific sarcoma. Confirmation by fluorescence in situ hybridization (FISH) or molecular testing, therefore, is recommended for questionable cases or to reach a definitive diagnosis.

Fluorescence In Situ Hybridization

FISH provides a powerful diagnostic method for demonstrating a specific gene fusion or chromosomal alteration. Metaphase chromosomal preparation from the tumor can be used to identify translocations by chromosomal painting using chromosome-specific probes or gene-specific probes. However, this is not always possible since cell culture of sarcoma tissue to obtain metaphase chromosomes may be unsuccessful. In these cases, interphase FISH provides an excellent alternative using touch preparations from fresh or frozen tumor specimens without the requirement for tissue culture. One major advantage of interphase FISH over traditional karyotyping is the ability to detect cryptic gene rearrangements. In fact, the chromosomes of interphase nuclei are much more extended than metaphase or prometaphase chromosomes. As a result, FISH analysis performed on interphase nuclei permits higher resolution and can help to determine the physical mapping order of large DNA probes. Dual-color DNA probes from the two rearranged genes (fusion probe) or breakpoint-flanking regions of one involved gene (break-apart probe) are most commonly used to assess sarcomas for the presence of a specific translocation (Fig. 37.3). Chromosomal centromeric probes and DNA probes spanning the translocation breakpoint also can be used. The interpretation of the FISH result depends on the types of hybridization probes.

The possibility of performing interphase FISH on formalin-fixed paraffin-embedded (FFPE) tissue, either on histology sections or on preparations of cell nuclei obtained from paraffin blocks, has recently increased its potential diagnostic applications [41, 42]. For interphase FISH of FFPE specimens, analysis of a nuclear preparation is superior to analysis of histological sections, although more labor intensive and seldom used in clinical practice. The most prevalent method for FISH detection of specific translocation in a sarcoma is the use of thin tissue sections of 4–5 μm

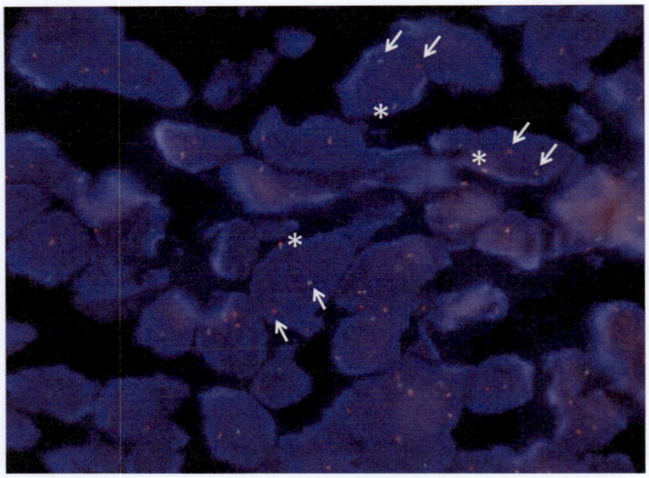

Figure 37.3 Interphase FISH detection of gene fusion in soft tissue sarcoma. Breakpoint-flanking probes of *SS18* (*SYT*), one red and one green, are hybridized to 4–5 μm thick sections from a formalin-fixed paraffin-embedded synovial sarcoma sample processed for routine histopathology. The juxtaposed *red* and *green* signals, which can appear *yellow* in some nuclei, represent undisturbed normal signal (*asterisks*). The translocation involving the *SS18* gene due to fusion with one of the *SSX* genes results in splitting the fused signal (juxtaposed *green* and *red*) into randomly disturbed single *red* and *green dots* (*arrows*)

thick. FISH detection of the specific translocation using the break-apart probes is most frequently used for the diagnosis of translocation-specific sarcomas (Fig. 37.3). Although dual-color fusion probe FISH can be used for the diagnosis of translocation-specific sarcomas, interpretation is not as easy as for break-apart probe FISH because of the presence of the truncation or overlap of tumor nuclei in a tissue section.

Other cytogenetic approaches like spectral karyotyping and comparative genomic hybridization (CGH), including conventional metaphase-based and array-based CGH, are suitable for genomic-wide analysis for detection of deletion, duplication, and copy-number changes. Although these methods may be diagnostically useful for the detection of specific regional chromosomal deletions, for example, the regional chromosomal loss of 22p11 in malignant rhabdoid tumor, they do not usually allow easy evaluation of balanced chromosomal translocations in sarcomas or other tumors.

Southern Blot

Southern blot analysis detects sarcoma-specific translocations using labeled DNA probes specific to the fusion genes. The procedure is highly specific and particularly useful in detecting translocations with frequently variable translocation breakpoints, as for ES/PNET. The main limitations of the Southern blot method are the labor intensiveness of the procedure and the requirement for fresh or frozen tissue to obtain high-molecular-weight genomic DNA. False-negative results may arise when DNA fragments surpass the upper limits of DNA length resolution (>15–20 kilobases [kb]) or with fusion genes encompassing large intron(s). Increasing the number of restriction enzymes to create shorter DNA fragments usually resolves this problem. False-positive results may be seen due to incomplete restriction enzyme digestion, contamination by a cloning vector or bacteria, structural polymorphism of the genes involved in the translocation, and restriction recognition site polymorphisms or variants.

Polymerase Chain Reaction

Polymerase chain reaction (PCR) amplification of the region encompassing the breakpoint of a fusion gene is often problematic. First, the breakpoint positions within the introns of the two rearranged genes are often variable, requiring selection of PCR primers within the adjacent exon and resulting in a variable size of the PCR product from case to case. Also, the introns can be very large, resulting in very large PCR products that may not be completely amplified and reducing the sensitivity of the test. Therefore, PCR of sarcoma-specific translocations using genomic DNA is not used for clinical testing.

Reverse Transcription-PCR

Chromosomal translocations in sarcomas give rise to aberrant fusion transcripts that are highly specific to a given tumor type (Table 37.1). More importantly, the structures of these fusion transcripts are highly consistent. Although the translocation breakpoint may involve various nucleotide positions of an intron at the DNA level, the resulting fusion transcript structure is the same due to RNA splicing. In a given sarcoma type, the gene fusion point at the messenger RNA (mRNA) level is highly precise to the single ribonucleotide. The tumor specificity and structural consistency of the fusion transcripts make reverse transcription-PCR (RT-PCR) the preferred method for molecular detection of specific translocations [43].

After reverse transcription of tumor mRNA into complementary DNA (cDNA), PCR primers complementary to the exons that flank the translocation breakpoint are used to amplify fusion transcript-specific RT-PCR products. Variations of RT-PCR methods have been used for the detection of sarcoma-specific fusion transcripts. Since the fusion-joining point may be far away from the poly(A) tail of the aberrant transcript, random hexamers or gene-specific downstream primers usually are used instead of oligo d(T) for the reverse transcription of RNA into cDNA. Instead of the traditional two-step RT-PCR method, reverse transcription and PCR can be performed in a single reaction, a procedure called one-step RT-PCR. The reverse transcriptase works first at low temperature to convert mRNA into cDNA, while the Taq DNA polymerase is inactive. The temperature is then raised to inactivate the reverse transcriptase, to activate the Taq DNA polymerase, and to initiate the amplification reaction at the same time. Reactions with multiple primer sets are difficult to optimize, but are very convenient for molecular testing of sarcomas with numerous fusion gene variants such as ES/PNET [44]. Nested PCR using an additional pair of primers to further amplify the first-round RT-PCR product can greatly increase sensitivity, although it also increases the likelihood of amplicon contamination.

Identification of a positive RT-PCR result usually relies on detection of the expected-sized product on a DNA-separating gel, such as agarose or acrylamide, or by capillary electrophoresis. When fresh or frozen tissue is the starting material, the target size of the RT-PCR product is designed carefully to be less than 500 bp and preferably around 200 bp. For fusion genes that have little size variation, such as *SS18–SSX* fusion of synovial sarcoma, the presence of a single RT-PCR product of the expected size generally is considered adequate for positive identification, although post-PCR confirmatory analysis of the product sequence can be performed. For fusion genes with molecular size variability, such as *FUS–DDIT3* in myxoid liposarcoma, additional analysis of the PCR products is mandatory to confirm the specificity of the PCR products. Confirmatory methods include blot transfer with subsequent hybridization with a fusion gene-specific probe, DNA sequencing of the PCR product, restriction endonuclease digestion, or an additional nested PCR step. Inclusion of positive, negative, and no-template (water) control reactions is necessary because of the high sensitivity of the amplification process and the risk of amplicon contamination with RT-PCR detection of fusion transcripts for clinical diagnosis.

Soft tissue tumor FFPE blocks may be used as the source of RNA, although with some caution [45]. As a result of the fixation and embedding processes, the RNA from tissue blocks is substantially degraded. RNA degradation requires that the size of the amplification product(s) be designed to be considerably smaller (around 100 bp) compared to assays designed for use of fresh or frozen tissue. RT-PCR from FFPE tissue blocks usually requires more amplification cycles, and a nested approach may be necessary for the detection of the aberrant transcript, both of which increase the risk of false-positive results due to carryover amplicon contamination. Very stringent conditions and additional control reactions are necessary to ensure test specificity.

Consideration must be given to the variability of fusion gene transcripts for each type of sarcoma (see Table 37.1) when interpreting RT-PCR test results. For instance, in ES/PNET, considerable variations occur among the different exons involved in the gene fusion [44]. Although the tumors may be cytogenetically indistinguishable, differences in the exon composition of the final fusion transcript can only be detected by a PCR-based method. Variant chromosomal translocations involving different chromosomal and gene partners also give rise to variability in up to approximately 10 % of ES/PNET cases. In fact, the t(21;22), instead of the far more common t(11;22), results in the fusion of *EWSR1* with *ERG* [46]. Very rarely, EWSR1 is fused with other loci including *ETV1* or *E1AF* in ES/PNET [47]. Awareness of these variants is very important when a negative RT-PCR result for the more common *EWSR1–FLI1* rearrangements occurs.

Real-Time RT-PCR

Although designed for quantitative measurements, real-time RT-PCR has become a reliable detection method for fusion gene transcripts [48, 49] because of three major advantages over the conventional endpoint RT-PCR. First, real-time RT-PCR greatly enhances the specificity of detection by incorporating a probe that is complementary to the region of the gene internal to the PCR primers. Second, real-time PCR measures the geometric (exponential) phase of a PCR reaction (cycles 20–25), allowing quantification of the fusion transcript. Third, the PCR product accumulation is measured in real time by fluorescence detection through the semitransparent plastic cap of the reaction tube, and therefore, post-PCR manipulation and possible PCR contamination are reduced. Real-time RT-PCR conclusively has very high specificity and sensitivity, which are important when analyzing very small samples or target genes with very low expression levels [48]. Simultaneous amplification of multiple targets by multiplex real-time RT-PCR is possible by using target-specific probes labeled with different fluorescent labels [50].

With careful optimization, real-time RT-PCR can be highly reliable for detection of fusion transcripts, using all types of tissue sources [49]. The early geometric-phase detection with enhanced specificity and elimination of post-PCR manipulation makes real-time RT-PCR ideal for detection of sarcoma fusion transcripts, even if the RNA source is FFPE tissue [51]. The specific and quantitative detection power of real-time RT-PCR for FFPE tissue is illustrated in Fig. 37.4, in which amplification of the *SS18–SSX* fusion transcript of synovial sarcoma is shown. Positive identification of fusion transcripts can be achieved using as little as 20 ng of RNA extracted from one paraffin block, making small specimens, such as core needle biopsies, suitable for definitive molecular diagnosis. The operating cost profile

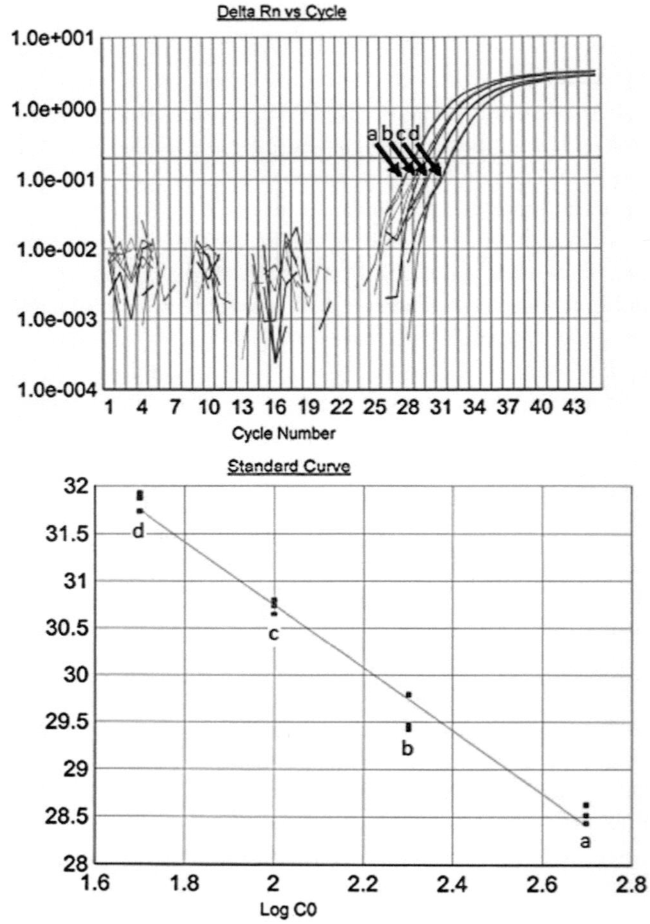

Figure 37.4 Real-time RT-PCR detection of *SS18–SSX* fusion transcripts in a synovial sarcoma. *Top panel*: Real-time RT-PCR plot of PCR cycle number vs fluorescence signal for *SS18–SSX* fusion transcript amplification in a synovial sarcoma with (a) 500 ng, (b) 200 ng, (c) 100 ng, and (d) 50 ng of total input RNA, each amplified in triplicate. The RNA was extracted from formalin-fixed paraffin-embedded tissue. *Bottom panel*: Log gradient plot of the data from the top panel, demonstrating linear quantitative amplification consistent with the amount of input RNA template. The *y*-axis represents the threshold cycle number, and the *x*-axis is the log of the RNA concentration (Log C0). The quantity of the specific RNA measured by real-time RT-PCR is inversely proportional to the threshold cycle number

and time to reporting also are in favor of real-time RT-PCR over conventional RT-PCR, and real-time RT-PCR is now commonly used for the routine diagnosis of sarcoma and minimal disease detection [48].

DNA Sequencing and Next-Generation Exome Sequencing

Sanger sequencing with capillary electrophoresis platforms will likely remain in significant use for targeted sequencing projects (biomarker identification and pathway analysis) and clinical molecular testing applications until next generation sequencing platforms become more standard for clinical molecular laboratories (see below). Technical advances in high-throughput next-generation sequencing (NGS), also known as massively parallel or multiplex cyclic sequencing, are key elements that are enabling the application of genomic knowledge into clinical practice, including the diagnosis of translocation-specific sarcomas [52]. NGS technologies have increased the speed and throughput capacities over Sanger sequencing while reducing cost and have significantly increased the possibility of detecting new gene fusions [7]. Detection of the sarcoma fusion genes may be accomplished by NGS platforms targeting the transcriptome in sarcoma cells. Through combination of hybridization capture of cDNAs and next-generation sequencing, targeted RNA sequencing (RNA-seq) provides an efficient and cost-effective method to analyze specific subsets of the transcriptome of a tumor simultaneously for mutations, fusion transcripts, and gene expression levels [53]. NGS technologies with appropriate assembly algorithms have facilitated the reconstruction of the entire transcriptome in the absence of a reference genome [54]. Targeted RNA-seq is also a powerful tool suitable for a wide range of large-scale tumor-profiling studies to identify sequence variations and novel fusion gene products [55].

Gene Expression Profiling

Gene expression profiling of many cancers, including sarcomas, has produced inconsistent results in predicting clinical drug or management response and prognosis and is not used for the detection of sarcoma-specific transcripts as an aid to the histological diagnosis. One constraint of gene expression profiling is the preference for use of fresh or frozen tissue. The limited availability of fresh or frozen tissue represents a drawback compared with other methods that can utilize routinely processed FFPE tissue. Nevertheless, gene expression profiling definitely represents a potentially powerful tool for molecular grading of sarcomas, and specific gene expression profiles predict metastatic outcome. Refinement of the methods to select the relevant genes and validation of the expression signatures proposed for clinical use may open new avenues to the management of patients with sarcoma [56].

Immunohistochemistry

Fusion protein-specific antibodies are not available for routine diagnostic purposes, but the detection of aberrant protein expression can be used to infer the occurrence of a tumor-specific translocation. Expression can be altered because by immunohistochemistry the protein is (1) no longer present (e.g., lack of expression of INI1 in malignant rhabdoid tumor); (2) detected in a cell type that does not normally express that protein (e.g., ALK expression in a mesenchymal cell in the case of inflammatory myofibroblastic tumor with *ALK* rearrangement or expression of MDM2 in atypical lipomatous tumors with 12q13–15 amplification); (3) detected at higher levels compared to normal tissues (TFE3 in alveolar soft part sarcoma); and (4) present in an inappropriate cellular compartment (e.g., nuclear localization of β-catenin in desmoid tumors with mutated *CTNNB1*).

Clinical Utility of Testing

The molecular characterization of human sarcomas has significantly changed, is still reshaping sarcoma classification and diagnosis, and is promoting rapid progress in disease monitoring, prediction of outcome, and design of novel therapeutic strategies.

Establishing a Definitive Diagnosis and Redefining Tumor Entities

Soft tissue tumors comprise a vast and heterogeneous group of neoplasms. Because different tumors often have different biological behaviors and respond differently to therapeutic strategies, precise classification is of great clinical importance. The majority of soft tissue tumors were first delineated on the basis of morphologic and clinical findings into homogeneous groups. However, many tumors with similar histological and pathological characteristics actually are heterogeneous groups that differ in their clinical behaviors and underlying pathogenesis. Correlation of cytogenetic and molecular characteristics with pathologic findings is essential for understanding both the biological significance and the clinical value of specific molecular changes.

A surprising correlation has emerged among chromosomal alterations, gene rearrangements, and distinct histopathologic entities. Morphologic and cytogenetic/molecular observations in fact have been validating each other, and a combined approach has resulted in a more rational classification of soft tissue tumors. This combined morphologic and molecular classification has been particularly helpful in understanding the so-called small round blue cell tumors. ES and PNET are essentially a single-tumor type defined by the characteristic translocation between chromosomes 11 and 22, resulting in an *EWSR1* gene rearrangement. Despite the morphologic similarities, typical olfactory neuroblastoma lacks *EWSR1* rearrangement that argues against the previously proposed inclusion of this tumor in the ES/PNET group [57]. The finding of *PAX3–FOXO1* chimeric products is of considerable value in defining ARMS. In fact, the small proportion of primitive embryonal-like RMS containing a *PAX3–FOXO1* gene fusion likely represents unrecognized solid ARMS [58]. Molecular testing also allows the identification of previously unrecognized variants of known tumors. One such example, illustrated in Fig. 37.5, is a poorly differentiated synovial sarcoma with rhabdoid features.

Another group of tumors that has significantly benefited by a combined morphologic and molecular approach is adipose tissue neoplasms. The finding of ring or giant marker chromosomes cytogenetically defines the group of atypical lipomatous tumors (well-differentiated liposarcoma) and justifies the distinction of atypical lipomatous tumors from spindle cell and pleomorphic lipomas. The finding of *FUS–DDIT3* fusion transcripts in both myxoid liposarcoma and round cell liposarcoma demonstrates that they represent a continuum, an observation nicely correlating with the not infrequent observation of cases with mixed histology [59]. The t(17;22), which produces the *COL1A1–PDGFB* fusion, is present in both dermatofibrosarcoma protuberans (DFSP) and giant cell fibroblastoma, indicating that these are adult and pediatric presentations, respectively, of a single tumor entity [10, 60]. Similarly, the identification of the t(7;16)(q34;p11), resulting in the *FUS–CREB3L2* fusion gene, in both low-grade fibromyxoid sarcoma and hyalinizing spindle cell tumor with giant rosettes has clarified that these tumors represent variants of the same biological entity [61]. The *FUS–CREB3L2* fusion gene is highly specific for this tumor type, since it is present in low-grade fibromyxoid sarcoma, but not in other sarcomas with similar histologic features [62] and is uncommon in sclerosing epithelioid fibrosarcoma [63].

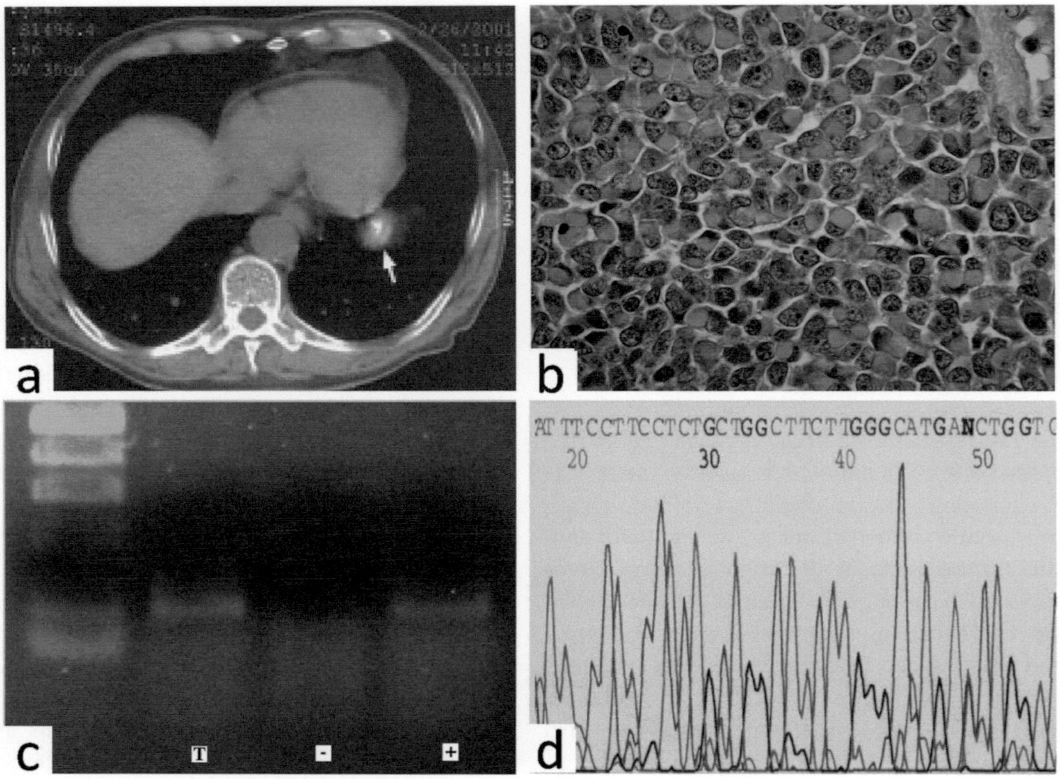

Figure 37.5 RT-PCR detection of *SS18–SSX2* fusion transcript in a primary poorly differentiated synovial sarcoma of the lung with rhabdoid features (courtesy of Dr. Thomas Ciesielski). (**a**) CT scan of a 72-year-old patient with a subpleural 2 cm nodule (*arrow*). An extensive physical and radiographic examination failed to reveal a separate primary lesion. (**b**) Proliferating tumor cells with rhabdoid cytoplasm. This histological variant of synovial sarcoma may be difficult to diagnose without molecular testing. (**c**) RT-PCR of formalin-fixed paraffin-embedded tumor tissue shows the presence of a 97 bp RT-PCR product from the *SS18–SSX2* fusion transcript in *lane 2* (*T* tumor). *Lanes 3* and *4* are the negative (−) and positive (+) controls, respectively. (**d**) Direct DNA sequencing of the RT-PCR product from *panel* (**c**) shows a *SS18–SSX2*-type fusion transcript

Providing Prognostic and Predictive Information

By allowing accurate diagnosis, molecular testing greatly contributes to defining both the therapy and prognosis for a patient with sarcoma. For patients with GIST, the mutational status correlates with both prognosis and response to treatment. GIST with *KIT* exon 11 mutations are more aggressive, but also respond better to treatment with imatinib, compared with tumors that have an exon 9 *KIT* mutation, no *KIT* mutation, or a *PDGFRA* mutation, and therefore have longer progression-free and overall survival [27, 31]. Specific mutations, like the *PDGFRA* D842V mutation, predict a lack of response (primary resistance) to imatinib. Other mutations, clustered in specific regions of the KIT kinase domain that is the target of imatinib, have been associated with disease progression after an initial treatment benefit (secondary resistance) [27]. Imatinib reduces the growth of *COL1A1–PDGFB*-transformed animal cells as well as primary cultures of DFSP tumor cells in vitro and in vivo [9, 64] and is an effective treatment for DFSP with the *COL1A1–PDGFB* fusion gene, including cases that have undergone progression to fibrosarcoma, with a response rate close to 50 % [65]. The *PAX3–FOXO1* fusion is an adverse prognostic factor in ARMS [66]. Therefore, not only is *PAX–FOXO1* fusion transcript the defining feature of ARMS, but also the specific type of gene fusion present in the tumor identifies a high-risk subgroup (with *PAX3–FOXO1*) and a favorable-outcome subgroup (with *PAX7–FOXO1*). The *SS18–SSX* fusion type is not prognostically significant [67–69]. Intensive treatment protocols for fusion-negative sarcomas have eliminated the better outcome previously reported in patients with *EWS–FLI1* fusion transcripts [70].

High-throughput analysis of gene expression can provide valuable prognostic information, even though this testing is not routinely used in clinical care yet. One example is the Complexity Index in Sarcoma (CINSARC) study that has produced a panel of 67 genes related to mitosis and chromosome management to define patient outcome. Remarkably, in this study, gene expression analysis performed better than conventional tumor grading in the identification of patients with a high risk of metastatic disease [56].

Minimal Disease Detection

Molecular detection of occult tumor cells can be a prognostic indicator important for clinical staging and selection of therapeutic strategies. Detection of low-level expression of *EWSR1–FLI* fusion transcripts in bone marrow and blood has been reported for patients with sarcomas [71, 72]. Micrometastases were detected in 31 % of patients with localized disease and 50 % of patients with clinically metastatic tumors. RT-PCR detection of specific fusion transcripts has been used to study the marrow and body fluids of patients with ES, ARMS, and desmoplastic small round cell tumors (DSRCT). Molecular evidence of metastasis was detected in all patients with clinically evident metastatic tumors but not in the patients with localized disease [73]. Although correlative studies are needed to validate the prognostic significance of occult tumor cells, molecular staging is an emerging field that may change the approach to the clinical management of patients with soft tissue sarcomas.

Developing Tumor-Specific Therapy

High-throughput molecular analysis integrating test results on DNA sequence, copy number, and mRNA expression has revealed genetic alterations in major types of sarcoma that can be used to identify specific targets for patient treatment [74]. The therapeutic implications of sarcoma-specific gene fusion events are tremendous, since each fusion is a potential target for tumor-specific therapies. A tumor-specific cytotoxic T cell response can be induced by peptides derived from the fusion point of the SS18–SSX chimeric protein in synovial sarcoma that may function in vitro as a neoantigen [75]. Other forms of tumor-specific immunotherapies are under development, and the opportunity exists to design tumor-specific drugs against specific fusion proteins present in soft tissue sarcomas, which may include targeting by RNA interference or other gene therapy approaches [76, 77].

Quality Control and Laboratory Issues

The availability of two or more unrelated test methods for the diagnosis of each sarcoma type can facilitate the confirmation of unexpected results or the resolution of discrepant results. One key issue regarding the accurate molecular diagnosis of sarcomas is the selection of the appropriate test. This is largely determined by the type of sarcoma under consideration, the specimen type, and the specimen quality and quantity. For fusion genes with limited structural variations, such as synovial sarcoma, ARMS, clear cell sarcoma of soft parts, extraskeletal myxoid chondrosarcoma, DSRCT, alveolar soft part sarcoma, and inflammatory myofibroblastic tumor, RT-PCR and real-time RT-PCR are the method of choice. Interphase FISH is the best testing method for sarcomas having fusion genes with chromosomal and intramolecular variations, such as myxoid/round cell liposarcoma, DFSP, and ES/PNET. Ideally, all specimens with a preliminary diagnosis of sarcoma should have viable tissue for karyotyping. A portion of the diagnostic specimen can be temporarily stored in culture medium at room temperature or 4 °C until a provisional histological diagnosis is made and then sent for karyotyping, if appropriate. Whenever possible, a portion of the tumor specimen should be frozen and stored, to provide the best source of nucleic acid suitable for virtually all types of molecular tests used for soft tissue sarcoma testing. Unfixed, fresh, or frozen tissue also is suitable for protein analysis, although this is rarely used clinically. Touch preparations for FISH should be made and stored for possible use. When only paraffin-embedded archival material is available, interphase FISH and real-time RT-PCR are the best testing choices.

Turnaround time varies significantly for the different testing methods. Cytogenetic karyotyping requires short-term culture (3–10 days). The length of time for culturing reflects the quality and the quantity of the specimen source, as well as the tumor proliferation rate in vitro. Turnaround time for interphase FISH also depends on specimen type. Touch preparation and frozen sections allow for rapid FISH analysis (1–2 days). For archival tissue sources, an additional 1 or 2 days are required to obtain the nuclear suspension or the tissue sections. RT- PCR has a 2- or 3-day turnaround time for common fusion gene detection but requires a longer time for more complex fusion variant detection. Real-time RT-PCR offers a shorter turnaround time (1 or 2 days) because it does not require post-PCR manipulation steps or confirmatory testing. Longer turnaround times may be expected if the laboratory batches specimens and only runs the test once per week, for example.

Conclusion

Cytogenetics and molecular cytogenetics have contributed significantly to the study of the pathobiology of soft tissue tumors. Identification of recurrent chromosomal changes has resulted in the definition of an increasing number of tumor-related molecular changes and is fostering a continual refinement of the classification of sarcomas and related mesenchymal tumors. The recognition of distinctive rearrangements in tumor subsets is providing powerful tools to refine the histological diagnosis in a field in which pathological diagnosis and clinical management are often difficult, due to both the variety of tumor phenotypes and their relative rarity. In this respect, interphase FISH, real-time RT-PCR, and multiplex RT-PCR testing for the detection of fusion products specific for different tumor types offer practical and cost-effective methods for complementing conventional histological diagnosis. Novel technical approaches, including NGS, may increase speed and throughput of molecular analysis, and the application of genomic knowledge into clinical practice may radically change the management of patients with sarcomas [7, 52, 56, 74].

References

1. Mitelman F, Johansson B, Mertens F. The impact of translocations and gene fusions on cancer causation. Nat Rev Cancer. 2007;7:233–45.
2. Kleihues P, Schauble B, Schauble B, zur Hausen A, et al. Tumors associated with p53 germline mutations: a synopsis of 91 families. Am J Pathol. 1997;150:1–13.
3. Antonescu CR, Dal Cin P. Promiscuous genes involved in recurrent chromosomal translocations in soft tissue tumours. Pathology. 2014;46:105–12.
4. Bennicelli JL, Barr FG. Chromosomal translocations and sarcomas. Curr Opin Oncol. 2002;14:412–9.
5. Fletcher CD. The evolving classification of soft tissue tumours – an update based on the new 2013 WHO classification. Histopathology. 2014;64:2–11.
6. Ladanyi M, Bridge JA. Contribution of molecular genetic data to the classification of sarcomas. Hum Pathol. 2000;31:532–8.
7. Mertens F, Tayebwa J. Evolving techniques for gene fusion detection in soft tissue tumours. Histopathology. 2014;64:151–62.
8. Coffin CM, Patel A, Perkins S, et al. ALK1 and p80 expression and chromosomal rearrangements involving 2p23 in inflammatory myofibroblastic tumor. Mod Pathol. 2001;14:569–76.
9. Greco A, Roccato E, Miranda C, et al. Growth-inhibitory effect of STI571 on cells transformed by the COL1A1/PDGFB rearrangement. Int J Cancer. 2001;92:354–60.
10. Simon MP, Pedeutour F, Sirvent N, et al. Deregulation of the platelet-derived growth factor B-chain gene via fusion with collagen gene COL1A1 in dermatofibrosarcoma protuberans and giant-cell fibroblastoma. Nat Genet. 1997;15:95–8.
11. Ladanyi M, Lui MY, Antonescu CR, et al. The der(17)t(X;17)(p11;q25) of human alveolar soft part sarcoma fuses the TFE3 transcription factor gene to ASPL, a novel gene at 17q25. Oncogene. 2001;20:48–57.
12. Koontz JI, Soreng AL, Nucci M, et al. Frequent fusion of the JAZF1 and JJAZ1 genes in endometrial stromal tumors. Proc Natl Acad Sci U S A. 2001;98:6348–53.
13. Chung DC, Rustgi AK. The hereditary nonpolyposis colorectal cancer syndrome: genetics and clinical implications. Ann Intern Med. 2003;138:560–70.
14. Fletcher CD, Fletcher JA, Dal Cin P, et al. Diagnostic gold standard for soft tissue tumours: morphology or molecular genetics? Histopathology. 2001;39:100–3.
15. Rosai J, Akerman M, Dal Cin P, et al. Combined morphologic and karyotypic study of 59 atypical lipomatous tumors. Evaluation of their relationship and differential diagnosis with other adipose tissue tumors (a report of the CHAMP Study Group). Am J Surg Pathol. 1996;20:1182–9.
16. Ladanyi M. Diagnosis and classification of small round-cell tumors of childhood. Am J Pathol. 1999;155:2181–2.
17. Antonescu CR, Dal Cin P, Nafa K, et al. EWSR1-CREB1 is the predominant gene fusion in angiomatoid fibrous histiocytoma. Genes Chromosomes Cancer. 2007;46:1051–60.
18. Rossow KL, Janknecht R. The Ewing's sarcoma gene product functions as a transcriptional activator. Cancer Res. 2001;61:2690–5.
19. Perez-Losada J, Sanchez-Martin M, Rodriguez-Garcia MA, et al. Liposarcoma initiated by FUS/TLS-CHOP: the FUS/TLS domain plays a critical role in the pathogenesis of liposarcoma. Oncogene. 2000;19:6015–22.
20. Barr FG. Gene fusions involving PAX and FOX family members in alveolar rhabdomyosarcoma. Oncogene. 2001;20:5736–46.
21. Fletcher CD, Akerman M, Dal Cin P, et al. Correlation between clinicopathological features and karyotype in lipomatous tumors. A report of 178 cases from the Chromosomes and Morphology (CHAMP) Collaborative Study Group. Am J Pathol. 1996;148:623–30.
22. Wunder JS, Eppert K, Burrow SR, et al. Co-amplification and overexpression of CDK4, SAS and MDM2 occurs frequently in human parosteal osteosarcomas. Oncogene. 1999;18:783–8.
23. Gisselsson D, Palsson E, Hoglund M, et al. Differentially amplified chromosome 12 sequences in low- and high-grade osteosarcoma. Genes Chromosomes Cancer. 2002;33:133–40.
24. Yoshida A, Ushiku T, Motoi T, et al. Immunohistochemical analysis of MDM2 and CDK4 distinguishes low-grade osteosarcoma from benign mimics. Mod Pathol. 2010;23:1279–88.
25. Dei Tos AP, Doglioni C, Piccinin S, et al. Coordinated expression and amplification of the MDM2, CDK4, and HMGI-C genes in atypical lipomatous tumours. J Pathol. 2000;190:531–6.
26. Meza-Zepeda LA, Berner JM, Henriksen J, et al. Ectopic sequences from truncated HMGIC in liposarcomas are derived from various amplified chromosomal regions. Genes Chromosomes Cancer. 2001;31:264–73.
27. Corless CL, Barnett CM, Heinrich MC. Gastrointestinal stromal tumours: origin and molecular oncology. Nat Rev Cancer. 2011;11:865–78.
28. Sommer G, Agosti V, Ehlers I, et al. Gastrointestinal stromal tumors in a mouse model by targeted mutation of the Kit receptor tyrosine kinase. Proc Natl Acad Sci U S A. 2003;100:6706–11.
29. Chen LL, Holden JA, Choi H, et al. Evolution from heterozygous to homozygous KIT mutation in gastrointestinal stromal tumor correlates with the mechanism of mitotic nondisjunction and significant tumor progression. Mod Pathol. 2008;21:826–36.
30. Demetri GD, Antonia S, Benjamin RS, et al. Soft tissue sarcoma. J Natl Compr Canc Netw. 2010;8:630–74.
31. Gastrointestinal-Stromal-Tumor-Meta-Analysis-Group. Comparison of two doses of imatinib for the treatment of unresectable or metastatic gastrointestinal stromal tumors: a meta-analysis of 1,640 patients. J Clin Oncol. 2010;28:1247–53.
32. Rubin BP, Blanke CD, Demetri GD, et al. Protocol for the examination of specimens from patients with gastrointestinal stromal tumor. Arch Pathol Lab Med. 2010;134:165–70.
33. Heinrich MC, Corless CL, Demetri GD, et al. Kinase mutations and imatinib response in patients with metastatic gastrointestinal stromal tumor. J Clin Oncol. 2003;21:4342–9.
34. Martin J, Poveda A, Llombart-Bosch A, et al. Deletions affecting codons 557–558 of the c-KIT gene indicate a poor prognosis in patients with completely resected gastrointestinal stromal tumors: a study by the Spanish Group for Sarcoma Research (GEIS). J Clin Oncol. 2005;23:6190–8.
35. Lazar AJ, Tuvin D, Hajibashi S, et al. Specific mutations in the beta-catenin gene (CTNNB1) correlate with local recurrence in sporadic desmoid tumors. Am J Pathol. 2008;173:1518–27.

36. Idowu BD, Al-Adnani M, O'Donnell P, et al. A sensitive mutation-specific screening technique for GNAS1 mutations in cases of fibrous dysplasia: the first report of a codon 227 mutation in bone. Histopathology. 2007;50:691–704.
37. Delaney D, Diss TC, Presneau N, et al. GNAS1 mutations occur more commonly than previously thought in intramuscular myxoma. Mod Pathol. 2009;22:718–24.
38. Jackson EM, Sievert AJ, Gai X, et al. Genomic analysis using high-density single nucleotide polymorphism-based oligonucleotide arrays and multiplex ligation-dependent probe amplification provides a comprehensive analysis of INI1/SMARCB1 in malignant rhabdoid tumors. Clin Cancer Res. 2009;15:1923–30.
39. Barr FG, Chatten J, D'Cruz CM, et al. Molecular assays for chromosomal translocations in the diagnosis of pediatric soft tissue sarcomas. JAMA. 1995;273:553–7.
40. Bridge JA, Sandberg AA. Cytogenetic and molecular genetic techniques as adjunctive approaches in the diagnosis of bone and soft tissue tumors. Skeletal Radiol. 2000;29:249–58.
41. Adem C, Gisselsson D, Dal Cin P, et al. ETV6 rearrangements in patients with infantile fibrosarcomas and congenital mesoblastic nephromas by fluorescence in situ hybridization. Mod Pathol. 2001;14:1246–51.
42. Hui P, Howe JG, Crouch J, et al. Real-time quantitative RT-PCR of cyclin D1 mRNA in mantle cell lymphoma: comparison with FISH and immunohistochemistry. Leuk Lymphoma. 2003;44:1385–94.
43. Athale UH, Shurtleff SA, Jenkins JJ, et al. Use of reverse transcriptase polymerase chain reaction for diagnosis and staging of alveolar rhabdomyosarcoma, Ewing sarcoma family of tumors, and desmoplastic small round cell tumor. J Pediatr Hematol Oncol. 2001;23:99–104.
44. Dagher R, Pham TA, Sorbara L, et al. Molecular confirmation of Ewing sarcoma. J Pediatr Hematol Oncol. 2001;23:221–4.
45. Guillou L, Coindre J, Gallagher G, et al. Detection of the synovial sarcoma translocation t(X;18) (SYT;SSX) in paraffin-embedded tissues using reverse transcriptase-polymerase chain reaction: a reliable and powerful diagnostic tool for pathologists. A molecular analysis of 221 mesenchymal tumors fixed in different fixatives. Hum Pathol. 2001;32:105–12.
46. Sorensen PH, Lessnick SL, Lopez-Terrada D, et al. A second Ewing's sarcoma translocation, t(21;22), fuses the EWS gene to another ETS-family transcription factor, ERG. Nat Genet. 1994;6:146–51.
47. Barr FG, Womer RB. Molecular diagnosis of ewing family tumors: too many fusions... ?. J Mol Diagn. 2007;9:437–40.
48. Cummings TJ, Brown NM, Stenzel TT. TaqMan junction probes and the reverse transcriptase polymerase chain reaction: detection of alveolar rhabdomyosarcoma, synovial sarcoma, and desmoplastic small round cell tumor. Ann Clin Lab Sci. 2002; 32:219–24.
49. Hill DA, Riedley SE, Patel AR, et al. Real-time polymerase chain reaction as an aid for the detection of SYT-SSX1 and SYT-SSX2 transcripts in fresh and archival pediatric synovial sarcoma specimens: report of 25 cases from St. Jude Children's Research Hospital. Pediatr Dev Pathol. 2003;6:24–34.
50. Peter M, Gilbert E, Delattre O. A multiplex real-time pcr assay for the detection of gene fusions observed in solid tumors. Lab Invest. 2001;81:905–12.
51. Hostein I, Menard A, Bui BN, et al. Molecular detection of the synovial sarcoma translocation t(X;18) by real-time polymerase chain reaction in paraffin-embedded material. Diagn Mol Pathol. 2002;11:16–21.
52. Voelkerding KV, Dames SA, Durtschi JD. Next-generation sequencing: from basic research to diagnostics. Clin Chem. 2009;55:641–58.
53. Gibbons JG, Janson EM, Hittinger CT, et al. Benchmarking next-generation transcriptome sequencing for functional and evolutionary genomics. Mol Biol Evol. 2009;26:2731–44.
54. Martin JA, Wang Z. Next-generation transcriptome assembly. Nat Rev Genet. 2011;12:671–82.
55. Levin JZ, Berger MF, Adiconis X, et al. Targeted next-generation sequencing of a cancer transcriptome enhances detection of sequence variants and novel fusion transcripts. Genome Biol. 2009;10:R115.
56. Chibon F, Lagarde P, Salas S, et al. Validated prediction of clinical outcome in sarcomas and multiple types of cancer on the basis of a gene expression signature related to genome complexity. Nat Med. 2010;16:781–7.
57. Kumar S, Perlman E, Pack S, et al. Absence of EWS/FLI1 fusion in olfactory neuroblastomas indicates these tumors do not belong to the Ewing's sarcoma family. Hum Pathol. 1999;30:1356–60.
58. Parham DM, Shapiro DN, Downing JR, et al. Solid alveolar rhabdomyosarcomas with the t(2;13). Report of two cases with diagnostic implications. Am J Surg Pathol. 1994;18:474–8.
59. Knight JC, Renwick PJ, Dal Cin P, et al. Translocation t(12;16)(q13;p11) in myxoid liposarcoma and round cell liposarcoma: molecular and cytogenetic analysis. Cancer Res. 1995;55:24–7.
60. Sandberg AA, Anderson WD, Fredenberg C, et al. Dermatofibrosarcoma protuberans of the breast. Cancer Genet Cytogenet. 2003;142:56–9.
61. Reid R, de Silva MV, Paterson L, et al. Low-grade fibromyxoid sarcoma and hyalinizing spindle cell tumor with giant rosettes share a common t(7;16)(q34;p11) translocation. Am J Surg Pathol. 2003;27:1229–36.
62. Mertens F, Fletcher CD, Antonescu CR, et al. Clinicopathologic and molecular genetic characterization of low-grade fibromyxoid sarcoma, and cloning of a novel FUS/CREB3L1 fusion gene. Lab Invest. 2005;85:408–15.
63. Wang WL, Evans HL, Meis JM, et al. FUS rearrangements are rare in 'pure' sclerosing epithelioid fibrosarcoma. Mod Pathol. 2012; 25(6):846–53.
64. Sjoblom T, Shimizu A, O'Brien KP, et al. Growth inhibition of dermatofibrosarcoma protuberans tumors by the platelet-derived growth factor receptor antagonist STI571 through induction of apoptosis. Cancer Res. 2001;61:5778–83.
65. Rutkowski P, Van Glabbeke M, Rankin CJ, et al. Imatinib mesylate in advanced dermatofibrosarcoma protuberans: pooled analysis of two phase II clinical trials. J Clin Oncol. 2010;28:1772–9.
66. Anderson J, Gordon T, McManus A, et al. Detection of the PAX3-FKHR fusion gene in paediatric rhabdomyosarcoma: a reproducible predictor of outcome? Br J Cancer. 2001;85:831–5.
67. Guillou L, Benhattar J, Bonichon F, et al. Histologic grade, but not SYT-SSX fusion type, is an important prognostic factor in patients with synovial sarcoma: a multicenter, retrospective analysis. J Clin Oncol. 2004;22:4040–50.
68. Kawai A, Woodruff J, Healey JH, et al. SYT-SSX gene fusion as a determinant of morphology and prognosis in synovial sarcoma. N Engl J Med. 1998;338:153–60.
69. Ladanyi M, Antonescu CR, Leung DH, et al. Impact of SYT-SSX fusion type on the clinical behavior of synovial sarcoma: a multi-institutional retrospective study of 243 patients. Cancer Res. 2002;62:135–40.
70. van Doorninck JA, Ji L, Schaub B, et al. Current treatment protocols have eliminated the prognostic advantage of type 1 fusions in Ewing sarcoma: a report from the Children's Oncology Group. J Clin Oncol. 2010;28:1989–94.
71. Fidelia-Lambert MN, Zhuang Z, Tsokos M. Sensitive detection of rare Ewing's sarcoma cells in peripheral blood by reverse transcriptase polymerase chain reaction. Hum Pathol. 1999;30:78–80.

72. Sumerauer D, Vicha A, Kucerova H, et al. Detection of minimal bone marrow infiltration in patients with localized and metastatic Ewing sarcoma using RT-PCR. Folia Biol (Praha). 2001;47: 206–10.
73. Schleiermacher G, Delattre O. Detection of micrometastases and circulating tumour cells using molecular biology technics in solid tumours. Bull Cancer. 2001;88:561–70.
74. Barretina J, Taylor BS, Banerji S, et al. Subtype-specific genomic alterations define new targets for soft-tissue sarcoma therapy. Nat Genet. 2010;42:715–21.
75. Worley BS, van den Broeke LT, Goletz TJ, et al. Antigenicity of fusion proteins from sarcoma-associated chromosomal translocations. Cancer Res. 2001;61:6868–75.
76. Tanaka K, Iwakuma T, Harimaya K, et al. EWS-Fli1 antisense oligodeoxynucleotide inhibits proliferation of human Ewing's sarcoma and primitive neuroectodermal tumor cells. J Clin Invest. 1997;99:239–47.
77. Uchida A, Seto M, Hashimoto N, et al. Molecular diagnosis and gene therapy in musculoskeletal tumors. J Orthop Sci. 2000;5: 418–23.

Gliomas

38

Ehud Lavi

Abstract

Many advances have been made in evaluating the molecular genetics of gliomas. For example, the presence of 1p and 19q deletions is associated with gliomas of oligodendroglial lineage, with oligodendrogliomas that have a better survival, and with oligodendrogliomas that respond to chemotherapy and radiation therapy. While prospective data are needed to confirm these associations, 1p and 19q deletion testing has become a part of routine neurooncology practice. Alterations of chromosome 10, *EGFR*, *PTEN*, *IDH1*, *MGMT*, *ATRX*, and *TP53* are associated with different grades of astrocytic gliomas and with patient survival. While their clinical utility requires further investigation, these markers (and others) will be increasingly used to stratify patients to current and new therapeutic approaches. In the future, it is likely that the survival rate of primary gliomas will be lengthened using molecularly targeted therapies.

Keywords

Astrocytoma • Oligodendroglioma • Glioblastoma • MGMT • EGFR • IDH-1 • IDH-2 • ATRX • p53 • PTEN

Introduction

Approximately 28,320 people in the US were diagnosed with malignant nervous system tumors in 2010 [1]. Primary brain tumors constitute approximately 2 % of all malignancies [2]. The most common of the primary brain tumors are gliomas. Depending on the grade and morphologic type of glioma, newly diagnosed patients are treated by watchful waiting, surgical resection, radiotherapy, or chemotherapy or some combination of these. Regardless of therapy, most gliomas will progress and patients with glioma have a high risk of mortality and reduced quality of life. Thus, there has been intense interest in understanding the biology and genetics of gliomas, to provide better diagnostic tools and new therapeutic approaches. Molecular pathology markers are being identified that have been or will soon prove to be clinically useful in the practice of clinical neurooncology (see Table 38.1).

E. Lavi, M.D. (✉)
Anatomic Pathology, Pathology and Laboratory Medicine, Weill Cornell Medical College,
525 E. 68th St., Starr 1043, New York, NY 10065, USA
e-mail: ehl2005@med.cornell.edu

Pathology Considerations

Gliomas are classified into tumors of astrocytic, oligodendroglial, ependymal, and mixed lineage. “Diffuse gliomas” is a descriptive general term that applies to all diffusely infiltrating tumors of glial lineages before a more specific determination of lineage can be determined based on molecular and immunohistochemical markers. Diffuse astrocytic tumors are divided into three different grades by the World Health Organization (WHO) system [3]: grade II (or astrocytoma [A]), grade III (or anaplastic astrocytoma [AA]), and grade IV (or glioblastoma, previously known as glioblastoma multiforme [GBM]). These tumors occur predominantly in adults. Diffuse astrocytic tumors can be subclassified

D.G.B. Leonard (ed.), *Molecular Pathology in Clinical Practice*, DOI 10.1007/978-3-319-19674-9_38

Table 38.1 Molecular markers of gliomas used in clinical practice

Marker	Indication
1p/19q deletion	Oligodendroglioma diagnosis and prognosis Prediction of oligodendroglioma therapeutic response Confirmation of an oligodendroglial component in oligoastrocytomas
MGMT promoter methylation	Response of glioblastoma to alkylating drugs (temozolomide) Small cell glioblastoma diagnosis Prognostic marker
IDH1 mutation	Diagnostic tool for low- and intermediate-grade astrocytomas and oligodendrogliomas Distinction from primary glioblastomas, pilocytic astrocytomas, and ependymomas Neoplastic glioma vs reactive gliosis Prognostic marker
EGFR amplification (overexpression)	Differentiation from oligodendroglioma Therapeutic response to novel EGFR pathway inhibitors
Chromosome 10 loss/*PTEN* mutation	Prognosis of anaplastic astrocytomas Response to EGFR pathway inhibitors
TP53 mutation	Secondary glioblastoma vs primary Neoplastic glioma vs reactive gliosis

into several histological types, including fibrillary, gemistocytic, small cell, and giant cell subtypes. Several of these histological types can be found within a single diffuse astrocytic tumor. Pilocytic astrocytomas are nondiffuse, well circumscribed, and localized. Pilocytic astrocytomas are often WHO grade I, and predominantly occur in children and young adults. Glioblastomas can be subclassified into two groups based on the duration of symptoms [4]. Primary glioblastoma presents de novo with a short duration of symptoms (often less than 3 months). Secondary glioblastoma presents with a longer duration of symptoms or with a preceding grade II or III glioma. Primary and secondary glioblastomas usually present in patients greater than 60 and less than 40 years of age, respectively.

Oligodendrogliomas most commonly are divided into two grades: grade II (oligodendroglioma) and grade III (anaplastic oligodendroglioma), although some neuropathologists have described a grade IV oligodendroglioma [5]. Ependymomas are also classified as low (WHO grade II) and high grade (anaplastic or WHO grade III).

One of the problems with the neuropathologic diagnosis of gliomas is their histologic heterogeneity. AA exhibits increased cellularity, nuclear atypia, and mitotic activity. Microvascular proliferation and necrosis are additional features of glioblastomas. Depending on the extent of surgical sampling, some of the histologic elements that distinguish AA and glioblastoma may not be present in the specimen submitted for pathological diagnosis, and some gliomas may be undergraded. Thus, molecular markers that assist in tumor grading are clinically useful.

In addition to histologic heterogeneity, diffuse gliomas often exhibit cell type heterogeneity. Both astrocytic and oligodendroglial elements may be present in diffuse gliomas. When both of these elements comprise a significant proportion of the tumor, the glioma used to be classified as a mixed oligoastrocytoma (MOA). However, this term no longer exists based on recent recommendations of the International Society of Neuropathology [6].

Molecular Pathology Tools for Glioma Analysis and Grading

Gliomas have been extensively characterized by cytogenetic, molecular cytogenetic, and molecular genetic methods (reviewed in Refs. 4, 7, 8). Figure 38.1 summarizes the major genetic alterations found in diffuse gliomas. Some of these alterations are highly correlated with the grade of gliomas, especially for astrocytic tumors.

Several genetic alterations have been associated with gliomas, especially primary glioblastoma and oligodendrogliomas. These alterations include chromosomal deletions of chromosome arms 1p and 19q, *MGMT* promoter methylation, loss of chromosome 10, *PTEN* mutations, *IDH1* mutations, and amplification of *EGFR* with resulting overexpression of the EGFR protein. While the clinical use of these markers has been validated only partially, growing evidence supports the usefulness of these molecular markers for glioma grading, prognosis, and treatment decisions. The presence of *EGFR* amplification, chromosome 10 loss, or *PTEN* mutation, or some combination of the three, in a glioma indicates that the tumor is likely a glioblastoma. Importantly, a small but significant proportion of tumors with the histologic features of AA have one or more of these alterations [9–13]. It is reasonable to hypothesize, though needs to be proven, that since patients with glioblastoma have a poor prognosis, then patients whose AA shares molecular characteristics with glioblastoma also may have poor survival.

One of the first and most significant molecular developments in the study of gliomas was the discovery of chromosomal alterations in chromosomes 1 and 19. Cairncross et al. demonstrated in 1994 that some anaplastic oligodendrogliomas respond to combination chemotherapy and radiation therapy [14]. Simultaneously, several investigators observed that approximately 70 % of oligodendrogliomas have deletions of 19q, 70 % have deletions of 1p, and 60 % have deletions of both 1p and 19q [7]. Usually, the entire chromosomal arms are deleted [15]. In contrast, about 40 %, 20 % and 10 % of astrocytomas have deletion of 19q, 1p, and both 1p and 19q, respectively [15]. The proportion of MOA with 1p and 19q deletions is intermediate, suggesting that some of these tumors can be grouped with oligodendrogliomas [15, 16]. A significant proportion of MOA also has *TP53*

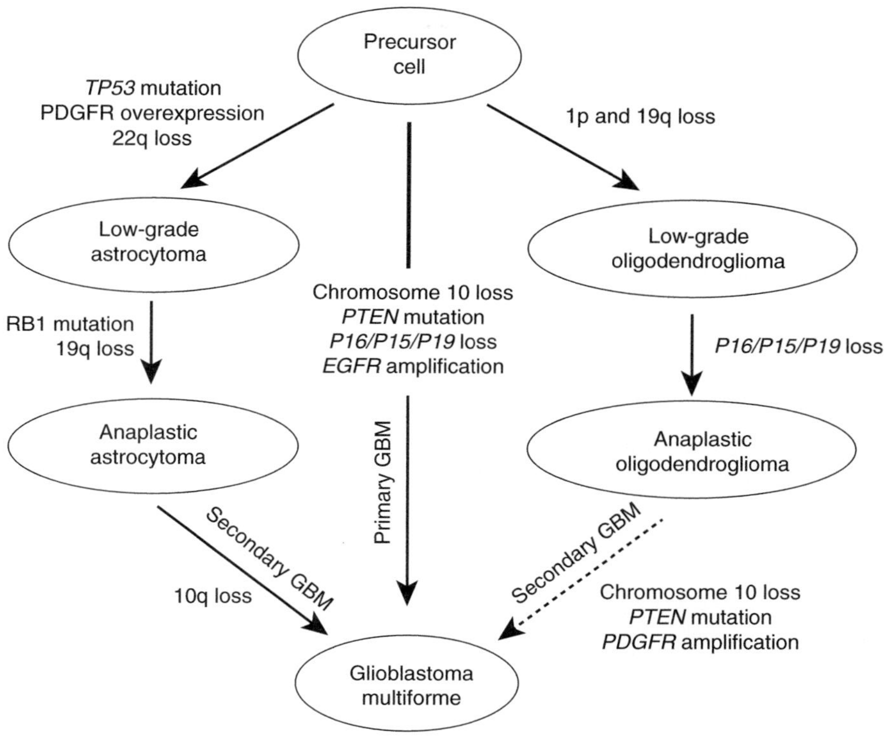

Figure 38.1 Possible genetic pathways of diffuse glioma formation and progression (modified from Refs. 7 and 8). Histologic classification is based on current WHO guidelines [3]. Although the molecular genetic evidence is increasing, it is still controversial whether anaplastic oligodendroglioma progresses to glioblastoma (GBm) (*dashed arrow*)

mutations and other genetic anomalies, suggesting that these tumors can be grouped with the astrocytomas [15, 16].

Two retrospective studies have provided evidence that the oligodendrogliomas with 1p deletions, 19q deletions, or both have a better prognosis and respond better to chemotherapy and radiation therapy [17, 18]. The data strongly suggest that 1p/19q deletions are associated with tumors of oligodendroglial lineage, with oligodendrogliomas that have a better prognosis, and with oligodendrogliomas that respond to chemotherapy and radiation therapy. Additional prospective studies provided evidence that the presence or absence of 1p/19q deletions suggests different treatment recommendations for oligodendrogliomas that require adjuvant therapy, especially anaplastic oligodendrogliomas [19, 20]. Patients with the deletion may receive chemotherapy first and delay radiation treatment, while patients without the deletion may receive radiation as first-line treatment.

Other alterations occur in oligodendrogliomas that lack 1p and 19q deletions. *CDKN2A–CDKN2B–ARF* (*P16*, *P15*, *P19*), *PTEN*, and chromosome 10 are frequently deleted in anaplastic oligodendrogliomas. The expression of *CDKN2A* and *CDKN2B* often is inactivated by promoter methylation. While the presence of these alterations is associated with a poorer prognosis [17, 21, 22], their detection has not become a part of standard clinical neurooncology.

MGMT is a DNA repair enzyme that normally counteracts the cell death effect of alkylating chemotherapy agents such as temozolomide, which is widely used in the treatment of glioblastoma. MGMT activity is downregulated and not fully expressed in about half of patients with glioblastoma due to *MGMT* gene promoter methylation and decreased gene expression and enzyme production. Thus, the presence of *MGMT* promoter methylation determines that the patient will be more responsive to chemotherapy. *MGMT* promoter methylation also correlates with better prognosis in general, suggesting that it might indicate a prognostically favorable molecular phenotype of the disease. In a study by Hegi et al., 46 % of the patients with *MGMT* methylation were alive at 2 years, while only 23 % of the patients with unmethylated *MGMT* were alive at 2 years [23]. Temozolomide provides some beneficial effect even in patients with unmethylated *MGMT* promoter; thus, both groups receive the same treatment. Since the methylation pattern might change over time, repeated testing at each tumor resection is justified.

Several growth factors are upregulated and involved in the pathogenesis of gliomas, especially the most malignant forms of glioblastoma. EGFR signaling is upregulated in approximately 30 % of gliomas and 60 % of glioblastomas. An even higher percentage of "small cell glioblastoma," which can be misdiagnosed and possibly confused for oligodendroglioma, has upregulated EGFR signaling. The presence of EGFR upregulation as opposed to 1p/19q deletion may help to distinguish between glioblastoma and malignant oligodendroglioma, respectively. Another scenario in which EGFR overexpression is diagnostically useful is when a biopsy is taken from the edge of a tumor that appears to be histologically consistent with a grade III glioma but radiographically appears as glioblastoma. The presence of EGFR overexpression in these tumor specimens may support a diagnosis of glioblastoma instead of AA.

In glioblastomas that overexpress EGFR, mutant forms of EGFR are present in about half of the cases. The most common variant is EGFR vIII, which has deletion of exons 2–7 of the *EGFR* gene and results in an EGFR protein that is active independently of ligand binding (reviewed in Ref. 24). Several other amplified and mutated EGFR proteins also have been identified (e.g., the C958 variant is truncated after amino acid 958), some of which remain ligand dependent. Current translational studies are investigating the prevalence of these different amplified and mutated EGFR variants in primary and secondary glioblastoma and in glioblastoma from patients of different ages [25].

Many glioblastomas have dysregulation of EGFR downstream signaling, such as *PTEN* tumor suppressor gene mutations, phosphoinositide 3-kinase pathway, and AKT. These findings suggested a rationale for drug treatments that target these pathways. Mellinghoff and colleagues showed that gliomas with an EGFR vIII mutation in the presence of an intact PTEN-AKT pathway had increased sensitivity to erlotinib, whereas tumors with loss of the PTEN-AKT signaling did not. However subsequent trials showed less response to EGFR-targeted therapies, so the use of these drugs remains controversial.

Mutations in the *IDH1* and *IDH2* genes occur in high frequency in primary low- and intermediate-grade diffuse gliomas (both in astrocytomas and in oligodendrogliomas) [7, 20, 26, 27], as well as secondary glioblastomas. The most common mutation is the R132H mutation of *IDH1*, with a frequency of over 80 % in grade II astrocytomas, oligodendrogliomas, anaplastic oligodendrogliomas, and mixed oligoastrocytomas, close to 70 % of AA, but only less than 0.5 % in primary glioblastoma. *IDH1* mutations also serve as a tool to distinguish astrocytomas and oligodendrogliomas from low-grade tumors that usually do not express this mutation such as ependymomas, pilocytic astrocytomas, and dysembryoplastic neuroepithelial tumors, as well as neoplastic glial proliferation from reactive gliosis. Gliomas with *IDH1* mutations have a better prognosis, with or without adjuvant therapy. Therefore, *IDH1* mutation serves as a prognostic and diagnostic marker (Fig. 38.2).

A Mayo Clinic/North Central Cancer Treatment Group (NCCTG) study indicated that AA with chromosome 10 loss or *PTEN* mutation, using full sequencing of the *PTEN* gene and exons 5–8 of the *TP53* gene, behaves like glioblastomas [10]. The median survival of patients with AA and chromosome 10 loss or *PTEN* mutation was approximately 4 months, a survival worse than that of patients with glioblastoma (median survival of approximately 12 months). The median survival of patients whose AA lacked these alterations was 34 months. This difference in survival was statistically significant even after adjustment for patient age, performance score, and extent of resection, all of which are important prognostic variables for patients with gliomas. Importantly, the patient survival for glioblastoma with and without chromosome 10 loss or *PTEN* mutations was very similar [10]. It is possible that sampling bias (in terms of the tissue available for histologic and molecular analysis) may have accounted for the differences. However, sampling bias is a difficult problem to overcome in routine clinical practice, and molecular testing for chromosome 10 loss or *PTEN* mutations in a sample of a tumor with the features of AA indicates that the tumor may be a glioblastoma.

Interestingly, the Mayo Clinic/NCCTG study did not show that AA with *EGFR* amplification behaved like

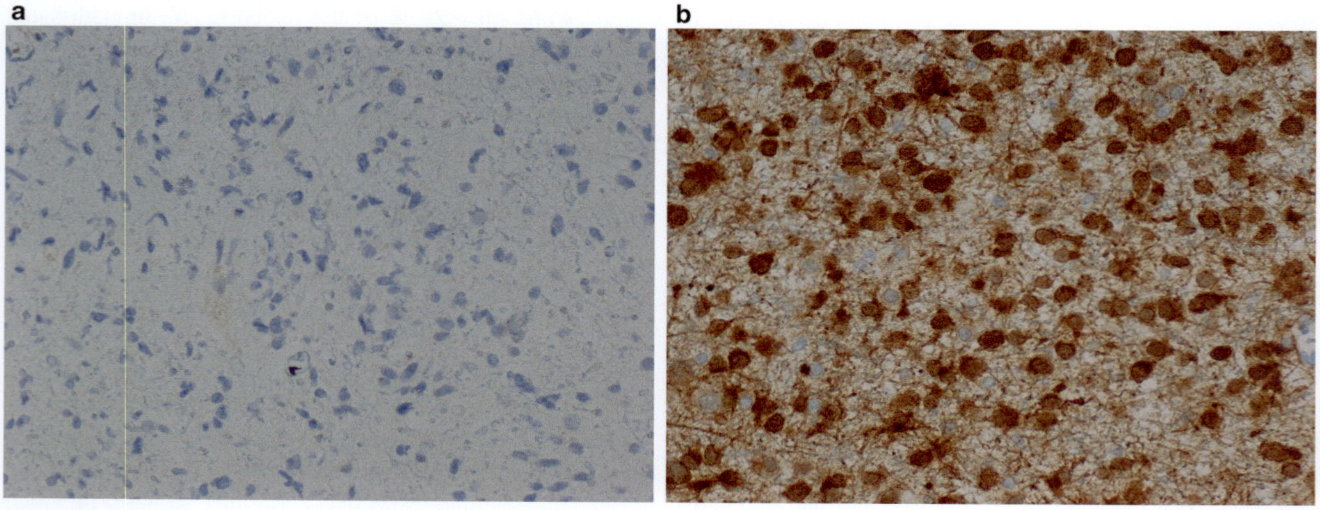

Figure 38.2 Immunohistochemistry images of low-grade glial neoplasms with negative (**a**) and positive (**b**) staining with antibody against the R132H mutations in *IDH1*

glioblastoma [10]. However, careful stratification indicated that AA and glioblastoma with *EGFR* amplification in young patients (i.e., <40 years old) progress much faster than AA and glioblastoma without *EGFR* amplification in this age group [10]. Conversely, AA and glioblastoma with *EGFR* amplification in older patients (i.e., >60 years old) had a better prognosis than those without this alteration. Importantly, this result has been confirmed by another group [28]. These differences in age-related prognosis may reflect the different biology of primary and secondary high-grade astrocytic tumors.

TP53 mutations are found in about half of astrocytomas and AA. About one quarter of glioblastomas have *TP53* mutations, and these tumors often have the clinical presentation of a secondary glioblastoma. Since *TP53* alterations usually are associated with low-grade tumors, it has been hypothesized that high-grade astrocytic tumors with *TP53* alterations may have a better prognosis. Except for the rare giant cell and gemistocytic variants (in which *TP53* mutations are especially prevalent) [29, 30], the presence or absence of *TP53* alterations does not seem to correlate with survival for glioblastoma [31–34]. However, in the Mayo Clinic/NCCTG series, the median survival of patients with AA with *TP53* mutations was 5 years [10]. This survival was significantly longer than for patients whose tumors did not have *TP53* mutations [10].

Although *PTEN*, chromosome 10, *TP53*, and *EGFR* alterations have been found to be correlated with clinical grade and thus with patient prognosis, they have yet to be routinely used in clinical practice for two reasons. First, the studies require broader validation. Second, and more importantly, the presence or absence of such alterations does not currently change the clinical management for these patients. High-grade glioma trials designed to specifically evaluate the clinical usefulness of these markers are needed to move these molecular markers into clinical practice.

A recent development in the field of molecular markers of gliomas has been the use of genetic mutations of the alpha-thalassemia/mental retardation syndrome X-linked (*ATRX*) gene. Loss of ATRX expression by immunohistochemistry, representing the presence of a mutated *ATRX* gene, is present in about half of all diffuse astrocytomas. *ATRX* mutations are essentially mutually exclusive with chromosomal deletions of 1p/19q and therefore indicate an astrocytic lineage. ATRX loss in glioma tumor cells also provides an indication of better prognosis than a preserved unmutated ATRX [35].

Available Assays

Despite intensive effort, the target genes on 1p and 19q that cause the differential treatment response have not been identified. However, molecular testing for 1p/19q deletion can be performed by loss of heterozygosity (LOH) analysis (currently by polymerase chain reaction [PCR] analysis of microsatellite loci or by high-throughput analysis of single-nucleotide polymorphisms) and by fluorescence in situ hybridization (FISH) with locus-specific bacterial artificial chromosome (BAC) probes. FISH can be performed on two formalin-fixed paraffin-embedded (FFPE) tissue sections and does not require microdissection, which is an advantage over the other methods. An advantage of FISH is that 1p/19q deletion can be focal [36], and normal cells are frequently present in gliomas. FISH can directly evaluate lesions and tumor cells of interest. An advantage of LOH analysis is detection of mitotic recombination (which is not detected by FISH). However, this LOH mechanism has been shown to be rare in gliomas [15].

FISH detection of 1p and 19q deletions has been described [15, 18]. Figure 38.3 illustrates typical 1p/19q FISH results for two anaplastic oligodendrogliomas, one with and one without 1p/19q deletion. Approximately 60 % of the nuclei in the tumor with 1p and 19q deletion contain one 1p36 or 19q13.3 probe signal and two 1q24 or 19p13 control probe signals (Fig. 38.3a). The remaining cells with two signals for each probe are likely contaminating normal glial, neuronal, or endothelial cells or tumor cells that lack deletion. The mean 1p/1q and 19q/19p signal ratios per nucleus are 0.62 and 0.71, respectively. Normal value studies and an evaluation of a large series of tumors by multiple methods indicate that ratios less than 0.80 are associated with 1p or 19q deletion. By comparison, approximately 60 % of the nuclei in the tumor without 1p and 19q deletion contain two signals for all four probes (Fig. 38.3b). The mean 1p/1q and 19q/19p signal ratios per nucleus are 1.04 and 1.01, respectively. The nuclei with one signal for each probe are likely a result of truncation of signals by paraffin sectioning. The nuclei with three or more signals are likely a result of nuclear overlap.

When used with appropriate control probes (e.g., the BAC probes on 1q42 and 19p13), FISH is able to detect 1p and 19q deletions in polyploid or aneuploid tumors. In addition, trisomy 19 is detected by this FISH method, an alteration long known to be associated with high-grade astrocytic tumors [37]. Based on normal value studies, chromosome 1 or 19 aneusomy is not reported unless the proportion of nuclei with three or more signals for each probe exceeds 30 % of the nuclei evaluated. Quantitative analysis of microsatellite alleles (QuMA) also detects 1p and 19q deletions (and trisomy 19) [38]. Both QuMA and current LOH analysis methods have the capacity for automation and rapid throughput. However, both require microdissection for accurate deletion detection, which increases turnaround time.

For similar reasons, FISH is the optimal method for the detection of chromosome 10 loss and *EGFR* amplification. In a careful method comparison study, semiquantitative PCR analysis and Southern blot analysis did not detect small foci

a

1q24 copy number	1p36 copy number: 0	1	2	3	4	Total
0	0	0	0	0	0	0
1	0	17	1	0	0	18
2	0	70	12	0	0	82
3	0	0	0	0	0	0
4	0	0	0	0	0	0
Total	0	87	13	0	0	100

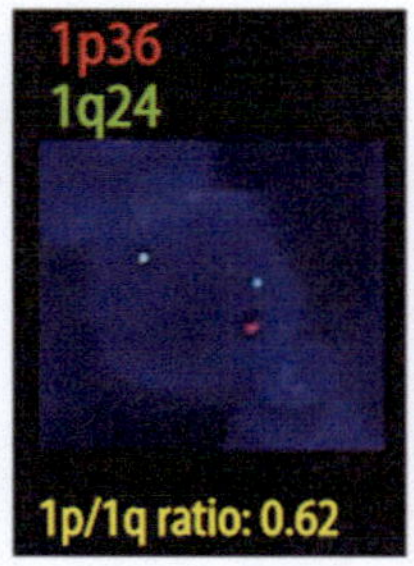

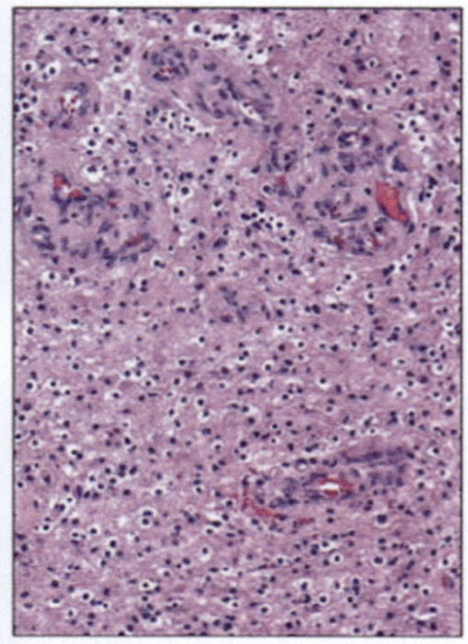

19p13 copy number	19q13.3 copy number: 0	1	2	3	4	Total
0	0	0	0	0	0	0
1	0	24	0	0	0	24
2	0	51	23	0	0	74
3	0	0	1	1	0	2
4	0	0	0	0	0	0
Total	0	75	24	1	0	100

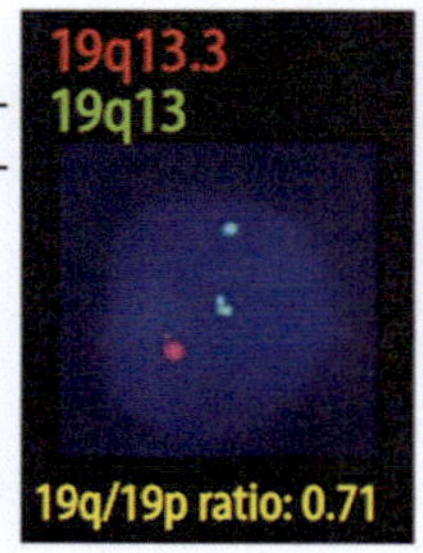

b

1q24 copy number	1p36 copy number: 0	1	2	3	4	Total
0	0	0	0	0	0	0
1	0	15	11	0	0	26
2	0	6	57	4	0	67
3	0	0	1	5	0	6
4	0	0	0	0	1	1
Total	0	21	69	9	1	100

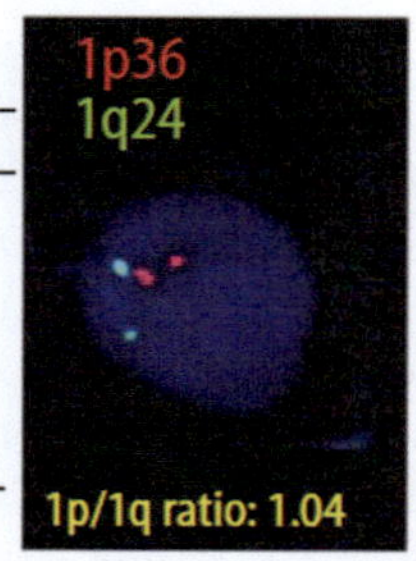

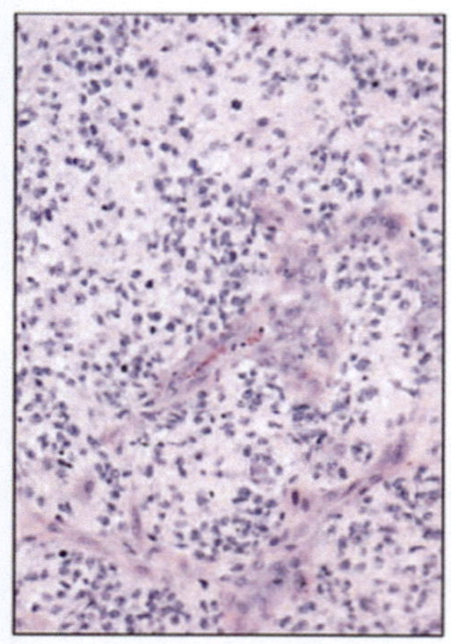

19p13 copy number	19q13.3 copy number: 0	1	2	3	4	Total
0	0	0	0	0	0	0
1	0	13	8	0	0	21
2	0	6	66	0	0	72
3	0	0	0	6	0	6
4	0	0	0	0	1	1
Total	0	19	74	6	1	100

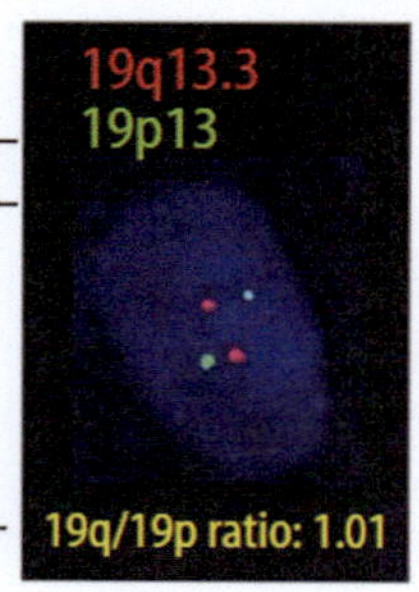

Figure 38.3 Representative histology and FISH results for two primary grade 3 anaplastic oligodendrogliomas. (**a**) An anaplastic oligodendroglioma with 1p and 19q deletion. (**b**) An anaplastic oligodendroglioma without 1p and 19q deletion. The values in the tables summarize the percent nuclei with the indicated number of 1p36 and 1q24 or 19p13 and 19q13.3 signals

of *EGFR* amplification compared to FISH [10]. The most accurate means to detect the EGFRvIII variant in gliomas is by immunohistochemistry with variant-specific antibodies [39]. The other *EGFR* variants can be detected by DNA sequencing of tumor specimens.

The *MGMT* promoter methylation test is currently done by PCR analysis using fresh, frozen, or FFPE tissue. Immunohistochemistry for assessment of MGMT expression, as a marker for *MGMT* promoter methylation, is inconsistent and currently not recommended. *TP53* and *PTEN* mutation detection is best performed by high-throughput DNA sequencing/alteration methods (see Chaps. 2, 59, and 60). TP53 immunohistochemistry is a surrogate marker for *TP53* mutations by analyzing the level of expression of the protein in tissue sections. Immunohistochemistry is now the standard tool for analyzing reliably the expression of IDH1 with the R132H mutation in tissue sections due to the development of useful antibodies that selectively recognize this mutation [27]. Immunohistochemistry is a reliable tool for detection of nuclear expression of ATRX. Immunohistochemistry is less reliable for the protein level of PTEN in tissue sections.

Laboratory Issues

The use of molecular markers in gliomas is heavily dependent on the availability of sufficient lesional tissue for the different immunohistochemical and molecular studies. Stereotactic needle biopsies may not always be able to provide the amount of tissue necessary for such studies, and therefore open biopsies may be required for these studies. The accuracy of the tests is also dependent on the use of proper controls as well as proficiency testing to assure continued proper performance.

Future Directions

Array-based gene expression, gene dosage analyses, and the cancer genome atlas have the potential to identify new molecular markers for many cancers, including gliomas. Several groups are currently evaluating these methods of analysis in selected gliomas. Using a 1,100-gene expression array, Watson et al. identified 196 transcripts associated with oligodendrogliomas of different grades [40]. Similarly, two groups have used 12,000-gene expression arrays to discover differential expression of a limited number of transcripts that can be used to classify high-grade gliomas [41, 42]. Array-based comparative genomic hybridization (aCGH) likely will lead to the discovery of novel gene dosage alterations that can be used to classify gliomas [43, 44]. Importantly, the markers (and marker panels) ascertained by these methods will have to be carefully validated. However, there is the exciting possibility that a limited number of protein or molecular markers could be developed to enhance the molecular identification of gliomas and potentially to standardize neuropathologic diagnosis.

Much of the current translational research in gliomas is focused on developing therapeutic approaches that target specific protein and/or molecular alterations. The aCGH studies described above have, as one goal, the identification of new drug targets, with several promising targets for novel therapeutic approaches already identified. For example, several components of the receptor tyrosine kinase pathway are altered in gliomas: EGFR is overexpressed, *PTEN* is mutated, and AKT2 is activated. Small-molecule inhibitors, immunotherapeutics, and viral therapeutic agents are being developed that target this pathway (for examples, see Refs. 45, 46) and are being tested in glioma patients.

The design of current and future trials will need to develop the concept that therapeutic approaches will be customized to the molecular alterations found in specific tumors. Clinical molecular pathology will play an important role in this customization of clinical neurooncology practice.

References

1. Gittleman HR, Ostrom QT, Rouse CD, Dowling JA, et al. Trends in central nervous system tumor incidence relative to other common cancers in adults, adolescents, and children in the United States, 2000 to 2010. Cancer. 2015;121:102–12.
2. Jemal A, Murray T, Samuels A, Ghafoor A, Ward E, Thun MJ. Cancer statistics. CA Cancer J Clin. 2003;53:5–26.
3. Louis DN, Ohgaki H, Wiestler OD, Cavenee WK. WHO classification of tumors of the central nervous system. Lyon, France: IARC Press; 2007.
4. Kleihues P, Ohgaki H. Primary and secondary glioblastomas: from concept to clinical diagnosis. Neuro-oncol. 1999;1:44–51.
5. Smith JS, Wang XY, Qian J, et al. Amplification of the platelet-derived growth factor receptor-A (PDGFRA) gene occurs in oligodendrogliomas with grade IV anaplastic features. J Neuropathol Exp Neurol. 2000;59:495–503.
6. Louis DN, Perry A, Burger P, et al. International Society of neuropathology—Haarlem consensus guidelines for nervous system tumor classification and grading. Brain Pathol. 2014;5:429–35.
7. Jansen M, Yip S, Louis DN. Molecular pathology in adult gliomas: diagnostic, prognostic, and predictive markers. Lancet Neurol. 2010;9:717–26.
8. Kitange GJ, Smith JS, Jenkins RB. Genetic alterations and chemotherapeutic response in human diffuse gliomas. Expert Rev Anticancer Ther. 2001;1:595–605.
9. Lin H, Bondy ML, Langford LA, et al. Allelic deletion analyses of MMAC/PTEN and DMBT1 loci in gliomas: relationship to prognostic significance. Clin Cancer Res. 1998;4:2447–54.
10. Smith JS, Tachibana I, Passe SM, et al. PTEN mutation, EGFR amplification, and outcome in patients with anaplastic astrocytoma and glioblastoma multiforme. J Natl Cancer Inst. 2001;93:1246–56.
11. Tada K, Shiraishi S, Kamiryo T, et al. Analysis of loss of heterozygosity on chromosome 10 in patient with malignant astrocytic tumors: correlation with patient age and survival. J Neurosurg. 2001;95:651–9.
12. Rasheed A, Herndon JE, Stenzel TT, et al. Molecular markers of prognosis in astrocytic tumors. Cancer. 2002;94:2688–97.
13. Terada K, Tamiya T, Daido S, et al. Prognostic value of loss of heterozygosity around three candidate tumor suppressor genes on chromosome 10q in astrocytomas. J Neurooncol. 2002;58:107–14.
14. Cairncross G, Macdonald D, Ludwin S, et al. Chemotherapy for anaplastic oligodendroglioma. National Cancer Institute of Canada Clinical Trials Group. J Clin Oncol. 1994;12:2013–21.
15. Smith JS, Alderete B, Minn Y, et al. Localization of common deletion regions on 1p and 19q in human gliomas and their association with histological subtype. Oncogene. 1999;18:4144–52.
16. Mueller W, Hartmann C, Hoffmann A, et al. Genetic signature of oligoastrocytomas correlates with tumor location and denotes distinct molecular subsets. Am J Pathol. 2002;161:313–9.

17. Cairncross JG, Ueki K, Zlatescu MC, et al. Specific genetic predictors of chemotherapeutic response and survival in patients with anaplastic oligodendrogliomas. J Natl Cancer Inst. 1998;90:1473–9.
18. Smith J, Perry A, Borell T, et al. Alterations of chromosome arms 1p and 19q as predictors of survival in oligodendrogliomas, astrocytomas, and mixed oligoastrocytomas. J Clin Oncol. 2000;18:636–45.
19. Kouwenhoven MC, Kros JM, French PJ, et al. 1p/19q loss within oligodendroglioma is predictive for response to first line temozolomide but not to salvage treatment. Eur J Cancer. 2006;42:2499–503.
20. Yan H, Parsons DW, Jin G, et al. IDH1 and IDH2 mutations in gliomas. N Engl J Med. 2009;360:765–73.
21. Sasaki H, Zlatescu MC, Betensky RA, Ino Y, Cairncross JG, Louis DN. PTEN is a target of chromosome 10q loss in anaplastic oligodendrogliomas and PTEN alterations are associated with poor prognosis. Am J Pathol. 2001;159:359–67.
22. Sanson M, Leuraud P, Aguirre-Cruz L, et al. Analysis of loss of chromosome 10q, DMBT1 homozygous deletions, and PTEN mutations in oligodendrogliomas. J Neurosurg. 2002;97:1397–401.
23. Hegi ME, Diserens AC, Gorlia T, et al. MGMT gene silencing and benefit from temozolomide in glioblastoma. N Engl J Med. 2005;352:997–1003.
24. Frederick L, Wang XY, Eley G, James CD. Diversity and frequency of epidermal growth factor receptor mutations in human glioblastomas. Cancer Res. 2000;60:1383–7.
25. Feldkamp MM, Roncari L, Lau N, Salhia B, Guha A. Expression of EGFRvIII is a better prognostic marker for GBM than either EGFR expression or the Ki-67 labeling index. Neuro-oncol. 2002;4:343.
26. Hartmann C, Meyer J, Balss J, et al. Type and frequency of IDH1 and IDH2 mutations are related to astrocytic and oligodendroglial differentiation and age: a study of 1,010 diffuse gliomas. Acta Neuropathol. 2009;118:469–74.
27. Capper D, Weissert S, Balss J, et al. Characterization of R132H mutation-specific IDH1 antibody binding in brain tumors. Brain Pathol. 2009;20:245–54.
28. Simmons ML, Lamborn KR, Takahashi M, et al. Analysis of complex relationships between age, p53, epidermal growth factor receptor, and survival in glioblastoma patients. Cancer Res. 2001;61:1122–8.
29. Peraud A, Watanabe K, Schwechheimer K, Yonekawa Y, Kleihues P, Ohgaki H. Genetic profile of the giant cell glioblastoma. Lab Invest. 1999;79:123–9.
30. Kosel S, Scheithauer BW, Graeber MB. Genotype-phenotype correlation in gemistocytic astrocytomas. Neurosurgery. 2001;48:187–93.
31. Nieder C, Petersen S, Petersen C, Thames HD. The challenge of p53 as prognostic and predictive factor in gliomas. Cancer Treat Rev. 2000;26:67–73.
32. Kraus JA, Glesmann N, Beck M, et al. Molecular analysis of the PTEN, TP53 and CDKN2A tumor suppressor genes in long-term survivors of glioblastoma multiforme. J Neurooncol. 2000;48:89–94.
33. Kraus JA, Wenghoefer M, Glesmann N, et al. TP53 gene mutations, nuclear p53 accumulation, expression of Waf/p21, Bcl-2, and CD95 (APO-1/Fas) proteins are not prognostic factors in de novo glioblastoma multiforme. J Neurooncol. 2001;52:263–72.
34. Shiraishi S, Tada K, Nakamura H, et al. Influence of p53 mutations on prognosis of patients with glioblastoma. Cancer. 2002;95:249–57.
35. Wiestler B, Capper D, Holland-Letz T, et al. ATRX loss defines the classification of anaplastic gliomas and identifies a subgroup of IDH mutant astrocytic tumors with better prognosis. Acta Neuropathol. 2013;126:443–51.
36. Randazzo L, Scarpace L, Lemke N, et al. Tumoral and chromosomal heterogeneity in oligodendrogliomas detected with medium-throughput 1p/19q LOH analysis. Neuro-oncol. 2002;4:346.
37. Bigner SH, Mark J, Burger PC, et al. Specific chromosomal abnormalities in malignant human gliomas. Cancer Res. 1988;48:405–11.
38. Nigro JM, Takahashi MA, Ginzinger DG, et al. Detection of 1p and 19q loss in oligodendroglioma by quantitative microsatellite analysis, a real-time quantitative polymerase chain reaction assay. Am J Pathol. 2001;158:1253–62.
39. Ohman L, Gedda L, Hesselager G, et al. A new antibody recognizing the vIII mutation of human epidermal growth factor receptor. Tumour Biol. 2002;23:61–9.
40. Watson MA, Perry A, Budhjara V, Hicks C, Shannon WD, Rich KM. Gene expression profiling with oligonucleotide microarrays distinguishes World Health Organization grade of oligodendrogliomas. Cancer Res. 2001;61:1825–9.
41. Mischel PS, Shai R, Choe GY, et al. Identification of distinctive subtypes of primary glioblastoma multiforme by gene expression profiling. Neuro-oncol. 2002;4:330.
42. Nutt CL, Mani DR, Betensky RA, et al. An accurate microarray class prediction model for high grade gliomas. Neuro-oncol. 2002;4:345.
43. Misra A, Pellarin M, Moore D, et al. A high-resolution genome wide map of genetic aberrations in human astrocytoma. Neuro-oncol. 2002;4:330.
44. Brennan C, Kim H, Cauwels C, et al. Identification of candidate genetic alterations from array-CGH in human glioblastomas. Neuro-oncol. 2002;4:327.
45. Lal A, Glazer CA, Martinson HM, et al. Mutant epidermal growth factor receptor up-regulates molecular effectors of tumor invasion. Cancer Res. 2002;62:3335–9.
46. Sausville EA, Elsayed Y, Monga M, Kim G. Signal transduction-directed cancer treatments. Annu Rev Pharmacol Toxicol. 2003;43:199–231.

Molecular Detection of Circulating Tumor Cells and Cell-Free Nucleic Acids

39

Nirali M. Patel and Karen Kaul

Abstract

One of the key roles performed by pathologists is determination of the presence or absence of tumor in clinical samples. This is the basis for most approaches to staging, monitoring response to treatment, and detecting relapse of neoplasia and, as such, is a critical step in determining the course of patient management. Pathologists have utilized a variety of methods, continually seeking to improve assay performance and thus patient outcome. The literature reflects this quest, including reports assessing the increased sensitivity afforded by immunohistochemistry (IHC), flow cytometry, and, more recently, molecular approaches for the detection of tumor cells and nucleic acids in blood and bone marrow samples. The goal is, of course, the more accurate detection of disease spread and, ultimately, better patient care.

This chapter addresses some of the recent work in tumor detection, focusing on molecular and, to some degree, immunofluorescent approaches for the detection of circulating tumor cells and free nucleic acids in clinical samples. A synopsis of the hundreds of articles published to date is beyond the scope of this chapter; instead, more general issues and findings are addressed, along with presentation of selected work. Several reviews are available for more detailed reading (Alix-Panabières and Pantel, Clin Chem 59:110–118, 2013; Pinzani et al., Methods 50:302–307, 2010; Pratt et al. Chem Eng Sci 66:1508–1522, 2011; Schwarzenbach et al., Nat Rev Clin Oncol 11:145–156, 2014).

Keywords

Circulating tumor cells • Circulating nucleic acids • Sequencing • Methods • Cancer • Monitoring • Staging

Introduction

One of the key roles performed by pathologists is determination of the presence or absence of tumor in clinical samples. This is the basis for most approaches to staging, monitoring response to treatment, and detecting relapse of neoplasia and, as such, is a critical step in determining the course of patient management. Pathologists have utilized a variety of methods, continually seeking to improve assay performance and thus patient outcome. The literature reflects this quest, including reports assessing the increased sensitivity afforded by immunohistochemistry (IHC), flow cytometry, and, more recently, molecular approaches for the detection of tumor

N.M. Patel, M.D. (✉)
Department of Pathology and Laboratory Medicine, Lineberger Comprehensive Cancer Center, University of North Carolina at Chapel Hill, Chapel Hill, NC, USA

Molecular Genetics Laboratory, UNC Hospitals,
101 Manning Dr., Room A1091, Anderson Pavilion, Chapel Hill, NC 27514, USA
e-mail: nirali_patel@med.unc.edu

K. Kaul, M.D., Ph.D.
Pathology and Laboratory Medicine, NorthShore University HealthSystem, Evanston, IL, USA

D.G.B. Leonard (ed.), *Molecular Pathology in Clinical Practice*, DOI 10.1007/978-3-319-19674-9_39

cells and nucleic acids in blood and bone marrow samples. The goal is, of course, the more accurate detection of disease spread and, ultimately, better patient care.

This chapter addresses some of the recent work in tumor detection, focusing on molecular and, to some degree, immunofluorescent approaches for the detection of circulating tumor cells and free nucleic acids in clinical samples. A synopsis of the hundreds of articles published to date is beyond the scope of this chapter; instead, more general issues and findings are addressed, along with presentation of selected work. Several reviews are available for more detailed reading [1–4].

Circulating Tumor Cells

Cancer metastasis occurs when tumor cells acquire the ability to escape their local environment, enter the circulation to reach distant sites, attach at the distant site, and proliferate to form a metastatic cancer lesion. Depending on the type of tumor, cells enter either the venous or lymphatic circulation (or both) and thus are spread to distant tissues (such as the lung, liver, or bone marrow) or local lymph nodes, respectively, prior to the development of clinically detectable metastatic lesions. The fact that significant proportions of patients with organ-confined tumors who undergo theoretically curative surgery later have recurrence of their disease argues that current approaches to cancer staging are, to some degree, inadequate. Sensitive detection of circulating tumor cells could lead to improved staging and monitoring of cancer patients. Such techniques can also be applied to the study of stem cell harvests and assessment of body fluids.

Available Assays

Methods for detection of circulating tumor cells (CTCs) incorporate multiple technologies and platforms. At their most basic, information can be obtained about the quantity of tumor cells in blood and the antigens they express. Some systems also allow for captured CTCs to be examined morphologically, be cultured in vitro, or be used for cytogenetic or molecular analysis. While only one assay is currently FDA-approved for CTC enumeration, work is being done to create simpler and more sensitive instruments for CTC detection that allow for additional analysis to be performed on isolated CTCs and their extracted nucleic acids.

Immunohistochemistry

IHC methods for tumor cell detection have been applied to preparations of cells from the bone marrow, lymph node aspirates, and peripheral blood mononuclear cells. Cells can be smeared or centrifuged by cytospin onto slides, or sections taken from frozen or formalin-fixed, paraffin-embedded (FFPE) tissue. IHC is performed using antibodies to specific proteins associated with tumor type and standardized methods. Slides can be scanned under the light microscope by the eye, though to achieve a high level of sensitivity, thousands to millions of cells must be screened, which is tedious and time consuming. Thus, image analysis has become a popular approach for screening [5]. Alternatively, flow cytometry is utilized to achieve assessment of high numbers of cells rapidly [6].

In general, the interpretation of occult disease detection assays consists of either a positive or negative result, given that the assay controls are appropriate. For IHC markers, nonspecific or aberrant expression of protein markers requires that careful evaluation of the cytologic characteristics of the positive cells be performed. The ability to visualize cell morphology with IHC can reduce false-positive results because the interpretation of a positive result can be limited to IHC positive cells with appropriate tumor cell morphology.

Reverse Transcription-Polymerase Chain Reaction

Reverse transcription-polymerase chain reaction (RT-PCR) was the earliest molecular method by which detection of circulating tumor cells was explored [7]. RT-PCR assays rely on the detection of mRNA transcripts specific to a tumor type, such as tyrosinase in melanoma [8] or prostate-specific antigen for prostate cancer [9]. Unfortunately, such methods detect all cells expressing the marker of interest, which may include benign circulating epithelial cells [10]. More specific RT-PCR detection of CTCs may be possible through detection of markers of malignancy such as chromosomal translocations or point mutations. However, translocations are more common in sarcomas and hematologic malignancies such as lymphoma and leukemia, limiting their utility when applied to the detection of carcinoma CTCs.

Antibody Capture

Normal hematopoietic cells do not express the surface epithelial cell proteins, such as epithelial cell adhesion molecule (EpCAM), seen on carcinoma-derived CTCs. Therefore, many methods rely on positive selection strategies based on CTC expression of antigen markers such as BER EP4 to facilitate separation and identification, as well as increase the sensitivity and specificity of detection. The most common techniques use magnetically labeled antibodies. While automated immunomagnetic cell separation is currently used clinically for applications such as chimerism testing after stem cell transplant [11], CTC detection requires a higher level of sensitivity due to the small numbers of CTCs present. The only assay currently FDA approved, the CellSearch® System (Janssen Diagnostics, LLC, Raritan, NJ) (Fig. 39.1) [12], utilizes antibody-coated ferrofluids to separate CTCs

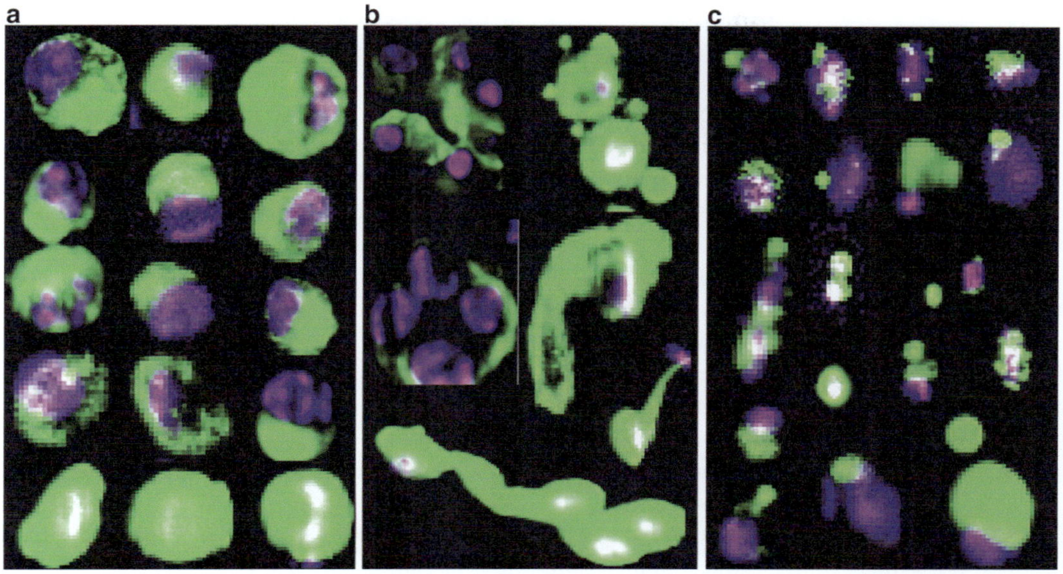

Figure 39.1 Gallery of CTC images from the CellSpotter Analyzer (Janssen Diagnostics LLC, Raritan, NJ) Diagnostics obtained from 7.5 mL of blood from cancer patients. (**a**) Examples of typical intact CTCs. (**b**) Examples of intact CTCs present as clusters or with odd shapes that are present less frequently. (**c**) Examples of CTC fragments and apoptotic CTCs. Images presented in **c** were not included in the CTC counts but are frequently observed in CTC analysis of carcinoma patients. From Allard WJ, Matera J, Miller MC et al. (2004) Tumor cells circulate in the peripheral blood of all major carcinomas but not in healthy subjects or patients with non-malignant diseases. Clin Cancer Res. 47:6897–6904. Reprinted with permission from American Association for Cancer Research

from normal blood components. To increase specificity, the isolated cells are then stained with 4′,6-diamidino-2-phenylindole (DAPI) and a fluorescently-labeled antitumor antibody prior to imaging. Automatically captured images are reviewed by a pathologist to determine the number of tumor cells present, based on a combination of fluorescent immunostaining and morphology [13].

To increase sensitivity, alternative methods of detection are being explored. One recently described ultrasensitive CTC detection device relies on detection of changes in electrical conductance caused by the presence of magnetic immunoparticles on cells instead of image analysis of separated cells to detect CTCs. Similar to flow cytometry, this system could allow multiple antigens to be simultaneously bound by multiple fluorescently labeled antibodies and detected on the same cell for increased specificity [14]. Such methods would require rigorous quality control and validation prior to clinical usage.

Negative cell selection strategies have successfully utilized CD45 immunomagnetic labeling to remove hematopoietic cells and enrich for CTCs in head and neck cancer patients [15]. These methods have possible advantages in that CTCs may express cytokeratins or other epithelial-specific markers weakly or not at all, limiting the ability to adequately tag CTCs for positive selection. Negative cell selection methods would allow for a wider spectrum of CTCs to be captured, including those that have undergone epithelial-to-mesenchymal transformation and thus might lack typical epithelial markers.

Size-Based Selection

CTCs of interest from solid tumors are often larger in size than normal blood components. This has led to the development of filter-based methods which collect larger cells for use in targeted analysis. One such device utilizes a parylene membrane to isolate possible CTCs from diluted blood. Once the blood has been passed through the filter, the trapped cells are analyzed directly on the membrane via light or electron microscopy, as well as by IHC [16]. These captured cells also are viable for cell culture, which is not possible for cells that have been fixed and stained [17]. Additional devices utilizing the principles of microfluidics have been successfully used to isolate CTCs [18, 19].

CTC chips combine the principles of both antibody capture and filter devices. Patient blood samples are filtered through silicon chips made up of microposts coated with antibodies to EpCAM; the chips are engineered to reduce cellular shear forces and allow a reasonable volume of blood to be analyzed. The captured epithelial cells are analyzed similarly to those captured on a filter and also remain viable for cell culture [20].

Clinical Utility

Blood

Many studies evaluating CTCs have been published. In a variety of tumor types, a correlation between the detection of blood-borne cells and tumor stage has been demonstrated [21–25]. Unfortunately, the data do not support the conclusion that the absence of CTCs indicates absence of metastatic disease with enough precision for clinical application [26]. Ultimately, the presence of CTCs may provide valuable information on the systemic spread of tumor in a manner different from conventional staging approaches. Small but aggressive tumors may shed cells into the circulation, while a more indolent but larger tumor may not; such a situation may appear to correlate poorly with tumor stage but may more accurately reflect tumor aggressiveness. The detection of circulating breast cancer cells is correlated with vascular invasion in the primary tumor. Larger studies using appropriate markers are needed to determine how to integrate these molecular test results for CTCs into cancer staging strategies.

While a relationship between CTCs and tumor stage is evident, studies demonstrating a correlation between circulating cells and cancer recurrence or progression have shown mixed results. A correlation between blood-borne cells and disease-free survival following radical prostatectomy has been reported [27]. Early studies correlated the presence of CTCs in patients with metastatic breast cancer to progression-free survival and overall survival [13]. However, in newly diagnosed breast cancer patients, the presence of CTCs prior to surgery was associated with an increased risk of cancer-associated death, but not a decreased risk of recurrence free survival [28]. Similar relationships have been established in colorectal [29] and prostate [30] cancers. These findings support the use of CTCs as prognostic markers that can help stratify patients into risk categories based on multiple clinical parameters.

CTC characterization may also be used to monitor response to chemotherapy. Prostate cancer patients treated with androgen deprivation therapy demonstrating the continuing presence or re-emergence of CTCs with androgen receptor signaling have poorer outcomes than those patients whose CTCs do not demonstrate androgen receptor signaling [31].

Bone Marrow

In general, better correlation has been observed between patient outcome and molecular or IHC detection of tumor cells in the bone marrow compared to blood [24, 25, 32, 33]. It is possible that circulating cells have the ability to get into the bloodstream but lack the ability to survive at a metastatic site, while cells in the marrow are at an "advanced" stage in the metastatic continuum, having acquired the capacity to survive in the circulation, attach, and grow in a remote environment. This, however, is a speculation until the molecular events underlying the metastatic process are better understood.

While few studies using single markers have shown results that correlate with clinical or pathologic parameters, correlation with survival/outcome was observed using IHC to detect cytokeratin-positive cells in bone marrow samples from breast cancer patients [32]. Similar findings have been reported for prostate [33] and colorectal cancer [34]. In the USA, such studies can be hampered by clinical practices that do not include bone marrow sampling as part of routine staging for many tumors.

Circulating Epithelial Cells in Benign Disease

While detection of CTCs has prognostic value when identified in cancer patients, CTC detection methods may show positivity in patients with benign diseases, particularly in disease processes in which the vascular integrity may be compromised, such as by inflammation, or by surgery. Patients with benign colonic diseases, including diverticulosis, Crohn disease, ulcerative colitis, endometriosis, and benign polyps, showed the presence of circulating epithelial cells identified as "circulating tumor cells" by the CellSearch (Janssen Diagnostics, LLC) and CK19-EPISPOT (Mabtech, Cincinnati, OH) assays in up to 18.9 % of patients. Up to 41 CTCs were detected in these patients, compared to no CTC detection in any of the healthy controls. Both platforms use antibodies to cytokeratin expression to identify circulating epithelial cells; again, these markers are not specific to malignant cells [35]. Further work is needed since patients with cancer may also be affected by benign disease of any organ and be falsely classified into poor prognosis groups based on circulating benign epithelial cells that are falsely identified as CTCs, regardless of the method used.

Circulating Nucleic Acids

Circulating tumor nucleic acids have multiple origins. They can exist as cell-free nucleic acids (cfNA) or be extracted from intact circulating tumor cells (see previous section). The presence of circulating nucleic acids has long been noted from peripheral blood samples [36], and the presence of circulating fetal DNA is routinely used for prenatal diagnosis [37, 38]. Increased levels of cfNA are often seen in patients with cancer [39]. In addition, since the advent of massively parallel sequencing, the molecular characterization of tumors has greatly expanded. Studies suggest that the majority of tumors carry somatic alterations [40, 41] that could be used to identify cfNA originating from tumors. This raises the possibility of "liquid biopsies," where peripheral blood is analyzed for the presence of tumor-specific mutations. This is particularly significant as cell-free tumor DNA can originate from the patient's primary tumor, metastases, and CTCs that have undergone apoptosis within vessels. The contribution of cfNA from each would then provide information about tumor heterogeneity that would be unable to be obtained from a traditional biopsy and at lower risk to the patient [42].

Detection Methods

Compared to CTCs, cfNA are relatively easy to extract. The cellular component of the blood is spun down and the acellular plasma or serum used for extraction of nucleic acids, using either manual or automated methods. However, this apparent ease of isolation may adversely impact the implementation of cfNA analysis. Because of the ubiquity of blood-based specimens, a wide variety of extraction methods are available, each with its own performance characteristics. While general increases in cfNA are observed in patients with cancer [43], no standards are available to determine the efficiency of a specific cfNA extraction process. In addition to varying quantities of cfNA, the length of cfNA varies, from 20 bp-long microRNAs to DNA fragments over 80,000 bp long [44].

Exosomes

A more recent finding of relevance to the detection and isolation of cfNA is the existence of exosomes, which are small membrane-encoated vesicles ranging from 40 to 100 nm in diameter. Exosomes contain mRNA, miRNA, and proteins and are able to influence cell function when taken up by the cells [45, 46]. Exosomes have been shown to be stable in various body fluids and can be separated intact from serum and their contents used for subsequent analysis [47]. Exosomes appear to have important functions in normal immune regulation and also appear to have a role in regulation of immunoreactivity to cancer cells, as well as intercellular communication between cancer cells and stroma [46]. A better understanding of exosomes will be critical to understanding the metastatic process as well as the potential use of exosomes as cancer biomarkers.

Clinical Utility

Three main categories of cfNA are being explored for utility in patients with cancer: DNA, mRNA, and microRNA.

Cell-Free DNA (cfDNA)

If tumor-specific mutations are known, the presence of detectable point mutations in patient plasma over time could be used to monitor relapse and/or progression. The percentage of total cfDNA that is derived from tumor has been seen to track with the amount of disease present [42, 48]. A recent study showed that the percentage of cfDNA with TP53 mutation detectable in ovarian carcinoma patients tracked over time with CA125 levels. The same study also demonstrated that levels of cfDNA with tumor-specific mutations tracked with clinical presentation in a breast cancer patient with relapsed disease [42]. Tumor-derived cfDNA may be present in large amounts, as up to 52 % of cfDNA from a patient with a 13 cm hepatocellular carcinoma originated from the tumor. In this study, patients with smaller tumors had lower fractional concentrations of tumor-derived DNA. When the tumors were resected, the amount of tumor DNA in the circulation decreased [48].

High-sensitivity assays could also be used to look for mutations to help guide therapy, as demonstrated by the ability to detect 56 % of patients positive for *BRAF* V600 mutations using amplification refractory mutation system (ARMS) PCR in cfDNA [49]. Copy number changes and chromosomal rearrangements can be detected in cfDNA by genome sequencing (Fig. 39.2) [50], as noted in case reports of maternal malignancies detected by the presence of multiple aneuploidies on noninvasive prenatal testing using cfDNA [51].

Cell-Free mRNA (cfmRNA)

Because cfmRNA must be transcribed from DNA, it may provide more specific information about the pathways activated in a patient's tumor. Multiple studies have associated cfmRNA detection with clinical outcomes. The presence of cyclin D1 mRNA in the plasma of tamoxifen-treated breast cancer patients has been associated with poorer overall survival and lack of response to tamoxifen [52]. Expression levels of circulating hTERT cfmRNA have been studied in multiple tumor types. Increased levels above those seen in healthy individuals are associated with reduced disease-free and overall survival in patients with gastric cancer [22]. Elevated values have also been associated with shorter recurrence-free survival in patients with prostatic carcinoma [53].

Cell-Free microRNA (cfmiRNA)

MicroRNAs are involved in regulation of gene expression and are frequently dysregulated in cancer [54], and miRNA expression profiles have been established for many tumor types, increasing their potential clinical utility [55]. While most biomarker studies utilize multiple cell-free microRNA (cfmiRNA) targets, such as the combination of miR-21, -210, -155, and 196a in pancreatic adenocarcinoma [56], a recent study found that patients with stage IV breast cancer had higher concentrations of miR-21 [57]. Of note, miR-16, which is often used as a normalizer when evaluating expression levels of cfmiRNA, is present in high quantities in red blood cells. Therefore, the presence of hemolysis may interfere with the interpretation of cfmiRNAs in the plasma [58]. While measurement of cell-free miRNA has

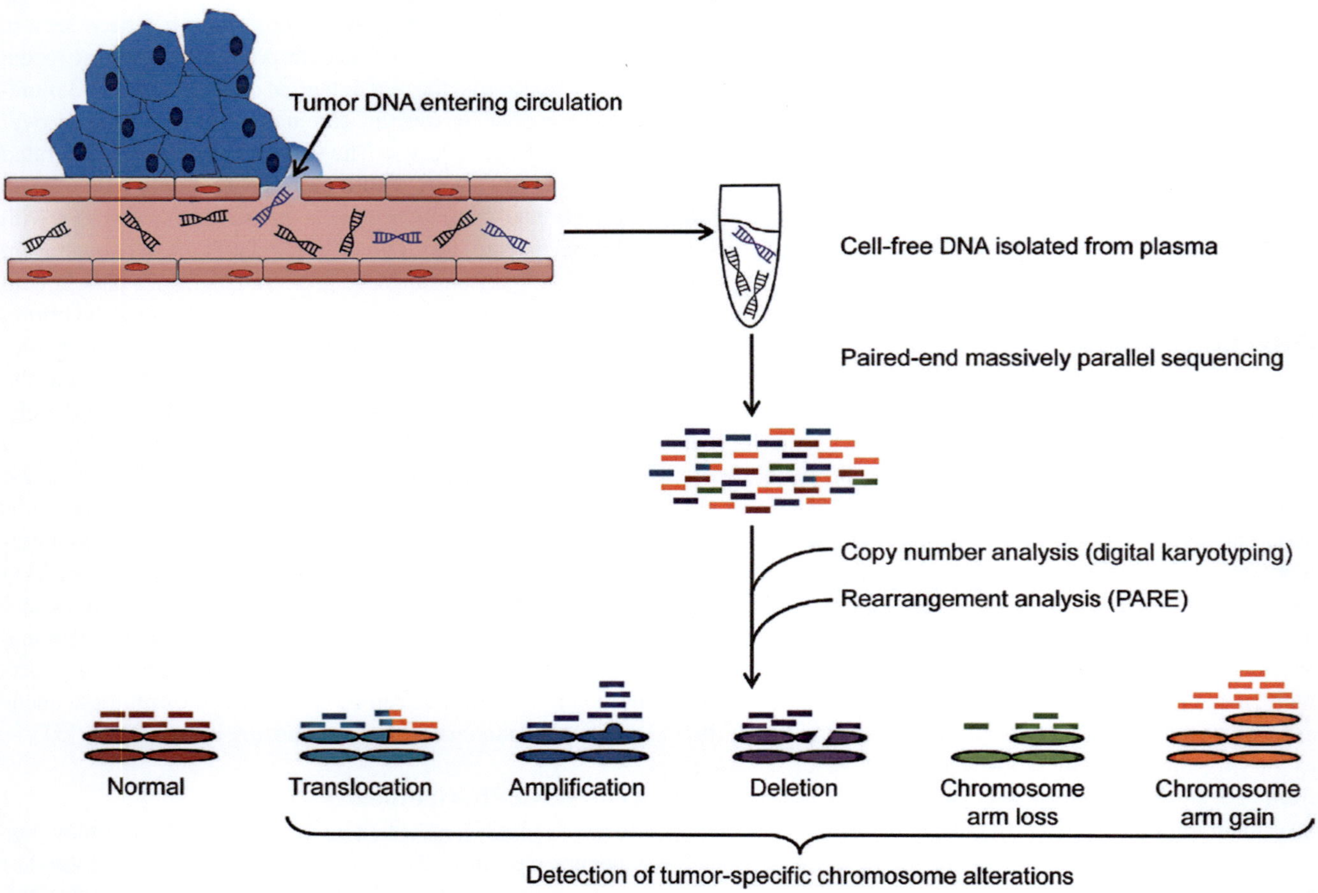

Figure 39.2 Schematic of analyses for direct detection of chromosomal alterations in plasma. The method uses next-generation paired-end sequencing of cell-free DNA isolated from plasma to identify chromosomal alterations characteristic of tumor DNA. Such alterations include copy number changes (gains and losses of chromosome arms) as well as rearrangements resulting from translocations, amplifications, or deletions. From Leary RJ, Sausen M, Kinde I, et al. (2012). Detection of chromosomal alterations in the circulation of cancer patients with whole-genome sequencing. *Sci Transl Med.* 4:162ra154. Reprinted with permission from AAAS

great potential, a more thorough understanding of normal and disease-related miRNA variation, as well as more straightforward analytic methods, will be needed.

Conclusions and Future Directions

Since 1991, when the first report of detection of circulating cells in melanoma was published [7], investigation of the clinical relevance of CTCs has been pursued by teams of investigators. To date, the only well-developed clinical parameter is the number of CTCs present in breast, colon, and prostate cancer patients, to be used for risk stratification. However, as the technology used for molecular analysis becomes capable of utilizing ever smaller quantities of input nucleic acids, the information that can be gained from cfNAs and isolated CTCs will continue to increase. In addition, these alternative tumor detection methods are beginning to be directly compared. For example, a recent study demonstrated a relationship between the amount of cfDNA in the serum of patients and overall survival, with those patients with higher levels of cfDNA demonstrating poorer survival. In addition, both levels of cfDNA and detection of CTCs are tracked with disease progression (Fig. 39.3) [30]. In addition, these more sensitive analysis methods will allow for elucidation of tumor heterogeneity, and it may therefore become possible to combine targeted therapies which block all of the oncogenic pathways utilized by a specific patient's cancer, much like antiretroviral therapies are currently tailored to the group phenotype of all HIV virions present in a patient, rather than one specific subclone.

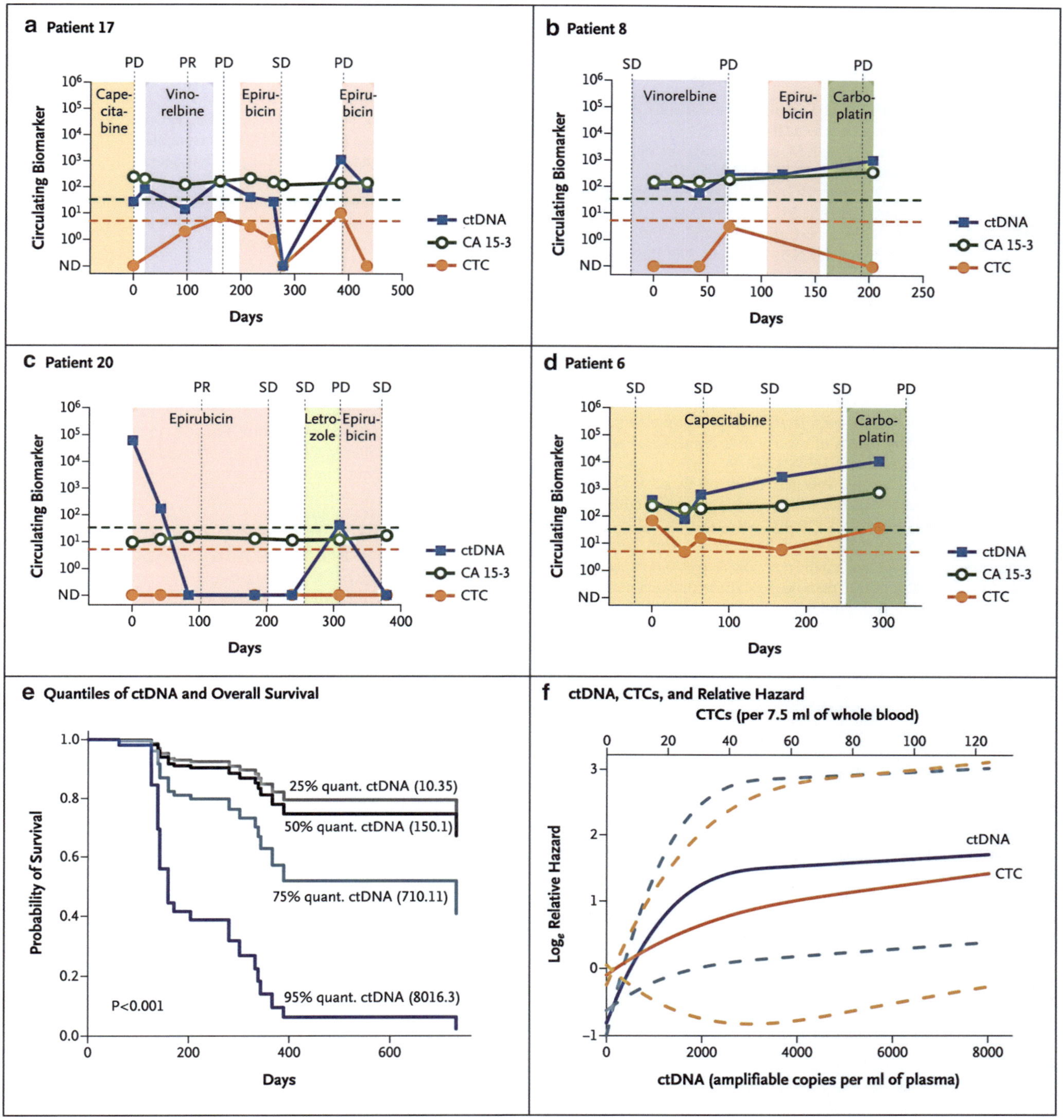

Figure 39.3 Comparison of circulating biomarkers to monitor tumor dynamics and predict survival. Panels **a**–**d** show serial circulating tumor DNA (ctDNA) levels (number of copies per milliliter of plasma), circulating tumor cell (CTC) numbers (per 7.5 ml of whole blood), CA15-3 levels (U per milliliter), and disease status as ascertained on computed tomography (*vertical dashed lines*) for four patients (one in each panel). Details of endocrine or cytotoxic therapy are indicated by *colored shading*. The *orange dashed line* indicates the threshold of five CTCs per 7.5 ml of whole blood. The *green dashed line* indicates the CA15-3 threshold of 32.4 U per milliliter. *ND* not detected, *PD* progressive disease, *PR* partial response, and *SD* stable disease. Panel **e** shows the results of a Cox regression model, which identified an inverse relationship between quantiles (quant.) of ctDNA (indicated in copies per milliliter of plasma) and overall survival, with increasing levels significantly associated with poor overall survival ($P<0.001$). At 200, 400, and 600 days, a total of 23, 8, and 3 patients were at risk, respectively. Panel **f** shows that increasing ctDNA levels (copies per milliliter), as indicated on the *bottom x* axis, and increasing numbers of CTCs (per 7.5 ml of whole blood), as indicated on the *top x* axis, were associated with an increased loge relative hazard. The prognostic discrimination power of circulating tumor DNA level was greatest with levels up to 2,000 copies per milliliter. Patients with levels of more than 2,000 copies per milliliter were uniformly found to have the worst prognosis. The prognostic power of CTCs increased according to the number of cells. *Dashed lines* represent 95 % confidence intervals. From New England Journal of Medicine, Dawson SJ et al., Analysis of circulating tumor DNA to monitor metastatic breast cancer, 368:1199–1209. Copyright © (2013) Massachusetts Medical Society. Reprinted with permission from Massachusetts Medical Society

References

1. Alix-Panabières C, Pantel K. Circulating tumor cells: liquid biopsy of cancer. Clin Chem. 2013;59:110–8.
2. Pinzani P, Salvianti F, Pazzagli M, et al. Circulating nucleic acids in cancer and pregnancy. Methods. 2010;50:302–7.
3. Pratt ED, Huang C, Hawkins BG, et al. Rare cell capture in microfluidic devices. Chem Eng Sci. 2011;66:1508–22.
4. Schwarzenbach H, Nishida N, Calin GA, et al. Clinical relevance of circulating cell-free microRNAs in cancer. Nat Rev Clin Oncol. 2014;11:145–56.
5. Bauer KD, de la Torre-Bueno J, Diel IJ, et al. Reliable and sensitive analysis of occult bone marrow metastases using automated cellular imaging. Clin Cancer Res. 2000;6:3552–9.
6. Tvasellas G, Huang A, McCullough T, et al. Flow cytometry correlates with RT-PCR for detection of spiked but not circulating colorectal cancer cells. Clin Exp Metastasis. 2002;19:495–502.
7. Smith B, Selby P, Southgate J, et al. Detection of melanoma cells in peripheral blood by means of reverse transcriptase and polymerase chain reaction. Lancet. 1991;338:1227–9.
8. Mellado B, del Carmen Vela M, Colomer D, et al. Tyrosinase mRNA in blood of patients with melanoma treated with adjuvant interferon. Clin Oncol. 2002;20:4032–9.
9. Katz AE, de Vries GM, Begg MD, et al. Enhanced reverse transcriptase-polymerase chain reaction for prostate specific antigen as an indicator of true pathologic stage in patients with prostate cancer. Cancer. 1995;75:1642–8.
10. Crisan D, Ruark DS, Decker DA, et al. Detection of circulating epithelial cells after surgery for benign breast disease. Mol Diagn. 2000;5:33–8.
11. Decot V, Latget-Cannard V, Lecompte T, et al. Chimerism analysis following nonmyeloablative stem cell transplantation using a new cell subset separation method: Robosep™. Biomed Mater Eng. 2000;18:19–36.
12. Allard WJ, Matera J, Miller MC, et al. Tumor cells circulate in the peripheral blood of all major carcinomas but not in healthy subjects or patients with non-malignant diseases. Clin Cancer Res. 2004;47:6897–904.
13. Cristofanelli M, Hayes DF, Budd GT, et al. Circulating tumor cells: a novel prognostic factor for newly diagnosed breast cancer. J Clin Oncol. 2005;23:1420–30.
14. Issadore D, Chung J, Shao H, et al. Ultrasensitive clinical enumeration of rare cells ex vivo using a micro-hall detector. Sci Transl Med. 2012;4:141ra92.
15. Yang L, Lang JC, Balasubramanian P, et al. Optimization of an enrichment process for circulating tumor cells from the blood of head and neck cancer patients through depletion of normal cell. Biotechnol Bioeng. 2008;102:521–34.
16. Lin HK, Zheng S, Williams AJ, et al. Portable filter-based microdevice for detection and characterization of circulating tumor cells. Clin Cancer Res. 2010;16:5011–8.
17. Zheng S, Lin HK, Lu B, et al. 3D microfilter device for viable circulating tumor cell (CTC) enrichment from blood. Biomed Microdevices. 2011;13:203–13.
18. Bhagat AAS, Hou HW, Li LD, et al. Pinched flow coupled shear-modulated inertial microfluidics for high-throughput rare blood cell separation. Lab Chip. 2011;11:1870–8.
19. Moon HS, Kwon K, Kim SI, et al. Continuous separation of breast cancer cells from blood samples using multi-orifice flow fractionation (MOFF) and dielectrophoresis (DEP). Lab Chip. 2011;11:1118–25.
20. Sequist LV, Nagrath S, Toner M, et al. The CTC-chip: an exciting new tool to detect circulating tumor cells in lung cancer patients. J Thorac Oncol. 2009;4:281.
21. Hoon DS, Wang Y, Dale PS, et al. Detection of occult melanoma cells in blood with a multiple marker polymerase chain reaction assay. J Clin Oncol. 1995;13:2109–16.
22. Kang Y, Zhang J, Sun P, et al. Circulating cell-free human telomerase reverse transcriptase mRNA in plasma and its potential diagnostic and prognostic value for gastric cancer. Int J Clin Oncol. 2012;18:478–86.
23. Olsson CA, de Vries GM, Benson MC, et al. The use of RT-PCR for prostate-specific antigen assay to predict potential surgical failures before radical prostatectomy: molecular staging of prostate cancer. Br J Urol. 1996;77:411–7.
24. Soeth E, Roder C, Juhl H, et al. The detection of disseminated tumor cells in bone marrow from colorectal cancer patients by a cytokeratin 20 specific nested reverse transcriptase—polymerase chain reaction is related to the stage of disease. Int J Cancer. 1996;69:278–82.
25. Vogel I, Kalthoff H. Disseminated tumour cells. Their detection and significance for prognosis of gastrointestinal and pancreatic carcinomas. Virchows Arch. 2001;439:109–17.
26. Riethdorf S, Müller V, Zhang L, et al. Detection and HER2 expression of circulating tumor cells: prospective monitoring in breast cancer patients treated in the neoadjuvant GeparQuattro Trial. Clin Cancer Res. 2010;10:2634–45.
27. Bianco Jr FJ, Powell IJ, Cher ML, et al. Presence of circulating prostate cancer cells in African American males adversely affects survival. Urol Oncol. 2002;7:147–52.
28. Franken B, de Groot MR, Mastboom WJB, et al. Circulating tumor cells, disease recurrence and survival in newly diagnosed breast cancer. Breast Cancer Res. 2012;14:R133.
29. Cohen SJ, Punt CJA, Ianotti N, et al. Relationship of circulating tumor cells to tumor response, progression-free survival, and overall survival in patients with metastatic colorectal cancer. J Clin Oncol. 2008;26:3213–21.
30. Dawson SJ, Tsui DWY, Murtaza M, et al. Analysis of circulating tumor DNA to monitor metastatic breast cancer. N Engl J Med. 2013;368:1199–209.
31. Miyamoto DT, Lee RJ, Stott SL, et al. Androgen receptor signaling in circulating tumor cells as a marker of hormonally responsive prostate cancer. Cancer Discov. 2012;2:995–1003.
32. Braun S, Pantel K, Muller P, et al. Cytokeratin-positive cells in the bone marrow and survival or patients with stage I, II, or III breast cancer. N Engl J Med. 2000;342:525–33.
33. Wood Jr DP, Banerjee M. Presence of circulating prostate cells in the bone marrow of patients undergoing radical prostatectomy is predictive of disease-free survival. J Clin Oncol. 1997;15:3451–7.
34. Liefers GJ, Cleton-Jansen AM, van de Velde CJH, et al. Micrometastases and survival in stage II colorectal cancer. N Engl J Med. 1998;339:223–8.
35. Pantel K, Deneve E, Nocca D, et al. Circulating epithelial cells in patients with benign colon diseases. Clin Chem. 2012;58:936–40.
36. Mandel P, Metais P. Les acides nucleiques du plasma sanguin chez l'homme. CR Acad Sci Paris. 1948;142:241–3.
37. Ariga H, Ohto H, Busch MP, et al. Kinetics of fetal cellular and cell-free DNA in the maternal circulation during and after pregnancy: implications for noninvasive prenatal diagnosis. Transfusion. 2002;41:1524–30.
38. Ehrich M, Deciu C, Zwielhofer T, et al. Noninvasive detection of fetal trisomy 21 by sequencing of DNA in maternal blood: a study in a clinical setting. Am J Obstet Gynecol. 2011;204:205.e1–11.
39. Taback B, O'Day SJ, Hoon DSB. Quantification of circulating DNA in the plasma and serum of cancer patients. Ann N Y Acad Sci. 2004;1022:17–24.
40. Thu KL, Vucic EA, Chari R, et al. Lung adenocarcinoma of never smokers and smokers harbor differential regions of genetic alteration

and exhibit different levels of genomic instability. PLoS One. 2012;7:e33003.
41. Welch JS, Link DC. Genomics of AML: clinical applications of next-generation sequencing. Hematology Am Soc Hematol Educ Program. 2011;2011:30–5.
42. Forshew T, Murtaza M, Parkinson C, et al. Noninvasive identification and monitoring of cancer mutations by targeted deep sequencing of plasma DNA. Sci Transl Med. 2012;4:136ra68.
43. Shapiro B, Chakrabarty M, Cohn EM, et al. Determination of circulating DNA levels in patients with benign or malignant gastrointestinal disease. Cancer. 1983;51:2116–20.
44. Giacona MB, Ruben GC, Iczkowski KA, et al. Cell-free DNA in human blood plasma: length measurements in patients with pancreatic cancer and healthy controls. Pancreas. 1998;17:89–97.
45. Peinado H, Aleckovic M, Lavotshkin S, et al. Melanoma exosomes educate bone marrow progenitor cells toward a pro-metastatic phenotype through MET. Nat Med. 2012;18:883–91.
46. Skog J, Wurdinger T, van Rijn S, et al. Glioblastoma microvesicles transport RNA and proteins that promote tumor growth and provide diagnostic biomarkers. Nat Cell Biol. 2008;10:1470–6.
47. Rani S, O'Brien K, Kelleher FC, et al. Isolation of exosomes for subsequent mRNA, MicroRNA, and protein profiling. Methods Mol Biol. 2011;784:181–95.
48. Chan KCA, Jiang P, Zheng YWL, et al. Cancer genome scanning in plasma: detection of tumor-associated copy number aberrations, single-nucleotide variants, and tumoral heterogeneity by massively parallel sequencing. Clin Chem. 2013;59:211–24.
49. Board RE, Eillison G, Orr MCM, et al. Detection of BRAF mutations in the tumor and serum of patients enrolled in the AZD6244 (ARRY-142886) advanced melanoma phase II study. Br J Cancer. 2009;101:1724–30.
50. Leary RJ, Sausen M, Kinde I, et al. Detection of chromosomal alterations in the circulation of cancer patients with whole-genome sequencing. Sci Transl Med. 2012;4:162ra154.
51. Osburne CM, Hardisty E, Devers P, et al. Discordant noninvasive prenatal testing results in a patient subsequently diagnosed with metastatic disease. Prenat Diagn. 2013;33:609–11.
52. García V, García JM, Peña C, et al. Free circulating mRNA in plasma from breast cancer patients and clinical outcome. Cancer Lett. 2008;263:312–20.
53. March-Villalba JA, Martinez-Jabaloyas JM, Herrero MJ, et al. Cell-free circulating plasma hTERT mRNA is a useful marker for prostate cancer diagnosis and is associated with poor prognosis tumor characteristics. PLoS One. 2012;78:e43470.
54. Croce CM. Causes and consequences of microRNA dysregulation in cancer. Nat Rev Genet. 2009;10:295–304.
55. Schwarzenbach H, Hoon DSB, Pantel K. Cell-free nucleic acids as biomarkers in cancer patients. Nat Rev Cancer. 2011;11:426–37.
56. Wang J, Chen J, Chang P, et al. MicroRNAs in plasma of pancreatic ductal adenocarcinoma patients as novel blood-based biomarkers of disease. Cancer Prev Res. 2009;2:807–13.
57. Asaga S, Kuo C, Nguyen T, et al. Direct serum assay for microRNA-21 concentrations in early and advanced breast cancer. Clin Chem. 2011;57:84–91.
58. Kirschner MB, Kao SC, Edelman JJ, et al. Haemolysis during sample preparation alters microRNA content of plasma. PLoS One. 2011;6:e24145.

Section IV

Neoplastic Hematopathology

Section Editor: Iris Schrijver

Acute Myeloid Leukemia

40

David Grimwade, Steven Knapper, and Krzysztof Mrózek

Abstract

The diagnostic entity of acute myeloid leukemia (AML) encompasses a heterogeneous group of diseases whose prognosis differs substantially according to the nature of the underlying molecular lesions and the age of the patient. AML is predominantly a disease of the elderly with a dramatic increase in incidence in individuals over 60 years of age. Traditionally, cases of AML have been classified as primary (de novo) or secondary including those arising following exposure to radiation and various chemotherapeutic agents (therapy-related AML), or occurring on a background of an antecedent hematologic disorder, particularly myelodysplasia.

Keywords

Acute myeloid leukemia • Cytogenetics • Fluorescence in situ hybridization (FISH) • FLT3 CEBPA • NPM1 • Risk stratification • Minimal residual disease (MRD) detection

Introduction

The diagnostic entity of acute myeloid leukemia (AML) encompasses a heterogeneous group of diseases whose prognosis differs substantially according to the nature of the underlying molecular lesions and the age of the patient. AML is predominantly a disease of the elderly with a dramatic increase in incidence in individuals over 60 years of age. Traditionally, cases of AML have been classified as primary (de novo) or secondary including those arising following exposure to radiation and various chemotherapeutic agents (therapy-related AML), or occurring on a background of an antecedent hematologic disorder, particularly myelodysplasia (Table 40.1).

Molecular Basis of Disease

Considerable progress has been made in understanding the cytogenetic and molecular basis of AML over the course of the last four decades. This has had a major impact on the laboratory workup of patients with suspected AML, with definition of the karyotype and mutational profile of the leukemic cells being of critical importance by serving to identify biologically distinct subsets of disease and predicting likely response to therapy and overall survival. Age of presentation has an important bearing on disease features, with balanced chromosomal translocations being relatively common in children and younger adults, while AML in older patients is characterized by a more common picture of whole chromosome losses (monosomy) and gains (e.g., trisomy) and losses (deletion) or gains (duplication, unbalanced translocation) of chromosomal segments that often occur in the context of a complex karyotype.

D. Grimwade, Ph.D., F.R.C.Path. (✉)
Department of Medical and Molecular Genetics, Cancer Genetics Laboratory, King's College London, Faculty of Life Sciences and Medicine, 8th Floor, Tower Wing, Guy's Hospital Campus, London SE1 9RT, UK
e-mail: david.grimwade@genetics.kcl.ac.uk

S. Knapper, D.M., B.M.B.Ch., F.R.C.Path.
Department of Haematology, Cardiff University, Cardiff, UK

K. Mrózek, M.D., Ph.D.
Comprehensive Cancer Center, The Ohio State University, Columbus, OH, USA

D.G.B. Leonard (ed.), *Molecular Pathology in Clinical Practice*, DOI 10.1007/978-3-319-19674-9_40

Cytogenetic Classification of AML

Balanced Chromosomal Rearrangements

Improved understanding of the molecular basis of AML was incorporated into the 2008 revision of the World Health Organization (WHO) Classification of Tumours of Haematopoietic and Lymphoid Tissues [1, 2], which necessitates application of a range of laboratory tests including cytogenetics and molecular testing to complement morphological and immunophenotypic assessment for disease diagnosis and categorization. The WHO classification is organized in a hierarchical fashion, with the first group being AML with particular balanced translocations or inversions (and their molecular counterparts), which are defined as "AML with recurrent genetic abnormalities" (Table 40.2). These include t(15;17)(q22;q12~21), the diagnostic hallmark of acute promyelocytic leukemia (APL), which accounts for approximately 12 % of AML cases. Cloning of the translocation breakpoints in the early 1990s [3–5] showed that t(15;17) leads to fusion of the gene that encodes the myeloid transcription factor, *r*etinoic *a*cid *r*eceptor *a*lpha (*RARA*), with a previously unknown gene designated *PML* (for promyelocytic leukemia), which has subsequently been found to be involved in growth suppression and regulation of apoptosis [6]. While the vast majority of APL cases have an underlying *PML–RARA* fusion, in approximately 1–2 % *RARA* is fused to an alternative partner [7] and classified as "AML with a variant *RARA* translocation." These rare subtypes of APL include involvement of *ZBTB16* (*PLZF*), *NPM1*, *NUMA*, *FIP1L1*, and *BCOR*, as a result of the t(11;17)(q23;q21), t(5;17)(q35;q21), t(11;17)(q13;q21), t(4;17)(q12;q21), and t(X;17)(p11;q21), respectively, and *PRKAR1A* and *STAT5B* in rearrangements involving 17q [8–14]. The nature of the fusion partner has an important bearing on disease biology, particularly the response to molecularly targeted therapies, i.e., all transretinoic acid (ATRA) and arsenic trioxide (ATO) [15]. ATRA targets the ligand-binding domain of the RARα moiety in the C-terminal region of the fusion proteins (as well as wild-type RARα). Sensitivity to ATRA has been documented in APL subtypes

Table 40.1 Factors predisposing to the development of AML

Genetic predisposition
Down syndrome
Fanconi anemia
Other inherited bone marrow failure syndromes:
Shwachman-Diamond
Diamond-Blackfan
Dyskeratosis congenita
Kostmann's
Familial platelet disorder (*RUNX1* mutation)
DNA repair defects, e.g., Bloom syndrome
Other germline mutations e.g., involving *CEBPA*, *DDX41*, *GATA2*
Prior hematologic disorder
Chronic myeloid leukemia
Myeloproliferative neoplasms
Myelodysplastic syndrome
Paroxysmal nocturnal hemoglobinuria
Exposure to environmental or therapeutic agents
Chronic exposure to benzene and derivatives
Ionizing radiation
Chemotherapeutic agents:
Alkylating agents
Topoisomerase II-targeting drugs

Table 40.2 Cytogenetic abnormalities used in the WHO classification of AML

Cytogenetic abnormalities used to define entities within the WHO category: "AML with recurrent genetic abnormalities"	
t(8;21)(q22;q22); *RUNX1-RUNX1T1*	t(6;9)(p23;q34); *DEK-NUP214*
inv(16)(p13.1q22) or t(16;16)(p13.1;q22); *CBFB-MYH11*	inv(3)(q21q26.2) or t(3;3)(q21;q26.2); *GATA2-EVI1*[b]
t(15;17)(q22;q12); *PML-RARA*	t(1;22)(p13;q13); *RBM15-MKL1*
t(9;11)(p22;q23); *MLLT3-MLL*	
Cytogenetic abnormalities sufficient to diagnose WHO category: "AML with myelodysplasia-related changes"	
Complex karyotype	
Defined as three or more unrelated abnormalities, none of which can be a translocation or inversion associated with "AML with recurrent genetic abnormalities"	
Unbalanced abnormalities	**Balanced abnormalities**
−7 or del(7q)	t(11;16)(q23;p13.3)[a]
−5 or del(5q)	t(3;21)(q26.2;q22.1)[a]
i(17q) or t(17p)	t(1;3)(p36.3;q21.1)
−13 or del(13q)	t(2;11)(p21;q23)[a]
del(11q)	t(5;12)(q33;p12)
del(12p) or t(12p)	t(5;7)(q33;q11.2)
del(9q)	t(5;17)(q33;p13)
idic(X)(q13)	t(5;10)(q33;q21)
	t(3;5)(q25;q34)

Data from Vardiman et al. (Blood 2009;114(5):937–51) [2]

[a]A translocation commonly occurring in therapy-related AML. Before this translocation can be used as evidence for diagnosis of "AML with myelodysplasia-related changes," therapy-related disease should be excluded [b]Based upon Gröschel et al. [231] and Yamazaki et al. [232]

involving PML, NPM1, NUMA, and FIP1L1 [15], whereas PLZF-RARα and STAT5B-RARα have both been associated with primary resistance to retinoids and a poorer prognosis [14, 16, 17]. To date, sensitivity to ATO has only been demonstrated in *PML-RARA*-positive APL, reflecting the capacity of ATO to bind directly to the PML moiety of the fusion protein inducing its degradation via the proteasome [18]. Therefore, ATO should not be used for the treatment of APL as part of front-line therapy or in the context of suspected relapse, unless positive for *PML–RARA*.

Approximately 10 % of patients with AML are classified as having core-binding factor (CBF) leukemia with balanced chromosomal rearrangements that disrupt genes that encode components of the heterodimeric transcription factor complex, comprising RUNX1 (AML1, CBFα) and CBFβ, which plays a critical role in hematopoiesis [19]. The CBFα subunit is targeted by the t(8;21)(q22;q22), which fuses *RUNX1* (*AML1*, *CBFA2*) to the gene encoding the RUNX1T1 (formerly *ETO* for *e*ight *t*wenty *o*ne) transcriptional repressor, thereby potentially silencing RUNX1 target genes [19, 20]. The β-subunit is targeted by the inv(16)(p13.1q22) or the less common t(16;16)(p13.1;q22), in which *CBFB* is fused to the gene encoding myosin heavy chain (*MYH11*). *RUNX1* is a recurrent translocation target in non-CBF acute leukemias, with fusions to *ETV6* (*TEL*) as a result of the cytogenetically cryptic t(12;21)(p13;q22) in pediatric acute lymphoblastic leukemia (ALL), or to a range of partners in AML [21, 22], including *MECOM* (*EVI1*/*MDS1*) as a result of t(3;21)(q26;q22) in "AML with myelodysplasia-related changes" (Table 40.2). *RUNX1* also has been implicated in therapy-related leukemias arising following exposure to drugs targeting topoisomerase II [23, 24].

The *MLL* (for *m*yeloid/*l*ymphoid or *m*ixed-*l*ineage *l*eukemia, at present named *KMT2A*) gene located at 11q23 is a further recurrent translocation target in acute leukemia, with almost 80 partner genes now characterized [25]. MLL is an epigenetic regulator that plays a critical role in hematopoiesis, modulating *HOX* gene expression [26]. The most common *MLL* translocation observed in AML is the t(9;11)(p22;q23), which occurs in approximately 2 % of cases and leads to fusion of *MLL* with *MLLT3* (formerly known as *AF9*). AML with t(9;11)(p22;q23) has been associated with a relatively favorable outcome in some pediatric [27] and adult [28] AML studies and is distinguished as a separate entity in the 2008 WHO classification. Apart from the t(9;11), the most frequent other *MLL* translocations observed in AML are t(6;11)(q27;q23) involving *MLLT4* (*AF6*), t(11;19)(q23;p13.3) involving *MLLT1* (*ENL*), t(11;19)(q23;p13.1) involving *ELL*, and complex rearrangements between 10p12 and 11q23 (e.g., a reciprocal translocation and an inversion of an 11q segment translocated to 10p12 or inverted insertion of an 11q segment into 10p12 or a 10p segment into 11q23), in which the fusion partner is *MLLT10* (*AF10*) [29, 30]. While translocations involving *MLL* are observed in de novo leukemia and account for the majority of leukemias presenting in infancy, the locus is also a recurrent translocation target in therapy-related leukemias [31], particularly those arising following exposure to the epipodophyllotoxin class of topoisomerase II inhibitors [32]. Such cases are classified within the WHO as "therapy-related AML."

The remaining subtypes of AML distinguished as separate disease entities on the basis of cytogenetics are those characterized by the t(6;9)(p23;q34), inv(3)(q21q26.2) or t(3;3)(q21;q26.2), and t(1;22)(p13;q13). The t(6;9)(p23;q34) is found in approximately 1 % of AML and leads to fusion of *DEK* at 6p23 with *NUP214* (*CAN*) at 9q34, which encodes a component of the nuclear pore complex [33, 34]. The inv(3) or t(3;3) occurs in a similar proportion of AML cases and is associated with upregulation of the zinc finger transcription factor MECOM (EVI1), which is involved in normal hematopoiesis. AML with inv(3) or t(3;3) may present de novo, or secondary to prior myelodysplastic syndrome (MDS), and is characterized by a normal or elevated presenting platelet count and abnormal megakaryopoiesis with micromegakaryocytes in the bone marrow (BM) [35]. *MECOM* has long been implicated in leukemogenesis, having been identified as a recurrent integration target in murine retroviral mutagenesis screens [36, 37]; further evidence has been provided by characterization of MDS associated with insertional activation of *MECOM* occurring as a complication of gene therapy for chronic granulomatous disease [38]. Interestingly, these have provided important insights into potential mechanisms underlying acquisition of additional cytogenetic abnormalities in AML, with both cases showing monosomy 7, which is well recognized as a frequent secondary abnormality in cases with inv(3) or t(3;3). Forced overexpression of *MECOM* was found to disrupt normal centrosome duplication, suggesting that activation of *MECOM* as a result of retroviral insertion or chromosomal translocation leads to genomic instability, giving rise to acquisition of additional changes such as monosomy 7 involved in progression to MDS and AML.

AML with t(1;22)(p13;q13) is extremely rare (only approximately 40 cases reported worldwide [39]) and is associated with acute megakaryoblastic leukemia occurring in infants and young children (<3 years of age), particularly those without Down syndrome. The translocation fuses *RBM15* (for RNA-binding motif protein 15, also known as *OTT*) with *MKL1* (for MegaKaryoblastic Leukemia [Translocation] 1, or *MAL*) [40, 41], which is involved in normal megakaryocyte maturation [42].

AML with Myelodysplasia-Related Cytogenetic Changes

Apart from distinguishing AML with recurrent genetic abnormalities (as described above) from cases lacking one of these aberrations (or their molecular counterparts), cytogenetics is also used in the 2008 WHO classification as a criterion (in conjunction with ≥20 % leukemic blasts in the bone marrow [BM]) to define a subgroup of "AML with myelodysplasia-related changes" (Table 40.2). Some of these cytogenetic entities are relatively common, such as monosomy 5 and 7 (−5 and −7) or deletion of the long arms of these chromosomes [del(5q) and del(7q)], which often occur as part of a complex karyotype. Noteworthy is the observation that while −7 is recurrently present both as a sole chromosome aberration and as part of a complex karyotype, −5 is very rare in patients with noncomplex karyotypes [43]. Moreover, most patients with a complex karyotype, with −5 detected using banding techniques (e.g., G-banding), do not harbor true monosomy 5, because segments from a seemingly missing chromosome 5 can be found using spectral karyotyping [44] or fluorescence in situ hybridization (FISH) [45] in marker chromosomes or unbalanced structural aberrations only partially identified by G-banding. While balanced translocations such as t(11;16)(q23;p13.3) involving *MLL*, t(3;21)(q26.2;q22.1) involving *RUNX1*, and t(3;5)(q25;q34) that generates the *NPM1–MLF1* fusion [46] may be initiating lesions in the development of leukemia, many of the changes considered as "myelodysplasia related" entail loss of chromosomal segments or whole chromosomes, which are poorly understood at the molecular level and may represent secondary and cooperating lesions in AML pathogenesis. Some of the aberrations designated "myelodysplasia related," especially balanced translocations and idic(X)(q13), are extremely rare [47], making characterization of their biological features and establishment of their impact on the clinical outcome challenging.

Mutations Involved in the Pathogenesis of AML

While balanced chromosomal rearrangements are considered to be primary lesions involved in the pathogenesis of AML, they are insufficient to mediate the full leukemic phenotype, requiring acquisition of additional cooperating mutations. Work is currently in progress to define the spectrum of such mutations in cytogenetically defined subsets of AML (Table 40.3), particularly using high-throughput sequencing technologies. In addition, a major focus of research in recent years has been the deciphering of the molecular events underlying the pathogenesis of AML with normal karyotype (CN-AML). Such strategies also carry the potential of generating important targets for molecular approaches to disease therapy.

Fms-Related Tyrosine Kinase 3 (*FLT3*)

The FLT3 tyrosine kinase has been an intense focus for research. Groups working in Japan in the late 1990s identified two major classes of receptor-activating mutations of *FLT3* that, cumulatively, are found in approximately 30 % of AML patients [127, 128]. In normal hematopoiesis, the membrane-spanning FLT3 receptor is expressed on early progenitor cells including CD34+ hematopoietic stem cells and plays an important role in proliferation, survival, and differentiation. High levels of abnormal FLT3 expression are seen in 70–100 % of AML [129].

FLT3 internal tandem duplication mutations (*FLT3*-ITDs) are in-frame palindromic duplications of exons 14 and 15 of the *FLT3* gene, between three and 400 bp in length, that disrupt the autoinhibitory function of the FLT3 juxtamembrane domain, leading to activation of signaling pathways downstream of FLT3. Pooled data show an overall *FLT3*-ITD incidence of 23 % in newly diagnosed AML, with a lower incidence in children [130]. Although ITD length has previously been thought not to influence prognosis, some longer ITDs, which integrate within the first tyrosine kinase domain of the receptor, are associated with lower complete remission (CR) rate and poor relapse-free survival [131]. *FLT3*-ITDs are accompanied by *NPM1* mutations in a significant proportion of CN-AML patients (see below) [58]. *FLT3*-ITDs are predominantly seen in CN-AML, being associated with proliferative disease with a high presenting white blood cell (WBC) count and poor prognosis in terms of significantly increased relapse rate and decreased survival in both adults and children [48, 132]. *FLT3*-ITD mutations at diagnosis are highly heterogeneous with respect to *FLT3*-ITD allelic ratio, ITD length, and cooperating partner mutations. Patients with a high "ITD mutant-to-wild-type *FLT3* allelic ratio," sometimes due to mitotic recombination leading to partial uniparental disomy, have an especially poor prognosis and usually relapse within 12 months of initial treatment [57]. Relapsed *FLT3*-ITD-mutated AML carries a particularly dismal prognosis; blasts in this setting are highly dependent on FLT3 kinase signaling, carrying a particularly high *FLT3*-mutant allelic burden with the wild-type *FLT3* allele often virtually absent [133].

A further 7–10 % of AML patients have mutations involving the activation loop within the tyrosine kinase domain of the FLT3 receptor (*FLT3*-TKDs), usually single base substitutions (most frequently D835Y) or small deletions. Although similarly FLT3 activating and associated with high presenting WBC levels, prognostic implications of *FLT3*-TKDs are less clear; patient series describe conflicting adverse, intermediate, and even favorable prognostic associations [51, 56, 134]. In contrast to *FLT3*-ITD mutations, *FLT3*-TKD mutations appear to frequently be "late genetic hits," are often lost at relapse, and have subtly different effects than ITDs on FLT3 downstream signaling [135].

Whether or not allogeneic stem cell transplantation (SCT) in first CR improves outcomes in *FLT3*-ITD AML patients remains controversial [136], although the presence of the mutation in the context of wild-type *NPM1* is considered an indication for SCT in the consensus document by the European LeukemiaNet [137]. The high incidence and clear

Table 40.3 Genes and their recurrent mutations in AML, with associated clinical characteristics and outcomes

Gene symbola/chromosome location	Gene name	Overall mutation frequency	Mutation frequency in CN-AML	Mutation frequency in other cytogenetic subsets	Associations of mutations with clinical and molecular characteristics	Clinical significance of the presence of mutations
FLT3 (*CD135*, *STK1*, *FLK2*)/13q12	Fms-related tyrosine kinase 3	*FLT3*-ITD: 21–30 % [48–50]	*FLT3*-ITD: 28–39 % [51–54]	*FLT3*-ITD: t(15;17): 30–37 % [48, 53, 54] t(8;21): 5–15 % [51, 53, 54] inv(16): 0–7 % [51, 53, 54] t(6;9): 90 % [54] inv(3)/t(3;3): 9 % [54] t(11;v)(q23;v): 3 % [51, 53] +8: 7–23 % [51] del(7q): 4 % [51] −5/del(5q): 3 % [54] CK: 2–3 % [51, 53, 54]	*FLT3*-ITD is associated with high WBC and high % of blood and BM blasts [48, 54, 57]	Pts with *FLT3*-ITD have worse DFS, EFS, and OS than those with no *FLT3*-ITD, but *FLT3*-ITD does not impact significantly on the CR achievement probability [53, 54] Outcome is particularly poor for pts with high *FLT3*-ITD mutant-to-FLT3-WT allelic ratio [54, 57, 58]
		FLT3-TKD: 5–11 % [49–51]	*FLT3*-TKD: 5–14 % [52, 54, 55] <60 years 9 % [56] 12 % [51]	*FLT3*-TKD: t(15;17): 8–9 % [54, 55] t(8;21): 2–7 % [51, 54, 55] inv(16): 14–24 % [51, 54] t(11;v)(q23;v): 6–7 % [51, 55] +8: 7–12 % [51, 54] del(5q): 9 % [51] −7: 5 % [51] del(7q): 9 % [51] −7/del(7q): 2–5 % [54, 55] CK: 1–4 % [51, 54, 55]	*FLT3*-TKD is associated with high WBC, % of blood, and BM blasts; rare in secondary AML [51, 56]	The prognostic significance of *FLT3*-TKD differs among studies [51, 55, 56]
CEBPA/19q13.1	CCAAT/enhancer-binding protein (C/EBP) alpha	7.5–9 % overall [49, 59] 3 % single mutations [59] 4 % double mutations [59]	13–18 % overall [52, 60, 61] 6–8 % double mutations [59, 60] 4–5 % single mutations [59, 60]	MRC favorable – 0 % mutation [59] MRC intermediate – 3 % single mutations – 5 % double mutations [59] MRC adverse – 3 % single mutations – 0 double mutations [59]	*CEBPA* double mutations are associated with younger age, FAB M1 and M2 BM morphology, low frequency of *FLT3*-ITD, and virtual absence of *NPM1* mutations [59, 62]	Among all AML pts, double *CEBPA* mutations are associated with better OS and RFS than those of pts with single *CEBPA* mutations and *CEBPA*-WT. On MVA, double *CEBPA* mutations have been an independent favorable prognostic factor for OS, RFS, and CIR. Double *CEBPA* mutations bestow longer OS also among pts in the MRC intermediate cytogenetic-risk group [59] In CN-AML pts, OS of pts with double *CEBPA* mutations was longer than OS of *CEBPA*-WT and single *CEBPA*-mutated pts. On MVA, double *CEBPA* mutations were an independent favorable factor for OS [62] In younger (<60 years) CN-AML pts, both single and double *CEBPA* mutations conferred longer OS than OS of *CEBPA*-WT pts, but only double *CEBPA* mutations retained favorable prognostic significance in MVA for OS, EFS, and RFS [60]

(continued)

Table 40.3 (continued)

Gene symbola/chromosome location	Gene name	Overall mutation frequency	Mutation frequency in CN-AML	Mutation frequency in other cytogenetic subsets	Associations of mutations with clinical and molecular characteristics	Clinical significance of the presence of mutations
NPM1 (*NPM*, *B23*)/5q35.1	Nucleophosmin (nucleolar phospho-protein B23, numatrin)	29–35 % [49, 63]	46–62 % [52, 63–65]	t(15;17): 0 % [66, 67] t(8;21): 0–3.5 % [66, 67] inv(16): 0–3 % [66, 67] +8: 10–21 % [66, 67] −7/del(7q): 0–4 % [66, 67] −5/del(5q): 3 % [67] t(11;v)(q23;v): 6 % [66] CK: 0–2 % [66, 67]	*NPM1* mutations are more frequent in women, associated with higher WBC, % of BM blasts and platelet counts; low or absent CD34 and high CD33 expression on blasts. *NPM1* mutated pts twice as often have *FLT3*-ITD and *FLT3*-TKD than *NPM1*-WT pts. *NPM1* mutations almost never coexist with double *CEBPA* mutations, *MLL*-PTD, R172 *IDH2*, and *BCOR* mutations [63–67]	In younger adults (<60 years), *NPM1* mutations confer superior CR rates, EFS, DFS, and OS in the absence of *FLT3*-ITD [52, 64–67] In older pts (≥60 years), *NPM1* mutations alone are an independent favorable prognostic factor [68]
IDH1/2q32-qter	Isocitrate dehydrogenase 1 (NADP+), soluble	7–10 % [49, 69, 70],	13–16 % [69–71],	CBF AML: 1.5 % [70] t(15;17): 1 % [69]	Among all AML pts, *IDH1* mutations are associated with higher platelet counts, higher % of BM blasts [69], FAB M1 BM morphology [70], and CN-AML [69, 70] In CN-AML, *IDH1* mutations are associated with higher platelet counts, lower frequency of *FLT3*-ITD [71] and *NPM1* mutations [70]	In CN-AML overall, *IDH1* mutations are not associated with outcome [70, 71] In CN-AML pts with *NPM1* mutations and no *FLT3*-ITD, *IDH1* mutations are associated with a higher relapse risk, shorter OS [70] and DFS [71]

IDH2/15q21-qter	Isocitrate dehydrogenase 2 (NADP+), mitochondrial	3–10 % [49, 69, 70, 72],	11–19 % [69, 71],	t(8;21): 0 % [69, 70] inv(16): 0 % [69, 70]	Among all AML pts, *IDH2* mutations are associated with older age, MRC cytogenetic intermediate-risk group and *NPM1* mutations [72]. Pts with *IDH2* mutations involving residue R172 have lower WBC and an abnormal, MRC intermediate-risk karyotype more often than pts with *IDH2* mutations involving R140, most of whom have CN-AML In CN-AML, *IDH2* mutations are associated with older age and higher platelet counts [69, 71] *IDH2* mutations involving R140 are associated with FAB M1 BM morphology [73] *IDH2* mutations involving R172 do not or very rarely occur together with *FLT3*-ITD, *FLT3*-TKD, *MLL*-PTD, or *NPM1*, *WT1*, and *CEBPA* mutations [70–72]	Among all AML pts, *IDH2* mutations involving R172 are associated with low CR rates and increased CIR *IDH2* mutations involving R140 constitute an independent favorable prognostic factor for relapse risk and OS [72] In CN-AML, *IDH2* mutations involving R172 are associated with lower CR rates [70, 71], increased relapse risk, and shorter OS [70]. *IDH2* mutations involving R140 are not associated with outcome [71]
TET2 (*FLJ*20032)/4q24	Tet methylcytosine dioxygenase 2	8–27 % overall [49, 74–76] 7 % in younger pts (≤60 years) [74] 24 % in older pts (>60 years) [74]	18–30 % overall [74, 76, 77] 15 % in younger pts (<60 years) [77] 29 % in older pts (≥60 years) [77]	+8: 35 % [74]	*TET2* mutations are associated with older age, higher WBC, lower platelet counts, and absence of *IDH1* and *IDH2* mutations [74–77]	*TET2* mutations have no impact on outcome of all AML pts [75] In CN-AML, *TET2* mutations are associated with lower CR rates and shorter DFS, OS, and EFS in the ELN Favorable Genetic Group [76, 77]

(continued)

Table 40.3 (continued)

Gene symbola/chromosome location	Gene name	Overall mutation frequency	Mutation frequency in CN-AML	Mutation frequency in other cytogenetic subsets	Associations of mutations with clinical and molecular characteristics	Clinical significance of the presence of mutations
DNMT3A/2p23	DNA (cytosine-5-)-methyltransferase 3 alpha	23 % [49, 78] 18 % in younger pts (<60 years) [79]	34 % overall [80] 27–35 % in younger pts (<60 years) [79–81] 33 % in older pts (≥60 years) [80]	CBF AML: 1 % [79]	Among all AML pts, *DNMT3A* mutations are associated with older age, higher WBC, % of BM blasts and platelet counts, CN-AML, *FLT3*-ITD, *NPM1*, and *IDH1* mutations, and higher *MLL5* expression [79] In CN-AML, *DNMT3A* mutations are associated with higher WBC and % of BM blasts and are found more often in pts with *NPM1* mutations, *FLT3*-ITD and *CEBPA*-WT [80]	In all AML pts, *DNMT3A* mutations independently predict a shorter OS, but are not associated with RFS or CR rate [79] *DNMT3A* mutations are associated with shorter OS and RFS in all pts and an intermediate cytogenetic-risk subset without *FLT3*-ITD and *NPM1* mutations [78] In CN-AML overall, *DNMT3A* mutations are associated with shorter DFS (but not OS [80]), with lower CR rates and shorter OS on MVA [79] and shorter EFS and OS, which remain significant on MVA [81] In CN-AML pts <60 years, non-R882-*DNMT3A* mutations confer shorter DFS and OS [80] In CN-AML pts ≥60 years, R882-*DNMT3A* mutations are associated with shorter DFS and OS [80]
ASXL1 (*KIAA0978*)/20q11	Additional sex combs like transcriptional regulator 1	3–19 % [49, 82–84]	5–10 % overall [82, 83] 3 % in younger pts (<60 years) [85] 16 % in older pts (≥60 years) [85]	t(15;17): 0–5 % [82, 83] t(8;21): 8–20 % [82, 83] inv(16): 0 % [82, 83] sole +8: 32 % [82]	*ASXL1* mutations are more frequent in men [82, 85], relatively rare in younger adults (<60 years) Among all pts, *ASXL1* mutations are associated with lower WBC [83], FAB M1 BM morphology, expression of HLA-DR and CD34 [82] and very rarely coexist with *NPM1* mutations and *FLT3*-ITD [83, 84] In CN-AML pts, *ASXL1* mutations are associated with lower WBC, % of BM and blood blasts, *CEBPA* mutations and low incidence of *NPM1* mutations and *FLT3*-ITD [85]	In all AML pts, *ASXL1* mutations confer lower CR rates and worse OS in univariable analyses and worse OS in MVA [83] In CN-AML pts ≥60 years, *ASXL1* mutations confer lower CR rates and worse DFS, OS, and EFS [85]

BCOR (*FLJ*20285, *KIAA*1575)/Xp11.4	BCL6 corepressor	2.5 % [86]	4 % [86]	None found among 131 pts with abnormal karyotypes [86]	In CN-AML, *BCOR* mutations very rarely coexist with *NPM1* mutations and *FLT3*-ITD; ~45 % of *BCOR*-mutated pts harbor *DNMT3A* and *RUNX1* mutations [86]	In CN-AML, *BCOR* mutations are associated with a shorter OS and EFS [86]
BCORL1 (*FLJ*11362)/Xq25-q26.1	BCL6 corepressor-like 1	6 % [87]	2 % [87]	NA	*BCORL1* mutations have not been detected together with *TP53*, *CEBPA*, or *NPM1* mutations [87]	Prognostic significance is not yet established
PHF6/Xq26	PHD finger protein 6	2–3 % [49, 88, 89],	NA	NA	*PHF6* mutations are seven times more common in men than women; associated with FAB M0, M1, and M2 BM morphology, detected mostly in pts with CN-AML and +8 [88]	Prognostic significance is not yet established
MLL (*ALL-1, CXXC7, HRX, HTRX1, TRX1, MLL1A, KMT2A*)/11q23	Myeloid/ lymphoid or mixed-lineage leukemia (trithorax homologue, *Drosophila*)	5–7 % [49, 50]	5–11 % [52, 90–92]	sole +11: 91 % [93]	In younger (<60 years) CN-AML pts, *MLL*-PTD is associated with lower WBC and less extramedullary involvement and negatively associated with *NPM1* mutations [52, 94] and mutually exclusive with *CEBPA* mutations [52] In older (≥60 years) CN-AML pts, *MLL*-PTD is associated with lower hemoglobin and incidence of *NPM1* mutations and absence of *CEBPA* and R172 *IDH2* mutations [95]	In earlier studies on CN-AML, *MLL*-PTD were associated with shorter CRD (but not CR rates or OS) [90–92] No prognostic significance was found in intensively treated younger (<60 years) [94] and older (≥60 years) CN-AML pts [95]

(continued)

Table 40.3 (continued)

Gene symbola/chromosome location	Gene name	Overall mutation frequency	Mutation frequency in CN-AML	Mutation frequency in other cytogenetic subsets	Associations of mutations with clinical and molecular characteristics	Clinical significance of the presence of mutations
RUNX1 (*AML1, CBFA2, AMLCR1, PEBP2A2*)/21q22.3	Runt-related transcription factor 1	5 % [49] 6 % in younger pts (<60 years) [96]	13–26 % overall [97, 98] 6–8 % in younger pts (<60 years) [96, 98] 16 % in older pts (≥60 years) [98]	t(15;17): 0 % [96] t(8;21): 0 % [96] inv(16): 0 % [96] +13: 90 % [97] +8: 30 % [97] +11: 31 % [97] +21: 36 % [97] −7/del(7q): 29 % [97]	Among all pts, *RUNX1* mutations are associated with FAB M0 and M2 BM morphology, *MLL*-PTD and *IDH1–IDH2* mutations and wild-type *NPM1* and *CEBPA* [96] In CN-AML, *RUNX1* mutations are associated with older age, lower hemoglobin, WBC and % blood blasts, *ASXL1* mutations, and wild-type *NPM1* and *CEBPA* [98]	Among all pts, *RUNX1* mutations associated with resistant disease and worse RFS, OS, and EFS [96, 97] In CN-AML, *RUNX1*-mutated pts had lower CR rates and worse DFS, OS, and EFS than wild-type *RUNX1* pts [97, 98]
KIT (*PBT, C-Kit, CD117, SCFR*)/4q11-q12	v-kit Hardy-Zucker-man 4 feline sarcoma viral oncogene homologue	6 % [49] 2 % (only *KIT* D816 mutations) [50]		t(8;21): 12–47 % [99–102] inv(16): 22–47 % [99, 101–103]		In t(8;21) pts, *KIT* mutations associated with inferior OS, EFS, RFS, RI, and CIR [99–102] In inv(16) pts, *KIT* mutations associated with worse RI, higher CIR, and shorter OS [102, 103]
TP53 (*p53, LFS1*)/17p13.1	Tumor protein p53	2–14 % [49, 104]	1 % [104]	CK-*TP53* mutation: 60–69 % [104, 105] CK-*TP53* mutation/loss: 70–78 % [104, 105] t(8;21): 7 % [104] t(15;17): 0 % [104] inv(16): 0 % [104] t(11;v)(q23;v) : 0 % [104] +13 sole: 10 % [104] +8 sole: 7 % [104] −7 sole: 0 % [104]	*TP53* mutation and loss are associated with older age and larger number of chromosome aberrations in CK pts [105]	*TP53* mutations and loss confer lower CR rates and worse EFS, RFS, and OS in pts with a complex karyotype [105]

WT1 (*GUD, AWT1, WAGR, WIT-2*)/11p13	Wilms tumor 1	5–8 % [49, 106]	8–10 % [106, 107] 11–13 % in younger pts (<60 years) [108, 109] 7 % in older pts (≥60 years) [110]		Among all AML pts, *WT1* mutations found in younger pts and those with *FLT3*-ITD [106] In CN-AML pts, *WT1* mutations are almost twice as common in younger (<60 years) than in older (≥60 years) pts, associated with higher WBC and % of blood blasts and lower hemoglobin [109, 110]. Mutually exclusive of *TET2* and *IDH1/2* mutations [233, 234]	In CN-AML pts, *WT1* mutations confer: worse DFS and OS (but not CR probability) [109] worse CR probability, CIR, DFS, and OS [106, 107] no impact on RFS or OS [108] CN-AML pts with *WT1* mutations and *FLT3*-ITD have lower CR rates and worse RFS and OS than pts with *WT1* mutations without *FLT3*-ITD [108]
NRAS (*N-ras*)/1p13.2	Neuroblastoma RAS viral (v-ras) oncogene homologue	10–11 % [49, 50, 112],	9–14 % [52, 113]	inv(16): 18–38 % [112, 113] t(8;21): 6–10 % [112, 113] t(15;17): 2–5 % [112, 113] inv(3): 18–27 % [112, 113] t(3;5): 63 % [112] t(11;v)(q23;v): 4–20 % [112, 113] +8: 17 % [112] −7/del(7q): 8 % [112] CK: 2–4 % [112, 113]	No significant associations, except for lower WBC in one study [113]	No significant impact on outcome [112, 113] *RAS* mutations reported to increase sensitivity of AML blasts to higher doses of cytarabine [114]
KRAS (*KRAS1, KRAS2*)/12p12.1	v-Ki-ras2 Kirsten rat sarcoma viral oncogene homologue	2–5 % [49, 112]	4 % [112]	inv(16): 17 % [112] t(8;21): 5 % [112] t(15;17): 4 % [112] inv(3): 10 % [112] t(3;5): 0 % [112] t(11;v)(q23;v): 6 % [112] +8: 3 % [112] −7/del(7q): 7 % [112] CK: 3 % [112]	No significant associations [112]	No significant impact on outcome [112]

(continued)

Table 40.3 (continued)

Gene symbola/chromosome location	Gene name	Overall mutation frequency	Mutation frequency in CN-AML	Mutation frequency in other cytogenetic subsets	Associations of mutations with clinical and molecular characteristics	Clinical significance of the presence of mutations
CBL (*CBL2*, *c-Cbl*, *RNF55*)/11q23.3-qter	Cbl proto-oncogene, E3 ubiquitin protein ligase	1–4 % [76, 115, 116]	0 % [115]	inv(16): 5 % [115] t(8;21): 5 % [115] abn(11q): 15 % [115]	Mutations are detected mainly in pts with inv(16), t(8;21), and abn(11q) [115]	Prognostic significance is not yet established
Genes of the cohesion complex: *STAG1* (SA-1, SCC3A)/3q22.2-q22.3 *STAG2* (*SA*, *SCC3B*)/Xq25 *SMC3* (*CSPG6*, *BAM*, *HCAP*, *SMC3L1*)/10q25 *RAD21* (*hHR21*, *KIAA0078*, *SCC1*)/8q24.11 *SMC1A* (*SMC1*, *SMC1L1*, *DXS423E*, *KIAA0178*, *SB1.8*, *Smcb*)/Xp11.22-p11.21	 Stromal antigen 1 Stromal antigen 2 Structural maintenance of chromosomes 3 RAD21 homologue (*S. pombe*) Structural maintenance of chromosomes 1A	6–13 % [117–119] 0–1.8 % [118] 1.3–6.4 % [117–119] 0.6–3.5 % [117–119] 1.0–4.5 % [117–119] 0.5–3.5 % [117–119]	8 % [118]	t(15;17): 0 % [119]	Cohesin complex mutations occur mainly in pts with intermediate-risk cytogenetics, mostly CN-AML, and are strongly correlated with lower expression of *BAALC* [118] and the presence of mutations in *NPM1* [117, 118], *DNMT3A* [117], *FLT3* [117], and genes encoding protein tyrosine phosphatases [117]	No significant impact on CR rates, RFS or OS in all AML pts, nor in all CN-AML pts, CN-AML pts with mutated *NPM1*, or CN-AML pts with mutated *NPM1* and wild-type *FLT3* [118]
Spliceosomal genes *SF3B1* (*Hsh155*, *Prp10*, *PRPF10*, *SAP155*, *SF3b155*)/2q33.1 *SRSF2* (*SFRS2*, *PR264*, *SC-35*, *SC35*, *SFRS2A*)/17q25.2 *U2AF1* (*U2AFBP*, *RN*, *RNU2AF1*, *U2AF35*)/21q22.3	Splicing factor 3b, subunit 1, 155 kDa Serine/arginine-rich splicing factor 2 U2 small nuclear RNA auxiliary factor 1	8–14 % [117, 120] 6 % in adult de novo AML [121] 0 % in pediatric AML [121] 28 % in AML evolved from MPN [122] 41 % in AML with 20–30 % BM blasts [120]		+13: 88 % [123]	*SF3B1*, *U2AF1*, and *SRSF2* mutations are associated with older age, lower WBC and % BM blasts, and higher % erythroblasts [120] Spliceosome mutations occur significantly more often in the presence of mutations in genes encoding serine/threonine kinases [117]	*SRSF2* mutations conferred worse OS in AML evolved from MPN [122]

GATA2 (*NFE1B*)/3q21	GATA binding protein 2	10–14 % [124, 125]	8.1–9.4 % [125, 126]		In CN-AML pts, mutations in *GATA2* are found in 39 % of pts with double *CEBPA* mutations, but in no pts with monoallelic *CEBPA* mutations or *CEBPA*-WT [126] In intermediate-risk AML, *GATA2* mutations are detected in 18–27 % [124, 125] of pts with double *CEBPA* mutations, in 0–16 % of pts with single *CEBPA* mutations [124, 125] and in 0–3 % of pts *CEBPA*-WT [124, 125]	Among pts with double *CEBPA* mutations, *GATA2* mutations had no significant impact on EFS or OS of CN-AML pts [126] and on EFS or OS of intermediate-risk AML pts [124] Among intermediate-risk AML pts with double *CEBPA* mutations and no *FLT3*-ITD, *GATA2* mutations had no significant impact on CIR and OS [125]

BM bone marrow, *CBF AML* core-binding factor AML with t(8;21) or inv(16)/t(16;16), *CIR* cumulative incidence of relapse, *CK* complex karyotype, *CN-AML* cytogenetically normal acute myeloid leukemia, *CR* complete remission, *CRD* CR duration, *DFS* disease-free survival, *EFS* event-free survival, *ELN* European Leukemia Net, *FLT3-ITD* internal tandem duplication of the *FLT3* gene, *FLT3–TKD* activating tyrosine kinase domain mutations of the *FLT3* gene, *MLL-PTD* partial tandem duplication of the *MLL* gene, *MPN* myeloproliferative neoplasms, *MRC* UK Medical Research Council, *MVA* multivariable analysis, *NA* not available, *OS* overall survival, *pts* patients, *RFS* relapse-free survival, *RI* relapse incidence, *WBC* white blood cell count, *WT* wild-type alleles

[a]In bold type, gene symbol approved by Human Genome Organization (HUGO), followed by previous gene symbols and aliases (in parentheses, non-bold type), and the gene's chromosome location

deleterious prognostic impact of *FLT3*-ITD mutations, however, coupled with the tangible clinical gains achieved through targeting dysregulated tyrosine kinase activity in other malignancies, such as chronic myeloid leukemia (CML) and breast cancer, have provided a strong rationale for the development of FLT3-targeted therapy in AML. Several multi-kinase inhibitors with FLT3-inhibitory activity, the most developed of which being midostaurin (PKC412), lestaurtinib (CEP701), and sorafenib, have been assessed in combination with chemotherapy in international phase III clinical trials, with results currently awaited. Newer and more potent FLT3-inhibitory molecules, most notably quizartinib (AC220) and ASP2215, are in earlier stages of clinical development [138].

Other molecular abnormalities that have been consistently shown to confer a poorer prognosis include mutations in the *RUNX1* gene [96–98, 139] and partial tandem duplications of the *MLL* gene (*MLL*-PTD) [52, 90–92], although recent data indicate that intensive consolidation therapy that includes autologous transplant in first CR may improve the outcome of CN-AML patients with the latter rearrangement [94].

CEBPA and *NPM1*

Major steps forward in understanding the molecular pathogenesis of AML were the discoveries of mutations in the genes encoding CCAAT/enhancer-binding protein-α (*CEBPA*) and nucleophosmin (*NPM1*) that serve to identify subsets of patients with relatively favorable prognosis [63, 140] and which were recognized as provisional disease entities in the 2008 WHO classification [1]. Mutations in *CEBPA*, which encodes a myeloid transcription factor, were first described in 2001 and occur in approximately 10 % of cytogenically normal AML (CN-AML) [141]. Mutations cluster in both the amino- and carboxy-terminal regions, with the former leading to expression of a truncated 30 kDa isoform of CEBPA (p30) and loss of the 42 kDa full-length protein (p42) [142]. Carboxy-terminal mutations affect regions involved in mediating dimerization and DNA binding. Interestingly, in the majority of patients with *CEBPA* mutations, both alleles are involved, combining an upstream mutation in one allele with a downstream mutation in the other [141, 142]. The analysis of patient samples has shown that *CEBPA* mutations can be inherited, with progression to AML in later life being associated with acquisition of additional mutations, which can include involvement of the other *CEBPA* allele [143, 144]. Significant insights into the biology of *CEBPA* mutations have been provided by murine models, which have shown how loss of p42 expression (mimicking biallelic N-terminal *CEBPA* mutations), or compound heterozygous mutations affecting amino- and carboxy-terminal regions in combination, affects hematopoiesis and gives rise to AML [145, 146]. While early studies reported that *CEBPA* mutation predicts a relatively favorable outcome in AML [52, 147–149], subsequent studies have shown that the more favorable prognosis is seen in the subset of patients with biallelic mutations, especially those who lack *FLT3*-ITD [59, 60, 150–152].

Mutations in *NPM1*, discovered by Brunangelo Falini and colleagues in 2005 [63], represent the most common molecular lesion identified in AML to date, occurring in a third of cases, including 50–60 % of those with CN-AML. Over 30 different mutations have been described, which involve the C-terminal region of the protein. These lead to loss of tryptophan residues and generation of a nuclear export signal resulting in delocalization of nucleophosmin from the nucleoli to the cytoplasm [153]. *NPM1* mutation is considered, an AML-defining lesion, being stable in the vast majority of cases over the disease course [154, 155]. Indeed, *NPM1* mutation has been shown to enhance self-renewal of hematopoietic progenitors, associated with expanded myelopoiesis leading to the development of AML in a murine model [156]. Patients with AML harboring an *NPM1* mutation in the absence of a *FLT3*-ITD have a relatively favorable prognosis [64–66]. *NPM1* mutations also have been shown to be strong, independent predictors of better outcome in older patients, especially those aged 70 years and older [68]. Whereas most studies have focused on CN-AML [157], patients with AML with cytogenetic abnormalities that would be considered to have a standard risk but who harbor an *NPM1* mutation also have a better outcome in the absence of *FLT3*-ITD; however, those with *FLT3*-ITD in the absence of the protective effect of an *NPM1* mutation have a very poor prognosis [43, 158]. Whether the combined *FLT3*-ITD/*NPM1*-mutated genotype is itself associated with an intermediate or adverse outcome remains open to debate.

Mutations Identified in Epigenetic Modifiers

Using a variety of high-throughput technologies, recurring mutations that affect regulation of gene expression, directly or through more indirect mechanisms, have been identified in recent years. In a landmark study, genome sequencing was undertaken to identify the presence of biologically relevant mutations in a case of *NPM1*-mutated CN-AML [159]. A mutation was identified in codon 132 of isocitrate dehydrogenase 1 (*IDH1*), which was already known to be involved in the pathogenesis of gliomas, with *IDH1* mutations predicting a relatively favorable prognosis in this group of solid tumors [160]. In the cytoplasm, IDH1 catalyzes the conversion of isocitrate to α-ketoglutarate, generating NADPH. The *IDH1* mutation that affects the arginine amino acid at codon 132 (R132) reduces α-ketoglutarate formation, but in addition alters enzyme function leading to generation of 2-hydroxyglutarate (2-HG), associated with increased reactive oxygen species (ROS) levels, HIF1α induction, and upregulation of VEGF [161, 162]. IDH1 mutations at R132 occur in approximately 7 % of AML, particularly in those with a normal karyotype and *NPM1* mutation (reviewed by

Löwenberg [163]). Based upon these findings, AMLs were screened for mutations in the mitochondrial homologue *IDH2*, which were identified in an additional 10 % of AML cases. The *IDH2* mutations cluster at codons R140 (8 %) and R172 (2 %) [69, 71, 163, 164]; these mutations are prognostically distinct, with the latter predicting a poor prognosis [71–73]. Interestingly, an inverse relationship has been observed between mutations occurring in the *IDH* genes and *TET2* [74–77, 165]. The latter was found to be a recurrent mutation target in a range of myeloid neoplasms including AML by array-based comparative genomic hybridization (aCGH) and single nucleotide polymorphism (SNP) profiling. TET2 has subsequently been shown to be involved in the regulation of hydroxylation of 5-methylcytosine, with disruption of TET2 leading to myeloid transformation in murine models [166, 167]. Methylation profiles of *IDH*- and *TET2*-mutated AMLs were found to be highly comparable, with evidence to suggest that accumulation of 2-HG secondary to *IDH* mutation inhibits TET2 function [165]. Moreover, it has recently been shown that TET2 binding to DNA is regulated by WT1, providing an explanation why WT1 mutations are also mutually exclusive of TET2 and IDH mutations [233, 234]. Consequently, this pathway is deregulated in a third of AML cases.

Studies examining the clinical significance of *TET2* mutations have yielded somewhat conflicting results. Gaidzik et al. [75] found no impact of *TET2* mutations on outcome of a cytogenetically heterogeneous patient population, and this was also true for the whole cohort of CN-AML patients analyzed by Metzeler et al. [77]. However, another study determined that *TET2* mutations confer worse outcome in AML patients with intermediate-risk cytogenetic findings (defined using the Southwest Oncology Group [SWOG] criteria) [74], and two studies demonstrated adverse impact of *TET2* mutations on the outcome of those CN-AML patients who are classified in the Favorable Genetic Group of the European LeukemiaNet (ELN) classification (i.e., CN-AML with mutated *CEBPA* and/or mutated *NPM1* without *FLT3*-ITD) [76, 77].

Re-sequencing of the index *NPM1*-mutated CN-AML case with *IDH1* mutation originally characterized by Mardis and colleagues [159] identified an additional acquired alteration in another gene involved in epigenetic regulation, namely, the DNA methyltransferase *DNMT3A* [168]. This gene was confirmed to be mutated in approximately 20 % of all AML patients and in approximately 30 % of those with a normal karyotype [79–81, 168–171]. Mutations in *DNMT3A* are associated with the presence of *NPM1* mutation and *FLT3*-ITD and are distributed throughout the gene, with a mutational hotspot at position R882. The presence of a *DNMT3A* mutation predicts a poorer outcome (Table 40.3).

High-throughput technologies have identified mutations in additional epigenetic modifiers in AML. These include *ASXL1* (*a*dditional *sex* combs *l*ike transcriptional regulator 1), which is involved in the regulation of histone methylation [82, 83, 85, 172], with mutations occurring 3–5 times more often in patients aged 60 years or older [83, 85] than in younger patients and being associated with the presence of *RUNX1* or *CEBPA* mutations, the absence of *NPM1* and *FLT3*-ITD mutations, and poorer clinical outcome [85]. Using exome sequencing, mutations in genes located on the X-chromosome encoding the related transcriptional repressors BCOR and BCORL1 have been identified [86, 87]. The former is a rare translocation target in APL [12]; is mutated in approximately 4 % of CN-AML, detected in cases with wild-type *NPM1*; and may also confer a poorer prognosis [86]. There are few data on *BCORL1* mutations, which were first identified in older adults with secondary AML and subsequently found to be mutated in 6 % of a cohort of unselected AML patients [87]. In addition, approximately 3 % of AML have mutations in the *PHF6* gene, which encodes a homeodomain protein and is frequently mutated in T-cell ALL [49, 88].

Indications for Testing

Thorough laboratory investigation of AML is fundamental to the optimal clinical management of the disease and is not only critical to establish the diagnosis but also to identify patients who may benefit from targeted therapies, to inform risk stratification and to guide post-remission therapy including the need for stem cell transplantation. Prognostic factors in AML can be subdivided into those defined at diagnosis (pretreatment) or following the start of antileukemic therapy (post-treatment) (Table 40.4). With the exception of age, patient performance status, and type of AML (de novo vs secondary), pretreatment determination of the likely outcome to therapy is dependent on laboratory investigation, with karyotype, *NPM1*, *CEBPA*, and *FLT3* mutation status being the most important factors identified to date. Predicting the likely outcome following initiation of therapy falls entirely within the realm of the laboratory and, for patients achieving morphological complete remission (CR), is dependent on the detection of minimal residual disease (MRD), for which flow cytometry and molecular diagnostic strategies have been developed.

Establishing a Diagnosis of AML

Morphological analysis of peripheral blood and BM smears stained with Wright Giemsa or May-Grünwald Giemsa is clearly the first step in establishing a diagnosis in patients with suspected leukemia. After confirmation that a patient has AML on the basis of morphology, cytochemistry, and immunophenotyping (for which standardized antibody panels have been published [173, 174]), cases may be classified further according to blast characteristics and degree of dif-

Table 40.4 Prognostic factors for relapse in patients with newly diagnosed AML

Pre-treatment predictors	
Major	**Other**
Age	Elevated WBC
Cytogenetics	Elevated LDH
Molecular:	Secondary disease[a]
FLT3-ITD	Dysplastic features[a]
NPM1 mutation	BCL2/BAX ratio
Biallelic *CEBPA* mutations	Resistance protein expression e.g., PGP[a]
	TP53 mutation[a]
	Autonomous growth of AML blasts in culture[a]
	Immunophenotype e.g. CD34 expression[a]
	Expression of chemotherapy metabolizing enzymes
	High expression of BAALC, MN1, MECOM, and ERG
	Mutations in WT1, DNMT3A, RUNX1, ASXL1
	MLL-PTD
	Absence of IDH2 mutation at R140
Post-treatment predictors	
Initial response (% BM blasts) MRD assessment	

BM bone marrow, *LDH* lactate dehydrogenase, *MRD* minimal residual disease, *PGP* P-glycoprotein, *WBC* presenting white blood cell count

[a] Many factors previously considered to confer adverse risk have been shown to be closely related to cytogenetic risk group

ferentiation in the BM. This initial workup may reveal features that are helpful in predicting the presence of particular cytogenetic and/or molecular subtypes of disease [e.g., APL with t(15;17)/*PML–RARA*, AML FAB-type M4Eo with inv(16)/t(16;16)/*CBFB–MYH11*], and may be especially valuable in situations in which the expected cytogenetic abnormality is lacking, yet the predicted fusion gene is formed as a result of a cryptic rearrangement, for example, an insertion event (Fig. 40.1), which may be detected by FISH or reverse transcription PCR (RT-PCR) [7, 175].

Rapid examination of the peripheral blood smear (and BM, once available) with immediate communication of results to the clinical team is essential for patients with a possible diagnosis of APL, which represents a medical emergency. A rapid and accurate diagnosis is critical for appropriate patient management, allowing ATRA and supportive care measures to be initiated promptly, to reduce the risk of induction death due to hemorrhage. Indeed, international disease guidelines recommend that ATRA therapy be initiated as soon as a diagnosis of APL is suspected and not delayed until the results of cytogenetic, FISH, or PCR analyses are available [176]. For the rapid diagnosis of APL, immunofluorescent methods using antibodies directed against the PML protein are of value, with the conversion from a normal pattern of 5–20 discrete dots to a microparticulate nuclear staining pattern (>30 microspeckles, Fig. 40.2) being indicative of expression of the PML-RARα fusion protein. Even if the diagnosis of APL is confirmed by the PML antibody test or other methods (i.e., cytogenetics, FISH), RT-PCR should still be performed on diagnostic samples to confirm the PML-RARα isoform type, which is important to define the most appropriate assay for subsequent monitoring for MRD [176].

Immunophenotyping is a valuable component of the routine workup of acute leukemia for a number of reasons, serving to (1) establish, confirm, and further refine a diagnosis of AML and (2) identify aberrant *l*eukemia-*a*ssociated *i*mmuno*p*henotypes (LAIPs), which can be used to monitor response to therapy. Although immunophenotypic studies are assuming a more important role in assessing remission status by informing risk-adapted treatment approaches in AML (reviewed by Freeman et al. [177]), they are not discussed in any great detail in this chapter, which is restricted to the role of molecular genetic analyses.

Role of Karyotype Assessment

Karyotype analysis is a mandatory component of the workup for all patients with AML, as emphasized in international ELN disease guidelines, by providing important diagnostic and prognostic information [173]. Apart from identifying patients with particular subtypes of AML who may benefit from molecularly targeted therapies [e.g., ATRA/ATO in t(15;17)/*PML–RARA*-associated APL and tyrosine kinase inhibitors for patients with t(9;22)(q34;q11.2)/*BCR–ABL1*-associated AML], karyotype analysis has been used to distinguish groups of patients with substantially different probabilities of achieving a remission and risks of relapse, particularly as a tool to guide SCT in first CR.

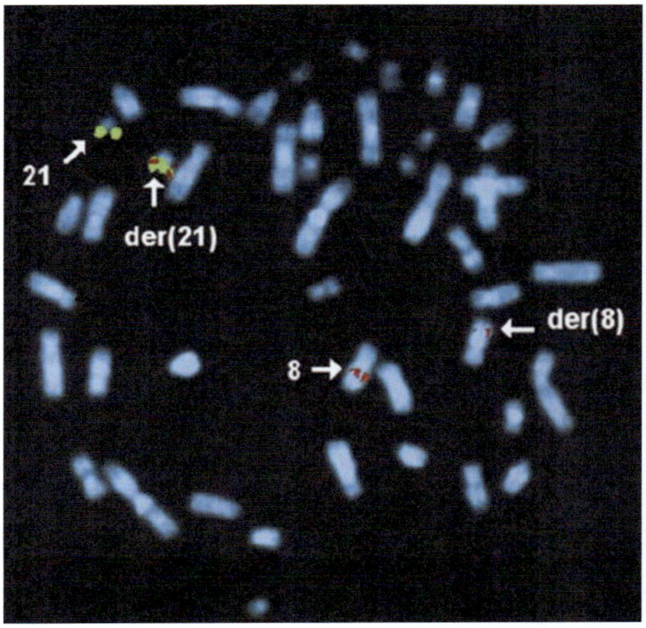

Figure 40.1 Characterization by FISH of AML with fusion gene formation due to cryptic rearrangements. Cryptic (8;21) rearrangement in an AML M2 case demonstrated by FISH with *RUNX1* (*green*) and *RUNX1T1* (*red*) probe set (Vysis, Downers Grove, IL). Fusion signals are seen on the derivative 21, and *RUNX1T1* signals are diminished on the derivative 8 (Figure prepared by Marina Lafage-Pochitaloff, Institut Paoli Calmettes, Marseille. From Grimwade D. The clinical significance of cytogenetic abnormalities in acute myeloid leukaemia. Baillieres Best Pract Res Clin Haematol. 2001;14:510. Reprinted with permission from Elsevier)

In multivariable analyses that take into account age, type of AML (de novo or secondary), and presenting WBC, the diagnostic karyotype emerges as the most significant prognostic factor and provides the framework for current risk-stratified treatment approaches applied in younger adults (reviewed by Grimwade and Hills [178]). Large multicenter studies have consistently reported that patients with APL with the t(15;17)(q22;q12~21) treated on ATRA- and anthracycline-based protocols, together with core-binding factor (CBF) AML with t(8;21)(q22;q22) or inv(16)(p13.1q22)/t(16;16)(p13.1;q22) treated with intensive chemotherapy involving high-dose cytarabine, are characterized by relatively favorable prognoses [176, 179, 180]. In this favorable risk group, relapse rates are too low and salvage rates too high for there to be any survival benefit for the routine application of allogeneic SCT in first remission [181–183]. Conversely, adults with adverse risk cytogenetics (Table 40.5) [43], including abnormalities of 3q [other than t(3;5)], del(5q), −5/−7, abnormalities of 17p, translocations involving 11q23 [apart from t(9;11)(p22;q23) and t(11;19)(q23;p13)], t(9;22)(q34;q11.2), and complex karyotype, have a very poor prognosis with conventional chemotherapy and therefore are considered candidates for SCT and experimental treatment approaches. The definition of a complex karyotype is inconsistent [178], with the WHO adopting a cutoff of three or more unrelated cytogenetic abnormalities [2]. However, subsequent large studies from the UK Medical Research Council (MRC) and Munich Leukemia Laboratory provide evidence that a threshold of four or more unrelated abnormalities is most prognostically relevant [43, 184]. Considering the outcome of cases of AML with more than one cytogenetic abnormality, in which the karyotype includes features that in their own right would confer favorable or adverse risk, respectively, has led to the definition of hierarchical risk groups, which are used to inform risk-stratified treatment approaches (Table 40.5).

Approximately half of the patients with adverse risk cytogenetic features have a so-called monosomal karyotype (MK+), as defined by the Dutch-Belgium Hemato-Oncology Cooperative (HOVON) group based on loss of an autosomal chromosome (i.e., excluding −Y and −X) in combination with at least one other autosomal monosomy (e.g., 44,XY,-7,-18) or one or more structural abnormality [e.g., 45,XY,inv(3)(q21q26.2),-7] [185]. Monosomal karyotypes almost invariably include at least one chromosomal abnormality that would independently be associated with adverse risk. Moreover, since up to 75 % of complex karyotypes are hypodiploid (i.e., have ≤45 chromosomes) and some pseudodiploid (46 chromosomes) and hyperdiploid complex karyotypes (≥47 chromosomes) also include at least one monosomy (Fig. 40.3) [186], the vast majority of patients with a complex karyotype are considered to have a monosomal karyotype. The MK+ cases have a particularly poor prognosis [43, 184, 187], which potentially could be improved by allogeneic SCT [188]. Although hitherto there has been little evidence that MK+ AML is biologically distinct from cases with other adverse risk cytogenetic abnormalities, a recent study has revealed that monosomal karyotype was more frequent among patients with a complex karyotype who also had *TP53* alterations (i.e., mutations and/or *TP53* gene losses) than among those who did not [105]. In multivariable analysis for overall survival (OS) of patients with a complex karyotype, *TP53* alterations constituted the most important prognostic factor, which outweighed other variables, including monosomal karyotype [105].

Prognostic Significance of Cytogenetics in Pediatric AML

Cytogenetics also comprises part of the routine workup for AML arising in children, although few large studies have considered its prognostic significance in the pediatric population. The Pediatric Oncology Group (POG) considered a cohort of 478 patients aged less than 21 years, reporting the best outcomes in those with inv(16), t(8;21) and normal karyotype [189]. Poorer outcome was reported in patients with 11q23 abnormalities and APL patients with t(15;17),

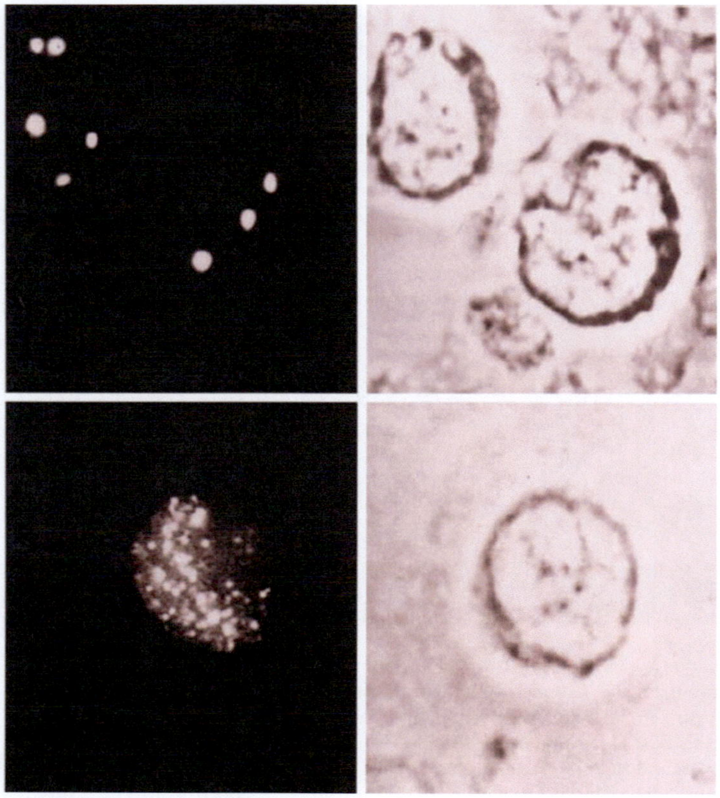

Figure 40.2 Rapid diagnosis of acute promyelocyte leukemia with the PML-RARα fusion by PML immunostaining. In leukemic blasts from cases of PML-RARα-negative AML and in normal cells, PML protein is localized within nuclear body structures (PML nuclear bodies). In such cells PML antisera detect a wild-type staining pattern comprising fewer than 30 (typically 5–20) discrete nuclear dots, e.g., a case of AML M1 (*upper left panel*). Whereas in APL cases with the PML-RARα fusion, PML nuclear bodies are disrupted, leading to a characteristic microspeckled/microparticulate nuclear staining pattern (>30 nuclear dots) with PML antisera, which detects PML-RARα and wild-type PML proteins (*lower left panel*). Nuclear integrity is confirmed by a nuclear stain or in this case by phase contrast microscopy (*right-hand panels*). These studies were performed with a PML polyclonal antibody, with FITC-conjugated secondary antibody

Table 40.5 Revised Medical Research Council AML cytogenetic classification applied in younger adults [43]

Risk group	Cytogenetic abnormality
Favorable	t(15;17)(q22;q12~q21) t(8;21)(q22;q22) inv(16)(p13.1q22)/t(16;16)(p13.1;q22)
Intermediate	Normal karyotype Cytogenetic abnormalities not classified as favorable or adverse
Adverse	In the absence of favorable risk cytogenetic abnormalities: abn(3q) [excluding t(3;5)(q21~25;q31~35)] inv(3)(q21q26.2)/t(3;3)(q21;q26.2) add(5q)/del(5q), −5 add(7q)/del(7q), −7 t(11q23) [excluding t(9;11)(p21~22;q23) and t(11;19)(q23;p13)] t(9;22)(q34;q11.2) −17/abn(17p) Complex karyotype (≥4 unrelated abnormalities other than favorable or adverse abnormalities)

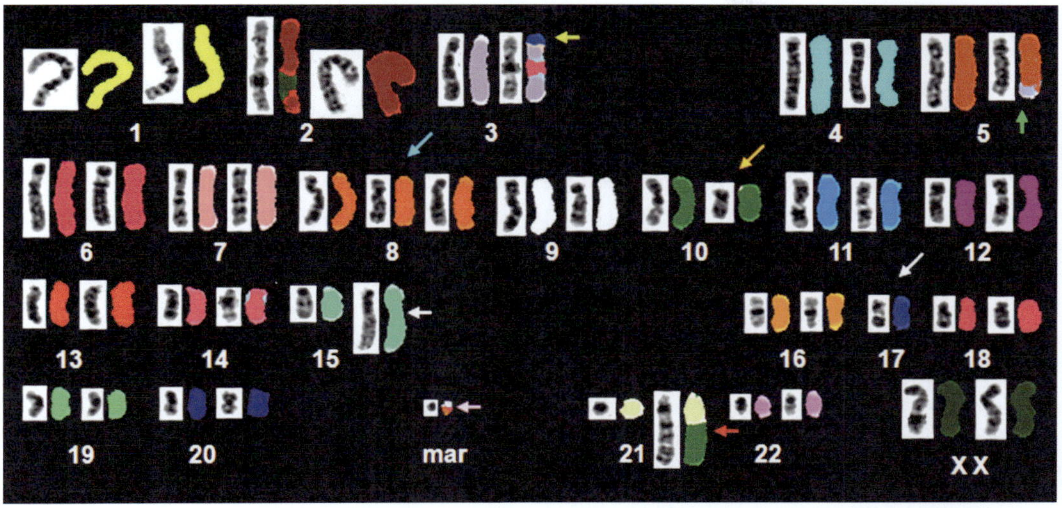

Figure 40.3 Complex karyotype containing eight chromosome abnormalities detected in a patient with AML, analyzed using spectral karyotyping (SKY). Each chromosome is represented twice, by G-banding-like inverted and contrast-enhanced 4′,6-diamidino-2-phenylindole (DAPI)-stained image on the left and SKY image shown in classification colors on the *right*. This karyotype contains several chromosome abnormalities relatively common in AML with a complex karyotype: an unbalanced translocation between chromosomes 3 and 17 leading to loss of material from 3p and chromosome 17 (*yellow arrow*), an unbalanced translocation between chromosomes 3 and 5 resulting in partial loss of 5q (*green arrow*), trisomy of chromosome 8 (*blue arrow*), loss of one copy of chromosome 17 (*gray arrow*), and a complex rearrangement between chromosomes 10 and 21 leading to gain of material from 21q (*red arrow*). Also present is a complex rearrangement of chromosome 15 resulting in amplification of 15q material (*white arrow*), abnormal chromosome 10 (*orange arrow*), and a small marker chromosome whose origin could not be established reliably by SKY technique (*pink arrow*). Had this case been analyzed using G-banding method only, the karyotype would have been classified as monosomal because chromosome 17 appeared to be lost entirely, with its part translocated to chromosome 3 not being recognizable without SKY. From Mrózek K. Cytogenetic, molecular genetic, and clinical characteristics of acute myeloid leukemia with a complex karyotype. Semin Oncol 2008;35(4):365–77. Reprinted with permission from Elsevier

with the caveat that most of the latter group did not receive ATRA. The findings of a more recent, similarly sized study (454 patients <18 years of age) published by the Berlin-Frankfurt-Münster (BFM) group were in accordance with most adult series, showing the best outcomes in patients with inv(16), t(8;21), and t(15;17) [190]. Significantly poorer outcomes were observed in patients with −7 and 11q23 aberrations [apart from t(9;11) as the sole abnormality and t(11;19)]. The largest study to date was conducted by the UK MRC group and considered the prognostic significance of 22 cytogenetically defined subgroups within a cohort of 729 children aged 0–15 years [191]. In this study, in which APL patients were excluded, the best outcomes were observed in CBF AML, with 10-year overall survival rates of approximately 80 %. In contrast to the POG and BFM studies, patients with 11q23 abnormalities ($n = 104$) had an intermediate prognosis (61 % OS at 10 years), with no evidence of heterogeneity according to the translocation partner. While this study did not analyze the prognostic significance of secondary aberrations accompanying 11q23 abnormalities, a recent large international effort identified trisomy 8 as an independent favorable prognostic factor and trisomy 19 as an adverse prognostic factor in pediatric 11q23/*MLL*-rearranged AML, whereas complex karyotype was found to be an unfavorable prognostic factor in univariable analysis only [192]. Interestingly, in the MRC series, some of the abnormalities that have been associated with adverse risk in adult patients, i.e., −5, 3q abnormalities, and complex karyotype, were not predictive of a worse outcome in children. However, significantly poorer survivals were observed in pediatric AML with 5q abnormalities, t(6;9), −7, trisomy 13, and 12p abnormalities, including translocations involving *ETV6*, with only 36 % of patients alive after 10 years [191].

Prognostic Significance of Cytogenetics in Older Adults with AML

The outcome of AML presenting in older adults is much poorer (7–15 % 5-year survival for adults >60 years), as compared to when the disease presents in younger individuals (with cure rates of 40–45 %). Nevertheless, cytogenetics is still prognostic in this age group and therefore recommended as part of the diagnostic workup. The largest study to date was conducted by the MRC group, studying 1,065 patients (aged >55 years) treated in the AML11 trial [193]. The best outcome was observed in APL patients with the t(15;17) and CBF AML patients, with a superior CR rate (72 %) associated with low rates of resistant disease, although favorable risk cytogenetics only accounted for 7 % of patients in this age group, as compared to 24 % of younger adults [193]. Overall survival rates were much poorer in the older age group than those observed in younger adults with the same cytogenetic abnormalities (only 34 % OS at 5 years vs >60 %). While the relapse rate in APL patients with the t(15;17) was low (26 % at 5 years), the relapse rates in the CBF AML patients were substantially higher (>80 % relapse risk at 5 years), as compared to 33 % in younger patients, which may reflect differences in disease biology as well being a consequence of less intensive therapy in older patients. Older patients with a complex karyotype (defined as five or more abnormalities) had an extremely poor prognosis, with relatively few achieving CR (26 %) due to high rates of resistant disease (56 %). The small proportion of elderly patients achieving remission almost invariably relapsed, leading to OS rates of only 2 % at 5 years [193]. Similar data have been published by other groups [194–196], raising the question as to whether elderly patients with high-risk cytogenetics might be most appropriately offered palliative non-intensive treatment approaches or supportive care. On the other hand, recent preliminary data indicate that at least some patients aged 60–70 years who achieve a CR may benefit from reduced-intensity allogeneic SCT [197]. Moreover, alternative, novel therapies are being investigated in older adults with AML [198]. In the MRC series, patients with normal karyotypes or noncomplex cytogenetic aberrations had marginally less poor outcomes, with 5-year survivals of 15 % and 10 %, respectively. The slightly better outcome in CN-AML occurring in older patients may reflect the influence of cases with *NPM1* gene mutation. Most recently, the Groupe Ouest -Est d'étude des Leucémies Aiguës et autres Maladies du Sang (GOELAMS) reported, in a study involving 186 older adults (>60 years) with unfavorable cytogenetic abnormalities, that the presence of a monosomal karyotype (found in 59 %) predicted a particularly poor prognosis [199].

Detection of Chromosomal Aberrations by Molecular Testing: Fluorescence In Situ Hybridization

Although karyotype assessment provides a valuable framework for design of risk-adapted treatment of AML, it has limitations as a means of determining the most suitable treatment approach for individual patients. Indeed, molecular analyses can serve to further refine the diagnosis of AML, reliably identify subgroups of patients that require a specific treatment approach (e.g., molecularly targeted therapies), and define targets for subsequent MRD assessment. Critical limitations of cytogenetic analysis include false-negative results due to sampling of residual normal BM elements and test failure in approximately 10 % of patients, with rates differing according to whether samples are analyzed in local or more remote laboratories, entailing substantial differences in transit time. In such cases, RT-PCR and/or FISH can be used to detect the presence of fusion genes corresponding to the favorable cytogenetic-risk group.

Even in AML with evaluable metaphases at diagnosis, patients may not necessarily be assigned to the most appropriate risk group on the basis of karyotype assessment alone due to cryptic rearrangements. Studies conducted by the European Working Party and UK MRC have established that almost 10 % of cases with morphologic APL and successful karyotype analysis actually lack the classical t(15;17) but nevertheless have an underlying *PML–RARA* fusion [7, 200]. This is most commonly the result of insertion events, in which chromosomes 15 and 17 are typically of normal appearance. Such cases share the beneficial response to targeted therapies, i.e., ATRA and ATO. This is supported by outcome data from the UK MRC ATRA trial, which showed that patients in whom *PML–RARA* was identified solely by molecular means had a comparable outcome to those with t(15;17) documented by karyotype [200]. This would suggest that cases of AML with cryptic rearrangement of *CBF* genes (i.e., with cryptic *RUNX1–RUNX1T1* or *CBFB–MYH11*) also are likely to be biologically equivalent to and share the favorable prognosis of those with karyotype-documented t(8;21) or inv(16)/t(16;16) [175]. This supports the adoption of routine molecular testing for *CBF* fusions in AML, which is most efficiently undertaken by RT-PCR. In CBF AML, testing for *KIT* mutations, which predict a poorer outcome, may be merited (reviewed by Döhner et al. [173]). Approximately 5 % of cases of CBF AML have a cryptic rearrangement and such cases cannot be reliably identified on the basis of distinct morphological features [175]. Where evidence of CBF AML is identified by RT-PCR testing in the absence of the typical cytogenetic lesion, the result should be independently confirmed using FISH to document fusion gene formation, for example, as a result of an insertion event (Fig. 40.1).

The most appropriate strategy for molecular screening for fusion genes depends upon the age group of the patient, with CBF AML representing a greater proportion of AML arising in children (approximately 17 %) and younger adults (approximately 12 %) than in the elderly, where they comprise less than 5 % of cases [193]. Molecular testing for CBF AML enables identification of additional patients informative for MRD assessment using a fusion gene marker, as well as distinguishing individuals who can potentially be spared an allogeneic SCT in first CR. Apart from undertaking molecular analysis for the *PML–RARA* fusion in cases with M3/M3v morphology, screening for this abnormality also is merited in patients presenting with severe coagulopathy (hemorrhage and/or thrombosis), an APL-like immunophenotype, or cases with cells suggestive of APL morphology even if occurring in a minor population.

In patients lacking molecular evidence of *PML–RARA*, CBF AML, or other favorable risk genotype (i.e., *NPM1*-mutated/*FLT3*-ITD-negative, biallelic *CEBPA* mutation), FISH may prove helpful in screening for chromosomal losses (e.g., −5/del(5q), −7/del(7q), −17/del(17p)) or complex patterns of losses and gains characteristic of the adverse cytogenetic group. In addition, RT-PCR and/or FISH can be used to diagnose rearrangements, which may distinguish subgroups of patients at different risk of relapse and identify targets for subsequent MRD testing. This includes the detection of cases with 11q23/*MLL* rearrangements, as well as those with the *BCR–ABL1* fusion, who could benefit from tyrosine kinase inhibitors. FISH and reverse transcription quantitative PCR (RT-qPCR) can be used to distinguish AML cases with cryptic 3q abnormalities associated with overexpression of *MECOM* (*EVI1*), which are characterized by very poor prognosis [201]. In addition, in children and younger adults, molecular analysis for the cytogenetically cryptic t(5;11)(q35;p15.5), which leads to the *NUP98–NSD1* fusion, may be clinically useful, occurring in approximately 4 % of pediatric AML, including 16 % of those with normal karyotype. These patients appear to have a poor prognosis, but may benefit from allogeneic SCT [202, 203].

Detection of Mutations Implicated in Leukemogenesis and/or Predictive of Outcome: An Integrated Approach to Molecular Testing in AML

Over the last two decades, increased understanding of the molecular basis of AML has resulted in marked improvements in the risk stratification of patients. In the late 1990s, the risk of relapse was defined largely in terms of pretreatment cytogenetics, with approximately 25 %, 60 %, and 15 % of younger adults falling within favorable, intermediate, and adverse risk groups, respectively. With refinement of cytogenetic classification and recognition of a wide spectrum of prognostically relevant molecular markers, the relative proportions of patients assigned to each group have markedly changed, with expansion of the favorable risk group to 45 % by inclusion of cases with the *NPM1*-mutated/*FLT3*-ITD-negative genotype and with biallelic *CEBPA* mutations (Fig. 40.4). As recognized by inclusion of these patients in the ELN genetic reporting system [173], this is important clinically, since the outcome of these molecularly defined subtypes of AML is comparable to that of CBF AML (Fig. 40.5). Hence, they represent a further group of patients who can be spared routine allogeneic SCT in first CR. Conversely, recent studies have led to better definition of patients with adverse risk cytogenetic and molecular genetic features, who now comprise over a third of AML arising in younger adults and in whom allogeneic SCT in first CR is the favored treatment approach, if feasible.

Taking into account the mutual exclusivity of *NPM1* mutations with balanced chromosomal rearrangements or biallelic *CEBPA* mutations, efficient algorithms for the diagnostic workup can be used to guide management of AML. However, it is anticipated that these algorithms will continue to evolve as more prognostically relevant biomarkers are identified and further targeted therapies become available that are specific to the various molecular subtypes of disease.

Rationale for Minimal Residual Disease Monitoring

Relapse remains a major cause of treatment failure for patients with AML. Since the group of patients destined to relapse cannot be reliably identified on the basis of pretreatment characteristics, MRD testing allows more accurate tailoring of therapy according to individual patient requirements. MRD assessment may prove useful in several clinical scenarios. Assessment of kinetics of response relatively early in the treatment course using RT-qPCR (e.g., detecting *WT1* transcripts) or flow cytometry provides independent prognostic information, distinguishing subgroups of patients with different risks of relapse, with an inverse relationship between decline in MRD and risk of subsequent disease recurrence (reviewed by Grimwade et al. [204]). While this remains to be formally tested, patients at low risk could potentially be spared excessive therapy with its inherent additional risk of treatment-related morbidity and mortality, including that related to subsequent development of secondary MDS or AML. Conversely, the outcome of patients at high risk of relapse could potentially be improved with the administration of additional consolidation therapy, possibly in the form of allogeneic SCT or more novel approaches. MRD assessment also may be of potential value in the management of patients undergoing allogeneic SCT, as a means of determining the most suitable type of transplant, as well as identifying the need for additional therapy in the posttransplant setting.

Various methods have been evaluated for the detection of MRD, including cytogenetics, FISH, immunophenotyping, and molecular approaches. Cytogenetics is too insensitive for MRD monitoring, although it may be of interest as a complement to morphological assessment to determine remission status following induction therapy [205–207]. Although FISH is applicable in at least half of AML cases, the number of nuclei or metaphases available for scoring limits its sensitivity, and interphase FISH is affected by the capacity to distinguish low levels of disease from background. Even with hypermetaphase FISH, which is extremely labor intensive, sensitivities achieved are inferior to immunophenotype or PCR-based methods, and hence, attention has been focused on these approaches.

The use of multiparameter flow cytometry to detect MRD takes advantage of differences between normal and leukemic BM, with the majority of AMLs characterized by an abnormal pattern of markers (designated LAIP) which distinguishes them from their normal counterparts. The technique is relatively sensitive (capable of detecting one leukemic cell

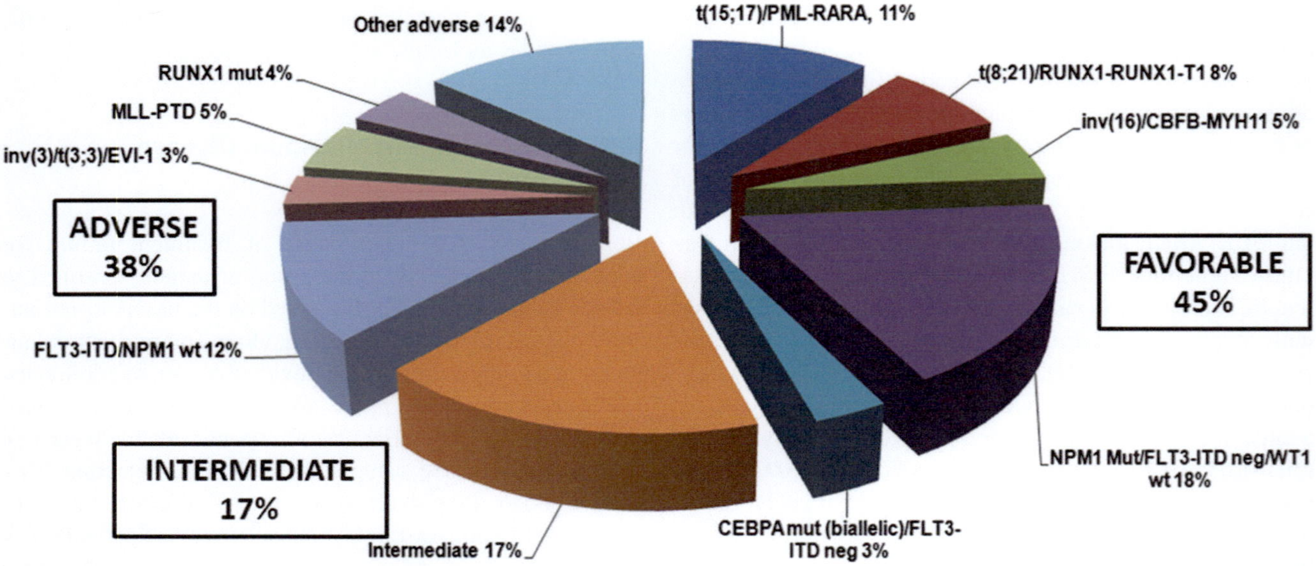

Figure 40.4 Integration of cytogenetic and molecular markers to refine risk groups in AML. From Smith ML, Hills RK, Grimwade D. Independent prognostic variables in acute myeloid leukaemia. Blood Rev 2011;25(1):39–51. Reprinted with permission from Elsevier

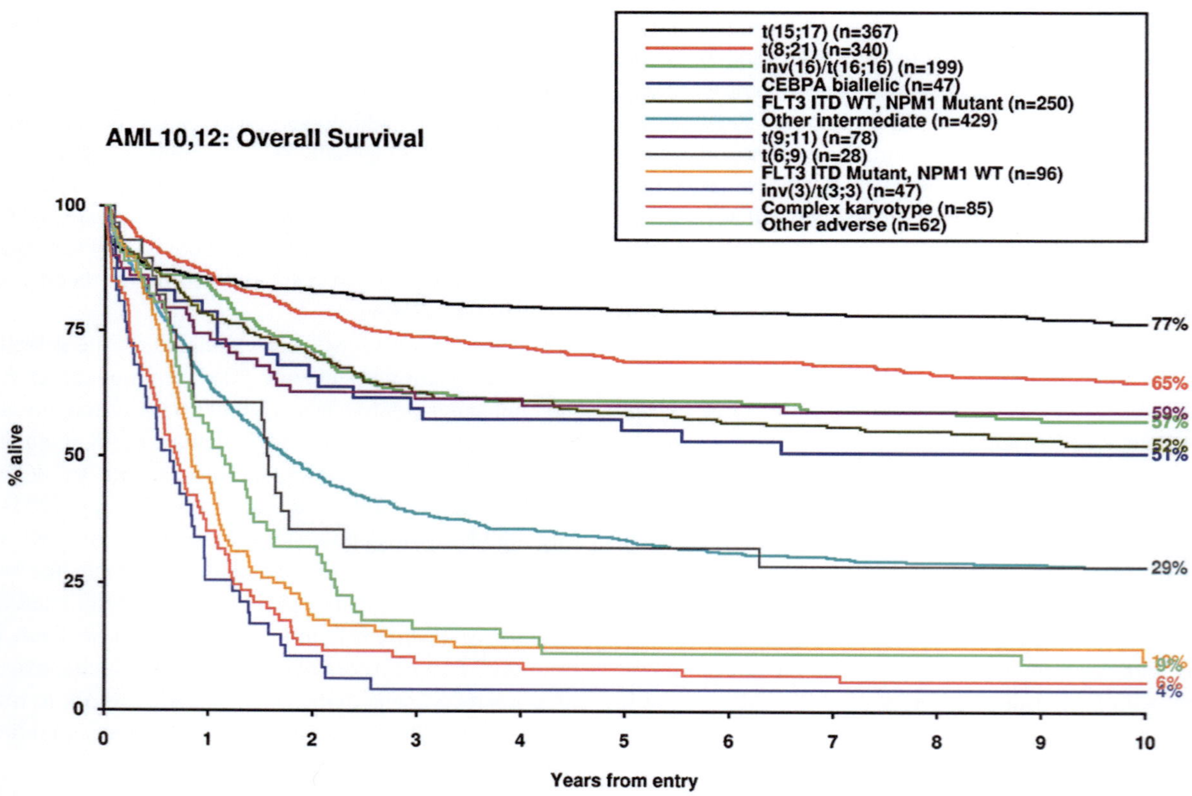

Figure 40.5 Outcome of younger adults with AML according to cytogenetic and molecular abnormalities. Overall survival for younger adults treated in the MRC AML10 and AML12 trials screened for *NPM1*, *CEBPA*, and *FLT3*-ITD mutations [58, 59] for whom cytogenetic data were available. Cases were classified in hierarchical fashion with t(15;17)(q22;q12~q21), t(8;21)(q22;q22), inv(16)(p13.1q22)/t(16;16)(p13.1;q22), t(9;11)(p21~22;q23), t(6;9)(p23;q34), and inv(3)(q21q26.2)/t(3;3)(q21;q26.2) at the top of the hierarchy, then *CEBPA* biallelic mutations, and *NPM1*-mutated/*FLT3*-ITD-negative, *NPM1*-wild-type/*FLT3*-ITD-positive, and other intermediate cytogenetic abnormalities, complex karyotypes, and other adverse cytogenetic abnormalities

in 10^3–10^5 normal BM cells) and has served to highlight the dynamic nature of disease response, which may differ between phenotypically distinct subclones, in which the surface markers that characterize leukemic blasts at relapse in some instances represent only a very minor population at the time of diagnosis [177]. These phenomena make the use of flow cytometry to track MRD extremely challenging and suggest that this approach is likely to be most informative relatively early during the disease course, rather than during longitudinal testing beyond completion of consolidation therapy. Flow cytometry has been used to inform risk-stratified therapy in pediatric AML [208]. Importantly, patients with evidence of MRD at the end of therapy, who otherwise have a very poor prognosis due to a high risk of relapse, can be salvaged by allogeneic SCT conducted in first CR [209]. Moreover, flow cytometric approaches may be used to identify and track leukemic stem cells which may prove more informative in measuring response to therapy compared to the use of LAIPs [204].

For AML characterized by chimeric fusion genes, numerous early studies investigated the use of nested RT-PCR assays for MRD detection to improve outcome prediction. Achievement of molecular remission (CRm) in the BM is a prerequisite for disease cure in APL, prompting inclusion of MRD assessment in standardized response criteria in this subset of AML patients [176, 210]. Importantly, patients in whom *PML–RARA* fusion transcripts are detectable at the end of consolidation, or reappear at a later stage, are destined to relapse rapidly unless additional therapy is given (reviewed by Sanz et al. [176]). Given the significant risk of fatal hemorrhage as a complication of clinical relapse of APL, there is a strong rationale for serial molecular MRD monitoring to identify patients with subclinical levels of leukemia, thus enabling early intervention to prevent progression. Studies conducted by the Gruppo Italiano Malattie EMatologiche dell'Adulto (GIMEMA) and Programa Español para el Tratamiento de Enfermedades Hematológicas (PETHEMA) suggested a benefit for administration of preemptive therapy at the point of molecular relapse as compared to patients treated in frank hematologic relapse [211, 212], although these studies predated the availability of ATO.

MRD monitoring is helpful in guiding treatment of relapse. APL patients with persistent evidence of MRD, in whom harvested stem cells or BM are also PCR positive, are unlikely to benefit from autologous transplant procedures, due to a high rate of relapse [213]. Nevertheless, if a suitable donor is available, such patients can potentially be cured by allogeneic SCT [214]. MRD assessment is also of value in the posttransplant setting to direct the need for additional therapy. While nested RT-PCR assays are still used by some laboratories for MRD detection in APL, they have been largely superseded by RT-qPCR assays, which afford significant advantages (see below). Importantly, the use of a housekeeping gene to normalize results indicates whether there is a falling or rising trend in disease-related transcripts, which is critical to determine whether patients are responding to therapy or are destined to relapse. The lack of capacity of conventional endpoint assays to assess a trend in transcript levels was particularly problematic in *RUNX1–RUNX1T1-associated* CBF leukemia, in which PCR positivity of patients in long-term remission limited test utility for clinical decision making (reviewed by Yin and Grimwade [215]).

Over the last 15 years, optimized RT-qPCR assays designed to detect a wide range of leukemia-specific transcripts (e.g., fusion genes, *NPM1* mutations) have been established through extensive international collaborative efforts, such as the Europe Against Cancer (EAC) [216] and European LeukemiaNet programs [217]. Studies using such assays have significantly extended those previously involving conventional nested RT-PCR, showing that MRD monitoring provides an independent prognostic factor among patients with a defined molecular lesion, who could not otherwise have been distinguished on the basis of pretreatment characteristics. The data are strongest in APL where MRD monitoring can be used to guide molecularly targeted therapies for a more tailored treatment approach. In the UK MRC AML15 trial, serial MRD monitoring with the standardized EAC assay predicted impending relapse of APL on the basis of a rising *PML–RARA* transcript level, and disease progression could be prevented in the majority of patients with early intervention with ATO [218]. This strategy led to a significant reduction in the frank relapse rate as compared to the previous MRC AML12 trial, in which patients received comparable therapy, but were not subject to MRD monitoring. Moreover, early intervention with ATO in the context of subclinical disease was associated with fewer treatment-related complications as compared to treatment in hematological relapse, with no induction of hyperleukocytosis or the associated differentiation syndrome. The analysis of the MRC AML15 data set has shown that longitudinal MRD monitoring beyond the posttreatment time point to direct preemptive therapy is most cost-effective in high-risk patients (i.e., presenting WBC > 10^{10}/l), associated with 10 % survival benefit at 5 years. However, in low-risk patients, documented to be in molecular remission following rapid clearance of *PML–RARA* fusion transcripts (i.e., PCR negative in BM following course two of ATRA + anthracycline therapy), there may be less clinical benefit in routine MRD monitoring beyond the posttreatment time point.

The MRC study also demonstrated that BM is the best sample source for MRD monitoring in APL patients. Peripheral blood (PB) had a 1.5 log inferior sensitivity compared to BM, thereby limiting its reliability to detect submicroscopic levels of disease and therefore significantly reducing the chance to successfully deliver preemptive therapy to prevent progression to overt relapse. In order to develop optimal molecular monitoring schedules, apart from measuring the maximal sensitivity with which MRD can be detected in any given patient (determined by the relative level of expression of leukemic transcripts in AML blasts as defined at diagnosis) and establishing the most appropriate sample source (PB vs BM), it is important to characterize the kinetics of disease relapse. In APL, *PML–RARA* transcripts typically rise by approximately one log per month in relapsing patients; therefore, taking into account the median assay sensitivity of approximately 1 in 10^4, patients registered in the UK National Cancer Research Institute (NCRI) trials are monitored by BM assessments every 3 months until 36 months post-consolidation, at which point MRD monitoring is discontinued (due to the low risk of subsequent relapse). The optimal sampling schedule for other molecularly defined subtypes of AML remains to be firmly established; however, some work has already been conducted in terms of defining the kinetics of disease relapse in CBF and *NPM1*-mutated AML [219].

Available Assays

Mutation Screening and Analysis

Many methods are available for the detection of mutations. The optimal testing method depends on the location and distribution of mutations within the gene of interest and the number of genes to be analyzed. Ideally, genomic DNA, RNA, and viable cells from the diagnostic specimen are stored for testing, once the testing needs are determined. Mutation analysis within the coding sequence of genes can be conducted using genomic DNA or complementary DNA (cDNA) generated from RNA, although for genes in which splice-site mutations have been described, genomic DNA may be preferable. Denaturing high-performance liquid chromatography (DHPLC) of PCR products from genes of interest has been widely used for mutation screening, followed by sequence analysis of amplicons with an abnormal DHPLC pattern suggestive of a mutation. Rapid screening for the presence of an *NPM1* mutation can now also be undertaken by antibody staining of NPM1 using cytospin preparations of leukemic blasts, with the presence of a mutation being indicated by delocalization of NPM1 to the cytoplasm [220]. However, the identification of the specific mutation is particularly useful in *NPM1*-mutated AML, to allow the use of an appropriate mutation-specific assay to track MRD by RT-qPCR. Clinical tests for *CEBPA* must take into consideration the high GC content of the gene sequence and should be able to distinguish biallelic mutations, which predict a relatively favorable outcome [59, 60, 150–152]. Tests to detect *FLT3*-ITD should include the capacity to quantify the relative level of the mutant allele, because patients with high mutant allele ratios associated with acquired disomy have a particularly poor prognosis [57, 58, 133]. Typically, *FLT3*-ITD mutations are detected by PCR using fluorescently labeled primers and GeneScan analysis software (Applied Biosystems). A major advance has been provided by targeted sequencing technology, which is becoming increasingly available, allowing the mutational profile of multiple genes to be rapidly tested in parallel with relatively little DNA. These assays can also provide information on clonal architecture of AML, based on the relative variant allele frequencies of the different mutations.

RT-PCR and RT-qPCR

RT-PCR is widely used for the detection of leukemia-associated fusion transcripts, by PCR amplification of cDNA. For diagnostic samples, a single round of PCR may suffice to detect the fusion transcript; however, to optimize specificity and sensitivity, two rounds of PCR with nested primers may be used. Some laboratories avoid nested RT-PCR due to concern about increased risk of PCR contamination. Standardized methods for the detection of AML-associated fusion transcripts by RT-PCR, most notably *PML–RARA*, *RUNX1–RUNX1T1*, *CBFB–MYH11*, and *BCR–ABL1*, have been developed by the European BIOMED1 group [221].

For the detection of leukemia-associated transcripts by RT-qPCR for MRD monitoring, RNA is initially converted to cDNA using RT protocols identical to those involved in conventional RT-PCR. However, in contrast to the latter technique, in which two rounds of PCR amplification are routinely performed, RT-qPCR approaches involve only a single round of PCR. Importantly, as compared to nested RT-PCR, RT-qPCR assays are more readily standardized and less labor intensive and yield more reproducible results with much shorter turnaround times. SYBR Green I detection during RT-qPCR is not favored for MRD detection, given its lack of sensitivity or specificity in comparison to the use of specific probes, which are, however, significantly more expensive.

RT-qPCR methods allow measurement of leukemic transcripts relative to the expression of endogenous control gene transcripts, which enables exact evaluation of the kinetics of molecular response to treatment and documentation of rising leukemia-associated transcripts prior to frank relapse. The method also allows identification of poor-quality samples (e.g., hypocellular, delayed shipment to the laboratory) or problems with initial sample processing (e.g., red cell lysis), RNA extraction, or the RT step which could give rise to "false-negative" results had conventional endpoint assays been used. Changes in leukemic target transcript level normalized to an endogenous control gene may be calculated on the basis of differences in cycle threshold (Ct) values, provided the efficiencies of the PCR reactions are comparable. Alternatively, normalized MRD data may be reported in terms of absolute copy numbers derived from plasmid standard curves run in parallel (reviewed by Flora and Grimwade [222]).

For reliable performance of RT-qPCR for MRD detection, testing of diagnostic material is critical to identify the optimal assay to use for each patient. For MRD detection in *NPM1*-mutated AML, in which over 30 different mutation types have been described [153], a mutation-specific reverse primer can be used in conjunction with a common probe and forward primer, which have been extensively tested [155, 223]. Variable breakpoints are observed in many balanced chromosomal rearrangements, e.g., t(15;17) and inv(16)/t(16;16) [216]. In some instances, a common primer and probe can be used in conjunction with a breakpoint-specific primer [216]. However, for patients with rare breakpoint patterns, design of a patient-specific assay may be required for subsequent MRD testing. Apart from molecular characterization to define the most appropriate assay for MRD detection, the analysis of diagnostic BM samples provides information on the maximal achievable sensitivity for MRD detection, based on the expression of leukemic transcripts relative to the endogenous control genes in the blast population, which has been shown to vary markedly both within and between molecular subtypes of AML [177]. Assay sensitivity for the detection of *PML–RARA* fusion transcripts is typically approximately 1 in 10^4, which is significantly lower than for cases with *RUNX1–RUNX1T1* and *NPM1*-mutated AML, in which MRD can be detected with at least one log greater sensitivity. In some patients with the latter subtype of AML, the *NPM1*-mutated allele is so highly expressed that sensitivities may reach 1 in 10^{6-7}.

Laboratory Issues

Transit of Samples to the Laboratory

A key issue in the provision of reliable molecular testing results relates to sample collection procedures and transit time to the laboratory. Heparin can potentially interfere with PCR, and PB or BM samples are more appropriately collected in ethylenediaminetetraacetic acid (EDTA). For assays that involve PCR amplification of genomic DNA, e.g., detection of *FLT3*-ITD/D835 mutations, relatively prolonged transit times are less problematic. However, for RNA-based assays, RT-qPCR has revealed degradation equivalent to approximately 0.5 log per 24 h delay in sample processing. Appropriate quantitation of fusion transcripts is feasible if endogenous control transcripts with a comparable degradation rate are amplified in parallel. However, it is important to bear in mind that the control transcript will not correct for the loss in sensitivity resulting from lower transcript levels due to degradation. Hence, there is interest in the use of RNA-stabilizing agents that reduce RNA degradation during specimen transit, which have been most extensively evaluated in MRD monitoring for CML.

Molecular Testing Using PCR-Based Methods

An important concern with RT-PCR is the potential for false-positive results due to PCR contamination. Specific steps to avoid PCR contamination include stringent process and sample controls as described elsewhere in this book. Less well appreciated is the potential of false-negative results in the presence of rare or atypical breakpoints. False-negative results are also a potential problem in the presence of poor-quality RNA or inefficiency of the RT step.

Quality Assurance and Reporting of RT-qPCR Results

Adherence to rigorous internal quality control (QC) and participation in external proficiency testing (PT) programs are essential for provision of high-quality and reliable clinical results. The College of American Pathologists PT surveys are available for myeloid malignancy genotyping, including *CBFB–MYH11*, *FLT3*-ITD and *FLT3*-TKD, *NPM1*, *PML–RARA*, and *RUNX1* testing. In Europe, initiatives including the BIOMED-1, Europe Against Cancer (EAC), and European LeukemiaNet programs have led to improved standardization of methods for the detection of leukemia-associated fusion transcripts by RT-PCR and RT-qPCR [216, 217, 221]. These programs are important to ensure reliability of diagnostic molecular testing and are absolutely fundamental if MRD data are to be used to predict outcome and to modify treatment approach.

The EAC QC exercises have highlighted variations in performance between laboratories that are ostensibly carrying out RT-qPCR assays according to a standardized protocol [216], which highlights the importance of developing and adhering to standard operating procedures for RT-qPCR tests and generating clear guidelines for reporting of RT-qPCR results. Such guidelines are established for the detection of *BCR–ABL1* transcripts for CML, with standardization efforts including the development of WHO reference reagents [224]. Ideally, RT-qPCR assays are performed in triplicate, so that the degree of reproducibility of individual results may be readily appreciated and outlying results disregarded. The EAC program [216] revealed that, in some instances, fusion gene assays yield an amplification signal in one of the triplicate wells of negative control samples. Given that, in many instances, the participating laboratories had not previously amplified the specific transcript; such results most likely reflect nonspecific amplification or cDNA carryover between adjacent wells. This is an intrinsic shortcoming of platforms using the 96-well plate format and has led to reporting of MRD analyses in which amplification is restricted to one of the three wells as PCR negative (but recommending earlier repeat testing, should the result reflect possible residual disease at the limits of assay detection). According to the criteria established by the EAC consortium [216], PCR positivity is defined by presence of specific amplification in at least two of the three replicate wells, with Ct values ≤40 (i.e., equivalent to at least one plasmid copy). Since PCR amplification of primary patient samples is less efficient than plasmid controls, reproducible amplification at Ct values of 40–45 occasionally can be observed in follow-up patient samples, which most likely indicates low-level MRD; however, these low-level positive results are of uncertain clinical significance and again would be seen as an indication for earlier repeat MRD assessment.

Conclusions and Future Directions

Over the course of the last few years, next-generation sequencing (NGS) has led to the identification of many gene mutations and fusions not previously identified in AML [117]. NGS can be applied to determine which lesions are likely to represent initiating events in the development of AML, as well as to decipher the spectrum of cooperating mutations involved in the pathogenesis of particular molecularly defined subsets of the disease. A key challenge is to distinguish the "driver" mutations from "passenger" mutations in the process of leukemic transformation, which will require further investigation using in vitro functional assays and in vivo models. It is hoped that establishing the mutational profile using high-throughput sequencing across a large number of AML cases will provide insights into common pathways that act in concert to induce the AML phenotype and to the development of new targeted therapies. For example, drugs targeting IDH mutations are now in clinical trial; moreover, a study that involved screening for interaction partners of MLL fusion proteins identified BET proteins as potential therapeutic targets [225]. Very encouraging results have been obtained with BET inhibitors in established murine models of leukemia with *MLL* fusions, providing a strong rationale for the evaluation of these compounds in early phase clinical trials in patients [225]. Likewise, very promising results have been seen using pharmacologic targeting of the lysine-specific demethylase KDM1A (also known as LSD1 or AOF2) by tranylcypromine analogs alone or in combination with ATRA, which are capable of abrogating clonogenic potential and inducing differentiation of both murine and human AML cells in vitro and in vivo [226, 227]. Another potential target for therapeutic intervention is autocrine activation of MET and compensatory upregulation of HGF expression [228]. The capacity for rapid molecular testing is crucial to identify patients who could benefit from such targeted treatment approaches. Clinical trials involving evaluation of FLT3 inhibitors in AML harboring *FLT3*-activating mutations or dasatinib in CBF leukemias with *KIT* mutations have shown that this is feasible.

AML is highly heterogeneous at the molecular level, with the average case harboring over ten mutations [117]. This degree of complexity presents a major challenge to establish the most informative and clinically relevant mutations; however, through advances in NGS, the analysis of extensive panels of genes is feasible in a single test [49]. The Interlaboratory Robustness of Next-generation sequencing (IRON) study demonstrated high rates of concordance for mutation detection using NGS platforms (testing for mutations in *TET2*, *CBL*, and *KRAS* genes) in leukemia samples analyzed in ten laboratories in eight countries [229]. As rapid sequencing methods become more affordable with appropriate bioinformatic methods and standards, as well as provision of constitutional DNA for comparison, high-throughput sequencing will be used in routine clinical testing, which would allow leukemia-specific mutations to be identified in any patient. This may help refine outcome prediction and inform management. The capacity to identify a range of novel somatic mutations presents a significant opportunity, providing potential targets for MRD detection using RNA- or DNA-based real-time quantitative PCR assays and digital PCR. Indeed, molecular methods may be useful to track treatment response in the majority of patients with AML in the future.

Wider availability of MRD monitoring, using molecular approaches in conjunction with advances in multicolor flow cytometry to define LAIPs and better definition of the leukemic stem cell population, may allow more informed decisions on the use of allogeneic SCT in first remission, distinguishing patients who are most and least likely to benefit. MRD monitoring may be helpful in identifying patients who are unlikely to be cured without dose intensification, as well as sparing patients from ineffective excessive therapy. In relatively favorable subsets of AML, deintensified protocols are being explored, which could achieve disease cure with less treatment-related toxicity, lower cost, and improved quality of life. In this context, MRD assessment may play an important role to guide therapy but also to rapidly identify those patients who need additional therapy to prevent disease relapse. MRD-based deintensified treatment approaches have been widely investigated in pediatric ALL and subsequently in *PML–RARA*-positive APL, taking advantage of available molecularly targeted therapies, i.e., ATRA and ATO [111, 230, 235]. Similar strategies will hopefully be investigated in other subsets of AML in future clinical trials.

Research developments, in terms of our understanding of the biology of AML and the clinical evaluation of novel targeted therapies, are clearly going to have an impact on the range of clinical tests that will need to be developed and offered by molecular laboratories in the future. Indeed, the pathology laboratory is set to play an increasingly important role in optimizing and individualizing the management of patients with AML.

Acknowledgments We are indebted to Alan Burnett, Nigel Russell, Robert Hills, Rosemary Gale, David Linch, and members of the UK National Cancer Research Institute (NCRI) AML Working Group for their assistance in providing relevant data. DG gratefully acknowledges the National Institute for Health Research (NIHR) for the support for molecular diagnostics and assessment of minimal residual disease in the UK NCRI AML17 trial. This paper presents independent research funded by the National Institute for Health Research (NIHR) under its Programme Grants for Applied Research (Grant Reference Number RP-PG-0108-10093). The views expressed are those of the authors and not necessarily those of the NHS, the NIHR, or the Department of Health. In addition, D.G. grateful acknowledges research funding from Leukaemia & Lymphoma Research of Great Britain, the Guy's and St. Thomas' Charity, and the MRD Workpackage (WP12) of the European LeukemiaNet. K.M. thanks Clara D. Bloomfield for her continuous help and encouragement and gratefully acknowledges the support from the Coleman Leukemia Research Foundation.

References

1. Swerdlow SH, Campo E, Harris NL, Jaffe ES, Pileri SA, Stein H, Thiele J, Vardiman JW. WHO classification of tumours of haematopoietic and lymphoid tissues. Lyon: IARC; 2008.
2. Vardiman JW, Thiele J, Arber DA, et al. The 2008 revision of the World Health Organization (WHO) classification of myeloid neoplasms and acute leukemia: rationale and important changes. Blood. 2009;114(5):937–51.
3. de Thé H, Chomienne C, Lanotte M, et al. The t(15;17) translocation of acute promyelocytic leukaemia fuses the retinoic acid receptor α gene to a novel transcribed locus. Nature. 1990; 347(6293):558–61.
4. Borrow J, Goddard AD, Sheer D, et al. Molecular analysis of acute promyelocytic leukemia breakpoint cluster region on chromosome 17. Science. 1990;249(4976):1577–80.
5. Goddard AD, Borrow J, Freemont PS, et al. Characterization of a zinc finger gene disrupted by the t(15;17) in acute promyelocytic leukemia. Science. 1991;254(5036):1371–4.
6. Brown NJ, Ramalho M, Pedersen EW, et al. PML nuclear bodies in the pathogenesis of acute promyelocytic leukemia: active players or innocent bystanders? Front Biosci. 2009;14:1684–707.
7. Grimwade D, Biondi A, Mozziconacci M-J, et al. Characterization of acute promyelocytic leukemia cases lacking the classic t(15;17): results of the European Working Party. Blood. 2000;96(4):1297–308.
8. Chen Z, Brand NJ, Chen A, et al. Fusion between a novel *Krüppel*-like zinc finger gene and the retinoic acid receptor-α locus due to a variant t(11;17) translocation associated with acute promyelocytic leukaemia. EMBO J. 1993;12(3):1161–7.
9. Redner RL, Rush EA, Faas S, et al. The t(5;17) variant of acute promyelocytic leukemia expresses a nucleophosmin-retinoic acid receptor fusion. Blood. 1996;87(3):882–6.
10. Wells RA, Catzavelos C, Kamel-Reid S. Fusion of retinoic acid receptor α to NuMA, the nuclear mitotic apparatus protein, by a variant translocation in acute promyelocytic leukaemia. Nat Genet. 1997;17(1):109–13.
11. Kondo T, Mori A, Darmanin S, et al. The seventh pathogenic fusion gene *FIP1L1-RARA* was isolated from a t(4;17)-positive acute promyelocytic leukemia. Haematologica. 2008;93(9): 1414–6.
12. Yamamoto Y, Tsuzuki S, Tsuzuki M, et al. BCOR as a novel fusion partner of retinoic acid receptor alpha in a t(X;17)(p11;q12) variant of acute promyelocytic leukemia. Blood. 2010;116(20): 4274–83.
13. Catalano A, Dawson MA, Somana K, et al. The *PRKAR1A* gene is fused to *RARA* in a new variant acute promyelocytic leukemia. Blood. 2007;110(12):4073–6.
14. Arnould C, Philippe C, Bourdon V, et al. The signal transducer and activator of transcription STAT5b gene is a new partner of retinoic acid receptor α in acute promyelocytic-like leukaemia. Hum Mol Genet. 1999;8(9):1741–9.
15. Grimwade D, Mistry AR, Solomon E, et al. Acute promyelocytic leukemia: a paradigm for differentiation therapy. Cancer Treat Res. 2010;145:219–35.
16. Licht JD, Chomienne C, Goy A, et al. Clinical and molecular characterization of a rare syndrome of acute promyelocytic leukemia associated with translocation (11;17). Blood. 1995; 85(4):1083–94.
17. Dong S, Tweardy DJ. Interactions of STAT5b-RARα, a novel acute promyelocytic leukemia fusion protein, with retinoic acid receptor and STAT3 signaling pathways. Blood. 2002;99(8): 2637–46.
18. Zhang X-W, Yan X-J, Zhou Z-R, et al. Arsenic trioxide controls the fate of the PML-RARα oncoprotein by directly binding PML. Science. 2010;328(5975):240–3.
19. Goyama S, Mulloy JC. Molecular pathogenesis of core binding factor leukemia: current knowledge and future prospects. Int J Hematol. 2011;94(2):126–33.
20. Martens JHA, Stunnenberg HG. The molecular signature of oncofusion proteins in acute myeloid leukemia. FEBS Lett. 2010;584(12):2662–9.
21. De Braekeleer E, Férec C, De Braekeleer M. *RUNX1* translocations in malignant hemopathies. Anticancer Res. 2009;29(4):1031–7.
22. Guastadisegni MC, Lonoce A, Impera L, et al. *CBFA2T2* and *C20orf112*: two novel fusion partners of *RUNX1* in acute myeloid leukemia. Leukemia. 2010;24(8):1516–9.
23. Slovak ML, Bedell V, Popplewell L, et al. 21q22 balanced chromosome aberrations in therapy-related hematopoietic disorders: report from an International Workshop. Genes Chromosomes Cancer. 2002;33(4):379–94.
24. Ottone T, Hasan SK, Montefusco E, et al. Identification of a potential "hotspot" DNA region in the *RUNX1* gene targeted by mitoxantrone in therapy-related acute myeloid leukemia with t(16;21) translocation. Genes Chromosomes Cancer. 2009; 48(3):213–21.
25. Meyer C, Hofmann J, Burmeister T, et al. The *MLL* recombinome of acute leukemias in 2013. Leukemia. 2013;27(11):2165–76.
26. Smith E, Lin C, Shilatifard A. The super elongation complex (SEC) and MLL in development and disease. Genes Dev. 2011;25(7):661–72.
27. Rubnitz JE, Raimondi SC, Tong X, et al. Favorable impact of the t(9;11) in childhood acute myeloid leukemia. J Clin Oncol. 2002;20(9):2302–9.
28. Mrózek K, Heinonen K, Lawrence D, et al. Adult patients with de novo acute myeloid leukemia and t(9;11)(p22;q23) have a superior outcome to patients with other translocations involving band 11q23: a Cancer and Leukemia Group B study. Blood. 1997; 90(11):4532–8.
29. Beverloo HB, Le Coniat M, Wijsman J, et al. Breakpoint heterogeneity in t(10;11) translocation in AML-M4/M5 resulting in

fusion of *AF10* and *MLL* is resolved by fluorescent *in situ* hybridization analysis. Cancer Res. 1995;55(19):4220–4.
30. Klaus M, Schnittger S, Haferlach T, et al. Cytogenetics, fluorescence in situ hybridization, and reverse transcriptase polymerase chain reaction are necessary to clarify the various mechanisms leading to an *MLL-AF10* fusion in acute myelocytic leukemia with 10;11 rearrangement. Cancer Genet Cytogenet. 2003;144(1):36–43.
31. Bloomfield CD, Archer KJ, Mrózek K, et al. 11q23 balanced chromosome aberrations in treatment-related myelodysplastic syndromes and acute leukemia: report from an International Workshop. Genes Chromosomes Cancer. 2002;33(4):362–78.
32. Felix CA, Kolaris CP, Osheroff N. Topoisomerase II and the etiology of chromosomal translocations. DNA Repair (Amst). 2006;5(9-10):1093–108.
33. Soekarman D, von Lindern M, Daenen S, et al. The translocation (6;9)(p23;q34) shows consistent rearrangement of two genes and defines a myeloproliferative disorder with specific clinical features. Blood. 1992;79(11):2990–7.
34. Xu S, Powers MA. Nuclear pore proteins and cancer. Semin Cell Dev Biol. 2009;20(5):620–30.
35. Secker-Walker LM, Mehta A, Bain B. Abnormalities of 3q21 and 3q26 in myeloid malignancy: a United Kingdom Cancer Cytogenetic Group study. Br J Haematol. 1995;91(2):490–501.
36. Morishita K, Parker DS, Mucenski ML, et al. Retroviral activation of a novel gene encoding a zinc finger protein in IL-3-dependent myeloid leukemia cell lines. Cell. 1988;54(6):831–40.
37. Du Y, Jenkins NA, Copeland NG. Insertional mutagenesis identifies genes that promote the immortalization of primary bone marrow progenitor cells. Blood. 2005;106(12):3932–9.
38. Stein S, Ott MG, Schultze-Strasser S, et al. Genomic instability and myelodysplasia with monosomy 7 consequent to *EVI1* activation after gene therapy for chronic granulomatous disease. Nat Med. 2010;16(2):198–204.
39. Mrózek K, Heinonen K, Bloomfield CD. Clinical importance of cytogenetics in acute myeloid leukaemia. Best Pract Res Clin Haematol. 2001;14(1):19–47.
40. Mercher T, Le Coniat MB, Monni R, et al. Involvement of a human gene related to the *Drosophila spen* gene in the recurrent t(1;22) translocation of acute megakaryocytic leukemia. Proc Natl Acad Sci USA. 2001;98(10):5776–9.
41. Ma Z, Morris SW, Valentine V, et al. Fusion of two novel genes, *RBM15* and *MKL1*, in the t(1;22)(p13;q13) of acute megakaryoblastic leukemia. Nat Genet. 2001;28(3):220–1.
42. Cheng E-C, Luo Q, Bruscia EM, et al. Role for MKL1 in megakaryocytic maturation. Blood. 2009;113(12):2826–34.
43. Grimwade D, Hills RK, Moorman AV, et al. Refinement of cytogenetic classification in acute myeloid leukemia: determination of prognostic significance of rare recurring chromosomal abnormalities amongst 5,876 younger adult patients treated in the UK Medical Research Council trials. Blood. 2010;116(3):354–65.
44. Mrózek K, Heinonen K, Theil KS, et al. Spectral karyotyping in patients with acute myeloid leukemia and a complex karyotype shows hidden aberrations, including recurrent overrepresentation of 21q, 11q, and 22q. Genes Chromosomes Cancer. 2002;34(2):137–53.
45. Galván AB, Mallo M, Arenillas L, et al. Does monosomy 5 really exist in myelodysplastic syndromes and acute myeloid leukemia? Leuk Res. 2010;34(9):1242–5.
46. Yoneda-Kato N, Look AT, Kirstein MN, et al. The t(3;5)(q25.1;q34) of myelodysplastic syndrome and acute myeloid leukemia produces a novel fusion gene, NPM-MLF1. Oncogene. 1996;12(2):265–75.
47. Mrózek K, Holland KB, Pettenati MJ, et al. Prognostic significance of unbalanced chromosome abnormalities used by 2008 World Health Organization (WHO) classification to define "acute myeloid leukemia (AML) with myelodysplasia-related changes" in adults: a Cancer and Leukemia Group B (CALGB) study. Blood. 2009;114(22):1021 (abstract 2602).
48. Kottaridis PD, Gale RE, Frew ME, et al. The presence of a FLT3 internal tandem duplication in patients with acute myeloid leukemia (AML) adds important prognostic information to cytogenetic risk group and response to the first cycle of chemotherapy: analysis of 854 patients from the United Kingdom Medical Research Council AML 10 and 12 trials. Blood. 2001;98(6):1752–9.
49. Patel JP, Gönen M, Figueroa ME, et al. Prognostic relevance of integrated genetic profiling in acute myeloid leukemia. N Engl J Med. 2012;366(12):1079–89.
50. Bacher U, Haferlach T, Kern W, et al. A comparative study of molecular mutations in 381 patients with myelodysplastic syndrome and in 4130 patients with acute myeloid leukemia. Haematologica. 2007;92(6):744–52.
51. Mead AJ, Linch DC, Hills RK, et al. FLT3 tyrosine kinase domain mutations are biologically distinct from and have a significantly more favorable prognosis than FLT3 internal tandem duplications in patients with acute myeloid leukemia. Blood. 2007;110(4):1262–70.
52. Schlenk RF, Döhner K, Krauter J, et al. Mutations and treatment outcome in cytogenetically normal acute myeloid leukemia. N Engl J Med. 2008;358(18):1909–18.
53. Schnittger S, Schoch C, Dugas M, et al. Analysis of FLT3 length mutations in 1003 patients with acute myeloid leukemia: correlation to cytogenetics, FAB subtype, and prognosis in the AMLCG study and usefulness as a marker for the detection of minimal residual disease. Blood. 2002;100(1):59–66.
54. Thiede C, Steudel C, Mohr B, et al. Analysis of FLT3-activating mutations in 979 patients with acute myelogenous leukemia: association with FAB subtypes and identification of subgroups with poor prognosis. Blood. 2002;99(12):4326–35.
55. Bacher U, Haferlach C, Kern W, et al. Prognostic relevance of *FLT3*-TKD mutations in AML: the combination matters – an analysis of 3082 patients. Blood. 2008;111(5):2527–37.
56. Whitman SP, Ruppert AS, Radmacher MD, et al. *FLT3* D835/I836 mutations are associated with poor disease-free survival and a distinct gene-expression signature among younger adults with de novo cytogenetically normal acute myeloid leukemia lacking *FLT3* internal tandem duplications. Blood. 2008;111(3):1552–9.
57. Whitman SP, Archer KJ, Feng L, et al. Absence of the wild-type allele predicts poor prognosis in adult *de novo* acute myeloid leukemia with normal cytogenetics and the internal tandem duplication of *FLT3*: a Cancer and Leukemia Group B study. Cancer Res. 2001;61(19):7233–9.
58. Gale RE, Green C, Allen C, et al. The impact of *FLT3* internal tandem duplication mutant level, number, size, and interaction with *NPM1* mutations in a large cohort of young adult patients with acute myeloid leukemia. Blood. 2008;111(5):2776–84.
59. Green CL, Koo KK, Hills RK, et al. Prognostic significance of *CEBPA* mutations in a large cohort of younger adult patients with acute myeloid leukemia: impact of double *CEBPA* mutations and the interaction with *FLT3* and *NPM1* mutations. J Clin Oncol. 2010;28(16):2739–47.
60. Taskesen E, Bullinger L, Corbacioglu A, et al. Prognostic impact, concurrent genetic mutations, and gene expression features of AML with *CEBPA* mutations in a cohort of 1182 cytogenetically normal AML patients: further evidence for *CEBPA* double mutant AML as a distinctive disease entity. Blood. 2011;117(8):2469–75.
61. Bienz M, Ludwig M, Oppliger Leibundgut E, et al. Risk assessment in patients with acute myeloid leukemia and a normal karyotype. Clin Cancer Res. 2005;11(4):1416–24.
62. Dufour A, Schneider F, Metzeler KH, et al. Acute myeloid leukemia with biallelic *CEBPA* gene mutations and normal karyotype

represents a distinct genetic entity associated with a favorable clinical outcome. J Clin Oncol. 2010;28(4):570–7.
63. Falini B, Mecucci C, Tiacci E, et al. Cytoplasmic nucleophosmin in acute myelogenous leukemia with a normal karyotype. N Engl J Med. 2005;352(3):254–66.
64. Schnittger S, Schoch C, Kern W, et al. Nucleophosmin gene mutations are predictors of favorable prognosis in acute myelogenous leukemia with a normal karyotype. Blood. 2005;106(12):3733–9.
65. Döhner K, Schlenk RF, Habdank M, et al. Mutant nucleophosmin (*NPM1*) predicts favorable prognosis in younger adults with acute myeloid leukemia and normal cytogenetics: interaction with other gene mutations. Blood. 2005;106(12):3740–6.
66. Verhaak RGW, Goudswaard CS, van Putten W, et al. Mutations in nucleophosmin (*NPM1*) in acute myeloid leukemia (AML): association with other gene abnormalities and previously established gene expression signatures and their favorable prognostic significance. Blood. 2005;106(12):3747–54.
67. Thiede C, Koch S, Creutzig E, et al. Prevalence and prognostic impact of *NPM1* mutations in 1485 adult patients with acute myeloid leukemia (AML). Blood. 2006;107(10):4011–20.
68. Becker H, Marcucci G, Maharry K, et al. Favorable prognostic impact of *NPM1* mutations in older patients with cytogenetically normal de novo acute myeloid leukemia and associated gene- and microRNA-expression signatures: a Cancer and Leukemia Group B study. J Clin Oncol. 2010;28(4):596–604.
69. Paschka P, Schlenk RF, Gaidzik VI, et al. *IDH1* and *IDH2* mutations are frequent genetic alterations in acute myeloid leukemia and confer adverse prognosis in cytogenetically normal acute myeloid leukemia with *NPM1* mutation without *FLT3* internal tandem duplication. J Clin Oncol. 2010;28(22):3636–43.
70. Boissel N, Nibourel O, Renneville A, et al. Prognostic impact of isocitrate dehydrogenase enzyme isoforms 1 and 2 mutations in acute myeloid leukemia: a study by the Acute Leukemia French Association group. J Clin Oncol. 2010;28(23):3717–23.
71. Marcucci G, Maharry K, Wu Y-Z, et al. *IDH1* and *IDH2* gene mutations identify novel molecular subsets within de novo cytogenetically normal acute myeloid leukemia: a Cancer and Leukemia Group B study. J Clin Oncol. 2010;28(14):2348–55.
72. Green CL, Evans CM, Zhao L, et al. The prognostic significance of *IDH2* mutations in AML depends on the location of the mutation. Blood. 2011;118(2):409–12.
73. Boissel N, Nibourel O, Renneville A, et al. Differential prognosis impact of *IDH2* mutations in cytogenetically normal acute myeloid leukemia. Blood. 2011;117(13):3696–7.
74. Chou W-C, Chou S-C, Liu C-Y, et al. *TET2* mutation is an unfavorable prognostic factor in acute myeloid leukemia patients with intermediate-risk cytogenetics. Blood. 2011;118(14):3803–10.
75. Gaidzik VI, Paschka P, Späth D, et al. *TET2* mutations in acute myeloid leukemia (AML): results from a comprehensive genetic and clinical analysis of the AML Study Group. J Clin Oncol. 2012;30(12):1350–7.
76. Weissmann S, Alpermann T, Grossmann V, et al. Landscape of *TET2* mutations in acute myeloid leukemia. Leukemia. 2012;26(5):934–42.
77. Metzeler KH, Maharry K, Radmacher MD, et al. *TET2* mutations improve the new European LeukemiaNet risk classification of acute myeloid leukemia: a Cancer and Leukemia Group B study. J Clin Oncol. 2011;29(10):1373–81.
78. Ribeiro AFT, Pratcorona M, Erpelinck-Verschueren C, et al. Mutant *DNMT3A*: a new marker of poor prognosis in acute myeloid leukemia. Blood. 2012;119(24):5824–31.
79. Thol F, Damm F, Ludeking A, et al. Incidence and prognostic influence of *DNMT3A* mutations in acute myeloid leukemia. J Clin Oncol. 2011;29(21):2889–96.
80. Marcucci G, Metzeler KH, Schwind S, et al. Age-related prognostic impact of different types of *DNMT3A* mutations in adults with primary cytogenetically normal acute myeloid leukemia. J Clin Oncol. 2012;30(7):742–50.
81. Renneville A, Boissel N, Nibourel O, et al. Prognostic significance of DNA methyltransferase 3A mutations in cytogenetically normal acute myeloid leukemia: a study by the Acute Leukemia French Association. Leukemia. 2012;26(6):1247–54.
82. Chou W-C, Huang H-H, Hou H-A, et al. Distinct clinical and biological features of de novo acute myeloid leukemia with additional sex comb-like 1 (*ASXL1*) mutations. Blood. 2010;116(20):4086–94.
83. Pratcorona M, Abbas S, Sanders MA, et al. Acquired mutations in *ASXL1* in acute myeloid leukemia: prevalence and prognostic value. Haematologica. 2012;97(3):388–92.
84. Rocquain J, Carbuccia N, Trouplin V, et al. Combined mutations of *ASXL1*, *CBL*, *FLT3*, *IDH1*, *IDH2*, *JAK2*, *KRAS*, *NPM1*, *NRAS*, *RUNX1*, *TET2* and *WT1* genes in myelodysplastic syndromes and acute myeloid leukemias. BMC Cancer. 2010;10:401.
85. Metzeler KH, Becker H, Maharry K, et al. *ASXL1* mutations identify a high-risk subgroup of older patients with primary cytogenetically normal AML within the ELN Favorable genetic category. Blood. 2011;118(26):6920–9.
86. Grossmann V, Tiacci E, Holmes AB, et al. Whole-exome sequencing identifies somatic mutations of *BCOR* in acute myeloid leukemia with normal karyotype. Blood. 2011;118(23):6153–63.
87. Li M, Collins R, Jiao Y, et al. Somatic mutations in the transcriptional corepressor gene *BCORL1* in adult acute myelogenous leukemia. Blood. 2011;118(22):5914–7.
88. Van Vlierberghe P, Patel J, Abdel-Wahab O, et al. *PHF6* mutations in adult acute myeloid leukemia. Leukemia. 2011;25(1):130–4.
89. Yoo NJ, Kim YR, Lee SH. Somatic mutation of *PHF6* gene in T-cell acute lymphoblatic leukemia, acute myelogenous leukemia and hepatocellular carcinoma. Acta Oncol. 2012;51(1):107–11.
90. Caligiuri MA, Strout MP, Lawrence D, et al. Rearrangement of *ALL1* (*MLL*) in acute myeloid leukemia with normal cytogenetics. Cancer Res. 1998;58(1):55–9.
91. Schnittger S, Kinkelin U, Schoch C, et al. Screening for MLL tandem duplication in 387 unselected patients with AML identify a prognostically unfavorable subset of AML. Leukemia. 2000;14(5):796–804.
92. Döhner K, Tobis K, Ulrich R, et al. Prognostic significance of partial tandem duplications of the *MLL* gene in adult patients 16 to 60 years old with acute myeloid leukemia and normal cytogenetics: a study of the Acute Myeloid Leukemia Study Group Ulm. J Clin Oncol. 2002;20(15):3254–61.
93. Caligiuri MA, Strout MP, Schichman SA, et al. Partial tandem duplication of *ALL1* as a recurrent molecular defect in acute myeloid leukemia with trisomy 11. Cancer Res. 1996;56(6):1418–25.
94. Whitman SP, Ruppert AS, Marcucci G, et al. Long-term disease-free survivors with cytogenetically normal acute myeloid leukemia and *MLL* partial tandem duplication: a Cancer and Leukemia Group B study. Blood. 2007;109(12):5164–7.
95. Whitman SP, Caligiuri MA, Maharry K, et al. The *MLL* partial tandem duplication in adults aged 60 years and older with *de novo* cytogenetically normal acute myeloid leukemia. Leukemia. 2012;26(7):1713–7.
96. Gaidzik VI, Bullinger L, Schlenk RF, et al. *RUNX1* mutations in acute myeloid leukemia: results from a comprehensive genetic and clinical analysis from the AML study group. J Clin Oncol. 2011;29(10):1364–72.
97. Schnittger S, Dicker F, Kern W, et al. *RUNX1* mutations are frequent in de novo AML with noncomplex karyotype and confer an unfavorable prognosis. Blood. 2011;117(8):2348–57.
98. Mendler JH, Maharry K, Radmacher MD, et al. *RUNX1* mutations associate with poor outcome in younger and older patients with cytogenetically normal acute myeloid leukemia and with distinct

gene- and microRNA-expression signatures. J Clin Oncol. 2012;30(25):3109–18.
99. Cairoli R, Beghini A, Grillo G, et al. Prognostic impact of *c-KIT* mutations in core binding factor leukemias. An Italian retrospective study. Blood. 2006;107(9):3463–8.
100. Schnittger S, Kohl TM, Haferlach T, et al. *KIT*-D816 mutations in *AML1-ETO*-positive AML are associated with impaired event-free and overall survival. Blood. 2006;107(5):1791–9.
101. Boissel N, Leroy H, Brethon B, et al. Incidence and prognostic impact of *c-Kit*, *FLT3*, and *Ras* gene mutations in core binding factor acute myeloid leukemia (CBF-AML). Leukemia. 2006;20(6):965–70.
102. Paschka P, Marcucci G, Ruppert AS, et al. Adverse prognostic significance of *KIT* mutations in adult acute myeloid leukemia with inv(16) and t(8;21): a Cancer and Leukemia Group B study. J Clin Oncol. 2006;24(24):3904–11.
103. Care RS, Valk PJM, Goodeve AC, et al. Incidence and prognosis of c-KIT and FLT3 mutations in core binding factor (CBF) acute myeloid leukaemias. Br J Haematol. 2003;121(5):775–7.
104. Haferlach C, Dicker F, Herholz H, et al. Mutations of the *TP53* gene in acute myeloid leukemia are strongly associated with a complex aberrant karyotype. Leukemia. 2008;22(8):1539–41.
105. Rücker FG, Schlenk RF, Bullinger L, et al. *TP53* alterations in acute myeloid leukemia with complex karyotype correlate with specific copy number alterations, monosomal karyotype, and dismal outcome. Blood. 2012;119(9):2114–21.
106. Renneville A, Boissel N, Zurawski V, et al. Wilms tumor 1 gene mutations are associated with a higher risk of recurrence in young adults with acute myeloid leukemia: a study from the Acute Leukemia French Association. Cancer. 2009;115(16):3719–27.
107. Virappane P, Gale R, Hills R, et al. Mutation of the Wilms' tumor 1 gene is a poor prognostic factor associated with chemotherapy resistance in normal karyotype acute myeloid leukemia: the United Kingdom Medical Research Council Adult Leukaemia Working Party. J Clin Oncol. 2008;26(33):5429–35.
108. Gaidzik VI, Schlenk RF, Moschny S, et al. Prognostic impact of *WT1* mutations in cytogenetically normal acute myeloid leukemia: a study of the German-Austrian AML Study Group. Blood. 2009;113(19):4505–11.
109. Paschka P, Marcucci G, Ruppert AS, et al. Wilms' tumor 1 gene mutations independently predict poor outcome in adults with cytogenetically normal acute myeloid leukemia: a Cancer and Leukemia Group B study. J Clin Oncol. 2008;26(28):4595–602.
110. Becker H, Marcucci G, Maharry K, et al. Mutations of the Wilms tumor 1 gene (WT1) in older patients with primary cytogenetically normal acute myeloid leukemia: a Cancer and Leukemia Group B study. Blood. 2010;116(5):788–92.
111. Ravandi F, Estey E, Jones D, et al. Effective treatment of acute promyelocytic leukemia with all-*trans*-retinoic acid, arsenic trioxide, and gemtuzumab ozogamicin. J Clin Oncol. 2009;27(4):504–10.
112. Bowen DT, Frew ME, Hills R, et al. *RAS* mutation in acute myeloid leukemia is associated with distinct cytogenetic subgroups but does not influence outcome in patients younger than 60 years. Blood. 2005;106(6):2113–9.
113. Bacher U, Haferlach T, Schoch C, et al. Implications of *NRAS* mutations in AML: a study of 2502 patients. Blood. 2006;107(10):3847–53.
114. Neubauer A, Maharry K, Mrózek K, et al. Patients with acute myeloid leukemia and *RAS* mutations benefit most from postremission high-dose cytarabine: a Cancer and Leukemia Group B study. J Clin Oncol. 2008;26(28):4603–9.
115. Reindl C, Quentmeier H, Petropoulos K, et al. CBL exon 8/9 mutants activate the FLT3 pathway and cluster in core binding factor/11q deletion acute myeloid leukemia/myelodysplastic syndrome subtypes. Clin Cancer Res. 2009;15(7):2238–47.
116. Ghassemifar R, Thien CB, Finlayson J, et al. Incidence of c-Cbl mutations in human acute myeloid leukaemias in an Australian patient cohort. Pathology. 2011;43(3):261–5.
117. Cancer Genome Atlas Research Network. Genomic and epigenomic landscapes of adult de novo acute myeloid leukemia. N Engl J Med. 2013;368(22):2059–74.
118. Thol F, Bollin R, Gehlhaar M, et al. Mutations in the cohesin complex in acute myeloid leukemia: clinical and prognostic implications. Blood. 2014;123(6):914–20.
119. Kon A, Shih LY, Minamino M, et al. Recurrent mutations in multiple components of the cohesin complex in myeloid neoplasms. Nat Genet. 2013;45(10):1232–7.
120. Taskesen E, Havermans M, van Lom K, et al. Two splice-factor mutant leukemia subgroups uncovered at the boundaries of MDS and AML using combined gene expression and DNA-methylation profiling. Blood. 2014;123(21):3327–35.
121. Je EM, Yoo NJ, Kim YJ, et al. Mutational analysis of splicing machinery genes *SF3B1*, *U2AF1* and *SRSF2* in myelodysplasia and other common tumors. Int J Cancer. 2013;133(1):260–5.
122. Zhang S-J, Rampal R, Manshouri T, et al. Genetic analysis of patients with leukemic transformation of myeloproliferative neoplasms shows recurrent *SRSF2* mutations that are associated with adverse outcome. Blood. 2012;119(19):4480–5.
123. Herold T, Metzeler KH, Vosberg S, et al. Isolated trisomy 13 defines a genetically homogenous AML subgroup with high frequency of mutations in spliceosome genes and poor prognosis. Blood. 2014;124(8):1304–11.
124. Fasan A, Eder C, Haferlach C, et al. *GATA2* mutations are frequent in intermediate-risk karyotype AML with biallelic *CEBPA* mutations and are associated with favorable prognosis. Leukemia. 2013;27(2):482–5.
125. Green CL, Tawana K, Hills RK, et al. *GATA2* mutations in sporadic and familial acute myeloid leukaemia patients with *CEBPA* mutations. Br J Haematol. 2013;161(5):701–5.
126. Greif PA, Dufour A, Konstandin NP, et al. *GATA2* zinc finger 1 mutations associated with biallelic *CEBPA* mutations define a unique genetic entity of acute myeloid leukemia. Blood. 2012;120(2):395–403.
127. Nakao M, Yokota S, Iwai T, et al. Internal tandem duplication of the flt3 gene found in acute myeloid leukemia. Leukemia. 1996;10(12):1911–8.
128. Yamamoto Y, Kiyoi H, Nakano Y, et al. Activating mutation of D835 within the activation loop of FLT3 in human hematologic malignancies. Blood. 2001;97(8):2434–9.
129. Rosnet O, Bühring HJ, Marchetto S, et al. Human FLT3/FLK2 receptor tyrosine kinase is expressed at the surface of normal and malignant hematopoietic cells. Leukemia. 1996;10(2):238–48.
130. Levis M, Small D. FLT3: ITDoes matter in leukemia. Leukemia. 2003;17(9):1738–52.
131. Kayser S, Schlenk RF, Londono MC, et al. Insertion of *FLT3* internal tandem duplication in the tyrosine kinase domain-1 is associated with resistance to chemotherapy and inferior outcome. Blood. 2009;114(12):2386–92.
132. Meshinchi S, Alonzo TA, Stirewalt DL, et al. Clinical implications of *FLT3* mutations in pediatric AML. Blood. 2006;108(12):3654–61.
133. Pratz KW, Sato T, Murphy KM, et al. FLT3-mutant allelic burden and clinical status are predictive of response to FLT3 inhibitors in AML. Blood. 2010;115(7):1425–32.
134. Fröhling S, Schlenk RF, Breitruck J, et al. Prognostic significance of activating *FLT3* mutations in younger adults (16 to 60 years) with acute myeloid leukemia and normal cytogenetics: a study of the AML Study Group Ulm. Blood. 2002;100(13):4372–80.
135. Choudhary C, Schwäble J, Brandts C, et al. AML-associated Flt3 kinase domain mutations show signal transduction differences compared with Flt3 ITD mutations. Blood. 2005;106(1):265–73.

136. Gale RE, Hills R, Kottaridis PD, et al. No evidence that FLT3 status should be considered as an indicator for transplantation in acute myeloid leukemia (AML): an analysis of 1135 patients, excluding acute promyelocytic leukemia, from the UK MRC AML10 and 12 trials. Blood. 2005;106(10):3658–65.
137. Cornelissen JJ, Gratwohl A, Schlenk RF, et al. The European LeukemiaNet AML Working Party consensus statement on allogeneic HSCT for patients with AML in remission: an integrated-risk adapted approach. Nat Rev Clin Oncol. 2012;9(10):579–90.
138. Knapper S. The clinical development of FLT3 inhibitors in acute myeloid leukemia. Expert Opin Investig Drugs. 2011;20(10):1377–95.
139. Tang J-L, Hou H-A, Chen C-Y, et al. *AML1/RUNX1* mutations in 470 adult patients with de novo acute myeloid leukemia: prognostic implication and interaction with other gene alterations. Blood. 2009;114(26):5352–61.
140. Pabst T, Mueller BU, Zhang P, et al. Dominant-negative mutations of *CEBPA*, encoding CCAAT/enhancer binding protein-α (C/EBPα), in acute myeloid leukemia. Nat Genet. 2001;27(3):263–70.
141. Nerlov C. C/EBPα mutations in acute myeloid leukaemias. Nat Rev Cancer. 2004;4(5):394–400.
142. Pabst T, Mueller BU. Complexity of CEBPA dysregulation in human acute myeloid leukemia. Clin Cancer Res. 2009;15(17):5303–7.
143. Smith ML, Cavenagh JD, Lister TA, et al. Mutation of *CEBPA* in familial acute myeloid leukemia. N Engl J Med. 2004;351(23):2403–7.
144. Pabst T, Eyholzer M, Haefliger S, et al. Somatic *CEBPA* mutations are a frequent second event in families with germline *CEBPA* mutations and familial acute myeloid leukemia. J Clin Oncol. 2008;26(31):5088–93.
145. Kirstetter P, Schuster MB, Bereshchenko O, et al. Modeling of C/EBPα mutant acute myeloid leukemia reveals a common expression signature of committed myeloid leukemia-initiating cells. Cancer Cell. 2008;13(4):299–310.
146. Bereshchenko O, Mancini E, Moore S, et al. Hematopoietic stem cell expansion precedes the generation of committed myeloid leukemia-initiating cells in C/EBPα mutant AML. Cancer Cell. 2009;16(5):390–400.
147. Preudhomme C, Sagot C, Boissel N, et al. Favorable prognostic significance of *CEBPA* mutations in patients with de novo acute myeloid leukemia: a study from the Acute Leukemia French Association (ALFA). Blood. 2002;100(8):2717–23.
148. Fröhling S, Schlenk RF, Stolze I, et al. *CEBPA* mutations in younger adults with acute myeloid leukemia and normal cytogenetics: prognostic relevance and analysis of cooperating mutations. J Clin Oncol. 2004;22(4):624–33.
149. Marcucci G, Maharry K, Radmacher MD, et al. Prognostic significance of, and gene and microRNA expression signatures associated with, *CEBPA* mutations in cytogenetically normal acute myeloid leukemia with high-risk molecular features: a Cancer and Leukemia Group B study. J Clin Oncol. 2008;26(31):5078–87.
150. Wouters BJ, Löwenberg B, Erpelinck-Verschueren CAJ, et al. Double *CEBPA* mutations, but not single *CEBPA* mutations, define a subgroup of acute myeloid leukemia with a distinctive gene expression profile that is uniquely associated with a favorable outcome. Blood. 2009;113(13):3088–91.
151. Pabst T, Eyholzer M, Fos J, et al. Heterogeneity within AML with CEBPA mutations; only CEBPA double mutations, but not single CEBPA mutations are associated with favourable prognosis. Br J Cancer. 2009;100(8):1343–6.
152. Renneville A, Boissel N, Gachard N, et al. The favorable impact of CEBPA mutations in patients with acute myeloid leukemia is only observed in the absence of associated cytogenetic abnormalities and FLT3 internal duplication. Blood. 2009;113(21):5090–3.
153. Falini B. Acute myeloid leukemia with mutated nucleophosmin (*NPM1*): molecular, pathological, and clinical features. Cancer Treat Res. 2010;145:149–68.
154. Schnittger S, Kern W, Tschulik C, et al. Minimal residual disease levels assessed by *NPM1* mutation-specific RQ-PCR provide important prognostic information in AML. Blood. 2009;114(11):2220–31.
155. Krönke J, Schlenk RF, Jensen K-O, et al. Monitoring of minimal residual disease in *NPM1*-mutated acute myeloid leukemia: a study from the German-Austrian Acute Myeloid Leukemia Study Group. J Clin Oncol. 2011;29(19):2709–16.
156. Vassiliou GS, Cooper JL, Rad R, et al. Mutant nucleophosmin and cooperating pathways drive leukemia initiation and progression in mice. Nat Genet. 2011;43(5):470–5.
157. Mrózek K, Marcucci G, Paschka P, et al. Clinical relevance of mutations and gene-expression changes in adult acute myeloid leukemia with normal cytogenetics: are we ready for a prognostically prioritized molecular classification? Blood. 2007;109(2):431–48.
158. Haferlach C, Mecucci C, Schnittger S, et al. AML with mutated *NPM1* carrying a normal or aberrant karyotype show overlapping biologic, pathologic, immunophenotypic, and prognostic features. Blood. 2009;114(14):3024–32.
159. Mardis ER, Ding L, Dooling DJ, et al. Recurring mutations found by sequencing an acute myeloid leukemia genome. N Engl J Med. 2009;361(11):1058–66.
160. Yan H, Parsons DW, Jin G, et al. *IDH1* and *IDH2* mutations in gliomas. N Engl J Med. 2009;360(8):765–73.
161. Ward PS, Patel J, Wise DR, et al. The common feature of leukemia-associated IDH1 and IDH2 mutations is a neomorphic enzyme activity converting α-ketoglutarate to 2-hydroxyglutarate. Cancer Cell. 2010;17(3):225–34.
162. Gross S, Cairns RA, Minden MD, et al. Cancer-associated metabolite 2-hydroxyglutarate accumulates in acute myelogenous leukemia with isocitrate dehydrogenase 1 and 2 mutations. J Exp Med. 2010;207(2):339–44.
163. Löwenberg B. Genetic markers in relation to the therapeutic management of acute myeloid leukemia. Hematology Education. 2011;5:36–41.
164. Thol F, Damm F, Wagner K, et al. Prognostic impact of *IDH2* mutations in cytogenetically normal acute myeloid leukemia. Blood. 2010;116(4):614–6.
165. Figueroa ME, Abdel-Wahab O, Lu C, et al. Leukemic IDH1 and IDH2 mutations result in a hypermethylation phenotype, disrupt TET2 function, and impair hematopoietic differentiation. Cancer Cell. 2010;18(6):553–67.
166. Moran-Crusio K, Reavie L, Shih A, et al. Tet2 loss leads to increased hematopoietic stem cell self-renewal and myeloid transformation. Cancer Cell. 2011;20(1):11–24.
167. Ko M, Huang Y, Jankowska AM, et al. Impaired hydroxylation of 5-methylcytosine in myeloid cancers with mutant *TET2*. Nature. 2010;468(7325):839–43.
168. Ley TJ, Ding L, Walter MJ, et al. *DNMT3A* mutations in acute myeloid leukemia. N Engl J Med. 2010;363(25):2424–33.
169. Shen Y, Zhu Y-M, Fan X, et al. Gene mutation patterns and their prognostic impact in a cohort of 1185 patients with acute myeloid leukemia. Blood. 2011;118(20):5593–603.
170. Hou H-A, Kuo Y-Y, Liu C-Y, et al. *DNMT3A* mutations in acute myeloid leukemia: stability during disease evolution and clinical implications. Blood. 2012;119(2):559–68.
171. Marková J, Michková P, Burčková K, et al. Prognostic impact of *DNMT3A* mutations in patients with intermediate cytogenetic risk profile acute myeloid leukemia. Eur J Haematol. 2012;88(2):128–35.
172. Gelsi-Boyer V, Trouplin V, Adélaïde J, et al. Mutations of polycomb-associated gene *ASXL1* in myelodysplastic syndromes

and chronic myelomonocytic leukaemia. Br J Haematol. 2009;145(6):788–800.
173. Döhner H, Estey EH, Amadori S, et al. Diagnosis and management of acute myeloid leukemia in adults: recommendations from an international expert panel, on behalf of the European LeukemiaNet. Blood. 2010;115(3):453–74.
174. Béné MC, Nebe T, Bettelheim P, et al. Immunophenotyping of acute leukemia and lymphoproliferative disorders: a consensus proposal of the European LeukemiaNet Work Package 10. Leukemia. 2011;25(4):567–74.
175. Grimwade D. Screening for core binding factor gene rearrangements in acute myeloid leukemia. Leukemia. 2002;16(5):964–9.
176. Sanz MA, Grimwade D, Tallman MS, et al. Management of acute promyelocytic leukemia: recommendations from an expert panel on behalf of the European LeukemiaNet. Blood. 2009;113(9):1875–91.
177. Freeman SD, Jovanovic JV, Grimwade D. Development of minimal residual disease-directed therapy in acute myeloid leukemia. Semin Oncol. 2008;35(4):388–400.
178. Grimwade D, Hills RK. Independent prognostic factors for AML outcome. Hematology Am Soc Hematol Edu Program. 2009;385–95.
179. Byrd JC, Dodge RK, Carroll A, et al. Patients with t(8;21)(q22;q22) and acute myeloid leukemia have superior failure-free and overall survival when repetitive cycles of high-dose cytarabine are administered. J Clin Oncol. 1999;17(12):3767–75.
180. Byrd JC, Ruppert AS, Mrózek K, et al. Repetitive cycles of high-dose cytarabine benefit patients with acute myeloid leukemia and inv(16)(p13q22) or t(16;16)(p13;q22): results from CALGB 8461. J Clin Oncol. 2004;22(6):1087–94.
181. Burnett AK. Current controversies: which patients with acute myeloid leukaemia should receive a bone marrow transplantation? An adult treater's view. Br J Haematol. 2002;118(2):357–64.
182. Cornelissen JJ, van Putten WLJ, Verdonck LF, et al. Results of a HOVON/SAKK donor versus no-donor analysis of myeloablative HLA-identical sibling stem cell transplantation in first remission acute myeloid leukemia in young and middle-aged adults: benefits for whom? Blood. 2007;109(9):3658–66.
183. Koreth J, Schlenk R, Kopecky KJ, et al. Allogeneic stem cell transplantation for acute myeloid leukemia in first complete remission: systematic review and metaanalysis of prospective clinical trials. JAMA. 2009;301(22):2349–61.
184. Haferlach C, Alpermann T, Schnittger S, et al. Prognostic value of monosomal karyotype in comparison to complex aberrant karyotype in acute myeloid leukemia: a study on 824 cases with aberrant karyotype. Blood. 2012;119(9):2122–5.
185. Breems DA, Van Putten WLJ, De Greef GE, et al. Monosomal karyotype in acute myeloid leukemia: a better indicator of poor prognosis than a complex karyotype. J Clin Oncol. 2008;26(29):4791–7.
186. Mrózek K. Cytogenetic, molecular genetic, and clinical characteristics of acute myeloid leukemia with a complex karyotype. Semin Oncol. 2008;35(4):365–77.
187. Medeiros BC, Othus M, Fang M, et al. Prognostic impact of monosomal karyotype in young adult and elderly acute myeloid leukemia: the Southwest Oncology Group (SWOG) experience. Blood. 2010;116(13):2224–8.
188. Fang M, Storer B, Estey E, et al. Outcome of patients with acute myeloid leukemia with monosomal karyotype who undergo hematopoietic cell transplantation. Blood. 2011;118(6):1490–4.
189. Raimondi SC, Chang MN, Ravindranath Y, et al. Chromosomal abnormalities in 478 children with acute myeloid leukemia: clinical characteristics and treatment outcome in a cooperative pediatric oncology group study-POG 8821. Blood. 1999;94(11):3707–16.
190. von Neuhoff C, Reinhardt D, Sander A, et al. Prognostic impact of specific chromosomal aberrations in a large group of pediatric patients with acute myeloid leukemia treated uniformly according to trial AML-BFM 98. J Clin Oncol. 2010;28(16):2682–9.
191. Harrison CJ, Moorman AV, Hills RK, et al. Cytogenetics of childhood acute myeloid leukemia: 753 patients in UK Medical Research Council treatment trials, AML 10 and 12. J Clin Oncol. 2010;28(16):2674–81.
192. Coenen EA, Raimondi SC, Harbott J, et al. Prognostic significance of additional cytogenetic aberrations in 733 de novo pediatric 11q23/*MLL*-rearranged AML patients: results of an international study. Blood. 2011;117(26):7102–11.
193. Grimwade D, Walker H, Harrison G, et al. The predictive value of hierarchical cytogenetic classification in older adults with acute myeloid leukemia (AML): analysis of 1065 patients entered into the United Kingdom Medical Research Council AML11 trial. Blood. 2001;98(5):1312–20.
194. Farag SS, Archer KJ, Mrózek K, et al. Pretreatment cytogenetics add to other prognostic factors predicting complete remission and long-term outcome in patients 60 years of age or older with acute myeloid leukemia: results from Cancer and Leukemia Group B 8461. Blood. 2006;108(1):63–73.
195. Fröhling S, Schlenk RF, Kayser S, et al. Cytogenetics and age are major determinants of outcome in intensively treated acute myeloid leukemia patients older than 60 years: results from AMLSG trial AML HD98-B. Blood. 2006;108(10):3280–8.
196. Schoch C, Haferlach T, Haase D, et al. Patients with de novo acute myeloid leukaemia and complex karyotype aberrations show a poor prognosis despite intensive treatment: a study of 90 patients. Br J Haematol. 2001;112(1):118–26.
197. Farag SS, Maharry K, Zhang M-J, et al. Comparison of reduced-intensity hematopoietic cell transplantation with chemotherapy in patients aged 60–70 years with acute myeloid leukemia in first remission. Biol Blood Marrow Transplant. 2011;17(12):1796–803.
198. Blum W, Garzon R, Klisovic RB, et al. Clinical response and *miR-29b* predictive significance in older AML patients treated with a 10-day schedule of decitabine. Proc Natl Acad Sci USA. 2010;107(16):7473–8.
199. Perrot A, Luquet I, Pigneux A, et al. Dismal prognostic value of monosomal karyotype in elderly patients with acute myeloid leukemia: a GOELAMS study of 186 patients with unfavorable cytogenetic abnormalities. Blood. 2011;118(3):679–85.
200. Burnett AK, Grimwade D, Solomon E, et al. Presenting white blood cell count and kinetics of molecular remission predict prognosis in acute promyelocytic leukemia treated with all-*trans* retinoic acid: result of the randomized MRC trial. Blood. 1999;93(12):4131–43.
201. Lugthart S, van Drunen E, van Norden Y, et al. High *EVI1* levels predict adverse outcome in acute myeloid leukemia: prevalence of *EVI1* overexpression and chromosome 3q26 abnormalities underestimated. Blood. 2008;111(8):4329–37.
202. Hollink IHIM, van den Heuvel-Eibrink MM, Arentsen-Peters STCJM, et al. *NUP98/NSD1* characterizes a novel poor prognostic group in acute myeloid leukemia with a distinct *HOX* gene expression pattern. Blood. 2011;118(13):3645–56.
203. Akiki S, Dyer SA, Grimwade D, et al. *NUP98-NSD1* fusion in association with *FLT3*-ITD mutation identifies a prognostically relevant subgroup of pediatric acute myeloid leukemia patients suitable for monitoring by real time quantitative PCR. Genes Chromosomes Cancer. 2013;52(11):1053–64.
204. Grimwade D, Vyas P, Freeman S. Assessment of minimal residual disease in acute myeloid leukemia. Curr Opin Oncol. 2010;22(6):656–63.
205. Grimwade D, Walker H, Oliver F, et al. What happens subsequently in AML when cytogenetic abnormalities persist at bone marrow harvest? Results of the 10th UK MRC AML trial. Bone Marrow Transplant. 1997;19(11):1117–23.

206. Marcucci G, Mrózek K, Ruppert AS, et al. Abnormal cytogenetics at date of morphologic complete remission predicts short overall and disease-free survival, and higher relapse rate in adult acute myeloid leukemia: results from Cancer and Leukemia Group B study 8461. J Clin Oncol. 2004;22(12):2410–8.
207. Chen Y, Cortes J, Estrov Z, et al. Persistence of cytogenetic abnormalities at complete remission after induction in patients with acute myeloid leukemia: prognostic significance and the potential role of allogeneic stem-cell transplantation. J Clin Oncol. 2011;29(18):2507–13.
208. Rubnitz JE, Inaba H, Dahl G, et al. Minimal residual disease-directed therapy for childhood acute myeloid leukaemia: results of the AML02 multicentre trial. Lancet Oncol. 2010;11(6): 543–52.
209. Maurillo L, Buccisano F, Del Principe MI, et al. Toward optimization of postremission therapy for residual disease-positive patients with acute myeloid leukemia. J Clin Oncol. 2008;26(30):4944–51.
210. Cheson BD, Bennett JM, Kopecky KJ, et al. Revised recommendations of the International Working Group for Diagnosis, Standardization of Response Criteria, Treatment Outcomes, and Reporting Standards for Therapeutic Trials in Acute Myeloid Leukemia. J Clin Oncol. 2003;21(24):4642–9.
211. Lo Coco F, Diverio D, Avvisati G, et al. Therapy of molecular relapse in acute promyelocytic leukemia. Blood. 1999;94(7): 2225–9.
212. Esteve J, Escoda L, Martín G, et al. Outcome of patients with acute promyelocytic leukemia failing to front-line treatment with all-*trans* retinoic acid and anthracycline-based chemotherapy (PETHEMA protocols LPA96 and LPA99): benefit of an early intervention. Leukemia. 2007;21(3):446–52.
213. Meloni G, Diverio D, Vignetti M, et al. Autologous bone marrow transplantation for acute promyelocytic leukemia in second remission: prognostic relevance of pretransplant minimal residual disease assessment by reverse-transcription polymerase chain reaction of the PML/RARα fusion gene. Blood. 1997;90(3): 1321–5.
214. Lo-Coco F, Romano A, Mengarelli A, et al. Allogeneic stem cell transplantation for advanced acute promyelocytic leukemia: results in patients treated in second molecular remission or with molecularly persistent disease. Leukemia. 2003;17(10):1930–3.
215. Yin JAL, Grimwade D. Minimal residual disease evaluation in acute myeloid leukaemia. Lancet. 2002;360(9327):160–2.
216. Gabert J, Beillard E, van der Velden VHJ, et al. Standardization and quality control studies of 'real-time' quantitative reverse transcriptase polymerase chain reaction of fusion gene transcripts for residual disease detection in leukemia—a Europe Against Cancer program. Leukemia. 2003;17(12):2318–57.
217. Hehlmann R, Grimwade D, Simonsson B, et al. The European LeukemiaNet: achievements and perspectives. Haematologica. 2011;96(1):156–62.
218. Grimwade D, Jovanovic JV, Hills RK, et al. Prospective minimal residual disease monitoring to predict relapse of acute promyelocytic leukemia and to direct pre-emptive arsenic trioxide therapy. J Clin Oncol. 2009;27(22):3650–8.
219. Ommen HB, Schnittger S, Jovanovic JV, et al. Strikingly different molecular relapse kinetics in *NPM1c*, *PML-RARA*, *RUNX1-RUNX1T1*, and *CBFB-MYH11* acute myeloid leukemias. Blood. 2010;115(2):198–205.
220. Falini B, Martelli MP, Tiacci E, et al. Immunohistochemical surrogates for genetic alterations of *CCDN1*, *PML*, *ALK*, and *NPM1* genes in lymphomas and acute myeloid leukemia. Best Pract Res Clin Haematol. 2010;23(3):417–31.
221. van Dongen JJM, Macintyre EA, Gabert JA, et al. Standardized RT-PCR analysis of fusion gene transcripts from chromosome aberrations in acute leukemia for detection of minimal residual disease. Report of the BIOMED-1 concerted action: investigation of minimal residual disease in acute leukemia. Leukemia. 1999;13(12):1901–28.
222. Flora R, Grimwade D. Real-time quantitative RT-PCR to detect fusion gene transcripts associated with AML. Methods Mol Med. 2004;91:151–73.
223. Gorello P, Cazzaniga G, Alberti F, et al. Quantitative assessment of minimal residual disease in acute myeloid leukemia carrying *nucleophosmin* (*NPM1*) gene mutations. Leukemia. 2006;20(6): 1103–8.
224. White HE, Matejtschuk P, Rigsby P, et al. Establishment of the first World Health Organization International Genetic Reference Panel for quantitation of BCR-ABL mRNA. Blood. 2010;116(22):e111–7.
225. Dawson MA, Prinjha RK, Dittmann A, et al. Inhibition of BET recruitment to chromatin as an effective treatment for MLL-fusion leukaemia. Nature. 2011;478(7370):529–33.
226. Harris WJ, Huang X, Lynch JT, et al. The histone demethylase KDM1A sustains the oncogenic potential of MLL-AF9 leukemia stem cells. Cancer Cell. 2012;21(4):473–87.
227. Schenk T, Chen WC, Göllner S, et al. Inhibition of the LSD1 (KDM1A) demethylase reactivates the all-*trans*-retinoic acid differentiation pathway in acute myeloid leukemia. Nat Med. 2012;18(4):605–11.
228. Kentsis A, Reed C, Rice KL, et al. Autocrine activation of the MET receptor tyrosine kinase in acute myeloid leukemia. Nat Med. 2012;18(7):1118–22.
229. Kohlmann A, Klein H-U, Weissmann S, et al. The Interlaboratory RObustness of Next-generation sequencing (IRON) study: a deep sequencing investigation of *TET2*, *CBL* and *KRAS* mutations by an international consortium involving 10 laboratories. Leukemia. 2011;25(12):1840–8.
230. Estey E, Garcia-Manero G, Ferrajoli A, et al. Use of all-*trans* retinoic acid plus arsenic trioxide as an alternative to chemotherapy in untreated acute promyelocytic leukemia. Blood. 2006;107(9): 3469–73.
231. Gröschel S, Sanders MA, Hoogenboezem R, et al. A single oncogenic enhancer rearrangement causes concomitant *EVI1* and *GATA2* deregulation in leukemia. Cell. 2014;157(2):369–81.
232. Yamazaki H, Suzuki M, Otsuki A, et al. A remote *GATA2* hematopoietic enhancer drives leukemogenesis in inv(3) (q21;q26) by activating *EVI1* expression. Cancer Cell. 2014; 25(4):415–27.
233. Rampal R, Alkalin A, Madzo J, et al. DNA hydroxymethylation profiling reveals that *WT1* mutations result in loss of TET2 function in acute myeloid leukemia. Cell Rep. 2014;9(5):1841–55.
234. Wang Y, Xiao M, Chen X, et al. WT1 recruits TET2 to regulate its target gene expression and suppress leukemia cell proliferation. Mol Cell. 2015;57(4):662–73.
235. Lo-Coco F, Avvisati G, Vignetti M, et al. Retinoic acid and arsenic trioxide for acute promyelocytic leukemia. N Engl J Med. 2013;369(2):111–21.

Acute Lymphoblastic Leukemia

41

Andrea Biondi, Carlos Alberto Scrideli, and Giovanni Cazzaniga

Abstract

Acute lymphoblastic leukemia (ALL) comprises a heterogeneous group of disorders which originate from various important genetic lesions in B and T progenitor cells, including mutations that lead to stage-specific developmental arrest and those that impart the capacity for unlimited self-renewal, resulting in clonal expansion of immature progenitor cells (Pui et al. Lancet 371:1030–43, 2008; Pui et al. Blood 120:1165–74, 2012; Morgolin et al. 2011). Different B- and T-cell ALLs can be recognized according to immunologic and molecular criteria (Pui et al. Blood 82:343–62, 1993; Yeoh et al. Cancer Cell 1:133–43, 2002; Pui et al. J Clin Oncol 29:551–65, 2011). The identification of the molecular events underlying the process of leukemia transformation has provided not only important biological information but also clinically significant genetic markers for the identification of prognostically relevant ALL subgroups and for the molecular monitoring of minimal residual disease (MRD). For ALL, immunoglobulin (*IG*) and T-cell receptor (*TCR*) gene rearrangement studies are used as markers of clonality and for MRD detection. In addition, the identification of different genetic variations is used to define different ALL subgroups and to refine treatment protocols tailored to the risk of relapse.

Keywords

B-lineage ALL • T-ALL • Chromosomal translocations • Minimal residual disease • Genetic abnormalities • IG and TCR gene rearrangements • Clonality

Introduction

Acute lymphoblastic leukemia (ALL) comprises a heterogeneous group of disorders which originate from various important genetic lesions in B and T progenitor cells, including mutations that lead to stage-specific developmental arrest and those that impart the capacity for unlimited self-renewal, resulting in clonal expansion of immature progenitor cells [1–3]. Different B- and T-cell ALLs can be recognized according to immunologic and molecular criteria [4–6]. The identification of the molecular events underlying the process of leukemia transformation has provided not only important biological information but also clinically significant genetic markers for the identification of prognostically relevant ALL subgroups and for the molecular monitoring of minimal residual disease (MRD). For ALL, immunoglobulin (*IG*) and

A. Biondi, M.D. (✉)
Department of Pediatrics, University of Milano-Bicocca, Monza, Italy
e-mail: abiondi.unimib@gmail.com

C.A. Scrideli, M.D., Ph.D.
Pediatrics, Pediatric Oncology and Hematology, Ribeirão Preto Medical School, University of Sao Paulo, Ribeirão Preto, SP, Brazil
e-mail: scrideli@fmrp.usp.br

G. Cazzaniga, Ph.D.
Pediatrics, Centro Ricerca Tettamanti, Università di Milano Bicocca, Fondazione MBBS/Ospedale San Gerardo, Monza, Italy
e-mail: gianni.cazzaniga@hsgerardo.org

D.G.B. Leonard (ed.), *Molecular Pathology in Clinical Practice*, DOI 10.1007/978-3-319-19674-9_41

T-cell receptor (*TCR*) gene rearrangement studies are used as markers of clonality and for MRD detection. In addition, the identification of different genetic variations is used to define different ALL subgroups and to refine treatment protocols tailored to the risk of relapse.

Molecular Basis of Disease

IG and *TCR* Gene Rearrangements in ALL

The immune system can specifically recognize and distinguish an enormous variety of specific antigens and antigenic epitopes (at least 10^{10}). Each lymphocyte has a unique membrane receptor, the immunoglobulin receptor (IG) on B lymphocytes and the T-cell receptor on T lymphocytes, that recognizes specific antigens [7–10].

Rearrangements of gene segments that encode the variable regions of the *IG* and *TCR* genes are responsible for the enormous diversity of antigen-specific lymphocyte receptors. This great variability of *IG* and *TCR* is mediated by several mechanisms: (1) the number of variable (V), diversity (D), and joining (J) segments (germline genome diversity); (2) the number of possible V(-D)-J combinations (combinatory diversity); (3) deletions of nucleotides at the ends of rearranging V, (D), and J gene segments, as well as random insertion of noncoded nucleotides (N-region nucleotides) between V–D and D–J segments (junctional diversity); and (4) somatic mutations in the V gene segments of the *IG* genes. This last process has not been observed for *TCR* genes [7–11]. The V, (D), and J segments of B and T precursor cells are rearranged during their differentiation, and each lymphocyte, in this way, contains a specific V-(D-)-J combination. Additional variability can be generated in the junctions V–D and D–J through the loss of nucleotides, as well as through insertion of new nucleotides. Insertion of nucleotides (insertion of N regions) in the junctional sites is mediated by the enzyme terminal deoxynucleotidyl transferase (TdT), which is present in the nucleus of immature B and T cells. N-region insertion occurs in rearranged immunoglobulin heavy chain genes (*IGH*), but is limited or absent in the immunoglobulin kappa and lambda light chain genes (*IGK* and *IGL*). Junctional diversity also occurs in *TCR* genes, primarily the T-cell receptor delta and gamma genes (*TRD* and *TRG*). The potential diversity introduced by the addition of N regions is very high and can increase the total combinatorial diversity to more than 10^{10} for the IGH molecules, 10^{12} for T-cell receptor alpha and beta (TRAB), and more than 10^{9} for T-cell receptor delta and gamma (TRDG) [8–10].

During the earliest stages of the B-cell differentiation, the *IGH* genes rearrange before the *IGL* genes, and of the light chain genes, *IGK* is the first to rearrange. If the *IGK* rearrangement is not functional, the *IGL* gene will rearrange. Another type of rearrangement of the *IGH* gene that can occur is class switching, from IgM and IgD to IgG, IgA, or IgE [8–10, 12]. During the earliest stages of the differentiation of T cells, the *TRD* gene is the first to rearrange, followed immediately by rearrangement of the *TRG* gene and in many cells also the rearrangement of the *TRB* gene. The *TRD* gene can be deleted when *TRA* rearrangement occurs [8–10, 13].

Because ALL is derived from a single transformed lymphoid precursor cell, all ALL cells of a patient should have the same *IG* and *TCR* gene rearrangements with identical junctional region sequences that can be regarded as leukemia-specific fingerprints. Such targets can be identified at initial diagnosis in more than 95 % of patients with ALL by using various polymerase chain reaction (PCR) primer sets [11, 14–17]. Studies of rearrangements of the *IG* genes in B-lineage ALL by Southern blot and PCR have shown that, despite an immature phenotype, more than 95 % of B-precursor ALL contain *IGH* rearrangements, approximately 60 % have *IGK* rearrangements or deletions, and approximately 20 % have *IGL* rearrangements [8, 9, 14, 18]. Cross-lineage rearrangements of the *TCR* gene also have been observed in approximately 90 % of B-lineage ALL pediatric patients [17]. Rearrangements of *TRA*, *TRB*, *TRD*, and *TRG* are found in 46–61 %, 29–35 %, 54–80 %, and 49–70 % of B-lineage ALL, respectively [19–25]. In B-precursor ALL, approximately 80 % of all *TRD* rearrangements are due to incomplete gene rearrangements *VD2-DD3* and *DD2-DD3* [20, 26, 27]. These *VD2-DD3* rearrangements also are prone to continuing rearrangements, particularly with *JA* gene segments. *V2-JA* rearrangements are detected in approximately 40 % of childhood B-precursor ALL and are rare or absent in normal lymphoid cells [23].

In T-lineage ALL, *TRA*, *TRB*, *TRD*, and *TRG* gene rearrangements have been described in 17–67 %, 85–89 %, 68–90 %, and 90–100 % of cases, respectively [8–10, 18, 21, 24, 25]. Cross-lineage *IG* gene rearrangements are not very common in T-lineage ALL, occurring in less than 20 % of cases, and involving only the *IGH* gene [8–10, 21].

Cross-lineage rearrangements of the *IG* and *TCR* genes in non-B and non-T cells, respectively, are probably due to the fact that the leukemic cells originate from a less-committed lymphoid precursor or even a more primitive pluripotent cell (lymphoid/myeloid), in which both *IG* and *TCR* genes are accessible to a common recombinase enzyme. Such rearrangements occur before the final determination of lineage; as soon as this determination for the B, T, or myeloid lineage occurs, the cell adopts the lineage-specific phenotype with expression or differentiation of the lineage-specific antigen, while the gene of cross lineage persists as an "artifact." Due to this, rearrangements in the *TCR* gene are relatively common in B- precursor cell ALL; however, they are very rare in B-ALL and mature B-cell neoplasia (B-cell chronic lymphocytic leukemia, multiple myeloma, and B-cell non-Hodgkin lymphoma. Similarly, rearrangements of *IG* genes are rare in mature T-cell neoplasms (T- cell chronic lymphocytic leukemia and T-cell non-Hodgkin lymphoma [8, 9, 17].

Chromosomal and Genetic Abnormalities in ALL

The genes involved in the most frequent leukemia chromosomal abnormalities have been identified, providing important insights into disease pathogenesis and normal cellular physiology. Molecular assays for leukemias have been developed and now permit a more accurate diagnosis of the leukemia subtypes with frequently recurring genetic and chromosomal alterations. Essentially, two types of chromosomal aberrations occur in ALL: alterations in the number of chromosomes and structural abnormalities. In childhood ALL, high hyperdiploidy (51–65 chromosomes) is associated with a favorable outcome, while hypodiploidy (fewer than 45 chromosomes) is associated with poor prognosis. Trisomies of each chromosome has been observed in ALL, but the most common are trisomy 4, 6, 14, 17, 18, 21, and X. Combined trisomies between chromosomes 4 and 10 and between chromosomes 10 and 17 are associated with good prognosis and low risk of relapse. Intrachromosomal amplification of chromosome 21 (iAMP21) has been identified as a recurrent abnormality in childhood ALL and is associated with older children, common/pre-B immunophenotypes, low white blood cell (WBC) count, and poor prognosis [3, 28–31].

Somatically acquired chromosomal translocations or inversions occur in up to 65 % of ALL. In most instances, the genes disrupted by these abnormalities have been identified, thus providing important insights into disease pathogenesis and normal cellular physiology. Chromosomal translocations have two main consequences: activation of a protooncogene brought under the regulation of the promoter and enhancer elements of another gene that normally is active in the leukemia progenitor cell, and creation of a fusion gene from two distinct genes with expression of a chimeric protein (Fig. 41.1). The products of the latter aberrant genes are most often transcription factors or tyrosine kinases [32]

These genetic alterations have important prognostic implications that can be used to classify precursor lymphoid neoplasms and to guide the selection of therapy [33] (Table 41.1).

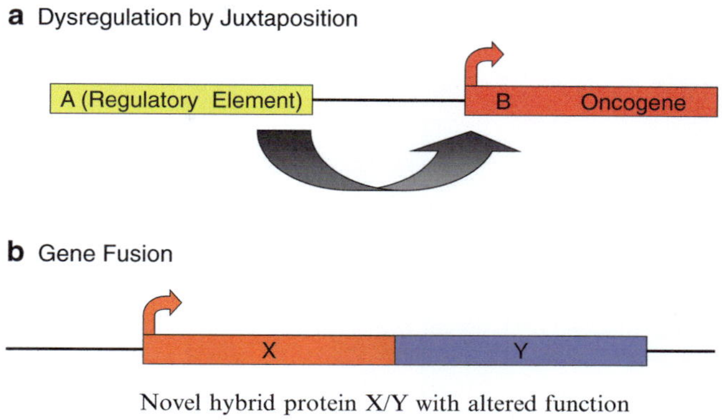

Figure 41.1 Schematic representation of two types of gene alterations generated by chromosomal translocations. (**a**) A protooncogene (B) is activated by the promoter and enhancer elements of a distinct translocation gene partner (A, Regulatory Element). (**b**) Discrete segments of two different genes (X and Y) are joined as a result of a translocation, creating a fusion gene that encodes a chimeric protein

Table 41.1 WHO Classification (2008) of acute lymphoblastic leukemia/lymphoma

B lymphoblastic leukemia/lymphoma
B lymphoblastic leukemia/lymphoma, NOS
B lymphoblastic leukemia/lymphoma with recurrent genetic abnormalities
B lymphoblastic leukemia/lymphoma with t(9;22)(q34;q11.2); *BCR-ABL1*
B lymphoblastic leukemia/lymphoma with t(v;11q23); *MLL* rearranged
B lymphoblastic leukemia/lymphoma with t(12;21)(p13;q22); *ETV6/RUNX1* (*TEL-AML1*)
B lymphoblastic leukemia/lymphoma with hyperdiploidy
B lymphoblastic leukemia/lymphoma with hypodiploidy
B lymphoblastic leukemia/lymphoma with t(5;14)(q31;q32); *IL3-IGH*
B lymphoblastic leukemia/lymphoma with t(1;19)(q23;p13.3); *TCF3/PBX1* (*E2A-PBX1*)
T lymphoblastic leukemia/lymphoma

NOS not otherwise specified

Genetic Abnormalities in B-Lineage ALL

B-lineage ALL is the most frequent acute leukemia in children, corresponding to 80–85 % of cases with about 80 % of these having cytogenetic alterations and characteristic genetic translocations (Table 41.2). The chromosomal translocation t(12;21)(p13;q22) results in the *ETV6/RUNX1* (*TEL/AML1*) fusion gene. This is a cryptic translocation, which cannot be detected by karyotyping. Thus, fluorescence in situ hybridization (FISH) or PCR must be used for detection. It is the most common chromosomal rearrangement in childhood ALL, occurring in about 25 % of cases [34]; by contrast, it is rarely found in adult ALL (1–3 %) [35]. The t(12;21) translocation is almost exclusively associated with a young age (<10 years) and a precursor B-cell phenotype [34]. Both *ETV6* and *RUNX1* are important regulators of normal hematopoiesis, and are involved in other translocations in both lymphoid and myeloid leukemias, which suggests

Table 41.2 Main genetic alterations involving B-lineage ALL

Translocation	Involved gene(s)	Frequency
Pre-B cell/early pre-B cell		
t(12;21)(p13;q22)	*ETV6/RUNX1*	20–25 % children/1–3 % adults
t(1;19)(q23;p13)	*TCF3/PBX1*	5 % children
t(4;11)(q21;q23)	*AF4/MLL*	2 %
t(11;19)(q23;p13)	*MLL/ENL*	<1 %
t(9;11)(p21;q23)	*AF9/MLL*	<1 %
t(9;22)(q34;q11)	*ABL1/BCR*	3–5 % children/25 % adults
t(17;19)(q22;p13)	*HLF/E2A*	<1 %
t(12;v)(p12-p13;V)	*ETV6* or *KIP1*	5–10 %
Dic(9;12) (9p11-p12;p12)	Unknown	1 %
Dic(9;20) dic(9;20) (p11-13;q11)	Unknown	2 %
t(5;14)(q35;q32)	*IL3/IGH*	<1 %
B-cell ALL		
t(8;14)(q24;q32)	*MYC/IGH*	95 %
t(8;22)(q24;q11)	*MYC/IGL*	<5 %
t(2;8)(p11;q24)	*IgK/MYC*	<5 %
New recurrent abnormalities		
Del9p	*CDKN2A/B*	30–35 %
Del9p	*PAX5*	30–35 %
iAMP21	*AML1*	2 %
CRLF2	*CRLF2*	5–7 % (50 % with Down syndrome)
IKZF1	*IKZF1*	15 %

that the resulting fusion proteins could deregulate normal hematopoietic development leading to leukemia [1, 31]. ETV6-RUNX1 also causes overexpression of the erythropoietin receptor and activation of JAK-STAT signaling [36, 37]. The t(12;21) can be present in blood cells at birth, 5–10 years before the leukemia becomes evident, as demonstrated by studies using neonatal blood spots. The leukemias induced by ETV6-RUNX require a second genetic event for their development. The loss of function of normal TEL protein, through the loss of the normal *TEL* allele as observed in patients with t(12;21), appears to be this second event [1, 38].

Whether t(12;21) is associated with a good prognosis or with only a marginally better outcome compared to other cytogenetic ALL subgroups remains controversial [34]. *ETV6/RUNX1* rearrangement has been observed in about 25 % of relapsing cases treated within European Berlin-Frankfurt-Munster (BFM) group protocols. These patients tend to have a longer duration of remission (>2 years) compared to other childhood ALL cytogenetic groups; however, early relapses have also been observed, illustrating a heterogeneous pattern of clinical behavior in this group of patients [34, 39].

The t(1;19)(q23;p13) translocation is one of the most frequently observed translocations in childhood ALL, occurring in approximately 25 % of pre-B cytoplasmic IG-positive cases and in 1 % of early pre-B cytoplasmic IG-negative cases. This translocation most frequently creates a fusion of *TCF3* (*E2A*), a helix-loop-helix (bHLH) protein-coding gene on chromosome 19, with *PBX1*, a homeobox-containing gene located on chromosome 1 [36, 37, 40]. A few molecular variants of the t(1;19), leading to different species of *TCF3/PBX1* mRNAs, have been described [41]. Both genes play a critical role in lymphocyte development and alteration of *HOX* genes has a clear role in leukemogenesis. Although this translocation has been associated with a poor clinical outcome, the current chemotherapy protocols have improved prognosis for this subgroup of patients [31, 36, 37, 42].

Another rare translocation, found in 1 % of B-precursor ALLs, is t(17;19)(q22;p13.3), which also involves the *TCF3* gene but creates a fusion with the *HLF* gene, resulting in a chimeric transcript and protein that could contribute to leukemogenesis by aberrant regulation in genes that control the fate of early lymphoid progenitors. This translocation has been associated with poor prognosis [3, 36, 37, 43].

Abnormalities of the q23 region of chromosome 11 are seen with relative frequency in childhood ALL (5 %), infant acute leukemia (70 %), and secondary leukemias in patients who received topoisomerase II inhibitors (85 %). Leukemias with translocations involving 11q23 have an early pre-B phenotype and express myeloid antigens. More than 40 different chromosomal loci have been identified as fusion partners in 11q23 translocations. In the majority of cases, the translocation partner is chromosome 4, and less frequently chromosome 1, 10, or 19. At the molecular level, the t(4;11) fuses *MLL* at 11q23 to *AF4* at 4q21, resulting in an *MLL/AF4* chimeric gene. *MLL*-rearranged leukemias exhibit an upregulation of HOX Class I genes. The ability of MLL to regulate expression of the *HOX* genes suggests a role in hematopoiesis and also in leukemogenesis [36, 37]. This translocation is related to aggressive clinical features such as hyperleukocytosis, organomegaly, frequent central nervous system involvement, and poor outcome [3, 6, 36, 37, 44–49].

The t(9;22) translocation is identified in 3–5 % of childhood ALL and approximately 25 % of adult ALL [47, 48, 50]. This translocation creates a novel chromosome (the Philadelphia chromosome, Ph+) and a fusion between the protooncogene *ABL1* on chromosome 9 and the "breakpoint cluster region" gene (*BCR*) on chromosome 22. Whereas the *ABL1* breakpoint on chromosome 9 is consistently between exons a1 and a2, the *BCR* breakpoints on chromosome 22 can occur in two different gene regions. The "minor" breakpoint cluster region (m-bcr), between exons e1 and e2, is present in approximately 90 % of childhood Ph+ ALL; by contrast, a "major" breakpoint cluster region (M-bcr), between exons 13 and 14 or 14 and 15 (formerly called b2 and b3 or b3 and b4, respectively), is a usual finding in chronic myelogenous leukemia [50] and occasionally present in Ph+ ALL. The m-bcr generates a fusion protein of

190 kDa (p190), whereas the M-bcr results in a fusion protein of 210 kDa (p210) [47, 48, 50–53]. The presence of t(9;22) is associated with a high risk of treatment failure in children and adults with ALL. However, Ph^+ childhood ALL is a heterogeneous disease with regard to treatment response. High leukocyte count, old age, and poor response to prephase treatment with prednisone and intrathecal methotrexate influence treatment outcome. Patients with a good prednisone response have a significantly lower risk of treatment failure compared to those with a poor prednisone response (PPR), when treated with intensive BFM protocol chemotherapy, whether associated with bone marrow transplantation (BMT) or not. These PPR children have a clinical response and prognosis as poor as that of Ph^+ ALL adults [47, 48, 54]. For the treatment of these patients, s elective tyrosine kinase inhibitors have been used in association with chemotherapy and/or BMT. The use of the ABL tyrosine kinase inhibitor imatinib, and derivatives of second generation (e.g., nilotinib, dasatinib) has transformed the treatment and outcome of ALL patients with the *BCR-ABL1* fusion gene [55, 56].

More recently, a group of childhood B-lineage ALLs termed "BCR-ABL1-like" has been described. These ALLs exhibit a similar gene expression profile as that observed in *BCR-ABL1* positive ALL patients. This subtype represents up to 15 % of all B-lineage cases and is frequently associated with deletion or mutation of *IKZF1*. In 50 % of the cases, the *CRLF2* gene is rearranged, which confers a very poor prognosis [6, 36, 37, 57, 58].

The t(8;14)(q24;q32), involving the *MYC* gene (8q24) and the *IGH* locus (14q32), occurs in 85–90 % of cases of surface immunoglobulin positive B-cell ALL. The dysregulation of *MYC* expression appears be responsible for the B-cell proliferation. Two other variants, t(2;8)(p11;q24) and t(8;22)(q24;q11), involving the *MYC* gene and *IGK* and *IGL*, respectively, are less commonly observed [3, 29, 59, 60]. The t(5;14)(q31;q32) is an uncommon translocation, observed in less than 1 % of ALL patients, and results in the fusion of the *IGH* gene with the interleukin-3 (*IL3*) gene. The overexpression of *IL3* appears be involved in the pathogenesis of the leukemia and hypereosinophilia in these patients [3].

Subgenetic alterations involving genes that regulate normal B lymphoid development are identified in 40 % of B-lineage ALL. The most commonly involved gene is *PAX5*, required for B-lineage maturation. Other regulating B-lymphoid development genes frequently involved include the IKAROS family of transcription factors *IKZF1*, *IKZF2*, *IKZF3*, as well as *EBF1*, *TCF3*, *LEF1*, *RAG1/2*, *BLNK*, and *VPREB1* [30, 57, 61]. Deletions or sequence alterations of the lymphoid development associated *IKZF1* gene and tumor suppressor gene *CDKN2A/B* have been associated with relapse risk, confirming that genetic alterations detected at diagnosis can predict the risk of relapse [6, 36, 37, 61]. Overexpression of *CRLF2*, associated or not with corresponding genomic lesions (*IGH-CRLF2*, *P2RY8-CRLF2* or the p.Phe232Cys mutation) occurs in 5–7 % of childhood B-lineage precursor ALL and in 50 % of individuals with Down syndrome and ALL. These alterations commonly are associated with *JAK1/2* mutations and, in patients who do not have Down syndrome, with *IKZF1* mutations and poor prognosis [6, 36, 37].

Genetic Abnormalities in T-Lineage ALL

T-lineage ALL accounts for approximately 15 % of all childhood ALL and in general is considered a high-risk category. This leukemia characteristically presents with chromosomal rearrangements involving T-cell receptor genes, proto-oncogenes, or transcription factor genes, or alterations of key genes or pathways related to T-cell lymphogenesis (Table 41.3).

Developmental genes abnormalities have been found in T-lineage ALL (T-ALL) comprising the basic helix-loop-helix (bHLH) gene family (*MYC*, *TAL1*, *LYL1*), the homeobox gene family (*HOX*) including the HOXA cluster, and the LIM gene family (*LMO1* and *LMO2*). When rearranged near enhancers with the loci 14q11.2, 7q34-q35 or 7p15, that contain the *TRA/TRD*, *TRB*, and *TRG* genes, respectively, these regulatory genes become active and lead to dysregulated expression of transcription factor genes. The *TAL1* gene can be involved due to t(1;14)(p32,q11), which occurs in 5 % of childhood T-ALL, or can be affected by a submicroscopic interstitial deletion between the *SIL* and *TAL1(SCL)* genes at 1p32. This "*TAL* deletion" occurs in 20–25 % of childhood T-ALL [3, 29–31, 60].

Different T-ALL signatures, based on gene expression profiles, indicate that the leukemic arrest in specific genetic subgroups (*LYL1*, *TLX1*, *TAL1*) occurs at particular stages of thymocyte development (i.e., at the pro-T, early cortical thymocytes, or late cortical thymocyte stage) [62–65] and seems to comprise at least four distinct molecular-cytogenetic subgroups: TAL/MLO, TLX3/HOX11L2, TLX1/HOX11, and HOXA subgroups [66, 64, 65, 67, 68]. A fifth subtype of T-ALL termed "early T precursor" (ETP) comprises approximately 15 % of T-ALL and is associated with a high risk of relapse. Inactivating alterations that disrupt hematopoietic development and cause histone-modification of genes are possible in ETP, as well as somatic activation of regulating cytokine receptors and RAS signaling [67, 69].

The *TAL* deletion leads to expression of a *SIL-TAL* chimeric transcript, resulting from the fusion of the 5′ part of *SIL* to the 5′ region of *TAL1*. In addition, high levels of *TAL1* have been observed in 40–60 % of T-ALL. The aberrant expression of TAL1 may activate a specific set of target genes that are normally quiescent in T-cell progenitors or could exert a negative effect through inhibition of E2A or E2A-HEB heterodimers, leading to a leukemogenic effect.

Table 41.3 Main genetic alterations involving T-cell ALL

	Involved gene(s)	Frequency
Translocation involving T-cell receptor genes		
t(7;10)(q34;q24) and t(10;14)(q24;q11)	*TLX1* (*HOX11*)	7 % children; 31 % adults
t(5;14)(q35;q32)	*TLX3* (*HOX11L2*)	20 % children; 13 % adults
inv(7)(p15q34), t(7;7)	*HOXA* genes	5 %
t(1;14)(p32;q11) and t(1;7)(p32;q34)	*TAL1*	3 %
t(7;9)(q34;q32)	*TAL2*	<1 %
t(7;19)(q34;p13)	*LYL1*	<1 %
t(14;21)(q11.2;q22)	*BHLHB1*	<1 %
t(11;14)(p15;q11)	*LMO1*	2 %
t(11;14)(p13;q11) and t(7;11)(q35;p13)	*LMO2*	3 %
t(1;7)(p34;q34)	*LCK*	<1 %
t (7;9)(q34;q34.3),	*NOTCH1*	<1 %
t(7;12)(q34;p13) and t(12;14)(p13;q11)	*CCND2*	<1 %
Translocation involving oncogenes		
1p32 deletion	*SIL-TAL1*	9–30 %
t(10;11)(p13;q14)	*CALM-AF10*	10 %
11q23	*MLL*	8 %
t(9;9)(q34;q34)	*NUP214-ABL1*	5 %
t(9;14)(q34;q32)	*EML1-ABL1*	<1 %
t(9;22)(q34;q11)	*BCR-ABL1*	<1 %
t(9;12)(p24;p13)	*ETV6-JAK2*	<1 %
Cryptic deletions		
9p21	*P16*	65 % children; 15 % adults
Del(6q)	Unknown	20–30 %
Mutations		
Notch1	*NOTCH1*	50 %
PTEN	*PTEN*	17 %
IL7R	*IL7R*	7–9 %

The *LYL1* gene is involved in the t(7;19)(q34;p13) leading to constitutive overexpression, usually in a more immature T-lineage phenotype. The *MYC* gene can be translocated to a *TCR* locus [t(8;14)(q24;q21)] in some cases of T-ALL [3, 29–31, 62].

In addition to genes encoding bHLH proteins, gene rearrangements of the LIM gene family (encoded by *LMO1* and *LMO2*) and the *TCR* loci have been described in T-ALL. The t(11;14)(p13;q11) (*LMO1/TCRD*) occurs in 7–13 % of T-ALL and has been associated with males, high WBC count and extramedullary disease. The t(11;14)(p15;q11) (*LMO2/TCRD*) is infrequent and found in <1 % of the cases [3, 29, 70, 71].

Translocations involving the *HOX* genes *TLX1* (*HOX11*) and *TLX3* (*HOX11L2*), complete the list of developmental genes that are inappropriately placed under control of the *TCR* loci. Activation of expression of the *HOX11* gene by chromosomal translocations t(10;14)(q24;q11) and t(7;10)(q34;q24) interferes with normal T-cell development and promotes malignant transformation. HOX11 expression is associated with a favorable prognosis in childhood T-ALL. *HOX11L2* is activated by t(5;14)(q35;q32) and (5;14)(q35;q11). Despite the fact that this finding has been associated with a poor prognosis, this does not seem to apply in children receiving more intensive chemotherapy [3, 29–31, 60].

Recurrent translocations involving the HOXA cluster have been described. This subgroup of T-ALL is characterized by elevated expression of the *HOXA* genes and includes *MLL* rearrangements, inv(7)(p15q34), t(10;11)(p13;q23), and *CALM-AF10* rearrangements as well as the cryptic del(9)(q34.11q34.13) deletion that results in a *SET-NUP214* fusion product. *MLL* fusions are found in 4–8 % of T-ALL. The t(11;19)(q23;p13) that involves *MLL/ENL* is the most frequent. Other identified translocations include t(6;11)(q27;q23) (*MLL/AF6*), t(10;11)(p13;q23) (*MLL/AF10*), t(X;11)(q13;q23) (*MLL/AFX1*), and t(4;11)(q12;q23) (*MLL/AF4*). T-ALL with an *MLL* fusion is characterized by a specific expression profile with differentiation arrest in early stage thymocyte development [29–31, 60, 61, 72].

Chromosomal translocations involving *NOTCH1*, a gene that regulates the normal embryologic development of

T-cells and other tissues, are rare in T-ALL. In contrast, activating *NOTCH1* mutations are present in more than 50 % of T-cell ALLs. *NOTCH1* regulates oncogenes including the *MYC* and *RAS*, and this is probably the mechanism by which aberrant NOTCH signaling causes T-ALL. This oncogenic mechanism is supported by experimental models, in which mutations of the *NOTCH1* gene can induce T-cell ALL [29–31]. Small molecule inhibitors of the NOTCH pathway thus have the potential to induce remission in T-cell ALL [31].

Cryptic deletions are common in T-ALL and may be concomitant with other changes. The most common cryptic deletion causes loss of the *INK4/ARF* locus at 9p21, important to cell cycle control. Del(6q) also has been observed, but the involved gene is unknown [29, 31]. Inactivating gene mutations in *PTEN* have been described in approximately 17 % of pediatric T-ALL and are associated with poor prognosis [73]. Somatic-gain mutations in *IL7R* have been observed in 7–9 % of pediatric T-ALL [74]. The main genetic alterations in T-ALL are summarized in Table 41.3.

Indications for Testing

Many genetic alterations have important prognostic implications that can guide the selection of therapy. Treatment of the acute leukemias has progressed from uniform strategies devised for large groups of patients to more refined protocols tailored to the risk of relapse in discrete subgroups. Although routinely recorded features such as blast cell immunophenotype and presenting WBC count provide useful criteria for risk assessment, molecular genetic changes are the most sensitive markers of potential leukemia aggressiveness. Hence, overall these are the best suited to guide treatment. *IG* and *TCR* gene rearrangement studies are useful for the diagnosis of childhood ALL, for detection of cerebrospinal involvement [24, 25, 51–53, 75], and for MRD assessment because they occur in the vast majority of ALL patients [16, 45, 46, 76–80].

Molecular detection of chromosomal abnormalities in blast cells of leukemia patients has important prognostic implications that can guide staging and selection of treatment. In addition, detection of specific translocations is used to MRD monitoring [81].

The term "minimal residual disease" has been used to define the lowest level of disease detected by conventional methods of analysis in patients who are in complete continuous remission. At clinical presentation, the number of leukemic cells is approximately 10^{11}–10^{12}; if the patient is not treated, the clone continues to expand, and death occurs with approximately 10^{13} leukemic cells. With cytotoxic treatment, the number of neoplastic cells is diminished and when less than 5 % of leukemic blasts are identified in the bone marrow (BM) by conventional cytology, the patient is considered to be in complete remission. Thus, patients in complete remission have from zero to 10^{10} leukemic cells. The detection of MRD, either after clinical remission was achieved or during treatment, can help direct adjustments to therapeutic strategies and identify patients who are at higher risk of relapse [16, 45, 46, 76–80]. The presence of MRD at the time of transplantation as well as in the post transplant period are also powerful, independent predictors of adverse outcome [82–87].

Available Assays

Detection of Clonality by PCR

Monoclonality in ALL is detected by PCR amplification of the *IG* and/or *TCR* V(D)J region, typically using consensus primers to conserved sequences within the framework regions of the V region and the D and/or J regions (Fig. 41.2). The V(D)J region varies in size and sequence across a population of B or T cells and allows for detection of a monoclonal leukemic cell population by PCR amplification of a unique PCR product specific to the leukemic clone. For a population of nonlymphoid cells, where the *IG* and *TCR* genes are in the germline configuration, amplification will not occur, due to the great distance between the closest V and J regions [8, 9, 11, 15, 17].

RT-PCR for Leukemia-Specific Translocations

PCR analysis of fusion genes is based on the design of oligonucleotide primers within exons at the opposite sides of the breakpoint fusion regions, so that the PCR product contains the tumor-specific fusion sequence. The exact breakpoint at the DNA level may be different from patient to patient and therefore difficult to determine. In the majority of ALL translocations, the breakpoint regions span greater than 2 kb, exceeding the conventional range for PCR. However, because the breakpoints are mostly intronic and spliced out at the messenger RNA (mRNA) level, the preferred target for detection of translocations is the chimeric mRNA [26].

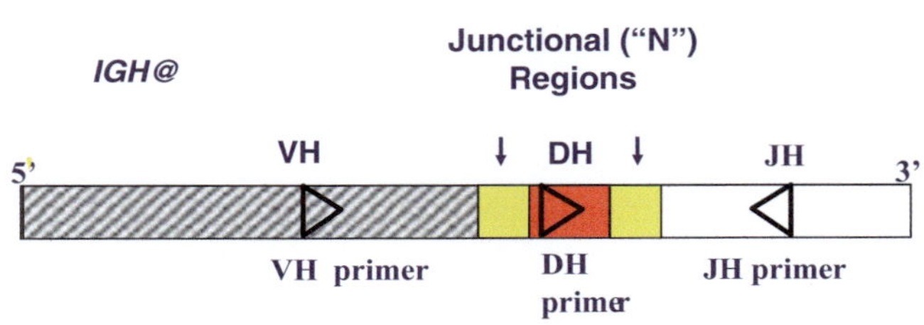

Figure 41.2 Schematic representation of an *IGH* VDJ recombination region and the strategy used to amplify the N regions. Probes for the N regions can be used as patient-specific probes (*boxes* with vertical *arrows* above them indicate N regions)

Reverse transcription-PCR (RT-PCR) requires extraction of total RNA or mRNA from mononuclear cells, reverse transcription of the RNA into complementary DNA (cDNA) and then PCR, followed by a method to detect the RT-PCR product, such as electrophoresis. The sensitivity of the method is specific for each target and can be assessed by amplification of serial dilutions of RNA from diagnostic specimens or cell lines containing the specific translocation into RNA from healthy individuals who do not have the translocation. The presence of a very small number of abnormal cells, in the range of 1 in 10^5 to 1 in 10^6, has been consistently detected using appropriate conditions [88]. This sensitivity is approximately 1000–10,000 times greater than with Southern blot analysis. A PCR test that is sufficiently sensitive to detect one leukemia cell in 10^2–10^3 normal cells is acceptable for diagnostic testing. A higher sensitivity of one leukemia cell in 10^4–10^5 normal cells is required for MRD assessment during follow-up testing [16]. More than one primer set may need to be used to detect all fusion transcripts when the translocation breakpoints can be in different introns of one or both of the fusion genes (Fig. 41.3).

MRD Quantification of *IG* and *TCR* Gene Rearrangements

Real time quantitative PCR (RT-qPCR) of *IG* and *TCR* gene rearrangements can be used to quantify MRD by using allele-specific oligonucleotide (ASO) probes. Sensitivities of one in 10^3–10^5 (Fig. 41.4) are achievable with this strategy [89–94]. Although initial assays used an ASO fluorescent probe to the junctional region, a more useful approach is to use a fluorescent probe complementary to the germline *IGH* and *TCR* gene segments, in combination with an ASO primer complementary to the junctional region [95, 96]. The ASO primer approach theoretically results in more sensitive MRD detection compared with the use of germline primers, because no competition can occur with the amplification of similar rearrangements in normal cells. Although specific amplification can be easily distinguished from incidental nonspecific amplification, conditions with higher stringency of amplification may need to be used to overcome nonspecific amplification while maintaining the efficiency of the method.

Quantification of Leukemia-Specific Translocations for MRD Assessment

Numerous publications have demonstrated the feasibility of the RT-qPCR method to quantify chimeric transcripts resulting from chromosomal translocations that occur in ALL [81, 91]. Although the principles of RT-qPCR are the same whether DNA or RNA is being analyzed, the RT step for RNA represents a major assay variable for accuracy of quantification and sensitivity. In fact, assays must be designed to correct for variations linked to differences in RNA input amount and, more importantly, in efficiency (or inhibition) during RT. For this reason, the number of target gene copies has to be normalized using a ubiquitously and constantly expressed housekeeping gene as a reference (e.g., *ABL1*, *B2M*, and *PBGD*) [97]. The number of chimeric transcripts are expressed in relation to the number of copies of the reference gene transcript.

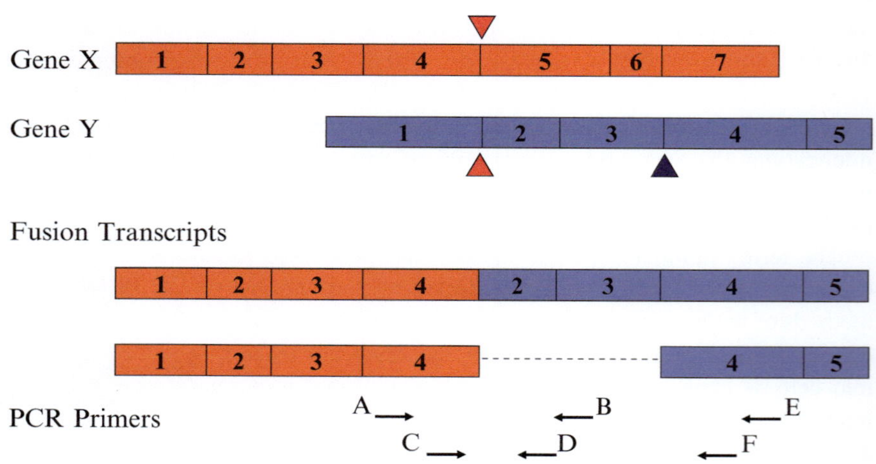

Figure 41.3 RT-PCR detection of different fusion transcripts generated by the same translocation. The possibility of different fusion transcripts requires the use of multiple primer pairs to detect fusion transcripts formed by breakpoints in different introns of the gene(s), depending on the size of the transcript

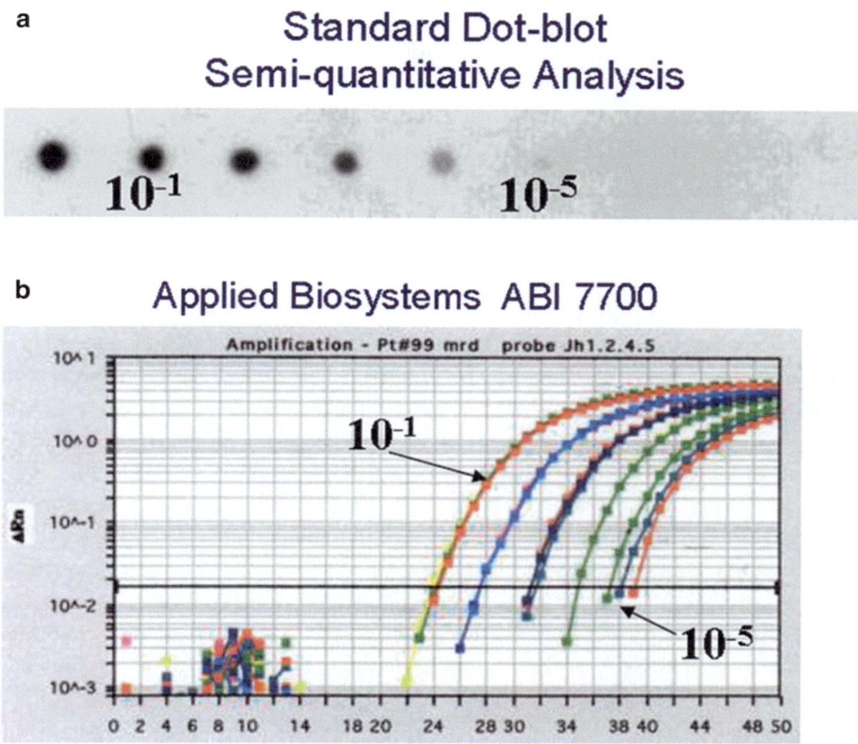

Figure 41.4 Assessement of assay sensitivity by two different methods of a patient-specific *IgH* clonotypic marker. (**a**) semiquantitative dot-blot analysis; (**b**) real-time quantitative PCR using Applied Biosystems ABI 7700

Interpretation of Test Results

PCR for *IG* and *TCR* Gene Rearrangements

Leukemia-specific *IG* and *TCR* gene rearrangements identified at diagnosis can be used for MRD assessment of BM or peripheral blood samples during and following treatment. However, similar *IG* and *TCR* gene rearrangements from normal lymphocytes in these specimens also are amplified. To discriminate between the leukemia-derived PCR products and PCR products of normal cells with rearrangements resulting in comparable size PCR products, the amplified bands are subjected either to "fingerprint" [98–100] or homo-heteroduplex analysis [18, 101, 102]. What was traditionally called fingerprint analysis consists of PCR amplification with a fluorescent primer and analysis by capillary electrophoresis. Clonal amplification results in a single peak, often in a background of polyclonal, constitutional amplification products. The homo-heteroduplex analysis takes advantage of the different migration properties in a polyacrylamide gel of V-J rearrangements containing a few mismatches (heteroduplex) compared with the fully matched V-J junctions (homoduplex) typical of a clone.

A variety of *IG* and *TCR* gene rearrangements can be present at diagnosis in childhood B-precursor ALL. Oligoclonal *IGH* rearrangements have been observed in 30–40 % of cases and *IGK* rearrangements in 5–10 % and are due to VH replacements, VH-DJH junctions, or de novo *IGH* gene rearrangements [18, 103–106]. Oligoclonality for *TRB* and *TRG* gene rearrangements is thought to be rare in B-lineage ALL [107–109, 111]. One exception was reported by Szczepanski et al., who found *TRG* oligoclonality in 38 % of B-lineage ALLs [17]. Oligoclonality of *TRD* is frequently observed in incomplete rearrangements, such as *VD2DD3* or *DD2DD3* [10, 109, 110]. In T-lineage ALL, oligoclonality is rarely seen at diagnosis [107, 111, 24, 25].

Clonal evolution, that is, different clone characteristics at relapse than the original clone characteristics, has been detected in rearrangements of both the *IG* and *TCR* genes. Rearrangements of the *IG* genes are particularly sensitive to clonal evolution, which occurs in more than 30 % of cases. Clonal evolution of rearranged *TCR* genes is less frequent, but observed in 10–25 % of cases. The likelihood of change in gene rearrangements seems to increase with time, but once they occur, further changes are not commonly observed during additional relapses [17, 112–114]. This clonal evolution may be due to the emergence of a new independent clone, due to secondary leukemia, or due to growth of subclones formed by continuous and secondary rearrangements of these genes [115–118].

RT-PCR for Leukemia-Specific Translocations

Several potential pitfalls must be avoided to prevent false-positive and false-negative results with translocation RT-

PCR assays. First, RNA degradation must be prevented by careful specimen handling, including prompt delivery to the laboratory and cooler temperatures. Second, a control mRNA from the same cDNA preparation used for amplification of the fusion transcript should be amplified to assess the integrity of the RNA, the efficiency of the RT step, and the presence of inhibitors.

A major concern has been raised about the clinical utility of RT-PCR MRD translocation testing in ALL patients because fusion transcripts can be detected in the hematopoietic tissues of healthy individuals. Low levels of *BCR/ABL1* transcripts have been detected in a sizable proportion of healthy individuals [119]. Using a two-round (nested) RT-PCR method, the *MLL/AF4* fusion transcript has been detected in the fetal liver and BM of normal infant samples and in 12 % of pediatric ALL with no cytogenetic or genomic evidence of 11q23 alterations [120]. The significance of these findings is still uncertain.

Molecular Detection of MRD and Clinical Studies

Sequential monitoring of MRD using sensitive and specific techniques with a detection power of one blast cell in 10^3–10^6 normal cells, has importantly refined the assessment of response to treatment [78, 121, 122, 89, 123, 124]. The study of MRD has drawn great interest in clinical oncology because of the potential for tailoring treatment and the possibility of gaining insight into the nature of a cure. Several parameters are critical for the interpretation of MRD studies, including the type of disease (ALL or acute myeloid leukemia [AML]), therapeutic context, timing of sampling, the target gene, sensitivity of the assay, interlaboratory standardization (particularly relevant in multicenter studies), the retrospective or prospective nature of the study, and the number of tests conducted for each patient.

Currently, highly sensitive and specific methods for MRD detection are available. Molecular assays have been applied to the identification of two types of "clone-specific" targets in ALL: breakpoint fusion regions arising from chromosomal translocations, especially fusion transcripts generated by the t(9;22), t(4;11), t(1;19), and t(12;21) translocations, and patient-specific sequences reflecting unique recombinations of *IG* and *TCR* genes [81, 90–93, 139]. Flow cytometry, using fluorescence-activated cell sorting analysis can detect abnormal immunophenotype patterns or combinations of these at diagnosis, which could distinguish leukemic cells from normal cells and be used to detect MRD [125–131].

Early response to treatment, based on the rate of disappearance of leukemic cells in the BM has proven to be an independent prognostic factor in childhood ALL and is being used by several groups as a criterion for the stratification of children in risk-adapted therapy. Morphological analysis, although useful and applicable at any center, has proven to be subjective, of limited sensitivity, and imprecise for the assessment of early response to treatment.

A prerequisite for applying MRD measurements in clinical studies is that the data should be available for all patients. In ALL, PCR-based MRD detection with *IG* and *TCR* gene rearrangements can be applied in more than 90 % of childhood and adult ALL cases. Accordingly, most of the clinical studies of MRD in ALL have used one of the different PCR approaches for the detection of *IG* and/or *TCR* gene rearrangements [16, 90–93]. Clinical application of MRD testing in the stratification and treatment of ALL requires reliable, reproducible, and quality-assured methods, including regular quality assessment to ensure the reproducibility and reliability of the MRD results [91, 92, 94, 132, 139, 93].

MRD has been significantly correlated with clinical prognosis, being particularly useful in the evaluation of an early response and thus permitting a refined stratification of treatment for both children and adults. Stratification into risk groups according to criteria not based on MRD has proven less accurate, especially for low-risk patients [45, 46, 133, 79, 80, 90, 134, 135].

During the initial induction treatment for ALL, the level of MRD is the most important independent prognostic factor regardless of age, risk group, or genetic translocations. The detection of high level MRD (10^{-2}–10^{-3}) on day 15 or day 19 of induction therapy is associated with an unfavorable prognosis, and lower levels with excellent prognosis. The "very good responder" patients could be candidates for less intensive treatment protocols. In contrast, children and adults with higher levels of MRD at the end of induction have very poor prognosis even with more intensive treatment protocols, including BMT [79, 80, 122, 136, 137, 138–141]. Reduction or intensification of treatment based on MRD results was investigated in different clinical trials [94, 139, 142].

Post-remission MDR assessments at different time points have been assessed in several clinical trials. The most important predictive time point for relapse in childhood ALL is the level of MRD measured at day 78 [80, 132]. The value of MRD detection at the end of treatment is questionable, because a negative result does not preclude subsequent relapse, thus reducing the utility of MRD detection as a criterion for elective cessation of treatment [113, 114, 137, 143].

MRD is an independent prognostic factor in relapsed patients and in those pre- and post-BMT [80, 82–87, 138, 144–146]. Reduction of MRD levels to less then 0.1 % prior the BMT is thought to be necessary to achieve a better outcome [82, 83, 87, 144]. Prospective studies are ongoing to better address these issues.

RT-qPCR of fusion transcripts generated by the t(9;22), t(4;11), t(1;19), and t(12;21) has been used to assess MRD [26, 81, 97, 147]. In theory, these fusion transcripts represent ideal targets for MRD assessment because they are very specific and absent in normal cells. However, they are present in only 30–40 % of B-lineage ALL and 10–20 % of T-ALL [94]. In addition, due to large breakpoint regions and a high number of potential fusion partners (e.g., *MLL*), fusion gene targets for MRD assessment are applicable only to a small number of patients [94]. The data reported so far have been controversial, leaving unanswered the question of whether MRD assessment based on tumor-specific translocations would help to identify patients with different outcomes within the same genetically defined subgroup and actually have been limited mainly to the quantitative detection of *BCR-ABL1* transcripts in Ph+ ALL [132]. Fusion transcripts almost invariably persist in chemotherapy-treated patients with ALL bearing the t(9;22), and detection of these transcripts correlates with the high relapse rate of this disease subtype in both adults and children [47, 48]. In studies of a large group of children, Ph^+ ALL appeared to be quite heterogeneous with regard to treatment response [54]. Thus, MRD evaluation may help to identify patients persistently negative for the *BCR/ABL1* fusion gene among those with good early responses to treatment, who can be cured with intensive chemotherapy alone. Absence of detectable *BCR/ABL1* transcripts could then be used as a surrogate marker to monitor in vivo response to new drugs in childhood Ph^+ ALL [55, 56].

Early conversion to persistently negative RT-qPCR results for the t(4;11) translocation involving the *MLL* and *AF4* oncogenes (particularly after three months) are associated with prolonged complete clinical remission (CCR). In the Interfant-99 protocol, the use of patient specific primers in combination with MLL probes to detect MRD was able to recognize different risk groups in infant ALL [148, 149].

In ALL patients with the t(1;19) translocation, persistently negative RT-qPCR tests are a good indicator of CCR, but positive tests are not necessarily an accurate predictor of relapse, thus reducing the utility of this test for clinical decision making [40, 41]. Continuous monitoring with accurate quantification may represent the most reliable approach.

Residual disease has been investigated in a limited number of patients with ALL carrying the t(12;21) and the results are controversial. Relapse was observed in cases with persistently positive MRD detection at greater than one in 10^3. However, relapse has been reported to occur even in patients with previously negative tests [47, 48, 150, 151]. Larger prospective studies are needed to fully assess the prognostic value of RT-qPCR testing for the t(12;21) translocation, as well as its value as an overall marker for monitoring MRD in childhood ALL [47, 48, 152].

Laboratory Issues

Although numerous methods to monitor MRD in acute leukemias have been developed in the past decade and new technologies are now being used, standardization and quality control still remain pertinent for clinical molecular testing in hematopathology. This is particularly true in efforts to assure reproducible results within multicenter international studies.

Standardization and quality control in the molecular approach for detection of antigen receptor gene rearrangements was addressed within the BIOMED-1 and BIOMED-2 frameworks and more recently in the EuroMRD effort, which developed and validated MRD strategies and provided guidelines to MRD interpretation [16, 91, 92, 94, 139, 153, 11]. One of the major problems resides in the fact that each patient's leukemia has a unique rearrangement, requiring the use of patient-specific primers and/or probes and individual optimization. Use of patient-specific assays represents a major challenge in uptake of this method in clinical molecular laboratories. In an effort to maximize detection of virtually all ALL patients and to prevent false-negative results, research PCR primers have been designed for multiple targets: *TRD*, *TRG*, and *IGK* rearrangements, as well as the *SIL/TAL* rearrangement [16]. The method uses a total of 54 primers with ASO probes in single or nested PCR for target identification at diagnosis, sequence analysis of junctional regions, and MRD detection in follow-up samples. A total of 25 PCRs are performed at diagnosis to identify the PCR targets. This standardized approach allows rapid detection of clonal *IG* and *TCR* rearrangements in ALL with high sensitivity and high specificity, and enables discrimination between monoclonal and oligoclonal gene rearrangements. The combination of the four PCR target types allowed PCR monitoring in more than 90 % of B-cell precursor ALL and 95 % of T-ALL cases. In the vast majority of childhood and adult ALL cases, two or more PCR targets were available for MRD monitoring. The sensitivity of detecting PCR targets depended at least partially on the size of the junctional region, with a sensitivity of one in 10^4 for most cases. To increase the percentage of cases successfully stratified by MRD, newly identified molecular targets have been incorporated. The monoclonal *VD2-JA* rearrangements in precursor B-ALL were used as patient-specific targets for MRD detection, because they show high sensitivity and good stability [23]. A sensitive *TRB* RT-qPCR assay was developed [154] with utility for MDR studies in those T-ALLs in which the repertoire of *IG* and *TCR* rearrangements is limited and therefore less sensitive.

Careful standardization and quality control of MRD techniques were also the aims of the European BIOMED-1

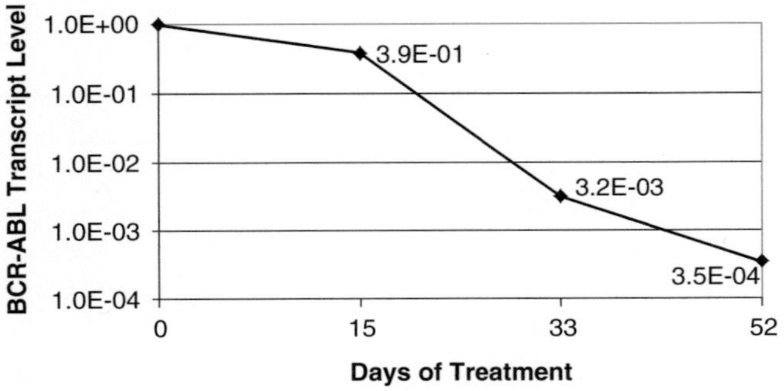

Figure 41.5 Minimal residual disease monitoring by real-time quantitative PCR (RT-qPCR) for a patient with ALL carrying the t(9;22) *BCR-ABL* translocation (p190 Ph+ALL) during the course of treatment

Concerted Action group, with participants from laboratories in several European countries [26]. The five most frequent, well defined ALL chromosomal aberrations with fusion gene transcripts were selected: t(1;19) with *E2A-PBX1*, t(4;11) with *MLL-AF4*, t(9;22) with *BCR-ABL1* (p190 and p210), t(12;21) with *ETV6-RUNX1*, and microdeletion 1p32 with *SIL-TAL1*. PCR primers, positioned to amplify several different transcript versions, were designed according to predefined criteria for single and nested PCR (Fig. 41.3).

The Europe Against Cancer program was established to achieve standardization and quality control for the RT-qPCR technique for detection and quantification of fusion gene transcripts. Twenty-five European laboratories in ten countries collaborated and established consensus standards for RT-qPCR (hydrolysis probe technology) for the main translocations seen in a spectrum of hematologic malignancies, including ALL. A set of 12 primers and nine probes has been selected to cover the most frequent chimeric transcripts, with a threshold of detection of 100 molecules and/or a one in 10^4 dilution [81]. This approach is anticipated to allow accurate quantitative measurement of fusion transcripts with an international consensus protocol for diagnosis and MRD assessment in follow-up samples.

A representative experiment of RT-qPCR detection of the fusion transcript generated by the translocation t(9;22) is shown in Fig. 41.5.

Conclusions and Future Directions

PCR amplification of fusion transcripts resulting from chromosomal translocations and of *IG* and *TCR* gene rearrangements has emerged as a sensitive and reproducible method to monitor MRD in ALL. The measure of the initial response to therapy in patients who have achieved complete remission by morphologic standards can dissect clinical heterogeneity within an apparently genetically homogeneous childhood ALL subgroup. Moreover, MRD monitoring can be applied to the appropriate patient subgroups for early prediction of impending relapses.

However, before any application in clinical decision making, the value of MRD monitoring must be studied in the context of clinical trials. Moreover, high levels of confidence in interpreting MRD results are needed to rule out false-positive and false-negative results, considering the problems and pitfalls of the current technology. In this context, the interpretation of MRD results that are produced by different studies would benefit from international standardization.

MRD analysis should be incorporated in any future clinical trials of ALL investigating a therapeutic question. Moreover, only the combination of simple and reliable MRD methods will allow the potential benefits of MRD monitoring to be extended to all children with leukemia. Finally, genome-based technologies such as microarrays and next generation sequencing will help to identify new genetic lesions in patients who are currently thought to represent the same genetic subtypes of ALL but who differ in MRD clearance and therapeutic response. With such new approaches, new specific markers for MRD monitoring hopefully will be identified.

References

1. Pui CH, Robison LL, Look AT. Acute lymphoblastic leukaemia. Lancet. 2008;371:1030–43.
2. Pui CH, Mullighan CG, Evans WE, et al. Pediatric acute lymphoblastic leukemia: where are we going and how do we get there? Blood. 2012;120:1165–74.
3. Margolin JF, Rabin KR, Steuber CP, et al. Acute lymphoblastic leukemia. In: Pizzo PA, Poplack DG, editors. Principles and practice of pediatric oncology. 6th ed. PA: Lippincott Williams & Wilkins; 2011. p. 518–65.
4. Pui CH, Behm FG, Crist WM. Clinical and biological relevance of immunologic marker studies in childhood acute lymphoblastic leukemia. Blood. 1993;82:343–62.
5. Yeoh EJ, Roos ME, Shurtleff AS, et al. Classification, subtype discovery, and prediction outcome in pediatric acute lymphoblastic leukemia by gene expression profile. Cancer Cell. 2002;1:133–43.
6. Pui CH, Carroll WL, Meshinchi S, et al. Biology, risk stratification, and therapy of pediatric acute leukemias: an update. J Clin Oncol. 2011;29:551–65.
7. Tonegawa S. Somatic generation of antibody diversity. Nature. 1983;302:575–81.
8. van Dongen JJM, Wolvers-Tettero ILM. Analysis of immunoglobulin and T cell receptor genes. Part I: basic and technical aspects. Clin Chim Acta. 1991;198:1–92.
9. van Dongen JJM, Wolvers-Tettero ILM. Analysis of immunoglobulin and T cell receptor genes. Part II: possibilities and limitations in the diagnosis and management of lymphoproliferative diseases and related disorders. Clin Chim Acta. 1991;198:93–174.
10. van Dongen JJM, Langerak AW. Immunoglobulin and T-cell receptor gene rearrangements. In: Pui CH, editor. Childhood leukemias. 2nd ed. Cambridge: Cambridge University Press; 2006. p. 210–34.

11. Langerak AW, Groenen PJ, Brüggemann M, et al. EuroClonality/BIOMED-2 guidelines for interpretation and reporting of Ig/TCR clonality testing in suspected lymphoproliferations. Leukemia. 2012;2012(26):2159–71.
12. van Zelm MC, van der Burg M, de Ridder D, et al. Ig gene rearrangement steps are initiated in early human precursor B cell subsets and correlate with specific transcription factor expression. J Immunol. 2005;175:5912–22.
13. Dik WA, Pike-Overzet K, Weerkamp F, et al. New insights on human T cell development by quantitative T cell receptor gene rearrangement studies and gene expression profiling. J Exp Med. 2005;201:1715–23.
14. Brisco MJ, Tan LW, Orsborn AM, et al. Development of a highly sensitive assay, based on the polymerase chain reaction, for rare B-lymphocyte clones in a polyclonal population. Br J Haematol. 1990;75:163–7.
15. Scrideli CA, Simoes AL, Defavery R, et al. Childhood B lineage acute lymphoblastic leukemia clonality study by the polymerase chain reaction. J Pediatr Hematol Oncol. 1997;19:516–22.
16. Pongers-Willemse MJ, Seriu T, Stolz F, et al. Primers and protocols for standardized MRD detection in ALL using immunoglobulin and T cell receptor gene rearrangements and TAL1 deletions as PCR targets. Report of the BIOMED-1 Concerted Action: Investigation of minimal residual disease in acute leukemia. Leukemia. 1999;13:110–8.
17. Szczepanski T, Beishuizen A, Pongers-Willemse MJ, et al. Crosslineage T-cell receptor gene rearrangements occur in more than ninety percent of childhood precursor-B-acute lymphoblastic leukaemias: alternative PCR targets for detection of minimal residual disease. Leukemia. 1999;13:196–205.
18. Assumpção JG, Ganazza MA, de Araújo M, et al. Detection of clonal immunoglobulin and T-cell receptor gene rearrangements in childhood acute lymphoblastic leukemia using a low-cost PCR strategy. Pediatr Blood Cancer. 2010;55:1278–86.
19. Tkachuck DC, Griesser H, Takirara Y, et al. Rearrangement of T-cell delta locus in lymphoproliferative disorders. Blood. 1988;72:353–7.
20. Biondi A, Francia de Celli P, Rossi V, et al. High prevalence of T-cell receptor V delta 2-(D)-D delta 3 or D delta 1/2-D delta 3 rearrangements in B-precursor acute lymphoblastic leukemias. Blood. 1990;75:1834–40.
21. Trainor KJ, Brisco MJ, Wan JH, et al. Gene rearrangement in B- and T-lymphoproliferative disease detected by the polymerase chain reaction. Blood. 1991;78:192–6.
22. Szczepanki T, LangeraK AW, Wolvers-Tettero IL, et al. Immunoglobulin and T cell receptor gene rearrangement patterns in acute lymphoblastic leukemia are less mature in adults than in children: implications for selection of PCR targets for detection of minimal residual disease. Leukemia. 1998;12:1081–8.
23. Szczepanski T, van der Velden VH, Hoogeveen PG, et al. Vdelta2-Jalpha rearrangements are frequent in precursor-B-acute lymphoblastic leukemia but rare in normal lymphoid cells. Blood. 2004;103:3798–804.
24. Scrideli CA, Queiroz RG, Kashima S, et al. T cell receptor gamma (TCRG) gene rearrangements in Brazilian children with acute lymphoblastic leukemia: analysis and implications for the study of minimal residual disease. Leuk Res. 2004;28:267–73.
25. Scrideli CA, Queiroz RP, Takayanagui OM, et al. Molecular diagnosis of leukemic cerebrospinal fluid cells in children with newly diagnosed acute lymphoblastic leukemia. Haematologica. 2004;89:1013–5.
26. van Dongen JJ, Macintyre EA, Gabert JA, et al. Standardized RT-PCR analysis of fusion gene transcripts from chromosome aberrations in acute leukemia for detection of minimal residual disease. Report of the BIOMED-1 Concerted Action: investigation of minimal residual disease in acute leukemia. Leukemia. 1999;13:1901–28.
27. Yano T, Pullman A, Andade R, et al. A common Vd2-Dd2-Dd3 T cell receptor gene rearrangement in precursor B acute lymphoblastic leukemia. Br J Haematol. 1991;79:44–9.
28. Heerema NA, Sather HN, Sensel MG, et al. Prognostic impact of trisomies of chromosomes 10, 17, and 5 among children with acute lymphoblastic leukemia and high hyperdiploidy (>50 chromosomes). J Clin Oncol. 2000;18:1876–87.
29. Harrison CJ. Cytogenetics of paediatric and adolescent acute lymphoblastic leukaemia. Br J Haematol. 2009;144:147–56.
30. Meijerink JP, den Boer ML, Pieters R. New genetic abnormalities and treatment response in acute lymphoblastic leukemia. Semin Hematol. 2009;46:16–23.
31. Armstrong SA, Look AT. Molecular genetics of acute lymphoblastic leukemia. J Clin Oncol. 2005;23:6306–15.
32. Look AT. Oncogenic transcription factors in the human acute leukaemias. Science. 1997;278:1059–64.
33. Vardiman JW, Thiele J, Arber DA, et al. The 2008 revision of the World Health Organization (WHO) classification of myeloid neoplasms and acute leukemia: rationale and important changes. Blood. 2009;114:937–51.
34. Borkhardt A, Cazzaniga G, Viehmann S, et al. Incidence and clinical relevance of TEL/AML1 fusion genes in children with acute lymphoblastic leukemia enrolled in the German and Italian multicenter therapy trials. Associazione Italiana Ematologia Oncologia Pediatrica and the Berlin-Frankfurt-Munster Study Group. Blood. 1997;90:571–77.
35. Raynaud S, Mauvieux L, Cayuela JM, et al. TEL/AML1 fusion gene is a rare event in adult acute lymphoblastic leukemia. Leukemia. 1996;10:1529–30.
36. Mullighan CG. Molecular genetics of B-precursor acute lymphoblastic leukemia. J Clin Invest. 2012;122:3407–15.
37. Mullighan CG. The molecular genetic makeup of acute lymphoblastic leukemia. Hematology Am Soc Hematol Educ Program. 2012;2012:389–96.
38. Greaves MF, Maia AT, Wiemels JL, et al. Leukemia in twins: lessons in natural history. Blood. 2003;102:2321–33.
39. Seeger K, Adams HP, Buchwald D, et al. TEL-AML1 fusion transcript in relapsed childhood acute lymphoblastic leukemia. The Berlin–Frankfurt–Munster Study Group. Blood. 1998;91:1716–22.
40. Hunger SP, Fall MZ, Camitta BM, et al. E2A-PBX1 chimeric transcript status at end of consolidation is not predictive of treatment outcome in childhood acute lymphoblastic leukemias with a t(1;19)(q23;p13): a Pediatric Oncology Group study. Blood. 1998;91:1021–8.
41. Privitera E, Luciano A, Ronchetti D, et al. Molecular variants of the 1;19 chromosomal translocation in pediatric acute lymphoblastic leukemia (ALL). Leukemia. 1994;8:554–9.
42. Pui CH, Sandlund JT, Pei D, et al. Results of therapy for acute lymphoblastic leukemia in black and white children. JAMA. 2003;290:2001–7.
43. Raimondi SC, Privitera E, Williams DL, et al. New recurring chromosomal translocations in childhood acute lymphoblastic leukemia. Blood. 1991;77:2016–22.
44. Behm FG, Raimondi SC, Frestedt JL, et al. Rearrangement of the MLL gene confers a poor prognosis in childhood acute lymphoblastic leukemia, regardless of presenting age. Blood. 1996;87:2870–7.
45. Biondi A, Cimino G, Pieters R, et al. Biological and therapeutic aspects of infant leukemia. Blood. 2000;96:24–33.
46. Biondi A, Valsecchi MG, Seriu T, et al. Molecular detection of minimal residual disease is a strong predictive factor of relapse in childhood B-lineage acute lymphoblastic leukemia with medium risk features. A case control study of the International BFM Study Group. Leukemia. 2000;14:1939–43.
47. Cazzaniga G, Lanciotti M, Rossi V, et al. Prospective molecular monitoring of BCR/ABL transcript in children with Ph+ acute

lymphoblastic leukaemia unravels differences in treatment response. BrJ Haematol. 2002;119:445–53.
48. Cazzaniga G, Rossi V, Biondi A. Monitoring minimal residual disease using chromosomal translocations in childhood ALL. Best Pract Res Clin Haematol. 2002;15:21–35.
49. Mann G, Attarbaschi A, Schrappe M, et al. Improved outcome with hematopoietic stem cell transplantation in a poor prognostic subgroup of infants with mixed-lineage-leukemia (MLL)-rearranged acute lymphoblastic leukemia: results from the Interfant-99 Study. Blood. 2010;116:2644–50.
50. Deininger MW, Goldman JM, Melo JV. The molecular biology of chronic myeloid leukemia. Blood. 2000;96:3343–56.
51. Scrideli CA, Cazzaniga G, Fazio G, et al. Gene expression profile unravels significant differences between childhood and adult Ph+ acute lymphoblastic leukemia. Leukemia. 2003;17:2234–7.
52. Scrideli CA, Queiroz RG, Bernardes JE, et al. PCR detection of clonal IgH and TCR gene rearrangements at the end of induction as a non-remission criterion in children with ALL: comparison with standard morphologic analysis and risk group classification. Med Pediatr Oncol. 2003;41:10–6.
53. Scrideli CA, Queiroz RP, Takayanagui OM, et al. Polymerase chain reaction on cerebrospinal fluid cells in suspected leptomeningeal involvement in childhood acute lymphoblastic leukemia: comparison to cytomorphological analysis. Diagn Mol Pathol. 2003;12:124–7.
54. Schrappe M, Arico M, Harbott J, et al. Philadelphia chromosome-positive (Ph+) childhood acute lymphoblastic leukemia: good initial steroid response allows early prediction of a favorable treatment outcome. Blood. 1998;92:2730–41.
55. Schultz KR, Bowman WP, Aledo A, et al. Improved early event-free survival with imatinib in Philadelphia chromosome-positive acute lymphoblastic leukemia: a children's oncology group study. J Clin Oncol. 2009;27:5175–81.
56. Biondi A, Schrappe M, De Lorenzo P, et al. Imatinib after induction for treatment of children and adolescents with Philadelphia-chromosome-positive acute lymphoblastic leukaemia (EsPhALL): a randomised, open-label, intergroup study. Lancet Oncol. 2012;13:936–45.
57. Mullighan CG, Su X, Zhang J, et al. Deletion of IKZF1 and prognosis in acute lymphoblastic leukemia. N Engl J Med. 2009;360:470–80.
58. Den Boer ML, van Slegtenhorst M, De Menezes RX, et al. A subtype of childhood acute lymphoblastic leukaemia with poor treatment outcome: a genome-wide classification study. Lancet Oncol. 2009;10:125–34.
59. Cline MJ. The molecular basis of leukaemia. N Engl J Med. 1994;330:328–36.
60. Scrideli CA, Tone LG. Molecular basis of acute lymphoblastic leukemia. In: Novak E, Rego EM, editors. Physiopathogenesis of hematological cancer. 1st ed. Sharjah: Bentham Science; 2012. p. 168–82.
61. Mullighan CG, Downing JR. Genome-wide profiling of genetic alterations in acute lymphoblastic leukemia: recent insights and future directions. Leukemia. 2009;23:1209–18.
62. Ferrando AA, Look AT. Gene expression profiling in T-cell acute lymphoblastic leukemia. Semin Hematol. 2003;40:274–80.
63. Ferrando AA, Look AT. DNA microarrays in the diagnosis and management of acute lymphoblastic leukemia. Int J Hematol. 2004;80:395–400.
64. Van Vlierberghe P, Pieters R, Beverloo HB, et al. Molecular-genetic insights in paediatric T-cell acute lymphoblastic leukaemia. Br J Haematol. 2008;143:153–68.
65. Van Vlierberghe P, van Grotel M, Tchinda J, et al. The recurrent SET-NUP214 fusion as a new HOXA activation mechanism in pediatric T-cell acute lymphoblastic leukemia. Blood. 2008;111: 4668–80.
66. Ferrando AA, Neuberg DS, Staunton J, et al. Gene expression signatures define novel oncogenic pathways in T cell acute lymphoblastic leukemia. Cancer Cell. 2002;1:75–87.
67. Meijerink JP. Genetic rearrangements in relation to immunophenotype and outcome in T-cell acute lymphoblastic leukaemia. Best Pract Res Clin Haematol. 2010;23:307–18.
68. Homminga I, Vuerhard MJ, Langerak AW, et al. Characterization of a pediatric T-cell acute lymphoblastic leukemia patient with simultaneous LYL1 and LMO2 rearrangements. Haematologica. 2012;97:258–61.
69. Zhang J, Ding L, Holmfeldt L, et al. The genetic basis of early T-cell precursor acute lymphoblastic leukaemia. Nature. 2012;481:157–63.
70. Heerema NA, Sather HN, Sensel MG, et al. Frequency and clinical significance of cytogenetic abnormalities in pediatric T-lineage acute lymphoblastic leukemia: a report from the Children's Cancer Group. J Clin Oncol. 1998;16:1270–8.
71. Karrman K, Forestier E, Heyman M, et al. Clinical and cytogenetic features of a population-based consecutive series of 285 pediatric T-cell acute lymphoblastic leukemias: rare T-cell receptor gene rearrangements are associated with poor outcome. Genes Chromosomes Cancer. 2009;48:795–805.
72. Soulier J, Clappier E, Cayuela JM, et al. HOXA genes are included in genetic and biologic networks defining human acute T-cell leukemia (T-ALL). Blood. 2005;106:274–86.
73. Jotta PY, Ganazza MA, Silva A, et al. Negative prognostic impact of PTEN mutation in pediatric T-cell acute lymphoblastic leukemia. Leukemia. 2010;24:239–42.
74. Zenatti PP, Ribeiro D, Li W, et al. Oncogenic IL7R gain-of-function mutations in childhood T-cell acute lymphoblastic leukemia. Nat Genet. 2011;43:932–9.
75. Biojone E, Queiróz Rde P, Valera ET, et al. Minimal residual disease in cerebrospinal fluid at diagnosis: a more intensive treatment protocol was able to eliminate the adverse prognosis in children with acute lymphoblastic leukemia. Leuk Lymphoma. 2012;53:89–95.
76. Cave H, van der Werff Ten Bosch J, Suciu S, et al. Clinical significance of minimal residual disease in childhood acute lymphoblastic leukemia. N Engl J Med. 1998;339:591–8.
77. van Dongen JJ, Seriu T, Panzer-Grumayer ER, et al. Prognostic value of minimal residual disease in acute lymphoblastic leukaemia in childhood. Lancet. 1998;352:1731–8.
78. Flohr T, Schrauder A, Cazzaniga G, et al. Minimal residual disease-directed risk stratification using real-time quantitative PCR analysis of immunoglobulin and T-cell receptor gene rearrangements in the international multicenter trial AIEOP-BFM ALL 2000 for childhood acute lymphoblastic leukemia. Leukemia. 2008;22:771–82.
79. Scrideli CA, Assumpção JG, Ganazza MA, et al. A simplified minimal residual disease polymerase chain reaction method at early treatment points can stratify children with acute lymphoblastic leukemia into good and poor outcome groups. Haematologica. 2009;94:781–9.
80. Conter V, Bartram CR, Valsecchi MG, et al. Molecular response to treatment redefines all prognostic factors in children and adolescents with B-cell precursor acute lymphoblastic leukemia: results in 3184 patients of the AIEOP-BFM ALL 2000 study. Blood. 2010;115:3206–14.
81. Gabert J, Beillard E, van der Velden VH, et al. Standardization and quality control studies of "real-time" quantitative reverse transcriptase polymerase chain reaction of fusion gene transcripts for residual disease detection in leukemia—a Europe Against Cancer program. Leukemia. 2003;17:2318–57.
82. Knechtli CJ, Goulden NJ, Hancock JP, et al. Minimal residual disease status as a predictor of relapse after allogeneic bone marrow transplantation for children with acute lymphoblastic leukaemia. Br J Haematol. 1998;102:860–71.

83. Knechtli CJ, Goulden NJ, Hancock JP, et al. Minimal residual disease status before allogeneic bone marrow transplantation is an important determinant of successful outcome for children and adolescents with acute lymphoblastic leukemia. Blood. 1998;92:4072–9.
84. van der Velden VHJ, Joosten SA, Willemse MJ, et al. Real-time quantitative PCR for detection of minimal residual disease before allogeneic stem cell transplantation predicts outcome in children with acute lymphoblastic leukemia. Leukemia. 2001;15:1485–7.
85. Paganin M, Zecca M, Fabbri G, et al. Minimal residual disease is an important predictive factor of outcome in children with relapsed 'high-risk' acute lymphoblastic leukemia. Leukemia. 2008;22:2193–200.
86. Ruggeri A, Michel G, Dalle JH, et al. Impact of pre-transplant minimal residual disease after cord blood transplantation for childhood acute lymphoblastic leukemia in remission. An Eurocord, PDWP-EBMT analysis. Leukemia. 2012;26:2455–61.
87. Buckley SA, Appelbaum FR, Walter RB. Prognostic and therapeutic implications of minimal residual disease at the time of transplantation in acute leukemia. Bone Marrow Transplant. 2013;48:630–41.
88. Sklar J. Polymerase chain reaction: the molecular microscope of residual disease. J Clin Oncol. 1991;1:1521–23.
89. Eckert C, Scrideli CA, Taube T, et al. Comparison between TaqMan and LightCycler technologies for quantification of minimal residual disease by using immunoglobulin and T-cell receptor genes consensus probes. Leukemia. 2003;17:2517–24.
90. Cazzaniga G, Biondi A. Molecular monitoring of childhood acute lymphoblastic leukemia using antigen receptor gene rearrangements and quantitative polymerase chain reaction technology. Haematologica. 2005;90:382–90.
91. van der Velden VH, Hochhaus A, Cazzaniga G, et al. Detection of minimal residual disease in hematologic malignancies by real-time quantitative PCR: principles, approaches, and laboratory aspects. Leukemia. 2003;17:1013–34.
92. van der Velden VH, Cazzaniga G, Schrauder A, et al. Analysis of minimal residual disease by Ig/TCR gene rearrangements: guidelines for interpretation of real-time quantitative PCR data. Leukemia. 2007;21:604–11.
93. Garand R, Beldjord K, Cavé H, et al. Flow cytometry and IG/TCR quantitative PCR for minimal residual disease quantitation in acute lymphoblastic leukemia: a French multicenter prospective study on behalf of the FRALLE, EORTC and GRAALL. Leukemia. 2013;27:370–6.
94. Brüggemann M, Gökbuget N, Kneba M. Acute lymphoblastic leukemia: monitoring minimal residual disease as a therapeutic principle. Semin Oncol. 2012;39:47–57.
95. Pongers-Willemse MJ, Verhagen OJ, Tibbe GJ, et al. Real-time quantitative PCR for the detection of minimal residual disease in acute lymphoblastic leukemia using junctional region specific TaqMan probes. Leukemia. 1998;12:2006–14.
96. Verhagen OJ, Willemse MJ, Breunis WB, et al. Application of germline IgH probes in real-time quantitative PCR for the detection of minimal residual disease in acute lymphoblastic leukemia. Leukemia. 2000;14:1426–35.
97. Beillard E, Pallisgaard N, van der Velden VH, et al. Evaluation of candidate control genes for diagnosis and residual disease detection in leukemic patients using "real-time" quantitative reverse- transcriptase polymerase chain reaction (RQ-PCR)—a Europe Against Cancer program. Leukemia. 2003;17:2474–86.
98. Guidal C, Vilmer E, Grandchamp B, et al. A competitive PCR-based method using TCRD, TCRG and IGH rearrangements for rapid detection of patients with high levels of minimal residual disease in acute lymphoblastic leukemia. Leukemia. 2002;16:762–4.
99. Landman-Parker J, Aubin J, Delabesse E, et al. Simplified strategies for minimal residual disease detection in B cell precursor acute lymphoblastic leukaemia. Br J Haematol. 1996;95: 281–90.
100. Evans PA, Short MA, Owen RG, et al. Residual disease detection using fluorescent polymerase chain reaction at 20 weeks of therapy predicts clinical outcome in childhood acute lymphoblastic leukemia. J Clin Oncol. 1998;16:3616–27.
101. Bottaro M, Berti E, Biondi A, et al. Heteroduplex analysis of T-cell receptor gamma gene rearrangements for diagnosis and monitoring of cutaneous T-cell lymphomas. Blood. 1994;83:3271–8.
102. Langerak AW, Szczepański T, van der Burg M, et al. Heteroduplex PCR analysis of rearranged T cell receptor genes for clonality assessment in suspect T cell proliferations. Leukemia. 1997;11:2192–9.
103. Kitchingman GR, Mirro J, Stass S, et al. Biologic and prognostic significance of the presence of more than two mu heavy-chain genes in childhood acute lymphoblastic leukemia of B precursor cell origin. Blood. 1986;67:698–703.
104. Kuang S, Gu L, Dong S, et al. Long-term follow-up of minimal residual disease in childhood acute lymphoblastic leukemia patients by polymerase chain reaction analysis of multiple clone-specific or malignancy-specific gene markers. Cancer Genet Cytogenet. 1996;88:110–7.
105. Green E, McConville CM, Powell JE, et al. Clonal diversity of Ig and T-cell-receptor gene rearrangements identifies a subset of childhood B-precursor acute lymphoblastic leukemia with increased risk of relapse. Blood. 1998;92:952–8.
106. Scrideli CA, Defavery R, Bernardes JE, et al. Prognostic significance of bi/oligoclonality in childhood acute lymphoblastic leukemia as determined by polymerase chain reaction. Sao Paulo Med J. 2001;119:175–80.
107. Brumpt C, Delabesse E, Beldjord K, et al. The incidence of clonal T-cell receptor rearrangements in B-cell precursor acute lymphoblastic leukemia varies with age and genotype. Blood. 2000;96:2254–61.
108. Beishuizen A, Verhoeven MA, Van Wering ER, et al. Analysis of Ig and T cell receptor genes in 40 childhood acute lymphoblastic leukemia at diagnosis and subsequent relapse: implications for the detection of minimal residual disease by polymerase chain reaction analysis. Blood. 1994;83:2238–47.
109. Steward CG, Goulden NJ, Katz F, et al. A polymerase chain reaction study of the stability of Ig heavy-chain and T cell receptor delta gene rearrangements between presentation and relapse of childhood B-lineage acute lymphoblastic leukemia. Blood. 1994;83:1355–62.
110. Ghali DW, Panzer S, Fischer S, et al. Heterogeneity of the T cell receptor delta gene indicating subclone formation in acute precursor B cell leukemias. Blood. 1995;85:2795–801.
111. Hara J, Benedict SH, Yumura K, et al. Rearrangement of variable region T cell receptor γ genes in acute lymphoblastic leukemia. Vγ gene usage differs in mature and immature T cells. J Clin Invest. 1999;83:1277–83.
112. Marshall GM, Kwan E, Haber M, et al. Characterization of clonal immunoglobulin heavy chain and I cell receptor gamma gene rearrangements during progression of childhood acute lymphoblastic leukemia. Leukemia. 1995;9:1847–50.
113. Scrideli CA, Kashima S, Cipolloti R, et al. Minimal residual disease in Brazilian children with acute lymphoid leukemia: comparison of three detection methods by PCR. Leuk Res. 2002;26:431–8.
114. Scrideli CA, Kashima S, Cipolloti R, et al. Clonal evolution as the limiting factor in the detection of minimal residual disease by polymerase chain reaction in children in Brazil with acute lymphoid leukemia. J Pediatr Hematol Oncol. 2002;24:364–7.

115. Steenbergen EJ, Verhagen OJ, Van Leeuwen EF, et al. Distinct ongoing Ig heavy chain rearrangement processes in childhood B-precursor acute lymphoblastic leukemia. Blood. 1993;82:581–9.
116. Lo Nigro L, Cazzaniga G, Di Cataldo A, et al. Clonal stability in children with acute lymphoblastic leukemia (ALL) who relapsed five or more years after diagnosis. Leukemia. 1999;13:190–5.
117. Choi Y, Greenberg SJ, Du TL, Ward PM, et al. Clonal evolution in B- lineage acute lymphoblastic leukemia by contemporaneous VH-VH gene replacements and VH-DJH gene rearrangements. Blood. 1996;87:2506–12.
118. Height SE, Swanbury GJ, Matute E, et al. Analysis of clonal rearrangements of the Ig heavy chain locus in acute leukemia. Blood. 1996;87:5242–50.
119. Bose S, Deininger M, Gora-Tybor J, et al. The presence of typical and atypical BCR-ABL fusion genes in leukocytes of normal individuals: biologic significance and implications for the assessment of minimal residual disease. Blood. 1998;92:3362–67.
120. Uckun FM, Herman-Hatten K, Crotty ML, et al. Clinical significance of MLL-AF4 fusion transcript expression in the absence of a cytogenetically detectable t(4;11)(q21;q23) chromosomal translocation. Blood. 1998;92:810–21.
121. Campana D, Pui CH. Detection of minimal residual disease in acute leukaemia: methodological and clinical significance. Blood. 1995;85:1416–34.
122. Szczepanski T. Why and how to quantify minimal residual disease in acute lymphoblastic leukemia? Leukemia. 2007;21:622–6.
123. Fronkova E, Mejstrikova E, Avigad S, et al. Minimal residual disease (MRD) analysis in the non-MRD-based ALL IC-BFM 2002 protocol for childhood ALL: is it possible to avoid MRD testing? Leukemia. 2008;22:989–97.
124. Moppett J, Burke GA, Steward CG, et al. The clinical relevance of detection of minimal residual disease in childhood acute lymphoblastic leukaemia. J Clin Pathol. 2003;56:249–53.
125. Bjorklund E, Mazur J, Soderhall S, et al. Flow cytometric follow-up of minimal residual disease in bone marrow gives prognostic information in children with acute lymphoblastic leukemia. Leukemia. 2003;17:138–48.
126. Coustan-Smith E, Sancho J, Behm FG, et al. Prognostic importance of measuring early clearance of leukemic cells by flow cytometry in childhood acute lymphoblastic leukemia. Blood. 2002;100:52–8.
127. Coustan-Smith E, Ribeiro RC, Stow P, et al. A simplified flow cytometric assay identifies children with acute lymphoblastic leukemia who have a superior clinical outcome. Blood. 2006;108:97–102.
128. Porwit-MacDonald A, Bjorklund E, Lucio P, et al. BIOMED-1 concerted action report: flow cytometric characterization of CD7+ cell subsets in normal bone marrow as a basis for the diagnosis and follow-up of T cell acute lymphoblastic leukemia (T-ALL). Leukemia. 2000;14:816–25.
129. Lucio P, Gaipa G, van Lochem EG, van Wering ER, Porwit-MacDonald A, Faria T, et al. BIOMED-I concerted action report: flow cytometric immunophenotyping of precursor B-ALL with standardized triple-stainings. BIOMED-1 Concerted Action Investigation of Minimal Residual Disease in Acute Leukemia: International Standardization and Clinical Evaluation. Leukemia. 2001;15:1185–92.
130. Malec M, van der Velden VH, Bjorklund E, et al. Analysis of minimal residual disease in childhood acute lymphoblastic leukemia: comparison between RQ-PCR analysis of Ig/TcR gene rearrangements and multicolor flow cytometric immunophenotyping. Leukemia. 2004;18:1630–6.
131. Kerst G, Kreyenberg H, Roth C, et al. Concurrent detection of minimal residual disease (MRD) in childhood acute lymphoblastic leukaemia by flow cytometry and real-time PCR. Br J Haematol. 2005;128:774–82.
132. Schrappe M. Minimal residual disease: optimal methods, timing, and clinical relevance for an individual patient. Hematology Am Soc Hematol Educ Program. 2012;2012:137–42.
133. Szczepanski T, Orfao A, van der Velden VH, et al. Minimal residual disease in leukaemia patients. Lancet Oncol. 2001;2:409–17.
134. Zhou J, Goldwasser MA, Li A, et al. Quantitative analysis of minimal residual disease predicts relapse in children with B-lineage acute lymphoblastic leukemia in DFCI ALL Consortium Protocol 95-01. Blood. 2007;110:1607–11.
135. Schultz KR, Pullen DJ, Sather HN, et al. Risk- and response-based classification of childhood B-precursor acute lymphoblastic leukemia: a combined analysis of prognostic markers from the Pediatric Oncology Group (POG) and Children's Cancer Group (CCG). Blood. 2007;109:926–35.
136. Panzer-Grumayer ER, Schneider M, Panzer S, et al. Rapid molecular response during early induction chemotherapy predicts a good outcome in childhood acute lymphoblastic leukemia. Blood. 2000;95:790–4.
137. Sutton R, Venn NC, Tolisano J, et al. Clinical significance of minimal residual disease at day 15 and at the end of therapy in childhood acute lymphoblastic leukaemia. Br J Haematol. 2009;146:292–9.
138. Borowitz MJ, Devidas M, Hunger SP, et al. Clinical significance of minimal residual disease in childhood acute lymphoblastic leukemia and its relationship to other prognostic factors: a Children's Oncology Group study. Blood. 2008;111:5477–85.
139. Bruggemann M, Raff T, Flohr T, et al. Clinical significance of minimal residual disease quantification in adult patients with standard-risk acute lymphoblastic leukemia. Blood. 2006;107:1116–23.
140. Raff T, Gokbuget N, Luschen S, et al. Molecular relapse in adult standard-risk ALL patients detected by prospective MRD monitoring during and after maintenance treatment: data from the GMALL 06/99 and 07/03 trials. Blood. 2007;109:910–5.
141. Specchia G, Liso A, Pannunzio A, et al. Molecular detection of minimal residual disease is associated with early relapse in adult acute lymphoblastic leukemia. Haematologica. 2004;89:1271–3.
142. Vora A, Goulden N, Wade R, et al. Treatment reduction for children and young adults with low-risk acute lymphoblastic leukaemia defined by minimal residual disease (UKALL 2003): a randomised controlled trial. Lancet Oncol. 2013;14:199–209.
143. Ryan J, Quinn F, Meunier A, et al. Minimal residual disease detection in childhood acute lymphoblastic leukaemia patients at multiple time-points reveals high levels of concordance between molecular and immunophenotypic approaches. Br J Haematol. 2009;144:107–15.
144. Bader P, Kreyenberg H, Henze GH, ALL-REZ BFM Study Group, et al. Prognostic value of minimal residual disease quantification before allogeneic stem-cell transplantation in relapsed childhood acute lymphoblastic leukemia: the ALL-REZ BFM Study Group. J Clin Oncol. 2009;27:377–84.
145. Eckert C, Biondi A, Seeger K, et al. Prognostic value of minimal residual disease in relapsed childhood acute lymphoblastic leukaemia. Lancet. 2001;358:1239–41.
146. Coustan-Smith E, Gajjar A, Hijiya N, et al. Clinical significance of minimal residual disease in childhood acute lymphoblastic leukemia after first relapse. Leukemia. 2004;18:499–504.
147. Pallisgaard N, Clausen N, Schroder H, et al. Rapid and sensitive minimal residual disease detection in acute leukaemia by quantitative real-time RT-PCR exemplified by t(12;21) TEL-AML1 fusion transcript. Genes Chromosomes Cancer. 1999;26:355–65.

148. Cimino G, Elia L, Rapanotti MC, et al. A prospective study of residual-disease monitoring of the ALL1/AF4 transcript in patients with t(4;11) acute lymphoblastic leukemia. Blood. 2000;95:96–101.
149. van der Velden VH, Corral L, Valsecchi MG, et al. Prognostic significance of minimal residual disease in infants with acute lymphoblastic leukemia treated within the Interfant-99 protocol. Leukemia. 2009;23(6):1073–9.
150. de Haas V, Breunis WB, Dee R, et al. The TEL-AML1 real-time quantitative polymerase chain reaction (PCR) might replace the antigen receptor-based genomic PCR in clinical minimal residual disease studies in children with acute lymphoblastic leukaemia. Br J Haematol. 2002;116:87–93.
151. Madzo J, Zuna J, Muzíková K, et al. Slower molecular response to treatment predicts poor outcome in patients with TEL/AML1 positive acute lymphoblastic leukemia: prospective real-time quantitative reverse transcriptase-polymerase chain reaction study. Cancer. 2003;97:105–13.
152. Taube T, Eckert C, Korner G, et al. Real-time quantification of TEL-AML1 fusion transcripts for MRD detection in relapsed childhood acute lymphoblastic leukaemia. Comparison with antigen receptor-based MRD quantification methods. Leuk Res. 2004;28:699–706.
153. van Dongen JJ, Langerak AW, Brüggemann M, et al. Design and standardization of PCR primers and protocols for detection of clonal immunoglobulin and T-cell receptor gene recombinations in suspect lymphoproliferations: report of the BIOMED-2 Concerted Action BMH4-CT98-3936. Leukemia. 2003;17:2257–317.
154. Bruggemann M, van der Velden VH, Raff T, et al. Rearranged T-cell receptor beta genes represent powerful targets for quantification of minimal residual disease in childhood and adult T-cell acute lymphoblastic leukemia. Leukemia. 2004;18:709–19.

B-Cell Malignancies

42

Jennifer B. Dunlap, Guang Fan, Nicky Leeborg, and Rita M. Braziel

Abstract

The mature B-cell neoplasms include numerous subtypes of B-cell leukemias and lymphomas (BCL), as well as plasma cell neoplasms. BCL represent 80–90 % of mature lymphoid leukemias and non-Hodgkin lymphomas (NHL) in the Western world. BCL subtypes include numerous distinct diseases, with different biologies, natural histories, morphologic characteristics, immunophenotypes, genetic features, prognoses, and responses to therapy. BCL also include the majority of immunodeficiency-associated lymphomas. Accurate subclassification of BCL has been a challenge for pathologists, resulting in early application of new techniques in molecular analysis to improve diagnostic accuracy. Today, the molecular features of BCL are used to aid in rendering an accurate diagnosis, to predict prognosis, to help determine optimal therapy, and to assess for minimal residual disease (MRD) after therapy. The molecular abnormalities in BCL have commonly been evaluated for clinical purposes, including those occurring in genes coding for antigen receptor (AgR) molecules and those occurring in oncogenes and tumor suppressor genes. This chapter will discuss current molecular testing methods for BCL, as well as some of the newer methods being developed for BCL.

Keywords

B-cell leukemia • B-cell lymphoma • Non-Hodgkin lymphoma • Molecular testing • Immunodeficiency-associated lymphoma • Oncogenes • Tumor suppressor genes • Immunoglobulin receptor gene rearrangement

Introduction

The mature B-cell neoplasms include numerous subtypes of B-cell leukemias and lymphomas (BCL), as well as plasma cell neoplasms. BCL represent 80–90 % of mature lymphoid leukemias and non-Hodgkin lymphomas (NHL) in the Western world. BCL subtypes include numerous distinct diseases, with different biologies, natural histories, morphologic characteristics, immunophenotypes, genetic features, prognoses, and responses to therapy. BCL also include the majority of immunodeficiency-associated lymphomas. The currently accepted subtypes of BCL are defined according to the World Health Organization (WHO) Classification of Tumours of Haematopoietic and Lymphoid Tissues [1] and are listed in Table 42.1. Accurate subclassification of BCL has been a challenge for pathologists, resulting in early application of new techniques in molecular analysis to improve diagnostic accuracy. Today, the molecular features of BCL are used to aid in rendering an accurate diagnosis, to predict prognosis, to help determine optimal therapy, and to assess for minimal residual disease (MRD) after therapy. The molecular abnormalities in BCL have commonly been

J.B. Dunlap, M.D.
Division of Hematopathology, Oregon Health & Sciences University, Portland, OR USA

G. Fan, M.D., Ph.D. • N. Leeborg, M.D. • R.M. Braziel, M.D. (✉)
Division of Hematopathology, Department of Pathology, Oregon Health & Science University, 3181 Sw Sam Jackson Pk Rd, Portland, OR 97239, USA
e-mail: braziel@ohsu.edu

D.G.B. Leonard (ed.), *Molecular Pathology in Clinical Practice*, DOI 10.1007/978-3-319-19674-9_42

Table 42.1 World Health Organization classification of B-cell malignancies

	Abbreviations used in text
Precursor B-cell lymphoblastic leukemia/lymphoma	Pre-B ALL/LBL
Mature B-cell neoplasms	
Chronic lymphocytic leukemia/small lymphocytic lymphoma	CLL/SLL
B-cell prolymphocytic leukemia	PLL
Hairy cell leukemia	HCL
Lymphoplasmacytic lymphoma	LPL
Plasma cell myeloma/plasmacytoma	PCM
Splenic marginal zone lymphoma	SMZL
Extranodal marginal zone lymphoma of mucosa-associated lymphoid tissue	MALToma
Nodal marginal zone lymphoma	NMZL
Follicular lymphoma	FL
Primary cutaneous follicle center lymphoma	PCFL
Mantle cell lymphoma	MCL
Diffuse large B-cell lymphoma	DLBCL
Lymphomatoid granulomatosis	LyG
Primary mediastinal (thymic) large B-cell lymphoma	PMLBCL
Intravascular large B-cell lymphoma	IBCL
ALK positive large B-cell lymphoma	ALK-DLBCL
Plasmablastic lymphoma	PBL
Large B-cell lymphoma arising in HHV-8-associated Castleman disease	HHV-8-DLBCL
Primary effusion lymphoma	PEL
Burkitt lymphoma	BL
B-cell lymphoma, unclassifiable, with features intermediate between DLBCL and BL	HGBCLU
B-cell lymphoma, unclassifiable, with features intermediate between DLBCL and classical Hodgkin lymphoma	
Immunodeficiency-associated B-cell lymphoproliferative disorders (LPD)	
LPD associated with primary immune disorders	
Lymphomas associated with HIV infection	
Post-transplant LPD	PTLD
Other iatrogenic immunodeficiency-associated LPD	

evaluated for clinical purposes, including those occurring in genes coding for antigen receptor (AgR) molecules and those occurring in oncogenes and tumor suppressor genes. However, it must be noted that the recent development of techniques such as microarray gene expression profiling, multiplex genetic mutation testing, and array-based comparative genomic hybridization (aCGH) has resulted in a significant expansion of knowledge about the biology of the different BCL and the number of clinically important molecular markers.

Molecular Basis of Disease

B-Cell Antigen Receptor Genes

AgRs are the primary effector molecules of the adaptive immune system and consist of multi-subunit glycoprotein molecules present on all T and B lymphocytes [2]. Each lymphocyte has a unique antigen receptor molecule on its membrane. B-cell AgRs are membrane-bound immunoglobulins (Ig), which include the heavy chain gene (*IGH*) at 14q32, the kappa light chain gene (*IGK*) at 2p11, and the lambda light chain gene (*IGL*) at 22q11. Each AgR gene in germline configuration consists of variable (V), joining (J), constant (C), and in the case of the *IGH* gene, diversity (D) regions. There are approximately 45 V, 23 D, and 6 J regions in the *IGH* gene. During B cell development, one *IGH* allele undergoes rearrangement, with deletion of large intervening DNA segments, followed by DNA repair at the site of recombination. This process is mediated by recombination activating genes (*RAG1/2*) which encode RAG1/2 proteins able to induce breaks in double stranded DNA. DNA damage response proteins then bring the separated AgR gene segments together and form a functional rearranged *IGH* gene [3]. AgR rearrangement occurs in a specific order: first, one *IGH* D segment is fused to one J segment, then this DJ segment is fused with a V segment to form a functional VDJ exon that encodes the variable antigen recognition site of the IGH protein. Following *IGH* rearrangement, the final product is a gene

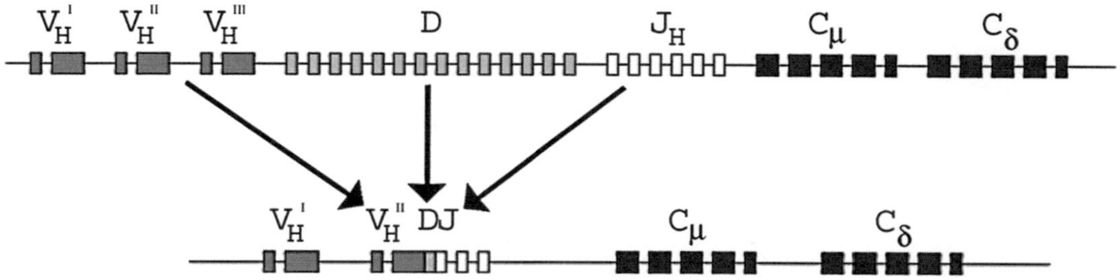

Figure 42.1 Configuration and rearrangement of the *IGH* gene on chromosome 14q32. DJ rearrangement occurs initially, followed by VD rearrangement. The rearrangements occur in a random fashion across B cells, resulting in unique rearrangement in each normal B cell. The rearranged *IGH* gene contains one V_H segment (plus all the upstream V_H segments), one D_H segment, one J_H segment (plus all the downstream J_H segments), and the C_H segments, in that order on the chromosome

containing one V region, one J region, one D region, and multiple C regions, arranged in the following order on the chromosome: V-(D)-J-C (Fig. 42.1). Ig gene rearrangement is an error-prone process and many attempted rearrangements result in nonfunctional AgR genes. If the first *IGH* rearrangement in a cell fails, the second *IGH* allele is rearranged. A single B cell may therefore have two *IGH* rearrangements, one nonfunctional and one functional. The *IGK* alleles rearrange in a similar fashion, but only after the successful rearrangement of one of the *IGH* alleles. The *IGL* alleles rearrange in most cases only if rearrangements of the *IGK* genes fail and both alleles are deleted [4]. Normal B cells that fail to produce a functional *IGH* or light chain rearrangement are usually eliminated through apoptosis.

After successful rearrangement, the Ig genes in mature B cells often undergo additional changes, including somatic hypermutation. In response to antigen exposure, somatic hypermutation occurs in the *IGH* V region (IGVH) of an already rearranged *IGH* gene in germinal center-derived B cells to enhance antigen affinity of the AgR. Somatic hypermutation occurs through point mutations, small insertions, small deletions, or some combination of these. The enzyme activation-induced cytidine deaminase (AID) mediates the process of both class-switching and somatic hypermutation. AID expression is upregulated in germinal centers in response to antigen stimuli [3, 4]. The term "postgerminal center" is used to refer to B cells that have been exposed to antigen in the germinal center and undergone additional somatic mutation of IGVH. Errors in class switch recombination, somatic hypermutation, and AID expression contribute to the pathogenesis of many B cell lymphomas [5].

Structurally and genetically unique AgR rearrangements occur in every B cell and are exploited as markers of cell lineage and clonality. B cells with these unique gene rearrangements may undergo limited clonal expansion as a part of a normal immune response, but uncontrolled clonal expansion occurs in BCL. In this setting, the unique AgR rearrangement can serve as a diagnostic marker of B-cell clonality and a marker for detection of MRD following therapy. Clonal rearrangements of *IGH* and *IGK* can be detected in essentially all malignancies of mature B cells, but many precursor B-cell malignancies will have only *IGH* rearrangements, since malignant transformation occurs before rearrangement of the *IGK* or *IGL* genes.

Recurrent Cytogenetic and Molecular Abnormalities in BCL and Plasma Cell Myeloma

Many, but not all BCL are associated with characteristic cytogenetic or molecular abnormalities that help to establish an accurate primary diagnosis, have specific prognostic significance, and/or serve as targets for MRD assessment. Most of the molecular abnormalities described below have been included under the National Comprehensive Cancer Network Guidelines (Version 3.2012) as "useful testing under certain circumstances for clarification of diagnosis." Table 42.2 provides a summary of most of the recurrent cytogenetic abnormalities identified thus far in subtypes of BCL. This list illustrates the large number of potential targets for molecular testing, but also highlights the increasing challenge for clinical laboratories to provide relevant molecular information to clinicians. There are many additional newly discovered mutations in different BCL, either not yet proven to have clinical relevance and/or not yet part of routine testing algorithms in BCL; some of these are listed in Table 42.3 for the different BCL subtypes. The most clinically relevant BCL subtype-specific cytogenetic and molecular abnormalities, namely those with currently known diagnostic or prognostic significance, are discussed in more detail under the individual BCL categories below. General considerations that are applicable to most or all BCL subtypes are discussed later in the sections on diagnostic and prognostic indications for molecular testing in BCL.

Chronic Lymphocytic Leukemia/Small Lymphocytic Lymphoma

Although morphologically and immunophenotypically similar, chronic lymphocytic leukemia/small lymphocytic lymphoma (CLL/SLL) is quite heterogeneous genetically, with different molecular abnormalities resulting in different natural histories and responses to therapy. New insights into the biology of CLL/SLL have improved the approach to treatment. Many of the relevant chromosomal abnormalities in CLL/SLL are not detected by karyotyping because the low proliferative capacity of most CLL/SLL limits the clinical utility of metaphase cytogenetics. The genetic abnormalities in CLL/SLL therefore usually are detected by interphase fluorescence in situ hybridization (FISH), which has become the clinical standard of care in CLL/SLL. Evaluation for these abnormalities is clinically indicated at diagnosis in most cases of CLL/SLL, because therapeutic decisions are affected by the molecular profile.

Table 42.2 Nonrandom chromosomal abnormalities in B-cell malignancies

Lymphoma subtype	Nonrandom chromosomal alterations	Genes involved
CLL/SLL	Del 13q14 Trisomy 12 Del 11q22-23 Del 17p13 Del 6 3q27	Unknown Unknown *ATM* *TP53*
LPL	Del 6q Trisomy 4	
MZL	t(11;18)(q21;q21) t(1;14)(p22;q32) t(14;18)(q32;q21) t(3;14)(q32) Trisomy 3 Trisomy 18	*API2–MALT1* *BCL10–IGH* *IGH–MALT1* *FOXP1–IGH*
FL	t(14;18)(q32;q21)	*IGH–BCL2*
MCL	t(11;14)(q13;q32)	*Cyclin D1*–IGH
DLBCL/BCLU	3q27 rearrangement t(14;18)(q32;q21) 8q24 rearrangement	BCL6 *IGH–BCL2* *MYC*
BL	t(8;14)(q24;q32) t(2;8)(p11;q24) t(8;22)(q24;q11)	*MYC–IGH* *IGLK–MYC* *MYC–IGLL*
PCM	t(11;14)(q13;q32) t(4;14)(p16;q32) t(14;16)(Q32;Q23) Monosomy 13	*Cyclin D1–IGH* *FGFR3+MMSET–IGH* *IGH–MUM1-IRF4*

See Table 42.1 for abbreviations.

Adverse molecular prognostic factors in CLL/SLL include lack of IGVH hypermutation and the presence of *TP53* or *ATM* gene mutations. Somatic hypermutation of IGVH is seen in approximately 50 % of CLL/SLL, and long-term progression-free and overall survival is better for patients with hypermutated IGVH. The explanation for this seems to be that unmutated CLL/SLL cells are genomically less stable than mutated CLL/SLL cells, are more likely to have acquired a *TP53* deletion at relapse than those with mutated IGVH, and therefore are more likely to be resistant to salvage chemotherapy. Patients with intact *TP53* gene function appear to have prolonged survival regardless of the extent of IGVH hypermutation [6]. Testing for IGVH hypermutation requires multiple PCR analyses and gene sequencing and is performed at only a few specialty laboratories and academic centers.

The *TP53* gene deletion at 17p13.3 is identified by FISH testing in 7–15 % of CLL/SLL cases at diagnosis (illustrated in Fig. 42.2), but is detected by karyotype at a much lower rate. Other types of *TP53* mutations also occur in many CLL/SLL including missense substitutions, frameshift mutations, and in frame deletions, and are highly correlated with 17p deletion; however, some *TP53* mutations occur in the absence of deletion of 17p [7, 8]. *TP53* maintains genome integrity by orchestrating the repair or elimination of cells with damaged DNA and contributes to the cytotoxicity of many anticancer agents. Both 17p deletion and inactivating mutations of *TP53*

Table 42.3 Common gene mutations and deletions in B-cell lymphomas

MZL	CLL/SLL	MCL	FL	DLBCL–GCB	DLBCL–ABC
TNFAIP3–A20	*TP53*	*TP53*	*TP53*	*TP53*	*CD79B*
NOTCH2	*ATM*	*ATM*	*BCL2*	*BCL2*	*CARD11*
	NOTCH1	*NOTCH1*	*EZH2*	*EZH2*	*MYD88*
	SF3B1	*Cyclin D1*	*CREBBP*	*CREBBP*	*TNFAIP3–A20*
	FBXW7	*p16*	*EP300*	*EP300*	*INK4A–ARF*
	MYD88	*TNFAIP3–A20*	*MLL2*	*MLL2*	*BLIMP1–PRDM1*
	BIRC3		*MEF2B*	*MEF2B*	*BCL6*
				SGK1	
				GNA13	
				TNFRSF14	

See Table 42.1 for abbreviations.

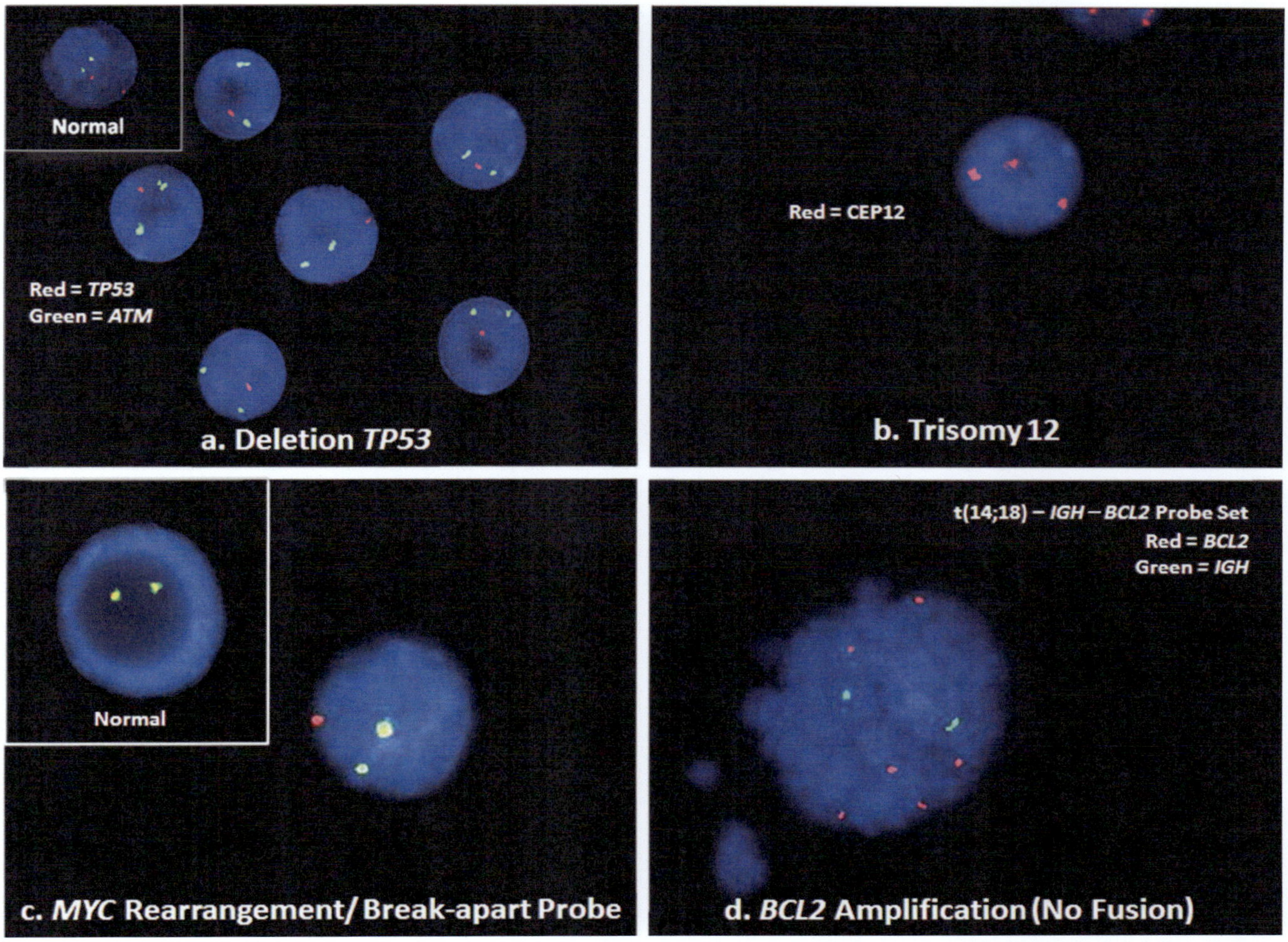

Figure 42.2 Illustrations of typical genetic abnormalities in BCL, detected by interphase FISH. (**a**) CLL/SLL lymphocytes with deletion of *TP53*. This case shows two *green ATM* (11q22.3) signals, but only one *red TP53* (17p13.1) signal (RGG). A normal cell would have two *red* and two *green* signals (RRGG), as seen in the *inset*. (**b**) A centromeric probe (CEP12) for chromosome 12 demonstrates trisomy 12 with 3 *red* signals (RRR) in this cell from the blood of a CLL/SLL patient. A normal cell would have two *red* signals (RR). (**c**) A break-apart probe for the *MYC* gene shows a *MYC* rearrangement with a *yellow* fusion signal for the normal *MYC* and separate *green* and *red* signals for the rearranged *MYC* gene (RGY). The pattern in a normal cell with the break-apart probe would be two *yellow* signals (YY), shown in the *inset*. (**d**) BCL cell with *BCL2* amplification. This FISH result does not show the t(14;18)–*IGH–BCL2* fusion signals (RGYY) typical of the translocation. Rather, the pattern of six *red* signals for the *BCL2* gene with only two signals for the *IGH* gene (6R2G) is consistent with *BCL2* amplification. See Table 42.1 for abbreviations

render patients resistant to chemotherapy [9]. *TP53* dysfunction is associated with an adverse clinical outcome in CLL/SLL patients, as well as in other BCL.

Deletions in 11q22-23 are detected by FISH in 14–20 % of CLL/SLL cases and are associated with inactivation of the ataxia telangiectasia (*ATM*) gene. The ATM protein kinase is involved in*TP53* regulation; therefore, *ATM* deletions produce *TP53* dysfunction in CLL/SLL cells. *ATM* deletions most often are detected by FISH and are associated with a poor prognosis, although not as poor as that of patients with *TP53* deletion/mutation. The addition of Rituximab monoclonal antibody therapy which targets CD20 on B cells to chemotherapy regimens appears to overcome the poor prognosis conferred by the 11q deletion [10, 11]. Mutations in *ATM* have been reported in approximately 10 % of CLL/SLL cases and only partially correlate with deletions in 11q. Approximately 18–30 % of cases with 11q deletion show concomitant *ATM* mutations. The significance of an *ATM* mutation in the absence of an 11q deletion is not well established.

As a single abnormality in CLL/SLL, 13q14 deletions convey the most favorable prognosis. CLL/SLL with 13q14 abnormalities usually has IGVH hypermutation. Detected by FISH, 13q14 deletions are seen in 40–55 % of CLL/SLL cases and are thought to affect one or more tumor suppressor genes. Frequent deletions and downregulation of microRNA genes miR15 and miR16 at 13q14 have been described in the majority of CLL/SLL cases with 13q14 deletions [12]. 13q14 deletions are sometimes seen in other BCL, but the specific gene(s) involved may not be the same.

Trisomy 12 can be detected by FISH or routine karyotyping and occurs in 16–20 % of CLL/SLL cases (FISH illustration in Fig. 42.2). Trisomy 12 usually is associated with unhypermutated IGVH and has been associated with atypical CLL/SLL morphology. Patients with trisomy 12 have an intermediate prognosis, with a median survival exceeded only by patients with single 13q14 abnormalities [10, 11].

Deletions of chromosome 6q are present in approximately 7 % of CLL/SLL cases and can be detected by FISH. The majority are identified at 6q21-23, with a smaller percentage documented at 6q25-27. Although limited, initial studies suggest that this class of cytogenetic abnormality is associated with an intermediate risk profile. Incorporation of FISH probes for 6q in clinical practice may improve our understanding of this molecular abnormality in risk stratification of patients with CLL/SLL.

In addition to the genetic abnormalities described above, exome and genome sequencing studies have identified additional recurrent gene mutations in CLL/SLL (Table 42.3) including those in *SF3B1*, *NOTCH1*, and others [13]. Frameshift mutations in the proline-glutamic acid-serine-threonine (PEST) degradation domain of *NOTCH1* are associated with unhypermutated IGVH, trisomy 12, and a poor prognosis. Missense mutations in *SF3B1*, a gene involved in RNA splicing, are relatively common in CLL/SLL (approximately 10 %) and whereas the data are preliminary, there is evidence that these mutations also confer a worse clinical outcome [13–15].

B-Cell Prolymphocytic Leukemia

B-cell prolymphocytic leukemia (B-PLL) is an aggressive mature B-cell leukemia characterized by splenomegaly with minimal to no lymphadenopathy and prolymphocytes comprising >55 % of circulating lymphoid cells. Complex karyotypes are common, as are *TP53* mutations, 13q14 deletions, and to a lesser extent, trisomy 12. Cases with t(11;14)(q13;q32) are generally excluded from this category and considered leukemic variants of mantle cell lymphoma (MCL). The *MYC* gene can be overexpressed in B-PLL [16] and, although rare, the t(8;14)(q24;q32) translocation that involves *MYC* and is characteristic of Burkitt lymphoma (BL) has been reported in B-PLL [17, 18]. The significance of *MYC* abnormalities in B-PLL is not entirely clear and additional study is needed to elucidate the genetic events underlying the pathophysiology of this disease.

Hairy Cell Leukemia

Hairy cell leukemia (HCL) is an indolent neoplasm of mature B cells characterized by circumferential "hairlike" projections of the B-cell cytoplasmic membrane, splenomegaly, diffuse marrow involvement, and peripheral cytopenias. The *BRAF* V600E point mutation is present in nearly all cases of HCL and has redefined a disease which previously had no known recurrent molecular abnormalities. The *BRAF* V600E mutation is rare in other mature BCL [19]. The apparent specificity of this mutation for HCL makes this a disease-defining mutation with clear diagnostic utility, in addition to possible implications for MRD detection and treatment.

Lymphoplasmacytic Lymphoma

In the 2008 WHO classification, lymphoplasmacytic lymphoma (LPL) is defined as a B-cell neoplasm composed of a mixture of small lymphocytes, plasmacytoid lymphocytes, and plasma cells, that does not fulfill the criteria for any of the other malignancies of small B lymphocytes, i.e., a diagnosis of exclusion [1]. LPL includes Waldenström macroglobulinemia (WM). There are several common cytogenetic abnormalities in LPL, but none are specific for this lymphoma subtype. These abnormalities include 6q deletion, which is seen in approximately 50 % of cases presenting in the bone marrow (BM), less often in cases presenting in lymph nodes, and may be associated with a worse prognosis [20]. Trisomy 4 is present in 20 % of WM [21]. The t(9;14) translocation previously reported in LPL has been reassessed and confirmed not to be associated with LPL [22]. Gene expression profiling studies using flow cytometric sorted cells have shown that WM B cells cluster with CLL/SLL B cells, whereas WM plasma cells segregate with plasma cell myeloma cells [23]. One of the upregulated genes in WM B cells is interleukin-6, a molecule that may be a therapeutic target in LPL. WM is sometimes associated with clonal expansions of cytotoxic T cells in the blood, which can confound diagnosis. These T-cell clones can be eliminated by chemotherapy for LPL [24]. A mutation in *MYD88* is present in almost all patients with WM. This mutation in *MYD88* at 3p22.2 results in an amino acid change (L265P), and triggers NFKB signaling. The *MYD88* L265P mutation is absent or only occasionally expressed in other subtypes of non-IgM LPL, as well as plasma cell myelomas and marginal zone lymphomas [25].

Plasma Cell Myeloma/Plasmacytoma

Plasma cell myeloma (PCM) and related plasma cell neoplasms have two major subgroups by cytogenetic and molecular characteristics with some overlap. The first group is hyperdiploid PCM, which comprises 55–60 % of cases and has trisomy or tetrasomy, predominantly of odd numbered chromosomes. The second group has chromosomal translocations that involve the *IGH* gene on 14q32, with a variety of partner genes. These translocations occur in approximately 50 % of PCM and the different translocations are sometimes associated with specific clinical features and outcome. Most cannot be identified by karyotyping, but are readily identified by FISH studies utilizing molecular probes for 14q32 and its translocation partners. Translocations involving the *IGH* locus in PCM are believed to occur at the time of isotype class switching, in contrast to other B-cell malignancies.

The t(11;14)(q13;q32) is the most common translocation, occurring in 20–25 % of all PCM. It involves the *CCND1* gene and is associated with a good prognosis and long survival. PCM with the t(11;14)—*CCND1–IGH* translocation often show considerable morphologic and immunophenotypic overlap with LPL. Detection of the translocation and cyclin D1 protein expression by immunohistochemistry (IHC) are important in making the appropriate diagnosis [26].

The t(4;14)(p16.3;q32) portends the worst prognosis in PCM and is seen in approximately 25 % of cases; it involves *IGH* and the fibroblast growth factor receptor-3 (*FGFR3*) and *MMSET* genes at 4p16.3. The t(14;16)(q32;q23) translocation involving the *MAF* gene occurs in approximately 20 % of PCM and conveys an intermediate prognosis, as does the t(6;14)(p25;q32) translocation involving the *MUM1* gene, also known as the *IRF4* gene.

Progressive disease with transformation to high grade variants of PCM with large cell anaplastic or plasmablastic morphology is associated with *MYC* rearrangements [27, 28], *TP53* mutations and deletions, mutations of *KRAS* and *NRAS*, 1p deletions, and amplifications of 1q21 [29, 30].

Cytogenetic abnormalities detected by karyotyping may show significantly different clinical outcomes compared to abnormalities detected by interphase FISH only [31]. For example, monosomy 13 detected by karyotyping is seen in approximately 50 % of PCM and is associated with poor survival, while chromosome 13 abnormalities detected by interphase FISH only are associated with intermediate survival. Multicolor FISH, also known as spectral karyotyping, can detect chromosomal abnormalities in PCM, including deletions, amplifications, and rearrangements that are missed or cryptic by conventional karyotyping, such as Xp11, 8q24, 11q13, 12q13, 13q21, 14q32, and 22q11.2 abnormalities [32]. New classification systems and stratification for treatment of PCM have been proposed due to these novel abnormalities, but further investigation into the clinical significance of this complex and expensive testing is needed before it can move into routine clinical care.

Marginal Zone B-Cell Lymphomas

The marginal zone lymphomas (MZL) are low grade B-cell lymphomas and include splenic marginal zone lymphoma (SMZL), extranodal marginal zone lymphomas of mucosa-associated lymphoid tissue (MALToma), and nodal marginal zone lymphoma (NMZL). Multiple molecular abnormalities occur in MZL, and MZL of different sites have different molecular abnormalities (Table 42.2). Testing for these abnormalities is helpful in confirmation of primary diagnosis and prognosis. Diagnostic and prognostic testing for these molecular abnormalities usually is performed by multicolor FISH.

The most common translocation in gastric, intestinal, and lung MALTomas is t(11;18)(q21;q21), which occurs in 30–50 % of cases [33–35]. The genes involved are the apoptosis inhibitor gene (*API2*) on 11q21, a member of the inhibitor of apoptosis (IAP) protein family with caspase-inhibitory functions, and the *MALT1* gene on 18q21, encoding a human paracaspase protein. The resulting *API2–MALT1* chimeric transcript and fusion protein leads to inhibition of apoptosis and confers a survival advantage on the MZL cells. T(11;18)(q21;q21) is associated with worse prognosis and occurs most frequently in *H. pylori*-positive antibiotic-resistant MZL or advanced gastric MZL, but not in nodal or splenic MZL, nor in extranodal MZL with increased large cells or large-cell transformation. FISH is the most sensitive and specific method for detection of this translocation; however, reverse transcription PCR (RT-PCR) is occasionally used for detection.

An apoptosis regulatory molecule, BCL10, is overexpressed as a result of the t(1;14)(p22;q32) translocation, which involves *BCL10* on 1p22 and the *IGH* gene on 14q32 [36]. Advanced MALTomas sometimes have both *API2–MALT1* and *BCL10–IGH* translocations, and BCL10 appears to interact with the API2–MALT1 fusion protein to synergize activation of NFKB, suggesting that they are part of a common pathway. The *BCL10–IGH* translocation is associated with a worse prognosis in low grade MALTomas and is typically detected by FISH.

The t(14;18)(q32;q21) translocation, also detected by FISH, involves *IGH* on 14q32 and *MALT1* on 18q21. The *IGH–MALT1* translocation occurs in most liver MALTomas, as well as some cutaneous, ocular adnexal, and salivary MALTomas, but is rare in MALTomas of the stomach, intestine, lung, thyroid, and breast, and does not occur in NMZL or SMZL. *IGH–MALT1* does not usually occur with the *API2–MALT1* translocation, but sometimes occurs with trisomy 3 or trisomy 18 or both [37]. The clinical significance of this translocation is not yet established. This translocation should not be confused with the cytogenetically identical, but molecularly distinct t(14;18)(q32;q21) translocation, resulting in an *IGH–BCL2* fusion, which is associated with follicular lymphoma.

Trisomy 3 occurs in more than 50 % of low-grade MZL, and aCGH studies have shown gains at 3q21-23 and 3q25-29, suggesting that *BCL6* is involved in some cases. Trisomy 18 occurs in approximately 30 % of MZL. The genes involved are not well understood and the clinical relevance is unknown.

The t(3;14)(p13;q32) involving *FOXP1* on chromosome 3 and the *IGH* gene on chromosome 14 is present in approximately 10 % of MALTomas. *IGH–FOXP1* is seen most commonly in MZL arising in the thyroid, ocular adnexa, and skin and is absent in MZL from the lung and stomach. The translocation results in overexpression of FOXP1, is associated with trisomy 3, and may have a more aggressive clinical behavior [38, 39].

A20 (also known as *TNFAIP3*), found at 6q23, is a negative regulator of the NFKB pathway and is inactivated in a subset of MALTomas via mutation, methylation, or deletion [40]. *A20* inactivation is preferentially seen in MALTomas arising from the ocular adnexa, salivary gland, and thyroid. Activating *MYD88* point mutations (L265P), identical to those identified in the activated B-cell-like subtype of diffuse large B-cell lymphoma (DLBCL), and WM have been reported in 9 % of MALTomas, although the clinical significance is not yet clear [41]. Both *A20* and *MYD88* mutations contribute to constitutive activation of the NFKB pathway mediating cell survival and growth.

Follicular Lymphoma

Follicular lymphoma (FL) is the second most common subtype of NHL, accounting for approximately 22 % of cases [42]. FL patients demonstrate a remarkably variable clinical course, with some patients surviving for less than 1 year while others live for more than 20 years [43]. Standard pathologic, immunologic, and genetic analyses of FL have failed to identify a reliable method for prediction of prognosis in newly diagnosed FL patients. Gene expression profiling of a large series of FL suggests that the length of survival of FL patients correlates with the features of nonmalignant cells present in the lymphoma at diagnosis [44]. However, gene expression profiling is not available yet for routine clinical diagnosis and no alternative immunohistochemical algorithm has yet been developed in FL.

The t(14;18)(q32;q21) translocation, detected in approximately 80 % of FL at the time of initial diagnosis, is the cytogenetic hallmark of FL and juxtaposes the *BCL2* oncogene on 18q21 with the *IGH* gene on 14q32. Overexpression of a normal BCL2 protein results from this translocation and protects the cells from apoptosis. Molecular analysis for *IGH–BCL2* translocation using FISH (Fig. 42.2) is often used for confirmation of the initial diagnosis of FL in cases with equivocal histologic and immunologic findings. Molecular testing for *IGH–BCL2* translocation by PCR in FL may be performed to evaluate the course of disease and the impact of therapy [45, 46]. Analysis to aid in evaluation of response to therapy is typically performed by PCR, because FISH is not sensitive enough for detection of a low level of MRD in BM or blood. *BCL2* breakpoints occur most commonly in a 150 base pair (bp) span termed the major breakpoint cluster region (MBR), but may occur in areas of the gene called the minor breakpoint cluster region (MCR) or the intermediate cluster region (3′MBR). The insertion of variable numbers of random extra nucleotides at the breakpoint junction during crossover and the variability of the breakpoints in the *BCL2* fusion gene and the six J_H fragments results in considerable variation in the length of PCR products when testing is performed for this translocation. PCR fragment length usually ranges from 120 to 270 bp for the MBR, but occasional breakpoints as much as 800 bp downstream of the MBR region have been detected with standard MBR primers, resulting in PCR products of more than 1,000 bp. The clustering of breakpoints on chromosome 18 and the high degree of sequence homology among the 3′ portions of the JH segments make the *IGH–BCL2* translocation very amenable to PCR detection and a good PCR target for MRD detection (see section on "Minimal Residual Disease Detection").

Histologic progression occurs in approximately 30 % of FL patients, but the genetic events that are involved in this progression are not completely defined. Studies of paired lymph node biopsy specimens derived from the same FL patient before and after transformation identify at least two mechanisms for transformation. One is associated with high proliferation and one with recurrent oncogenic abnormalities. Mutations in *TP53* occur in 20 % of transformed FL. *MYC* gene expression is markedly increased in 70 % of transformed FL, but appears to be a surrogate marker for the gene expression profiling high proliferation signature [47]. The frequency of *MYC* mutations and translocations in transformed FL is low [48]. Copy number variability in two regions (1p36.22-p36.33 and 6q21-q24.3) are predictors of transformation risk in FL, independent of the International Prognostic Index (IPI) score. These prognostic features may be useful to identify high-risk patients as candidates for risk-adapted therapies [49].

Genes encoding proteins involved with histone modification are frequent targets of somatic hypermutation in both DLBCL and FL and may play an important role in B-cell lymphomagenesis. Both DLBCL and FL may have mutations in these genes, but the frequency of mutation is highest in FL, with *MLL2* mutation in 89 % and *MEF2B* mutation in 13 % of FL [50]. *MLL2* encodes a histone methyltransferase and *MEF2b* cooperates with *CREBBP* and *EP300* to acetylate histones.

Mantle Cell Lymphoma

Molecular testing is performed at initial diagnosis in most patients with MCL as the diagnosis confers a very poor prognosis and mandates aggressive therapy in most cases [51]. Diagnostic testing targets the t(11;14)(q13;q32) translocation, which juxtaposes the *BCL1* or *CCND1* gene on chromosome 11q13 with an *IGH* enhancer, resulting in overexpression of normal cyclin D1 protein and increased cell cycling. This translocation is not completely specific for

MCL, as it also occurs in many plasma cell myelomas. However, no diagnostic problems are caused by this overlap as the *CCND1–IGH* translocation does not occur in the subtypes of BCL with which MCL shows significant morphologic or immunophenotypic overlap. Multiple methods have been used to detect the *CCND1–IGH* translocation, including karyotyping, PCR, RT-PCR for *CCND1* mRNA, and FISH [52]. The optimal diagnostic method has proven to be FISH (Fig. 42.3), which detects >90 % of cases, even in formalin-fixed paraffin-embedded (FFPE) biopsy tissue. PCR detection is less successful because the 11q13 breakpoints are widely distributed; approximately 30–50 % are localized to a 1 kb DNA segment called the major translocation cluster (MTC), but the remaining translocations involve many different sites not easily detectable by PCR analysis. There is little application for the PCR assay when FISH is faster, more specific, and can be performed on FFPE tissue.

The proliferation signature by gene expression profiling can identify MCL patients with the poorest prognosis [53]. The evaluation of Ki-67 by IHC is often used as a surrogate for the gene expression proliferation signature in the routine diagnostic workup of MCL, but is difficult to interpret and is less predictive in the intermediate range. However, a high level of Ki-67 expression is likely associated with poor outcome, independent of the morphologic variant. The mitotic index (counting the number of mitotic figures/mm2) may be superior to Ki-67 expression [54]. Gene expression profiling has identified the transcription factor *SOX11* as a specific marker for MCL and IHC analysis demonstrates strong nuclear staining with SOX11 in >90 % of MCL cases including those that are cyclin D1-negative [55]. While this is potentially a diagnostically useful marker, the prognostic significance remains controversial.

ATM deletions like those in CLL/SLL also are seen in many MCL cases, and progression or aggressive clinical behavior in MCL is associated with *P16* and *TP53* abnormalities [56]. Additionally, recurrent *NOTCH1* mutations occur in MCL; similarly to CLL/SLL, *NOTCH1* mutations are associated with poor prognosis [57]. MCLs rarely have somatic hypermutation of IGVH.

Diffuse Large B-Cell Lymphoma

DLBCL is the most common subtype of lymphoma and this category of the WHO classification represents another clinically and biologically heterogeneous group of BCL. Over the past decade, promising new technologies have been applied to the problem of identification of prognostic subgroups of DLBCL. Microarray gene expression profiling has identified three molecularly and prognostically distinct subtypes of DLBCL: a germinal center B-cell-like DLBCL subgroup (GCB) with a favorable prognosis; an activated B-cell-like DLBCL subgroup (ABC) with a poorer prognosis; and a favorable primary mediastinal large B-cell lymphoma subgroup (PMBL) [58–60].

In addition to distinct gene expression patterns, these DLBCL subgroups have different cytogenetic and molecular abnormalities and utilize different oncogenic pathways. The GCB type of DLBCL derives from the germinal center B cell. *IGH–BCL2* translocations [t(14;18)] identical to those seen in FL are specific to GCB DLBCL and are not seen in the other DLBCL subtypes. GCB DLBCL may also have amplification of the *REL* locus on chromosome 2p,

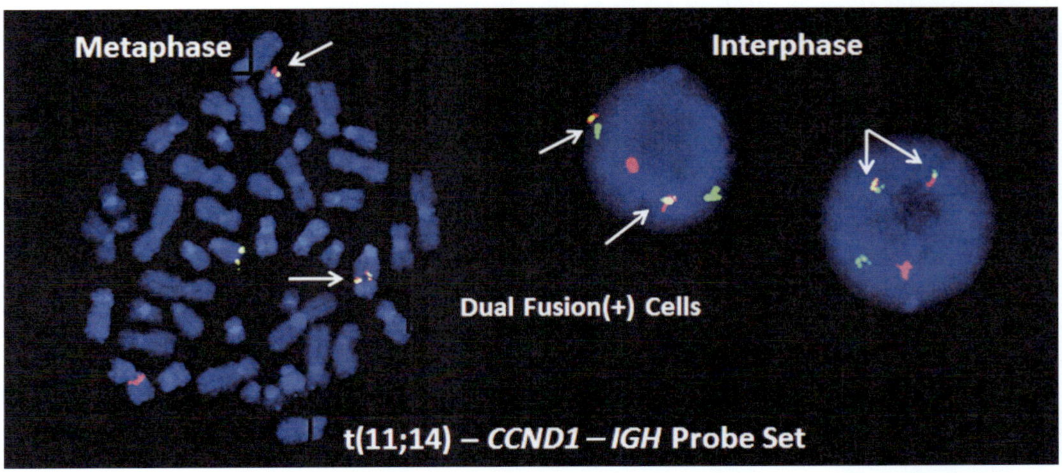

Figure 42.3 FISH analysis for the t(11;14) *CCND1–IGH* translocation in a mantle cell lymphoma (MCL). On the *left* is a single metaphase spread and on the *right* are two interphase cells, all with two *yellow*, one *red* and one *green* signal called a dual fusion signal pattern (RGYY). These probes detect both derivative chromosomes resulting from the translocation. Both derivative chromosomes produce a *yellow* fusion signal, whereas the normal alleles produce separate *red* and *green* signals

deletion of *PTEN* on chromosome 10, and amplification of microRNA cluster mir-17-92 [61], as well as mutations in genes involved in chromatin/histone modification such as *EZH2* and *CREBBP* [50, 62] (Table 42.3).

ABC DLBCL originates from a post germinal center B cell, has a gene expression profile similar to that of activated peripheral blood B cells [58], and is characterized by constitutive activation of the NFKB pathway. Mutations in *A20*, *MYD88* and *CARD11* are thought to contribute to deregulation of the NFKB pathway [63]. Also typical of ABC DLBCL are trisomy 3, increased FOXP1 mRNA expression, deletion of chromosome 6q, deletion of the *INK4a–ARF* tumor suppressor locus on chromosome 9, and gain or amplification of part of chromosome 19 [61] (Table 42.3).

PMBL represents a distinct entity in the 2008 WHO classification, which is more frequent in young adults and typically presents as a mediastinal mass without involvement of lymph nodes or BM. PMBL is thought to be derived from a thymic medullary B cell. The gene expression profile more closely resembles that of classical Hodgkin lymphoma than the other subtypes of DLBCL. aCGH has demonstrated amplification of chromosome 9p24 in up to 75 % of cases and 2p15 in approximately 50 % of cases. Candidate genes include *REL* and *BCL11A* at 2p and *JAK2*, *PDL1*, and *PDL2* at 9p [64]. *SOCS1* mutations and upregulation of NFKB are also genetic hallmarks of PMBL [65].

Mutations or translocations in *BCL6* (3q27) are common abnormalities in DLBCL, occurring in approximately 30 % of cases and not associated with a specific subgroup [66, 67]. Translocations involve both *IGH* and non *IGH* gene partners. The particular translocation partner may dictate the prognostic significance of the *BCL6* translocation, with translocations involving the *IGH* locus having a more favorable prognosis than those with other partner genes. *MYC* translocations are present in approximately 10 % of DLBCL. In contrast to BL, *MYC* rearrangements in DLBCL often are present in the context of a complex karyotype, and in 30–40 % of cases, *MYC* is rearranged with a non-Ig gene. FISH using a *MYC* break-apart probe is useful in the detection of these cases (Fig. 42.2). *MYC* translocations in DLBCL have a worse prognosis with poor response to therapy [68, 69]. Of note, FISH analysis does not detect all cases with significant expression of MYC. IHC for MYC protein identifies a subset of *MYC* FISH-negative DLBCL cases with high levels of MYC protein expression. These IHC-positive, FISH-negative cases have a very poor clinical prognosis, but only if there is also high expression of BCL2 protein [70, 71].

Burkitt Lymphoma

BL is a high grade BCL that is characteristically associated with the t(8;14)(q24;q32) translocation involving the *MYC* gene on 8q24 and the *IGH* gene on 14q32 [72]. Occasional BL demonstrates variant t(2;8)(p11;q24) or t(8;22)(q24;q11) translocations involving *MYC* and the kappa and lambda light chain loci, respectively [73]. These translocations result in increased expression of MYC and markedly increased cell proliferation. The site of translocation of *MYC* is reported to vary between sporadic and endemic BL. In endemic disease, the 8q24 breakpoint occurs up to 300 kb 5′ from the coding region of the *MYC* gene, while sporadic BL characteristically involves a breakpoint in *MYC* exon 1 [74]. The site of translocation in the *IGH* gene also is variable, with endemic cases involving the J region and sporadic cases involving the C regions. The degree of molecular variability in these translocations is the reason they are not amenable to detection by standard PCR assays. Routine karyotyping and FISH analysis using *MYC* probes are successful in detecting almost all *MYC* translocations in BL. BL typically do not have other chromosomal abnormalities. Gene expression profiling of BL and DLBCL has identified typical gene signatures for BL vs DLBCL [75]. The MYC protein and its target genes, as well as some genes expressed in normal germinal center B cells are more highly expressed in BL than GCB DLBCL, while major histocompatibility complex (MHC) class I genes and NFKB target genes are expressed at lower levels in BL than in DLBCL. Some of the recurrently mutated genes in DLBCL (*EZH2*, *SGK1*, *BCL2*, *CD79B*, and *MYD88*) are rarely mutated in BL [76].

B-Cell Lymphoma, Unclassifiable, with Features Intermediate Between DLBCL and BL

A subset of B-cell lymphomas shows morphologic and immunologic overlap with both BL and DLBCL. In some but not all of these cases, the gene expression profile is similar to BL [75]. Historically, these have been called “atypical Burkitt” or “Burkitt-like” lymphomas, but in the 2008 WHO classification, they were put into the category of BCL, unclassifiable, with features intermediate between DLBCL and BL (BCLU) [1]. Unlike classical BL, *MYC* translocations in BCLU frequently involve a non-Ig gene partner and may occur in the background of a complex karyotype. Most of the so-called “double hit lymphomas,” defined by the presence of a *MYC* rearrangement and another genetic abnormality, most commonly *BCL2* gene rearrangement, are included in this category. However, some double hit lymphomas may be morphologically and phenotypically indistinguishable from DLBCL or even FL. Identification of double hit lymphomas at diagnosis is clinically important because, regardless of how they are subclassified morphologically, double hit lymphomas have a particularly aggressive clinical course and are often refractory to conventional chemotherapeutic regimens used for DLBCL. In rare cases of “triple hit lymphoma,” *MYC*, *BCL2*, and *BCL6* are all rearranged and the clinical outcome is particularly dismal. FISH analysis is typically used at diagnosis for detection of these cytogenetic abnormalities, but will not detect all cases, particularly those with other mechanisms of overexpression of MYC. Because of the possible overlap with typical DLBCL, some institutions now routinely use a diagnostic FISH panel for detection of *MYC* rearrangements plus *IGH–BCL2* and *BCL6* rearrangements at the time of initial diagnosis for all new DLBCLs and BCLUs.

ALK-Positive Large B-Cell Lymphoma

ALK-positive large B-cell lymphoma (ALK-positive LBCL) is a rare subtype of DLBCL that is typically composed of a monomorphic proliferation of large, immunoblastic-appearing B cells. These malignant B cells may show plasmacytic differentiation and must be distinguished from plasmablastic lymphomas (PBL) and T- and NK-cell anaplastic large cell lymphomas. ALK-positive LBCL is characterized by strong and homogeneous immunostaining with the ALK antibody, usually with a restricted granular cytoplasmic pattern. Despite the fact that they express the ALK protein, the t(2;5)(p23;q35) *NPM–ALK* translocation that is characteristic of T- and NK-cell anaplastic large cell lymphomas, is seen only in rare cases; these cases also show an unusual combined cytoplasmic, nuclear, and nucleolar staining pattern with the ALK antibody. The key genetic abnormality in ALK-positive DLBCL is the genetic alteration of the ALK locus on chromosome 2, with the most frequent abnormality being the t(2;17)(p23;q23)–*ALK–CLTCL1* fusion. FISH analysis with the *ALK* gene break-apart probe is the typical method used to detect *ALK–CLTCL1* translocation in these lymphomas. Approximately 50 cases of ALK-positive DLBCL, which is not associated with immunosuppression or Epstein-Barr Virus (EBV), have been reported [77, 78].

Immunodeficiency-Associated B-Cell Lymphoproliferative Disorders

Immunodeficiency-associated lymphoproliferative disorders (LPD) are heterogeneous and arise in the clinical context of primary (congenital or genetic defect) or acquired immune deficiency. Four types of immunodeficiency-associated LPD are recognized in the current WHO classification: (1) LPD associated with primary immune disorders (PID), (2) lymphomas associated with HIV infection, (3) post-transplant lymphoproliferative disorders (PTLD), and (4) other iatrogenic immunodeficiency-associated LPD [1]. As a group, immunodeficiency-associated LPD are typically of B-cell type, tend to occur at extranodal sites, and range from nonneoplastic proliferations to aggressive malignancies [79]. Morphologically, they range from reactive-appearing lymphoid or plasmacytic hyperplasia to overt lymphoma. LPD are frequently associated with EBV infection. The disease may regress upon restoration of host immune integrity, such as by withdrawal of an immunosuppressive medication, but the presence of lymphoma often requires treatment as a malignancy [80]. The development of B cell monoclonality and the accumulation of molecular alterations causing microsatellite instability, cell cycle dysregulation, or mutations in oncogenes, accompany the progression to lymphoma [81, 82].

EBV and human herpesvirus-8 (HHV-8) are both double-stranded DNA gamma herpesviruses, linked to the pathogenesis of multiple neoplasms arising in immunocompromised hosts. Common to herpesviruses, after a primarily lytic phase (production and release of new virions), latent infection is established with virus persisting in infected cells for the life of the host. Oncogenesis is associated with the latent phase, and in the case of EBV infection, different patterns of latent protein expression are seen in different hematolymphoid neoplasms [83]. Loss of T-cell antiviral immunity increases the risk of uncontrolled proliferation and development of LPD [84]. EBV is commonly implicated in LPD associated with primary immunodefeciency (PID) (subtypes of PID listed in Table 42.4). PID with a particular propensity for the development of EBV-associated lymphomas include X-linked LPD, severe combined immunodeficiency, hyper IgM syndrome (CD40 ligand and CD40 deficiencies), common variable immunodeficiency, and Wiskott-Aldrich syndrome [85]. In patients with an EBV-positive LPD and no apparent cause of acquired immune deficiency, an underlying primary immunodeficiency should be considered, especially in the pediatric population.

BCL in HIV-Positive Patients

Despite the decreasing frequency of lymphoma in HIV patients since the advent of highly active antiretroviral therapy (HAART), there remains a 70-fold increased incidence of NHL in HIV-infected individuals as compared to the general population [86]. Hodgkin lymphomas also are increasing in the HIV-infected population [87]. The frequency of EBV-positivity in AIDS-related lymphomas is approximately 50 % overall, but varies depending on the type of lymphoma. Approximately 30 % of BL, 75 % of

Table 42.4 Primary immunodeficiencies with increased risk of B-cell lymphoma

Immunodeficiency subtype	Genes with mutations
Severe combined immunodeficiency (SCID)	*IL-2RA, RAG1/2, JAK3*
X-linked agammaglobulinemia (XLA)	*BTK*
Common variable immune deficiency (CVID)	*ICOS*
	CD19
	TACI
Hyper IgM syndrome	*CD154 (CD40L)*
	CD40
	IKK-gamma/NEMO
	UNG
	AID
Hyper IgE syndrome	*STAT3*
Familial hemophagocytic lymphohistiocytosis (HLH)	*SH2D1A, XIAP, PRF1, MUNC13-4, STX*
Ataxia telangiectasia (A-T)	*ATM*
Mijmegen breakage syndrome (NBS)	*NMN*
Wiskott-Aldrich syndrome (WAS)	*WASP*
Autoimmune lymphoproliferative syndrome (ALPS)	*FAS/FASL*

PBL, and almost 100 % of Hodgkin and primary central nervous system lymphomas are EBV positive [79]. HHV-8 is seen in nearly all cases of multicentric Castleman disease in HIV-positive patients and dual infection of tumor cells with EBV and HHV-8 is seen in primary effusion lymphoma (PEL). Interestingly, there is also an inverse relationship between EBER-positivity and BCL6 protein expression, with the theory that EBV microRNAs suppress *BCL6* transcription [88, 89]. Chronic antigenic stimulation in HIV patients triggers somatic hypermutation and class switch recombination in B cells, increasing the chance of oncogenic mutations and translocations [5]. Most AIDS-related lymphomas are aggressive BCL (BL and DLBCL), but some additional lymphoma subtypes have a particular association with HIV infection, including PEL, PBL, and DLBCL arising in HHV8-associated Castleman disease [90].

PBL is a rare, highly aggressive neoplasm defined as a diffuse proliferation of large B cells morphologically resembling immunoblasts with an immunophenotype similar to that of plasma cells [91, 92]. PBL classically presents in the oral cavity of HIV-infected patients, though cases in immunocompetent patients and extraoral manifestations are described [91–94]. EBV, most frequently latency type 1 pattern, is present in 75 % of cases overall and increases to nearly 100 % in HIV-associated PBL of the oral cavity. *MYC* rearrangements are the most common recurrent chromosomal abnormality in PBL and 85 % involve rearrangement with an Ig gene partner, usually *IGH*. Those with *MYC* rearrangements are significantly more likely to be EBV-positive (74 % vs 43 %) [95].

PEL is a very rare, but highly aggressive large B-cell lymphoma that typically involves body cavities of HIV patients and is associated with HHV-8 infection. PEL is composed of large immunoblastic or plasmablastic cells, often with an immunophenotype similar to that of PBL. Approximately 70–80 % of cases are associated with EBV; however, EBV is not absolutely required for the diagnosis of PEL and is likely only a cofactor, offering survival advantage in the HHV-8 infected cells [96]. Mutations in the *BCL6* gene are described in PEL, but rearrangements involving the *CCND1*, *BCL2*, and *MYC* genes have not been described [97].

DLBCL arising in HHV-8-associated Castleman disease primarily occurs in HIV-positive patients. These lymphomas are sometimes referred to as plasmablastic because the cells morphologically resemble plasma cells but must not be confused with PBL described above. Unlike PBL, the abnormal B cells in this entity are infected with HHV-8 rather than EBV. The neoplastic B cells show uniform expression of one Ig heavy chain (typically IgM) and are typically Ig lambda positive. PCR analysis for *IGH* gene rearrangements almost always shows a polyclonal pattern.

Mutational analysis of lymphomas arising in the setting of HIV infection shows heterogeneous molecular lesions, with many containing hypermutations in IGVH and mutations in *BCL6* [97]. The most common molecular alteration in AIDS-related lymphomas is mutation of the 5′ noncoding region of *BCL6* [98]. Approximately 50 % of cases have at least one mutation involving the *PAX5*, *RHO–TTF*, *PIM1*, or *MYC* oncogenes, and 23 % of cases show mutations in two or more of these genes [82].

Post-transplant Lymphoproliferative Disorders

PTLD represent a spectrum of lymphoid and plasmacytic proliferations arising in immunocompromised hosts after solid organ, BM, or peripheral blood stem cell transplant. The majority of PTLD arise in the first year after transplant and the risk depends on the type of transplant, degree of immunosuppression, and EBV seropositivity at the time of transplant. PTLDs are characteristically EBV-positive and of B-cell type, although EBV-negative BCL and T-cell lymphomas can occur [1]. The morphology of PTLD varies from polymorphic to a monomorphic population of cells which may be polyclonal or monoclonal. Early lesions resemble infectious mononucleosis but can progress to overt lymphoma, with increasing numbers of large B cells. The neoplastic B cells commonly show a non-germinal center immunophenotype, with the majority having IGVH (as in CLL/SLL) but not somatic hypermutation [81]. Peripheral blood EBV viral DNA levels correlate with PTLD development; although an individual value cannot supplant a tissue biopsy for diagnosis, trends in EBV DNA levels can be used for disease monitoring and guiding therapy [99]. Transition from a reactive morphology to an overt monomorphic, monoclonal malignancy is the natural history of PTLD; however, early recognition may allow alterations in immunosuppressive regimens and regression of disease, avoiding aggressive chemotherapy. Molecular abnormalities associated with progression of PTLD include microsatellite instability, DNA mismatch repair defects, accumulation of mutations in proapoptotic factors *BAX* and caspase genes and DNA repair gene *RAD50,* aberrant somatic hypermutation, and mutations in *MYC*, *BCL6*, and *TP53*. DNA hypermethylation has been described in 60 % of monomorphic PTLD [81].

Indications for Testing

Testing strategies for the molecular abnormalities of BCL are evolving as the number of genes important for diagnosis and prognosis of BCL increases. Thus, the molecular testing performed to confirm a primary diagnosis, predict BCL prognosis, or identify appropriate targeted therapies for subtypes of BCL will not be the same as testing performed for detection of MRD after therapy. At initial diagnosis or relapse of BCL, the laboratory often needs to rapidly evaluate multiple genetic targets, but with only a low level of assay sensitivity. This is in distinct contrast to testing for MRD after therapy, for which a very sensitive assay is needed.

Several major clinical indications for molecular testing in BCL include: (1) to distinguish between a reactive and neoplastic proliferation of B cells, (2) to identify specific chromosomal abnormalities to aid in accurate subclassification of BCL, (3) for prognosis within a BCL subtype when alternative therapies are related to specific molecular abnormalities, and (4) to evaluate response to therapy by molecular analysis for detection of MRD. When there is a need to distinguish between reactive and neoplastic B-cell proliferations, assays for detection of B-cell clonality are most frequently used because they are applicable to virtually all BCL. The *IGH* gene is the most common target evaluated for confirmation of B-cell clonality at diagnosis. The *IGH* gene is also the most common target for detection of persistent BCL following therapy.

Because substantial morphologic and immunologic overlap exists between different BCL subtypes, accurate subclassification by routine histologic and phenotypic evaluation alone is sometimes difficult and may require evaluation for characteristic molecular abnormalities. Assays for specific BCL-associated molecular alterations have more limited clinical utility than clonality testing in that they are applicable to only a subset of BCL patients, but they often provide essential information for accurate subclassification at diagnosis. Assessment of BCL for molecular features related to adverse prognosis is being performed on a more frequent basis than in the past, due to an increased number of significant molecular factors as well as the development of new targeted therapies. Some prognostic factors for poor outcome appear to be relevant only to a particular subtype of BCL, but other factors, such as *TP53* dysfunction and *MYC* rearrangement, seem to be associated with poor prognosis or progressive disease in many BCL subtypes. Patients with BCL manifesting molecular markers of poor prognosis often are treated more aggressively at the time of initial diagnosis. The use of FISH assays for molecular evaluation of BCL at diagnosis and relapse has expanded remarkably over the past several years and will likely continue to expand as new molecular probes are identified. However, it must be stressed that the sensitivity of even the best FISH assay is not sufficient for detection of MRD in treated BCL patients. MRD testing requires the development and implementation of standardized, sensitive, and quantitative testing.

Minimal Residual Disease Detection

In the past, assessment of therapeutic response by molecular testing for MRD was infrequently performed outside of clinical trials. However, recent use of new therapeutic modalities such as monoclonal antibodies and vaccine therapies for treatment of BCL has resulted in improved clinical outcomes, and multiple large prospective studies in Europe have clearly demonstrated the high prognostic value of MRD monitoring in children with acute lymphoblastic leukemia [100]. Molecular remissions associated with prolongation of progression-free and overall survival also have been seen in multiple clinical trials with MRD monitoring in CLL/SLL [101–103]. MRD detection is used in clinical practice for FL. The finding of a persistent positive MRD test is associated with a higher risk of disease relapse [104]. However, the optimal methodology and timing for detection of MRD has yet to be determined for all subtypes of BCL. The consensus for MRD detection of CLL/SLL by multicolor flow cytometry was published in 2007, with comparison to standard flow cytometry and allele-specific PCR [105].

In general, techniques used for MRD detection have a sensitivity to detect one BCL cell in 10^3–10^5 normal cells, depending on the assay method. Flow cytometry analysis can reach a sensitivity of 1 in 10^4 and patient-specific PCR analysis for *IGH* gene arrangements can reach a sensitivity of 1 in 10^5 [106, 107]. An ideal MRD assay would be applicable to all patients with the disease, provide some quantification of the target, be rapid, inexpensive, readily standardized, and disease-specific, as well as demonstrating good intralaboratory and interlaboratory reproducibility. In fact, current MRD assays lack many of these features.

As mentioned above, the most sensitive and specific method of testing for MRD in BCL is patient/clone-specific (allele-specific) PCR analysis for *IGH* gene rearrangements. This method takes advantage of the fingerprint-like sequences of the junctional regions of the rearranged *IGH* gene, which differ in length and composition for each B-cell clone. *IGH* PCR analysis of a BCL is performed and the PCR products (junctional regions of the clonal *IGH* rearrangement) are then sequenced. The *IGH* rearrangement sequence is subsequently used for the design of patient-specific PCR primers, which are used in PCR assays to assess MRD. The usual target for MRD detection is a VH-JH rearrangement. The use of two MRD targets also has been recommended for reliable and sensitive MRD detection [108, 109]. In patient-specific *IGH* PCR, the background signal from polyclonal B cells does not obscure the clonal PCR products, resulting in significantly more sensitivity compared to *IGH* gene rearrangement PCR, which is only approximately one in 10^2 cells, and is not sufficient for MRD detection [110]. The major problem, however, is that patient-specific *IGH* PCR is extremely labor-intensive and currently impractical for routine clinical testing.

Quantitative PCR (qPCR) detection of specific molecular abnormalities is useful in follow-up of patients with BCL. A standard curve is made from a dilution series of either a diagnostic lymphoma sample for patient-specific PCR or a cell-line dilution if patient-specific sequences are not known, and the amount of residual lymphoma cells relative to normal cells in a sample can be calculated by using this standard curve [111]. The qPCR method may be used with fusion gene translocation targets as well as the *IGH* gene, and is amenable to interlaboratory standardization. The determination of the trend in the quantitative copy numbers of residual BCL signals over time may provide important therapeutic information during and after treatment of BCL patients. PCR analysis using patient-specific primers is extensively used in Europe for molecular monitoring of MRD in patients with precursor B-lymphoblastic leukemia (pre-B-ALL), treated on different clinical trials. In addition, the Europe Against Cancer Program has reported a standardized testing approach for the most common fusion gene transcripts in clinical trials for patients with ALL and BCL [112]. Optimal primer sequences and methods have been reported by the European BIOMED-2 Concerted Action for detection of MRD in patients with pre-B-ALL group. A concise review about why and how to quantify MRD in ALL was published in 2007 [113]. This type of MRD testing is currently performed mainly in specific research laboratories for patients in BCL clinical trials, but as therapeutic options increase, quantitative and sensitive MRD testing is expected to become routine.

Flow cytometric analysis has largely replaced qPCR testing for routine clinical analysis for MRD in CLL/SLL and pre-B-ALL patients, because it provides a faster turn-around-time and is much less labor intensive. The comparability of multicolor flow cytometry and qPCR methods for detection of MRD at the 10^{-4} level has been demonstrated in a CLL/SLL study, in patients treated with fludarabine/cyclophosphamide or fludarabine/cyclophosphamide/rituximab [101].

Other than *IGH* PCR, the only significant molecular target that has been used for MRD detection in BCL is the t(14;18)(q32;q21) in FL. This testing has traditionally been performed on follow-up BM specimens, because the majority of FL patients have detectable disease in the BM at the time of initial diagnosis. With newer therapies that include monoclonal antibodies, a molecular remission in the marrow is desirable and can be achieved in the majority of patients. However, although the durability of clinical remission correlates with the attainment of molecular remission [114, 115], some patients with negative MRD in the BM after therapy have subsequent relapse in peripheral lymph nodes or other tissues. The clinical utility of this testing therefore has been called into question as it is clear that a negative monitoring result in BM does not necessarily predict progression-free survival [116]. Previously involved lymph nodes may serve as a reservoir of neoplastic cells in FL patients [117]. Additional studies are needed to resolve some of these questions.

Another issue with routine clinical testing for MRD in FL is the lack of test standardization across laboratories [118]. In older studies, nested PCR assays were used because they provide the highest level of sensitivity, detecting one FL cell in 10^5–10^6 normal cells. However, nested PCR assays are labor intensive with a high risk of PCR contamination compared with non-nested techniques, so standard PCR or reverse transcription-qPCR (RT-qPCR) assays have been used instead. The analytical sensitivity of PCR and RT-qPCR assays for the *IGH–BCL2* translocation is less than that of nested PCR techniques; at best, sensitivity is one positive cell in 10^4 normal cells [119]. The clinical relevance of the differences in sensitivity between nested PCR and standard PCR analyses for FL is not clear. With a highly sensitive test like nested PCR, the analysis will detect occasional benign *IGH–BCL2* translocation-carrying cells that are known to exist in many unaffected individuals. Therefore, this assay may produce more false-positive MRD results. A slightly less sensitive test using PCR or RT-qPCR may not detect these rare events but also may miss very low level MRD. The best compromise and optimal clinical approach may be the serial measurement of the *IGH–BCL2* translocation by RT-qPCR to trend the quantitative levels of FL cells over time.

Available Assays

Several methods are used by clinical laboratories to detect the known molecular abnormalities in BCL. These include PCR, RT-PCR, RT-qPCR, and FISH. Routine PCR testing in B-cell malignancies today is largely restricted to testing for B-cell clonality, as many of the PCR analyses for other abnormalities have been supplanted by FISH assays, but some testing is still done for specific fusion transcripts [120]. There are multiple other methodologies in development, but not in general clinical usage yet.

Polymerase Chain Reaction Analyses

PCR amplification of genomic DNA is used for detection of AgR rearrangements and can be used for many BCL-associated translocations. However, in genes with numerous translocation partners, such as *IGH* and *MYC*, FISH is more effective than PCR. Translocations involving variable sites over an area of a chromosome too large for the typical PCR may be amenable to RT-PCR due to removal of the intronic regions that results in a smaller amplification region. Typically, RT-PCR cannot reliably be performed on FFPE tissue because RNA is often degraded during tissue processing. PCR using DNA as a substrate can be performed on fresh, frozen, and most FFPE tissue, as well as microdissected and cytology specimens. PCR requires fairly small amounts of DNA and can be performed relatively rapidly, providing a clinically useful result in 1–3 days.

IGH PCR amplifies only rearranged *IGH* alleles because germline alleles have too great a distance between the PCR primer binding sites to allow for amplification. PCR detection of IGVH rearrangements uses V- and J- region primers and relies on the V, D, and J segments being brought into close proximity during rearrangement so that the PCR reaction can amplify across these segments. The closest V and J segments are too far apart in the germline configuration for PCR amplification to occur. *IGH* clonality analysis by PCR uses consensus primers designed to anneal to sequences conserved across the multiple *IGH* V- and J-regions. For *IGH* PCR, one J-region primer will recognize all six J segments because there is a single well-conserved region among the six J regions, but there is no single V-region primer that will recognize all V segments. V regions have three more highly conserved framework regions (FR I, II, and III) and highly variable intervening sequences called complementarity-determining regions (CDR I and II). Because the FR sequences are more conserved across the different V regions, the V-region primers are designed to bind to FR sequences. The FR III region is closest to the J region in the rearranged state, resulting in a smaller PCR product than for the other FR regions. FR III- and J-region primers amplify the highly variable V-D junction (CDR III) and detect 60–70 % of IGVH rearrangements. The sequence of the FR III V-region primer also affects the detection rate. One interlaboratory comparison showed a difference of 55–70 % based on the specific sequence used for the V-region primer [121]. PCR amplification for all three FR regions with a J-region consensus primer achieves a detection rate of 80–90 % in most BCL.

IGH PCR amplifies any rearranged *IGH* allele, producing a background signal from the polyclonal B cells present in a specimen. The polyclonal background may obscure the signal from a monoclonal B-cell population. Numerous strategies are used for PCR product detection, including gel electrophoresis with colorimetric, fluorescent, or chemiluminescent labeling. Capillary electrophoresis with fluorescently labeled primers is most commonly used and provides slightly enhanced sensitivity and higher throughput, with improved resolution.

Standardized multiplex PCR reagents developed by the European BIOMED-2 collaborative study group are available commercially for AgR PCR clinical testing [112]. These patented reagents simultaneously amplify multiple targets in a single PCR reaction using multiple primer pairs to amplify gene targets within a single DNA sample. Primer length, melting temperature, and specificity are important considerations when developing a multiplex assay to ensure robust amplification of each of the target regions. Additionally, primers must be screened to exclude the possibility of primer dimer formation and nonspecific amplification reactions. The amplified DNA products are designed to be different lengths that can be resolved by conventional gel techniques. The European BIOMED-2 group has published standardized methods for detection of clonal Ig gene and T-cell receptor (*TR*) gene rearrangements (Table 42.5) [112], which has aided comparisons between laboratories.

Table 42.5 BIOMED-2 multiplex PCR for B-cell clonality [122]

Multiplex PCR tube	Expected size range (bp)	Common nonspecific bands (bp)
IGH: V_H-J_H	Tube A: 310–360 Tube B: 250–295 Tube C: 100–170	Tube A: ~85 Tube B: ~228 Tube C: ~211
IGH: D_H-J_H	Tube D: 110–290 (D_H1/2/4/5/6-J_H) 390–420 (D_H3-J_H) Tube E: 100–130	Tube D: ~350 Tube E: ~211
IGK	Tube A: 120–160 (Vκ1f/6/Vκ7-Jκ) 190–210 (Vκ3f-Jκ) 260–300 (Vκ2f/Vκ4/Vκ5-Jκ) Tube B: 210–250 Vκ1f/6/Vκ7-Kde 270–300 (Vκ3f/intron-de) 350–390 (Vκ2f/Vκ4/Vκ5-Kde)	Tube A: ~217 Tube B: ~404
IGL	Tube A: 140–165	

Fluorescence In Situ Hybridization

FISH is a very useful technique for detection of targeted BCL-associated chromosomal abnormalities and can detect both structural and numerical chromosomal abnormalities. Poor growth of BCL cells in culture, which is needed for metaphase cells for routine karyotyping, makes routine cytogenetics difficult for BCL. FISH overcomes the need for metaphase cells, because it can be done with either metaphase or interphase preparations. Genomic probes for the breakpoints of many different BCL translocations and for gene deletions are now readily available and the analyses are routinely performed. FISH assays are particularly useful in detection of chromosomal translocations in which the breakpoints are widely dispersed, because FISH probes are much larger than probes and primers used in PCR analysis. For example, FISH probes can detect almost all of the *MYC* 8q24 breakpoints in the t(8;14)(q24;q32) translocations associated with BL. FISH also can detect some genetic abnormalities that cannot be detected by karyotyping.

Interpretation of Test Results

The relative ease of performing the analytical phase of AgR clonality testing using the BIOMED-2 multiplex PCR reagents and protocols [112, 120], has resulted in many laboratories implementing the procedures. However, interpretation of the BIOMED-1 multiplex clonality test results is considerably more difficult than with previous single primer pair assays. Recognition of this problem in interpretation led to a large study by the EuroClonality Consortium to develop recommendations for interpretation and reporting of the multiplex BIOMED-2 AgR clonality assays [122]. These address not only the complicated types of profiles seen on readout systems, but also propose standardized terminology for the technical descriptions of the assays and for the ultimate molecular conclusions reported.

A synopsis of the proposed EuroClonality uniform system for technical description is provided in Table 42.6. Examples of the different patterns that can be seen in AgR clonality assays are shown in Fig. 42.4. A polyclonal B-cell population produces multiple small peaks with a Gaussian curve pattern

Table 42.6 EuroClonality system for standardized technical description of BIOMED-2 Ig or T-cell receptor multiplex PCR [122]

Type of profile per tube (in duplicate)	Technical descriptions
No peaks but poor DNA quality	No specific product; poor DNA quality
No peaks (without background)	No specific product
Gaussian curve (with or without minor reproducible peaks)	Polyclonal or irregular polyclonal
One or two reproducible clonal peaks	Clonal Weak clonal Clonal + polyclonal background (Gaussian curve or irregular polyclonal)
One or two non-reproducible (clear) peaks	Pseudoclonal
Multiple (>2) non-reproducible peaks	Pseudoclonal
Multiple (>2) reproducible peaks	Multiple products (can be compatible with oligoclonal or may still be compatible with clonal)
Pattern not one of above	Not evaluable

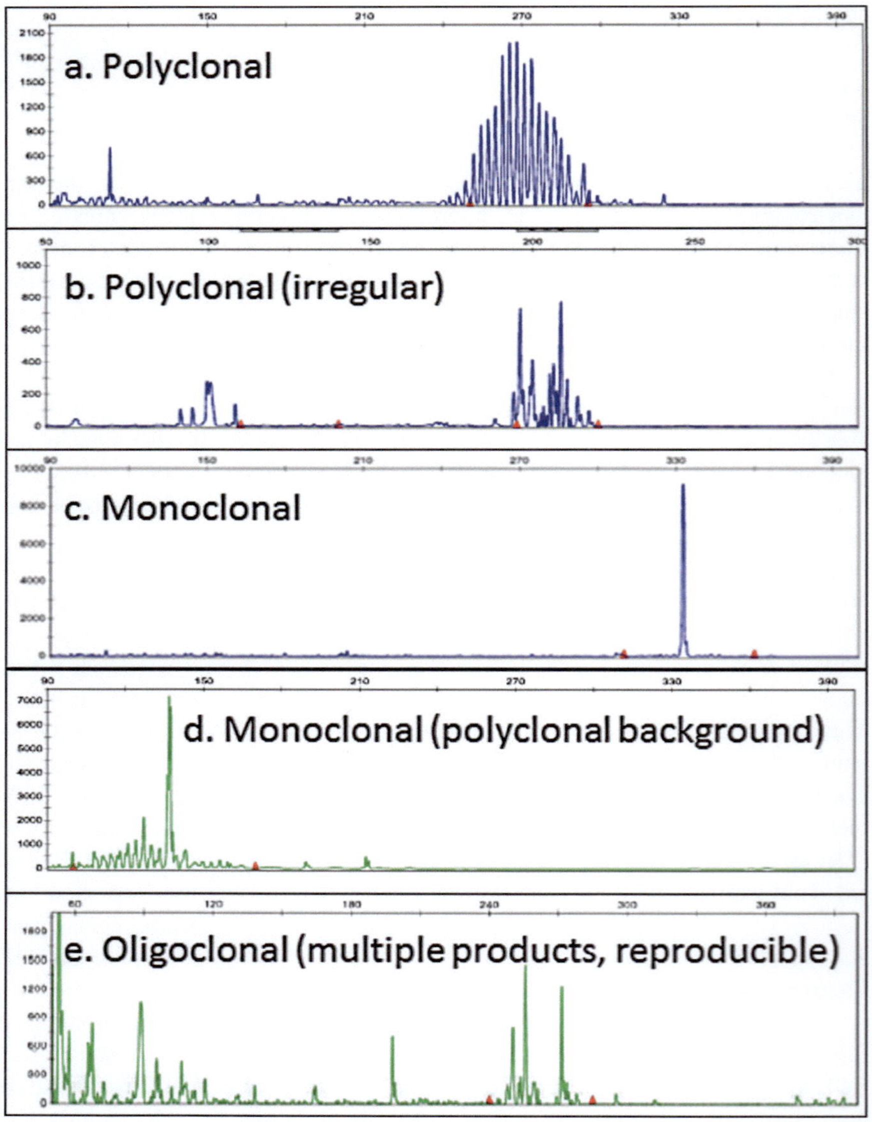

Figure 42.4 Examples of different possible patterns in B cell clonality assays using BIOMED-2 primer sets. (**a**) A polyclonal pattern with a Gaussian distribution of peaks is shown. (**b**) The irregular pattern of multiple peaks is interpreted as a polyclonal B cell population. (**c**) The single peak without a polyclonal background is interpreted as a monoclonal B cell population. (**d**) The single peak with a polyclonal background is interpreted as a monoclonal B cell population. (**e**) An oligoclonal pattern is demonstrated by the multiple distributed peaks of irregular height

(Fig. 42.4a) or an irregular pattern (Fig. 42.4b), while monoclonal B-cell populations typically produce one or two sharp peaks, with or without a polyclonal background (Fig. 42.4d and 42.4c, respectively). To assist with interpretation, various algorithms have been proposed, particularly in the USA. One algorithm used for determining whether a peak is monoclonal compared to the background polyclonal peaks is to require that a monoclonal peak be more than two to three times the height of the adjacent polyclonal peaks [123]; however, these criteria are clearly not useful in all cases. Application of these algorithms can be difficult, so considerable variability in interpretation remains. Adoption of the recommended EuroClonality guidelines for interpretation may improve the consistency of interlaboratory reporting of these assays.

Pitfalls in Interpretation of BCL Testing

Molecular studies of BCL should always be interpreted in conjunction with routine histologic and immunophenotypic information and always with the knowledge of the range of molecular features found in normal and hyperplastic lymphoid populations. Interpretation in this larger clinical and histopathologic context will avoid erroneous interpretations with the potential for adverse clinical consequences. Our knowledge of the molecular events occurring in benign and malignant lymphoid populations is rapidly expanding in this era of genomics and proteomics, such that the interpretation of a particular genetic finding may well change as the field evolves. There are various potential technical and biological pitfalls in the interpretation of molecular analyses for BCL that may result in false-positive or false-negative results.

Reproducible Nonspecific Bands in BIOMED-2 Multiplex PCR Analysis

Accurate interpretation of multiplex PCR AgR clonality results requires knowledge of the location and appearance of certain nonspecific peaks/bands that have been identified and described by the BIOMED-2/EuroClonality consortium (Fig. 42.5c and Table 42.5) [122]. Failure to recognize these nonspecific peaks could result in generation of an erroneous interpretation of clonality, as they are usually reproducible on repeat analyses.

Non-reproducible Clonal Bands in BIOMED-2 Multiplex PCR Analysis

Factitious apparent clonal bands that do not repeat can be seen in AgR clonality testing (Fig. 42.5b). To avoid misinterpretation of these non-reproducible non-clonal peaks/bands, multiplex PCR analyses for AgR clonality should be performed in duplicate [122]. Failure to recognize these non-reproducible non-clonal peaks by duplicate analysis could result in generation of an erroneous interpretation of clonality.

Molecular Abnormalities in Benign Lymphoid Proliferations

The presence of a clonal B-cell population, by itself, does not establish a diagnosis of B-cell malignancy. B-cell clones can be detected by *IGH* PCR in benign lymphoid hyperplasias and aberrant immune responses in the absence of other criteria for malignancy [124–126]. Benign B-cell clonality occurs most frequently in the setting of immune deficiencies, autoimmune diseases, and immunosuppression, and reinforces the critical necessity for interpretation of tests for B-cell clonality in conjunction with clinical, morphologic, and immunophenotypic information. The fact that patients with immune dysfunction have an increased risk of NHL, in particular BCL, further confounds the issue.

Other types of BCL-associated genetic alterations also have been described in benign settings and could result in a false interpretation of malignancy. For example, rare B cells carry a t(14;18)(q32;q21)–*IGH–BCL2* translocation in individuals without FL [127–129]. Nested PCR assays capable of detecting one *IGH–BCL2* translocation-carrying cell in 10^5–10^6 normal cells will be positive in up to half of the tissue biopsies, BM aspirates, and peripheral blood specimens from normal individuals. To date, there is no evidence that these individuals are at higher risk for development of FL. Therefore, diagnostic tests for FL should have a lower sensitivity to avoid detection of the *IGH–BCL2* translocation in unaffected individuals.

Lineage Infidelity or Promiscuity

A potential pitfall in interpretation of molecular tests for AgR rearrangements in BCL is the occurrence of so-called lineage infidelity or promiscuity, which includes the rearrangement of the *TR* genes in BCL. This is particularly common in precursor B-cell malignancies but also may be seen in malignancies of mature B cells. The majority of precursor B-cell malignancies will have rearrangement of the *TRG* gene, and 5–10 % of mature B-cell malignancies also show *TR* gene rearrangements [110, 111, 113]. This finding could lead to erroneous conclusions about cell lineage if not interpreted in conjunction with other clinical and laboratory parameters associated with the case.

Oligoclonality and Clonal Evolution

An oligoclonal pattern is defined as the presence of more bands or peaks than would be expected from a single monoclonal B-cell population, specifically, more than two reproducible bands/peaks per PCR. An oligoclonal pattern can be seen when there is expansion of several B-cell clones in reactive processes or in immunocompromised individuals with a reduced B-cell repertoire, as well as in specimens with very few B-cells. Oligoclonal patterns must be interpreted with care.

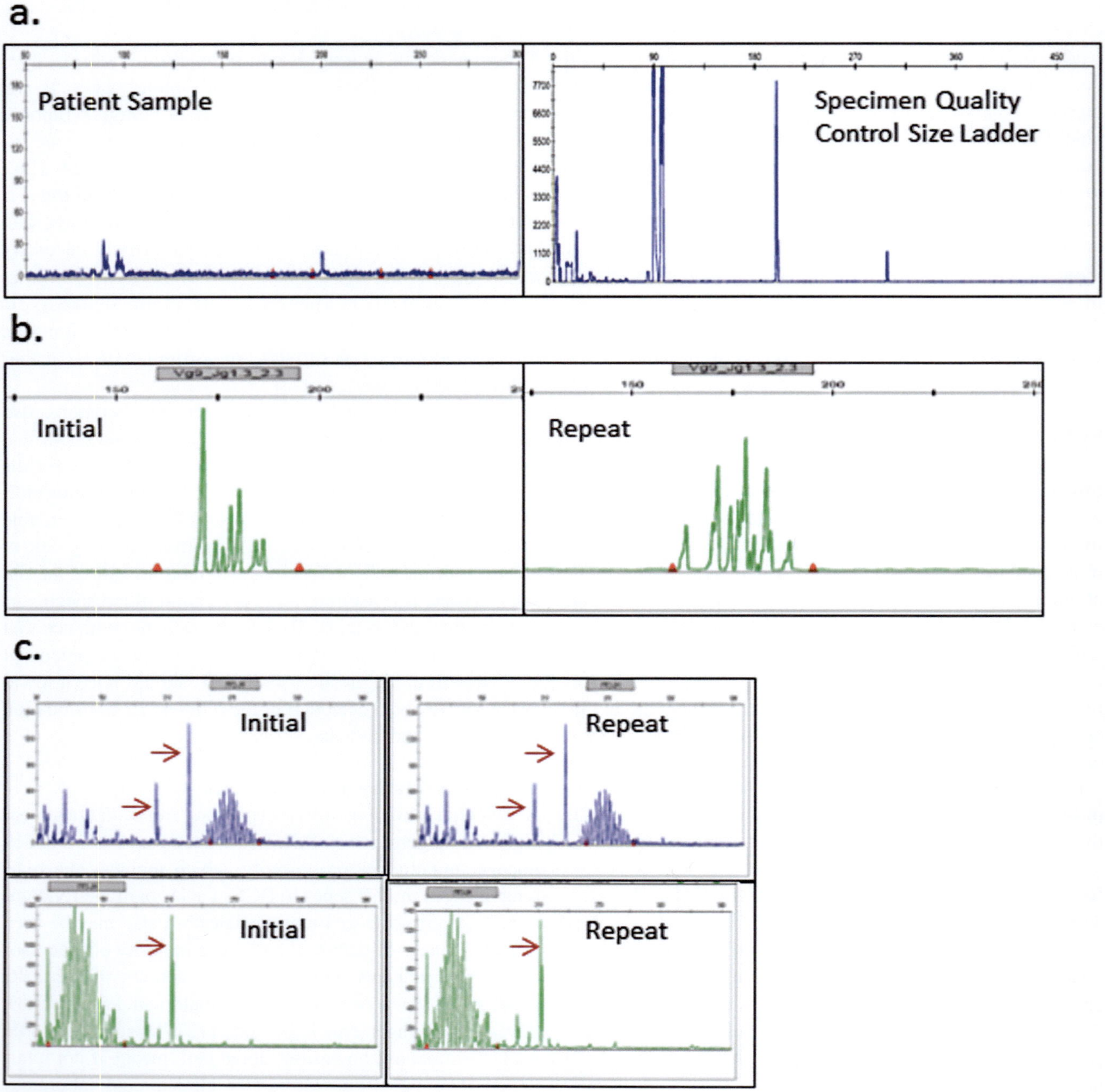

Figure 42.5 Pitfalls in interpretation of PCR assays for Ig clonality assessment using BIOMED-2 primer sets. (**a**) Poor sample quality. The patient sample shows no specific product in the *left panel* but the results are not reliable because the specimen quality control size ladder (*right panel*) illustrates that larger amplicons (> 200 bp) are not amplified well. (**b**) Non-reproducible peaks. Apparent clonal peaks detected initially (*arrows* in *left panel*) were not present on repeat analysis (*right panel*), underscoring the benefit of duplicate analyses. (**c**) Reproducible nonspecific peaks. Well-known, but nonspecific amplicons (*arrows*) are reproducibly detected but do not indicate clonality. Knowledge of the sizes of these nonspecific reproducible peaks is essential to avoid erroneous diagnoses of clonality. (See Table 42.5)

Although it is rare, occasional patients will have two separate monoclonal B-cell populations, resulting in more than two clonal peaks/bands. Specific documentation of two separate B-cell populations by flow cytometry or immunophenotyping is required to support the interpretation of two monoclonal B-cell populations, i.e., a biclonal process.

During the course of disease in some BCL patients, the monoclonal population may develop additional *IGH* rearrangements that may alter the size of peaks/bands seen by *IGH* PCR (so-called clonal evolution). If *IGH* PCR is used for MRD testing, clonal evolution may change or eliminate the diagnostic PCR band(s) and lead to false-negative results. *IGLK* gene rearrangements involving the kappa-deleting element (Kde) appear to be more stable than *IGH* gene rearrangements, possibly because they usually delete the two enhancers for the *IGLK* gene [106, 129]. However, these *IGLK*-Kde rearrangements are present in only a minority of BCL, limiting their clinical utility.

Inadequate Test Sensitivity

Molecular assays never achieve 100 % analytical sensitivity, so a false-negative result must always be considered. Actual sensitivity will vary between laboratories, but a standard *IGH* PCR of fresh or frozen tissue will usually detect one clonal cell in 10^2–10^3 normal cells. *IGH* PCR using FFPE tissue may have much lower sensitivity, sometimes as low as 40–60 %, and is highly subject to the conditions used for tissue fixation and processing. Every assay for *IGH* clonality must include appropriate sensitivity controls, based on the purpose of the clonality testing for each case. A test sensitivity of one positive cell in 20 normal cells (5 %) is adequate for diagnostic or prognostic testing of almost all BCL, but 5 % assay sensitivity is inadequate for MRD assessment testing. The minimal sensitivity for a test offered for MRD assessment should be one positive cell in 10^4 normal cells, and a sensitivity of one positive cell in 10^5–10^6 normal cells is achievable and desirable for some assays. The *IGH* AgR and *IGH–BCL2* PCR assays usually have different sensitivities, which may lead to discrepant results when both tests are performed for the same specimen.

Poor Specimen Quality

The absence of a polyclonal Gaussian distribution of peaks/bands and/or a clonal signal may be due to poor DNA quality or a paucity of lymphoid cells in the specimen and should result in a check of DNA quality in the control PCR (Fig. 42.5a), as well as evaluation of the T- and B-cell content by IHC or flow cytometry. The quality of extracted DNA or RNA is not usually a problem with fresh or frozen tissue or cells, if viable tissue has been obtained. However, poor DNA quality is a known problem with PCR assays of FFPE tissue which is even less suitable for RNA extraction and testing due to RNA degradation. Different fixatives will affect the success of DNA and RNA extraction. Formalin fixation allows adequate DNA and RNA preservation for PCR in most cases, but adequate DNA or RNA for PCR is difficult to obtain from paraffin-embedded tissue fixed with mercury-based (B5), Zenker, or Bouin fixatives.

Primer Failure

Clearly, the most common cause of false-negative *IGH* PCR results for BCL is the failure of primer binding due to sequence alteration of the primer binding site by somatic hypermutation of IGVH regions in post-germinal center BCL. The false-negative rate with *IGH* PCR ranges from less than 5 % (MCL) to greater than 50 % (MZL, FL, plasma cell dyscrasias). In the BCLs that give false-negative results by *IGH* PCR, clonality may be demonstrated on a PCR analysis for *IGK* rearrangements. The possibility of a false-negative *IGH* clonality result, particularly in post-germinal center BCL (FL and MZL) must always be considered in the interpretation of *IGH* PCR results.

Unusual or Complex *IGH* Rearrangements

Occasional BCL have very complex rearrangements of *IGH* and other associated genes that may confound standard *IGH* PCR testing. This has been seen most frequently in FL, but similar genetic events undoubtedly occur with other *IGH* translocation partners. For example, most FL have a single *IGH–BCL2* rearrangement involving one chromosome 14 *IGH* allele, which is then unable to participate in a functional *IGH* rearrangement. An additional clonal rearrangement of the untranslocated *IGH* allele on the other chromosome 14 usually occurs and can be detected by *IGH* PCR. However, occasional FL will have translocations of both *IGH* alleles to chromosome 18, resulting in the absence of a detectable clonal *IGH* rearrangement by PCR.

Laboratory Issues

Differences across clinical molecular laboratories in PCR testing for *IGH* rearrangements and *IGH–BCL2* translocations has been documented repeatedly by the proficiency testing surveys of the College of American Pathologists [130], as well as by other, independent interlaboratory surveys [131]. The reasons for the lack of reproducibility among laboratories are multiple and not easily overcome. Some strategies for PCR testing and interpretation that improve test performance are discussed below.

Use of Appropriate Controls

Appropriate controls for PCR tests include positive, negative, sensitivity, and no DNA reactions. Laboratories may not know or overestimate the diagnostic sensitivity of their *IGH* and *IGH–BCL2* PCR assays if the sensitivity of the assay was established at the time of test validation, but sensitivity controls are not included in every run because the sensitivity may decline over time or be variable from run to run.

Interlaboratory surveys indicate that some laboratories may not use adequate controls. Apart from the controls mentioned above, an additional important PCR control, particularly with FFPE tissue, is the amplification of a non-rearranging gene to document the presence of adequate DNA in the tested sample and the absence of inhibitors of the DNA polymerase, to avoid a false-negative result.

Amplification of Duplicate Aliquots of DNA

Small samples or samples with few B cells may have insufficient B cells to produce a polyclonal background. In this setting, *IGH* PCR may amplify rare B cells, producing a misleading monoclonal or oligoclonal pattern. Likewise, a sensitive *IGH–BCL2* assay capable of detecting MRD could also amplify a rare benign translocation-carrying cell, as previously discussed. Over-interpretation of a single band or peak on *IGH* and *IGH–BCL2* PCR assays by laboratories not performing the assays in duplicate may cause false-positive results. With amplification of duplicate DNA aliquots for each specimen, only clearly visible bands or peaks of identical size in each duplicate should be interpreted as a positive clonal result. Peaks/bands seen in analyses of specimens containing rare B cells, or rare normal translocation-carrying cells, will not be replicated in both reactions.

Adherence to Strict Criteria for Interpretation and Reporting

The interpretation of assays for *IGH* rearrangements, the *IGH–BCL2* translocation, and other BCL-associated translocations must be performed with caution. The interpretation of even the most commonly performed PCR assays for *IGH* is quite challenging. Therefore, PCR results should be very carefully interpreted and reported, preferentially in conjunction with clinical history, morphology, and immunophenotyping data. Reports should clearly indicate that a false-negative result is a possibility. False-positive PCR results largely can be avoided by performing the assay in duplicate. Parallel analysis of BCL from different sites or pre- and post-treatment in a given patient will allow comparison of PCR product sizes, which can provide very helpful information for interpretation. Testing for MRD assessment is usually done in association with specific clinical trials. Widespread use of the BIOMED-2 multiplex PCR reagents and protocols for AgR clonality testing, together with the adoption of the recommended EuroClonality guidelines for interpretation and reporting, will likely improve interlaboratory consistency over the next few years.

Conclusions and Future Directions

Clinical demand for genetic characterization of BCL at the time of primary diagnosis has intensified as our understanding of NHL biology has increased and therapies targeting specific BCL subgroups have been developed. Today, genetic features of NHL are used to aid in rendering an accurate primary diagnosis, to predict prognosis, to evaluate for MRD during and after therapy, and to help determine optimal therapy. The rapid acquisition of knowledge about BCL biology and translation of this knowledge into targeted therapeutic strategies is occurring at an unprecedented rate. New testing strategies and technologies are essential for clinical laboratories to keep up with the growing information on BCL obtained from research methods such as gene expression profiling, aCGH, proteomics, and exome and genome sequencing.

The role of the hematopathologist is clearly changing and expanding. As gene expression profiling, aCGH, and other genome-wide research identifies novel genes and biologic mechanisms that play important roles in the therapeutic responsiveness and overall survival of lymphoma patients, clinicians are beginning to incorporate this new knowledge into the selection of more targeted therapies. Clinical molecular laboratories today must provide input at the time of initial diagnosis and during and after treatment. Laboratories must ensure the proper performance of molecular tests and the accurate interpretation and clinical use of the results. Testing for initial diagnosis and prognosis for BCL is not the same testing needed for MRD assessment during and after therapy. Furthermore, the lines between classical cytogenetic laboratories and molecular laboratories are blurring due to the marked increase in the use of FISH analysis. Hematopathologists increasingly need to be knowledgeable about both lymphoma biology and different therapies for lymphoma, and to interact closely with clinicians to ensure that appropriate testing is performed and appropriately used for clinical decisions.

Clinical laboratories that perform molecular testing on BCL are faced with two daunting tasks. First and foremost is the necessity of expanding test menus to meet the increasing clinical demand of testing for new molecular markers for NHL. Expanding test menus to meet clinical needs will require implementation of new technologies. These technical advances are essential for rapid testing for a broad panel of relevant genes at a reasonable cost. Several approaches show promise for diagnostic implementation and could alleviate the technological bottleneck that slows down the translation of new molecular knowledge into clinical tests. However, the lack of a reasonable level of reimbursement for molecular testing in general is a major roadblock to successful implementation of new techniques for important new genetic markers in BCL.

The second and equally important task is the urgent need for standardization of molecular testing methods to reduce the differences in test results and their interpretation across clinical molecular laboratories. Lessons learned from the European studies to standardize molecular testing and reporting for BCL are being used to standardize BCL molecular testing in the USA. It is likely that utilization of the BIOMED-2 reagents and protocols, together with the development of optimal proficiency testing materials and consensus interpretation guidelines will make strides towards a comparable level of laboratory standardization of molecular testing in the USA.

References

1. Swerdlow SH, Campom E, Harris NL, Jaffe ES, Pileri SA, Stein H. WHO classification of tumours of haematopoietic and lymphoid tissues. Lyon, France: IARC press; 2008.
2. Pan L, Cesarman E, Knowles DM. Antigen receptor genes: structure, function, and genetic analysis of their rearrangements. In: Knowles DM, editor. Neoplastic hematology. Philadelphia: Lippincott Williams & Wilkins; 2001. p. 307–28.
3. LeBien TW, Tedder TF. B lymphocytes: how they develop and function. Blood. 2008;112(5):1570–80.
4. Korsmeyer SJ, et al. Developmental hierarchy of immunoglobulin gene rearrangements in human leukemic pre-B-cells. Proc Natl Acad Sci U S A. 1981;78(11):7096–100.
5. Vendrame E, Martinez-Maza O. Assessment of pre-diagnosis biomarkers of immune activation and inflammation: insights on the etiology of lymphoma. J Proteome Res. 2011;10(1):113–9.
6. Lin KI, et al. Relevance of the immunoglobulin VH somatic mutation status in patients with chronic lymphocytic leukemia treated with fludarabine, cyclophosphamide, and rituximab (FCR) or related chemoimmunotherapy regimens. Blood. 2009;113(14):3168–71.
7. Zenz T, et al. TP53 mutation profile in chronic lymphocytic leukemia: evidence for a disease specific profile from a comprehensive analysis of 268 mutations. Leukemia. 2010;24(12):2072–9.
8. Zenz T, et al. Importance of genetics in chronic lymphocytic leukemia. Blood Rev. 2011;25(3):131–7.
9. Zenz T, et al. TP53 mutation and survival in chronic lymphocytic leukemia. J Clin Oncol. 2010;28(29):4473–9.
10. Dohner H, et al. Genomic aberrations and survival in chronic lymphocytic leukemia. N Engl J Med. 2000;343(26):1910–6.
11. Tsimberidou AM, et al. Chemoimmunotherapy may overcome the adverse prognostic significance of 11q deletion in previously untreated patients with chronic lymphocytic leukemia. Cancer. 2009;115(2):373–80.
12. Calin GA, et al. Frequent deletions and down-regulation of micro-RNA genes miR15 and miR16 at 13q14 in chronic lymphocytic leukemia. Proc Natl Acad Sci U S A. 2002;99(24):15524–9.
13. Wang L, et al. SF3B1 and other novel cancer genes in chronic lymphocytic leukemia. N Engl J Med. 2011;365(26):2497–506.
14. Rossi D, et al. Mutations of the SF3B1 splicing factor in chronic lymphocytic leukemia: association with progression and fludarabine-refractoriness. Blood. 2011;118(26):6904–8.
15. Quesada V, et al. Exome sequencing identifies recurrent mutations of the splicing factor SF3B1 gene in chronic lymphocytic leukemia. Nat Genet. 2012;44(1):47–52.
16. Del Giudice I, et al. B-cell prolymphocytic leukemia and chronic lymphocytic leukemia have distinctive gene expression signatures. Leukemia. 2009;23(11):2160–7.
17. Kuriakose P, et al. Translocation (8;14)(q24;q32) as the sole cytogenetic abnormality in B-cell prolymphocytic leukemia. Cancer Genet Cytogenet. 2004;150(2):156–8.
18. Crisostomo RH, Fernandez JA, Caceres W. Complex karyotype including chromosomal translocation (8;14) (q24;q32) in one case with B-cell prolymphocytic leukemia. Leuk Res. 2007;31(5):699–701.
19. Tiacci E, et al. BRAF mutations in hairy-cell leukemia. N Engl J Med. 2011;364(24):2305–15.
20. Chang H, et al. Prognostic relevance of 6q deletion in Waldenstrom's macroglobulinemia: a multicenter study. Clin Lymphoma Myeloma. 2009;9(1):36–8.
21. Terre C, et al. Trisomy 4, a new chromosomal abnormality in Waldenstrom's macroglobulinemia: a study of 39 cases. Leukemia. 2006;20(9):1634–6.
22. Cook JR, et al. Lack of PAX5 rearrangements in lymphoplasmacytic lymphomas: reassessing the reported association with t(9;14). Hum Pathol. 2004;35(4):447–54.
23. Gutierrez NC, et al. Gene expression profiling of B lymphocytes and plasma cells from Waldenstrom's macroglobulinemia: comparison with expression patterns of the same cell counterparts from chronic lymphocytic leukemia, multiple myeloma and normal individuals. Leukemia. 2007;21(3):541–9.
24. Li J, et al. Clonal expansions of cytotoxic T cells exist in the blood of patients with Waldenstrom macroglobulinemia but exhibit anergic properties and are eliminated by nucleoside analogue therapy. Blood. 2010;115(17):3580–8.
25. Treon SP, et al. MYD88 L265P somatic mutation in Waldenstrom's macroglobulinemia. N Engl J Med. 2012;367(9):826–33.
26. Hoyer JD, et al. The (11;14)(q13;q32) translocation in multiple myeloma. A morphologic and immunohistochemical study. Am J Clin Pathol. 2000;113(6):831–7.
27. Shou Y, et al. Diverse karyotypic abnormalities of the c-myc locus associated with c-myc dysregulation and tumor progression in multiple myeloma. Proc Natl Acad Sci U S A. 2000;97(1):228–33.
28. Chiecchio L, et al. Frequent upregulation of MYC in plasma cell leukemia. Genes Chromosomes Cancer. 2009;48(7):624–36.
29. Fonseca R, et al. International Myeloma Working Group molecular classification of multiple myeloma: spotlight review. Leukemia. 2009;23(12):2210–21.
30. Hose D, et al. Proliferation is a central independent prognostic factor and target for personalized and risk-adapted treatment in multiple myeloma. Haematologica. 2011;96(1):87–95.
31. Dewald GW, et al. Relationship of patient survival and chromosome anomalies detected in metaphase and/or interphase cells at diagnosis of myeloma. Blood. 2005;106(10):3553–8.
32. Saez B, et al. Identification of recurrent chromosomal breakpoints in multiple myeloma with complex karyotypes by combined G-banding, spectral karyotyping, and fluorescence in situ hybridization analyses. Cancer Genet Cytogenet. 2006;169(2):143–9.
33. Remstein ED, James CD, Kurtin PJ. Incidence and subtype specificity of API2-MALT1 fusion translocations in extranodal, nodal, and splenic marginal zone lymphomas. Am J Pathol. 2000;156(4):1183–8.
34. Ye H, et al. High incidence of t(11;18)(q21;q21) in Helicobacter pylori-negative gastric MALT lymphoma. Blood. 2003;101(7):2547–50.
35. Liu H, et al. T(11;18)(q21;q21) is associated with advanced mucosa-associated lymphoid tissue lymphoma that expresses nuclear BCL10. Blood. 2001;98(4):1182–7.
36. Zhang Q, et al. Inactivating mutations and overexpression of BCL10, a caspase recruitment domain-containing gene, in MALT lymphoma with t(1;14)(p22;q32). Nat Genet. 1999;22(1):63–8.
37. Streubel B, et al. T(14;18)(q32;q21) involving IGH and MALT1 is a frequent chromosomal aberration in MALT lymphoma. Blood. 2003;101(6):2335–9.

38. Streubel B, et al. T(3;14)(p14.1;q32) involving IGH and FOXP1 is a novel recurrent chromosomal aberration in MALT lymphoma. Leukemia. 2005;19(4):652–8.
39. Sagaert X, et al. Forkhead box protein P1 expression in mucosa-associated lymphoid tissue lymphomas predicts poor prognosis and transformation to diffuse large B-cell lymphoma. J Clin Oncol. 2006;24(16):2490–7.
40. Honma K, et al. TNFAIP3/A20 functions as a novel tumor suppressor gene in several subtypes of non-Hodgkin lymphomas. Blood. 2009;114(12):2467–75.
41. Ngo VN, et al. Oncogenically active MYD88 mutations in human lymphoma. Nature. 2011;470(7332):115–9.
42. Armitage JO, Weisenburger DD. New approach to classifying non-Hodgkin's lymphomas: clinical features of the major histologic subtypes. Non-Hodgkin's Lymphoma Classification Project. J Clin Oncol. 1998;16(8):2780–95.
43. Horning SJ. Follicular lymphoma: have we made any progress? Ann Oncol. 2000;11 Suppl 1:23–7.
44. Dave SS, et al. Prediction of survival in follicular lymphoma based on molecular features of tumor-infiltrating immune cells. N Engl J Med. 2004;351(21):2159–69.
45. Gribben JG, et al. Detection by polymerase chain reaction of residual cells with the bcl-2 translocation is associated with increased risk of relapse after autologous bone marrow transplantation for B-cell lymphoma. Blood. 1993;81(12):3449–57.
46. Lopez-Guillermo A, et al. Molecular response assessed by PCR is the most important factor predicting failure-free survival in indolent follicular lymphoma: update of the MDACC series. Ann Oncol. 2000;11 Suppl 1:137–40.
47. Davies AJ, et al. Transformation of follicular lymphoma to diffuse large B-cell lymphoma proceeds by distinct oncogenic mechanisms. Br J Haematol. 2007;136(2):286–93.
48. Lossos IS, et al. Transformation of follicular lymphoma to diffuse large-cell lymphoma: alternative patterns with increased or decreased expression of c-myc and its regulated genes. Proc Natl Acad Sci U S A. 2002;99(13):8886–91.
49. Cheung KJ, et al. Genome-wide profiling of follicular lymphoma by array comparative genomic hybridization reveals prognostically significant DNA copy number imbalances. Blood. 2009;113(1):137–48.
50. Morin RD, et al. Frequent mutation of histone-modifying genes in non-Hodgkin lymphoma. Nature. 2011;476(7360):298–303.
51. Weisenburger DD, et al. Mantle cell lymphoma. A clinicopathologic study of 68 cases from the Nebraska Lymphoma Study Group. Am J Hematol. 2000;64(3):190–6.
52. Belaud-Rotureau MA, et al. A comparative analysis of FISH, RT-PCR, PCR, and immunohistochemistry for the diagnosis of mantle cell lymphomas. Mod Pathol. 2002;15(5):517–25.
53. Rosenwald A, et al. The proliferation gene expression signature is a quantitative integrator of oncogenic events that predicts survival in mantle cell lymphoma. Cancer Cell. 2003;3(2):185–97.
54. Tiemann M, et al. Histopathology, cell proliferation indices and clinical outcome in 304 patients with mantle cell lymphoma (MCL): a clinicopathological study from the European MCL Network. Br J Haematol. 2005;131(1):29–38.
55. Mozos A, et al. SOX11 expression is highly specific for mantle cell lymphoma and identifies the cyclin D1-negative subtype. Haematologica. 2009;94(11):1555–62.
56. Greiner TC, et al. Mutation and genomic deletion status of ataxia telangiectasia mutated (ATM) and p53 confer specific gene expression profiles in mantle cell lymphoma. Proc Natl Acad Sci U S A. 2006;103(7):2352–7.
57. Kridel R, et al. Whole transcriptome sequencing reveals recurrent NOTCH1 mutations in mantle cell lymphoma. Blood. 2012;119(9):1963–71.
58. Alizadeh AA, et al. Distinct types of diffuse large B-cell lymphoma identified by gene expression profiling. Nature. 2000;403(6769):503–11.
59. Shipp MA, et al. Diffuse large B-cell lymphoma outcome prediction by gene-expression profiling and supervised machine learning. Nat Med. 2002;8(1):68–74.
60. Rosenwald A, et al. The use of molecular profiling to predict survival after chemotherapy for diffuse large-B-cell lymphoma. N Engl J Med. 2002;346(25):1937–47.
61. Lenz G, et al. Molecular subtypes of diffuse large B-cell lymphoma arise by distinct genetic pathways. Proc Natl Acad Sci U S A. 2008;105(36):13520–5.
62. Pasqualucci L, et al. Analysis of the coding genome of diffuse large B-cell lymphoma. Nat Genet. 2011;43(9):830–7.
63. Compagno M, et al. Mutations of multiple genes cause deregulation of NF-kappaB in diffuse large B-cell lymphoma. Nature. 2009;459(7247):717–21.
64. Bentz M, et al. Gain of chromosome arm 9p is characteristic of primary mediastinal B-cell lymphoma (MBL): comprehensive molecular cytogenetic analysis and presentation of a novel MBL cell line. Genes Chromosomes Cancer. 2001;30(4):393–401.
65. Lenz G, Staudt LM. Aggressive lymphomas. N Engl J Med. 2010;362(15):1417–29.
66. Barrans SL, et al. Rearrangement of the BCL6 locus at 3q27 is an independent poor prognostic factor in nodal diffuse large B-cell lymphoma. Br J Haematol. 2002;117(2):322–32.
67. Lossos IS, et al. Expression of a single gene, BCL-6, strongly predicts survival in patients with diffuse large B-cell lymphoma. Blood. 2001;98(4):945–51.
68. Savage KJ, et al. MYC gene rearrangements are associated with a poor prognosis in diffuse large B-cell lymphoma patients treated with R-CHOP chemotherapy. Blood. 2009;114(17):3533–7.
69. Barrans S, et al. Rearrangement of MYC is associated with poor prognosis in patients with diffuse large B-cell lymphoma treated in the era of rituximab. J Clin Oncol. 2010;28(20):3360–5.
70. Johnson NA, et al. Concurrent expression of MYC and BCL2 in diffuse large B-cell lymphoma treated with rituximab plus cyclophosphamide, doxorubicin, vincristine, and prednisone. J Clin Oncol. 2012;30(28):3452–9.
71. Green TM, et al. Immunohistochemical double-hit score is a strong predictor of outcome in patients with diffuse large B-cell lymphoma treated with rituximab plus cyclophosphamide, doxorubicin, vincristine, and prednisone. J Clin Oncol. 2012;30(28):3460–7.
72. Neri A, et al. Different regions of the immunoglobulin heavy-chain locus are involved in chromosomal translocations in distinct pathogenetic forms of Burkitt lymphoma. Proc Natl Acad Sci U S A. 1988;85(8):2748–52.
73. Konigsberg R, et al. Predictive role of interphase cytogenetics for survival of patients with multiple myeloma. J Clin Oncol. 2000;18(4):804–12.
74. Bellan C, et al. Burkitt's lymphoma: new insights into molecular pathogenesis. J Clin Pathol. 2003;56(3):188–92.
75. Dave SS, et al. Molecular diagnosis of Burkitt's lymphoma. N Engl J Med. 2006;354(23):2431–42.
76. Schmitz R, et al. Burkitt lymphoma pathogenesis and therapeutic targets from structural and functional genomics. Nature. 2012;490(7418):116–20.
77. Beltran B, et al. ALK-positive diffuse large B-cell lymphoma: report of four cases and review of the literature. J Hematol Oncol. 2009;2:11.
78. Li HL, et al. Correlation of seven biological factors (Hsp90a, p53, MDM2, Bcl-2, Bax, Cytochrome C, and Cleaved caspase3) with clinical outcomes of ALK+ anaplastic large-cell lymphoma. Biomed Environ Sci. 2011;24(6):630–41.
79. Tran H, et al. Immunodeficiency-associated lymphomas. Blood Rev. 2008;22(5):261–81.
80. Hasserjian RP, et al. Immunomodulator agent-related lymphoproliferative disorders. Mod Pathol. 2009;22(12):1532–40.

81. Capello D, Rossi D, Gaidano G. Post-transplant lymphoproliferative disorders: molecular basis of disease histogenesis and pathogenesis. Hematol Oncol. 2005;23(2):61–7.
82. Gaidano G, et al. Aberrant somatic hypermutation in multiple subtypes of AIDS-associated non-Hodgkin lymphoma. Blood. 2003;102(5):1833–41.
83. Judde JG, et al. Monoclonality or oligoclonality of human herpesvirus 8 terminal repeat sequences in Kaposi's sarcoma and other diseases. J Natl Cancer Inst. 2000;92(9):729–36.
84. Cesarman E. Gammaherpesvirus and lymphoproliferative disorders in immunocompromised patients. Cancer Lett. 2011;305(2):163–74.
85. Chaganti S, et al. Epstein-Barr virus persistence in the absence of conventional memory B cells: IgM+IgD+CD27+ B cells harbor the virus in X-linked lymphoproliferative disease patients. Blood. 2008;112(3):672–9.
86. Grulich AE, et al. Incidence of cancers in people with HIV/AIDS compared with immunosuppressed transplant recipients: a meta-analysis. Lancet. 2007;370(9581):59–67.
87. Simard EP, Pfeiffer RM, Engels EA. Spectrum of cancer risk late after AIDS onset in the United States. Arch Intern Med. 2010;170(15):1337–45.
88. Martin-Perez D, et al. Epstein-Barr virus microRNAs repress BCL6 expression in diffuse large B-cell lymphoma. Leukemia. 2012;26(1):180–3.
89. Carbone A, et al. BCL-6 protein expression in AIDS-related non-Hodgkin's lymphomas: inverse relationship with Epstein-Barr virus-encoded latent membrane protein-1 expression. Am J Pathol. 1997;150(1):155–65.
90. Epeldegui M, et al. Elevated expression of activation induced cytidine deaminase in peripheral blood mononuclear cells precedes AIDS-NHL diagnosis. AIDS. 2007;21(17):2265–70.
91. Colomo L, et al. Diffuse large B-cell lymphomas with plasmablastic differentiation represent a heterogeneous group of disease entities. Am J Surg Pathol. 2004;28(6):736–47.
92. Suzuki Y, et al. CD3- and CD4-positive plasmablastic lymphoma: a literature review of Japanese plasmablastic lymphoma cases. Intern Med. 2010;49(16):1801–5.
93. Borenstein J, Pezzella F, Gatter KC. Plasmablastic lymphomas may occur as post-transplant lymphoproliferative disorders. Histopathology. 2007;51(6):774–7.
94. Kim JE, et al. Human immunodeficiency virus-negative plasmablastic lymphoma in Korea. Leuk Lymphoma. 2009;50(4):582–7.
95. Valera A, et al. IG/MYC rearrangements are the main cytogenetic alteration in plasmablastic lymphomas. Am J Surg Pathol. 2010;34(11):1686–94.
96. Trivedi P, et al. Infection of HHV-8+ primary effusion lymphoma cells with a recombinant Epstein-Barr virus leads to restricted EBV latency, altered phenotype, and increased tumorigenicity without affecting TCL1 expression. Blood. 2004;103(1):313–6.
97. Carbone A. Emerging pathways in the development of AIDS-related lymphomas. Lancet Oncol. 2003;4(1):22–9.
98. Gaidano G, et al. Frequent mutation of the 5' noncoding region of the BCL-6 gene in acquired immunodeficiency syndrome-related non-Hodgkin's lymphomas. Blood. 1997;89(10):3755–62.
99. Rickinson A. Epstein-Barr virus. Virus Res. 2002;82(1–2):109–13.
100. Eckert C, et al. Potential of LightCycler technology for quantification of minimal residual disease in childhood acute lymphoblastic leukemia. Leukemia. 2000;14(2):316–23.
101. Bottcher S, et al. Standardized MRD flow and ASO IGH RQ-PCR for MRD quantification in CLL patients after rituximab-containing immunochemotherapy: a comparative analysis. Leukemia. 2009;23(11):2007–17.
102. Bosch F, et al. Fludarabine, cyclophosphamide, and mitoxantrone as initial therapy of chronic lymphocytic leukemia: high response rate and disease eradication. Clin Cancer Res. 2008;14(1):155–61.
103. Kay NE, et al. Combination chemoimmunotherapy with pentostatin, cyclophosphamide, and rituximab shows significant clinical activity with low accompanying toxicity in previously untreated B chronic lymphocytic leukemia. Blood. 2007;109(2):405–11.
104. Tysarowski A, et al. Usefulness of real-time PCR in long-term follow-up of follicular lymphoma patients. Acta Biochim Pol. 2007;54(1):135–42.
105. Rawstron AC, et al. International standardized approach for flow cytometric residual disease monitoring in chronic lymphocytic leukaemia. Leukemia. 2007;21(5):956–64.
106. van der Velden VH, et al. Detection of minimal residual disease in hematologic malignancies by real-time quantitative PCR: principles, approaches, and laboratory aspects. Leukemia. 2003;17(6):1013–34.
107. Stow P, et al. Clinical significance of low levels of minimal residual disease at the end of remission induction therapy in childhood acute lymphoblastic leukemia. Blood. 2010;115(23):4657–63.
108. Campana D. Minimal residual disease in acute lymphoblastic leukemia. Hematology Am Soc Hematol Educ Program. 2010;2010:7–12.
109. Guggemos A, et al. Assessment of clonal stability of minimal residual disease targets between 1st and 2nd relapse of childhood precursor B-cell acute lymphoblastic leukemia. Haematologica. 2003;88(7):737–46.
110. Szczepanski T, et al. Vdelta2-Jalpha rearrangements are frequent in precursor-B-acute lymphoblastic leukemia but rare in normal lymphoid cells. Blood. 2004;103(10):3798–804.
111. Szczepanski T, et al. Comparative analysis of Ig and TCR gene rearrangements at diagnosis and at relapse of childhood precursor-B-ALL provides improved strategies for selection of stable PCR targets for monitoring of minimal residual disease. Blood. 2002;99(7):2315–23.
112. van Dongen JJ, et al. Design and standardization of PCR primers and protocols for detection of clonal immunoglobulin and T-cell receptor gene recombinations in suspect lymphoproliferations: report of the BIOMED-2 concerted action BMH4-CT98-3936. Leukemia. 2003;17(12):2257–317.
113. Szczepanski T. Why and how to quantify minimal residual disease in acute lymphoblastic leukemia? Leukemia. 2007;21(4):622–6.
114. Colombat P, et al. Rituximab (anti-CD20 monoclonal antibody) as single first-line therapy for patients with follicular lymphoma with a low tumor burden: clinical and molecular evaluation. Blood. 2001;97(1):101–6.
115. Mandigers CM, et al. Dynamics of circulating t(14;18)-positive cells during first-line and subsequent lines of treatment in follicular lymphoma. Ann Hematol. 2003;82(12):743–9.
116. Schmitt C, et al. One single dose of rituximab added to a standard regimen of CHOP in primary treatment of follicular lymphoma appears to result in a high clearance rate from circulating bcl-2/IgH positive cells: Is the end of molecular monitoring near? Leuk Res. 2006;30(12):1563–8.
117. Janikova A, et al. The persistence of t(14;18)-bearing cells in lymph nodes of patients with follicular lymphoma in complete remission: the evidence for 'a lymphoma stem cell'. Leuk Lymphoma. 2009;50(7):1102–9.
118. Darby AJ, et al. Variability of quantitative polymerase chain reaction detection of the bcl-2-IgH translocation in an international multicenter study. Haematologica. 2005;90(12):1706–7.
119. Kornacker M, et al. Commercial LightCycler-based quantitative real-time PCR compared to nested PCR for monitoring of Bcl-2/IgH rearrangement in patients with follicular lymphoma. Ann Hematol. 2009;88(1):43–50.

120. Gabert J, et al. Standardization and quality control studies of 'real-time' quantitative reverse transcriptase polymerase chain reaction of fusion gene transcripts for residual disease detection in leukemia - a Europe against cancer program. Leukemia. 2003; 17(12):2318–57.
121. Bagg A, et al. Immunoglobulin heavy chain gene analysis in lymphomas: a multi-center study demonstrating the heterogeneity of performance of polymerase chain reaction assays. J Mol Diagn. 2002;4(2):81–9.
122. Langerak AW, et al. EuroClonality/BIOMED-2 guidelines for interpretation and reporting of Ig/TCR clonality testing in suspected lymphoproliferations. Leukemia. 2012;26(10):2159–71.
123. Miller JE, et al. An automated semiquantitative B and T cell clonality assay. Mol Diagn. 1999;4(2):101–17.
124. Elenitoba-Johnson KS, et al. PCR analysis of the immunoglobulin heavy chain gene in polyclonal processes can yield pseudoclonal bands as an artifact of low B cell number. J Mol Diagn. 2000; 2(2):92–6.
125. Nihal M, Mikkola D, Wood GS. Detection of clonally restricted immunoglobulin heavy chain gene rearrangements in normal and lesional skin: analysis of the B cell component of the skin-associated lymphoid tissue and implications for the molecular diagnosis of cutaneous B cell lymphomas. J Mol Diagn. 2000; 2(1):5–10.
126. Lee SC, et al. Pseudo-spikes are common in histologically benign lymphoid tissues. J Mol Diagn. 2000;2(3):145–52.
127. Summers KE, et al. Frequency of the Bcl-2/IgH rearrangement in normal individuals: implications for the monitoring of disease in patients with follicular lymphoma. J Clin Oncol. 2001;19(2): 420–4.
128. van der Velden VH, et al. Immunoglobulin kappa deleting element rearrangements in precursor-B acute lymphoblastic leukemia are stable targets for detection of minimal residual disease by real-time quantitative PCR. Leukemia. 2002;16(5):928–36.
129. Limpens J, et al. Lymphoma-associated translocation t(14;18) in blood B cells of normal individuals. Blood. 1995;85(9): 2528–36.
130. Hsi ED, et al. Detection of bcl-2/J(H) translocation by polymerase chain reaction: a summary of the experience of the Molecular Oncology Survey of the College of American Pathologist. Arch Pathol Lab Med. 2002;126(8):902–8.
131. Johnson PW, et al. Variability of polymerase chain reaction detection of the bcl-2-IgH translocation in an international multicentre study. Ann Oncol. 1999;10(11):1349–54.

T-Cell Lymphomas

43

Jason D. Merker and Daniel A. Arber

Abstract

Mature T-cell and natural killer (NK)-cell neoplasms account for a small proportion of non-Hodgkin lymphomas (NHL). Despite the fact that they are relatively uncommon, T-cell lymphoproliferations often are submitted to the clinical molecular laboratory for testing. The diagnostic need for molecular testing is because T cells do not have a definitive immunophenotypic marker of clonality, like kappa and lambda antigen receptor immunophenotyping in B cells, so molecular methods can be used. A variety of molecular assays are available to evaluate T-cell receptor (*TR*) gene rearrangements, structural and numeric chromosomal abnormalities, and viral sequences associated with mature T- and NK-cell neoplasms. However, many of these molecular tests, especially PCR-based *TR* gene rearrangement testing, have important caveats that must be considered when interpreting the assays. Therefore, molecular results must be considered in the context of available clinical information, histology, immunophenotype, and other laboratory data for proper interpretation and clinical use.

Keywords

ALK • BIOMED-2 • EBV • HTLV-1 • In situ hybridization • IRF4 • Oligoclonal • Pseudoclonality • Southern blot • TCL

Molecular Basis of Disease

T-cell and natural killer (NK)-cell neoplasms are relatively rare entities, collectively accounting for approximately 12 % of non-Hodgkin lymphomas (NHL) [1]. Subtypes of mature T- and NK-cell neoplasms are defined according to the World Health Organization (WHO) classification system [2], listed in Table 43.1. Despite the fact that they are relatively uncommon, most T-cell lymphoproliferations are assessed in the clinical molecular laboratory. The diagnostic need for molecular testing is because T cells do not have a definitive immunophenotypic marker of clonality, like kappa and lambda antigen receptor immunophenotyping in B cells, so molecular methods can be used. More specifically, two broad categories of molecular changes are used for clinical testing of T-cell lymphomas (TCL): T-cell receptor (*TR*) gene rearrangements and chromosomal alterations such as translocations, insertions, or deletions.

J.D. Merker, M.D., Ph.D. (✉)
Department of Pathology, Stanford University School of Medicine, 300 Pasteur Drive, L235, Stanford, CA 94305-5324, USA
e-mail: jdmerker@stanford.edu

D.A. Arber, M.D.
Department of Pathology, Stanford University Medical Center, 300 Pasteur Drive, H1507, MC 5627, Stanford, CA 94305, USA
e-mail: darber@stanfordmed.org

TR Gene Rearrangements

Pluripotent bone marrow (BM) stem cells give rise to progenitor T cells, which migrate to the thymus for primary ontogeny. There, early in T lymphocyte development *TR* genes undergo somatic rearrangement of germline gene sequences, similar to the process that occurs with immunoglobulin

D.G.B. Leonard (ed.), *Molecular Pathology in Clinical Practice*, DOI 10.1007/978-3-319-19674-9_43

Table 43.1 2008 WHO classification of mature T- and NK-cell neoplasms [2]

T-cell prolymphocytic leukemia
T-cell large granular lymphocytic leukemia
Chronic lymphoproliferative disorders of NK cells
Aggressive NK-cell leukemia
Epstein-Barr virus (EBV) positive T-cell lymphoproliferative disorders of childhood
Systemic EBV-positive T-cell lymphoproliferative disease of childhood
Hydroa vacciniforme-like lymphoma
Adult T-cell leukemia/lymphoma
Extranodal NK/T-cell lymphoma, nasal type
Enteropathy-associated T-cell lymphoma
Hepatosplenic T-cell lymphoma
Subcutaneous panniculitis-like T-cell lymphoma
Mycosis fungoides
Sézary syndrome
Primary cutaneous CD30-positive T-cell lymphoproliferative disorders
Primary cutaneous peripheral T-cell lymphomas, rare subtypes
Primary cutaneous gamma-delta T-cell lymphoma
Primary cutaneous CD8-positive aggressive epidermotropic cytotoxic T-cell lymphoma
Primary cutaneous CD4-positive small/medium T-cell lymphoma
Peripheral T-cell lymphoma, NOS
Angioimmunoblastic T-cell lymphoma
Anaplastic large cell lymphoma, ALK-positive
Anaplastic large cell lymphoma, ALK-negative

heavy chain (*IGH*) and kappa and lambda light chain (*IGK* and *IGL*) genes. The four *TR* genes are: *TR* delta (*TRD*) at chromosome 14q11, *TR* gamma (*TRG*) at 7p14, *TR* beta (*TRB*) at 7q34, and *TR* alpha (*TRA*) at 14q11. In the germline configuration, *TRD* and *TRB* contain multiple variable (V), diversity (D), and joining (J) region segments. The *TRG* and *TRA* loci do not contain D segments. Depending on the locus, the number of segments is 8–67 V segments, 2–3 D segments, and 4–61 J segments [3]. For *TRD* and *TRB*, the somatic rearrangement initially involves the joining of one D to one J segment, followed by the joining of one V segment to the DJ segment (Fig. 43.1). For *TRG* and *TRA*, the V segment is joined to the J segment. The rearrangement process results in the deletion of the intervening coding and noncoding DNA sequences between the linked V, D, and J segments. Thus, the *TRD* and *TRB* gene rearrangements result in V-D-J juxtaposition similar to *IGH*, and *TRG* and *TRA* rearrangements result in V-J rearrangements similar to *IGK* and *IGL*. In all cases, the V-(D)-J segment is joined to the downstream constant (C) region by mRNA splicing. The *TR* genes are ultimately translated into two types of receptors, which exist as heterodimers (αβ or γδ). Of note, the *TR* genes do not undergo somatic hypermutation as occurs with antigen stimulation for the immunoglobulin (Ig) genes.

The *TR* genes generally rearrange in the following order: *TRD*, *TRG*, *TRB*, and finally *TRA* [4]. The *TRD* genes are located within the *TRA* locus, so rearrangement of *TRA* will result in *TRD* deletion on that allele. Also of note for clonal-

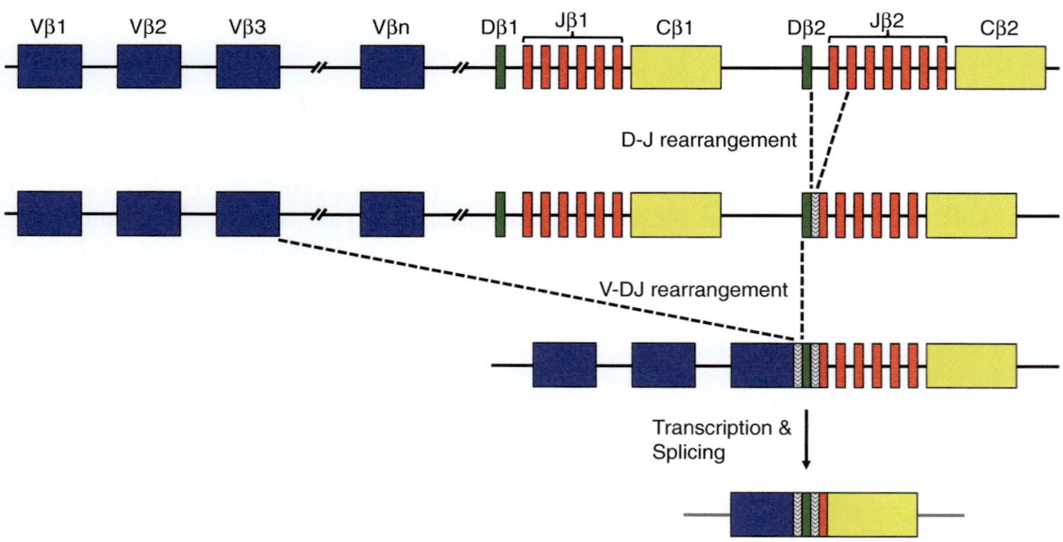

Figure 43.1 The *TRB* locus is used as an example to demonstrate the rearrangement of the variable (V), diversity (D), joining (J), and constant (C) region gene segments. The *hashed white boxes* between the rearranged V-D and D-J gene segments represent variable regions of nucleotide deletion and addition that occur during *TR* gene rearrangement

ity assessment, this hierarchical order of rearrangements results in both αβ- and γδ-T cells containing *TRG* rearrangements. For this and other reasons, *TRG* is commonly used for PCR-based clonality assessment.

The numerous different V, (D), and J segments present within each *TR* locus enable a large number of different V-(D)-J segments to be generated. The *TR* repertoire is further expanded by deletion and addition of nucleotides between the D-J and V-D junctions by terminal deoxynucleotidyl transferase (TdT), and by the combinations of different α–β or γ–δ chains. Collectively, these mechanisms generate extensive diversity of TRs with varying antigen specificity.

More than 95 % of mature, circulating T cells express the αβ receptor. In contrast, γδ T cells are mainly found in the skin, spleen, gastrointestinal tract, and other extranodal sites, which are often sites of origin for γδ T-cell lymphomas. T-cell neoplasms ensue after maturation arrest at one of the stages of T-cell development, such as from immature T cells in T lymphoblastic leukemia/lymphoma, or from more mature T cells in peripheral TCL and mycosis fungoides. Due to a common progenitor as well as some shared functional and immunophenotypic features, NK-cell neoplasms often are classified with mature T-cell neoplasms. Since NK cells do not rearrange the *TR* genes, neoplasms derived from these cells do not demonstrate *TR* gene rearrangements. The mature T- and NK-cell neoplasms of the WHO classification are listed in Table 43.1 [2].

Somatic Chromosomal Abnormalities

A variety of somatic structural and numeric chromosomal abnormalities have been observed in mature TCL, and a subset of these is listed in Table 43.2. ALK-positive anaplastic large cell lymphoma (ALCL), is associated with translocations involving the anaplastic lymphoma receptor tyrosine kinase (*ALK*) gene on chromosome 2. The most common *ALK* translocation is t(2;5)(p23;q35), which occurs in approximately 75 % of ALK-positive ALCL cases and results in the fusion of nucleophosmin (*NPM1*) on chromosome 5 with *ALK* [5, 6]. The t(1;2)(q21;p23) occurs in approximately 15 % of ALK-positive ALCL cases and results in the fusion of the tropomyosin 3 (*TPM3*) gene on chromosome 1 with *ALK* [5, 7]. The numerous other less common *ALK* fusion partners include *ATIC* at 2q35, *TFG* at 3q12, *CLTC* at 17q23, *MSN* at Xq12, *TPM4* at 19p13, *MYH9* at 22q12, and *RNF213* (*ALO17*) at 17q25 [5, 8]. The various translocations result in the activation of ALK, which is not normally expressed in lymphocytes, with subsequent oncogenic actions [5, 6].

Table 43.2 Select somatic chromosomal abnormalities associated with mature T-cell neoplasms

WHO classification	Chromosomal abnormality
T-cell prolymphocytic leukemia	inv(14)(q11q32); *TRA–TCL1*
Enteropathy-associated T-cell lymphoma	Chromosome 9q gains
Hepatosplenic T-cell lymphoma	i(7)(q10)
Primary cutaneous anaplastic large cell lymphoma	*IRF4* (6p25) rearrangements
Anaplastic large cell lymphoma, ALK-positive	t(2;5)(p23;q35); *NPM1–ALK*

Other somatic structural chromosomal abnormalities commonly associated with mature TCL include an inversion of chromosome 14 [inv(14)(q11q32)] associated with T-cell prolymphocytic leukemia [9], and an isochromosome involving the long arm of chromosome 7 [i(7)(q10)] often present with trisomy 8 and associated with hepatosplenic TCL [10]. In addition, amplification of oncogenes and loss of tumor suppressor genes can contribute to the development of mature TCL. As an example, gains involving the long arm of chromosome 9 are observed in more than half of enteropathy-associated TCL [11]. Likewise, loss of function of the *CDKN2B* (*P15*) and *CDKN2A* (*P16*) genes on the short arm of chromosome 9 due to allelic loss and aberrant promoter methylation occurs in mycosis fungoides and Sézary syndrome [12].

Indications for Testing

The diagnosis of a mature T- or NK-cell neoplasm is primarily based on histology, immunophenotype, and clinical information. For a subset of cases, distinguishing between a reactive and neoplastic process is difficult. Furthermore, in contrast to restricted Ig light-chain expression in mature B-cell lymphomas, T cells do not have a definitive immunophenotypic marker of clonality. Therefore, detection of a clonal *TR* gene rearrangement can assist in classifying the suspected lymphoproliferation as reactive or neoplastic. Due to specimen and test availability, clonality assessment most commonly involves PCR-based analysis of the *TRG* locus, or less frequently the *TRB* locus. If sufficient fresh or frozen neoplastic specimen is available, Southern blot analysis of the *TRB* locus may be considered.

Another potential application of *TR* gene rearrangement assays includes determination of clonal relatedness of multiple lesions derived from the same patient. T-cell neoplasms that share the same clonal origin will generally demonstrate identical *TR* gene rearrangement; however, ongoing and secondary rearrangements of the *TR* loci may result in alteration

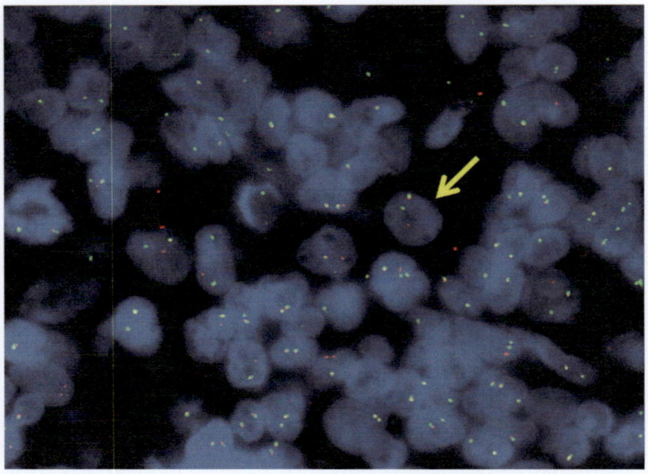

Figure 43.2 Interphase fluorescence in situ hybridization (FISH) image demonstrating rearrangement of the *IRF4* locus with an *IRF4* break-apart probe. The *yellow arrow* points to a cell with an *IRF4* rearrangement with one overlapping green and red fusion signal (indicating a normal unrearranged *IRF4* locus) and separate red and green signals (indicating an abnormal rearranged *IRF4* locus) (Image provided by Andrew Feldman, Mayo Clinic.)

or loss of this initial *TR* rearrangement. Evolution of the *TR* rearrangement has primarily been observed with precursor lymphoid neoplasms [13]. Other reported applications of *TR* gene rearrangement assays include staging, minimal residual disease (MRD) monitoring, and lineage assignment, but most clinical assays do not have sufficient sensitivity for the first two applications and cross-lineage rearrangements are observed at a high enough rate to limit the utility of use for lineage assignment.

Although it is less commonly applied in routine clinical practice, demonstration of somatic chromosomal structural or numeric abnormalities by molecular or cytogenetic methods can assist in classifying the suspected lymphoproliferation as reactive or neoplastic. Only a few T-cell neoplasms are associated with specific chromosomal structural abnormalities, but these may assist with subclassification. As an example, the t(2;5)(p23;q35) involving *NPM1* and *ALK*, as well as other *ALK* rearrangements, are found in ALK-positive ALCL. More recently, data from multiple groups collectively indicate that *IRF4* rearrangements (Fig. 43.2) are found in 25–30 % of primary cutaneous anaplastic large cell lymphomas, but are uncommon in T-cell neoplasms considered in the differential diagnosis, including cutaneous involvement by systemic ALK-negative ALCL, lymphomatoid papulosis, and transformed mycosis fungoides [14–16]. Consequently, testing for *IRF4* rearrangements by fluorescence in situ hybridization (FISH) may assist with the classification of cutaneous CD30-positive T-cell lymphoproliferative disorders in the context of histology, immunophenotype, and clinical information.

Detection of certain viruses can assist with the subclassification of mature T- and NK-cell neoplasms. Epstein-Barr virus (EBV) is strongly associated with aggressive NK-cell leukemia, EBV-positive T-cell lymphoproliferative disorders of childhood, nasal-type extranodal NK/TCL, and angioimmunoblastic TCL [2]. In situ hybridization (ISH) for EBV-encoded RNA (EBER) is the preferred method of testing paraffin-embedded tissue sections. In addition, the retrovirus human T-cell lymphotropic virus type 1 (HTLV-1) is involved in the pathogenesis of adult T-cell leukemia/lymphoma (ATLL) [17], and demonstration of HTLV-1 infection in ATLL cases is performed by HTLV-1 serology and PCR [18].

Available Assays

Clonality assessment is broadly available to assist in the classification of suspected lymphoproliferative disorders. Likewise, other molecular methods are available for the detection of chromosomal abnormalities and viral sequences associated with mature TCL and NK-cell lymphomas.

PCR-Based Clonality Assessment

Clonality assessment is much more frequently performed by PCR methods in clinical practice than by Southern blot analysis. Advantages of PCR-based assays include good sensitivity, short turnaround time, minimal quantity of required DNA, and the ability to utilize partially degraded DNA such as that derived from formalin-fixed, paraffin-embedded (FFPE) tissues. In addition, genomic DNA from fresh or frozen tissues, blood, BM, or body fluids can be used for assessment of T-cell clonality.

PCR-Based Clonality Assessment Using *TRG*

The majority of laboratories that perform PCR-based assessment of T-cell clonality examine the *TRG* locus. The *TRG* contains nine commonly rearranged V segments, which are further grouped into four V gene families based on sequence homology, and 5 J segments [19, 20]. The *TRG* locus is less complex than the *TRB* locus, making primer design to detect all rearrangements simpler. Because the *TRG* locus is rearranged prior to *TRB*, clonal rearrangements involving *TRG* can be detected in both αβ and γδ T cells.

Multiple approaches are used for PCR primer design for the detection of *TRG* rearrangements. Consensus V and J segment primers can amplify the majority of *TRG* rearrangements observed in lymphoid cells [21, 22]. Alternatively, primers directed against the four Vγ families coupled with a group of J-region primers can be multiplexed [3, 23, 24],

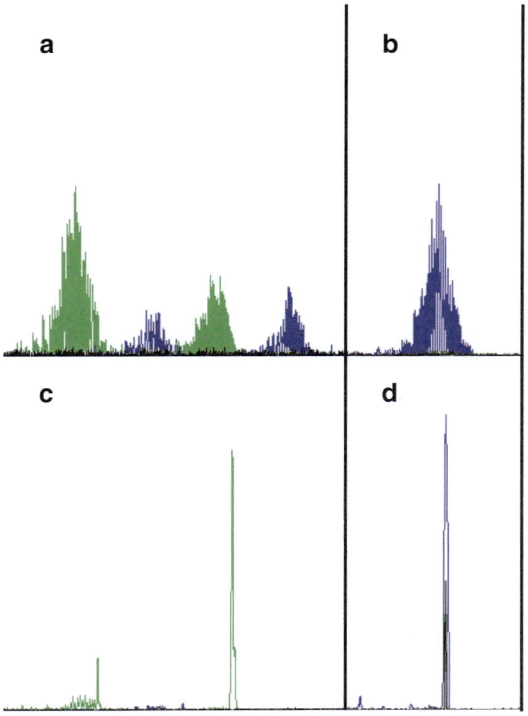

Figure 43.3 Examples of capillary electropherograms for PCR-based analysis of the *TRG* locus with two different primer sets. The assays show polyclonal results for a normal lymph node specimen (**a**, **b**) and clonal results for a T-cell neoplasm (**c**, **d**), using two different methods. The assay depicted in panels (**a**) and (**c**) is based on the BIOMED-2 Concerted Action, and the resulting PCR products are distributed among multiple size ranges. This assay uses two multiplex reactions, and the results from one multiplex reaction are shown. In contrast, the assay depicted in (**b**) and (**d**) uses a single multiplex reaction and results in PCR products distributed within a single size range. The T-cell neoplasm specimen was derived from a patient with mycosis fungoides, and multiple lesions from this patient demonstrated a dominant peak at the size shown. Note that for illustrative purposes, the vertical axes have been rescaled; the dominant clonal peaks in (**c**) and (**d**) are actually tenfold higher than the peak of the corresponding Gaussian distribution in (**a**) and (**b**), respectively

which is currently the most common primer design for PCR-based detection of *TRG* rearrangements. Even with this common approach, significant differences in the assays used by different laboratories affect assay interpretation and performance. After PCR amplification, the products can be visualized by methods including capillary electrophoresis, heteroduplex analysis, or denaturing gradient gel electrophoresis. Examples of two different PCR-based *TRG* assays using capillary electrophoresis are shown in Fig. 43.3.

PCR-Based Clonality Assessment Using *TRB*

Although it is less commonly examined for PCR-based assessment of T-cell clonality than *TRG*, the *TRB* locus may be assessed as an adjunct or alternative to *TRG*. The *TRB* locus is significantly more complex than the *TRG* locus, containing approximately 65 V segments, two D segments, and 13 J segments [25]. The most common primer set used for analysis of *TRB* was developed by the BIOMED-2 study [3] and contains 23 Vβ, two Dβ, and 13 Jβ primers divided among three reaction tubes. The resulting PCR products are examined by capillary electrophoresis or heteroduplex analysis to detect the majority of *TRB* rearrangements.

Southern Blot Analysis Clonality Assessment

Although it is much less frequently performed than the PCR-based assays described above, Southern blot analysis can be a valuable tool for diagnostically challenging lymphoproliferative cases when sufficient fresh or frozen tissue is available. In general, Southern blot analysis of *TR* loci has better inter-observer agreement and fewer issues with false-positive results than PCR-based analysis. However, most biopsies for suspected lymphoproliferative disorders are small and preserved as FFPE blocks, and thus yield neither sufficient quantity nor quality of DNA for Southern blot analysis. In addition, Southern blot analysis is both time consuming and technically demanding.

Southern blot analysis for T-cell clonality most commonly examines the *TRB* locus. Although Southern blot analysis detects a clonal rearrangement in >90 % of T-cell neoplasms, it is generally unable to detect a clonal rearrangement in NK-cell or γδ T-cell neoplasms. Southern blot analysis of the *TRB* locus uses a probe directed against the *TRB* constant regions (Cβ) or probes directed against one or both of the *TRB* J segments (Jβ1 and Jβ2) [26]. An example of a *TRB* Southern blot is shown in Fig. 43.4. Even though numerous rearrangements derived from T lymphocytes are present in a lane, only the clonal rearrangement reaches the detection level.

Guidelines suggest using at least three different restriction enzymes for digestion of the genomic DNA [27]. The presence of up to two non-germline bands in at least two of the three digests is considered definitive evidence of a clonal rearrangement. One or two non-germline bands in only one of the three digests may represent a clonally rearranged allele or a benign germline polymorphism, and performing digestion with an additional restriction endonuclease may assist in distinguishing between these possibilities. Only two of the three digests are required to demonstrate non-germline bands because one of the digests may have a rearrangement that is a similar size to and obscured by the germline band. The allowance for up to two rearranged bands per digest accounts for rearrangement of both *TRB* alleles or for the creation of a new restriction site in the rearranged allele within the probe region. The presence of more than two non-germline bands may indicate oligoclonality or a chromosomal abnormality, but incomplete digestion of

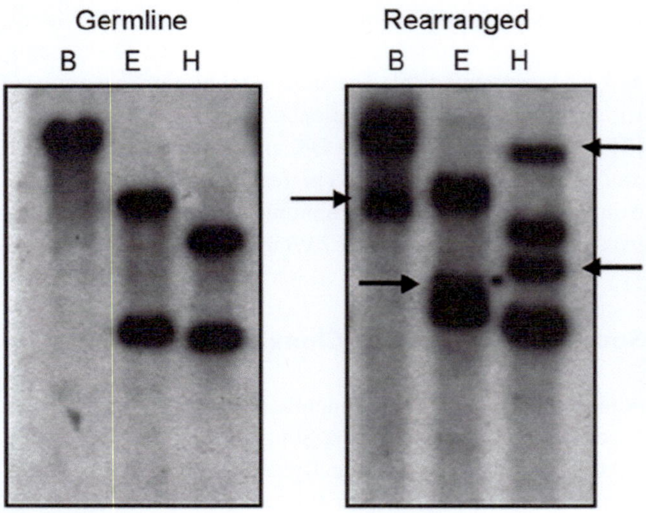

Figure 43.4 Example of a *TRB* Southern blot. Three restriction enzymes (B, *Bam*HI; E, *Eco*RII; H, *Hind*III) were used to digest genomic DNA from germline (*left panel*) and TCL (*right panel*) specimens. The lymphoma specimen demonstrates one or two additional rearrangements (*arrows*) compared to the germline specimen with all three restriction enzymes

genomic DNA or germline polymorphisms also may lead to multiple rearranged bands and must be excluded.

Detection of Chromosomal Abnormalities

Reverse transcription PCR (RT-PCR) and real-time quantitative PCR (RT-qPCR) can be used for the detection or detection and quantitation, respectively, of fusion transcripts such as *NPM1–ALK* found in the majority of cases of ALK-positive ALCL. *NPM1–ALK* and other fusion transcripts involving *ALK* result in the expression of the ALK protein, which is not normally expressed in lymphocytes. ALK expression is a favorable prognostic marker, and patients with ALK-positive ALCL have improved overall survival compared to patients with ALK-negative ALCL [28, 29]. This association appears to be independent of the translocation partner [30]. Furthermore, up to 25 % of ALK-positive ALCL cases involve translocation partners other than *NPM1*, and some *NPM1–ALK* translocations will not be detected by RT-PCR. For these and other reasons, ALK immunohistochemistry is the most widely used test for examining ALK expression in ALCL (Fig. 43.5). RT-PCR and RT-qPCR for *NPM1–ALK* may provide prognostic information or allow MRD monitoring in select patients with ALK-positive ALCL and the *NPM1–ALK* fusion [31]. These sensitive methods should be used with caution in diagnostic situations because low levels of *NPM1–ALK* fusion transcripts have been reported in ALK-negative ALCL, Hodgkin lymphoma, reactive tissue, and even peripheral blood from healthy individuals [32, 33].

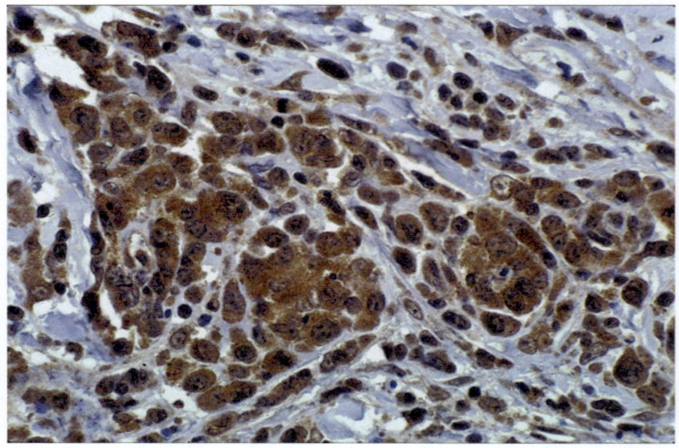

Figure 43.5 Immunohistochemistry demonstrating nuclear and cytoplasmic ALK staining in an ALK-positive anaplastic large cell lymphoma secondarily involving the skin

FISH on fresh or FFPE tissues also can be used to detect *NPM1–ALK* fusions and other *ALK* rearrangements, and FISH for *ALK* rearrangements correlates well with ALK immunohistochemistry [34]. Likewise, FISH can be performed for other structural and numeric chromosomal abnormalities, but FISH testing for mature T- and NK-cell lymphomas is offered in only a few clinical laboratories.

Detection of Viral Sequences Associated with T-Cell Lymphomas

ISH is commonly used for the detection and localization of EBV in tumor cells of the various EBV-positive mature T- and NK-cell neoplasms, especially nasal-type extranodal NK/T-cell lymphoma. ISH can be performed on FFPE tissue sections and identifies EBV RNA within the nuclei of virtually all tumor cells. EBER RNA is most commonly targeted due to the very high copy number in EBV-infected tumor cells. PCR detection of EBV in lymphoid tissue specimens is less useful because the vast majority of adults have been infected with EBV and the assay may detect latently infected background B cells that are not associated with the tumor.

The diagnosis of ATLL involves the demonstration of HTLV-1 infection. This may be performed by HTLV-1 serology or PCR.

Interpretation of PCR-Based T-Cell Clonality Assays

Interpretation of PCR-based T-cell clonality assays is a challenging and commonly debated area of molecular pathology. Interpretation is dependent on assay design and the method used to evaluate the PCR products. Different interpretive criteria are required depending on assay design [35]. Key features of assay design that influence choice of interpretive criteria include primer selection, multiplexing strategy, use of one or multiple different fluorescently labeled primers, and whether the resulting PCR products result in a single or multiple Gaussian regions. In gel-based assays, interpretation as a clonal rearrangement is based on the finding of a discrete band of an appropriate size in contrast to a smear or ladder of bands derived from polyclonal T cells. With capillary electrophoresis-based assays, a wide variety of interpretive criteria is used, and each laboratory must establish and validate its own criteria for a positive result while considering the many issues described in this section. Commonly applied interpretive criteria for the detection of a clonal T-cell rearrangement include observing a reproducible peak above baseline or establishing a cutoff ratio based on the height of the peak in question relative to that of the polyclonal background [3, 36–38]. Computer-aided algorithms also are used to identify peaks that deviate from the normal distribution curve [39]. Less-stringent criteria can be applied with capillary electrophoresis in follow-up specimens when the size of the expected clonal PCR product is known from prior testing.

Oligoclonal proliferations should be differentiated from monoclonal proliferations. The number of bands on a gel or prominent peaks on a capillary electrophoresis tracing necessary to define an oligoclonal vs monoclonal proliferation depends on the assay design and locus examined. In general, the presence of more than two bands or prominent peaks is considered compatible with an oligoclonal proliferation when examining the *TRG* locus.

Clonality Assay Limit of Detection

The limit of detection for *TR* gene rearrangements by Southern blot analysis has been generally reported to vary from 1–10 % clonal cells [40, 41], with 5 % representing a reasonable estimate in standard clinical practice [26]. The limit of detection for PCR-based *TR* gene rearrangement assays depends on the assay design, extent of polyclonal background, and detection method. As an example, commonly used primer sets developed by the BIOMED-2 study are reported to have limits of detection of 1–10 % when heteroduplex analysis is used and 0.5–5 % when capillary electrophoresis is used [3]. Lower limits of detection can be achieved with patient-specific primers, in the range of 0.01–0.001 %. However, this approach is labor and time intensive, and is not generally utilized for mature TCL outside of the research or clinical trial setting.

Clinical Sensitivity

In principle, virtually all *TR* gene rearrangements can be detected by Southern blot analysis if a sufficiently large clonal T-cell population is present in the specimen. In practice, low tumor burden is a major cause of false-negative *TR* Southern blot analysis of T-cell neoplasms, and consequently PCR-based assays have higher clinical sensitivity [42]. A clonal *TRG* rearrangement is detected in >90 % of mature T-cell neoplasms when family-specific V-region primers are used, and a clonal *TRB* rearrangement is detected in >75 % of mature T-cell neoplasms [43–45]. Rates of detection >95 % in fresh/frozen and FFPE tissues have been reported when both *TRG* and *TRB* loci are examined. False-negative results may occur when the family or consensus primers fail to efficiently anneal to the rearranged V, D, or J segments due to limited homology or alteration of the targeted gene region caused by the rearrangement. False-negative results also may be attributed to primer design. As an example, the BIOMED-2 study did not include a Jγ1.2 (JγP) primer to avoid false-positive *TRG* results from canonical rearrangements [3]. This J segment is used in approximately 3 % of T-cell neoplasms [46]. Consequently, a false-negative *TRG* result may rarely occur if the other *TRG* allele has not rearranged. Finally, specimen sampling issues may result in a false-negative *TR* gene rearrangement if an insufficient number of clonal T cells are present within the tested specimen. An appropriately trained pathologist must review and select the tissue for testing to ensure sufficient abnormal cells are present.

Clinical Specificity

Lack of clinical specificity is a major limitation of PCR-based clonality studies, especially involving the *TR* loci. Clonal rearrangement of *TR* loci has been reported in a variable percentage of myeloid and B-cell neoplasms as well as in a variety of nonneoplastic conditions. In some cases, the detected clonal rearrangement represents a true cross-lineage rearrangement within the neoplastic cell population (e.g., detection of a *TR* rearrangement in B lymphoblastic leukemia/lymphoma [B-ALL]). In many other cases, the detected clonal *TR* gene rearrangement represents either a limited number or a restricted repertoire of T cells in the specimen.

TR gene rearrangements generally should not be used for lineage determination due to lineage infidelity, which is the rearrangement of *TR* genes in non-T cells (or the rearrangement of Ig genes in non-B cells). Clonal rearrangements involving *TRD* or *TRG* occur in approximately 10 % of acute myeloid leukemia cases [47, 48]. Cross-lineage *TR* gene rearrangements are very common in B-ALL, with over half of cases demonstrating *TRG* rearrangements [49]. In contrast, cross-lineage *TR* gene rearrangements are relatively rare in mature B-cell neoplasms when examined by Southern blot analysis, generally observed in <10 % of cases [50–53]. However, a large study by the BIOMED-2 group using their PCR-based assays examined 369 mature B-cell neoplasms and identified a clonal *TR* gene rearrangement in approximately 25 % of cases [54]. They noted that these cases could be divided into two groups based on the pattern of *TR* gene rearrangements. In approximately 10 % of the cases, the rearrangement involved a single locus and exhibited a strong clonal pattern, probably representing true cross-lineage rearrangements present within the malignant B-cell population. In approximately 15 % of cases, *TR* gene rearrangements were observed at two or more loci and exhibited a weak clonal pattern, probably representing a coexisting restricted or small T-cell population. This underscores that such weak bands or small peaks observed in clonality assays should be interpreted with caution to avoid false-positive results. Subsequent work further illustrates that application of more stringent interpretive criteria to this primer set may improve the clinical specificity of the assay [35].

Detection of Ig gene rearrangements in mature T-cell neoplasms has been observed, but generally at a lower rate than *TR* rearrangements in B-cell neoplasms [51, 52]. In a study of 188 mature T-cell neoplasms by the BIOMED-2 study, 10 % demonstrated clonal Ig gene rearrangements by PCR, but most of these cases exhibited a weak clonal pattern probably representing a coexisting restricted or small B-cell population [44]. Of the different mature T-cell neoplasm classifications examined, the highest level of Ig gene rearrangements was found in angioimmunoblastic T-cell lymphoma (AITL). In this and other studies, up to one-third of AITL cases have clonal Ig gene rearrangements [44, 55]. Likewise, a high percentage of clonal Ig rearrangements have been reported in peripheral TCL, NOS with rates of 10–35 % [44, 55, 56].

TR gene rearrangement studies are typically performed to distinguish monoclonal from polyclonal lymphoproliferations, but the detection of a monoclonal *TR* gene rearrangement is not always indicative of malignancy. *TR* gene rearrangements have been reported in nonneoplastic conditions. Clonal T-cell populations are observed in peripheral blood specimens, especially from older individuals [57–59]. Likewise, oligoclonal and clonal *TR* gene rearrangements occur in individuals with autoimmune disorders, viral infections, reactive lymphoproliferations, and benign cutaneous lesions [60, 61]. As an example, lymphomatoid papulosis (LyP), a benign primary cutaneous CD30-positive T-cell lymphoproliferative disorder, is associated with the development of a malignant lymphoma in approximately 20 % of cases [62]. Over 40 % of LyP cases are associated with clonally rearranged *TR* genes, but this is not indicative of malignancy or predictive of progression to lymphoma [63, 64]. Consequently, in LyP cases, *TR* gene rearrangement studies are of little value.

Pseudoclonality

Pseudoclonality refers to the artifactual detection of an apparently clonal or oligoclonal lymphoid population and is a common problem in PCR-based clonality assessment of certain specimen types. PCR can result in the selective amplification of one or a limited number of *TR* gene rearrangements when there are a limited number of T cells. Small numbers of T cells and consequently pseudoclonal results are commonly encountered in small skin biopsy specimens, needle biopsies, and B-cell malignancies with very high tumor burdens. Duplicate or triplicate testing of these specimen types often will demonstrate different size gene rearrangements, indicating pseudoclonality. If available, testing of other lesions from the patient can assist in distinguishing clonality from pseudoclonality. This approach appears to be particularly useful in distinguishing inflammatory dermatoses from cutaneous TCL [65, 66].

Oligoclonality

Oligoclonal proliferations have a restricted *TR* gene repertoire and occur in processes such as antigen-stimulated expansion of distinct subclones, immune reconstitution, or immunosenescence. The number of predominant peaks or bands required to distinguish monoclonality from oligoclonality depends on the assay and locus examined. For *TRG*, the presence of more than two predominant peaks or bands generally is interpreted as an oligoclonal proliferation. As noted previously, oligoclonal proliferations are commonly observed in individuals with autoimmune disorders, viral infections, reactive lymphoproliferations, and benign cutaneous lesions [60]. Likewise, reduced diversity of the *TR* repertoire and *TR* gene oligoclonality is observed in older adults and during immune reconstitution after chemotherapy or stem cell transplantation [67, 68]. If selective amplification of one of the clones occurs in these oligoclonal proliferations, the result may appear clonal (i.e., pseudoclonality). Replicate testing or testing of multiple neoplastic specimens from the same patient will frequently reveal different sized gene rearrangements, indicating pseudoclonality in these cases.

PCR Products Outside of Size Range

In T-cell clonality assessment by PCR, bands outside the defined size range may represent true *TR* gene rearrangements, but these must be distinguished from nonspecific PCR products. For size ranges established between the 5th and 95th percentiles, bands or peaks just outside of this size range likely represent true rearrangements. Likewise, significantly oversized or undersized bands or peaks also may represent true rearrangements due to amplification from downstream J segments or partial V segment deletions, respectively [69]. In cases in which the peaks or bands are outside of the size range, sequencing the potential rearrangement product allows definitive characterization.

Weak Clonal Results

Weak bands or small peaks in PCR-based *TR* gene rearrangement assays must be interpreted with caution to avoid false-positive results. Such results should be repeated to ensure that the results are reproducible. In addition, examination of other loci and other involved specimens from the same patient, as well as using an orthogonal detection method, can assist in determining the significance of these weak clonal results. At this time, specific criteria for interpretation of PCR-based clonality testing have not been universally embraced, although (as is discussed above) multiple approaches have been proposed. Each laboratory is required to design, validate, and establish interpretive criteria for their specific assay given the issues and limitations discussed in this section.

Laboratory Issues

Appropriate controls for PCR-based *TR* gene rearrangement assays include positive, negative, sensitivity, and no DNA template reactions. Positive controls can be derived from previously positive patient specimens or characterized cell lines [70, 71]. A polyclonal control is typically derived from tonsillar tissue processed in the same way as clinical specimens. Sensitivity controls can be made by dilution of DNA from a positive cell line in DNA from a specimen with a polyclonal T-cell population, such as tonsil, to determine and then monitor the limit of detection of the assay. The limit of detection for a clonal population in a non-lymphoid background will be lower than in the presence of a polyclonal lymphoid background and may lead to inaccurate assessment of sensitivity. Finally, no DNA template control reactions, which include all PCR primers and reagents but no DNA, should be included to monitor for exogenous DNA or PCR product contamination. For Southern blot analysis, control germline DNA may be obtained from a variety of non-lymphoid cells, such as placenta [26].

In many laboratories, the majority of specimens will be FFPE tissues. Although some DNA degradation is inherent to formalin fixation, the extracted DNA is usually of sufficient quality for PCR-based *TR* gene rearrangement testing. However, some cases, approximately 20 % of cases in one study [45], will not have sufficient DNA quality for successful analysis. Consequently, a non-*TR* or -*IG* control gene must be amplified for each specimen to prevent a false-negative interpretation due to inadequate DNA quality (or the presence of a PCR inhibitor such as heparin). Furthermore, the control gene should be the same size or larger than the largest amplicon in the assay.

Conclusions and Future Directions

A variety of molecular pathology assays are available to evaluate *TR* gene rearrangements, structural and numeric chromosomal abnormalities, and viral sequences associated with mature T- and NK-cell neoplasms. In a subset of TCL, these molecular studies are important for disease classification or determining prognosis. However, many of these molecular studies, especially PCR-based *TR* gene rearrangement studies, have important caveats that must be considered during validation and subsequent clinical use and interpretation of the assays. Therefore, molecular test results must be considered in the context of available clinical information, histology, immunophenotype results, and other laboratory data to ensure proper clinical use of the results.

With the widespread application of genomic and other high-throughput methodologies such as massively parallel sequencing in the research setting, the amount of data regarding the genetics underlying hematolymphoid neoplasms is rapidly increasing. Recurrent somatic mutations as well as structural chromosomal alterations have been identified in lymphoid malignancies. Most of this work has focused on B-cell neoplasms, but projects involving mature T-cell neoplasms are underway. Recently, massively parallel sequencing has led to identification of a recurrent translocation in ALK-negative ALCL [72]. In addition, massively parallel sequencing strategies are being applied to analysis of *TR* loci [73], and clinical assays based on these methods are now in use. These data and new methods have the potential to improve the diagnosis, determination of prognosis, and ability to monitor response to therapy in mature T- and NK-cell neoplasms.

References

1. A clinical evaluation of the International Lymphoma Study Group classification of non-Hodgkin's lymphoma. The Non-Hodgkin's Lymphoma Classification Project. Blood 1997; 89 (11):3909–18
2. Swerdlow SH, Campo E, Harris NL, Jaffe ES, Pileri SA, Stein H, Thiele J, Vardiman JW, editors. WHO classification of tumours of haematopoietic and lymphoid tissues. 4th ed. Lyon: IARC Press; 2008.

3. van Dongen JJ, Langerak AW, Bruggemann M, Evans PA, Hummel M, Lavender FL, Delabesse E, Davi F, Schuuring E, Garcia-Sanz R, van Krieken JH, Droese J, Gonzalez D, Bastard C, White HE, Spaargaren M, Gonzalez M, Parreira A, Smith JL, Morgan GJ, Kneba M, Macintyre EA. Design and standardization of PCR primers and protocols for detection of clonal immunoglobulin and T-cell receptor gene recombinations in suspect lymphoproliferations: report of the BIOMED-2 Concerted Action BMH4-CT98-3936. Leukemia. 2003;17(12):2257–317.
4. Dik WA, Pike-Overzet K, Weerkamp F, de Ridder D, de Haas EFE, Baert MRM, van der Spek P, Koster EEL, Reinders MJT, van Dongen JJM, Langerak AW, Staal FJT. New insights on human T cell development by quantitative T cell receptor gene rearrangement studies and gene expression profiling. J Exp Med. 2005;201(11):1715–23.
5. Chiarle R, Voena C, Ambrogio C, Piva R, Inghirami G. The anaplastic lymphoma kinase in the pathogenesis of cancer. Nat Rev Cancer. 2008;8(1):11–23.
6. Morris SW, Kirstein MN, Valentine MB, Dittmer KG, Shapiro DN, Saltman DL, Look AT. Fusion of a kinase gene, ALK, to a nucleolar protein gene, NPM, in non-Hodgkin's lymphoma. Science. 1994;263(5151):1281–4.
7. Lamant L, Dastugue N, Pulford K, Delsol G, Mariame B. A new fusion gene TPM3-ALK in anaplastic large cell lymphoma created by a (1;2)(q25;p23) translocation. Blood. 1999;93(9):3088–95.
8. Delsol G, Falini B, Muller-Hermelink HK, Campo E, Jaffe ES, Gascoyne RD, Stein H, Kinney MC. Anaplastic large cell lymphoma (ALCL), ALK-positive. In: Swerdlow SH, Campo E, Harris NL, et al., editors. WHO classification of tumours of haematopoietic and lymphoid tissues. 4th ed. Lyon: IARC Press; 2008. p. 312–6.
9. Brito-Babapulle V, Catovsky D. Inversions and tandem translocations involving chromosome 14q11 and 14q32 in T-prolymphocytic leukemia and T-cell leukemias in patients with ataxia telangiectasia. Cancer Genet Cytogenet. 1991;55(1):1–9.
10. Alonsozana EL, Stamberg J, Kumar D, Jaffe ES, Medeiros LJ, Frantz C, Schiffer CA, O'Connell BA, Kerman S, Stass SA, Abruzzo LV. Isochromosome 7q: the primary cytogenetic abnormality in hepatosplenic gammadelta T cell lymphoma. Leukemia. 1997;11(8):1367–72.
11. Zettl A, Ott G, Makulik A, Katzenberger T, Starostik P, Eichler T, Puppe B, Bentz M, Muller-Hermelink HK, Chott A. Chromosomal gains at 9q characterize enteropathy-type T-cell lymphoma. Am J Pathol. 2002;161(5):1635–45.
12. Scarisbrick JJ, Woolford AJ, Calonje E, Photiou A, Ferreira S, Orchard G, Russell-Jones R, Whittaker SJ. Frequent abnormalities of the p15 and p16 genes in mycosis fungoides and sezary syndrome. J Invest Dermatol. 2002;118(3):493–9.
13. Pongers-Willemse MJ, Seriu T, Stolz F, d'Aniello E, Gameiro P, Pisa P, Gonzalez M, Bartram CR, Panzer-Grumayer ER, Biondi A, San Miguel JF, van Dongen JJ. Primers and protocols for standardized detection of minimal residual disease in acute lymphoblastic leukemia using immunoglobulin and T cell receptor gene rearrangements and TAL1 deletions as PCR targets: report of the BIOMED-1 CONCERTED ACTION: investigation of minimal residual disease in acute leukemia. Leukemia. 1999;13(1):110–8.
14. Wada DA, Law ME, Hsi ED, Dicaudo DJ, Ma L, Lim MS, Souza A, Comfere NI, Weenig RH, Macon WR, Erickson LA, Ozsan N, Ansell SM, Dogan A, Feldman AL. Specificity of IRF4 translocations for primary cutaneous anaplastic large cell lymphoma: a multicenter study of 204 skin biopsies. Mod Pathol. 2011;24(4):596–605.
15. Pham-Ledard A, Prochazkova-Carlotti M, Laharanne E, Vergier B, Jouary T, Beylot-Barry M, Merlio JP. IRF4 gene rearrangements define a subgroup of CD30-positive cutaneous T-cell lymphoma: a study of 54 cases. J Invest Dermatol. 2010;130(3):816–25.
16. Feldman AL, Law M, Remstein ED, Macon WR, Erickson LA, Grogg KL, Kurtin PJ, Dogan A. Recurrent translocations involving the IRF4 oncogene locus in peripheral T-cell lymphomas. Leukemia. 2009;23(3):574–80.
17. Mortreux F, Gabet AS, Wattel E. Molecular and cellular aspects of HTLV-1 associated leukemogenesis in vivo. Leukemia. 2003;17(1):26–38.
18. Tsukasaki K, Hermine O, Bazarbachi A, Ratner L, Ramos JC, Harrington Jr W, O'Mahony D, Janik JE, Bittencourt AL, Taylor GP, Yamaguchi K, Utsunomiya A, Tobinai K, Watanabe T. Definition, prognostic factors, treatment, and response criteria of adult T-cell leukemia-lymphoma: a proposal from an international consensus meeting. J Clin Oncol. 2009;27(3):453–9.
19. Chen Z, Font MP, Loiseau P, Bories JC, Degos L, Lefranc MP, Sigaux F. The human T-cell V gamma gene locus: cloning of new segments and study of V gamma rearrangements in neoplastic T and B cells. Blood. 1988;72(2):776–83.
20. Quertermous T, Strauss WM, Van Dongen JJ, Seidman JG. Human T cell gamma chain joining regions and T cell development. J Immunol. 1987;138(8):2687–90.
21. Benhattar J, Delacretaz F, Martin P, Chaubert P, Costa J. Improved polymerase chain reaction detection of clonal T-cell lymphoid neoplasms. Diagn Mol Pathol. 1995;4(2):108–12.
22. Bourguin A, Tung R, Galili N, Sklar J. Rapid, nonradioactive detection of clonal T-cell receptor gene rearrangements in lymphoid neoplasms. Proc Natl Acad Sci U S A. 1990;87(21):8536–40.
23. Greiner TC, Raffeld M, Lutz C, Dick F, Jaffe ES. Analysis of T cell receptor-gamma gene rearrangements by denaturing gradient gel electrophoresis of GC-clamped polymerase chain reaction products. Correlation with tumor-specific sequences. Am J Pathol. 1995;146(1):46–55.
24. Theodorou I, Bigorgne C, Delfau MH, Lahet C, Cochet G, Vidaud M, Raphael M, Gaulard P, Farcet JP. VJ rearrangements of the TCR gamma locus in peripheral T-cell lymphomas: analysis by polymerase chain reaction and denaturing gradient gel electrophoresis. J Pathol. 1996;178(3):303–10.
25. Rowen L, Koop BF, Hood L. The complete 685-kilobase DNA sequence of the human beta T cell receptor locus. Science. 1996;272(5269):1755–62.
26. van Dongen JJ, Wolvers-Tettero IL. Analysis of immunoglobulin and T cell receptor genes. Part I: basic and technical aspects. Clin Chim Acta. 1991;198(1-2):1–91.
27. Enns RK, Altmiller DH, Hinkel CS, Madej RM, O'Leary TJ. Immunoglobulin and T-cell receptor gene rearrangement assays; approved guideline, second edition, NCCLS document MM2-A2, 2002
28. Falini B, Pileri S, Zinzani PL, Carbone A, Zagonel V, Wolf-Peeters C, Verhoef G, Menestrina F, Todeschini G, Paulli M, Lazzarino M, Giardini R, Aiello A, Foss HD, Araujo I, Fizzotti M, Pelicci PG, Flenghi L, Martelli MF, Santucci A. ALK+ lymphoma: clinico-pathological findings and outcome. Blood. 1999;93(8):2697–706.
29. Gascoyne RD, Aoun P, Wu D, Chhanabhai M, Skinnider BF, Greiner TC, Morris SW, Connors JM, Vose JM, Viswanatha DS, Coldman A, Weisenburger DD. Prognostic significance of anaplastic lymphoma kinase (ALK) protein expression in adults with anaplastic large cell lymphoma. Blood. 1999;93(11):3913–21.
30. Falini B, Pulford K, Pucciarini A, Carbone A, De Wolf-Peeters C, Cordell J, Fizzotti M, Santucci A, Pelicci PG, Pileri S, Campo E, Ott G, Delsol G, Mason DY. Lymphomas expressing ALK fusion protein(s) other than NPM-ALK. Blood. 1999;94(10):3509–15.
31. Damm-Welk C, Busch K, Burkhardt B, Schieferstein J, Viehmann S, Oschlies I, Klapper W, Zimmermann M, Harbott J, Reiter A, Woessmann W. Prognostic significance of circulating tumor cells in bone marrow or peripheral blood as detected by qualitative and quantitative PCR in pediatric NPM-ALK-positive anaplastic large-cell lymphoma. Blood. 2007;110(2):670–7.

32. Maes B, Vanhentenrijk V, Wlodarska I, Cools J, Peeters B, Marynen P, de Wolf-Peeters C. The NPM-ALK and the ATIC-ALK fusion genes can be detected in non-neoplastic cells. Am J Pathol. 2001;158(6):2185–93.
33. Trumper L, Pfreundschuh M, Bonin FV, Daus H. Detection of the t(2;5)-associated NPM/ALK fusion cDNA in peripheral blood cells of healthy individuals. Br J Haematol. 1998;103(4):1138–44.
34. Cataldo KA, Jalal SM, Law ME, Ansell SM, Inwards DJ, Fine M, Arber DA, Pulford KA, Strickler JG. Detection of t(2;5) in anaplastic large cell lymphoma: comparison of immunohistochemical studies, FISH, and RT-PCR in paraffin-embedded tissue. Am J Surg Pathol. 1999;23(11):1386–92.
35. Cushman-Vokoun AM, Connealy S, Greiner TC. Assay design affects the interpretation of t-cell receptor gamma gene rearrangements: comparison of the performance of a one-tube assay with the BIOMED-2-based TCRG gene clonality assay. J Mol Diagn. 2010; 12(6):787–96.
36. Greiner TC, Rubocki RJ. Effectiveness of capillary electrophoresis using fluorescent-labeled primers in detecting T-cell receptor gamma gene rearrangements. J Mol Diagn. 2002;4(3):137–43.
37. Sprouse JT, Werling R, Hanke D, Lakey C, McDonnel L, Wood BL, Sabath DE. T-cell clonality determination using polymerase chain reaction (PCR) amplification of the T-cell receptor gamma-chain gene and capillary electrophoresis of fluorescently labeled PCR products. Am J Clin Pathol. 2000;113(6):838–50.
38. Lee SC, Berg KD, Racke FK, Griffin CA, Eshleman JR. Pseudo-spikes are common in histologically benign lymphoid tissues. J Mol Diagn. 2000;2(3):145–52.
39. Kuo FC, Hall D, Longtine JA. A novel method for interpretation of T-cell receptor gamma gene rearrangement assay by capillary gel electrophoresis based on normal distribution. J Mol Diagn. 2007;9(1):12–9.
40. Minden MD, Toyonaga B, Ha K, Yanagi Y, Chin B, Gelfand E, Mak T. Somatic rearrangement of T-cell antigen receptor gene in human T-cell malignancies. Proc Natl Acad Sci U S A. 1985;82(4): 1224–7.
41. Aisenberg AC, Wilkes BM, Jacobson JO, Harris NL. Immunoglobulin gene rearrangements in adult non-Hodgkin's lymphoma. Am J Med. 1987;82(4):738–44.
42. Sandberg Y, van Gastel-Mol EJ, Verhaaf B, Lam KH, van Dongen JJ, Langerak AW. BIOMED-2 multiplex immunoglobulin/T-cell receptor polymerase chain reaction protocols can reliably replace Southern blot analysis in routine clonality diagnostics. J Mol Diagn. 2005;7(4):495–503.
43. van Krieken JH, Langerak AW, Macintyre EA, Kneba M, Hodges E, Sanz RG, Morgan GJ, Parreira A, Molina TJ, Cabecadas J, Gaulard P, Jasani B, Garcia JF, Ott M, Hannsmann ML, Berger F, Hummel M, Davi F, Bruggemann M, Lavender FL, Schuuring E, Evans PA, White H, Salles G, Groenen PJ, Gameiro P, Pott C, Dongen JJ. Improved reliability of lymphoma diagnostics via PCR-based clonality testing: report of the BIOMED-2 Concerted Action BHM4-CT98-3936. Leukemia. 2007;21(2):201–6.
44. Bruggemann M, White H, Gaulard P, Garcia-Sanz R, Gameiro P, Oeschger S, Jasani B, Ott M, Delsol G, Orfao A, Tiemann M, Herbst H, Langerak AW, Spaargaren M, Moreau E, Groenen PJ, Sambade C, Foroni L, Carter GI, Hummel M, Bastard C, Davi F, Delfau-Larue MH, Kneba M, van Dongen JJ, Beldjord K, Molina TJ. Powerful strategy for polymerase chain reaction-based clonality assessment in T-cell malignancies Report of the BIOMED-2 Concerted Action BHM4 CT98-3936. Leukemia. 2007;21(2): 215–21.
45. Liu H, Bench AJ, Bacon CM, Payne K, Huang Y, Scott MA, Erber WN, Grant JW, Du MQ. A practical strategy for the routine use of BIOMED-2 PCR assays for detection of B- and T-cell clonality in diagnostic haematopathology. Br J Haematol. 2007;138(1):31–43.
46. Lawnicki LC, Rubocki RJ, Chan WC, Lytle DM, Greiner TC. The distribution of gene segments in T-cell receptor gamma gene rearrangements demonstrates the need for multiple primer sets. J Mol Diagn. 2003;5(2):82–7.
47. Boeckx N, Willemse MJ, Szczepanski T, van der Velden VH, Langerak AW, Vandekerckhove P, van Dongen JJ. Fusion gene transcripts and Ig/TCR gene rearrangements are complementary but infrequent targets for PCR-based detection of minimal residual disease in acute myeloid leukemia. Leukemia. 2002;16(3):368–75.
48. Przybylski G, Oettle H, Ludwig WD, Siegert W, Schmidt CA. Molecular characterization of illegitimate TCR delta gene rearrangements in acute myeloid leukaemia. Br J Haematol. 1994;87(2):301–7.
49. Szczepanski T, Flohr T, van der Velden VH, Bartram CR, van Dongen JJ. Molecular monitoring of residual disease using antigen receptor genes in childhood acute lymphoblastic leukaemia. Best Pract Res Clin Haematol. 2002;15(1):37–57.
50. Kneba M, Bergholz M, Bolz I, Hulpke M, Batge R, Schauer A, Krieger G. Heterogeneity of immunoglobulin gene rearrangements in B-cell lymphomas. Int J Cancer. 1990;45(4):609–13.
51. Pelicci PG, Knowles 2nd DM, Dalla Favera R. Lymphoid tumors displaying rearrangements of both immunoglobulin and T cell receptor genes. J Exp Med. 1985;162(3):1015–24.
52. Griesser H, Feller A, Lennert K, Minden M, Mak TW. Rearrangement of the beta chain of the T cell antigen receptor and immunoglobulin genes in lymphoproliferative disorders. J Clin Invest. 1986;78(5): 1179–84.
53. Chen Z, Le Paslier D, Dausset J, Degos L, Flandrin G, Cohen D, Sigaux F. Human T cell gamma genes are frequently rearranged in B-lineage acute lymphoblastic leukemias but not in chronic B cell proliferations. J Exp Med. 1987;165(4):1000–15.
54. Evans PA, Pott C, Groenen PJ, Salles G, Davi F, Berger F, Garcia JF, van Krieken JH, Pals S, Kluin P, Schuuring E, Spaargaren M, Boone E, Gonzalez D, Martinez B, Villuendas R, Gameiro P, Diss TC, Mills K, Morgan GJ, Carter GI, Milner BJ, Pearson D, Hummel M, Jung W, Ott M, Canioni D, Beldjord K, Bastard C, Delfau-Larue MH, van Dongen JJ, Molina TJ, Cabecadas J. Significantly improved PCR-based clonality testing in B-cell malignancies by use of multiple immunoglobulin gene targets. Report of the BIOMED-2 Concerted Action BHM4-CT98-3936. Leukemia. 2007;21(2):207–14.
55. Tan BT, Warnke RA, Arber DA. The frequency of B- and T-cell gene rearrangements and epstein-barr virus in T-cell lymphomas: a comparison between angioimmunoblastic T-cell lymphoma and peripheral T-cell lymphoma, unspecified with and without associated B-cell proliferations. J Mol Diagn. 2006;8(4):466–75.
56. Tan BT, Seo K, Warnke RA, Arber DA. The frequency of immunoglobulin heavy chain gene and T-cell receptor gamma-chain gene rearrangements and Epstein-Barr virus in ALK+ and ALK- anaplastic large cell lymphoma and other peripheral T-cell lymphomas. J Mol Diagn. 2008;10(6):502–12.
57. Posnett DN, Sinha R, Kabak S, Russo C. Clonal populations of T cells in normal elderly humans: the T cell equivalent to "benign monoclonal gammapathy". J Exp Med. 1994;179(2):609–18.
58. Delfau-Larue MH, Laroche L, Wechsler J, Lepage E, Lahet C, Asso-Bonnet M, Bagot M, Farcet JP. Diagnostic value of dominant T-cell clones in peripheral blood in 363 patients presenting consecutively with a clinical suspicion of cutaneous lymphoma. Blood. 2000;96(9):2987–92.
59. Fitzgerald JE, Ricalton NS, Meyer AC, West SG, Kaplan H, Behrendt C, Kotzin BL. Analysis of clonal CD8+ T cell expansions in normal individuals and patients with rheumatoid arthritis. J Immunol. 1995;154(7):3538–47.
60. Hodges E, Krishna MT, Pickard C, Smith JL. Diagnostic role of tests for T cell receptor (TCR) genes. J Clin Pathol. 2003; 56(1):1–11.

61. Langerak AW, Molina TJ, Lavender FL, Pearson D, Flohr T, Sambade C, Schuuring E, Al Saati T, van Dongen JJ, van Krieken JH. Polymerase chain reaction-based clonality testing in tissue samples with reactive lymphoproliferations: usefulness and pitfalls. A report of the BIOMED-2 Concerted Action BMH4-CT98-3936. Leukemia. 2007;21(2):222–9.
62. Bekkenk MW, Geelen FA, van Voorst Vader PC, Heule F, Geerts ML, van Vloten WA, Meijer CJ, Willemze R. Primary and secondary cutaneous CD30(+) lymphoproliferative disorders: a report from the Dutch Cutaneous Lymphoma Group on the long-term follow-up data of 219 patients and guidelines for diagnosis and treatment. Blood. 2000;95(12):3653–61.
63. Kadin ME. Pathobiology of CD30+ cutaneous T-cell lymphomas. J Cutan Pathol. 2006;33 Suppl 1:10–7.
64. el-Azhary RA, Gibson LE, Kurtin PJ, Pittelkow MR, Muller SA. Lymphomatoid papulosis: a clinical and histopathologic review of 53 cases with leukocyte immunophenotyping, DNA flow cytometry, and T-cell receptor gene rearrangement studies. J Am Acad Dermatol. 1994;30(2 Pt 1):210–8.
65. Thurber SE, Zhang B, Kim YH, Schrijver I, Zehnder J, Kohler S. T-cell clonality analysis in biopsy specimens from two different skin sites shows high specificity in the diagnosis of patients with suggested mycosis fungoides. J Am Acad Dermatol. 2007;57(5):782–90.
66. Ponti R, Fierro MT, Quaglino P, Lisa B, Paola F, Michela O, Paolo F, Comessatti A, Novelli M, Bernengo MG. TCR[gamma]-chain gene rearrangement by PCR-based GeneScan: diagnostic accuracy improvement and clonal heterogeneity analysis in multiple cutaneous T-cell lymphoma samples. J Invest Dermatol. 2007;128(4):1030–8.
67. Sarzotti M, Patel DD, Li X, Ozaki DA, Cao S, Langdon S, Parrott RE, Coyne K, Buckley RH. T cell repertoire development in humans with SCID after nonablative allogeneic marrow transplantation. J Immunol. 2003;170(5):2711–8.
68. Mariani S, Coscia M, Even J, Peola S, Foglietta M, Boccadoro M, Sbaiz L, Restagno G, Pileri A, Massaia M. Severe and long-lasting disruption of T-cell receptor diversity in human myeloma after high-dose chemotherapy and autologous peripheral blood progenitor cell infusion. Br J Haematol. 2001;113(4):1051–9.
69. Langerak AW. Undersized, oversized? It is not one-size-fits-all in lymphoid clonality detection. Leuk Res. 2008;32(2):203–4.
70. Yao R, Rich SA, Schneider E. Validation of sixteen leukemia and lymphoma cell lines as controls for molecular gene rearrangement assays. Clin Chem. 2002;48(8):1344–51.
71. Sandberg Y, Verhaaf B, van Gastel-Mol EJ, Wolvers-Tettero IL, de Vos J, Macleod RA, Noordzij JG, Dik WA, van Dongen JJ, Langerak AW, Lam KH. Human T-cell lines with well-defined T-cell receptor gene rearrangements as controls for the BIOMED-2 multiplex polymerase chain reaction tubes. Leukemia. 2007;21(2):230–7.
72. Feldman AL, Dogan A, Smith DI, Law ME, Ansell SM, Johnson SH, Porcher JC, Ozsan N, Wieben ED, Eckloff BW, Vasmatzis G. Discovery of recurrent t(6;7)(p25.3;q32.3) translocations in ALK-negative anaplastic large cell lymphomas by massively parallel genomic sequencing. Blood. 2011;117(3):915–9.
73. Benichou J, Ben-Hamo R, Louzoun Y, Efroni S. Rep-Seq: uncovering the immunological repertoire through next-generation sequencing. Immunology. 2012;135(3):183–91.

Myeloproliferative Neoplasms and Myelodysplastic Syndromes

44

Albert K. Ho and Daniel M. Jones

Abstract

Myeloproliferative neoplasms (MPNs) and myelodysplastic syndromes (MDS) represent primary clonal hematopoietic disorders that affect the range of immature and maturing blood cell types. This chapter summarizes the distinguishing molecular and cytogenetic features between MDS and MPNs and the most useful clinical molecular tests. An overview is given on the impact of new methods, such as massively parallel sequencing, on our knowledge of pathogenesis. The role of minimal residual disease testing, particularly in MPNs, is discussed in detail.

Keywords

Myeloproliferative neoplasm • Myelodysplastic syndrome • MPN • MDS • JAK2 • BCR-ABL1 • CML • CALR • Calreticulin

Molecular Basis of Disease

Myeloproliferative neoplasms (MPNs) and myelodysplastic syndromes (MDS) represent primary clonal hematopoietic disorders that were among the first neoplasms to be diagnosed and monitored using molecular methods. From the discovery of the Philadelphia chromosome as the causative genomic change in chronic myelogenous leukemia (CML) in 1960 [1], to the recent identification of a common set of mutations producing epigenetic modulation in both MDS and MPN, molecular and cytogenetic testing have been central to the diagnosis of these neoplasms for the last 30 years. Most cases of MPN now have a diagnostic genetic alteration linked to pathogenesis (Table 44.1), whereas the classification of MDS remains tied to blast count and hematologic features (Table 44.2), with certain genetic changes common to several MDS entities.

Besides affecting the myeloid compartment of the hematopoietic system, MPN and MDS share many overlapping morphologic, genetic, and immunophenotypic features (Table 44.3), with the distinction based on the dominant presenting feature. MPNs have increased numbers of blood components due to abnormal proliferation. In contrast, MDS typically presents with decreased numbers of blood components due to ineffective hematopoiesis. An overlap category of myelodysplastic/myeloproliferative neoplasms is recognized when there are features of both entities. Molecular testing in MPNs has become established as the standard of care for diagnosis, monitoring for residual disease, establishing prognosis, and therapeutic decision making. In MDS, the role of molecular testing is currently more limited with cytogenetic studies representing the primary modality used for subclassification and prognostic stratification. However, mutational and epigenetic studies are poised to become part of the routine workup of MDS in the near future.

A.K. Ho, M.D., Ph.D. (✉)
Quest Diagnostics, Nichols Institute,
14225 Newbrook Dr., Chantilly, VA 20151, USA
e-mail: Albert.K.Ho@questdiagnostics.com

D.M. Jones, M.D., Ph.D.
School of Health Professions, University of Texas MD Anderson Cancer Center, Houston, TX, USA

Box 223355, Chantilly, VA 20191, USA
e-mail: dan.jones.gm@gmail.com

D.G.B. Leonard (ed.), *Molecular Pathology in Clinical Practice*, DOI 10.1007/978-3-319-19674-9_44

Table 44.1 Categories of myeloproliferative neoplasms and their molecular alterations

Type	Cytogenetic change(s)	Genes affected	Pathway type
CML	t(9;22)	*BCR–ABL1*	TK growth
	+8, del17p (CE)		
PV, PMF, ET	XY/XX	*JAK2*	Cytokine receptors
	+9, +1/1q (CE)		
CEL/MPN-U	XY/XX	*FIP1L1–PDGFRA*	RTK
	t(8p11;var)	*FGFR1*-various	
CMML, MPN-U	t(5;12)(q31-q33;p12)	*ETV6–PDGFRB*	
	t(5q33;var)	*PDGFRB*-various	

CE clonal evolution, *CEL* chronic eosinophilic leukemia, *CML* chronic myelogenous leukemia, *CMML* chronic myelomonocytic leukemia, *ET* essential thrombocythemia, *MPN-U* myeloproliferative neoplasm, unclassifiable, *PMF* primary myelofibrosis, *PV* polycythemia vera, *(R)TK* (receptor) tyrosine kinase

Table 44.2 Categories of myelodysplastic syndrome and their molecular alterations

Type	Definition
Refractory cytopenia with unilineage dysplasia, including refractory anemia, neutropenia, and thrombocytopenia	Cytopenia and marrow morphologic dysplasia limited to one of the three primary lineages
	Blasts: <5 % BM, <1 % blood
Refractory Anemia with ringed sideroblasts (RS)	Anemia, ≥15 % BM erythroid precursors meeting definition of RS
	Blasts: <5 % BM, <1 % blood
Myelodysplastic syndrome with isolated del(5q)	Anemia, high platelet count and isolated deletion(s) of chromosome 5q
	Blasts: <5 % BM, <1 % blood
Refractory cytopenias with multilineage dysplasia +/– RS	Cytopenias, morphologic dysplasia identified in two or more lineages
	Blasts: <5 % BM, <1 % blood
Refractory anemia with excess blasts-I	Cytopenias
	Blasts: 5–9 % BM and <5 % blood
Refractory anemia with excess blasts-II	Cytopenias
	Blasts: 10–19 % BM and/or >5 % blood, Auer rods can be present
Myelodysplasia, unclassifiable	Cytopenias
	Blasts: <5 % BM, <1 % blood
	Often used for those cases showing some features of myeloproliferative neoplasms, e.g., increased basophils, eosinophils, and/or fibrosis
Chronic myelomonocytic leukemia	1×10^9/L monocytes in blood, with marrow dysplasia
	Mixed disorder with more of a myeloproliferative pattern in some cases

BM bone marrow

Table 44.3 Shared features between MDS and MPNs

Immunophenotypic similarities	Loss/decreased expression of pan-myeloid antigens
	Aberrant upregulation of adhesion molecules (e.g., CD56)
Cytogenetic similarities	Acquisition of +8 with progression
	Acquisition of TP53 mutations with progression
	LOH/UPD involving myeloid regulatory loci
Molecular similarities	Mutations in the epigenetic regulators including *IDH1*, *IDH2*, *TET2*, and *DNMT3A*
	Mutations in *RAS* genes and myeloid transcriptional regulators such as *ASXL1*

LOH loss of heterozygosity, *UPD* uniparental disomy

Indications for Testing

Myeloproliferative Disorders

Elevated white blood cells (leukocytosis), red blood cells (erythrocytosis), or platelets (thrombocytosis), and/or splenomegaly are the hallmarks of MPNs. However, these changes also can represent reactive phenomena, as a manifestation of the normal bone marrow (BM) stress response to infection, trauma, or other types of injury. Because distinction of reactive and neoplastic expansions can be difficult on clinical and morphologic features, molecular and cytogenetic

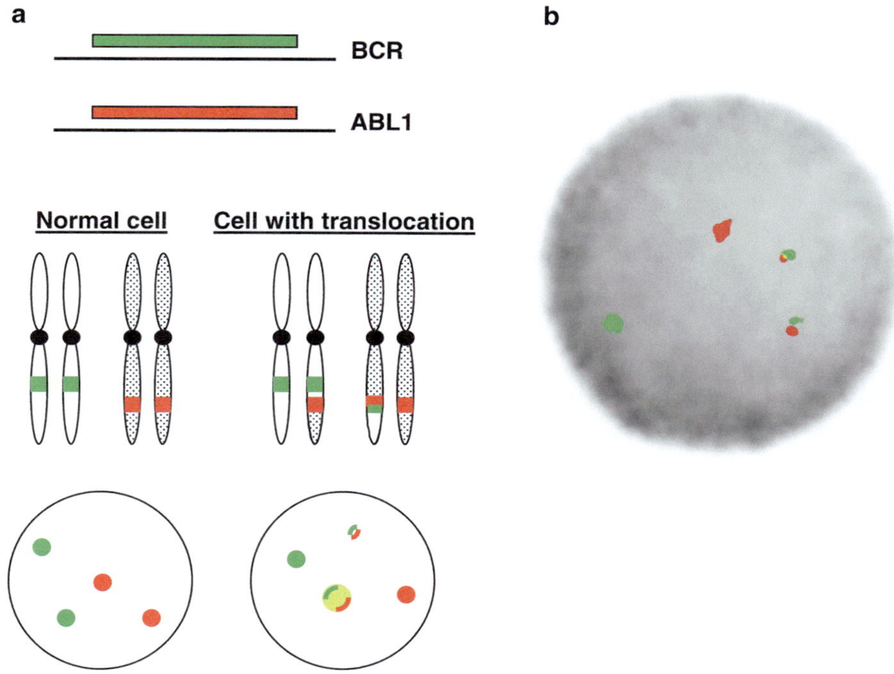

Figure 44.1 *BCR–ABL1* gene rearrangement detected by fluorescence in situ hybridization (FISH). (**a**) Schematic of fusion FISH with orange-labeled probes for *ABL1* gene on chromosome 9 and green-labeled probes on the *BCR* gene on chromosome 22. (**b**) Image from a CML cell showing the t(9;22)

testing can lead to a definitive diagnosis (Table 44.1). The most common MPNs are CML, essential thrombocythemia (ET), polycythemia vera (PV), and primary myelofibrosis (PMF). These entities can have overlapping morphologic and clinical characteristics [2]. A variety of less common MPNs have been recognized in recent years and can be definitively diagnosed by the presence of characteristic cytogenetic or molecular changes.

Chronic Myelogenous Leukemia

Patients with CML typically present with neutrophilia and variable basophilia and eosinophilia. Although some patients are asymptomatic and diagnosed following routine blood work, presentations with fatigue and/or splenomegaly are common. Left untreated, many patients with CML eventually progress to an accelerated phase and then to blast crisis which can be indistinguishable from acute myeloid leukemia (AML).

The medical advances made in the diagnosis and treatment of CML represent some of the greatest achievements in molecular medicine to date. CML was the first malignancy noted to have a defining genetic abnormality when the Philadelphia chromosome (Ph), a translocation between chromosomes 9 and 22, t(9;22) (q34;q11), was identified [1]. Subsequently, the Ph chromosome was identified as the juxtaposition of the breakpoint cluster region (*BCR*) gene on chromosome 22 with the Abelson tyrosine kinase (*ABL1*) gene on chromosome 9 (Fig. 44.1a), resulting in relocalization of an altered ABL1 protein from the nucleus to the cytoplasm, which produces constitutive activation of the ABL growth signaling pathway. The *BCR–ABL1* gene fusion is found in all cases of CML and in about 20–30 % of adult and 2–10 % of childhood B lymphoblastic leukemia (B-ALL) [3].

The differential diagnosis of CML includes benign leukocytosis/leukemoid reaction and the rare chronic neutrophilic leukemia (CNL) and its related atypical chronic myeloid leukemia (aCML). Although CNL and aCML typically lack the basophilia associated with CML other features may be similar. In 2013, cases of CNL/aCML were shown to have a high frequency of activating and truncation mutations in the colony-stimulating factor 3 receptor gene (*CSF3R*) [4].

Essential Thrombocythemia, Primary Myelofibrosis, and Polycythemia Vera

Based on clinical features, ET, PMF, and PV are closely related MPNs, distinguished primarily by their dominant presenting features and clinical course. This close clinical relationship was explained in 2005 when several groups independently identified a point mutation in the *JAK2* tyrosine kinase gene as a recurrent abnormality in these three MPNs, and some cases of chronic myelomonocytic leukemia (CMML). The activating *JAK2* mutation, V617F, is

Table 44.4 Frequency of mutations in different MPNs

Mutation type	PV	ET	PMF	CMML
JAK2 V617F	95 %	50 %	40 %	5 %
JAK2 exon 12/13	5 %	ND	ND	<1 %
MPL codon 505 or 515	ND	5 %	5 %	ND
KRAS–NRAS codons 12/13/61	ND	ND	<1	30–40 %

CMML chronic myelomonocytic leukemia, *ET* essential thrombocythemia, *MPNs* myeloproliferative neoplasms, *ND* not detected, *PMF* primary myelofibrosis, *PV* polycythemia vera

detected in up to 95 % of cases of PV, and approximately 50 % of ET and PMF cases (Table 44.4). A subset of PV, but not PMF or ET, has activating point mutations or in-frame duplications in exon 12 of *JAK2*. Among PMF and ET without V617F, activating mutations in the thrombopoietin receptor gene (*MPL*) are seen in approximately 10 % of cases. Because the JAK2 kinase links multiple cytokine receptors, including the erythropoietin receptor, the thrombopoietin receptor (MPL) and the granulocyte-monocyte cytokine colony stimulating factor receptor (CD116), these mutations define this group of MPNs as having JAK-linked dysregulated cytokine growth factor receptor pathways.

Differences in the features and behavior of *JAK2–MPL*-mutated MPNs are related to the spectrum of other coexisting somatic mutations in any particular case [5], to genetic polymorphisms in the cytokine genes of the affected individual [6], and to the varying gene dosage and level of expression of the mutated *JAK2* or *MPL*. As a result of loss of heterozygosity or mutation of both alleles, *JAK2* V617F can be present in up to several copies per cell, and cases with a higher V617F allele burden often manifest as PV or PMF rather than as ET. In contrast to patients with the V617F mutation, PV patients with *JAK2* exon 12 mutations tend to present at a younger age, and with higher hematocrit, lower platelet count, and lower white blood cell (WBC) count. ET and PMF patients with *MPL* mutations tend to show different patterns of clonal evolution than *JAK2*-mutated cases, with the common karyotypic findings of gains of chromosome 1 in ET with *MPL* mutations and chromosome 9 in PMF with *MPL* mutations [7]. Germline *JAK2* and *MPL* mutations continue to be discovered in families with predisposition to the development of MPNs [8].

Calreticulin gene (*CALR*) mutations occur in 50–71 % of ET cases, and 56–88 % of PMF cases that are negative for *JAK2* and *MPL* mutations [9–12]. These mutations include a variety of insertion and deletions located in exon 9 of *CALR* that shift the translational reading frame and produce a common novel C-terminal peptide sequence. Mutated CALR may differentially influence signaling through the JAK-STAT pathway. *CALR* mutations are largely mutually exclusive with *JAK2* and *MPL* mutations and are not found in PV, CML, AML, or most cases of MDS. *CALR*-mutated PMF is prognostically distinct from *MPL*- and *JAK2*-mutated MPNs and from those cases that lack all three mutations [9–14]. Therefore, testing for *CALR* mutations can assist in the diagnosis of MPN, and provide a genetic marker for monitoring response to therapy.

Myeloproliferative Neoplasms Associated with Eosinophilia

Most causes of significant eosinophilia are reactive or secondary to chronic parasitic infections or due to cytokine-producing malignancies, particularly T-cell lymphoma, Hodgkin lymphoma, and some carcinomas. However, a group of rare MPNs present with eosinophilia and immature/dysplastic myelopoiesis and are characterized by gene fusions involving a variety of growth factor genes (Table 44.1). The majority show fusion of the *FGFR1* gene to a variety of other genes, thereby producing ligand-independent FGFR1 activation. Another type has a chromosome 4 interstitial cryptic *FIP1L1–PDGFRA* fusion that activates the PDFRA kinase, with the neoplasms showing dramatic response to imatinib treatment, similar to CML. A very rare *PDGFRB*-translocation syndrome produces a similar MPN due to fusion with *ETV6* or a variety of other partner genes.

Myelodysplastic/Myeloproliferative Neoplasms

The most common of the mixed myeloid disorders is CMML, which can present with a high WBC count resembling acute monocytic leukemia, or with a low WBC count associated with dyspoietic BM findings. This variability in presentation underlies a heterogeneous molecular pathogenesis. *RAS* gene mutations are identified in the vast majority of cases with hyperproliferative presentations, and a variety of cytogenetic and somatic mutations, including *TET2* and *JAK2* V617F, are seen in other cases [15].

Myelodysplastic Syndromes

Decreased numbers of WBCs (leukopenia), platelets (thrombocytopenia), and erythrocytes (anemia) are among the most common abnormal laboratory findings in patients with MDS. In younger patients, these cytopenias often have a nonneoplastic etiology such as immune-mediated marrow suppression, autoimmune disease, acute bacterial and viral infections, nutritional deficiency (e.g., B12, folate or iron), or toxin exposure. However, with advancing age, cytopenias are increasingly related to genetically mediated BM failure or MDS. The dysplastic changes of MDS can be superimposed upon other causes of marrow suppression, exacerbating the ineffective hematopoiesis. In these cases, abnormal blood cells show impaired maturation and are destroyed by apoptosis before being released into the bloodstream. These genetically abnormal marrow components often have an atypical morphology (dysplasia) that can be recognized in a BM aspirate smear.

Available Assays and Laboratory Issues

Chronic Myelogenous Leukemia

BCR–ABL1 Detection

In CML, most of the *BCR–ABL1* translocations involve the major breakpoint cluster region (M-bcr) adjacent to exons 12–16 of *BCR* (formerly called exons b1–b5) and result in either the e13a2 or e14a2 *BCR–ABL1* gene fusions (or both transcripts), which encode closely related 210 kD fusion proteins (p210). In contrast, in Ph chromosome-positive (Ph+) B-ALL, 50–65 % of the *BCR* breakpoints arise at the minor breakpoint cluster region (m-bcr), adjacent to exons 1 and 2 of *BCR*, with the *BCR–ABL1* transcript containing the e1a2 junction, which is translated into the p190 BCR-ABL1 fusion protein. Rarely, usually in CML with monocytosis and neutrophilia, the breakpoint occurs in the μ-BCR region (exons 17–20), resulting in a larger p230 fusion BCR-ABL1 protein.

The *BCR–ABL1* fusion gene can be detected by several methods. The Ph chromosome can be visualized by conventional G-banded karyotyping with a false-negative rate of <10 %, which is usually related to more complex fusions that obscure the breakpoints involved. However, karyotyping has a low sensitivity that is not acceptable for minimal residual disease (MRD) monitoring given that only 20 metaphases are usually analyzed (i.e., a maximal sensitivity of 5 %).

Fluorescence in situ hybridization (FISH) on interphase cells is another method to detect the *BCR–ABL1* fusion (Fig. 44.1). Dual-color, dual-fusion probes are typically used and can identify variant breakpoints or three-way translocations that do not result in recognizable Ph+ metaphases. Given an adequate sample, the false-negative rate for FISH is much less than 1 %. The use of FISH for MRD monitoring after completion of therapy is more limited given that the maximal sensitivity is approximately 1 % Ph+ cells, given that only several hundred cells are typically counted [16].

Other molecular methods can be used for detecting *BCR–ABL1* fusions, including PCR from genomic DNA, Southern blotting, or northern blotting. However, the vast majority of clinical molecular laboratories detect the *BCR–ABL1* fusion gene by reverse transcription polymerase chain reaction (RT-PCR). Qualitative RT-PCR has been largely replaced by quantitative/real-time PCR (RT-qPCR) methods using an allele-specific PCR approach with primers directed separately against the M-bcr and m-bcr regions (p210 and p190 isoforms, respectively).

BCR–ABL1 RT-PCR Assay Standardization and the International Scale

Essentially all RT-qPCR *BCR–ABL1* assays normalize the amount of fusion transcript to the level of a control transcript to allow comparison across different levels of input positive cells. This approach also permits assessment of RNA quality, because low levels of the control gene likely indicate a degraded sample. Commonly used genes for normalization include *GAPDH*, *ACTB*, *BCR*, *GUSB*, and *ABL1* [17]. These control genes are expressed at very different levels resulting in highly variable *BCR–ABL1* fusion to control transcript values. This variability between assays using different control transcripts makes comparison of results from different laboratories difficult. Additionally, laboratories use a variety of RNA extraction methods, different reverse transcription protocols, and have different reporting criteria.

Standardization of RT-qPCR assays has become a high priority because molecular milestones of *BCR–ABL1* transcript levels are now the basis of treatment decision-making for CML. The first advance in standardization, led by the Europe Against Cancer (EAC) initiative, was the development of well-validated RT-qPCR primers and probes, as well as standardized PCR conditions for *BCR–ABL1* assays [18]. The second effort, beginning with the European LeukemiaNet collaborative, developed consensus on measurement of therapeutic milestones in CML (Table 44.5) [19]. This effort reached fruition in 2012 and established the International Scale (IS) whereby individual laboratories could adjust their internal *BCR–ABL1*/control transcript ratios to the molecular milestones based on standard calibrators [20, 21].

Table 44.5 Definitions and therapeutic milestones for *BCR–ABL1* disease response

Definitions		
Complete hematologic response (CHR)	WBC count < 10×10^9/L	
	Normal WBC differential	
	≤1% circulating immature cells	
	Platelet count < 450×10^9/L	
	No signs and symptoms of CML	
Major molecular response (MMR)	>3-log reduction in *BCR–ABL1* transcript levels (0.1 % IS)	
Complete molecular response (CMR)	PCR negative	
Complete cytogenetic response (CCyR)	No Ph detected	
Partial/major cytogenetic response (PCyR)	1–35 % Ph+ cells	
Therapeutic milestones	**Suboptimal**	**Failure**
3 months on therapy	Less than CHR	No HR
6 months	Less than PCyR	Less than CHR
12 months	Less than CCyR	Less than PCyR
	Not approaching MMR	
18 months	Less than MMR	Less than CCyR

Ph Philadelphia chromosome, *WBC* white blood cell
Guidelines as reported in [19]

Therapy and Treatment Response Monitoring in CML

With an understanding of the molecular basis of CML, the design and synthesis of small molecules that could inhibit the kinase activity of ABL1 was attempted. This resulted in US Food and Drug Administration (FDA) approval of the kinase inhibitor imatinib mesylate (also called ST1571) in 1999. Before the discovery of imatinib, the widely used therapeutic options for CML were interferon-α with or without cytarabine, hydroxyurea, or allogeneic stem cell transplant (ASCT). With results first published in 2003, the pivotal International Randomized Interferon vs ST1571 (IRIS) study established imatinib as the frontline therapy for newly diagnosed CML, with superior responses and compliance rates compared to interferon/cytarabine [22, 23]. Subsequently, second generation tyrosine kinase inhibitors (TKI) that successfully target BCR-ABL1 were introduced, particularly nilotinib and dasatinib that were both approved as frontline therapy by the FDA in 2010.

Most patients with CML show excellent response to imatinib, with progression-free survival rates at 5 years of >90 %. However, periodic RT-qPCR *BCR–ABL1* testing every 3–6 months during treatment is warranted to monitor for primary or secondary drug resistance. In patients with CML, blood and BM samples show similar levels of *BCR–ABL1* transcript, but testing of blood is preferred due to the ease of collection. While receiving imatinib, most patients quickly show hematologic remission, defined as resolution of leukocytosis, as indicated by a WBC count below 10×10^9/L with a normal differential and ≤1 % circulating immature cells, a platelet count below 450×10^9/L, and disappearance of signs and symptoms of disease, including splenomegaly. On standard dose imatinib, most patients experience hematologic remission within 4–12 weeks. For those patients being monitored by karyotyping, complete cytogenetic response, defined as 0 % Ph+ metaphases when at least 20 cells have been examined, is usually achieved before 12 months. Partial (1–35 % Ph+ metaphases), and especially minor cytogenetic responses (36–95 % Ph+ metaphases) are indicative of suboptimal therapy or drug resistance (Table 44.5).

The primary therapeutic endpoint for CML treatment is a major molecular remission (MMR) defined as a *BCR–ABL1*/control transcript IS ratio below 0.1 %. This IS target was originally established by the IRIS study in which optimal response was defined as at least a three-log decrease in the *BCR–ABL1*/*ABL1* transcript ratio from the 100 % value that was the median pretreatment level. With the advent of IS calibration, patient-specific responses can now be defined. In many patients on imatinib, complete molecular response can be achieved, such that no *BCR–ABL1* transcripts are detected with an assay that has a diagnostic sensitivity of at least 0.005 % (IS).

Optimally, MMR is achieved within 12–18 months of beginning a TKI. During this initial period, RT-qPCR using peripheral blood is recommended every 3 months, and is usually performed less frequently (every 6–12 months) after MMR is achieved. Cytogenetic testing should be performed at 6 months, 12 months, and possibly 18 months if Ph+ chromosomes are still detected. FISH may serve as a useful surrogate marker of disease level when chromosome analysis does not yield adequate metaphase preparations. Recent studies, including a follow-up on the IRIS trial, have demonstrated that attaining MMR at earlier time points results in improved outcomes in CML [23, 24].

Resistance in CML and Detection of ABL1 Kinase Domain Mutations

When a patient with CML does not meet the milestones for optimal therapeutic response, changes to the treatment regimen must be considered. The first step in the workup of TKI resistance is usually to repeat the RT-qPCR test to confirm the level of residual *BCR–ABL1* transcript, followed by DNA sequencing of the ABL1 kinase domain to assess for the presence of mutations. While ABL1 kinase mutations are the most common cause of resistance, other *BCR–ABL1*-dependent mechanisms of resistance include amplification or additional copies of the Ph chromosome, which can be detected by FISH, and pharmacodynamic factors which inhibit drug effects. Overcoming these factors may be achieved by TKI dose escalation [25]. Imatinib resistance also can be due to *BCR–ABL1* mutation-independent mechanisms (Table 44.6) such as clonal evolution due to *ASXL1*, *IZKF1*, or *RUNX1* mutations [29, 30], *TP53* deletion, or acquisition of AML-type genetic changes [31], which may be detected by a BM karyotyping.

Approximately 50 % of patients displaying secondary TKI resistance in CML, as shown by increasing RT-qPCR

Table 44.6 Testing indicated for drug-resistant CML

Test	Findings	Reference/guidelines
Bone marrow morphology	Increased blasts, basophils, fibrosis	[19]
Karyotype	Secondary genetic changes, especially del17p/TP53	[26]
ABL kinase domain sequencing	>70 different amino acids in kinase domain, lead to variable upregulation or insensitivity to kinase inhibition	[27, 28]
BCR–ABL1 FISH	Amplification/extra copies of Philadelphia chromosome	[26]
RUNX1, *IZKF1*, or *ASXL1* mutation status	Maturation arrest with blast crisis	[29, 30]

FISH fluorescence in situ hybridization

levels after achieving MMR, will have a mutation in the ABL1 kinase domain [28]. More than 150 different mutations involving over 60 different amino acid residues have been documented in the ABL1 kinase domain. However, 15 *ABL1* mutations account for >85 % of cases [32], with mutations in the T315I gatekeeper and in the P-loop domain most consistently associated with adverse outcomes (Fig. 44.2). The in vivo sensitivity to different kinase inhibitors is largely predicted by response of model cell lines harboring these mutations [33]. Studies of this type have identified the common G250E mutation as being resistant to imatinib, but not to the second generation inhibitors dasatinib and nilotinib, whereas other mutations tend to be resistant to dasatinib but not nilotinib (e.g., T315A, F317L/I/V, and V299L) or to nilotinib but not dasatinib (e.g., Y253H, E255K/V, and F359V/C). The T315I ABL1 kinase domain mutation is resistant to most small molecule inhibitors [34]. Patients with T315I-mutated CML often progress to blast phase and require chemotherapy and ASCT, although some biologic therapies, such as homoharringtonine [35], and third generation kinase inhibitors, such as ponatinib/AP24534 [36], show promise.

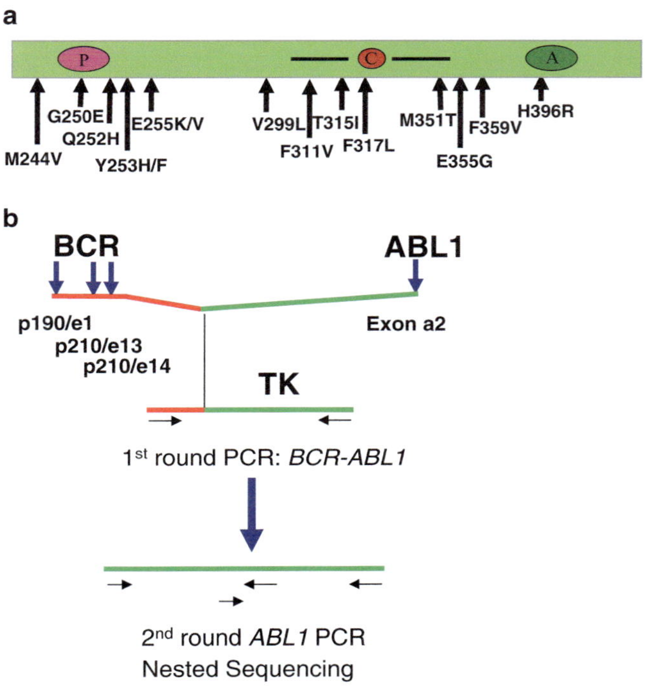

Figure 44.2 *ABL1* mutation in drug-resistant CML. (**a**) Schematic of the ABL1 kinase domain, with P-loop (P), catalytic domain (C), and activation domain (A) indicated. The locations of the 15 most commonly mutated amino acid residues are indicated. (**b**) Schematic of t(9;22) translocation breakpoints with a strategy for two step PCR amplification of the *BCR–ABL1* fusion transcript, followed by amplification of the *ABL1* tyrosine kinase (TK) domain using several primer sets (*black arrows*) prior to sequencing

Several molecular tests detect ABL1 mutations, with the most common being Sanger sequencing to assess the entire kinase domain in one or two cycling reactions [27]. As an initial step, the *BCR–ABL1* fusion gene is specifically amplified (Fig. 44.2b), because residual leukemic cells may only represent a small portion of leukocytes, and Sanger sequencing is not sufficiently sensitive to detect rare mutated transcripts. A more sensitive but more directed approach is to perform mutation-specific real-time PCR reactions to detect the most commonly observed mutations.

Recommendations for when to perform mutation testing of the ABL1 kinase domain vary between different centers. A conservative approach is to trigger testing whenever there is loss of hematologic or complete cytogenetic remission, unexpected cytopenias, or a greater than ten-fold rise in *BCR–ABL1* transcript levels above MMR [27].

Essential Thrombocythemia, Primary Myelofibrosis, and Polycythemia Vera

Both qualitative and quantitative methods are used to detect the common V617F mutation (Fig. 44.3), whereas Sanger sequencing is used to detect the less common *JAK2* exon 12 mutations as well as mutations in *CALR*, *MPL* and *CSF3R*. Testing for *JAK2* V617F is recommended in the initial workup of all suspected MPNs, along with erythropoietin levels for suspected PV, *BCR–ABL1* testing for all cases with

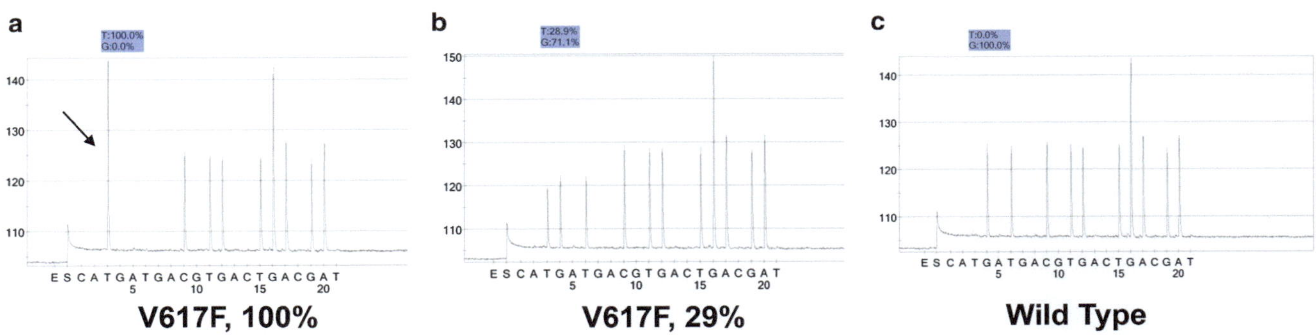

Figure 44.3 *JAK2* mutation detection by pyrosequencing assay. Cases with homozygous V617F mutations (**a**, *arrow* showing T allele), heterozygous mutated and wild type sequences (**b**, both T and G alleles), and wild type results (**c**, only G allele) are illustrated

neutrophilia (especially if accompanied by basophilia or eosinophilia), and BM evaluation for suspected ET or PMF.

Although some therapies for *JAK2*-mutated MPNs, such as lenalidomide and interferon, produce selective decreases in the *JAK2* mutation burden, monitoring *JAK2* mutation levels after therapy is not yet as routine as for CML. Quantitative *JAK2* testing is probably most useful for monitoring for relapse of MPNs after ASCT, and in monitoring of *JAK2* kinase inhibitors [7], most of which are still investigational. Because pathogenic mutations in *JAK2*, *CALR*, *MPL*, and *CSF3R* all affect signaling through the JAK-STAT pathway and may all be candidates for JAK inhibitor therapies, a panel approach for testing has been proposed for newly diagnosed MPNs [37]. Advanced sequencing technologies would thus be an appealing approach for such multigene testing.

Myelodysplastic Syndrome

Cytogenetic Analysis for Diagnosis and Prognosis in MDS

With the exception of one distinctive cytogenetically defined entity (refractory anemia with isolated 5q-), MDS is currently classified in the WHO system based on the number of myeloblasts and whether one or several of the myeloid, monocytic, erythroid, or megakaryocytic lineages are clearly dysplastic (Table 44.2). Because appreciation of morphologic changes in the BM can be difficult, cytogenetic studies are always done to identify the complex genomic changes associated with MDS and to support the diagnosis. Recently, multiprobe FISH panels, which assess the presence or absence of common changes such as del5q/-5, del7q/-7, +8, and del20q, are increasingly being used to supplement karyotyping although their added value remains unclear [38, 39].

Common and less common cytogenetic aberrations in MDS have been used along with hematologic criteria to stratify cases of MDS into low, moderate, and high risk for poor outcome and progression to high-grade MDS/AML (Table 44.7). The most commonly used schema is the International Prognostic Scoring System (IPSS), which was recently revised to add several additional cytogenetic changes (Table 44.8). Although FISH assays are becoming more common for MDS (Fig. 44.4), detection of these aberrations by FISH (especially at low percentages) rather than karyotype may not have the same prognostic significance for the IPSS. Genomic microarrays provide additional gene-based information compared to karyotype and may soon supplement conventional karyotyping in the workup of MDS [41].

Common Somatic Mutations in MDS

At least half of suspected MDS cases have no cytogenetic abnormalities identified by chromosome analysis. In such cases FISH panels typically detect only a few, if any, additional aberrations. Many of these cases will have only mild dysplasia. In these instances, the distinction between a reactive condition and MDS can be difficult, and may only be established after extensive testing and exclusion of all other possible etiologies. Demonstration of clonality within blood or BM cells could more rapidly and definitively offer a diagnosis of MDS.

Several genes that are commonly mutated in MDS have been identified by genomic sequencing. These genes include *TET2*, *IDH1*, *IDH2*, *ASXL1*, *SF3B1*, *DNMT3A*, *EZH2*, and *LNK* (Table 44.9). The mutation types vary and include

Table 44.7 Cytogenetic prognostic subgroups in the revised International Prognostic Scoring System (IPSS-R)

Risk group	Karyotypic findings
Very good	del(11q), -Y
Good	XX/XY, del(20q), del(5q) alone and double, del(12p)
Intermediate	+8, 7q-, i(17q),+19,+21, any other single or double, independent clones
Poor	der(3)q21/q26, -7, double including 7q-, complex changes (3 abnormalities)
Very poor	complex changes (>3 abnormalities)

Table adapted from Ref. 40

Table 44.8 Criteria for scoring using the revised International Prognostic Scoring System (IPSS-R)

	Score for individual parameter						
Variable	0	1	1.5	1.5	2.5	3.5	5
Cytogenetic findings	Very good		Good		Int	Poor	Very poor
% BM blasts	<5 %			5–10 %	11–30 %		
Hemoglobin (g/dL)	≥10			<10			
Platelets ($x\,10^9$/L)	≥100		<100				
ANC ($x\,10^9$/L)	≥0.8	0.8					
Cumulative score		1	2	3	4	5	
		Very good	Good	Int	Poor	Very poor	
Overall survival[a]		8.7	5.3	3.0	1.6	0.8	

ANC absolute neutrophil count, *BM* bone marrow, *Int* intermediate
[a]Overall survival represents median survival in years
Table adapted from Ref. 40

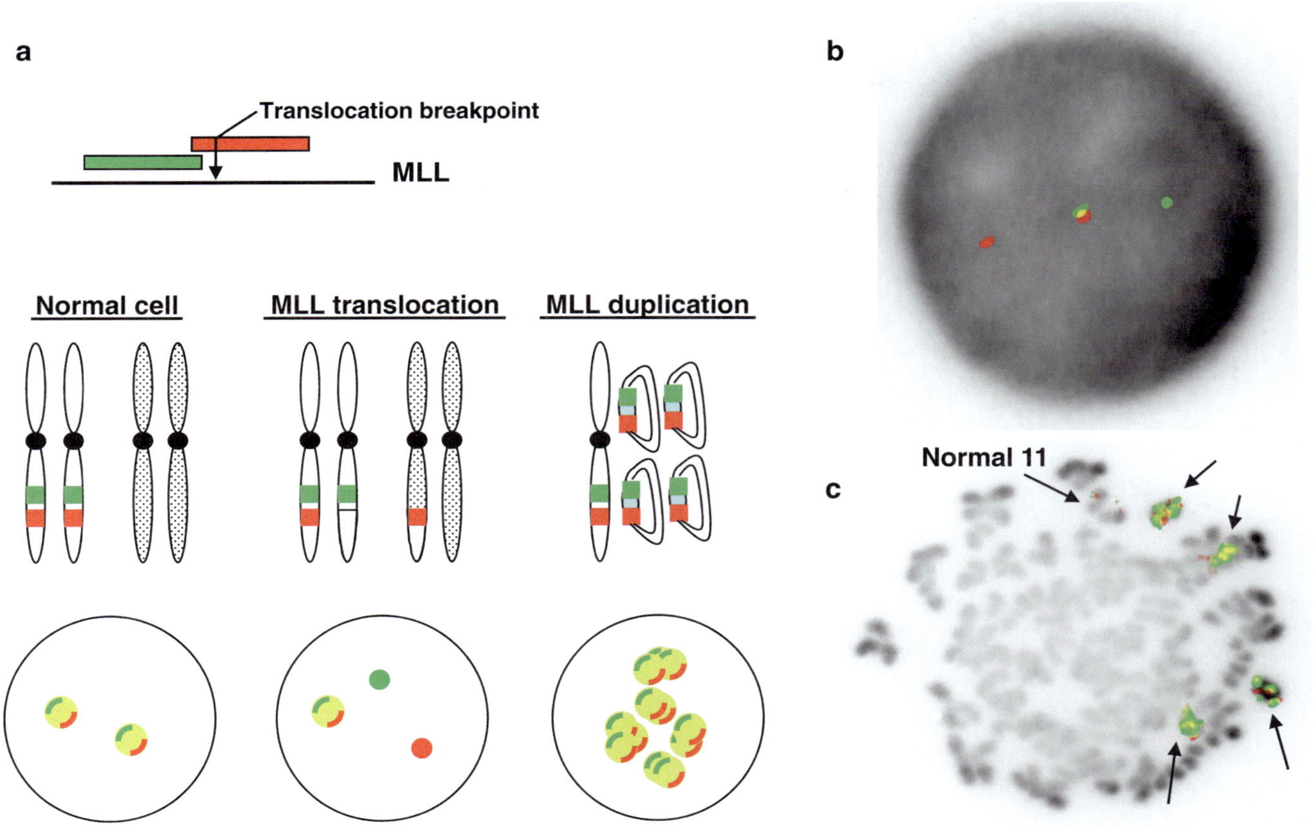

Figure 44.4 *MLL* alterations in MDS and AML. (**a**) Schematic of dual break-apart fluorescence in situ hybridization (FISH) strategy for *MLL* at chromosome 11q23. A green-labeled probe is used for the 5′ exons of *MLL*, with an orange-labeled probe for the 3′ exons with an overlap at exon 6. (**b**) Findings in an interphase cell in an MDS case with a split probe for one copy of the *MLL* gene, indicative of an *MLL* translocation. (**c**) FISH performed on a metaphase spread in a case of AML reveals *MLL* gene amplification associated with ring chromosomes

Table 44.9 Divergent and common molecular pathogenesis of MPNs and MDS

Gene	Mutation % in MPNs (excluding CML)	Mutation % in MDS	Function
Growth regulators			
JAK2	50 %, including ~100 % of PV	2–3 %	Kinase downstream of cytokine receptors
MPL	2–3 %	<1 %	Cytokine receptor
PGFRA	2 %	ns	RTK
PGFRB	<1 %	<1 %	RTK
FGFR1	1–2 %	ns	RTK
CBL	ns	ns	RTK negative regulator
Transcriptional and epigenetic regulators			
TET2	10–30 %; 50 % of CMML, 30 % of SM	25–30 %	Catalyzes conversion of 5-methylcytosine to 5-hydroxymethylcytosine
IDH1–IDH2	1–5 %	5–10 %	Isocitrate dehydrogenase; converts isocitrate to 2-ketoglutarate, TET2 co-regulation
DNMT3A	5–10 %	5–10 %	DNA cytosine methyltransferase
EZH2	3–7 %	5–10 %	Histone methyltransferase complex protein
ASXL1	3–15 %	10–15 %	Transcriptional repression of HOX genes

CML chronic myelogenous leukemia, *CMML* chronic myelomonocytic leukemia, *MDS* myelodysplastic syndrome, *MPN* myeloproliferative neoplasm, *ns* not present or insufficient data, *PV* polycythemia vera, *RTK* receptor tyrosine kinase inhibitor, *SM* systemic mastocytosis

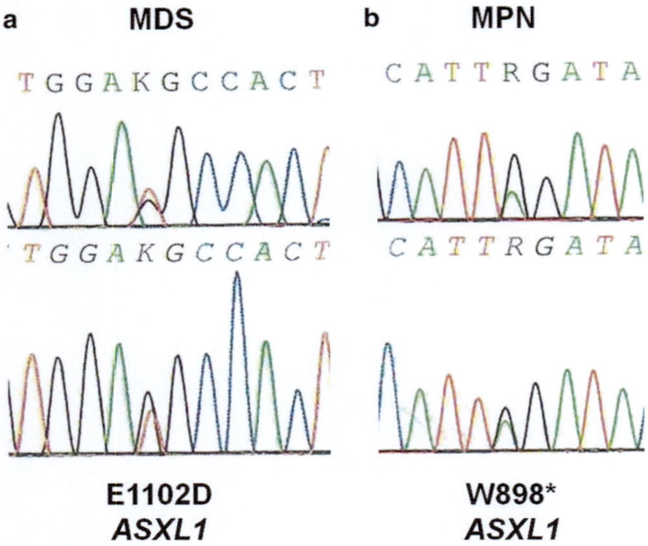

Figure 44.5 Similar mutation profiles in myelodysplastic syndrome and myeloproliferative neoplasms. (**a**) A sequence tracing of the E1102D heterozygous missense mutation in the *ASXL1* gene, in a patient with myelodysplastic syndrome (MDS). (**b**) A nonsense mutation in *ASXL1* (W898*) in a myeloproliferative neoplasm (MPN)

deletions, insertions, missense mutations (Fig. 44.5a), nonsense mutations (Fig. 44.5b), as well as frameshift mutations, and can either be clustered in hotspots or distributed throughout the gene. Detection of any of these mutations can help establish a diagnosis of MDS in patients who otherwise have negative tests. The next generation of risk stratification for MDS has begun to incorporate gene mutations into multivariate outcome prediction models [42–44].

Conclusions and Future Directions

The function of many of the most frequently mutated genes in MDS involves the epigenetic regulation of transcriptional complexes involved in hematopoiesis. For these genes, mutations at several different loci, such as *EZH2*, *TET2*, and *DNMT3A*, can be found in the same tumor. This is in contrast to the essentially mutually exclusive nature of mutations involving cytokine and growth factor genes, such as *BCR–ABL1* or *JAK2*. Another feature of the epigenetic class of genes is that they are commonly mutated in AML as well as in MDS and MPNs (Table 44.9). Taken together; these findings suggest that myeloid neoplasms have a shared pathogenesis involving multifocal dysregulation of the epigenetic program. Given that many new classes of therapeutic agents, including deacetylase inhibitors and hypomethylating agents, target these complexes, it seems likely that detection of these mutations will become critical to individualizing therapy in both MDS and MPNs.

References

1. Druker BJ. Translation of the Philadelphia chromosome into therapy for CML. Blood. 2008;112:4808–17.
2. Tefferi A. The history of myeloproliferative disorders: before and after Dameshek. Leukemia. 2008;22:3–13.
3. Jones D, Luthra R, Cortes J, Thomas D, O'Brien S, Bueso-Ramos C, Hai S, Ravandi F, de Lima M, Kantarjian H, Jorgensen JL. BCR-ABL fusion transcript types and levels and their interaction with secondary genetic changes in determining the phenotype of Philadelphia chromosome-positive leukemias. Blood. 2008;112:5190–2.
4. Maxson JE, Gotlib J, Pollyea DA, Fleischman AG, Agarwal A, Eide CA, Bottomly D, Wilmot B, McWeeney SK, Tognon CE, Pond JB, Collins RH, Goueli B, Oh ST, Deininger MW, Chang BH, Loriaux MM, Druker BJ, Tyner JW. Oncogenic CSF3R mutations in chronic neutrophilic leukemia and atypical CML. N Engl J Med. 2013;368:1781–90.
5. Bacher U, Weissmann S, Kohlmann A, Schindela S, Alpermann T, Schnittger S, Kern W, Haferlach T, Haferlach C. TET2 deletions are a recurrent but rare phenomenon in myeloid malignancies and are frequently accompanied by TET2 mutations on the remaining allele. Br J Haematol. 2012;156:67–75.
6. Tefferi A, Lasho TL, Patnaik MM, Finke CM, Hussein K, Hogan WJ, Elliott MA, Litzow MR, Hanson CA, Pardanani A. JAK2 germline genetic variation affects disease susceptibility in primary myelofibrosis regardless of V617F mutational status: nullizygosity for the JAK2 46/1 haplotype is associated with inferior survival. Leukemia. 2010;24:105–9.
7. Millecker L, Lennon PA, Verstovsek S, Barkoh B, Galbincea J, Hu P, Chen SS, Jones D. Distinct patterns of cytogenetic and clinical progression in chronic myeloproliferative neoplasms with or without JAK2 or MPL mutations. Cancer Genet Cytogenet. 2010;197:1–7.
8. Goldin LR, Bjorkholm M, Kristinsson SY, Samuelsson J, Landgren O. Germline and somatic JAK2 mutations and susceptibility to chronic myeloproliferative neoplasms. Genome Med. 2009;1:55.
9. Klampfl T, Gisslinger H, Harutyunyan AS, Nivarthi H, Rumi E, Milosevic JD, Them NC, Berg T, Gisslinger B, Pietra D, Chen D, Vladimer GI, Bagienski K, Milanesi C, Casetti IC, Sant'antonio E, Ferretti V, Elena C, Schischlik F, Cleary C, Six M, Schalling M, Schonegger A, Bock C, Malcovati L, Pascutto C, Superti-Furga G, Cazzola M, Kralovics R. Somatic mutations of calreticulin in myeloproliferative neoplasms. N Engl J Med. 2013;369:2379–90.
10. Nangalia J, Massie CE, Baxter EJ, Nice FL, Gundem G, Wedge DC, Avezov E, Li J, Kollmann K, Kent DG, Aziz A, Godfrey AL, Hinton J, Martincorena I, Van LP, Jones AV, Guglielmelli P, Tarpey P, Harding HP, Fitzpatrick JD, Goudie CT, Ortmann CA, Loughran SJ, Raine K, Jones DR, Butler AP, Teague JW, O'Meara S, McLaren S, Bianchi M, Silber Y, Dimitropoulou D, Bloxham D, Mudie L, Maddison M, Robinson B, Keohane C, Maclean C, Hill K, Orchard K, Tauro S, Du MQ, Greaves M, Bowen D, Huntly BJ, Harrison CN, Cross NC, Ron D, Vannucchi AM, Papaemmanuil E, Campbell PJ, Green AR. Somatic CALR mutations in myeloproliferative neoplasms with nonmutated JAK2. N Engl J Med. 2013;369:2391–405.
11. Rotunno G, Mannarelli C, Guglielmelli P, Pacilli A, Pancrazzi A, Pieri L, Fanelli T, Bosi A, Vannucchi AM. Impact of calreticulin mutations on clinical and hematological phenotype and outcome in essential thrombocythemia. Blood. 2014;123:1552–5.
12. Tefferi A, Lasho TL, Finke CM, Knudson RA, Ketterling R, Hanson CH, Maffioli M, Caramazza D, Passamonti F, Pardanani A. CALR vs JAK2 vs MPL-mutated or triple-negative myelofibrosis: clinical, cytogenetic and molecular comparisons. Leukemia. 2014;28:1472.

13. Sirhan S, Lasho TL, Hanson CA, Mesa RA, Pardanani A, Tefferi A The presence of JAK2V617F in primary myelofibrosis or its allele burden in polycythemia vera predicts chemosensitivity to hydroxyurea. Am J Hematol. 2008;83:363–5.
14. Tefferi A, Guglielmelli P, Lasho TL, Rotunno G, Finke C, Mannarelli C, Belachew AA, Pancrazzi A, Wassie EA, Ketterling RP, Hanson CA, Pardanani A, Vannucchi AM. CALR and ASXL1 mutations-based molecular prognostication in primary myelofibrosis: an international study of 570 patients. Leukemia. 2014;28:1494.
15. Kohlmann A, Grossmann V, Klein HU, Schindela S, Weiss T, Kazak B, Dicker F, Schnittger S, Dugas M, Kern W, Haferlach C, Haferlach T. Next-generation sequencing technology reveals a characteristic pattern of molecular mutations in 72.8% of chronic myelomonocytic leukemia by detecting frequent alterations in TET2, CBL, RAS, and RUNX1. J Clin Oncol. 2010;28:3858–65.
16. Kantarjian H, Schiffer C, Jones D, Cortes J. Monitoring the response and course of chronic myeloid leukemia in the modern era of BCR-ABL tyrosine kinase inhibitors: practical advice on the use and interpretation of monitoring methods. Blood. 2008;111:1774–80.
17. Wang YL, Lee JW, Cesarman E, Jin DK, Csernus B. Molecular monitoring of chronic myelogenous leukemia: identification of the most suitable internal control gene for real-time quantification of BCR-ABL transcripts. J Mol Diagn. 2006;8:231–9.
18. van Dongen JJ, Macintyre EA, Gabert JA, Delabesse E, Rossi V, Saglio G, Gottardi E, Rambaldi A, Dotti G, Griesinger F, Parreira A, Gameiro P, Diaz MG, Malec M, Langerak AW, San Miguel JF, Biondi A. Standardized RT-PCR analysis of fusion gene transcripts from chromosome aberrations in acute leukemia for detection of minimal residual disease. Report of the BIOMED-1 Concerted Action: investigation of minimal residual disease in acute leukemia. Leukemia. 1999;13:1901–28.
19. Baccarani M, Castagnetti F, Gugliotta G, Palandri F, Soverini S. Response definitions and European Leukemianet Management recommendations. Best Pract Res Clin Haematol. 2009;22:331–41.
20. Branford S, Fletcher L, Cross NC, Muller MC, Hochhaus A, Kim DW, Radich JP, Saglio G, Pane F, Kamel-Reid S, Wang YL, Press RD, Lynch K, Rudzki Z, Goldman JM, Hughes T. Desirable performance characteristics for BCR-ABL measurement on an international reporting scale to allow consistent interpretation of individual patient response and comparison of response rates between clinical trials. Blood. 2008;112:3330–8.
21. White HE, Matejtschuk P, Rigsby P, Gabert J, Lin F, Lynn WY, Branford S, Muller MC, Beaufils N, Beillard E, Colomer D, Dvorakova D, Ehrencrona H, Goh HG, El HH, Jones D, Kairisto V, Kamel-Reid S, Kim DW, Langabeer S, Ma ES, Press RD, Romeo G, Wang L, Zoi K, Hughes T, Saglio G, Hochhaus A, Goldman JM, Metcalfe P, Cross NC. Establishment of the first World Health Organization International Genetic Reference Panel for quantitation of BCR-ABL mRNA. Blood. 2010;116:e111–7.
22. Hughes TP, Kaeda J, Branford S, Rudzki Z, Hochhaus A, Hensley ML, Gathmann I, Bolton AE, van Hoomissen IC, Goldman JM, Radich JP. Frequency of major molecular responses to imatinib or interferon alfa plus cytarabine in newly diagnosed chronic myeloid leukemia. N Engl J Med. 2003;349:1423–32.
23. Hughes TP, Hochhaus A, Branford S, Muller MC, Kaeda JS, Foroni L, Druker BJ, Guilhot F, Larson RA, O'Brien SG, Rudoltz MS, Mone M, Wehrle E, Modur V, Goldman JM, Radich JP. Long-term prognostic significance of early molecular response to imatinib in newly diagnosed chronic myeloid leukemia: an analysis from the International Randomized Study of Interferon and STI571 (IRIS). Blood. 2010;116:3758–65.
24. Quintas-Cardama A, Kantarjian H, Jones D, Shan J, Borthakur G, Thomas D, Kornblau S, O'Brien S, Cortes J. Delayed achievement of cytogenetic and molecular response is associated with increased risk of progression among patients with chronic myeloid leukemia in early chronic phase receiving high-dose or standard-dose imatinib therapy. Blood. 2009;113:6315–21.
25. Zhang WW, Cortes JE, Yao H, Zhang L, Reddy NG, Jabbour E, Kantarjian HM, Jones D. Predictors of primary imatinib resistance in chronic myelogenous leukemia are distinct from those in secondary imatinib resistance. J Clin Oncol. 2009;27:3642–9.
26. Kantarjian HM, Talpaz M, Giles F, O'Brien S, Cortes J. New insights into the pathophysiology of chronic myeloid leukemia and imatinib resistance. Ann Intern Med. 2006;145:913–23.
27. Jones D, Kamel-Reid S, Bahler D, Dong H, Elenitoba-Johnson K, Press R, Quigley N, Rothberg P, Sabath D, Viswanatha D, Weck K, Zehnder J. Laboratory practice guidelines for detecting and reporting BCR-ABL drug resistance mutations in chronic myelogenous leukemia and acute lymphoblastic leukemia: a report of the Association for Molecular Pathology. J Mol Diagn. 2009;11:4–11.
28. Soverini S, Hochhaus A, Nicolini FE, Gruber F, Lange T, Saglio G, Pane F, Muller MC, Ernst T, Rosti G, Porkka K, Baccarani M, Cross NC, Martinelli G. BCR-ABL kinase domain mutation analysis in chronic myeloid leukemia patients treated with tyrosine kinase inhibitors: recommendations from an expert panel on behalf of European LeukemiaNet. Blood. 2011;118:1208–15.
29. Grossmann V, Kohlmann A, Zenger M, Schindela S, Eder C, Weissmann S, Schnittger S, Kern W, Muller MC, Hochhaus A, Haferlach T, Haferlach C. A deep-sequencing study of chronic myeloid leukemia patients in blast crisis (BC-CML) detects mutations in 76.9% of cases. Leukemia. 2011;25:557–60.
30. Roche-Lestienne C, Deluche L, Corm S, Tigaud I, Joha S, Philippe N, Geffroy S, Lai JL, Nicolini FE, Preudhomme C. RUNX1 DNA-binding mutations and RUNX1-PRDM16 cryptic fusions in BCR-ABL+ leukemias are frequently associated with secondary trisomy 21 and may contribute to clonal evolution and imatinib resistance. Blood. 2008;111:3735–41.
31. Merzianu M, Medeiros LJ, Cortes J, Yin C, Lin P, Jones D, Glassman A, Kantarjian H, Huh Y. inv(16)(p13q22) in chronic myelogenous leukemia in blast phase: a clinicopathologic, cytogenetic, and molecular study of five cases. Am J Clin Pathol. 2005;124:807–14.
32. Jones D, Chen SS, Jabbour E, Rios MB, Kantarjian H, Cortes J. Uncommon BCR-ABL kinase domain mutations in kinase inhibitor-resistant chronic myelogenous leukemia and Ph+ acute lymphoblastic leukemia show high rates of regression, suggesting weak selective effects. Blood. 2010;115:5428–9.
33. Jabbour E, Jones D, Kantarjian HM, O'Brien S, Tam C, Koller C, Burger JA, Borthakur G, Wierda WG, Cortes J. Long-term outcome of patients with chronic myeloid leukemia treated with second-generation tyrosine kinase inhibitors after imatinib failure is predicted by the in vitro sensitivity of BCR-ABL kinase domain mutations. Blood. 2009;114:2037–43.
34. Jabbour E, Kantarjian H, Jones D, Breeden M, Garcia-Manero G, O'Brien S, Ravandi F, Borthakur G, Cortes J. Characteristics and outcomes of patients with chronic myeloid leukemia and T315I mutation following failure of imatinib mesylate therapy. Blood. 2008;112:53–5.
35. Quintas-Cardama A, Kantarjian H, Cortes J. Homoharringtonine, omacetaxine mepesuccinate, and chronic myeloid leukemia circa 2009. Cancer. 2009;115:5382–93.
36. O'Hare T, Shakespeare WC, Zhu X, Eide CA, Rivera VM, Wang F, Adrian LT, Zhou T, Huang WS, Xu Q, Metcalf III CA, Tyner JW, Loriaux MM, Corbin AS, Wardwell S, Ning Y, Keats JA, Wang Y, Sundaramoorthi R, Thomas M, Zhou D, Snodgrass J, Commodore L, Sawyer TK, Dalgarno DC, Deininger MW, Druker BJ, Clackson T. AP24534, a pan-BCR-ABL inhibitor for chronic myeloid leukemia, potently inhibits the T315I mutant and overcomes mutation-based resistance. Cancer Cell. 2009;16:401–12.

37. Tefferi A, Thiele J, Vannucchi AM, Barbui T. An overview on CALR and CSF3R mutations and a proposal for revision of WHO diagnostic criteria for myeloproliferative neoplasms. Leukemia. 2014;28:1407.
38. Cherry AM, Brockman SR, Paternoster SF, Hicks GA, Neuberg D, Higgins RR, Bennett JM, Greenberg PL, Miller K, Tallman MS, Rowe J, Dewald GW. Comparison of interphase FISH and metaphase cytogenetics to study myelodysplastic syndrome: an Eastern Cooperative Oncology Group (ECOG) study. Leuk Res. 2003;27:1085–90.
39. Coleman JF, Theil KS, Tubbs RR, Cook JR. Diagnostic yield of bone marrow and peripheral blood FISH panel testing in clinically suspected myelodysplastic syndromes and/or acute myeloid leukemia: a prospective analysis of 433 cases. Am J Clin Pathol. 2011;135:915–20.
40. Schanz J, Tuchler H, Sole F, Mallo M, Luno E, Cervera J, Granada I, Hildebrandt B, Slovak ML, Ohyashiki K, Steidl C, Fonatsch C, Pfeilstocker M, Nosslinger T, Valent P, Giagounidis A, Aul C, Lubbert M, Stauder R, Krieger O, Garcia-Manero G, Faderl S, Pierce S, Le Beau MM, Bennett JM, Greenberg P, Germing U, Haase D. New comprehensive cytogenetic scoring system for primary myelodysplastic syndromes (MDS) and oligoblastic acute myeloid leukemia after MDS derived from an international database merge. J Clin Oncol. 2012;30:820–9.
41. Kolquist KA, Schultz RA, Furrow A, Brown TC, Han JY, Campbell LJ, Wall M, Slovak ML, Shaffer LG, Ballif BC. Microarray-based comparative genomic hybridization of cancer targets reveals novel, recurrent genetic aberrations in the myelodysplastic syndromes. Cancer Genet. 2011;204:603–28.
42. Damm F, Kosmider O, Gelsi-Boyer V, Renneville A, Carbuccia N, Hidalgo-Curtis C, Della Valle V, Couronne L, Scourzic L, Chesnais V, Guerci-Bresler A, Slama B, Beyne-Rauzy O, Schmidt-Tanguy A, Stamatoullas-Bastard A, Dreyfus F, Prebet T, de Botton S, Vey N, Morgan MA, Cross NC, Preudhomme C, Birnbaum D, Bernard OA, Fontenay M. Mutations affecting mRNA splicing define distinct clinical phenotypes and correlate with patient outcome in myelodysplastic syndromes. Blood. 2012;119:3211–8.
43. Haferlach T, Nagata Y, Grossmann V, Okuno Y, Bacher U, Nagae G, Schnittger S, Sanada M, Kon A, Alpermann T, Yoshida K, Roller A, Nadarajah N, Shiraishi Y, Shiozawa Y, Chiba K, Tanaka H, Koeffler HP, Klein HU, Dugas M, Aburatani H, Kohlmann A, Miyano S, Haferlach C, Kern W, Ogawa S. Landscape of genetic lesions in 944 patients with myelodysplastic syndromes. Leukemia. 2014;28:241–7.
44. Patnaik MM, Padron E, Laborde RR, Lasho TL, Finke CM, Hanson CA, Hodnefield JM, Knudson RA, Ketterling RP, Al-Kali A, Pardanani A, Ali NA, Komrokji RS, Tefferi A. Mayo prognostic model for WHO-defined chronic myelomonocytic leukemia: ASXL1 and spliceosome component mutations and outcomes. Leukemia. 2013;27:1504–10.

Section V

Infectious Diseases

Section Editor: Angela M. Caliendo

Human Immunodeficiency Virus Type 1

45

Angela M. Caliendo and Colleen S. Kraft

Abstract

HIV-1 quantitative viral load testing and genotypic resistance testing comprise the core aspects of the monitoring of HIV-infected patients on a longitudinal basis. The development of these assays and the clinical interpretation and use of these assays has evolved over decades since 1996 into the current state of practice. Initial uses of viral load testing involved prognostication, followed by the use of viral loads as a marker of response to antiretroviral therapy. Qualitative viral load testing can be used for diagnosis, and proviral DNA assays are used in the diagnosis of HIV in newborns born to HIV-infected mothers. Mutations in the HIV-1 genome were determined to imply resistance or susceptibility to antiretroviral treatment. Genotypic resistance testing correlates these mutations with previously known drug mutations. Phenotypic testing involves the creation of a pseudoviral vector and its performance in the presence of different antiretroviral drugs. Issues surrounding these diagnostic tests, including sample types, assay characteristics, and interpretation of results are delineated in this chapter.

Keywords

HIV-1 • Viral load • Quantitative • Genotypic resistance testing • Resistance testing

Description of the Pathogen

Human immunodeficiency virus types 1 and 2 (HIV-1 and HIV-2), the causative agents of the acquired immunodeficiency syndrome (AIDS), are RNA viruses belonging to the genus *Lentivirus* of the family *Retroviridae* [1]. The replication of all retroviruses involves reverse transcription of the RNA genome into a double-stranded DNA molecule, with subsequent integration into the host genome as proviral DNA. Given this replicative cycle, molecular tests used in the diagnosis and management of HIV-1 infection target either HIV-1 RNA or proviral DNA.

HIV-1 is classified into three distinct genetic groups: M (major), O (outlier), and N (nonmajor and nonoutlier). Viruses in the M group are further divided into eight subtypes (formerly called clades), A–G, H–K, and N–P, and at least 55 circulating recombinant forms (CRFs) as described by the Los Alamos National Laboratory based on the

A.M. Caliendo, M.D., Ph.D. (✉)
Department of Medicine, Alpert Medical School of Brown University, Providence, RI, USA

Rhode Island Hospital,
Jane Brown 054, 593 Eddy St., Providence, RI 02903, USA
e-mail: acaliendo@Lifespan.org

C.S. Kraft, M.D., M.Sc.
Pathology and Laboratory Medicine, Medicine, Infectious Diseases, Emory University,
1364 Clifton Rd., NE, F145C, Atlanta, GA 30322, USA
e-mail: colleen.kraft@emory.edu

D.G.B. Leonard (ed.), *Molecular Pathology in Clinical Practice*, DOI 10.1007/978-3-319-19674-9_45

sequence diversity within the HIV-1 *gag* and *env* genes [1, 2]. The nucleotide sequence of the *env* gene may differ by as much as 25 % among the different subtypes, while viruses within the same subtype generally differ by less than 15 % [1]. Group M virus is found worldwide, with subtype B predominating in Europe and North America, while subtype C predominates in Africa and India. The genetic diversity of HIV-1 plays an important role in the design and interpretation of RNA viral load and genotypic resistance tests.

Clinical Utility

The uses of molecular tests in the clinical management of individuals with HIV-1 infection include the diagnosis of HIV-1 infection, and monitoring response to antiretroviral therapy (ART). The clinical utility of HIV-1 viral load testing, which refers to the quantification of HIV-1 RNA in the blood of infected individuals, has been well studied. Given the availability of commercial test kits, HIV-1 RNA viral load testing has become the standard of care in the clinical management of HIV-infected individuals. HIV-1 RNA viral load is a strong predictor of the rate of progression to AIDS that is independent of CD4 cell count and other factors. Regression models have shown that HIV-1 RNA viral load alone explains half of the variability in prediction of the onset of AIDS and death [3, 4].

Diagnosis of Acute HIV-1 Infection

HIV-1 RNA testing is useful in the diagnosis of acute HIV-1 infection, and a qualitative RNA assay (Aptima, Gen-Probe Incorporated, San Diego) has been approved by the US Food and Drug Administration (FDA) for diagnostic use. Quantitative HIV-1 RNA viral load tests are not approved for the diagnosis of acute HIV-1 infection, and should be specifically validated by the individual laboratory for diagnosis of acute infection, if used for this indication. Acute HIV-1 infection, also referred to as acute retroviral syndrome, has a "window period" after exposure to the virus and prior to seroconversion, when the ELISA and western blot tests are negative or indeterminate [5]. During the window period, patients often are symptomatic with a mononucleosis-type syndrome, which may include fever, fatigue, rash, lymphadenopathy, and oral ulcers [5]. During acute HIV-1 infection, RNA levels are very high in the peripheral blood, usually 10^5–10^7 copies/ml of plasma, making viral load measurement a very useful diagnostic tool; however, if an individual is tested within days to weeks of exposure to HIV-1, the RNA levels may be lower.

The updated algorithm for HIV diagnosis from the Centers for Disease Control and Prevention (CDC) will include initial screening with a third or fourth generation serologic test (HIV1/HIV2 enzyme immunoassay, EIA), followed by an HIV1/HIV2 discriminatory test. In this algorithm, if the initial EIA is positive, but the discriminatory test is negative, the recommended follow up is HIV-1 RNA testing. The fourth generation EIA tests simultaneously detect both p24 antigen and HIV-1 antibody, which narrows the window period and yields a positive test 20 days prior to western blot. The third generation EIA tests detect antibody only and are positive approximately 15 days prior to western blot. The downside of using nucleic acid amplification testing to diagnose acute HIV-1 infection is the potential for false-positive results, which should be suspected if the viral load is <10,000 copies/ml in an individual thought to be acutely infected. To minimize the likelihood of reporting a false-positive result, an HIV1/2 EIA also should be obtained at the time of HIV-1 RNA testing, and repeat RNA and EIA testing should be obtained on all patients within 1–2 weeks. Requiring laboratory approval for using HIV-1 quantitative RNA viral load testing for diagnosis of acute HIV-1 infection is a prudent approach to ensure that the patient has signs and symptoms consistent with acute HIV-1 infection prior to testing.

Diagnosis of HIV-1 Infection in Neonates

Molecular tests are crucial for the diagnosis of HIV-1 infection in neonates, since all infants born to HIV-1 infected mothers remain seropositive into the second year of life due to transfer of maternal immunoglobulin G (IgG) across the placenta. Studies have established the utility of both qualitative proviral DNA and RNA viral load testing for the diagnosis of HIV-1 infection in newborns [6–8]. Current guidelines for the diagnosis of neonatal HIV-1 infection recommend that the molecular testing be performed at ages 14–21 days, 1–2 months, and 4–6 months, with two positive tests obtained separately providing confirmation of HIV-1 infection [9]. Virologic testing also should be performed at birth if the infant is considered at high risk of HIV-1 infection (e.g., mother's HIV-1 viral load not suppressed, or mother is not on ART).

Antiretroviral Therapy Initiation and Monitoring

Clinical guidelines have been established for the initiation of ART [9], and viral load levels are among the parameters used in this decision. After initiation of ART, the goal is to achieve the lowest RNA viral load (usually below the limit of detection of the assay), as this has been shown to correlate with better clinical and virologic outcomes [10, 11].

The classes of antiretroviral drugs that are used in clinical care include: nucleoside reverse transcriptase inhibitors (NRTIs), non-nucleoside reverse transcriptase inhibitors (NNRTIs), protease inhibitors (PIs), entry inhibitors, integrase inhibitors (INSTI), fusion inhibitors, and CCR5 inhibitors (http://www.aidsmeds.com/). The current standard from the Department of Health and Human Services (DHHS) Panel on Antiretroviral Guidelines for treating HIV-1 infected individuals is two NRTIs in combination with either a PI, NNRTI, or integrase inhibitor [9]. In general, a plasma HIV-1 RNA level should be measured at baseline, immediately before beginning therapy, and 2–8 weeks after the start of therapy to determine the initial response [9]. In order to evaluate continued effectiveness of the regimen, testing should be repeated every 3–4 months.

Antiretroviral Therapy Regimen Selection

The replication cycle of HIV-1 is error prone because the reverse transcriptase (RT) does not have proofreading activity [12]. As a result, about one error occurs with each replicative cycle. This error rate coupled with a replication rate that produces about one billion viral particles per day gives rise to a viral "quasispecies." The virus that an individual acquires during transmission may be a strain of HIV-1 with multiple resistance mutations resulting in treatment resistance even prior to initiation of their own treatment with ART [13]. HIV-1 drug resistance also occurs in patients on ART when viral replication is not maximally suppressed to undetectable. These scenarios have led to the recommendations that individuals undergo HIV-1 genotypic resistance testing prior to initiation of therapy and with virologic failure (HIV-1 viral load >1,000 copies/ml) while on ART [9].

The clinical utility of genotypic resistance testing in the management of HIV-1-infected individuals has been studied in several clinical trials [14–16]. These studies demonstrated that genotypic resistance testing is a useful tool in selecting active drugs when changing ART due to virologic failure [9]. The two main types of HIV-1 resistance testing are genotypic resistance testing and phenotypic resistance testing. The regions of the viral genome that are sequenced for HIV-1 genotypic testing include portions of the RT and protease (PR) genes, which correspond to regions with mutations induced in response to therapy with NRTIs, NNRTIs, and PIs. Typically for ART-naive individuals, sequencing of these regions is adequate to detect the important mutations; however, if the patient is on a newer drug, such as an INSTI, then the standard genotypic resistance testing should be supplemented with sequencing of the integrase gene for mutations related to INSTI. HIV-1 phenotypic resistance testing also can be performed on patients with virologic failure on ART to determine which new ART is predicted to be most effective. Phenotypic resistance testing is less preferred given the longer turnaround time and increased expense of this test that involves the creation of a laboratory-modified virus containing portions of the patient's virus that is cultured in the presence of various antiretroviral drug concentrations. Therefore, phenotypic resistance testing is typically reserved for use for individuals with complex mutations where HIV-1 genotypic resistance testing is difficult to interpret for prediction of drug response.

The class of drugs known as CCR5 inhibitors are effective in individuals if their HIV-1 uses CCR5 (and not CXCR4) as a co-receptor to CD4 for entry into target cells [17]. Prior to initiating treatment with a CCR5 inhibitor, the patient's virus must be analyzed to determine whether it is tropic for CCR5, CXCR4, or both. A tropism assay is performed and the results are used to determine whether the patient is a candidate for use of this drug class. If a patient's virus utilizes both, or only CXCR4, the patient would not be a candidate for the CCR5 inhibitor class of ART.

Available Assays

Qualitative HIV-1 RNA and DNA Assays

The APTIMA® HIV-1 RNA Qualitative Assay (Genprobe, San Diego, CA), is the first nucleic acid test US FDA-approved for the diagnosis of HIV-1 infection and can be used to diagnose neonatal HIV-1 infection and acute HIV-1 infection, confirm a repeatedly positive antibody screen, or resolve indeterminate western blots results. The test requires 500 μl of plasma that can be collected in EDTA, acid citrate dextrose, sodium citrate, or in plasma preparation tubes (PPTs). The test is manual, and amplifies and detects the 5′ long terminal repeat (LTR) and pol gene of the HIV-1 genome. This assay detects all HIV-1 group M, N, and O viruses, has a limit of detection (LOD) of 30 copies/ml with a specificity of 99.8 %. An advantage of the APTIMA test is detection of RNA 12 days earlier than EIA detection of antibody and 6 days earlier than testing for p24 antigen (package insert).

Qualitative proviral DNA assays can be used primarily for the diagnosis of neonatal or acute HIV-1 infections. Due to the limited availability of commercial proviral DNA assays, many laboratories have developed their own tests using either standard or real-time amplification methods. The performance characteristics of laboratory developed assays can vary, and performance characteristics to consider include sensitivity, specificity, reproducibility, and the ability to detect non-B subtypes of HIV-1 proviral DNA. A qualitative test is also available that is Research Use Only by Roche, which detects both HIV RNA and DNA, the COBAS® AmpliPrep/COBAS® TaqMan® HIV-1 Qualitative Test, version 2.0. This can detect HIV-1 RNA and proviral DNA in plasma, anticoagulated fresh whole blood, and dried blood spots.

Table 45.1 US FDA-approved HIV-1 viral load tests

Test	Method	Target	Specimen volume[a]	Range
Amplicor HIV-1 Monitor® version 1.5 (Roche Diagnostics Indianapolis, IN)	RT-PCR	HIV-1 *gag* gene		
Standard			200 μl	400–750,000 copies/mL
Ultrasensitive			500 μl	50–100,000 copies/mL
COBAS® Amplicor HIV-1 Monitor version 1.5 (Roche Diagnostics, Indianapolis, IN)	RT-PCR	HIV-1 *gag* gene		
Standard			200 μl	400–750,000 copies/mL
Ultrasensitive			500 μl	50–100,000 copies/mL
COBAS® AmpliPrep/COBAS® Amplicor HIV-1 Monitor version 1.5	RT-PCR	HIV-1 *gag* gene		
Standard			250 μl	500–1,000,000 copies/mL
Ultrasensitive			750 μl	50–100,000 copies/mL
Versant® HIV-1 RNA 3.0 (bDNA) (Siemens Healthcare Diagnostics)	Branched DNA	HIV-1 *pol* gene	1 mL	75–500,000 copies/mL
COBAS® AmpliPrep/COBAS® TaqMan® HIV-1 Test (Roche Diagnostics, Indianapolis, IN)	RT-qPCR			
v 1.0		HIV-1 *gag* gene	1 mL	48–10,000,000 copies/mL
v 2.0		HIV-1 *gag* gene and LTR	1 mL	20–10,000,000 copies/mL
RealTime Taqman® HIV-1 (Abbott Molecular)	RT-qPCR	HIV-1 integrase gene	1 mL	40–10,000,000 copies/mL

RT-PCR reverse transcription-polymerase chain reaction, *RT-qPCR* reverse transcription-quantitative polymerase chain reaction
[a]For tests that use an automated extraction instrument (AmpliPrep and RealTime), the specimen volume listed refers to the volume of sample that is loaded on the instrument, which is greater than the actual volume of specimen taken through the extraction

Viral Load Assays

Currently, six US FDA-approved tests are available for the quantification of HIV-1 RNA from plasma specimens. These assays differ in their limit of detection, linear range, gene target, and input plasma volume (Table 45.1). The earliest available viral load tests (Amplicor Monitor and Versant bDNA) have essentially been replaced by the real-time quantitative reverse-transcriptase PCR (RT-qPCR) tests. The RT-qPCR assays that are approved by the US FDA offer several advantages over the earliest available viral load assays, including more extensive automation, broader linear range, and decreased risk of carryover amplicon contamination due to their automation and closed tube system. The lower limit of quantification is an important characteristic of all viral load assays and is defined as the lowest amount of nucleic acid that can be quantified with "acceptable precision." RT-qPCR tests can have a LOD as low as 20–40 copies/mL; this is achieved due to a larger sample input plasma volume, usually approximately 1 mL. The two US FDA-approved RT-qPCR tests have good correlation and agreement between viral load values, with mean/median differences in viral load values ranging from 0.22 to 0.56 $\log_{10}$copies/ml depending on the subtype of the samples [18–20]. On average, there is very good agreement between the different viral load tests, but caution should be used when switching viral load tests for management of an individual patient since the differences in viral load values may be significant and could lead to different management decisions [21]. For example, a patient whose viral load becomes detectable upon switching tests when they were previously suppressed would be considered to have failed therapy, when in fact the change in viral load was due to a difference in the test sensitivity. Although agreement in viral load values with the different tests is improving, the same viral load test should be used when monitoring patients over time, and, if the viral load test is changed, then a new baseline viral load should be obtained.

Increasing genetic diversity of HIV-1 isolates from individuals in the USA has been reported, primarily from those who have immigrated from Africa and Asia [22, 23], so detection of non-B subtypes is taking on increased importance. The RT-qPCR tests were intentionally designed to detect not only non-B subtypes but also many CRFs. The COBAS Taqman version 1 test measures all subtypes of group M and N viruses and many CRFs [24], while the recently approved version 2 test has improved quantification of CRFs and of Group O virus. The Abbott RealTime test quantifies all group M, N, and O viruses, and CRFs [25, 26].

Ongoing international surveillance of HIV-1 isolates ensures that these assays maintain their ability to detect evolving viral genetic diversity, which occurs because of the high recombination activity within the HIV-1 subtypes and CRFs [27].

Proper collection and processing of blood samples are essential to ensure accurate assessment of viral load levels; the key is to minimize RNA degradation. For conventional and RT-qPCR assays, EDTA is the preferred anticoagulant for blood collection, and the plasma must be separated from blood cells within 4–6 h of collection, as delays in processing may lead to a falsely decreased viral load value. Plasma specimens can be stored at 4 °C for several days without significant degradation of RNA, and HIV-1 RNA has been shown to remain stable after three cycles of freezing (−70 °C) and thawing [28]. For long term storage, plasma samples should be frozen at or below −70 °C [29]. Vacutainer PPTs may be acceptable for the collection of blood specimens for viral load testing, but this specimen type must be validated by the individual laboratory. The PPTs contain a gel barrier which, after centrifugation, physically separates plasma from the cellular components [30]. Whole blood collected in PPTs can be held at room temperature for as long as 6 h after collection and shipped as plasma (in the original tube) at ambient temperature or on wet or dry ice without affecting the HIV-1 viral load [31]. Freezing PPTs (after separating the plasma) prior to testing can give higher viral load values compared to those obtained when the plasma is separated and stored at 4 °C which is thought to be due to the lysis of cells releasing proviral DNA as well as virions adherent to platelets [32–36]. For this reason freezing specimens in PPTs in situ is not recommended, although Fernandes et al. showed that it could be done when using the Abbott platform, and this is likely due to the additional centrifugation prior to testing [37]. The PPTs provide a closed sample collection system, which is a safe, convenient, and practical approach to shipping specimens collected at sites remote from the laboratory.

Although measuring viral load in plasma is the standard of care in clinical practice, these tests have been adapted for use with other specimens, most notably serum, dried blood spots, cerebrospinal fluid (CSF), seminal fluid or semen, and cervical secretions. When serum specimens are used, the viral load is decreased approximately 50 % compared to plasma [38]. Both whole blood and plasma dried spots can be used for viral load testing; in fact, viral load levels from dried plasma spots are equivalent to those obtained from fresh frozen plasma specimens [39]. Similarly, HIV-1 RNA from dried whole blood spots, corrected for hematocrit (number of spot RNA copies per milliliter of blood)/([100-hematocrit]/100), yields viral load results comparable to those obtained from plasma [40]. HIV-1 RNA in dried plasma spots remains stable for up to 16 days when stored at 4 °C or ambient temperature [41]. RNA from dried blood spots has been shown to be stable up to 1 year at room temperature or cooler [42]. Viral load levels in CSF have been used in the evaluation of patients with AIDS dementia, and if virus is quantified, ART that penetrates into the CSF compartment is chosen for treatment [43].

Drug Resistance Assays

Antiretroviral resistance can be detected using either genotypic or phenotypic assays. HIV-1 genotypic assays identify mutations or changes in the nucleotide sequence known to confer decreased susceptibility to antiretroviral drugs. Phenotypic resistance testing, on the other hand, refers to a viral trait or behavior resulting from the expression of a specific genotype. HIV-1 phenotypic assays measure viral replication in the presence of antiretroviral drugs. Results of phenotypic assays are typically reported as the inhibitory concentration of a drug that reduces in vitro HIV-1 replication by 50 % (IC_{50}). The IC_{50} is usually reported as the fold change in IC_{50} relative to a wild-type strain. A "virtual phenotype" is a test where the results of the genotypic assay are entered into a database containing matching genotypic and phenotypic results from thousands of clinical specimens, and the closest matching phenotypic results are averaged and reported as the virtual phenotype. Studies have demonstrated that the virtual phenotype is equivalent to conventional phenotyping for clinical decision making regarding changes in drug therapy. The virtual phenotype, while useful clinically, is not longer available [44, 45].

Two US FDA-cleared genotypic tests are available that include reagents for sequencing and software programs to assist with sequence alignment and interpretation (Trugene HIV-1 Genotyping Kit and OpenGene DNA Sequencing System, Siemens Healthcare Diagnostics, Tarrytown, NY; ViroSeq HIV-1 Genotyping System, Abbott Molecular, Des Plaines, IL) (Table 45.2). Though the Trugene HIV-1 assay has been widely used and much of our understanding of the clinical utility of HIV genotypic testing has come from studies with this test, effective December 2014 Trugene HIV-1 test is no longer available. HIV-1 RNA is extracted followed by reverse transcription and PCR amplification of the entire PR gene and most of the RT gene, which are sequenced using automated dideoxynucleotide terminator cycle sequencing. The PR and RT gene sequences are analyzed by comparison to a reference sequence (wild type HIV-1 strain) to identify mutations. For patients who have been exposed to INSTI, the HIV-1 integrase genotype (HIV-1 Integrase Inhibitor Resistance by Sequencing; GeneSeq® for Integrase Inhibitors Assay) can be performed by reference laboratories, since the typical genotypic tests only detect mutations in the PR and RT genes not the integrase gene where the INSTI resistance mutations reside.

Table 45.2 Available assays for resistance testing

Assay	Method	Comments
Trugene® HIV-1 Genotyping Kit and Open Gene DNA Sequencing System (Siemens Healthcare Diagnostics)*	Genotypic	US FDA-cleared; Detects protease and reverse transcriptase mutations
Viroseq® HIV-1 Genotyping System (Abbott Molecular)	Genotypic	US FDA-cleared; Detects protease and reverse transcriptase mutations
GeneSeq® for Reverse Transcriptase and Protease Inhibitors Assay (Monogram Biosciences)	Genotypic	Detects protease and reverse transcriptase mutations
GenoSure® MG (Monogram Biosciences)	Genotypic	Detects protease and reverse transcriptase mutations
HIV-1 Genotype, RT and Protease Genes (Quest Diagnostics Nichols Institute)	Genotypic	Detects protease and reverse transcriptase mutations
GeneSeq® for Integrase Inhibitors Assay (Monogram Biosciences)	Genotypic	Detects integrase mutations
HIV-1 Integrase Inhibitor Resistance by Sequencing (ARUP, Salt Lake City, UT)	Genotypic	Detects integrase mutations
PhenoSense®GT (Monogram Biosciences)	Combined genotypic and Phenotypic	Detects protease and reverse transcriptase mutations
PhenoSense™ HIV (for Reverse Transcriptase and Protease Inhibitors) (Monogram Biosciences)	Phenotypic	Detects protease and reverse transcriptase mutations
PhenoSense™ for Entry Inhibitor Susceptibility (Monogram Biosciences)	Phenotypic	Measures susceptibility to entry inhibitors (Fuzeon®)
PhenoSense™ Integrase (Monogram Biosciences)	Phenotypic	Measures susceptibility to integrase inhibitors
Trofile™ Co-receptor Tropism (Monogram Biosciences)	Tropism	Used prior to initiating therapy with maraviroc

*This test is no longer commercially available

Phenotypic assays measure the ability of HIV-1 to replicate in the presence of various concentrations of an antiretroviral drug using high-throughput automated assays based on recombinant DNA technology. The single commercially available assay, PhenoSense (Monogram Biosciences, South San Francisco, CA) (Table 45.2) amplifies the PR and RT genes using RT-PCR and the amplified product is inserted into a modified HIV-1 vector which lacks RT and PR genes and has a luciferase reporter gene inserted into the viral envelope gene. Viral replication, in the presence of various drugs, is measured by quantification of luciferase expression [46] and results are reported as fold-change in IC_{50} compared to a wild-type control. Increases in IC_{50} of greater than 2.5-fold can be reliably detected by this assay.

Prior to initiating therapy with a CCR5 inhibitor (maraviroc), the patient's virus must be assessed for use of the CCR5 as a co-receptor, as viruses that use CXCR4 as a co-receptor will not be susceptible to this drug. The commercially available Trofile assay (Monogram Biosciences, South San Francisco, CA) generates pseudoviruses using full-length *env* genes amplified from the patient's virus. Co-receptor tropism is then determined by measuring the ability of the pseudoviral population to infect CD4+ U87 cells that express either CXCR4 or CCR5. Depending on which cells are infected, the patient's virus is then designated X4-tropic, R5-tropic, or dual-tropic [47]. Patients are candidates for a CCR5 inhibitor if their virus is solely CCR5-tropic. Patients with CCR5-tropic virus that are treated with maraviroc may develop resistance to the drug due to either (1) mutations that allow the virus to adapt and use CXCR4 co-receptors or (2) structural changes in the envelope of a R5-tropic virus that prevent the drug from being effective [48, 49].

The currently available range of resistance testing (genotype and phenotype) provides clinicians with tools to better assess how to tailor the ART regimen, as well as determine whether drugs that are considered "resistant" by genotype may be usable in a salvage regimen after analysis by phenotypic testing.

Little data directly address specimen collection and processing for HIV-1 resistance testing which are very sensitive to RNA degradation because the methods require the amplification of a large portion of the 9 kilobase viral genome (1,200–1,600 base pairs). Current recommendations for resistance testing are to follow guidelines established for HIV-1 RNA viral load testing regarding collection, processing, and storage of specimens. Considering the cost of these assays and the variability of viral load measurements near the limit of quantification, resistance testing is not recommended until the viral load in the plasma is >1,000 copies/ml. Both the Trugene and ViroSeq assays successfully genotype non-B subtypes of HIV-1 [50].

Interpretation

Qualitative HIV-1 RNA Assays

CDC guidelines recommend use of HIV-1 RNA testing for the diagnosis of HIV infection when the screening result (by EIA) is not confirmed by the HIV-1/2 discriminatory test. This raises important issues regarding the implementation of the algorithm, as laboratory directors will need to determine whether to use plasma or serum samples, and assess if the same sample used for screening/discriminatory testing should be used for RNA testing. Testing for RNA after the serologic tests raises concerns of cross contamination between samples, as serologic testing is not routinely performed with the same precautions to prevent carryover of RNA between samples, as is needed for molecular testing. An assessment of the specimen integrity, including contamination prevention and storage conditions, following serologic testing is needed to assess the specimen adequacy for RNA testing. Removing an aliquot of plasma/serum prior to serologic testing for RNA testing, would reduce the risk of cross contamination and assure proper specimen storage, but this would be very labor intensive, particularly for laboratories with a low positivity rate, and risk misidentification. Asking for a second specimen to be collected for RNA testing requires an additional visit for the patient and may decrease the likelihood that testing is done, plus increases the turnaround time for final results. Consideration of these issues and discussions with healthcare providers prior to implementation of the testing algorithm for HIV-1 diagnosis should increase the likelihood of a successful adoption of the algorithm.

Viral Load Assays

HIV-1 RNA viral load assays have become the standard of care for monitoring response to ART. In order to effectively use HIV-1 viral load assays in clinical practice, the changes in viral load that represent a clinically important change in viral replication must be defined. This requires knowledge of both viral biology and assay performance. The available HIV-1 viral load assays have an intra-assay variability of 0.12–0.2 $\log_{10}$ on repeated testing of individual samples [38, 51]. Biologically, HIV-1 RNA levels are fairly stable in individuals who are not receiving ART; the biological variation is approximately 0.3 $\log_{10}$ [52]. Therefore, changes in HIV-1 RNA levels must exceed 0.5 $\log_{10}$ (three-fold) to represent biologically relevant changes in viral replication. For all the viral load assays, the intra-assay variability is even greater near the lower limit of quantification, so for HIV-1 RNA values less than 3 $\log_{10}$ (1,000 copies/ml), small changes in viral load should not be overinterpreted. Reporting viral load levels as $\log_{10}$-transformed data may assist in preventing clinicians from over-interpreting small changes in viral load.

Several clinical illnesses, including herpes simplex virus infections, acute infections, and opportunistic infections, as well as vaccinations for influenza, tetanus, or pneumonococcal infection, can lead to transient increases in HIV-1 RNA levels [53–55]. For some individuals these increases in viral load may be quite dramatic, even greater than 1 $\log_{10}$ change; however, HIV-1 RNA levels usually return to baseline within a month of the acute event. For this reason viral load measurements should be avoided during acute illness or within a month of vaccination.

False-positive results can occur with HIV-1 viral load assays and are attributed to carryover contamination with amplicons, limitations in assay chemistry, or cross-contamination of specimens during specimen processing. Carryover contamination has been essentially eliminated with the automated RT-qPCR tests (TaqMan and RealTime) since the test reaction is not open to the air after the amplification step. An advantage of the Versant bDNA assay is that carryover contamination does not occur with this signal amplification method. However, the Versant bDNA assay chemistry involves complex hybridization of nucleic acid probes which can result in nonspecific hybridization leading to false-positive results. The assay has a specificity of approximately 98 % when testing specimens from HIV-1-negative individuals [56]. Most of the false-positive samples have viral load values of less than 2,000 copies/ml. Contamination with HIV-1 RNA during specimen processing can lead to false-positive results with any of the assays, although this risk is reduced with the automated extraction systems used in the RT-qPCR tests.

Drug Resistance Assays

Interpretation of genotypic resistance testing is very complex and requires a detailed understanding of the genetics of resistance. For many drugs, the mutations associated with resistance have been well characterized when used as monotherapy. However, when drugs are used in combination, as is the standard of care for HIV-1-infected individuals, interactions may occur, which may increase or decrease individual drug efficacy. These interactions, although they are complex, must be understood to accurately interpret genotypic results. A current and comprehensive discussion of the specific mutations associated with each antiretroviral drug and the interactions of mutations is available from a variety of sources, including Los Alamos National Laboratory HIV Databases (http://hiv-web.lanl.gov), International AIDS Society-USA (http://www.iasusa.org), and Stanford University HIV Drug Resistance Database (http://hivdb.stanford.edu).

The proper interpretation of genotypic drug resistance assays involves (1) identification of resistance mutations and (2) interpretation of how these mutations alter viral susceptibility to specific antiretroviral drugs. While establishing appropriate quality control guidelines for the technical aspect of an assay is common practice, the complex interpretation of HIV-1 genotyping assays represents a challenge for molecular pathologists. Since interpretation of genotypic assays is so complex and critical to patient care, FDA-cleared assays provide software programs that assist in base calling, sequence alignment, and identification of the resistance mutations by comparing the sequence to a wild-type HIV-1 sequence.

After identifying the resistance mutations, a "rules-based" software program is used to interpret the implications of the various mutations for response to different drugs. For example, with the OpenGene system (Siemens Healthcare Diagnostics Inc, Tarrytown, NY), the manufacturer provides regular interpretation software updates which are cleared by the US FDA prior to release. In addition to listing the mutations identified in the RT and PR genes, an interpretive report is provided that lists each drug and provides a designation of either "no evidence of resistance," "possible resistance," "resistance," or "insufficient evidence." A similar approach is used in the ViroSeq assay (Abbott Molecular), though the interpretation of all mutations may not be identical for both systems. These rules-based interpretation systems are essential for providing clinicians with results in a user friendly format that is easily understood and clinically useful without the need for an extensive knowledge of the genetics of HIV-1 resistance. Clinically, resistance results must be interpreted in the context of the treatment history of each patient, which usually means avoiding drugs previously used to treat the patient when possible.

Mutations in HIV-1 are reported with a specific nomenclature in which amino acids are reported using single letter abbreviations. The wild-type amino acid encoded by the nucleotide triplet is followed by the location of the mutation (codon number) and then the mutant amino acid. For example, K103N indicates that the lysine (wild type) at codon 103 is replaced by an asparagine (mutant). Genotyping reports include a list of the mutations identified as well as the effect of the mutations on antiretroviral drug susceptibility (Table 45.3).

An important issue for the interpretation of HIV-1 phenotypic assays is defining the cutoff change in IC_{50} that is associated with resistance. Initially, this cutoff was established based on the technical performance of the assays, which is the increase in IC_{50} that could be reliably detected when compared to wild-type virus. Clinically important increases in IC_{50} have been defined for most drugs, and these cutoffs can vary with different drugs. For example, with abacavir, stavudine, and lopinavir, the fold change in IC_{50} that is clinically important is 4.5, 1.7, and 10, respectively [57]. However, with NNRTIs, four- to ten-fold increases in IC_{50} values in therapy-naive subjects were not associated with a poor virologic outcome [58]. Reports of phenotypic assay results include not only the change in IC_{50} value but also an interpretation of whether there is an increase or decrease in susceptibility compared to wild-type HIV-1.

Table 45.3 Example of a genotypic resistance report

Resistance associated RT mutations: A62V, K65R, A98G, L100I, V179D, M184V	
Nucleoside and nucleotide RT inhibitors	***Resistance interpretation***
Abacavir (ABC)	**Resistance**
Didanosine (ddI)	Possible resistance
Zidovudine (AZT)	No evidence of resistance
Lamivudine (3TC)/emtricitabine (FTC)	**Resistance**
Stavudine (d4T)	Possible resistance
Tenofovir (TDF)	**Resistance**
Nonnucleoside RT inhibitors	***Resistance interpretation***
Efavirenz (EFV)	Possible resistance
Etravirine (ETR)	Possible resistance
Nevirapine (NVP)	Possible resistance
Resistance associated PR mutations: L10V, I13V, L63P	
Protease inhibitors	***Resistance interpretation***
Amprenavir (APV)/fosamprenavir (FPV)	No evidence of resistance
Atazanavir (ATV)	No evidence of resistance
Darunavir + ritonavir (DRV/r)	No evidence of resistance
Indinavir (IDV)	No evidence of resistance
Lopinavir + ritonavir (LPV/r)	No evidence of resistance
Nelfinavir (NFV)	No evidence of resistance
Saquinavir + ritonavir (SQV/r)	No evidence of resistance
Tipranavir + ritonavir (TPV/r)	No evidence of resistance

RT reverse transcriptase

The DHHS guidelines recommend genotypic resistance testing for individuals who are not ART-experienced [9], and phenotypic testing is typically reserved for those individuals who have resistance in all of the classes of drugs by genotyping tests. Phenotypic testing can take 1–2 weeks and is significantly more expensive than genotypic testing. If both tests are used, it is key to remember that the results of the assays may not agree, as the presence of a resistance mutation does not obviate its expression in a phenotypic assay. Interpretation of these assays depend on the patient's drug regimen history, and so the genotypic and phenotypic testing may actually provide complementary information which explains the reasons for virologic failure [57].

The currently available genotypic and phenotypic methods can detect a mutant virus only if it comprises at least 20 % of the total viral population. Therefore, resistance testing is best used to predict failure of a regimen rather than ensure success, because a mutant may be present at a concentration below the detection limit of the assay. Detection of these minor mutants is important because, in the presence of drug selection pressure, these minority populations will quickly predominate. Likewise, drug selection pressure is required for mutations to persist, and in the absence of drug selection pressure the viral population can revert back to wild type. One study showed that this reversion back to wild type can occur within weeks to months of withdrawing the antiretroviral drug [59]. Although the virus may appear susceptible to the specific drug, reintroducing the drug will select for resistant virus again. For this reason, it is recommended that specimens for resistance testing be obtained while the patient is on ART.

Laboratory Issues

With the proven clinical utility and the availability of commercial assays, HIV-1 RNA viral load testing is performed routinely in many clinical laboratories. The appropriate choice of a viral load assay will vary depending on the laboratory. Issues to consider include available space, volume of testing, turnaround time requirements, expertise of technologists, and cost of reportable result. Each of the viral load assays has its strengths and weaknesses. The Amplicor Monitor assay has largely been replaced by the RT-qPCR tests due to the automation which reduces technologist time and the closed system which prevents carryover and contamination.

Since the initial step in some genotypic and all phenotypic assays involves amplification of viral RNA, genetic fingerprinting programs within the resistance testing platforms are a very important tool to assist the laboratory in detecting contamination or sample mix-up. Each sequence that is generated is compared to a laboratory specific database that contains the sequences of other specimens and controls. Due to the variation in the HIV-1 sequence (due to its frequent mutation rate), an exact or a highly similar match should not be present in the database unless it is an earlier specimen from the same patient. Identification of different patients with highly similar sequences can be a clue to problems with contamination in the laboratory. Rarely, highly similar sequences may be evidence that transmission has occurred between two patients within a healthcare system and has been used for contact tracing in some contexts [60]. This genetic fingerprinting function is included in the Trugene System, allowing all sequenced specimens to be checked against the fingerprinting database. The ViroSeq system uses UTP and uracil *N*-glycosylase (UNG), which is a very effective method to control for contamination of amplified products. As with viral load testing, extreme care must be taken to avoid cross contamination of specimens during processing for resistance testing.

The College of American Pathologists (CAP) Surveys Program offers proficiency testing for HIV-1 viral load measurements and HIV-1 genotypic testing (for the PR and RT genes only), with challenges provided three times per year. A similar program is offered through the Quality Control for Molecular Diagnostics (QCMD, http://www.qcmd.org/), which provides challenges for qualitative HIV-1 DNA testing, qualitative and quantitative HIV-1 viral load testing, and HIV-1 genotypic resistance testing.

Phenotypic resistance testing, which requires culture of HIV-1, is not performed in clinical laboratories but is available from one commercial laboratory through Monogram Biosciences.

There are specific CPT codes available for HIV-1 RNA viral load testing as well as resistance testing. Reimbursement rates vary greatly from state to state and in some states may be below the cost of performing the tests. Adequate reimbursement is essential to assure access to resistance testing for all HIV-1 infected individuals.

The Future

The use of ART in combination with HIV-1 RNA viral load and drug resistance testing has revolutionized the clinical care for HIV-1-infected persons. Future advancements for these tests will likely focus on improved test performance and automation. The COBAS® AmpliPrep/COBAS® TaqMan® HIV-1 Test is the most sensitive of the RT-qPCR tests with an lower limit of quantification (LLOQ) of 20 copies/ml. Continued modification of these tests may further reduce the LOD, although it is unclear how much more sensitivity can be obtained with current technologies, without increasing the input sample volume to levels that are not practical. Newer technologies such as digital PCR may allow a further lowering of the LOD. If more sensitive tests become available, clinical trials will be needed to determine if patients with viral load values suppressed to these low levels (<20 copies/ml) have an improved outcome compared to those suppressed to 40–50 copies/ml. Current resistance testing technology will not allow assessment of mutations in patients with viral load values below 500–1,000 copies/ml, making best alternative therapy selection difficult in this group.

Digital PCR is a new technology that is currently under development for the quantification of infectious pathogens. The technology involves partitioning the reaction mixture by the generation of thousands of droplets, each of which is amplified by PCR and determined to be positive or negative. By counting the number of positive droplets, the absolute concentration of virus (target nucleic acid) in the initial reaction is determined. Digital PCR is still in the development phase, and has yet to demonstrate adequate sensitivity for viral load testing. One possible role of digital PCR is to serve as a method to better correlate the concentrations of different lots of the World Health Organization (WHO) HIV-1 international standards, since digital PCR is an independent method to determine viral load values.

The advent of next-generation sequencing has allowed researchers to evaluate the HIV-1 quasispecies much more closely, evaluating variants that exist in 1–5 % of the HIV-1 population, which is much improved over the 20 % that can be detected with traditional sequencing. Several research groups have assessed individuals failing ART and found that some patients had low-level resistance mutations that explained why the patient's viral load was less likely to become undetectable on therapy [61]. This is promising technology, although more clinical data on outcomes in these individuals are needed [62], as well as determining the clinical relevance of mutations found in very low concentration (<1 % of the quasispecies) [63]. These issues will need to be resolved for next-generation sequencing to be used routinely in the clinical laboratory.

One clear unmet need for the future is the development of viral load and resistance testing that is appropriate for use in resource-constrained areas. For molecular testing to be performed routinely in resource-constrained laboratories, the test must be simple, reliable, and inexpensive. The test should be able to be performed without electricity or refrigeration. In these settings, the absolute viral load is less important, and viral loads in $\log_{10}$ increments are acceptable. Besides withstanding a potentially uncontrolled storage environment, the test should be easy to maintain and troubleshoot, with appropriate quality assurance features. Development of microfluidic devices that can be used in such settings [64, 65] are promising advances, but the clinical implementation of these has lagged behind the technical development.

References

1. Richman DD, Whitley RJ, Hayden FG. Clinical virology. 3rd ed. Washington, DC: ASM Press; 2009.
2. Taylor BS, Sobieszczyk ME, McCutchan FE, Hammer SM. The challenge of HIV-1 subtype diversity. N Engl J Med. 2008; 358(15):1590–602.
3. Mellors JW, Kingsley LA, Rinaldo Jr CR, Todd JA, Hoo BS, Kokka RP, Gupta P. Quantitation of HIV-1 RNA in plasma predicts outcome after seroconversion. Ann Intern Med. 1995;122(8):573–9.
4. Mellors JW, Margolick JB, Phair JP, Rinaldo CR, Detels R, Jacobson LP, Munoz A. Prognostic value of HIV-1 RNA, CD4 cell count, and CD4 Cell count slope for progression to AIDS and death in untreated HIV-1 infection. JAMA. 2007;297(21):2349–50.
5. Kahn JO, Walker BD. Acute human immunodeficiency virus type 1 infection. N Engl J Med. 1998;339(1):33–9.
6. Cunningham CK, Charbonneau TT, Song K, Patterson D, Sullivan T, Cummins T, Poiesz B. Comparison of human immunodeficiency virus 1 DNA polymerase chain reaction and qualitative and quantitative RNA polymerase chain reaction in human immunodeficiency virus 1-exposed infants. Pediatr Infect Dis J. 1999; 18(1):30–5.
7. Steketee RW, Abrams EJ, Thea DM, Brown TM, Lambert G, Orloff S, Weedon J, Bamji M, Schoenbaum EE, Rapier J, Kalish ML. Early detection of perinatal human immunodeficiency virus (HIV) type 1 infection using HIV RNA amplification and detection. New York City Perinatal HIV Transmission Collaborative Study. J Infect Dis. 1997;175(3):707–11.
8. Young NL, Shaffer N, Chaowanachan T, Chotpitayasunondh T, Vanparapar N, Mock PA, Waranawat N, Chokephaibulkit K, Chuachoowong R, Wasinrapee P, Mastro TD, Simonds RJ. Early diagnosis of HIV-1-infected infants in Thailand using RNA and DNA PCR assays sensitive to non-B subtypes. J Acquir Immune Defic Syndr. 2000;24(5):401–7.
9. AIDSinfo | Information on HIV/AIDS treatment, prevention and research. http://www.aidsinfo.nih.gov. Accessed 17 Feb 2012.
10. Demeter LM, Hughes MD, Coombs RW, Jackson JB, Grimes JM, Bosch RJ, Fiscus SA, Spector SA, Squires KE, Fischl MA, Hammer SM. Predictors of virologic and clinical outcomes in HIV-1-infected patients receiving concurrent treatment with indinavir, zidovudine, and lamivudine. AIDS Clinical Trials Group Protocol 320. Ann Intern Med. 2001;135(11):954–64.
11. Raboud JM, Montaner JS, Conway B, Rae S, Reiss P, Vella S, Cooper D, Lange J, Harris M, Wainberg MA, Robinson P, Myers M, Hall D. Suppression of plasma viral load below 20 copies/ml is required to achieve a long-term response to therapy. AIDS. 1998;12(13):1619–24.
12. Zhuang J, Jetzt AE, Sun G, Yu H, Klarmann G, Ron Y, Preston BD, Dougherty JP. Human immunodeficiency virus type 1 recombination: rate, fidelity, and putative hot spots. J Virol. 2002;76(22): 11273–82.
13. Little SJ, Holte S, Routy JP, Daar ES, Markowitz M, Collier AC, Koup RA, Mellors JW, Connick E, Conway B, Kilby M, Wang L, Whitcomb JM, Hellmann NS, Richman DD. Antiretroviral-drug resistance among patients recently infected with HIV. N Engl J Med. 2002;347(6):385–94.
14. Baxter JD, Mayers DL, Wentworth DN, Neaton JD, Hoover ML, Winters MA, Mannheimer SB, Thompson MA, Abrams DI, Brizz BJ, Ioannidis JP, Merigan TC. A randomized study of antiretroviral management based on plasma genotypic antiretroviral resistance testing in patients failing therapy. CPCRA 046 Study Team for the Terry Beirn Community Programs for Clinical Research on AIDS. AIDS. 2000;14(9):F83–93.
15. Durant J, Clevenbergh P, Halfon P, Delgiudice P, Porsin S, Simonet P, Montagne N, Boucher CA, Schapiro JM, Dellamonica P. Drug-resistance genotyping in HIV-1 therapy: the VIRADAPT randomised controlled trial. Lancet. 1999;353(9171):2195–9.
16. Tural C, Ruiz L, Holtzer C, Schapiro J, Viciana P, Gonzalez J, Domingo P, Boucher C, Rey-Joly C, Clotet B. Clinical utility of HIV-1 genotyping and expert advice: the Havana trial. AIDS. 2002;16(2):209–18.
17. Macarthur RD, Novak RM. Maraviroc: the first of a new class of antiretroviral agents. Clin Infect Dis. 2008;47(2):23641.
18. Crump JA, Scott LE, Msuya E, Morrissey AB, Kimaro EE, Shao JF, Stevens WS. Evaluation of the Abbott m2000rt RealTime HIV-1 assay with manual sample preparation compared with the ROCHE COBAS AmpliPrep/AMPLICOR HIV-1 MONITOR v1.5 using specimens from East Africa. J Virol Methods. 2009;162(1-2):218–22.
19. Scott LE, Noble LD, Moloi J, Erasmus L, Venter WD, Stevens W. Evaluation of the Abbott m2000 RealTime human immunodeficiency virus type 1 (HIV-1) assay for HIV load monitoring in South Africa compared to the Roche Cobas AmpliPrep-Cobas Amplicor, Roche Cobas AmpliPrep-Cobas TaqMan HIV-1, and BioMerieux NucliSENS EasyQ HIV-1 assays. J Clin Microbiol. 2009;47(7):2209–17.

20. van Rensburg EJ, Tait K, Watt A, Schall R. Comparative evaluation of the Roche Cobas AmpliPrep/Cobas TaqMan HIV-1 version 2 test using the TaqMan 48 analyzer and the Abbott RealTime HIV-1 assay. J Clin Microbiol. 2011;49(1):377–9.
21. Braun P, Ehret R, Wiesmann F, Zabbai F, Knickmann M, Kuhn R, Thamm S, Warnat G, Knechten H. Comparison of four commercial quantitative HIV-1 assays for viral load monitoring in clinical daily routine. Clin Chem Lab Med. 2007;45(1):93–9.
22. Cartwright CP. The changing epidemiology of HIV/AIDS at a Minnesota hospital: impact of demographic change and viral diversity. J Med Virol. 2006;78 Suppl 1:S19–21.
23. Lin HH, Gaschen BK, Collie M, El-Fishaway M, Chen Z, Korber BT, Beatrice ST, Zhang L. Genetic characterization of diverse HIV-1 strains in an immigrant population living in New York City. J Acquir Immune Defic Syndr. 2006;41(4):399–404.
24. Schumacher W, Frick E, Kauselmann M, Maier-Hoyle V, van der Vliet R, Babiel R. Fully automated quantification of human immunodeficiency virus (HIV) type 1 RNA in human plasma by the COBAS AmpliPrep/COBAS TaqMan system. J Clin Virol. 2007; 38(4):304–12.
25. Gueudin M, Plantier JC, Damond F, Roques P, Mauclere P, Simon F. Plasma viral RNA assay in HIV-1 group O infection by real-time PCR. J Virol Methods. 2003;113(1):43–9.
26. Swanson P, Holzmayer V, Huang S, Hay P, Adebiyi A, Rice P, Abravaya K, Thamm S, Devare SG, Hackett Jr J. Performance of the automated Abbott RealTime HIV-1 assay on a genetically diverse panel of specimens from London: comparison to VERSANT HIV-1 RNA 3.0, AMPLICOR HIV-1 MONITOR v1.5, and LCx HIV RNA quantitative assays. J Virol Methods. 2006;137(2): 184–92.
27. Thomson MM, Najera R. Molecular epidemiology of HIV-1 variants in the global AIDS pandemic: an update. AIDS Rev. 2005;7(4):210–24.
28. Sebire K, McGavin K, Land S, Middleton T, Birch C. Stability of human immunodeficiency virus RNA in blood specimens as measured by a commercial PCR-based assay. J Clin Microbiol. 1998;36(2):493–8.
29. Johnson JA, Li JF, Wei X, Lipscomb J, Irlbeck D, Craig C, Smith A, Bennett DE, Monsour M, Sandstrom P, Lanier ER, Heneine W. Minority HIV-1 drug resistance mutations are present in antiretroviral treatment-naive populations and associate with reduced treatment efficacy. PLoS Med. 2008;5(7):e158.
30. Ginocchio CC, Wang XP, Kaplan MH, Mulligan G, Witt D, Romano JW, Cronin M, Carroll R. Effects of specimen collection, processing, and storage conditions on stability of human immunodeficiency virus type 1 RNA levels in plasma. J Clin Microbiol. 1997;35(11):2886–93.
31. Holodniy M, Rainen L, Herman S, Yen-Lieberman B. Stability of plasma human immunodeficiency virus load in VACUTAINER PPT plasma preparation tubes during overnight shipment. J Clin Microbiol. 2000;38(1):323–6.
32. Kraft CS, Binongo JN, Burd EM, Eaton ME, McCloskey CB, Fernandes H, Hill CE, Caliendo AM. Successful use of Plasma Preparation Tubes (PPTs) in the COBAS(R) AmpliPrep/COBAS(R) TaqMan(R) HIV-1 test. J Clin Virol. 2013;57(1):77–9.
33. Lee TH, Stromberg RR, Heitman JW, Sawyer L, Hanson CV, Busch MP. Distribution of HIV type 1 (HIV-1) in blood components: detection and significance of high levels of HIV-1 associated with platelets. Transfusion. 1998;38(6):580–8.
34. Lee TH, Stromberg RR, Henrard D, Busch MP. Effect of platelet-associated virus on assays of HIV-1 in plasma. Science. 1993;262(5139):1585–6.
35. Sabino EC, Gaburo Jr N, Leite JP, Viecili M, Rosenfeld LG. Platelets may affect detection and quantitation of HIV RNA in plasma samples with low viral loads. J Acquir Immune Defic Syndr. 2004;37(3):1432–3.
36. Wan H, Seth A, Rainen L, Fernandes H. Coamplification of HIV-1 proviral DNA and viral RNA in assays used for quantification of HIV-1 RNA. J Clin Microbiol. 2010;48(6):2186–90.
37. Fernandes H, Morosyuk S, Abravaya K, Ramanathan M, Rainen L. Evaluation of effect of specimen-handling parameters for plasma preparation tubes on viral load measurements obtained by using the Abbott RealTime HIV-1 load assay. J Clin Microbiol. 2010; 48(7):2464–8.
38. Lew J, Reichelderfer P, Fowler M, Bremer J, Carrol R, Cassol S, Chernoff D, Coombs R, Cronin M, Dickover R, Fiscus S, Herman S, Jackson B, Kornegay J, Kovacs A, McIntosh K, Meyer W, Michael N, Mofenson L, Moye J, Quinn T, Robb M, Vahey M, Weiser B, Yeghiazarian T. Determinations of levels of human immunodeficiency virus type 1 RNA in plasma: reassessment of parameters affecting assay outcome. TUBE Meeting Workshop Attendees. Technology Utilization for HIV-1 Blood Evaluation and Standardization in Pediatrics. J Clin Microbiol. 1998;36(6): 1471–9.
39. Lofgren SM, Morrissey AB, Chevallier CC, Malabeja AI, Edmonds S, Amos B, Sifuna DJ, von Seidlein L, Schimana W, Stevens WS, Bartlett JA, Crump JA. Evaluation of a dried blood spot HIV-1 RNA program for early infant diagnosis and viral load monitoring at rural and remote healthcare facilities. AIDS. 2009;23(18):2459–66.
40. Fiscus SA, Brambilla D, Grosso L, Schock J, Cronin M. Quantitation of human immunodeficiency virus type 1 RNA in plasma by using blood dried on filter paper. J Clin Microbiol. 1998;36(1):258–60.
41. Cassol S, Salas T, Gill MJ, Montpetit M, Rudnik J, Sy CT, O'Shaughnessy MV. Stability of dried blood spot specimens for detection of human immunodeficiency virus DNA by polymerase chain reaction. J Clin Microbiol. 1992;30(12):3039–42.
42. Brambilla D, Jennings C, Aldrovandi G, Bremer J, Comeau AM, Cassol SA, Dickover R, Jackson JB, Pitt J, Sullivan JL, Butcher A, Grosso L, Reichelderfer P, Fiscus SA. Multicenter evaluation of use of dried blood and plasma spot specimens in quantitative assays for human immunodeficiency virus RNA: measurement, precision, and RNA stability. J Clin Microbiol. 2003;41(5):1888–93.
43. Christo PP, Greco DB, Aleixo AW, Livramento JA. Factors influencing cerebrospinal fluid and plasma HIV-1 RNA detection rate in patients with and without opportunistic neurological disease during the HAART era. BMC Infect Dis. 2007;7:147.
44. Mazzotta F, Lo Caputo S, Torti C, Tinelli C, Pierotti P, Castelli F, Lazzarin A, Angarano G, Maserati R, Gianotti N, Ladisa N, Quiros-Roldan E, Rinehart AR, Carosi G. Real versus virtual phenotype to guide treatment in heavily pretreated patients: 48-week follow-up of the Genotipo-Fenotipo di Resistenza (GenPheRex) trial. J Acquir Immune Defic Syndr. 2003;32(3):268–80.
45. Perez-Elias MJ, Garcia-Arota I, Munoz V, Santos I, Sanz J, Abraira V, Arribas JR, Gonzalez J, Moreno A, Dronda F, Antela A, Pumares M, Marti-Belda P, Casado JL, Geijos P, Moreno S. Phenotype or virtual phenotype for choosing antiretroviral therapy after failure: a prospective, randomized study. Antivir Ther. 2003;8(6):577–84.
46. Petropoulos CJ, Parkin NT, Limoli KL, Lie YS, Wrin T, Huang W, Tian H, Smith D, Winslow GA, Capon DJ, Whitcomb JM. A novel phenotypic drug susceptibility assay for human immunodeficiency virus type 1. Antimicrob Agents Chemother. 2000;44(4):920–8.
47. Whitcomb JM, Huang W, Fransen S, Limoli K, Toma J, Wrin T, Chappey C, Kiss LD, Paxinos EE, Petropoulos CJ. Development and characterization of a novel single-cycle recombinant-virus assay to determine human immunodeficiency virus type 1 coreceptor tropism. Antimicrob Agents Chemother. 2007;51(2):566–75.
48. MacArthur RD, Novak RM. Reviews of anti-infective agents: maraviroc: the first of a new class of antiretroviral agents. Clin Infect Dis. 2008;47(2):236–41.
49. Tsibris AM, Sagar M, Gulick RM, Su Z, Hughes M, Greaves W, Subramanian M, Flexner C, Giguel F, Leopold KE, Coakley E, Kuritzkes DR. In vivo emergence of vicriviroc resistance in a

human immunodeficiency virus type 1 subtype C-infected subject. J Virol. 2008;82(16):8210–4.
50. Mracna M, Becker-Pergola G, Dileanis J, Guay LA, Cunningham S, Jackson JB, Eshleman SH. Performance of Applied Biosystems ViroSeq HIV-1 Genotyping System for sequence-based analysis of non-subtype B human immunodeficiency virus type 1 from Uganda. J Clin Microbiol. 2001;39(12):4323–7.
51. Brambilla D, Leung S, Lew J, Todd J, Herman S, Cronin M, Shapiro DE, Bremer J, Hanson C, Hillyer GV, McSherry GD, Sperling RS, Coombs RW, Reichelderfer PS. Absolute copy number and relative change in determinations of human immunodeficiency virus type 1 RNA in plasma: effect of an external standard on kit comparisons. J Clin Microbiol. 1998;36(1):311–4.
52. Saag MS, Holodniy M, Kuritzkes DR, O'Brien WA, Coombs R, Poscher ME, Jacobsen DM, Shaw GM, Richman DD, Volberding PA. HIV viral load markers in clinical practice. Nat Med. 1996;2(6):625–9.
53. Donovan RM, Bush CE, Markowitz NP, Baxa DM, Saravolatz LD. Changes in virus load markers during AIDS-associated opportunistic diseases in human immunodeficiency virus-infected persons. J Infect Dis. 1996;174(2):401–3.
54. O'Brien WA, Grovit-Ferbas K, Namazi A, Ovcak-Derzic S, Wang HJ, Park J, Yeramian C, Mao SH, Zack JA. Human immunodeficiency virus-type 1 replication can be increased in peripheral blood of seropositive patients after influenza vaccination. Blood. 1995;86(3):1082–9.
55. Staprans SI, Hamilton BL, Follansbee SE, Elbeik T, Barbosa P, Grant RM, Feinberg MB. Activation of virus replication after vaccination of HIV-1-infected individuals. J Exp Med. 1995;182(6):1727–37.
56. Daar ES, Little S, Pitt J, Santangelo J, Ho P, Harawa N, Kerndt P, Glorgi JV, Bai J, Gaut P, Richman DD, Mandel S, Nichols S. Diagnosis of primary HIV-1 infection. Los Angeles County Primary HIV Infection Recruitment Network. Ann Intern Med. 2001;134(1):25–9.
57. Parkin N, Chappey C, Maroldo L, Bates M, Hellmann NS, Petropoulos CJ. Phenotypic and genotypic HIV-1 drug resistance assays provide complementary information. J Acquir Immune Defic Syndr. 2002;31(2):128–36.
58. Van Houtte M. Update on resistance testing. J HIV Ther. 2001;6(3):61–4.
59. Devereux HL, Youle M, Johnson MA, Loveday C. Rapid decline in detectability of HIV-1 drug resistance mutations after stopping therapy. AIDS. 1999;13(18):F123–7.
60. Blick G, Kagan RM, Coakley E, Petropoulos C, Maroldo L, Greiger-Zanlungo P, Gretz S, Garton T. The probable source of both the primary multidrug-resistant (MDR) HIV-1 strain found in a patient with rapid progression to AIDS and a second recombinant MDR strain found in a chronically HIV-1-infected patient. J Infect Dis. 2007;195(9):1250–9.
61. Fisher R, van Zyl GU, Travers SA, Kosakovsky Pond SL, Engelbrech S, Murrell B, Scheffler K, Smith D. Deep sequencing reveals minor protease resistance mutants in patients failing a protease inhibitor regimen. J Virol. 2012;86:6231. doi:10.1128/JVI.06541-11. JVI.06541-11 [pii].
62. Kozal MJ, Chiarella J, St John EP, Moreno EA, Simen BB, Arnold TE, Lataillade M. Prevalence of low-level HIV-1 variants with reverse transcriptase mutation K65R and the effect of antiretroviral drug exposure on variant levels. Antivir Ther. 2011;16(6):925–9.
63. Stekler JD, Ellis GM, Carlsson J, Eilers B, Holte S, Maenza J, Stevens CE, Collier AC, Frenkel LM. Prevalence and impact of minority variant drug resistance mutations in primary HIV-1 infection. PLoS One. 2011;6(12):e28952. doi:10.1371/journal.pone.0028952. PONE-D-11-14045 [pii].
64. Chen D, Mauk M, Qiu X, Liu C, Kim J, Ramprasad S, Ongagna S, Abrams WR, Malamud D, Corstjens PL, Bau HH. An integrated, self-contained microfluidic cassette for isolation, amplification, and detection of nucleic acids. Biomed Microdevices. 2010;12(4):705–19.
65. Liu C, Geva E, Mauk M, Qiu X, Abrams WR, Malamud D, Curtis K, Owen SM, Bau HH. An isothermal amplification reactor with an integrated isolation membrane for point-of-care detection of infectious diseases. Analyst. 2011;136(10):2069–76.

Hepatitis B and C Viruses

46

Frederick S. Nolte

Abstract

Hepatitis due to infections with hepatitis B virus (HBV) and hepatitis C virus (HCV) are major global public health problems. Molecular diagnostic methods are now standard of care for the diagnosis, management and monitoring therapy of patients with chronic hepatitis B and C. After a brief description of the viruses and clinical manifestations of infection, the clinical utility of viral load testing and genotyping for HBV and HCV are reviewed. The relative advantages and limitations of the commercially available methods for performing these tests will be compared and key laboratory issues affecting the results are highlighted. The chapter also provides guidance for interpretation of these test results and insight into future directions for molecular diagnostic testing in patients with hepatitis B and C.

Keywords

Hepatitis B • Hepatitis C • Hepatitis B virus • Hepatitis C virus • Viral load • Genotyping • Molecular diagnostics

Introduction

Viral hepatitis is believed to have existed in antiquity, with references traced back to the fifth century BC. Over time, research led to the understanding that the disease was caused by more than one virus. Understanding of the pathogenesis began with the landmark discovery of the Australia antigen, subsequently renamed hepatitis B surface antigen (HbsAg) by Blumberg and coworkers in 1965 [1]. What followed was a rapid growth in information about the hepatitis B virus (HBV), development of serologic and molecular tests for HBV, understanding of the natural history and pathogenesis of infection, development and approval of antiviral therapies, and, most importantly, the development of effective vaccines for prevention of HBV infection.

Although non-A, non-B hepatitis has been thought to have a viral etiology since 1974, the virus eluded investigators for more than a decade. In 1989, a brute force application of molecular cloning techniques through the joint efforts of the Centers for Disease Control and Prevention (CDC) and Chiron Corporation led to the identification of the hepatitis C virus (HCV) [2]. This discovery led rapidly to the development of serologic screening assays for HCV infection prior to blood donation, which dramatically reduced the incidence of post-transfusion chronic hepatitis. Sequencing of the HCV genome also provided impetus for the development of molecular assays for detection, quantification, and characterization of HCV. Although there has been explosive growth in information about this medically important virus since its discovery, much remains to be learned about its pathogenesis, treatment, and prevention.

The key characteristics of HBV and HCV are summarized in Table 46.1. Both viruses represent major global public health problems, with an estimated 350 million and

F.S. Nolte, Ph.D. (✉)
Molecular Pathology, Pathology and Laboratory Medicine,
Medical University of South Carolina,
171 Ashley Ave., MSC908, Charleston, SC 29425-9080, USA
e-mail: nolte@musc.edu

D.G.B. Leonard (ed.), *Molecular Pathology in Clinical Practice*, DOI 10.1007/978-3-319-19674-9_46

Table 46.1 Characteristics of hepatitis B virus and hepatitis C virus

Characteristic	Hepatitis B virus	Hepatitis C virus
Type of virus	Hepadnavirus	Hepacivirus
Viral genome	3.2 kb, relaxed circular, partially double-stranded DNA	9.5 kb, positive-sense, single-stranded RNA
Routes of transmission	Parenteral Sexual Injection drug use Perinatal	Parenteral Injection drug use Blood products before 1990 Perinatal (infrequent) Sexual (infrequent)
Frequency of acute icteric disease	Common in adults Uncommon in children	Uncommon
Frequency of evolution to chronic disease	Infrequent (<10 %) in adults Common in children	Frequent (>80 %)
Estimated number of acute infections/year in the USA	185,000	38,000
Estimated number of chronically infected persons in the USA	1,250,000	2,700,000
Estimated number of chronically infected persons in the world	350,000,000	170,000,000
Treatment	Interferon pegylated interferon-α Nucleoside/nucleotide analogs	Pegylated interferon-α with: Ribavirin and Protease inhibitors or RNA polymerase inhibitors or NS5A inhibitors RNA polymerase inhibitor and Ribavirin alone
Prophylaxis	Recombinant Hepatitis B vaccine Immune globulin	None

Source: Adapted from Lauer GM, Walker BD. Hepatitis C virus infection. *N Engl J Med*. 2001;345:41–52

170 million persons chronically infected with HBV and HCV, respectively. Although clinical characteristics and risk factors for infection may give some indication of the specific etiology of viral hepatitis, the diagnosis is laboratory based. Laboratory diagnosis is based on serologic and molecular tests because cell culture techniques for isolation of HBV and HCV are not effective. This chapter reviews the molecular tests that are available to detect, quantify, and characterize HBV and HCV and how these tests can be used for effective diagnosis and clinical management of patients.

Hepatitis B Virus

Description of the Pathogen

The HBV genome is a 3.2 kilobase relaxed circular, partially double-stranded DNA molecule. It has four partially overlapping open reading frames encoding the viral envelope (pre-S and S), nucleocapsid (precore and core), polymerase, and X proteins. After binding to hepatocytes, the virion is taken up into the cell by endocytosis and uncoated. The partially double-stranded DNA genome is converted to a covalently closed circular DNA (cccDNA) in the cell nucleus. The cccDNA is used as a template for transcription of the pregenomic RNA (pgRNA) and messenger RNA in the cell nucleus. The pgRNA moves into the host cell cytoplasm and serves as the template for translation of the HBV reverse transcriptase (RT) as well as the core protein by the cellular translational proteins. Concurrently, the HBV RT reverse transcribes the pgRNA to a new circular DNA molecule. Early in the replication cycle, some of the newly synthesized genomes will circulate back to the nucleus to maintain and increase the pool of cccDNA [3].

Although HBV is a DNA virus, it replicates by a RT that lacks proofreading activity and, as a result, is prone to errors. The overlapping open reading frames of the genome limit the types of mutations that can be tolerated. However, variations in HBV sequences have been detected in almost all regions of the genome. Consequently, HBV exists as quasispecies, and different patients may be infected with different strains and genotypes.

Seven phylogenetic genotypes (A through H) of HBV have been identified, most of which have distinct geographic distribution. Genotypes are defined by intergroup divergence of greater than 8 % in the complete genome nucleotide sequence. All known genotypes have been found in the USA with the prevalence of A, B, C, D, and E–G being 35 %, 22 %, 31 %, 10 %, and 2 %, respectively [4]. Recent data suggest that HBV genotype plays an important role in the progression of HBV-related liver disease as well as response to interferon alpha (IFN-α) and pegylated IFN-α; however, HBV genotyping is not necessary in routine clinical practice [5].

Clinical Utility

Serologic assays with high levels of sensitivity, specificity, and reproducibility have been developed to detect HBV antigens and their respective antibodies. This complicated system of serologic markers is used for diagnosis of HBV infection and to define the phase of infection, degree of infectivity, prognosis, and the patient's immune status. The presence of HBV DNA in the serum is a marker of viral replication in the liver and has replaced hepatitis B e antigen (HBeAg) as the most sensitive marker of viral replication. HBeAg is the extracellular form of the hepatitis B core protein. Molecular assays to quantify blood levels HBV DNA are useful for the initial evaluation of HBV infections, monitoring of patients with chronic infections, and assessing the efficacy of antiviral treatment [3, 5]. In addition, US blood donors are routinely screened for HBV DNA by qualitative tests to detect donors in the early stage of infection [6]. Antiviral resistance mutations are detected by molecular methods that identify known mutations associated with drug resistance.

The initial evaluation of patients found to have HBsAg in serum should include routine liver tests and a variety of virologic tests including HBV DNA tests [5]. Chronic HBV infection is a disease of variable course, and establishing baseline laboratory values at the time of diagnosis is important clinically for the tracking of disease progression over time and to evaluate candidates for liver biopsy. Monitoring disease activity in chronically HBV-infected patients is best done by measuring aminotransferase (ALT) levels at regular intervals in HBeAg-positive patients. However, serial HBV DNA testing is recommended in HBeAg-negative patients. The determination of serum HBV DNA levels (viral load) is important in the pretreatment evaluation and monitoring of therapeutic response in patients with chronic infection [5]. Currently, therapy for chronic HBV infection does not eradicate the virus and has limited long-term efficacy. The decision to treat should be based on ALT elevations, the presence of HBeAg or HBV DNA viral load of >2,000 IU/ml or both, the presence of moderate disease activity and fibrosis on liver biopsy, and virologic testing to exclude concurrent infections with hepatitis D virus (HDV), HCV, and human immunodeficiency virus (HIV). The goals of treatment of chronic hepatitis B are to achieve sustained suppression of HBV replication and to prevent further progression of liver disease. Parameters used to indicate treatment response include normalization of serum ALT, decrease in serum HBV DNA level, and loss of HBeAg with or without detection of anti-HBeAg. Currently, eight US Federal Drug Administration (FDA)-approved therapies are available for treatment of chronic HBV infection: IFN-α, pegylated IFN-α2a, four nucleoside analogs (NS; lamivudine, telbivudine, entecavir, and emtricitabine) and two nucleotide analogs (NT; adefovir and tenofovir). Several factors predict a favorable response to IFN treatment with the most important being high ALT and low serum HBV DNA viral load, which are indirect markers of immune clearance.

Therapy usually does not eradicate the virus because of the difficulty of eliminating the covalently closed circular form of the HBV genome from the liver and the existence of extrahepatic reservoirs of HBV. Endpoints of treatment have traditionally been clearance of HBeAg, development of anti-HBe antibodies, and undetectable serum HBV DNA using insensitive hybridization assays with detection limits of approximately 10^6 genome copies/ml. Achieving these endpoints usually is accompanied by resolution of liver disease as evidenced by normalization of the ALT level and decreased histologic activity on liver biopsy. The response usually is sustained at long-term follow-up. Nevertheless, most responders continue to have detectable HBV DNA when sensitive nucleic acid amplification tests are used. Responses to antiviral therapy are categorized as biochemical, virologic, or histologic and as on-therapy, or sustained off-therapy (Table 46.2) [5].

Table 46.2 Definitions of response and time of assessments for antiviral therapy for chronic hepatitis B virus (HBV) infection

Response definitions	
Biochemical response	Decrease in serum ALT to within normal range
Virologic response	Decrease in serum HBV DNA to undetectable levels by nucleic acid amplification assay, and loss of HBeAg in patients who were initially HBeAg positive
Primary non-response (NS and NT analogs only)	Decrease in serum HBV DNA by <2 $\log_{10}$ IU/ml after at least 24 weeks of therapy
Virologic relapse	Increase in serum HBV DNA of ≥1 $\log_{10}$ IU/ml after discontinuation of treatment by at least two tests performed >4 weeks apart
Histologic response	Decrease in histology activity index by at least 2 points and no worsening of fibrosis score compared to pretreatment biopsy
Complete response	Fulfill criteria of biochemical and virologic response and loss of HBsAg
Time of assessment definitions	
On-therapy	During therapy
Maintained	Persists throughout the course of treatment
Off-therapy	At the end of a defined course of therapy
Sustained-6	6 months after discontinuation of therapy
Sustained-12	12 months after discontinuation of therapy

ALT aminotransferase, *NS* nucleoside, *NT* nucleotide

Several variations in the nucleotide sequence of HBV have important clinical consequences. An important mutation in the S gene is a glycine-to-arginine substitution at codon 145 (G145R) in the conserved "a" determinant, which causes decreased affinity of the HBsAg for anti-HBs antibodies [7]. HBV with this mutation has been found in children of HBsAg-positive mothers who develop HBV infection despite vaccination and an adequate anti-HBs antibody response after vaccination, as well as in liver transplant recipients who have recurrent infection despite administration of HBV immune globulin [8, 9]. These immune escape mutants have raised concern about vaccine efficacy and serologically silent infections. The G145R mutation has been reported in many countries and is responsible for 2–40 % of vaccine failures. Although there is diminished binding to anti-HBs antibodies, the vast majority of S mutants can be readily detected with the current generation of HBsAg tests. Thus, an initial concern that widespread use of HBV immune globulin and vaccination would result in HBV mutants that would escape detection in the HBsAg test was unfounded.

Mutations in the basal core promoter and the precore genes affect the synthesis of HBeAg and commonly arise under immune pressure [10]. The most common basal core promoter mutation has a dual change of A to T at nucleotide (nt) 1,762 (T1762) and G to A at nt 1,764 (A1764) that diminishes the amount of mRNA and hence HBeAg secretion [11]. The predominant precore mutation is a G to A change at nt 1,896 (A1896), which leads to premature termination of the precore protein at codon 28, thus preventing the production of HBeAg [12]. The A1896 mutation is infrequent in North America and Western Europe but is geographically widespread. This geographic variability in frequency is related to the predominant genotypes in a geographic region because the mutation is found only in genotypes B, C, D, and E.

The A1896 mutation was first reported in patients with chronic active hepatitis or fulminant hepatitis. However, the A1896 mutation also can be present in asymptomatic carriers and viruses with this mutation replicate no more efficiently than wild-type HBV. Thus, the pathophysiologic significance of this mutation is unclear [13]. However, the clinical picture of persistent HBV replication and active liver disease in HBeAg-negative patients appears to be increasingly prevalent, and in some regions the A1896-mutant virus may be more prevalent than wild-type virus.

Therapy for chronic hepatitis B requires long courses of treatment with NS or NT analogs. A major concern with long-term therapy is the development of antiviral resistance. The rate at which resistant mutants are selected is related to pretreatment serum HBV DNA viral load, rapidity of viral suppression, duration of treatment, and prior antiviral exposure. The incidence of genotypic resistance also varies with the sensitivity of the methods used to detect resistance mutations and the patient population tested. The definitions of terms used to describe resistance to NS and NT analogs are summarized in Table 46.3 [5].

Table 46.3 Definitions of terms used to describe antiviral resistance of HBV

Term	Definition
Virologic breakthrough	Increase in serum HBV DNA >1 $\log_{10}$ above nadir after achieving a virologic response during continued treatment
Viral rebound	Increase in serum HBV DNA >20,000 IU/ml or above pretreatment level after achieving a virologic response during continued treatment
Biochemical breakthrough	Increase in ALT above upper limit of normal after achieving normalization during continued treatment
Genotypic resistance	Detection of mutations that have been shown in vitro to confer resistance to drug being administered
Phenotypic resistance	In vitro confirmation that a mutation decreases the susceptibility to the drug as demonstrated by an increase in the inhibitory concentration

ALT aminotransferase

Table 46.4 Antiviral agents and the HBV mutations associated with resistance

Antiviral agent	Description of agent	Mutations associated with resistance
Lamivudine	Nucleoside analog (cytidine)	(L180M+M204V/I/S), A181V/T, S202G/I
Telbivudine	Nucleoside analog (dTTP)	M204I, A181T/V
Entecavir	Nucleoside analog (2-deoxyguanosine)	T184S/C/G/A/I/L/F/M, S202G/C/I, M250V/I/L
Emtricitabine	Nucleoside analog (cytidine)	M204V/I
Adefovir	Nucleotide analog (dATP)	A181V/T, N236T
Tenofovir	Nucleotide analog (dATP)	A194T, N236T, A181V/T

Typically, when a patient experiences a virologic breakthrough, HBV resistance genotyping should be performed. The standardized nomenclature of HBV antiviral resistance mutations is shown Table 46.4 [3, 14, 15]. No HBV mutations are associated with resistance to IFN-α or pegylated IFN-α2a.

Available Assays

HBV DNA Detection and Quantification

The commercially available tests for quantification of HBV DNA in serum and plasma are listed in Table 46.5. These tests employ either branched DNA or real-time PCR for

Table 46.5 Commercial assays for quantification of HBV DNA

Assay (manufacturer)	Method	Dynamic range
COBAS Taqman HBV test (Roche Diagnostics, Indianapolis, IN)[a]	Real-time PCR	1.7×10^2–8.5×10^8 copies/ml[b]
Real-time HBV (Abbott Laboratories, Abbott Park, IL)[a]	Real-time PCR	1.0×10^1–1×10^9 IU/ml
Versant HBV DNA (Siemens Corp., Washington, DC)	Branched DNA	3.3×10^3–1×10^8 copies/ml
Artus HBV PCR (Qiagen, Valencia, CA)	Real-time PCR	2×10^2–1×10^8 IU/ml
Affigene HBV Trender (Cepheid, Sunnyvale, CA)	Real-time PCR	1.7×10^2–1.7×10^8 IU/ml

[a]US FDA-cleared
[b]COBAS Ampliprep/COBAS Taqman test v2.0 dynamic range is 54–1.1×10^8 copies/ml

amplification and differ in their limits of detection and dynamic ranges. The COBAS Taqman (Roche Diagnostics, Indianapolis, IN) and the real-time (Abbott Laboratories, Abbott Park, IL) HBV tests are approved for in vitro diagnostic use by the US FDA. The others are available as research use only (RUO) kits or analyte specific reagents (ASRs). All of the quantitative HBV DNA test formats have been used in monitoring the status of HBV infection before and after treatment.

Qualitative assays for detection of HBV DNA in blood donations are produced by Gen-Probe Inc. (San Mateo, CA) (using transcription-mediated amplification) and Roche Diagnostics (using PCR) with limits of detection of 11 IU/ml and 15 IU/ml, respectively. However, the value of nucleic acid testing compared to serology for HBV screening of blood donors remains controversial and has not been universally adopted [6].

HBV Genotyping

Two commercial HBV genotyping systems are available as RUO kits. Innogenetics Inc. (Alpharetta, CA) offers three different line probe assays for HBV phylogenetic genotyping, detection of precore mutations, and detection of all relevant lamivudine, emtricitabine, telbivudine, adefovir, and entecavir resistance mutations as well as known compensatory mutations [16, 17]. All assays use PCR to amplify portions of the relevant genes to produce a biotinylated product. The PCR products are denatured and hybridized to a series of informative probes immobilized on a nitrocellulose strip. The hybrids are visualized on the strip after addition of streptavidin–alkaline phosphatase and colorimetric substrate. The mutations are identified by the colored patterns of PCR product hybridization to the probes. The line probe assays typically have better sensitivity for detection of sequence variants than direct Sanger sequencing.

Interpretation of Test Results

A major dilemma in the interpretation of serum HBV viral load results is what values should be used to define treatment indications and response. Because HBV DNA may persist in individuals who have serological recovery from acute infection, low levels may not be associated with progressive liver disease and viral clearance is an unrealistic treatment endpoint. An arbitrary value of 20,000 IU/ml (>10^5 copies/ml) was chosen as a diagnostic criterion for chronic hepatitis B at the 2000 NIH conference [18]. However, progressive liver disease can be found in individuals with lower levels. In addition, wide fluctuations in HBV viral load from undetectable to >2 million IU/ml are observed in some patients with chronic hepatitis B [19, 20]. Consequently, serial monitoring is more important than reliance on a single cutoff value in determining prognosis and the need for treatment.

The first manifestation of antiviral resistance is an increase in HBV viral load >1 $\log_{10}$ from nadir during treatment in a patient who had an initial virologic response. Virologic breakthroughs often are related to therapy noncompliance, so compliance should be assessed before testing for genotypic resistance. HBV viral load levels tend to be low initially because antiviral-resistant mutants have decreased replication fitness. However, compensatory mutations that can restore replication fitness often emerge during continued therapy leading to progressive increases in HBV viral load followed by biochemical breakthrough. Antiviral resistant mutations can be detected months to years prior to biochemical breakthrough. Thus early detection of these mutations can prevent hepatitis flares and liver decompensation. Cross-resistance mutations do occur that limit future treatment options and multidrug-resistant mutants in patients who have received sequential monotherapies have been described [21].

Laboratory Issues

A World Health Organization (WHO) international HBV standard was created in 2001 in response to the recognized need to standardize HBV DNA quantification assays [22]. The WHO HBV standard is a high-titer, genotype A virus preparation (code 97/746) which was assigned a potency of 10^6 IU/ml. A second standard (code 97/750) was established in 2006 and is quantitatively equivalent to the first standard. The standard established that 1 IU was equivalent to 5.4 genome equivalents by testing the pooled material with a range of commercially available and laboratory-developed tests. However, despite the availability of HBV DNA standards, the various quantitative assays usually have different conversion factors for copies to IU/ml, which may reflect their different amplification and detection chemistries. Laboratories should report HBV viral load test results in IU/ml as both $\log_{10}$ transformed and arithmetic values.

As with any viral load test, some of the variability in quantification may be attributable to sample processing. Either serum or plasma can be used for most tests. Whole blood should be centrifuged within 6 h of collection and the serum or plasma removed from the cells. Short-term storage of serum or plasma is safe at refrigerator temperatures (4 °C). Freezing at temperatures ≤20 °C is recommended for long-term storage of samples.

The standardized nomenclature for reporting of HBV antiviral resistance mutations shown Table 46.4 should be used when resistance genotyping is performed. The inability of genotyping assays to detect minor populations of circulating HBV is a significant technical issue. In general, direct sequencing is limited to resolution of populations which are ≥20 % of the viral population. HBV is included in the hepatitis viral load proficiency testing surveys available from the College of American Pathologists.

Future Directions

Molecular assays for quantification and genotyping of HBV will become more fully integrated in the testing strategies for the diagnosis and management of patients with chronic hepatitis B. Clinical practice guidelines now reflect the importance of HBV viral load and genotyping tests in improving patient outcomes and this is likely to create more demand for these tests. The current generation of real-time PCR viral load assays meets the clinical needs and development and adoption of the WHO international standard has improved the agreement between results of different assays. Improved HBV treatment will depend on development of better laboratory tools for assessing genotypic resistance. Genotyping beyond individual mutation detection to a more comprehensive genomic analysis to predict fitness and other polymutational phenotypes, and detection of minor resistant populations will be possible with next-generation sequencing methods [22, 24].

Hepatitis C Virus

Description of the Pathogen

HCV is an RNA virus with a positive-sense, single-stranded genome of approximately 9,500 nt encoding a single polyprotein of about 3,000 amino acids. The long open reading frame is flanked at each end by short untranslated regions (UTR). The genome structure is most similar to viruses of the family *Flaviviridae*, which includes many of the arthropod-borne viruses. As in other flaviviruses, the three N-terminal proteins of HCV (core, envelope 1 [E1], and envelope 2 [E2]) are probably structural and the four C-terminal proteins (nonstructural 2, 3, 4, and 5) are thought to function in viral replication. HCV is classified within the family *Flaviviridae* in its own genus, *Hepacivirus*.

The 5′ UTR is a highly conserved region of 341 nt and has a complex secondary structure. It contains an internal ribosome entry site and is important in the translation of the long open reading frame. The 3′ UTR contains a short region that varies in sequence and length, followed by a polypyrimidine stretch of variable length, and finally a highly conserved sequence of 98 nt, which constitutes the terminus of the genome. The function of the 3′ UTR is not known but is thought to be essential for viral replication.

The E1 and E2 regions of HCV are the most variable regions within the genome at both the nucleotide and amino acid levels. Two regions in E2, called hypervariable regions 1 and 2 (HVR1 and HRV2, respectively), show extreme sequence variability, which is thought to result from selective pressure by antiviral antibodies. E2 also contains the binding site for CD81, one of the putative cell receptors or coreceptors for HCV.

The nonstructural regions 2 (NS2) and 3 (NS3) contain a zinc-dependent autoprotease that cleaves the polyprotein at the NS2-NS3 junction. The aminoterminal portion of the NS3 protein also is a serine protease that cleaves the polyprotein at several sites. The carboxyterminal portion of the NS3 protein has helicase activity, which is important for HCV replication. The NS4A protein is a cofactor for NS3 serine protease. The NS5B region encodes the RNA-dependent RNA polymerase, which replicates the viral genome. A region in NS5A has been linked to IFN-α response and therefore is called the IFN-α-sensitivity determining region (ISDR).

HCV Genotypes

The first complete HCV genome sequence was reported by Choo et al. in 1991 [25]. As additional genome sequences from isolates from different parts of the world were determined and compared, it was evident that HCV exists as distinct genotypes with as much as 35 % sequence diversity over the whole viral genome [26]. Much of the early literature on genotyping is confusing because investigators developed and used their own classification schemes. However, a consensus nomenclature system was developed in 1994. In this system, the genotypes are numbered using Arabic numerals in order of their discovery, and the more closely related strains within some types are designated as subtypes with lowercase letters. The complex of genetic variants found within an individual isolate is termed the “quasispecies.” The quasispecies results from the accumulation of mutations that occur during viral replication in the host.

The genotype and subtype assignments and nomenclature rules for HCV have recently been updated [27]. Seven major genotypes and 67 subtype of HCV are now recognized with another 20 provisional subtypes. HCV strains belonging to different genotypes differ at 30–35 % of nucleotides and those that belong to the same subtype differ at <15 % of nucleotides at the genome level.

HCV genotypes 1, 2, and 3 are found throughout the world, but there are clear differences in their distribution [28]. HCV subtypes 1a, 1b, 2a, 2b, 2c, and 3a are responsible for more than 90 % of infections in North and South America, Europe, and Japan. In the USA, type 1 accounts for approximately 70 % of the infections with equal distribution between subtypes 1a and 1b. In Japan, subtype 1b causes more than 70 % of HCV infections. Although subtypes 2a and 2b have wide distributions in North America, Europe, and Japan, subtype 2c is widespread in a region of northern Italy. HCV subtype 3a is common among intravenous drug users in the USA and Europe. The other subtypes of genotype 3 are common in Nepal, Bangladesh, India, and Pakistan. Genotype 4 is prevalent in North Africa and the Middle East, and genotypes 5 and 6 are limited to South Africa and Hong Kong, respectively [29]. Subtype 4a constitutes the majority of infections in Egypt, and this and other subtypes of genotype 4 are found in Zaire and Gabon. Subtype 5a is predominant in South Africa, where some reports indicate that it is responsible for more than 50 % of infections. Subtype 6a infections are common in Hong Kong. To date, only 2 genotype 7 infections has been reported in patients from Central Africa [30].

The retrospective nature of most of the genotype studies has not allowed determination of the role of genotype as a risk factor for disease progression nor separation of genotype from other known risk factors for severe disease, such as older age at infection, male gender, alcohol consumption, and concurrent viral infection. However, in two prospective studies, viral genotype did not correlate with disease progression [31, 32].

Clinical Utility

HCV RNA Detection and Quantification

Detection of HCV RNA in serum or plasma by nucleic acid amplification methods is important for confirming the diagnosis of HCV, distinguishing active from resolved infection, assessing the virologic response to therapy, and screening the blood supply. These tests are incorporated into diagnostic algorithms for hepatitis C proposed by the CDC [33], American Association for the Study of Liver Diseases [34], and National Academy of Clinical Biochemistry [35].

The detection of HCV RNA in the plasma or serum is the earliest marker of infection, appearing 1–2 weeks after infection and weeks before elevation of liver enzyme levels or the appearance of anti-HCV antibodies. Approximately 80 % of individuals infected with HCV will be chronically infected with the virus. In antibody-positive individuals, HCV RNA tests can distinguish active from resolved infections. In patients with a high pretest probability of infection, a positive serologic screening test is usually confirmed with a test for HCV RNA rather than the recombinant immunoblot assay (RIBA). This strategy is cost-effective and more informative than using the RIBA to confirm positive antibody screening tests in a diagnostic setting [36]. However, with the discontinuation of the HCV RIBA by the manufacturer in 2012, all reactive HCV antibody screening tests should be followed by US FDA-approved HCV RNA testing [37].

HCV RNA testing also is helpful for the diagnosis of infection in infants born to HCV-infected mothers due to persistence of maternal antibody, and in immunocompromised or debilitated patients who may have blunted serologic responses. An HCV RNA test also should be used for patients suspected of having an acute infection and in patients with hepatitis of no identifiable cause.

HCV RNA tests are the most reliable means of identifying patients with active HCV infection. A negative HCV RNA test in a serologically positive individual may indicate that the infection has resolved or that the viremia is intermittent. Up to 15 % of chronically infected individuals have intermittent viremia and, as a result, a single negative HCV RNA determination may not be sufficient to exclude active infection when the index of clinical suspicion is high [38]. In these individuals a second specimen should be collected and tested.

The use of anti-HCV antibody tests to screen the blood supply has dramatically reduced the risk of transfusion-associated HCV infection in developed countries. The risk in the USA from blood that is negative for anti-HCV antibodies is less than 1 in 103,000 transfused units [39]. To drive the risk of infection from transfusion even lower, blood donor pools currently are tested for the presence of HCV RNA [40]. The serologic screening tests for HCV have a 70-day window period of seronegativity, and antigen detection tests are not yet available for blood product screening. HCV RNA testing is estimated to reduce the detection window by 25 days and reduce the number of transfused infectious units from 116 to 32 per year [41].

Assays for the detection and quantification of HCV core antigen in serum have recently been commercially developed but are not yet US FDA-cleared for diagnostic use (Ortho Clinical Diagnostics, Rochester, NY; Bio-Rad, Hercules, CA; and Abbott Laboratories, Abbott Park, IL) [42–46]. These tests significantly shorten the serologically silent window period using seroconversion panels, and their performance correlates closely with RNA detection tests in blood donors. However, the analytical sensitivity is less than most RNA tests, at approximately 10,000 IU/ml. The analytical sensitivity of the core antigen test is too high to be used in the monitoring of late events during and after treatment. Antigen detection may represent a cost-effective alternative to HCV RNA testing to distinguish active from resolved infections in resource-poor settings.

HCV viral load testing is useful in pretreatment evaluations of patients being considered for therapy, since a viral load of less 600,000 IU/ml is one of several predictors of achieving a sustained virologic response [47, 48]. Other factors associated with achieving a sustained response to therapy include the absence of cirrhosis, age <40 years, female gender, white race, viral genotype 2 or 3, and presence of C or T at position rs12979860 near the gene for lambda IFN 3 (*IL28B*) [49, 50].

HCV viral load does not predict disease progression and is not associated with severity of liver disease [51]. This is in sharp contrast to HIV-1, in which the viral load is the principal factor determining the rate of disease progression. Monitoring HCV viral load in untreated patients is not warranted and should be discouraged. Until recently, the standard therapy for patients with chronic HCV infection was pegylated IFN-α in combination with ribavirin administered for either 48 weeks for HCV genotype 1, 4, 5, and 6 infections, or for 24 weeks for HCV genotype 2 and 3 infections. Sustained virologic response (SVR) rates were attained in 40–50 % of patients with genotype 1 and in 80 % or more of those with genotype 2 and 3 infections. SVR is defined as the absence of detectable HCV RNA in plasma or serum as determined with a test that has a limit of detection of ≤50 IU/ml and is considered a virologic cure.

The first direct acting antivirals (DAA) for treatment of hepatitis C were approved by the US FDA in 2011. Both are NS3/4A serine protease inhibitors, boceprevir (BOC) (Merck, Kenilworth, NJ) and telaprevir (TVR) (Vertex, Boston, MA). These DAA agents are used in combination with pegylated IFN-α and ribavirin. Triple therapy for genotype 1 infections has led to approximately a 30 % increase in SVR over the previous standard of care therapy in all patient subgroups. Limited phase 2 testing has shown that TVR also has activity against genotype 2 infections but not against genotype 3 infections. BOC appears to have activity against both genotypes 2 and 3 infections. However, neither drug should be used to treat patients with genotype 2 and 3 infections [52].

The algorithms for monitoring HCV viral load in patients receiving triple therapy and the stopping rules are shown in Fig. 46.1 [52]. The important time points for response-guided therapy are at 8, 12, and 24 weeks for BOC and 4, 12, and 24 weeks for TVR. Treatment with all three drugs should be stopped if HCV RNA level is >100 IU/ml at week 12 or detectable at week 24 for BOC triple therapy and if HCV RNA level is >1,000 IU/ml at weeks 4 or 12 and/or detectable at week 24 with TVR.

The goal of treatment is a SVR, defined as no detectable HCV RNA in serum or plasma by a highly sensitive assay (limit of detection ≤10–15 IU/ml) 6 months after the end of treatment. Patients who achieve a SVR have little or no chance of virologic relapse of their disease.

In 2013, two more potent DAAs were approved by the US FDA: sofosbuvir (Gilead Sciences, Inc., Foster City, CA), a NS5B polymerase inhibitor [53], and simeprevir (Johnson &

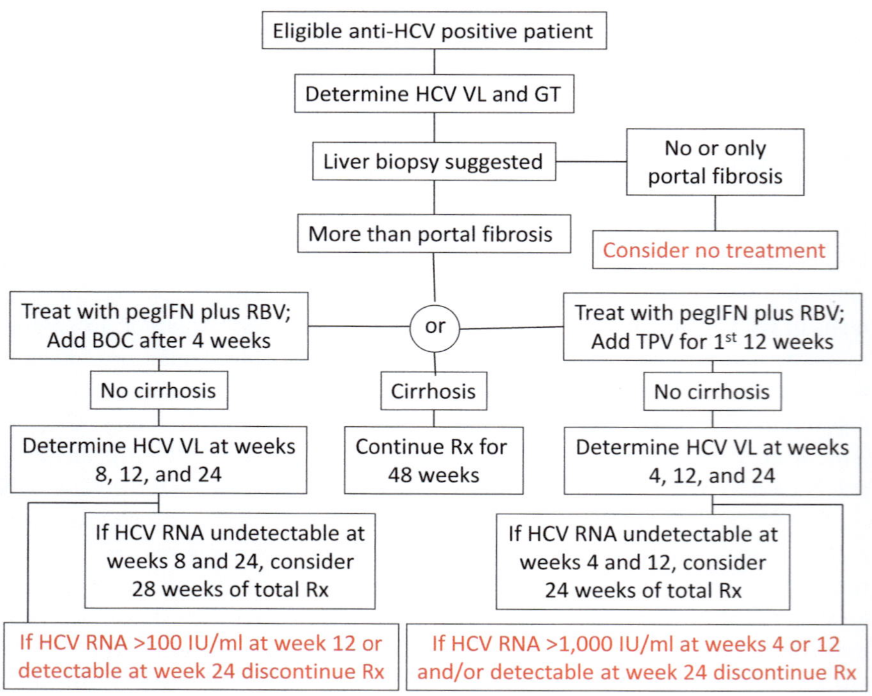

Figure 46.1 Triple therapy algorithms for treatment-naive patients with chronic HCV genotype 1 infections. Stopping rules in *red* (Adapted from Ref. 53). *BOC* boceprevir, *GT* genotype, *IU* international units, *pegIFN* pegylated interferon-α, *RBV* ribavirin, *Rx* treatment, *TVP* telaprevir, *VL* viral load

Johnson, New Brunswick, NJ), a second generation protease inhibitor [54]. Sofosbuvir was approved in combination with pegylated IFN-α and ribavirin for treatment of genotypes 1 and 4 and in combination with ribavirin alone for genotypes 2 and 3. Simeprevir was approved by the US FDA for treatment of genotype 1 infections in combination with pegylated IFN-α and ribavirin, but only for patients with genotype 1 who have not failed therapy with first generation protease inhibitors.

Monitoring of on-treatment viral load levels does not affect management decisions with a sosobuvir-based regimen since treatment failure is almost exclusively due to relapse [53]. However, given the expense of the drugs and the potential risk of viral resistance with inappropriate use, viral load testing at week 4 and end of treatment at either week 12 or 24 depending on the regimen seems prudent.

Viral load levels should be determined at weeks 4, 12, and 24 to assess treatment response and for stopping rules in patients treated with simeprevir, pegylated IFN-α, and ribavirin. Discontinuation is warranted for patients who are unlikely to achieve a SVR based on the on-treatment virologic response. If HCV RNA level is >25 IU/ml at week 4, the entire regimen should be discontinued. If the HCV RNA level is >25 IU/ml at week 12 or 24 after the simeprevir has been completed, the pegylated IFN-α and ribavirin should be discontinued [54].

Numerous other DAAs have been developed and are currently in clinical trials. These include NS3/4A protease inhibitors, NS5B polymerase inhibitors, and inhibitors of host cell proteins required for HCV replication. The most current recommendations for all aspects of HCV treatment can be found at http://www.hcvguidelines.org/.

HCV Genotyping

Sequence analysis of variable regions of the HCV genome has been used to investigate outbreaks of infection and to study modes of transmission. Two large outbreaks of infection associated with contaminated lots of anti-rhesus D immunoglobulin (anti-D) in Ireland and Germany were investigated using molecular typing [55, 56]. In both studies, sequence analysis showed that the HCV infecting the women was the same as that found in the implicated batches of anti-D. In another report, sequencing part of the NS3 region provided evidence of patient-to-patient transmission during colonoscopy [57]. Sequence analysis also has been used as part of investigations of HCV infections associated with blood transfusions. In addition, molecular genotyping has been used to study vertical and sexual transmission of HCV [58–61].

Although a number of baseline factors are predictive of response to treatment of chronic hepatitis C infection, HCV genotype is a strong and consistent predictor for achieving a SVR to pegylated IFN-α and ribavirin. In the large clinical trials of combination therapy with pegylated IFN-α and ribavirin, only 30 % of patients infected with genotype 1 had a SVR compared to 65 % of patients infected with genotypes 2 or 3 [47, 48].

Several studies focused on the identification of isolates within a genotype with different responses to IFN, and led to the definition of the ISDR. For example, Enomoto et al. found that genotype 1b isolates in Japan identical to the HCV-J prototype strain within the carboxyterminal part of the NS5A protein were resistant to IFN [62]. In contrast, patients infected with genotype 1b strains with mutations within this region had a better response to IFN. This region of amino acids 2,209–2,248 in the NS5A protein is the ISDR. The same group recently confirmed and extended their observations. They found that sustained response rates correlated with the number of mutations in the ISDR with a larger group of patients and identified the mutation sites within the ISDR that were significantly associated with sustained response [63]. Although these results have been confirmed for Japanese isolates, in studies of patients from other countries the majority of IFN-sensitive isolates showed no or only a few mutations in the ISDR [64, 65]. The reasons for the different findings are not clear but may involve racial, virologic, or other factors.

The determination of HCV subtypes has no clinical relevance in patients treated with IFN and ribavirin, while different treatment durations based on viral load kinetics are recommended for patients with different HCV genotypes. However, the emergence of resistant variants and virologic breakthrough were more common in patients infected with HCV subtype 1a than 1b when treated with TVR triple therapy [66]. HCV subtyping may play a role in helping to select treatment regimens and predict the development of resistance to DAA drugs. In addition, triple therapy with a protease inhibitor is not recommended for patients infected with genotypes 2 and 3.

Antiviral-resistance mutations that cluster around the catalytic site of the NS3/4A serine protease emerge during protease inhibitor therapy and are associated with failure and relapse [52]. Similar resistant variants are detected in both BOC- and TVR-treated patients, suggesting that cross-resistance occurs with these protease inhibitors. Also antiviral-resistant variants are found in about 5 % of patients prior to treatment, but do not appear to impact response to either protease inhibitor. Currently there is no role for antiviral resistance genotyping at baseline or during treatment with the protease inhibitors [67].

Several mutations in the NS3/4A protease are associated with reduced susceptibility to simeprevir. One of the most common and clinically relevant mutations is the substitution Q80K. This mutation may be present at baseline in approximately 30 % of patients with genotype 1a and is associated with lower SVR rates. For patients with genotype 1a, Q80K mutation testing is recommended and patients with this variant should be offered other treatment options [68].

IL28B Genotyping

Human genome wide association studies identified multiple single nucleotide polymorphisms (SNPs) in a region 3 kilobases upstream of the human INF-λ-3 or *interleukin-28B* (*IL28B*) gene on chromosome 19 that are associated with spontaneous clearance of HCV infection and treatment response to pegylated IFN-α and ribavirin. A SNP at position rs129779860 T/C is associated with an approximately twofold change in response to treatment in both patients of European and African ancestry. Because the favorable C/C genotype is in substantially greater frequency than the unfavorable T/T genotype in European than in African populations, this genetic polymorphism also explains approximately half the difference in response rates between the two populations [69]. The C/C genotype also strongly enhances spontaneous HCV clearance in a natural history setting among individuals of both European and African ancestry [70].

A second SNP in the same region of *IL28*, rs80999117 T/G, has been implicated in both treatment-induced viral clearance rates and spontaneous clearance of HCV infection in Japanese, Australian, and Swiss populations [71, 72]. The rs129779860 and rs80999117 polymorphisms are approximately 4,000 base pairs apart and show high levels of linkage disequilibrium, resulting in distinct haplotypes in the studied populations. INF-λ-3 is a type III IFN that shares many characteristics with IFN-α, a type I IFN. However, INF-λ-3 has less antiviral activity against HCV than IFN-α, but the unique INF-λ-3 receptor is more liver cell-specific than the IFN-α receptor.

The predictive value of rs129779860*IL28B* genotyping for a SVR to treatment with pegylated IFN-α and ribavirin is superior to baseline viral load, HCV, fibrosis stage, age, and gender, and is higher for HCV genotype 1 than for genotypes 2 or 3. The IL28B C/C genotype is also a robust pretreatment predictor of a SVR to protease inhibitor triple therapy. However, as new more potent direct acting antiviral agents are developed, *IL28B* genotype will discriminate responders and non-responders less well. Currently there are no US FDA-cleared tests for *IL28B* genotyping.

Available Assays

Many test kits for detection or quantification of HCV RNA are commercially available. These tests are based on traditional reverse transcription-polymerase chain reaction (RT-PCR), transcription-mediated amplification (TMA), branched-DNA (bDNA) assay, or, most recently, real-time RT-PCR methods.

Qualitative Detection HCV Assays

Two US FDA-approved qualitative HCV RNA test kits are available for diagnostic use: the Amplicor HCV test v2.0 (Roche Diagnostics) and the Versant HCV RNA qualitative test (Siemens Corp.). The Amplicor HCV test v2.0 is based on RT-PCR amplification of a portion of the 5′ UTR and has an analytical sensitivity of 50 IU/ml [73]. The test incorporates an internal control to detect PCR inhibitors and deoxyuridine triphosphate (dUTP) and uracil-N-glycosylase in the reaction mixture to prevent false positives due to amplicon carryover. The test is available in two formats, a manual microwell plate assay and a semiautomated assay designed for the COBAS instrument. The performance characteristics of the Amplicor HCV tests are well established [74].

The Versant HCV RNA qualitative test also targets the 5′ UTR but uses TMA to amplify the targeted region. The analytical sensitivity of the Versant HCV RNA assay is 5 IU/ml. The increase in analytical sensitivity over the Amplicor tests is due in part to the larger sample volume (500 μl vs 200 μl) and the use of a specific target capture step to isolate HCV RNA rather than total RNA precipitation. This test also uses an internal control RNA to detect the presence of amplification inhibitors.

The Versant HCV RNA assay can detect residual serum HCV RNA in some patients with no detectable HCV RNA determined by the Amplicor v2.0 assay at the end of treatment with IFN and who subsequently have a virologic relapse [75, 76]. However, this difference was not observed with end-of-treatment samples from patients treated with pegylated IFN-α [77]. The two qualitative HCV RNA assays demonstrate excellent concordance with specimens submitted for HCV diagnosis [78]. The difference in analytical sensitivity between the two tests does not result in any meaningful difference in clinical sensitivity when the tests are used diagnostically, because typically patients with chronic hepatitis C infection to present for initial evaluation with very high viral loads.

The Procleix HIV-1/HCV test (Gen-Probe Inc.) also uses TMA technology and is approved by the US FDA for the screening of blood products [79]. The Ampliscreen HCV RNA test v2.0 is an RT-PCR assay (Roche Diagnostics) designed for blood screening that is based on the Amplicor HCV test. Both assays have analytical sensitivities of less than 50 IU/ml.

Quantitative HCV Assays

Several assays are commercially available for quantification of HCV RNA levels in patients. These assays use conventional RT-PCR, bDNA, or real-time RT-PCR to amplify the HCV RNA. Most clinical laboratories use one of the US FDA-approved real-time RT-PCR (RT-qPCR) assays for determining HCV viral loads. The Amplicor HCV Monitor test v2.0 (Roche Diagnostics) is a quantitative RT-PCR assay that amplifies the same target region as the qualitative Amplicor HCV test. The assay uses an internal quantification standard to calculate the amount of HCV RNA in a sample. The assay has a sensitivity of 600 IU/ml and a 2.9 $\log_{10}$ dynamic range. Specimens with values greater than the upper limit of quantification (500,000 IU/ml) can be diluted 100-fold and retested as recommended by the manufacturer. The Amplicor HCV Monitor test is available in both manual microwell plate and semiautomated COBAS instrument (Roche Diagnostics) formats.

The Versant HCV RNA Assay v3.0 (Gen-Probe, Inc.) uses bDNA technology. The sensitivity of the Versant HCV RNA Assay v3.0 is 615 IU/ml, with a 4.1 $\log_{10}$ dynamic range. A number of changes to the design of the v3.0 test improved both the sensitivity and specificity over the v2.0 test. These include an increased number of capture probes, improved probe design, the use of non-natural synthetic nucleotides in detection probes, and redesigned label extenders. The System 340 bDNA analyzer (Gen-Probe, Inc.) automates all incubations, wash steps, readings, and data analysis. The instrument can process two 96-microwell plates per run.

Overall, the results of the Versant HCV RNA Assay v3.0 and the Amplicor HCV Monitor Test v2.0 have been found to be in substantial agreement [80, 81]. The results of the Amplicor Monitor test are reported as IU/ml and those of the Versant assay are reported as either copies/ml or IU/ml. Both tests have minimal HCV genotype bias and have similar analytical sensitivities. The Versant results tend to be more precise than the Amplicor Monitor results, but the Amplicor Monitor test is better able to discriminate low-positive from negative specimens. The Versant assay has a much greater dynamic range than the Amplicor Monitor test; however, a pretest sample dilution permits quantification of high viral load specimens by the Amplicor Monitor test. The throughput and level of automation are much greater with the Versant assay than with the Amplicor Monitor test.

The two US FDA-approved RT-qPCR assays for HCV viral load both amplify 5′UTR sequences but employ different amplicon detection probes. The probe in the Abbott RealTime HCV assay (Abbott Laboratories) is labeled with a 5′ fluorophore and a 3′ quencher. In the unhybridized state the probe assumes a random coil configuration that keeps the quencher in close proximity to the fluorophores and inhibits fluorescence. Upon hybridization to the target sequence the fluorophore and quencher are separated and fluorescent signal is produced. Reduced genotype bias is achieved by annealing the probe to the target at a relatively low temperature that permits probe binding despite mismatches between the probe and the target. Quantification is performed using an internal calibrator. The assay has a very low limit of detection (12 IU/ml) and quantification (12 IU/ml), and a 7 $\log_{10}$ dynamic range [82].

The Roche RT-qPCR assays (Roche Diagnostics) employ 5′ exonuclease probes from which the fluorophore and quencher are released as the probe is hydrolyzed by the action of the *Taq*Man DNA polymerase as it extends the primer during amplification. The assays are calibrated externally by the manufacturer and lot specific calibration coefficients are used by the system software to calculate the HCV RNA concentrations. An internal quantification standard is added prior to nucleic acid extraction to correct for the presence of any amplification inhibitors that may be present in the samples. The earlier versions of these assays had significant genotype bias, particularly with regard to genotype 4 [83–85]. The second versions of these assays were modified to improve genotype inclusivity by using a smaller sample input volume and redesigning the primer set [86]. The manual and fully automated versions of the assay differ in their limits of quantification and dynamic ranges (Table 46.6).

RT-qPCR assays have broader dynamic ranges than conventional RT-PCR and bDNA assays and limits of detection that are comparable to the available qualitative assays. Diagnostic testing and therapeutic monitoring therefore can be performed with a single test, greatly simplifying nucleic

Table 46.6 Commercial HCV RNA tests

Test (company)	Method	Lower limit of detection (IU/ml)	Dynamic range
Qualitative			
Amplicor HCV Test v2.0 (Roche Diagnostics, Indianapolis, IN)[a]	RT-PCR	50	NA
Versant HCV RNA Assay (Siemens Corp., Washington, DC)[a]	TMA	5	NA
Ampliscreen HCV Test v2.0 (Roche Diagnostics)[a]	RT-PCR	<50	NA
Procleix HIV-1/HCV Assay (Gen-Probe, Inc., San Mateo, CA)[a]	TMA	<50	NA
Quantitative			
Amplicor HCV Monitor Test v2.0 (Roche Diagnostics)	RT-PCR	600	$600–5\times10^5$
Versant HCV RNA Assay v3.0 (Siemens Corp.)[a]	bDNA	615	$615–7.7\times10^6$
CobasTaqMan HCV with High Pure System (Roche Diagnostics)[a]	Real-time RT-PCR	15	$25–3\times10^8$
CobasAmpliPrep/Cobas Taqman (Roche Diagnostics)[a]	Real-time RT-PCR	18	$43–6.9\times10^7$
RealTime HCV (Abbott Laboratories, Abbott Park, IL)[a]	Real-time RT-PCR	12	$12–1\times10^8$

NA not applicable
[a]US FDA-approved tests

acid testing. If conventional RT-PCR or bDNA assays are used, then an additional more sensitive qualitative test is needed to adequately assess treatment response. The package inserts for the protease inhibitors BOC and TVR include statements that an HCV assay with a lower limit of quantification ≤25 IU/ml should be used to monitor response to therapy.

HCV Genotyping Assays

A variety of laboratory-developed and commercial assays are used for HCV genotyping. The methods include nucleic acid sequencing, reverse hybridization, subtype-specific PCR, DNA fragment length polymorphism, heteroduplex mobility analysis, melting curve analysis, and serologic genotyping. Currently there is only one US FDA-approved HCV genotyping assay, the Abbott RealTime HCV Genotype II assay (Abbott Laboratories).

A commercially available reverse hybridization line probe assay is the most commonly used method for genotyping HCV among clinical laboratories participating in the HCV proficiency-testing surveys of the College of American Pathologists. This reverse hybridization assay was developed by Innogenetics and is now marketed as the Versant HCV Genotype 2.0 Assay (Siemens Corp.). In this line probe assay (LiPA), biotinylated PCR products from the 5′ UTR and core regions of the HCV genome are hybridized under stringent conditions with oligonucleotide probes attached to a nitrocellulose strip: 19 type- and subtype-specific probes interrogate the 5′UTR and an additional three probes interrogate the core region. The core region probes were added to provide better discrimination of subtypes 1a and 1b and genotype 6 [87]. Hybridized PCR products are detected with a streptavidin-alkaline phosphatase conjugate. The pattern of reactive lines defines the genotype and in some cases the subtype. The second-generation assay discriminates among genotypes 1a, 1b, 2a/c, 2b, 3a, 3b, 3c, 3k, 4a/c/d, 4b, 4e, 4h, 5a, and 6a/b. The results from the Versant HCV Genotype 2.0 Assay correlate well with results obtained by direct sequencing assays of the 5′ UTR and other genes at the genotype level and at distinguishing subtypes 1a and 1b, but may not be able to adequately identify the other subtypes [88]. Mixed genotype infections can be recognized as unusual patterns of hybridization signals. However, the LiPA requires a considerable amount of amplicon for typing, and the assay may regularly fail when the viral load is less than 10^4 copies/ml.

A DNA enzyme immunoassay (Sorin Biomedica, Irvine, CA) for HCV genotyping is based on hybridization of denatured amplicon from the core region to genotype-specific probes that are bound to the wells of a microtiter plate. Mouse monoclonal antibodies to double-stranded DNA are used to detect the hybrids. The results of the DNA enzyme immunoassay were highly concordant with the results of other genotyping methods in two evaluations [89, 90].

Sequence analysis of amplified subgenomic sequences is the most definitive way to genotype HCV strains. Genotyping schemes based on sequencing variable genes such as E1, C, and NS5B provide enough resolution to determine types and subtypes [29, 91]. The 5′ UTR is too highly conserved to discriminate all subtypes reliably. Genotyping methods targeting highly variable regions have higher failure rates due to primer mismatches and failed amplification reactions. Sequencing reactions can be performed directly on PCR products or on cloned amplicons. Mixed infections with multiple genotypes may be missed by sequence analysis. Definitive detection of mixed infections requires analysis of a large number of clones. Cloning may, however, emphasize artifactual nucleotide substitutions introduced by the DNA polymerase during amplification or by selection during the cloning procedure, and is generally not practical for the clinical laboratory.

The practice of using sequence analysis of a single subgenomic region for HCV genotyping has been challenged by the description of naturally occurring intergenotypic recombinants of two HCV genotypes [92–95]. The recombinant forms have been detected in patients in Russia (genotypes 2k and 1b), Vietnam (genotypes 2 and 6), and France (genotypes 2 and 5), as well as in experimentally infected chimpanzees (genotypes 1a and 1b).

A novel HCV genotyping method using a solid phase electrochemical array was developed by GenMark Diagnostics (Carlsbad, CA). The method uses sequence specific capture of a PCR amplicon from the HCV 5′UTR by surface-bound oligonucleotide capture probes formed within a preassembled monolayer with electrochemical detection using ferrocene-labeled oligonucleotide signal probes. High concordance between the GenMark and LiPA HCV genotyping (Siemens Corp.) tests were observed at the HCV genotype level; however, there were minor discrepancies in genotype 1 subtype identifications by the two tests due to differences in the regions of the HCV genome interrogated [96].

Laboratory-developed methods also are used to genotype HCV, including subtype-specific PCR [26], primer-specific and mispair extension analysis [97], nested restriction site-specific PCR [98], restriction fragment length polymorphism [99], heteroduplex mobility analysis [100], and melting-curve analysis with fluorescence resonance energy transfer probes [101, 102].

Interpretation of Test Results

The presence of HCV RNA in serum or plasma defines active infection, and HCV RNA is usually detectable within the first week after exposure. However, a single negative HCV RNA test result does not exclude the possibility of active infection because viremia may be intermittent in some chronically infected patients [103]. An HCV RNA test may be the only evidence of infection in individuals with false-negative antibody tests. False-negative HCV antibody tests can occur in HIV-1 infected individuals, patients undergoing hemodialysis, and patients with HCV-associated essential mixed cryoglobulinemia [104–106].

A negative HCV RNA test at the completion of therapy defines an end-of-treatment response (ETR), and a negative test 6 months after the completion of therapy defines a SVR. The test used to assess these treatment endpoints must have an analytical sensitivity or lower limit of detection of ≤10–15 IU/ml because the use of less sensitive tests can lead to misidentification of responders [107, 108].

HCV RNA quantitation is useful in planning duration of therapy and in predicting the likelihood of response to treatment. Patients with high HCV RNA levels tend to respond less well to IFN and ribavirin, but lengthening the course of therapy from 24 to 48 weeks more than doubles the response rate. Patients with viral loads greater than 600,000 IU/ml are considered to have high HCV RNA levels. HCV viral load does not predict disease progression, is not correlated with disease severity, and, consequently, should not be routinely monitored in untreated patients. Viral load testing can be used in an early assessment of viral kinetics in patients undergoing treatment with IFN and ribavirin. Patients who fail to achieve at least a 2 $\log_{10}$ decline in viral load after 12 weeks of treatment have little chance of an SVR and therapy should be discontinued. Viral genotyping helps inform the choice of therapy, predict the outcome of therapy and determine its duration as described above (Fig. 46.1). No association between genotype and disease progression or severity has been proven, so genotyping should be reserved for those patients being considered for treatment.

Laboratory Issues

The use of internal controls increases the confidence in negative HCV RNA test results and eliminates concerns that the test is falsely negative because of the presence of amplification inhibitors in the sample or poor recovery of the viral RNA. False-negative HCV RNA results also may occur if the specimen was not processed or stored appropriately due to the lability of the viral RNA. Serum or plasma should be separated from the cellular components of blood within 6 h of collection to avoid significant loss of HCV RNA. Once separated, the sample is stable for 3 days at 4 °C. Storage for longer periods should be at −70 °C.

False-positive HCV RNA tests can result from contamination of the sample with HCV target RNA or amplicon. However, widespread use of real-time PCR methods which combine target amplification and detection in a single tube has eliminated amplicon contamination as potential source of false-positive test results.

HCV RNA tests should be used for follow-up of low-positive HCV antibody screening tests if the RIBA is not available. Only the qualitative HCV RNA tests are US FDA approved for diagnosis but are not widely available in clinical laboratories. Although the quantitative tests are not intended for diagnostic use, the newer real-time PCR-based assays have similar sensitivity as the qualitative tests and should work well to diagnose both acute and chronic HCV infections.

Much has been written about the lack of agreement and the genotype bias of early commercially available versions of the HCV quantitative assays. The development the WHO First International HCV RNA standard and its acceptance by the manufacturers of these assays as a calibrator was a significant advance in HCV RNA quantification [109]. However, despite the implementation of an international standard, HCV RNA measurements are not equivalent between the different assays [85, 110]. Therefore, patients should be tested with the same assay during the course of their treatment to minimize the potential for patient management errors [111]. The major sources of this variability are differences in genotype bias between the assays and the fact that the WHO standard is an imperfect standard. Its value was derived from a consensus concentration obtained by diverse viral load assays in numerous laboratories rather than by an independent chemical method.

The widespread use of tests not cleared by the US FDA for HCV genotyping has placed an increased burden on clinical laboratories to verify the performance characteristics of these tests prior to clinical use. When validating HCV genotyping tests, laboratories should take advantage of the published evaluations and commercially available genotype panels to streamline the verification process.

The College of American Pathologists has a well-established proficiency testing program for laboratories performing tests for detection, quantification, and characterization of HCV RNA. These surveys have shown a steady improvement in the performance of laboratories over time that probably reflects progress in both the available technologies and laboratory practices.

Future Directions

Although the incidence of new HCV infections in the USA is declining, the number of individuals infected for more than 20 years who are at risk for serious complications is expected to increase until about the year 2015. In the 23 years since the discovery of HCV, the major route of transmission through blood transfusion has all but been eliminated, improvements in therapy have resulted in better response rates, and molecular tests have proven invaluable in the diagnosis and management of patients with HCV.

The CDC has expanded its previous recommendations for prevention and control of HCV infection to include antibody screening all persons born between 1945 and 1965.

Consequently, more infected individuals will be identified and many will be candidates for therapy. Several new classes of direct acting antiviral agents for HCV infection will be available soon, further increasing the number of candidates for therapy [112]. As new testing guidelines and therapies evolve, the number of molecular tests performed will increase and the test menu may change to include not only HCV viral load testing and taxonomic genotyping but analysis of mutations leading to antiviral resistance and predicting patients' responses to therapy. Refer to the website http://www.hcvguidelines.org/ for the latest recommendations. On the technology front, next-generation sequencing will become increasingly important in the analysis virus populations with applications in epidemiology, viral evolution, and antiviral resistance testing.

References

1. Blumberg BS, Alter HJ, Visnich S. A "New" antigen in leukemia sera. JAMA. 1965;191:541–6.
2. Choo QL, Kuo G, Weiner AJ, Overby LR, Bradley DW, Houghton M. Isolation of a cDNA clone derived from a blood-borne non-A, non-B viral hepatitis genome. Science. 1989;244:359–62.
3. Horvath R, Tegtmeier GE. Hepatitis B and D viruses. In: Versalovic J et al., editors. Manual of clinical microbiology. 10th ed. Washington, DC: ASM Press; 2011.
4. Chu CJ, Keeffe EB, Han SH, Perrillo RP, Min AD, Soldevila-Pico C, Carey W, Brown Jr RS, Luketic VA, Terrault N, Lok AS. Hepatitis B virus genotypes in the United States: results of a nationwide study. Gastroenterology. 2003;125:444–51.
5. Lok AS, McMahon BJ. Chronic hepatitis B: update 2009. Hepatology. 2009;50:661–2.
6. Kuhns MC, Busch MP. New strategies for blood donor screening for hepatitis B virus: nucleic acid testing versus immunoassay methods. Mol Diagn Ther. 2006;10:77–91.
7. Carman WF, Zanetti AR, Karayiannis P, Waters J, Manzillo G, Tanzi E, Zuckerman AJ, Thomas HC. Vaccine-induced escape mutant of hepatitis B virus. Lancet. 1990;336:325–9.
8. Hsu HY, Chang MH, Ni YH, Lin HH, Wang SM, Chen DS. Surface gene mutants of hepatitis B virus in infants who develop acute or chronic infections despite immunoprophylaxis. Hepatology. 1997;26:786–91.
9. McMahon G, Ehrlich PH, Moustafa ZA, McCarthy LA, Dottavio D, Tolpin MD, Nadler PI, Ostberg L. Genetic alterations in the gene encoding the major HBsAg: DNA and immunological analysis of recurrent HBsAg derived from monoclonal antibody-treated liver transplant patients. Hepatology. 1992;15:757–66.
10. Hillyard DR. Molecular detection and characterization of hepatitis B virus. In: Persing DH et al., editors. Molecular microbiology: diagnostic principles and practice, vol. 2. 2nd ed. Washington, DC: ASM Press; 2011. p. 579.
11. Okamoto H, Tsuda F, Akahane Y, Sugai Y, Yoshiba M, Moriyama K, Tanaka T, Miyakawa Y, Mayumi M. Hepatitis B virus with mutations in the core promoter for an e antigen-negative phenotype in carriers with antibody to e antigen. J Virol. 1994;68:8102–10.
12. Carman WF, Jacyna MR, Hadziyannis S, Karayiannis P, McGarvey MJ, Makris A, Thomas HC. Mutation preventing formation of hepatitis B e antigen in patients with chronic hepatitis B infection. Lancet. 1989;2:588–91.
13. Miyakawa Y, Okamoto H, Mayumi M. The molecular basis of hepatitis B e antigen (HBeAg)-negative infections. J Viral Hepat. 1997;4:1–8.
14. Degertekin B, Lok AS. Indications for therapy in hepatitis B. Hepatology. 2009;49:S129–37.
15. Andersson KL, Chung RT. Monitoring during and after antiviral therapy for hepatitis B. Hepatology. 2009;49:S166–73.
16. Hussain M, Chu CJ, Sablon E, Lok AS. Rapid and sensitive assays for determination of hepatitis B virus (HBV) genotypes and detection of HBV precore and core promoter variants. J Clin Microbiol. 2003;41:3699–705.
17. Osiowy C, Giles E. Evaluation of the INNO-LiPA HBV genotyping assay for determination of hepatitis B virus genotype. J Clin Microbiol. 2003;41:5473–7.
18. Lok AS, McMahon BJ. Chronic hepatitis B. Hepatology. 2001;34:1225–41.
19. Chu CJ, Lok AS. Clinical utility in quantifying serum HBV DNA levels using PCR assays. J Hepatol. 2002;36:549–51.
20. Chu CJ, Hussain M, Lok AS. Quantitative serum HBV DNA levels during different stages of chronic hepatitis B infection. Hepatology. 2002;36:1408–15.
21. Yim HJ, Hussain M, Liu Y, Wong SN, Fung SK, Lok AS. Evolution of multi-drug resistant hepatitis B virus during sequential therapy. Hepatology. 2006;44:703–12.
22. Saldanha J, Gerlich W, Lelie N, Dawson P, Heermann K, Heath A. An international collaborative study to establish a World Health Organization international standard for hepatitis B virus DNA nucleic acid amplification techniques. Vox Sang. 2001;80:63–71.
23. Solmone M, Vincenti D, Prosperi MC, Bruselles A, Ippolito G, Capobianchi MR. Use of massively parallel ultradeep pyrosequencing to characterize the genetic diversity of hepatitis B virus in drug-resistant and drug-naive patients and to detect minor variants in reverse transcriptase and hepatitis B S antigen. J Virol. 2009;83:1718–26.
24. Margeridon-Thermet S, Shulman NS, Ahmed A, Shahriar R, Liu T, Wang C, Holmes SP, Babrzadeh F, Gharizadeh B, Hanczaruk B, Simen BB, Egholm M, Shafer RW. Ultra-deep pyrosequencing of hepatitis B virus quasispecies from nucleoside and nucleotide reverse-transcriptase inhibitor (NRTI)-treated patients and NRTI-naive patients. J Infect Dis. 2009;199:1275–85.
25. Choo QL, Richman KH, Han JH, Berger K, Lee C, Dong C, Gallegos C, Coit D, Medina-Selby R, Barr PJ, et al. Genetic organization and diversity of the hepatitis C virus. Proc Natl Acad Sci U S A. 1991;88:2451–5.
26. Okamoto H, Kurai K, Okada S, Yamamoto K, Lizuka H, Tanaka T, Fukuda S, Tsuda F, Mishiro S. Full-length sequence of a hepatitis C virus genome having poor homology to reported isolates: comparative study of four distinct genotypes. Virology. 1992; 188:331–41.
27. Smith DB, Bukh J, Kuiken C, Muerhoff S, Rice CM, Stapleton JT, Simmonds P. Expanded classification of hepatitis C virus into 7 genotypes and 67 subtypes: updated criteria and genotype assignment web resource. Hepatology. 2014;59:318–27.
26. Dusheiko G, Schmilovitz-Weiss H, Brown D, McOmish F, Yap PL, Sherlock S, McIntyre N, Simmonds P. Hepatitis C virus genotypes: an investigation of type-specific differences in geographic origin and disease. Hepatology. 1994;19:13–8.
29. Simmonds P, Holmes EC, Cha TA, Chan SW, McOmish F, Irvine B, Beall E, Yap PL, Kolberg J, Urdea MS. Classification of hepatitis C virus into six major genotypes and a series of subtypes by phylogenetic analysis of the NS-5 region. J Gen Virol. 1993; 74:2391–9.
30. Murphy DG, Willems B, Deschênes M, Hilzenat N, Mousseau R, Sabbah S. Use of sequence analysis with reference to C/E1 and 5′ untranslated region sequences. J Clin Microbiol. 2007;45: 1102–12.

31. Benvegnu L, Pontisso P, Cavalletto D, Noventa F, Chemello L, Alberti A. Lack of correlation between hepatitis C virus genotypes and clinical course of hepatitis C virus-related cirrhosis. Hepatology. 1997;25:211–5.
32. Poynard T, Bedossa P, Opolon P. Natural history of liver fibrosis progression in patients with chronic hepatitis C. The OBSVIRC, METAVIR, CLINIVIR, and DOSVIRC groups. Lancet. 1997;349: 825–32.
33. Centers for Disease Control and Prevention. Recommendations for prevention and control of hepatitis C virus (HCV) infection and HCV-related chronic disease. MMWR Recomm Rep. 1998;47:1–39.
34. Ghany MG, Strader DB, Thomas DL, Seeff LB. Diagnosis, management, and treatment of hepatitis C: an update. Hepatology. 2009;49:1335–74.
35. Dufour DR, Lott JA, Nolte FS, Gretch DR, Koff RS, Seeff LB. Diagnosis and monitoring of hepatic injury. II. Recommendations for use of laboratory tests in screening, diagnosis, and monitoring. Clin Chem. 2000;46:2050–68.
36. Alter MJ, Kuhnert WL, Finelli L. Guidelines for laboratory testing and result reporting of antibody to hepatitis C virus. Centers for Disease Control and Prevention. MMWR Recomm Rep. 2003; 52(1-13):15.
37. Centers for Disease Control and Prevention. Testing for HCV infection: an update of Guidance for Clinicians and Laboratorians. MMWR Recomm Rep. 2013;62:362–5.
38. Fanning L, Kenny-Walsh E, Levis J, Choudhury KR, Cannon B, Sheehan M, Whelton M, Shanahan F. Natural fluctuations of hepatitis C viral load in a homogeneous patient population: a prospective study. Hepatology. 2000;31:225–9.
39. Schreiber GB, Busch MP, Kleinman SH, Korelitz JJ. The risk of transfusion-transmitted viral infections. The Retrovirus Epidemiology Donor Study. N Engl J Med. 1996;334:1685–90.
40. Legler TJ, Riggert J, Simson G, Wolf C, Humpe A, Munzel U, Uy A, Kohler M, Heermann KH. Testing of individual blood donations for HCV RNA reduces the residual risk of transfusion-transmitted HCV infection. Transfusion. 2000;40:1192–7.
41. Kolk DP, Dockter J, Linnen J, Ho-Sing-Loy M, Gillotte-Taylor K, McDonough SH, Mimms L, Giachetti C. Significant closure of the human immunodeficiency virus type 1 and hepatitis C virus preseroconversion detection windows with a transcription-mediated-amplification-driven assay. J Clin Microbiol. 2002;40:1761–6.
42. Icardi G, Ansaldi F, Bruzzone BM, Durando P, Lee S, de Luigi C, Crovari P. Novel approach to reduce the hepatitis C virus (HCV) window period: clinical evaluation of a new enzyme-linked immunosorbent assay for HCV core antigen. J Clin Microbiol. 2001;39: 3110–4.
43. Bouvier-Alias M, Patel K, Dahari H, Beaucourt S, Larderie P, Blatt L, Hezode C, Picchio G, Dhumeaux D, Neumann AU, McHutchison JG, Pawlotsky JM. Clinical utility of total HCV core antigen quantification: a new indirect marker of HCV replication. Hepatology. 2002;36:211–8.
44. Veillon P, Payan C, Picchio G, Maniez-Montreuil M, Guntz P, Lunel F. Comparative evaluation of the total hepatitis C virus core antigen, branched-DNA, and amplicor monitor assays in determining viremia for patients with chronic hepatitis C during interferon plus ribavirin combination therapy. J Clin Microbiol. 2003;41:3212–20.
45. Mederacke I, Wedemeyer H, Ciesek S, Steinmann E, Raupach R, Wursthorn K, Manns MP, Tillmann HL. Performance and clinical utility of a novel fully automated quantitative HCV-core antigen assay. J Clin Virol. 2009;46:210–5.
46. Morota K, Fujinami R, Kinukawa H, Machida T, Ohno K, Saegusa H, Takeda K. A new sensitive and automated chemiluminescent microparticle immunoassay for quantitative determination of hepatitis C virus core antigen. J Virol Methods. 2009;157:8–14.
47. McHutchison JG, Gordon SC, Schiff ER, Shiffman ML, Lee WM, Rustgi VK, Goodman ZD, Ling MH, Cort S, Albrecht JK. Interferon alfa-2b alone or in combination with ribavirin as initial treatment for chronic hepatitis C. Hepatitis Interventional Therapy Group. N Engl J Med. 1998;339:1485–92.
48. Poynard T, Marcellin P, Lee SS, Niederau C, Minuk GS, Ideo G, Bain V, Heathcote J, Zeuzem S, Trepo C, Albrecht J. Randomised trial of interferon alpha2b plus ribavirin for 48 weeks or for 24 weeks versus interferon alpha2b plus placebo for 48 weeks for treatment of chronic infection with hepatitis C virus. International Hepatitis Interventional Therapy Group (IHIT). Lancet. 1998;352:1426–32.
49. Thompson AJ, Muir AJ, Sulkowski MS, Ge D, Fellay J, Shianna KV, Urban T, Afdhal NH, Jacobson IM, Esteban R, Poordad F, Lawitz EJ, McCone J, Shiffman ML, Galler GW, Lee WM, Reindollar R, King JW, Kwo PY, Ghalib RH, Freilich B, Nyberg LM, Zeuzem S, Poynard T, Vock DM, Pieper KS, Patel K, Tillmann HL, Noviello S, Koury K, Pedicone LD, Brass CA, Albrecht JK, Goldstein DB, McHutchison JG. Interleukin-28B polymorphism improves viral kinetics and is the strongest pretreatment predictor of sustained virologic response in genotype 1 hepatitis C virus. Gastroenterology. 2010;139(120-129):e118.
50. Mangia A, Thompson AJ, Santoro R, Piazzolla V, Tillmann HL, Patel K, Shianna KV, Mottola L, Petruzzellis D, Bacca D, Carretta V, Minerva N, Goldstein DB, McHutchison JG. An IL28B polymorphism determines treatment response of hepatitis C virus genotype 2 or 3 patients who do not achieve a rapid virologic response. Gastroenterology. 2010;139:821–7. 827.e821.
51. McCormick SE, Goodman ZD, Maydonovitch CL, Sjogren MH. Evaluation of liver histology, ALT elevation, and HCV RNA titer in patients with chronic hepatitis C. Am J Gastroenterol. 1996;91:1516–22.
52. Ghany MG, Nelson DR, Strader DB, Thomas DL, Seeff LB. An update on treatment of genotype 1 chronic hepatitis C virus infection: 2011 practice guideline by the American Association for the Study of Liver Diseases. Hepatology. 2011;54:1433–44.
53. Lawitz E, Mangia A, Wyles D, Rodriguez-Torres M, Hassanien T, Gordon SC, Schultz M, Davis MN, Kayali Z, Reddy KR, et al. Sofosbuvir for previously untreated chronic hepatitis C. N Engl J Med. 2013;368:1878–87.
54. Fried MW, Buti M, Dore GJ, Flisiak R, Ferenci P, Jacobson I, Marcellin P, Manns M, Nitkin I, Poordad F, et al. Once-daily simeprevir (TMC435) with pegylated interferon and ribavirin in treatment-naïve genotype 1 Hepatitic C: the randomized PILLAR study. Hepatology. 2013;58:1918–29.
55. Hohne M, Schreier E, Roggendorf M. Sequence variability in the env-coding region of hepatitis C virus isolated from patients infected during a single source outbreak. Arch Virol. 1994; 137:25–34.
56. Power JP, Lawlor E, Davidson F, Holmes EC, Yap PL, Simmonds P. Molecular epidemiology of an outbreak of infection with hepatitis C virus in recipients of anti-D immunoglobulin. Lancet. 1995;345:1211–3.
57. Bronowicki JP, Venard V, Botte C, Monhoven N, Gastin I, Chone L, Hudziak H, Rihn B, Delanoe C, LeFaou A, Bigard MA, Gaucher P. Patient-to-patient transmission of hepatitis C virus during colonoscopy. N Engl J Med. 1997;337:237–40.
58. Aizaki H, Saito A, Kusakawa I, Ashiwara Y, Nagamori S, Toda G, Suzuki T, Ishii K, Matsuura Y, Miyamura T. Mother-to-child transmission of a hepatitis C virus variant with an insertional mutation in its hypervariable region. J Hepatol. 1996;25:608–13.
59. Chayama K, Kobayashi M, Tsubota A, Koida I, Arase Y, Saitoh S, Ikeda K, Kumada H. Molecular analysis of intraspousal transmission of hepatitis C virus. J Hepatol. 1995;22:431–9.
60. Healey CJ, Smith DB, Walker JL, Holmes EC, Fleming KA, Chapman RW, Simmonds P. Acute hepatitis C infection after sexual exposure. Gut. 1995;36:148–50.

61. Weiner AJ, Thaler MM, Crawford K, Ching K, Kansopon J, Chien DY, Hall JE, Hu F, Houghton M. A unique, predominant hepatitis C virus variant found in an infant born to a mother with multiple variants. J Virol. 1993;67:4365–8.
62. Enomoto N, Sakuma I, Asahina Y, Kurosaki M, Murakami T, Yamamoto C, Ogura Y, Izumi N, Marumo F, Sato C. Mutations in the nonstructural protein 5A gene and response to interferon in patients with chronic hepatitis C virus 1b infection. N Engl J Med. 1996;334:77–81.
63. Watanabe H, Enomoto N, Nagayama K, Izumi N, Marumo F, Sato C, Watanabe M. Number and position of mutations in the interferon (IFN) sensitivity-determining region of the gene for nonstructural protein 5A correlate with IFN efficacy in hepatitis C virus genotype 1b infection. J Infect Dis. 2001;183:1195–203.
64. Hofgartner WT, Polyak SJ, Sullivan DG, Carithers Jr RL, Gretch DR. Mutations in the NS5A gene of hepatitis C virus in North American patients infected with HCV genotype 1a or 1b. J Med Virol. 1997;53:118–26.
65. Sarrazin C, Berg T, Lee JH, Teuber G, Dietrich CF, Roth WK, Zeuzem S. Improved correlation between multiple mutations within the NS5A region and virological response in European patients chronically infected with hepatitis C virus type 1b undergoing combination therapy. J Hepatol. 1999;30:1004–13.
66. Sarrazin C, Kieffer TL, Bartels D, Hanzelka B, Muh U, Welker M, Wincheringer D, Zhou Y, Chu HM, Lin C, Weegink C, Reesink H, Zeuzem S, Kwong AD. Dynamic hepatitis C virus genotypic and phenotypic changes in patients treated with the protease inhibitor telaprevir. Gastroenterology. 2007;132:1767–77.
67. Pawlotsky JM. Treatment failure and resistance with direct-acting antiviral drugs against hepatitis C virus. Hepatology. 2011;53:1742–51.
68. Olysio prescribing information. Janssen Therapeutics, Titusville, NJ. Reference ID 3412095, 2013
69. Ge D, Fellay J, Thompson AJ, Simon JS, Shianna KV, Urban TJ, Heinzen EL, Qiu P, Bertelsen AH, Muir AJ, Sulkowski M, McHutchison JG, Goldstein DB. Genetic variation in IL28B predicts hepatitis C treatment-induced viral clearance. Nature. 2009;461:399–401.
70. Thomas DL, Thio CL, Martin MP, Qi Y, Ge D, O'Huigin C, Kidd J, Kidd K, Khakoo SI, Alexander G, Goedert JJ, Kirk GD, Donfield SM, Rosen HR, Tobler LH, Busch MP, McHutchison JG, Goldstein DB, Carrington M. Genetic variation in IL28B and spontaneous clearance of hepatitis C virus. Nature. 2009;461:798–801.
71. Suppiah V, Moldovan M, Ahlenstiel G, Berg T, Weltman M, Abate ML, Bassendine M, Spengler U, Dore GJ, Powell E, Riordan S, Sheridan D, Smedile A, Fragomeli V, Muller T, Bahlo M, Stewart GJ, Booth DR, George J. IL28B is associated with response to chronic hepatitis C interferon-alpha and ribavirin therapy. Nat Genet. 2009;41:1100–4.
72. Tanaka Y, Nishida N, Sugiyama M, Kurosaki M, Matsuura K, Sakamoto N, Nakagawa M, Korenaga M, Hino K, Hige S, Ito Y, Mita E, Tanaka E, Mochida S, Murawaki Y, Honda M, Sakai A, Hiasa Y, Nishiguchi S, Koike A, Sakaida I, Imamura M, Ito K, Yano K, Masaki N, Sugauchi F, Izumi N, Tokunaga K, Mizokami M. Genome-wide association of IL28B with response to pegylated interferon-alpha and ribavirin therapy for chronic hepatitis C. Nat Genet. 2009;41:1105–9.
73. Lee SC, Antony A, Lee N, Leibow J, Yang JQ, Soviero S, Gutekunst K, Rosenstraus M. Improved version 2.0 qualitative and quantitative AMPLICOR reverse transcription-PCR tests for hepatitis C virus RNA: calibration to international units, enhanced genotype reactivity, and performance characteristics. J Clin Microbiol. 2000;38:4171–9.
74. Nolte FS, Fried MW, Shiffman ML, Ferreira-Gonzalez A, Garrett CT, Schiff ER, Polyak SJ, Gretch DR. Prospective multicenter clinical evaluation of AMPLICOR and COBAS AMPLICOR hepatitis C virus tests. J Clin Microbiol. 2001;39:4005–12.
75. Comanor L, Anderson F, Ghany M, Perrillo R, Heathcote EJ, Sherlock C, Zitron I, Hendricks D, Gordon SC. Transcription-mediated amplification is more sensitive than conventional PCR-based assays for detecting residual serum HCV RNA at end of treatment. Am J Gastroenterol. 2001;96:2968–72.
76. Sarrazin C, Teuber G, Kokka R, Rabenau H, Zeuzem S. Detection of residual hepatitis C virus RNA by transcription-mediated amplification in patients with complete virologic response according to polymerase chain reaction-based assays. Hepatology. 2000;32:818–23.
77. Sarrazin C, Hendricks DA, Sedarati F, Zeuzem S. Assessment, by transcription-mediated amplification, of virologic response in patients with chronic hepatitis C virus treated with peginterferon alpha-2a. J Clin Microbiol. 2001;39:2850–5.
78. Krajden M, Ziermann R, Khan A, Mak A, Leung K, Hendricks D, Comanor L. Qualitative detection of hepatitis C virus RNA: comparison of analytical sensitivity, clinical performance, and workflow of the Cobas Amplicor HCV test version 2.0 and the HCV RNA transcription-mediated amplification qualitative assay. J Clin Microbiol. 2002;40:2903–7.
79. Jackson JB, Smith K, Knott C, Korpela A, Simmons A, Piwowar-Manning E, McDonough S, Mimms L, Vargo JM. Sensitivity of the Procleix HIV-1/HCV assay for detection of human immunodeficiency virus type 1 and hepatitis C virus RNA in a high-risk population. J Clin Microbiol. 2002;40:2387–91.
80. Beld M, Sentjens R, Rebers S, Weegink C, Weel J, Sol C, Boom R. Performance of the New Bayer VERSANT HCV RNA 3.0 assay for quantitation of hepatitis C virus RNA in plasma and serum: conversion to international units and comparison with the Roche COBAS Amplicor HCV Monitor, Version 2.0, assay. J Clin Microbiol. 2002;40:788–93.
81. Germer JJ, Heimgartner PJ, Ilstrup DM, Harmsen WS, Jenkins GD, Patel R. Comparative evaluation of the VERSANT HCV RNA 3.0, QUANTIPLEX HCV RNA 2.0, and COBAS AMPLICOR HCV MONITOR version 2.0 Assays for quantification of hepatitis C virus RNA in serum. J Clin Microbiol. 2002;40:495–500.
82. Caliendo AM, Valsamakis A, Zhou Y, Yen-Lieberman B, Andersen J, Young S, Ferreira-Gonzalez A, Tsongalis GJ, Pyles R, Bremer JW, Lurain NS. Multilaboratory comparison of hepatitis C virus viral load assays. J Clin Microbiol. 2006;44:1726–32.
83. Chevaliez S, Bouvier-Alias M, Pawlotsky JM. Performance of the Abbott real-time PCR assay using m2000sp and m2000rt for hepatitis C virus RNA quantification. J Clin Microbiol. 2009;47:1726–32.
84. Germer JJ, Kathrotiya JD, Bouse CF, Mitchell PS, Yao JD. Anomalous quantitation standard growth curves in a laboratory-developed hepatitis C virus (HCV) RNA quantification assay using the TaqMan HCV analyte-specific reagent. J Clin Microbiol. 2009;47:2317–20.
85. Pyne MT, Konnick EQ, Phansalkar A, Hillyard DR. Evaluation of the Abbott investigational use only RealTime hepatitis C virus (HCV) assay and comparison to the Roche TaqMan HCV analyte-specific reagent assay. J Clin Microbiol. 2009;47:2872–8.
86. Vermehren J, Colucci G, Gohl P, Hamdi N, Abdelaziz AI, Karey U, Thamke D, Zitzer H, Zeuzem S, Sarrazin C. Development of a second version of the Cobas AmpliPrep/Cobas TaqMan hepatitis C virus quantitative test with improved genotype inclusivity. J Clin Microbiol. 2011;49:3309–15.

87. Verbeeck J, Stanley MJ, Shieh J, Celis L, Huyck E, Wollants E, Morimoto J, Farrior A, Sablon E, Jankowski-Hennig M, Schaper C, Johnson P, Van Ranst M, Van Brussel M. Evaluation of Versant hepatitis C virus genotype assay (LiPA) 2.0. J Clin Microbiol. 2008;46:1901–6.
88. Bouchardeau F, Cantaloube JF, Chevaliez S, Portal C, Razer A, Lefrere JJ, Pawlotsky JM, De Micco P, Laperche S. Improvement of hepatitis C virus (HCV) genotype determination with the new version of the INNO-LiPA HCV assay. J Clin Microbiol. 2007;45:1140–5.
89. Viazov S, Zibert A, Ramakrishnan K, Widell A, Cavicchini A, Schreier E, Roggendorf M. Typing of hepatitis C virus isolates by DNA enzyme immunoassay. J Virol Methods. 1994;48:81–91.
90. Ross RS, Viazov SO, Holtzer CD, Beyou A, Monnet A, Mazure C, Roggendorf M. Genotyping of hepatitis C virus isolates using CLIP sequencing. J Clin Microbiol. 2000;38:3581–4.
91. Bukh J, Miller RH, Purcell RH. Genetic heterogeneity of hepatitis C virus: quasispecies and genotypes. Semin Liver Dis. 1995;15: 41–63.
92. Kalinina O, Norder H, Mukomolov S, Magnius LO. A natural intergenotypic recombinant of hepatitis C virus identified in St. Petersburg. J Virol. 2002;76:4034–43.
93. Noppornpanth S, Lien TX, Poovorawan Y, Smits SL, Osterhaus AD, Haagmans BL. Identification of a naturally occurring recombinant genotype 2/6 hepatitis C virus. J Virol. 2006;80: 7569–77.
94. Legrand-Abravanel F, Claudinon J, Nicot F, Dubois M, Chapuy-Regaud S, Sandres-Saune K, Pasquier C, Izopet J. New natural intergenotypic (2/5) recombinant of hepatitis C virus. J Virol. 2007;81:4357–62.
95. Gao F, Nainan OV, Khudyakov Y, Li J, Hong Y, Gonzales AC, Spelbring J, Margolis HS. Recombinant hepatitis C virus in experimentally infected chimpanzees. J Gen Virol. 2007;88:143–7.
96. Sam SS, Steinmetz HB, Tsongalis GJ, Tafe LJ, Lefferts JA. Validation of a solid-phase electrochemical array for genotyping hepatitis C virus. Exp Mol Pathol. 2013;95:18–22.
97. Hu YW, Balaskas E, Kessler G, Issid C, Scully LJ, Murphy DG, Rinfret A, Giulivi A, Scalia V, Gill P. Primer specific and mispair extension analysis (PSMEA) as a simple approach to fast genotyping. Nucleic Acids Res. 1998;26:5013–5.
98. Krekulova L, Rehak V, Wakil AE, Harris E, Riley LW. Nested restriction site-specific PCR to detect and type hepatitis C virus (HCV): a rapid method to distinguish HCV subtype 1b from other genotypes. J Clin Microbiol. 2001;39:1774–80.
99. Davidson F, Simmonds P, Ferguson JC, Jarvis LM, Dow BC, Follett EA, Seed CR, Krusius T, Lin C, Medgyesi GA, et al. Survey of major genotypes and subtypes of hepatitis C virus using RFLP of sequences amplified from the 5′ non-coding region. J Gen Virol. 1995;76:1197–204.
100. White PA, Zhai X, Carter I, Zhao Y, Rawlinson WD. Simplified hepatitis C virus genotyping by heteroduplex mobility analysis. J Clin Microbiol. 2000;38:477–82.
101. Bullock GC, Bruns DE, Haverstick DM. Hepatitis C genotype determination by melting curve analysis with a single set of fluorescence resonance energy transfer probes. Clin Chem. 2002;48:2147–54.
102. Schroter M, Zollner B, Schafer P, Landt O, Lass U, Laufs R, Feucht HH. Genotyping of hepatitis C virus types 1, 2, 3, and 4 by a one-step LightCycler method using three different pairs of hybridization probes. J Clin Microbiol. 2002;40:2046–50.
103. Busch MP. Insights into the epidemiology, natural history and pathogenesis of hepatitis C virus infection from studies of infected donors and blood product recipients. Transfus Clin Biol. 2001;8:200–6.
104. Agnello V, Chung RT, Kaplan LM. A role for hepatitis C virus infection in type II cryoglobulinemia. N Engl J Med. 1992;327: 1490–5.
105. Cribier B, Rey D, Schmitt C, Lang JM, Kirn A, Stoll-Keller F. High hepatitis C viraemia and impaired antibody response in patients coinfected with HIV. AIDS. 1995;9:1131–6.
106. Fabrizi F, Poordad FF, Martin P. Hepatitis C infection and the patient with end-stage renal disease. Hepatology. 2002;36:3–10.
107. Morishima C, Morgan TR, Everhart JE, Wright EC, Apodaca MC, Gretch DR, Shiffman ML, Everson GT, Lindsay KL, Lee WM, Lok AS, Dienstag JL, Ghany MG, Curto TM. Interpretation of positive transcription-mediated amplification test results from polymerase chain reaction-negative samples obtained after treatment of chronic hepatitis C. Hepatology. 2008;48:1412–9.
108. Carlsson T, Quist A, Weiland O. Rapid viral response and treatment outcome in genotype 2 and 3 chronic hepatitis C: comparison between two HCV RNA quantitation methods. J Med Virol. 2008;80:803–7.
109. Saldanha J, Lelie N, Heath A. Establishment of the first international standard for nucleic acid amplification technology (NAT) assays for HCV RNA. WHO Collaborative Study Group. Vox Sang. 1999;76:149–58.
110. Michelin BD, Muller Z, Stelzl E, Marth E, Kessler HH. Evaluation of the Abbott RealTime HCV assay for quantitative detection of hepatitis C virus RNA. J Clin Virol. 2007;38:96–100.
111. Laperche S, Bouchardeau F, Thibault V, Pozzetto B, Vallet S, Rosenberg AR, Roque-Afonso AM, Gassin M, Stoll-Keller F, Trimoulet P, Gault E, Chanzy B, Mercier B, Branger M, Pawlotsky JM, Henquell C, Lunel F, Gaudy-Graffin C, Alain S, Chaix ML, Duverlie G, Izopet J, Lefrere JJ. Multicenter trials need to use the same assay for hepatitis C virus viral load determination. J Clin Microbiol. 2007;45:3788–90.
112. Rice CM, Saeed M. Hepatitis C treatment triumphs. Nature. 2014;510:43–4.

Viral Infections in Transplant Recipients

47

Raymund R. Razonable and Randall T. Hayden

Abstract

Viruses are major opportunistic pathogens that cause significant morbidity and mortality after transplantation. They do not only cause direct clinical illness, but have indirect effects that increase the risk of graft failure and mortality. The clinical presentation of viral infections is very nonspecific, and hence, the role of the clinical laboratory is essential in confirming diagnosis. There have been remarkable improvements in the laboratory diagnosis and monitoring of viral infections, with the evolution from conventional culture methods to more sensitive molecular assays. A number of nucleic acid-based detection assays are currently used in clinical practice for the diagnosis, surveillance, and monitoring of viral infections in transplant patients. Some have the ability to quantify viral load, which is useful for differentiating latent from active infection, for differentiating mild from potentially severe disease, and for monitoring therapeutic response.

The majority of molecular tests for viral diagnosis in transplantation lack standardization, and their clinical uses across different testing sites have been difficult. Variability in specimen type, nucleic acid extraction methods, target sequence, limit of detection, and quantitative and calibration standard are some of the reasons for varying viral load reports from different assays. This lack of standardization not only complicates management of individual patients, but also hampers the development of consensus interpretive and treatment guidelines. This book chapter discusses the clinical application of molecular tests for the diagnosis of adenovirus, BK virus, parvovirus B19, cytomegalovirus, Epstein Barr virus, and the other members of the herpes virus family.

Keywords

Viral infections • Transplantation • Herpes viruses • Polyomaviruses • Parvovirus • Adenovirus • Cytomegalovirus

Introduction

Transplantation is a standard treatment modality for many end-stage clinical illnesses that would otherwise be fatal. The use of immunosuppressive drugs, which are essential to prevent and treat graft rejection after solid organ transplantation (SOT) and graft-vs-host disease (GVHD) after allogeneic hematopoietic stem cell transplantation (HSCT), increases the risk of opportunistic infections.

R.R. Razonable, M.D., F.I.D.S.A.
Division of Infectious Diseases, Department of Internal Medicine, Mayo Clinic, Rochester, MN, USA

R.T. Hayden, M.D. (✉)
Department of Pathology, St. Jude Children's Research Hospital, 262 Danny Thomas Place, Room C5025, Mailstop #250, Memphis, TN, 38105-3678, USA
e-mail: Randall.Hayden@stjude.org

D.G.B. Leonard (ed.), *Molecular Pathology in Clinical Practice*, DOI 10.1007/978-3-319-19674-9_47

Viruses are major opportunistic pathogens that cause significant morbidity and mortality after SOT and HSCT [1]. Viruses not only cause clinical syndromes directly, but also have indirect effects that increase the risk of graft failure and mortality [1]. The clinical presentation of viral diseases in transplant recipients can be classic or atypical with non-specific manifestations. Hence, the role of the clinical laboratory is essential in confirming clinical suspicions of viral infection [2]. In this regard, the last decade has seen remarkable improvements in the laboratory diagnosis and monitoring of viral infections. Test methods have evolved (and continue to evolve) from conventional culture methods to more sensitive molecular assays. Conventional methods have slow turnaround time and poor sensitivity, while molecular tests, which rely on the detection of viral nucleic acids, provide rapid turnaround time and improved sensitivity.

A number of nucleic acid-based detection assays (also known as nucleic acid tests [NATs]) are currently used in clinical practice for the diagnosis, surveillance, and monitoring of viral infections in transplant patients, but the most widely used are based on the polymerase chain reaction (PCR) (Table 47.1) [2]. Other molecular methods used in the clinical laboratory are based on RNA amplification (nucleic acid sequence based amplification and transcription-mediated amplification) and on signal amplification. Some NATs quantify the amount of virus in a sample (defined as the viral load), which is useful for differentiating latent from active infection, for differentiating mild from potentially severe disease, and for monitoring therapeutic response.

The increased sensitivity of molecular tests for viral detection has posed an important challenge in differentiating active from latent infection. A number of viruses that cause clinical disease in transplant recipients exist in a latent state, and there is concern that highly sensitive molecular assays may detect nucleic acid from such latent, non-replicating viruses in the absence of active disease. If not interpreted in the proper clinical context, this may lead to unnecessary treatment.

Table 47.1 Clinical utility of molecular diagnostic tests for viruses in transplantation

Clinical use	General assay characteristics	Specific clinical applications
Diagnosis	Rapid turnaround time thereby facilitating targeted antiviral therapy Highly specific for the pathogen of interest More sensitive than conventional methods such as culture High sensitivity may detect latent virus: viral quantification or detection of viral RNA may aid in the differentiation of replicating from latent virus	Nucleic acid tests for adenovirus, BK virus, parvovirus B19, herpes simplex virus, varicella zoster virus, cytomegalovirus, Epstein Barr virus, and other herpesviruses are sensitive and rapid methods for confirming clinical suspicion of specific viral diseases
Surveillance	Guide initiation of preemptive therapy strategy Identifies patients at high risk of clinical disease (risk stratification) Identifies patients at high risk of treatment failure and relapse (prognosis)	Surveillance for cytomegalovirus infection by nucleic acid testing guides the initiation of antiviral treatment prior to the onset of clinical disease Surveillance for BK virus in kidney transplant recipients identifies infection prior to the onset of nephropathy, thereby allowing preemptive reduction in immunosuppression as treatment Surveillance for Epstein Barr virus infection identifies patients at high risk of post-transplant lymphoproliferative disease High cytomegalovirus and Epstein Barr virus viral loads indicate high risk of clinical disease, although widely applicable viral thresholds have been difficult to define due to lack of assay standardization
Monitor treatment responses	Guide the duration of antiviral therapy Early indicator of risk of treatment failure Early indicator of disease relapse Early indicator of the emergence of resistant viruses	Treatment of cytomegalovirus disease is generally continued until the virus is undetectable by a sensitive PCR test Viral load testing for cytomegalovirus, Epstein Barr virus, and BK virus generally decline following initiation of a successful treatment strategy Rise in cytomegalovirus, Epstein Barr virus, and BK virus viral load during treatment indicates relapse, an over-immunosuppressed state, or the possible emergence of drug resistance

Table 47.2 Factors contributing to the variability in viral load reporting among different laboratories

Assay platform
Clinical specimen type
Pipetting technique
Nucleic acid extraction method
Molecular amplification target gene
Probes
Detection method
Frequency of assay calibration
Quantitative calibrator
Number of amplification cycles for PCR-based methods

The majority of molecular tests for viral diagnosis in transplantation lack standardization, and their clinical use across different testing sites has been difficult, if not impossible [3, 4]. Most viral laboratory-developed tests (LDTs) do not use international standards, and hence, the performance characteristics vary widely and the results are not directly comparable. Variability in specimen type (plasma, whole blood, or peripheral blood leukocytes), nucleic acid extraction methods, target sequence, limit of detection, and quantitative standard are just some of the reasons why values obtained from different LDTs are not directly comparable (Table 47.2). This lack of standardization not only complicates management of individual patients, but also hampers the development of consensus interpretive and treatment guidelines.

This chapter discusses the clinical application of molecular tests for the diagnosis of viral infections in transplant recipients. Although many viruses can infect transplant recipients, this chapter will focus on more commonly encountered pathogens, including adenovirus, BK virus (BKV), parvovirus B19, cytomegalovirus (CMV), Epstein Barr virus (EBV), and the other members of the herpes virus family.

Adenovirus

Description of Pathogen and Clinical Utility of Testing

Adenoviruses are a family of 57 immunologically distinct, non-enveloped, double-stranded DNA viruses that cause a variety of clinical syndromes in humans [5, 6]. Each adenovirus serotype, termed groups A through G, is associated with a distinct clinical illness, which in immunocompetent hosts can manifest as self-limited respiratory, gastrointestinal, or conjunctival disease [5]. Infection with adenovirus occurs throughout the year, although a predominance of cases is observed during fall and winter months [7]. Adenovirus infections occur most commonly in children, those living in close quarters, and immunocompromised patients including transplant recipients [5].

The incidence of adenovirus infection after transplantation is estimated at 5–15 % of patients [8, 9]. In a large prospective study of 263 adult SOT recipients, adenovirus DNA was detected in the blood of 7.2 % of patients during the first year after transplantation [8]. However, this study may have underestimated the true incidence of adenoviral disease since it did not capture localized and non-viremic infections. Children have a higher incidence of adenoviral infection compared to adult patients. Adenovirus was detected in 10 % of 484 pediatric liver recipients [10], compared to only 5.8 % of 191 adult liver recipients [11]. In a cohort of pediatric allogeneic HSCT recipients, the probability of developing adenovirus infection was 12.3 % [12], while the incidence was 2.5 % in adult allogeneic HSCT recipients [13].

Adenovirus infection after transplantation may or may not be associated with clinical symptoms [5]. The clinical manifestations, rate, and severity of infection may vary based on immunosuppression level, the type of SOT or HSCT, and the time to onset since transplantation [5]. Since immunosuppression is most intense during the early period after transplantation, clinical disease is most often seen during the first 3 months after transplantation [5]. In a prospective study, 60 % of SOT patients with adenovirus DNA detectable in blood after transplantation had no clinical symptoms [8]. For the remaining 40 % of SOT patients, symptoms were related to gastrointestinal and respiratory tract infections [8]. Nonspecific symptom of fever also was observed in SOT recipients. In liver transplant recipients, infection with adenovirus serotype 5 was associated with hepatitis while serotypes 1 and 2 were associated with pneumonia [10, 11]. Adenovirus may involve the allograft, which can manifest as allograft dysfunction and may be mistaken for rejection. Adenoviral pneumonia may contribute to bronchiolitis obliterans, graft loss, or even death in lung transplant patients [14]. Adenovirus infection can cause hemorrhagic cystitis and graft dysfunction after kidney transplantation [15]. In highly immunosuppressed patients, such as allogeneic stem cell transplant recipients, adenovirus infection may manifest as disseminated disease with involvement of the liver, gastrointestinal tract, and lungs [12]. Adenovirus infection is reported as one of the most significant risk factors for death in allogeneic HSCT recipients [12].

Available Assays and Interpretation of Results

The gold standard for the diagnosis of invasive adenoviral disease is histological evaluation of a tissue specimen [5], which demonstrates typical cytopathic inclusions known as "smudge cells." The presence of adenovirus within the tissue sample may be confirmed through the use of immunohistochemistry or in situ hybridization. Less invasive approaches to diagnosis are (1) antigen detection, (2) culture, and (3) molecular assays using blood and other fluids from affected organs. A single diagnostic test may not be able to detect all adenovirus serotypes. Enzyme immunoassays (EIAs) are typically the basis of rapid antigen detection kits. Rapid antigen detection kits are commercially available but their performance characteristics in the transplant population have not been rigorously studied. Moreover, while most EIAs can detect serotypes associated with ocular or gastrointestinal disease, they are not able to detect all adenovirus types and some have been associated with a low sensitivity of detection [5]. Rapid detection of adenovirus also can be done by immunofluorescence, using either polyclonal or monoclonal antibodies [5]. Culture techniques suffer from prolonged turnaround time. Although time to detection has improved with the introduction of the shell vial assay [5], sensitivity remains an issue.

PCR Tests for the Detection of Adenovirus

Nucleic acid detection using PCR has emerged as the preferred diagnostic tool for identification of adenoviral infections in transplant recipients [16]. Adenovirus PCR testing is generally more sensitive than culture-based methods [17]. In a study of HSCT recipients, adenovirus NAT had a higher sensitivity compared to viral culture and antigen detection [18, 19]. Numerous molecular assays are available, including commercial reagents and LDTs, with widely variable performance characteristics. The assay performance differences are (at least in part) dependent on the specimen type, primers used, and extraction method, among other factors. Whole blood, plasma, stool, urine, respiratory secretions (e.g., bronchoalveolar lavage), and other body fluids have been used. Comparability of tests is complicated by the fact that very few are cleared by the US Federal Drug Administration (FDA) for clinical in vitro diagnostic use. Some qualitative assays are US FDA cleared, but only for use with respiratory samples. Compounding the problem is the lack of internationally standardized quantitative calibrators. Many NATs will not detect all adenovirus serotypes, although a few have been developed to detect all known adenovirus serotypes [17, 20]. Some multiplex PCR systems include adenovirus in a test for simultaneous detection of many respiratory viruses [21]. However, multiplexed PCR can reduce the sensitivity of viral detection. Some of the broadly multiplexed viral tests have diminished sensitivity for adenovirus compared to adenovirus-specific tests. The large number of adenovirus serotypes and their genetic heterogeneity can complicate adequate validation of these assays. Hence, verification of NAT assay performance should include a wide variety of adenovirus serotypes, with assessment of both sensitivity and quantitative accuracy.

Quantitative Adenovirus Tests

Quantitative NAT for adenovirus can be used for risk stratification and prognostication [16, 18, 19]. Serial surveillance of the blood for adenovirus DNA in transplant recipients may identify the infection prior to the onset of clinical illness. Detection of adenoviral DNA in asymptomatic patients can allow for preemptive therapy for patients with a high risk of progression to clinical disease, such as those with high viral load, severe lymphopenia, and receiving intense immunosuppression for GVHD or allograft rejection [16]. Recent guidelines have recommended serial adenovirus surveillance of blood of high-risk allogeneic HSCT recipients to identify and predict the onset of invasive adenoviral disease [9, 17]; however, the clinical utility of this approach remains uncertain [22]. In one prospective study of 97 allogeneic HSCT recipients, surveillance of the blood identified adenovirus in five patients (5 % incidence, including one with a very high viral load), although this did not have an impact on the clinical outcome of these patients [23].

Some groups have even demonstrated the clinical utility of quantitative adenovirus PCR surveillance of stool samples to predict subsequent adenovirus viremia [16, 20]. In these studies, the detection of high levels of adenoviral DNA in the stool preceded the onset of viremia by at least 11 days [16, 18, 20]. The incidence of viremia was 73 % for those with $>1 \times 10^6$ copies of adenovirus DNA per gram of stool, while patients with lower values did not develop adenoviral viremia [20]. Serial stool surveillance predicted invasive adenoviral disease with 100 % sensitivity and 83 % specificity [20].

Adenovirus may be shed asymptomatically for prolonged periods of time, and thus, recovery of adenovirus from urine, upper respiratory secretions, or stool sites by culture does not necessarily confirm adenovirus as the cause of a specific disease [24, 25]. Indeed, the detection of adenovirus in one site, such as the urine alone, has poor predictive value and, therefore is not recommended for routine surveillance. However, the detection of adenovirus at two or more sites is highly predictive of invasive disease [24, 25]. Quantitation of viral load may help differentiate true infection from subclinical shedding, although the viral load threshold for discriminating a clinically relevant infection is not defined due to a lack of studies using standardized assays.

Quantitative adenovirus NAT can be used for monitoring treatment response. Treatment of established adenovirus disease consists of cautious reduction of immunosuppression and supportive care. There is no US FDA-approved antiviral drug for the treatment of established adenoviral disease, although cidofovir (CDV) has been used most frequently [5]. Treatment responses may be monitored by quantitative adenovirus PCR. Failure of the viral load to decline by 1 log within 2 weeks of treatment, or a persistent rise in viral load has been associated with mortality [26]. Generally, a higher adenoviral DNA level in the blood is associated with poor prognosis and a higher rate of treatment failure [6]. In a study of 27 adult allogeneic HSCT recipients, the peak adenovirus DNA load was significantly higher among seven patients who died of adenovirus disease compared to those without adenovirus-related death (1×10^8 vs 3×10^5; $p < 0.001$) [6].

BK Virus

Description of Pathogen and Clinical Utility of Testing

BKV is a non-enveloped, double-stranded DNA virus that belongs to the family *Polyomaviridae*, together with JC virus (JCV) [27]. Both BKV and JCV are named by the initials of the patients from which the viruses were originally identified. Primary BKV infection is common during childhood and is typically asymptomatic. More than 90 % of adults have serologic evidence of past BKV infection. BKV is transmitted through oral or respiratory routes. After primary infection, BKV remains latent in urothelial cells and leukocytes [27]. Reactivation of latent virus resulting in asymptomatic urinary shedding may occur in up to 10 % of healthy individuals [27].

In transplant recipients, BKV reactivation is more common and may lead to cytopathic changes in the urothelium. BKV viruria has been detected in up to 40 % of kidney transplant recipients and up to 75 % of allogeneic HSCT recipients [27]. The vast majority of BKV viruria in transplant recipients is subclinical, but kidney transplant and HSCT patients with viruria at very high levels may have clinical manifestations [28–31]. High levels of urinary tract BKV replication may result in sloughing of altered epithelial cells with nuclear inclusions (known as “decoy cells”), which are excreted in the urine and may be detected by urine cytologic examination [32, 33]. Inflammation elicited by necrosis and denudation of the tubular basement membrane is followed by infiltration of lymphocytes, tubular atrophy, and fibrosis. In the absence of therapeutic intervention, approximately 30–50 % of kidney transplant patients with high-level BKV viruria progress to viremia and end organ disease.

The two major clinical syndromes associated with BKV after transplantation are BKV-associated nephropathy (BKAN; in kidney transplant recipients) [29, 34, 35] and hemorrhagic cystitis (primarily in allogeneic HSCT recipients) [28, 36]. BKAN occurs in 1–10 % of kidney transplant recipients, while recipients of other solid organ allografts rarely develop BKAN. BKAN is most commonly manifested by a rise in serum creatinine with corresponding renal histopathologic findings of varying severity, including inflammation, tubular atrophy, and fibrosis, together with viral inclusions that can be identified by electron microscopy, immunohistochemistry, or in situ hybridization. Hemorrhagic cystitis, often of late onset, affects 5–15 % of allogeneic HSCT patients [37]. Occurring in the post-engraftment period, hemorrhagic cystitis may be characterized by abdominal pain, dysuria, frequent micturition, and microscopic or gross hematuria [28, 37]. Severe hematuria leading to clot formation, ureteral obstruction, and renal failure has been reported. The other diseases associated with BKV infection are ureteric stenosis, pneumonitis, and hemophagocytic syndrome [27].

Antiviral drug treatment is not established for BKAN or for hemorrhagic cystitis [27]. Cidofovir has been used anecdotally for the treatment of BKV infection in transplant patients [27], although data to convincingly support this antiviral therapy in transplant patients is not available. A randomized controlled clinical trial comparing CDV to placebo for the treatment of BKAN has been halted due to poor enrollment of study subjects. In the absence of the proven effectiveness of antiviral therapy, reduction in immunosuppressive therapy is regarded as the first line of treatment [27], since the pathogenesis of BKAN involves an imbalance between BKV replication and BKV-specific immune control.

Available Assays and Interpretation of Results

Histopathology for BKV

Histopathology is the gold standard for diagnosis of BKAN [38]. Early and accurate diagnosis of BKAN is essential to prevent graft failure. However, often no clear clinical symptoms of BKV infection are present, and the only clinical sign may be a gradual rise in serum creatinine. Histopathology of allograft biopsy specimens with BKAN shows extensive viral cytopathic effect, necrosis of the cells of the tubules and collecting ducts, and varying degrees of interstitial inflammation [38]. The pathology is focal and patchy, and, thus, this invasive procedure may yield false-negative results due to sampling error [32]. Likewise, in HSCT patients with late onset hemorrhagic cystitis, a biopsy of the bladder epithelium is needed to demonstrate the potential role of BKV infection [37].

A noninvasive alternative for diagnosis of BKV infection is to examine the urine for the presence of decoy cells, which contain characteristic intracellular viral inclusion bodies [39]. Identification of decoy cells confirms active BKV replication, but this finding is not highly specific for BKAN or hemorrhagic cystitis. Several studies have demonstrated that the sensitivity of urinary decoy cell detection in kidney transplant recipients with BKAN is modest (and comparatively less than molecular methods). In one study, urine decoy cell detection had 25 % sensitivity and 84 % specificity in identifying four patients with BKAN among a cohort of 114 kidney transplant patients [39]; the corresponding positive predictive value for concurrent BKAN was only 5 % and the negative predictive value was 97 % [39]. Decoy cell detection has been used to support the diagnosis of late-onset hemorrhagic cystitis due to BKV in HSCT recipients, but this is nonspecific, since decoy cells can be detected in other viral infections, such as adenovirus, and may be confused with malignancy [37].

Molecular Tests for BKV

Molecular tests are the most common method for diagnosis of BKV infection in kidney transplant recipients. Diagnosis of active BKV infection is most commonly achieved using quantitative PCR (qPCR) for BKV DNA, which has been demonstrated to have better predictive value than urinary decoy cell detection for the diagnosis of BKAN. BKV qPCR can be performed using urine or blood samples of transplant recipients, with urine samples providing higher sensitivity and blood samples providing higher specificity for probable BKAN. A positive relationship between BKV DNA levels in blood and impairment of renal allograft function has been shown, suggesting that viremic patients are at high risk for BKAN [27].

BKV viral load in the blood and urine has been demonstrated to be significantly higher in patients with biopsy-proven BKAN compared to those without BKAN [34]. In a study of 78 kidney transplant recipients, including ten patients who developed BKV viremia at a median of 23 weeks after transplantation, the mean BKV viral load in plasma was significantly higher in the five patients with BKAN than patients without histologic evidence of nephropathy (2×10^4 copies/ml vs 2×10^3 copies/ml, respectively; $p < 0.001$) [40]. Furthermore, the plasma BKV level increased over time to as high as 1×10^7 copies/ml in all patients who developed BKAN. BKV plasma viral load had 100 % sensitivity, 88 % specificity, 50 % positive predictive value, and 100 % negative predictive value for histologically proven BKAN [39, 40]. In another study, a BKV viremia threshold of $>1.6 \times 10^4$ copies/ml had 100 % sensitivity, 96 % specificity, 50 % positive predictive value, and 100 % negative predictive value of diagnosing BKAN [39]. In this same study, a BKV viruria threshold of $>2.5 \times 10^7$ copies/ml had 100 % sensitivity, 92 % specificity, 31 % positive predictive value, and 100 % negative predictive value for diagnosis of BKAN [39].

Molecular assays are the most common method for diagnosis of BKV infection in allogeneic HSCT recipients with hemorrhagic cystitis. BKV often is considered in the differential diagnosis of late onset hemorrhagic cystitis in HSCT recipients. The optimal test for detecting BKV in the urine is PCR for viral DNA. However, demonstrating BKV DNA by PCR alone has low specificity since even healthy individuals and HSCT recipients without hemorrhagic cystitis may shed and excrete BKV DNA in the urine. To improve the specificity, other features of reactivated BKV should be demonstrated including high peak BKV DNA (usually in the range higher than 10^9–10^{10} copies/ml or greater, a three log rise in BKV viral load from baseline that coincides with the onset of late onset hemorrhagic cystitis, or the presence of significant BKV viremia (usually higher than 10^4 copies/ml) [37]. If BKV DNA is not demonstrated by PCR in patients with hemorrhagic cystitis with decoy cells, other viral etiologies should be considered, such as adenovirus and CMV.

Molecular tests are the most common method for screening kidney transplant patients for BKV infection. The results of prospective studies indicate that BKV replication, as measured by BKV DNA qPCR tests of the urine, precedes BKV viremia by a median of 4 weeks [29, 30], and histologically proven BKAN by a median of 12 weeks [29]. Current guidelines recommend screening kidney transplant recipients for BKV infection by urine and/or plasma BKV qPCR at least once every 3 months during the first 2 years after transplantation [27, 41], and then annually until the fifth year after transplantation [27, 41]. In high-risk individuals, such as those who received intense immunosuppression for the treatment of acute rejection, other experts recommend monthly screening during the first 6 months after kidney transplantation [27, 41]. Using this strategy, at least 80–90 % of patients who develop BKAN can be identified before significant histopathology and functional renal impairment occurs [27, 41]. All patients with high-level urinary BKV viral load ($>10^7$ copies/mL) should have follow-up plasma BKV viral load testing [27, 41]. In patients with sustained plasma BKV viral load of $>10^4$ log 10 copies/ml for more than 3 weeks, a presumptive diagnosis of BKAN is made [27, 30]. The positive predictive value for BKAN in patients with high-level urinary BKV viral loads ($>10^7$ copies/ml or decoy cells) persisting for more than 2 months [30, 31, 35], or plasma BKV viral loads of $>10^4$ copies/ml is more than 50 % [27, 41]. Moreover, in patients with allograft dysfunction, the positive predictive value of plasma BKV viral load may exceed 90 % [42]. If definitive diagnosis of BKAN is sought in patients with suggestive urine and blood BKV viral loads, allograft biopsy and histopathology may be performed.

Molecular tests can be used to monitor response to treatment. BKV viral load testing is used for monitoring the response to antiviral therapy or reduction of immunosuppressive therapy in patients with BKV infection and disease [27, 41, 42]. An effective treatment response following reduction in immunosuppression, treatment with CDV or leflunomide, or allograft nephrectomy in kidney transplant recipients with BKAN is indicated by a decline in BKV viral load in the blood and urine, although the rate of decline over time is not uniform or defined [27, 41, 42]. A similar decline in BKV viral load should be seen following CDV or leflunomide therapy in HSCT recipients with late onset hemorrhagic cystitis [37].

The caveat in the clinical utility of molecular tests for the diagnosis and monitoring of BKV-associated disease is the lack of standardization (Table 47.2). The performance of these LDTs can vary widely due to differences in the specimen type used (for blood samples: whole blood or plasma; for urine samples: cell pellets, supernatants, or resuspended urine samples), the methodology, and the limits of detection, among others. Methodologies vary widely in terms of nucleic acid extraction, molecular amplification target gene (large T gene or VP-1 gene), quantitative calibrators, and detection reagents [43]. As a result, values obtained by different LDTs may not be comparable, which makes development of interpretive clinical guidelines difficult. The planned establishment of a WHO international quantitative standard for BKV should dramatically improve test standardization and may have a substantial impact on our ability to monitor and treat patients in a more uniform manner.

The Herpes Viruses

Cytomegalovirus

Description of Pathogen and Clinical Utility of Testing

Cytomegalovirus (CMV), a large, enveloped, double-stranded DNA virus belonging to the *Betaherpesvirinae* subfamily, is the most common herpes infection in SOT and HSCT recipients [44, 45]. A ubiquitous infection in humans, about 60–80 % of adults have serologic evidence of previous CMV infection [46–49]. Primary CMV infection may occur during infancy, preschool age, or sexually active years. Primary CMV infection in immunocompetent individuals often has a subclinical presentation, although it also may manifest with an infectious mononucleosis-like illness characterized by fever and lymphadenopathy. After the resolution of the primary infection, CMV becomes latent in various cells, with episodic subclinical reactivation throughout life that is controlled by a functioning immune system [46–49]. In transplant recipients, however, CMV reactivation and infection may result in a potentially severe clinical illness.

Transplant recipients may acquire CMV as a primary infection, reactivation, or reinfection (or superinfection) with a new strain [46–48]. Primary CMV infection occurs when a CMV-seronegative transplant candidate receives an allograft, hematopoietic stem cells, or blood products from a CMV-seropositive donor (CMV D+/R− transplant) [46–48]. Primary CMV infection is often characterized by severe illness due to the inability of immunosuppressed transplant patients to mount an effective immune response. Reactivation CMV infection occurs in a CMV-seropositive transplant recipient (CMV R+) when endogenous latent virus reactivates from latency. Reactivation of CMV often is associated with milder clinical illness among SOT recipients. However, reactivation of CMV may lead to severe and recurrent disease for allogeneic HSCT CMV R+ patients, especially if they receive hematopoietic stem cells from a CMV-seronegative donor (CMV D−). Reinfection or superinfection occurs when a CMV R+ patient receives an allograft from a CMV D+, and the infection is due to donor-transmitted virus. Genetic analysis demonstrates that the majority of CMV infection in CMV D+/R+ patients originates from donor-transmitted virus [50].

The clinical manifestations of CMV disease after transplantation can be classified either as CMV syndrome or tissue invasive disease. CMV syndrome, which occurs in approximately 70 % of CMV disease cases, is characterized by fever, arthralgias, and myelosuppression [47–49]. In 30 % of cases, CMV disease presents with end-organ involvement, such as interstitial pneumonia, hepatitis, esophagitis, gastritis, colitis, and rarely chorioretinitis [47–49]. In addition, CMV is associated with numerous indirect effects such as increased risk of allograft rejection, graft failure, and concomitant opportunistic infections due to bacteria, viruses, or fungi [47–49].

The incidence and severity of CMV disease in transplant recipients is influenced by the type of organ transplant, CMV status of the donor and recipient, and the overall level of immunosuppression [47–49]. The highest risk groups are lung and intestinal transplant recipients and allogeneic HSCT recipients, especially those who receive a haploidentical transplant and cells from unrelated donors. Individuals with no preexisting CMV-specific immunity, such as CMV D+/R− SOT patients, are at highest risk of CMV disease. CMV R+ patients who received allogeneic HSCT from a CMV D− are at high risk of CMV disease due to the lack of CMV-specific immunity in the transplanted hematopoietic stem cells. Symptomatic disease may occur in any transplant patient if there is severe suppression of the immune system, such as following treatment of rejection or GVHD.

Due to the negative impact of CMV disease on transplant outcome, prevention is a key component in the management of all SOT and HSCT recipients [45, 51]. The two approaches used to prevent CMV disease in transplant patients are antiviral prophylaxis and preemptive therapy. Antiviral prophylaxis is accomplished by the administration of antiviral drugs, most commonly oral valganciclovir, for a defined period of time to all patients at risk for CMV disease [45, 51]. The major disadvantage of this approach is delayed-onset CMV disease, which occurs in high risk CMV D+/R− SOT patients after they complete antiviral prophylaxis [52]. In preemptive therapy, transplant recipients are monitored using CMV PCR or antigenemia tests to detect early CMV replication; and antiviral treatment, usually valganciclovir or intravenous ganciclovir (GCV), is administered as soon as viremia or antigenemia is detected but prior to the onset of clinical symptoms [53]. The strategy of preemptive therapy is dependent on the availability of CMV NAT or antigenemia assays to guide treatment decisions (see discussion below) [2].

Available Assays and Interpretation of Results

Histopathology and Serology

Laboratory tests are essential to confirm the clinical suspicion of CMV disease in transplant patients. Histopathology with or without immunohistochemistry or in situ hybridization may be required to confirm tissue-invasive CMV disease. Because of the impaired and delayed ability of transplant patients to mount an effective immune response, CMV serologic testing to demonstrate IgM and IgG antibodies against CMV is rarely useful for the diagnosis of CMV disease after transplantation. Instead, serologic testing is used mainly prior to transplantation for CMV disease risk stratification. Depending on the donor and recipient CMV immune status, patients may be classified as high risk (e.g., CMV D+/R− SOT recipients) or low risk (CMV D−/R− patients) [45].

Viral Culture

Viral culture is a highly specific method that confirms the clinical suspicion of CMV disease. Viral culture can be done of blood and other body fluids such as respiratory secretions and cerebrospinal fluid (CSF). Viral culture of urine specimens is of low sensitivity and specificity for active CMV disease, since it often indicates urinary shedding, and therefore is not recommended for routine use in adult transplant recipients [2, 45, 51]. While viral culture of blood is highly specific and predictive of CMV disease and its severity, its major drawbacks are poor sensitivity and slow turnaround time [2]. The turnaround time for conventional culture results is between 2 and 3 weeks, thereby rarely affecting clinical care. The rapid centrifugation shell vial method has reduced the time for virus detection, with results obtained in 24–48 h, but this method still lacks sensitivity (compared to antigenemia or molecular techniques) [2]. Because of this, viral blood culture is no longer commonly used in clinical practice, although it remains helpful for end-organ viral detection in respiratory secretions and tissue samples.

CMV Antigenemia Tests

Antigenemia assays are based on detection of CMV proteins such as pp65 in peripheral leukocytes [2]. CMV antigenemia was used by many transplant centers for CMV surveillance and diagnosis because it is much more sensitive than viral culture [45]. Numerous studies have demonstrated the clinical utility of CMV antigenemia assays for rapid diagnosis of CMV disease, for surveillance of patients at high risk of infection (and to guide preemptive therapy), and for monitoring treatment response [54, 55]. However, the antigenemia assay is a labor-intensive test and lacks standardization. Since it relies on the presence of peripheral leukocytes, the assay must be performed within a relatively short period after sample collection and prior to leukocyte degradation in clinical samples [2]. The reliance on leukocytes may limit the applicability of the CMV antigenemia test in certain patient populations such as those with leukopenia, including HSCT recipients.

Molecular Tests for CMV Detection and Quantitation

Molecular testing methods have revolutionized the laboratory diagnosis of CMV disease in transplant recipients [2]. Laboratories have increasingly relied on NAT for CMV detection and quantitation, with the vast majority of CMV NAT being LDTs [56]. Commercial primers and probes are available as analyte specific reagents (ASRs). Most qualitative NATs that detect CMV DNA are difficult to interpret due to the potential detection of latent virus. Hence, the vast majority of CMV NATs rely on quantitative viral DNA detection [2, 56]. Assays that target RNA are more specific for active viral infection, although they suffer from modest sensitivity [57].

As with other quantitative assays described in this chapter, the major drawback to quantitative CMV NAT was the lack of standardization until recently [2, 3]. A wide range of factors may affect the performance characteristics of CMV NATs, including result accuracy and precision (Table 47.2). Difference in specimen type (i.e., whole blood, plasma, serum, leukocytes) is a common contributor to assay performance variability between laboratories. For example, NATs using whole blood are more sensitive than use of plasma samples, especially at lower viral load values, but less specific [58]. Nucleic acid extraction methods (e.g., manual vs automated, or liquid phase, magnetic bead or silica membrane/column), molecular amplification target gene (DNA polymerase gene, glycoprotein B gene, immediate early gene, major immediate early gene, or other CMV genes), and primer sequences and detection reagents (commercial vs noncommercial), quantitative calibrators (Roche, Acrometrix, Advanced Biotechnologies, and Qiagen), number of PCR cycles, and the range and limits of detection are some of the other factors that cause variability in the results of CMV NATs [43]. For example, the mean CMV viral load reported by laboratories that used Roche calibrators (4.32 log 10) was significantly lower than those that utilized Acrometrix (4.87 log 10, $p=0.0003$), ABI (5.06 log 10, $p<0.0001$), and Qiagen (5.03 log 10, $p<0.0001$) calibrators [43]. Result variability using Roche calibrators were lower compared to Acrometrix and ABI calibrators [43]. Accordingly, the results of CMV NATs vary widely and are not directly comparable. The lack of standardization among the various CMV NATs was highlighted by a paper comparing the results of samples sent to 33 different laboratories across North America and Europe [3]. In this study, wide inter-assay variability in viral load was reported by the participating laboratories [3]. For example, one sample had a four-log difference in viral load reported from two laboratories [3].

In 2011, the World Health Organization developed an international quantitative CMV standard, with the goals of adoption by commercial manufacturers and individual laboratories for CMV NATs. The COBAS Ampliprep/COBAS Taqman CMV test (Roche) has been calibrated according to this international standard, and was approved by the US FDA for viral load monitoring of SOT patients with CMV disease [59]. This specific CMV test has a limit of detection of 137 IU/ml up to 9.1×10^6 IU/ml [56, 59]. Reporting of all quantitative CMV results in international units (IU) should allow portability of results (comparable results achieved irrespective of laboratory or method), assisting in care of individual patients and in the effort to develop uniform guidelines for treatment [56].

CMV NATs are the most commonly used method to establish the diagnosis of CMV disease in transplant recipients [45, 56]. Numerous studies established the clinical utility of LDTs and commercially available quantitative PCR assays for the diagnosis of CMV disease in transplant patients [45, 47, 48, 51, 60, 61]. Generally, transplant patients with CMV disease have higher viral load values than those with asymptomatic infection [53]. For example, a single-center study demonstrated that compared to those without detectable viremia, the risk of CMV disease is increased 50-fold in liver transplant recipients with viral loads greater than 2,860 copies/10^6 peripheral blood leukocytes [53]. However, the specific quantitative thresholds to signify clinically relevant disease from asymptomatic infection have been difficult to define, largely due to the lack of assay standardization noted above. Numerous authors have suggested that quantitative viral threshold values associated with active disease vary depending on the sample type (plasma vs whole blood vs leukocytes), type of transplant (lung vs kidney, and SOT vs HSCT), the overall net state of immunosuppression (T-cell depleted vs non T-cell depleted), whether CMV infection is primary vs reactivation, and the assay used for detection, among other factors. Moreover, there may be cases of compartmentalized (or localized) tissue-invasive CMV disease that have no detectable level of viremia. In these cases, demonstration of CMV in tissue by histopathology may be required [47, 48, 53].

CMV NATs are useful in predicting the risk of CMV disease in transplant recipients [45, 56]. Using CMV PCR assays, transplant patients are monitored for evidence of CMV replication so that antiviral therapy can be administered prior to the development of clinical symptoms [53, 62]. This is the principle behind the "preemptive therapy" approach to CMV disease prevention, which is the most common strategy for the prevention of CMV disease in allogeneic HSCT recipients. Preemptive therapy also can be used in SOT recipients at moderate risk of CMV disease, such as CMV R+ kidney and liver transplant recipients. Using this approach, blood samples for CMV detection are collected at least once weekly during the first 12 weeks (or 100 days) after transplantation; some centers may monitor highest risk allogeneic HSCT recipients more frequently (e.g., twice weekly). Early studies evaluating the clinical utility of qualitative CMV PCR using cell-based samples demonstrated high sensitivity, poor specificity, and poor positive predictive value [2].

Several more contemporary approaches have been developed to improve the clinical specificity of CMV NAT, including the use of quantitative PCR assays, detection of CMV DNA in plasma (instead of leukocytes), and detection of CMV messenger RNA (mRNA) rather than DNA. Detection of CMV DNA in plasma rather than in leukocytes provides better correlation with clinical disease [2]. Quantitative CMV NAT methods have the potential to define a viral threshold that distinguishes asymptomatic infection from active CMV disease. For example, in a single center study that evaluated 97 liver transplant recipients by quantitative CMV PCR testing, a viral load threshold between 2,000 and 5,000 copies/ml of plasma was defined as the optimal cut off for predicting CMV disease with a sensitivity of 86 %, specificity of 87 %, positive predictive value of 64 % and a negative predictive value of 96 % [62]. However, for reasons discussed above, the lack of assay standardization has limited the generation of a viral load threshold that is widely applicable across populations and laboratories.

CMV viral load testing is useful in assessing therapeutic response in patients with CMV disease [45, 56]. Three antiviral drugs are US FDA-approved for the treatment of CMV disease: GCV, CDV, and foscarnet (phosphonoformic acid [FOS]); of these three, GCV is the most widely used in clinical practice. Current guidelines recommend that the duration of treatment of CMV disease should be guided by the clinical resolution of symptoms and clearance of the virus from the blood [44, 45]. Accordingly, CMV viral load testing is performed weekly to document virologic response and clearance during antiviral treatment. Several studies have reported >90 % or about one log reduction in viral load during the first 1–2 weeks after initiation of antiviral therapy in the vast majority of patients [63, 64]. In a minority of patients, the viral load decline may be delayed for up to 2 weeks. Moreover, the rate of viral load decline varies by individual patient, as influenced by the underlying immunosuppression, preexisting virus-specific immunity, and potentially viral strain variation [65, 66]. Patients with low pretreatment viral loads will generally achieve an undetectable viral load sooner than those with high pretreatment viral loads [59, 64]; hence, more prolonged antiviral therapy generally is given for patients with higher initial viral loads. Thus, molecular tests allow an individualized approach to management. In general, antiviral therapy is continued until the CMV viral load is below the limit of detection [51, 59]. Discontinuation of antiviral treatment in patients with detectable viremia is a risk factor for CMV disease relapse [67]. However, an overly sensitive CMV viral load test may lead to over-treatment if the assay can detect "non-clinically relevant" virus [61].

CMV viral load testing is a useful marker of CMV disease relapse. The optimal duration of antiviral treatment for CMV infection and disease, as discussed above, should be individualized based on clinical and virologic resolution of infection. Hence, sequential monitoring of CMV viral load after initiation of therapy allows the identification of patients at risk of recurrent infection. Up to 30 % of transplant patients treated for CMV infection and disease will develop relapse of viremia or clinical symptoms after discontinuation of antiviral therapy. In clinical practice, CMV relapse is heralded by the reappearance of CMV DNA in the blood following initial successful viral load suppression. Patients generally are monitored by CMV viral load testing weekly for up to 4 weeks following an antiviral treatment course to monitor for relapse. Retreatment with intravenous GCV or oral valganciclovir is generally effective for treatment of relapse.

CMV relapse is most common in patients with severe immunosuppression and without CMV-specific immunity. Early laboratory predictors of CMV relapse are a high peak CMV viral load and a slow rate of decline in CMV viral load (also known as viral decay) [62, 68, 69]. In a study of 52 SOT recipients with CMV disease who were monitored with the Amplicor CMV Monitor test (Roche) [68, 69], the time to clearance of CMV DNA from plasma was 33.8 days in the 12 patients with relapsing CMV disease compared to 17.2 days in the group without recurrent disease ($p=0.002$). The viral load half-life with treatment was 8.8 days compared to 3.2 days ($p=0.001$) in the group with and without recurrent disease, respectively [62]. Moreover, those with very high pretreatment viral load values had higher risk of CMV relapse [67]. In a prospective study of 24 SOT patients with CMV infection or disease who received a 14-day course of IV GCV, the CMV viral load prior to the initiation of antiviral therapy was statistically higher in eight patients who had CMV relapse compared to the 14 who did not relapse (80,150 copies/10^6 leukocytes vs 5,500 copies/10^6 leukocytes, respectively, $p=0.007$) [67]. As discussed above, transplant patients who discontinue antiviral therapy with ongoing viremia have a higher risk of clinical relapse, compared to those who have attained viral load suppression, even if they have resolution of clinical symptoms [67]. In this study, those who had CMV infection relapse had a detectable viral load at the end of treatment (mean 18,800 copies/10^6 leukocytes), while viral load was undetectable in the non-relapsing group [67].

CMV Drug Resistance Testing

Failure of viral load to decline to an undetectable level, or a rise in viral load after an initial decline, following initiation of antiviral therapy suggests potential drug resistance [45, 51, 70]. Risk factors for CMV drug resistance are (1) prolonged exposure to antiviral drugs, (2) severe immunosuppression, (3) lack of CMV-specific immunity (i.e., CMV D+/R−), and (4) suboptimal antiviral drug concentrations [45, 51, 70]. Fortunately, resistance to GCV and other drugs is uncommon, with rates estimated at less than 5 % of all CMV disease cases [45, 51, 70].

CMV drug resistance can be confirmed by either phenotypic or molecular (genotypic) testing [71]. Phenotypic assays rely on analysis of growth characteristics of viral isolates in the presence of different concentrations of antiviral drugs and therefore require viable virus. Phenotypic assays are biologically more relevant for detection of drug resistance. However, phenotypic assays are labor intensive with subjective test result interpretation, and require at least 1 month to obtain results, which is generally not timely for clinical care.

Molecular assays can detect the presence of nucleotide sequence changes associated with drug resistance [71]. Genotypic results generally correlate with clinical drug resistance and provide rapid results that can guide clinical therapeutic selection. Drug resistance is indicated by mutations in the UL97 gene (which encodes viral kinase) and/or the UL54 gene (which encodes the CMV DNA polymerase) [71]. UL97 mutations are more common and confer resistance to GCV, while UL54 mutations are less common but confer resistance to any or all of the three anti-CMV drugs (GCV, FOS, and CDV). GCV resistance mutations are most frequently mapped to the UL97 gene within codons 460 and 520 and either point mutations or deletions within the codon range 590–607 [71]. One caveat for genotypic assays is the presence of some normal baseline sequence variability in the UL97 and UL54 genes in drug-sensitive CMV strains [71].

Epstein Barr Virus

Description of Pathogen and Clinical Utility of Testing

EBV is an oncogenic gamma-herpesvirus that causes B-cell proliferation in humans [72]. A common infection in humans, EBV frequently is acquired by exposure to infected body fluids, such as saliva. In healthy individuals, primary EBV infection can be asymptomatic or can cause infectious mononucleosis, which is characterized by fever, sore throat, and lymphadenopathy. Following primary infection, EBV establishes lifelong latency in various organs which serve as reservoirs and vehicles for transmission to susceptible EBV-seronegative transplant recipients.

EBV infection after transplantation can occur either as a primary infection (in an EBV-seronegative transplant recipient who received an organ from an EBV-positive donor) or as a reactivation infection (in EBV-seropositive transplant recipients). EBV infection can manifest as an asymptomatic infection or as post-transplant lymphoproliferative disorder (PTLD) [72]. The term PTLD encompasses a heterogeneous spectrum of lymphoproliferative disorders, typically of B cell origin, from benign reactive hyperplasia to mononucleosis-like illness and fulminant non-Hodgkin lymphoma. The EBV genome is found in >90 % of B-cell origin PTLD, especially during the first 2 years after transplantation [72]. In contrast, a large number of late-onset PTLD (those occurring 2 or more years after transplantation) may be EBV-negative and may not involve B cells. The median time to the development of PTLD in SOT patients is 6 months, whereas in HSCT patients, signs and symptoms could appear within 70–90 days after transplantation. The clinical features of PTLD are similar in both SOT and HSCT patients.

The incidence of EBV-induced PTLD varies widely from 0.8 % – 20 % depending on the EBV donor and recipient pre-transplant immune status, type of SOT or HSCT, patient age, and the type of immunosuppression [72]. The highest risk factor for PTLD after transplantation is primary EBV infection [72, 73]. Hence, an EBV-naive and seronegative transplant recipient who receives an organ allograft from an EBV-seropositive donor (referred to as EBV D+/R–) is at highest risk of PTLD [72, 73]. Children are at high risk of PTLD likely due to a lack of prior EBV immunity [74]. Primary EBV infection in an EBV D+/R– transplant patient generally leads to massive B cell proliferation [73]. Mutant cells that are produced during massive B cell proliferation may not be eliminated optimally in patients with severe immunosuppression and ineffective T cell function, resulting in progression to PTLD [72]. This risk is augmented in the presence of CMV disease and the use of lymphocyte-depleting immunosuppressive drugs for treatment of rejection after SOT [75]. Because of the role of T cells in EBV control, allogeneic HSCT recipients who received T cell-depleted grafts, and those receiving intense immunosuppression for GVHD are at highest risk of developing PTLD [76].

Available Assays and Interpretation of Results

Histopathology for EBV

The definitive diagnosis of PTLD is established by histopathology [72]. A variety of special studies are used to complement the histopathologic diagnosis of PTLD, including immunophenotyping by flow cytometry, immunohistochemical stains, and molecular tests [72]. Documenting the presence of EBV-specific nucleic acids in the affected tissues establishes the diagnosis of EBV-associated PTLD, and suggests the role of EBV infection in the pathogenesis of PTLD. In this regard, in situ hybridization that targets the EBV-encoded small nuclear RNA is the preferred approach and is more sensitive for detecting EBV-infected cells than in situ hybridization directly targeting EBV DNA [72].

Serology for EBV

The challenge for clinicians and the clinical laboratory is to predict patients that are at highest risk of developing PTLD. Serology may be performed to demonstrate IgM and IgG antibodies to viral capsid antigen (VCA) or antibody to the Epstein Barr nuclear antigen (EBNA) [72]. The most important role of EBV serology in transplantation is the pre-transplant assessment of donor and recipient EBV immune status by serologic testing for PTLD risk stratification [72]. The presence of anti-VCA IgM antibody and the absence of EBNA antibody suggest acute or recent infection, and this may indicate increased risk of developing PTLD in a transplant recipient. Serology, however, is generally unreliable as a diagnostic tool for either PTLD or primary EBV infection in immunocompromised patients due to delayed or absent humoral immune responses. Moreover, transplant patients often receive blood products, and the passive transfer of antibodies may render EBV IgG antibody assays difficult to interpret [72].

Molecular Tests for Detection of EBV

EBV PCR testing is the most common test to diagnose EBV infection after transplantation. A multitude of EBV PCR LDTs and commercial tests have been developed over the past decade, and have been used clinically to quantitatively detect active EBV infection in the post-transplant setting [77, 78]. Generally, EBV PCR can be used (1) to demonstrate the presence of EBV infection in patients with PTLD [72, 77, 78], (2) for surveillance of EBV replication in high-risk EBV D+/R– transplant patients [72, 77, 78], and (3) for surveillance of treatment efficacy in EBV-associated PTLD [72, 77].

The optimal approach for utilization of quantitative EBV PCR assays remains uncertain [77]. As with other quantitative molecular tests, the lack of assay standardization is one of the major impediments to optimal use of EBV viral load in the clinical care of transplant patients [77]. While there has been remarkable progress in the development of various EBV PCR assays, their clinical utility and comparability has been hampered by the lack of an international reference standard [77]. Moreover, differences in nucleic acid extraction methods (liquid phase, magnetic beads, or silica membrane/column), quantitative calibrators (Qiagen, Roche, Abbott, Acrometrix, or Advanced Biotechnologies), detection reagents (commercial or noncommercial reagents), and molecular amplification target gene (EBNA gene, DNA polymerase gene, or LMP-1 gene) are among some of the factors that contribute to the widely variable EBV viral load results obtained with different assays [43]. Because of these variables, commercial and LDT EBV PCR assays are not standardized and cannot be directly compared.

In turn, no interpretative guidelines exist, nor are there clinically relevant EBV viral load thresholds to guide management of EBV infection and PTLD across centers. One large study that compared 28 laboratories in Europe and North America showed wide interlaboratory variation in detection and reporting of EBV viral load values from the same specimen [4]. Significant and extreme interlaboratory variability exists in both qualitative and quantitative EBV PCR results, raising questions regarding the validity of interinstitutional result comparison in the absence of formal cross-referencing of assays between institutions [4, 43]. In contrast, within most laboratories, intralaboratory result reproducibility and result linearity are reasonable. Hence, trends in the EBV viral load of patients over time using the same assay are a more useful test compared to single values or compared to serial testing performed at multiple institutions [4, 77]. There are now efforts to harmonize commercial and LDTs with the recent introduction of an international calibration standard for EBV PCR tests.

The optimal sample for EBV PCR testing is not defined, and this further contributes to the variability of results between assays performed in different laboratories (Table 47.2). Some laboratories prefer whole blood while others use plasma, serum, or lymphocytes [4, 77]. Detecting EBV in other body fluids may be useful in specific situations, such as the demonstration of EBV DNA in the CSF of a patient with PTLD involving the central nervous system [79, 80], or in bronchoalveolar lavage fluid of a patient with PTLD involving the lungs [77]. Cell-containing samples such as whole blood and lymphocytes are generally more sensitive compared to plasma and serum, but may more often contain latent EBV. EBV viral load testing using plasma improves specificity for the diagnosis of EBV-positive PTLD, while not significantly lowering sensitivity relative to assessments in cell-containing blood compartments [4, 77]. In the absence of widely accepted treatment thresholds (due to lack of assay standardization), serial detection using quantitative methods may afford the greatest clinical predictive value.

PTLD may be heralded several weeks before clinical symptoms by the presence of EBV infection in peripheral blood [72]. Based on this natural history, EBV qPCR testing has been used in the clinical setting to detect EBV infection in high-risk transplant patients, including EBV D+/R− and pediatric transplant recipients [72]. The frequency for monitoring patients is not standardized. Weekly monitoring may be used during the early post-transplant period. Monthly monitoring for EBV infection may be used during the first year since most EBV disease will occur during this period [72]. Demonstration of EBV DNA in the blood should trigger a reduction in immunosuppression (as first-line treatment of EBV infection and possible PTLD) and evaluation for PTLD [72]. In one study of a cohort of 1,131 SOT and HSCT patients, 66 (5.6 %) patients developed PTLD [78]. PTLD developed in 53 of 376 patients (14 %) who had at least one positive EBV PCR in a whole blood sample, compared to 13 of 755 patients (2 %) who had repeatedly negative samples [78]. The risk of PTLD was directly correlated with the degree of viremia, with PTLD occurring in 11 % of patients with EBV PCR viral loads between 10^3 and 10^5 copies/ml, compared to 37 % of patients with EBV viral loads higher than 10^5 copies/ml of whole blood [78].

As a result of wide variability in assay methods, no consensus threshold for prediction of EBV-positive PTLD has been defined. In general, however, a low EBV viral load that may be observed even in healthy EBV-seropositive transplant recipients can be clinically relevant in EBV D+/R− transplant recipients. In contrast, a high or increasing EBV viral load should trigger evaluation for possible PTLD in all transplant recipients. Screening for EBV by qPCR should permit early diagnosis of PTLD that will then allow institution of a therapeutic strategy, which typically consists of reductions in immunosuppression and the administration of anti-CD20 monoclonal antibodies (Rituximab). Cytotoxic chemotherapy is reserved for established PTLD that does not respond to initial reduction in immunosuppression and anti-CD20 monoclonal antibody therapy.

Herpes Simplex Virus Types 1 and 2

Description of Pathogen and Clinical Utility of Testing

The alpha-herpesviruses, herpes simplex virus types 1 and 2 (HSV-1, HSV-2), are important causes of mucocutaneous illness, aseptic lymphocytic meningitis, encephalitis, fulminant hepatitis, and disseminated disease in humans [81]. Classically associated with oro-labial ulcerative diseases, HSV-1 infection is acquired early in life. The prevalence of HSV-1 infection increases with age, reaching 80 % by 60 years of age [82]. HSV-2 infection, which is associated with genital herpes, occurs less frequently. The prevalence of HSV-2 infection increases with sexual activity and age, and reaches 26.3 % by 49 years of age [83].

Following primary infection, HSV-1 and HSV-2 establish latency in dorsal nerve root ganglia. Periodic HSV-1 and HSV-2 reactivation from latency occurs throughout life with clinical and subclinical manifestations. The majority of HSV infections in transplant recipients result from reactivation of latent virus, especially during the early post-transplant period and during periods of severe immunosuppression [81]. In some cases, primary HSV infection may be acquired from the transplanted organ (donor-transmitted HSV) [84] or acquired naturally as a result of intimate contacts during the post-transplant period.

The most common clinical manifestations of HSV disease after transplantation, whether primary infection or reactivation, are oro-labial, genital, or perianal disease [81, 85]. Classically, HSV lesions are vesicular or ulcerative and localized. In severe cases, particularly among highly immunocompromised transplant patients, HSV infection can disseminate to develop organ-invasive manifestations such as hepatitis [81]. Fever, leukopenia, and hepatitis are the most common presenting signs and symptoms of disseminated disease [81]. CNS involvement may occur in the form of encephalitis or meningitis. HSV reactivation occurs most commonly during the first month after transplantation [81]. Hence, standard clinical practice is prophylactic treatment of transplant recipients with antiviral therapy (usually with acyclovir, valacyclovir, or valganciclovir) during the first 4–6 weeks after transplantation [81]. Thereafter, risk of HSV disease decreases dramatically, though it remains higher than that in immunocompetent hosts.

The clinical presentation of mucocutaneous HSV disease in transplant recipients is often typical, with vesicles and ulcers, such that the diagnosis may be made on clinical criteria. Occasionally, clinical manifestations may be atypical, and other pathogens may be suspected. In these cases, clinical laboratory confirmation of HSV infection is helpful. The clinical laboratory is also helpful in the diagnosis of invasive HSV disease, such as those with suspected CNS involvement and those with herpes hepatitis.

Available Assays and Interpretation of Results

The laboratory methods available for the diagnosis of HSV infection are (1) direct fluorescent antibody (DFA) testing of mucocutaneous lesions, bronchoalveolar lavage, and other samples, (2) histopathology of biopsy specimens, (3) serologic testing, (4) viral culture, and (5) HSV PCR testing.

Direct Fluorescent Antibody Testing for HSV

Serologic detection of HSV antibodies is rarely useful for diagnosing acute HSV infection in transplant recipients since HSV seropositivity is very common, and generation of antibodies during primary HSV infection may be delayed due to the effects of immunosuppression. HSV antigens can be detected on scrapings of ulcerative mucocutaneous lesions by immunofluorescent microscopy. The Tzanck smear, which demonstrates viral cytopathic effects, can be done on scrapings obtained from herpetic ulcers. However, the Tzanck smear is not very specific for HSV since similar findings can be demonstrated in other herpes virus infections.

Viral Culture for HSV Identification

Viral culture of the vesicular fluid is very sensitive for the diagnosis of HSV disease since vesicles typically contain very high concentrations of HSV during the first 48 h of clinical disease. Indeed, viral culture is a reference standard for HSV detection in body fluids, although it has now been largely supplanted by HSV PCR as the diagnostic test of choice for CSF specimens [86]. HSV PCR is increasingly used, but has not supplanted viral culture for the detection of HSV in body fluids other than CSF [87].

Molecular Tests for HSV

HSV PCR assays provide high sensitivity and specificity, and a more rapid turnaround time compared to culture [87–89]. In one study that compared HSV PCR to viral culture in 200 dermal, ocular, and genital samples, HSV PCR detected the virus in 88 samples whereas the shell vial culture was positive only in 69 samples [87]; there were 19 samples that were detected by HSV PCR alone while no sample was positive by viral culture alone [87]. Molecular assays can be optimized to distinguish HSV-1 from HSV-2, which is important epidemiologically and for patient counseling regarding disease acquisition [89]. HSV PCR can be multiplexed for the detection of other viruses that may present similarly with vesicular lesions such as VZV. In one study, HSV and VZV were co-detected in 1.3 % of dermal, ocular, and genital specimens over 8 years [90].

HSV PCR is especially useful for identifying HSV in blood or other sterile fluids, as viral cultures have poor sensitivity in detecting HSV in these samples. If disseminated disease is suspected in transplant patients, detection of HSV by PCR in any blood compartment will confirm the clinical suspicion, and signifies a poor prognosis [91]. Histopathology with immunocytochemistry for HSV may be needed to document tissue-invasive disease in patients suspected to have fulminant herpes hepatitis, although in these cases, the HSV PCR of a blood specimen will almost certainly be diagnostic [92].

Quantification of HSV in a clinical sample, such as the CSF, genital secretions, or blood, has been suggested as a prognostic indicator of severity of infection and as a guide for duration of treatment. In one study, the quantity of HSV DNA in cervicovaginal secretions was directly correlated with the signs and symptoms of HSV disease [93]. Likewise, there was a strong correlation between HSV viral load and the presence of histopathologically proven HSV esophagitis [94]; in this study, an HSV viral load in the blood greater than 2.5×10^4 copies had 83 % sensitivity and 100 % specificity for a diagnosis of HSV esophagitis. A significant association between initial HSV viral load and the duration of treatment course was demonstrated in a study of patients with HSV encephalitis [95]; hence, quantitative HSV PCR may assist in the monitoring of response to antiviral therapy in these patients [96]. However, HSV PCR tests in clinical use are predominantly qualitative assays (i.e., reported as positive or negative); and the potential value and optimal use of viral load testing in guiding clinical decisions, while promising, remains uncertain.

Varicella Zoster Virus

Description of Pathogen and Clinical Utility of Testing

Varicella zoster virus (VZV) is a highly infectious alphaherpesvirus that causes "chickenpox" during primary infection. VZV primary infection is characterized by fever, other constitutional symptoms, and a vesicular, pruritic, widely disseminated rash that starts on the face and spreads down the trunk. The distinctive feature of VZV infection is the evolution of the rash so that papules, vesicles, and crusted lesions may all be seen at the same time. Moreover, the rash typically spares the palms and the soles. Primary infection is typically a self-limited illness in the immunocompetent patient. However, primary VZV infection may infrequently lead to hepatitis, pneumonitis, encephalitis, retinal necrosis, and purpura fulminans [97].

Following primary infection, VZV establishes latency in cranial nerve and dorsal root ganglia. Latent VZV can reactivate later in life as herpes zoster (known as shingles), which is characterized by a vesicular exanthem with a dermatomal distribution [98]. Some patients, especially those who are immunocompromised, such as transplant patients, may develop severe, disseminated zoster. These cases may include visceral involvement [98], such as fulminant hepatitis [99]. Cutaneous lesions may become secondarily infected with bacteria, and patients with herpes zoster may have long-term sequelae, including painful and debilitating postherpetic neuralgia [98].

VZV infection in transplant recipients is mainly due to reactivation, since the vast majority of older adults are seropositive for VZV due to childhood infection. Children also are typically vaccinated against VZV using live-attenuated virus vaccine, and possess vaccine-induced immunity. Accordingly, over 90 % of transplant recipients are seropositive and have immunity against VZV. VZV reactivation, which manifests as mono- or multi-dermatomal herpes zoster, occurs in approximately 8–11 % of transplant patients [98]. The peak incidence of herpes zoster occurs during the first year after SOT or allogeneic HSCT [98]. While the majority of herpes zoster remains localized to one or a few adjacent dermatomes, severely immunocompromised transplant patients may have disseminated disease with visceral involvement [98], including fulminant VZV hepatitis [100].

Since the vast majority of patients are immune to VZV prior to transplantation, primary VZV infection is rarely seen after transplantation. Chickenpox, however, may be seen in unvaccinated pediatric transplant recipients and in the minority of adults who are VZV-seronegative. The clinical manifestations of VZV infection in these patients are typical but can be especially severe, sometimes with visceral involvement [98].

The diagnosis of primary VZV infection and herpes zoster is usually clinical due to their classic clinical presentation. However, transplant patients may have atypical presentations or may have disseminated zoster that can mimic other disease states. Therefore, in transplant patients who may develop rash from a multitude of other infectious and noninfectious causes, laboratory testing for VZV can be an important tool to establish a definitive diagnosis.

Available Assays and Interpretation of Results

For the definitive diagnosis of VZV infection and herpes zoster, rapid DFA or PCR diagnostic assays are preferred [101]. PCR is currently the most sensitive test for the detection of VZV and may be used for detecting VZV in vesicle fluid, blood (in case of suspected disseminated or tissue-invasive disease), other body fluids such as CSF, or tissues [102]. Most of the assays are LDTs and provide qualitative results, although some clinical laboratories offer VZV quantification tests [101, 102]. The potential clinical applications of quantitative VZV PCR assays include prognosis of disease severity (higher viral load is associated with more severe disease) and in guiding treatment strategies (higher viral load may require a more intensified and longer duration of treatment). However, these potential applications have not been widely utilized in clinical practice. Some VZV PCR assays have been incorporated into multiplexed PCR tests for viral illnesses [103]. Viral culture is much less sensitive than PCR and has a slower turnaround time [98]. Serologic testing is rarely helpful in the diagnosis of VZV infection and herpes zoster in transplant recipients [98].

Human Herpesviruses 6 and 7

Description of Pathogens and Clinical Utility of Testing

Human herpesvirus 6 (HHV-6) and 7 (HHV-7) are lymphotropic β-herpesviruses that infect the majority of humans during the first few years of life [104, 105]. Primary HHV-6 and HHV-7 infections may be asymptomatic or manifest clinically as a febrile illness associated with rash, diarrhea, respiratory symptoms, or seizures [106]. HHV-6 is comprised of two different variants, HHV-6A and HHV-6B [107]. HHV-6B is responsible for the majority of documented primary infections in children [106]. Primary HHV-6 and HHV-7 infections result in lifelong latency in mononuclear cells [107]. In less than 1 % of infected individuals, HHV-6 persistence occurs as a result of the integration of the virus into the host chromosome [108].

HHV-6 and HHV-7 infections occur either as primary infections or reactivations in transplant recipients [104–106]. The reported rates of HHV-6 infection after transplantation have varied widely from 20–55 %, while HHV-7 infection has been reported in up to 46 % of transplant patients [104, 106]. Because the virus exists in latent form in >95 % of adults, the vast majority of post-transplant infections are due to reactivation of latent virus. Reactivation of both viruses occurs relatively early, generally within the first 2–4 weeks after transplantation [104, 106]. Primary HHV-6 and HHV-7 infections occur rarely, and are seen mainly among HHV-6 and HHV-7 seronegative children who may have acquired the infection from seropositive donors or as a result of natural transmission in the community [104, 106].

While HHV-6 and HHV-7 reactivations are common, clinical disease associated with these viruses is uncommon, and hence, routine surveillance in transplant recipients is not recommended [105]. There have only been a few sporadic cases of symptomatic HHV-7 infection reported, including patients presenting with fever, myelitis, and myelosuppression [106]. Clinical disease due to HHV-6 occurs in only 1 % of transplant patients, and most reported cases have been due to HHV-6B [104, 106]. In a study of 200 liver transplant recipients, HHV-6 infection was demonstrated by PCR in 51 % of patients at a median of 27 days after transplantation [68, 69]. However, HHV-6 associated disease was documented only in two patients (incidence, 1 %) [68, 69]. HHV-6 may manifest as a febrile syndrome accompanied by some degree of bone marrow suppression, an illness similar to CMV infection [104, 106]. HHV-6 also has been reported as a cause of febrile dermatosis, hepatitis, gastroduodenitis, colitis, pneumonitis, and encephalitis after transplantation [104, 106]. HHV-6 infection in liver or renal transplant patients is an independent risk factor for CMV disease [109]. CMV viral load was significantly higher in HHV-6 positive patients compared to those without HHV-6 infection (median viral load 1,560 copies/ml vs undetectable, respectively; $p<0.001$). An increase in HHV-6 viral load was significantly associated with the development of opportunistic infections, including invasive fungal disease [109].

Available Assays and Interpretation of Results

Clinical laboratory tests available for the detection of HHV-6 and HHV-7 infection are serology, culture, antigen detection, histopathology with immunohistochemistry, and PCR tests [104–106]. Among them, PCR testing with the use of LDTs has emerged as the diagnostic method of choice in transplant recipients [104–106]. In contrast, HHV-6 and HHV-7 IgM and IgG may identify acute or previous infections, but serologic testing is not routinely performed in clinical practice due to poor sensitivity and specificity in identifying acute infection in transplant patients with impaired ability to mount an effective immune response. Moreover, high seroprevalence rates limit the potential utility of serology in the diagnosis of acute HHV-6 or HHV-7 disease after transplantation. Viral culture for these agents is not typically performed in clinical laboratories.

Molecular methods using LDTs are preferred for detection of HHV-6 or HHV-7 in active disease (Table 47.1) [104–106]. HHV-6 and HHV-7 PCR can be performed using whole blood, plasma, peripheral blood leukocytes, or other body fluids such as CSF and bronchoalveolar lavage fluid [104, 106]. PCR of peripheral blood mononuclear cells is the most sensitive technique for detecting these viruses, but the use of this specimen type may not distinguish latent from active infection. To increase specificity for active infection, quantitative PCR is preferred over qualitative assays. In addition, methods that utilize noncellular samples (such as plasma) or those that detect mRNA may increase specificity for active HHV-6 or HHV-7 infection [104, 106]. A clinically relevant viral load threshold has been difficult to define due to lack of standardized assays, but a level of more than 1,000 copies/ml has been demonstrated in one study to be associated with mortality after allogeneic HSCT [110].

Surveillance for HHV-6 and HHV-7 by PCR is not routinely performed nor recommended after transplantation because of the low rate of clinical disease and the high rate of subclinical viral reactivations [104, 106]. The role of HHV-6 and HHV-7 PCR is in the diagnosis of active infection and in guiding antiviral treatment responses [104, 106]. A decline in HHV-6 and HHV-7 viral load should be anticipated during effective therapies with GCV, CDV, or foscarnet.

The interpretation of HHV-6 PCR results should consider the potential detection of chromosomally integrated HHV-6 [111, 112]. In approximately 1 % of individuals, HHV-6 latency exists in the form of chromosomal integration, and hence, every nucleated cell in the body will have detectable HHV-6 DNA. In a cohort of 548 liver transplant patients, chromosomally integrated HHV-6 was detected in seven patients (1.3 %) [111]. When HHV-6 is chromosomally integrated in germ cells (eggs or sperm), the viral genome is inherited in a Mendelian pattern [112]. Accordingly, clinical samples containing nucleated cells will always have detectable HHV-6 DNA, but without discernible clinical effect. Patients with chromosomally integrated HHV-6 are characterized by extremely high levels of HHV-6 DNA in whole blood [112]. In a consensus report, chromosomally integrated HHV-6 should be suspected when the viral load exceeds 5.5 logs in whole blood [112]. Such high levels have been mistaken as active infection and have led to unnecessary antiviral treatment. Chromosomally integrated HHV-6 can be confirmed by demonstrating persistently elevated levels on subsequent serial testing, the presence of one viral DNA per nucleated cell, and testing of hair follicle samples for HHV-6 [112].

Human Herpesvirus 8

Description of Pathogen and Clinical Utility of Testing

Human herpesvirus 8 (HHV-8) is a gamma-herpesvirus that primarily infects CD19+ B cells and endothelial-derived spindle cells [109, 113]. Primary HHV-8 infection in immunocompetent individuals is associated with mild nonspecific symptoms of diarrhea, fatigue, rash, and lymphadenopathy [109]. In immunocompromised individuals, however, HHV-8 is associated with neoplastic diseases. Unlike most of the human herpes viruses, HHV-8 infection is geographically restricted [114]. Hence, seroprevalence rates vary widely by geographic region with estimates of 0–5 % in North America, northern Europe, and Asia, 5–20 % in the Mediterranean and Middle East, and >50 % in parts of Africa [114].

HHV-8 is the etiologic agent of Kaposi's sarcoma (KS), a multicentric neoplasm of lymphatic endothelium-derived cells, which manifests clinically in individuals with compromised immunity as multifocal progressive mucocutaneous lesions with dissemination to the visceral organs, including transplanted allografts [114]. Other less common malignant diseases associated with HHV-8 are primary effusion lymphoma (PEL) and Castleman's disease (CD) [114]. HHV-8 has been reported as a potential cause of bone marrow suppression and monoclonal gammopathy after transplantation [114].

HHV-8 disease may occur in the transplant setting either as a primary infection in HHV-8 seronegative recipients of allografts from HHV-8 seropositive donors [115–117] or as a secondary reactivation of endogenous latent HHV-8 [118]. The incidences of these clinical diseases mirror the geographic distribution of the virus. Hence, the incidence of KS after transplantation is as low as 0.5 % among transplant recipients from North America, Asia, and northern Europe to as high as 28 % among HHV-8 seropositive transplant recipients from the Middle East [114]. The median time to the onset of KS is 30 months after transplantation [114].

Risk factors for HHV-8-associated disease, specifically KS, include older age, male gender, and residence or exposure in an HHV-8 endemic area. For example, in Saudi Arabia, KS was the most common tumor in kidney transplant recipients [119]. Both pre-transplant HHV-8 seronegativity and seropositivity have been associated with the development of KS, suggesting that both primary HHV-8 infection and reactivation can result in clinical disease [114]. Because control of HHV-8 infection is mediated by T cells, the intensity of pharmacologic immunosuppression and the use of anti-lymphocyte agents may play a role in HHV-8 pathogenesis after transplantation [120]. HHV-8 T-cell responses were notably absent in transplant patients at the onset of KS, and these responses were restored following reduction in immunosuppression, which coincided clinically with remission of KS [120]. Sirolimus may have a protective role against KS, potentially due to antiproliferative effects. There have been reports of KS regression following a change in the immunosuppressive regimen from cyclosporine to the mTOR inhibitor sirolimus [114].

Available Assays and Interpretation of Results

HHV-8 infection can be diagnosed serologically or by molecular testing [114, 121]. Demonstration of HHV-8 seroconversion or an IgM response can indicate acute HHV-8 infection, but the clinical utility of this in the transplant setting is limited [114]. Serological assays are non-standardized and methodologies are directed against different antigens [121]. Accordingly, the sensitivity of serology is highly variable and ranges from <80 %–>90 % [121, 122]. As noted previously in this chapter, the utility of serologic testing is also severely limited in the post-transplant setting. In some centers located in endemic regions, HHV-8 serological screening of the donors and recipients may be done to stratify the risk of HHV-8 infection and clinical disease after transplantation.

HHV-8 PCR testing offers high sensitivity and specificity for detecting active HHV-8 infection [114]. Quantification of HHV-8 viral load in clinical samples has the potential utility of predicting subsequent occurrence of KS [114, 123, 124]. In a case study of a liver transplant patient who developed KS, retrospective analysis of clinical specimens indicated that HHV-8 was detected in the serum more than 3 months prior to KS onset [124]. HHV-8 viral load testing can be used to monitor patients with KS and assess their response to therapy [114, 125–127]. For example, HHV-8 viral load peaked at the time of diagnosis and declined to undetectable levels during treatment of KS [128]. HHV-8 viremia was associated with the stage and progression of KS, and hence, quantification of HHV-8 DNA load could be a useful tool for monitoring transplant patients with KS [114, 121, 125, 126]. In a cross-sectional study of 43 patients who developed KS after transplantation, progression of the disease was associated with higher viral load, defined as >1,000 copies/μg of DNA [126].

The diagnosis of KS requires histopathology to demonstrate the pathognomonic findings of spindle-shaped cells with vascular channels lined by abnormal endothelial cells [105]. Immunohistochemistry using monoclonal antibodies against HHV-8 antigens or in situ hybridization can be a useful adjunct to demonstrate the presence of HHV-8 in KS and other angiogenic proliferative diseases [105, 114, 129].

Parvovirus B19

Description of Pathogen and Clinical Utility of Testing

Parvovirus B19 is a small, single-stranded, linear, non-enveloped, DNA virus that commonly infects humans. Most people are infected between the ages of 5 and 15 years [130].

Up to 80 % of older adults have antibodies against parvovirus B19 [131]. The virus is primarily spread person-to-person by infected respiratory droplets. However, vertical transmission and transmission via blood products and organ transplantation has been reported [131]. During active infection, the virus replicates most efficiently and preferentially in human erythrocyte precursors. Infection appears to confer lifelong immunity among immunocompetent individuals, although reinfection is possible. Parvovirus B19 can persist in the bone marrow and other tissues, supporting reactivation as a mechanism for disease after transplantation [132].

Parvovirus B19 infection can be either symptomatic or asymptomatic depending on the patient's age and immunologic status [130]. Nonspecific flu-like symptoms may occur during primary infection, but distinctive clinical entities attributed to parvovirus B19 infection have been well-described in immunocompetent and immunocompromised hosts, including erythema infectiosum, hydrops fetalis, polyarthralgia syndrome, and aplastic anemia [130]. Parvovirus B19 occurs in <1–2 % of transplant recipients [131]. However, some studies have reported that up to 30 % of organ transplant recipients develop parvovirus B19 viremia, with or without clinical manifestations [133]. In transplant recipients, the most common presentation of parvovirus B19 infection is recurrent and progressive aplastic anemia, which is reported in 99 % of all cases in the literature [134]. Fever, arthralgia, and rash were observed in 25 %, 7 %, and 6 % of patients, respectively [134].

Available Assays and Interpretation of Results

Parvovirus B19 infection should be specifically suspected in transplant recipients with otherwise unexplained anemia. Diagnostic testing can be performed by serology or direct viral detection in clinical specimens, such as blood, bone marrow, and organ biopsies or resections (i.e., liver, lung, or kidney). In immunocompromised patients, parvovirus B19 serology may not be reliable due to inadequate or delayed antibody-mediated immune response [134]. In one study, parvovirus B19 IgM antibody was present in only 75 % of transplant recipients at the time of disease onset [134].

Molecular testing offers higher sensitivity and specificity for the detection of parvovirus B19 infection compared to serologic testing, although all tests are LDTs [134]. The positive predictive value of a positive parvovirus B19 PCR test for the diagnosis of parvovirus B19 disease in an immunocompromised host with red cell aplasia is high. Hence, the detection of parvovirus B19 by PCR is highly suggestive of the diagnosis in a patient with unexplained anemia after transplantation [134]. In contrast, the detection of parvovirus B19 DNA in an asymptomatic patient with no anemia is of questionable significance, and likely represents subclinical reactivation. Most molecular assays are qualitative tests and detect low-level parvovirus B19 that characteristically persists long after the clinical resolution of the illness. Parvovirus B19 DNA can be detected by PCR in the serum of some patients for a prolonged period after acute infection [134]. Thus, a positive parvovirus B19 PCR test must be carefully interpreted in the context of the clinical setting and other laboratory test results.

Confirmation of parvovirus B19 disease may require bone marrow examination [131]. The classic bone marrow findings include overall hypercellularity, the presence of giant pronormoblasts with finely granulated cytoplasm and glassy intranuclear inclusions with a clear central halo (lantern cells), and the absence of late normoblasts. Histopathologic findings can be complemented by in situ hybridization or immunohistochemical staining to demonstrate the presence of parvovirus B19 in the bone marrow [131]. While these histopathologic findings are characteristic of parvovirus B19 disease, PCR testing may be performed to demonstrate the presence of the virus in the bone marrow [134].

Laboratory Issues and Future Directions

Clinical laboratories face many challenges with viral testing in transplant and other severely immunocompromised patients. These challenges encompass virtually every aspect of testing and stem not only from the wide number of viruses and their classic and atypical clinical presentations, but also from a lack of consensus regarding optimal testing practices and result interpretation, a near absence of US FDA-cleared, standardized assays, and a scarcity of material for test validation and proficiency testing.

Important considerations for viral testing in the transplant setting include optimal specimen type, collection (technique and frequency), preservation, and storage depending on the potential viral infection, the clinical question being asked (surveillance, diagnosis, or treatment response), and the site of potential involvement. Assay selection, required performance characteristics, and test interpretation are interrelated to these issues. However, the literature for many or most relevant viral pathogens remains clouded by a lack of standardization. In the absence of commercially available, automated test kits, test results can vary tremendously, particularly between different laboratories. Even with the recent availability of quantitative standards for some viruses, unanswered questions remain related to the clinical use of standardized results, and unified quantitative treatment thresholds have not yet been developed. Most laboratories with transplant programs must develop both the appropriate viral LDTs as well as the interpretive guidelines for their patient populations. Further complicating clinical viral testing is that most of these viruses have a high rate of latency in the general population. Detection may not correspond to disease or risk of progression. Risk stratification using viral load results may be based on factors such as underlying disease, transplant type, graft relatedness, presence of GVHD, and the degree of immune suppression. However, an absence of clear, uniform interpretive guidelines may lead to questions of appropriate test utilization, both from clinical utility and cost perspectives.

Despite substantial challenges, progress in understanding the clinical usefulness of viral testing in the transplant setting has been impressive. A growing body of literature supports the use of aggressive, quantitative surveillance to reduce morbidity and mortality due to CMV and other viruses. The number of published viral genome, primer, and probe sequences has mushroomed, as has the number of available platforms and amplification chemistries. The recent introduction of international quantitative standards for CMV and EBV promises to allow some degree of normalization between assays and laboratories. Such standardization should spill over to other viruses such as BKV, adenovirus, and others. In their absence, those involved in such testing must navigate an increasingly complex landscape to select and properly interpret the methods best suited to improving care of their transplant patient populations and patient care settings.

References

1. Razonable RR, Eid AJ. Viral infections in transplant recipients. Minerva Med. 2009;100(6):479–501.
2. Razonable RR, Paya CV, et al. Role of the laboratory in diagnosis and management of cytomegalovirus infection in hematopoietic stem cell and solid-organ transplant recipients. J Clin Microbiol. 2002;40(3):746–52.
3. Pang XL, Fox JD, et al. Interlaboratory comparison of cytomegalovirus viral load assays. Am J Transplant. 2009;9(2):258–68.
4. Preiksaitis JK, Pang XL, et al. Interlaboratory comparison of Epstein-Barr virus viral load assays. Am J Transplant. 2009;9(2): 269–79.
5. Ison MG, Green M. Adenovirus in solid organ transplant recipients. Am J Transplant. 2009;9 Suppl 4:S161–5.
6. Ganzenmueller T, Buchholz S, et al. High lethality of human adenovirus disease in adult allogeneic stem cell transplant recipients with high adenoviral blood load. J Clin Virol. 2011;52(1):55–9.
7. Bil-Lula I, Ussowicz M, et al. PCR diagnostics and monitoring of adenoviral infections in hematopoietic stem cell transplantation recipients. Arch Virol. 2010;155(12):2007–15.
8. Humar A, Kumar D, et al. A surveillance study of adenovirus infection in adult solid organ transplant recipients. Am J Transplant. 2005;5(10):2555–9.
9. Gustafson I, Lindblom A, et al. Quantification of adenovirus DNA in unrelated donor hematopoietic stem cell transplant recipients. J Clin Virol. 2008;43(1):79–85.
10. Michaels MG, Green M, et al. Adenovirus infection in pediatric liver transplant recipients. J Infect Dis. 1992;165(1):170–4.
11. McGrath D, Falagas ME, et al. Adenovirus infection in adult orthotopic liver transplant recipients: incidence and clinical significance. J Infect Dis. 1998;177(2):459–62.
12. George D, El-Mallawany NK, et al. Adenovirus infection in paediatric allogeneic stem cell transplantation recipients is a major independent factor for significantly increasing the risk of treatment related mortality. Br J Haematol. 2012;156(1):99–108.
13. Yilmaz M, Chemaly RF, et al. Adenoviral infections in adult allogeneic hematopoietic SCT recipients: a single center experience. Bone Marrow Transplant. 2013;48(9):1218–23.
14. Ohori NP, Michaels MG, et al. Adenovirus pneumonia in lung transplant recipients. Hum Pathol. 1995;26(10):1073–9.
15. Yagisawa T, Takahashi K, et al. Adenovirus induced nephropathy in kidney transplant recipients. Transplant Proc. 1989;21(1 Pt 2):2097–9.
16. Jeulin H, Salmon A, et al. Comparison of in-house real-time quantitative PCR to the Adenovirus R-Gene kit for determination of adenovirus load in clinical samples. J Clin Microbiol. 2010;48(9):3132–7.
17. Huang ML, Nguy L, et al. Development of multiplexed real-time quantitative polymerase chain reaction assay for detecting human adenoviruses. Diagn Microbiol Infect Dis. 2008;62(3):263–71.
18. Jeulin H, Salmon A, et al. Diagnostic value of quantitative PCR for adenovirus detection in stool samples as compared with antigen detection and cell culture in haematopoietic stem cell transplant recipients. Clin Microbiol Infect. 2011;17(11):1674–80.
19. Lee JH, Jang JH, et al. Respiratory viral infections during the first 28 days after transplantation in pediatric hematopoietic stem cell transplant recipients. Clin Transplant. 2012;26:736–40.
20. Lion T, Kosulin K, et al. Monitoring of adenovirus load in stool by real-time PCR permits early detection of impending invasive infection in patients after allogeneic stem cell transplantation. Leukemia. 2010;24(4):706–14.
21. Funahashi Y, Iwata S, et al. Multiplex real-time PCR assay for simultaneous quantification of BK polyomavirus, JC polyomavirus, and adenovirus DNA. J Clin Microbiol. 2010;48(3):825–30.
22. Schonberger S, Meisel R, et al. Prospective, comprehensive, and effective viral monitoring in children undergoing allogeneic hematopoietic stem cell transplantation. Biol Blood Marrow Transplant. 2010;16(10):1428–35.
23. Ohrmalm L, Lindblom A, et al. Evaluation of a surveillance strategy for early detection of adenovirus by PCR of peripheral blood in hematopoietic SCT recipients: incidence and outcome. Bone Marrow Transplant. 2011;46(2):267–72.
24. Suparno C, Milligan DW, et al. Adenovirus infections in stem cell transplant recipients: recent developments in understanding of pathogenesis, diagnosis and management. Leuk Lymphoma. 2004;45(5):873–85.
25. Ison MG. Adenovirus infections in transplant recipients. Clin Infect Dis. 2006;43(3):331–9.
26. Leruez-Ville M, Minard V, et al. Real-time blood plasma polymerase chain reaction for management of disseminated adenovirus infection. Clin Infect Dis. 2004;38(1):45–52.
27. Hirsch HH, Randhawa P. BK virus in solid organ transplant recipients. Am J Transplant. 2009;9 Suppl 4:S136–46.
28. Arthur RR, Shah KV, et al. Association of BK viruria with hemorrhagic cystitis in recipients of bone marrow transplants. N Engl J Med. 1986;315(4):230–4.
29. Hirsch HH, Knowles W, et al. Prospective study of polyomavirus type BK replication and nephropathy in renal-transplant recipients. N Engl J Med. 2002;347(7):488–96.
30. Brennan DC, Agha I, et al. Incidence of BK with tacrolimus versus cyclosporine and impact of preemptive immunosuppression reduction. Am J Transplant. 2005;5(3):582–94.
31. Funk GA, Gosert R, et al. Polyomavirus BK replication dynamics in vivo and in silico to predict cytopathology and viral clearance in kidney transplants. Am J Transplant. 2008;8(11):2368–77.
32. Drachenberg CB, Beskow CO, et al. Human polyoma virus in renal allograft biopsies: morphological findings and correlation with urine cytology. Hum Pathol. 1999;30(8):970–7.
33. Drachenberg RC, Drachenberg CB, et al. Morphological spectrum of polyoma virus disease in renal allografts: diagnostic accuracy of urine cytology. Am J Transplant. 2001;1(4):373–81.
34. Nickeleit V, Klimkait T, et al. Testing for polyomavirus type BK DNA in plasma to identify renal-allograft recipients with viral nephropathy. N Engl J Med. 2000;342(18):1309–15.

35. Drachenberg CB, Hirsch HH, et al. Polyomavirus BK versus JC replication and nephropathy in renal transplant recipients: a prospective evaluation. Transplantation. 2007;84(3):323–30.
36. Bedi A, Miller CB, et al. Association of BK virus with failure of prophylaxis against hemorrhagic cystitis following bone marrow transplantation. J Clin Oncol. 1995;13(5):1103–9.
37. Dropulic LK, Jones RJ. Polyomavirus BK infection in blood and marrow transplant recipients. Bone Marrow Transplant. 2008;41(1):11–8.
38. Drachenberg CB, Papadimitriou JC, et al. Histological patterns of polyomavirus nephropathy: correlation with graft outcome and viral load. Am J Transplant. 2004;4(12):2082–92.
39. Viscount HB, Eid AJ, et al. Polyomavirus polymerase chain reaction as a surrogate marker of polyomavirus-associated nephropathy. Transplantation. 2007;84(3):340–5.
40. Nickeleit V, Hirsch HH, et al. Polyomavirus infection of renal allograft recipients: from latent infection to manifest disease. J Am Soc Nephrol. 1999;10(5):1080–9.
41. Hirsch HH, Brennan DC, et al. Polyomavirus-associated nephropathy in renal transplantation: interdisciplinary analyses and recommendations. Transplantation. 2005;79(10):1277–86.
42. Hirsch HH, Drachenberg CB, et al. Polyomavirus-associated nephropathy in renal transplantation: critical issues of screening and management. Adv Exp Med Biol. 2006;577:160–73.
43. Hayden RT, Yan X, et al. Factors contributing to variability of quantitative viral PCR results in proficiency testing samples: a multivariate analysis. J Clin Microbiol. 2012;50(2):337–45.
44. Kotton CN, Kumar D, et al. Updated international consensus guidelines on the management of cytomegalovirus in solid-organ transplantation. Transplantation. 2013;96(4):333–60.
45. Razonable RR, Humar A. Cytomegalovirus in solid organ transplantation. Am J Transplant. 2013;13 Suppl 4:93–106.
46. Eid AJ, Razonable RR. New developments in the management of cytomegalovirus infection after solid organ transplantation. Drugs. 2010;70(8):965–81.
47. Razonable R. Direct and indirect effects of cytomegalovirus: can we prevent them? Enferm Infecc Microbiol Clin. 2010;28(1):1–5.
48. Razonable RR. Strategies for managing cytomegalovirus in transplant recipients. Expert Opin Pharmacother. 2010;11(12): 1983–97.
49. Razonable RR. Management of viral infections in solid organ transplant recipients. Expert Rev Anti Infect Ther. 2011;9(6): 685–700.
50. Manuel O, Pang XL, et al. An assessment of donor-to-recipient transmission patterns of human cytomegalovirus by analysis of viral genomic variants. J Infect Dis. 2009;199(11):1621–8.
51. Humar A, Snydman D. Cytomegalovirus in solid organ transplant recipients. Am J Transplant. 2009;9 Suppl 4:S78–86.
52. Razonable RR, Rivero A, et al. Allograft rejection predicts the occurrence of late-onset cytomegalovirus (CMV) disease among CMV-mismatched solid organ transplant patients receiving prophylaxis with oral ganciclovir. J Infect Dis. 2001;184(11):1461–4.
53. Razonable RR, van Cruijsen H, et al. Dynamics of cytomegalovirus replication during preemptive therapy with oral ganciclovir. J Infect Dis. 2003;187(11):1801–8.
54. Kanda Y, Yamashita T, et al. A randomized controlled trial of plasma real-time PCR and antigenemia assay for monitoring CMV infection after unrelated BMT. Bone Marrow Transplant. 2010;45(8):1325–32.
55. Park SY, Lee SO, et al. Paradoxical rising cytomegalovirus antigenemia during preemptive ganciclovir therapy in hematopoietic stem cell transplant recipients: incidence, risk factors, and clinical outcomes. J Clin Microbiol. 2011;49(12):4179–84.
56. Razonable RR, Hayden RT. Clinical utility of viral load in management of cytomegalovirus infection after solid organ transplantation. Clin Microbiol Rev. 2013;26(4):703–27.
57. Hebart H, Lengerke C, et al. Prospective comparison of PCR-based vs late mRNA-based preemptive antiviral therapy for HCMV infection in patients after allo-SCT. Bone Marrow Transplant. 2011;46(3):408–15.
58. Lisboa LF, Asberg A, et al. The clinical utility of whole blood versus plasma cytomegalovirus viral load assays for monitoring therapeutic response. Transplantation. 2011;91(2):231–6.
59. Razonable RR, Asberg A, et al. Virologic suppression measured by a cytomegalovirus (CMV) DNA test calibrated to the World Health Organization international standard is predictive of CMV disease resolution in transplant recipients. Clin Infect Dis. 2013;56(11):1546–53.
60. Eid AJ, Arthurs SK, et al. Clinical predictors of relapse after treatment of primary gastrointestinal cytomegalovirus disease in solid organ transplant recipients. Am J Transplant. 2010;10(1):157–61.
61. Lisboa LF, Preiksaitis JK, et al. Clinical utility of molecular surveillance for cytomegalovirus after antiviral prophylaxis in high-risk solid organ transplant recipients. Transplantation. 2011;92(9): 1063–8.
62. Humar A, Gregson D, et al. Clinical utility of quantitative cytomegalovirus viral load determination for predicting cytomegalovirus disease in liver transplant recipients. Transplantation. 1999;68(9):1305–11.
63. Razonable RR, Brown RA, et al. Comparative quantitation of cytomegalovirus (CMV) DNA in solid organ transplant recipients with CMV infection by using two high-throughput automated systems. J Clin Microbiol. 2001;39(12):4472–6.
64. Asberg A, Humar A, et al. Oral valganciclovir is noninferior to intravenous ganciclovir for the treatment of cytomegalovirus disease in solid organ transplant recipients. Am J Transplant. 2007;7(9):2106–13.
65. Asberg A, Jardine AG, et al. Effects of the intensity of immunosuppressive therapy on outcome of treatment for CMV disease in organ transplant recipients. Am J Transplant. 2010;10(8):1881–8.
66. Emery VC, Manuel O, et al. Differential decay kinetics of human cytomegalovirus glycoprotein B genotypes following antiviral chemotherapy. J Clin Virol. 2012;54(1):56–60.
67. Sia IG, Wilson JA, et al. Cytomegalovirus (CMV) DNA load predicts relapsing CMV infection after solid organ transplantation. J Infect Dis. 2000;181(2):717–20.
68. Humar A, Kumar D, et al. Cytomegalovirus (CMV) virus load kinetics to predict recurrent disease in solid-organ transplant patients with CMV disease. J Infect Dis. 2002;186(6):829–33.
69. Humar A, Kumar D, et al. Clinical impact of human herpesvirus 6 infection after liver transplantation. Transplantation. 2002;73(4): 599–604.
70. Eid AJ, Arthurs SK, et al. Emergence of drug-resistant cytomegalovirus in the era of valganciclovir prophylaxis: therapeutic implications and outcomes. Clin Transplant. 2008;22(2):162–70.
71. Lurain NS, Chou S. Antiviral drug resistance of human cytomegalovirus. Clin Microbiol Rev. 2010;23(4):689–712.
72. Allen U, Preiksaitis J. Epstein-Barr virus and posttransplant lymphoproliferative disorder in solid organ transplant recipients. Am J Transplant. 2009;9 Suppl 4:S87–96.
73. Walker RC, Paya CV, et al. Pretransplantation seronegative Epstein-Barr virus status is the primary risk factor for posttransplantation lymphoproliferative disorder in adult heart, lung, and other solid organ transplantations. J Heart Lung Transplant. 1995;14(2):214–21.
74. Gross TG, Savoldo B, et al. Posttransplant lymphoproliferative diseases. Pediatr Clin North Am. 2010;57(2):481–503. table of contents.
75. Walker RC, Marshall WF, et al. Pretransplantation assessment of the risk of lymphoproliferative disorder. Clin Infect Dis. 1995;20(5):1346–53.
76. Weinstock DM, Ambrossi GG, et al. Preemptive diagnosis and treatment of Epstein-Barr virus-associated post transplant lymphoproliferative disorder after hematopoietic stem cell transplant:

an approach in development. Bone Marrow Transplant. 2006;37(6):539–46.
77. Gulley ML, Tang W. Using Epstein-Barr viral load assays to diagnose, monitor, and prevent posttransplant lymphoproliferative disorder. Clin Microbiol Rev. 2010;23(2):350–66.
78. Holman CJ, Karger AB, et al. Quantitative Epstein-Barr virus shedding and its correlation with the risk of post-transplant lymphoproliferative disorder. Clin Transplant. 2012;26:741–7.
79. Terasawa T, Ohashi H, et al. Failure to detect Epstein-Barr virus (EBV) DNA in plasma by real-time PCR in a case of EBV-associated posttransplantation lymphoproliferative disorder confined to the central nervous system. Int J Hematol. 2002;75(4):416–20.
80. Volpi A. Epstein-Barr virus and human herpesvirus type 8 infections of the central nervous system. Herpes. 2004;11 Suppl 2:120A–7.
81. Zuckerman R, Wald A. Herpes simplex virus infections in solid organ transplant recipients. Am J Transplant. 2009;9 Suppl 4:S104–7.
82. Schillinger JA, Xu F, et al. National seroprevalence and trends in herpes simplex virus type 1 in the United States, 1976–1994. Sex Transm Dis. 2004;31(12):753–60.
83. Xu F, Sternberg MR, et al. Trends in herpes simplex virus type 1 and type 2 seroprevalence in the United States. JAMA. 2006;296(8):964–73.
84. Dummer JS, Armstrong J, et al. Transmission of infection with herpes simplex virus by renal transplantation. J Infect Dis. 1987;155(2):202–6.
85. Wald A, Zeh J, et al. Reactivation of genital herpes simplex virus type 2 infection in asymptomatic seropositive persons. N Engl J Med. 2000;342(12):844–50.
86. Strick LB, Wald A. Diagnostics for herpes simplex virus: is PCR the new gold standard? Mol Diagn Ther. 2006;10(1):17–28.
87. Espy MJ, Uhl JR, et al. Diagnosis of herpes simplex virus infections in the clinical laboratory by LightCycler PCR. J Clin Microbiol. 2000;38(2):795–9.
88. Wald A, Huang ML, et al. Polymerase chain reaction for detection of herpes simplex virus (HSV) DNA on mucosal surfaces: comparison with HSV isolation in cell culture. J Infect Dis. 2003;188(9):1345–51.
89. Issa NC, Espy MJ, et al. Sequencing and resolution of amplified herpes simplex virus DNA with intermediate melting curves as genotype 1 or 2 by LightCycler PCR assay. J Clin Microbiol. 2005;43(4):1843–5.
90. Dhiman N, Wright PA, et al. Concurrent detection of herpes simplex and varicella-zoster viruses by polymerase chain reaction from the same anatomic location. Diagn Microbiol Infect Dis. 2011;70(4):538–40.
91. Roubalova K, Suchankova A, et al. Presence of herpes simplex virus (HSV) in peripheral leukocytes of patient who developed active HSV infection after bone marrow transplantation. J Clin Virol. 2000;17(1):37–42.
92. Levitsky J, Duddempudi AT, et al. Detection and diagnosis of herpes simplex virus infection in adults with acute liver failure. Liver Transpl. 2008;14(10):1498–504.
93. Aumakhan B, Hardick A, et al. Genital herpes evaluation by quantitative TaqMan PCR: correlating single detection and quantity of HSV-2 DNA in cervicovaginal lavage fluids with cross-sectional and longitudinal clinical data. Virol J. 2010;7:328.
94. Jazeron JF, Barbe C, et al. Virological diagnosis of herpes simplex virus 1 esophagitis by quantitative real-time PCR assay. J Clin Microbiol. 2012;50(3):948–52.
95. Ziyaeyan M, Alborzi A, et al. Diagnosis and quantitative detection of HSV DNA in samples from patients with suspected herpes simplex encephalitis. Braz J Infect Dis. 2011;15(3):211–4.
96. Chaillon A, Schnepf N, et al. Case report: benefits of quantitative polymerase chain reaction in the clinical management of herpes simplex virus 1 infection with prominent hepatitis and unusual secondary progression. J Med Virol. 2012;84(3):457–61.
97. Fluri S, Kaczala GW, et al. Chickenpox is not always benign: postvaricella purpura fulminans requires prompt and aggressive treatment. Pediatr Emerg Care. 2010;26(12):932–4.
98. Pergam SA, Limaye AP. Varicella zoster virus (VZV) in solid organ transplant recipients. Am J Transplant. 2009;9 Suppl 4:S108–15.
99. Roque-Afonso AM, Bralet MP, et al. Chickenpox-associated fulminant hepatitis that led to liver transplantation in a 63-year-old woman. Liver Transpl. 2008;14(9):1309–12.
100. Alvite-Canosa M, Paniagua-Martin MJ, et al. Fulminant hepatic failure due to varicella zoster in a heart transplant patient: successful liver transplant. J Heart Lung Transplant. 2009;28(11):1215–6.
101. Ishizaki Y, Tezuka J, et al. Quantification of circulating varicella zoster virus-DNA for the early diagnosis of visceral varicella. J Infect. 2003;47(2):133–8.
102. Watzinger F, Suda M, et al. Real-time quantitative PCR assays for detection and monitoring of pathogenic human viruses in immunosuppressed pediatric patients. J Clin Microbiol. 2004;42(11):5189–98.
103. Sawada A, Koyama-Sato M, et al. Multiplex polymerase chain reaction for six herpesviruses after hematopoietic stem cell transplantation. Pediatr Int. 2011;53(6):1010–7.
104. Lautenschlager I, Razonable RR. Human herpesvirus-6 infections in kidney, liver, lung, and heart transplantation: review. Transpl Int. 2012;25(5):493–502.
105. Razonable RR. Human herpesviruses 6, 7 and 8 in solid organ transplant recipients. Am J Transplant. 2013;13 Suppl 3:67–77. quiz 77-68.
106. Razonable RR, Zerr DM. HHV-6, HHV-7 and HHV-8 in solid organ transplant recipients. Am J Transplant. 2009;9 Suppl 4:S97–100.
107. Grossi PA, Costa AN, et al. Infections and organ transplantation: new challenges for prevention and treatment – a colloquium. Transplantation. 2012;93(5 Suppl):S4–39.
108. Lee SO, Brown RA, et al. Chromosomally integrated human herpesvirus-6 in transplant recipients. Transpl Infect Dis. 2012.
109. Abdel Massih RC, Razonable RR. Human herpesvirus 6 infections after liver transplantation. World J Gastroenterol. 2009;15(21):2561–9.
110. de Pagter PJ, Schuurman R, et al. Human herpes virus 6 plasma DNA positivity after hematopoietic stem cell transplantation in children: an important risk factor for clinical outcome. Biol Blood Marrow Transplant. 2008;14(7):831–9.
111. Lee SO, Brown RA, et al. Clinical significance of pretransplant chromosomally integrated human herpesvirus-6 in liver transplant recipients. Transplantation. 2011;92(2):224–9.
112. Pellett PE, Ablashi DV, et al. Chromosomally integrated human herpesvirus 6: questions and answers. Rev Med Virol. 2011;22(3):144–55.
113. Antman K, Chang Y. Kaposi's sarcoma. N Engl J Med. 2000;342(14):1027–38.
114. Ariza-Heredia EJ, Razonable RR. Human herpes virus 8 in solid organ transplantation. Transplantation. 2011;92(8):837–44.
115. Luppi M, Barozzi P, et al. Molecular evidence of organ-related transmission of Kaposi sarcoma-associated herpesvirus or human herpesvirus-8 in transplant patients. Blood. 2000;96(9):3279–81.

116. Marcelin AG, Roque-Afonso AM, et al. Fatal disseminated Kaposi's sarcoma following human herpesvirus 8 primary infections in liver-transplant recipients. Liver Transpl. 2004;10(2): 295–300.
117. Boulanger E, Afonso PV, et al. Human herpesvirus-8 (HHV-8)-associated primary effusion lymphoma in two renal transplant recipients receiving rapamycin. Am J Transplant. 2008;8(3):707–10.
118. Barozzi P, Luppi M, et al. Post-transplant Kaposi sarcoma originates from the seeding of donor-derived progenitors. Nat Med. 2003;9(5):554–61.
119. Qunibi W, Akhtar M, et al. Kaposi's sarcoma: the most common tumor after renal transplantation in Saudi Arabia. Am J Med. 1988;84(2):225–32.
120. Barozzi P, Bonini C, et al. Changes in the immune responses against human herpesvirus-8 in the disease course of posttransplant Kaposi sarcoma. Transplantation. 2008;86(5):738–44.
121. Spira TJ, Lam L, et al. Comparison of serologic assays and PCR for diagnosis of human herpesvirus 8 infection. J Clin Microbiol. 2000;38(6):2174–80.
122. Laney AS, Peters JS, et al. Use of a multiantigen detection algorithm for diagnosis of Kaposi's sarcoma-associated herpes virus infection. J Clin Microbiol. 2006;44(10):3734–41.
123. Mendez JC, Procop GW, et al. Relationship of HHV8 replication and Kaposi's sarcoma after solid organ transplantation. Transplantation. 1999;67(8):1200–1.
124. Pozo F, Tenorio A, et al. Persistent human herpesvirus 8 viremia before Kaposi's sarcoma development in a liver transplant recipient. Transplantation. 2000;70(2):395–7.
125. Farge D, Lebbe C, et al. Human herpes virus-8 and other risk factors for Kaposi's sarcoma in kidney transplant recipients. Groupe Cooperatif de Transplantation d' Ile de France (GCIF). Transplantation. 1999;67(9):1236–42.
126. Pellet C, Chevret S, et al. Prognostic value of quantitative Kaposi sarcoma-associated herpesvirus load in posttransplantation Kaposi sarcoma. J Infect Dis. 2002;186(1):110–3.
127. Pietrosi G, Vizzini G, et al. Primary and reactivated HHV8 infection and disease after liver transplantation: a prospective study. Am J Transplant. 2011;11(12):2715–23.
128. Lock MJ, Griffiths PD, et al. Development of a quantitative competitive polymerase chain reaction for human herpesvirus 8. J Virol Methods. 1997;64(1):19–26.
129. Lebbe C, Legendre C, et al. Kaposi sarcoma in transplantation. Transplant Rev. 2008;22(4):252–61.
130. Young NS, Brown KE. Parvovirus B19. N Engl J Med. 2004;350(6):586–97.
131. Eid AJ, Posfay-Barbe KM. Parvovirus B19 in solid organ transplant recipients. Am J Transplant. 2009;9 Suppl 4:S147–50.
132. Corcioli F, Zakrzewska K, et al. Tissue persistence of parvovirus B19 genotypes in asymptomatic persons. J Med Virol. 2008;80(11):2005–11.
133. Ki CS, Kim IS, et al. Incidence and clinical significance of human parvovirus B19 infection in kidney transplant recipients. Clin Transplant. 2005;19(6):751–5.
134. Eid AJ, Brown RA, et al. Parvovirus B19 infection after transplantation: a review of 98 cases. Clin Infect Dis. 2006; 43(1):40–8.

Viral Infections of the Central Nervous System

48

Duane W. Newton and Christine C. Ginocchio

Abstract

Although relatively rare and typically benign, viral infections of the central nervous system (CNS) can have a significant impact on affected patients. This chapter provides a description of the epidemiology and diagnosis of a variety of important pathogens associated with CNS infections, including enteroviruses, herpesviruses, and arboviruses, as well as viral agents which cause CNS infections in immunocompromised patients.

Keywords

Infection • Central nervous system • Enterovirus • HSV • VZV • HHV-6 • Arbovirus • Immunocompromised • Cytomegalovirus • JC virus • HIV

Introduction

Viral infections of the central nervous system (CNS) are relatively infrequent and usually result in a benign, self-limiting disease [1–4]. However, in a small percentage of cases, these infections can have extremely serious consequences that result in a spectrum of permanent neurologic sequelae or death. Viral agents gain access to the CNS by either neuronal or hematogenous spread, and infections can occur at many sites throughout the CNS including the spinal cord, leptomeninges, dorsal nerve roots, nerves, and brain parenchyma. Viral CNS infections are classified clinically as either meningitis or encephalitis, although a close interrelationship exists between the two disease states [1–4]. Host factors (age, sex, immune status, genetic differences) and viral factors (serotype, receptor preference, cell tropism, viral load) in concert with geographic and seasonal factors contribute to the potential for the development of CNS disease [1–4].

D.W. Newton, Ph.D., D.(A.B.M.M.) (✉)
Clinical Microbiology Laboratory, Division of Clinical Pathology, University of Michigan,
1500 E. Medical Center Drive, UH2G332, Ann Arbor, MI 48109-5054, USA
e-mail: dnewton@med.umich.edu

C.C. Ginocchio, Ph.D., M.T.(A.S.C.P.)
Department of Pathology and Laboratory Medicine Hofstra North Shore-LIJ School of Medicine Hempstead, NY 11549, USA

Scientific and Medical Affairs, BioMérieux, Durham, NC 22717, USA

Scientific and Medical Affairs, BioFire Diagnostics, Salt Lake City, UT 84108, USA

Epidemiology of Viral CNS Disease

Viral meningitis, meningoencephalitis, and encephalitis frequently occur in epidemics and as seasonal outbreaks (late spring through autumn) in temperate climates, and account for the majority of viral CNS infections [1–4]. The most common viral agents responsible for CNS disease are listed in Table 48.1. In the USA and in countries that immunize against mumps, enteroviruses account for approximately 80–92 % of all cases of meningitis in which a causative agent is identified [3–6]. In addition, the recently characterized human parechoviruses are the agents of a portion of viral meningitides whose etiology was previously unrecognized [5, 6]. In countries that do not immunize against mumps, mumps virus accounts for up to 30 % of viral meningitis cases [7]. Arthropod-borne viruses (arboviruses) (Table 48.2) account for the majority of the remaining cases of meningitis in the USA [8–10].

D.G.B. Leonard (ed.), *Molecular Pathology in Clinical Practice*, DOI 10.1007/978-3-319-19674-9_48

Table 48.1 Primary viral agents causing central nervous system disease

Herpesviruses	Herpes simplex 1 and 2
	Varicella-zoster
	Epstein-Barr
	Cytomegalovirus
	Human herpesvirus 6
Enteroviruses	Poliovirus
	Coxsackievirus
	Echovirus
	Numbered enteroviruses
Parechoviruses	Human parechovirus 1–14
Arboviruses	See Table 48.2
Childhood illness associated	Measles
	Mumps
	Rubella
Rabies	
Vesicular stomatitis virus	
JC polyoma virus	
Human immunodeficiency virus type 1	

Table 48.2 Arthropod-borne viruses (arboviruses) and endemic areas

Family	Genus	Virus	Predominant regions
Togaviridae	*Alphavirus*	Eastern equine	Eastern, southern USA; Canada; Central, South America
		Western equine	Western, central USA; Central, South America
		Venezuelan equine	Central, South America; eastern, western USA
Flaviviridae	*Flavivirus*	St Louis	USA; South America
		Powassan	Canada; USA; Russia
		Tick-borne	Central Europe; Russia
		Japanese	Asia; Russia; India; Sri Lanka
		Murray Valley	USA
		West Nile	North America; Europe; Middle East; Africa; Asia; Australia; Oceania
Bunyaviridae	*Bunyavirus*	California group[a]	California; upper Midwest; West Virginia; Virginia; Kentucky; Tennessee;
			North Carolina; Alabama
Reoviridae	*Coltivirus*	Colorado tick fever	Western mountain USA

[a]La Crosse, Cache Valley, Jamestown Canyon, and Snowshoe hare

Encephalitis occurs at a lower frequency than meningitis, with arboviruses being the leading cause both worldwide and in the USA [8–10]. Flaviviruses and alphaviruses are the most frequent arboviruses causing encephalitis and are responsible for the majority of mosquito and tick-borne encephalitis that cause epidemic and endemic disease in Asia, Europe, and the Americas [8–10]. Case fatality rates vary greatly, ranging from 5–70 %. Human immunodeficiency virus (HIV) and rabies virus (genus *Lyssavirus*) are other important causes of encephalitis worldwide [1, 2]. Herpes simplex virus (HSV) CNS infections affect all ages, occur at all times of the year, and have the highest encephalitis mortality rate in the USA [1–4]. In a small number of cases, childhood viral diseases including rubella, measles, varicella-zoster virus (VZV), mumps, and human herpes virus 6 (HHV-6) can progress to neurologic disease during primary infection or with viral reactivation (VZV and HHV-6). Cytomegalovirus (CMV) [11–13] and JC polyomavirus (JCV) [14] are responsible for encephalitides in immunocompromised patients.

Overview of Diagnostic Testing for Viral CNS Disease

Traditionally, the diagnosis of viral CNS infection has been based on laboratory findings in conjunction with patient history, clinical manifestations, and geographic and epidemiologic factors [1–4, 8, 9]. The diagnosis of viral encephalitis requires supplemental tests, including lumbar puncture, radiographic imaging such as computed tomography (CT) scans and magnetic resonance imaging (MRI) studies, and in some cases brain biopsy.

In general, patients with viral meningitis typically have a cerebrospinal fluid (CSF) pleocytosis with 10–500 leukocytes/mm^3, a slightly elevated protein (<100 mg/dL), and a glucose level greater than 40 % of a simultaneously drawn serum sample [1, 2]. However, there can be a tremendous range of values that often overlap with those indicative of bacterial meningitis. Patients with viral meningitis or encephalitis may or may not have a CSF pleocytosis [15]. Therefore, normal CSF cell counts should not be used as a sole exclusion criterion for both diagnosis and determining which samples should be tested by molecular methods for viral pathogens. CSF glucose levels can be normal or low, as seen with bacterial meningitis. Encephalitis can lead to hemorrhagic necrosis with elevated protein levels and the presence of red blood cells.

Negative cultures for bacterial, fungal, and mycobacterial pathogens can aid in the diagnosis of viral CNS infections but can take several weeks for definitive results. However, bacterial cultures may be falsely negative if patients have been treated with antibiotics prior to sample collection. Traditionally, the identification of the specific virus relied on viral culture, serologic detection of virus-specific IgM and IgG antibodies (either systemic or intrathecal), or both [3, 4, 16–18]. However, the ability to isolate the virus is highly dependent on the viral species, time of sample collection, sample handling and processing, and prior treatment of the patient with antiviral agents. In only approximately 10–16 % of viral meningitis cases is the causative agent identified using viral culture [3, 4, 7, 16–19]. Serologic diagnosis can be made from serum in certain cases as early as 5 days after infection with the development of specific IgM antibodies, but often takes weeks to demonstrate a diagnostic rise in IgG antibody titers between acute and convalescent serum samples [3, 4, 14, 16–18, 20, 22]. Some patients with West Nile viral infections have detectable IgM antibodies in the serum for up to 500 days after infection, making the distinction between recent and past infection difficult [22]. In addition, immune status of the patient can affect the development of virus-specific antibodies. Since CNS infection may compromise the integrity of the blood–brain barrier, interpretation of CSF serology can be problematic.

Currently, molecular amplification methods that detect viral pathogens in CSF play a critical role in the rapid and accurate diagnosis of viral CNS infections [16, 18, 19]. This approach has largely abrogated the need for brain biopsy for the diagnosis of encephalitis and, in cases where biopsy is needed, can be used to detect viral pathogens in tissue specimens. In most cases, CSF is easily obtained, especially compared to brain biopsy. CSF should be stored frozen, preferably at ≤70 °C, to maintain the stability of viral nucleic acids. Isolation of the nucleic acids is achieved using a variety of extraction methods (described in Chap. 2) that also remove amplification inhibitors and neutralize any DNases or RNases present in the sample. The volume of CSF required can vary significantly and is dependent on the viral target, relative levels of virus present in the CSF, and the sensitivity of the testing method.

Results from molecular tests can be available within 24 h and possibly as soon as 2 h for applications utilizing real-time PCR technologies that incorporate amplification and detection in one step. This is in contrast to viral culture and serology, which can require up to 28 days for a final result. In the case of enteroviral infections, rapid detection of this pathogen has been shown to direct the selection of appropriate therapy, decrease the number of patients unnecessarily placed on empiric antibiotic therapy, shorten length of hospitalization, and save medical costs [23–26]. Overall, molecular amplification assays are highly sensitive and, depending on the virus and amplification target, can detect as low as one viral particle per reaction. High assay specificity is obtained by gene-specific targeting and often is significantly more sensitive and specific than serologic testing, which can demonstrate cross-reactivity among related viruses. Multiplex assays offer the versatility of screening for several pathogens in one test. Quantitative assays are useful for differentiating active from latent infection for herpesviruses and for monitoring response to antiviral therapy.

The last decade has seen a significant increase in the availability of commercially developed systems, assays, and reagents for molecular detection of viral infections. Table 48.3 lists the currently available US Food and Drug Administration (FDA)-cleared systems/assays and a representative selection of commercially available analyte-specific reagents (ASRs) that can be used in laboratory-developed tests (LDTs). This is not intended to be an exhaustive list, but represents several that are available in the US market. In addition, many types of reagents and kits are available from other manufacturers, including many that are Conformité Européenné (CE)-marked and not available in the USA.

This chapter reviews the advances in the molecular testing for the most common causes of viral meningitis and encephalitis, including the enteroviruses, herpesviruses, and arboviruses. In addition, viruses affecting persons with immune suppression, including human immunodeficiency virus type 1 (HIV-1), JCV, and CMV are briefly discussed.

Enteroviruses and Parechoviruses

Epidemiology and Disease

Human enteroviruses are small, nonenveloped, single-stranded RNA viruses that are distributed into seven species (human enteroviruses A, B, C, and D and human rhinoviruses A, B, and C) of the Picornaviridae family (www.picornaviridae.com; accessed June 2014). The non-polio enteroviruses, including the coxsackieviruses, echoviruses, and numbered enteroviruses, are responsible for approximately 50 million infections per year in the USA and possibly more than a billion worldwide [4, 27, 28]. Enteroviruses cause an array of illnesses in both adults and children, including respiratory, ocular, cardiac, gastrointestinal, and neurologic diseases, as well as skin and oral eruptions [27, 28]. In the neonate, enteroviruses can cause a sepsis-like picture or meningoencephalitis, which can be severe. Outside the neonatal period, children under 5 years of age appear to be the most susceptible to infection, partly due to a lack of acquired immunity and poor hygienic habits. Encephalitis is uncommon and meningitis is rarely associated with complicated disease and poor clinical outcome; enteroviral meningitis may be more severe in adults than in children. Although enteroviral infections can occur year-round, the majority of the infections in temperate climates occur during the summer through autumn months.

Human parechoviruses are related but molecularly distinct members of the *Picornaviridae* that were originally classified as additional serotypes of enteroviruses (echovirus 22 and 23) because of similarities in clinical and laboratory

Table 48.3 Commercial molecular assays and reagents available in the USA for detection of relevant viral agents

Target	Manufacturer	Test name	Method
US FDA-cleared[a] for CSF			
Enterovirus (EN)	bioMérieux, Inc.	NucliSENS EasyQ Enterovirus	Real-time NASBA
	Cepheid	Xpert EV	Real-time PCR
Herpes simplex virus	Focus Diagnostics	Simplexa HSV 1 and 2	Scorpion probes, real-time PCR
Analyte-specific reagents[b]			
Cytomegalovirus (CMV)	Epoch Biosciences/Nanogen	CMV primers and probes	MGB Alert, real-time PCR
	EraGen Biosciences	CMV primers ASR	Multicode bases, real-time PCR
	Focus Diagnostics	Simplexa CMV ASR	Scorpion probes, real-time PCR
	bioMérieux/Argene	Herpes Generic Consensus and Identification Assays	Hybridization probes, PCR
Enterovirus (EV)	Epoch Biosciences/Nanogen	Enterovirus	MGB Alert, real-time PCR
	EraGen Biosciences	Enterovirus primers ASR	Multicode bases, real-time PCR
	Focus Diagnostics	Simplexa Enterovirus ASR	Scorpion probes, real-time PCR
Herpes simplex virus (HSV)	Cepheid	HSV 1 and 2	TaqMan hydrolysis probes, real-time PCR
	Epoch Biosciences/Nanogen	HSV 1 and 2	MGB Alert, real-time PCR
	EraGen Biosciences	HSV primers ASR	Multicode bases, real-time PCR
	Roche Diagnostics	HSV 1 and 2 ASR	FRET probes, real-time PCR
	bioMérieux/Argene	Herpes Generic Consensus and Identification Assays	Hybridization probes, PCR
Human herpes virus 6 (HHV-6)	bioMérieux/Argene	Herpes Generic Consensus and Identification Assays	Hybridization probes, PCR
Varicella-zoster virus (VZV)	EraGen Biosciences	VZV primers ASR	Multicode bases, real-time PCR
	Focus Diagnostics	Simplexa VZV 1 and 2 ASR	Scorpion probes, real-time PCR
	bioMérieux/Argene	Herpes Generic Consensus and Identification Assays	Hybridization probes, PCR

ASR analyte-specific reagents, *CSF* cerebrospinal fluid, *FRET* fluorescence resonance energy transfer, *MGB* minor groove binder, *NASBA* nucleic acid sequence-based amplification, *PCR* poymerase chain reaction
[a]www.amp.org, accessed Jan 2012
[b]Not US FDA-cleared for diagnosis of CNS infections

characteristics [6]. However, parechovirus has now been established as its own genus based on extensive molecular studies. Increased surveillance and molecular phylogenetic studies have identified 16 distinct types [6]. The epidemiology and clinical presentation of parechovirus infection overlap with enteroviruses. While neonates and young children are primarily affected by both viruses, parechovirus infections in persons over age 10 have rarely been reported [6].

Laboratory Diagnosis

Many enteroviruses can be cultured in human and primate cell lines [27]. No single cell line is optimal for all enteroviral types, and therefore several different cell lines susceptible to enteroviral infection typically are used for clinical testing. Viral CSF culture has a sensitivity of approximately 65–75 %, in part because of the lability of the virus and possible low levels in the CSF. Furthermore, not all enteroviral serotypes are able to be recovered in tissue culture, including several coxsackievirus A strains that require mouse inoculation for detection. Isolation of enteroviruses in culture can take 3–8 days and therefore is generally not rapid enough to affect either treatment options or length of hospitalization, resulting in unnecessary antibiotic therapy until bacterial CSF cultures are negative at 48–72 h. Several serologic assays can be used to diagnose enteroviral infections, but are not clinically useful because they can be cross-reactive, nonspecific, and difficult to interpret due to the extended incubation and prodromal periods found with many enteroviral illnesses. In addition, culture of parechoviruses is also difficult, so the detection of both enteroviruses and parechoviruses is primarily performed using molecular methods.

Molecular Tests

To increase the sensitivity of enterovirus detection and to reduce the diagnostic turnaround time, molecular tests have been developed [19, 24, 29–36]. The molecular testing methods utilize either reverse transcription-polymerase chain reaction (RT-PCR) amplification combined with enzyme-linked immunosorbent assay (ELISA) [24, 29, 31–34, 36], real-time RT-PCR [35], or nucleic acid sequence-based amplification (NASBA) combined with molecular beacon technology [30]. The assays utilize primer sequences selected from the conserved 5′ untranslated region (5′ UTR) of the enteroviral genome. Sequence variations are present in this region, and the scope of detection of the various enteroviral serotypes is dependent on primer sequence selection [24, 29–36]. Since different serotypes circulate in distinct areas of the world, assays should be validated using local clinical isolates and reference strains known to be endemic in the region. Overall, enterovirus molecular tests are highly sensitive, some detecting the majority of enteroviral isolates at as low as 0.1 tissue culture infectious dose 50 ($TCID_{50}$) [24, 29–36]. The molecular enterovirus tests are generally very specific, but have been shown to cross-react with rhinovirus [29, 35]. The significance of this cross-reactivity is discussed later in this chapter.

The availability of commercial reagents for molecular detection of enteroviruses has increased substantially in recent years. Two systems for the detection of enteroviruses from CSF samples are US FDA-cleared: Xpert EV (Cepheid, Sunnyvale, CA; 2007) and NucliSENS EasyQ Enterovirus (bioMérieux, Durham, NC; 2008) (Table 48.3). Cepheid's Xpert platform is a closed, integrated extraction and real-time amplification and detection system using TaqMan hydrolysis probe chemistry. This platform is capable of single unit testing, with a total testing time of approximately 1.5 h. bioMérieux's NucliSENS EasyQ system is based on NASBA isothermal RNA amplification with real-time target detection using molecular beacons, with a total testing time of 5 h. Both assays target 5′ UTR of the enterovirus genome.

A representative list of ASRs available commercially is presented in Table 48.3. These ASRs can be used on different amplification and detection platforms, providing flexibility for the design of LDTs. Analytical assessments of the Xpert assay have demonstrated very good performance characteristics. In a multicenter study comparing Xpert to a combined standard of clinical and laboratory data to define true infection, Xpert demonstrated 94.7 % sensitivity and 100 % specificity, with an overall accuracy of 98.6 % [37]. When used in a point of care test setting to maximize clinical impact of the results, Xpert also performed well (100 % sensitivity, 98.9 % specificity) for samples for which a result was obtained [38]. However, the authors reported a 16 % invalid rate for Xpert EV on initial testing, and these samples were not included in the calculations of performance. This invalid rate was similar to an 8 % rate from a previous study that assessed the performance of Xpert during routine use [39]. These authors reported that the invalid rate could be reduced by sample dilution or a single freeze–thaw without impacting the assay performance characteristics.

Although US FDA-cleared in 2008, comparatively fewer studies have been published evaluating the performance of the EasyQ system (bioMérieux). One study conducted by Landry et al. prior to US FDA clearance of this system compared an early version of the real-time NASBA assay to the original NASBA assay combined with electrochemiluminescence (ECL) detection of enterovirus in CSF and stool samples [30]. The real-time NASBA assay was 91 % sensitive and 100 % specific compared to NASBA-ECL upon initial testing of 160 samples, with an indeterminate rate of 2.5 %. A more recent report assessing the CE-marked version of the real-time NASBA EasyQ assay demonstrated a 90 % sensitivity and 100 % specificity compared to an LDT using a conventional RT-PCR method [40]. Marlowe et al. evaluated the Xpert assay compared to both the EasyQ assay and a TaqMan-based LDT, with 25/25 positive samples detected by Xpert, 24/25 detected by the LDT, and 21/25 detected by EasyQ [41]. These authors also showed an initial 7.2 % (10/138) invalid rate for Xpert EV, which was attributed to a single lot of reagents, with eight of ten resolved upon repeat testing with a new reagent lot.

CE-marked assays for the detection of enteroviruses in CSF are available from bioMérieux/Argene Biosoft (Varilhes, France). Enterovirus Consensus Assay utilizes RT-PCR and stair primer technology that was designed to overcome the problems associated with sequence divergence in the primer-binding regions, thus ensuring the detection of all enteroviral serotypes [29]. The assay was shown to be more sensitive than assays using the original Rotbart [32, 33] and Zoll [36] primers, and only exhibited cross-reactivity with rhinovirus type 3. Studies have determined that the sensitivity of the assay is <0.4 $TCID_{50}$ and can detect approximately six RNA copies per input reaction.

Implementation of molecular testing for enteroviruses into routine use can positively impact the management of patients with suspected meningitis. Multiple studies have shown shorter duration of hospitalization, decreased use of inappropriate antibiotics, reduced ordering of ancillary laboratory tests, and overall decreases in health-care costs when enterovirus results are rapidly available [23–26]. These benefits have the potential to be maximized with systems such as Xpert, and should continue to improve with the increased development of more on-demand, near-patient platforms.

Molecular detection of parechoviruses has been limited to the use of RT-PCR LDTs in a limited number of clinical laboratories. Similar to assays for detection of enteroviruses, most assays for the detection of parechoviruses target the 5′ UTR, with recently described assays capable of detecting all known parechovirus types [42]. Several studies which have retrospectively analyzed stored CSF specimens have demonstrated an overall prevalence for parechoviruses of 2–3 % in CNS infections, but prevalence in individual years can vary widely from 0–10 % [6, 43–46].

Herpesviruses

The herpesviruses, including herpes simplex virus types 1 and 2 (HSV-1, HSV-2), VZV, CMV, and HHV-6, are large (150–200 nm), enveloped viruses with a linear, double-stranded DNA genome packaged in an icosahedral capsid. These viruses cause a broad spectrum of viral CNS disease including meningitis, encephalitis, meningoencephalitis, myelitis, and polyradiculitis [1, 2]. Epstein-Barr virus (EBV) DNA has been detected in virtually all AIDS-related cases of primary CNS lymphomas [47]. CMV is discussed briefly under diseases associated with immunosuppression and in detail in Chap. 47. The role of HHV-7 in CNS disease remains unclear.

Herpes Simplex Virus

Epidemiology and Disease

HSV-2 is the usual cause of HSV meningitis and accounts for approximately 1–5 % of all cases of viral meningitis and 4–6 % of cases of viral encephalitis overall (adult and pediatric) [1–4, 48, 49]. The clinical course of the disease usually is self-limiting and generally not associated with permanent neurological damage. HSV-2 also causes Mollaret's meningitis, a benign recurrent meningitis [50].

HSV-1 is responsible for the majority of HSV-associated encephalitis and for 10–20 % (approximately 1,250 cases per year in the USA) of all viral encephalitis cases (adult and pediatric). Approximately 30 % are primary HSV-1 infections, and the remaining cases are due to HSV reactivation. In contrast to HSV meningitis, HSV encephalitis can be a devastating disease, resulting in persistent focal neurologic disease due to damage to one or both temporal lobes [1–4, 48, 49]. Encephalitis occurs in approximately 60–75 % of babies with disseminated HSV disease, and the mortality rate for cases of HSV-2 encephalitis can be as high as 80 % without appropriate antiviral therapy [51].

Diagnosis

CSF viral cultures are positive only in approximately 15 % of HSV meningitis cases due to primary infection and, with the exception of neonatal infection, are rarely positive in cases of HSV encephalitis [1–3, 32, 33, 48, 49, 51]. Traditionally, the diagnosis of HSV encephalitis was dependent on obtaining tissue by brain biopsy for viral culture, electron microscopy, immunohistochemical staining, and the demonstration of intrathecal production of HSV-specific antibodies [1–3, 16–18, 49, 51].

Over the last decade, studies comparing HSV CSF PCR with brain biopsy and/or intrathecal HSV-specific antibody production for the diagnosis of HSV CNS infections have demonstrated sensitivities and specificities ranging from 96–98 % and 96–99 %, respectively [16, 51–53]. HSV PCR can identify infected persons who fail to either seroconvert with primary infection or demonstrate significant rises in antibody titers after reactivation. Finally, HSV PCR can aid in differentiating HSV antibody increases due to active HSV CNS infection from reactivation in persons with concomitant CNS disease not related to HSV. Another advantage of PCR assays for diagnosis of HSV encephalitis is that the assay sensitivity remains high (95 %) up to approximately 1 week after initiating therapy [52]. However, CSF samples collected early after symptom onset may be negative in some patients with HSV CNS disease, so repeating the lumbar puncture and HSV PCR testing is recommended in such cases when HSV infection is strongly suspected [54]. Caution should be exercised if using CSF PCR for test of cure since DNA can be slow to clear from the CSF (as many as 21 % of CSF specimens can remain PCR positive for more than 15 days after successful completion of therapy) [52]. Although HSV viral loads are not correlated with prognosis [55, 56], persistent detection of HSV in the CSF of neonates with encephalitis has been shown to be a poor prognostic indicator [56, 57].

Varicella-Zoster Virus

Epidemiology and Disease

The most common manifestation of VZV resulting from primary infection is chickenpox and generally occurs in early childhood [58]. VZV-associated neurologic syndromes include acute cerebellar ataxia, diffuse or focal encephalitis, meningitis, transverse myelitis, and Reye syndrome [1, 2, 58]. Herpes zoster (also known as shingles), resulting from the reactivation of latent VZV infection, occurs in approximately 20 % of immunocompetent persons (generally 45 years or older) and the incidence is approximately 15 % higher in persons with immunosuppression [58, 59]. In a small percentage of all zoster cases, severe complications can occur, including meningitis, encephalitis, myelitis, Ramsay Hunt syndrome, Guillain-Barre syndrome, and contralateral hemiplegia [58–60]. Ocular manifestations are more common in reactivation disease, such as herpes zoster opthalmicus and acute retinal necrosis, especially in immunocompromised individuals and those not treated with antiviral therapy [61, 62]. Interestingly, concomitant herpes zoster rash may only be present in less than half of patients with VZV CNS disease [63].

Diagnosis

Studies have demonstrated that the recovery of VZV in culture is poor (20 % positive), as is serologic diagnosis (48 % positive) [64]. Antigen detection by immunofluorescent staining improves detection from vesicular lesions (82 % positive), whereas PCR was the most sensitive, with a detection rate of approximately 95 % [64]. Based on improved detection with PCR assays, VZV accounts for 6–30 % of all herpesviruses detected from CSF [20, 21, 64–71]. However, results need to be interpreted cautiously since VZV DNA has been detected in CSF without overt disease, particularly in immunosuppressed individuals.

Human Herpes Virus 6

Epidemiology and Disease

HHV-6 is generally acquired early in life and is manifested as exanthem subitum (more commonly known as roseola), or as a non-exanthemous febrile illness, sometimes accompanied by severe neurologic manifestations, including febrile seizures, meningitis, meningoencephalitis, and encephalitis [72]. Detection of HHV-6 in children with febrile seizures is important for identifying children with a potential for the recurrence of seizure episodes due to ongoing HHV-6 infection. Immunocompromised patients can manifest severe HHV-6 reactivation infections, including encephalitis [72].

Diagnosis

Culture confirmation of HHV-6 infection is not routinely performed in clinical virology laboratories due to the complexity of the testing, which requires purification and culture of patient lymphocytes or co-cultivation of activated patient lymphocytes and activated human umbilical cord blood lymphocytes [72]. Serologic confirmation of the disease depends on the detection of IgM in primary infection or conversion from either a negative to a positive IgG antibody response or a fourfold or greater rise in IgG antibody titer [72]. However, antibody titers can be difficult to interpret for several reasons: IgM antibodies may not develop in some children, can be positive with HHV-6 reactivation, and can remain positive for extended periods of time; and significant rises in HHV-6-specific IgG antibody titers can be found during infections with other herpesviruses. The detection of HHV-6 DNA in the CNS by PCR can support the diagnosis; however, in a percentage of cases, HHV-6 DNA can be found in normal brain tissue and in the CSF of children without evidence of CNS disease [72]. Although rare, chromosomal integration of HHV-6 can complicate the interpretation of positive molecular tests from body fluids, and may result in the misdiagnosis of acute CNS infection [73]. Quantitative methods may be more accurate for correlating the presence of HHV-6 with active disease [74, 75].

Molecular Tests for Herpesviruses

Comparisons of the sensitivity of HSV PCR to viral culture, antibody detection, and direct immunofluorescence assays have clearly established the utility of PCR as a first-line diagnostic test in the clinical laboratory [7, 16, 18, 19]. Most PCR assays are applicable to the majority of conventional or real-time PCR instruments. The assays for herpesviruses use different primer sets targeting a number of genes including: DNA polymerase gene (HSV-1, HSV-2, CMV, EBV, VZV, HHV-6); UL42, glycoprotein B (gB), glycoprotein D (gD), or thymidine kinase (TK) genes (HSV); genes 28 and 29 (VZV); and major capsid protein, U89/U90 (HHV-6). Identification of the specific herpesvirus is achieved using either traditional methods, including the use of species-specific primers, hybridization with species specific probes, agarose gel electrophoresis, restriction enzyme analysis, ELISA-based colorimetric detection methods [20, 21, 64, 66–68, 70], or fluorescent probe technologies that permit real-time detection [65, 69, 71]. One commercial assay has been US FDA-cleared for the detection of herpesviruses in CSF (Table 48.3, Simplexa™ HSV 1 and 2 Direct Kit, Focus Diagnostics, Cypress, CA). Two assays are US FDA-cleared for the detection of HSV from oral and anogenital lesions: the Multicode—RTx HSV 1 and 2 kit (EraGen Biosciences, Madison, WI) and the IsoAmp HSV assay (Biohelix, Beverly, MA). A third assay is US FDA-cleared for the detection of HSV from anogenital lesions: the BD ProbeTec™ Herpes Simplex Viruses (HSV 1 and 2) Q*x* Assay (Becton Dickinson, Sparks, MD). None of these US FDA-cleared HSV tests for lesions should be used for the diagnosis of HSV CNS infections.

Several commercial test kits or ASRs are available for the detection of herpesviruses in CSF (Table 48.3). Roche Diagnostics (Indianapolis, IN) has developed ASRs for CMV, HSV-1, HSV-2, VZV, and EBV identification using the LightCycler instrument [65, 69, 71]. A single-tube amplification and detection step allows the identification of both HSV-1 and HSV-2 and the differentiation of subtype by melting-curve analysis [65]. The manufacturer's claim of sensitivity is approximately 12.5 copies or 2.5–6.3 genome equivalents per reaction.

ASRs for several herpesviruses are available from Cepheid (Sunnyvale, CA), Epoch Biosciences/Nanogen (Bothell, WA), EraGen Biosciences (Madison, WI), and Focus Diagnostics (Cypress, CA). Although not available for sale in the USA, Artus Biotech (Artus GmbH, Hamburg, Germany) has CE-marked systems and assays for the detection of herpesviruses. Easy*artus* HSV 1 and 2, EBV, VZV, and CMV PCR kits are approved for use with BioRobot EZ1 DSP for specimen extraction, and LightCycler (Roche), ABI PRISM 700 and 7900HT SDS (Applied Biosystems Foster City, CA), and the Rotor-Gene 3000 (Corbett Research, San Francisco, CA) for amplification and detection. Real-time PCR for the same viruses can be accomplished using the *artus* Herpes Virus LC-PCR kits. Assays with these reagents have been optimized for use on the LightCycler (Roche) with manufacturer-claimed limits of detection (copies/PCR) of

5.0 for HSV-1 and -2, 28.9 for EBV, 4.0 for VZV, and 4.9 for CMV. Assessments of clinical and analytical performance of the commercially available reagents has been limited; however, a recent study evaluating the performance of ASRs from Cepheid, EraGen, and Roche for the detection of HSV-1 and -2 from pediatric CSF samples demonstrated comparable clinical and analytical sensitivities among the assays [76].

Multiplex assays that can simultaneously screen for the six major herpesviruses (HSV-1, HSV-2, CMV, VZV, EBV, and HHV-6) offer some distinct advantages including the identification of a herpesvirus that may not have been considered in the original diagnosis and the detection of co-infections in the CNS [77]. However, caution must be used in determining the significance of detecting more than one herpesvirus because low level reactivation may occur in the presence of immune suppression due to the primary infection.

Several LDTs targeting herpesviruses have been validated for CSF specimens and/or brain tissue using either traditional or real-time PCR methods [16, 21, 65–71]. Herpes Generic Consensus kit (bioMérieux/Argene Biosoft, Varilhes, France) uses the same stair primer technology as in their enterovirus assay to compensate for sequence divergence in the primer binding regions of the six herpesviruses [66]. After PCR amplification and generic colorimetric detection of the herpesvirus, the Herpes Identification Hybridoma well kit (bioMérieux/Argene Biosoft, Varilhes, France) is used to identify the specific herpesvirus present. All primers, probes, an internal control, external controls, and all PCR reagents, with the exception of amplification enzyme, are provided in the test kit. Assay sensitivity varies between 5–50 copies per PCR reaction, with EBV being the least sensitive. This assay is available as a research use only (RUO) kit in the USA and is CE-marked kit outside of the USA.

Microarray-based technology offers the opportunity to expand the detection capabilities of multiplex real-time PCR assays, and has been applied to the development of LDTs [78] and commercially available assays [79] for detection of viral CNS infections. Clart Entherpex kit (Genomica, Coslada, Spain) is a CE-marked multiplex real-time PCR DNA microarray allowing the simultaneous detection of HSV-1 and -2, VZV, CMV, EBV, HHV-6, HHV-7, HHV-8, and human enteroviruses in CSF, and has demonstrated similar clinical and analytical sensitivity compared to single-endpoint PCR for detection of these viral targets [79].

Arboviruses

Epidemiology and Disease

Alphaviruses, flaviviruses, and bunyaviruses are responsible for the majority of the arboviral encephalopathies (Table 48.2) and are found throughout the world [1, 2, 10]. Arboviruses have an RNA genome, with the exception of African Swine Fever Virus which has a DNA genome. The arboviral encephalitides are zoonotic, and transmission of the viruses occurs between susceptible amplifier vertebrate hosts (such as birds, squirrels, and chipmunks) via blood feeding arthropods (including mosquitoes, psychodids, ticks, and ceratopogonids). Peak incidence occurs in summer and continues through the fall months when arthropods are most active, but cases can continue to occur in the winter months in warmer regions. Humans, horses, and domestic animals can develop a clinical illness, with the majority of human arboviral infections being either asymptomatic or manifesting as a flu-like self-limiting illness. Arboviruses can occasionally enter the brain by mechanisms not clearly understood, with productive infection of brain cells occurring, resulting in encephalitis, often with a fatal outcome or permanent neurologic damage in the affected individual [1, 2, 10].

The mosquito-borne viruses were first discovered in the 1930s [10]. Until 1999 and the emergence of West Nile virus (WNV) in Queens, New York [80], the most important cause of epidemic and endemic encephalitis in the USA was St Louis encephalitis virus (SLE), which is found throughout the lower 48 states. From 1964 to 2009, confirmed cases of SLE averaged approximately 100 cases per year, and over 4,500 cases of neuroinvasive disease have been reported to the Centers for Disease Control and Prevention (CDC; Atlanta, GA) since 1964 [8]. Less than 1 % of the SLE cases are clinically apparent, with a case fatality rate of 5–25 % for symptomatic persons [8].

Since the initial outbreak in 1999, WNV has migrated across the USA, and through 2011 all but two states (Alaska and Hawaii) have reported bird, mosquito, vertebrate, or human cases [8, 9]. WNV is responsible for neuroinvasive disease (encephalitis and meningitis) and what is termed West Nile fever, which is typically less severe and does not show signs of neuroinvasion [80]. Through 2014, over 18,000 cases of neuroinvasive WNV infections with over 1,200 deaths have been reported to the CDC [8, 9]. Approximately one in 150 WNV cases progress to meningitis or encephalitis, which is the most common neurological manifestation. Case fatality rates remain constant at approximately 10 %, with advanced age being the most important risk factor for death [8–10]. In addition, WNV has been transmitted to persons receiving either transfusions or transplanted organs from asymptomatic donors infected with WNV [9, 80, 81]. Phylogenetic analysis has shown that WNV can be separated into two lineages [82], with lineage 2 being associated with recent outbreaks in Europe.

La Crosse virus is found in several midwestern and mid-Atlantic states, and an average of 80–100 cases are reported per year, usually in children under the age of 16 years. Since 1964, eastern equine encephalitis virus and western equine encephalitis virus have been responsible for 270 and 639 cases, respectively [8]. In the northern USA, Powassan virus is a minor cause of encephalitis and is transmitted by ticks

[8]. Japanese encephalitis virus, found mainly in Asia and the Pacific, is the leading cause of encephalitis worldwide, with more than 45,000 cases reported annually [1, 2, 10]. Venezuelan encephalitis virus remains the third most common cause of equine encephalitides and the most common cause of epidemic encephalitis in Central and South America [1, 2, 10].

Diagnosis

By the time persons present with encephalitic symptoms, the viremic phase of the disease often has ceased and infected persons have developed serum and intrathecal IgM or IgG antibodies or both [10, 80]. Since IgM antibodies do not cross the blood–brain barrier, the identification of virus-specific IgM antibodies in the CSF is strongly suggestive of CNS infection. A variety of assays, including hemagglutination inhibition, complement fixation, plaque reduction neutralization test (PRNT), IgM antibody capture ELISA (MAC-ELISA), IgG antibody ELISA, indirect immunofluorescence (IFA), and antigen capture ELISA, have been useful in the identification of arboviral infections [10, 20, 80, 83]. The identification of virus-specific IgM antibodies or the demonstration of a four-fold or greater rise in neutralizing IgG antibodies in either CSF or serum is achieved by PRNT using multiple arboviruses. Commercially available MAC-ELISAs are more reliable, rapid, and reproducible compared to LDTs [20, 80, 83]. In persons with immunosuppressive disorders or who are very early in the course of the infection, antibody titers can be negative and the diagnosis is dependent on isolation of the virus. However, due to the transient nature of the viremic stage and probably low levels of virus in the CSF and serum, virus isolation using cell culture generally has been unsuccessful and not practical for most clinical laboratories.

Although serological confirmation of disease remains the gold standard, molecular tests are important for identifying early infection prior to seroconversion, infection in transplant tissues and blood [80, 81], infection in immunocompromised patients, and confirmation of a clinical diagnosis [80, 84–87]. A positive result with a nucleic acid amplification assay is diagnostic of an arboviral infection; however, a negative result does not exclude the possibility of an arboviral infection. For example, up to 55 % of CSF samples and only approximately 10 % of serum samples are positive using a molecular test in patients with serologically confirmed cases of WNV disease [80]. Nevertheless, the molecular detection of arboviral nucleic acids is standard for vector-borne disease surveillance studies and control programs [80, 84–86, 88] and for monitoring both the blood supply and transplantation tissues [80, 81].

Molecular Tests

Several assays using traditional RT-PCR, nested RT-PCR, real-time RT-PCR, and NASBA combined with either ECL or molecular beacon detection have been developed for the identification of arboviral infections [80, 84–88]. Assay methods are highly sensitive, specific, and rapid, with results available in as little as 2 h for real-time RT-PCR and NASBA molecular beacon assays. Primers usually target the NS1, NS3, NS5, and 3′ NC regions of the genomes of the flaviviruses. Primer-probe sets may be virus specific [84–86], or universal primers can be used for the detection of all flaviviruses [87]. Although commercially available reagents are limited for the molecular detection of WNV in Europe, there are none available in the USA. Furthermore, proficiency testing (PT) performed with early versions of commercial tests and LDTs showed good performance in the ability to detect WNV lineage 1, but an inability of more than 40 % of participating laboratories to detect lineage 2 [89]. Although the performance in detecting lineage 2 improved slightly in a recent assessment [90], one-third of testing laboratories were unable to detect both lineages. Accommodations for sequence variation must be incorporated into assay design to ensure the optimal detection of both WNV lineages 1 and 2.

Viral Agents Associated with Immunosuppression

Cytomegalovirus

Epidemiology and Disease

CMV is an enveloped, double-stranded DNA virus with particles ranging in diameter from 120–200 nm. CMV disease may be due to primary infection but generally is related to CMV reactivation in association with progressive immune deficiency [11–13]. Neurological syndromes associated with CMV include peripheral neuropathy, ventriculoencephalitis, myelitis/polyradiculopathy, and diffuse micronodular encephalitis with dementia [11–13].

Diagnosis

The presumptive diagnosis of CMV CNS disease has been based primarily on clinical presentation, serologic testing, neuroradiologic studies including CT scan and MRI, CSF chemistries, and the magnitude and types of CSF pleocytosis [11–13]. CSF viral culture is positive in only approximately 50 % of patients with CMV CNS disease, and culture is relatively slow, requiring 1–4 weeks for a final result [11–13].

Molecular Tests

Molecular methods are used to more accurately and rapidly detect CMV in patients with active CMV CNS disease [91]. The detection of CMV DNA by PCR in CSF of acquired immunodeficiency syndrome (AIDS) patients was highly sensitive (100 % negative predictive value for CNS disease) but did not always correlate with active CMV CNS disease

(68.4 % positive predictive value for CNS disease) [91]. Sensitive qualitative PCR may detect non-replicating virus, which could clearly limit the use of these tests in the differentiation of asymptomatic infection from active CNS disease. Quantitative PCR assays with established cut-off values for differentiating infection from active disease may provide a superior alternative to qualitative PCR. For example, CSF from AIDS patients with autopsy-proven CMV encephalitis had a median value of 3,333 CMV genomes/10^5 cells compared to a median value of 125 CMV genomes/10^5 cells for AIDS patients with neurologic symptoms not related to CMV, and a median value of 19 CMV genomes/10^5 cells for HIV-1 seronegative controls [91]. High levels of cellular CMV correlated with marked histopathologic changes in AIDS patients. Additional studies are necessary to determine the level of CMV DNA that would be considered indicative of active CNS disease.

Several manufacturers produce commercially available ASRs for real-time PCR-based detection and quantification of CMV DNA from a variety of clinical specimen types (Table 48.3). A different approach, used in both transplant recipients and HIV-1-infected persons for diagnosing active disease vs asymptomatic CMV infection, is based on detection of CMV mRNA transcripts (immediate-early and early, UL83, pp150, and pp67 gene transcripts) [91, 92]. Although commercial assays are not available, CMV transcript detection can be a useful target for the differentiation of active infection from latent infection. The detection of pp67 mRNA in CSF is most accurate for the diagnosis of active CMV CNS disease (100 % positive predictive value [PPV], 97 % negative predictive value [NPV]), when compared to viral culture (100 % PPV, 82.7 % NPV) and qualitative DNA PCR (68.4 % PPV, 100 % NPV) [92]. In addition to diagnostic utility, quantitative PCR and pp67 mRNA assays have been effective for monitoring response to therapy for CMV infections [91].

Human JC Polyomavirus

Epidemiology and Disease

Human JCV is a small (40 nm) nonenveloped DNA virus with an icosahedral capsid. Primary infection with human JCV generally occurs early in life, is usually asymptomatic, and results in a latent infection of both renal tissues and B lymphocytes [14]. Reactivation occurs during cell-mediated immune deficiency and can lead to progressive multifocal leukoencephalopathy (PML), a rapidly evolving severe demyelinating disease of the CNS that is usually fatal. This disease is primarily but not exclusively seen in patients with AIDS and, prior to the era of highly active antiretroviral therapy (HAART), was a serious cause of infection in 2–10 % of AIDS patients. A review of cases over a 10-year period also showed that approximately 20 % of non-AIDS patients with PML had hematologic malignancies or were bone marrow transplant recipients [93].

Diagnosis

The diagnosis of PML can be difficult, is generally presumptive, and typically based on recognition of characteristic multifocal white matter lesions using imaging techniques (CT or MRI) in patients manifesting subacute neurologic deficits. Although laboratory tools such as serology, virus isolation, and electron microscopy have been used to aid in diagnosis [14], these tests have had limited utility due to poor specificity (serology), labor intensiveness (cell culture), or impracticality (EM). Histopathologic analysis of brain biopsies often has been required to confirm the diagnosis and remains the gold standard for diagnosis [94].

Molecular Tests

Several PCR-based strategies have been used for detection of JCV in CSF for the diagnosis of PML and to monitor patients with AIDS who achieved a PML remission as a result of HAART [14, 95–97]. Testing has been performed using unique or sequential CSF samples, with assays using single or nested PCR combined with conventional or real-time detection technologies. Primers target different noncoding and coding (VP1, VP2, small T-antigen, large T-antigen) regions, often with variable results, presumably due to the large amount of sequence variation within the various subtypes of JCV [14]. PCR detection of all JCV genotypes can be improved if primers that target the more conserved regions of the genome or degenerate primers are used; however, care must be taken in assay design to prevent cross-reaction with other polyomaviruses. PCR assays have a rate of detection of JCV in CSF from patients with PML ranged from 30–89.5 % [95–97]. Specificity of PCR for identifying viral isolates of JCV was 100 %, while specificity for the diagnosis of confirmed PML was generally about 95 % [95–97]. However, in patients with PML on HAART, the sensitivity of PCR for detection of JCV in CSF is considerably lower than in patients with PML not on HAART [98]. In summary, CSF examination for JCV DNA was shown to be useful for confirming the diagnosis of PML. However, a negative test does not exclude the possibility of PML and brain biopsy is necessary to confirm such cases.

Human Immunodeficiency Virus

Human immunodeficiency viruses are enveloped, plus-stranded RNA retroviruses. Early in the course of infection, HIV-1 enters the CNS [99, 100]. A complex interaction between the virus and host immune responses leads to neurological damage that is manifested by several syndromes including meningitis, encephalitis, peripheral neuropathies, and AIDS dementia complex (ADC) [99, 100].

Molecular Tests

High HIV-1 RNA levels in CSF correlate with an increased incidence of ADC and with the presence of cerebral atrophy [99]. Most persons with high CSF viral load have concomitant high plasma viral load. However, there are patients on HAART with either low-level or undetectable plasma viral load (<50 copies/ml) who have signs of neurologic disease and high CSF viral load (>50,000 copies/ml). Suppression of plasma viral load does not always correspond with HIV-1 suppression in other body compartments, and the monitoring of such compartments may be indicated in certain clinical situations. Therefore, when neurological symptoms are evident, measurement of HIV-1 RNA levels in the CSF becomes important. Detectable viral load in the CSF can affect the selection of HAART, since not all drugs penetrate the CSF to the same degree. In addition, due to the large overlap of neurological symptoms associated with the AIDS-related neurological disorders, such as CMV encephalopathies and PML, CSF viral load can aid in the differential diagnosis of ADC [92]. The measurement of CSF viral load, using commercially available methods described in Chap. 45, can be performed once the laboratory has validated this off-label sample type.

Interpretation of Results

The enhanced performance of molecular assays compared to conventional methods has significantly improved diagnosis of viral CNS infections, and detection of specific viral nucleic acid targets in the CSF most often represents true positive results. Potential scenarios for false-positive results could include analytical cross-reactivity of primers/probes due to homology between related viruses. Assays for the detection of enteroviruses can cross-react with some rhinovirus types, which provides challenges in the interpretation of results from respiratory specimens, but should not impact interpretation of CSF results because rhinoviruses are not CNS pathogens. Clinical false-positive results may also occur in the detection of CMV nucleic acid in the CSF which may represent latent rather than reactivated infection. As mentioned above, quantitative or viral mRNA-targeted assays may be more useful than DNA-targeted qualitative assays in identifying reactivation. False-negative molecular results are possible and can be due to analytical factors related to specimen quality and integrity (collection, transport, storage). In addition, assay limitations due to mutation or sequence variation should be recognized, and processes for assessing and monitoring these components of assay performance over time should be included in the laboratory's quality assurance program. Furthermore, timing of specimen collection (within the first week of an arboviral infection), and prior therapy (impact of HAART in detection of JCV) must be considered in interpreting negative results.

Laboratory Issues

A major limitation in the use of molecular assays for the diagnosis of viral CNS infections is the relative lack of US FDA-cleared options available for US laboratories. Although several assays/systems have recently reached the market, these have been limited to the detection of enteroviral infections. Due to the extreme difficulty in performing clinical trials of an appropriate scope to obtain US FDA clearance, it is unlikely that US FDA-cleared products for other targets in the CSF (notably HSV) will be available in the near future. This will compel laboratories either to verify alternative specimen types on currently available US FDA-cleared assays or utilize ASRs or LDTs, both of which may limit widespread utilization of the technology. In addition, the number and diversity of commercially available PT panels has not kept pace with the growth in utilization of molecular assays for the diagnosis of CNS infections. Regulatory compliance through the use of in-house PT panels or specimen exchange programs causes additional challenges to the laboratory. Finally, operational attention in the design of the laboratory, including when, where, and on which platforms certain assays are being performed, also needs to be taken into consideration. For example, separation by time, location, and potentially even platforms for extraction, amplification and detection steps, as well as CSF samples and lesion samples submitted for detection of HSV. Lesion samples are a high volume specimen type, generally contain a high viral titer, and demonstrate high positivity rates for most laboratories. These factors can present an unwanted, but controllable opportunity for environmental cross-contamination of CSF samples.

Conclusions and Future Directions

Currently, the application of molecular testing for the detection of clinically relevant viral CNS infections is considered an essential component in standard of care clinical testing for many viral infections. For certain viral pathogens, such as HSV and enteroviruses, molecular tests are considered the new gold standard. For other viruses, correlation of molecular results with other laboratory findings, such as serologic status, clinical presentation, and patient management is still an active area of study. Nevertheless, molecular tests are rapid, accurate and significantly impact patient management and outcome. The selection of the best method or target must be carefully considered, as variations in both can affect the overall performance of the assays. In certain cases, where latent viruses may be detected, quantitative assays or assays that target mRNA rather than DNA may provide more useful clinical correlation for CNS disease. Laboratories must thoroughly evaluate and validate the tests, continue to monitor technical performance, and maintain strict environmental precautions to prevent cross-contamination of samples. Standardization of test methods, cooperative participation in PT programs, and support by the laboratory community for the development of commutable molecular standards will improve performance and correlation of intralaboratory and interlaboratory results.

References

1. Cassady KA, Whitley RJ. Pathogenesis and pathophysiology of viral central nervous system diseases. In: Scheld WM, Whitley RJ, Durack DT, editors. Infections of the central nervous system. Philadelphia, PA: Lippincott-Raven; 2004.
2. Cassady KA, Whitley RJ. Viral central nervous system infections. In: Richman DD, Whitley RJ, Hayden FG, editors. Clinical virology. Washington, DC: ASM Press; 2009.
3. Hammer SM, Connolly KJ. Viral aseptic meningitis in the United States: clinical features, viral etiologies, and differential diagnosis. Curr Clin Top Infect Dis. 1992;12:1–25.
4. Rotbart HA. Viral meningitis. Semin Neurol. 2000;20:277–92.
5. CDC. Nonpolio enterovirus and human parechovirus surveillance – United States, 2006–2008. MMWR Morb Mortal Wkly Rep. 2010;59:1577–80.
6. Harvala H, McLeish N, Kondracka J, et al. Comparison of human parechovirus and enterovirus detection frequencies in cerebrospinal fluid samples collected over a 5-year period in edinburgh: HPeV type 3 identified as the most common picornavirus type. J Med Virol. 2011;83:889–96.
7. Hosoya M, Honzumi K, Sato M, et al. Application of PCR for various neurotropic viruses on the diagnosis of viral meningitis. J Clin Virol. 1998;11:117–24.
8. CDC. Arboviral encephalitides. 2012. http://www.cdc.gov/ncidod/dvbid/index.htm. Accessed Feb 2012.
9. CDC. West Nile virus. 2012. http://www.cdc.gov/ncidod/dvbid/westnile/index.htm. Accessed Feb 2012.
10. Gubler DJ. Human arbovirus infections worldwide. Ann N Y Acad Sci. 2001;951:13–24.
11. Cinque P, Marenzi R, Ceresa D. Cytomegalovirus infections of the nervous system. Intervirology. 1997;40:85–97.
12. Hibberd PL, Snydman DR. Cytomegalovirus infection in organ transplant recipients. Infect Dis Clin North Am. 1995;9:863–77.
13. Ives DV. Cytomegalovirus disease in AIDS. AIDS. 1997;11:1791–7.
14. Safak M, Khalili K. An overview: human polyomavirus JC virus and its associated disorders. J Neurovirol. 2003;9 Suppl 1:3–9.
15. Landry ML. Frequency of normal cerebrospinal fluid protein level and leukocyte count in enterovirus meningitis. J Clin Virol. 2005;32:73–4.
16. Cinque P, Cleator GM, Weber T, et al. The role of laboratory investigation in the diagnosis and management of patients with suspected herpes simplex encephalitis: a consensus report. The EU concerted action on virus meningitis and encephalitis. J Neurol Neurosurg Psychiatry. 1996;61:339–45.
17. Reiber H, Lange P. Quantification of virus-specific antibodies in cerebrospinal fluid and serum: sensitive and specific detection of antibody synthesis in brain. Clin Chem. 1991;37:1153–60.
18. Thomson Jr RB, Bertram H. Laboratory diagnosis of central nervous system infections. Infect Dis Clin North Am. 2001;15:1047–71.
19. Cinque P, Bossolasco S, Lundkvist A. Molecular analysis of cerebrospinal fluid in viral diseases of the central nervous system. J Clin Virol. 2003;26:1–28.
20. Johnson AJ, Martin DA, Karabatsos N, et al. Detection of anti-arboviral immunoglobulin G by using a monoclonal antibody-based capture enzyme-linked immunosorbent assay. J Clin Microbiol. 2000;38:1827–31.
21. Johnson G, Nelson S, Petric M, et al. Comprehensive PCR-based assay for detection and species identification of human herpesviruses. J Clin Microbiol. 2000;38:3274–9.
22. Roehrig JT, Nash D, Maldin B, et al. Persistence of virus-reactive serum immunoglobulin M antibody in confirmed West Nile virus encephalitis cases. Emerg Infect Dis. 2003;9:376–9.
23. Hamilton MS, Jackson MA, Abel D. Clinical utility of polymerase chain reaction testing for enteroviral meningitis. Pediatr Infect Dis J. 1999;18:533–7.
24. Ramers C, Billman G, Hartin M, et al. Impact of a diagnostic cerebrospinal fluid enterovirus polymerase chain reaction test on patient management. JAMA. 2000;283:2680–5.
25. Robinson CC, Willis M, Meagher A, et al. Impact of rapid polymerase chain reaction results on management of pediatric patients with enteroviral meningitis. Pediatr Infect Dis J. 2002;21:283–6.
26. Stellrecht KA, Harding I, Woron AM, et al. The impact of an enteroviral RT-PCR assay on the diagnosis of aseptic meningitis and patient management. J Clin Virol. 2002;25 Suppl 1:S19–26.
27. Pallansch MA, Roos RP. Enteroviruses: polioviruses, coxsackieviruses, echoviruses, and newer enteroviruses. In: Knipe DM, Howley PM, editors. Fields virology. Philadelphia, PA: Lippincott, Williams, and Wilkins; 2007.
28. Rotbart HA. Enteroviral infections of the central nervous system. Clin Infect Dis. 1995;20:971–81.
29. Bourlet T, Caro V, Minjolle S, et al. New PCR test that recognizes all human prototypes of enterovirus: application for clinical diagnosis. J Clin Microbiol. 2003;41:1750–2.
30. Landry ML, Garner R, Ferguson D. Real-time nucleic acid sequence-based amplification using molecular beacons for detection of enterovirus RNA in clinical specimens. J Clin Microbiol. 2005;43:3136–9.
31. Oberste MS, Maher K, Flemister MR, et al. Comparison of classic and molecular approaches for the identification of untypeable enteroviruses. J Clin Microbiol. 2000;38:1170–4.
32. Rotbart HA. Diagnosis of enteroviral meningitis with the polymerase chain reaction. J Pediatr. 1990;117:85–9.
33. Rotbart HA. Enzymatic RNA amplification of the enteroviruses. J Clin Microbiol. 1990;28:438–42.
34. Stellrecht KA, Harding I, Hussain FM, et al. A one-step RT-PCR assay using an enzyme-linked detection system for the diagnosis of enterovirus meningitis. J Clin Virol. 2000;17:143–9.
35. Verstrepen WA, Bruynseels P, Mertens AH. Evaluation of a rapid real-time RT-PCR assay for detection of enterovirus RNA in cerebrospinal fluid specimens. J Clin Virol. 2002;25 Suppl 1:S39–43.
36. Zoll GJ, Melchers WJ, Kopecka H, et al. General primer-mediated polymerase chain reaction for detection of enteroviruses: application for diagnostic routine and persistent infections. J Clin Microbiol. 1992;30:160–5.
37. Nolte FS, Rogers BB, Tang YW, et al. Evaluation of a rapid and completely automated real-time reverse transcriptase PCR assay for diagnosis of enteroviral meningitis. J Clin Microbiol. 2011;49:528–33.

38. Ninove L, Nougairede A, Gazin C, et al. Comparative detection of enterovirus RNA in cerebrospinal fluid: GeneXpert system vs. real-time RT-PCR assay. Clin Microbiol Infect. 2011;17:1890–4.
39. Sefers SE, Raymer AK, Kilby JT, et al. Prevalence and management of invalid GeneXpert enterovirus results obtained with cerebrospinal fluid samples: a 2-year study. J Clin Microbiol. 2009;47: 3008–10.
40. Capaul SE, Gorgievski-Hrisoho M. Detection of enterovirus RNA in cerebrospinal fluid (CSF) using NucliSens EasyQ Enterovirus assay. J Clin Virol. 2005;32:236–40.
41. Marlowe EM, Novak SM, Dunn JJ, et al. Performance of the GeneXpert enterovirus assay for detection of enteroviral RNA in cerebrospinal fluid. J Clin Virol. 2008;43:110–3.
42. Nix WA, Maher K, Johansson ES, et al. Detection of all known parechoviruses by real-time PCR. J Clin Microbiol. 2008;46: 2519–24.
43. Noordhoek GT, Weel JF, Poelstra E, et al. Clinical validation of a new real-time PCR assay for detection of enteroviruses and parechoviruses, and implications for diagnostic procedures. J Clin Virol. 2008;41:75–80.
44. Renaud C, Kuypers J, Ficken E, et al. Introduction of a novel parechovirus RT-PCR clinical test in a regional medical center. J Clin Virol. 2011;51:50–3.
45. Walters B, Penaranda S, Nix WA, et al. Detection of human parechovirus (HPeV)-3 in spinal fluid specimens from pediatric patients in the Chicago area. J Clin Virol. 2011;52:187–91.
46. Wolthers KC, Benschop KS, Schinkel J, et al. Human parechoviruses as an important viral cause of sepsislike illness and meningitis in young children. Clin Infect Dis. 2008;47:358–63.
47. International Agency for Research on Cancer, IARC. Proceedings of the IARC working group on the evaluation of carcinogenic risks to humans. Epstein-Barr virus and Kaposi's sarcoma herpesvirus/human herpesvirus 8. Lyon, France, 17–24 June 1997. IARC Monogr Eval Carcinog Risks Hum. 1997;70:1–492.
48. Jackson AC. Acute viral infections. Curr Opin Neurol. 1995; 8:170–4.
49. Roizman B, Knipe DM, Whitley RJ. Herpes simplex viruses. In: Knipe DM, Howley PM, editors. Fields virology. Philadelphia, PA: Lippincott, Williams, and Wilkins; 2007.
50. Tedder DG, Ashley R, Tyler KL, et al. Herpes simplex virus infection as a cause of benign recurrent lymphocytic meningitis. Ann Intern Med. 1994;121:334–8.
51. Kimberlin DW, Whitley RJ. Neonatal herpes: what have we learned. Semin Pediatr Infect Dis. 2005;16:7–16.
52. Lakeman FD, Whitley RJ. Diagnosis of herpes simplex encephalitis: application of polymerase chain reaction to cerebrospinal fluid from brain-biopsied patients and correlation with disease. National Institute of Allergy and Infectious Diseases Collaborative Antiviral Study Group. J Infect Dis. 1995;171:857–63.
53. Sauerbrei A, Eichhorn U, Hottenrott G, et al. Virological diagnosis of herpes simplex encephalitis. J Clin Virol. 2000;17:31–6.
54. Tyler KL. Update on herpes simplex encephalitis. Rev Neurol Dis. 2004;1:169–78.
55. Murphy RF, Caliendo AM. Relative quantity of cerebrospinal fluid herpes simplex virus DNA in adult cases of encephalitis and meningitis. Am J Clin Pathol. 2009;132:687–90.
56. Schloss L, Falk KI, Skoog E, et al. Monitoring of herpes simplex virus DNA types 1 and 2 viral load in cerebrospinal fluid by real-time PCR in patients with herpes simplex encephalitis. J Med Virol. 2009;81:1432–7.
57. Mejias A, Bustos R, Ardura MI, et al. Persistence of herpes simplex virus DNA in cerebrospinal fluid of neonates with herpes simplex virus encephalitis. J Perinatol. 2009;29:290–6.
58. Cohen JI, Straus SE, Arvin AM. Varicella zoster virus. In: Knipe DM, Howley PM, editors. Fields virology. Philadelphia, PA: Lippincott, Williams, and Wilkins; 2007.
59. Gnann Jr JW, Whitley RJ. Clinical practice. Herpes zoster. N Engl J Med. 2002;347:340–6.
60. Gilden DH, Kleinschmidt-DeMasters BK, LaGuardia JJ, et al. Neurologic complications of the reactivation of varicella-zoster virus. N Engl J Med. 2000;342:635–45.
61. Hillenkamp J, Nolle B, Bruns C, et al. Acute retinal necrosis: clinical features, early vitrectomy, and outcomes. Ophthalmology. 2009;116(1971–1975), e1972.
62. Liesegang TJ. Herpes zoster ophthalmicus natural history, risk factors, clinical presentation, and morbidity. Ophthalmology. 2008;115:S3–12.
63. Pahud BA, Glaser CA, Dekker CL, et al. Varicella zoster disease of the central nervous system: epidemiological, clinical, and laboratory features 10 years after the introduction of the varicella vaccine. J Infect Dis. 2011;203:316–23.
64. Sauerbrei A, Eichhorn U, Schacke M, et al. Laboratory diagnosis of herpes zoster. J Clin Virol. 1999;14:31–6.
65. Espy MJ, Uhl JR, Mitchell PS, et al. Diagnosis of herpes simplex virus infections in the clinical laboratory by LightCycler PCR. J Clin Microbiol. 2000;38:795–9.
66. Minjolle S, Michelet C, Jusselin I, et al. Amplification of the six major human herpesviruses from cerebrospinal fluid by a single PCR. J Clin Microbiol. 1999;37:950–3.
67. Quereda C, Corral I, Laguna F, et al. Diagnostic utility of a multiplex herpesvirus PCR assay performed with cerebrospinal fluid from human immunodeficiency virus-infected patients with neurological disorders. J Clin Microbiol. 2000;38:3061–7.
68. Read SJ, Kurtz JB. Laboratory diagnosis of common viral infections of the central nervous system by using a single multiplex PCR screening assay. J Clin Microbiol. 1999;37:1352–5.
69. Read SJ, Mitchell JL, Fink CG. LightCycler multiplex PCR for the laboratory diagnosis of common viral infections of the central nervous system. J Clin Microbiol. 2001;39:3056–9.
70. Rowley AH, Whitley RJ, Lakeman FD, et al. Rapid detection of herpes-simplex-virus DNA in cerebrospinal fluid of patients with herpes simplex encephalitis. Lancet. 1990;335:440–1.
71. Weidmann M, Meyer-Konig U, Hufert FT. Rapid detection of herpes simplex virus and varicella-zoster virus infections by real-time PCR. J Clin Microbiol. 2003;41:1565–8.
72. Braun DK, Dominguez G, Pellett PE. Human herpesvirus 6. Clin Microbiol Rev. 1997;10:521–67.
73. Ward KN, Leong HN, Thiruchelvam AD, et al. Human herpesvirus 6 DNA levels in cerebrospinal fluid due to primary infection differ from those due to chromosomal viral integration and have implications for diagnosis of encephalitis. J Clin Microbiol. 2007;45:1298–304.
74. Secchiero P, Zella D, Crowley RW, et al. Quantitative PCR for human herpesviruses 6 and 7. J Clin Microbiol. 1995;33:2124–30.
75. Van den Bosch G, Locatelli G, Geerts L, et al. Development of reverse transcriptase PCR assays for detection of active human herpesvirus 6 infection. J Clin Microbiol. 2001;39:2308–10.
76. Selvaraju SB, Wurst M, Horvat RT, et al. Evaluation of three analyte-specific reagents for detection and typing of herpes simplex virus in cerebrospinal fluid. Diagn Microbiol Infect Dis. 2009;63:286–91.
77. Tang YW, Espy MJ, Persing DH, et al. Molecular evidence and clinical significance of herpesvirus coinfection in the central nervous system. J Clin Microbiol. 1997;35:2869–72.
78. Shi J, Wu Y, Cai M, et al. Rapid diagnosis of herpetic encephalitis in children by PCR-microarray technology for simultaneous detection of seven human herpes viruses. Eur J Pediatr. 2010;169:421–5.
79. Leveque N, Van Haecke A, Renois F, et al. Rapid virological diagnosis of central nervous system infections by use of a multiplex reverse transcription-PCR DNA microarray. J Clin Microbiol. 2011;49:3874–9.

80. Campbell GL, Marfin AA, Lanciotti RS, et al. West Nile virus. Lancet Infect Dis. 2002;2:519–29.
81. Harrington T, Kuehnert MJ, Kamel H, et al. West Nile virus infection transmitted by blood transfusion. Transfusion. 2003;43: 1018–22.
82. Bakonyi T, Ivanics E, Erdelyi K, et al. Lineage 1 and 2 strains of encephalitic West Nile virus, central Europe. Emerg Infect Dis. 2006;12:618–23.
83. Martin DA, Muth DA, Brown T, et al. Standardization of immunoglobulin M capture enzyme-linked immunosorbent assays for routine diagnosis of arboviral infections. J Clin Microbiol. 2000;38:1823–6.
84. Lambert AJ, Martin DA, Lanciotti RS. Detection of North American eastern and western equine encephalitis viruses by nucleic acid amplification assays. J Clin Microbiol. 2003;41:379–85.
85. Lanciotti RS, Kerst AJ. Nucleic acid sequence-based amplification assays for rapid detection of West Nile and St. Louis encephalitis viruses. J Clin Microbiol. 2001;39:4506–13.
86. Lanciotti RS, Kerst AJ, Nasci RS, et al. Rapid detection of west nile virus from human clinical specimens, field-collected mosquitoes, and avian samples by a TaqMan reverse transcriptase-PCR assay. J Clin Microbiol. 2000;38:4066–71.
87. Scaramozzino N, Crance JM, Jouan A, et al. Comparison of flavivirus universal primer pairs and development of a rapid, highly sensitive heminested reverse transcription-PCR assay for detection of flaviviruses targeted to a conserved region of the NS5 gene sequences. J Clin Microbiol. 2001;39:1922–7.
88. White DJ, Kramer LD, Backenson PB, et al. Mosquito surveillance and polymerase chain reaction detection of West Nile virus, New York State. Emerg Infect Dis. 2001;7:643–9.
89. Niedrig M, Linke S, Zeller H, et al. First international proficiency study on West Nile virus molecular detection. Clin Chem. 2006;52:1851–4.
90. Linke S, Mackay WG, Scott C, et al. Second external quality assessment of the molecular diagnostic of West Nile virus: are there improvements towards the detection of WNV? J Clin Virol. 2011;52:257–60.
91. Ginocchio CC. Laboratory diagnosis of human cytomegalovirus (HCMV) central nervous system disease in AIDS patients. Int J Antimicrob Agents. 2000;16:447–53.
92. Zhang F, Tetali S, Wang XP, et al. Detection of human cytomegalovirus pp 67 late gene transcripts in cerebrospinal fluid of human immunodeficiency virus type 1-infected patients by nucleic acid sequence-based amplification. J Clin Microbiol. 2000;38:1920–5.
93. Koralnik IJ, Schellingerhout D, Frosch MP. Case records of the Massachusetts General Hospital. Weekly clinicopathological exercises. Case 14-2004. A 66-year-old man with progressive neurologic deficits. N Engl J Med. 2004;350:1882–93.
94. Koralnik IJ, Boden D, Mai VX, et al. JC virus DNA load in patients with and without progressive multifocal leukoencephalopathy. Neurology. 1999;52:253–60.
95. Garcia de Viedma D, Alonso R, Miralles P, et al. Dual qualitative-quantitative nested PCR for detection of JC virus in cerebrospinal fluid: high potential for evaluation and monitoring of progressive multifocal leukoencephalopathy in AIDS patients receiving highly active antiretroviral therapy. J Clin Microbiol. 1999;37:724–8.
96. Hammarin AL, Bogdanovic G, Svedhem V, et al. Analysis of PCR as a tool for detection of JC virus DNA in cerebrospinal fluid for diagnosis of progressive multifocal leukoencephalopathy. J Clin Microbiol. 1996;34:2929–32.
97. Whiley DM, Mackay IM, Sloots TP. Detection and differentiation of human polyomaviruses JC and BK by LightCycler PCR. J Clin Microbiol. 2001;39:4357–61.
98. Marzochetti A, Di Giambenedetto S, Cingolani A, et al. Reduced rate of diagnostic positive detection of JC virus DNA in cerebrospinal fluid in cases of suspected progressive mulitfocal leukoencephalopathy in the era of potent antiretroviral therapy. J Clin Microbiol. 2005;43:4175–7.
99. Albright AV, Soldan SS, Gonzalez-Scarano F. Pathogenesis of human immunodeficiency virus-induced neurological disease. J Neurovirol. 2003;9:222–7.
100. McArthur JC, Haughey N, Gartner S, et al. Human immunodeficiency virus-associated dementia: an evolving disease. J Neurovirol. 2003;9:205–21.

Bacterial Infections

49

Kevin Alby and Melissa B. Miller

Abstract

Molecular techniques have revolutionized the detection and identification of microorganisms. Real-time PCR has allowed for the rapid and accurate detection of MRSA, VRE, and group B *Streptococcus*. The identification of difficult and slow-growing organisms has been expedited by sequence-based methods such as 16S rRNA gene sequencing. Rapid identification of organisms and detection of resistance markers directly from positive blood culture bottles has become a reality. Finally, a transformation is taking place with the introduction of MALDI-TOF into clinical laboratories that promises to improve the accuracy and speed of bacterial and fungal identifications by days. The advantages of these methodologies and their associated clinical applications, along with their inherent pitfalls and problems, are elucidated in this chapter.

Keywords

MRSA • *Staphylococcus aureus* • VRE • *Enterococcus* • Group B *Streptococcus* • Antimicrobial resistance • Mass spectrometry • MALDI-TOF • 16S rRNA • Tuberculosis • Sepsis • Molecular epidemiology

Introduction

As the general population ages, the incidence of chronic conditions rises, the prevalence of antimicrobial resistance increases, and emerging pathogens arise, the laboratory diagnosis of infectious diseases has evolved and become more complex. As the complexity of diagnostic microbiology has increased, so have the methods employed to detect infectious agents. The implementation of molecular technology in the clinical microbiology laboratory in some cases has augmented traditional methods, such as culture and serology, while in other circumstances it has completely replaced traditional methods. For routine bacteriology (i.e., blood cultures, urine cultures, and respiratory cultures), culture has remained the gold standard primarily based on a lower cost and the potential complex nature of infections. However, in situations where low quantities of the pathogen may be present, the patient may have received antibiotics prior to specimen collection, the etiologic agent may require unusual culture conditions, or a more rapid turnaround time is needed, molecular testing approaches are particularly beneficial.

Currently, the optimal use of molecular techniques in microbiology resides with specimens in which a limited number of pathogenic organisms are sought (i.e., detection of methicillin-resistant *Staphylococcus aureus* from nares or vancomycin-resistant *Enterococcus* from rectal swabs) and in cases where the enhanced sensitivity, decreased turnaround time, and/or patient impact of molecular methods outweighs the increased cost to the laboratory

K. Alby, Ph.D.
Department of Pathology and Laboratory Medicine, Perelman School of Medicine, University of Pennsylvania, Philadelphia, Pennsylvania

M.B. Miller, Ph.D. (✉)
Department of Pathology and Laboratory Medicine, University of North Carolina School of Medicine, Campus Box 7525, Chapel Hill, NC 27599, USA
e-mail: mbmiller@unch.unc.edu

D.G.B. Leonard (ed.), *Molecular Pathology in Clinical Practice*, DOI 10.1007/978-3-319-19674-9_49

(i.e., molecular identification of organisms directly from positive blood cultures). A particularly exciting transition in clinical microbiology is the use of mass spectrometry (MS) for the identification of a wide spectrum of bacterial and fungal organisms as well as the detection of antimicrobial resistance. This chapter discusses the most common molecular methods and their applications in clinical bacteriology laboratories, including the associated advantages and disadvantages.

Bacterial Identification

Probe Hybridization

The molecular methods used for the identification of bacterial organisms cultured from patient specimens include direct probe hybridization and sequencing. Direct probe hybridization can be used for culture confirmation as well as direct detection of organisms from clinical material. Both nucleic acid probes and peptide nucleic acid (PNA) probes are commercially available.

Probes are single-stranded oligonucleotides that vary in size from 20 base pairs (bp) to a few kilobases, but are generally less than 50 bp. Probe specificity is defined by the nucleic acid sequence of the probe. Bacterial identification using probes to 16S rRNA or 23S rRNA are commonly used due to the relatively high copy number of rRNAs in bacteria which increases the sensitivity of direct detection. Further, rRNA sequences contain conserved regions in addition to hypervariable regions allowing for the level of identification to be varied depending on the probe sequence. Commercially available probes for culture confirmation include Group B *Streptococcus*, *Listeria monocytogenes*, *Neisseria gonorrhoeae*, *Staphylococcus aureus*, *Streptococcus pneumoniae*, and several mycobacteria including *M. tuberculosis* (Hologic, San Diego, CA). In addition, probes for direct detection of group A *Streptococcus* from throat swabs are available (Hologic). Although more expensive than conventional culture and identification methods, probe-based detection and identification methods have moderately increased sensitivity and specificity and decreased turnaround time [1]. However, both false-negative and false-positive results may occur. Bacterial strains may possess polymorphisms that prevent probe hybridization [2, 3] or different strains may contain similar sequences that result in cross-reactivity [4, 5]. Additional disadvantages of probe hybridization methods are the limited number of commercial probes and the inability to probe clinical specimens directly.

In situ hybridization (ISH) allows for the detection of nucleic acid sequences in cells or tissues fixed to glass slides. Probes, which can be DNA, RNA, or PNA, are typically short (15–30 bps) allowing for easier penetration and access to the target sequence. Both colorimetric and fluorescent ISH (FISH) probes are used in histopathology and clinical microbiology. Advantages of ISH in histopathology are the ability to evaluate the host tissue response and identification of the specific cells containing the infectious agent(s). In addition, "non-culturable" or difficult to culture organisms can be detected by ISH, i.e., *Tropheryma whipplei* for Whipple's disease. Disadvantages include autofluorescence by some microorganisms (including *Pseudomonas*, *Legionella*, many yeasts, and molds), specificity and reliability of certain probe sequences, insufficient probe penetration of sample material, secondary structure of target sequence, low target content, and photobleaching [6].

In clinical microbiology, the direct identification of microbial organisms in patient samples or cultures often is determined using commercial PNA-FISH probes (AdvanDx, Woburn, MA). PNA probes have a neutral peptide-like backbone, as opposed to the negatively charged sugar–phosphate backbone of DNA probes [7]. However, like DNA probes, PNA probes hybridize to DNA and RNA in a sequence-specific manner and can be fluorescently labeled for ease of detection. Reported advantages of PNA probes include stronger and faster hybridization, discrimination of one bp difference, resistance to nucleases and proteases, survival under stringent conditions (e.g., high temperature) that allow for access to regions with secondary structure, and increased hydrophobicity that allows for penetration of cell membranes during ISH [7]. Commercial PNA probes include many multi-labeled probe kits for the discrimination of morphologically similar organisms including *Staphylococcus aureus*/coagulase-negative *Staphylococcus*, *Enterococcus faecalis*/other enterococci, *Escherichia coli*/*Pseudomonas aeruginosa*, gram-negative rods (*E. coli*, *P. aeruginosa*, *Klebsiella pneumoniae*), yeast (*C. albicans*/*parapsilosis*, *C. tropicalis*, and *C. glabrata*/*krusei*), and Group B *Streptococcus* (AdvanDx, Inc., Woburn, MA). PNA-FISH probes are used by clinical laboratories for the identification of organisms from positive blood culture bottles in less than 2.5 h, which has a significant positive impact on patient care and institutional cost savings [8–11].

Sequencing

In many larger laboratories, sequencing is used to rapidly and accurately identify organisms. Sequencing is more rapid than conventional methods, but initial growth of an isolate is still required prior to sequencing. Ideal applications of sequencing for organism identification include *Mycobacterium* spp., aerobic actinomycetes including *Nocardia* spp., select anaerobes and gram-positive bacteria, which are organisms that are typically slow-growing or difficult to identify by routine methods. Sequencing can also be used to identify organisms that cannot be cultured because they are inherently difficult to grow or as a result of antibiotic therapy. In this situation, sequencing would need to be performed directly from the clinical specimen, but this practice must be used with caution and only for specimens from sterile sites. A substantial body of evidence exists for direct sequencing from explanted heart valves for the identification of organisms causing endocarditis [12, 13].

Many bacterial genome regions are used for sequence-based identification in clinical laboratories, but the 16S rRNA gene is the most common target. The 16S rRNA gene encodes for the highly conserved rRNA associated with the small subunit of the ribosome and is often used for taxonomic purposes and species identification. While 16S rRNA is highly conserved among bacteria, nucleotide variations unique to each species are concentrated in specific regions. The entire gene is 1,550 bp including the conserved and variable regions, but discriminatory sequence can generally be obtained using 500 bp [14]. Universal primers complementary to the conserved regions on either side of the variable region permit amplification from all bacterial species and the resulting amplicon contains unique sequence for identification. Commercial research use only kits are available for sequencing of 16S rRNA (MicroSeq; Applied Biosystems) (Thermo Fisher Scientific, Waltham, MA), but many clinical laboratories use laboratory-developed protocols. Notably, some organisms are identical by 16S rDNA sequencing (e.g., *M. chelonae* and *M. abscessus*, *S. pneumoniae* and *S. mitis*). However, some of the identical organisms by 16S rDNA sequencing can be differentiated by sequencing other genes, such as those of the internal transcribed space (ITS) region, *rpoB*, *secA*, or *hsp65* [15–17].

Sequence results are more robust than conventional culture methods because they are less subjective if a comprehensive and accurate database is used for sequence comparison. Analysis of the sequence data involves evaluating the quality of the sequence obtained and subsequent comparison of the sequence with known sequences through public and/or commercial databases, such as NCBI GenBank, MicroSeq, Integrated Database Network System (SmartGene, Raleigh, NC), or RipSeq (Isentio, Palo Alto, CA). Once an isolate is growing in culture, the entire procedure can be done in about 1.5 work days. Beyond the relatively long time to result compared to mass spectrometry, other limitations are the quality of public databases or the expense of access to curated databases, and the similarity of 16S rRNA sequences of some organisms.

Mass Spectrometry

A major advancement in bacterial identification is the routine use of mass spectrometry (MS) in clinical microbiology laboratories [18]. Traditionally, bacterial identification is achieved by performing a number of biochemical reactions to identify the unique combination of phenotypic properties that are specific to a particular microorganism. Originally performed individually, these phenotypic tests have been streamlined and are now performed on automated instruments. Although automated systems have reduced the time to identification relative to traditional methods, there is still room for improvement.

The use of MS to identify organisms was first described in the mid-1970s [19], but not until the advent of using matrix assisted MS was the reliability and reproducibility sufficient for clinical applications [20]. The type of MS most commonly used in clinical microbiology is *M*atrix *A*ssisted *L*aser *D*esorption/*I*onization *T*ime *O*f *F*light (MALDI-TOF) MS. As illustrated in Fig. 49.1, the core of MALDI-TOF MS for bacterial identification is that differences in DNA lead to

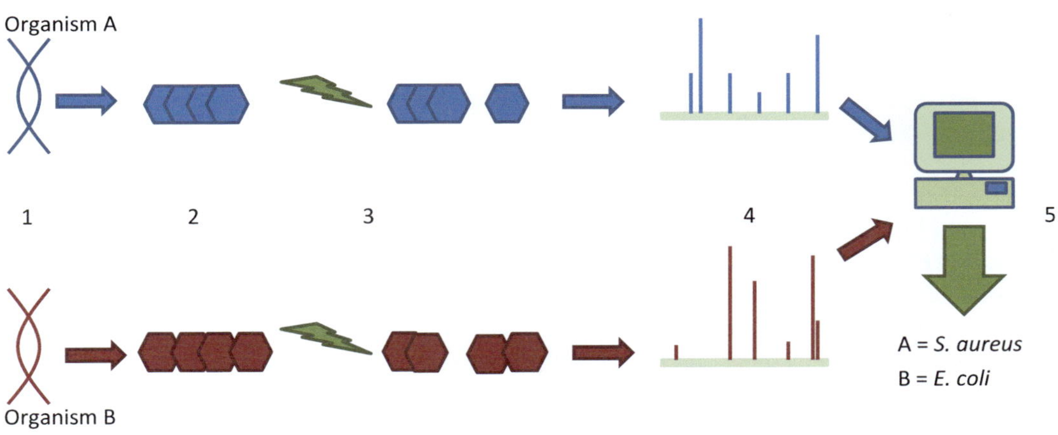

Figure 49.1 Schematic of MALDI-TOF mass spectrometry for differentiation of two organisms (A and B). Differences in DNA (*1*) encode for different protein products (*2*) which are differentially fragmented under laser excitation (*3*). These fragmented proteins produce organism-specific spectra (*4*), which are compared against a reference database of spectra (*5*) for organism identification

differences in the protein composition of an organism, and the differences in protein composition can be resolved by MALDI-TOF MS. The technology works by using the laser to create a cloud of ions to which a current is applied and released into a flight chamber. The ions are generated from the bacterial isolate that has been smeared onto a target slide and overlaid with a matrix solution (typically α-cyano-4-hydroxycinnamic acid). The matrix solution is critical for even distribution of the laser energy, generation of primarily singly charged ions, and reproducible results. The process of using smeared bacterial isolates is often referred to as whole cell or intact cell MS (WCMS or ICMS) [21, 22]. As the ions travel through the flight chamber they are separated according to their size and charge, with the smallest and most highly charged particles moving fastest through the chamber. The ions strike a detector at the end of the chamber, and a spectrum is generated that provides the relative quantity of ions of a particular mass–charge ratio. These spectra are algorithmically compared to a reference database with identity and confidence values assigned.

Much like 16S rRNA gene sequencing, the strength of this application relies on a robust reference database for comparison [18]. Several studies have shown that identification rates significantly increase after database augmentation [23–25]. Also, much as quality sequence reads are necessary for identification, high quality spectra are a must for good reference matching and identification. Ideal spectra for identification typically consist of proteins in the 2–20 kDa range, which is rich in ribosomal and other cytoplasmic proteins. Obtaining quality spectra using WCMS can be difficult with organisms such as mycobacteria, filamentous fungi, and yeasts, due to their rigid cell walls [18, 26]. Therefore, these organisms must undergo an additional extraction step to make the internal cellular proteins more accessible for ionization. The most basic extraction step is to apply a formic acid solution to the smeared spot and allow it to dry before adding the matrix solution. Higher order bacteria, such as mycobacteria and *Nocardia* spp., and filamentous fungi require a more rigorous extraction, typically involving bead beating, formic acid, and acetonitrile treatments [27]. In general, MALDI-TOF MS performs well, typically identifying >90 % of routine organisms to the correct species [18, 28, 29]. Two MALDI-TOF MS platforms currently are used in clinical microbiology laboratories: the MALDI Biotyper (Bruker Daltronics, Billerica, MA) and VITEK MS (bioMerieux, Durham, NC) each offering FDA-cleared databases. Additional developments in MALDI-TOF MS for the clinical microbiology laboratory include detection of antimicrobial resistance and direct pathogen detection from blood cultures (see below).

Another emerging technology for the identification of microorganisms is the use of PCR electrospray-ionization mass spectrometry (ESI/MS). This methodology uses conserved primers to generate PCR amplicons directly from a specimen source as well as MS to generate an approximation of the base content of the amplicons. This information is unique enough to develop spectral signatures for different organisms. These spectra are then compared to a database which provides likely identifications based on the primer sets used as well as the relative abundance of the organism(s) identified [30]. PCR ESI/MS has several advantages: (1) direct detection of a wide variety of potential pathogens (viruses, bacteria, and fungi) from specimens; (2) more rapid and cost-effective testing compared to sequencing technologies such as next-generation sequencing; and (3) to provide information outside the constraints of array-based technologies such as only being able to query a limited number of predefined organisms [30]. In fact, this technology can be used in pathogen discovery as new pathogens will not be identified but will group with similar known organisms. This was done successfully during the Sudden Acute Respiratory Syndrome (SARS) pandemic [31]. Still, as with all new technologies, work remains to be done to optimize the process for routine clinical use including further optimization of extraction methods as well as the development of additional primer sets.

Antimicrobial Resistance Detection

The increased emphasis on faster turnaround times for results combined with availability of more targeted therapeutics has created a niche for rapid molecular detection of resistance determinants in clinical microbiology laboratories. Antimicrobial resistance can be detected by probe hybridization, nucleic acid amplification (NAA) technologies such as PCR, and sequencing. However, the use of molecular methods to detect microbial resistance is not without its limitations. Multifactorial resistance mechanisms, polyclonal or polymicrobial infections, phenotypic synergism, and unknown genotype–phenotype relationships can prevent accurate determination of resistance using molecular methods.

Amplification Methods

Methicillin-Resistant *Staphylococcus aureus*

The most established application of molecular bacterial resistance testing is the detection of methicillin-resistant *Staphylococcus aureus* (MRSA). Resistance to methicillin in staphylococci is almost exclusively caused by a single mechanism, the alteration of the penicillin binding protein PBP2 to the conformer PBP2a. This change is mediated by a well-defined genetic component, the *mecA* gene. The altered PBP2a has a lower affinity for methicillin and other penicillinase-stable β-lactams such that resistance is conferred.

Traditional detection methods include chromogenic agars, oxacillin screening agars, and traditional disk diffusion for cefoxitin and minimum inhibitory concentration testing for oxacillin. These methods require 12–24 h of incubation. Decreasing the time to differentiate methicillin-susceptible staphylococcus aureus (MSSA) and MRSA by use of either protein-based methods (PBP2a latex; Oxoid, Cambridge, UK) or molecular methods for the detection of the *mecA* gene (see below) is associated with improved patient outcomes and institutional cost savings [9, 32].

Vancomycin-Resistant *Enterococcus*

First detected nearly 30 years after the introduction of vancomycin, vancomycin-resistant enterococci (VRE) developed in part due to increasing use of vancomycin for *Clostridium difficile* colitis and MRSA infections [33, 34]. Vancomycin acts by blocking the transglycosylation and transpeptidation steps of cell wall biosynthesis. The resistance phenotype is based on lowering the affinity of vancomycin for its target peptidoglycan precursors and is encoded by the *van* genes. High-level resistance (MIC, ≥64 μg/ml) is encoded *vanA* and *vanB* which are typically found on transposons, or the chromosomally associated *vanD*, and is generally found in *Enterococcus faecium* and *Enterococcus faecalis* [35–37]. Also chromosomally encoded are the *vanC* genes of *Enterococcus gallinarum*, *Enterococcus casseliflavus*, and *Enterococcus flavescens*, which are associated with low-level resistance (MIC, 2–32 μg/ml). Because *vanA* and *vanB* tend to reside on mobile elements and confer high-level resistance, detection of enterococci containing these resistance determinants is critical for effective infection control measures.

Although numerous laboratory-developed NAA assays and commercial analyte specific reagents (ASRs) are available, only a few assays for the molecular detection of VRE from rectal sites are cleared by the US Food and Drug Administration (FDA) (Xpert *vanA* test, Cepheid, Sunnyvale, CA; BD GeneOhm VanR, Becton Dickinson, Sparks, MD; and IMDX VanR, Intelligent Medical Devices, Beverly, MA). Although VRE in the USA and Europe most commonly contains *vanA*, *vanB* should also be considered due to its lower but significant prevalence. The main advantages to the molecular detection of VRE are increased sensitivity, increased specificity (exclusion of *vanC* mediated resistance), and decreased time-to-result [38–40].

Mycobacterium tuberculosis

Although resistance to antituberculosis drugs is not a new phenomenon, new methods have been developed to identify resistant strains. Due to the slow growth of *M. tuberculosis* (TB), molecular techniques are well suited to not only detect TB directly from patient specimens but also screen for resistance (see Chap. 53). Several test kits have been CE-marked for clinical use in Europe. These include the Genotype MTBDR system (Hain Lifescience, Germany), the Innogenetics INNO-LiPA Rif.TB (Gent, Belgium), and the Xpert MTB/RIF cartridge for the Cepheid GeneXpert platform, with the latter also receiving FDA clearance. All the systems detect rifampin resistance as it is the most common resistance found among the first-line TB drugs. In addition, rifampin resistance can be a marker for multidrug-resistant (MDR) TB in geographic regions with endemic MDR-TB [41]. Rifampin resistance is determined by analyzing the *rpoB* gene for specific mutations in the 81 bp rifampin resistance determining region using hybridization probes [42]. The Genotype MTBDR system also determines isoniazid resistance by screening the *katG* and *inhA* genes [43, 44]. An expanded Genotype MTBDRsl panel adds detection of resistance to fluoroquinolones, aminoglycosides, and ethambutol. Additional information on mycobacterial detection and resistance can be found in Chap. 53.

Mass Spectrometry

Much like the revolutionary impact on bacterial identifications, MS will likely impact resistance testing. Preliminary studies have demonstrated the rapid identification of MRSA, extended spectrum beta lactamase (ESBL) organisms, and carbapenemase-producing organisms by MALDI-TOF MS. Resistant organisms can be identified in two ways using MS. Similar to genetic approaches, resistant organisms can be identified by the presence or absence of characteristic mass peaks. This approach has been most widely used in the identification of MRSA by MS, though there are conflicting reports as to its effectiveness [45–47]. The other approach to identifying resistant organisms using MS is to apply a phenotypic approach such as measurement of substrate modification. For example, to determine the presence of a microbial carbapenemase, a carbapenem and test organism can be co-incubated followed by MS detection of native carbapenem drug peaks and/or peaks of its hydrolyzed products in the supernatant [48, 49]. Although this approach only detects resistance mechanisms that modify the substrate, it has the distinct advantage of looking for a phenotype instead of a particular resistance determinant. This can be especially useful in the cases of ESBLs and carbapenemases which have many genetic determinants that cause the same phenotype [50].

Specific Applications

Staphylococcus aureus/MRSA

Screening patients for MRSA nasal colonization is a central strategy for preventing the spread of this organism in health care settings. The reference method used to accurately detect resistance due to altered PBP2 in *S. aureus* is NAA and detection of the *mecA* gene. Conventional and real-time PCR have been used to detect *mecA* both on bacterial isolates and directly on patient specimens. However, direct specimen testing has limitations, often including a lower positive predictive value than conventional methods based on the possible co-detection of MSSA and methicillin-resistant coagulase-negative staphylococci [51, 52]. Manufacturers have circumvented this problem through the detection of the SCC*mec-orf* junction in the *S. aureus* genome. However, strains that contain the SCC*mec* cassette but have a non-functional or deleted *mecA* (so-called "*mecA*-dropouts") will be falsely positive. In addition, MRSA strains that carry *mecC*, a *mecA* homologue, will be falsely negative in these assays, though the prevalence of these strains is still low [53]. Several FDA-cleared molecular assays are available for the detection of MRSA with or without MSSA detection from nasal swabs and clinical specimens, such as positive blood cultures and swabs obtained from skin and soft tissue infections (Table 49.1). NAA detection of MRSA is at least equal in sensitivity to culture-based methods, but has the advantage of offering a faster turnaround time, which, when combined with appropriate infection control interventions, may significantly decrease hospital costs by decreasing the number of health-care-associated MRSA infections [54].

Group B *Streptococcus* (*S. agalactiae*)

Although the incidence of Group B *Streptococcus* (GBS) neonatal disease has been declining since the 1990s due to enhanced prevention efforts, it is still the leading infectious cause of morbidity and mortality in neonates in the USA. In 2002, the Centers for Disease Control and Prevention (CDC), with the American College of Obstetricians and Gynecologists and the American Academy of Pediatrics, first published guidelines to perform vaginal–rectal screening of all pregnant women at 35–37 weeks gestation. Women who are colonized should be given intrapartum prophylactic treatment. Thus, accurate GBS results are critical to ensure appropriate antibiotic administration. Additionally, if a woman's GBS colonization status is not known due to lack of prenatal care or premature delivery, she should receive prophylactic antibiotics based on risk assessment, specifically for gestation less than 37 weeks, membrane rupture more than 18 h prior to delivery, or a fever of greater than 38 °C [55]. Since antibiotic administration is not without risks to the mother and newborn, intrapartum rapid molecular tests for GBS colonization are beneficial.

The first molecular technique used for routine GBS screening was direct probe hybridization either to colonies or swab-inoculated Lim broth. Although this provided the advantage of decreased turnaround time and reduced technologist time [56], it is not cost-effective for routine antepartum screening. Further development of molecular technologies in GBS detection has resulted in seven FDA-cleared molecular tests (Table 49.2) and numerous laboratory-developed tests (LDTs). Notably, the BD GeneOhm StrepB test (BD GeneOhm Sciences, San Diego, CA) and the Cepheid Smart GBS and Xpert GBS offer detection of GBS directly from rectovaginal swabs for antepartum or intrapartum detection of GBS colonization. FDA-cleared in 2006, Xpert GBS performed on the GeneXpert (Cepheid) is a moderate-complexity test that is self-contained from extraction to result. This technology makes random access testing for intrapartum screening feasible. Given that approximately 10 % of women with negative cultures at 35–37 weeks' gestation are GBS positive at the time of delivery [57],

Table 49.1 FDA-cleared molecular tests for the detection of methicillin-resistant *Staphylococcus aureus* (MRSA) directly from patient specimens

Test name	Manufacturer	Organism(s) detected	Specimen types	References
Screening tests				
GeneOhm MRSA ACP	BD Diagnostics	MRSA	Nasal swab	[77]
IDI-MRSA	BD Diagnostics	MRSA	Nasal swab	[78–81]
LightCycler MRSA Advanced	Roche Molecular Diagnostics	MRSA	Nasal swab	[82]
NucliSens EasyQ MRSA	bioMérieux	MRSA	Nasal swab	–
Xpert MRSA	Cepheid	MRSA	Nasal swab	[79, 83]
Xpert SA Nasal Complete	Cepheid	MRSA/SA	Nasal swab	[84]
Diagnostic tests				
GeneOhm StaphSR	BD Diagnostics	MRSA	Positive blood cultures	[85, 86]
Filmarray BCID	BioFire	MRSA/SA	Positive blood culture bottles	[101]
Verigene BC-GP Nucleic Acid	Nanosphere		Positive blood cultures	[87–89]
Xpert MRSA/SA BC	Cepheid	MRSA/SA	Positive blood cultures	[90–92]
Xpert MRSA/SA SSTI	Cepheid	MRSA/SA	Skin/soft tissue swabs	[92, 93]

Table 49.2 FDA-cleared molecular tests for detection of group B *Streptococcus*

Test name	Manufacturer	Methodology	Specimen tested	Sensitivity[a]	Specificity[a]	References
BD Max GBS	BD GeneOhm	Real-time PCR	Enrichment broth, antepartum swabs	95 %*	96.7 %*	[94]
Strep B (IDI-Strep B)	BD GeneOhm	Real-time PCR	Direct swab, antepartum and intrapartum	94 %* 86.8–95 %	96 %* 92.5–99.1 %	[59, 95–97]
Smart GBS	Cepheid	Real-time PCR	Direct swab, antepartum and intrapartum	81.6–98.7 %* 98.6–100 %	90.4–96.3 %* 90.4–100 %	[98, 99]
Xpert GBS	Cepheid	Real-time PCR	Direct swab, antepartum and intrapartum	88.6 %* 83.3–98.5 %	96.7 %* 64.5–99.6 %	[58, 100]
Illumigene GBS	Meridian Bioscience	Loop-mediated isothermal amplification	Enrichment broth of antepartum swabs	97.4 %*	92.3 %*	[102]
Group B AccuProbe	Gen-Probe	Hybridization Protection Assay	Enrichment broth or cultured isolate	97.7 %* 86.5–95.6 %	99.1 %* 97.5–100 %	[56, 97, 101]
GBS PNA FISH	AdvanDx	Fluorescent in situ hybridization	Enrichment broth of antepartum swabs	89.2 %* 98.4 %	98.1 %* 100 %	[99]

[a]Sensitivities and specificities were calculated using culture as the gold standard and vary depending on whether used for antepartum or intrapartum screening in the cited reference. Package insert data are indicated by an asterisk (*)

intrapartum testing is the most accurate test for colonization at the time of delivery. As an intrapartum screening test at one institution, the Xpert GBS had a sensitivity of 95.8 % and specificity of 64.5 %, whereas the antenatal culture was 83.3 % sensitive and 80.6 % specific, when intrapartum culture was used as the gold standard [58]. In a multicenter study of the IDI-StrepB assay (BD GeneOhm), when intrapartum culture was the gold standard, molecular detection at the time of labor was 94 % sensitive and 95.9 % specific [59]. Relative to either the sensitivity of antenatal cultures (54 %) or risk factor analysis (42 %), the sensitivity of the IDI-StrepB assay was superior [59]. The advantage in all these applications is the decreased turnaround time relative to culture in the intrapartum setting. Additional data regarding the sensitivity and specificity of molecular tests for GBS detection is shown in Table 49.2.

Sepsis

The use of molecular methods for the diagnosis of sepsis has been a challenging endeavor. Only one FDA-approved test is available for the identification of potential pathogens directly from blood obtained from septic patients, and this test is limited to candidemia. The gold standard remains automated blood cultures, and this reference method may be difficult to match owing to the large amount of blood that is cultured (typically 40 ml). Nonetheless, research use only products are available for direct testing of blood. Roche Molecular Systems SeptiFast (Branchburg, NJ) uses multiplex real-time PCR and melt curve analysis, while the Molzym SepsiTest (Bremen, Germany) uses multiplex PCR followed by sequencing, and the SIRS-Lab Vyoo (Jena, Germany) uses multiplex PCR followed by gel electrophoresis. These products vary in both the organisms and the resistance determinants detected, as well as analytical performance characteristics [60–64]. In general, these products suffer from both a lack of sensitivity and specificity, as well as requiring additional optimization before routine clinical use is possible.

Other shortcomings of NAA-based diagnosis of sepsis include the inconclusive clinical significance of the detection of pathogen DNA in the blood stream and the inability to obtain full antimicrobial susceptibility results [62]. However, blood culture is an imperfect reference method, suffering from a number of limitations including a prolonged time to pathogen identification, effects of variable blood volume, and lack of growth for fastidious pathogens or in the presence of prior antimicrobial therapy [62]. One limitation that can be addressed by molecular methods is the time to definitive identification.

A number of commercial molecular testing products are available for the identification of organisms and resistant determinants directly from positive blood culture bottles. This approach takes advantage of the culture amplification of bacteria from blood while adding molecular methods to lessen the time to identification. FDA-cleared tests for use directly with positive blood culture bottles include AdvanDx PNA-FISH (Woburn, MA), Cepheid (Sunnyvale, CA), Biofire FilmArray BC-ID (Salt Lake City, UT) and Nanosphere BC-GP and BC-GN panels (Northbrook, IL). The molecular targets for each of these products are listed in Table 49.3. The use of MALDI-TOF MS in direct pathogen detection directly from positive blood cultures also is being investigated [65, 66]. Recent data show identification rates of

Table 49.3 FDA-cleared molecular tests for identification of potential pathogens from positive blood culture bottles

Test name	Manufacturer	Methodology	Organisms detected	Resistance detected
AdvanDx	Separate tests as listed in Organisms Detected column	PNA-FISH	*Candida albicans*	Not directly; inferred from some species identifications
			C. albicans/glabrata	
			Yeast Traffic Light[a]	
			Enterococcus faecalis/OE[b]	
			E. coli/P. aeruginosa	
			EK/*P. aeruginosa*	
			GNR Traffic Light[c]	
Becton Dickinson	StaphSR	Real-time PCR	*Staphylococcus aureus*	*mecA* (MRSA)
Cepheid	Xpert MRSA/SA BC	Real-time PCR	*Staphylococcus aureus*	*mecA* (MRSA)
Nanosphere	Verigene BC-GP	Multiplex gold nanoparticle probes	*Staphylococcus* spp.	*mecA* (MRSA) *vanA* (VRE) *vanB* (VRE)
			Streptococcus spp.	
			Listeria spp.	
			Staphylococcus aureus	
			Staphylococcus epidermidis	
			Staphylococcus lugdunensis	
			Streptococcus pneumonia	
			Streptococcus anginosus group	
			Streptococcus agalactiae	
			Streptococcus pyogenes	
			Enterococcus faecalis	
			Enterococcus faecium	
Nanosphere	Verigene BC-GN		*Escherichia coli*	
			Klebsiella pneumoniae	
			Klebsiella oxytoca	
			Pseudomonas aeruginosa	
			Serratia marcescens	
BioFire	Filmarray BCID		*Escherichia coli K1*	
			Haemophilus influenzae	
			Listeria monocytogenes	
			Neisseria meningitidis	
			Streptococcus agalactiae	
			Streptococcus pneumoniae	

[a]*Candida albicans/parapsilosis, Candida tropicalis, Candida glabrata/krusei*
[b]Other enterococci
[c]*Escherichia coli, Klebsiella pneumoniae, Pseudomonas aeruginosa*

approximately 85 %, while reducing time to identification by more than a day [67]. Several studies have demonstrated the cost-effectiveness of utilizing rapid detection of organisms from positive blood culture bottles [8, 9, 11].

Molecular Epidemiology

Pulsed field gel electrophoresis (PFGE) is the gold standard for molecular epidemiology studies of the majority of organisms [68]. In brief, bacterial cells are immobilized in agarose and subjected to proteolytic degradation followed by restriction endonuclease digestion. The resulting genomic fragments are separated by PFGE which allows for better resolution of high molecular weight products [69]. PFGE is a critical tool for infection control and public health specialties, as a proven reproducible method to show strain relatedness and identify outbreaks. Other common approaches to molecular epidemiology include amplified fragment length polymorphism (AFLP) analysis and multi locus sequence typing (MLST) [70]. AFLP analysis is based on the same theory as PFGE: differences in DNA sequence can be identified by differences in restriction endonuclease patterns. The major difference between AFLP analysis and PFGE is that PFGE looks at the entire genome of an organism, while AFLP analysis emphasizes regions of the genome known to have high rates of polymorphisms. MLST analysis is done by amplifying and sequencing a small set of known housekeeping genes (usually 7–14) that have a standard rate of genetic variability.

These labor-intensive, and often expensive, approaches to molecular epidemiology have their disadvantages. Although PFGE has high discriminatory power, it is not very reproducible even amongst members of the same laboratory. This variability makes longitudinal comparisons difficult and often requires the same strains to be run repeatedly and/or implementation of a standard strain to normalize banding patterns. Although MLST analysis is very reproducible, it lacks the discriminatory power that more genome wide approaches such as AFLP analysis and PFGE offer. AFLP analysis tries to combine the discriminatory power of PFGE with the reproducibility of MLST analysis, with some success, but this approach is not applicable to all organisms [68].

MALDI-TOF MS represents a promising development for the field of molecular epidemiology, providing a relatively fast and easy method of comparing strain relatedness, with minimal hands-on time. MALDI-TOF MS has the advantage of interrogating the entire proteome of a microorganism, although the protein size range analyzed is typically only 2–20 kDa. Researchers have looked at the ability of MALDI-TOF MS to distinguish bacterial subspecies of organisms such as *Salmonella* [71, 72]. Only a few studies have been performed that compare the ability of a MALDI-TOF MS system directly to PFGE and assess its ability to determine absolute strain relatedness [73]. MALDI-TOF MS has been used to identify clonal populations of MRSA with some success [74], but the accuracy of this has been debated [75]. It remains to be seen, however, if the level of resolution of MALDI-TOF MS fingerprinting is enough to allow this technology to replace PFGE in the epidemiologic investigations of microorganisms.

Future Perspectives

Advances in molecular biology in the last 10–15 years have made an astounding impact on clinical laboratory testing for infectious diseases. Notably, TB can be confirmed in 24 h as opposed to 6–8 weeks, sexually transmitted infections such as those caused by *C. trachomatis* and *N. gonorrhoeae* can be rapidly and accurately identified improving treatment and prevention of transmission, and organisms with important infection control implications such as *B. pertussis*, MRSA, and VRE, can be quickly identified leading to appropriate therapy and/or precautions. The applications of molecular technology in clinical microbiology are endless, but disadvantages also abound. A molecular infectious disease laboratory is established only with considerable cost and expertise. Further, we are still learning what many NAA test results mean in terms of infectious etiology and clinical significance [76]. Is the mere presence of a microorganism's DNA convincing evidence of disease causation? Additional clinical and scientific evidence may be needed to validate the clinical relevance molecular-based results.

Though there is still much to be learned about the appropriate application and interpretation of molecular infectious disease testing, numerous exciting opportunities are on the horizon. The use of real-time PCR testing in the clinical laboratory has revolutionized diagnostic microbiology. The expanding capacity of multiplex technologies is allowing the simultaneous detection of over 20 analytes in just over an hour (BioFire Diagnostics). Perhaps the technology with the greatest impact on clinical microbiology is the use of MALDI-TOF MS not only for the identification of organisms, but also their potential resistance profiles and strain typing. Lastly, as next-generation sequencing becomes more affordable and accessible to clinical laboratories, clinical investigators will be able to ask questions about pathogenesis and microbiome changes in real time. Never before has clinical microbiology changed at the rapid pace we are currently experiencing. We must remember that the power of molecular technologies should be coupled with well-controlled and clinically relevant diagnostic approaches to have the greatest impact on patient care.

References

1. Tenover FC. DNA hybridization techniques and their application to the diagnosis of infectious diseases. Infect Dis Clin North Am. 1993;7(2):171–81.
2. Lebrun L, Espinasse F, Poveda JD, Vincent-Levy-Frebault V. Evaluation of nonradioactive DNA probes for identification of mycobacteria. J Clin Microbiol. 1992;30(9):2476–8.
3. Lumb R, Lanser JA, Lim IS. Rapid identification of mycobacteria by the Gen-Probe Accuprobe system. Pathology. 1993;25(3): 313–5.
4. Butler WR, O'Connor SP, Yakrus MA, Gross WM. Cross-reactivity of genetic probe for detection of *Mycobacterium tuberculosis* with newly described species *Mycobacterium celatum*. J Clin Microbiol. 1994;32(2):536–8.
5. Ford EG, Snead SJ, Todd J, Warren NG. Strains of *Mycobacterium terrae* complex which react with DNA probes for *M. tuberculosis* complex. J Clin Microbiol. 1993;31(10):2805–6.
6. Moter A, Gobel UB. Fluorescence in situ hybridization (FISH) for direct visualization of microorganisms. J Microbiol Methods. 2000;41(2):85–112.
7. Perry-O'Keefe H, Rigby S, Oliveira K, Sorensen D, Stender H, Coull J, Hyldig-Nielsen JJ. Identification of indicator microorganisms using a standardized PNA FISH method. J Microbiol Methods. 2001;47(3):281–92.
8. Forrest GN, Mankes K, Jabra-Rizk MA, Weekes E, Johnson JK, Lincalis DP, Venezia RA. Peptide nucleic acid fluorescence in situ hybridization-based identification of *Candida albicans* and its impact on mortality and antifungal therapy costs. J Clin Microbiol. 2006;44(9):3381–3.
9. Forrest GN, Mehta S, Weekes E, Lincalis DP, Johnson JK, Venezia RA. Impact of rapid in situ hybridization testing on coagulase-negative staphylococci positive blood cultures. J Antimicrob Chemother. 2006;58(1):154–8.
10. Heil EL, Daniels LM, Long DM, Rodino KG, Weber DJ, Miller MB. Impact of a rapid peptide nucleic acid fluorescence in situ hybridization assay on treatment of *Candida* infections. Am J Health Syst Pharm. 2012;69(21):1910–4.

11. Ly T, Gulia J, Pyrgos V, Waga M, Shoham S. Impact upon clinical outcomes of translation of PNA FISH-generated laboratory data from the clinical microbiology bench to bedside in real time. Ther Clin Risk Manag. 2008;4(3):637–40.
12. Fournier PE, Thuny F, Richet H, Lepidi H, Casalta JP, Arzouni JP, Maurin M, Celard M, Mainardi JL, Caus T, Collart F, Habib G, Raoult D. Comprehensive diagnostic strategy for blood culture-negative endocarditis: a prospective study of 819 new cases. Clin Infect Dis. 2010;51(2):131–40.
13. Miyazato A, Ohkusu K, Tabata M, Uwabe K, Kawamura T, Tachi Y, Ezaki T, Niinami H, Mitsutake K. Comparative molecular and microbiological diagnosis of 19 infective endocarditis cases in which causative microbes were identified by PCR-based DNA sequencing from the excised heart valves. J Infect Chemother. 2012;18(3):318–23.
14. Clarridge III JE. Impact of 16S rRNA gene sequence analysis for identification of bacteria on clinical microbiology and infectious diseases. Clin Microbiol Rev. 2004;17(4):840–62.
15. Conville PS, Zelazny AM, Witebsky FG. Analysis of *secA1* gene sequences for identification of *Nocardia* species. J Clin Microbiol. 2006;44(8):2760–6.
16. Roth A, Fischer M, Hamid ME, Michalke S, Ludwig W, Mauch H. Differentiation of phylogenetically related slowly growing mycobacteria based on 16S–23S rRNA gene internal transcribed spacer sequences. J Clin Microbiol. 1998;36(1):139–47.
17. Zelazny AM, Root JM, Shea YR, Colombo RE, Shamputa IC, Stock F, Conlan S, McNulty S, Brown-Elliott BA, Wallace Jr RJ, Olivier KN, Holland SM, Sampaio EP. Cohort study of molecular identification and typing of *Mycobacterium abscessus*, *Mycobacterium massiliense*, and *Mycobacterium bolletii*. J Clin Microbiol. 2009;47(7):1985–95.
18. Patel R. Matrix-assisted laser desorption ionization-time of flight mass spectrometry in clinical microbiology. Clin Infect Dis. 2013;57(4):564–72.
19. Anhalt JP, Fenselau C. Identification of bacteria using mass spectrometry. Anal Chem. 1975;47(2):219–25.
20. Cain TC, Lubman DM, Weber WJ, Vertes A. Differentiation of bacteria using protein profiles from matrix-assisted laser desorption/ionization time-of-flight mass spectrometry. Rapid Commun Mass Spectrom. 1994;8(12):1026–30.
21. Holland RD, Wilkes JG, Rafii F, Sutherland JB, Persons CC, Voorhees KJ, Lay Jr JO. Rapid identification of intact whole bacteria based on spectral patterns using matrix-assisted laser desorption/ionization with time-of-flight mass spectrometry. Rapid Commun Mass Spectrom. 1996;10(10):1227–32.
22. Claydon MA, Davey SN, Edwards-Jones V, Gordon DB. The rapid identification of intact microorganisms using mass spectrometry. Nat Biotechnol. 1996;14(11):1584–6.
23. Couturier MR, Mehinovic E, Croft AC, Fisher MA. Identification of HACEK clinical isolates by matrix-assisted laser desorption ionization-time of flight mass spectrometry. J Clin Microbiol. 2011;49(3):1104–6.
24. Fedorko DP, Drake SK, Stock F, Murray PR. Identification of clinical isolates of anaerobic bacteria using matrix-assisted laser desorption ionization-time of flight mass spectrometry. Eur J Clin Microbiol Infect Dis. 2012;31(9):2257–62.
25. Wybo I, Soetens O, De Bel A, Echahidi F, Vancutsem E, Vandoorslaer K, Pierard D. Species identification of clinical *Prevotella* isolates by matrix-assisted laser desorption ionization-time of flight mass spectrometry. J Clin Microbiol. 2012;50(4):1415–8.
26. Chen JH, Yam WC, Ngan AH, Fung AM, Woo WL, Yan MK, Choi GK, Ho PL, Cheng VC, Yuen KY. Advantages of using matrix-assisted laser desorption ionization-time of flight mass spectrometry as a rapid diagnostic tool for identification of yeasts and mycobacteria in the clinical microbiological laboratory. J Clin Microbiol. 2013;51(12):3981–7.
27. Saleeb PG, Drake SK, Murray PR, Zelazny AM. Identification of mycobacteria in solid-culture media by matrix-assisted laser desorption ionization-time of flight mass spectrometry. J Clin Microbiol. 2011;49(5):1790–4.
28. Cherkaoui A, Hibbs J, Emonet S, Tangomo M, Girard M, Francois P, Schrenzel J. Comparison of two matrix-assisted laser desorption ionization-time of flight mass spectrometry methods with conventional phenotypic identification for routine identification of bacteria to the species level. J Clin Microbiol. 2010;48(4):1169–75.
29. Martiny D, Busson L, Wybo I, El Haj RA, Dediste A, Vandenberg O. Comparison of the Microflex LT and Vitek MS systems for routine identification of bacteria by matrix-assisted laser desorption ionization-time of flight mass spectrometry. J Clin Microbiol. 2012;50(4):1313–25.
30. Ecker DJ, Sampath R, Massire C, Blyn LB, Hall TA, Eshoo MW, Hofstadler SA. Ibis T5000: a universal biosensor approach for microbiology. Nat Rev Microbiol. 2008;6(7):553–8.
31. Sampath R, Hofstadler SA, Blyn LB, Eshoo MW, Hall TA, Massire C, Levene HM, Hannis JC, Harrell PM, Neuman B, Buchmeier MJ, Jiang Y, Ranken R, Drader JJ, Samant V, Griffey RH, McNeil JA, Crooke ST, Ecker DJ. Rapid identification of emerging pathogens: coronavirus. Emerg Infect Dis. 2005;11(3): 373–9.
32. Andersen BM, Tollefsen T, Seljordslia B, Hochlin K, Syversen G, Jonassen TO, Rasch M, Sandvik L. Rapid MRSA test in exposed persons: costs and savings in hospitals. J Infect. 2010;60(4):293–9.
33. Aubry-Damon H, Soussy CJ, Courvalin P. Characterization of mutations in the *rpoB* gene that confer rifampin resistance in *Staphylococcus aureus*. Antimicrob Agents Chemother. 1998; 42(10):2590–4.
34. Luber AD, Jacobs RA, Jordan M, Guglielmo BJ. Relative importance of oral versus intravenous vancomycin exposure in the development of vancomycin-resistant enterococci. J Infect Dis. 1996;173(5):1292–4.
35. Cetinkaya Y, Falk P, Mayhall CG. Vancomycin-resistant enterococci. Clin Microbiol Rev. 2000;13(4):686–707.
36. Courvalin P. Vancomycin resistance in gram-positive cocci. Clin Infect Dis. 2006;42 Suppl 1:S25–34.
37. Depardieu F, Reynolds PE, Courvalin P. VanD-type vancomycin-resistant *Enterococcus faecium* 10/96A. Antimicrob Agents Chemother. 2003;47(1):7–18.
38. Espy MJ, Uhl JR, Sloan LM, Buckwalter SP, Jones MF, Vetter EA, Yao JD, Wengenack NL, Rosenblatt JE, Cockerill III FR, Smith TF. Real-time PCR in clinical microbiology: applications for routine laboratory testing. Clin Microbiol Rev. 2006;19(1):165–256.
39. Zirakzadeh A, Patel R. Epidemiology and mechanisms of glycopeptide resistance in enterococci. Curr Opin Infect Dis. 2005;18(6):507–12.
40. Sloan LM, Uhl JR, Vetter EA, Schleck CD, Harmsen WS, Manahan J, Thompson RL, Rosenblatt JE, Cockerill III FR. Comparison of the Roche LightCycler *vanA*/*vanB* detection assay and culture for detection of vancomycin-resistant enterococci from perianal swabs. J Clin Microbiol. 2004;42(6):2636–43.
41. Boehme CC, Nabeta P, Hillemann D, Nicol MP, Shenai S, Krapp F, Allen J, Tahirli R, Blakemore R, Rustomjee R, Milovic A, Jones M, O'Brien SM, Persing DH, Ruesch-Gerdes S, Gotuzzo E, Rodrigues C, Alland D, Perkins MD. Rapid molecular detection of tuberculosis and rifampin resistance. N Engl J Med. 2010;363(11):1005–15.
42. Somoskovi A, Parsons LM, Salfinger M. The molecular basis of resistance to isoniazid, rifampin, and pyrazinamide in *Mycobacterium tuberculosis*. Respir Res. 2001;2(3):164–8.
43. Caws M, Duy PM, Tho DQ, Lan NT, Hoa DV, Farrar J. Mutations prevalent among rifampin- and isoniazid-resistant *Mycobacterium tuberculosis* isolates from a hospital in Vietnam. J Clin Microbiol. 2006;44(7):2333–7.

44. Lavender C, Globan M, Sievers A, Billman-Jacobe H, Fyfe J. Molecular characterization of isoniazid-resistant *Mycobacterium tuberculosis* isolates collected in Australia. Antimicrob Agents Chemother. 2005;49(10):4068–74.
45. Bernardo K, Pakulat N, Macht M, Krut O, Seifert H, Fleer S, Hunger F, Kronke M. Identification and discrimination of *Staphylococcus aureus* strains using matrix-assisted laser desorption/ionization-time of flight mass spectrometry. Proteomics. 2002;2(6):747–53.
46. Du Z, Yang R, Guo Z, Song Y, Wang J. Identification of *Staphylococcus aureus* and determination of its methicillin resistance by matrix-assisted laser desorption/ionization time-of-flight mass spectrometry. Anal Chem. 2002;74(21):5487–91.
47. Edwards-Jones V, Claydon MA, Evason DJ, Walker J, Fox AJ, Gordon DB. Rapid discrimination between methicillin-sensitive and methicillin-resistant *Staphylococcus aureus* by intact cell mass spectrometry. J Med Microbiol. 2000;49(3):295–300.
48. Burckhardt I, Zimmermann S. Using matrix-assisted laser desorption ionization-time of flight mass spectrometry to detect carbapenem resistance within 1 to 2.5 hours. J Clin Microbiol. 2011; 49(9):3321–4.
49. Hrabak J, Walkova R, Studentova V, Chudackova E, Bergerova T. Carbapenemase activity detection by matrix-assisted laser desorption ionization-time of flight mass spectrometry. J Clin Microbiol. 2011;49(9):3222–7.
50. Sparbier K, Schubert S, Weller U, Boogen C, Kostrzewa M. Matrix-assisted laser desorption ionization-time of flight mass spectrometry-based functional assay for rapid detection of resistance against beta-lactam antibiotics. J Clin Microbiol. 2012;50(3):927–37.
51. Becker K, Pagnier I, Schuhen B, Wenzelburger F, Friedrich AW, Kipp F, Peters G, von Eiff C. Does nasal cocolonization by methicillin-resistant coagulase-negative staphylococci and methicillin-susceptible *Staphylococcus aureus* strains occur frequently enough to represent a risk of false-positive methicillin-resistant *S. aureus* determinations by molecular methods? J Clin Microbiol. 2006;44(1):229–31.
52. Desjardins M, Guibord C, Lalonde B, Toye B, Ramotar K. Evaluation of the IDI-MRSA assay for detection of methicillin-resistant *Staphylococcus aureus* from nasal and rectal specimens pooled in a selective broth. J Clin Microbiol. 2006;44(4): 1219–23.
53. Paterson GK, Harrison EM, Holmes MA. The emergence of *mecC* methicillin-resistant *Staphylococcus aureus*. Trends Microbiol. 2014;22(1):42–7.
54. Robicsek A, Beaumant JL, Paule SM, et al. Universal surveillance for methicillin-resistant Staphylococcus aureus in 3 affiliated hospitals. Ann Int Med. 2008;148(6):409–18.
55. Centers for Disease Control and Prevention. Prevention of perinatal group B Streptococcal disease. Morb Mortal Wkly Rep. 2010;59(RR-10):1–32.
56. Bourbeau PP, Heiter BJ, Figdore M. Use of Gen-Probe AccuProbe Group B *Streptococcus* test to detect group B streptococci in broth cultures of vaginal-anorectal specimens from pregnant women: comparison with traditional culture method. J Clin Microbiol. 1997;35(1):144–7.
57. Asrat T, Rumney P, Towers C, Preslicka C. The accuracy of late third trimester antenatal screening for group B Streptococcus in predicting GBS colonization at delivery. Am J Obstet Gynecol. 2006;195(6):S40.
58. Gavino M, Wang E. A comparison of a new rapid real-time polymerase chain reaction system to traditional culture in determining group B *Streptococcus* colonization. Am J Obstet Gynecol. 2007;197(4):388. e381–4.
59. Davies HD, Miller MA, Faro S, Gregson D, Kehl SC, Jordan JA. Multicenter study of a rapid molecular-based assay for the diagnosis of group B *Streptococcus* colonization in pregnant women. Clin Infect Dis. 2004;39(8):1129–35.
60. Fitting C, Parlato M, Adib-Conquy M, Memain N, Philippart F, Misset B, Monchi M, Cavaillon JM, Adrie C. DNAemia detection by multiplex PCR and biomarkers for infection in systemic inflammatory response syndrome patients. PLoS One. 2012; 7(6):e38916.
61. Josefson P, Stralin K, Ohlin A, Ennefors T, Dragsten B, Andersson L, Fredlund H, Molling P, Olcen P. Evaluation of a commercial multiplex PCR test (SeptiFast) in the etiological diagnosis of community-onset bloodstream infections. Eur J Clin Microbiol Infect Dis. 2011;30(9):1127–34.
62. Mancini N, Carletti S, Ghidoli N, Cichero P, Burioni R, Clementi M. The era of molecular and other non-culture-based methods in diagnosis of sepsis. Clin Microbiol Rev. 2010;23(1):235–51.
63. Pasqualini L, Mencacci A, Leli C, Montagna P, Cardaccia A, Cenci E, Montecarlo I, Pirro M, di Filippo F, Cistaro E, Schillaci G, Bistoni F, Mannarino E. Diagnostic performance of a multiple real-time PCR assay in patients with suspected sepsis hospitalized in an internal medicine ward. J Clin Microbiol. 2012;50(4):1285–8.
64. Wellinghausen N, Kochem AJ, Disque C, Muhl H, Gebert S, Winter J, Matten J, Sakka SG. Diagnosis of bacteremia in whole-blood samples by use of a commercial universal 16S rRNA gene-based PCR and sequence analysis. J Clin Microbiol. 2009;47(9):2759–65.
65. Martinez RM, Bauerle ER, Fang FC, Butler-Wu SM. Evaluation of three rapid diagnostic methods to directly identify microorganisms from positive blood cultures. J Clin Microbiol. 2014;52(7):2521–9.
66. Jamal W, Saleem R, Rotimi VO. Rapid identification of pathogens directly from blood culture bottles by Bruker matrix-assisted laser desorption laser ionization-time of flight mass spectrometry versus routine methods. Diagn Microbiol Infect Dis. 2013; 76(4):404–8.
67. Buchan BW, Riebe KM, Ledeboer NA. Comparison of the MALDI Biotyper system using Sepsityper specimen processing to routine microbiological methods for identification of bacteria from positive blood culture bottles. J Clin Microbiol. 2012;50(2):346–52.
68. Westbrook G, Holmes H. Epidemiologic strain typing. In: Garcia LS, editor. Clinical microbiology procedures handbook. 3rd ed. Washington, DC: ASM Press; 2010. p. 1–6.
69. Schwartz DC, Cantor CR. Separation of yeast chromosome-sized DNAs by pulsed field gradient gel electrophoresis. Cell. 1984;37(1):67–75.
70. Li W, Raoult D, Fournier PE. Bacterial strain typing in the genomic era. FEMS Microbiol Rev. 2009;33(5):892–916.
71. Dieckmann R, Malorny B. Rapid screening of epidemiologically important *Salmonella enterica* subsp. enterica serovars by whole-cell matrix-assisted laser desorption ionization-time of flight mass spectrometry. Appl Environ Microbiol. 2011;77(12):4136–46.
72. Kuhns M, Zautner AE, Rabsch W, Zimmermann O, Weig M, Bader O, Gross U. Rapid discrimination of *Salmonella enterica* serovar typhi from other serovars by MALDI-TOF mass spectrometry. PLoS One. 2012;7(6):e40004.
73. Fujinami Y, Kikkawa HS, Kurosaki Y, Sakurada K, Yoshino M, Yasuda J. Rapid discrimination of *Legionella* by matrix-assisted laser desorption ionization time-of-flight mass spectrometry. Microbiol Res. 2011;166(2):77–86.
74. Wolters M, Rohde H, Maier T, Belmar-Campos C, Franke G, Scherpe S, Aepfelbacher M, Christner M. MALDI-TOF MS fingerprinting allows for discrimination of major methicillin-resistant *Staphylococcus aureus* lineages. Int J Med Microbiol. 2011; 301(1):64–8.
75. Lasch P, Fleige C, Stammler M, Layer F, Nubel U, Witte W, Werner G. Insufficient discriminatory power of MALDI-TOF mass spec-

trometry for typing of *Enterococcus faecium* and *Staphylococcus aureus* isolates. J Microbiol Methods. 2014;100:58–69.
76. Fredericks DN, Relman DA. Sequence-based identification of microbial pathogens: a reconsideration of Koch's postulates. Clin Microbiol Rev. 1996;9(1):18–33.
77. Patel PA, Ledeboer NA, Ginocchio CC, Condon S, Bouchard S, Qin P, Karchmer T, Peterson LR. Performance of the BD GeneOhm MRSA achromopeptidase assay for real-time PCR detection of methicillin-resistant *Staphylococcus aureus* in nasal specimens. J Clin Microbiol. 2011;49(6):2266–8.
78. Bischof LJ, Lapsley L, Fontecchio K, Jacosalem D, Young C, Hankerd R, Newton DW. Comparison of chromogenic media to BD GeneOhm methicillin-resistant *Staphylococcus aureus* (MRSA) PCR for detection of MRSA in nasal swabs. J Clin Microbiol. 2009;47(7):2281–3.
79. Hombach M, Pfyffer GE, Roos M, Lucke K. Detection of methicillin-resistant *Staphylococcus aureus* (MRSA) in specimens from various body sites: performance characteristics of the BD GeneOhm MRSA assay, the Xpert MRSA assay, and broth-enriched culture in an area with a low prevalence of MRSA infections. J Clin Microbiol. 2010;48(11):3882–7.
80. Paule SM, Mehta M, Hacek DM, Gonzalzles TM, Robicsek A, Peterson LR. Chromogenic media vs. real-time PCR for nasal surveillance of methicillin-resistant *Staphylococcus aureus*: impact on detection of MRSA-positive persons. Am J Clin Pathol. 2009;131(4):532–9.
81. Snyder JW, Munier GK, Johnson CL. Comparison of the BD GeneOhm methicillin-resistant *Staphylococcus aureus* (MRSA) PCR assay to culture by use of BBL CHROMagar MRSA for detection of MRSA in nasal surveillance cultures from intensive care unit patients. J Clin Microbiol. 2010;48(4):1305–9.
82. Peterson LR, Liesenfeld O, Woods CW, Allen SD, Pombo D, Patel PA, Mehta MS, Nicholson B, Fuller D, Onderdonk A. Multicenter evaluation of the LightCycler methicillin-resistant *Staphylococcus aureus* (MRSA) advanced test as a rapid method for detection of MRSA in nasal surveillance swabs. J Clin Microbiol. 2010; 48(5):1661–6.
83. Wolk DM, Picton E, Johnson D, Davis T, Pancholi P, Ginocchio CC, Finegold S, Welch DF, de Boer M, Fuller D, Solomon MC, Rogers B, Mehta MS, Peterson LR. Multicenter evaluation of the Cepheid Xpert methicillin-resistant *Staphylococcus aureus* (MRSA) test as a rapid screening method for detection of MRSA in nares. J Clin Microbiol. 2009;47(3):758–64.
84. Patel PA, Schora DM, Peterson KE, Grayes A, Boehm S, Peterson LR. Performance of the Cepheid Xpert(R) SA Nasal Complete PCR assay compared to culture for detection of methicillin-sensitive and methicillin-resistant *Staphylococcus aureus* colonization. Diagn Microbiol Infect Dis. 2014;80(1):32–4.
85. Frey AB, Wilson DA, LaSalvia MM, Tan CD, Rodriguez ER, Shrestha NK, Hall GS, Procop GW. The detection and differentiation of methicillin-resistant and methicillin-susceptible *Staphylococcus aureus* endocarditis by using the BD GeneOhm StaphSR Assay. Am J Clin Pathol. 2011;136(5):686–9.
86. Stamper PD, Cai M, Howard T, Speser S, Carroll KC. Clinical validation of the molecular BD GeneOhm StaphSR assay for direct detection of *Staphylococcus aureus* and methicillin-resistant *Staphylococcus aureus* in positive blood cultures. J Clin Microbiol. 2007;45(7):2191–6.
87. Buchan BW, Ginocchio CC, Manii R, Cavagnolo R, Pancholi P, Swyers L, Thomson Jr RB, Anderson C, Kaul K, Ledeboer NA. Multiplex identification of gram-positive bacteria and resistance determinants directly from positive blood culture broths: evaluation of an automated microarray-based nucleic acid test. PLoS Med. 2013;10(7):e1001478.
88. Wojewoda CM, Sercia L, Navas M, Tuohy M, Wilson D, Hall GS, Procop GW, Richter SS. Evaluation of the Verigene Gram-positive blood culture nucleic acid test for rapid detection of bacteria and resistance determinants. J Clin Microbiol. 2013;51(7): 2072–6.
89. Samuel LP, Tibbetts RJ, Agotesku A, Fey M, Hensley R, Meier FA. Evaluation of a microarray-based assay for rapid identification of Gram-positive organisms and resistance markers in positive blood cultures. J Clin Microbiol. 2013;51(4):1188–92.
90. Kelley PG, Grabsch EA, Farrell J, Xie S, Montgomery J, Mayall B, Howden BP. Evaluation of the Xpert MRSA/SA Blood Culture assay for the detection of *Staphylococcus aureus* including strains with reduced vancomycin susceptibility from blood culture specimens. Diagn Microbiol Infect Dis. 2011;70(3):404–7.
91. Spencer DH, Sellenriek P, Burnham CA. Validation and implementation of the GeneXpert MRSA/SA blood culture assay in a pediatric setting. Am J Clin Pathol. 2011;136(5):690–4.
92. Wolk DM, Struelens MJ, Pancholi P, Davis T, Della-Latta P, Fuller D, Picton E, Dickenson R, Denis O, Johnson D, Chapin K. Rapid detection of *Staphylococcus aureus* and methicillin-resistant *S. aureus* (MRSA) in wound specimens and blood cultures: multicenter preclinical evaluation of the Cepheid Xpert MRSA/SA skin and soft tissue and blood culture assays. J Clin Microbiol. 2009;47(3):823–6.
93. Dubouix-Bourandy A, de Ladoucette A, Pietri V, Mehdi N, Benzaquen D, Guinand R, Gandois JM. Direct detection of *Staphylococcus* osteoarticular infections by use of Xpert MRSA/SA SSTI real-time PCR. J Clin Microbiol. 2011;49(12):4225–30.
94. Riedlinger J, Beqaj SH, Milish MA, Young S, Smith R, Dodd M, Hankerd RE, Lebar WD, Newton DW. Multicenter evaluation of the BD Max GBS assay for detection of group B streptococci in prenatal vaginal and rectal screening swab specimens from pregnant women. J Clin Microbiol. 2010;48(11):4239–41.
95. Atkins KL, Atkinson RM, Shanks A, Parvin CA, Dunne WM, Gross G. Evaluation of polymerase chain reaction for group B *Streptococcus* detection using an improved culture method. Obstet Gynecol. 2006;108(3 Pt 1):488–91.
96. Goodrich JS, Miller MB. Comparison of culture and 2 real-time polymerase chain reaction assays to detect group B *Streptococcus* during antepartum screening. Diagn Microbiol Infect Dis. 2007;59(1):17–22.
97. Scicchitano LM, Bourbeau PP. Comparative evaluation of the AccuProbe Group B *Streptococcus* Culture Test, the BD GeneOhm Strep B assay, and culture for detection of group B streptococci in pregnant women. J Clin Microbiol. 2009;47(9):3021–3.
98. Jordan JA, Hall G, Davis T. Multicenter study evaluating performance of the Smart Group B *Streptococcus* (GBS) assay using an enrichment protocol for detecting GBS colonization in patients in the antepartum period. J Clin Microbiol. 2010; 48(9):3193–7.
99. Wilson DA, Hall GS, Procop GW. Detection of group B *Streptococcus* bacteria in LIM enrichment broth by peptide nucleic acid fluorescent in situ hybridization (PNA FISH) and rapid cycle PCR. J Clin Microbiol. 2010;48(5):1947–8.
100. El Helali N, Nguyen JC, Ly A, Giovangrandi Y, Trinquart L. Diagnostic accuracy of a rapid real-time polymerase chain reaction assay for universal intrapartum group B *Streptococcus* screening. Clin Infect Dis. 2009;49(3):417–23.
101. Williams-Bouyer N, Reisner BS, Woods GL. Comparison of Gen-Probe AccuProbe group B *Streptococcus* culture identification test with conventional culture for the detection of group B streptococci in broth cultures of vaginal-anorectal specimens from pregnant women. Diagn Microbiol Infect Dis. 2000;36(3): 159–62.

Gastrointestinal Infections

50

Eileen M. Burd and Benjamin H. Hinrichs

Abstract

Establishing a specific etiology for gastrointestinal infections can be challenging because of the common clinical features and wide variety of causative microorganisms. In many cases, the etiologic agent cannot be determined using traditional diagnostic methods and may result in unnecessary antibiotic use or prolonged periods of illness. Molecular tests provide many advantages over traditional laboratory methods but, with the exception of a few analytes, are still largely in the developmental phase for gastrointestinal pathogens and are not widely used. The main advantages of molecular tests include increased sensitivity and the ability to detect agents which will not grow in culture. To test for all possible gastrointestinal pathogens at one time would require a large panel that would include a variety of bacterial, viral and parasitic agents. Challenges inherent in developing diagnostic molecular panels include ensuring that all variants of a particular microorganism can be detected as well as the rapid evolution of pathogens. In this chapter, the diagnostic merit of molecular tests as well as available tests will be presented for the major groups of gastrointestinal pathogens.

Keywords

Infectious gastroenteritis • Diarrhea • Bacterial gastroenteritis • Viral gastroenteritis • Parasitic gastroenteritis • Laboratory diagnosis • Polymerase chain reaction • Gastrointestinal pathogens panel

Introduction

Gastrointestinal infections are a common global health problem. They most often affect the stomach or intestines and generally result in diarrhea. Most gastrointestinal infections are not serious and resolve without treatment after a few days. In select populations, however, diarrheal diseases carry a high degree of morbidity and mortality. The elderly, young children, and people with chronic illnesses or compromised immune systems can become acutely dehydrated and require medical attention.

Many bacteria, viruses, and parasites can infect the gastrointestinal system. Since symptoms are similar, differentiation among the various etiologies is difficult. The microorganisms that cause gastrointestinal infections vary with the geographic region, degree of economic development, level of sanitation, and hygienic standards. In developed countries like the USA, outbreaks of diarrhea are most often a result of food poisoning. Many common gastrointestinal infections are caused by bacteria, including *Bacillus cereus*, *Campylobacter*, *Salmonella*, and enterotoxigenic *Escherichia coli* that are commonly acquired by eating undercooked foods.

E.M. Burd, Ph.D. (✉)
Pathology and Laboratory Medicine, Microbiology Emory University, Atlanta, GA, USA
e-mail: eburd@emory.edu

B.H. Hinrichs, M.D.
Pathology and Laboratory Medicine, Gastrointestinal Pathology, Emory University, Atlanta, GA, USA

D.G.B. Leonard (ed.), *Molecular Pathology in Clinical Practice*, DOI 10.1007/978-3-319-19674-9_50

Highly infectious viruses, such as norovirus, can cause gastroenteritis and account for many foodborne illness outbreaks. Gastrointestinal viruses are relatively stable in the environment and can spread rapidly through person-to-person or fomite contact, particularly in enclosed communities, such as hospitals, dormitories, daycare centers, and cruise ships.

Gastrointestinal parasite infections are typically acquired from ingestion of contaminated food or water. The parasite *Giardia lamblia* is often consumed by hikers who drink untreated stream water. *Cryptosporidium* has been associated with drinking water or recreational water. Outbreaks of *Cyclospora* and *Cystoisospora* (formerly *Isospora*) have been associated with consumption of contaminated food or water. These parasites are more common in tropical and subtropical areas of the world and people traveling to countries where the disease is endemic may be at increased risk for infection.

Identification of the causative agent in clinically significant gastrointestinal infections is important so that appropriate treatment, if any, can be provided. Most gastrointestinal infections will resolve without treatment other than rehydration to replenish lost fluids. Antibiotics are not normally prescribed unless a person is immunocompromised since using any antibiotic or the wrong antibiotic can worsen some infections, prolong the infection, or increase the risk of relapse. Antibiotics may be given for certain bacteria, specifically *Campylobacter*, *Shigella*, and *Vibrio cholerae*, but are not used for uncomplicated cases of *Salmonella* or toxigenic *E. coli*. Gastrointestinal parasitic infestations are treated with appropriate antiparasitic medication to help eliminate the parasite.

Molecular methods can provide rapid and sensitive detection of gastrointestinal pathogens. Molecular amplification is greatly complicated by the presence of a complex and abundant gut microflora and high concentrations of potential PCR inhibitors in diarrheal stool specimens [1]. Approaches to reduce PCR inhibition include dilution of extracted nucleic acids, treatment of samples with chelating agents (Chelex 100, Bio-Rad Laboratories, Hercules, CA), or adding detergents or denaturing chemicals during extraction. Inclusion of amplification facilitators such as bovine serum albumin or betaine also can increase amplification and overcome low levels of contaminants that co-purify with nucleic acids. Due to the high number of possible enteric pathogens with common clinical presentations, multiplexed molecular tests are advantageous. US Food and Drug Administration (FDA)-approved or -cleared molecular tests are available for some gastrointestinal pathogens in single test or multiplex formats.

For some analytes, reference materials are commercially available and can be used for development of molecular tests, limit of detection studies, cross-reactivity studies, positive and negative controls, training, lot-to-lot comparison of reagent test kits, and other purposes. When reference materials are not commercially available, characterized organisms recovered in clinical or research laboratories may be used. Similarly, proficiency testing surveys are available for many gastrointestinal pathogens, including from the College of American Pathologists (Northfield, IL), the Wisconsin State Laboratory of Hygiene (Madison, WI), and the American Proficiency Institute (Traverse City, MI). When proficiency testing surveys are not commercially available, the laboratory director is responsible for arranging at least semi-annual alternative assessment to evaluate the reliability of analytic testing. Appropriate alternative assessment procedures include split sample analysis with a reference or other laboratory, split samples with an established in-house method such as histology, or clinical validation by chart review. In addition to defining the alternative assessment procedures, the laboratory director must set the criteria for successful performance and ensure documentation of all activities.

Bacterial Pathogens

Bacterial Gastroenteritis

Description of Pathogens

Bacterial gastroenteritis is very common and can affect adults and children. Isolated cases of bacterial gastroenteritis can be seen, but illness usually occurs in outbreaks associated with a group of people who ate the same contaminated food. Bacterial diarrhea is particularly common among people from industrialized countries who travel to developing countries. In developing countries, epidemics of bacterial gastroenteritis with significant associated mortality often arise in areas where sanitation and hygienic practices are poor.

Many bacterial pathogens are well-recognized causes of gastroenteritis. In industrialized countries, *Campylobacter*, *Salmonella*, *Shigella*, and Shiga-toxin producing *Escherichia coli* are the leading causes of bacterial gastroenteritis. Other etiologic agents include *Aeromonas*, *Plesiomonas*, *Listeria*, *Clostridium*, *Staphylococcus aureus*, *Yersinia*, *Vibrio*, and others.

Some enteric pathogens produce characteristic symptoms (e.g., "rice water" stools produced by *Vibrio cholerae*) and the clinical features and pathogenic aspects of a gastrointestinal illness can sometimes be suggestive of a specific etiology. Most often, however, the presenting clinical features do not reliably suggest a particular etiology and laboratory tests are needed to identify the specific pathogen.

In general, these bacterial pathogens can be readily cultured from freshly collected stool specimens of infected patients using a variety of selective and specialized media. Clinical laboratories generally use a limited set of media to recover the most common bacterial pathogens (e.g., *Salmonella*, *Shigella*, and *Campylobacter*) and other culture media are used to identify less common agents on special request (e.g., based on travel history, exposure, etc.). Culture and identification of enteric pathogens is cost-effective but can take several days to provide a diagnosis. Culture has some limitations and it is especially difficult to distinguish nonpathogenic from pathogenic strains of *E. coli*. Recent recommendations suggest that, because of the variety of serotypes and difficulty of distinguishing pathogenic forms from normal flora, laboratories should detect enterotoxigenic *E. coli* using immunoassays that detect the toxin in addition to culture [2].

Clinical Utility of Testing

Bacterial gastroenteritis usually is self-limited, but treatment is required in some cases and improper management can lead to a prolonged course. Identification of an etiologic agent allows for more effective targeted treatment which can reduce overall medical costs, and is useful to differentiate bacterial gastroenteritis from other diseases, such as malabsorption syndromes, inflammatory bowel disease, appendicitis, Crohn's disease, diverticulitis, and other enteropathies, that can present with similar symptoms. Since bacterial gastroenteritis can involve groups of people and a common food source, definitive identification of an etiologic agent can be helpful in prompting epidemiologic investigation and testing of potentially contaminated food by public health laboratories. Current stool culture-based tests for bacterial gastrointestinal pathogens typically require several day turnaround times and may yield poor results, especially if a patient has received antibiotic therapy. Molecular tests, especially multiplexed panels, provide accurate diagnosis of at least the most common causes of bacterial diarrhea from a single specimen in one day.

Available Assays

The ProGastro® SSCS® Assay (Hologic Gen-Probe, San Diego, CA) is an US FDA-cleared multiplex real-time PCR test for five common bacterial gastrointestinal pathogens. The test detects *Salmonella*, *Shigella*, *Campylobacter* (*C. jejuni* and *C. coli* only) nucleic acids and Shiga Toxin 1 (stx1) and Shiga Toxin 2 (stx2) genes. The test includes internal controls and is run on a SmartCycler II (Cepheid, Sunnyvale, CA) real-time PCR instrument with results delivered in 4 h.

The xTAG® Gastrointestinal Pathogen Panel (xTAG® GPP, Luminex Corporation, Austin, TX) is another US FDA-cleared, qualitative, multiplex test that simultaneously detects and identifies some viral and parasitic gastrointestinal pathogens in addition to the major bacterial pathogens in a single sample. The bacterial pathogens and toxins that can be detected using the panel include *Salmonella*, *Shigella*, *Campylobacter*, enterotoxigenic *E. coli*, Shiga-like toxin, and toxigenic *Clostridium difficile*. The assay also detects rotavirus A, norovirus GI/GII, *Giardia*, and *Cryptosporidium*. Results are interpreted as presumptive and must be confirmed by US FDA-cleared tests or other acceptable methods. The CE-marked panel available in Canada and Europe detects *Yersinia enterocolitica*, *Vibrio cholera*, adenovirus 40/41, and *Entamoeba histolytica* in addition to those available in the US FDA-cleared panel.

The BioFire FilmArray™ (bioMerieux, Durham, NC) Gastrointestinal (GI) Panel is US FDA-cleared and detects 23 bacterial, viral, and protozoal pathogens, including some not present on other panels. Analytes on the panel include *Aeromonas*, *Campylobacter*, *Clostridium difficile* (Toxin A/B), *Plesiomonas shigelloides*, *Salmonella*, *Yersinia enterocolitica*, *Vibrio*, *Vibrio cholera*, Enteroaggregative *E. coli*, Enteropathogenic *E. coli*, Enterotoxigenic *E. coli*, Shiga-like toxin-producing *E. coli*, *E. coli* O157, *Shigella*/Enteroinvasive *E. coli*, Adenovirus F 40/41, Astrovirus, Norovirus GI/GII, Rotavirus A, Sapovirus, *Cryptosporidium*, *Cyclospora cayetanensis*, *Entamoeba histolytica*, and *Giardia lamblia* along with internal controls to ensure that all processes have been performed successfully. A stool sample collected in Cary Blair transport medium is inoculated into a reaction pouch that contains all of the reagents necessary for the entire reaction. Separate nucleic acid extraction is not required. The pouch is placed in the FilmArray instrument and nucleic acids are extracted and purified, followed by nested multiplex PCR. The first-stage PCR is a single, highly multiplexed reaction and the second-stage PCR reactions detect the products from the first stage PCR. Endpoint melt curve analysis is used to identify the products that are generated. The instrument tests one sample at a time with hands-on time of approximately 2 min and results available in approximately 1 h.

Diatherix Laboratories, an independent CLIA-certified clinical reference laboratory located in the Hudson-Alpha Institute for Biotechnology in Huntsville, Alabama, offers testing for gastrointestinal pathogens using a proprietary technology called target enriched multiplex polymerase chain reaction (Tem-PCR). The bacterial pathogens included in the panel include *Clostridium difficile*, *Clostridium difficile* toxin B gene, *Campylobacter jejuni*, *Escherichia coli* strain 0157, *Listeria monocytogenes*, *Salmonella enterica*, *Staphylococcus aureus*, *Vibrio cholera*, and *Vibrio parahaemolyticus*.

Molecular tests are expected to play an increasingly important role in the diagnosis of gastrointestinal illnesses. Because of the complexity of gastrointestinal pathogens and the emergence of variants of these pathogens, future clinical molecular tests will likely include new approaches such as bead-based microarrays, microfluidic systems, and other methods that simultaneously target many more pathogens than current methods allow.

Interpretation of Results

Interpretation of positive results is not generally problematic. Because the asymptomatic carriage rate is extremely low, detection of specific bacterial pathogens in stool in the absence of other enteric pathogens can be considered diagnostic.

Laboratory Issues

Bacterial culture may still be needed for cases where antibiotic susceptibility testing is required. Antimicrobial therapy is indicated for some cases of gastrointestinal illness due to *Salmonella*, *Shigella*, *Aeromonas*, *Yersinia*, and *Vibrio* and some others, but not for *Pseudomonas*, *S. aureus*, or toxigenic *E. coli* [3]. Because of increasing resistance and strain variability, susceptibility testing is recommended to guide therapy.

Reference materials are available from several vendors. Previously characterized positive stool samples or negative samples spiked with well-characterized organisms recovered in the clinical laboratory can be used. Dried genomic nucleic acids are available for some analytes from the American Type Culture Collection (ATCC) (43504D, Manassas, VA) or BEI Resources (Manassas, VA) which is managed by ATCC. The NATtrol™ (ZeptoMetrix Corp, Buffalo, NY) verification set contains all of the analytes in the BioFire GI panel.

Proficiency testing programs that are compatible with molecular methods and accommodate most of the analytes on gastrointestinal pathogen panels are available from several organizations. A combination of programs might be needed to fully accommodate entire testing panels. The College of American Pathologists (Northfield, IL) offers a Gastrointestinal Panel for Molecular Multiplex Testing (GIP) survey that includes *Campylobacter*, *Clostridium difficile* toxin AB, *Cryptosporidium*, Enterotoxigenic *E. coli*, *Giardia*, Norovirus GI/GII, Rotavirus A, *Salmonella*, Shiga-like toxin producing *E. coli* SXT-1 and SXT-2, and *Shigella*. The Wisconsin State Laboratory of Hygiene (Madison, WI) offers a Comprehensive (MC) Bacteriology survey that includes *C. difficile* toxin or antigen as well as enteric pathogen identification. Separate surveys include *C. difficile* (CD), Shiga Toxin (SHG), and Enteric Pathogens (NP) including *Aeromonas*, *Campylobacter*, *E. coli* O157:H7, *Plesiomonas*, *Salmonella*, *Shigella*, *Vibrio*, and *Yersinia*. The American Proficiency Institute (Traverse City, MI) has several programs available that include *Campylobacter*, toxigenic *Clostridium difficile*, Rotavirus, *Giardia*, and *Cryptosporidium* in addition to bacteriology and virology programs.

As molecular tests become more widely used, accommodation will need to be made for reporting of positive results to public health departments. Most state public health departments require notification when certain infectious agents, including many gastrointestinal pathogens, are suspected or identified. This reporting allows public health departments to investigate outbreaks and conduct surveillance studies to assess changes and trends in disease occurrence. For some gastrointestinal bacteria such as *Salmonella* and Shiga-toxin-producing *E. coli*, health departments usually require a culture of the organism to be submitted for definitive identification, typing studies, etc. that help identify common foodborne sources. This policy will need to be modified if molecular testing for bacterial gastrointestinal pathogens becomes widely used in clinical laboratories.

Clostridium difficile

Description of Pathogen

Clostridium difficile is a spore-forming, Gram-positive anaerobic bacillus that is carried by some individuals as a component of the normal intestinal microbiota. Pathogenic strains produce toxin A and/or toxin B, which damage the intestinal mucosa. Toxigenic *C. difficile* is associated with nearly all cases of antibiotic-related colitis and 15–20 % of antibiotic related diarrhea [4, 5].

C. difficile infection (CDI) has become a scourge of hospitals worldwide and is estimated to account for an excess $1 billion to $3.2 billion per year of healthcare costs in the USA [6, 7]. While advanced age and length of hospitalization are directly related to increased risk of CDI, exposure to antibiotics remains the most significant modifiable risk factor [8]. Exposure to antibiotics and subsequent loss of endogenous enteric microbiota is believed to create a favorable environment for the growth of *C. difficile*. While reports of *C. difficile* colonization in both healthy children and adults suggests the possibility of an endogenous source of infection [9, 10], epidemiologic studies have established the significance of the organism as a transmissible nosocomial pathogen [8, 11].

Disease is caused by the production of toxins A and B, which are encoded by the genes *tcdA* and *tcdB*, respectively. Not all strains carry these genes, and demonstration of the ability to produce toxin is an essential criterion for the diagnosis of CDI. Recent studies highlight the importance of toxin B over toxin A in disease pathogenesis [12], and most clinical assays focus on the detection of *tcdB* gene sequences. Two regulatory genes, *tcdC* and *tcdD*, are hypothesized to negatively influence the expression of *tcdA* and *tcdB*, and together with the toxin genes are part of the chromosomally encoded region known as the pathogenicity locus (PaLoc) [8].

Since 2001, several US and Canadian hospitals reported outbreaks of CDI associated with increased disease severity [13, 14]. Epidemiologic studies revealed a high percentage of cases were caused by a strain referred to as BI/NAP1/027, named in reference to typing results for restriction endonuclease analysis (REA), pulsed field gel electrophoresis (PFGE), and PCR-ribotyping, respectively. The BI/NAP1/027 strain carries 18-bp and 1-bp (nt 117) deletions within the *tcdC* gene, and these deletions are speculated to result in the formation of an abnormal *tcdC* protein with a loss of regulatory function [13]. The resultant loss of negative regulation may lead to an increase in toxin formation and greater virulence [13]. Supporting this theory is the observation that isolates of the BI/NAP1/027 strain produce increased amounts of toxin A and B in vitro [15]. An additional toxin known as the binary toxin CDT is present in the BI/NAP1/027 strain as well as 6 % of *C. difficile* isolates, and is encoded by two chromosomal genes, *cdtA* and *cdtB*, located outside of the PaLoc [13]. Although production of the binary toxin is associated with the more virulent BI/NAP1/027 strain, its role in pathogenesis is not well established [8, 16].

Clinical Utility of Testing

Rapid and accurate diagnosis of CDI is critical not only for the timely treatment of individual patients, but also for preventing the spread of nosocomial disease. The diversity of tests available makes possible a number of diagnostic algorithms. None of these testing strategies has performed optimally to date, leading a number of investigators to suggest the adoption of the highly sensitive and specific PCR-based assays. Several studies have evaluated the effects of implementing nucleic acid testing. Algorithms examined include PCR assays as confirmatory tests of glutamate dehydrogenase (GDH)-positive samples, as reflex tests for GDH-positive, toxin-enzyme immunoassays (EIA) negative samples, and as stand-alone assays for direct testing of stool samples. A comparison of these testing algorithms to those using toxin-EIA only, GDH followed by toxin-EIA, and GDH/toxin-EIA followed by cell culture cytotoxin neutralization (CCCN) testing of toxin-EIA negative samples indicates a clear trade-off between sensitivity and cost [17]. The cost per test for all strategies using PCR-based assays was significantly greater than the most expensive non-PCR-based testing algorithm ($35.22 vs $24.41, respectively) [17]. However, strategies using PCR as confirmation of GDH-positive samples or as a reflex test for GDH-positive, toxin-EIA negative samples detected an additional 89 toxigenic *C. difficile* samples over a 1 year period that were missed by algorithms using traditional testing methods [17]. Furthermore, stand-alone, direct PCR testing of stool samples detected an additional 138 positive specimens missed by even the most sensitive non-PCR-based testing algorithm. Importantly, all diagnostic strategies using PCR provided results for the majority of samples (>83.7 %) in less than 1 h and in less than 5 h for the remainder [17]. These rapid turnaround times are in contrast to algorithms relying on CCCN as a reflex test for GDH-positive, toxin-EIA negative samples, which required as long as 48 h for 12.3 % of samples tested [17].

An optimal testing strategy balances the number of CDI cases detected with total costs and turnaround time. Although the additional costs of algorithms employing PCR are significant, use of these assays would likely allow for the earlier detection of disease. In turn, earlier detection of disease could prevent the spread of nosocomial infection and decrease the total number of CDI cases. In addition, rapid detection allows for the timely institution of treatment and possibly shortened hospital stays. The assessment of total cost, therefore, must consider both expenses related directly to testing in addition to costs savings realized as a result of lowering the incidence of nosocomial disease and decreasing time of hospitalization.

In an effort to determine how different diagnostic algorithms might affect isolation practices of patients with suspected CDI, Tenover et al. applied the findings of several studies to a theoretical model of 1,000 patients with 10 % disease prevalence [16]. The results confirm the poor performance of strategies relying solely on GDH/toxin-EIA testing as the number of patients placed in isolation with true CDI nearly matches the numbers of patients without the disease [16]. Furthermore, 45 patients with CDI are not identified, and therefore, are not placed into proper infection control isolation [16]. Algorithms that reflex to toxigenic culture or CCCN after GDH/toxin-EIA testing detect more cases of CDI, but still produce high numbers of false-positive results (55 patients). Using toxigenic culture as a reflex test produced values for sensitivity and specificity statistically equivalent to PCR-based reflex testing; however, the length of time required to produce final results would likely lead to excessive costs. Using PCR-based assays as stand-alone tests detected the greatest number of CDI cases (95 %), and led to the unnecessary isolation of only 36 patients [16]. While these results further confirm the superior diagnostic performance of nucleic acid testing either as a reflex test for GDH-positive, toxin-EIA negative samples or as a stand-alone method, the authors of the study recommend additional investigations examining the cost-effectiveness of these strategies [16].

A potential concern for diagnostic algorithms using GDH as a screening test is highlighted by a report from Larson et al who identified four (1.9 %) of 211 GDH-negative samples with the *tcdB* gene by direct PCR testing [17]. These four apparent false-negative samples also were negative by CCCN, but confirmed as containing toxigenic *C. difficile* by toxigenic culture. The results are consistent with studies demonstrating lower sensitivities and negative predictive values for an algorithm combining GDH and PCR compared to utilizing just PCR [18].

While not contributing directly to patient care, typing methods have provided important insights into CDI epidemiology. In addition to aiding determinations of infection source, reservoir, and mode of transmission, typing methods allow investigators to correlate abnormally severe clinical behavior with putative virulence factors. Both phenotypic and genotypic methods are used; however, phenotypic methods are generally less reproducible and some strains have not been able to be phenotyped [19].

Available Assays

The optimal means of diagnosing CDI is still evolving, and current recommendations put forth by several professional organizations are conflicting [8, 20]. In the past, CCCN was regarded as the gold standard because of the ability to directly identify the presence of toxin B. However, the inability of CCCN to detect a large number of CDI cases is well documented, and the clinical utility is further diminished by a lengthy turnaround time (24–48 h) [17, 21]. Bacterial culture followed by a sensitive and specific toxin assay performed on the isolated organism (toxigenic culture) has replaced CCCN as a reference method in many studies [8, 20, 22]. Toxigenic culture has demonstrated superior sensitivity compared to CCCN, but because toxin production is assessed only after the organism has been grown in vitro, the clinical meaning is not clear [20]. Unfortunately, similar to CCCN, toxigenic culture requires considerable technical expertise, and has an average turnaround time of 3–7 days [23].

EIA for the detection of toxins A and B (toxin-EIA) are rapid and easy to use alternatives to culture-based testing, and are currently the most commonly used tests in the USA [8, 21]. However, recent studies comparing their performance to toxigenic culture indicate sensitivities ranging from 32–67 % [24, 25], thus preventing their use as a reliable screening or stand-alone test [8, 20]. EIA tests are available for the detection of GDH, a constitutively expressed enzyme produced by nearly all *C. difficile* strains as well as some non-*C. difficile Clostridium* sp. [16, 26]. These GDH EIAs demonstrate sensitivities of greater than 90 %, and diagnostic algorithms often use these assays as initial screening tests [26]. However, GDH EIAs detect both toxigenic and non-toxigenic strains, and GDH-positive samples must be confirmed with an assay demonstrating toxin production. Options for confirmation include toxigenic culture, CCCN, and toxin-EIAs. However, due to the low sensitivities of CCCN and toxin-EIAs, a number of cases would likely be missed.

Molecular tests have emerged as additional options for both confirmatory and stand-alone testing. These methods generally demonstrate excellent sensitivities and specificities, and most assays are capable of delivering results in 1–3 h [16]. Several tests are US FDA-cleared, and additional assays will likely become commercially available in the near future. At this time all US FDA-cleared assays are qualitative, although quantitative testing is technologically possible with real-time PCR. Most US FDA-cleared assays are based on real-time PCR. However, other novel methods such as helicase-dependent amplification (HDA) and loop-mediated isothermal amplification (LAMP) also are employed. In addition, the majority of commercially available real-time PCR assays target solely the *tcdB* gene. US FDA-cleared multiplex PCR assays target *tcdB* as well as variable *tcdA*, *tcdC*, and *cdt* gene sequences and the single base pair deletion at nucleotide 117 in the *tcdC* gene associated with the 027/NAP1/B1 strain. Initial studies evaluating these US FDA-cleared assays are promising; however, the 2010 Update by the Society for Healthcare Epidemiology of America and the Infectious Diseases Society of America stated the need for further studies before recommending molecular assays for routine testing [8]. Lastly, CDI screening also may be performed using the US FDA-cleared xTAG® Gastrointestinal Pathogen Panel (Luminex Corporation), a multiplex test that simultaneously detects 11 gastrointestinal pathogens including *C. difficile* and other major bacterial, viral, and parasitic pathogens. Published reports evaluating the US FDA-cleared version of this assay are currently lacking.

As stated above, most real-time PCR assays target *tcdB*; however, interest in detecting the hypervirulent BI/NAP1/027 strain has spurred the development of assays that evaluate *tcdC* [12]. Some investigators contend that *tcdC* may be used as a surrogate target for *tcdA* and *tcdB*, and excellent correlation between the presence of *tcdC* and *tcdA* and/or *tcdB* has been demonstrated [25]. The authors also report the ability to detect deletions in *tcdC*, including the 18-bp deletion associated with the BI/NAP1/027 strain. Nevertheless, the assay was unable to discriminate the 18-base pair (bp) deletion from a 39-bp *tcdC* deletion not currently associated with an epidemic strain, and therefore, cannot be used to reliably detect the presence of the BI/NAP1/027 strain [25].

The US FDA has cleared assays using non-PCR amplification methods such as LAMP and HDA. LAMP assays amplify target DNA isothermally, and identify successful amplification by detecting an increase in turbidity due to the build-up of a reaction by-product. HDA assays also amplify isothermally and use helicase enzymes to separate DNA strands rather than thermal denaturation [27]. These assays are attractive to laboratories that are not able to purchase expensive thermal cyclers or detection systems. Like real-time PCR methods, LAMP- and HDA-based assays are rapid and demonstrate excellent sensitivities and specificities [27–29]. The *illumi*gene *C. difficile* assay is US FDA-cleared for testing of symptomatic children ages 1–2 years. Other US FDA-cleared nucleic acid detection assays have not received clearance for this age group. As asymptomatic colonization of children under the age of two is well documented [9], testing of this age group is controversial.

Finally, genetic typing methods for epidemiologic analysis may be broadly categorized into methods using REA, PCR, or direct sequencing [19]. These methods require DNA extracted from a single clone, and therefore, culture should be obtained when there is concern either of an outbreak or of a particularly virulent toxigenic strain [19]. Genetic typing techniques have the ability to discriminate and characterize a broad range of epidemic and non-epidemic *C. difficile* strains; however, currently there is focused interest in the epidemiology of the BI/NAP1/027 strain. Two multiplex PCR assays that detect the single bp deletion at nucleotide 117 in the *tcdC* gene associated with this hypervirulent strain have recently been US FDA-cleared. In both cases, detection of the BI/NAP1/027 strain is US FDA-cleared for epidemiologic investigations only.

Interpretation

A positive real-time PCR test is generally diagnostic of toxigenic *C. difficile* in a patient displaying typical signs and symptoms of CDI. While it is possible that a patient may be colonized with toxigenic *C. difficile* and suffer diarrhea caused by a different etiology, this situation is likely to be rare [16].

PCR may detect toxigenic *C. difficile* even though non-toxigenic *C. difficile* or negative growth is reported by culture. Many of these cases are positive by GDH EIA, toxin-EIA, or CCCN, and thus are regarded as true positives. Culture may fail to detect growth because of significant time delays between sample collection and testing, concurrent antibiotic treatment at time of collection, or laboratory issues as discussed below [18].

Positive predictive values for real-time PCR assays may be as low as 84 %, and demonstrate that not all positive results are indicative of CDI [18]. Studies reporting the occurrence of isolated PCR-positive results also suggest PCR-based assays may be too sensitive. Additional studies correlating the clinical outcomes of patients who test negative by conventional methods but positive by PCR are needed to improve diagnostic accuracy.

The occurrence of a positive PCR result in an asymptomatic patient indicates colonization with toxigenic *C. difficile* and is well documented [10]. For this reason the testing of asymptomatic patients, except for epidemiologic purposes, is not recommended [9].

Negative PCR results generally indicate the absence of CDI, as evidenced by high negative predictive values for these assays. Recommendations made by the European Society of Clinical Microbiology and Infectious Diseases state that a single negative result from a *tcdB* PCR assay, a GDH EIA, or toxin-EIA may be used to rule out the presence of toxigenic *C. difficile* [20]. While negative PCR results may occur in samples testing positive by conventional detection methods, this is an uncommon occurrence and may be due to one of the reasons discussed below.

Laboratory Issues

The sensitivity of real-time PCR assays may be as low as 77.3 % and negative results are speculated to occur for a number of reasons [22]. Samples negative by PCR, but positive for toxigenic isolates may contain substances inhibitory to PCR amplification. The detection of PCR inhibitors is aided by the incorporation of internal controls into all US FDA-cleared real-time PCR assays. Other investigators propose that negative PCR tests may be due to sampling error of stool, a known heterogeneous testing medium, when low numbers of organisms are present [18, 30].

A concern regarding the clinical significance of PCR stems from the fact that PCR merely detects the presence of a gene and does not evaluate gene expression. While it is theoretically possible for PCR to detect *C. difficile* carrying *tcdB* that is not expressed, testing only unformed stool specimens from patients with a clinical suspicion of CDI may help avoid this issue [16]. So far, no published studies have evaluated this point directly.

Real-time PCR assays targeting *tcdB* are believed to comprehensively detect all current strains of toxigenic *C. difficile* as *tcdB* negative strains or strains with significant deletions in *tcdB* do not exist naturally [12, 31]. Strain-to-strain *tcdB* sequence variability resulting in poor primer binding is occasionally cited as a concern for the ability of toxin B PCR assays to sensitively detect the wide range of *C. difficile* strains. While significant sequence variation within the *tcdB* gene is reported [31], most currently targeted *tcdB* sequences appear conserved across the range of strain types [16]. Therefore, the effect of *tcdB* sequence variation on sensitivity of toxin B PCR assays is expected to be minimal [16].

Also of concern is the potential evolution of a novel toxigenic *C. difficile* strain with an altered *tcdB* sequence as a result of genetic drift. Although most toxigenic *C. difficile* strains contain an intact *tcdB* gene, the detection of a strain deficient in at least a portion of the *tcdB* gene is reported in a case of recurrent CDI [32, 33]. While the report of a clinically significant *tcdB* deficient strain reinforces the need to be vigilant for the development of *tcdB*-negative, *tcdA-positive* strains affecting the clinical performance of toxin B PCR assays, the occurrence of such variant strains is currently rare [22, 33]. Multiplex real-time PCR assays, with the ability to simultaneously detect several different sequence targets (e.g., *tcdA* and *tcdB*, *cdtA*, *cdtB*, and *tcdC*) may decrease the likelihood of detection failure due to primer sequence mismatches [23].

The recognition of clinically significant toxin A negative, toxin B positive strains also is cited as a concern for the ability of LAMP assays to comprehensively detect all CDI cases.

Although four toxin A negative, toxin B positive strains are currently recognized, only one strain, toxinotype VIII, has been associated with significant numbers of CDI cases [34]. The *tcdA* gene of toxinotype VIII contains both a 1.8 kb deletion in addition to a nonsense mutation resulting in a truncated toxin A protein [31, 34]. Despite the modified toxin A gene sequence of toxinotype VIII, a recent study found that three strains of toxinotype VIII tested on the *illumi*gene *C. difficile* assay were detected [35]. Several studies report samples that are PCR-positive, but negative by toxigenic culture.

Although toxigenic culture is a more sensitive reference method than CCCN, instances of detection failure are documented [18]. Reasons for detection failure may be clinical as mentioned above, but also may involve factors related to laboratory handling of specimens. Results of toxigenic culture for *C. difficile* may be adversely affected by long delays between collection and testing of specimens, the failure to enrich for spores, or the loss of spore viability during the spore enrichment process affecting only particular strains [18, 22]. In addition, culture is speculated to occasionally fail to detect toxigenic strains as a result of overgrowth by a non-toxigenic strain, as studies have reported the presence of multiple strain types in patient samples [22, 36].

A *C. difficile* verification panel that includes ribotype 027 and *C. sordellii* as a negative control is commercially available (ZeptoMetrix Corp, Buffalo, NY). A panel of 8 *C. difficile* strains, each with a different toxinotype as well as freeze-dried, well-characterized *C. difficile* strains and genomic DNA from those strains are available from ATCC (Manassas, VA). The ACCURUN 501 *C. difficile* Control (SeraCare Life Sciences, Gaithersburg, MD) contains inactivated organisms in a human synthetic stool matrix. The control set contains *C. difficile* NAP1/027/B1 hypervirulent strain, two toxigenic *C. difficile* strains, and *C. sordelli* as a negative control. Proficiency testing samples for *C. difficile* molecular tests are available from the College of American Pathologists, the Wisconsin State Laboratory of Hygiene, and the American Proficiency Institute.

Tropheryma whipplei

Description of Pathogen

The etiological agent of Whipple's disease is *Tropheryma whipplei*, a bacterium present in the environment, sewage, human stool, and saliva, but whose entire ecological distribution is yet to be characterized [37, 38]. In accordance with these findings, a fecal-oral route of transmission has been proposed [38]. Evidence also exists for the ability of the organisms to asymptomatically colonize the upper gastrointestinal tract, as PCR has identified *T. whipplei* DNA in the saliva and gastric juice of 35 % and 11.4 % of individuals, respectively, without evidence of Whipple's disease [39, 40].

Whipple's disease, however, is rare, and only an estimated 1,000 cases have been described [38]. Its pathogenesis is poorly understood, and while genetic risk factors have been proposed, none have been confirmed [38]. The most common presentation of disease includes symptoms related to malabsorption such as diarrhea and weight loss, although a long history of nonspecific complaints, often including arthralgias, is typical [38, 40]. These vague and chronic symptoms may last an average of 6 years before clinical signs more characteristic of the disease appear [38]. Atypical cases lacking classic gastrointestinal symptoms and involving the cardiovascular system and the central nervous system (CNS) as well as other organ sites may occur in up to 15 % of those affected [38]. The long time period before typical symptoms are manifested in addition to the high percentage of unusual presentations often results in a delay of treatment. Early diagnosis and the initiation of antibiotics are critical to avoiding long-term morbidity, and, therefore, improved detection methods are needed.

Clinical Utility of Testing

The diagnosis of Whipple's disease is made primarily by histological examination of tissue biopsies; however, since the 1990s, PCR has played an increasing role in diagnosis. Culture and serological methods have recently been developed as diagnostic tools; however, their availability is limited [37, 38]. In the past, electron microscopy (EM) was commonly used to demonstrate the characteristic trilaminar bacterial cell wall; however, its utilization is declining [41].

The optimal use of PCR in establishing a diagnosis of Whipple's disease is debated. Some reports recommend PCR testing in parallel with the procurement of biopsies, citing the lack of optimal specificity of histology and PCR when used alone [38]. Others advocate the use of PCR only when biopsies fail to indicate disease, although this is not supported by the low rate of PCR positivity in histologically negative duodenal biopsies [42].

Intestinal biopsies from patients without gastrointestinal symptoms may be negative by PCR, and thus clinical symptoms in atypical cases should guide the selection of samples for PCR analysis [42]. In addition to duodenal biopsies, PCR testing has proven useful when performed on a number of different specimen types including lymph nodes, cardiac valves, synovial fluid, cerebrospinal fluid (CSF), and vitreous humor [37]. CSF has tested positive by PCR methods in several patients without CNS symptoms, and may indicate the need for antibiotics with good CNS penetration [41]. While saliva, feces, and blood may be positive in patients with Whipple's disease, higher rates of background positivity makes the utility of testing these specimens uncertain [37, 43, 44].

No biological marker or test is currently available to determine the required duration of treatment for Whipple's disease [38]. Nevertheless, monitoring response to treatment using PCR appears to have utility for predicting outcome [41, 44]. PCR positivity after treatment correlated with a higher likelihood of relapse; however, the positive predictive value was only 58 % [45]. Likewise, while negative post-treatment PCR results have been associated with remission, a significant number of patients without detectable *T. whipplei* DNA in intestinal biopsies have developed recurrent disease [46].

Molecular methods for genetic subtyping of *T. whipplei* are limited to the research setting, as currently no correlations are established between subtype and geographic location or specific clinical manifestations [44].

Available Assays

Duodenal biopsies demonstrating expansion of the lamina propria by macrophages filled with Periodic acid-Schiff (PAS)-positive bacterial fragments is the classic histological finding of Whipple's disease, and is observed in the majority of Whipple's disease patients [40]. While relatively specific when identified in a patient with typical Whipple's symptomatology, the protean symptoms of this pathogen necessitate the consideration of other infectious diseases, such as *Mycobacterium avium* complex and *Rhodococcus equi*, as well as noninfectious disorders, all of which may have overlapping histological appearances [41, 44]. Biopsies obtained from other anatomic sites demonstrating macrophages filled with PAS-positive material are even less specific, and must be interpreted with caution [37, 40, 44]. Immunohistochemistry for *T. whipplei* performed on paraffin-embedded tissues has recently been developed and has greatly improved both the sensitivity and specificity of histological diagnosis [38]. Lastly, intestinal biopsies may be non-contributory due to the patchy nature of disease and the possibility for diagnostic material to be confined deep within the submucosa and not usually evaluated in superficial mucosal biopsies [41, 44].

The existence of disorders with overlapping histological findings and the possibility for biopsies to miss disease supports the diagnostic role of PCR-based methods. While reports of sensitivity are limited, several studies document PCR positivity in nearly all cases of histologically proven disease [42, 45]. Detection of *T. whipplei* DNA from negative intestinal biopsies by PCR-based tests highlights the diagnostic sensitivity and utility of molecular methods [42, 44].

Molecular detection of *T. whipplei* is primarily using PCR methods including conventional [45], nested [39], semi-nested [47], and real-time PCR [48–50]. Primers targeting 16S rDNA, 16S-23S rDNA intergenic spacer, 23S rDNA, and *rpo*B sequences are commonly used [44]. Assay sensitivity and specificity varies according to the amplification target and the PCR method.

Conventional PCR assays provide qualitative results, and detection techniques are time consuming, requiring 2 or more days to perform. Ethidium bromide-stained gel electrophoresis may be used to detect amplified bands of characteristic size; however, an additional confirmatory identification step is recommended [38]. Options include Southern hybridization using sequence-specific fluorescent oligonucleotide probes or direct sequencing techniques [38]. Nevertheless, these assays can perform adequately, and a study evaluating a conventional PCR assay using paraffin-embedded tissue from patients with histologically confirmed Whipple's disease demonstrated a sensitivity and specificity of 96.6 % and 100 % respectively [45].

Semi-nested or nested PCR methods generally allow for a lower limit of detection than conventional PCR assays; however, these methods are associated with a higher risk of contamination due to the required handling of amplification products [44]. An additional disadvantage of these methods includes their longer turnaround time compared to real-time PCR methods.

Real-time PCR methods are more rapid and less prone to contamination than conventional, semi-nested, and nested PCR assays. In addition, real-time PCR assays provide quantitative results, which help differentiate true infection from contamination or low-level colonization [49]. A study comparing the performance of a LightCycler® (Roche Molecular Systems, Branchburg, NJ) real-time PCR assay to a conventional PCR assay demonstrated good correlation of results; however, the turnaround time was significantly shorter for the real-time PCR assay (3.5 h vs 2–3 days) [48].

No tests are FDA-cleared or -approved for the detection of *T. whipplei*; however, amplification of *T. whipplei* DNA by PCR in blood, CSF and tissues is available from some reference laboratories.

Interpretation of Results

A positive PCR result in the setting of classic Whipple's disease symptoms and biopsy findings is generally confirmatory. Correlating positive PCR results with clinical findings is especially important in atypical presentations and when histology is non-contributory. The need for clinical correlation is highlighted by occasional studies identifying the presence of organisms in asymptomatic adults. Most of these studies produced results using nested and semi-nested PCR assays [39, 43], which are associated with a high contamination risk [44]. Such unexpected positive results could be due to environmental contamination, asymptomatic colonization, or nonspecific amplification of non-*T. whipplei* DNA. These findings have not been confirmed as several other studies have found that PCR performed on intestinal biopsies is consistently negative in patients undergoing endoscopy to investigate conditions other than Whipple's disease [42, 49]. The ability for real-time PCR to produce quantitative results may allow differentiation of true infection from contamination or asymptomatic colonization [49]; however, specific ranges have not been determined.

Negative PCR results in patients diagnosed with Whipple's disease histologically may be due to DNA degradation as a result of the DNA extraction process, the presence of PCR inhibitors, or damaged DNA from formalin-fixation [44]. In addition, negative PCR results may prompt consideration of other infectious etiologies capable of producing histological findings similar to Whipple's disease [44].

Laboratory Issues

As mentioned above, DNA degradation during extraction from tissues and other clinical samples may cause false-negative results. Choosing and validating an appropriate extraction method, therefore, is critical, and commercial extraction kits include chaotropic lysis (Isoquick Kit, Orca Research, Bothell, WA, USA), Pure-Gene protocol (PureGene Kit, Flowgen Instruments Ltd., Lichfield, UK), and QIAamp DNA binding columns (QIAGEN, Hilden, Germany) [44]. Extraction efficiency may be evaluated using primers targeting human gene sequences as internal controls.

PCR inhibitors may cause false-negative results. Similar to the evaluation of extraction efficiency, the presence of PCR inhibitors may be identified using primers targeting ubiquitous human genes as internal controls [44].

PCR testing can be performed retrospectively on paraffin-embedded tissue biopsies; however, the use of fresh or frozen specimens provides more sensitive results [42].

Suspensions of organism are often used as reference material but are not currently commercially available. Proficiency testing surveys also are not commercially available.

Helicobacter pylori

Description of Pathogen

Helicobacter pylori is a spiral-shaped and flagellated, Gram-negative bacterium that can be found in the stomach of some individuals. The *H. pylori* genome is approximately 1.64–1.67 million bp with 1,515–1,590 predicted protein-coding sequences. *H. pylori* has unusually high levels of genetic variation between strains due to a natural DNA uptake system that can incorporate very large fragments of exogenous DNA into the *H. pylori* genome.

H. pylori infection is a leading cause of gastric and duodenal ulcers, and is strongly associated with gastric malignancies such as gastric adenocarcinoma and gastric mucosa-associated lymphoid tissue (MALT) lymphoma [51]. While the clinical course of infection may be variable and depends on both host and microbial factors, the organism most often produces a chronic infection manifested as chronic gastritis [51, 52]. Treatment aims to completely eliminate the organism, and eradication cures the majority of both duodenal and gastric ulcers. Although treatment results in regression of most low-grade gastric MALT lymphomas [53, 54], treatment effectiveness in reducing the risk of gastric adenocarcinoma is less clear [51, 53].

H. pylori infection rates are greatest in developing countries due to lower socioeconomic conditions; however, prevalence estimates in the USA are high, reaching 30–40 % [55]. Strains demonstrating antibiotic resistance limit the effectiveness of standard eradication regimens, which usually include clarithromycin, either amoxicillin or metronidazole, and a proton-pump inhibitor (PPI) [51, 56]. Prevalence of clarithromycin resistance is estimated to be 10–15 % in the USA, and resistance results in a 70 % reduction in the eradication rate [56]. While resistance to metronidazole occurs more frequently (20–40 %), eradication rates of resistant strains are decreased by only 25 % [56]. Strains resistant to amoxicillin and second-line antibiotics such as tetracycline are much less common, but their presence could alter the effectiveness of rescue therapies [56].

The high prevalence of *H. pylori* infection and antibiotic resistance, in addition to the clear benefit of eradication therapy necessitates the use of reliable diagnostic tests. Molecular methods consisting primarily of PCR-based assays are both rapid and sensitive, and while useful for the general diagnosis of *H. pylori* infection may also play an important role in special clinical situations such as acute bleeding. Furthermore, although antibiotic resistance may be detected effectively using conventional phenotypic testing of *H. pylori* cultures, genotypic susceptibility testing of cultures and biopsy specimens offers a fast and reliable alternative.

Clinical Utility of Testing

Diagnostic testing for *H. pylori* is indicated in patients with either active or previously documented peptic ulcer disease, low-grade gastric MALT lymphoma, and in certain cases of dyspepsia not yet investigated by endoscopy [57]. The diagnosis of *H. pylori* infection may be established using a wide variety of diagnostic tests and the choice of test is largely determined by clinical factors such as whether or not the patient requires upper gastrointestinal endoscopy [57].

Tests utilized with endoscopy and regarded as invasive include culture, histology, rapid urease tests (RUTs), and PCR assays performed on biopsy material. Noninvasive tests not requiring endoscopy include serology, the urea-breath test (UBT), and stool tests such as antigen assays and PCR. Each test has particular disadvantages and comparing diagnostic performance is made difficult by the fact that no single test method is regarded as the gold standard. As a substitute for a gold standard, studies comparing different assays often designate true positives as those samples yielding positive results with two or more testing methods.

While certain non-molecular methods such as the UBT, histology, and RUTs offer sufficient sensitivity for routine testing, PCR-based molecular methods performed on tissue biopsies offer even greater sensitivity and may identify true positives missed by RUT and histology [58–62]. This increased sensitivity has the greatest utility in evaluating patients with bleeding peptic ulcers where non-molecular assays perform poorly [58, 63, 64]. Real-time PCR assays may also improve patient care by offering quantitative results. High bacterial densities are associated with lower eradication rates, and, therefore, quantitative measurements by real-time PCR may be used to identify patients who could benefit from a modified, more intense treatment regimen [65]. In addition, PCR-based assays for the detection of *H. pylori* DNA in fecal specimens represent potentially simple and noninvasive methods for establishing the existence of infection and for proving successful eradication. However, interpreting results of these tests requires the clinician to be aware of complicating factors that are specific to assays performed on stool. These issues are discussed in detail below.

While culture is currently the gold standard for antibiotic susceptibility testing, the sensitivity of these methods may be reduced due to the fastidious nature of *H. pylori*, overgrowth of cultures by bacterial contaminants, and by low numbers of viable *H. pylori* organisms in the post-treatment period [66]. In addition, cultures may take several days for growth. Fortunately, effective and rapid genotypic susceptibility testing methods are available and may be applied to both culture and biopsy specimens.

Numerous studies have looked for an association between the presence of virulence or pathogenic factors and severity of disease. The *cagA* and *vacA* genes are most commonly implicated, and certain alleles of these genes are associated with more severe gastritis as well as higher rates of peptic or duodenal ulcer disease and gastric adenocarcinoma [67–69]. While these pathogenic factors can be detected by molecular methods, including conventional and multiplex PCR, the clinical utility of testing is questionable [70–72]. Confounding variation in host genetic and environmental factors, in addition to discrepant results when comparing different geographic regions and ethnicities, undermines a clear relationship between the presence of pathogenic factors and disease severity [73, 74]. The lack of a clear association has prevented development of clinical guidelines recommending testing of these pathogenic factors for patient care [75].

Available Assays

Several laboratory developed tests (LDTs) for the detection of *H. pylori* DNA in tissue biopsies and stool have been described and include amplification methods such as conventional, nested, multiplex, and real-time PCR, as well as FISH. No US FDA-cleared tests are available. Amplification targets include genes related to the production of virulence factors such as urease (*ureA*), phosphoglucomutase (*glmM*, formerly named urease C (*ureC*)), and *vacA*, as well as species-specific sequences of 16S rRNA and 23S rRNA. Other genes targeted include the sequences encoding the 26-kDa species-specific protein antigen (SSA) and heat shock protein (HSP60), as well as random *H. pylori* genome sequences. Sensitivity and specificity of the assays are determined largely by target gene and primer choice, but also depend on the type of PCR method. Conventional PCR assays provide qualitative results and perform the same or better than conventional detection methods [58]. Detection of PCR amplicons is usually achieved with ethidium bromide-stained gel electrophoresis. Such detection methods require the open handling of PCR products, and, therefore, have a greater risk of contamination than real-time PCR methods.

Real-time PCR methods provide quantitative results, are generally more rapid and sensitive than conventional PCR assays, and also involve less contamination risk [60]. Assays using a hemi-nested or nested design generally allow for a lower limit of detection than conventional PCR assays [76, 77], and achieve similar levels of detection when compared to quantitative RT-PCR (RT-qPCR) assays [61]. Disadvantages of nested and semi-nested designs compared with RT-qPCR include more technologist time and a higher risk of contamination due to handling of amplification products [61].

Multiplex PCR methods combining several different primer targets demonstrate greater sensitivity than conventional testing methods [59]. In addition, a multiplex assay for the detection of both *H. pylori* and *Helicobacter heilmannii-like* organisms may be useful for determining prevalence of disease due to the latter, less common organism [78].

PCR-based assays for the detection of *H. pylori* DNA in fecal specimens frequently use in-house developed capture-probe systems or QIAamp DNA extraction stool kits (Qiagen, Germantown, MD) to obtain purified DNA and to reduce PCR inhibitors [56]. Capture-probe techniques use biotinylated oligonucleotide probes targeting the *H. pylori* 16S rRNA gene [56]. After overnight incubation, the desired gene fragment is harvested using paramagnetic polystyrene beads coated with streptavidin [56, 79]. Gene-capture methods used with conventional PCR targeting 16S rRNA *H. pylori*-specific sequences have demonstrated sensitivities ranging from 75 to 100 % [79, 80]. The QIAamp DNA stool kit has been shown to perform well when used in a semi-nested PCR assay targeting 23S rRNA gene sequences, but results have varied when detecting other genes [56, 81]. Lastly, a filtration-based extraction technique used by Russo et al. demonstrated excellent sensitivity (95.6 %) and specificity (100 %) using a conventional PCR assay with *ureA* primers [82].

Most antibiotic resistance among *H. pylori* strains is due to chromosomal mutations, and therefore, amenable to detection

Table 50.1 *H. pylori* antibiotic resistance mutations detectable by described assays

Antibiotic	Resistance gene	Nucleotide change	Amino acid change
Clarithromycin	23S rRNA	A2142G	NA
		A2143G	NA
Ciprofloxacin	gyrA	C(T) to A	N87K
		C(T) to G	N87K
		A to G	D91G
		G to T	D91Y
		G to A	D91N
Tetracycline	16S rRNA	A926G	NA
		A926C	NA
		A926T	NA
		A928C	NA

NA not applicable

by molecular means (see Table 50.1). *H. pylori* resistance to clarithromycin and other macrolides is caused by point mutations at two nucleotide sites (A2142G and A2143G) within the 23S rRNA gene resulting in decreased ribosomal binding of the antibiotic [52]. Clarithromycin resistance mutations may be detected using several different molecular methods such as restriction fragment length polymorphism (RFLP), pyrosequencing, fluorescence in situ hybridization (FISH), and real-time PCR [56]. PCR followed by RFLP and real-time PCR methods are used most often [56].

RFLP-based assays for the detection of clarithromycin resistance take advantage of the fact that antibiotic resistance mutations create restriction sites within the 23S rRNA gene not present in susceptible strains. Conventional PCR using 23S rRNA specific primers produces amplicons, which when cleaved with restriction endonucleases and visualized by agarose gel electrophoresis create a pattern composed of two bands instead of one. While conceptually simple, these methods are more time consuming than real-time PCR assays.

Real-time PCR methods can detect clarithromycin resistance mutations directly from biopsy specimens with excellent sensitivity and rapid turnaround times of 1–4 h [66, 83–85]. An assay described by Gibson et al. uses fluorescent-labeled probes complementary to the clarithromycin-sensitive 23S rRNA gene sequence [86]. Resistance mutations result in mismatched bases between the probe and target, and melting curve analysis reveals a lower peak melting temperature for the mismatched hybrid than a fully complementary probe and target hybrid [86]. This assay has good concordance with culture-based methods [66, 84], but also identified susceptibilities for an additional 28 patients whose cultures were negative. Of the 28 additional susceptibility results rendered, 21 had resistance genotypes. Another assay design using a biprobe system was tested on 200 patients who failed eradication therapy. The assay detected resistance genotypes with a sensitivity and specificity of 98.4 % and 94.1 %, respectively, when compared to culture-based testing [85]. Clarithromycin-resistant genotypes can also be detected in stool samples using real-time PCR methods; however, the sensitivity is lower [87]. Real-time PCR assays have also been developed to detect point mutations in the quinolone resistance-determining region of the *gyrA* gene resulting in resistance to ciprofloxacin and point mutations in the 16S rRNA gene conferring decreased susceptibility and resistance to tetracyclines [88, 89]. The assay for determining fluoroquinolone resistance identifies mutations using two hybridization biprobes designed to detect the most frequently occurring mutations at amino acid positions 87 or 91 [88]. Tetracycline resistance is detected using 16S rDNA primers and a fluorescently labeled probe complementary to the wild-type 16S rDNA allele. In both assays, melting curve analysis differentiates amplicons with resistance mutations from those with wild-type sequences [89]. While various mutations in the NADPH nitroreductase gene (*rdxA*) are associated with metronidazole resistance, detection of these mutations is not a reliable indicator of resistance [90].

Histopathologic diagnosis of *H. pylori* infection is a sensitive and specific method (>95 % and 100 %, respectively) under optimal conditions, yet ancillary molecular techniques such as FISH may help in difficult cases [56]. Visualization of the characteristic bacterial forms may be difficult when reduced numbers of bacteria are present, such as when biopsies are obtained after eradication therapy or if the patient has been on long-term acid suppression therapy with PPIs. These same conditions may change the typical morphology of *H. pylori* from a comma or S-shaped bacillus to a coccoidal form, obscuring a visual diagnosis. Several studies using fluorescently labeled, species-specific probes have demonstrated the ability of FISH to reliably detect *H. pylori* [91, 92]. Additionally, clarithromycin-resistant strains also can be detected using FISH performed on formalin-fixed tissue sections [92]. Fluorescent-labeled oligonucleotide probes designed to detect the most common mutations determining clarithromycin resistance are both sensitive and specific when compared to culture-based susceptibility testing [91]. FISH testing, however, may produce results more rapidly than culture.

Interpretation of Results

PCR tests can achieve equal or better performance when compared to non-molecular tests [58–62]. The sensitivity is highly dependent on the target gene and is discussed in greater detail in the "Laboratory Issues" section below.

The specificity of different PCR test methods varies and determining specificity is complicated by the lack of gold standard. Real-time PCR assays applied to tissue biopsies have detected *H. pylori* at low densities that were missed by histology, UBT, and RUT suggesting that the poorer sensitivity of these non-molecular assays is due to low numbers of organisms [61]. However, due to the high sensitivity of PCR-based methods and the amplification of DNA from nonviable organisms, isolated positive PCR results in the post-treatment period must be interpreted with caution. Positive results in this setting may represent continued presence of organisms at low levels or nonviable organisms, and, therefore, PCR may not have utility in determining eradication failures in the post-treatment period. Isolated positive PCR results in untreated patients may reflect true infection with a low *H. pylori* density, but may also be due to nonspecific amplification of non-*H. pylori* bacterial DNA [93]. Due to these factors, PCR-based methods should not be used as the sole diagnostic test.

Like PCR testing of biopsy specimens, the specificity of results obtained from PCR testing of stool samples may be decreased due to amplification of nonviable organisms. Studies examining the use of PCR-based testing of stool for determining eradication success rates in the early post-treatment period are conflicting [80, 94]. While negative PCR results within 12 days of treatment were obtained for a small group of infected patients, another study demonstrated false-positive results occurring in half the patients 1 month after treatment [94, 95]. False-positive PCR results decrease after longer follow-up periods, and approach zero after 12 weeks of therapy [94]. In addition, analytical specificity of PCR testing on stool samples may be reduced due to the presence of non-*pylori Helicobacter* species present in fecal material [56]. While clinical specificity for PCR-based assays is determined by comparison with UBT, culture, and RUTs, determinations of analytical specificity by testing of non-*pylori Helicobacter* species is rarely performed [96].

Antibiotic resistance genotype testing using real-time PCR can produce results indicating the presence of more than one genotype [85]. These results are interpreted as representing a mixed population and combinations of one or more distinct mutant strains among wild-type strains have been detected [85]. While some studies have detected mutant strains in the presence of wild-type strains down to a level of 10 % [85], other studies cite failed resistance detection due to high levels of susceptible strains [87].

Laboratory Issues

Sensitivity and specificity of PCR-based methods are greatly dependent on primer choice and target gene. Additionally, significant inter-study variation in sensitivity and specificity exists for several of the commonly used primers. Nucleotide differences among distinct *H. pylori* strains may partly explain this test performance variability [77]. A study comparing the diagnostic performance of several different primers demonstrated poor specificity for SSA gene primers and unsatisfactory sensitivity for the *ureA* gene and random *H. pylori* genome sequences [76]. While this study concluded that *glmM* gene PCR performed best, other studies have reported lower specificities [60, 77]. Assays using 16S rRNA sequences generally report excellent sensitivities, but the specificity of these primers is questionable. Several authors argue that 16S rRNA primers are inappropriate because of sequence conservation among different bacterial genera as well as the possibility for nonspecific amplification of human DNA [76, 77]. Assays targeting *vacA* have reported moderate sensitivity (89.5 %) but excellent specificity (99.0 %) [84]. The HSP60 gene is thought to be both well conserved and demonstrates species-specific variation [77]. A nested assay design using primers targeting HSP60 claims to have sensitivity and specificity approaching 100 % [77].

Determining whether tissue to be used for PCR assays is preserved by formalin fixation or cryopreservation represents an important variable in testing, but may ultimately be decided by proximity of laboratory and endoscopy suite. Both formalin-fixed and frozen tissue specimens may be used for PCR-based testing, although frozen samples are far superior [56]. Formalin fixation causes DNA to fragment; however, assays using formalin-fixed tissues may still perform acceptably if short DNA sequences are targeted.

PCR assays applied to stool specimens suffer from inconsistent results attributable to substances inhibitory to PCR amplification, low numbers of *H. pylori* organisms within fecal samples, as well as degradation of DNA during intestinal transit [53, 56]. To avoid false-negative results, complex purification and extraction steps to eliminate PCR inhibitors are required before DNA amplification. Performance of the different biochemical, immunologic, and physical purification methods varies due to degradation of target DNA and incomplete removal of inhibitors [96]. Frozen stocks of *H. pylori* strain NCTC 11637 and dried genomic DNA from that strain (American Type Culture Collection 43504D, Manassas, VA) as well as titered cultures of *H. pylori* (ZeptoMetrix Corp, Buffalo, NY) are commercially available reference materials. Proficiency testing exercises are not commercially available.

Viral Agents

The most common causes of viral gastroenteritis include adenovirus serotypes 40 and 41, rotavirus, astrovirus, and caliciviruses (noroviruses, sapoviruses). Conventional detection of these viruses is based on antigen detection and EM. Molecular methods have been primarily used for epidemiologic or research purposes but have also demonstrated significant improvement in the diagnosis of viral gastroenteritis and are becoming available in clinical laboratories.

Other viruses less frequently implicated as causes of acute gastroenteritis include coronaviruses and toroviruses.

In addition, viruses such as cytomegalovirus and herpes simplex virus are opportunistic causes of enteric disorders in patient infected with the human immunodeficiency virus (HIV) or with compromised immunity but are diagnosed by examination or testing of gastric or intestinal biopsy tissues rather than examination of stool.

Adenovirus

Description of Pathogen

Adenoviruses are nonenveloped viruses with a linear, nonsegmented, double-stranded DNA genome surrounded by an icosahedral protein capsid. The genome size varies among adenoviral groups and is between 26,000 and 45,000 nucleotides which theoretically provides the capacity for 22–40 genes. The genome consists of immediate early (E1A), early (E1-E4), intermediate, and late genes (L1-L5).

Adenoviruses are classified into five genera including Atadenovirus, Aviadenovirus, Ichtadenovirus, Mastadenovirus, and Siadenovirus. The adenoviruses that infect humans belong to the genus *Mastadenovirus*. Seven species of human adenovirus (A through G) within the genus *Mastadenovirus* are currently recognized. Species designations are determined by immunologic properties as well as DNA homology and oncogenicity [97]. Each species group contains several serotypes classified by neutralization reactions to specific antisera [97]. At present, over 50 serotypes have been described [98]. Serotype groups may be further subdivided into genomic types. Genotypes are assigned lowercase letters to differentiate them from the prototype strain as indicated by the letter "p" [97]. Interspecies DNA sequence variation may be as low as 4 % whereas genotypes within an adenovirus species may be 50 % to nearly 100 % homologous [99, 100]. Intraspecies recombination resulting in intermediate strains has been reported [101].

Species F serotypes 40 and 41 are the most frequent adenovirus serotypes isolated from patients with gastroenteritis and are referred to as the "enteric adenoviruses." These serotypes are second only to rotavirus as the most common cause of acute diarrheal illness in children [102]. Adenoviruses of all serotypes are implicated in approximately 5–15 % of childhood diarrhea cases [97]. Gastroenteritis due to adenovirus occurs worldwide and the incidence does not demonstrate significant seasonal variation [103]. More than one serotype or species may be isolated in a given patient [104]. Serotypes infrequently associated with gastroenteritis include 1, 2, 3, 5, 7, 12–18, 21, 25, 26, 29, 31, and 52 [102].

Transmission is thought to occur by fecal-oral spread and the mean incubation period for gastroenteritis is 3–10 days [97, 103]. After clinical symptoms improve, enteric adenoviruses are shed in stool rarely for longer than a few days compared to patients with respiratory infections not involving enteric adenoviruses who may shed for 3–6 weeks and as long as 18 months [97]. The duration of viral shedding in the gastrointestinal tract may be prolonged in immunocompromised individuals [97]. Adenoviruses can also be shed in the stool of individuals with asymptomatic infections which are common, particularly in children [97].

Clinical symptoms include watery, non-bloody diarrhea accompanied by mild fever, vomiting, and abdominal pain. Gastroenteritis in immunocompetent patients usually resolves without complication; however, rare fatalities are documented [97].

Gastrointestinal infections in immunocompromised patients occur most often in hematopoietic stem cell (HSCT), bone marrow (BMT), and solid organ (SOT) transplant patients. Infections in these patients are frequently severe and can become disseminated. In pediatric allogeneic HSCT patients, detectable virus in stool almost always precedes systemic adenovirus infection [105]. Adenovirus species isolated most frequently in HSCT and BMT patients with gastrointestinal disease include species A (serotype 31), B (serotype 7), and C (serotype 2) [106]. The incidence of adenovirus infections in patients with HIV infection or acquired immunodeficiency syndrome (AIDS) has dropped due to effective treatment of the HIV infection with highly active antiretroviral therapy [10]. Serotypes within species D cause the majority of gastroenteritis in HIV-positive patients and include serotypes 9, 17, 20, 22, 23, 26, 27, and 42–51 [106].

Clinical Utility of Testing

Diagnosis of adenovirus gastroenteritis is primarily determined through testing of stool samples although tissue biopsy specimens also may be used. Conventional methods used to identify the presence of adenovirus in stool samples include shell vial cultures, direct fluorescent antibody assays, EIAs, and EM. Disadvantages of culture methods include delays of up to weeks and false-negative results with difficult to culture AV serotypes such as 40 and 41 [99]. Immunofluorescent and immunochromatographic methods, while rapid, are insensitive [107]. EM also is insensitive and is not routinely used in clinical laboratories. Indirect diagnosis using serology is limited by poor sensitivity especially in immunocompromised patients and by high seroprevalence among children preventing the ability to identify acute disease [107, 108]. Despite these diagnostic limitations, conventional methods may be sufficient to detect infection in immunocompetent patients with localized or benign gastrointestinal symptoms [109].

Adenovirus infection may become severe in immunocompromised patients and the ability to begin early treatment, such as reduction of immunosuppression or cidofovir therapy, requires rapid and sensitive diagnostic techniques [107]. Several PCR-based assays have been validated for stool specimens and are comparable or better than conventional methods [110–112]. Both qualitative and quantitative PCR assays are used. Qualitative assays vary in serotype detection of all or only some serotypes. While qualitative PCR methods are sensitive, quantitative assays assess stool viral load and proliferation kinetics. These parameters may become important in assessing the need for preemptive treatment of adenovirus infection in pediatric HSCT patients by detection of significant levels of virus in stools before the onset of viremia and disseminated infection in the majority of these patients [105, 113].

Multiplex assays differ in their clinical application. One particular assay provides qualitative, yet species-specific results [114], while others offer quantitative results and detect adenovirus in combination with other important gastrointestinal pathogens. Quantitative assays may be useful for determining which pathogen is responsible for disease in cases of mixed infections [115, 116].

In most cases, determination of adenovirus serotype is unnecessary for clinical management [117]. By contrast, serotyping is important for epidemiology studies, when investigating an especially severe infection, and in predicting clinical outcome [106]. Isolation of specific adenovirus serotypes from the gastrointestinal tract, such as 1, 2, 5, and 6, may raise concern for the possibility of disseminated disease since these serotypes have been documented to cause systemic infections in immunocompromised patients [107]. On the other hand, serotypes 40 and 41, while frequently isolated in cases of gastroenteritis, have not been recovered from immunocompromised patients with disseminated infections [107]. While conventional serotyping methods may take up to several weeks [97], molecular methods such as PCR have improved turnaround times and allow for the characterization of isolates at the species, serotype, and genotype level [107]. Molecular and serological typing results usually are concordant [97].

Available Assays

Tissue biopsies may be submitted for culture or for histological examination using hematoxylin-and-eosin or Wright-Giemsa stains and immunohistochemistry. Molecular techniques such as in situ hybridization may aid diagnosis by confirming characteristic microscopic findings [118]. Alternatively, biopsy specimens may be submitted directly for molecular testing using conventional or real-time PCR [102, 119].

Molecular methods offer increased sensitivity and shorter turnaround time compared with conventional methods [110–112]. Different PCR methods for the detection of adenovirus in stool or tissue biopsies include conventional PCR, real-time PCR, and multiplex PCR. Most clinical laboratories use LDTs because no US FDA-cleared tests are available for stool testing. Regardless of the PCR method, degenerate or non-degenerate primers and probes targeting the hexon or fiber genes or the VA RNA-encoding regions are typically used. These regions display homology across serotypes for consistent binding of primers and probes, yet also include hypervariable regions suitable for differentiating serotypes.

Conventional PCR assays range in their detection abilities. Some systems detect and report specific serotypes [110, 120, 121], while others report genus- or species-specific results and purport to detect all serotypes [107, 117]. These assays are qualitative and usually have a 1–2 day turnaround time. Methods used to detect PCR amplicons include ethidium bromide-stained gel electrophoresis, Southern blotting, or liquid phase hybridization quantitated by time resolved fluorometry [122]. These detection methods are time- and labor-intensive and necessitate handling of PCR products, thus potentiating the risk of contamination.

Real-time PCR methods offer quantitative results and are more rapid and involve less contamination risk than conventional PCR assays [102, 119, 123, 124]. Several LDTs and one commercial assay are validated for use on stool specimens. While some methods rely on a single probe and primer pair, most utilize more than one set of primers and multiple probes. Weighing of stool specimens before DNA extraction allows results to be quantitated in copies per gram of stool. This standardization permits assessment of serial stool specimens for viral load kinetics and facilitates comparison of results between assays.

Several multiplex PCR assays have been validated for stool testing and differ in their clinical applications and detection methods. One particular method allows for identification of all six adenoviral species in a single reaction mixture using species-specific hexon primers [110]. Species-specific results are visualized by agarose gel electrophoresis, which shows a different amplicon length for each species [110]. Other multiplex assays offer quantitative results and combine adenovirus detection with other common gastrointestinal viral pathogens [115, 116]. Detection techniques differ and involve either fluorescent-labeled sequence-specific probes or sequence-specific capture probes bound to microspheres, which are interrogated by flow cytometry.

Conventional typing may take weeks making such methods impractical for clinical use. Molecular typing methods greatly improve turnaround time and several assays have been tested for use with stool samples. Strategies for producing serotype or genotype specific results vary by assay, and may be performed from cultured isolates or directly from clinical specimens [125, 126]. Traditional molecular typing methods rely on REA and may be performed on adenoviral genome DNA or following PCR amplification of specific regions [117, 127]. Genotype or serotype is inferred from the band pattern on agarose gel electrophoresis. REA methods are still used to identify new strains or for type identification of an isolate causing severe disease [106]. Sequence-based typing may be used to determine both serotype and genotype and is usually performed after PCR amplification of hypervariable regions [128]. Generated sequences are compared to banked sequences of known serotypes.

Interpretation of Results

Similar to other clinical situations where highly sensitive molecular assays are applied, PCR methods used in the diagnosis of adenovirus gastroenteritis offer improved sensitivity over conventional methods, but may provide positive results in the absence of disease. The ability for adenoviruses to cause asymptomatic infection and the tendency for nonenteric adenoviruses to be shed in the stool for weeks to months after resolution of clinical symptoms make interpretation of positive results in patients without symptoms difficult [97, 103].

Diagnosis of adenovirus gastroenteritis in immunocompetent patients is straightforward when PCR results are positive for an enteric adenovirus species or serotype in the presence of characteristic symptoms. Viral shedding in the absence of symptoms is unusual for enteric adenoviruses, especially in immunocompetent individuals.

Shedding of nonenteric serotypes for long periods of time occurs more frequently in immunocompromised patients and makes it difficult to determine conclusively that a detected adenovirus serotype is the cause of the patient's symptoms. Persistent viral shedding from a previous adenovirus infection may be difficult to distinguish from a newly acquired asymptomatic infection, which occurs often in the immunocompromised patient population. Further complicating interpretation in immunocompromised individuals is the frequent occurrence of coinfections.

The ability to determine serotype by sequencing is limited by incomplete reference databases containing sequence information for only certain serotypes [107]. The completeness of the reference database depends on the genome region sequenced. Serotype determination by methods relying on enzyme restriction patterns is limited to serotypes whose restriction patterns have been previously described. These methods are further hampered by the genetic variability created over time by recombination events between viruses of different serotypes. Such variation may alter cleavage sites and create unrecognizable restriction enzyme patterns. Infections caused by one or more serotypes may also create uninterpretable results.

As mentioned above, quantitative testing of stool allows clinicians to monitor stool viral load and proliferation kinetics. The mere presence of adenovirus in stool is common in pediatric HSCT patients, and does not necessitate treatment, as the majority will clear the virus spontaneously [129]. Quantitative measurements, however, have allowed investigators to identify rising stool viral loads in the majority of pediatric HSCT patients who go on to develop adenovirus viremia and disseminated disease [105, 113]. Quantitative serial stool measurements, therefore, may serve as a useful tool for predicting when early treatment is warranted and could prevent the overuse of the nephrotoxic antiviral drug cidofovir [113].

Laboratory Issues

Detection of all adenovirus serotypes is important because serotypes other than enteric adenoviruses cause a significant number of gastroenteritis cases in immunocompromised patients. The high degree of genetic heterogeneity among adenovirus serotypes makes detection of all known serotypes by a generic PCR assay difficult [106]. Genetic diversity also complicates identification of regions with sufficient homology to allow for uniform annealing of primers and probes in all serotypes. Currently, most assays use primers and probes that bind to the highly conserved hexon gene, which has only approximately 50 % nucleotide homology between serotypes (NCBI database, [105]). Uniform annealing of primers and probes is even more important for quantitative assays, to ensure equal amplification efficiency of all serotypes [108]. Concern that nucleotide mismatches between target and primer or probe would result in decreased sensitivity of detection for many serotypes has led to more optimal assay designs utilizing multiple primer and probe sets [123]. Lastly, multiplex assays that detect multiple viral pathogens can detect coinfections, although the test performance for adenovirus was occasionally negatively affected by coamplification of other viruses [116].

DNA from both adenovirus 40 and adenovirus 41 is available from ATCC (Manassas, VA). The Zeptometrix NATtrol™ gastrointestinal pathogens verification panel includes adenovirus among the other analytes. The Stool Pathogen Panel (SP) proficiency survey from the College of American Pathologists includes challenges for adenovirus 40/41.

Rotavirus

Description of Pathogen

Rotaviruses are non-enveloped viruses in the *Reoviridae* family, named because of their characteristic wheel-like appearance by EM. Rotaviruses are very stable in the environment and can remain infectious for several weeks. They have a triple-layered structure with concentric capsid layers that surround a core which contains the genome. The surface of the outermost capsid layer contains two major structural viral proteins, VP4, a protease-cleaved protein (P protein), and VP7, a glycoprotein (G protein). The middle layer of the capsid contains structural protein VP6. The inner capsid layer contains proteins VP1, VP2, and VP3. The rotavirus genome consists of 11 segments of double-stranded RNA with a complete genome length of 16,500–21,000 nucleotides. The genomes can reassort during dual infection of a single cell which results in co-circulation of a wide variety of strains.

Rotaviruses are classified into serogroups A through G based on the antigenic characteristics the VP6 protein. Only groups A, B, and C infect humans and animals. The remaining rotavirus groups have been found only in animals. The Group A human rotaviruses cause the majority of viral gastrointestinal infections in children. Group B rotaviruses were first identified as causing adult diarrhea in a large waterborne epidemic in China. Serologic evidence indicates that Group B rotavirus is also present in the UK and the US, and genome profiles consistent with Group B rotavirus have been detected as causes of diarrhea in India [130]. Group C rotaviruses are an emerging cause of gastroenteritis in both children and adults and have been identified in sporadic cases and outbreaks worldwide. The Group A rotaviruses are further classified into serotypes based on neutralizing serologic reactions against the P (VP4) and G (VP7) proteins. Also, because the two gene segments that encode the P and G proteins segregate independently, a genotyping system has been developed based on the sequences of both genes. The most prevalent Group A rotavirus genotypes in humans are G1P[8], G2P[4], G3P[8], G4P[8], and G9P[8]. A Rotavirus Classification Working Group has been formed to assist in classification of any newly described rotavirus genotypes based on sequence information for all 11 genomic RNA segments.

Rotavirus is endemic worldwide and is the single most common cause of diarrhea among infants and young children [131]. Most rotavirus infections are self-limiting but some children become very ill with severe vomiting, diarrhea, and life-threatening loss of fluids that requires hospitalization. Death due to rotavirus infection is relatively rare in the USA but is a significant concern in developing countries. Rotaviruses are estimated to cause more than half a million infant and young children deaths worldwide every year [131].

In the USA and other countries with temperate climates, annual outbreaks of rotavirus infection occur during winter and spring, with fewer cases in summer. However, with the introduction of rotavirus vaccines, the seasonality has shifted and the winter–spring trend in peak rotavirus activity is no longer consistently observed [132]. Seasonal variation is not seen in tropical climates.

Rotaviruses are shed in large quantities in the stools of infected children beginning 2 days before the onset of diarrhea and for up to about 10 days after the onset of symptoms. Immunocompromised individuals may shed detectable rotavirus for more than 30 days after infection. Rotaviruses are highly communicable, with a small infectious dose of less than 100 virus particles [133]. Rotaviruses are spread by fecal-oral transmission, both through close person-to-person contact and through fomites, and are common causes of diarrheal outbreaks in families, in childcare centers, and other institutions, and among hospitalized children [134]. The incubation period for rotavirus illness is about 2–3 days. Immunity after infection is incomplete, but repeat infections tend to have milder signs and symptoms than the initial infection.

A rotavirus vaccine is now included in the American Academy of Pediatrics recommended immunization schedule for infants. Two vaccines, RotaTeq® (Merck & Co., Inc., West Point, PA) and Rotarix® (GlaxoSmithKline, London, UK) were introduced in 2006 and 2008, respectively, and are currently licensed for use in the USA. A previous rotavirus vaccine was taken off the market in 1999 because of an increased risk for intussusception, which does not occur with either RotaTeq or Rotarix.

Adults and older children also can be infected with rotaviruses. Infection in adults is often subclinical or very mild. Clinically evident cases are most often seen in immunocompromised patients, the elderly, and travelers to developing countries [135].

Clinical Utility of Testing

Rotavirus infection cannot be diagnosed by clinical presentation because the clinical features of rotavirus gastroenteritis do not differ from those of gastroenteritis caused by other pathogens. Confirmation of rotavirus infection by laboratory testing is used for surveillance but also is useful in clinical settings to avoid inappropriate use of antimicrobial therapy.

Since rotavirus is present in high concentrations in the stool of infected children, stool is the preferred specimen for diagnosis. Rotaviruses can be cultured in Madin-Darby bovine kidney (MDBK), fetal African green monkey kidney cells (MA104 cell line), and some other cell lines in media containing trypsin or pancreatin, but culture is relatively inefficient and not performed in clinical laboratories. The most widely available method for detection of rotavirus antigen in stool is EIA directed at the VP6 antigen common to all group A rotaviruses. Several commercial EIA kits are available, which are inexpensive, easy to use, rapid, and sensitive (approximately 90–100 %). Latex agglutination is less sensitive and specific than EIA but is still used in some settings. Immunochromatographic point of care tests have reported sensitivities of 94–100 % and specificities of 96–100 % compared with clinical laboratory tests [136]. Other techniques, including EM, reverse transcription-polymerase chain reaction, nucleic acid hybridization, sequence analysis, and culture are used primarily in research settings.

Molecular methods have been used primarily for characterization of G and P genotypes in epidemiologic studies and to evaluate the impact of vaccination [137, 138]. RT-PCR has increased detection rates for rotavirus A by up to 48 % compared to EIA or EM [139]. Sensitivity of RT-PCR tests is estimated at 10^4 rotavirus particles per milliliter of stool, while EIA methods detect 10^6 rotavirus particles per milliliter of stool. While increased sensitivity is usually seen as a benefit, some have considered RT-PCR assays too sensitive for the detection of rotaviruses due to their ability to detect asymptomatic infections, which are common in infants and young children [140, 141].

Available Assays

Some commercial tests designed for testing food sources or environmental samples are available as research use only kits. Most reports of molecular tests used for diagnosis of human rotavirus infections are LDTs. The xTAG GPP gastrointestinal pathogen panel test kit (Luminex Corp., Austin, TX) is an US FDA-cleared qualitative RT-PCR multiplexed test that can be performed in about 5 h and simultaneously detects the most common parasitic, bacterial and viral gastrointestinal pathogens, including rotavirus Group A.

Interpretation of Results

Asymptomatic carriage of rotavirus can be detected by molecular tests and needs to be considered when interpreting positive results in clinical specimens [140, 141]. Asymptomatic carriage vs true mixed infection also needs to be considered in the rare event that rotavirus is detected in combination with another gastrointestinal pathogen in the same clinical sample or during an episode of diarrhea. Laboratories should be aware that rotaviruses can be detected by RT-PCR in clinical specimens for about 10 days after resolution of an acute diarrheal episode in healthy children [137].

Laboratory Issues

Ideally, diagnostic RT-PCR tests would be able to detect all three genogroups of human rotaviruses. Except for epidemiologic purposes, identification of the specific genogroup is probably not necessary. Laboratories should be aware that rotavirus RNA has been detected in serum, CSF, and throat swab specimens [142, 143].

The NATtrol™ (ZeptoMetrix Corp, Buffalo, NY) verification set includes reference material for rotavirus among other analytes. Human rotavirus in diarrheal stool samples is available from ATCC (Manassas, VA). The Gastrointestinal Panel for Molecular Multiplex Testing (GIP) and the Stool Pathogens (SP) survey, both from the College of American Pathologists, include proficiency testing challenges for rotavirus among other gastrointestinal pathogens.

Astrovirus

Description of Pathogen

Astroviruses are small, round, non-enveloped viruses with icosahedral cubic capsids that have a characteristic five or six-point star-like surface structure when viewed by EM. Astroviruses contain three structural proteins (VP26, VP29, and VP32). The genome is composed of non-segmented, positive-sense, single-stranded RNA. The total genome length is 6,800–7,900 nucleotides, excluding the poly (A) tract at the 3′ end and the genome has been sequenced.

The family *Astroviridae* contains two genera: *Mamastroviruses* which infect numerous types of mammals and *Avastroviruses* which infect birds (e.g., ducks, chickens, turkeys). Within each genus are species of astroviruses, which, according to International Committee on Taxonomy of Viruses guidelines, are named based on the host in which they replicate. The astroviruses are further subclassified within each species into serotypes. Three species of astroviruses are found in human stool: HAstV (serotypes 1–8), AstV-MLB, and HMOAstV (serotypes A to C). These species are more closely related to animal astroviruses than to each other, indicating phylogenetically separate origins of human astroviruses [144].

Simultaneous circulation of multiple types of astrovirus is not rare [144]. Human astrovirus serotype 1 (HAstV-1) is the most prevalent serotype detected worldwide. However, serotype 3 produces higher quantities of virus in stool and appears to cause a larger proportion of cases of persistent gastroenteritis [145].

Human astroviruses are endemic worldwide. Studies using sensitive detection techniques, such as RT-PCR, have demonstrated that astrovirus infection is a more common and important cause of viral gastroenteritis than previously known. Symptomatic illness is most common in children <2 years of age, although infection in immunocompromised individuals and outbreaks among adults and the elderly have also been reported. Astroviruses are highly stable in the environment and are resistant to a wide range of detergents and lipid solvents. The fecal-oral route is thought to be the most common means of transmission and contaminated food, water, and fomites are common sources of virus. As with many other viral causes of gastroenteritis, astrovirus infection has a peak incidence in winter in temperate climates and is associated with the rainy season in tropical regions. Astrovirus is thought to replicate in the intestinal tissue of the jejunum and ileum and generally causes mild, self-limiting illness of short duration. Prevalence is likely under-estimated since surveillance and seroprevalence studies have demonstrated that astrovirus infection is common and is largely asymptomatic.

Immunity to astrovirus infection is not well understood. Prevalence of symptomatic infection among young children and institutionalized elderly populations suggests that antibody is acquired early in childhood, provides protection through adult life, and begins to decline later in life [146]. Heterologous protection does not occur across the human astrovirus serotypes [147].

Clinical Utility of Testing

No vaccine or anti-viral treatment is available for prevention or treatment of astrovirus infection, but diagnosis may be important to avoid unnecessary antibiotic use. Establishing an etiology also may be important in hospitalized patients for infection control purposes to prevent nosocomial spread [148, 149]. Further, diagnosing astrovirus gastroenteritis in patients with malnutrition, immunodeficiency, and underlying gastrointestinal disease, may be important because of the increased likelihood of complications that require hospitalization in these populations. The impact of astrovirus infection on the morbidity of infants and children may become increasingly important as the rotavirus vaccine becomes more widely used and the burden of rotavirus is reduced.

Available Assays

Astroviruses have been adapted to cell culture using CaCo-2 human colonic carcinoma cells in some research settings, but are not cultured for clinical diagnostic purposes. EM and immune EM (IEM) have been effectively used to detect astroviruses in clinical stool specimens but are not available in many clinical laboratories. Also, identification by EM can be difficult since only a small portion of astrovirus particles (about 10 %) display the characteristic star-like morphology [150].

EIA tests have been developed for the qualitative detection of astrovirus antigen in clinical specimens and are commercially available in Europe (e.g., RIDASCREEN® Astrovirus test, R-biopharm AG, Darmstadt, Germany, IDEIA™ Astrovirus, Dako Diagnostics Ltd, Ely, UK) but are not US FDA-cleared for diagnostic use in the USA.

Commercial real-time RT-PCR kits are available for testing environmental and food samples. Molecular assays are considered to be an improved diagnostic method over EM and EIA [151], but US FDA-cleared diagnostic tests for astrovirus are not available. Specifications for LDTs for detection of astrovirus in clinical samples using highly sensitive group-specific RT-PCR primers targeted to conserved genomic regions coding for the nonstructural proteins and untranslated regions are available [151]. Reported detection limits for these assays vary from 1 to 10 viral copies depending of the quality of the analyzed nucleic acid. Some tests utilize primers from the capsid coding region which can be less sensitive, but provide type information [151].

Interpretation of Results

Shedding of astrovirus is generally limited to about 1 week in immunocompetent individuals, but as with other viruses that cause gastroenteritis, prolonged shedding of astrovirus (e.g., 4 weeks) has been observed in immunocompromised patients [148, 152]. Although asymptomatic infection is common, determining the significance of astrovirus detection should not be problematic in most clinical settings since presumably only diarrheal stools from symptomatic patients would be tested.

Laboratory Issues

Astrovirus infections are generally limited to the gastrointestinal tract; however, astroviruses have been detected in plasma as a cause of febrile illness and in brain tissue of an immunocompromised patient [153]. Human gastrointestinal astrovirus infections have been limited to the eight closely related serotypes described above. Recently, several highly divergent astrovirus serotypes (MLB1, MLB2, VA1, VA2, and VA3) have been detected in stool samples from patients with and without diarrhea [153]. An association with gastrointestinal disease has not been definitively made for these newly described astroviruses [153]. Reference material and proficiency testing challenges are not currently commercially available.

Caliciviridae (*Noroviruses, Sapoviruses*)

Description of Pathogen

Human caliciviruses belong to the family *caliciviridae* and are small, round, non-enveloped viruses with a single-stranded, positive-sense RNA genome. The family currently includes the genera *Norovirus* (previously Norwalk and Norwalk-like viruses), *Sapovirus* (previously Sapporo and Sapporo-like viruses), *Lagovirus*, *Vesivivirus*, and the newly proposed *Becovirus* and *Recovirus*. The noroviruses and sapoviruses have recognized roles as causes of acute gastroenteritis in humans. Within each genus, strains are further grouped into genogroups and genotypes or clusters.

The noroviruses are partitioned into genogroups GI to GVII, each further subdivided into genotypes and subgenotypes. Porcine, bovine, and murine noroviruses belong to genogroups II, III, and V, respectively. The majority of human norovirus outbreaks are caused by genogroup II genotype 3 (GII-3) and genogroup II genotype 4 (GII-4) viruses. Human norovirus are thought to be specific to humans and transmission from an animal reservoir has not been described. However, at least three clusters of porcine noroviruses in genogroup II are genetically closely related to the human noroviruses in genogroup II, introducing the potential for zoonotic transmission [154].

The sapoviruses are similarly partitioned into five genogroups (GI to GV) with genotypes in each group. Human sapoviruses belong to genogroups GI, GII, GIV, and GV. GIII contains the porcine strains. Caliciviruses appear to naturally undergo recombination during normal replication of the virus, leading to the emergence of a continuous array of new variants [155].

Human caliciviruses are cannot be grown in standard in vitro cell culture assays and their role as agents of gastrointestinal diseases was under appreciated because clinical tests for the detection of caliciviruses were not commonly available. Molecular methods such as RT-PCR have revealed that caliciviruses are broadly distributed worldwide and are very common causes of epidemic and sporadic gastroenteritis in both children and adults [156]. The study of noroviruses is significantly more advanced than that of sapoviruses. Noroviruses are recognized as the leading cause of epidemic gastroenteritis, often causing large water- or food-borne outbreaks in all ages, while sapoviruses are implicated mainly in pediatric gastroenteritis [157].

Caliciviruses are presumed to replicate primarily in the upper intestinal tract and histopathologic lesions are seen in the jejunum of infected individuals. Symptoms of calicivirus infection are popularly known as "stomach flu" and include vomiting, abdominal cramps, diarrhea, headache, and fever. Symptoms generally last 1–4 days and most people recover completely without treatment. Infants, older adults and people with underlying disease can become severely dehydrated and require medical attention. Asymptomatic infections with shedding of virus are common, and could be the source of some outbreaks [158]. Protective immunity is thought to be short-lived and individuals who have been infected may or may not be immune to reinfection. Studies of immune response are complicated by the ability of the virus to produce naturally occurring variants which are difficult for the immune system to recognize.

Caliciviruses are stable in the environment and can survive freezing, heating to 60 °C, and in chlorinated water up to 10 ppm. They can also survive for several days on many types of surfaces (e.g., door knobs, counter tops, pens, and telephones). Caliciviruses are highly contagious with an estimated infectious dose as low as 10–100 virus particles [159]. These characteristics facilitate rapid spread of caliciviruses, especially in households and institutional settings such as schools, day care centers, hospitals, nursing homes, restaurants, and cruise ships [160]. Calicivirus infections occur year round, although a winter seasonal peak is frequently observed [161].

Transmission is thought to occur mainly through fecal-oral routes. Evidence also suggests that caliciviruses may be transmitted by close exposure to aerosols generated during vomiting episodes in infected individuals. The most frequent cause of norovirus infection appears to be consumption of food or beverages that are contaminated either at their source or by infected food handlers. Uncooked shellfish, particularly oysters, as well as raspberries and precooked foods, such as salad, ham, and sandwiches, are among the common foods that have been responsible for outbreaks [161]. Outbreaks resulting from contamination of municipal water are rare, but water-borne outbreaks associated with community or family water systems have been documented. Sapoviruses have been associated with food-borne outbreaks, but much less frequently than noroviruses. Sapovirus infections are not associated with eating seafood. Nosocomial infections due to caliciviruses are increasingly recognized and may be quite common.

Clinical Utility of Testing

Laboratory diagnosis of calicivirus infection is difficult and clinical diagnosis is often used, especially when other agents of gastroenteritis have been ruled out. Detection of caliciviruses may be important because of their biologic, physicochemical, and epidemiologic features, which present significant challenges for infection control in hospital environments. The regular turnover of patients leaving the hospital and being replaced by new patients provides an opportunity for introduction of the virus from the community and subsequent transmission within the hospital environment.

Available Assays

Although Norovirus has been adapted to grow in a complex 3D culture system in research settings, attempts to culture human caliciviruses in routine cell lines have failed to yield replicating virus, even with addition of a wide variety of culture supplements.

Caliciviruses can be detected fairly rapidly in stool specimens from patients with diarrhea using direct EM. Detection by direct EM requires virus concentrations of at least 10^6 virus particles per milliliter of stool, making EM relatively insensitive, even after processing of the specimen to concentrate the virus particles [158]. IEM improves the sensitivity of direct EM by 10- to 100-fold, but this technique is infrequently used. False-negative results can occur if antibody is present in excess and masks detection of the virus [160]. Use of EM is limited due to the need for expensive equipment, experienced technologists and a significant amount of labor per specimen [162].

The cloning of the Norwalk virus genome and subsequently of other human caliciviruses has allowed the development of other methods for diagnosis. EIAs to detect virus in stool specimens using polyclonal hyperimmune animal sera can detect the presence of 10^4–10^6 intact virus particles/ml of stool [160, 163], but are considered to have inadequate sensitivity to be used for diagnosis, especially of sporadic cases [164]. Serologic EIAs to detect specific antiviral antibodies generally are used to detect a fourfold increase in antibody levels between acute and convalescent serum specimens. The hyperimmune antisera and recombinant antigens needed to produce these EIAs are not widely accessible and US FDA-approved diagnostic assays have not been produced. The assays are available at some public health laboratories and are primarily used for epidemiologic purposes.

Since caliciviruses cannot be grown in vitro, EM is available only in highly specialized facilities, and serology assays are insensitive, the potential utility of RT-PCR-based techniques is considerable. The highly variable nature of calicivirus genomes presents a significant challenge to designing molecular assays for diagnostic use. The literature contains details of a variety of RT-PCR assays that have been used for the detection of human caliciviruses in diagnostic studies as well epidemiologic investigations of food, water, and other environmental samples. Some of the assays are designed to detect sapoviruses without cross-reactivity with noroviruses or rotaviruses. Among them is a quantitative real-time PCR assay using primers against the junction of the RNA-dependent RNA polymerase/capsid genes that has been described to detect sapovirus genogroups I, II, and IV with an analytical sensitivity of ten copies of viral cDNA per reaction [165]. Conventional qualitative RT-PCR assays that detect all genogroups of human sapoviruses have also been developed [166]. Nested RT-PCR assays that claim to be more sensitive than conventional PCR that detect and differentiate all genogroups of human sapovirus have been reported using primers against the RNA-dependent RNA polymerase region [167] or the capsid-protein coding region [168]. Molecular assays using various protocols and primer sets to detect noroviruses have been similarly described. Only a small region of approximately 50 base pairs at the polymerase (ORF-1)/capsid (ORF2) junction of the norovirus genome appears to be sufficiently conserved to detect all within-genogroup variants [169–171]. Additional assays have been published that use multiple primers in a multiplex format to amplify the capsid region of the respective viral targets to simultaneously detect norovirus genogroups I and II, sapoviruses, and astroviruses [172].

The public health laboratories in all 50 states of the US, are able to test for norovirus RNA by RT-PCR in stool and emesis specimens, as well as environmental samples. The public health laboratories sponsor CaliciNet, a national network that tracks the different sequences of norovirus strains found in clinical and environmental samples to aid in assessment of relationships between strains in epidemiologic investigations and provide identification of emerging strains.

Several CE-marked molecular tests are available in Europe for the specific detection of Norovirus genogroups I and II in stool samples, including the MutaPLEX® Norovirus real-time RT-PCR kit (Immundiagnostik AG, Bensheim, Germany), the RealStar® Norovirus RT-PCR kit (Altona Diagnostics, Hamburg, Germany), the AmpliSens® *Norovirus* genotypes 1, 2-EPh PCR kit (Ecoli s.r.o., Slovak Republic), the SmartNorovirus (Cepheid, Maurens–Scopont, France) and the Xpert® Norovirus (Cepheid, Sunnyvale, CA). The xTAG GPP gastrointestinal pathogen panel test kit (Luminex Corp., Austin, TX and Milan, Italy) is a qualitative multiplex molecular test that uses the Luminex xTAG® Technology and the xMAP® Technology platform to simultaneously detect the most clinically important bacterial, viral, and parasitic gastrointestinal pathogens, including Norovirus types I and II from a single specimen. The xTAG GPP panel is US FDA-cleared for use in clinical laboratories in the USA and also has regulatory approval in Europe and Canada. The BioFire GI Panel (bioMerieux, Durham, NC) fully automated GI panel also includes detection of Norovirus genogroups I and II as well as sapoviruses.

Interpretation of Results

The increased sensitivity afforded by RT-PCR may make interpretation of results confusing, especially during the management of outbreaks. Norovirus can be detected in stool samples before symptoms occur and continue to be detected for a few days to several weeks after symptoms resolve.

Laboratory Issues

Ideally, diagnostic RT-PCR tests would be able to detect and distinguish the clinically significant genera of human caliciviruses. False-negative results may occur due to the sequence diversity of newly emergent variants which existing primer pairs may not detect. Identification of the specific genogroup is helpful for epidemiologic investigations but is probably not necessary in clinical laboratories. Norovirus is most easily detected in stool specimens obtained during the acute phase of illness (48–72 h after the onset of symptoms) when large numbers of virus are present. Norovirus RNA also has been reported in human serum [173] and in CSF [174].

Quantified, synthetic Norovirus GI and GII RNA standards are available from ATCC (Manassas, VA). The NATtrol™ (ZeptoMetrix Corp., Buffalo, NY) verification set contains reference material for noroviruses and sapoviruses in addition to a variety of bacteria and parasites.

The Gastrointestinal Panel for Molecular Multiplex Testing (GIP), as well as the Stool Pathogens (SP) survey, both from the College of American Pathologists, have Norovirus GI/GII as analytes on the panel, but do not currently include sapoviruses.

Parasitic Pathogens

Protozoa and helminth parasites can infest the gastrointestinal tract and are typically shed in the stool. Parasitic infections are prevalent in Central and South America, Africa, and Asia but are much less common in Australia, Canada, Europe, Japan, New Zealand, and the USA. In developed countries, parasitic infections are most frequently encountered among immigrants and travelers returning from endemic regions and occasionally among individuals who have not traveled, particularly those with AIDS or other causes of immunodeficiency.

Description of Pathogens

Many intestinal parasites may need to be considered in the differential diagnosis of gastrointestinal disease depending on the geographic area visited, specific history of exposure, and individual risk. The most common pathogenic protozoan parasites in developed countries are *Giardia lamblia* and *Cryptosporidium hominis*/*C. parvum* and are seen in travelers returning from endemic areas. *Entamoeba histolytica* is a much less common cause of gastrointestinal illness but early diagnosis is important because of the potential to cause dysentery and invasive extraintestinal disease. Many other intestinal parasites such as *Enterobius vermicularis*, *Cyclospora* sp., *Ascaris* sp., *Cystoisospora* sp., microsporidia, *Trichuris* sp., hookworms, *Strongyloides* sp., tapeworms, flukes, and others are associated with acute and chronic illness in the USA, particularly in socioeconomically poor areas and among immunocompromised individuals. Surveillance using molecular assays is causing reconsideration of the role of some parasites such as *Blastocystis hominis*, *Dientamoeba fragilis*, *Entamoeba coli*, and *E. hartmanii* that were previously considered to be associated with harmless asymptomatic infection but are now thought to have the potential to cause symptomatic illness [175].

Clinical Utility of Testing

Gastrointestinal parasitic infections are not common but cause significant morbidity and mortality, particularly in developing countries and in individuals who are immunocompromised or have other underlying medical conditions. Diagnosis of parasitic disease often is delayed when patients present with vague gastrointestinal symptoms or because of the inability of existing diagnostic methods to detect the causative organism when there is irregular morphology, a low parasite load, or intermittent shedding. When diagnosis is delayed, patients are more likely to have developed more severe symptoms at the time of diagnosis. Delayed diagnosis also allows for increased opportunity to spread infection to others. Prompt diagnosis permits initiation of effective treatment and implementation of infection control measures.

Available Assays

Clinical laboratory detection is routinely performed by microscopic examination of stool specimens using wet mounts and permanent stained slides. Because there is marked fluctuation in the shedding of parasites from day to day, the diagnostic yield of examining a single stool specimen is low (50–60 %); therefore, to improve sensitivity, a total of three stool specimens should be collected every other day or at least on separate days within a period of no more than 10 days [176]. Some parasitic enteropathogens (i.e., *Cyclospora*, *Cystoisospora*, and microsporidia) are difficult to detect in stool and require the use of special stains.

The specificity of microscopic examination is theoretically perfect, but depends on the skill of the microscopist. The sensitivity of microscopic examination also depends largely on the skill of the microscopist and can be low for some parasitic diseases. Concentration techniques are used routinely and improve sensitivity. Since microscopy is very labor-intensive, US FDA-approved immunoassays are available for detecting *Entamoeba histolytica*, *Giardia*, or *Cryptosporidium* antigens in stool, and numerous studies confirm that antigen immunoassays are more sensitive than microscopic examination [177]. Antigen immunoassays have added benefits of being rapid and are technically simple to perform. The sensitivity of microscopy and immunoassay examinations for ova and parasites is low enough that empiric treatment is often given when clinical suspicion is high but tests are negative. Use of X-ray contrast material, laxatives, antacids, or antibiotics (especially tetracyclines and metronidazole), and various other substances can interfere with detection of parasites and delay the diagnosis by as much as several weeks. Due to the nature of the infection, sigmoidoscopy or colonoscopy to obtain duodenal aspirates or biopsy specimens may be necessary for detection of some parasites such as *Cryptosporidium*, microsporidia, or *Giardia*. Even these invasive methods of testing can give false-negative results due the patchy nature of organism distribution in the gastrointestinal tract.

Molecular tools similar to those used for other pathogens are increasingly being used to study parasite polymorphisms and the epidemiology of parasitic diseases. Molecular tests are slowly entering the diagnostic arena and may become more commonly used when US FDA-approved or -cleared tests become available. Current non-molecular diagnostic processes for detection of gastrointestinal parasites can be slow and confusing, while molecular tests have the potential to greatly facilitate diagnosis.

Commercially developed laboratory tests beyond microscopy have been limited to a few well-recognized parasitic pathogens. Individual assays using PCR amplification of parasite DNA sequences extracted from stool or biopsy specimens have been developed for a number of specific gastrointestinal parasites, but are largely research tools and are not commercially available. Molecular detection of *Cryptosporidium* sp., *Cyclospora cayetanensis*, *Giardia lamblia*, microsporidia, *Entamoeba histolytica*, and *E. dispar* is performed at the Centers for Disease Control and Prevention and may be available at some public health or other reference laboratories.

Multiplex tests are more practical for routine clinical laboratory use and assays for various combinations of parasitic targets have been described in the literature for successful detection of the target organisms in diarrheal stool specimens. The US FDA-cleared xTAG® Gastrointestinal Pathogen Panel (xTAG GPP, Luminex Corporation, Austin, TX) contains primers for the amplification of *Giardia* and *Cryptosporidium* along with other nonparasitic gastrointestinal pathogens. The version of the test marked for diagnostic use in Canada and Europe also detects *Entamoeba histolytica*. The US FDA-cleared BioFire FilmArray™ (bioMerieux, Durham, NC) Gastrointestinal (GI) Panel includes detection of *Cryptosporidium*, *Cyclospora cayetanensis*, *Entamoeba histolytica*, and *Giardia lamblia* in addition to bacterial and viral gastrointestinal pathogens.

Interpretation of Results

In most cases, positive molecular test results in symptomatic patients will correlate with disease. Whereas microscopic examination requires the presence of whole intact parasite for visualization, PCR can only detect the presence of the parasite DNA and cannot distinguish between live, damaged, or dead organisms. Also, the length of time that parasite DNA can be detected after clearance of the organism from the body has not been studied for gastrointestinal parasites, and the possibility that positive results obtained by PCR analysis might be due to lingering parasite DNA may need to be considered, depending on the clinical situation. In addition, asymptomatic carriage is common and must be considered when drawing conclusions about positive results if molecular tests are being used for screening purposes, such as for travelers returning from endemic regions or foreign adopted children.

Laboratory Issues

Stool specimens submitted for microscopic ova and parasite examination are generally placed in preservatives to stabilize parasite morphology and prevent further development of certain helminth eggs and larvae. Preservatives can interfere with PCR-based tests since they act by producing cross-links between nucleic acids and proteins which can obstruct DNA extraction and block PCR amplification. Preservatives also have the potential to cause fragmentation of nucleic acids which could interfere with target amplification. Specimens for molecular tests must be collected without preservatives and kept refrigerated or frozen prior to testing.

Microscopic examination is the most comprehensive method for detection of parasites and has the advantage of allowing detection of any parasite that might be present. Molecular tests are more sensitive but are not developed to the point where microscopy will be completely replaced by PCR. The introduction of real-time PCR assays, especially those that combine several targets into multiplex assays, offers the possibility of using DNA-based detection techniques as a component of a diagnostic approach. However, one of the constraints of multiplex assays is the restriction in the number of parasitic targets that can be detected simultaneously. Additional pathogenic parasites that are not targeted in the molecular assays will still need to be tested for by traditional microscopy or antigen detection methods.

Native genomic DNA and/or whole organisms for culture are available for *Giardia*, *Cryptosporidium* and *Entamoeba histolytica* from ATCC (Manassas, VA) and BEI Resources (Manassas, VA). The NATtrol™ (ZeptoMetrix Corp, Buffalo, NY) verification set contains those same protozoan analytes and also includes *Cyclospora*. Challenges for the molecular detection of *Giardia* and *Cryptosporidium* are available as part of the GIP proficiency survey from the College of American Pathologists.

Future Directions

Since the methods used for pathogen discovery have dramatically improved, emerging gastrointestinal pathogens, such as parechoviruses [178], as well as variants of known pathogens are being recognized at a rapid rate. The rapidly changing catalogue of clinically relevant gastrointestinal pathogens makes development of US FDA-approved/cleared tests difficult.

Clinical laboratories may have difficulty determining when to bring a molecular test into the laboratory. Higher cost is sometimes a deterrent but other considerations are whether a laboratory diagnosis would change patient management, improve outcomes, improve workflow, and/or lower associated healthcare costs. Sometimes molecular tests are so far superior to existing diagnostic tests that the issue is not whether a clinical laboratory can afford to offer a molecular test, but rather whether the laboratory can afford not to when the total cost of healthcare is considered.

References

1. Monteiro L, Bonnemaison D, Vekris A, et al. Complex polysaccharides as PCR inhibitors in feces: Helicobacter pylori model. J Clin Microbiol. 1997;35:995–8.
2. Gould LH, et al. Recommendations for diagnosis of shiga toxin-producing Escherichia coli infections by clinical laboratories. MMWR Recomm Rep. 2009;58:1–14.

3. Garcia LD. Fecal culture for aerobic pathogens of gastroenteritis, Ch. 3.8.1. In: Garcia LD, editor. Clinical microbiology procedures handbook. 3rd ed. Washington, DC: American Society for Microbiology; 2010.
4. Bartlett JG. Clinical practice. Antibiotic-associated diarrhea. N Engl J Med. 2002;346:334–49.
5. Kelly CP, Pothoulakis C, LaMont JT. Clostridium difficile colitis. N Engl J Med. 1994;330:257–62.
6. Kyne L, Hamel MB, Polavaram R, et al. Health care costs and mortality associated with nosocomial diarrhea due to Clostridium difficile. Clin Infect Dis. 2002;34:346–53.
7. O'Brien JA, Lahue BJ, Caro JJ, et al. The emerging infectious challenge of Clostridium difficile–associated disease in Massachusetts hospitals: clinical and economic consequences. Infect Control Hosp Epidemiol. 2007;28:1219–27.
8. Cohen SH, Gerding DN, Johnson S, et al. Clinical practice guidelines for Clostridium difficile infection in adults: 2010 update by the Society for Healthcare Epidemiology of America (SHEA) and the Infectious Diseases Society of America (IDSA). Infect Control Hosp Epidemiol. 2010;31:431–55.
9. Viscidi R, Willey S, Bartlett JG. Isolation rates and toxigenic potential of Clostridium difficile isolates from various patient populations. Gastroenterology. 1981;81:5–9.
10. Nakamura S, Mikawa M, Nakashio S, et al. Isolation of Clostridium difficile from the feces and the antibody in sera of young and elderly adults. Microbiol Immunol. 1981;25:345–51.
11. Svenungsson B, Burman LG, Jalakas-Pörnull K, et al. Epidemiology and molecular characterization of Clostridium difficile strains from patients with diarrhea: low disease incidence and evidence of limited cross-infection in a Swedish teaching hospital. J Clin Microbiol. 2003;41:4031–7.
12. Lyras D, O'Connor JR, Howarth PM, et al. Toxin B is essential for virulence of Clostridium difficile. Nature. 2009;458:1176–9.
13. McDonald LC, Killgore GE, Thompson A, et al. An epidemic, toxin gene-variant strain of Clostridium difficile. N Engl J Med. 2005;353:2433–41.
14. Loo VG, Poirier L, Miller MA, et al. A predominantly clonal multi-institutional outbreak of Clostridium difficile–associated diarrhea with high morbidity and mortality. N Engl J Med. 2005;353:2442–9.
15. Warny M, Pepin J, Fang A, et al. Toxin production by an emerging strain of Clostridium difficile associated with outbreaks of severe disease in North America and Europe. Lancet. 2005;366: 1079–84.
16. Tenover FC, Baron EJ, Peterson LR, et al. Laboratory diagnosis of Clostridium difficile infection. Can molecular amplification methods move us out of uncertainty? J Mol Diagn. 2011;13:573–82.
17. Larson AM, Fung AM, Fang FC. Evaluation of tcdB real-time PCR in a three-step diagnostic algorithm for detection of toxigenic Clostridium difficile. J Clin Microbiol. 2010;48:124–30.
18. Novak-Weekley SM, Marlowe EM, Miller JM, et al. Clostridium difficile testing in the clinical laboratory by use of multiple testing algorithms. J Clin Microbiol. 2010;48:889–93.
19. Cohen SH, Tang YJ, Silva J. Molecular typing methods for the epidemiological identification of Clostridium difficile strains. Expert Rev Mol Diagn. 2001;1:61–70.
20. Crobach MJ, Dekkers OM, Wilcox MH, et al. European Society of Clinical Microbiology and Infectious Diseases (ESCMID): data review and recommendations for diagnosing Clostridium difficile-infection (CDI). Clin Microbiol Infect. 2009;15:1053–66.
21. Eastwood K, Else P, Charlett A, et al. Comparison of nine commercially available Clostridium difficile toxin detection assays, a real-time PCR assay for C. difficile tcdB, and a glutamate dehydrogenase detection assay to cytotoxin testing and cytotoxigenic culture methods. J Clin Microbiol. 2009;47:3211–7.
22. Stamper PD, Alcabasa R, Aird D, et al. Comparison of a commercial real-time PCR assay for tcdB detection to a cell culture cytotoxicity assay and toxigenic culture for direct detection of toxin-producing Clostridium difficile in clinical samples. J Clin Microbiol. 2009;47:373–8.
23. Stevens DL, Bryant AE, Berger A, et al. Clostridium. In: Versalovic J, Carroll KC, Funke G, Jorgensen JH, Landry ML, Warnock DW, editors. Manual of clinical microbiology, vol. 1. 10th ed. Washington: American Society for Microbiology; 2011. p. 834–57.
24. Alcala L, Sanchez-Cambronero L, Catalan MP, et al. Comparison of three commercial methods for rapid detection of Clostridium difficile toxins A and B from fecal specimens. J Clin Microbiol. 2008;46:3833–5.
25. Sloan LM, Duresko BJ, Gustafson DR, et al. Comparison of real-time PCR for detection of the tcdC gene with four toxin immunoassays and culture in diagnosis of Clostridium difficile infection. J Clin Microbiol. 2008;46:1996–2001.
26. Shetty N, Wren MW, Coen PG. The role of glutamate dehydrogenase for the detection of Clostridium difficile in faecal samples: a meta-analysis. J Hosp Infect. 2011;77:1–6.
27. Hicke B, Pasko C, Groves B, et al. Automated detection of toxigenic Clostridium difficile in clinical samples: isothermal tcdB amplification coupled to array-based detection. J Clin Microbiol. 2012;50:2681–7.
28. Norén T, Alriksson I, Andersson J, et al. Rapid and sensitive loop-mediated isothermal amplification test for Clostridium difficile detection challenges cytotoxin B cell test and culture as gold standard. J Clin Microbiol. 2011;49:710–1.
29. Pancholi P, Kelly C, Raczkowski M, et al. Detection of toxigenic Clostridium difficile: comparison of the cell culture neutralization, Xpert C. difficile, Xpert C. difficile/Epi and the Illumigene C. difficile assays. J Clin Microbiol. 2012. doi:10.1128/JCM.06597-11.
30. Eltringham IJ. Diagnosis of Clostridium difficile infection by toxin detection kits. Lancet Infect Dis. 2008;12:777–84.
31. Rupnik M. Heterogeneity of large clostridial toxins: importance of Clostridium difficile toxinotypes. FEMS Microbiol Rev. 2008;32:541–55.
32. Cohen SH, Yajarayma JT, Hansen B, et al. Isolation of a toxin B-deficient mutant strain of Clostridium difficile in a case of recurrent C. difficile-associated diarrhea. Clin Infect Dis. 1998;26:410–2.
33. Kvach EJ, Ferguson D, Riska PF, et al. Comparison of BD GeneOhm Cdiff real-time PCR assay with a two-step algorithm and a toxin A/B enzyme-linked immunosorbent assay for diagnosis of toxigenic Clostridium difficile infection. J Clin Microbiol. 2010;48:109–14.
34. Drudy D, Fanning S, Kyne L. Toxin A-negative, toxin B-positive Clostridium difficile. Int J Infect Dis. 2007;11:5–10.
35. Couturier B, She RC. The illumigene C. difficile assay detects both A+B+ and A-B+ toxin-producing strains of Clostridium difficile. Abstract ID55, 16th Annual Meeting of the Association for Molecular Pathology. Bethesda, MD: Association for Molecular Pathology; 2010. p. 34.
36. van den Berg RJ, Ameen HA, Furusawa T, et al. Coexistence of multiple PCR-ribotype strains of Clostridium difficile in faecal samples limits epidemiological studies. J Med Microbiol. 2005;54:173–9.
37. Marth T. Tropheryma. In: Versalovic J, Carroll KC, Funke G, Jorgensen JH, Landry ML, Warnock DW, editors. Manual of clinical microbiology, vol. 1. 10th ed. Washington: American Society for Microbiology; 2011. p. 1035–9.
38. Fenollar F, Puéchal X, Raoult D. Whipple's disease. N Engl J Med. 2007;356:55–66.

39. Ehrbar HU, Bauerfeind P, Dutly F, et al. PCR-positive tests for Tropheryma whippelii in patients without Whipple's disease. Lancet. 1999;353:2214.
40. Dobbins 3rd WO. The diagnosis of Whipple's disease. N Engl J Med. 1995;332:390–2.
41. Misbah SA, Mapstone NP. Whipple's disease revisited. J Clin Pathol. 2000;53:750–5.
42. Maiwald M, von Herbay A, Persing DH, et al. Tropheryma whippelii DNA is rare in the intestinal mucosa of patients without other evidence of Whipple disease. Ann Intern Med. 2001;134:115–9.
43. Street S, Donoghue HD, Neild GH. Tropheryma whippelii DNA in saliva of healthy people. Lancet. 1999;354:1178–9.
44. Fenollar F, Raoult D. Molecular techniques in Whipple's disease. Expert Rev Mol Diagn. 2001;1:299–309.
45. Ramzan NN, Loftus Jr E, Burgart LJ, et al. Diagnosis and monitoring of Whipple disease by polymerase chain reaction. Ann Intern Med. 1997;126:520–7.
46. von Herbay A, Ditton HJ, Mailwald M. Diagnostic application of a polymerase chain reaction assay for the Whipple's disease bacterium to intestinal biopsies. Gastroenterology. 1996;110:1735–43.
47. Dutly F, Hinrikson HP, Seidel T, et al. Tropheryma whippelii DNA in saliva of patients without Whipple's disease. Infection. 2000;28:219–22.
48. Sloan LM, Rosenblatt JE, Cockerill 3rd FR. Detection of Tropheryma whipplei DNA in clinical specimens by Lightcycler real-time PCR. J Clin Microbiol. 2005;43:3516–8.
49. Fenollar F, Fournier PE, Raoult D, et al. Quantitative detection of Tropheryma whipplei DNA by real-time PCR. J Clin Microbiol. 2002;40:1119–20.
50. Fenollar F, Fournier PE, Robert C, et al. Use of genome selected repeated sequences increases the sensitivity of PCR detection of Tropheryma whipplei. J Clin Microbiol. 2004;42:401–3.
51. Suerbaum S, Michetti P. Helicobacter pylori infection. N Engl J Med. 2002;347:1175–86.
52. Lawson AJ. Helicobacter. In: Versalovic J, Carroll KC, Funke G, Jorgensen JH, Landry ML, Warnock DW, editors. Manual of clinical microbiology, vol. 2. 10th ed. Washington, DC: American Society for Microbiology; 2011. p. 900–15.
53. McColl KE. Helicobacter pylori infection. N Engl J Med. 2010;362:1597–604.
54. Fischbach W, Goebeler-Kolve ME, Dragosics B, et al. Long term outcome of patients with gastric marginal zone B cell lymphoma of mucosa associated lymphoid tissue (MALT) following exclusive Helicobacter pylori eradication therapy: experience from a large prospective series. Gut. 2004;53:34–7.
55. Parsonnet J. Helicobacter pylori and gastric cancer. Gastroenterol Clin North Am. 1993;22:89–104.
56. Mégraud F, Lehours P. Helicobacter pylori detection and antimicrobial susceptibility testing. Clin Microbiol Rev. 2007;20:280–322.
57. Chey WD, Wong BC, et al. American College of Gastroenterology guideline on the management of Helicobacter pylori infection. Am J Gastroenterol. 2007;102:1808–25.
58. Lo CC, Lai KH, Peng NJ, et al. Polymerase chain reaction: a sensitive method for detecting Helicobacter pylori infection in bleeding peptic ulcers. World J Gastroenterol. 2005;11:3909–14.
59. Weiss J, Tsang TK, Meng X, et al. Detection of Helicobacter pylori gastritis by PCR and CLOtest findings. Am J Clin Pathol. 2008;129:89–96.
60. Shukla SK, Prasad KN, Tripathi A, et al. Quantitation of Helicobacter pylori ureC gene and its comparison with different diagnostic techniques and gastric histopathology. J Microbiol Methods. 2011;86:231–7.
61. Kobayashi D, Eishi Y, Ohkusa T, et al. Gastric mucosal density of Helicobacter pylori estimated by real-time PCR compared with results of urea breath test and histological grading. J Med Microbiol. 2002;51:305–11.
62. He Q, Wang JP, Osato M, et al. Real-time quantitative PCR for detection of Helicobacter pylori. J Clin Microbiol. 2002;40:3720–8.
63. Ramírez-Lázaro MJ, Lario S, Casalots A, et al. Real-time PCR improves Helicobacter pylori detection in patients with peptic ulcer bleeding. PLoS One. 2011;6:e20009.
64. Gisbert JP, Abraira V. Accuracy of Helicobacter pylori diagnostic tests in patients with bleeding peptic ulcer: a systematic review and meta-analysis. Am J Gastroenterol. 2006;101:848–63.
65. Moshkowitz M, Konikoff FM, Peled Y, et al. High Helicobacter pylori numbers are associated with low eradication rate after triple therapy. Gut. 1995;36:845–7.
66. Chisholm SA, Owen RJ. Application of polymerase chain reaction-based assays for rapid identification and antibiotic resistance screening of Helicobacter pylori in gastric biopsies. Diagn Microbiol Infect Dis. 2008;61:67–71.
67. Panayotopoulou EG, Sgouras DN, Papadakos KS, et al. CagA and VacA polymorphisms are associated with distinct pathological features in Helicobacter pylori-infected adults with peptic ulcer and non-peptic ulcer disease. J Clin Microbiol. 2010;48:2237–9.
68. Van Doorn LJ, Figueiredo C, Sanna R, et al. Clinical relevance of the cagA, vacA, and iceA status of Helicobacter pylori. Gastroenterology. 1998;115:58–66.
69. Blaser MJ, Perez-Perez GI, Kleanthous H, et al. Infection with Helicobacter pylori strains possessing cagA is associated with an increased risk of developing adenocarcinoma of the stomach. Cancer Res. 1995;55:2111–5.
70. Atherton JC, Cover TL, Twellis RJ, et al. Simple and accurate PCR-based system for typing vacuolating cytotoxin alleles of Helicobacter pylori. J Clin Microbiol. 1999;37:2979–82.
71. Chisholm SA, Teare EL, Patel B, et al. Determination of Helicobacter pylori vacA allelic types by single-step multiplex PCR. Lett Appl Microbiol. 2002;35:42–6.
72. Scholte GH, Van Doorn LJ, Quint WG, et al. Genotyping of Helicobacter pylori strains in formalin-fixed or formaldehyde-sublimate-fixed paraffin-embedded gastric biopsy specimens. Diagn Mol Pathol. 2001;10:166–70.
73. Yamaoka Y. Mechanisms of disease: Helicobacter pylori virulence factors. Nat Rev Gastroenterol Hepatol. 2010;7:629–41.
74. El-Omar EM, Carrington M, Chow WH, et al. Interleukin-1 polymorphisms associated with increased risk of gastric cancer. Nature. 2000;404:398–402.
75. Malfertheiner P, Megraud F, O'Morain C, et al. Current concepts in the management of Helicobacter pylori infection: the Maastrict III consensus report. Gut. 2007;56:772–81.
76. Lu JJ, Perng CL, Shyu RY, et al. Comparison of five PCR methods for detection of Helicobacter pylori DNA in gastric tissues. J Clin Microbiol. 1999;37:772–4.
77. Singh V, Mishra S, Rao GR, et al. Evaluation of nested PCR in detection of Helicobacter pylori targeting a highly conserved gene: HSP60. Helicobacter. 2008;13:30–4.
78. Chisholm SA, Owen RJ. Development and application of a novel screening PCR assay for direct detection of 'Helicobacter heilmannii'-like organisms in human gastric biopsies in Southeast England. Diagn Microbiol Infect Dis. 2003;46:1–7.
79. MacKay WG, Williams CL, McMillan M, et al. Evaluation of protocol using gene capture and PCR for detection of Helicobacter pylori DNA in feces. J Clin Microbiol. 2003;41:4589–93.
80. Shuber AP, Ascaño JJ, Boynton KA, et al. Accurate, noninvasive detection of Helicobacter pylori DNA from stool samples: potential usefulness for monitoring treatment. J Clin Microbiol. 2002;40:262–4.
81. Fontana C, Favaro M, Pietroiusti A, et al. Detection of clarithromycin-resistant Helicobacter pylori in stool samples. J Clin Microbiol. 2003;41:3636–40.

82. Russo F, Notarnicola M, Di Matteo G, et al. Detection of Helicobacter pylori cagA gene by polymerase chain reaction in faecal samples. Eur J Gastroenterol Hepatol. 1999;11:251–6.
83. Matsumura M, Hikiba Y, Ogura K, et al. Rapid detection of mutations in the 23S rRNA gene of Helicobacter pylori that confers resistance to clarithromycin treatment to the bacterium. J Clin Microbiol. 2001;39:691–5.
84. Chisholm SA, Owen RJ, Teare EL, et al. PCR-based diagnosis of Helicobacter pylori infection and real-time determination of clarithromycin resistance directly from human gastric biopsy samples. J Clin Microbiol. 2001;39:1217–20.
85. Oleastro M, Ménard A, Santos A, et al. Real-time PCR assay for rapid and accurate detection of point mutations conferring resistance to clarithromycin in Helicobacter pylori. J Clin Microbiol. 2003;41:397–402.
86. Gibson JR, Saunders NA, Burke B, et al. Novel method for rapid determination of clarithromycin sensitivity in Helicobacter pylori. J Clin Microbiol. 1999;37:3746–8.
87. Schabereiter-Gutner C, Hirschl AM, Dragosics B, et al. Novel real-time PCR assay for detection of Helicobacter pylori infection and simultaneous clarithromycin susceptibility testing of stool and biopsy specimens. J Clin Microbiol. 2004;42:4512–8.
88. Glocker E, Kist M. Rapid detection of point mutations in the gyrA gene of Helicobacter pylori conferring resistance to ciprofloxacin by a fluorescence resonance energy transfer-based real-time PCR approach. J Clin Microbiol. 2004;42:2241–6.
89. Lawson AJ, Elviss NC, Owen RJ. Real-time PCR detection and frequency of 16S rDNA mutations associated with resistance and reduced susceptibility to tetracycline in Helicobacter pylori from England and Wales. J Antimicrob Chemother. 2005;56:282–6.
90. Chisholm SA, Owen RJ. Mutations in Helicobacter pylori rdxA gene sequences may not contribute to metronidazole resistance. J Antimicrob Chemother. 2003;51:995–9.
91. Trebesius K, Panthel K, Strobel S, et al. Rapid and specific detection of Helicobacter pylori macrolide resistance in gastric tissue by fluorescent in situ hybridization. Gut. 2000;46:608–14.
92. Jüttner S, Vieth M, Miehlke S, et al. Reliable detection of macrolide-resistant Helicobacter pylori via fluorescence in situ hybridization in formalin-fixed tissue. Mod Pathol. 2004; 17:684–9.
93. El-Zaatari FA, Oweis SM, Graham DY. Uses and cautions for use of polymerase chain reaction for detection of Helicobacter pylori. Dig Dis Sci. 1997;42:2116–9.
94. Makristathis A, Barousch W, Pasching E, et al. Two enzyme immunoassays and PCR for detection of Helicobacter pylori in stool specimens from pediatric patients before and after eradication therapy. J Clin Microbiol. 2000;38:3710–4.
95. Makristathis A, Pasching E, Schütze K, et al. Detection of Helicobacter pylori in stool specimens by PCR and antigen enzyme immunoassay. J Clin Microbiol. 1998;36:2772–4.
96. Kabir S. Detection of Helicobacter pylori DNA in feces and saliva by polymerase chain reaction: a review. Helicobacter. 2004;9:115–23.
97. Robinson C, Echavarria M. Adenoviruses. In: Versalovic J, Carroll KC, Funke G, Jorgensen JH, Landry ML, Warnock DW, editors. Manual of clinical microbiology, vol. 2. 10th ed. Washington: American Society for Microbiology; 2011. p. 1601–11.
98. Robinson CM, Singh G, Henquell C, et al. Computational analysis and identification of an emergent human adenovirus pathogen implicated in a respiratory fatality. Virology. 2011;409:141–7.
99. Horowitz MS. Adenoviruses. In: Knipe DM, Howley PM, Griffin DE, Lamb RA, Martin MA, Roizman B, Straus SE, editors. Fields virology, vol. 2. 4th ed. Philadelphia: Lippincott Williams & Wilkins; 2001. p. 2301–26.
100. Shenk TE. Adenoviridae: the viruses and their replication. In: Knipe DM, Howley PM, Griffin DE, Lamb RA, Martin MA, Roizman B, Straus SE, editors. Fields virology, vol. 2. 4th ed. Philadelphia: Lippincott Williams & Wilkins; 2001. p. 2265–300.
101. Kajon AE, Dickson LM, Murtagh P, et al. Molecular characterization of an adenovirus 3-16 intertypic recombinant isolated in Argentina from an infant hospitalized with acute respiratory infection. J Clin Microbiol. 2010;48:1494–6.
102. Heim A, Ebnet C, Harste G, et al. Rapid and quantitative detection of human adenovirus DNA by real-time PCR. J Med Virol. 2003;70:228–39.
103. Uhnoo I, Svensson L, Wadell G. Enteric adenoviruses. Baillieres Clin Gastroenterol. 1990;4:627–42.
104. Echavarria M, Maldonado D, Elbert G, Videla C, Rappaport R, Carballal G. Use of PCR to demonstrate presence of adenovirus species B, C, or F as well as coinfection with two adenovirus species in children with flu-like symptoms. J Clin Microbiol. 2006;44:625–7.
105. Lion T, Baumgartinger R, Watzinger F, et al. Molecular monitoring of adenovirus in peripheral blood after allogeneic bone marrow transplantation permits early diagnosis of disseminated disease. Blood. 2003;102:1114–20.
106. Echavarria M. Adenoviruses in immunocompromised hosts. Clin Microbiol Rev. 2008;21:704–15.
107. Sarantis H, Johnson G, Brown M, et al. Comprehensive detection and serotyping of human adenoviruses by PCR and sequencing. J Clin Microbiol. 2004;42:3963–9.
108. Gu Z, Belzer SW, Gibson CS. Multiplexed, real-time PCR for quantitative detection of human adenovirus. J Clin Microbiol. 2003;41:4636–41.
109. Storch GA. Diagnostic virology. In: Knipe DM, Howley PM, Griffin DE, Lamb RA, Martin MA, Roizman B, Straus SE, editors. Fields virology, vol. 1. 4th ed. Philadelphia: Lippincott Williams & Wilkins; 2011. p. 493–531.
110. Pring-Akerblom P, Adrian T. Type- and group-specific polymerase chain reaction for adenovirus detection. Res Virol. 1994;145:23–5.
111. Vabret A, Gouarin S, Joannes M, et al. Development of a PCR-and hybridization-based assay (PCR Adenovirus Consensus) for the detection and the species identification of adenoviruses in respiratory specimens. J Clin Virol. 2004;31:116–22.
112. Echavarria M, Forman M, Ticehurst J. PCR method for detection of adenovirus in urine of healthy and human immunodeficiency virus-infected individuals. J Clin Microbiol. 1998;36:3323–6.
113. Lion T, Kosulin K, Landlinger C, et al. Monitoring of adenovirus load in stool by real-time CPR permits early detection of impending invasive infection in patients after allogeneic stem cell transplantation. Leukemia. 2010;24:706–14.
114. Pring-Akerblom P, Trijssenaar J, Adrian T, et al. Multiplex polymerase chain reaction for subgenus-specific detection of human Adenoviruses in clinical specimens. J Med Virol. 1999;58:87–92.
115. Liu J, Kibiki G, Maro V, et al. Multiplex reverse transcription PCR Luminex assay for detection and quantitation of viral agents of gastroenteritis. J Clin Virol. 2011;50:308–13.
116. van Maarseveen NM, Wessels E, de Brouwer CS, et al. Diagnosis of viral gastroenteritis by simultaneous detection of Adenovirus group F, Astrovirus, Rotavirus group A, Norovirus genogroups I and II, and Sapovirus in two internally controlled multiplex real-time PCR assays. J Clin Virol. 2010;49:205–10.
117. Kidd AH, Jonsson M, Garwicz D, et al. Rapid subgenus identification of human Adenovirus isolates by a general PCR. J Clin Microbiol. 1996;34:622–7.
118. Guarner J, de Leon-Bojorge B, Lopez-Corella E, et al. Intestinal intussusception associated with Adenovirus infection in Mexican children. Am J Clin Pathol. 2003;120:845–50.
119. Jeulin H, Salmon A, Bordigoni P, et al. Comparison of in-house real-time quantitative PCR to the Adenovirus R-Gene kit for

determination of Adenovirus load in clinical samples. J Clin Microbiol. 2010;48:3132–7.
120. Allard A, Girones R, Juto P, et al. Polymerase chain reaction for detection of Adenoviruses in stool samples. J Clin Microbiol. 1990;28:2659–67.
121. Rousell J, Blair Zajdel ME, Howdle PD, et al. Rapid detection of enteric Adenoviruses by means of the polymerase chain reaction. J Infect. 1993;27:271–5.
122. Hierholzer JC, Halonen PE, Dahlen PO, et al. Detection of Adenovirus in clinical specimens by polymerase chain reaction and liquid-phase hybridization quantitated by time-resolved fluorometry. J Clin Microbiol. 1993;31:1886–91.
123. Ebner K, Suda M, Watzinger F, et al. Molecular detection and quantitative analysis of the entire spectrum of human Adenoviruses by a two-reaction PCR assay. J Clin Microbiol. 2005;43:3049–53.
124. Damen M, Minnaar R, Glasius P, et al. Real-time PCR with an internal control for detection of all known human adenovirus serotypes. J Clin Microbiol. 2008;46:3997–4003.
125. Buitenwerf J, Louwerens JJ, De Jong JC. A simple and rapid method for typing adenoviruses 40 and 41 without cultivation. J Virol Methods. 1985;10:39–44.
126. Johansson ME, Brown M, Hierholzer JC, et al. Genome analysis of Adenovirus type 31 strains from immunocompromised and immunocompetent patients. J Infect Dis. 1990;163:293–9.
127. Allard A, Albinsson B, Wadell G, et al. Rapid typing of human Adenoviruses by a general PCR combined with restriction endonuclease analysis. J Clin Microbiol. 2001;39:498–505.
128. Quan-Gen L, Henningsson A, Juto P, et al. Use of restriction fragment analysis and sequencing of a serotype-specific region to type Adenovirus isolates. J Clin Microbiol. 1999;37:844–7.
129. Baldwin A, Kingman H, Darvill M, et al. Outcome and clinical course of 100 patients with adenovirus infection following bone marrow transplantation. Bone Marrow Transplant. 2000;26:1333–8.
130. Krishnan T, Sen A, Choudhury JS, et al. Emergence of adult diarrhoea rotavirus in Calcutta, India. Lancet. 1999;353:380–1.
131. Parashar UD, Gibson CJ, Bresse JS, et al. Rotavirus and severe childhood diarrhea. Emerg Infect Dis. 2006;12:304–6.
132. Curns AT, Panozzo CA, Tate JE, et al. Remarkable postvaccination spatiotemporal changes in US rotavirus activity. Pediatr Infect Dis J. 2011;30:S54–5.
133. Ward RL, Bernstein DI, Young EC, et al. Human rotavirus studies in volunteers: determination of infectious dose and serological response to infection. J Infect Dis. 1986;154:871–80.
134. Butz AM, Fosarelli P, Kick J, et al. Prevalence of rotavirus on high-risk fomites in daycare facilities. Pediatrics. 1993;92:202–5.
135. Hardy D. Epidemiology of rotaviral infection in adults. Rev Infect Dis. 1987;9:461–9.
136. Dennehy PH, Hartin M, Nelson SM, et al. Evaluation of the ImmunoCardSTAT! rotavirus assay for detection of group A rotavirus in fecal specimens. J Clin Microbiol. 1999;37:1977–9.
137. Argüelles MH, Villegas GA, Castello A, et al. VP7 and VP4 genotyping of human group A rotavirus in Buenos Aires, Argentina. J Clin Microbiol. 2000;38:252–9.
138. Patel MM, Tate JE, Selvarangan R, et al. Routine laboratory testing data for surveillance of rotavirus hospitalizations to evaluate the impact of vaccination. Pediatr Infect Dis J. 2007;26:914–9.
139. Gunson RN, Miller J, Leonard A, et al. Importance of PCR in the diagnosis and understanding of rotavirus illness in the community. Commun Dis Public Health. 2003;6:63–5.
140. O'Ryan ML, Lucero Y, Prado V, et al. Symptomatic and asymptomatic rotavirus and norovirus infections during infancy in a Chilean birth cohort. Pediatr Infect Dis J. 2009;28:879–84.
141. Zhang S, Chen TH, Wang J, et al. Symptomatic and asymptomatic infections of rotavirus, norovirus, and adenovirus among hospitalized children in Xi'an, China. J Med Virol. 2011;83:1476–84.
142. Blutt SE, Matson DO, Crawford SE, et al. Rotavirus antigenemia in children is associated with viremia. PLoS Med. 2007;4:e121.
143. Ushijima H, Xin KQ, Nishimura S, et al. Detection and sequencing of rotavirus VP7 gene from human materials (stools, sera, cerebrospinal fluids, and throat swabs) by reverse transcription and PCR. J Clin Microbiol. 1994;32:2893–7.
144. Kapoor A, Li L, Victoria J, et al. Multiple novel astrovirus species in human stool. J Gen Virol. 2009;90:2965–72.
145. Caballero S, Guix S, Morsy El-Senousy W, et al. Persistent gastroenteritis in children infected with astrovirus: association with serotype-3 strains. J Med Virol. 2003;71:245–50.
146. Glass RI, Noel J, Mitchell D, et al. The changing epidemiology of astrovirus-associated gastroenteritis: a review. Arch Virol. 1996;12:287–300.
147. Koopmans MP, Bijen MH, Monroe SS, et al. Age-stratified seroprevalence of neutralizing antibodies to astrovirus types 1 to 7 in humans in The Netherlands. Clin Diagn Lab Immunol. 1998;5:33–7.
148. Rodriguez-Baez N, O'Brien R, Qiu S-Q, et al. Astrovirus, adenovirus, and rotavirus in hospitalized children: prevalence and association with gastroenteritis. J Pediatr Gastroenterol Nutr. 2002;35:64–8.
149. Aitken C, Jeffries DJ. Nosocomial spread of viral disease. Clin Microbiol Rev. 2001;14:528–46.
150. Walter JE, Mitchell DK. Astrovirus infection in children. Curr Opin Infect Dis. 2003;16:247–53.
151. Guix S, Bosch A, Pinto RM. Human astrovirus diagnosis and typing: current and future prospects. Lett Appl Microbiol. 2005;41:103–5.
152. Wunderli W, Meerbach A, Guengoer T, et al. Astrovirus infection in hospitalized infants with severe combined immunodeficiency after allogeneic hematopoietic stem cell transplantation. PLoS One. 2011;6:e27483.
153. Holtz LR, Wylie KM, Sodergren E, et al. Astrovirus MLB2 viremia in febrile child. Emerg Infect Dis. 2011;17:2050–2.
154. Scipioni A, Mauroy A, Vinjé J, Thiry E. Animal noroviruses. Vet J. 2008;178:32–45.
155. Bull RA, Tanaka MM, White PA. Norovirus recombination. J Gen Virol. 2007;88:3347–59.
156. Dove W, Cunliffe NA, Gondwe JS, et al. Detection and characterization of human caliciviruses in hospitalized children with acute gastroenteritis in Blantyre, Malawi. J Med Virol. 2005;77:522–7.
157. Farkas T, Deng X, Ruiz-Palacios G, et al. Development of an enzyme immunoassay for detection of sapovirus-specific antibodies and its application in a study of seroprevalence in children. J Clin Microbiol. 2006;44:3674–9.
158. Atmar RL, Estes MK. Diagnosis of noncultivatable gastroenteritis viruses, the human caliciviruses. Clin Microbiol Rev. 2001;14:15–37.
159. Schaub SA, Oshiro RK. Public health concerns about caliciviruses as waterborne contaminants. J Infect Dis. 2000;181:S374–80.
160. Parashar U, Parashar U, Quiroz ES, et al. Norwalk-like viruses. Public health consequences and outbreak management. MMWR Recomm Rep. 2001;50:1–17.
161. Moreno-Espinosa S, Farkas T, Jiang X. Human caliciviruses and pediatric gastroenteritis. Semin Pediatr Infect Dis. 2004;15:237–45.
162. Rabenau HF, Sturmer M, Buxbaum S, et al. Laboratory diagnosis of norovirus: which method is the best? Intervirology. 2003;46:232–8.
163. Richards AF, Lopman B, Gunn A, et al. Evaluation of a commercial ELISA for detecting Norwalk-like virus antigen in faeces. J Clin Virol. 2003;26:109–15.
164. Burton-MacLeod JA, Kane EM, Beard RS, et al. Evaluation and comparison of two commercial enzyme-linked immunosorbent

assay kits for detection of antigenically diverse human noroviruses in stool samples. J Clin Microbiol. 2004;42:2587–95.
165. Chan MC, Sung JJ, Lam RK, et al. Sapovirus detection by quantitative real-time RT-PCR in clinical stool specimens. J Virol Methods. 2006;134:146–53.
166. Oka T, Katayama K, Hansman GS, et al. Detection of human sapovirus by real-time reverse transcription-polymerase chain reaction. J Med Virol. 2006;78:1347–53.
167. Honma S, Nakata S, Sakai Y, et al. Sensitive detection and differentiation of Sapporo virus, a member of the family Caliciviridae, by standard and booster nested polymerase chain reaction. J Med Virol. 2001;65:413–7.
168. Okada M, Yamashita Y, Oseto M, Shinozaki K. The detection of human sapoviruses with universal and genogroup-specific primers. Arch Virol. 2006;151:2503–9.
169. Kojima S, Kageyama T, Fukushi S, et al. Genogroup-specific PCR primers for detection of Norwalk-like viruses. J Virol Methods. 2003;100:107–14.
170. Kageyama T, Kojima S, Shinohara M, et al. Broadly reactive and highly sensitive assay for Norwalk-like viruses based on real-time quantitative reverse transcription-PCR. J Clin Microbiol. 2003;41:1548–57.
171. Hansman GS, Katayama K, Maneekarn N, et al. Genetic diversity of norovirus and sapovirus in hospitalized infants with sporadic cases of acute gastroenteritis in Chiang Mai, Thailand. J Clin Microbiol. 2004;42:1305–7.
172. Yan H, Yagyu F, Okitsu S, et al. Detection of norovirus (GI, GII), Sapovirus and astrovirus in fecal samples using reverse transcription single-round multiplex PCR. J Virol Methods. 2003;114:37–44.
173. Takanashi S, Hashira S, Matsunaga T, et al. Detection, genetic characterization, and quantification of norovirus RNA from sera of children with gastroenteritis. J Clin Virol. 2009;44:161–3.
174. Ito S, Takeshita S, Nezu A, et al. Norovirus-associated encephalopathy. Pediatr Infect Dis J. 2006;25:651–2.
175. Amin OM. Seasonal prevalence of intestinal parasites in the United States during 2000. Am J Trop Med Hyg. 2002;66:799–803.
176. Marti H, Koella JC. Multiple stool examinations for ova and parasites and rate of false-negative results. J Clin Microbiol. 1993;31:3044–5.
177. Polage CR, Stoddard GJ, Rolfs RT, et al. Physician use of parasite tests in the United States from 1997 to 2006 and in a Utah Cryptosporidium outbreak in 2007. J Clin Microbiol. 2011;49:591–6.
178. Pineiro L, Vicente D, Montes M, et al. Human parechoviruses in infants with systemic infection. J Med Virol. 2010;82:1790–6.

Sexually Transmitted Diseases

51

Jeanne A. Jordan

Abstract

Sexually transmitted infections are a major public health problem. The Centers for Disease Control and Prevention estimates over 20 million new infections occur each year in the USA alone, resulting in medical costs of $16 billion. Successful screening programs and accurate assays are therefore key to identifying infected individuals so that treatment and partner notification can be conducted to prevent the further spread of STIs. This chapter on STIs focuses on four of the most prevalent infections: *Chlamydia trachomatis*, *Neisseria gonorrhoeae*, *Trichomonas vaginalis*, and human papillomavirus.

Keywords

Sexually transmitted diseases • *Chlamydia trachomatis* • *Neisseria gonorrhoeae* • *Trichomonas vaginalis* • Human papillomavirus • Clinical molecular testing • Nucleic acid amplification testing

Introduction

Sexually transmitted infections (STIs) are a major public health problem. The Centers for Disease Control and Prevention (CDC) estimates over 20 million new infections occur each year in the USA alone, resulting in medical costs of $16 billion. Successful screening programs and accurate assays are therefore key to identifying infected individuals so that treatment and partner notification can be conducted to prevent the further spread of STIs. This chapter on STIs will focuses on four of the most prevalent infections: *Chlamydia trachomatis*, *Neisseria gonorrhoeae*, *Trichomonas vaginalis*, and human papillomavirus.

J.A. Jordan, Ph.D. (✉)
Epidemiology and Biostatistics, School of Public Health and Health Services, The George Washington University, 2300 Eye Street, Washington DC, USA
e-mail: jajordan@gwu.edu

C. trachomatis and *N. gonorrhoeae*

C. trachomatis (CT) and *N. gonorrhoeae* (NG; also abbreviated GC for gonococcus) are presented together, not because of their similarities in disease presentation, but because of the current trend in screening samples for both simultaneously. Historically, these organisms were identified using very different laboratory methods: CT by tissue culture and NG by growth on specialized bacterial medium. However, today these two STIs are primarily diagnosed using nucleic acid amplification testing (NAT), the focus of this chapter, rather than by culture or immunoassay.

C. trachomatis

Description of the Organism

C. trachomatis is a gram-negative, obligate intracellular bacterium of global public health significance. Infection with CT is associated with three different disease presentations: (1) trachoma, an infection of the eye, which if left untreated causes irreversible blindness (associated with infections of

D.G.B. Leonard (ed.), *Molecular Pathology in Clinical Practice*, DOI 10.1007/978-3-319-19674-9_51

CT serovars A, B, B1, and C); (2) genital infections in both women and men, which can cause serious complications in both sexes (associated with serovars D-K); and (3) lymphogranuloma venereum (LV), also considered an STI, which if untreated can lead to enlargement and ulceration of the external genitalia as well as lymphatic obstruction (associated with serovars L1, L2, and L3) [1]. This chapter focuses on the diagnosis of those serovars causing genital infections.

Clinical Utility

Worldwide, genital CT causes more cases of STI than any other bacterial pathogen, and as such, represents a major reproductive health problem. The World Health Organization (WHO) estimates that annually there are 89 million new cases of genital CT globally, with more than 4 million cases occurring annually in North America alone. In 2010, the CDC reported regional positivity rates in US women ≤25 year old being tested in family planning clinics that ranged from 5.5 to 11.3 %. In that same 2010 report, the rate of CT infection in US women was 610.6 per 100,000 [2].

In the USA alone, the CDC estimates that there were over 1.3 million new cases of CT in 2010. The population most affected by these STIs is young women ≤25 years of age. However, rates of CT and/or NG infection are also on the rise in men who have sex with men (MSM). In the MSM population, the infection can present in genital, anal, and/or pharyngeal sites, and as such non-urine based samples must be considered if infections are to be detected and treated.

CT is a major cause of secondary infertility in females, due to its association with cervicitis, endometritis, and urethritis, which can lead to scarring of the affected tissues. Between 10–40 % of CT infections in females will result in pelvic inflammatory disease (PID), with sequelae including ectopic pregnancy, tubal factor infertility, and chronic pelvic pain [3]. The risk of developing any one of these sequelae increases with the number of PID episodes that an individual experiences. Additionally, pregnant women infected with CT are at risk of transmitting the infection to their newborn infants resulting in newborn conjunctivitis or pneumonia. In males, genital CT infection is associated with nongonococcal urethritis (NGU), epididymitis, prostatitis, proctitis, and Reiter syndrome [1, 4]. Reiter syndrome is an inflammatory disease usually following an infection and affecting the joints, urinary tract, and eyes, as well as ulceration of the skin and mouth.

The individuals at greatest risk of genital CT infections are adolescents and young adults, ages 15–24 years, which is similar to the age of prevalence for human papillomavirus (HPV). Intervention based on selective screening for genital CT infection has reduced its prevalence, as well as the incidence of PID and ectopic pregnancy. These improved outcomes have occurred with the implementation of NAT, use of less-invasive and better-tolerated collection techniques, and development of transport systems that stabilize nucleic acid. Molecular testing for STIs is an advantageous approach, especially in the high-prevalence or high-risk patient populations.

CT infections commonly are asymptomatic in both women and men, with up to 70 % of infected females and 50 % of infected males lacking symptoms. This results in a significant number of individuals not seeking treatment, further transmitting the infection, and at risk of developing complications from the infection. Mass screening programs in Europe have led to a significant reduction in CT prevalence. However, to be successful, these programs must be practical and acceptable to the targeted patient populations. Acceptable screening programs include using self-collected vaginal specimens or first-void urines that can be stably shipped at ambient temperatures. This strategy has the advantage of limiting the number of physician office visits for individuals, thereby increasing compliance.

Urine samples are recommended when screening men for CT. However, other sites including rectal and pharyngeal screening also should be obtained if there is a history of anal and/or oral sex practices. The CDC recommends NAT for CT screening of all non-genital sites. Because this practice may be off-label use of an FDA-cleared test, the laboratory is responsible for validation of the test performance with non-genital site specimens prior to clinical use.

N. gonorrhoeae

Description of the Organism

N. gonorrhoeae (NG) is a gram-negative, oxidase-positive, intracellular diplococcus. Microscopically, the microorganism has a characteristic kidney or coffee bean appearance.

NG is a fastidious organism, being highly susceptible to temperature extremes and desiccation, which results in less-than-satisfactory isolation by culture, especially when off-site specimen transportation is required before culture [5].

Clinical Utility

The fastidious nature of NG has led to a transition from culture toward molecular testing [6]. Interestingly, experiences with NG testing have led some investigators to conclude that NAT for NG does not appreciably increase the number of positive specimens compared to culture methods, if optimal transport conditions have been maintained. However, NAT allows for the use of alternative, less-invasive specimens such as urine and self-collected vaginal swabs for NG detection. This strategy avoids the need to collect urethral or endocervical specimens, which should increase compliance for testing.

Like CT, the incidence of NG is highest among adults < 25 years of age. NG remains second only to CT infection in the number of bacterial cases of a reportable STI. Worldwide, approximately 62 million new cases of NG occur annually. In the USA in 2010, there were 100.8 cases of NG per 100,000 population, with an overall 309,341 cases reported to the CDC [2]. NG-associated urogenital tract infections, as for CT, can be silent and lack symptoms altogether, or the infection can present with mild-to-severe symptoms. In men, symptoms include acute urethritis and discharge, which if left untreated can lead to the following complications: epididymitis, prostatitis, or urethral strictures. In women infected with NG, symptoms can include endocervical inflammation and discharge, which if not treated can lead to abscess formation, salpingitis, or PID. In women, complications of NG infection include risk of infertility and ectopic pregnancy. Disseminated NG infection, although uncommon (approximately 1 % of cases), usually has a poor outcome, which includes bacteremia, skin rash, and asymmetrical septic polyarthritis. Over time, NG has developed resistance to antibiotics, including fluoroquinolone [7, 8], leaving the cephalosporins as the only class of recommended antibiotics remaining for treatment of NG infections.

Available Tests

Prior to the introduction of molecular testing, CT and NG were detected from clinical specimens primarily by culture. For CT, more rapid tests were developed to facilitate shorter turnaround times and included enzyme immunoassays (EIA) to detect either the lipopolysaccharide or major outer membrane protein antigen and direct fluorescence assays that used genus-specific or species-specific monoclonal antibodies [1]. For NG, direct gram stain and culture have been used routinely. Guidelines for CT and NG screening now include molecular testing as a recommended test method [2].

More molecular test platforms have been cleared by the US Food and Drug Administration (FDA) for detecting CT and/or NG than for any other infectious pathogen. These platforms include both non-amplified (e.g., the PACE DNA probe assay, Gen-Probe, San Diego, CA) and amplified testing methods. The non-amplified probe-based assays are not discussed further in this chapter.

The popularity of using NAT for CT and NG can be partially explained by market pressures; the sheer volume of STI testing performed annually drives commercial interests. In addition, a wide variety of validated specimen types have been approved for use with these testing platforms, both in symptomatic individuals and in asymptomatic individuals, which helps to facilitate compliance in high-risk groups for this ever-growing public health concern.

Table 51.1 lists seven FDA-cleared NAT platforms for CT and NG; four use target amplification and one uses signal amplification methods. The table summarizes the test methods, purification strategies, amplification and detection schemes, and types of contamination controls and internal amplification controls included in the test kit. The sample preparation protocols vary widely for these kits and range from using crude cell lysates to purified nucleic acid for testing. The different sample types used and the extent of sample purification affect the rates of inhibition and thus the need to include an internal amplification control.

Interpretation of Test Results

Tables 51.2, 51.3, 51.4, 51.5, 51.6, 51.7, and 51.8 describe in detail NAT platforms for CT and NG, including the genes targeted, the recommended clinical specimens, optimal specimen transport and storage conditions, specimen processing requirements, test interpretations, workflow issues, and other features of these test methods. Many investigators have published performance data using these platforms [9–22].

Laboratory Issues

Recommended Specimens for Testing

The recommended specimen types for NAT testing for CT/NG include vaginal swabs from women and urine specimens from men; both specimens are collected non-invasively, which improves testing acceptability in the at-risk populations [2].

Inhibitors and Internal Controls

Amplification inhibition is common for urogenital specimens, with consequent negative effects on test results [23]. The percentage of specimens containing amplification inhibitors ranges from 1 – 5 % for urines and as much as 20 % for cervical swabs. Initial studies found that inhibition could be reduced or eliminated if specimens were first refrigerated overnight or frozen and thawed before testing, pointing to the labile nature of some inhibitors. However, other inhibitors are quite stable and thus more difficult to neutralize. Many of the commercially available platforms include an internal control (IC) to identify specimens containing inhibitors. Testing algorithms state that when the internal control fails, the results of a specimen without detectable CT and/or NG cannot be reported as negative due to the likelihood that amplification inhibitors are present in the specimen.

Table 51.1 Characteristics of selected NAT platforms for *Chlamydia trachomatis* and *Neisseria gonorrhoeae*

Manufacturer	Assay method	Sample preparation	Amplification strategy	Detection strategy	Contamination controls	IC
Becton Dickinson	SDA	DNA extraction via para-magnetic particle technology	Target	Fluorescence	Closed System	Yes
					Routine environmental monitoring suggested for detecting contamination	
					Clean area using fresh 1 % (v/v) sodium hypochlorite, DNA AWAY, or 3 % (w/v) hydrogen peroxide	
Qiagen	Digene HC2	Hybrid capture from crude cell lysate	Signal	Chemiluminescence	Clean wash apparatus and tubing with 0.5 % sodium hypochlorite solution to prevent contamination from alkaline phosphatase. Check wash buffer and Reagent 2 for contamination	No
Hologic Gen-Probe	TMA and DKA	Target capture from crude cell lysate	Target	Chemiluminescence	Separate the various working areas; use unidirectional work-flow; decontaminate surfaces and pipettors with 2.5–3.5 % sodium hypochlorite; establish intervals for contamination monitoring	No
Roche Diagnostics	PCR	Crude cell lysate	Target	Colorimetric	AmpErase enzyme pre-amplification treatment to destroy previously generated amplicons; dUTP incorporation during amplification; unidirectional workflow; clean area using 0.5 % sodium hypochlorite	Yes
Roche Diagnostics	PCR	DNA extraction via magnetic glass particles	Target	Fluorescence	AmpErase enzyme pre-amplification treatment to destroy previously generated amplicons; dUTP incorporation during real-time PCR amplification	Yes
Abbott	PCR	DNA extraction via magnetic particle extraction technology on m2000sp	Target	Fluorescence	Routine environmental monitoring suggested for detecting contamination, if detected use 0.1 % v/v sodium hypochlorite followed by 70 % ethanol	Yes
Cepheid	PCR	DNA extraction performed within cartridge across a glass fiber affinity column	Target	Fluorescence	Individual, self-contained cartridges minimize cross-contamination	Yes

DKA dual kinetic assay, *HC2* hybrid capture 2, *IC* internal control, *NASBA* nucleic acid sequence-based amplification, *NAT* nucleic acid amplification testing, *PCR* polymerase chain reaction, *SDA* strand displacement amplification, *TMA* transcription-mediated amplification

Table 51.2 BectonDickinson ProbeTec™ ET CT/NG SDA assays run on viper system with XTR technology: parameters and test interpretation for CT/NG detection

Target	CT: Cryptic plasmid	
	NG: PivNg gene	
Specimens	Female and male urine	
	Endocervical, vaginal, and male urethral swabs	
	Endocervical liquid-based cytology	
Specimen handling	Urines: if collected unpreserved, store at 2–8 °C and process within 7 days of collection. If transferred to Q^X UPT within 8 h of collection, store at 2–30 °C and process within 30 days.	
	Endocervical swabs and male urethral swabs: transport swabs at 2–30 °C and process within 30 days.	
	Dry vaginal swabs: transport at 2–30 °C and process within 14 days of collection.	
	Vaginal swabs expressed in Q^X swab diluent: transport at 2–30 °C and process within 30 days.	
	Liquid based cytology specimens: transport and stored in original vials for up to 30 days at 2–30 °C.	
Test interpretation	CT/NG Q^X MaxRFU	Interpretation
CT/NG Q^X Pos control	≥125	QC Pass
CT/NG Q^X Pos control	<125	QC Fail
CT/NG Q^X Neg control	<125	QC Pass
CT/NG Q^X Neg control	≥125	QC Fail
CT/NG test result	≥125	CT Pos
CT/NG test result	<125	CT Neg
Other features	Positive control tubes contain approximately 2,400 copies each of pCTB4 and pNGint3 linearized plasmids. If the CT-specific signal is ≥125 MaxRFU then the extraction control value is ignored, but if it is <125 MaxRFU then the extraction control value is utilized by the algorithm for test result interpretation.	
Issues	Two *N. cinerea* and 2 *N. lactamica* strains cross-react in the NG Q^X assay. Blood in swab-based specimens exceeding 60 % may cause extraction control failures.	

MaxRFU maximum relative fluorescent units, *Neg* negative, *Pos* positive, *SDA* strand displacement amplification, *CT Chlamydia trachomatis*, *NG Neisseria gonorrhoeae*

Table 51.3 Qiagen HC2 assays (CT/NG dual ID HC2 DNA test, CT ID HC2 DNA test, and NG ID HC2 DNA test): parameters and test interpretation for CT/NG detection

Target	CT: 4 % of genome by CT RNA probe cocktail and 100 % of cryptic plasmid		
	NG: 0.5 % of genome by NG RNA probe cocktail and 100 % of cryptic plasmid		
Specimens	Cervical specimens (cervical brush in Specimen Transport Medium), or female swab specimen collection kit (Dacron swab and Specimen Transport Medium)		
Specimen handling	Cervical brush: Can be held for up to 2 weeks at room temperature and ship unrefrigerated to the laboratory. At the laboratory, specimens can be stored at 2–8 °C if testing is to be completed within 1 week, or stored at −20 °C for up to 3 months.		
	Swabs: Transport swabs at 2–27 °C; process within 4 days.		
Test interpretation	<1.00 RLU	Negative	CT and/or NG not detected
	≥1.00 RLU	Positive	CT and/or NG detected
Workflow issues	Positive results with the CT/NG Dual ID HC2 DNA test require follow up testing of the same specimen with the individual CT ID HC2 DNA Test and the NG ID HC2 DNA Test.		
Other features	Specimens may be tested manually or using the Rapid Capture System instrument for high-volume testing.		
	Cervical brush used with non-pregnant women only. Collect specimens from pregnant women using the HC Female Swab Collection Kit only.		
Issues	Presumptive cross-reactivity to certain other DNA sequences, such as pBR322 or pGEM in high concentration. Cross-reactivity observed with *C. psittaci, N. lactamica, N. meningitis, N. cuniculi*, and *N. mucosa.*		

HC2 hybrid capture 2, *ID* identification, *RLU* relative light units

Table 51.4 Hologic Gen-Probe Aptima Combo 2 assays run on Tigris DTS or panther system (TMA and DKA Technologies): parameters and test interpretation for CT/NG detection

Target	CT: 23S rRNA		
	NG: 16S rRNA		
Specimens	Female and male urine		
	Endocervical, vaginal, and male urethral swab		
	Liquid-based cytology (LBC) samples		
Specimen Handling	Swab-based specimens: transport at 2–30 °C and process within 60 days of collection.		
	Urines: transport urine in APTIMA urine transport tube at 2–30 °C and test within 30 days of collection.		
	LBC samples: once the LBC solution has been transferred to an APTIMA specimen transfer tube, test within 30 days of collection when stored at 2–8 °C or within 14 days when stored at 15–30 °C.		
	Transport all specimen types in the proper collection devices.		
Test interpretation	Signals in relative light units (RLU ×1,000)		
CT Test results	Negative	Equivocal	Positive
CT only	1 to <25	25 to <100	100 to <4,500
CT and NG	1 to <85	85 to <250	250 to <4,500
CT indeterminate	1 to <85	85 to <4,500	NA
NG test results	Negative	Equivocal	Positive
NG only	1 to <60	60 to <150	150 to <4,500
NG and CT	1 to <85	85 to <250	250 to <4,500
NG indeterminate	1 to <85	85 to <4,500	NA
Workflow issues	Simultaneous amplification and detection of CT and NG via differences in kinetic profiles of the probes; CT signal has rapid "flasher" kinetics, while NG signal has slower "glower" kinetics.		
	DTS options include manual assay or Tecan-assisted assay, or use of the TIGRIS DTS System.		
Other features	No known cross-reactivity with nongonococcal *Neisseria species.*		
Issues	Assay was not evaluated in low CT prevalence populations. Performance of vaginal swab specimens has not been evaluated in pregnant women or in women <16 years of age.		

CT Chlamydia trachomatis, *DKA* dual kinetic assay, *DTS* direct tube sampling, *LBC* liquid-based cytology, *NA* not applicable, *NG Neisseria gonorrhoeae*, *RLU* relative light units, *TMA* transcription-mediated amplification

False-negative NAT results

A new strain of *C. trachomatis* containing a 377 base pair deletion within its cryptic plasmid was described [24]. The deletion was found to be located within the target sequence of the Roche Cobas assay, resulting in false-negative results for this CT strain [24]. This would impact the epidemiologic surveillance data in areas where this strain circulated. Once identified, several manufacturers, including Roche, altered the design of their NAT, incorporating dual targets for CT detection.

Cross-Reactivity with Nongonococcal Neisseria Species and False-Positive Results

The specificity for some NAT platforms is problematic due to cross-reactivity with certain nongonococcal species of Neisseria [21, 25, 26]. This problem was thought to arise from the intraspecies and interspecies genetic recombination that occurs between Neisseria species, which can result in false-positive NAT results with certain of the commensal Neisseria species [19]. Of eight nongonococcal species tested, false-positive results were seen with *N. cinerea* and *N. lactamica* using the BD ProbeTec assay, with *N. subflava* and *N. cinerea* using the Roche Cobas assay, and with *N. lactamica*, *N. meningitis*, *N. cuniculi*, and *N. mucosa* using the Qiagen assay. Since *N. cinerea*, *N. lactamica*, *N. subflava*, and *N. sicca* isolates have been recovered from genital mucosa, genital specimens may result in false-positive results as is also true for pharyngeal specimens. A recent study evaluated the cross-reactivity patterns of six NAT tests designed to detect *N. gonorrhoeae* to nongonococcal strains. The study clearly demonstrated cross-reactivity from all six NATs, with false-positive reactions for the 234 isolates tested ranging from 1–14.1 %. The Cobas amplicor and ProbeTec tests showed the highest number of false-positive results at 14.1 % and 11 %, respectively [21].

Confirmatory Testing

When selecting a testing platform, the prevalence of infection in the population being tested is of significance. The analytical performance of any test is dependent on the prevalence of infection, with the risk of generating false-positive results being inversely related to the prevalence. These issues have fueled the debate over the need for confirmatory testing for positive test results for CT and NG, as both are reportable infections, with the potential for psy-

Table 51.5 Roche Cobas Amplicor CT/NG test and Cobas CT/NG test: parameters and test interpretation for CT/NG detection

Targets	CT: Cryptic plasmid				
	NG: M-Ngo PII (Cytosine DNA methyltransferase)				
Specimens	Female and male urine (CT only)				
	Endocervical and male urethral swabs (CT/NG)				
Specimen handling	Transport swabs and urine at 2–8 °C. Store swabs and urine at: 2–8 °C, process within 7 days of collection; –20 °C, process within 30–60 days of collection.				
Test interpretation					
For CT	IC	A450, A660	CT result	IC result	Interpretation
	Without	<0.2	NA	NA	Negative
		>0.2 to <2.0	NA	NA	Equivocal
		>2.0	NA	NA	Positive
	With	<0.2, ≥0.2	Negative	Positive	CT not detected
		<0.2, <0.2	Negative	Negative	Inhibitory specimen
		>0.2 to <2.0	Equivocal	Any	Equivocal
		≥2.0, Any value	Positive	Any	CT detected
For NG	IC	A450, A660	NG result	IC result	Interpretation
	Without	<0.2, NA	NA	NA	Negative
		≥0.2 to <3.5, NA	NA	NA	Equivocal[a]
		≥3.5, NA	NA	NA	Positive
	With	<0.2, ≥0.2	Negative	Positive	NG not detected
		<0.2, <0.2	Negative	Negative	Inhibition
		≥0.2 to <3.5, 0.2-3.5	Equivocal	Any	Equivocal[a]
		≥3.5, any	Positive	Any	NG detected
Workflow issues	Simultaneous amplification of CT/NG/IC with separate detection reactions.				
Other issues	IC is a plasmid-containing CT primer binding site and randomized internal sequence. The IC test was designed to permit detection of substances interfering with PCR if present at >20 copies/test. Reactions containing substances at lower concentrations may still result in inhibition, but not at detectable levels, and therefore result in a false-negative result for the target.				
	May detect nonpathogenic isolates of *N. subflava* and *N. cinerea*.				

[a]Equivocal result: Another aliquot is to be tested in duplicate and an interpretation made based on the results of at least 2 of 3 results using 2.0 A660 as the cutoff. See packet insert for details

A450 Absorbance 450, *A660* Absorbance 660, *CT Chlamydia trachomatis*, *DTS* direct tube sampling, *IC* internal control, *LBC* liquid-based cytology, *NA* not applicable, *NG Neisseria gonorrhoeae*, *PCR* polymerase chain reaction, *RLU* relative light units

Table 51.6 Roche Cobas 4800 System CT/NG Real-time PCR Test: Parameters and Test Interpretation for CT/NG Detection

Targets	CT: 2 targets used : one cryptic plasmid common to all CT serovars and one chromosomal DNA target in the *ompA* gene
	NG: 2 targets within the highly conserved DR-9 region
Specimens	Females: Self-collected vaginal swab collected in a clinical setting
	Males: urine specimen
Specimen handling	Transport self-collected vaginal swabs and male urine specimens stored in manufacturer's specific collection devices at 2–30 °C, stable for 12 months. Transport neat urine specimen at 2–30 °C, stable for 24 h.
Test interpretation	
CT POS, NG POS	Positive for both CT and NG DNA
CT NEG, NG NEG	Neither CT nor NG DNA was detected
CT POS, NG NEG	Positive for CT, NG DNA not detected
CT POS, NG invalid	Positive for CT, retest original specimen for NG
CT NEG, NG POS	CT DNA not detected, positive for NG
CT invalid, NG POS	Retest original specimen for CT, positive for NG
CT invalid, NG NEG	Retest original specimen for CT, NG not detected
CT NEG, NG invalid	CT DNA not detected, retest original specimen for NG
Invalid	Retest original specimen for both CT and NG
Failed	Retest original specimen for both CT and NG
Workflow issues	Batch sizes can either be 24/run or 96/run
Other issues	CT/NG IC consists of 2 recombinant plasmid DNAs one each specific for CT or NG genomic target sequences. The IC is also the sample processing control.
	Visibly bloody or dark brown-appearing vaginal swab samples or urine samples should not be processed. Highly viscous vaginal swab samples should have the swab removed and the sample vortexed before processing.

CT Chlamydia trachomatis, *NEG* negative, *NG Neisseria gonorrhoeae*, *POS* positive

Table 51.7 Abbott real-time CT/NG assay run on the m2000 System: parameters and test interpretation for CT/NG detection

Target	CT: Two DNA probes targeting the cryptic plasmid	
	NG: One DNA probe targeting the Opa gene	
Specimens	From symptomatic individuals: female endocervical swab, clinician-collected vaginal swab, and self-collected vaginal swab; male urethral swab; female and male urine specimen.	
	From asymptomatic individuals: clinician-collected vaginal swab and self-collected vaginal swab; female and male urine specimen.	
Specimen handling	Specimens must be collected using the Multi-Collect Specimens Collection Kit and may be stored and transported at 2–30 °C for up to 14 days. Longer storage requires storage at ≤ −10 °C for up to 90 days.	
Test interpretation	CT samples with no evidence of amplification	Negative for CT
	CT samples with a cycle number ≤ the assay CO	Positive for CT
	CT samples with a cycle number > than the assay CO	Equivocal for CT
	NG samples with no evidence of amplification, or with a cycle number > than the assay CO	Negative for NG
	NG samples with a cycle number ≤ to the assay CO	Positive for NG
Workflow issues	A sample with an initial interpretation of "Equivocal" for CT must be retested. An "Equivocal" interpretation does not apply to NG samples.	
Other features	The second set of CT-specific primers recognizes the new variant of CT (nvCT) [24]. The NG primers used do not cross-react with non-NG strains of Neisseria. The Abbott RealTime CT/NG assay will not detect plasmid-free *C. trachomatis* variants. Treatment success or failure should not be determined using this test. A negative result does not exclude the possibility of an infection, as results are dependent upon sample adequacy and absence of inhibitors.	

CO cutoff, *CT Chlamydia trachomatis*, *NG Neisseria gonorrhoeae*

Table 51.8 Cepheid Xpert real-time CT/NG assay

Target	CT: One chromosomal sequence	
	NG: Two chromosomal sequences	
Specimens	Symptomatic and asymptomatic females: first catch urine specimen, endocervical swab, self-collected vaginal swab collected in clinical setting.	
	Symptomatic and asymptomatic males: first catch urine specimen.	
Specimen Handling	Specimens must be collected in the specific manufacturer's transport devices	
	Swabs can be transported at 2–30 °C and are stable for up to 60 days at that temperature range	
	Urine specimen can be transported at 2–15 °C and are stable for up to 45 days, or transported at 2–30 °C and are stable for up to 3 days	
Test interpretation	CT detected; NG detected	Positive for CT1, NG2, and NG4 targets
	CT detected; NG not detected	Positive for CT1 target, Negative for NG2 and/or NG4 targets
	CT not detected; NG detected	Positive for NG2 and NG4 targets, Negative for CT1 target
	CT and NG not detected	Negative for CT1, and NG2 or NG4 targets
	Invalid	Sample adequacy control and/or sample processing control failed
	Error	Probe check control failed
	No result	Insufficient data collected
Other features	Built-in controls within each cartridge include a sample processing control, sample adequacy control and a probe check control.	
Workflow issues	Extraction, amplification and detection all occur within the cartridge.	

CT Chlamydia trachomatis, *NG Neisseria gonorrhoeae*

chosocial and/or medicolegal consequences for a false-positive or a true-positive result [27]. The newest 2010 CDC Guidelines for STI testing do not contain language recommending routine repeat testing of initial positive results [2]. NAT testing for CT/NG is the preferred diagnostic method of choice in evaluating adults and adolescents as victims of sexual assault [2].

Contamination Controls

The advent of NAT, with its exquisite sensitivity, has given birth to a whole new mind-set for cleanliness in the molecular testing laboratory. No longer is disinfection of the benchtop after a day's work adequate. New standards strive to remove or prevent amplicon contamination in the laboratory environment. Strategies includes daily cleaning of laboratory surfaces with a dilute bleach solution, and frequently replacing disposable gloves and gowns while working in the pre- and post-amplification area(s). Create and enforce a regular schedule for performing wipe testing to monitor for amplicon contamination. For many of the current NAT platforms, pre- and post-amplification steps should be performed, if possible, in separate rooms with positive and negative airflow, respectively. Alternatively, contamination can be greatly reduced when using a fully automated, closed real-time NAT system that incorporates sample preparation, nucleic acid amplification, and detection in a single closed reaction.

Validating Off-Label Use of CT/NG Tests

In at-risk populations, it is important to be able to detect rectal and/or oropharyngeal CT/NG infections using a NAT platform. To date, manufacturers of NAT tests for CT/NG have not included rectal and/or oropharyngeal specimens in their evaluations or clinical trials. Therefore, these applications are not described in the manufacturer's packet insert and must be validated by individual laboratories.

Future Directions

Continued Use of Self-Collected, Noninvasive Specimen Types

Reaching high-risk populations for STI screening will improve with policies that emphasize the use of noninvasively collected specimens, including self-collected vaginal swabs and first-void urine specimen [28]. This is especially true when attempting to reach the young adult patient population, age range from 14 – 24 years, where the prevalence of CT and NG infections is highest and the willingness to undergo a pelvic examination or urethral swab collection is lowest.

Liquid-Based Cytology Cervical Specimens for CT/NG NAT Testing

Testing for STIs using Pap smear specimens has become more common but only after critical issues were addressed that enabled liquid-based cytology samples to be used for STI testing [14]. One of the most important solutions developed was the concept of using a "pre-aliquot," prior to handling of the specimen in cytology, which solved the issue of cross-contamination from other specimens, as well as the ethical issue of waiting to perform the infectious disease testing until after the cytology screening is completed. Successful implementation of this strategy was not easy and required dialogue and cooperation between laboratories, pathologists, manufacturers, and regulatory bodies.

Antibiotic Resistance Testing Using NAT for Cephalosporin-Resistant *N. gonorrhoeae*

Resistance to penicillin, tetracycline, and fluoroquinolones is now common among *N. gonorrhoeae* isolates [7, 8, 29]. Now emergence of cephalosporin-resistant *N. gonorrhoeae* has been described in several countries around the world. Being able to screen for antimicrobial resistance using a NAT platform would be very useful from a public health perspective.

Trichomonas Vaginalis

Description of the Organism

Trichomonas vaginalis (TV) is a flagellated protozoan and the only species within its genus that can infect squamous epithelial cells of the human urogenital tract [30]. TV infection is considered to be a nonulcerative STI but is associated with severe local inflammation. In women, symptoms may include vulvar irritation and vaginal discharge, which appears frothy, mucopurulent, and yellow-green in color. During a TV infection, the vaginal pH is often abnormally elevated ($pH > 4.5$). Complications of TV infection in untreated women include endometritis, infertility, and cervical erosion. In men infected with TV, symptoms may include profuse purulent urethritis and a form of NGU, with complications including chronic prostatitis, urethral strictures, epididymitis, and/or infertility if the infection is untreated [31, 32].

Clinical Utility

Detection of TV infections in males has received far less attention than these infections in females. However, with the advent of NAT, this understudied infection in men has become more appreciated, and thus research studies have provided important information on its prevalence, clinical symptoms, sequelae, and the most appropriate specimen to collect for proper diagnosis. TV has a greater role in NGU than previously thought [33]. As with diagnosing TV infections in female patients, direct microscopic examination of urethral discharge has poor sensitivity for detecting TV in male patients.

Worldwide, TV infection accounts for approximately 276.4 million cases annually [34], which is greater than the number of cases of *C. trachomatis*, *N. gonorrhoeae*, and syphilis combined. In the USA, the annual incidence of TV infection is estimated to be approximately 8 million cases [2]. However, because TV infection is not a reportable disease, this number may be an underestimate. Unlike CT and NG, where prevalence is higher in adolescents and young adults, TV is more equally distributed among all age groups.

Detecting TV in an individual is considered by health-care providers to be a red flag for high-risk sexual behavior and is frequently present along with other STIs in the same individual. Diagnosing TV is difficult, because 50–70 % of all infected individuals are asymptomatic. Without a sensitive assay, infected individuals left untreated continue to act as a reservoir for ongoing disease transmission within the community.

TV infection is associated with two important sequelae: (1) an increased risk of acquiring human immunodeficiency virus (HIV); and (2) an increased risk of perinatal morbidity and mortality [35–38]. HIV transmission is enhanced by the local inflammatory reaction containing CD4-positive T cells within the genital tract that is present with TV infections. In women, TV infection is strongly associated with an abnormal vaginal ecology. Harboring TV may contribute to the change in vaginal flora, which is associated with decreased lactic acid production and subsequent increase in vaginal pH. Lactic acid production and the normally low pH of the genital tract environment help to inactivate HIV. Therefore, a change in the vaginal environment to a less hostile environment promotes an increased survival of HIV. If this hypothesis is correct, then controlling TV infections could lower HIV acquisition.

The increased risk of perinatal morbidity and mortality with TV infection is associated with premature rupture of membranes, preterm delivery, and low-birth-weight infants in pregnant women infected with TV [39]. Although controversial, these associations suggest a need for increased efforts to detect and treat this infection in pregnant women [40].

Screening for TV infection is less common than screening for CT and NG infections; often the practice is limited to public health clinics and obstetrical practices. Successful control of TV infections would be aided greatly by increased screening of high-risk populations, performing contact follow-ups with sexual partners, and using a more sensitive diagnostic assay. Improved detection of TV by using NAT, as is the case for CT, would be predicted to reduce the incidence of TV infection and assist in reducing HIV transmission and possibly even poor pregnancy outcomes [41].

Available Tests

Historically, the most common diagnostic method for TV in urogenital discharge was direct microscopic examination, broth culturing, or both. Direct microscopic examination of genital discharge material on a slide is certainly the most rapid and inexpensive method to use, but lacks adequate sensitivity, which is reported to be approximately 40–70 % [42]. The low level of sensitivity with microscopic examination may be due in part to the rapid loss of the characteristic protozoan motility once the organism is removed from a 37 °C environment. Loss of motility is accompanied by change in morphology; non-motile TV organisms round up and are difficult to differentiate from leukocytes, being similar in size.

Currently, broth culturing is the gold standard for detecting TV [43]. Successful growth in culture can be achieved with as few as 300–500 TV organisms per milliliter of vaginal fluid, but culturing requires 2–7 days of incubation and daily microscopic examination. Culture methods have sensitivities that range between 50 - 80 % but require specialized medium such as Diamond's broth, Tricosel medium, or the In-Pouch system (Biomed Diagnostics, Inc. White City, OR). These specialized media may not be available in the physician's office. In addition, some TV isolates do not grow in culture due to strain requirements, low numbers of organisms, or damaged/nonviable organisms.

These limitations led laboratories to develop NAT for TV DNA using a range of testing platforms, including conventional and real-time NAT assays [44–51]. To date, the most commonly cited NAT tests are laboratory-developed tests (LDTs). Table 51.9 lists the more common targets for LDT TV-specific assays, with the most sensitive assays being those targeting repetitive DNA sequences.

Interpretation of Test Results

Currently, a single FDA-cleared TV NAT test is available, the Hologic Gen-Probe APTIMA Trichomonas vaginalis assay that can be run on both the TIGRIS DTS and the PANTHER System. In 2011, one commercially available TV-specific NAT was FDA cleared. The Aptima *Trichomonas vaginalis* test (developed at Gen-Probe Inc.) detects 16S rRNA using TMA [52–54]. This assay fills a significant void in NAT STI screening algorithms. Tables 51.10 and 51.11 describe the details of this assay including interpretation of the test results.

Table 51.9 Summary of common laboratory-developed tests for *Trichomonas vaginalis* specific targets using NAT

Primer pair [Reference]	DNA target	Amplicon (bp)
TVK3, TVK7 [97]	Repetitive DNA	312
TVK3, TVK4 [97]	Repetitive DNA	350
BTUB2, BTUB9 [98]	Beta Tubulin	112
TV1, TV2 [99]	18S rRNA gene	312
TV-E650 [100]	E650	650
TVA5, TVA6 [99]	Ferredoxin gene	102

NAT nucleic acid testing

If a TV LDT generates a numerical value, then the rationale for establishing the positive and negative cutoff values for the assay as well as possibly an equivocal zone are required. The LDT standard operating procedure must define when to perform repeat testing on the original specimen and when to report a result as indeterminate. If culture-based testing is performed as the "gold standard" test, culture-negative, NAT-positive results for the same specimen must be assessed by an independent method. Lastly, an alternative proficiency testing program is required when external programs are not available.

Laboratory Issues

Before 2011, laboratories wanting to perform TV NAT would need to develop, validate, and implement diagnostic testing, as no commercial test was available. This would include establishing interpretation criteria for an LDT. Several important issues should be addressed when developing and validating a NAT for TV. Validating an LDT should include establishing the limit of detection (LOD), as well as determining the analytical performance characteristics including sensitivity, specificity, and positive and negative predictive values.

Target Selection

For TV NAT LDTs, the primers and probes should be assessed with specimens containing other organisms or specimen spiked with specific organisms similar to TV, which may cross-hybridize and result in a false-positive result. Specifically, other *Trichomonas* species, such as *T. tena*, as well as other organisms that may be present within the urogenital tract specimen, including human genomic DNA, should be tested. The TV-specific primer pairs and probes described in the literature recognize different gene targets that vary in their copy number. In general, choosing a gene target that is present in multiple copies per genome is usually preferable to choosing a single-copy gene target to improve the sensitivity of the test.

Internal Control

Both vaginal swabs and urine specimens can contain significant levels of inhibitors that interfere with the NAT reaction.

Table 51.10 Summary of the APTIMA *Trichomonas vaginalis* assay run on the TIGRIS DTS system

Manufacturer	Assay method	Sample preparation	Amplification strategy	Detection strategy	Contamination controls	IC
Hologic GenProbe	TMA and HPA	Target capture via capture oligomer	16S rRNA Target	Chemiluminescence	Closed System	No
					Routine environmental monitoring suggested for detecting contamination	

DTS direct tube sampling, *HPA* hybridization protection assay, *IC* internal control, *TMA* transcription mediated amplification

Table 51.11 Hologic Gen-Probe APTIMA *Trichomonas vaginalis* assay (target capture, transcription-mediated amplification (TMA) and hybridization protection assay (HPA) technologies): parameters and test interpretation for TV detection

Target	16S ribosomal RNA		
Specimens	Female urine specimen		
	Endocervical or vaginal swab		
	Endocervical sample collected in PreservCyt solution		
Specimen handling	Swab-based specimen: Transport at 2–30 °C and process within 60 days of collection.		
	Urine specimen: Transport urine specimen in APTIMA urine transport tube at 2–30 °C and test within 30 days of collection. Urine specimen still in primary collection containers must be transported to laboratory at 2–30 °C and transferred into the APTIMA urine specimen transport tube within 24 h of collection.		
	LBC samples: Transport and store LBC samples at 2–30 °C for up to 30 days. LBC samples must be transferred into an APTIMA specimen transfer tube, after transfer, specimens may be stored an additional 14 days at 15–30 °C or 30 days at 2–8 °C.		
Test interpretation	Signals in relative light units (RLU ×1,000)		
TV test results	Negative for TV	Positive for TV	Invalid Results
	0 to <100	100 to <2,400	0 or ≥2,400
Other features	DTS options include manual assay, Tecan-assisted assay, or TIGRIS DTS System		
	No cross-reactivity was observed with any of the organisms tested. Sensitivity of the assay to detect *T. vaginalis* at 2.5 TV/ml was negatively affected by the presence of *T. tenax* and *P. hominis*. Assay performance has not been evaluated in the presence of *Dientamoeba fragilis*. Assay has not been validated for use with self-collected vaginal swab samples. Performance of vaginal swab specimens has not been evaluated in pregnant women or in women <14 years of age. Therapeutic success or failure cannot be determined using this assay.		

DTS direct tube sampling, *LBC* liquid-based cytology, *RLU* relative light units, *TV* Trichomonas vaginalis

For interpreting negative results, an IC is important to include in the assay, especially if the input material being tested is a crude cell lysate. More details on inhibitors can be found within the CT and NG section of this chapter.

Specimen Collection

The optimal specimen to collect differs for women and men. For women, the specimen of choice is vaginal discharge collected using a Dacron-tipped, plastic-shaft swab, while for men the sediment from the first-void urine is superior to a urethral swab specimen. For increased analytical sensitivity, only the first 20–30 ml of the first void urine should be collected. Each specimen type to be tested needs to be validated prior to clinical testing. Validating the specific sample processing methods is crucial for ensuring good sensitivity.

Specimen Transport

Trichomonas vaginalis expresses and secretes numerous proteases. For greatest target stability, specimens should be transported at temperatures below room temperature (2–8 °C) or in a specimen transport device that stabilizes the nucleic acid. Each specimen transportation system or device used as well as the specimen storage conditions need to be validated prior to clinical testing.

Future Directions

Multiplex Testing for CT, NG, and TV

Multiplex testing for CT and NG has been available for years. Recently, increased attention has been given to including TV as a target. With the prevalence of TV being greater than that of CT and NG combined in many regions, along with the association of TV infection with increased risk of HIV acquisition, inclusion of TV in a multiplex STI panel is a reasonable idea. Depending on the prevalence of other STIs within a patient population or geographic area, additional targets may be considered applicable for a multiplex STI panel.

Greater Use of Noninvasive Specimens

As with CT and NG detection, collection of first-void urines or self-collected vaginal swab specimens may improve patient compliance for TV testing [28]. This approach may in turn help to identify the asymptomatic, infected individuals and reduce transmission to sexual partners.

Monitoring Trends in Developing Metronidazole Resistance in TV Isolates

Metronidazole and tinidazole are the only recommended drugs for treating individuals infected with TV. Routine testing of TV isolates for antimicrobial drug resistance is not available in most clinical laboratories, but is available through the Centers for Disease Control and Prevention (CDC). Recently, the CDC assessed the prevalence of in vitro drug resistance in six US cities and found low-level resistance to metronidazole in 4.3 % of isolates and no tinidazole resistance [55]. Because of the reliance on a single class of antimicrobial drugs to treat TV infection, the CDC recommends that periodic surveillance for TV drug resistance be carried out and that in vitro, culture-based antimicrobial resistance testing be considered for TV isolates from women having a history of failed treatments [2].

Human Papillomavirus

Description of the Organism

HPVs are small, non-enveloped viruses with a double-stranded, circular DNA (approximately 8 kilobases [kb]) genome and very limited cell tropism. To date, approximately 120 different types of HPV have been identified [56]. HPV can infect and replicate in the nuclei of only certain squamous epithelial cells, which are classified as either cutaneous or mucosal in nature. In general, the cutaneous types of HPV infect keratinizing epithelium, while mucosal types infect non-keratinizing epithelium. This section focuses on the approximately 60 types of anogenital HPV, which can be spread through sexual contact.

Clinical Utility

HPV is one of the most common sexually transmitted infections. More than 5 million new cases are estimated annually in the USA, with more than 20 million men and women currently infected. The prevalence of HPV is highest among sexually active young women ages 15–25 years [2].

The sexually transmitted HPV types can be further classified by their risk of disease progression. Infection with a low-risk HPV is commonly associated with condyloma acuminata or genital warts, and is considered benign or low-risk for progression to malignancy [57, 58]. In contrast, infection with a high-risk HPV can be associated with cervical cancer in women and penile cancer in men [59]. To a lesser extent high-risk HPV has been associated with anal, vulvar, and vaginal cancers (http://apps.who.int/hpvcentre). High-risk (HR) HPV types play a major role in the pathogenesis of epithelial cell cancers of the anogenital tract, due to viral induction of epithelial cell proliferation [60, 61]. Currently, most commercial assays include 14 HR HPV types (16, 18, 31, 33, 35, 39, 45, 51, 52, 56, 58, 59, 66, and 68). The first 12 of these 14 HPV types are considered oncogenic, with the latter 2 HPV types along with HPV 26, 53, and 72 being considered possible oncogenic types [57, 58]. The International Agency for Research on Cancer (IARC) designates HR HPV types.

While most men and women infected with anogenital HPV types will not develop cancer, a small subset will; a process that may take decades to occur [62, 63]. Certain cofactors may be important in disease progression as well, including the individual's immune status, certain human leukocyte antigen (HLA) types, smoking, nutritional status, or possibly coinfection with HIV type 1, herpes simplex virus, or CT [64–68]. Women 30 years of age or older who are persistently infected within the cervix with HR HPV are at an increased risk for developing cervical cancer. Thus, HPV acquisition during adolescence may have long-term consequences for health later in adulthood [69, 70].

Most high-grade cervical lesions are caused by persistent infection with one of the HR HPV types, with HPV 16 and HPV 18 being associated with at least 70 % of cases in the USA [71] Based on these findings, the 2009 American Society for Colposcopy and Cervical Pathology (ASCCP) consensus conference approved a strategy that included HPV 16/18 genotyping when managing women ≥ 30 years of age who are positive for HR HPV upon routine screening with negative cytology [72].

Worldwide, cervical cancer is the second most common female cancer, with approximately 529,828 women developing cervical cancer each year [59, 73]. In the USA in 2010, the American Cancer Society estimated that there were approximately 12,200 new cases of cervical cancer and 4,210 deaths [74]. Cervical cancer is a highly preventable disease if detected and treated early. Infection with HR HPV is associated with the appearance of clinical lesions. HPV is considered to be a necessary requirement for invasive cervical cancer [75]. Abnormal cell growth or cervical dysplasia is an early manifestation of HPV infection. The characteristic cellular changes caused by HPV infection can be detected on Pap smear evaluations or in cervical biopsies. The morphologic changes of dysplasia are classified as atypical squamous cells of undetermined significance (ASCUS), low-grade squamous intraepithelial lesion, or high-grade squamous intraepithelial lesion [76, 77].

Annually, approximately 2 million Pap tests performed in the USA are interpreted as an ASCUS-grade result. ASCUS rates typically fall within the range of 5–10 % but can be as high as 20 % in younger women. Current recommendations include reflex testing of Pap specimens for HR HPV with an ASCUS-grade result; patients testing negative for HPV DNA can be followed according to routine practice, while those testing positive for HR HPV should be referred to colposcopy, as progression to high-grade disease is probable [78, 79]. Patients with abnormal Pap smears whose specimens contain HR HPV DNA require close medical follow up [80–83].

In 2009, the Cytopathology and Technology Education Consortium developed a consensus statement that includes wording for the appropriate and inappropriate uses of HPV testing [84]. Laboratory directors of laboratories performing HPV testing should utilize these valuable guidelines. Currently in the USA, most laboratories performing HR HPV testing commonly receive specimens for the following two appropriate indications:

1. As a reflex test when managing women ≥21 years of age with cytologic result of ASCUS.
2. During routine cervical cancer screening for women ≥30 years of age in conjunction with cervical cytology testing.

In general, HR HPV testing during routine screening in women <30 years of age is considered inappropriate, and there is no role for low-risk HPV testing in routine cervical cancer screening or when evaluating women with abnormal cervical cytology.

Available Tests

In 2003, the FDA approved the Digene Hybrid Capture 2 (hc2) assay [85] with indicated uses that included (1) screening specimens from patients with an ASCUS-grade Pap test result to determine the need for colposcopy [78, 83]; and (2) primary screening tool in conjunction with a Pap test for women 30 years and older [81]. Recommended specimen types for this assay include cervical swabs and liquid-based cytology specimens. The recommended collection devices and transport media include cervical brushes and cervical biopsies transported in specimen transport medium, or a cervical broom transported in Cytyc Preserv-Cyt solution.

Since the Digene HC2 test was first approved, several other tests have been approved by the FDA and introduced into the market. These include one additional signal amplification assay for detecting HPV DNA (Cervista HV test from Hologic), and two target amplification assays that detect either DNA (Roche Cobas HPV test) or RNA (GenProbe Aptima HPV test). Tables 51.12, 51.13, 51.14, 51.15, and 51.16 illustrate the chemistries used, and the HR HPV types detected. Most of these molecular HR HPV tests have been evaluated and found to have excellent clinical sensitivities and negative predictive values, but perform less well in terms of clinical specificity and positive predictive value [86–90].

HPV 16/18 Genotyping

Genotyping has increasingly become a recommendation since studies published by the National Cancer Institute described a 20 % risk of progressing to cervical intraepithelial neoplasia level 3 (CIN3) over 10 years in women infected with HPV 16 and/or HPV 18 [72]. Two of the currently available, FDA-approved HPV NATs have the ability to genotype

Table 51.12 Summary of selected NAT platforms for HPV testing

Manufacturer	Assay method	Sample preparation	Amplification strategy	Detection strategy	Contamination control	IC
Qiagen	Hybrid capture 2 technology	Crude cell lysate	DNA target-RNA probe hybridization with signal amplification	Chemiluminescent detection using AP-labeled antibody specific to RNA-DNA hybrids	Wear powder free gloves; do not contaminate Detection Reagent 2; avoid touching pipette tips on any work surfaces	No
Hologic Cervista	Isothermal	DNA extraction	Invader chemistry, Signal amplification	Cleavase based fluorescence	Recommend using ART, clean lab surfaces	Yes
Hologic Gen-Probe	Isothermal	Target capture via magnetic microparticles	Transcription mediated target amplification E6/E7 mRNA	HPA with DNA probes, DKA via chemiluminescence	Use of 2.5–3.5 % sodium hypochlorite to clean surfaces, racks and pipettes, avoid ribonuclease contamination; use good laboratory practices	Yes
Roche	Real-time PCR	DNA extraction via magnetic glass particles	Target amplification	Fluorescent oligonucleotide probes	Uracil-N-glycosylase and dUTP	Yes

AP alkaline phosphatase, *ART* aerosol-resistant pipette tips, *DKA* dual kinetic assay, *FRET* fluorescence resonance energy transfer, *HPA* hybridization protection assay, *IC* internal control, *HPV* human papillamavirus, *NAT* nucleic acid testing

Table 51.13 Roche Cobas HPV assay

Target	Portion of HPV L1 DNA
Specimens	Cervical specimens collected using an endocervical brush/spatula in PreservCyt solution
Specimen handling	Transport and storage at 20–30 °C for up to 6 months
Test interpretation	Positive-cutoff not given; performed by cobas 4800 software Negative-cutoff not given; performed by cobas 4800 software All HPV negative specimens must have a positive beta globin signal to be valid Invalid-cutoff not given; performed by cobas 4800 software Repeat testing necessary if invalid
High-Risk (HR) HPV types included	14 HR types Separate detection of 16 and 18 Combined detection of 31, 33, 35, 39, 45, 51, 52, 56, 58, 59, 66, and 68
Genotyping	Separate detection of HPV types 16 and 18
Workflow issues	33 min hands-on time, 94 tests completed in <300 min. HPV testing should be performed on PreservCyt specimens prior to automated cytology processing
Other features	No cross-reactivity with Low-Risk HPV types and no gray zone

HPV human papillamavirus

HPV 16/18. The Roche assay provides individual data on the presence of HPV 16 and HPV 18 genotypes, while the Cervista HPV assay provides pooled genotyping information for HPV 16/18. Genotyping recommendations have been intended for clinical management of women > 30 years of age who have HR HPV positive/cytology negative results [91, 92]. Genotyping is not meant for screening younger women. However, based on clinical trial data, several groups are now suggesting that HPV 16/18 genotyping could play an important role in women ≥21 years of age with ASCUS [93–95].

Historically, the Roche Linear Array (LA) HPV Genotyping test (Research Use Only) has been used frequently in studies to resolve discordant results from comparator nucleic acid-based HPV tests. This assay detects and differentiates a total of 37 HPV types; 14 HR HPV types (16, 18, 31, 33, 35, 39, 45, 51, 52, 56, 58, 59, 66, and 68), and 23 low-risk HPV types (6, 11, 26, 40, 42, 53, 54, 55, 61, 62, 64, 67, 69, 70, 71, 72, 73, 81, 82, 83, 84, IS39, and CP6108). The Roche LA HPV Genotyping test incorporates the PGMY primers, which amplify a smaller region internal to the MY09/11 sequence of the HPV L1 gene for improved detection of HPV DNA in genital samples [96].

Table 51.14 Hologic Cervista HPV HR Test

Target	DNA, HPV gene not specified
Specimens	Cervical specimens collected using broom or brush/spatula device and placed in PreservCyt
Specimen handling	20–30 °C for up to 18 weeks
Test interpretation	Positive HR HPV Test FOZ ≥1.525 and HPV 16/18 Genotype FOZ >2.13 Negative FOZ <1.5 Invalid results if: (1) % CV >25 % (2) When all 3 FOZ values <0.7 (3) genomic DNA FOZ of a negative sample <1.5 Uses 3 separate HPV oligonucleotide mixtures, each containing different but related HPV types
High-Risk (HR) HPV types included	14 HR types Pooled 16, 18, 31, 33, 35, 39, 45, 51, 52, 56, 58, 59, 66, and 68
Genotyping	A separate genotyping assay is available for HR HPV 16/18
Workflow issues	129 min hands-on time, 48 test results in ~500 min. Each sample is tested in 3 reaction mixes.
Other features	No cross-reactivity with Low-Risk HPV types HPV HR test shows cross-reactivity with HPV 67 and 70 HPV 16/18 Genotyping test shows cross-reactivity with high levels of HPV 31

HPV human papillamavirus, *HR* high risk, *FOZ* fold over zero

Table 51.15 Hologic Gen-Probe Aptima HPV assay run on Tigris DTS system

Target	HPV E6/E7 mRNA	
Specimens	Cervical specimens collected with broom or cytobrush/spatula device and placed in PreservCyt solution	
Specimen handling	PreservCyt specimens should be transported at 2–30 °C, with *no more than* 30 days at temperatures above 8 °C; transfer into Aptima specimen transfer tubes can be stored at 2–30 °C ≤60 days	
Test interpretation	Positive:	Analyte S/CO ≥0.50, IC < 2,000,000 RLU and Analyte ≤ 13,000,000 RLU
	Negative:	Analyte S/CO < 0.50, IC ≥ IC cutoff and IC ≤ 2,000,000 RLU
	Invalid:	Analyte S/CO < 0.50 and IC < IC cutoff OR IC > 2,000,000 RLU OR Analyte > 13,000,000 RLU
HR HPV types Included	14 HR types; 16, 18, 31, 33, 35, 39, 45, 51, 52, 56, 58, 59, 66, and 68	
Genotyping	Not available	
Workflow issues	Automated using Tigris DTS system	
Other features	False-positive results may occur with this test from in vitro transcripts of LR HPV types 26, 67, 70, 82	

DTS direct tube sampling, *HPV* human papillamavirus, *IC* internal control, *RLU* relative light units, *S/CO* signal-to-cutoff

Table 51.16 Qiagen Digene hybrid capture 2 high-risk HPV DNA test

Target	Whole HPV DNA genome	
Specimens	Cervical specimens collected using hc2 DNA collection device with STM, or using a broom-type collection device and placed in PreservCyt solution.	
Specimen handling	Cervical brush and STM may be transported and held for up to 2 week at room temperature, with an additional week at 2–8 °C, or for 3 months at −20 °C. Cervical specimens in PreservCyt solution may be transported and stored at 2–30 °C for 3 months.	
Test interpretation	Positive:	RLU/CO ≥1.0
	Negative:	RLU/CO <1.0
	Invalid:	Mean value of the negative control must be <250 RLU with a %CV < 5 % for at least 2 of 3 values PreservCyt samples with RLU/CO value of ≥1.0 and <2.5
HR HPV types included	13 HR types; 16, 18, 31, 33, 35, 39, 45, 51, 52, 56, 58, 59, and 68[a]	
Genotyping	Not available	
Workflow issues	149 min hands-on time, 88 test results in <500 min	
Issues	Cross-reactivity occurs when high levels (≥4 ng/ml) of HPV 6 or 42 are present. False-positive results have been reported with HPV types 11, 40, 53, 54, 66, MM4, MM7, MM8, or MM9, as well as the plasmid pBR322. False-negative results can occur if no cell pellet is visible when processing PreservCyt solution. False-positive results can occur with inadequate denaturation, inadequate washing, or exogenous alkaline phosphatase	

[a]Detection of HPV types 39, 58, 59, and 68 has not been statistically confirmed due to low prevalence of these types in the general population
CO cutoff, *HPV* human papillamavirus, *HR* high risk, *RLU* relative light units, *STM* specimen transport medium

Interpreting the Roche Linear Array HPV Genotyping Test takes into account the PCR results of both the HPV and the internal control beta globin (BG) targets for each test strip being run. As a sensitivity control, the absence of one or both BG results in this assay indicates inadequate sample collection, failure to adequately extract DNA, or presence of inhibitors. A positive HPV result regardless of the BG results is interpreted as having detectable HPV DNA. A negative HPV result in the presence of positive results for both the BG low and high internal controls are interpreted as HPV DNA not detected. HPV test results are considered invalid if the HPV results are negative along with negative BG low and/or BG high results. Note that other HPV genotypes may be present in samples that were not detected because the type-specific primers were not included.

Future Directions

Much research is being conducted in the area of HPV and cancer and new diagnostic assay developments may arise from these findings. Research may lead to the development of newer technologies like quantum dots or superparamagnetic nanoparticle-based testing methods that may allow for easier and less expensive mass epidemiological screening for HR HPV. Because the vast majority of cervical cancers affect women in resource-limited settings, it is important to consider the impact that developing and implementing simple, affordable, and accurate testing for HR-HPV would have globally. Diagnostic tests such as point of care tests may be developed that allow for simple, affordable yet accurate screening of women who now have no access to cervical cancer screening.

Other assays may be developed to look at persistence and/or disease prognosis and may include those to detect HR HPV E6/E7 mRNA or protein expression. Determining the usefulness of measuring HPV viral load also may be considered as a means of predicting risk of disease progression. Further studies on the level of CpG methylation of HR-HPV DNA and/or the association of promoter methylation patterns of tumor suppressor genes linked to cervical cancers may develop into clinically useful tests. A research gap has been identified that could have important prognostic value which is the discovery and characterization of new biomarkers with strong association with cervical dysplasia and progression to cancer.

Evidence also links HR HPV with the development of non-cervical cancers. As such, it would be important to consider initiating studies to validate HR-HPV testing from other specimen types, including other female gynecologic cancers, anal or penile cancers, or oropharyngeal cancers. Lastly, with the increased adoption of HPV vaccination around the world post-vaccine studies will be important for tracking the prevalence of specific HR-HPV types associated with cervical cancer.

References

1. Moss T, editor. International handbook of chlamydia. Exeter, UK: Polestar Wheatons Ltd; 2001.
2. Workowski KA, Berman S, Centers for Disease Control and Prevention (CDC). Sexually transmitted diseases treatment guidelines 2010. MMWR Recomm Rep. 2010;59:1–116. No. RR-12.
3. Scholes D, Stergachis A, Heidrich FE, et al. Prevention of pelvic inflammatory disease by screening for cervical chlamydial infection. N Engl J Med. 1996;334:1362–6.
4. Burstein GR, Zenilman JM. Nongonococcal urethritis—a new paradigm. Clin Infect Dis. 1999;28 suppl 1:S66–73.
5. Judson FN. Gonorrhoeae. Med Clin North Am. 1990;74:1353–66.
6. Koumans EH, Johnson RE, Knapp JS, et al. Laboratory testing for *Neisseria gonorrhoeae* by recently introduced nonculture tests: a performance review with clinical and public health considerations. Clin Infect Dis. 1998;27:1171–80.
7. Centers for Disease Control and Prevention (CDC). Cephalosporin susceptibility among *Neisseria gonorrhoeae* isolates---United States 2000-2010. MMWR Morb Mortal Wkly Rep. 2011;60:873–7.
8. Centers for Disease Control and Prevention (CDC). Increases in fluoroquinolone-resistant *Neisseria gonorrhoeae*—Hawaii and California, 2001. MMWR Morb Mortal Wkly Rep. 2002;51(46):1041–4.
9. Chernesky MA, Martin DH, Hook EW, et al. Ability of new APTIMA CT and APTIMA GC assays to detect *Chlamydia trachomatis* and *Neisseria gonorrhoeae* in male urine and urethral swabs. J Clin Microbiol. 2005;43:127–31.
10. Gaydos CA, Quinn TC, Willis D, et al. Performance of the APTIMA combo 2 assay for detection of *Chlamydia trachomatis* and *Neisseria gonorrhoeae* in female urine and endocervical swab specimens. J Clin Microbiol. 2003;41:304–9.
11. Modarress KJ, Cullen AP, Jaffurs Sr WJ, et al. Detection of *Chlamydia trachomatis* and *Neisseria gonorrhoeae* in swab specimens by the Hybrid Capture II and PACE 2 nucleic acid probe tests. Sex Transm Dis. 1999;26:303–8.
12. Van Der Pol B. COBAS Amplicor: an automated PCR system for detection of *C. trachomatis* and *N. gonorrhoeae*. Expert Rev Mol Diagn. 2002;2:379–89.
13. Van Der Pol B, Ferrero DV, Buck-Barrington L, et al. Multicenter evaluation of the BDProbeTec ET System for detection of *Chlamydia trachomatis* and *Neisseria gonorrhoeae* in urine specimens, female endocervical swabs, and male urethral swabs. J Clin Microbiol. 2001;39:1008–16.
14. Bianchi A, Moret F, Desrues JM, et al. PreservCyt transport medium used for the ThinPrep Pap test is a suitable medium for detection of *Chlamydia trachomatis* by the COBAS Amplicor CT/NG test: results of a preliminary study and future implications. J Clin Microbiol. 2002;40:1749–54.
15. Chong S, Jang D, Song X, et al. Specimen processing and concentration of *Chlamydia trachomatis* added can influence false-negative rates in the LCx assay but not in the APTIMA Combo 2 assay when testing for inhibitors. J Clin Microbiol. 2003;41:778–82.
16. Diemert DJ, Libman MD, Lebel P. Confirmation by 16S rRNA PCR of the COBAS AMPLICOR CT/NG test for diagnosis of *Neisseria gonorrhoeae* infection in a low-prevalence population. J Clin Microbiol. 2002;40:4056–9.
17. Farrell DJ. Evaluation of AMPLICOR *Neisseria gonorrhoeae* PCR using cppB nested PCR and 16S rRNA PCR. J Clin Microbiol. 1999;37:386–90.
18. Livengood 3rd CH, Wrenn JW. Evaluation of COBAS AMPLICOR (Roche): accuracy in detection of *Chlamydia tracho-*

matis and *Neisseria gonorrhoeae* by coamplification of endocervical specimens. J Clin Microbiol. 2001;39:2928–32.
19. Palmer HM, Mallinson H, Wood RL, et al. Evaluation of the specificities of five DNA amplification methods for the detection of *Neisseria gonorrhoeae*. J Clin Microbiol. 2003;41:835–7.
20. Darwin LH, Cullen AP, Arthur PM, Long CD, Smith KR, Girdner JL, Hook 3rd EW, Quinn TC, Lorincz AT. Comparison of Digene hybrid capture 2 and conventional culture for detection of *Chlamydia trachomatis* and *Neisseria gonorrhoeae* in cervical specimens. J Clin Microbiol. 2002;40(2):641–4.
21. Tabrizi SN, Unemo M, Limnios AE, Hogan TR, Hjelmevoll SO, Garland SM, Tapsall J. Evaluation of six commercial nucleic acid amplification tests for detection of *Neisseria gonorrhoeae* and other species. J Clin Microbiol. 2011;49(10):3610–5. Epub 2011 Aug 3.
22. Cheng A, Qian Q, Kirby JE. Evaluation of the Abbott RealTime CT/NG assay in comparison to the Roche Cobas Amplicor CT/NG assay. J Clin Microbiol. 2011;49(4):1294–300. Epub 2011 Feb 16.
23. Rosenstraus M, Wang Z, Chang SY, et al. An internal control for routine diagnostic PCR: design, properties, and effect on clinical performance. J Clin Microbiol. 1998;36:191–7.
24. Ripa T, Nilsson PA. A *Chlamydia trachomatis* strain with a 377-bp deletion in the cryptic plasmid causing false-negative nucleic acid amplification tests. Sex Transm Dis. 2007;34:255–6.
25. Hagblom P, Korch C, Jonsson AB, et al. Intragenic variation by site-specific recombination in the cryptic plasmid of *Neisseria gonorrhoeae*. J Bacteriol. 1986;167:231–7.
26. Miyada CG, Born TL. A DNA sequence for the discrimination of *Neisseria gonorrhoeae* from other Neisseria species. Mol Cell Probes. 1991;5:327–35.
27. Van Der Pol B, Martin DH, Schachter J, et al. Enhancing the specificity of the COBAS AMPLICOR CT/NG test for *Neisseria gonorrhoeae* by retesting specimens with equivocal results. J Clin Microbiol. 2001;39:3092–8.
28. Wiesenfeld HC, Lowry DL, Heine RP, et al. Self-collection of vaginal swabs for the detection of chlamydia, gonorrhea, and trichomoniasis: opportunity to encourage sexually transmitted disease testing among adolescents. Sex Transm Dis. 2001;28:321–5.
29. Centers for Disease Control and Prevention (CDC). Update to CDC's sexually transmitted diseases treatment guideline, 2006: Fluoroquinolones no longer recommended for treatment of gonococcal infections. MMWR Morb Mortal Wkly Rep. 2007;56(14):332–6.
30. Petrin D, Delgaty K, Bhatt R, et al. Clinical and microbiological aspects of Trichomonas vaginalis. Clin Microbiol Rev. 1998;11:300–17.
31. Graves A, Gardner Jr WA. Pathogenicity of Trichomonas vaginalis. Clin Obstet Gynecol. 1993;36:145–52.
32. Schwebke JR. Update of trichomoniasis. Sex Transm Infect. 2002;78:378–9.
33. Krieger JN. Trichomoniasis in men: old issues and new data. Sex Transm Dis. 1995;22:83–96.
34. Global incidence and prevalence of selected curable sexually transmitted infections 2008. World Health Organization. http://www.who.int/reproductivehealth/publications/rtis/2008_STI_estimates.pdf
35. Laga M, Manoka A, Kivuvu M, et al. Non-ulcerative sexually transmitted diseases as risk factors for HIV-1 transmission in women: results from a cohort study. AIDS. 1993;7:95–102.
36. Moodley P, Connolly C, Sturm AW. Interrelationships among human immunodeficiency virus type 1 infection, bacterial vaginosis, trichomoniasis, and the presence of yeasts. J Infect Dis. 2002;185:69–73.
37. Rendon-Maldonado J, Espinosa-Cantellano M, Soler C, et al. Trichomonas vaginalis: in vitro attachment and internalization of HIV-1 and HIV-1-infected lymphocytes. J Eukaryot Microbiol. 2003;50:43–8.
38. Sorvillo F, Kerndt P. Trichomonas vaginalis and amplification of HIV-1 transmission. Lancet. 1998;351:213–4.
39. Cotch MF, Pastorek 2nd JG, Nugent RP, et al. Trichomonas vaginalis associated with low birth weight and preterm delivery. The vaginal infections and prematurity study group. Sex Transm Dis. 1997;24:353–60.
40. Klebanoff MA, Carey JC, Hauth JC, et al. Failure of metronidazole to prevent preterm delivery among pregnant women with asymptomatic Trichomonas vaginalis infection. N Engl J Med. 2001;345:487–93.
41. Sutton MY, Sternberg M, Nsuami M, et al. Trichomoniasis in pregnant human immunodeficiency virus-infected and human immunodeficiency virus-uninfected Congolese women: prevalence, risk factors, and association with low birth weight. Am J Obstet Gynecol. 1999;181:656–62.
42. McCann JS. Comparison of direct microscopy and culture in the diagnosis of trichomoniasis. Br J Vener Dis. 1974;50:450–2.
43. Garber GE, Sibau L, Ma R, et al. Cell culture compared with broth for detection of Trichomonas vaginalis. J Clin Microbiol. 1987;25:1275–9.
44. Caliendo AM, Jordan JA, Green AM, et al. Real-time PCR improves detection of Trichomonas vaginalis infection compared with culture using self-collected vaginal swabs. Infect Dis Obstet Gynecol. 2005;13:145–50.
45. Heine RP, Wiesenfeld HC, Sweet RL, et al. Polymerase chain reaction analysis of distal vaginal specimens: a less invasive strategy for detection of Trichomonas vaginalis. Clin Infect Dis. 1997;24:985–7.
46. Jordan JA, Lowery D, Trucco M. TaqMan-based detection of Trichomonas vaginalis DNA from female genital specimens. J Clin Microbiol. 2001;39:3819–22.
47. Kengne P, Veas N, Vidal J, et al. Trichomonas vaginalis: repeated DNA target for highly sensitive and specific polymerase chain reaction diagnosis. Cell Mol Biol. 1994;40:819–31.
48. Madico G, Quinn TC, Rompalo A, et al. Diagnosis of Trichomonas vaginalis infection by PCR using vaginal swab samples. J Clin Microbiol. 1998;36:3205–10.
49. Mayta H, Gilman RH, Calderon MM, et al. 18S ribosomal DNA-based PCR for diagnosis of Trichomonas vaginalis. J Clin Microbiol. 2000;38:2683–7.
50. Paces J, Urbankova V, Urbanek P. Cloning and characterization of a repetitive DNA sequence specific for Trichomonas vaginalis. Mol Biochem Parasitol. 1992;54:247–55.
51. Riley DE, Roberts MC, Takayama T, et al. Development of a polymerase chain reaction-based diagnosis of Trichomonas vaginalis. J Clin Microbiol. 1992;30:465–72.
52. Ginocchio CC, Chapin K, Smith JS, Aslanzadeh J, Snook J, Hill CS, Gaydos CA. Prevalence of Trichomonas vaginalis and coinfection with *Chlamydia trachomatis* and *Neisseria gonorrhoeae* in the United States as determined by the Aptima Trichomonas vaginalis nucleic acid amplification assay. J Clin Microbiol. 2012;50(8):2601–8.
53. Schwebke JR, Hobbs MM, Taylor SN, Sena AC, Catania MG, Weinbaum BS, Johnson AD, Getman DK, Gaydos CA. Molecular testing for Trichomonas vaginalis in women: results from a prospective U.S. clinical trial. J Clin Microbiol. 2011;49(12):4106–11.
54. Chapin K, Andrea S. Aptima Trichomonas vaginalis, a transcription-mediated amplification assay for the detection of Trichomonas vaginalis in urogenital specimens. Expert Rev Mol Diagn. 2011;11(7):679–88.

55. Kirkcaldy RD, Augostini P, Asbel LE, Bernstein KT, Kerani RP, Mettenbrink CJ, Pathela P, Schwebke JR, Secor WE, Workowski KA, Davis D, Braxton J, Weinstock HS. Trichomonas vaginalis antimicrobial resistance in 6 US cities, STD Surveillance System 2009-2010. Emerg Infect Dis. 2012;18(6):939–43. doi:10.3201/eid1806.111590.
56. Bernard HU, Burk RD, Chen Z, et al. Classification of papillomaviruses (PVs) based on 189 PV types and proposal of taxonomic amendments. Virology. 2010;401:70–9.
57. Shiffman M, Clifford G, Buonaguro FM. Classification of weakly carcinogenic human papillomavirus types: addressing the limits of epidemiology at the borderline. Infect Agent Cancer. 2009;4:8.
58. Munoz N, et al. Epidemiologic classification of human papillomavirus types associated with cervical cancer. N Engl J Med. 2003;348:518–27.
59. Bosch FX, Manos MM, Munoz N, et al. Prevalence of human papillomavirus in cervical cancer: a worldwide perspective. International biological study on cervical cancer (IBSCC) Study Group. J Natl Cancer Inst. 1995;87:796–802.
60. Crum CP, Ikenberg H, Richart RM, et al. Human papillomavirus type 16 and early cervical neoplasia. N Engl J Med. 1984;310:880–3.
61. Herrero R. Epidemiology of cervical cancer. J Natl Cancer Inst Monogr. 1996;21:1–6.
62. Ellerbrock TV, Chiasson MA, Bush TJ, et al. Incidence of cervical squamous intraepithelial lesions in HIV-infected women. JAMA. 2000;283:1031–7.
63. Svare EI, Kjaer SK, Worm AM, et al. Risk factors for genital HPV DNA in men resemble those found in women: a study of male attendees at a Danish STD clinic. Sex Transm Infect. 2002;78:215–8.
64. Behbakht K, Friedman J, Heimler I, et al. Role of the vaginal microbiological ecosystem and cytokine profile in the promotion of cervical dysplasia: a case–control study. Infect Dis Obstet Gynecol. 2002;10:181–6.
65. Chin-Hong PV, Palefsky JM. Natural history and clinical management of anal human papillomavirus disease in men and women infected with human immunodeficiency virus. Clin Infect Dis. 2002;35:1127–34.
66. Goedert JJ, Cote TR, Virgo P, et al. Spectrum of AIDS-associated malignant disorders. Lancet. 1998;351:1833–9.
67. Smith JS, Herrero R, Bosetti C, et al. Herpes simplex virus-2 as a human papillomavirus cofactor in the etiology of invasive cervical cancer. J Natl Cancer Inst. 2002;94:1604–13.
68. Wallin KL, Wiklund F, Luostarinen T, et al. A population-based prospective study of *Chlamydia trachomatis* infection and cervical carcinoma. Int J Cancer. 2002;101:371–4.
69. Cothran MM, White JP. Adolescent behavior and sexually transmitted diseases: the dilemma of human papillomavirus. Health Care Women Int. 2002;23:306–19.
70. Ressel GW. CDC releases 2002 guidelines for treating STDs: Part II. Human papillomavirus and hepatitis. Am Fam Physician. 2002;66:1996, 1999.
71. Khan MJ, Castle PE, Lorincz AT, et al. The elevated 10-year risk of cervical precancer and cancer in women with human papillomavirus (HPV) type 16 or 18 and the possible utility of type-specific HPV testing in clinical practice. J Natl Cancer Inst. 2005;97:1072–9.
72. http://www.asccp.org/Portals/9/docs/pdfs/Consensus%20Guidelines/clinical_update_20090408.pdf
73. WHO/ICO HPV Information centre. WHO/ICO Information Centre on HPV and Cervical Cancer (HPV Information Centre). Human Papillomavirus and Related Cancers in World. Summary Report 2010. www.who.int/hpvcentre. Accessed 21 Jan 2012
74. American Cancer Society. Cancer Facts and Figures 2011. Atlanta, GA: American Cancer Society; 2011.
75. Walboomers JM, Jacobs MV, Manos MM, et al. Human papillomavirus is a necessary cause of invasive cervical cancer worldwide. J Pathol. 1999;189:12–9.
76. Ronnett BM, Manos MM, Ransley JE, et al. Atypical glandular cells of undetermined significance (AGUS): cytopathologic features, histopathologic results, and human papillomavirus DNA detection. Hum Pathol. 1999;30:816–25.
77. Schenck U, Herbert A, Solomon D, et al. Terminology. International Academy of Cytology Task Force summary. Diagnostic cytology towards the 21st century: an international expert conference and tutorial. Acta Cytol. 1998;42:5–15.
78. Cox JT, Lorincz AT, Schiffman MH, et al. Human papillomavirus testing by hybrid capture appears to be useful in triaging women with a cytologic diagnosis of atypical squamous cells of undetermined significance. Am J Obstet Gynecol. 1995;172:946–54.
79. Solomon D, Schiffman M, Tarone R. Comparison of three management strategies for patients with atypical squamous cells of undetermined significance: baseline results from a randomized trial. J Natl Cancer Inst. 2001;93:293–9.
80. Berkova Z, Kaufmann RH, Unger ER, et al. The effect of time interval between referral and colposcopy on detection of human papillomavirus DNA and on outcome of biopsy. Am J Obstet Gynecol. 2003;188:932–7.
81. Kulasingam SL, Hughes JP, Kiviat NB, et al. Evaluation of human papillomavirus testing in primary screening for cervical abnormalities: comparison of sensitivity, specificity, and frequency of referral. JAMA. 2002;288:1749–57.
82. Nobbenhuis MA, Walboomers JM, Helmerhorst TJ, et al. Relation of human papillomavirus status to cervical lesions and consequences for cervical-cancer screening: a prospective study. Lancet. 1999;354:20–5.
83. Wang SS, Walker JL, Schiffman M, et al. Evaluating the risk of cervical precancer with a combination of cytologic, virologic, and visual methods. Cancer Epidemiol Biomarkers Prev. 2005;14:2665–8.
84. Solomon D. Statement on HPV DNA test utilization: Cytopathology education and technology consortium. Diagn Cytopathol. 2009;37(7):542–3.
85. Peyton CL, Schiffman M, Lorincz AT, et al. Comparison of PCR- and hybrid capture-based human papillomavirus detection systems using multiple cervical specimen collection strategies. J Clin Microbiol. 1998;36:3248–54.
86. Wong AA, Fuller J, Pabbaraju K, et al. Comparison of the hybrid capture 2 and cobas 4800 tests for detection of high-risk human papillomavirus in specimens collected in preservCyt medium. J Clin Microbiol. 2012;50(1):25–9.
87. Quigley NB, Potter NT, Chivukula M, et al. Rate of detection of high-risk HPV with two assays in women ≥ 30 years of age. J Clin Virol. 2011;52(1):23–7.
88. Ratnam S, Coutlee F, Fontaine D, et al. Aptima HPV E6/E7 mRNA test is as sensitive as hybrid capture 2 assay but more specific at detecting cervical precancer and caner. J Clin Microbiol. 2011;49(2):557–64.
89. Clad A, Reuschenbach M, Weinschenk J, et al. Performance of the Aptima high-risk human papillomavirus mRNA assay in a referral population in comparison with hybrid capture 2 and cytology. J Clin Microbiol. 2011;49(3):1071–6.
90. Kroupis C, Vourlidis N. Human papilloma virus (HPV) molecular diagnostics. Clin Chem Lab Med. 2011;49(11):1783–99.
91. Wright TC, Stoler MH, Sharma A, et al. Evaluation of HPV-16 and HPV-18 genotyping for the triage of women with high-risk HPV+ cytology-negative results. Am J Clin Pathol. 2011;136:578–86.
92. Castle PE, Stoler MH, Wright TC, et al. Performance of carcinogenic human papillomavirus (HPV) testing and HPV16 or HPV18 genotyping for cervical cancer screening of women aged 25 years and older: a subanalysis of the ATHENA study. Lancet Oncol. 2011;12(9):880–90.

93. Stoler MH, Wright TC, Sharma A, et al. High-risk Human Papillomavirus testing in women with ASC-US cytology. Am J Clin Pathol. 2011;135:468–75.
94. Einstein MH, Martens MG, Garcia FAR, et al. Clinical validation of the Cervista HPV HR ad 16/18 genotyping tests for use in women with ASC-US cytology. Gynecol Oncol. 2010;118:116–22.
95. Wong AK, Chan RC, Nichols WS, et al. Invader human papillomavirus (HPV) type 16 and 18 assays as adjuncts to HPV screening of cervical papanicolaou smears with atypical squamous cells of undetermined significance. Cancer. 2009;115(4):823–32.
96. Coutlee F, Gravitt P, Kornegay J, et al. Use of PGMY primers in L1 consensus PCR improves detection of human papillomavirus DNA in genital samples. J Clin Microbiol. 2002;40:902–7.
97. Kengne P, Veas F, Vidal N, Rey JL, Cuny G. Trichomonas vaginalis: repeated DNA target for highly sensitive and specific polymerase chain reaction diagnosis. Cell Mol Biol. 1994; 40(6):819–31.
98. Katiyar SK, Edlind TD. Beta-tubulin genes of Trichomonas vaginalis. Mol Biochem Parasitol. 1994;64(1):33–42.
99. Crucitti T, Van Dyck E, Tehe A, Abdellati S, Vuylsteke B, Buve A, Laga M. Comparison of culture and different PCR assays for detection of Trichomonas vaginalis in self collected vaginal swab specimens. Sex Transm Infect. 2003;79(5):393–8.
100. Ryu JS, Min DY. Diagnosis of trichomoniasis by polymerase chain reaction. Yonsei Med J. 1999;40(1):56–60.

Respiratory Infections

52

Christine C. Ginocchio

Abstract

The majority of respiratory tract infections (RTIs) are community acquired and are the single most common cause of physician office visits and among the most common causes of hospitalizations. The morbidity and mortality associated with RTIs are significant and the financial and social burden high due to lost time at work and school. The scope of clinical symptoms can significantly overlap among the respiratory pathogens, and the severity of disease can vary depending on patient age, underlying disease, and immune status, thereby leading to inaccurate presumptions about disease etiology. The rapid and accurate diagnosis of the causative agent of RTIs improves patient care, reduces morbidity and mortality, promotes effective hospital bed utilization and antibiotic stewardship, and reduces length of stay. This chapter focuses on the clinical utility, advantages, and disadvantages of viral and bacterial tests cleared by the Food and Drug Administration (FDA), and new promising technologies for the detection of bacterial agents of pneumonia currently in development or in US FDA clinical trials are briefly reviewed.

Keywords

Respiratory infections • Viral respiratory pathogens • Bacterial respiratory pathogens • Lower respiratory tract infections • Upper respiratory tract infections • Community-acquired pneumonia • Hospital-acquired pneumonia • Molecular tests

Introduction

The majority of respiratory tract infections (RTIs) are community-acquired and are the single most common cause of physician office visits and among the most common causes of hospitalizations [10, 68, 146, 182, 194]. The morbidity and mortality associated with RTIs are significant and the financial and social burden high due to lost time at work and school. Viral infections cause between 65–80 % of respiratory tract diseases with mixed viral infections present in 5–20 % of viral RTIs in adults and as high as 62 % in studies of children $\geq$6 years of age [66, 80, 132, 172, 182, 194]. In Europe and in the USA the incidence of pneumonia due to a bacterial pathogen is 1–10 cases per 10,000 inhabitants, depending on various factors such as age. The differentiation of viral from bacterial RTIs can be assisted considering the rate of onset of illness, patient age, symptoms, radiographic changes, biomarkers, response to treatment, and the presence of documented viral epidemics in the community. However, the scope of clinical symptoms can significantly overlap among the respiratory pathogens, and the severity of disease can vary depending on patient age, underlying disease, and immune status, thereby leading to inaccurate presumptions about disease etiology.

C.C. Ginocchio, Ph.D., M.T.(A.S.C.P.) (✉)
Department of Pathology and Laboratory Medicine, Hofstra North Shore-LIJ School of Medicine, Hempstead, NY 11549, USA

Scientific and Medical Affairs, Biomerieux, Durham, NC 22717, USA

Scientific and Medical Affairs BioFire Diagnostics, Salt Lake City, UT 84108, USA
e-mail: cginocch@gmail.com

D.G.B. Leonard (ed.), *Molecular Pathology in Clinical Practice*, DOI 10.1007/978-3-319-19674-9_52

Numerous studies have demonstrated that a rapid and accurate diagnosis of the causative agent of RTIs improves patient care, reduces morbidity and mortality, promotes effective hospital bed utilization and antibiotic stewardship, and reduces length of stay [9, 20, 22, 82, 92, 106, 115, 120, 121, 142, 160, 170, 191, 227, 229, 234]. Pathogen etiology may need to be considered in the clinical management of certain patients, such as immunocompromised patients or young infants, if there is a potential for the development of more severe disease [13, 65, 68, 80, 81, 86, 194]. In health care settings, the identification of a viral RTI prompts the initiation of appropriate infection control measures, thereby reducing morbidity and mortality associated with nosocomial transmission [19, 39, 40, 62, 126, 155, 217, 219].

Over the last several years great advances have been made in obtaining USA Food and Drug Administration (FDA) clearance for a variety of nucleic acid amplification tests (NAATS) that detect single or multiple viral respiratory pathogens and three bacterial pathogens (*Mycoplasma pneumoniae*, *Chlamydophila pneumoniae*, *Bordetella pertussis*). This chapter focuses on the clinical utility, advantages, and disadvantages of these tests. Unfortunately, no FDA-cleared assays are available for the detection of the majority of bacterial and fungal pathogens associated with community-acquired pneumonia (CAP), hospital-associated pneumonia (HAP), and ventilator-associated pneumonia (VAP). New promising technologies for the detection of bacterial agents of pneumonia currently in development or US FDA clinical trials are briefly reviewed. Although sensitive, accurate fungal diagnostics is an area of importance, the development of new diagnostic assays has been significantly delayed. Hence, for the detection of the vast majority of the nonviral pathogens, laboratory developed tests (LDTs) are the mainstay of molecular testing and will not be discussed. The importance of new rapid diagnostics for CAP, VAP, and HAP has been highlighted by a workshop conducted in November 2009 by the Infectious Diseases Society of America (IDSA) in collaboration with the FDA, the proceedings of which have been published in a special supplement of Clinical Infectious Diseases [102]. The IDSA, in an executive summary of the workshop, states that there is "a need to develop and implement modern molecular technologies to advance microbiological diagnostic testing."

Epidemiology

The common viruses that cause both lower RTIs (LRTIs) and upper RTIs (URTIs) are listed in Table 52.1. Overall, viruses are the most common cause of URTIs and the second most common etiologic cause of CAP (behind *Streptococcus pneumoniae*), ranging from 13–50 % of diagnosed cases [10, 146, 132, 172, 182, 194]. CAP in children is predominately of viral etiology, with the majority of the infections caused by respiratory syncytial virus (RSV), human rhinovirus (HRV), human metapneumovirus (HMPV), and parainfluenza viruses 1, 2, 3, 4 (PIV) [99, 194]. Influenza A (FluA) and influenza B (FluB), adenovirus (ADV), and the coronaviruses (CoVs) are additional causes of CAP in children. RTIs in non-immune compromised hospitalized children (especially <5 years of age), are mainly due to infection with one or multiple viruses without a secondary bacterial infection. Viral CAP decreases in frequency in healthy young and

Table 52.1 Common viral and bacterial respiratory pathogens

Virus: RTI and CAP	Bacteria: RTI and CAP	Bacteria: VAP and HAP
Adenovirus (ADV)	*Bordetella pertussis* and *Bordetella parapertussis*	*Acinetobacter* spp.,
Human bocavirus (HBoV)[a]	*Chlamydophila pneumoniae*	*Corynebacterium* spp.
Coronavirus (CoV) (OC43, 229E, NL63, HKU-1) SARS, MERS	*Haemophilus influenzae*	*Enterobacteriaceae* (MDRO)
Enterovirus (EV)	*Legionella pneumophila*	*Legionella pneumophila*
Human metapneumovirus (HPMV)	*Moraxella cattharalis*	*Pseudomonas* spp.
Influenza A (seasonal H1 [A/H1], seasonal H3 [A/H3], (H1N1)pdm09 [A/2009 H1])	*Mycoplasma pneumoniae*	*Stenotrophomonas maltophilia*
Influenza B	*Neisseria meningitidis*	*Staphylococcus aureus* (MSSA and MRSA)
Parainfluenza virus 1, 2, 3, 4 (PIV)	*Staphylococcus aureus* (MSSA and MRSA)	
Human rhinovirus (HRV)	*Streptococcus pneumoniae*	
Respiratory syncytial virus (RSV)		

[a]Pathogenic status not fully determined

RTI respiratory tract infection, *CAP* community-acquired pneumonia, *VAP* ventilator-associated pneumonia, *HAP* hospital-associated pneumonia, *MSSA* methicillin-sensitive *Staphylococcus aureus*, *MRSA* methicillin-resistant *Staphylococcus aureus*, *MDRO* multidrug-resistant organism

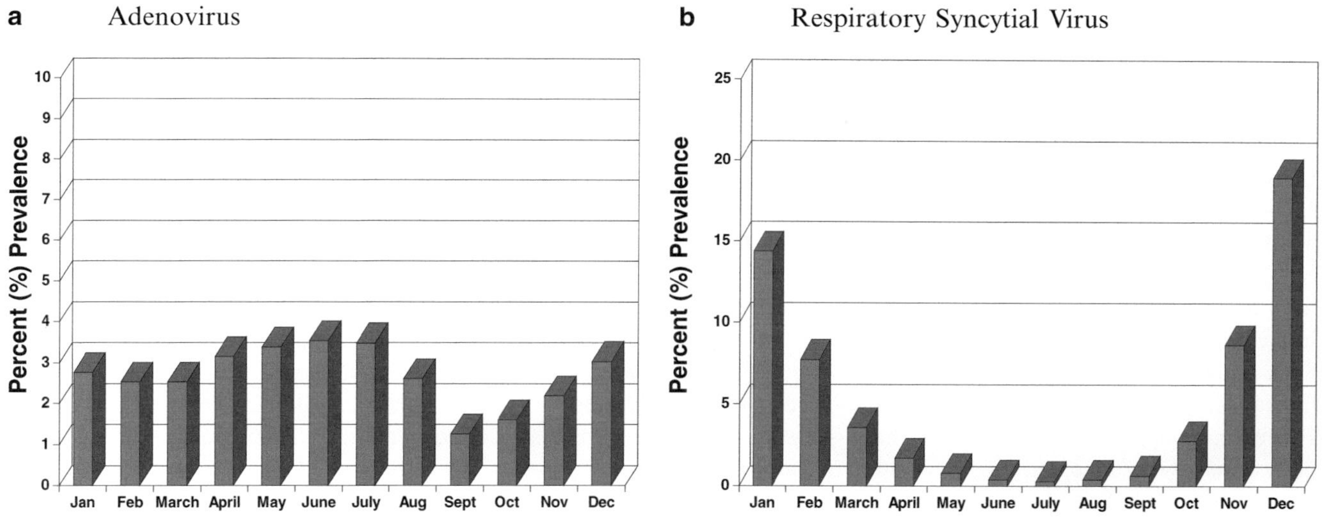

Figure 52.1 Mean prevalence of adenovirus (a) and respiratory syncytial virus (b) by month for the years 2000 through 2011. Adenovirus causes infections throughout the year, while respiratory syncytial virus infections are more seasonal

middle-aged adults to about one-third of the cases, with influenza, HRV, and CoV being the most common agents. Viral CAP rates substantially increase among the elderly, often complicated by secondary bacterial infection. The most common viral causes of CAP in the elderly are influenza and RSV; however, HMPV, PIVs, CoVs, and HRV cause both URTIs and LRTIs [66, 194].

Since 2008 several clusters of respiratory illness associated with human enterovirus 68 (HEV68) were reported in Asia, Europe, and the USA (MMWR [29]). HEV68, a unique enterovirus with similar biologic features to HRV, was associated with RTIs ranging from relatively mild illness to severe illness requiring intensive care and mechanical ventilation. Severe disease was particularly pronounced in children (MMWR [29]). Although human bocavirus (HBoV) has been implicated as a cause of RTI, in the majority of cases HBoV is detected in conjunction with other viral pathogens and the clinical significance of HBoV is still debated [105, 200]. HBoV is more commonly found in children; however, HBoV can affect persons of all ages. Underlying disease, such as cancer, is associated with severe infections requiring hospitalization.

Generally the CoVs (NL-63, OC43, HKU-1, 229E) cause mild, self-limiting URTIs such as the common cold. However, in the last decade, two CoVs—Severe Acute Respiratory Syndrome (SARS-CoV) and the Middle East Respiratory Syndrome (MERS-CoV) have emerged with a potential pandemic threat due to person-to-person communicability [33]. Both viruses can cause severe lower respiratory tract disease with extrapulmonary involvement and are associated with high case-fatality rates. Although SARS-CoV is currently not circulating, since 2012 MERS-CoV continues to cause outbreaks in the Middle East with secondary spread to Europe, Africa, Asia, and North America.

The prevalence of each viral pathogen can vary depending on environmental conditions (climate, season, geographic location). For example, in the New York City area, adenovirus (ADV) tends to circulate with the same prevalence year round (Fig. 52.1a), while RSV can be detected sporadically year round with the peak season in October through February (Fig. 52.1b) (unpublished data provided by author). The "classic" influenza season begins generally in late October and wanes during April. HMPV prevalence tends to rise as RSV season wanes in February and peaks in the spring, PIV-1 and PIV-4 are most prevalent in the summer through fall, while PIV-3 prevails in the spring and PIV-2 in the fall. Virus prevalence also can be patient population driven (e.g., pediatric, adult, geriatric, outpatient, or inpatient). For example, RSV and HMPV are primarily found in children <5 years of age, but can cause severe disease in all age groups [64, 65, 94, 97]. In the immunosuppressed population, other less common respiratory viral pathogens, such as herpes simplex virus (HSV) and cytomegalovirus (CMV), must be considered as a potential cause of RTIs.

The major bacterial pathogens responsible for CAP (Table 57.1) include *S. pneumoniae* (20–60 %), *Staphylococcus aureus* (methicillin-susceptible [MSSA] and methicillin-resistant [MRSA]) (3–5 %), *Haemophilus influenzae* (3–10 %), variable gram-negative rods (3–10 %), and rarely *Neisseria meningitidis* (<1 %) depending on the patient and underlying diseases such as chronic obstructive pulmonary disease (COPD) or asthma [10, 146]. *Moraxella cattharalis* is generally associated with otitis media in children and exacerbation of asthma and COPD in adults. The classic atypical pathogens that cause CAP include *C. pneumoniae*, *M. pneumoniae*, and *Legionella pneumophila*, which also can be nosocomially acquired in institutional settings [10, 17, 46, 67, 222].

The majority of RTIs (up to 70 %) caused by C. *pneumoniae* are asymptomatic or have minimal symptoms. *C. pneumoniae* accounts for 6–20 % of CAP and 5 % of cases of sinusitis, pharyngitis, tracheitis, bronchiolitis, bronchitis, and exacerbations of chronic bronchitis and asthma in both immunocompetent and immunosuppressed persons [17, 42]. *C. pneumoniae* can be present with other bacterial pathogens in up to 30 % of adult cases of CAP. *C. pneumoniae* infection can present with varied clinical courses from mild, self-limiting disease to severe forms of pneumonia, particularly in patients with cardiopulmonary disease and in the elderly [17]. All age groups are affected; however, *C. pneumoniae* infections are rarely found in young children <5 years of age. However, by age 20, 50 % of persons have detectable antibody levels, with the elderly demonstrating a seropositivity rate between 70–80 % [221].

M. pneumoniae is estimated to cause 6–20 % of the cases of CAP [222]. Although most infections are asymptomatic, mild, and often self-limiting, approximately 1–5 % of infections may require hospitalization and can lead to serious extrapulmonary complications. LRTIs are more common in school age children and adolescents, with the prevalence in pediatric LRTI ranging from 10–40 %. *M. pneumoniae* infection can cause outbreaks in the community and institutions such as schools, prisons, and hospitals.

Legionella spp. causes two distinct clinical entities. Pontiac Fever is a self-limiting flu-like illness and Legionaire's disease is a severe multisystem disease involving pneumonia. Cases can be sporadic or part of outbreaks due to environmental exposure [51, 67]. *L. pneumophila* is responsible for 2–8 % of CAP and is responsible for 2–15 % of all CAP that require hospitalization. *L. pneumophila* (serogroup 1) is responsible for 90 % of the diagnosed disease, most probably because the major diagnostic tests are specific for this serogroup. Risk factors for contracting Legionellosis include smoking, immunosuppression, age ≥65, chronic lung disease such as emphysema, diabetes, kidney disease, cancer, or contact with environmental systems such as air conditioning cooling towers, evaporative condensers, whirlpools, and hot spring baths.

Coxiella burnetii, an obligate gram-negative intracellular bacterium has primary reservoirs in cattle, sheep, and goats. Transmission to humans occurs primarily through inhalation of aerosols from contaminated soil or animal waste. Most *C. burnetti* infections are manifested as Q Fever, a self-limited, influenza-like febrile illness (88–100 %) of abrupt onset, manifested by chills, headache, myalgia, fatigue, and sweats; ([150], CDC MMWR [30]). However, pneumonia is predominant in North America and usually mild in nature. Patients have dyspnea, pleuritic chest pain, and a dry, nonproductive cough. Rarely, *C. burnetti* infection occasionally can progress to acute respiratory distress syndrome (ARDS) ([150], CDC MMWR [30]).

B. pertussis is the cause of whooping cough [43, 119]. Pertussis-like illness can be attributed to *Bordetella parapertussis*, *Bordetella holmseii*, and rarely *Bordetella bronchioseptica* infections. Overall, *Bordetella* infections have increased dramatically over the last 10 years due to waning immunity, incomplete antibody response to vaccination with acellular vaccines, or lack of vaccination. Recent epidemics have occurred between 2010 and 2014. In 2010, more than 27,000 cases were reported, of which over 9,000 occurred in California. Nationwide by 2013 more than 28,000 cases were reported to the CDC (http://www.cdc.gov/pertussis/surv-reporting.html). The highest incidence was noted in infants <1 year of age, but a significant amount of disease occurred among children aged 7–10 years. One large outbreak of pertussis-like illness in Ohio from 2010 to 2011 was attributed to both *B. pertussis* (68 % of the cases) and *B. holmseii* (29 % of the cases) [190]. Outbreaks of pertussis continue, highlighting the need for primary vaccination and the administration of "Tdap" booster immunizations.

HAP and VAP are more often associated with drug-resistant, multidrug-resistant, or pan-resistant bacteria, such as MRSA, extended-spectrum beta-lactamase (ESBL)-producing *Enterobacteriacae*, or carbapenemase-producing *Enterobacteriacae*, *Pseudomonas* spp., *Acinetobacter* spp., and *Stenotrophomonas maltophilia* [4]. For patients in the intensive care unit (ICU) or immunocompromised patients, other pathogens such as *Nocardia* spp, *Corynebacterium* spp., *Pneumocystis jiroveci*, *Fusarium* spp., *Aspergillus* spp, *Cryptococcus* spp., and the zygomycetes need to be considered in the differential diagnosis.

Clinical Utility

Limitations of Conventional Diagnostic Procedures

Conventional virus detection methods include rapid antigen detection tests (RADTs), direct fluorescent antibody tests (DFAs), rapid cell culture, and traditional tube culture [125]. Although these methods are acceptable diagnostic tools in certain clinical settings, they are often inferior in the breadth of pathogens identified, assay sensitivity, and result turnaround time, when compared to NAATs [18, 28, 39, 73, 74, 79, 125, 157]. The sensitivity and specificity of all the diagnostic tests, but in particular the conventional tests, are highly dependent on the viral target, age of the patient, duration of symptoms prior to sample collection, sample collection methods, and the transport and storage conditions [1, 39, 48, 49, 85, 95, 118, 127, 131, 164].

RADTs are generally the simplest tests to perform, many are waived tests under the Clinical Laboratory Improvement Amendments (CLIA), and results are generally available within 15–30 min. Despite these benefits, RADTS have limited utility due to the narrow scope of pathogens detected (RSV, FluA, and FluB) [125], and modest to poor sensitivities [21, 39, 45, 61, 75, 79, 125, 199] which can range from 50–90 % for RSV [47] and 10–85 % for influenza viruses depending on the comparator method. Overall, the specificities of RADTs are good [21, 39, 45, 61, 75, 79, 125, 199]; however, the specificity for the detection of influenza A (H1N1) pdm09 was significantly lower than previously reported [197, 198]. RADTs generally perform better when testing pediatric samples since children shed higher titers of virus and for longer time periods than adults, especially the elderly [28, 85, 93].

DFAs detect a broader range of viruses (ADV, FluA, FluB, HMPV, PIV-1, PIV-2, PIV-3, and RSV) and can be performed in 30–60 min. The sensitivities of DFAs vary by virus, ranging from a high of approximately 60–85 % for RSV to a low of 50 % for ADV when compared to NAATs [116, 125]. DFAs are generally very specific, although specificity can be dependent on the level of technical expertise of the reader.

Rapid cell culture (Quidel/Diagnostic Hybrids, Athens, OH) can detect ADV, FluA, FluB, PIV-1, PIV-2, PIV-3, and RSV and has demonstrated sensitivities that range from a high of >80 % for some FluA strains to a low of 50 % for RSV [125, 130, 152] and excellent specificities of greater than 95 % when compared to NAATs. Rapid cell culture is generally positive within 48 h for >90 % of the seven viruses detected.

Depending on the cell lines used and antibodies available for confirmation, traditional tube culture can have a broader scope of pathogen detection when compared to RADTs, DFAs, and rapid cell culture [125]. Traditional culture will identify ADV, enterovirus (EV), HMPV, FluA, FluB, PIV-1, PIV-2, PIV-3, RSV, and HRV, plus additional viruses associated with lower RTIs in immunocompromised patients, including CMV, HSV-1, HSV-2, varicella zoster virus (VZV). Often laboratories do not specifically screen for HRV by culture, although HRV is the most common respiratory virus detected and has been shown to cause significant and serious disease in young, elderly, immunosuppressed patients, as well as patients with underlying chronic lung disease such as COPD and asthma [83]. In addition, many additional important viruses (229E-CoV, OC43-CoV, NL63-CoV, HKU-1-CoV, SARS-CoV, MERS-CoV), PIV-4, and potentially HBoV) that cause both URTIs and LRTIs are not routinely identified by traditional culture [83, 105, 200]. Finally, due to time-to-virus-detection by traditional culture (generally 3–7 days for most respiratory viruses and 3–4 weeks for slow-growing viruses such as CMV), results are usually not available within a time frame (48 h) that could affect patient management (i.e., initiate appropriate antiviral therapy and/or discontinue inappropriate antibiotic therapy). In summary, RADTs, DFAs, and rapid cell culture may provide results within a clinically relevant time frame but with limited pathogen scope and reduced sensitivity compared to NAATs. In addition, RADTs, DFAs, and rapid/traditional cell culture rarely detect more than one virus from a single sample.

The standard methods for the detection of bacterial pathogens causing pneumonia are gram stain in combination with microbiological culture of lower respiratory tract specimens and blood. Often culture of respiratory specimens is not ordered on hospitalized patients and rarely performed in the outpatient setting. A gram stain result can be available within a few hours but results do not always correlate with culture [10]. Culture and antibiotic susceptibility results are usually available in 2–5 days after sample collection, and detection rates for pathogens are relatively low. A meta-analysis that evaluated 122 reports on CAP for the time period of 1966–1995 showed that a bacterial pathogen was only identified in 18 % of the samples tested [68]. A urinary antigen test for *S. pneumoniae* offers a substantial improvement over culture, with a sensitivity of 82 % and a specificity of 97 % in bacteremic adults [209, 210]. However, in non-bacteremic adults and in children, both the sensitivity and specificity are lower [210]. False-positive *S. pneumoniae* antigen tests have been reported relating to antibiotic interference. *Legionella* spp. are identified by growth on buffered charcoal yeast extract agar [158]. The sensitivity of *Legionella* culture can vary significantly from <10–80 % and DFA sensitivity from 25–70 % [158]. A urinary antigen test for *L. pneumophila* improves detection but is suboptimal since detection is limited to serogroup 1. For *L. pneumophila* serogroup 1 the sensitivity of the test varies from 70–100 %. Most laboratories do not culture for *Mycoplasma* or *Chlamydophila* [140].

Traditionally, *B. pertussis* was identified using culture on Bordet–Gengou media and/or DFA. However, the sensitivity of culture ranges from 12–60 %, the sensitivity of DFA ranges from 11–68 % [119]. Additionally, culture can take many days. Therefore, NAATS have become the gold standard for the rapid and sensitive (70–99 %) identification of pertussis [119].

Serologic antibody testing is available for some of the respiratory pathogens and can provide supplemental information. However, due to a delay in the development of detectable IgM or IgG antibodies for certain pathogens (e.g., *L. pneumophila*, *C. pneumoniae*, *B. pertussis*), usefulness for diagnosis in a clinically relevant time frame is very limited [17, 151, 158, 221]. Shortcomings of serological testing include the timing of the serum samples, difficulty in obtaining appropriately paired serum samples, and the high background of IgG antibody prevalence in some adult populations [140]. Serologic diagnosis can be misinterpreted due to prior immunization or infections, such as in the case of influenza, and require demonstration of a significant rise in antibody titers from initial to convalescent samples.

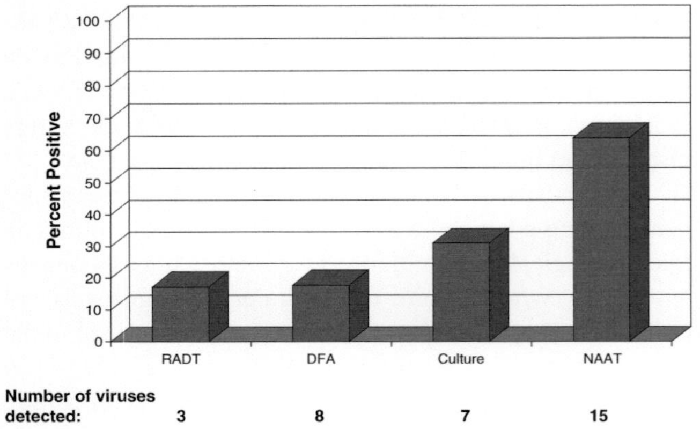

Figure 52.2 Comparison of viral test methods for identification of respiratory pathogens. Percentage of respiratory samples (n = 35,456) positive by each test methods: RADT (rapid antigen detection test) detects three viruses [influenza A (FluA), influenza B (FluB), and respiratory syncytial virus (RSV)]; DFA (direct fluorescent antibody assay) detects eight viruses [adenovirus (ADV), FluA, FluB, human metapneumovirus (HMPV), parainfluenza viruses (PIV) 1, 2, and 3, and RSV]; Culture (R-Mix rapid cell culture) detects seven viruses (ADV, FluA, FluB, PIV-1, PIV-2, PIV-3, and RSV); NAAT (nucleic acid amplification testing) detects 15 viruses (ADV, coronaviruses (CoV: OC43, NL63, HKU1, 229E), enterovirus/rhinovirus group (EV/HRV), FluA (A/H1, A/H3), FluB, HMPV, PIV (1–4), and RSV

Finally, persons with immune suppression may not develop antibodies or they may be of an insufficient level for detection, limiting the functionality of serology for monitoring vaccine response and for epidemiology studies to determine prevalence rates.

Application of Molecular Assays for the Detection of Respiratory Pathogens

Clinical Utility of NAAT for Respiratory Pathogens

Prior to the 2009 FluA(H1N1) pandemic, the infectious causes of CAP were mostly inferred based on clinical presentation which can be highly inaccurate since some bacteria, atypical pathogens, and many of the respiratory viruses cause illnesses with similar clinical symptoms [177, 194]. One study demonstrated that physicians recognized influenza in only 28 % of hospitalized children and 17 % of non-hospitalized children with laboratory-confirmed influenza when the diagnosis was based only on clinical symptoms [177]. Most diagnostic testing was limited to RADTs for FluA, FluB, and RSV as few hospitals offered comprehensive DFAs, viral culture, or laboratory-developed NAATs.

The superior ability of NAATs to rapidly and accurately detect both known and novel pathogens was best exemplified during the chaos of the 2009 FluA H1N1 pandemic [18, 39, 79, 197, 198]. Fortunately, at the start of the pandemic two NAATs were FDA-cleared for the detection of influenza viruses, the Prodesse PROFLU+ (Hologic, San Diego, CA) for the detection and differentiation of FluA and FluB ([124]; and one highly multiplexed NAAT: the Luminex xTAG RVP Respiratory Virus Panel (Luminex Molecular Diagnostics, Toronto, Canada) [113, 114, 143]. The xTAG assay enabled laboratories to detect FluA(H1N1)pdm09 and differentiate the seasonal FluA H1N1 (FluA-H1) and seasonal FluA H3N2 (FluA-H3), but also identify many other circulating viruses [79, 78]. As shown in Fig. 52.2, the number of samples positive for a respiratory virus increased dramatically with the use of the highly multiplexed xTAG RVP assay (64 %) compared to traditional test methods, including RADTS (17 %), DFA (18 %), and rapid cell culture (31 %) [79]. Interestingly, mixed viral infections containing up to four viral pathogens were identified in hospitalized patients [79]. Similarly, other studies have shown that when broad test panels are used more than one virus will be identified in 3–30 % of respiratory samples [8, 166]. Although the significance of mixed viral infections needs to be more clearly defined, the clinical impact needs to be considered as potentially severe in patients with comorbidities, immunosuppression, or other critical illnesses. During respiratory virus seasons with high influenza rates, patients with the same pathogen often are placed in hospital rooms together (cohorting) due to limited private rooms [19, 39, 40, 62, 126, 155, 165, 217, 219]. The consequences of a second viral infection in an already seriously ill hospitalized patient could be substantial, indicating that comprehensive test panels are essential in this setting.

Consequently, there has been a major shift in testing practices as numerous FDA-cleared single-and multi-analyte molecular tests for the detection of respiratory pathogens have become available (Table 52.2). Viral respiratory pathogens are particularly suited for detection using NAATs since the number of targets is relatively limited and the detection of a respiratory virus is generally considered diagnostic, although asymptomatic carriage of certain respiratory viruses has been reported in several studies [2, 14, 104, 181]. For the majority of viral and atypical bacterial respiratory pathogens, NAATs offer enhanced sensitivity over culture, RADTs and DFAs (see Tables 52.2 and 52.3 for references), and the specificity varies with the target and assay design but is generally very high. NAATs also are suited for detection of respiratory pathogens that are not routinely or easily cultured (e.g., *C. pneumoniae*, *M. pneumoniae*, HBoV, HMPV, and PIV-4), for pathogens dangerous to culture (e.g., SARS-CoV, MERS-CoV), and for pathogens where the time-to-detection by traditional testing is often too delayed to impact patient care (e.g., influenza and CMV by cell culture).

The expanded scope of pathogen detection from a previous low of three viral pathogens detected by RADTs to 17 viral and three bacterial pathogens detected by NAATs greatly enhances the clinical laboratory's diagnostic capabilities.

Table 52.2 FDA cleared tests for the detection of bacterial and viral respiratory pathogens[a,b]

Manufacturer/test[c]	Amplification and detection platform(s)[d]	Extraction Platforms	Targets[e]	Specimen types approved[f]	Method(s)[g]	References
Alere i NAT Flu A/B	Alere i Instrument	Included	FluA, FluB	NS	Isothermal amplification, Fluorescence detection	[11, 12, 35, 91, 98, 162]
Argene/bioMerieux Argene R-Gene Adenovirus Assay	Cepheid SmartCycler	bioMerieux NucliSENS easyMAG	ADV	NPS	Real-Time PCR, Fluorescence detection	[148]
BioFire/bioMerieux Film Array Respiratory Virus Panel	BioFire Film Array	Included	ADV, CoV (OC43, NL63, 229E, HKU-1), HMPV, FluA (H1, H3, 2009-H1N1), HRV/EV, PIV 1,2,3,4, *M. pneumoniae*, *C. pneumoniae*, *B. pertussis*	NPS	Real-Time RT-PCR/PCR, Fluorescence detection	[7, 23, 26, 57, 87, 90, 133, 174, 176, 179, 180, 183, 188, 193, 220, 230]
CDC Influenza Division[g] CDC Human Influenza Virus Real-Time RT-PCR Diagnostic Panels 1. Influenza A/B typing Kit 2. Influenza A subtyping Kit 3. Influenza A /H5 (Asian lineage) Kit 4. Influenza B lineage genotyping assay	ABI 7500 Fast Dx	Qiagen QIAamp, Qiagen QIAcube, Roche Magna Pure compact, Roche Magna Pure LC, bioMerieux NucliSENS easyMAG	1. FluA, FluB 2. A/H1, A/H3, A/2009 H1 3. A/H5N1 (Asian lineage) 4. B/Victoria, B/Yamagata lineages	Varies by test including: NPS, NS, NA, NW, NPS/TS, BAL, TA, BW, VC	Real-Time RT-PCR, Fluorescence detection	NA
Cepheid 1. XpertFlu Assay 2. Xpert Flu/RSV XC Assay	Cepheid GeneXpert	Included	1. FluA (A/2009 H1), FluB 2. FluA, FluB, RSV	1. NPS, NA, NW NPS, NW, NA (in VTM)	Real-Time RT-PCR, Fluorescence detection	[35, 56, 59, 107, 129, 163, 178, 195, 196, 198, 199]
Focus Diagnostics 1. Simplexa Influenza A H1N1 2. Simplexa FluA/B and RSV 3. Simplexa Flu A/B Direct	3 M Integrated Cycler	1 and 2: Qiagen QIAamp Viral RNA 3: Included	1. FluA (A/2009 H1) 2. FluA, FluB, RSV 3. FluA, FluB, RSV	1. NPS, NA, NPA 2. NPS, NA, NPA 3. NPS	Real-Time RT-PCR, Fluorescence detection	[3, 111, 117, 204, 205, 212, 229]
GenMark eSensor Respiratory Viral Panel	Thermocycler GenMark eSensor XT-8	bioMerieux NucliSENS easyMAG	FluA, (A/H1, A/H3, A/2009 H1), FluB, RSV (A, B), ADV (B/E, C), PIV (1–3), HMPV, HRV	NPS	RT-PCR/PCR, Electrochemical detection of bound signal probes	[175, 179, 193]
Hologic/Gen-Probe/Prodesse 1. ProFlu+ 2. ProFAST+ 3. ProAdeno+ 4. ProParaFlu+ 5. ProhMPV+	Cepheid Smartcycler II	bioMerieux NucliSENS easyMAG, Roche Magna Pure LC, Roche Magna Pure Total NA	1. FluA, FluB, RSV 2. A/H1, A/H3, A/2009 H1 3. ADV 4. PIV 1,2,3 5. HMPV	All NPS	Real-Time RT-PCR/PCR, Fluorescence detection	[26, 71, 124, 130, 133, 174, 202, 205, 220, 221]
IntelligentMDx IMDx FluA/B and RSV	Abbott m2000*rt*	Abbott m2000*sp*	FluA (A/H1, A/H3, A/2009 H1), FluB, RSV	NPS	Real-Time RT-PCR, Fluorescence detection	NA
Iquum/Roche Liat Influenza A and B	Iquum/Roche Liat Analyzer	Included	FluA, FluB	NPS	Real-Time RT-PCR, Fluorescence detection	NA

(continued)

Table 52.2 (continued)

Manufacturer/test[c]	Amplification and detection platform(s)[d]	Extraction Platforms	Targets[e]	Specimen types approved[f]	Method(s)[g]	References
Luminex 1. xTag Respiratory Virus Panel 2. xTag RVP *Fast*	Thermocyclers Luminex Lx100/200	bioMerieux NucliSENS easyMAG, bioMerieux NucliSENS miniMAG, Roche MagnaPure	1. ADV, hMPV, HRV, FluA (A/H1, A/H3), FluB, PIV 1,2,3, RSV (A, B) 2. AdV, HMPV, HRV, FluA (A/H1, A/H3), FluB, RSV (A, B)	1. NPS 2. NPS	RT-PCR/PCR Primer extension xTAG Bead Array Fluorescent detection	[5, 7, 8, 34, 47, 60, 72, 74, 78, 79, 88, 101, 108, 113, 114, 143, 144, 149, 151, 153, 157, 166–168, 179, 183, 185, 202, 203, 208, 213, 227]
Meridian Bioscience 1. *illumi*gene Pertussis 2. *illumi*gene Mycoplasma	Meridian Illumipro-10	1. Heat 2. Qiagen QIAmp DSP DNA miniKit	1. *B. pertussis* 2. *M. pneumoniae*	1. NPS 2. NPS, TS	Isothermal amplification with turbimetric detection	[184]
Nanosphere Verigene Respiratory Virus Nucleic Acid Test Plus	Nanosphere Verigene Processor SP Verigene Reader	Included	FluA (A/H1, A/H3, A/2009 H1), FluB, RSV (A, B)	NPS	RT-PCR Gold nanoparticle detection	[3, 20, 26, 41, 101, 160, 221]
Qiagen Artus Influenza A/B Rotor-gene RT-PCR Kit	Qiagen Roto-Gene Q MDx	Qiagen QIAsymphony RGQ	FluA, FluB	NPS	Real-Time RT-PCR, Fluorescent detection	[73]
Quidel 1. Lyra Influenza A+B Assay 2. Lyra RSV+HMPV Assay 3. Lyra Parainfluenza Virus Assay 4. Lyra Adenovirus Assay 5. Amplivue Bordetella Assay	1. and 2. Cepheid SmartCycler II, ABI 7500 Fast Dx, Life Technologies QuantStudio 3. and 4. ABI 7500 Fast Dx 5. Thermocycler and Amplivue Cassette	1–4: bioMerieux NucliSENS easyMAG Heat treatment	1. FluA, FluB 2. HMPV, RSV 3. PIV-1,2,3 4. ADV 5. *B. pertussis*	1. and 2. NPS, NS, NA, NW 3 and 4. NPS, NS 5. NPS	1–4. Real-Time RT-PCR/PCR, Fluorescent detection 5. Helicase dependent amplification, Lateral flow	NA
US Army JBAIDS 1. Influenza A/H5[g] 2. Influenza A&B Detection Kit[g] 3. Influenza A Subtyping Kit[g]	Idaho Technologies JBAIDS	Included	1. H5N1 (Asian lineage) 2. FluA and FluB 3. A/H1, A/H3, A/2009 H1	1. NPS, TS 2. NPS, NPW 3. NPS, NPW	Real-Time RT-PCR, Fluorescent detection	NA

[a]Adapted from FDA website

[b]Test methods and availability of products may change by publication date

[c]BioFire/bioMerieux, Salt Lake City, Utah; CDC: Centers for Disease Control and Prevention, Atlanta, GA; Cepheid, Sunnyvale, CA; Focus Diagnostics, Cypress, CA; Gen-Probe, San Diego, CA; Roche Molecular Diagnostics/Iquum, Marlborough, MA; Luminex, Austin TX; Nanosphere, Northbrook, IL; Qiagen, Valencia, CA; Quidel, San Diego, CA, JBAIDS: US Army: Joint Biological Agent Identification and Diagnostic System

[d]ABI: Applied Biosystems

[e]Abbreviations: RT: reverse transcriptase; PCR: polymerase chain reaction; NA: none available; ADV: adenovirus; CoV: coronavirus; FluA: all influenza A types; A/H1: seasonal H1N1; A/H3: seasonal H3N2; A/2009 H1: influenza A (H1N1)pdm09; H5N1: avian influenza A H5N1: FluB: influenza B; HMPV: human metapneumovirus: EV: enterovirus; HRV: human rhinovirus; PIV: parainfluenza virus; RSV; respiratory syncytial virus; *M. pneumoniae*: *Mycoplasma pneumoniae*; *C. pneumoniae*: *Chlamydophila pneumoniae*: *B. pertussis*: *Bordetella pertussis*

[f]These specimen types are specified in product package information and cleared by the Food and Drug Administration (FDA). Abbreviations: NPS; nasopharyngeal swab; NPW: nasopharyngeal wash; NPA: nasopharyngeal aspirate; NS: nasal swab; TS: throat swab; NA: nasal aspirate; NW: nasal wash; NPS/TS: dual specimen consisting of nasopharyngeal swab and throat swab; BAL: bronchial alveolar lavage; BA: bronchial aspirate; BW: bronchial wash; EA: endotracheal aspirate; EW: endotracheal wash; TA: tracheal aspirate; VC: viral culture

[g]Available only to qualified Department of Defense (DoD) Laboratories, US Public Health Laboratories, and National Respiratory and Enteric Virus Surveillance System (NREVSS) collaborating laboratories

Table 52.3 Research use only, investigational use only, or CE marked tests for the detection of respiratory pathogens[a]

Manufacturer/test[b]	Amplification and detection platform(s)	Extraction platforms	Targets[c]	Specimen types	Method(s)[d]	References
Abbott Ibis PLEX-ID/Flu assay PLEX-ID Respiratory Virus Assay	Abbott Ibis T5000 platform	Thermo King-Fisher	Pan-influenza (PB1) Five pan-FluA (NP, M1, PA, PB2, NS1) ADV (A-F), CoV HMPV, FluA, FluB, PIV (1–3), RSV	Respiratory samples (not specified) NPA	Broad range RT-PCR, Electrospray Ionization Mass Spectrometry, (RT-PCR/ ESI-MS)	[36, 37, 44, 55, 69, 88, 100, 159, 207, 214, 215]
Autogenomics 1. Infiniti RVP Plus 2. Infiniti Flu A-sH1N1	Thermocycler Autogenomics Infiniti Analyzer	Not specified	1. ADV (A, B, C, E) FluA (A/2009-H1N1), FluB, RSV, PIV (1–4), HRV (A, B), EV (A, B, C, D), CoV (HKU1, OC43, NL63, 229E), HMPV (A, B) 2. FluA, A/2009 H1	Respiratory samples (not specified)	RT-PCR BioFilmChip Microarray	NA
bioMerieux 1. NucliSENS Influenza A+B 2. NucliSENS RSV A+B 3. NucliSENS HMPV 4. NucliSENS *Mycoplasma* 5. NucliSENS *Chlamydophila*	bioMerieux NucliSENS easyQ	bioMerieux NucliSENS easyMAG	1. FluA and FluB 2. RSV (A, B) 3. HMPV 4. *M. pneumoniae*, *C. pneumoniae*	NPA, NPS, NS, NA, BAL	NASBA, Fluorescence detection	[15, 32, 50, 76, 134–138, 147, 154, 218]
Curetis Pneumonia Panel Bacterial	Curetis Unyvero System	Included	*A. baumanii*, *E. coli* *Enterobacter* spp., *M. morganii* *K. oxytoca*, *K. pneumoniae* *H. influenzae*, *Proteus* spp. *M. catarrhalis*, *S. aureus* *P. aeruginosa*, *S. marcescens* *S. maltophilia*, *S. pneumoniae* *C. pneumoniae*, *L. pneumophila* *P. jiroveci*, Plus 18 antibiotic resistance markers	BAL, TA, BW, BB, PB	Multiplex End Point PCR	[103, 201]
Hologic/Gen-Probe ProPneumo-1	Smartcycler II Qiagen Roto-Gene Applied Biosystems GeneAmp PCR 7500	bioMerieux NucliSENS easyMag	*C. pneumoniae* *M. pneumoniae*	NPS, NPW, BAL, sputum	Real-Time RT-PCR, Fluorescence detection	[96]
Icubate 1.Respiratory Panel V (viral) 2.Flu Typing 3. Respiratory Panel B (Bacterial)	Icubate Processor Incubator	Included	1. FluA (A/2009 H1), FluB, PIV (1–4), RSV (A,B), HMPV (A,B), HRV, ADV (3/7, 4), Cox A, B, Echo, HRV, Corona (OC43, NL63, 229E, HKU-1), HBoV 2. FluA (A/H1, A/H3, A/2009 H1, A/H5 (avian), N1 (shared), N2 (seasonal), FluB *H. influenzae* (non-typeable) *H. influenzae* (a, b, c, d) *H. influenzae* (e, f), *S. aureus* *N. meningitidis*, *S. pneumoniae* *C. pneumoniae*, *L. pneumophila* *M. pneumoniae*	Respiratory samples (not specified)	ARM-PCR technology (Amplicon Rescued Multiplex PCR), End point detection	NA

(continued)

Table 52.3 (continued)

Manufacturer/test[b]	Amplification and detection platform(s)	Extraction platforms	Targets[c]	Specimen types	Method(s)[d]	References
Luminex FluA/B, RSV Assay	Aries	included	FluA/B and RSV	NPS	Multi-code Real-Time RT-PCR, Fluorescence detection	NA
Pathofinder 1. Respifinder 15 2. Respifinder 19 3. Respifinder Smart 22	Thermocycler ABI310, ABI3100, ABI3130, ABI3730, ABI3500 Beckman CEQ Roche Lightcycler 480 Corbett RotorGgene 3000/6000 Qiagen RotorGene Q	Not specified	1. FluA (H5N1), FluB, PIV (1–4), RSV (A,B), hMPV, HRV, ADV, CoV (OC43, NL63, 229E) 2. 15 plus: *B. pertussis*, *M. pneumoniae*, *C. pneumoniae*, *L. pneumophila* 3. FluA (H1N1-2009), FluB, PIV (1–4), RSV (A,B), hMPV, EV/HRV, ADV, CoV (OC43, NL63, 229E, HKU-1), HBoV *B. pertussis*, *C. pneumoniae*, *L. pneumophila*, *M. pneumoniae*	NPW, NPA, NPW, BAL, Sputum	RT-PCR/PCR, Capillary electrophoresis, Multiplex PCR, Melt curve analysis	[24, 47, 141, 185, 186]
Qiagen Resplex II	GeneAmp PCR system 9700 LiquiChip 200 Workstation	QIAamp viral RNA QIAamp MiniElute QIASymphony QIAxtractor	FluA, FluB, PIV (1–4), RSV (A,B), HMPV, HRV, Cox/Echo Pan-ADV (B,E), CoV (OC43, NL63, 229E, HKU-1), HBoV	Respiratory Samples (not specified)	RT-PCR/PCR, Bead Array, Hybridization detection	[8, 69, 74, 90, 128, 129, 141, 145, 224, 227]
Seegene 1. Seeplex Respiratory Assay Group of 12: 2. Seeplex Respiratory Assay Group of 15: 3. Seeplex Typing Influenza A Virus	Variety including: Qiagen Rotor-gene Applied Biosystems GeneAmp PCR system 9700	Variety including: NucliSENS easyMAG Qiagen BioRobot MDx iNtRON Biotechnology Viral Gene-spin Kit	1. Set A: ADV, CoV (229E/NL63), PIV (1–3) 1. Set B: FluA/B, RSV (A,B), HRV A, CoV (OC43) 2. Set A: ADV (A/B/C/D/E), PIV (1–3), CoV (229E/NL63) 2. Set B: CoV (OC43), HRV (A/B/C), FluA, RSV (A, B) 2. Set C: HBoV (1/2/3/4), FluB, HMPV, EV, PIV 4 3. FluA (generic), A/H1, A/H3, A/2009-H1	Respiratory Samples (not specified)	Real-Time RT-PCR, Fluorescence detection	[16, 58, 74, 109, 110, 122, 192, 211, 231, 232]

[a]Test methods and availability of products may change by publication date

[b]Abbott, Chicago, IL; Autogenomics, Vista, CA; bioMérieux, Marcy, France, Curetis, Stutgart, GR; Luminex, Austin, TX; Hologic/Gen-Probe, San Diego, CA; GenMark Diagnostics, Carlsbad, CA; Icubate, Huntsville, AL; Qiagen, Valencia, CA; Pathofinder, Maastricht, NL; Seegene, Seoul, Korea, Thermo King-Fisher (Waltham, MA)

[c]Abbreviations: ADV: adenovirus; HBoV: human bocavirus; CoV: coronavirus; FluA: all influenza A types; H1: seasonal H1N1; H3: seasonal H3N2; 2009-H1: Influenza A(H1N1)pmd09; FluB: influenza B; HMPV: human metapneumovirus: EV: enterovirus; HRV: human rhinovirus; PIV: parainfluenza virus; RSV; respiratory syncytial virus; *M. pneumoniae*: *Mycoplasma pneumoniae*; *C. pneumoniae*: *Chlamydophila pneumoniae*: *L. pneumophila*: *Legionella pneumophila*, *M. morganii*: *Morganella morganii*, *N. meningitidis*: *Neisseria meningitidis*; *Strep. pneumoniae*: *Streptococcus pneumoniae*; *S. aureus*; *Staphylococcus aureus*

[d]Specimen types listed were identified either on manufacturer websites or from publications. Respiratory Samples (not specified): no specific information available. Abbreviations: NPS; nasopharyngeal swab; NPW: nasopharyngeal wash; NPA: nasopharyngeal aspirate; NS: nasal swab; NA: nasal aspirate; BAL: bronchial alveolar lavage; BB: bronchial brush; BW: bronchial wash; PB: protected brush; TA: tracheal aspirate

[e]RT: reverse transcriptase; PCR: polymerase chain reaction

The data derived from studies utilizing comprehensive viral and bacterial NAATs has and will continue to provide invaluable insights into the clinical manifestations of viral and bacterial infections, significance of mixed viral infections, and surprisingly the realization that viruses can colonize a host without overt disease.

Impact on Antimicrobial Selection and Stewardship

Aside from the use of RADTs during influenza season, RTI diagnostic testing including viral DFAs and culture, bacterial culture, NAATs, serologic testing for the atypical pathogens, and urinary antigen testing for *S. pneumoniae* and *L. pneumophila* are still underutilized in the outpatient setting [10, 189]. Therefore, treatment of patients with CAP is generally empiric and based on guidelines by the American Thoracic Society and IDSA [146] rather than on a confirmed laboratory diagnosis. Antibiotic selection must cover both the most prevalent bacterial pathogens and the atypical pathogens.

Despite the high prevalence of viral infections, approximately 22.6 million (55 %) out of 41 million antibiotic prescriptions were prescribed for viral lower and upper RTIs, despite the fact that a bacterial etiology was highly unlikely [82]. Conversely the identification of the viral pathogen can lead to the administration of an appropriate antiviral. For example, during the early weeks of the 2009 influenza A H1N1 pandemic, four different influenza viruses were circulating with varying antiviral susceptibility patterns. According to surveillance data provided by the Center for Disease Control and Prevention (CDC, Atlanta, GA), FluA-H1 strains demonstrated >99 % resistance to the first line therapeutic oseltamivir, a neuraminidase inhibitor, and susceptibility to adamantine, FluA-H3 was oseltamivir-susceptible and >99 % adamantine-resistant, FluA(H1N1)pdm09 was oseltamivir-susceptible and >99 % adamantine-resistant; FluB was oseltamivir-susceptible and adamantine-resistant. Therefore, the identification of what specific strain of influenza virus was causing the infection of specific patients was essential to ensure proper drug selection, especially in high-risk or critically ill patients. Additionally, the more appropriate use of influenza antivirals can be achieved when an accurate, rapid diagnosis is made. Recent studies demonstrated that rapid testing permitted the timely administration of oseltamivir [229] and allowed for a more rapid discontinuation of treatment in persons without documented influenza [191]. Finally, new viral therapeutic agents for respiratory viruses other than influenza are in development and/or in clinical trials [171, 233]. Proper administration of these new agents will depend on the laboratory providing accurate tests that detect a broad range of viral pathogens [189].

For HAP and VAP, initial empiric therapy choices may be standardized and initiated based on patient clinical status, underlying disease, and/or risk for infection with a multidrug-resistant pathogen. Initial therapy often is inadequate, thereby extending the course of the disease and increasing morbidity, mortality, and hospital length of stay. The mortality rate in ICU pneumonia cases ranges from 20–30 % when initial therapy was adequate, to 50–80 % when initial therapy was inappropriate and changed after culture results were obtained [112]. Furthermore, inadequate and/or unnecessary broad spectrum antibiotic therapy can enhance the spread of drug-resistant pathogens within institutional settings and increase the risk of hospital-acquired infections such as *Clostridium difficile*, MRSA, and vancomycin-resistant enterococci.

Comprehensive NAATs provide key information not only for antiviral therapy selection but can also aid in restricting antibiotic use to those circumstances where antibiotic therapy is appropriate and in promoting switches to targeted specific therapies, thus reducing the use of broad spectrum antibiotics when not indicated [170, 142, 189]. This practice is in keeping with the goals of antibiotic stewardship, especially considering the steady and critical rise of antibiotic resistance and limited or no options available for the treatment of multidrug or pan-resistant bacterial infections.

Prevention of Nosocomial Infections

The burden of nosocomial infections can be significant, incurring additional costs for supplemental diagnostic tests, extended hospitalization, and increased morbidity and mortality [19, 40, 62, 126, 155, 217, 219]. Therefore, rapid diagnostic tests are needed to identify infected patients upon admission, thereby preventing nosocomial transmission by facilitating isolation and appropriate cohorting decisions [165, 206]. Studies have documented significant nosocomial transmission of ADV, influenza, RSV, HMPV, PIV, and HRV in hospital units, chronic care facilities, and pediatric units [19, 40, 62, 126, 155, 217, 219, 232]. During the height of RSV season, when prevalence can be >50 %, high numbers of hospital admissions often require the cohorting of RSV-positive children due to a lack of private rooms. However, limiting diagnostic testing to RSV alone in a cohorting scenario could put other seriously ill children at risk for acquisition of a second viral infection with other pathogens such as HMPV or HRV [80]. The rapid identification of health care facility-acquired *Legionella* infection is essential so that the environment source can be identified and eradicated, thus preventing further transmission. In addition, PCR techniques are used to proactively routinely screen potential environmental sources.

Epidemiologic Surveillance and Outbreak Investigation

The identification of a wide range of viral pathogens is essential for epidemiologic surveillance and establishes both seasonal and population patterns which can serve as excellent indicators for predicting immunization scheduling (e.g., influenza), or for administering preventive measures (e.g., RSV immune globulin). Previously, such surveillance was done by state Departments of Health or on a national level by the CDC. Comprehensive NAATs now enable local laboratories to monitor in real time viral prevalence and provide to their clinicians and health care facilities regular updates on circulating viruses. Testing decisions should use local data and additional resources and epidemiology information provided on the CDC web site (http://www.cdc.gov/flu/).

A study by S. Wong et al. demonstrated that the use of a multiplex NAAT (17 viruses) identified a virus in 59 % of the outbreaks and 29 % of the outbreak specimens that were negative using DFAs and a limited number of individual NAATs (ten viruses) [226]. Overall, the detection rate increased from 72–91 % for outbreaks and from 47–56 % for outbreak specimens. Comprehensive testing can identify reemerging or new emerging viral pathogens, as was the case during the influenza A H1N1 2009 pandemic.

Additionally, NAATs have been a key component in understanding both the epidemiology and features of large outbreaks of pertussis-like illness [190]. For example the large percentage of cases (29 %) of *B. holmseii* identified in an outbreak in Ohio in 2010–2011 was in contrast to some previous reports where the frequency of detection was very low [190]. The USA has seen peaks of pertussis activity every 3–5 years, with increasing cases since 1980. Accurate detection of pertussis is essential to better control the spread of disease from a public health standpoint through antimicrobial prophylaxis of asymptomatic household contacts, children less than 1 year of age, pregnant women in their third trimester, persons with preexisting conditions that are at risk for the development of severe respiratory failure, and all contacts in high-risk settings (http://www.cdc.gov/pertussis/outbreaks/pep.html).

Available Assays

Sample Types, Transport, and Storage

The recovery of respiratory pathogens is highly dependent on using the appropriate sample type and collection methods [139]. Laboratories using commercial FDA-cleared assays should refer to the manufacturer's package information to determine what sample types have been validated for use with the specific test (Table 52.2). The use of alternate samples types is permitted after the laboratory has performed their own validation studies that establish acceptable performance characteristics when testing the alternate sample type.

Applicable upper respiratory tract specimens for viral, *C. pneumoniae*, and *M. pneumoniae* testing include nasopharyngeal (NP) washes, NP aspirates, NP swabs, and midturbinate swabs placed in viral transport media [1, 48, 49, 95, 118, 131, 164, 223]. Oropharyngeal swab specimens are less sensitive (54 %) than either NP swabs (73 %) or NP wash specimens (85 %) due to the substantially lower levels of virus present in the oropharynx than the nasopharynx [131]. However, the combined use of nasal-oropharyngeal swabs can enhance the recovery of both avian influenza and SARS-CoV [49]. NP flocked synthetic swabs should be used in lieu of traditional synthetic NP swabs since flocked NP swabs yield a greater recovery of viral pathogens, with sensitivity comparable to NP wash specimens [1, 48, 95]. The rates of positivity for *B. pertussis* by real-time PCR were shown to be comparable when specimens were collected with either NP rayon swabs on aluminum shafts in Amies gel with charcoal or NP flocked swabs in universal transport media [6].

Lower respiratory tract (LRT) samples appropriate for viral pathogens, *C. pneumoniae*, *M. pneumoniae*, *L. pneumophila*, and bacterial pathogens include induced sputum, bronchial alveolar lavages, bronchial washings, protected brushes, and Combicath specimens. Studies that examined the detection of FluA(H1N1)pdm09 found that in seriously ill patients requiring intensive care, upper respiratory tract samples can be negative while LRT samples are positive [120, 123, 156, 230].

Additional factors that influence pathogen recovery include the time of sample collection after the onset of clinical symptoms and the age of the patient (children tend to shed higher titers of virus and for longer periods of time than adults). Therefore, for optimal detection, samples should be collected within 3 days for adults and within 5 days for children after the onset of symptoms [39, 85, 95, 120, 123]. Samples should be transported to the laboratory as soon as possible, preferentially on wet ice or refrigerated (2–8 °C) if testing will be performed within 48 h. If testing is delayed, the samples should be stored at −80 °C. Multiple freeze-thaws should be avoided as this process can decrease pathogen titers.

Nucleic Acid Extraction

Target lysis in a stabilizing matrix to prevent target degradation by deoxyribonucleases (DNases) and/or ribonucleases (RNases), followed by isolation and purification of the nucleic acids (NAs) are essential and critical steps of every NAAT. This is particularly important for respiratory samples that can be highly viscous and contain inhibitory substances and enzymes that destroy the target NAs. Some sample types may require a pretreatment with proteinase K or a similar enzyme. Highly efficient commercial NA extraction systems ensure sufficient NA recovery and the removal of inhibitory substances that could result in inefficient or no amplification of the target NAs. Presently, the majority of NA extraction systems use a chaotropic agent to lyse viral particles or bacterial cells, silica particles or a membrane to capture the released NAs, and a series of wash steps to remove inhibitory substances. NAs are generally eluted in either RNase/DNase free water or a stabilizing buffer such as EDTA-Tris. Although NA extraction can be performed manually using for example spin columns, the majority of laboratories currently use automated platforms that can extract as few as one sample at a time or more than 96 samples in microwell plate formats. Many NAATs have been FDA-cleared with specific extraction platforms or methods and laboratories should be aware that the substitution of another extraction platform or method constitutes a major change in the assay protocol. From a regulatory perspective, if the extraction procedure is modified or changed then the entire test is now considered an LDT. Laboratories must be compliant with all applicable state and federal CLIA standards, and may choose to comply with the College of American Pathologists regulations to meet state or federal regulatory requirements.

Amplification and Detection of Nucleic Acids

Many amplification and detection methods are used in the current FDA-cleared assays (Table 52.2) and additional assays that are not FDA cleared but may be Conformité Européenne (CE) marked for use as an in vitro diagnostic device (IVD) in Europe (Table 52.3). Amplification methods include traditional reverse transcription polymerase chain reaction (RT-PCR), PCR, real-time RT-PCR and PCR, RT-PCR and primer extension, nested PCR, amplicon rescued multiplex PCR (ARM-PCR), and isothermal amplification such as nucleic acid sequence based amplification (NASBA), helicase-dependent amplification (HAD), nicking enzyme amplification reaction (NEAR), and loop mediated amplification (LAMP). Primers sets can be broad range (e.g., family), short range (e.g., genus), or pathogen-specific (e.g., genus and species). Targets may be single or multiple copy and include genomic RNA, or DNA, or messenger RNA. Detection technologies utilize fluorogenic intercalating dyes, fluorogenic probes (Taqman, fluorescence resonance energy transfer [FRET] hydridization, molecular beacons, scorpions, locked nucleic acid [LNA]), arrays (liquid bead, gold nanoparticles, or solid chip), electrochemical-based methods, melt curve analysis, lateral flow, or simple turbidity.

Tests vary considerably with the number of targets detected, ranging from one pathogen target plus an internal control (IC) to 20 targets plus an IC. They differ in which targets are detected (viral and/or bacterial) and if the tests are able to detect and differentiate various types within a virus family (e.g., PIV-1, -2, -3, and -4) (Tables 52.2 and 52.3). Platforms can be all inclusive with NA extraction, amplification, and detection performed in one cartridge (e.g., GeneXpert, Cepheid, Sunnyvale, CA; cobas Liat System, Roche Molecular Systems/Iquum, Marlborough, MA), in one pouch (Film Array, BioFire/bioMérieux, Salt Lake City, UT), or one chamber of a multi-test wheel cartridge (Simplexa Direct, Focus Diagnostics, Cypress, CA). Testing can be performed using modular systems that incorporate NA extraction with amplification but a separate unit for detection (e.g., Verigene, Nanosphere, Northbrook, IL), modular systems that separate isolation, from amplification combined with detection (Simplexa, Focus Diagnostics,; ProFlu+, Gen-Probe, San Diego, CA; Lyra, Quidel, San Diego, CA) and systems where isolation, amplification, and detection are all performed separately (xTag RVP, Luminex, Austin, TX; eSensor XT-8 System, GenMark Diagnostics, Carlsbad, CA; Infiniti RVP Plus, Autogenomics, Vista, CA; Resplex II, Qiagen, Valencia, CA).

Only a limited number of tests are FDA-cleared for the detection of bacterial pathogens. One highly multiplexed test, the FilmArray Respiratory Panel (BioFire/bioMérieux) tests for 17 viral pathogens and three bacterial pathogens, *C. pneumoniae*, *M. pneumoniae*, and *B. pertussis*. One additional assay is FDA-cleared for the detection of *M. pneumoniae*, the *illumi*gene Mycoplasma Assay (Meridian Biosciences, Inc, Cincinnati, OH). Two addition assays are FDA-cleared for the detection of *B. pertussis*, the *illumi*gene Pertussis assay (Meridian) and the Amplivue *Bordetella* assay (Quidel, San Diego, CA).

Time-to-results for the FDA-cleared assays ranges from 15 min to approximately 12 h depending on the platform, with the most rapid results (< 1.5 h) for the all-inclusive cartridge/pouch based tests. Technical hands-on time varies from < 2 min to approximately 3 h. Currently, most NAATs are rated as CLIA moderate to high complexity. In January 2015, the first waived NAAT under CLIA was cleared by the FDA, the Alere i Influenza A&B test (Alere Scarborough, Scarborough, ME). To perform the test, a sample receiver and test base are inserted into the Alere i instrument (Alere). After a 3 min heating step, the sample is eluted from the nasal collection swab directly into the sample receiver buffer. The transfer cartridge is used to transfer the sample to the test cartridge, where NEAR-amplification and detection occur in approximately 10 min [11, 12, 35, 162].

For comprehensive diagnosis of CAP and to rapidly identify pathogens associated with HAP and VAP, additional tests are needed that target the main bacterial pathogens [63]. The Research Use Only (RUO) Unyvero System (Curetis, Stutgart, GR) has an assay developed as an aid for the diagnosis of bacterial pneumonia. The specimen is preprocessed in Unyvero L4 Lysator, and then added to the assay-specific cartridge which is then inserted into the Unyvero A50 analyser. All steps are controlled by the Unyvero C8 Cockpit. The assay detects the major bacterial pathogens (*Acinetobacter baumanii*, *Enterobacter* spp. *Escherichia coli*, *Klebsiella oxytoca*, *Klebsiella pneumoniae*, *Haemophilus influenzae*, *Moraxella. catarrhalis*, *Morganella morganii*, *Proteus* spp., *S. aureus*, *Pseudomonas aeruginosa*, *Serratia marcescens*, *S. maltophilia*, *S. pneumoniae*), the atypical pathogens

(*C. pneumoniae*, *L. pneumophila*), and one fungal pathogen (*Pneumocystis jiroveci*) known to cause CAP, HAP, and VAP. In addition, the assay will detect 18 genes associated with the major categories of antibiotic resistance. Time-to-results is approximately 4–5 h. The assay serves as a preliminary screen to be followed by culture and traditional antimicrobial susceptibility testing. Preliminary studies demonstrated that the assay detected more pathogens than routine culture. The Unyvero system detected numerous resistance markers and allowed for a change in empiric antibiotic therapy within 5–6 h for 67 % of the patients tested [103, 201].

The RUO Abbott Plex-ID system (Abbott, Abbott Park, IL) is comprised of broad range PCR or RT-PCR and Electrospray Ionization Mass Spectrometry (PCR/ESI-MS) for pathogen detection [36, 37, 44, 55]. Following NA extraction, PCR and/or RT-PCR is performed in a microwell plate using multiple primer pairs, with one primer set per well. Following amplification, the automated platform performs post-PCR desalting, purification, and high-resolution mass spectrometry using ESI-MS. The raw spectra are analyzed and calibrated with an internal mass standard. Spectral analysis determines the nucleotide base composition of the single-stranded oligonucleotides complementary to the initial target. To evaluate the relative concentration of the target or targets present, a semiquantitative value can be obtained by comparing the peak heights with the internal PCR calibration internal mass standard present in every well. The initial Plex-ID (Ibis T5000) system has been replaced by the Abbott IRIDICA RUO system (Abbott) that is comprised of PLEX-ID SP (nucleic acid extraction platform), PLEX-ID FH (liquid handler for assay setup), and a new version of the PLEX-ID PCR/ESI-MS platform. Time-to-results is <8 h. PCR- or RT-PCR/ESI-MS has been used to detect and identify a variety of respiratory viruses, influenza subtypes, bacteria, and fungi associated with RTIs ([88, 159, 207, 214, 215]; Huttner et al. 2014).

NAAT Performance

Overall, NAATs for respiratory viral and the atypical bacterial pathogens are highly sensitive (85–100 %) and very specific (>95 %) when samples are collected shortly after the onset of clinical symptoms (see references in Tables 52.2 and 52.3). Assays can detect mixed infections [79] and a broad range of viral types within a family [34]. Performance results from clinical trials for FDA clearance and from investigator-initiated studies need to be reviewed carefully when evaluating an assay because many factors can affect the overall results, such as patient population and age, testing conditions, specimen collection factors, storage time from sample collection to testing, and comparator method used in the analysis. Similarly, results obtained in different studies can vary significantly for assays and targets, depending on the study design (see references in Tables 52.2 and 52.3). Numerous studies have demonstrated that not all targets within a particular assay are detected with the same sensitivity. NAATs also have certain limitations. Due to the complexity of primer and probe designs and interactions, highly multiplexed NAATs can sometimes be less sensitive than individual NAATs [70, 166, 167]. Reduced analytical sensitivity, however, does not always correlate with reduced clinical sensitivity since viral quantity in clinical samples, depending on the virus and timing of sample collection, are often much higher than the limit of detection of the assays. NAATs often are less sensitive for viruses with multiple serotypes, such as ADV [37, 74, 113, 133]. Decreased performance for the detection of ADV can be clinically significant, particularly when testing samples from immunosuppressed patients (e.g., transplant patients) for whom ADV infection has a high mortality rate if not treated. For high-risk patients, laboratories may elect to supplement testing with either a more sensitive, broadly reactive ADV-specific assay or with cell culture [25, 62, 148, 173]. Many of the assays cannot distinguish between HRV and EV due to the fact that the assays target the 5′ UTR which is genetically similar for the two viruses [113]. The performance of the assays, in particular for RNA viruses, also may be affected by sequence mutations that occur over time. These mutations can result in primer/probe mismatches that decrease assay sensitivity, result in a total lack of target amplification and detection, or result in cross reactivity [153]. Any modifications to the assays to accommodate such genetic changes would have to be cleared by the FDA. In highly multiplexed assays, revalidation can require extensive assessment of all target interactions, thus making changes extremely difficult.

The FDA-cleared assays for the detection of *B. pertussis* target the multicopy IS481 gene. This gene is found not only in *B. pertussis* (50–238 copies/cell) but also in *B. holmseii* (8-10 copies.cell) and in 1–5 % of the strains of *B. brochioseptica* [190]. Therefore, the assays are not specific for *B. pertussis* and alternative targets must be tested to differentiate the three species and also to detect *B. parapertussis* [89, 190, 216, 225]. Additionally, pseudo-outbreaks of pertussis have been described, indicating that great caution must be used not only in performing the NAAT but also in the collection of test samples, particularly in areas where vaccine is administered. Finally, due to the short time of localization of the atypical bacterial pathogens to the URT, the detection of these pathogens may require a combination of various sample types and various test methods, including NAATs, serology, and antigen testing, to provide the most sensitive results.

Interpretation of Test Results

The advantages of NAATs compared with traditional testing methods include improved sensitivity, not needing a viable organism for detection, broader scope of pathogens identified, and the ability to detect mixed infections. These same advantages can also raise issues with the interpretation of results. Until recently the detection of any respiratory virus had been considered significant. Several studies have shown that respiratory viruses can be detected in asymptomatic patients [2, 14, 104, 181]. One study found that NAATs identified a virus in 83 % of specimens from symptomatic children, but also detected a virus in 42 % of specimens from children without symptoms [2]. Another study demonstrated similar colonization with CoV (7.6 %) in symptomatic hospitalized children versus (7.1 %) in an asymptomatic outpatient control population. The overall prevalence of CoV or the types of CoV was not significantly higher among hospitalized children than controls. Respiratory viruses in NP swabs were identified from both asymptomatic and symptomatic solid organ transplant recipients early after transplantation [14]. The data suggest that due to the high prevalence of positive results in children and immunocompromised patients without symptoms, results should be interpreted cautiously, and in the context of clinical presentation, radiographic findings, and other laboratory tests. Additionally, clinicians must be aware that NAATs will detect nucleic acids lingering from a previous infection and that samples submitted for assessment of therapeutic response may remain positive for days to weeks after treatment due to the presence of nonviable organisms and not due to treatment failure. In these situations culture or quantitative NAATs (see Future Directions below) may provide the best option. With the increased use of highly multiplexed respiratory virus assays, a variety of mixed viral infections are detected and the clinical importance of each virus is not always evident. Nonviable virus from a previous infection may be detected, making it impossible to determine which or if all viruses contribute to the current illness. Test reports need to explain what viruses are included in the NAAT panel, sensitivity and specificity of the test, and that a negative result does not preclude infection with a specific pathogen due to many factors that can lead to decreased assay sensitivity.

Aside from the detection of the atypical pathogens and *Bordetella* spp. the detection of other bacterial pathogens, such as those included in the Unyvero test, directly from clinical samples raises several interesting questions that need to be addressed: (1) How do we differentiate between colonization and infection so as not to promote overuse of antibiotics? Are quantitative assays necessary or can assay cut off values be established at clinically relevant thresholds? (2) How many pathogens need to be included in a screening test? The detection of the broad scope of potential gram-positive and gram-negative bacterial pathogens is limited by multiplexing capabilities. Should these assays detect at a minimum those pathogens with the highest clinical impact or those difficult to treat? (3) How can we detect a broad range of resistance mechanisms, some of which do not have genetic markers (such as porin down-regulation in *Pseudomonas* spp.)? (4) Can we trust a positive result to direct antibiotic therapy? (5) Can we trust a negative result when there is the possibility of the presence of unknown resistance mechanisms? (6) Do we need to link a resistance marker to a specific bacterial target? For example, how do we interpret a result positive for a specific resistance gene when we do not detect the organism in which it would reside? (7) Will this type of testing provide actionable results, i.e., will this change clinical practice? The answers to these questions will only be resolved during clinical trials that compare NAAT results to classic microbiology testing, clinical practice, and patient outcomes. However, the future of testing may be a combination of multiplexed NAAT viral and bacterial screens.

Laboratory Issues

Laboratories must consider multiple factors in selecting the most appropriate NAAT or in developing testing algorithms (Table 52.4) [60]. Considerations include patient population(s), FDA status of the NAAT and the implications for regulatory issues, platform type, test complexity and technical expertise required, turnaround time, testing volumes, batch vs single unit testing, and the number and type of pathogens detected. The higher costs of NAATs can easily be offset by replacing the less sensitive test methods or by testing on site in lieu of referral to a reference laboratory [60, 144]. Additionally costs can be offset by other demonstrated benefits, such as improvements in patient care and financial outcomes, including 30 % reduction in antibiotic use, up to 20 % reduction in unnecessary diagnostic tests and procedures, and 50 % reduction in hospital days [9, 22, 82, 92, 115, 120, 123, 142, 170, 191, 227, 229]. To achieve these benefits NAATs should be performed within 24 h of sample collection so that results are available within a clinically relevant time frame. With the advent of single unit cartridge/pouch based tests that require minimal hands-on time and very minimal molecular technical expertise, all size laboratories can perform NAATs on all shifts. Considering the impact of global travel, comprehensive and highly specific NAATS should be performed year round and not limited to specific seasons. Although the positive predictive value of these tests remains high during times of low viral prevalence, laboratories should consider confirmatory testing when a virus is detected during an unusual time period. Some pathogens are more prevalent in specific groups

Table 52.4 Factors to consider in selecting an appropriate NAAT

Topic	Parameter	Factors to consider
Patient population	Age	Neonates, children, elderly
	Immune status	BMT, SOC, oncology, HIV
	Underlying disease	COPD, asthma, CHF, CF
	Health care inpatient setting	Risk of mixed infections, infection control
	Health care outpatient setting	Risk to family members
Regulatory issues	FDA status/CE marked	IVD, RUO, IUO, ASRs
	Regulatory requirements	CLIA, CAP, State, Federal
Laboratory issues	Test complexity	Technical expertise required, training
	Turnaround time	STAT (ED) versus routine, number of times tested per day
	Volume	Single unit cartridge versus larger batch testing
	Instrumentation/space	Complexity, cost, number of units
Assay performance	Appropriate sample types	Applicable for patient population(s)
	Sensitivity	Clinically relevant level (>90 %)
	Specificity	No cross reactivity (>95 %)
	Reactivity	Detect all subtypes (100 %)
	Consistent results	Reproducible, rare failures
Cost	Implementation	Assay validation or verification, training
	Instrumentation	Number of units
	Cost per test	Assessed by clinical benefit
	Quality	Quality control, proficiency testing

ASRs analyte specific reagents, *BMT* bone marrow transplant, *CAP* College of American Pathologists, CE cConformite Européenne, *CF* cystic fibrosis, *CHF* congestive heart failure, *CLIA* Clinical laboratory Improvement Act, *COPD* chronic obstructive pulmonary disease, asthma, *ED* emergency department, *HIV* human immunodeficiency virus, *IUO* investigational use only, *IVD* in vitro diagnostic, *NAAT* nucleic acid amplification test *RUO* research use only, *SOC* solid organ transplant,

(e.g., RSV and HMPV in children and the elderly), but limiting testing to specific age groups will miss clinically relevant disease in other patient populations [64, 83]. Infections with these pathogens can also sometimes have atypical presentations, such as pericarditis due to HMPV in an otherwise healthy adult [97]. Therefore, age may be useful in triaging initial testing but should not govern the final scope of what viruses are included in diagnostic testing. In addition, if step wise testing is considered based on risk factors such as age or immune status, coinfections that could lead to serious nosocomial transmission in health care settings should not be missed. Unexpected local, national, and international events, such as the H1N1-2009 pandemic can change our testing algorithms and laboratories must be prepared to adapt quickly to such events.

Quality Control

Kit positive and negative controls, ICs, and external controls should be used to verify the performance of the reagents and to ensure no inhibitory substances remain after extraction that could lead to poor amplification, reduced assay sensitivity, and false-negative results [77]. Controls should be tested in accordance with regulatory requirements as outlined by CLIA, CAP, and state or other federal regulatory agencies, and in accordance with the manufacturer's instructions. Ideally all controls should go through the same process as the patient sample. ICs are best added at the NA extraction step to ensure efficient recovery of NAs. ICs added after extraction will just confirm the amplification efficiency and an external extraction control must be used unless the extraction method has demonstrated negligible inhibition (generally <1 %) for the sample types tested. During amplification and detection, the IC is essential to demonstrate a lack of amplification failure or decreased efficiency. External positive and negative controls (not provided in the kit) must be used to verify each new lot and/or shipment of reagents. Each analyte of the multiplex must be verified individually in either a single reaction or as a component of a pooled control. Daily positive (individual or pooled) and negative controls must be run thereafter if batch testing is performed. Rotating controls after lot/shipment validation is acceptable. Tests using a single unit cartridge/pouch that contain a procedural control (IC or process control) do not require external controls to be run with each individual cartridge/pouch once the performance of the procedural control has been verified. External positive controls for each analyte and negative controls are only required for verification of each new lot/shipment or at a minimum once per month.

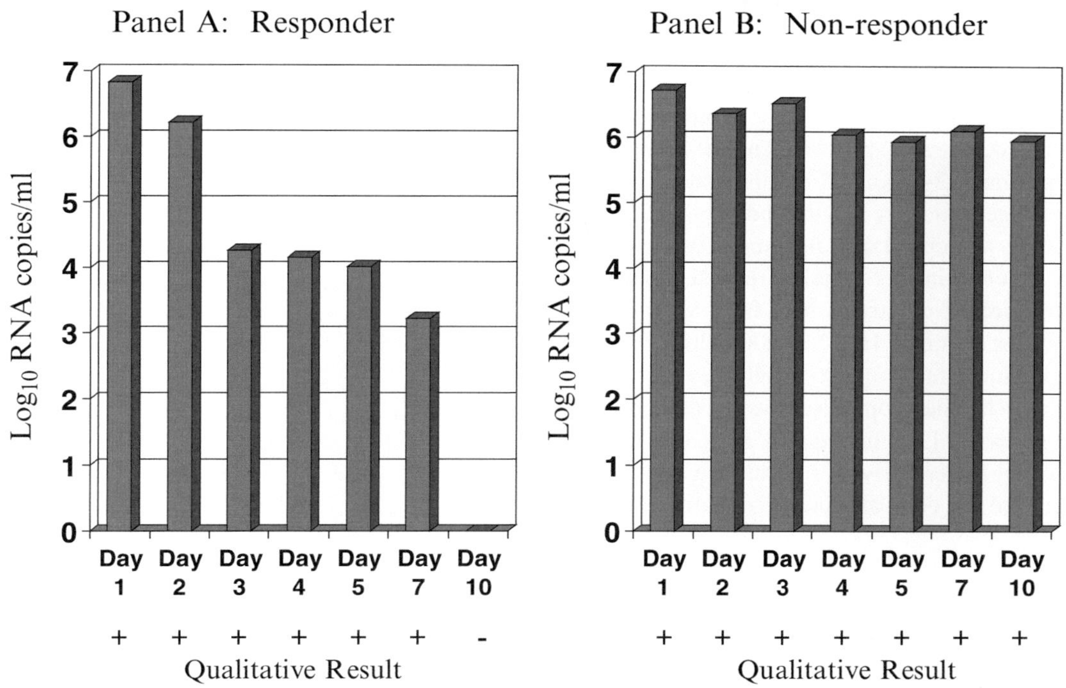

Figure 52.3 Quantitative versus qualitative testing for assessing antiviral response. Panel A: Influenza A viral load results over time in a patient with oseltamivir-susceptible influenza A virus. Panel B: Influenza A viral load results over time in a patient with oseltamivir-susceptible influenza A virus. +, positive for Influenza A detection; -, negative for influenza A detection

Laboratories must ensure proper procedures to prevent both sample and amplicon cross contamination that could cause false-positive results. Laboratories need to interpret negative results and IC values in the context of the presence or absence of potential nucleic acid degradation and amplification inhibition. Laboratories are responsible to continually assess the performance of their assays to ensure that over time, the performance has not declined due to factors such as genetic shifts in the target analytes. Finally, ongoing assessment of technical competency and participation in proficiency testing programs are essential to ensure high-quality performance and results.

Future Directions

Quantitative Viral Assays

Both virus type and the amount of virus present (viral load) can significantly impact the clinical characteristics and clinical course of RTIs. Quantitative detection of viral respiratory pathogens can help to assess the dynamics of viral proliferation, better understand viral pathogenesis, and permits a means to evaluate the significance of coinfections. Since NAATs detect both viable and nonviable virus, monitoring patients for treatment response with qualitative testing provides little information as tests may remain positive for days even with successful therapy. Quantitative tests that demonstrate a decline in viral load during therapy more accurately assess patient response (Fig. 52.3a) and the failure to see a decline (Fig. 52.3b) would potentially indicate earlier a need to consider alternative therapies. This information is especially important for critically ill patients and immunosuppressed patients. Finally, viral load assays provide important information in the assessment of new antiviral agents in FDA clinical trials. Future assay development should consider quantification of the viral targets.

Influenza Resistance Testing

Antiviral resistance to neuraminidase inhibitors can be assessed both phenotypically and genotypically [84, 161, 187]. Neuraminidase inhibition assays detect decreases in susceptibility by determining the 50 % inhibitory concentration (IC_{50}). However, these assays require growth of the virus and the presence of quasi-species can lead to unreliable results. Alternatively, genotypic assays are easier and identify known resistance mutations. However, newly identified mutations require phenotypic confirmation. Although no molecular assays are FDA-cleared for influenza resistance testing, several methods are used including traditional Sanger sequencing, pyrosequencing, PCR genotyping assays, and next-generation sequencing (NGS) [84, 161].

Pyrosequencing is currently the method of choice since the method is fast, has a high throughput, is sensitive (can detect a mutation if present in 10 % of the population), can assess multiple known mutations (e.g., H275Y mutation found in resistant H1N1-2009 strains) as well as unknown mutations and polymorphisms [52–54]. NGS has the added advantage of generating longer sequence lengths and has identified new genetic mutations associated with neuraminidase resistance. Laboratories should consider offering resistance testing in seasons where circulating strains may have varying resistance patterns (for example, H1N1 in 2007–2008 that demonstrated variable oseltamivir susceptibility), especially for patients at high risk to develop severe disease (e.g., pregnant or immunosuppressed) [38]. In addition, screening for resistance is indicated in seriously ill patients who continue to shed virus and are not clinically improving after prolonged antiviral therapy.

Next-Generation Sequencing

Over the last decade the development of NGS has transformed a labor-intensive slow process into a real-time method with applicability to respiratory diagnostics. The complexity of NGS is beyond the scope of this chapter but the use of NGS will continue to evolve in the clinical laboratory, particularly in light of easy-to-use bench top sequencers such as the Ion Torrent Personal Genome Machine (PGM) (Life Technologies, Carlsbad, CA) and the MiSeq (Illumina, San Diego, CA). Already NGS is used to detect and identify respiratory pathogens, resistance and pathogenicity markers, genetically characterize viruses, explore the respiratory microbiome, and understand the epidemiology of respiratory pathogens [169]. With new emerging technologies and simple methods to perform the required bioinformatics, this testing will increasingly become part of routine diagnostics.

Summary

The IDSA Diagnostics Task Force report: "Better Tests: Better Care: Improved Diagnostics for Infectious Diseases" highlighted the importance of diagnostic testing in the management of infectious diseases [27]. Likewise, the 2013 CDC [31] report "Antibiotic Resistance Threats in the US" states that both the development of new drugs and new diagnostics are essential to combat the threat of multiple-drug-resistant pathogens [30]. The incorporation of NAATs into routine practice for the diagnosis of infectious diseases will continue to grow, bringing new advanced technologies that allow the rapid and accurate detection of viral, bacterial, and fungal respiratory pathogens.

References

1. Abu-Diab A, Azzeh M, Ghneim R, et al. Comparison between pernasal flocked swabs and nasopharyngeal aspirates for detection of common respiratory viruses in samples from children. J Clin Microbiol. 2008;46:2414–7.
2. Advani S, Sengupta A, Forman M, et al. Detecting respiratory viruses in asymptomatic children. Pediatr Infect Dis J. 2012;31:1221–6.
3. Alby K, Popowitch EB, Miller MB. Comparative evaluation of the nanosphere verigene RV+ assay and the Simplexa Flu A/B & RSV kit for detection of influenza and respiratory syncytial virus. J Clin Microbiol. 2013;51:352–3.
4. American Thoracic Society and Infectious Diseases Society of America. Guidelines for the management of adults with hospital acquired, ventilator associated, and hospital associated pneumonia. Am J Respir Crit Care Med. 2005;171:388–416.
5. Anderson TP, Werno AM, Barratt K, et al. Comparison of 4 PCR assays for the detection of viral pathogens in respiratory specimens. J Virol Methods. 2013;191:118–21.
6. Arbefeville S, Ferrieri P. Comparison of rates of positivity for *Bordetella pertussis* by real-time PCR between specimens collected with rayon swabs on aluminum wire shafts in Aimes gel with charcoal and specimens collected with flocked swabs in universal viral transport medium during an epidemic. J Clin Microbiol. 2014;52:2656–8.
7. Babady NE, Mead P, Stiles J, et al. Comparison of the Luminex xTAG RVP Fast assay and the Idaho Technology FilmArray RP assay for detection of respiratory viruses in pediatric patients at a cancer hospital. J Clin Microbiol. 2012;50:2282–8.
8. Balada-Llasat JM, LaRue H, Kelly C, et al. Evaluation of commercial ResPlex II v2.0, MultiCode-PLx and xTAG respiratory viral panels for the diagnosis of respiratory viral infections in adults. J Clin Virol. 2011;50:42–5.
9. Barenfanger J, Drake C, Leon N, et al. Clinical and financial benefits of rapid detection of respiratory viruses: an outcomes study. J Clin Microbiol. 2000;38:2824–8.
10. Bartlett JG. Diagnostic tests for agents of community acquired pneumonia. Clin Infect Dis. 2011;52(S4):S296–304.
11. Bell J, Bonner A, Cohen DM, et al. Multicenter clinical evaluation of the novel Alere i Influenza A&B isothermal nucleic amplification test. J Clin Virol. 2014;61:81–6.
12. Bell JJ, Selvarangan R. Evaluation of the Alere i Influenza A&B nucleic acid amplification test by use of respiratory specimens collected in viral transport medium. J Clin Microbiol. 2014;52:3992–5.
13. Beneri C, Ginocchio CC, Manji R, et al. Comparison of clinical features of pediatric RSV and human metapneumovirus infections. Infect Control Hosp Epidemiol. 2009;30:1240–1.
14. BenMarzouk-Hidalgo OJ, Molina J, Cordero E, et al. Asymptomatic and symptomatic respiratory virus infection detected in naso-pharyngeal swabs from solid organ transplant recipients early after transplantation. J Clin Virol. 2011;52:276–7.
15. Béssède E, Renaudin H, Clerc M, et al. Evaluation of the combination of the NucliSENS easyMAG and the EasyQ applications for the detection of *Mycoplasma pneumoniae* and *Chlamydia pneumoniae* in respiratory tract specimens. Eur J Clin Microbiol Infect Dis. 2010;29:187–90.
16. Bibby DF, McElarney I, Breuer J, et al. Comparative evaluation of the Seegene Seeplex RV15 and real-time PCR for respiratory virus detection. J Med Virol. 2011;83:1469–75.
17. Blasi F, Tarsia P, Aliberti S. *Chlamydophila pneumoniae*. Clin Microbiol Infect. 2009;15:29–35.
18. Blyth CC, Iredell JR, Dwyer DE. Rapid-test sensitivity for novel swine-origin influenza A (H1N1) virus in humans. N Engl J Med. 2009;361:2493.

19. Boivin G, De Serres G, Hamelin ME, et al. An outbreak of severe respiratory tract infection due to human metapneumovirus in a long-term care facility. Clin Infect Dis. 2007;44:1152–8.
20. Boku S, Naito T, Murai K, et al. Near-point-of-care administration by the attending physician of the rapid influenza antigen detection immunochromatography test and the fully automated respiratory virus nucleic acid test: contribution to patient management. Diagn Microbiol Infect Dis. 2013;76:445–9.
21. Borek AP, Clemens SH, Gaskins VK, et al. Respiratory syncytial virus detection by Remel Xpect, Binax Now RSV, direct immunofluorescent staining, and tissue culture. J Clin Microbiol. 2006;44:1105–7.
22. Bourgeois FT, Valim C, McAdam AJ, et al. Relative impact of influenza and respiratory syncytial virus in young children. Pediatrics. 2009;124:e1072–80.
23. Branche AR, Walsh EE, Formica MA, et al. Detection of respiratory viruses in sputum from adults by use of automated multiplex PCR. J Clin Microbiol. 2014;52:3590–6.
24. Bruijnesteijn van Coppenraet LES, Swanink CMA, van Zwet AA, et al. Comparison of two commercial molecular assays for simultaneous detection of respiratory viruses in clinical samples using two automated electrophoresis detection systems. J Virol Methods. 2010;169:188–92.
25. Buckwalter SP, Teo R, Espy MJ, et al. Real-time qualitative PCR for 57 human adenovirus types from multiple specimen sources. J Clin Microbiol. 2012;50:766–71.
26. Butt SA, Maceira VP, McCallen ME, et al. Comparison of three commercial RT-PCR systems for the detection of respiratory viruses. J Clin Virol. 2014;61:406–10.
27. Caliendo AM, Gilbert DN, Ginocchio CC, et al. Better tests, better care: improved diagnostics for infectious diseases. Clin Infect Dis. 2013;57 Suppl 3:S139–70.
28. Casiano-Colón AE, Hulbert BB, Mayer TK, et al. Lack of sensitivity of rapid antigen tests for the diagnosis of respiratory syncytial virus infection in adults. J Clin Virol. 2003;28:169–74.
29. Centers for Disease Control and Prevention. Clusters of acute respiratory illness associated with human enterovirus 68 – Asia, Europe, and United States, 2008–2010. Weekly MMWR. 2011;60:1301–4.
30. Centers for Disease Control and Prevention. Diagnosis and management of Q fever – United States, 2013: recommendations from CDC and the Q Fever Working Group. MMWR Recom Rep. 2013;62:1–30.
31. Centers for Disease Control and Prevention. US Department of Health and Human Services. Antibiotic resistance threats in the United States, 2013.
32. Chan AB, Fox JD. NASBA and other transcription-based amplification methods for research and diagnostic microbiology. Rev Med Microbiol. 1999;10:185–96.
33. Chan JF, Lau SK, To KK, et al. Middle east respiratory syndrome coronavirus: another zoonotic betacoronavirus causing SARS-like disease. Clin Microbiol Rev. 2015;28:465–522.
34. Chandrasekaran A, Manji R, Joseph A, et al. Broad reactivity of the Luminex xTAG Respiratory Virus Panel (RVP) assay for the detection of human rhinoviruses. J Clin Virol. 2012;53:272–3.
35. Chapin KC, Flores-Cortez EJ. Performance of the molecular Alere i Influenza A&B test compared to Xpert Flu A/B. J Clin Microbiol. 2014;53:706–9.
36. Chen KF, Blyn L, Rothman RE, et al. Reverse transcription polymerase chain reaction and electrospray ionization mass spectrometry for identifying acute viral upper respiratory tract infections. Diagn Microbiol Infect Dis. 2011;69:179–86.
37. Chen KF, Rothman RE, Ramachandran P, et al. Rapid identification viruses from nasal pharyngeal aspirates in acute viral respiratory infections by RT-PCR and electrospray ionization mass spectrometry. J Virol Methods. 2011;173:60–6.
38. Chen LF, Dailey NJ, Rao AK, et al. Cluster of oseltamivir-resistant 2009 pandemic influenza A (H1N1) virus infections on a hospital ward among immunocompromised patients – North Carolina, 2009. J Infect Dis. 2011;203:838–46.
39. Cheng PK, Wong KK, Mak GC, et al. Performance of laboratory diagnostics for the detection of influenza A(H1N1)v virus as correlated with the time after symptom onset and viral load. J Clin Virol. 2010;47:182–5.
40. Cheng VC, Wu AK, Cheung CH, et al. Outbreak of human metapneumovirus infection in psychiatric inpatients: implications for directly observed use of alcohol hand rub in prevention of nosocomial outbreaks. J Hosp Infect. 2007;67:336–43.
41. Cho HJ, Jang JW, Ko SY, et al. Evaluation and verification of the nanosphere Verigene RV+ assay for detection of influenza A/B and H1/H3 subtyping. J Med Virol. 2015;87:18–24.
42. Choroszy-Król I, Magdalena Frej-Mądrzak M, Martyna Hober M, et al. Infections caused by *Chlamydophila pneumoniae*. Adv Clin Exp Med. 2014;23:123–6.
43. Clark TA. Changing *Pertussis* epidemiology: everything old is new again. J Infect Dis. 2014;209:979–81.
44. Cordey S, Thomas Y, Suter P, et al. Pilot evaluation of RT-PCR/electrospray ionization mass spectrometry (PLEX-ID/Flu assay) on influenza-positive specimens. Virol J. 2012;6:64–76.
45. Cruz AT, Cazacu AC, Greer JM, et al. Performance of a rapid assay (Binax NOW) for detection of respiratory syncytial virus at a children's hospital over a 3-year period. J Clin Microbiol. 2007;45:1993–5.
46. Cunha B. The atypical pneumonias: clinical diagnosis and importance. Eur Soc Clin Microbiol. 2006;12 Suppl 3:12–24.
47. Dabisch-Ruthe M, Vollmer T, Adams O, et al. Comparison of three multiplex PCR assays for the detection of respiratory viral infections: evaluation of xTAG respiratory virus panel fast assay, RespiFinder 19 assay and RespiFinder SMART 22 assay. BMC Infect Dis. 2012;12:163.
48. Daley P, Castriciano S, Chernesky M, et al. Comparison of flocked and rayon swabs for collection of respiratory epithelial cells from uninfected volunteers and symptomatic patients. J Clin Microbiol. 2006;44:2265–7.
49. de la Tabla VO, Masiá M, Antequera P, et al. Comparison of combined nose-throat swabs with nasopharyngeal aspirates for detection of pandemic influenza A/H1N1 2009 virus by real-time reverse transcriptase PCR. J Clin Microbiol. 2010;48:3492–5.
50. Deiman B, Schrover C, Moore C, et al. Rapid and highly sensitive qualitative real-time assay for detection of respiratory syncytial virus A and B using NASBA and molecular beacon technology. J Virol Methods. 2007;146:29–35.
51. Den Boer JW, Yzerman EPF, Schellekens J, et al. A large outbreak of Legionnaires' disease at a flower show, the Netherlands, 1999. Emerg Infect Dis. 2002;8(1):37–43. http://wwwnc.cdc.gov/eid/article/8/1/01-0176.htm.
52. Deyde VM, Gubareva LV. Influenza genome analysis using pyrosequencing method: current applications for a moving target. Expert Rev Mol Diagn. 2009;9:493–509.
53. Deyde VM, Nguyen T, Bright RA, et al. Detection of molecular markers of antiviral resistance in influenza A (H5N1) viruses using a pyrosequencing method. Antimicrob Agents Chemother. 2009;53:1039–47.
54. Deyde VM, Sheu TG, Trujillo AA, et al. Detection of molecular markers of drug resistance in 2009 pandemic influenza A (H1N1) viruses by pyrosequencing. Antimicrob Agents Chemother. 2010;54:1102–10.
55. Deyde VM, Sampath R, Gubareva LV. RT-PCR/electrospray ionization mass spectrometry approach in detection and characterization of influenza viruses. Expert Rev Mol Diagn. 2011;11:41–52. Review.

56. DiMaio MA, Sahoo MK, Waggoner J, et al. Comparison of Xpert Flu rapid nucleic acid testing with rapid antigen testing for the diagnosis of influenza A and B. J Virol Methods. 2012;186: 137–40.
57. Doern CD, Lacey D, Huang R, et al. Evaluation and implementation of FilmArray version 1.7 for the improved detection of adenovirus respiratory tract infection. J Clin Microbiol. 2013;51: 4036–9.
58. Drews SJ, Blair J, Lombos E, et al. Use of the Seeplex RV Detection kit for surveillance of respiratory viral outbreaks in Toronto, Ontario, Canada. Ann Clin Lab Sci. 2008;38:376–9.
59. Dugas AF, Valsamakis A, Gaydos CA, et al. Evaluation of the Xpert Flu rapid PCR assay in high-risk emergency department patients. J Clin Microbiol. 2014;52:4353–5.
60. Dundas NE, Ziadie MS, Revell PA, Brock E, Mitui M, Leos NK, Rogers BB, et al. A lean laboratory: operational simplicity and cost effectiveness of the Luminex xTAG™ respiratory viral panel. J Mol Diagn. 2011;13:175–9.
61. Dunn JJ, Ginocchio CC. Can newly developed, rapid immunochromatographic antigen detection tests be reliably used for the laboratory diagnosis of influenza virus infections? J Clin Microbiol. 2014;pii:JCM.02739-14.
62. Echavarria M, Kolavic SA, Cersovsky S, et al. Detection of adenoviruses (AdV) in culture-negative environmental samples by PCR during an AdV-associated respiratory disease outbreak. J Clin Microbiol. 2000;38:2982–4.
63. Endimiani A, Hujer KM, Hujer AM, et al. Are we ready for novel detection methods to treat respiratory pathogens in hospital-acquired pneumonia? Clin Infect Dis. 2011;52 Suppl 4:S373–83.
64. Falsey AR, Walsh EE. Respiratory syncytial virus infection in adults. Clin Microbiol Rev. 2000;13:371–84.
65. Falsey AR, Erdman D, Anderson LJ, et al. Human metapneumovirus infections in young and elderly adults. J Infect Dis. 2003;187: 785–90.
66. Falsey AR, Walsh EE. Viral pneumonia in older adults. Clin Infect Dis. 2006;42:518–24.
67. Fields BS, Benson RF, Besser RE. *Legionella* and Legionnaires' disease: 25 years of investigation. Clin Microbiol Rev. 2002;15: 506–26.
68. Fine MJ, Smith MA, Carson CA, et al. Prognosis and outcomes of patients with community-acquired pneumonia: a meta-analysis. JAMA. 1996;275:134–41.
69. Forman MS, Advani S, Newman C, et al. Diagnostic performance of two highly multiplexed respiratory virus assays in a pediatric cohort. J Clin Virol. 2012;55:168–72.
70. Fox JD. Nucleic acid amplification tests for detection of respiratory viruses. J Clin Virol. 2007;40 Suppl 1:15–23.
71. Fuenzalida L, Fabrega J, Blanco S, et al. Usefulness of two new methods for diagnosing metapneumovirus infections in children. Clin Microbiol Infect. 2010;16:1663–8.
72. Gadsby NJ, Hardie A, Claas EC, et al. Comparison of the luminex respiratory virus panel fast assay with in-house real-time PCR for respiratory viral infection diagnosis. J Clin Microbiol. 2010;48:2213–6.
73. Gharabaghi F, Tellier R, Cheung R, et al. Comparison of a commercial qualitative real-time RT-PCR kit with direct immunofluorescence assay (DFA) and cell culture for detection of influenza A and B in children. J Clin Virol. 2008;42:190–3.
74. Gharabaghi F, Hawan A, Drews SJ, et al. Evaluation of multiple commercial molecular and conventional diagnostic assays for the detection of respiratory viruses in children. Clin Microbiol Infect. 2011;17:1900–6.
75. Gimeno C, Costa E, Navalpotro D, et al. Sensitivity of a marketed immunochromatographic assay specifically targeting the pandemic influenza A/H1N1 2009 virus. Diagn Microbiol Infect Dis. 2010;68:80–2.
76. Ginocchio CC, Manji R, Lotlikar M, et al. Clinical evaluation of NucliSENS magnetic extraction and NucliSENS analyte-specific reagents for real-time detection of human metapneumovirus in pediatric respiratory specimens. J Clin Microbiol. 2008;46:1274–80.
77. Ginocchio CC. Quality assurance in clinical virology. In: Specter S, Hodinka R, Young SA, Wiedbrauk DL, editors. Clinical virology manual. 4th ed. Washington, DC: American Society for Microbiology; 2009.
78. Ginocchio CC, St George K. Likelihood that an unsubtypeable influenza A result in the Luminex xTAG Respiratory Virus Panel is indicative of novel A/H1N1 (swine-like) influenza. J Clin Microbiol. 2009;47:2347–8.
79. Ginocchio CC, Zhang F, Manji R, et al. Evaluation of multiple test methods for the detection of the novel 2009 influenza A (H1N1) during the New York City outbreak. J Clin Virol. 2009;45:191–5.
80. Goka EA, Vallely PJ, Kenneth J, Mutton KJ, et al. Single and multiple respiratory virus infections and severity of respiratory disease: a systematic review. Paediatr Respir Rev. 2014;15:363–70.
81. Gonçalves MA, de Vries AA. Adenovirus: from foe to friend. Rev Med Virol. 2006;16:167–86.
82. Gonzales R, Malone DC, Maselli JH, et al. Excessive antibiotic use for acute respiratory infections in the United States. Clin Infect Dis. 2001;33(6):757–62.
83. Greenberg SB. Update on rhinovirus and coronavirus infections. Semin Respir Crit Care Med. 2011;32(4):433–46.
84. Gubareva LV, Trujillo AA, Okomo-Adhiambo M, et al. Comprehensive assessment of 2009 pandemic influenza A (H1N1) virus drug susceptibility in vitro. Antivir Ther. 2010;15:1151–9.
85. Hall CB, Douglas Jr RG, Geiman JM. Quantitative shedding patterns of respiratory syncytial virus in infants. J Infect Dis. 1975;132:151–6.
86. Hall CB. Respiratory syncytial virus and parainfluenza virus. N Engl J Med. 2001;344:1917–28.
87. Hammond SP, Gagne LS, Stock SR, et al. Respiratory virus detection with FilmArray respiratory panel compared to conventional methods in immunocompromised patients. J Clin Microbiol. 2012;50:3216–21.
88. Hardick J, Sadyan S, Perelstein E, et al. A case-control study evaluating RT-PCR/ESI-MS technology compared to direct fluorescent antibody and xTAG RVP PCR. Diagn Microbiol Infect Dis. 2014;79:187–9.
89. Hasan MR, Tan R, Al-Rawahi GN, et al. Evaluation of amplification targets for the specific detection of Bordetella pertussis using real-time polymerase chain reaction. Can J Infect Dis Med Microbiol. 2014;25:217–21.
90. Hayden RT, Gu Z, Rodriguez A, et al. Comparison of two broadly multiplexed PCR systems for viral detection in clinical respiratory tract specimens from immunocompromised children. J Clin Virol. 2012;53:308–13.
91. Hazelton B, Gray T, Ho J, et al. Detection of influenza A and B with the Alere i Influenza A&B: a novel isothermal nucleic acid amplification assay. Influenza Other Respir Viruses. 2015;9(3): 151–4. doi:10.1111/irv.12303.
92. Hendrickson KJ. Cost-effective use of rapid diagnostic techniques in the treatment and prevention of viral respiratory infections. Pediatr Ann. 2005;34:24–31.
93. Henrickson KJ, Hall CB. Diagnostic assays for respiratory syncytial virus. Pediatr Infect Dis J. 2007;26:S36–40.
94. Hermos CR, Vargas SO, McAdam AJ. Human metapneumovirus. Clin Lab Med. 2010;30:131–48.
95. Hernes SS, Quarsten H, Hagen E, et al. Swabbing for respiratory viral infections in older patients: a comparison of rayon and nylon flocked swabs. Eur J Clin Microbiol Infect Dis. 2011;30:159–65.
96. Higgins RR, Lombos E, Tang P, et al. Verification of the ProPneumo-1 assay for the simultaneous detection of *Mycoplasma pneumoniae* and *Chlamydophila pneumoniae* in clinical respiratory specimens. Ann Clin Microbiol Antimicrob. 2009;8:10.

97. Hirschwerk DP, Goldberg S, Ginocchio C. Acute pericarditis caused by human metapneumovirus. Infect Dis Clin Pract. 2009;17:283–5.
98. Hurtado J, Mosquera M, de Lazzari E, et al. Evaluation of a new, rapid, simple test for the detection of influenza virus. BMC Infect Dis. 2015;15(1):44.
99. Hustedt JW, Vazquez M. The changing face of pediatric respiratory tract infections: how human metapneumovirus and human bocavirus fit into the overall etiology of respiratory tract infections in young children. Yale J Biol Med. 2010;83:193–200.
100. Hutter A, Emonet S, Harbarth S, et al. Polymerase-chain reaction/electrospray ionization-mass spectrometry for the detection of bacteria and fungi in brochoalveolar lavage fluids: a prospective observational study. Clin Microbiol Infect. 2014;20:1059–66.
101. Hwang SM, Lim MS, Han M, et al. Comparison of xTAG Respiratory Virus Panel and Verigene Respiratory Virus Plus for detecting influenza virus and respiratory syncytial virus. J Clin Lab Anal. 2014;29:116–21.
102. Infectious Diseases Society of America. An unmet medical need: Rapid molecular diagnostics for respiratory infections. Clin Infect Dis. 2011;52 Suppl 4:S384–95.
103. Jamal W, Al Roomi E, AbdulAziz LR, et al. Evaluation of Curetis Unyvero, a multiplex PCR-based testing system, for rapid detection of bacteria and antibiotic resistance and impact of the assay on management of severe nosocomial pneumonia. J Clin Microbiol. 2014;52:2487–92.
104. Jansen RR, Joannewieringa J, Sylvie M, Koekkoek SM, et al. Frequent detection of respiratory viruses without symptoms: toward defining clinically relevant cutoff values. J Clin Microbiol. 2012;49:2631–6.
105. Jartti T, Hedman K, Jartti L, et al. Human bocavirus-the first 5 years. Rev Med Virol. 2012;22:46–64.
106. Jartti T, Soderlund-Venermo M, Hedman K, et al. New molecular virus detection methods and their clinical value in lower respiratory tract infections in children. Paediatr Respir Rev. 2013;14:38–45.
107. Jenny SL, Hu Y, Overduin P, et al. Evaluation of the Xpert Flu A Panel nucleic acid amplification-based point-of-care test for influenza A virus detection and pandemic H1 subtyping. J Clin Virol. 2010;49:85–9.
108. Jokela P, Piiparinen H, Mannonen L, et al. Performance of the Luminex xTAG Respiratory Viral Panel Fast in a clinical laboratory setting. J Virol Methods. 2012;182:82–6.
109. Kanashiro TM, Vilas Boas LS, Thomaz AM, et al. Identification of respiratory virus in infants with congenital heart disease by comparison of different methods. Rev Inst Med Trop Sao Paulo. 2011;53:241–6.
110. Kim SR, Ki CS, Lee NY. Rapid detection and identification of 12 respiratory viruses using a dual priming oligonucleotide system-based multiplex PCR assay. J Virol Methods. 2009;156:111–6.
111. Ko SY, Jang JW, Dong DJ, et al. Evaluation of the Simplexa Flu A/B and RSV test for the rapid detection of influenza viruses. J Med Virol. 2013;85:2160–4.
112. Kollef ME, Kollef KE. Antibiotic utilization and outcomes for patients with clinically suspected ventilator-associated pneumonia and negative quantitative BAL culture results. Chest. 2005;128:2706–13.
113. Krunic N, Yager TD, Himsworth D, et al. xTAG RVP assay: analytical and clinical performance. J Clin Virol. 2007;40 Suppl 1:S39–46. Review.
114. Krunic N, Merante F, Yaghoubian S, et al. Advances in the diagnosis of respiratory tract infections: role of the Luminex xTAG respiratory viral panel. Ann N Y Acad Sci. 2011;1222:6–13.
115. Lambert SB, Allen KM, Carter RC, et al. The cost of community-managed viral respiratory illnesses in a cohort of healthy preschool-aged children. Respir Res. 2008;9:11.
116. Landry ML. Developments in immunologic assays for respiratory viruses. Clin Lab Med. 2009;29:635–47.
117. Landry ML, Ferguson D. Comparison of the Simplexa Flu A/B & RSV PCR with cytospin-immunofluorescence and laboratory-developed TaqMan PCR in predominately adult hospitalized patients. J Clin Microbiol. 2014;52:3057–9.
118. Larios OE, Coleman BL, Drews SJ, et al. Self-collected mid-turbinate swabs for the detection of respiratory viruses in adults with acute respiratory illnesses. PLoS One. 2011;6(6), e21335.
119. Leber AL, Salamon DP, Prince HE. Pertussis diagnosis in the 21st century: progress and pitfalls, part 1. Clin Microbiol Newl. 2011;33:111–5.
120. Lee BE, Mukhi SN, May-Hadford J, et al. Determination of the relative economic impact of different molecular-based laboratory algorithms for respiratory viral pathogen detection, including Pandemic (H1N1), using a secure web based platform. Virol J. 2011;8:277.
121. Lee BY, McGlone SM, Bailey RR, et al. To test or to treat? An analysis of influenza testing and antiviral treatment strategies using economic computer modeling. PLoS One. 2010;5, e11284.
122. Lee JH, Chun JK, Kim DS, et al. Identification of adenovirus, influenza virus, parainfluenza virus, and respiratory syncytial virus by two kinds of multiplex polymerase chain reaction (PCR) and a shell vial culture in pediatric patients with viral pneumonia. Yonsei Med J. 2010;51:761–7.
123. Lee N, Chan PK, Wong CK, et al. Viral clearance and inflammatory response patterns in adults hospitalized for pandemic 2009 influenza A(H1N1) virus pneumonia. Antivir Ther. 2011;16:237–47.
124. LeGoff J, Kara R, Moulin F, et al. Evaluation of the one-step multiplex real-time reverse transcription-PCR ProFlu-1 assay for detection of influenza A and influenza B viruses and respiratory syncytial viruses in children. J Clin Microbiol. 2008;46:789–91.
125. Leland D, Ginocchio CC. Role of cell culture for virus detection in the age of technology. Clin Microbiol Rev. 2007;20:49–78.
126. Leruez-Ville M, Chardin-Ouachée M, Neven B, et al. Description of an adenovirus A31 outbreak in a paediatric haematology unit. Bone Marrow Transplant. 2006;38:23–8.
127. Lessler J, Reich NG, Brookmeyer R, et al. Incubation periods of acute respiratory viral infections: a systematic review. Lancet Infect Dis. 2009;9:291–300.
128. Li H, McCormac MA, Estes RW, et al. Simultaneous detection and high-throughput identification of a panel of RNA viruses causing respiratory tract infections. J Clin Microbiol. 2007;45:2105–9.
129. Li M, Brenwald N, Bonigal S, et al. Rapid diagnosis of influenza: an evaluation of two commercially available RT-PCR assays. J Infect. 2012;65:60–3.
130. Liao RS, Tomalty LL, Majury A, et al. Comparison of viral isolation and multiplex real-time reverse transcription-PCR for confirmation of respiratory syncytial virus and influenza virus detection by antigen immunoassays. J Clin Microbiol. 2009;47:527–32.
131. Lieberman D, Shimoni A, Keren-Naus A, et al. Identification of respiratory viruses in adults: nasopharyngeal versus oropharyngeal sampling. J Clin Microbiol. 2009;47:3439–43.
132. Lieberman D, Shimoni A, Shemer-Avni Y, et al. Respiratory viruses in adults with community-acquired pneumonia. Chest. 2010;138:811–6.
133. Loeffelholz MJ, Pong DL, Pyles RB, et al. Comparison of the FilmArray Respiratory Panel and Prodesse real-time PCR assays for detection of respiratory pathogens. J Clin Microbiol. 2011;49:4083–8.
134. Loens K, Ieven M, Ursi D, et al. Detection of *Mycoplasma pneumoniae* by real-time nucleic acid sequence-based amplification. J Clin Microbiol. 2003;41:4448–50.
135. Loens K, Beck T, Goossens H, et al. Development of conventional and real-time nucleic acid sequence-based amplification assays for detection of *Chlamydophila pneumoniae* in respiratory specimens. J Clin Microbiol. 2006;44:1241–4.

136. Loens K, Beck T, Ursi D, et al. Development of real-time multiplex nucleic acid sequence-based amplification for detection of *Mycoplasma pneumoniae*, *Chlamydophila pneumoniae*, and *Legionella* spp. in respiratory specimens. J Clin Microbiol. 2008;46:185–91.
137. Loens K, Beck T, Ursi D, et al. Evaluation of different nucleic acid amplification techniques for the detection of *M. pneumoniae*, *C. pneumoniae* and *Legionella* spp. in respiratory specimens from patients with community-acquired pneumonia. J Microbiol Methods. 2008;73:257–62.
138. Loens K, Ursi D, Goossens H, et al. Evaluation of the NucliSens miniMAG RNA extraction and real-time NASBA applications for the detection of *Mycoplasma pneumoniae* and *Chlamydophila pneumoniae* in throat swabs. J Microbiol Methods. 2008;72: 217–9.
139. Loens K, Van Heirstraeten L, Malhotra-Kumar S, et al. Optimal sampling sites and methods for detection of pathogens possibly causing community-acquired lower respiratory tract infections. J Clin Microbiol. 2009;47:21–31.
140. Loens K, Goossens H, Ieven M. Acute respiratory infection due to *Mycoplasma pneumoniae*: current status of diagnostic methods. Eur J Clin Microbiol Infect Dis. 2010;29:1055–69.
141. Loens K, van Loon AM, Coenjaerts F, et al. Performance of different mono- and multiplex nucleic acid amplification tests on a multipathogen external quality assessment panel. J Clin Microbiol. 2012;50:977–87.
142. MacDougall K, Polk C. Antimicrobial stewardship programs in health care systems. Clin Microbiol Rev. 2005;18:638–56.
143. Mahony J, Chong S, Merante F, et al. Development of a respiratory virus panel test for detection of twenty human respiratory viruses by use of multiplex PCR and a fluid microbead-based assay. J Clin Microbiol. 2007;45:2965–70.
144. Mahony JB, Blackhouse G, Babwah J, et al. Cost analysis of multiplex PCR testing for diagnosing respiratory virus infections. J Clin Microbiol. 2009;47:2812–7.
145. Mak GC, Cheng PK, Lim W. Evaluation of Qiagen Resplex II for the detection of pandemic influenza A (H1N1) 2009 and influenza A (H3N2) virus. J Clin Virol. 2011;51:88–9.
146. Mandell LA, Wunderink RG, Anzueto A. Infectious Diseases Society of America/American Thoracic Society consensus guidelines on the management of community-acquired pneumonia in adults. Clin Infect Dis. 2007;44 Suppl 2:S27.
147. Manji R, Lotlikar M, Zhang F, et al. Clinical evaluation of NucliSENS magnetic extraction and NucliSENS analyte specific reagents for the real-time detection of respiratory syncytial virus (RSV) in paediatric respiratory specimens. J Clin Pathol. 2009;62:998–1002.
148. Manji R, Zheng X, Patel A, et al. Multi-center evaluation of the adenovirus R-gene US assay for the detection of adenovirus in respiratory samples. J Clin Virol. 2014;60:90–5.
149. Mansuy JM, Mengelle C, Da Silva I, et al. Performance of a rapid molecular multiplex assay for the detection of influenza and picornaviruses. Scand J Infect Dis. 2012;44:963–8.
150. Marrie TJ. Q fever pneumonia. Infect Dis Clin North Am. 2010;24:27–41.
151. Martınez MA, Ruiz M, Zunino E, et al. Detection of *Mycoplasma pneumoniae* in adult community-acquired pneumonia by PCR and serology. J Med Microbiol. 2008;57:1491–5.
152. McAdam AJ, Riley AM. Developments in tissue culture detection of respiratory viruses. Clin Lab Med. 2009;29:623–34.
153. McCloskey CB, Kraft CS, Ingersoll JM, et al. Characterization of 2009 pandemic influenza A (H1N1) virus specimens with a positive hemagglutinin 1 signal in the Luminex xTAG respiratory viral panel assay. J Clin Microbiol. 2011;49:1657–8.
154. Moore C, Valappil M, Corden S, et al. Enhanced clinical utility of the NucliSens EasyQ RSV A+B assay for rapid detection of respiratory syncytial virus in clinical samples. Eur J Clin Microbiol Infect Dis. 2006;25:167–74.
155. Moore C, Galiano M, Lackenby A, et al. Evidence of person-to-person transmission of oseltamivir-resistant pandemic influenza A(H1N1) 2009 virus in a hematology unit. J Infect Dis. 2011;203:18–24.
156. Mulrennan S, Tempone SS, Ling IT, et al. Pandemic influenza (H1N1) 2009 pneumonia: CURB-65 score for predicting severity and nasopharyngeal sampling for diagnosis are unreliable. PLoS One. 2010;5, e12849.
157. Murdoch DR. Nucleic acid amplification tests for the diagnosis of pneumonia. Clin Infect Dis. 2003;36:1162–70.
158. Murdoch DR. Diagnosis of *Legionella* infection. Clin Infect Dis. 2003;36:64–9.
159. Murillo L, Hardick J, Jeng K, et al. Evaluation of the pan influenza detection kit utilizing the PLEX-ID and influenza samples from the 2011 respiratory season. J Virol Methods. 2013;193:173–6.
160. Nakao A, Hisata K, Matsunaga N, et al. The clinical utility of a near patient rapid microarray based diagnostic tests for influenza and respiratory syncytial virus infections in a pediatric setting. Diagn Microbiol Infect Dis. 2014;78:363–7.
161. Nguyen HT, Fry AM, Gubareva LV. Neuraminidase inhibitor resistance in influenza viruses and laboratory testing methods. Antivir Ther. 2012;17(1 Pt B):159–73.
162. Nie S, Roth RB, Stiles J, et al. Evaluation of Alere i influenza A&B for rapid detection of influenza viruses A and B. J Clin Microbiol. 2014;52:3339–44.
163. Novak-Weekley SM, Marlowe EM, Poulter M, et al. Evaluation of the Cepheid Xpert Flu Assay for rapid identification and differentiation of influenza A, influenza A 2009 H1N1, and influenza B viruses. J Clin Microbiol. 2012;50:1704–10.
164. Ohrmalm L, Wong M, Rotzén-Östlund M, et al. Flocked nasal swab versus nasopharyngeal aspirate for detection of respiratory tract viruses in immunocompromised adults: a matched comparative study. BMC Infect Dis. 2010;10:340.
165. Ong GM, Wyatt DE, O'Neill HJ, et al. A comparison of nested polymerase chain reaction and immunofluorescence for the diagnosis of respiratory infections in children with bronchiolitis, and the implications for a cohorting strategy. J Hosp Infect. 2001;49:122–8.
166. Pabbaraju K, Tokaryk KL, Wong S, et al. Comparison of the Luminex xTAG respiratory viral panel with in-house nucleic acid amplification tests for diagnosis of respiratory virus infections. J Clin Microbiol. 2008;46:3056–62.
167. Pabbaraju K, Wong S, Lee B, et al. Comparison of a singleplex real-time RT-PCR assay and multiplex respiratory viral panel assay for detection of influenza "A" in respiratory specimens. Influenza Other Respi Viruses. 2011;5:99–103.
168. Pabbaraju K, Wong S, Tokaryk KL, et al. Comparison of the Luminex xTAG respiratory viral panel with xTAG respiratory viral panel fast for diagnosis of respiratory virus infections. J Clin Microbiol. 2011;49:1738–44.
169. Padmanabhan R, Mishra AK, Raoult D, et al. Genomics and metagenomics in medical microbiology. J Microbiol Methods. 2013;95:415–24.
170. Paterson DL. The role of antimicrobial management programs in optimizing antibiotic prescribing within hospitals. Clin Infect Dis. 2006;42:S90–5.
171. Patick AK. Rhinovirus chemotherapy. Antiviral Res. 2006;71:391–6.
172. Pavia AT. Viral infections of the lower respiratory tract: old viruses, new viruses, and the role of diagnosis. Clin Infect Dis. 2011;52 Suppl 4:284–9.
173. Pehler-Harrington K, Khanna M, Waters CR, et al. Rapid detection and identification of human adenovirus species by adenoplex, a multiplex PCR-enzyme hybridization assay. J Clin Microbiol. 2004;42:4072–6.
174. Pierce VM, Elkan M, Leet M, et al. Comparison of the Idaho Technology FilmArray system to real-time PCR for detection of

respiratory pathogens in children. J Clin Microbiol. 2012;50:364–71.
175. Pierce VM, Hodinka RL. Comparison of the GenMark diagnostics esensor respiratory virus panel to real-time PCR for the detection of respiratory viruses in children. J Clin Microbiol. 2012;50:3458–65.
176. Piralla A, Lunghi G, Percivalle E, et al. FilmArray Respiratory Panel performance of respiratory samples from neonatal care units. Diagn Microbiol Infect Dis. 2014;79:183–6.
177. Poehling KA, Edwards KM, Weinberg GA, et al. The underrecognized burden of influenza in young children. N Engl J Med. 2006;355:31–40.
178. Popowitch EB, Rogers E, Miller MB. Retrospective and prospective verification of the Cepheid Xpert influenza virus assay. J Clin Microbiol. 2011;49:3368–9.
179. Popowitch EB, O'Neill SS, Miller MB. Comparison of the BioFire FilmArray RP, GenMark eSensor RVP, Luminex xTAG RVPv1, and Luminex xTAG RVP Fast multiplex assays for the detection of respiratory viruses. J Clin Microbiol. 2013;51: 1528–33.
180. Poritz MA, Blaschke AJ, Byington CL, et al. FilmArray, an automated nested multiplex PCR system for multi-pathogen detection: development and application to respiratory tract infection. PLoS One. 2011;6, e26047.
181. Prill MM, Iwane MK, Edwards KM, et al. Human coronavirus in young children hospitalized for acute respiratory illness and asymptomatic controls. Pediatr Infect Dis J. 2012;31:235–40.
182. Proud D. Upper airway viral infections. Pulm Pharmaco Therap. 2008;21:468–73.
183. Rand KH, Rampersaud H, Houck HJ. Comparison of two multiplex methods for detection of respiratory viruses: FilmArray RP and xTAG RVP. J Clin Microbiol. 2011;49:2449–53.
184. Ratliff AE, Duffy LB, Waites KB. Comparison of the *illumi*gene mycoplasma DNA amplification assay and culture for detection of *Mycoplasma pneumonia*e. J Clin Microbiol. 2014;52:1060–3.
185. Raymaekers M, de Rijke B, Pauli I, et al. Timely diagnosis of respiratory tract infections: evaluation of the performance of the Respifinder assay compared to the xTAG respiratory viral panel assay. J Clin Virol. 2011;52:314–6.
186. Reijans M, Dingemans G, Klaassen CH, et al. Respifinder: a new multiparameter test to differentially identify fifteen respiratory viruses. J Clin Microbiol. 2008;46:1232–40.
187. Renaud C, Kuypers J, Englund JA. Emerging oseltamivir resistance in seasonal and pandemic influenza A/H1N1. J Clin Virol. 2011;52:70–8. Review.
188. Renaud C, Crowley J, Jerome KR, et al. Comparison of FilmArray Respiratory Panel and laboratory-developed real-time reverse transcription-polymerase chain reaction assays for respiratory virus detection. Diagn Microbiol Infect Dis. 2012;74:379–83.
189. Rice L. Rapid diagnostics and appropriate antibiotic use. Clin Infect Dis. 2011;52 Suppl 4:S357–60.
190. Rodgers L, Martin SW, Cohn A, et al. Epidemiologic and laboratory features of a large outbreak of Pertussis-like illnesses associated with cocirculating *Bordetella holmesii* and *Bordetella pertussis* – Ohio, 2010–2011. Clin Infect Dis. 2013;56:322–31.
191. Rogers BB, Shankar P, Jerris RC, et al. Impact of a rapid respiratory test panel on patient outcomes. Arch Pathol Lab Med. 2014;139(5):636–41. 10.5858/arpa.2014-0257-OA.
192. Roh KH, Kim J, Nam MH, et al. Comparison of the Seeplex reverse transcription PCR assay with the R-mix viral culture and immunofluorescence techniques for detection of eight respiratory viruses. Ann Clin Lab Sci. 2008;38:41–6.
193. Ruggiero P, McMillen T, Tang Y-W, et al. Evaluation of the BioFire FilmArray respiratory panel and the GenMark eSensor respiratory viral panel on lower respiratory tract specimens. J Clin Microbiol. 2014;52:288–90.
194. Ruuskanen O, Lahti E, Jennings LC, et al. Viral pneumonia. Lancet. 2011;377:1264–75.
195. Salez N, Ninove L, Thirion L, et al. Evaluation of the Xpert Flu test and comparison with in-house real-time RT-PCR assays for detection of influenza virus from 2008 to 2011 in Marseille, France. Clin Microbiol Infect. 2012;18:E81–3.
196. Salez N, de Lamballerie X, Zandotti C, et al. Improved sensitivity of the novel Xpert Flu test for detection of influenza B virus. J Clin Microbiol. 2013;51:4277–8.
197. Sambol AR, Abdalhamid B, Lyden ER, et al. Use of rapid influenza diagnostic tests under field conditions as a screening tool during an outbreak of the 2009 novel influenza virus: practical considerations. J Clin Virol. 2010;47:229–33.
198. Sambol AR, Iwen PC, Pieretti M, et al. Validation of the Cepheid Xpert Flu A real time RT-PCR detection panel for emergency use authorization. J Clin Virol. 2010;48:234–8.
199. Sandora TJ, Smole SC, Lee GM, et al. Test characteristics of commercial influenza assays for detecting pandemic influenza A (H1N1) in children. Pediatr Infect Dis J. 2010;29:261–2.
200. Schildgen O. Human bocavirus lessons learned to date pathogens. Pathogens. 2013;2(1):1–12.
201. Schulte B, Eickmeyer H, Heininger A, et al. Detection of pneumonia associated pathogens using a prototype multiplexed pneumonia test in hospitalized patients with severe pneumonia, 9(11): e110566. PLoS One. 2014;9(11):E110566.
202. Selvaraju SB, Selvarangan R. Evaluation of three influenza A and B real-time reverse transcription-PCR assays and a new 2009 H1N1 assay for detection of influenza viruses. J Clin Microbiol. 2010;48:3870–5.
203. Selvaraju SB, Selvarangan R. Evaluation of xTAG Respiratory Viral Panel FAST and xTAG Human Parainfluenza Virus Analyte-Specific Reagents for detection of human parainfluenza viruses in respiratory specimens. Diagn Microbiol Infect Dis. 2012;72: 278–81.
204. Selvaraju SB, Tierney D, Leber AL, et al. Influenza and respiratory syncytial virus detection in clinical specimens without nucleic acid extraction using FOCUS direct disc assay is substantially equivalent to the traditional methods and the FOCUS nucleic acid extraction-dependent RT-PCR assay. Diagn Microbiol Infect Dis. 2014;78:232–6.
205. Selvaraju SB, Bambach AV, Leber AL, et al. Comparison of the Simplexa Flu A/B and RSV kit (nucleic acid extraction-dependent assay) and the Prodesse ProFlu+assay for detecting influenza and respiratory syncytial viruses. Diagn Microbiol Infect Dis. 2014;80:50–2.
206. Serwint JR, Miller RM. Why diagnose influenza in hospitalized pediatric patients? Pediatr Infect Dis J. 1993;12:200–4.
207. Shin JH, Ranken R, Sefers SE, et al. Detection, identification and distribution of fungi in bronchoalveolar lavage specimens by use of multilocus PCR coupled with electrospray ionization/mass spectrometry. J Clin Microbiol. 2013;51:136–41.
208. Smith J, Sammons D, Toennis C, et al. Semi-quantitative analysis of influenza samples using the Luminex xTAG(®) respiratory viral panel kit. Toxicol Mech Methods. 2012;22:211–7.
209. Smith MD, Derrington P, Evans R, et al. Rapid diagnosis of bacteremic pneumococcal infections in adults by using the Binax NOW *Streptococcus pneumoniae* urinary antigen test: a prospective, controlled clinical evaluation. J Clin Microbiol. 2003;41:2810–3.
210. Smith MD, Sheppard CL, Hogan A, et al. Diagnosis of *Streptococcus pneumoniae* infections in adults with bacteremia and community-acquired pneumonia: clinical comparison of pneumococcal PCR and urinary antigen detection. J Clin Microbiol. 2009;47:1046–9.
211. Sung H, Park SJ, Woo YD, et al. Evaluation of Seeplex RV detection kit for detecting rhinovirus, human metapneumovirus, and coronavirus]. Korean J Lab Med. 2008;28:109–17.

212. Svensson MJ, Lind I, Zweygberg Wirgart B, et al. Performance of the Simplexa Flu A/B & RSV Direct kit on respiratory samples collected in saline solution. Scand J Infect Dis. 2014;46:825–31.
213. Takao S, Hara M, Okazaki T, et al. Simultaneous multiple assay (Luminex xTAG respiratory viral panel FAST assay) efficacy in human respiratory virus detection. Kansenshogaku Zasshi. 2011;85:31–6.
214. Taliaferro LP, Galvin TA, Ma H, et al. Evaluation of the broad-range PCR-electrospray ionization mass spectrometry (PCR/ESI-MS) system and virus microarrays for virus detection. Viruses. 2014;6:1876–96.
215. Tang Y-W, Lowery KS, Valsamakis A, et al. Clinical accuracy of a Plex-ID Flu device for simultaneous detection and identification of influenza viruses A and B. J Clin Microbiol. 2013;51:40–5.
216. Templeton KE, Scheltinga SA, van der Zee A, et al. Evaluation of real-time PCR for detection and discrimination between *Bordetella pertussis*, *Bordetella parapertussis*, and *Bordetella holmesii* for clinical diagnosis. J Clin Microbiol. 2003;41:4121–6.
217. Thorburn K, Kerr S, Taylor N, et al. RSV outbreak in a paediatric intensive care unit. J Hosp Infect. 2004;57:194–201.
218. Tillmann RL, Simon A, Müller A, et al. Sensitive commercial NASBA assay for the detection of respiratory syncytial virus in clinical specimen. PLoS One. 2007;2(12):e1357.
219. Valenti WM, Clarke TA, Hall CB, et al. Concurrent outbreaks of rhinovirus and respiratory syncytial virus in an intensive care nursery: epidemiology and associated risk. J Pediatr. 1982;100:722–6.
220. Van Wesenbeeck L, Meeuws H, Van Immerseel A, et al. Comparison of the FilmArray RP, Verigene RV+, and Prodesse ProFLU+/FAST+ multiplex platforms for detection of influenza viruses in clinical samples from the 2011–2012 influenza season in Belgium. J Clin Microbiol. 2013;51:2977–85.
221. Villegas E, Sorlozano A, Gutie J. Serological diagnosis of *Chlamydia pneumoniae* infection: limitations and perspectives. J Med Microbiol. 2010;59:1267–74.
222. Waites KB, Talkington DF. *Mycoplasma pneumoniae* and its role as a human pathogen. Clin Microbiol Rev. 2004;17:697–728.
223. Walsh P, Overmyer CL, Pham K, et al. Comparison of respiratory virus detection rates for infants and toddlers by use of flocked swabs, saline aspirates, and saline aspirates mixed in universal transport medium for room temperature storage and shipping. J Clin Microbiol. 2008;46:2374–6.
224. Wang W, Ren P, Sheng J, et al. Simultaneous detection of respiratory viruses in children with acute respiratory infection using two different multiplex reverse transcription-PCR assays. J Virol Methods. 2009;162:40–5.
225. Williams MM, Taylor TH, Warshauer DM, et al. Harmonization of *Bordetella pertussis* real-time PCR diagnostics in the United States in 2012. J Clin Microbiol. 2015;53:118–23.
226. Wong S, Pabbaraju K, Lee BE, et al. Enhanced viral etiological diagnosis of respiratory system infection outbreaks by use of a multitarget nucleic acid amplification assay. J Clin Microbiol. 2009;47:3839–45.
227. Woo PC, Chiu SS, Seto WH, et al. Cost-effectiveness of rapid diagnosis of viral respiratory tract infections in pediatric patients. J Clin Microbiol. 1997;35:1579–81.
228. Woodberry MW, Shanker R, Cent A, et al. Comparison of the Simplexa Flu A/B & RSV Direct assay and laboratory-developed real-time PCR assays for detection of respiratory viruses. J Clin Microbiol. 2013;51:3883–5.
229. Xu M, Qin X, Astion ML, et al. Implementation of FilmArray Respiratory Viral Panel in a core laboratory improves testing turnaround time and patient care. Am J Clin Pathol. 2013;139:118–23.
230. Yeh E, Luo RF, Dyner L, et al. Preferential lower respiratory tract infection in swine-origin 2009 A(H1N1) influenza. Clin Infect Dis. 2010;50:391–4.
231. Yoo SJ, Kuak EY, Shin BM. Detection of 12 respiratory viruses with two-set multiplex reverse transcriptase-PCR assay using a dual priming oligonucleotide system. Korean J Lab Med. 2007;27:420–7.
232. Zambon M, Bull T, Sadler CJ, et al. Molecular epidemiology of two consecutive outbreaks of parainfluenza 3 in a bone marrow transplant unit. J Clin Microbiol. 1998;36:2289–93.
233. Zhang XN, Song ZG, Jiang T, et al. Rupintrivir is a promising candidate for treating severe cases of Enterovirus-71 infection. World J Gastroenterol. 2010;16:201–9.
234. Vallières E, Renaud C. Clinical and economical impact of multiplex respiratory virus assays. Diagn Microbiol Infect Dis. 2013;76(3):255–61.

Mycobacterial Infections

53

Betty A. Forbes

Abstract

The genus *Mycobacterium* includes roughly 200 species. Some of these species are well recognized human and/or animal pathogens such as *Mycobacterium tuberculosis* complex. In addition, numerous other species of mycobacteria, referred to as nontuberculous mycobacteria (NTM), are present in the environment; certain NTMs possess moderate pathogenic potential and cause opportunistic infections in humans at a variety of body sites. Since all members of the genus *Mycobacterium*, by virtue of the high content of complex lipids in their cell wall, are acid-fast and are also slow growing compared to other bacteria, this group of organisms present significant challenges for timely and accurate laboratory diagnoses; in addition, chest X-ray and other clinical findings are nonspecific. In light of these challenges, molecular-based assays have been developed resulting in a dramatic improvement in the direct detection, identification, and susceptibility testing in particular for *M. tuberculosis*; however, numerous questions remain unanswered regarding the clinical utility of these various assays.

This chapter reviews current molecular-based assays for the direct detection of *M. tuberculosis* in respiratory and non-respiratory specimens as well as their use in identification of *M. tuberculosis* complex and NTMs. In addition, the use of various molecular methods to determine susceptibility of *M. tuberculosis* isolates to primary drugs used to treat tuberculosis and molecular epidemiology methods are discussed. Of significance, various laboratory issues associated with molecular-based assays are reviewed. And, finally, future directions and strategies for continued advances in nucleic acid testing technologies are reviewed.

Keywords

Mycobacterium tuberculosis • Mycobacteria • Nontuberculous mycobacteria • Nucleic acid amplification • Molecular-based assays • Direct detection

Introduction

The genus *Mycobacterium* includes roughly 200 species. Some of these species are well recognized human and/or animal pathogens such as *Mycobacterium tuberculosis* complex (*Mycobacterium tuberculosis*, *Mycobacterium bovis*, *Mycobacterium bovis* BCG, *Mycobacterium africanum*, *Mycobacterium caprae*, *Mycobacterium microti*,

B.A. Forbes, Ph.D. (✉)
Division of Clinical Pathology, Pathology Department, Virginia Commonwealth University Medical Center, Clinical Support Center, Medical College of Virginia Campus, Room 515, 403 North 13th St., PO Box 980210, Richmond, VA, 23298, USA
e-mail: baforbes@vcu.edu

D.G.B. Leonard (ed.), *Molecular Pathology in Clinical Practice*, DOI 10.1007/978-3-319-19674-9_53

Mycobacterium canetti, and *Mycobacterium pinnipedii*) and *Mycobacterium leprae*. In addition, numerous other species of mycobacteria, referred to as nontuberculous mycobacteria (NTM), are present in the environment. Certain NTMs possess moderate pathogenic potential and cause opportunistic infections in humans at a variety of body sites such as the respiratory tract, skin, lymph nodes, as well as bone and joint involvement; infections in humans caused by these organisms are increasing on a worldwide level [1]. Nevertheless, all members of the genus *Mycobacterium*, by virtue of the high content of complex lipids in their cell wall, are acid-fast and are also slow-growing compared to other bacteria.

Mycobacterium tuberculosis, transmitted via minute aerosol droplets that remain suspended in air for prolonged periods of time, is a significant human pathogen and public health problem. 2010 World Health Organization (WHO) estimates revealed 8.8 million incident cases of tuberculosis (TB), with about 13 % of these cases occurring among people infected with human immunodeficiency virus (HIV) [2]. Given the infectious nature of pulmonary TB, rapid and accurate diagnosis is a principal aim of TB control programs. Although worldwide TB incidence rates are estimated to have peaked in 2004, the overall worldwide burden continues to rise as a result of the rapid growth of the world population, the HIV epidemic, the growing challenge of drug resistance, and other epidemiological factors [3].

Clinical Utility

Despite the enormous global burden of TB and the overall low rates of case detection, conventional approaches to diagnosis continue to rely on tests that have major limitations: sputum smear microscopy is relatively insensitive, ranging from as low as 22–92 % [4–7]; culture is technically challenging and slow; determination of drug susceptibilities is even more technically challenging and slower yet; and chest X-ray and other clinical findings are nonspecific. In addition to further technological innovation, epidemiologic and operational research is needed to develop algorithms for optimal use of molecular-based assays for patient management, particularly in light of their expense. In developed countries, TB remains a low-prevalence disease, and the most rapid way to improve test performance is to select patients for testing in whom results will have the greatest predictive value. Towards this end, well-designed studies are needed to determine the clinical utility of nucleic amplification tests (NAATs). Numerous questions need to be answered regarding the effectiveness of NAATs for previously treated individuals, children, and other subpopulations, for detection of paucibacillary forms of TB, as well as how to assess the infectiousness of individual patients, when to isolate a patient, and when to begin contact investigations [8]. Nevertheless, a dramatic improvement in the direct detection, identification, and susceptibility testing of *M. tuberculosis* has been greatly facilitated in recent years using molecular techniques. Table 53.1 provides an overview of the commercial NAATs for *M. tuberculosis*.

Direct Detection

The limitations of routine acid-fast bacilli (AFB) smear and culture are well known. Although culture of sputum is positive in the majority of patients with pulmonary TB if multiple specimens are obtained, almost 30 % of patients reported to have TB, including 22 % of patients with pulmonary TB, are not culture-confirmed [2]. Similarly, childhood TB, drug-resistant TB, and smear-negative pulmonary and extrapulmonary TB in adults remain diagnostic challenges. Moreover, due to the slow growth rate of mycobacteria, cultures usually take at least a week, and in some instances, as long as 6–8 weeks to become positive.

Respiratory Specimens

While PCR is a common test method, alternative amplification techniques have been developed and patented by companies employing different enzymes and strategies, all based on reiterative reactions. The most commonly employed target amplified in *M. tuberculosis* is the IS*6110* insertion element, which is present in 10–16 copies in most clinical isolates. However, a number of other regions, either specific for *M. tuberculosis* or in conjunction with *M. tuberculosis*-specific probes, also are used as targets, such as the 16S rRNA gene, 65-kDa antigen, various regions of the β-subunit of the RNA polymerase (*rpoB* gene), and protein antigen b. Today, both commercial and laboratory-developed NAATs are available. Commercial direct amplification tests that are US Food and Drug Administration (FDA) approved include COBAS TaqMan *Mycobacterium tuberculosis* test (Roche Diagnostic Systems, Inc., Indianapolis, IN) based on PCR of 16S rRNA and the Amplified Mycobacterium Tuberculosis Direct (AMTD) Test (Hologic Gen-Probe, Inc., San Diego, CA) based on transcription-mediated amplification of rRNA. Both assays are US FDA-approved for direct detection of TB in AFB smear-positive sputum specimens from patients who have not received antituberculosis drugs for seven or more days, or have not been treated for TB within the last 12 months. However, only the Gen-Probe AMTD test is commercially available in the USA and is US FDA-approved for smear-negative specimens.

US FDA approved in 2013, the Xpert MTB/RIF test on the GeneXpert platform (Cepheid, Sunnyvale, CA) is an automated molecular-beacons test to diagnose *M. tuberculosis* and rifampin resistance. The Xpert MTB/RIF test is

Table 53.1 Commercially available, molecular-based amplification assays for the diagnosis and treatment of mycobacterial infections

Test (manufacturer)	Method	Applications/comments
Amplified *Mycobacterium tuberculosis* Direct Test (Gen Probe, Inc.)	TMA	US FDA-approved for testing smear-positive and smear-negative respiratory specimens. Target: rRNA. Direct detection of *M. tuberculosis* in broth cultures.
AMPLICOR *Mycobacterium tuberculosis* Test (Roche Diagnostics Systems, Inc.)	PCR	US FDA-approved for testing AFB smear-positive respiratory specimens only. Automated version: COBAS AMPLICOR MTB. Target: 16S rDNA. Direct detection of *M. tuberculosis* in broth cultures. No longer available in the USA
BDProbe Tec (Becton Dickinson Diagnostic Instrument Systems)	SDA	Fully automated. Targets: IS6110 and 16S rDNA.
INNO-LiPA Mycobacteria v2 (Innogenetics)	PCR with reverse hybridization	Identifies genus *Mycobacterium* and 16 mycobacterial species. Target: 16S-23S ribosomal spacer gene region.
INNO-LiPA Rif. TB (Innogenetics)	PCR with reverse hybridization	Detects *M. tuberculosis* complex plus rifampin resistance. Target: region of the *rpoB* gene.
GenoType Mycobacteria Direct (Hain Lifescience GmbH)	Nucleic acid sequenced-based amplification with reverse hybridization	Identifies 5 mycobacterial species. Target: 23S rRNA gene. Can be performed directly from decontaminated pulmonary and extrapulmonary specimens.
GenoType Mycobacterium CM/AS (Hain Lifescience GmbH)	Nucleic acid sequenced-based amplification with reverse hybridization	Identifies *M. tuberculosis* complex and 40 of the most common NTM species from culture and samples.
GenoType MTBDR*plus* (Hain Lifescience GmbH)	Nucleic acid sequenced-based amplification with reverse hybridization	Directly detects *M. tuberculosis* complex and 4 clinically important NTMs in smear-positive and smear-negative pulmonary and extrapulmonary TB or culture specimens. Detects isoniazid and rifampin resistance. Targets: region of the *rpoB* gene, *katG* gene and *inhA* gene.
GenoType MTBDR*sl* (Hain Lifescience GmbH)	Nucleic acid sequenced-based amplification with reverse hybridization	Identifies drug resistance of *M. tuberculosis* to second-line drugs (fluoroquinolone, amikacin-capreomycin and ethambutol).
Xpert MTB/RIF (Cepheid)	Semiquantitative, nested real-time PCR amplification	US FDA-approved for testing concentrated sediments from smear-positive and smear-negative induced and expectorated sputa for the presence of *M. tuberculosis* complex and detects genetic mutations associated with resistance to rifampin. Target: 81-base-pair region of the RNA polymerase (*rpoB*) Results are available in less than 2 h.

NTM nontuberculous mycobacteria
PCR polymerase chain reaction, *SDA* strand displacement amplification, *TMA* transcription-mediated amplification

approved for both AFB smear-positive and smear-negative induced or expectorated sputa obtained from untreated patients for whom there is clinical suspicion of TB. This commercial test integrates sample processing and PCR in a disposable plastic cartridge containing all reagents required for bacterial lysis, nucleic acid extraction, amplification, and amplicon detection; specimen processing is simplified to a non-precise step that both liquefies and inactivates sputum, which results in a reduction in viable tubercle bacilli of 6–8 logs and thereby eliminates the need for a biosafety cabinet. For culture-positive patients, a single direct Xpert MTB/RIF test identified 551 of 561 patients (98 %) with sputum smear-positive TB; sensitivities were 72.5 %, 85.1 %, and 90.2 % when processing one, two, or three AFB smear-negative specimens, respectively [9]. The Xpert MTB/RIF test also identified 98 % of organisms that were resistant to rifampin. This NAAT has been endorsed by the WHO for use as the initial diagnostic test for individuals suspected of having multidrug-resistant *M. tuberculosis* (MDR-TB) or HIV-associated TB (strong recommendation), and may also be considered as an add on test in settings where MDR-TB or HIV is of less concern, especially for further testing of smear-negative specimens (conditional recommendation acknowledging major resource limitations) [42]. Finally, the GeneXpert MTB/RIF detected *M. tuberculosis* in 521 non-respiratory specimens with a combined sensitivity and specificity of 77.3 % and 98.2 %, respectively [10].

Subsequent clinical trials following US FDA approval of the AMTD test on both AFB smear-positive and -negative specimens demonstrated the importance of using not only mycobacterial culture results but also multiple other parameters including clinical signs and symptoms, response to therapy, and other laboratory results to interpret the results of NAATs [11–13]. In one study [11], enrolling physicians were asked to quantify their degree of clinical suspicion for TB using a scale from 0–100 %; subjects were separated into three major groups (Table 53.2). In addition, a conservative consensus standard for the diagnosis of pulmonary TB was established and an independent expert panel reviewed all cases with a clinical suspicion < 80 % and only one culture or no cultures positive for *M. tuberculosis* (Table 53.2). Data from this and other studies support the use of the AMTD test as a rapid method for the diagnosis of pulmonary TB in patients for whom there is a moderate to high suspicion of TB, regardless of the AFB smear result.

Another commercially available NAAT is manufactured by Hain Lifescience Gmb (Nehren, Germany). This assay employs amplification followed by reverse hybridization of amplicon(s) to immobilized, membrane-bound probes, also referred to as a line probe assay (LPA). Hain Lifescience's first commercially available LPA, the GenoType Mycobacteria Direct assay, directly detects *M. tuberculosis* complex, *M. avium*, *M. malmoense*, *M. kansasii*, and *M. intracellulare* in clinical specimens [14].

Table 53.2 Evaluation of the enhanced AMTD test based on comprehensive clinical diagnosis [11]

Clinical suspicion of TB	AFB smear PPV and NPV (%)	AMTD test Sensitivity, specificity, PPV, NPV (%)
Low (<10 %)	36, 96	83, 97, 59, 99
Intermediate (10–80 %)	30, 71	75, 100, 100, 91
High (>80 %)	94, 37	87, 100, 100, 91

AFB acid-fast bacilli, *AMTD* Amplified Mycobacterium Tuberculosis Direct Test (Hologic Gen-Probe, Inc.), *NPV* negative predictive value, *PPV* positive predictive value, *TB* tuberculosis

More simplified versions of NAATs have been developed or are under development, particularly for peripheral laboratory facilities in resource-limited settings. A manual NAAT that uses loop-mediated, isothermal amplification (LAMP) with a simple visual colorimetric readout is being assessed in a joint development agreement between the Foundation for Innovative New Diagnostics and Eiken Chemical Company. The inherent properties of LAMP are particularly attractive for resource-poor settings, including the speed of reaction (40 min), lack of need for a thermal cycler, ease of use, and visual readout. A study in microscopy centers of developing countries using this assay to diagnose pulmonary TB demonstrated its operational feasibility [15]. In 2012, Fang et al. developed a portable integrated microchip of LAMP with sample-in/answer out capability [16]. This chip performed rapid DNA release, exponential signal amplification with a naked-eye result readout in single or multiplex format, and was able to detect 10–100 copies of *M. tuberculosis* and other bacteria. Noncommercial assays using LAMP have been reported for use with non-pulmonary specimens [17].

As more studies are published, optimal use of NAATs in conjunction with clinical information and other test methods will become manifest, allowing NAATs to be utilized in a cost-effective manner with positive impact on patient management. Clearly, based on recent studies, decisions about when and how to use NAATs for TB diagnosis should be individualized according to the clinical setting, and NAAT results interpreted within the context of the clinical suspicion for TB and on the basis of test performance. To help laboratories and clinicians in this regard, updated guidelines (Table 53.3) for the use of NAATs in the diagnosis of TB were set forth by the Centers for Disease Control and Prevention (CDC) in 2009 [18]. In 2013, the CDC published

Table 53.3 Guidelines for the use of nucleic acid amplification testing on respiratory specimens for TB

AFB smear	Specimen #	NAAT result	Action
Positive	1	Positive	Presumed to have TB and begin anti-TB treatment while awaiting culture results.
Positive	1	Negative	Test for inhibitors. If detected, NAAT is not informative. Clinician must rely on clinical judgment regarding the need for anti-TB therapy and further diagnostic workup while awaiting culture results. If inhibition not detected, repeat NAAT on an additional specimen.
	2	Negative	Presumed to have NTM if no inhibitors detected.
Negative	1	Positive	Use clinical judgment whether to begin anti-TB therapy while awaiting culture results and determine if additional diagnostic testing is needed. Consider testing an additional specimen using NAAT to confirm the NAAT result.
	2	Positive	Presumed to have TB pending culture results.
Negative	1	Negative	Clinician must rely on clinical judgment regarding the need for anti-TB therapy and further diagnostic workup while awaiting culture results.

Source: Data from [18]. *NAAT* nucleic acid amplification test, *TB* tuberculosis considerations to use specifically with the Xpert MTB/RIF assay [19]. In this document, a decisional analysis of combinations of sputum AFB smear result(s) and NAAT test results was provided as well as interpretation and minimal laboratory reports for results from the Xpert MTB/RIF assay.

Non-respiratory Specimens

Both laboratory-developed and commercial NAATs have been used to test non-respiratory specimens, although no commercial assay is approved for this purpose. Because a clinical diagnosis of TB often is uncertain and AFB smear and culture lack sensitivity, NAATs are particularly attractive for suspected cases of extrapulmonary TB. In particular, NAATs have been evaluated in patients suspected of having tuberculous meningitis [20–22]. Signs and symptoms of this disease are nonspecific, and AFB smears in patients with TB meningitis are positive in only 10 % of cases. Isolation of *M. tuberculosis* is positive in only approximately 50 % of adults [23], and is insufficiently timely to aid treatment decisions. Although promising, results of these studies have varied with respect to sensitivity, while specificity was >98 % for most NAATs.

Similar results with other extrapulmonary specimens have been obtained. In many studies, the performance of NAATs with extrapulmonary specimens has been similar to their performance with respiratory specimens [12, 24, 25]; in other studies, the sensitivity was quite low for respiratory specimens [26]. Based on studies published to date, more studies are needed to establish optimal sample volume, nucleic acid extraction and amplification procedures, and uniform criteria for interpretation of results for each specimen type, including formalin-fixed, paraffin-embedded tissues. However, based on current data, a negative NAAT test result does not rule out extrapulmonary TB, particularly if the AFB smear for the specimen is negative.

NAATs are useful for early identification of *M. tuberculosis* complex for all specimen types grown in liquid cultures, except for blood [27]. Sensitivity and specificity of NAATs used to test positive broth cultures are both greater than 98 %. In addition, the INNO-LiPA Mycobacteria assay (Innogenetics NV, Ghent, Belgium) (Table 53.1) successfully identifies mycobacteria directly from aliquots of culture medium from the MB/BacT ALERT 3D System (MB/BacT) (Organon Teknika, Boxtel, The Netherlands) [28].

NAATs have also been evaluated for their usefulness in monitoring therapeutic efficacy. Although beneficial to initial diagnosis, most NAATs are unsuitable for monitoring treatment of TB patients since nucleic acid targets persist long after AFB smears and cultures become negative [29]. However, detection of *M. tuberculosis* mRNA may prove to be a potentially useful method for monitoring therapeutic efficacy [30, 31], although more studies are required to determine its clinical utility.

Identification

Mycobacterial isolates traditionally have been identified to the species level based on phenotypic and biochemical tests. These methods are slow and cumbersome and often fail to obtain an identification, with results varying among different isolates of the same species. Therefore, laboratories are increasingly using molecular methods for identification. Rapid identification of *M. tuberculosis* is of paramount importance for therapeutic and public health reasons. Rapid detection and identification of the approximately 200 species of NTM is becoming more important. Lung disease is caused by many NTM species with a range of clinical presentations and different treatment recommendations [32]. Importantly, since treatment differs among the various NTM species, including slowly and rapidly growing NTMs, and susceptibility testing results may not be available for up to 14 days, accurate species identification is a prerequisite for treatment [33, 34]. Towards this goal, numerous publications describe different molecular approaches to identify not only *M. tuberculosis* complex organisms, but NTM as well [35–38]). Finally, two commercially available systems have been used to identify mycobacteria by amplification of the spacer region of the 16S-23S rRNA genes or the 23S rRNA gene with subsequent hybridization to a membrane strip containing probes specific for the most commonly isolated mycobacterial species [39, 40].

Susceptibility Testing

To successfully control the spread of TB, cases must be detected and treated in a timely manner. At best, conventional susceptibility testing methods for *M. tuberculosis* are available within 7–14 days, after a culture result is positive, already 7–14 days from specimen collection. Thus, molecular methods that can rapidly detect drug resistance can improve the clinical timeliness of test results. Mutations responsible for resistance to the primary drugs used to treat TB have been delineated, including rifampin (RIF), isoniazid (INH), ethambutol (EMB), streptomycin (STR), pyrazinamide (PZA), fluoroquinolones, ethambutol, and amikacin-capreomycin. Because RIF resistance is an excellent marker for multidrug-resistant TB and 95 % of all RIF-resistant strains have mutations localized in an 81 bp region of the bacterial RNA polymerase gene, *rpoB*, which encodes the active site of the enzyme [41], numerous molecular strategies have been developed to detect RIF resistance. In contrast, more than a single gene mutation is frequently responsible for resistance to other drugs, such as INH, EMB, and STR. The complexity of the drug resistance mechanisms for other drugs combined with the complexity of the technology has hampered their broader acceptance of broader resistance testing in the clinical laboratory setting. Nevertheless, relevant mutations for resistance to most of the primary and some secondary antituberculosis drugs have been described; most commonly, conventional or real-time polymerase chain reaction (PCR) in conjunction with analysis for specific mutations of the amplicon using a variety of methods are used to detect drug resistance mutations. Of note, to enhance the rapid diagnosis of MDR-TB, WHO in 2008 approved the use of LPAs for rapid molecular detection of drug resistance in smear-positive specimens or culture isolates [42]. Nevertheless, LPAs require routine specimen processing, DNA extraction, and conventional PCR analysis in a multiroom facility, and thus are limited to use in reference laboratories and not in resource-poor settings. Pyrosequencing also is used to detect resistance [43, 44]. More recently, a LPA has been used to detect resistance to second-line drugs and EMB in MDR-TB strains and clinical specimens [45, 46].

Epidemiology

Molecular epidemiology methods have made significant contributions to our understanding of the pathogenesis and transmission of TB within populations. For example, molecular fingerprinting techniques provided epidemiological evidence of exogenous reinfection as well as quantification of the level of infectiousness among AFB smear-negative patients [47]. Of great significance has been the use of DNA fingerprinting of *M. tuberculosis* isolates to determine the occurrence of laboratory cross contamination of cultures. Laboratory cross contamination represents a significant problem which can result in unnecessary treatment and drug toxicity for a patient. Molecular typing also provided insight as to the pathogenesis of cavitary and non-cavitary disease caused by NTM [32].

Available Tests

Hundreds of publications describe molecular methods, using a variety of formats, to directly detect mycobacteria in clinical specimens, identify mycobacteria, and detect drug resistance mutations in *M. tuberculosis*. Examples of NAATs used for mycobacteria are provided in Tables 53.1 and 53.4. The clinical use of many of these NAATs is described above in the "Clinical Utility" section.

Interpretation of Results

As with any laboratory test, prior to the interpretation of results of molecular assays on patient specimens or AFB clinical isolates, results of controls included with each run must first be interpreted. Selection and use of appropriate controls is an essential feature of any NAAT. Regardless of the format, positive and negative controls must be run in parallel with patient samples. If the assay is a laboratory-developed test (LDT) to directly detect *M. tuberculosis*, the concentration of the positive control should be near the lower limit of detection of the assay. If the run is large, multiple negative controls should be interspersed among the patient samples to monitor for cross contamination. If controls do not perform as expected, the run must be repeated. Optimally, an internal control with upstream and downstream primer recognition sequences the same as those used for detection of the organism should be added to each patient sample reaction to monitor for inhibition. If an internal control is not included (some commercial assays do not include an inhibition control, e.g., the AMTD test), a second reaction should be performed with addition and amplification of a known human target nucleic acid. If inhibition is detected, test results are reported as indeterminate or no amplification due to inhibition. For assays using gel or capillary electrophoresis, molecular weight markers are used.

Inherent problems and limitations associated with NAATs are false-positive results due to cross contamination, as well as false-negative results due to inhibition or inadequate sample collection, transport, and processing. In addition, sampling error due to low numbers of mycobacteria (paucibacillary) or inadequate sample volumes can lead to false-negative test results. Results should be interpreted in the context of the patient's history, physical examination, and clinical course. Thus, both clinicians as well as clinical microbiologists must have a thorough understanding of the advantages and limitations of the particular NAAT used for patient testing as well as the specific microbiology and pathogenesis of the identified mycobacteria.

Sequencing methods or PCR followed by restriction fragment length polymorphism (PCR-RFLP) analysis for identification of NTM provide a rapid tool for identification of this vast group of organisms. However, paradoxically, the identification of mycobacteria has become even more complex with the introduction of these techniques, since these methods have uncovered greater complexity of mycobacterial species. Further complicating the interpretation of molecular identification results were findings that specific species identification was not always successful by analysis of the 16S rRNA gene of patient strains [48]. Based on these results, identification of mycobacteria will mandate attention to quality control of available databases used for mycobacterial identification, coupled with the realization that the taxonomy of the genus *Mycobacterium* is far from elucidated. Thus, interpretation of identification results using molecular methods will require constant changes and updates to available databases [49].

In conclusion, molecular tests for mycobacteria should be interpreted within the context of clinical information and test

Table 53.4 Examples of laboratory-developed tests for mycobacterial infections

Application	Methods	Comments
Direct detection	PCR: single of multiplex Real-time PCR Peptide nucleic acids LAMP	Targets include *IS6110*, *MPB64* and protein antigen B.
Identification	PCR-RFLP with agarose gel or CE SSCP High-density DNA probe arrays Pyrosequencing	Targets include *hsp65*, 16S rDNA, *recA*, *rpoB*, *dnaJ*, and 32-kDa protein. Numerous techniques and targets for identification of *M. tuberculosis* complex.
Drug susceptibility	PCR-RFLP Heteroduplex analysis RT-PCR Real-time PCR Sequencing SSCP High-density DNA probe arrays Oligonucleotide arrays	To date, DNA sequencing is a more successful method for detecting RIF resistance.
Epidemiology	*IS6110* RFLP Secondary markers: Polymorphic guanine-cytosine-rich repetitive RFLP typing Spoligotyping (PCR-based) Mixed-linker PCR Variable number tandem repeat analysis Mycobacterial interspersed repetitive units analysis	*IS6110* RFLP has high discriminatory power. Spoligotyping is useful when discriminating isolates of *M. tuberculosis* with few *IS6110* bands, and is economical, easy to perform, and rapid.

CE capillary electrophoresis, *LAMP* loop-mediated isothermal amplification, *PCR* polymerase chain reaction, *PCR-RFLP* PCR restriction fragment length polymorphism, *RT-PCR* reverse transcription PCR, *SSCP* single strand conformation polymorphism

performance characteristics. Of great importance is strict adherence to guidelines for method validation that include the determination of clinical utility for accurate interpretation of results.

Laboratory Issues

Numerous laboratory issues pertain to the development, introduction, and performance of any clinical molecular test. To date, only guidelines, not universal standards, currently exist for the validation and subsequent quality control and assurance of commercial and/or laboratory-developed molecular tests; many of these guidelines are published by the Clinical Laboratory Standards Institute (Wayne, PA). For all NAATs, adequate and appropriately designed space, as well as other measures, is required to minimize cross contamination of samples [50]. This section will address those laboratory issues that are specific to the diagnosis of mycobacterial infections by molecular tests.

False-positive amplification results can occur from carryover of amplicon while setting up and performing the molecular assay, as well as from cross contamination of clinical specimens during processing for AFB smear and culture [51]. A review of 14 studies revealed a median false-positive rate of 3.1 % for AFB culture [52]. Of 236 patients reported with false-positive cultures, 67 % of patients were subsequently treated, and some had toxicity from therapy as well as unnecessary hospitalizations, tests, and contact investigations. Thus, performance of NAATs to directly detect and identify *M. tuberculosis*, with their inherent potential for false-positive results, underscores the critical need for adherence to strict laboratory technique, inclusion of appropriate negative controls, and careful interpretation of results within the context of the clinical presentation.

As is the case with other infectious agents, the lack of a perfect gold standard further complicates the interpretation of a positive amplification result with a negative culture for the same specimen or from different specimens from the same patient. Likewise, as previously discussed, false-negative amplification results can occur. The theoretical detection of one AFB has not been achieved in reality, which is a particular issue for the diagnosis of *M. tuberculosis* infection where there are often few organisms present in the clinical sample. This low pathogen burden coupled with the tendency of mycobacteria to clump and thereby cause an uneven distribution of organisms in a sample can result in duplicate tests with discrepant results that are difficult to interpret.

Owing to the nature of NAATs, quality control is essential for these procedures. A quality control program should consist of an internal quality control program, as well as participation in an external proficiency testing program such as offered by the CDC. Although performance of NAATs for the detection of *M. tuberculosis* has improved over the years, a recent, multicenter quality control study demonstrated that a large number of procedures still lack sufficient sensitivity for application to AFB smear-negative samples [53].

Specific to molecular identification methods, laboratories performing these techniques must be aware of the multiple problems with present sequence repositories such as base errors, ambiguous base designations, and incomplete sequences [48]. Visual inspection of sequence results is becoming more cumbersome and challenging due to the growing number of *hsp65* alleles described in the literature [54]. Another issue slowly arising from PCR-RFLP analysis for identification is the lack of standardization for electrophoresis conditions, which makes comparison of data from different laboratories challenging. For example, difficulties in PCR-RFLP interpretation stemming from similarities in a number of band sizes needed to discriminate species via agarose gel electrophoresis could be alleviated using 10 % polyacrylamide gel electrophoresis [35].

As previously mentioned, the complexity of drug resistance in *M. tuberculosis* has hindered the utility of molecular assays. However, this limitation may be ultimately overcome by development of other molecular approaches (see Future Directions). Another caveat to testing is that the presence of a resistance gene does not always imply expression of that gene and phenotypic resistance.

Cost-effectiveness is another laboratory issue associated with the performance of NAATs for the diagnosis of TB and identification of mycobacteria. Since NAATs cannot currently replace conventional methods for the diagnosis and management of TB, a NAAT is an additional test with associated costs. Although cost savings may be realized because of possibly preventing more invasive and costly diagnostic procedures (e.g., bronchoalveolar lavage), limiting unnecessary or potentially toxic empiric antituberculous therapy, shortening hospital stays in costly isolation rooms, and limiting transmission, this type of outcomes research has yet to be systematically done. Our understanding of the natural history of infection caused by *M. tuberculosis* will continue to evolve as different applications are explored and evaluated in the clinical setting.

Many questions must be answered in order to fully exploit and utilize the potential of molecular tests for the diagnosis of mycobacterial infections. Towards this end, continued objective evaluation of the analytic and clinical performance of molecular tests, and the impact on patient outcomes, is imperative. However, published studies are often plagued by limitations such as bias in test evaluation due to inadequate blinding. Other errors in the design or reporting of TB diagnostic agent evaluations include failure to describe methods for selection and enrollment of patients, inadequate sample size, declaration of positive predictive values and negative predictive values even when the test population does not resemble the population for which the test was intended, use of inadequate gold standards for clinical case definition and microbiology, and failure to state a specific research question or test indication under study [55]. Also, a case–control study design often is used that tends to have higher bias risk than prospective, cohort-designed studies. Therefore, results from published studies evaluating the performance of NAATs are difficult to compare because of the different bias in study designs as well as in the analysis among the studies. Other contributing factors to this dilemma are failure to demonstrate statistical power, failure to appropriately evaluate and resolve indeterminate and/or discrepant results, and failure to show reproducibility of test results [55]. Another limitation of existing NAAT studies is lack of data on whether these assays have an impact on patient outcomes and how much value NAATs contribute over and above the information already obtained by conventional methods [56].

Systematic reviews of diagnostic test evaluations have been published regarding the ability of NAATs to directly detect *M. tuberculosis* complex in clinical specimens (e.g., [56–58]). The overwhelming majority of the individual studies included in the systematic reviews reported very high estimates of specificity of NAATs for pulmonary and extrapulmonary tuberculosis. However, the systematic reviews report sensitivities were generally lower and highly variable across most studies. Overall, the accuracy of NAATs for the direct detection of *M. tuberculosis* complex was far superior when applied to pulmonary samples as opposed to extrapulmonary specimens. In addition, the sensitivity of NAATs was optimal in smear-positive pulmonary tuberculosis. As proposed by Nahid et al. [59], a NAAT should not be performed if sputum smears are negative and the clinical suspicion is low; by the same token, a negative NAAT in a patient with a high index of clinical suspicion should not preclude continued investigation. Finally, meta-analyses have shown that LPAs are highly accurate, and the GenoType assay, in particular, performs well for rapid detection of RIF resistance in smear-positive specimens [60].

Future Directions

Continued advances in nucleic acid testing technologies will only serve to enhance capabilities for the diagnosis of mycobacterial infections. Efforts employing a variety of strategies already are underway.

Miscellaneous Methods

Different strategies and formats for easier and more rapid means to detect and identify mycobacteria are continually being published. To illustrate, DNAs extracted directly from slides of AFB smears (AFB smear-positive and -negative) made from specimens submitted for AFB smear and culture were tested for *M. tuberculosis* by PCR and sequence analysis for RIF resistance. This approach was 100 % sensitive and specific for the detection of *M. tuberculosis* and RIF resistance [61].

Another approach is the use of fluorescently labeled peptide nucleic acids (PNAs) to directly detect *M. tuberculosis* microscopically [62]. PNAs are DNA-like molecules in which the sugar phosphate backbone is replaced with a peptide-like structure that can hybridize to specific DNA sequences with specific base pairing. PNAs can be labeled with a fluorescent dye to allow for visualization of PNA binding to specific DNA sequences present on a slide. Of significance, the PNA can easily pass through an intact cell wall and bind specifically to intracellular nucleic acid sequences. This strategy for the direct microscopic identification of *M. tuberculosis* and NTM appears to hold some promise.

Finally, new rapid phenotypic methods employing reporter phages avoid some pitfalls associated with genotypic methods for detecting drug resistance in *M. tuberculosis* [63]. A high-intensity mycobacterium-specific fluorophage (NGFP10) was recently reported that allowed direct visualization of *M. tuberculosis* in clinical sputum samples that also detected drug resistance [64]. In addition, efforts are underway to expand the coverage of polymorphic alleles associated with drug-resistance in order to detect MDR-TB. New strategies will continue to be developed and evaluated in direct detection and identification of mycobacteria as well as drug susceptibility testing.

Automation and Miniaturization

The development of real-time PCR assays and other amplification methods in which single or multiple nucleic acid targets can be amplified and analyzed in a single closed tube in minutes rather than hours is particularly suited for subsequent automation. A new generation of mismatch-tolerant probes, referred to as sloppy molecular beacons, can identify mutations in *M. tuberculosis* in clinical samples that contain both drug-susceptible and drug-resistant nucleic acid [65]. This approach allows for homogeneous, closed systems which avoid carryover amplification contamination, are amenable to multiplexing, and are easily amenable to a high-throughput format. Instruments that automate the extraction of either RNA or DNA have been introduced allowing for the performance of a greater number of molecular tests while also providing a more consistent quality of nucleic acid for analysis.

In addition to automation of NAATs for the diagnosis of mycobacterial infections, miniaturization of analytical devices by micromachining technology will be developed to perform PCR in micro-reactors consisting of either silicon or silicon and glass microchips [16, 60, 66]. Although several new diagnostic tests recently have been endorsed by the WHO, a point-of-care (POC) testing device has remained elusive. Developing POC tests with sample-to-answer capability is much needed, particularly in those countries with the highest incidence of TB coupled with limited resources. Advances in this area will have a major impact on the ability to diagnose TB in the field and in poorly resourced regions.

Microarrays

High-density oligonucleotide arrays can rapidly examine large numbers of DNA sequences with a single hybridization step. DNA microarrays can be used in two modes: (1) DNA-based comparison of the genomic content of different strains, and (2) RNA-based monitoring of gene expression. Work has begun for species identification and drug resistance profiling, and strain genotyping of mycobacteria involved in human disease [66]. For example, a commercial, rapid microarray system for the identification of mycobacteria was reported to have correctly identified 100 % of *M. tuberculosis* complex and 98.4 % of NTM clinical isolates [67]. Moreover, an overall sensitivity of 52.5 % for direct detection and identification of mycobacteria in clinical specimens was achieved with 100 % detection and identification of mycobacteria from sputum specimens, albeit the sample size was small ($n=40$). A commercial oligonucleotide microarray to detect RIF resistance in *M. tuberculosis*, the TB-Biochip (Engelhardt Institute of Molecular Biology, Moscow, Russia), was evaluated in a small study in which results obtained with the TB-Chip were compared with conventional susceptibility testing results; the microarray had a diagnostic sensitivity of 80 % [68]. Of note, the spoligotyping assay format for *M. tuberculosis* was converted to a DNA microarray format [69]. As *M. tuberculosis* drug resistance determinants are gradually delineated, this type of platform could be expanded, even with the addition of epidemiological markers.

References

1. Tortoli E. Microbiological features and clinical relevance of new species of the genus *Mycobacterium*. Clin Microbiol Rev. 2014; 27:727–52.
2. McNerney R, Maeurer M, Abubakar I, et al. Tuberculosis diagnostics and biomarkers: needs, challenges, recent advances, and opportunities. J Infect Dis. 2012;205:S147–S158.37.
3. Lawn SD, Zumla A. Tuberculosis. Lancet. 2011;378:52–72.
4. Boyd JC, Marr J. Decreasing reliability of acid-fast smear techniques for detection of tuberculosis. Ann Intern Med. 1975;82: 489–92.
5. Strumpf IJ, Tsang AY, Sayre JW. Re-evaluation of sputum staining for the diagnosis of pulmonary tuberculosis. Am Rev Respir Dis. 1979;119:599–602.
6. Lipsky BA, Gates J, Tenover FC, et al. Factors affecting the clinical value of microscopy for acid-fast bacilli. Rev Infect Dis. 1984;6:214–22.
7. Perera J, Arachchi DM. The optimum relative centrifugal force and centrifugation time for improved sensititivity of smear and culture for detection of Mycobacterium tuberculosis from sputum. Trans R Soc Trop Med Hyg. 1999;93:405–9.
8. American Thoracic Society Workshop: rapid diagnostic tests for tuberculosis. What is the appropriate use? Am J Respir Crit Care Med. 1997; 155:1804–14.
9. Boehme CC, Nabeta P, Hillemann D, et al. Rapid molecular detection of tuberculosis and rifampin resistance. N Engl J Med. 2010;363:1005–15.
10. Hillemann D, Rüsch-Gerdes S, Boehme CC, et al. Rapid molecular detection of extrapulmonary tuberculosis by the automated GeneXpert MTB/IF system. J Clin Microbiol. 2011;49:1201–5.
11. Cantanzaro A, Perry S, Clarridge JE, et al. The role of clinical suspicion in evaluating a new diagnostic test for active tuberculosis. JAMA. 2000;283:639–45.
12. O'Sullivan CE, Miller DR, Schneider PS, et al. Evaluation of Gen-Probe Amplified *Mycobacterium tuberculosis* Direct Test by using respiratory and nonrespiratory specimens in a tertiary care center laboratory. J Clin Microbiol. 2002;40:1723–7.
13. Peirsimoni C, Callegaro A, Scarparo C, et al. Comparative evaluation of the new Gen-Probe *Mycobacterium tuberculosis* Direct Test and the semiautomated Abbott LCx *Mycobacterium tuberculosis* assay for the direct detection of *Mycobacterium tuberculosis* complex in respiratory and extrapulmonary specimens. J Clin Microbiol. 1998;36:3601–4.
14. Franco-Álvarez de Luna F, Ruiz P, Gutiérrez J, et al. Evaluation of the GenoType Mycobacteria Direct Assay for detection of *Mycobacterium tuberculosis* complex and four atypical mycobacterial species in clinical samples. J Clin Microbiol. 2006;44:3025–7.
15. Boehme CC, Nabeta P, Henostroza G, et al. Operational feasibility of using loop-mediated isothermal amplification for diagnosis of pulmonary tuberculosis in microscopy centers of developing countries. J Clin Microbiol. 2007;45:1936–40.
16. Fang X, Chen H, Lingjia X, et al. A portable and integrated nucleic acid amplification microfluidic chip for identifying bacteria. Lab Chip. 2012;12:1495–9.
17. Nagdev KJ, Kashyap RS, Parida MM, et al. Loop-mediated isothermal amplification for rapid and reliable diagnosis of tuberculous meningitis. J Clin Microbiol. 2011;49:1861–5.
18. Centers for Disease Control and Prevention. Updated guidelines for the use of nucleic acid amplification tests for tuberculosis. MMWR Morb Mortal Wkly Rep. 2009;58:7–10.
19. Centers for Disease Control and Prevention. Availability of an assay for detecting Mycobacterium tuberculosis, including rifampin-resistant strains, and considerations for its use – United States, 2013. MMWR Morb Mortal Wkly Rep. 2013;62:821–4.
20. Baker CA, Cartwright CP, Williams DN, et al. Early detection of central nervous system tuberculosis with the Gen-Probe nucleic acid amplification assay: utility in an inner city hospital. Clin Infect Dis. 2002;35:339–42.
21. Bonington A, Strang JIG, Klapper PE, et al. Use of Roche AMPLICOR *Mycobacterium tuberculosis* PCR in early diagnosis of tuberculous meningitis. J Clin Microbiol. 1998;36:1251–4.
22. Lang AM, Feris-Iglesias J, Pena C, et al. Clinical evaluation of the Gen-Probe Amplified Direct Test for detection of *Mycobacterium tuberculosis* complex organisms in cerebrospinal fluid. J Clin Microbiol. 1998;36:2191–4.
23. Roos KL. *Mycobacterium tuberculosis* meningitis and other etiologies of the aseptic meningitis syndrome. Semin Neurol. 2000;20:329–35.
24. Peirsimoni C, Scarparo C, Piccoli P, et al. Performance assessment of two commercial amplification assays for direct detection of *Mycobacterium tuberculosis* complex from respiratory and extrapulmonary specimens. J Clin Microbiol. 2002;40:4138–42.
25. Scarparo C, Piccoli P, Rigon A, et al. Comparison of enhanced *Mycobacterium tuberculosis* Amplified Direct Test with COBAS AMPLICOR *Mycobacterium tuberculosis* assay for direct detection of *Mycobacterium tuberculosis* complex in respiratory and extrapulmonary specimens. J Clin Microbiol. 2000;38:1559–62.
26. Moon JW, Chang YS, Kim SK, et al. The clinical utility of polymerase chain reaction for the diagnosis of pleural tuberculosis. Clin Infect Dis. 2005;41:660–6.
27. Katila ML, Katila P, Erkinjuntti-Pekkanen R. Accelerated detection of mycobacteria with MGIT 960 and COBAS AMPLICOR systems. J Clin Microbiol. 2000;38:960–4.
28. Scarparo C, Piccoli P, Rigon A, et al. Direct identification of mycobacteria from MB/BacT Alert 3D bottles: comparative evaluation of two commercial probe assays. J Clin Microbiol. 2001;39: 3222–7.
29. Desjardin LE, Chen Y, Perkins MD, et al. Comparison of the ABI 7700 System (TaqMan) and competitive PCR for quantitation of IS6110 DNA in sputum during treatment of tuberculosis. J Clin Microbiol. 1998;36:1964–8.
30. Hellyer TJ, Desjardin LE, Hehman GL, et al. Quantitative analysis of mRNA as a marker for viability of *Mycobacterium tuberculosis*. J Clin Microbiol. 1999;37:290–5.
31. Li L, Mahan CS, Palaci M, et al. Sputum *Mycobacterium tuberculosis* mRNA as a marker of bacteriologic clearance in response to antituberculous therapy. J Clin Microbiol. 2010;48:46–51.
32. Griffith DE, Brown-Elliott BA, Wallace RJ. Diagnosing nontuberculous mycobacterial lung disease. Infect Dis Clin North Am. 2002;16:235–49.
33. Harada T, Akiyama Y, Kurashima A, et al. Clinical and microbiological differences between *M. abscessus* and *M. massiliense* lung diseases. J Clin Microbiol. 2012;50:3556–61.
34. De Groote MA, Huitte G. Infections due to rapidly growing mycobacteria. Clin Infect Dis. 2006;42:1756–63.
35. Brunello F, Ligozzi M, Cristelli E, et al. Identification of 54 mycobacterial species by PCR-restriction fragment length polymorphism analysis of the hsp65 gene. J Clin Microbiol. 2001;39:2799–806.
36. Clarridge JE. Impact of 16S rRNA gene sequence analysis for identification of bacteria on clinical microbiology and infectious diseases. Clin Microbiol Rev. 2004;17:840–62.
37. Adékambi T, Drancourt M, Raoult D. The *rpoB* gene as a tool for clinical microbiologists. Trends Microbiol. 2008;17:37–45.
38. Kahla IB, Henry M, Boukadida J, et al. Pyrosequencing assay for rapid identification of *Mycobacterium tuberculosis* complex species. BMC Res Notes. 2011;4:1–6.
39. Padilla E, Gonzalez V, Manterola JM, et al. Comparative evaluation of the new version of the INNO-LiPA mycobacteria and GenoType *Mycobacterium* assays for identification of *Mycobacterium* species from MB/BacT liquid cultures artificially inoculated with Mycobacterial strains. J Clin Microbiol. 2004;42:3083–8.

40. Lebrun L, Gönüllü N, Boutros N, et al. Use of the INNO-LiPA assay for rapid identification of mycobacteria. Diagn Microbiol Infect Dis. 2003;46:151–3.
41. Ramaswamy S, Musser JM. Molecular genetic basis of antimicrobial agent resistance in *Mycobacterium tuberculosis*: update. Tuber Lung Dis. 1998;79:3–29.
42. World Health Organization (2008) New laboratory diagnostic tools for tuberculosis control. WHO. Available at http://www.who.int/tb/laboratory/line_probe_assays/en/. Accessed Jan 4, 2013.
43. Garcia-Sierra N, Lacoma A, Prat C, et al. Pyrosequencing for rapid molecular detection of rifampin and isoniazid resistance in *Mycobacterium tuberculosis* strains and clinical specimens. J Clin Microbiol. 2011;49:3683–6.
44. Jureen P, Engstrand L, Eriksson S, et al. Rapid detection of rifampin resistance in *Mycobacterium tuberculosis* by pyrosequencing technology. J Clin Microbiol. 2006;44:1925–9.
45. Brossier F, Veziris N, Aubry A, et al. Detection by GenoType MTBDR*sl* test of complex mechanisms of resistance to second-line drugs and ethambutol in multidrug-resistant *Mycobacterium tuberculosis* complex isolates. J Clin Microbiol. 2010;48:1683–9.
46. Hillemann D, Rüsch-Gerdes S, Richter E. Feasibility of the GenoType MTBDR*sl*assay for fluoroquinolone, amikacin-capreomycin, and ethambutol resistance testing of *Mycobacterium tuberculosis* strains and clinical specimens. J Clin Microbiol. 2009;47:1767–72.
47. Burgos MV. Molecular epidemiology of tuberculosis. Eur Respir J. 2002;20 suppl 36:54s–65.
48. Turenne CY, Tschetter L, Wolfe J, et al. Necessity of quality-controlled 16S rRNA gene sequence databases: identifying nontuberculous *Mycobacterium* species. J Clin Microbiol. 2001;39: 3637–48.
49. Underwood A, Green J. Call for a quality standard for sequence-based assays in clinical microbiology: necessity for quality assessment of sequences used in microbial identification and typing. J Clin Microbiol. 2011;49:23–6.
50. Wolk D, Mitchell S, Patel R. Principles of molecular biology testing methods. Infect Dis Clin North Am. 2001;15:1157–204.
51. Chang CL, Kim HH, Son HC, et al. False-positive growth of *Mycobacterium tuberculosis* attributable to laboratory contamination confirmed by restriction fragment length polymorphism analysis. Int J Tuberc Lung Dis. 2001;5:861–7.
52. Burman WJ, Reves RR. Review of false-positive cultures for *Mycobacterium tuberculosis* and recommendations for avoiding unnecessary treatment. Clin Infect Dis. 2000;31:1390–5.
53. Noordhoek GT, Mulder S, Wallace P, et al. Multicentre quality control study for the detection of *Mycobacterium tuberculosis* in clinical samples by nucleic amplification methods. Clin Microbiol Infect. 2004;10:295–301.
54. da Silva Rocha A, Barreto AM, Campos CED, et al. Novel allelic variants of mycobacteria isolated in Brazil as determined by PCR-restriction enzyme analysis of hsp65. J Clin Microbiol. 2002;40: 4191–6.
55. Small PM, Perkins MD. More rigour needed in trials of new diagnostic agents for tuberculosis. Lancet. 2000;354:1048–9.
56. Ling DI, Flores LL, Riley LW, et al. Commercial nucleic-acid amplification tests for diagnosis of pulmonary tuberculosis in respiratory specimens: meta-analysis and meta-regression. PLoS One. 2008;3:e1536.
57. Greco S, Rulli M, Girardi E, et al. Diagnostic accuracy of in-house PCR for pulmonary tuberculosis in smear-positive patients: meta-analysis and metaregression. J Clin Microbiol. 2009;47: 569–76.
58. Sarmiento OL, Weigle KA, Alexander J, et al. Assessment by meta-analysis of PCR for diagnosis of smear-negative pulmonary tuberculosis. J Clin Microbiol. 2003;41:3233–40.
59. Nahid P, Pai M, Hopewell PC. Advances in the diagnosis and treatment of tuberculosis. Proc Am Thorac Soc. 2006;3:103–10.
60. Pai M, Minion J, Sohn H, et al. Novel and improved technologies for tuberculosis diagnosis: progress and challenges. Clin Chest Med. 2009;30:701–16.
61. Patnaik M, Liegmann K, Peter JB. Rapid detection of smear-negative *Mycobacterium tuberculosis* by PCR and sequencing for rifampin resistance with DNA extracted directly from slides. J Clin Microbiol. 2001;39:51–2.
62. Stender H, Lund K, Petersen KH, et al. Fluorescence in situ hybridization assay using peptide nucleic acid probes for differentiation between tuberculous and nontuberculous *Mycobacterium* species in smears of *Mycobacterium* cultures. J Clin Microbiol. 1999;37:2760–5.
63. Jain P, Thaler DS, Maiga M, et al. Reporter phage and breath tests: emerging phenotypic assays for diagnosing active tuberculosis, antibiotic resistance, and treatment efficacy. J Infect Dis. 2011; 204:S1142–50.
64. Jain P, Hartman TE, Eisenberg N, et al. ΦGFP10, a high-intensity fluorophage, enables detection and rapid drug susceptibility testing of *Mycobacterium tuberculosis* directly from sputum specimens. J Clin Microbiol. 2012;50:1362–9.
65. Chakravorty S, Kothari H, Aladegbami B, et al. *Rapid, high throughput detection of rifampin resistance and heteroresistance in Mycobacterium tuberculosis* by use of sloppy molecular beacon melting temperature coding. J Clin Microbiol. 2012;50: 2194–202.
66. Schneegass I, Kohler JM. Flow-through polymerase chain reactions in chip thermocyclers. J Biotechnol. 2001;82:101–21.
67. Liu J, Yue J, Yan Z, et al. Performance assessment of the CapitalBio *Mycobacterium* Identification Array System for identification of mycobacteria. J Clin Microbiol. 2012;50:76–80.
68. Caoili JC, Mayorova M, Farajzadeh A, et al. Evaluation of the TB-Biochip oligonucleotide microarray system for rapid detection of rifampin resistance in *Mycobacterium tuberculosis*. J Clin Microbiol. 2006;44:2378–81.
69. Ruettger A, Nieter J, Skrypnyk A, et al. Rapid spoligotyping of *Mycobacterium tuberculosis* complex bacteria by use of a microarray system with automatic data processing and assignment. J Clin Microbiol. 2012;50:2492–5.

Section VI

Identity Testing

Section Editor: Vivianna M. Van Deerlin

Forensic DNA Typing

54

Victor W. Weedn and David R. Foran

Abstract

Forensic DNA typing is generally dated to 1985 and has become the most commonly performed analysis in the modern forensic science laboratory. The technology and methods have evolved and continue to evolve. Analysis of Short Tandem Repeats (STRs) following polymerase chain reaction amplification is used routinely, but other genetic markers, such as Y chromosome STRs, single nucleotide polymorphisms, and mitochondrial DNA, are also tested. These technologies can be applied to a wide variety of evidentiary specimens and powerfully discriminate individuals. They are commonly introduced into court. In fact, forensic DNA is now considered the "gold standard" of forensic science technologies.

Keywords

Forensic DNA typing • Forensic molecular biology • Forensic genetics • STRs • Biological evidence

Introduction

The person on the street when asked about DNA testing will generally first envision a crime laboratory rather than a hospital laboratory. Still today, most criminal perpetrators are caught and prosecuted based upon eye witnesses or confessions, although increasingly scientific evidence comes into play. Forensic DNA typing has become the queen of the forensic sciences and is looked to as the most scientifically grounded of the forensic sciences [1]. The bulk of forensic evidence links an evidential item to the crime scene, but does not identify the perpetrator. Other than videocapture, only fingerprint friction ridge analysis and DNA typing identify the perpetrator per se. Fingerprints came into widespread use for forensic purposes in the late nineteenth century and were admitted into US courts as evidence in the 1930s. The Federal Bureau of Investigation (FBI) owes its origins to the need for a centralized database of fingerprints. Today, millions of fingerprints are filed for criminal and civil purposes. Likewise, millions of convicted offenders' DNA profiles, and in many states, arrestees', are also databased. Thus, DNA tests not only confirm a detective's hunch but, due to the DNA databases, also have become a powerful investigatory tool to identify otherwise unsuspected perpetrators [2].

Serology tests (blood group and type testing and then serum protein isoenzyme electrophoresis) were the forerunners to forensic DNA identity testing of biological materials. Unfortunately, these tests required specimens with a significant amount of high-quality blood serum and they did not have a very strong discriminatory power. Advantages of DNA typing over serologic methods include greater discriminatory power, species specificity, tissue independence, greater sensitivity, and less susceptibility to degradation [3].

The Bureau of Justice Statistics (BJS) first surveyed US crime laboratories in 1998, focusing exclusively on agencies

V.W. Weedn, M.D., J.D. (✉)
Department of Forensic Sciences, George Washington University, 2100 Foxhall Rd., NW, Washington, DC 20007, USA
e-mail: vweedn@gwu.edu

D.R. Foran, Ph.D.
Forensic Science Program, School of Criminal Justice, Michigan State University, 560 Baker Hall, East Lansing, MI 48824, USA
e-mail: foran@msu.edu

D.G.B. Leonard (ed.), *Molecular Pathology in Clinical Practice*, DOI 10.1007/978-3-319-19674-9_54

that performed DNA analysis, and found that there were 120 public forensic DNA laboratories, which had a median staff of 5 and faced substantial backlogs [4]. According to the 2005 *BJS Census of Publicly Funded Forensic Crime Laboratories*, about half the public crime laboratories were performing DNA testing [5]. Although there is no corresponding contemporary study, it seems clear that the size and number of forensic DNA laboratories have substantially increased, with most of the 450–500 public crime laboratories now performing DNA testing. The National Institute of Justice (NIJ), beginning with a 2003 *Advancing Justice Through DNA Technology* initiative, has spent hundreds of millions of dollars on forensic DNA capacity building [6].

Forensic Testing and Sample Considerations

Forensic v. Clinical Specimens and Tests

Forensic tests differ from clinical tests in several respects. First, whereas clinical samples can be standardized, forensic samples vary substantially. An analyst may routinely encounter cigarette butts as evidence, but then must be prepared to face a completely new challenge for the first time, such as a partially eaten piece of food. Second, clinical samples are relatively substantial, whereas forensic laboratories routinely receive trace evidence, permitting testing only once (although routine practice is to attempt to save a portion, if possible, for potential testing by the defense). Third, unlike clinical specimens, evidentiary materials are usually neither fresh nor pristine. For example, semen samples are generally admixed with vaginal cells and microbial flora in a rape swab (Fig. 54.1), spit on a sidewalk has been exposed to the sun and rain, and blood on the floor may have been there for months. Furthermore, forensic testing is performed with an eye to court challenges. Thus, the forensic scientist uses only well-validated protocols, documents all aspects of laboratory processing, and must be ready to defend the science, the procedures, and the testing against legal attack. Chain-of-custody must always be maintained in forensic laboratories. Moreover, clinical laboratory staff are generally not familiar with the regulations, standards, and quality assurance practices of forensic laboratories. Thus, clinical laboratories, though technically capable, are normally not prepared to conduct forensic identity testing. Nevertheless, since clinical laboratories use identity testing for other applications, an understanding of forensic identity testing is useful as an introduction to the methodology and for the historical background.

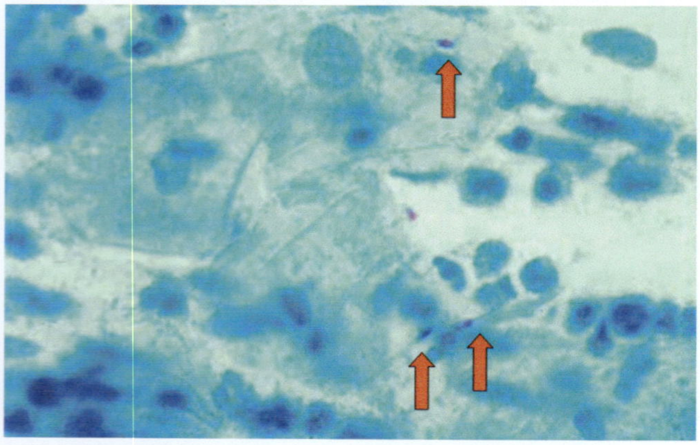

Figure 54.1 The most common DNA evidence in US crime laboratories is a vaginal swab from a rape kit. This photomicrograph is a stained vaginal smear from a rape kit. The *arrows* indicate spermatozoa. In addition to the DNA from the male contributor, there is DNA from the female epithelial squamous and white blood cells, as well as that of the microbial flora

Sexual Assaults (Swabs)

In the USA, rape kits have dominated the evidential submissions to forensic DNA laboratories (Fig. 54.1). Often, the demand for DNA testing on rape kits outstrips the ability of crime laboratories' testing capacity and large backlogs may exist despite substantial NIJ grant programs to reduce them [7]. Typical rape kits include vaginal, anal, and oral evidentiary swabs, buccal reference swabs, pubic combings, and exemplars of pubic and scalp hairs. If a condom was used by a rapist and later found, it may yield semen from the male perpetrator on the inside and vaginal epithelial cells from the female victim on the outside. Vaginal swab specimens are inherently mixed samples. Most commonly the DNA of the spermatozoa is partially purified by a differential extraction procedure in which the female fraction is released using a gentle lysis medium, after which male DNA is released from the sperm using a solution containing a strong reducing agent (dithiothreitol) to break the disulfide bonds in the capsules of the spermatozoan heads [8]. Laser capture of spermatozoa from microscopic slides has also been successfully used, while immunologic affinity methods have thus far been disappointing. Y-chromosome DNA markers (described below) are an alternative method of capturing male identity information.

Other Violent Crimes (Blood, Other Evidence)

Blood and similar specimens from homicides and other violent crimes are the next-most-common evidentiary materials submitted to forensic laboratories [9]. In an early study of biological evidence at crime scenes, blood was found to be present in 60 % of murders, assaults, and batteries [10]. The DNA can come from myriad items and materials. Saliva may

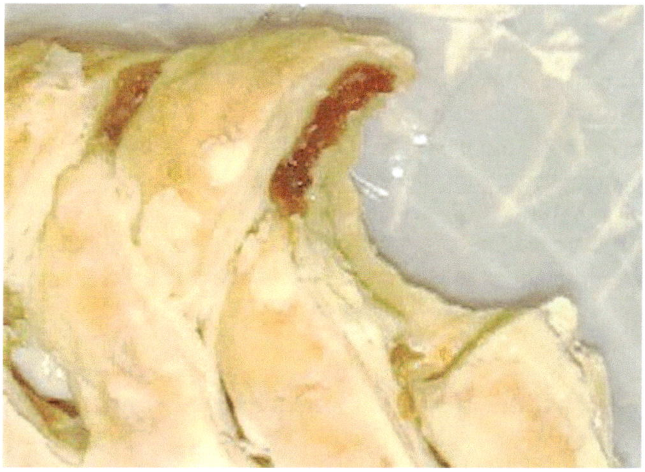

Figure 54.2 DNA testing identified a masked bandit when his peach strudel that was left at the scene of an armed robbery was used for DNA testing

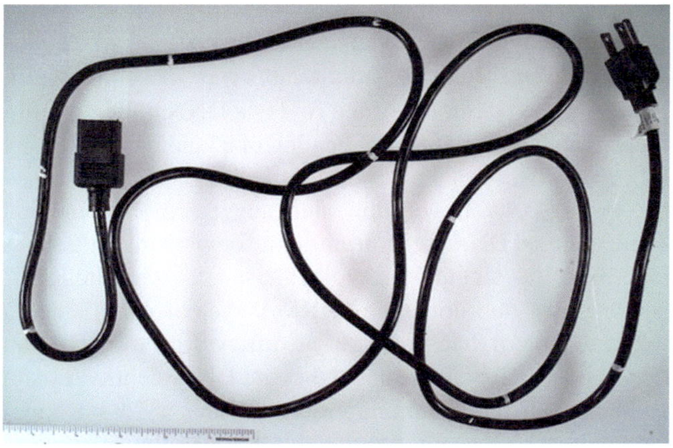

Figure 54.3 This vacuum cleaner cord was used as a ligature for a strangulation murder. Swabbings of the cord along its length revealed the victim's DNA in the center and a mixture of victim and accused DNA on outer areas of the cord

be deposited on beverage containers, envelope seals, gum, cigarettes, or food (Fig. 54.2). Investigators have followed suspects to obtain "abandoned" specimens, such as facial tissues, cigarette butts, gum, or drinking glass. Cords used as a murder weapon for strangulation can yield both victim and perpetrator DNA (Fig. 54.3). Shed hairs, which contain little or no nuclear DNA (nDNA), still harbor mitochondrial DNA (mtDNA), which also can be used for identification purposes. Fingernail swabbing or scrapings occasionally yield foreign DNA if a victim struggled and scratched the perpetrator, and similarly bite marks can be swabbed for DNA. Reference samples may come from toothbrushes, razors, combs, clothing, and medical specimens. One of the authors (DF) has shown DNA to be useful to identify the bombmaker of deflagrated improvised explosive devices [11].

Property Crimes (Touch DNA)

Increasingly, jurisdictions are performing DNA testing in property crimes, including theft, burglary, robbery, and arson, among others. The vast majority of US crimes are property crimes: 9.3 million property crimes compared to 1.3 million violent crimes in 2009 [12]. The case closure (clearance) rate for property crimes is <20 % [13] and DNA testing for such crimes has been found to be cost-effective [14]. Furthermore, it is generally thought that some individuals progress from nonviolent to violent crimes; often from petty theft to burglary to rape, and thus interdiction of a criminal career progression may break the cycle and prevent major crimes [15, 16]. In general, DNA testing for property crimes involves "touch DNA" from handled objects. The possibility of testing such trace or "low copy number" (LCN) DNA was introduced in 1997 when Dr. van Oorschot reported that minute quantities of DNA can be recovered from fingerprints [17]. Conventional laboratory testing will successfully type DNA from approximately 100 cells (0.5–1 ng at 6.5 pg/diploid cell), although many forensic laboratories may be successful down to as few as 15–20 cells (approximately 100 pg). LCN DNA is generally defined as <100 pg, but 35 pg is often considered an analytical threshold. LCN DNA testing for property crimes was pioneered by Drs. Peter Gill and Dave Werrett at the Forensic Science Service (now disbanded) in the UK [18] and later in the USA by Dr. Mechthild Prinz and Theresa Caragine in the New York City Office of the Chief Medical Examiner's Department of Forensic Biology [19]. Such testing involves minimizing reaction volumes and increasing polymerase chain reaction (PCR) cycling (see below). However, only a portion of the specimens yield a useful profile (perhaps 10–20 %). LCN DNA testing is problematic due to detection of contamination from prior handling, in-laboratory contamination, and inconsistent results that stem from random sampling of one or both alleles when both exist at very small levels (so-called stochastic sampling effects). These difficulties are compounded by the destructive nature of DNA testing, which may negate the possibility of retesting. For these reasons, some have suggested that LCN analysis should only be used for investigative purposes, and not as probative evidence in court. No national standards are yet in place and the FBI has generally recommended against such testing [20]. Nonetheless, LCN testing is increasingly used. The object is swabbed and resultant DNA extracts may be amplified two or three times, wherein analysts hope to obtain pure (single) profile results that are assumed to be from the last person who pulled the trigger of a gun or handled a knife. Forensic laboratories performing this testing will generally simply disregard any results other than clear single profiles.

Other Forensic DNA Testing Applications

Forensic DNA identity testing also can be used in other forensic and non-forensic contexts. For example, urine samples from drug testing may be analyzed to confirm that the sample is truly from the person who allegedly generated it [21]. DNA testing is used for disaster victim identification [22]. In cases involving nonhuman DNA (discussed below), individual, group (clade), or species may be determined, linking items such as a plant leaf or animal hair to a criminal case, or proving illegal poaching activity [23]. "Microbial forensics" has been developed for source attribution of terrorist pathogens, such as the anthrax letter attacks [24, 25]. Genetic analyses can identify the type of body fluid or tissue (e.g., urine, semen, saliva) based on the RNAs expressed. DNA testing can be used for investigatory purposes by supplying information about the perpetrator using phenotypic markers (described below), as well as through partial ("low stringency") matches that may detect relatives who represent investigatory leads (described below). In non-criminalistic applications, the same tests used in forensic identity testing can be used for determinations of parentage and sample switch disputes [26].

Genetic Systems and Methods for DNA Typing

Genetic Variation

In everyday life, we easily recognize individuals through obvious biological variation among individuals. Positive identification or individualization is a statement of uniqueness, which is theoretically impossible to prove. However, forensic identity testing harnesses the extraordinary statistical discriminatory power of genetic variation to support a policy-based, administrative, or judicial determination of identity [27]. Indeed, forensic DNA testing often is thought of as tantamount to positive identification. Genetic variation occurs in a continuum of biological classification, from kingdom to genus, clades, and individuals. Specifically, forensic DNA identity testing is based on the detection and comparison of polymorphisms (poly—many; morphs—types) in the DNA among individuals. Statistically, there is variation at approximately one in every thousand base pairs (bp) between every two unrelated humans. However, this variation is not random; many protein-coding regions are highly conserved, as mutations in genes succumb to natural selection. Most polymorphisms occur in the noncoding DNA, which predominates in the human genome (>98 %) and is more tolerant of mutation than the protein-coding DNA regions. Differences between individuals can be due to single nucleotide polymorphisms (SNPs) or variations in length of a specific region or locus in the genome; that is, length polymorphisms. Such polymorphisms result in different forms, or alleles, of genetic markers. All individuals have two copies of each autosomal chromosome: one inherited maternally and the other paternally. Routine forensic DNA testing, using short tandem repeat (STR) typing, (described below) involves length polymorphisms in repetitive DNA from noncoding regions of the chromosomes, although it employs only a small fraction of the differences in the human genome among individuals.

Restriction Fragment Length Polymorphisms

Historical Context

In the mid-1980s, most DNA-based forensic analysis involved restriction fragment length polymorphism (RFLP) testing, first described by Dr. Edwin Southern in 1975 [28]. Such testing merely gave a binary result and was too little information for too much work. Drs. Wyman and White detailed a polymorphic RFLP marker in 1980, in which variation between human individuals was observed [29]. However, the beginning of the forensic DNA typing revolution began with the 1985 publication of a landmark article by Dr. Alec Jeffreys of Leicester, England, in which he coined the term "DNA fingerprint" and suggested the potential application of DNA fingerprinting in forensic investigations [30, 31]. His technique involved use of "minisatellites," which was a multilocus probe RFLP system that yielded a bar code pattern that seemed to be different for every person (Fig. 54.4). Jeffreys conducted the first DNA identity tests in 1986 in a disputed immigration case and a double rape-homicide, which resulted in the 1987 exoneration of Richard Bucklin and then the 1988 conviction of Colin Pitchfork [32, 33]. In the USA, single-locus probe RFLP analysis was pioneered by Dr. Arthur Eisenberg (then at Lifecodes Corporation), that was more robust and permitted statistical evaluation (Fig. 54.5). In 1986–1987, commercial laboratories, particularly involving Dr. Edward Blake of the Serologic Research Institute, Drs. Michael Baird and Arthur Eisenberg of Lifecodes Corporation, and Dr. Robin Cotton of Cellmark Diagnostics, undertook forensic DNA testing in the USA, and in 1987 Tommy Lee Andrews became the initial American to be convicted of a crime (rape) using DNA data [34]. The FBI, led by Dr. Bruce Budowle, began performing DNA typing casework in December 1988. A few months later, in March 1989, Virginia became the first state crime laboratory with an operational DNA unit, directed by Dr. Paul Ferrara. RFLP testing was the mainstay of most criminalistic DNA typing for a decade. At the same time, Dr. Henry Erlich and coworkers of Cetus Corporation, developed a faster PCR-based (see below) HLA DQ-alpha dot-blot system (and later the Polymarker system, Fig. 54.6), but

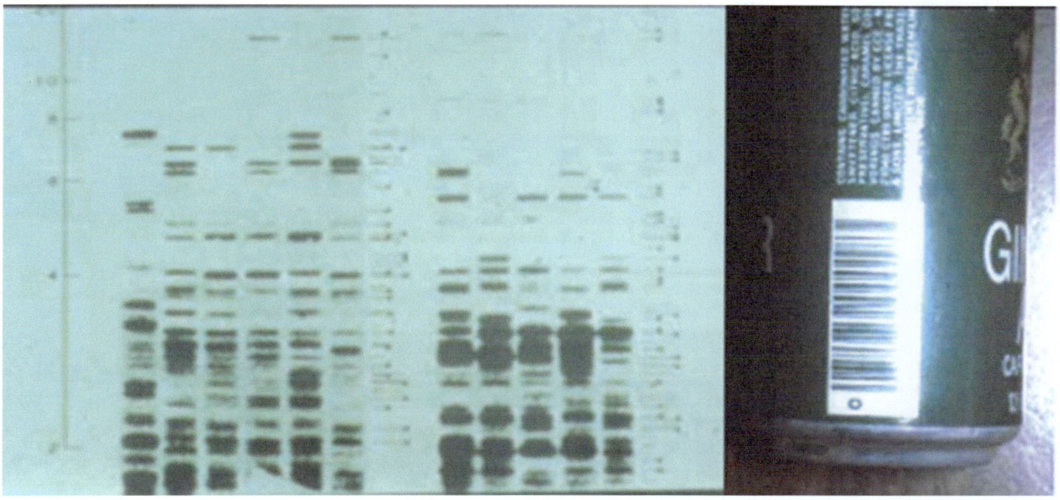

Figure 54.4 In 1985, Alec Jeffreys first described a DNA fingerprint. He used a multilocus minisatellite probe that resulted in a band pattern similar to a bar code, such as the one shown on the can to the *right*. The various lanes of the autoradiograph are from different individuals, demonstrating that each shows a unique pattern of bands. This multilocus probe method of DNA typing is no longer used in forensic identification

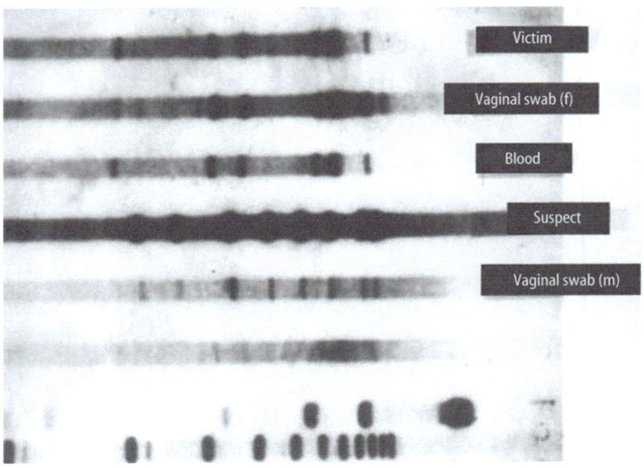

Figure 54.5 RFLP autoradiograph with five analytical lanes and three control lanes. The DNA profile of the reference sample from a female rape victim matches the DNA profile of blood found at the scene and that of the female fraction of a vaginal swab. The DNA profile of the suspect reference specimen matches the male fraction of a vaginal swab but does not match the DNA profile of the female victim

it did not have sufficient discriminatory power for widespread adoption by the forensic community. Nevertheless, the first use of DNA tests in litigation in the USA was in 1986, in the case of *Commonwealth v. Pestinikas*, using HLA DQ-alpha to show that organs had not been switched in an autopsy [35]. In the early 1990s, PCR-based STR systems (described below) were developed and eventually became the standard forensic DNA test worldwide. STR methods replaced RFLP systems due to robustness, sensitivity, statistically discrete systems, ease of automation, and economy. Other systems, such as Y-chromosome markers, mtDNA sequencing, and phenotypic markers also are sometimes used (described below) (see Table 54.1).

Early Cases Using DNA Testing

Queen v Pitchfork

The first criminal investigation using DNA typing was in a double rape-homicide (of Linda Mann in 1983 and of Dawn Ashworth in 1986) on a deserted footpath in the English countryside, known as the "Black Pad Murders." Richard Buckland, a person of low intelligence and sexual fetishes, became the focus of early suspicion and was charged but then exonerated by the new Jeffreys DNA tests. Males in the community between 13 and 30 years of age were asked to volunteer blood samples for DNA testing. There were no matches despite 4,500 "bloodings." However, police discovered that a man named Ian Kelly had substituted his blood for Colin Pitchfork's sample. Pitchfork was subsequently DNA matched and then convicted of both homicides.

Pennsylvania v Pestinikas

The first use of DNA typing in the USA was in a 1986 nursing home negligent homicide case. Forensic Science Associates performed DNA tests to prove that organs in the autopsy had not been switched as was alleged by one expert. The DNA in this case had become highly degraded, averaging fragments of approximately 100 bp.

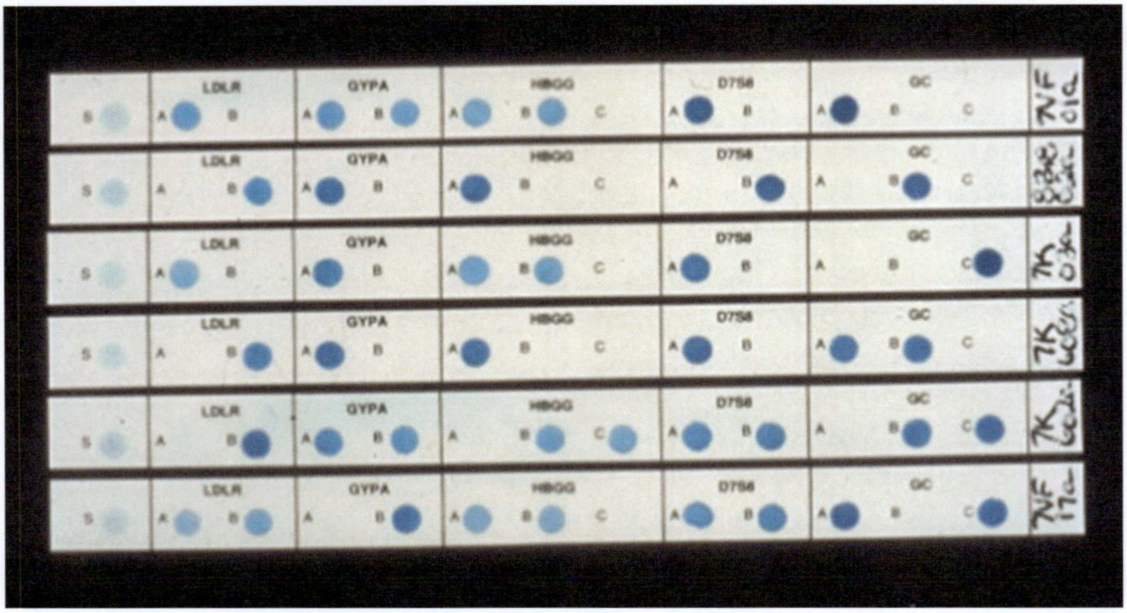

Figure 54.6 Polymarker strips from different individuals using five genetic systems detected by PCR amplification and reverse dot-blot hybridization probes. *GC* group-specific component, *GYPA* glycophorin A, *HBGG* hemoglobin gamma-globin chain, *LDLR* low-density lipoprotein receptor,

Table 54.1 Summary of DNA typing system usage in crime laboratories

Typing method	PCR-based	Late 1980s	1990s	2000s	Utility
RFLP	No	*Dominates*	*Dominates*	Abandoned	Routine casework
Dot blots	Yes	Used	Used	Abandoned	Routine casework
STRs	Yes	In research	Used	*Dominates*	Routine casework
mtDNA	Yes	In research	Used	Used	Hairs, degraded samples
Y-STRs	Yes		In research	Used	Vaginal swabs in rape cases
SNPs	Yes			In research	Very degraded samples

mtDNA mitochondrial DNA, *RFLP* restriction fragment length polymorphism, *SNPs* single nucleotide polymorphisms, *STRs* short tandem repeats, *Y-STRs* Y chromosome short tandem repeats

Florida v Andrews

The first US criminal conviction based on DNA typing was of a serial rapist, Tommy Lee Andrews (1987). A series of breaking and entering women's homes and rapes began in 1986 in Orlando, Florida. A stakeout resulted in an arrest, and Lifecodes Corporation matched the suspect's DNA to vaginal swabs of two of the rape victims.

PCR Amplification as Sample Preparation

Today, all major methods for routine forensic DNA testing begin with amplification of the DNA target by PCR. Dr. Kary Mullis shared the 1993 Nobel Prize in Chemistry for PCR development in 1983. Forensically valuable human leukocyte antigen (HLA) polymorphisms were among the earliest targets to be amplified by PCR in the laboratory [36]. PCR amplification is relatively easy to perform, inexpensive, quick, and amenable to automation. It also permits chemical labeling of the amplified fragments, as well as simultaneous amplification of several loci in a single reaction (multiplex). PCR amplification allows the routine testing of nanogram quantities of DNA, and can be optimized for testing of even picogram quantities, enabling the use of new classes of evidentiary specimens. However, such sensitivity requires extreme care to prevent contamination, including laboratory facilities with separate pre- and post-amplification areas, unidirectional handling of evidence intake through final analysis, limited laboratory access by untrained personnel, and knowledge of each analyst's DNA profile to identify any contamination. Lastly, PCR can be successful on evidentiary material in which the DNA has become degraded and only a few fragments with the intact target sequence remain. Although amplification methods other than PCR exist, the conservative forensic community will not likely be quick to adopt an alternative to PCR unless there is a very good reason.

Short Tandem Repeats

STRs are repeat length polymorphisms that have become the mainstay of current forensic identity profiling around the world. Core repeat units in STR systems are tetranucleotide or pentanucleotide elements (i.e., have four or five nucleotides in each core repeat, respectively), with resulting amplicon sizes of approximately 100–450 bp (see Fig. 54.7). STR analysis is robust, amenable to automation, highly sensitive, relatively insensitive to degraded DNA, and yields discrete alleles. Multiplexed amplification of multiple STR loci achieves extraordinary discriminatory powers (typically $>10^{-12}$) (see Fig. 54.8). As a result, PCR-based STR testing has become dominant in forensic DNA laboratories (Table 54.1).

In the late 1980s, Dr. C. Thomas Caskey working with Holly Hammond, then at Baylor College of Medicine in Houston, Texas, was funded by NIJ to develop STR systems for forensic applications [37]. Subsequently, in 1991, STRs were first used in casework by one of the authors (VW) at the US Armed Forces DNA Identification Laboratory (AFDIL), through a subcontract with Cellmark Diagnostics, to identify service members who died in the first Persian Gulf War. However, it was Drs. Peter Gill and David Werrett at UK's Forensic Science Service who, in the mid-1990s, began applying STR analysis (using in-house systems) to routine criminal casework [38, 39].

Recognizing the importance of cross-jurisdictional matches, the FBI convened a panel of forensic scientists in 1998 to select a panel of STR loci for use in their National DNA Index System (NDIS). Thirteen loci, all containing tetranucleotide repeats, were chosen: D3S1358, D5S818, D7S820, D8S1179, D13S317, D16S539, D18S51, D21S11, CSF1PO, FGA, THO1, TPOX, and vWA (Table 54.2) [40, 41]. These 13 core loci have become standard for forensic casework in much of the world and are referred to as the "CODIS" loci, after the Combined DNA Index System (CODIS) software into which DNA profiles are entered [42]. Databases are maintained of the STR alleles of convicted felons, casework profiles, and missing persons, although exactly which profiles can or must be uploaded varies based on state requirements. The commonality of genetic systems (i.e., STR loci) used in forensic casework enables computer searches for matches across jurisdictions.

All CODIS STR loci are tetranucleotide repeats. In general, smaller fragments are preferred for amplification of potentially degraded samples. Additionally, preferential amplification, where smaller target DNA fragments are

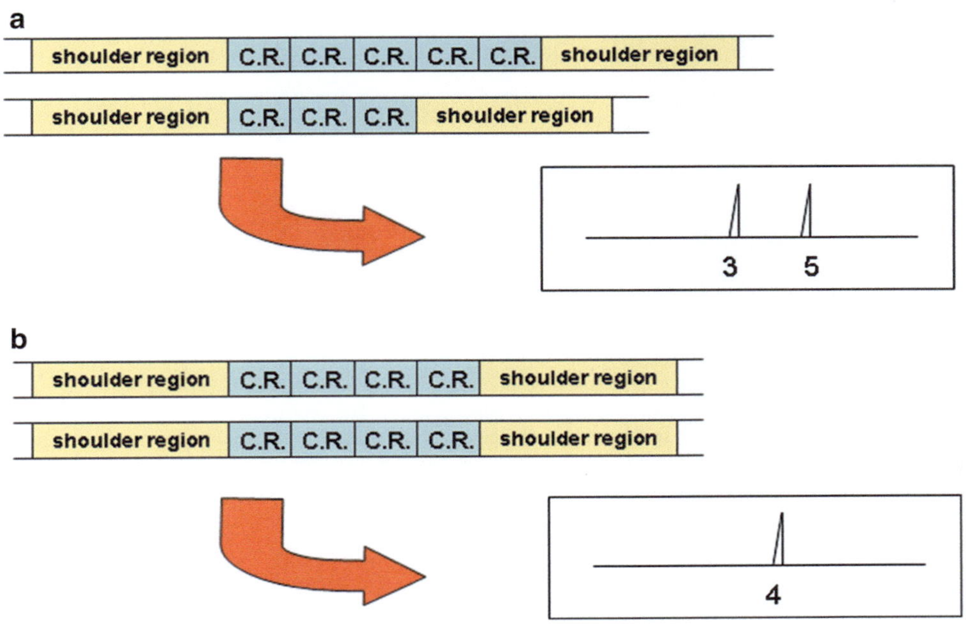

Figure 54.7 Diagram of short tandem repeat DNA segments composed of varying numbers of core repeats (C.R.) and accompanying electropherograms showing the corresponding allele peaks: (**a**) heterozygous pattern with alleles of 3 and 5 repeats, (**b**) homozygous pattern with allele of 4 repeats. The shoulder region is the flanking constant region to which PCR primers hybridize

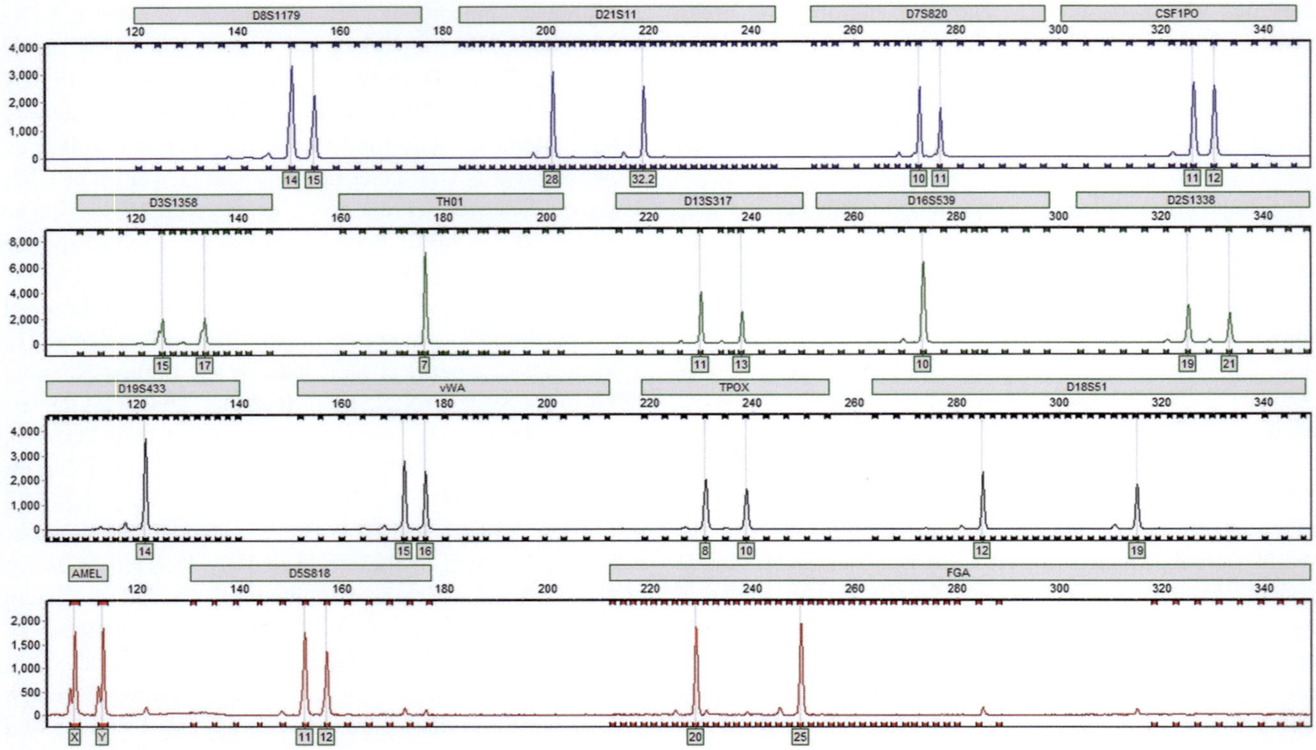

Figure 54.8 Electropherogram of multiplexed fluorescently labeled PCR amplicons of STR loci demonstrating the allelic determinations (*boxes*). The *X*-axis reflects time and the *Y*-axis reflects fluorescence intensity. Four fluorophore colors permit separate analysis of genetic loci with overlapping sizes. A fifth dye channel is used for a size standard that is not shown. This person is a 15,16 genotype at the vWA locus, a 7,7 genotype (7 phenotype) at the TH01 locus, has a 32.2 variant allele in the D21S11 locus, and is a male according to the amelogenin locus

Table 54.2 Nationally indexed "13 CODIS STR Core Loci"*

Locus	Location	GenBank#	Alleles	Repeats	Motif	*H*	Mut %
D3S1358	3p21.31	AC099539	25	8–21	Compound TCTG/TCTA	0.795	0.12
D5S818	5q23.2	AC008512	15	7–18	Simple AGAT	0.682	0.11
D7S820	7q21.11	AC004848	30	5–16	Simple GATA	0.806	0.1
D8S1179	8q24.13	AF216671	15	7–20	Compound TCTA/TCTG	0.78	0.14
D13S317	13q31.1	AL353628	17	5–16	Simple TATC	0.771	0.14
D16S539	16q24.1	AC024591	19	5–16	Simple GATA	0.767	0.11
D18S51	18q21.33	AP001534	51	7–40	Simple AGAA	0.876	0.22
D21S11	21q21.1	AP000433	89	12–41.2	Complex TCTA/TCTG	0.853	0.19
CSF1PO	5q33.1	X14720	20	5–16	Simple TAGA	0.734	0.16
FGA	4q31.3	M64982	80	12.2–51.2	Compound CTTT/TTCC	0.86	0.28
THO1	11p15.5	D00269	20	3–14	Simple TCAT	0.783	0.01
TPOX	2p25.3	M68651	15	4–16	Simple GAAT	0.621	0.01
vWA	12p13.31	M25858	29	10–25	Compound TCTG/TCTA	0.811	0.17

The STR systems are named by their designated genetic locus. The physical location is their chromosomal site. The number of alleles is the observed number rather than the theoretical potential number of alleles. The range of repeats includes non-whole number integers which represent partial repeats. The heterozygosity (H) is the gene diversity (sometimes designated as D) calculated as 1 minus the sum of the population frequencies squared for each allele. The mutation rate (Mut %) is expressed as a percentage.

amplified preferentially over larger targets, becomes an issue with large core repeats as the size discrepancy between overall allele lengths increases substantially. However, "stutter" can become problematic if the core repeat size (for example, dinucleotide and trinucleotide repeats) is too small. Stutter peaks are produced when the DNA polymerase slips during amplification, resulting in PCR products that have fewer or more repeat units than the starting template, with the major stutter product generally one repeat unit less than the template. Dinucleotide and trinucleotide repeats have substantial stutter, while pentanucleotide or larger repeats have almost none.

Commercial kits for amplification of the CODIS core STR loci are available in various combinations of multiplex primer sets from two companies: Promega Corporation and Applied Biosystems Inc. (ABI, a subsidiary of Life Technologies, Cartsbad, CA). ABI sells the Identifiler series, which includes all 13 core loci as well as amelogenin (below), D2S1338, and D19S433 in a single reaction. Promega offers the PowerPlex series, such as PowerPlex 16 that includes the 13 core loci, plus amelogenin and two pentanucleotide repeat loci, Penta D and Penta E. These two companies regularly produce new products that add loci to the multiplex, increasing discriminatory power. Mini-STRs, such as Applied Biosystem's Minifiler, are traditional STRs with primers designed to reduce the flanking regions and thus the amplicon size, so that typing results can be obtained from more substantially degraded specimens.

The 13 CODIS core STR loci are being expanded to a likely set of 24 loci. The impetus for this expansion is to reduce the likelihood of adventitious matches in large databases, to increase the compatibility with international databases, and to increase the discrimination power for missing person cases [43]. The putative additional loci include loci from the European Standard Set (ESS). ABI has responded with the Global Filer kit and Promega with the Powerplex Fusion kit. These new kits have been engineered to be more sensitive as well as capable of more rapid amplification (see discussion below).

Amelogenin and Other Sex Markers

An amelogenin assay is included in current commercial STR amplification kits as a sex marker [44]. The amelogenin gene is present as homologs on both the X and Y chromosomes, but there are a number of sequence differences in the noncoding regions. The locus used in forensic testing involves a 6 bp deletion on the X chromosome; thus, the X marker is shorter than the Y marker and males manifest two peaks whereas females manifest a single peak of twice the intensity (Fig. 54.9). The amelogenin sex marker system is robust and reliable, although in very rare instances, sex-typing discrepancies have been noted [45]. Other sex markers have been described, including ones that exist at higher copy number and are thus more sensitive than the single copy amelogenin.

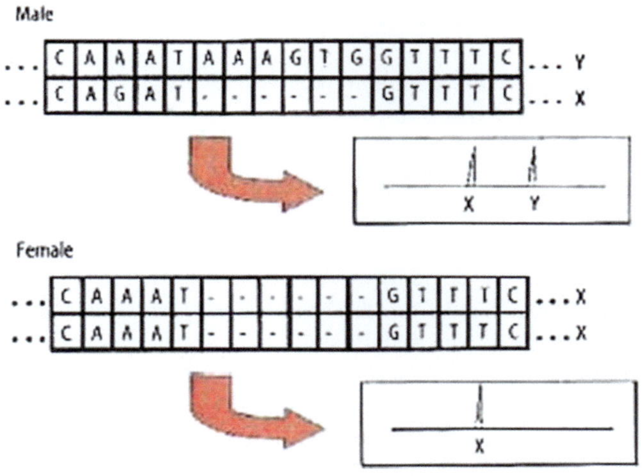

Figure 54.9 The amelogenin locus is 6 bp longer on the Y chromosome than on the X chromosome. Thus, a male will have two peaks and a female will have only one peak in the electropherogram

Male-Specific DNA Typing with Y-Chromosome Markers

Y-chromosome markers are not sex markers, but rather are male-specific identity systems that permit typing of the male DNA in mixed male/female specimens (e.g., vaginal swabs following rape or fingernail scrapings after assault). Y-chromosome markers are useful due to their strict paternal inheritance and can be helpful in lineage studies. The absence of recombination means that the exact same Y chromosome DNA alleles are present in distant paternal relatives of an individual. For example, Y-chromosome markers were used in determining the paternity of US President Thomas Jefferson among his distant descendants [46]. Y-chromosome markers are inherited together, and are reported together as a haplotype. Since they are not genetically independent, the population frequencies of each allele cannot be multiplied together; instead the counting method is used, where the number of times the haplotype is seen in a population database generates the frequency statistic. This means that the discriminatory power is much less than autosomal STRs and that a large number of loci is necessary to achieve substantial discrimination. Current commercial Y-chromosome markers are STRs that can be analyzed on the same equipment as standard STRs. More information on Y-STR haplotypes is available from various websites [47].

Single Nucleotide Polymorphisms

By far the most common polymorphisms in the human genome are SNPs [48–50]. It is estimated that there are approximately 15 million SNP sites out of the more than six billion bps of the diploid human genome. Very small DNA fragments can be interrogated for SNP alleles; thus, SNP genotyping can be applied for forensic identification despite extreme DNA degradation. The identification of human remains recovered from the World Trade Center disaster is one scenario in which SNPs showed an advantage over other DNA typing (Orchid-GeneScreen, now LabCorp, Burlington, NC), since the DNA was severely degraded in a large percentage of the specimens. Most SNPs are biallelic; that is, there are only two alleles, despite the fact that there are four possible nucleotide bases. Most SNPs are base substitutions; however, a smaller number are insertions or deletions ("indels"). Therefore, a large set of SNPs must be used to obtain decisive discriminatory values. In forensics, SNP analysis is not currently commercially available, but it is particularly amenable to automation and analysis with chip technologies. Indels are compatible with more standard fragment length technologies. SNPs may prove to be particularly valuable with Y chromosome or phenotypic markers (described below).

Mitochondrial DNA Sequencing

MtDNA is useful for forensic typing in tissues lacking a nucleus (e.g., shed [telogen] hairs), when specimens are greatly degraded (e.g., old skeletal remains), and in some cases of distant maternal relatives or to clarify kindred relations. Human mtDNA is a histone-free, circular, double-stranded DNA of approximately 16,569 bp (Fig. 54.10). MtDNA is useful for testing highly degraded specimens because it is present at a high copy number in each cell. Mitochondria are thought to be derived from ancient cellular symbionts, explaining the presence of their own DNA and modified genetic code. Each cell contains tens to thousands of mitochondria and each mitochondrion contains 1–10 copies of mtDNA; as a result there are a total of 500–2,000 copies per cell, compared to the single set of diploid nuclear chromosomes [51]. Furthermore, each mtDNA particle appears to be more resistant to degradation than nDNA [52], possibly because it is circular or because it is enveloped within the mitochondrion. The non-recombinant maternal inheritance pattern of mtDNA (Fig. 54.11) also can be of use in certain cases. Any paternal mtDNA that may pass into the fertilized egg from the sperm is thought to be destroyed by the ubiquitin pathway, leaving only the maternal egg-derived mtDNA intact. Thus, all mitochondria are derived from the mother's egg. MtDNA, unlike the paired nuclear DNA, does not undergo meiosis and does not participate in genetic

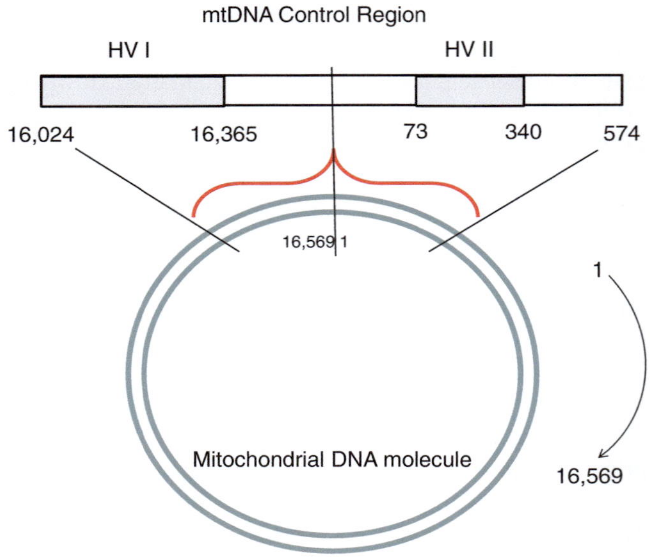

Figure 54.10 Mitochondrial DNA (mtDNA) is a circular DNA with 16,569 bp. The "control" region is a segment that encompasses the site used for the arbitrary numbering system and that contains two hypervariable regions (HVI and HVII) that are used for forensic purposes

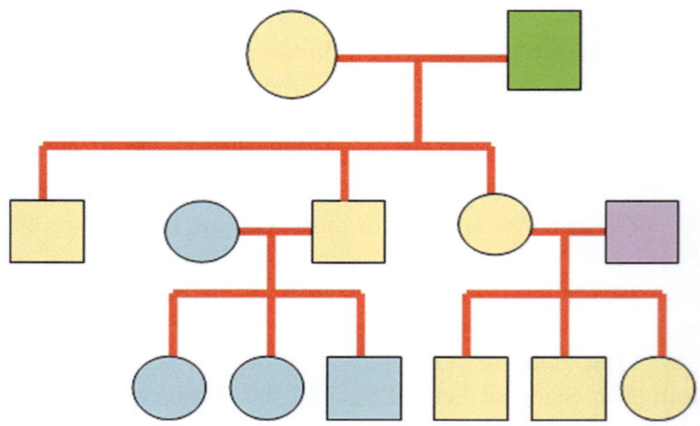

Figure 54.11 Mitochondrial DNA (mtDNA) is maternally inherited without recombination. The mtDNA sequence is exactly the same in all children of the grandmother and all children of her daughters. In contrast, grandchildren inherit only approximately 25 % of the nuclear DNA of their grandmother. The mtDNA sequence of the maternal grandmother (*top left*) represented by a tan color is transmitted to her male and female children (*middle row*) and her daughter's male and female children (*bottom row* on *right*)

recombination events, remaining unchanged through generations, until a mutational event occurs. In this regard, mtDNA analysis can be important when only a distant maternal relative is available as a reference specimen.

For identity testing, only nucleotide polymorphisms in mtDNA are of practical utility, since no STR-like repetitive DNA is present. The mtDNA sequence obtained from a sample is compared to the first complete human mtDNA sequence generated by Anderson et al. [53], or its Revised Cambridge Reference Sequence [54]. Using standard nomenclature, only the differences between the aligned sequence and the reference sequence are noted by the position and base (e.g., 16311C), with insertions designated by a period after the preceding base and the number of bases inserted (e.g., 16192.2T), deletions designated by D or minus sign (e.g., 249–), and ambiguous bases coded using an N. Human mtDNA is densely coding, specifically coding for 37 genes, and is thus generally highly conserved. The sequence polymorphisms are concentrated in two hypervariable regions that are located in the noncoding control region [55]. The control region is a 1.2 kb segment, which includes a cloning site that Anderson et al. arbitrarily set as base pair 1. Hypervariable region I (HVI) spans positions 16,024–16,365 and hypervariable region II (HVII) spans positions 73–340 (Fig. 54.10). Homopolymorphic C-stretch regions around positions 16,189 of HVI and 310 of HVII may complicate sequencing. MtDNA does not provide definitive identification due to maternal kindred sharing the same sequence and its relatively low discriminatory power. Common haplotypes exist (e.g., the 263G, 315.1C haplotype occurs in 7 % of Caucasians), but most haplotypes are rare. Polymorphisms in the rest of the molecule exist, but are too infrequent to be practically interrogated by traditional sequencing [56].

In the late 1970s, Dr. Wesley Brown brought mtDNA analysis techniques to Dr. Allan Wilson's molecular evolution laboratory at UC Berkeley, which eventuated in the beginnings of forensic mtDNA testing through Drs. Mary-Claire King, Mark Stoneking, and Svante Pääbo. In 1984, Dr. King began to use mtDNA for the "disappeared" in Argentina, which allowed lost children to be reunited with their grandparents [57]. Dr. Peter Gill at the Forensic Science Service (now disbanded) working with Erika Hagelberg of Cambridge University in the UK took the lead in mtDNA casework in 1992, and at about the same time AFDIL in the USA began to identify skeletal remains from the Vietnam War using this method [58, 59].

In crime laboratories, mtDNA is most commonly used to analyze shed hairs from pubic combings or those found at scenes, because such hairs lack roots and the hair shaft contains little or no nDNA. On average, an individual loses 200 hairs per day, and thus it is not surprising that shed hairs constitute an important trace evidential specimen. MtDNA may also be used on fingernails and keratotic skin, which also lack nDNA. The first recorded mtDNA case was in the successfully prosecuted 1996 case, *Tennessee v Ware*, involving a single hair found in the throat of a victim [60].

Occasionally, more than one mtDNA sequence exists in the same organism or tissue, a condition termed heteroplasmy. Although heteroplasmy was well known in plants and nonhuman animals, it was first seen in human mtDNA by Dr. Peter Gill of the Forensic Science Service [61] and

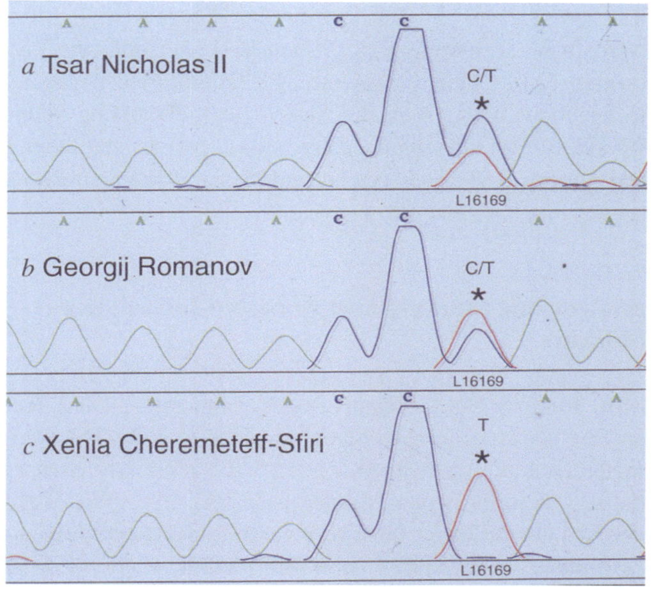

Figure 54.12 The first description of mtDNA heteroplasmy in humans was in the case of Czar Nicholas Romanov II, the last imperial Russian monarch. DNA sequence analysis shows that the czar (**a**) shares the heteroplasmy (C/T marked with an *asterisk*) at position 16,169 with his brother Georgij (**b**), but not with his distant relative Xenia Cheremeteff-Sfiri (**c**) (five generations removed) who has only the T nucleotide

then confirmed by one of the authors (VW) [62] during the identification of Czar Nicholas Romanov II (Fig. 54.12). Paternal leakage, recombination, and high mutation rates may contribute to heteroplasmy. The rate of mutations in noncoding mtDNA is 10–20 times greater than that in nuclear DNA, possibly due to the exposure of mtDNA to oxygen-free radicals or DNA polymerase with a higher error rate [63]. Thus single base differences between presumed maternal relatives must be viewed with caution. A low level of heteroplasmy may, in fact, be present in all individuals. To be detected using standard DNA sequencing, the level of heteroplasmy must be above approximately 30 % of the mtDNA sequence; otherwise, it is not distinguishable from background noise. Heteroplasmy is not uniform throughout the body and appears to be somewhat tissue specific. In addition, heteroplasmy may be rapidly lost (reversion to a homoplasmic state) in family lineages because of the bottleneck phenomenon that occurs during reproduction from a single egg. Heteroplasmy can complicate forensic analysis. For example, two hairs cannot be assumed to be from different individuals if they differ by a single nucleotide.

MtDNA testing is not performed by most forensic laboratories because the standard analytical method is DNA sequencing, which is expensive, labor-intensive, relatively slow, and, owing to how ubiquitous and prevalent the molecule is, may be susceptible to contamination. The exquisite sensitivity of the testing mandates special laboratory facilities and procedures. Also, interpretation is less straightforward than for routine STR results [64]. In 2006, the FBI created four regional state mtDNA laboratories (Arizona, Connecticut, Minnesota, and New Jersey), expanding forensic mtDNA sequencing capacity beyond private and federal laboratories. The number of laboratories performing mtDNA sequencing has since increased.

Phenotypic Markers and Ancestry-Informative Markers

Most forensic DNA systems involve noncoding DNA loci and are not associated with phenotypic traits [65]. The amelogenin marker is a major exception in that it directly assesses the sex of an individual. Some of the loci, like vWA of the von Willebrand locus, have very weak associations with disease states or other phenotypic information; of course older serologic testing was phenotype-based.

In some instances use of descriptive traits of an individual may be desirable, particularly if no eye-witnesses exist. Phenotypic markers have been and continue to be developed for use in forensic investigations. Markers have been established for eye color and weaker ones exist for hair and skin pigmentation [66, 67]. DNA Print Genomics (which ceased operations in 2009) had claimed their RETINOME system could predict eye color with 96 % accuracy. Generally, such tests are SNP assays for a set of informative but widely disparate loci. A genetic version of "driver's license" data would be useful for investigations, even if it were not to be used as probative evidence in court. A danger of misdirection from an incorrect prediction would have to be considered, since the accuracy is less than perfect [68].

Ancestry-informative markers are used to suggest a geo-ethnic origin [69, 70]. DNA Print Genomics "DNA Witness" appeared to have used them successfully in some investigations, but the technique was controversial [71]. Other groups, most notably the National Geographic Genographic Project [72], with various sets of markers and analyses, claim to be able to make statements of various proportions regarding ancestry background. Of course, admixture and modern travel greatly limit the value of such efforts. Some would derisively characterize these trials as genetic profiling [73].

Species Identification

Animal, plant, and microbial identification is sometimes important in a forensic investigation and can be accomplished using DNA analysis [23]. Typical forensic specimens include animal hair and fly larvae. Animals are generally examined by forensic scientists using the cytochrome b [74], 12S ribosomal RNA [75], or other mtDNA loci [76], and plants through their chloroplast DNA [77, 78]. This interrogated sequence is then entered into the online bioinformatics program BLAST (*B*asic *L*ocal *A*lignment *S*earch *T*ool), hosted by the US National Institutes of Health. The utility of a BLAST search is that today almost all DNA sequences produced by scientists are entered into the database (often required for journal publication) meaning virtually every species ever studied at the molecular level is represented. BLAST undertakes a query of the questioned sequence and in a few seconds produces a list of the most similar sequences in the database (often 100 % matches), complete with sequence alignment and appropriate references. For instance, a questioned hair may have a 100 % match to dozens or hundreds of dog sequences, followed by 99 % matches to more dog sequences, and will then begin to be interspersed with wolf sequences, coyote, etc. Except for extremely closely related, or highly exotic and rare species, BLAST queries typically result in an exact match, and the questioned speciation is identified. However, there is often a need for further strain (clade) or individualizing analysis. For instance, strain testing is used to trace marijuana plant sources [79]. Source attribution at the specific individual level is accomplished by DNA methodologies similar to human identity testing.

Tissue Identification

Occasionally, determination of the tissue origin of a specimen is required. Since the DNA from an individual is the same in all tissues, forensic scientists assay either messenger RNA (mRNA), as certain genes are expressed in some tissues and not others, or using immunoassays of the protein products [80, 81]. Commercial human gene expression microarrays have been used to determine tissue origin, but this is not a capability of crime laboratories.

Instruments and Technologies for DNA Typing

Since STRs replaced manual RFLP slab gel methods in the 1990s, capillary electrophoresis (CE) of amplified DNA, pioneered by Drs. John Butler and Bruce McCord, then at the FBI, has become the mainstay of forensic DNA laboratory operations around the world. CE instruments have replaced slab gel electrophoresis systems because of automation, faster run times, smaller sample volumes, and greater resolution. Typical casework calls for on-demand instrumentation that can handle relatively few specimens but with fast run times. High-throughput CE instruments are used as batch instruments for DNA data-banking operations. The ABI series of CE instruments (310, 3100, 3130 "Genetic Analyzers") from ABI are predominant and virtually exclusively used with the forensic community; the new ABI 3500 instrument is to supplant older models and features an ability to detect 6 dyes.

The forensic community is investigating other technologies for DNA analysis and NIJ has funded development [82]. Commercial "Rapid ID" DNA (rDNA) instruments (GE Healthcare Life Sciences [Pittsburgh, PA] and NetBio [Waltham, MD] ANDE; IntegenX [Pleasanton, CA] RapidHIT; and Lockheed Martin Corp [Bethseda, MA] and Zygem [Solana Beach, CA] RapiD; LGC [London, UK] RapiDNA) were introduced in 2012 to perform sample preparation, amplification, and electrophoresis to produce typing results within 2 h [83]. Their technology involves integrated microfluidic systems. Such systems are designed to be used at police booking stations to permit searches while persons of interest are in custody. These systems may also make crime-scene field-testing practical. Next-generation sequencers vary in their technologies, but also have microfluidics in common. They are designed for genomic/exomic applications for which they are incredibly rapid and relatively inexpensive for the amount of DNA sequenced. Analysis requires a specimen with a large quantity of DNA, relative to forensic evidentiary specimens, and is relatively expensive on a per run cost compared to current STR kits. However, if the next-generation sequencing assay is focused on targeted areas of interest, then less specimen DNA would be required and possibly multiple specimens could be processed in batch mode. In fact, the massively parallel sequence reads resulting from next-generation sequencing may be a benefit in analysis of degraded and low copy number DNA specimens.

Interpretation of Results

US crime laboratories will typically use the CODIS software ("popstats") to generate their statistics based on the FBI's allelic frequency data for Caucasian, African-American, and Hispanic racial groupings. STR systems are powerfully discriminating with an average random match probability of less than one in a trillion using the 13 core loci. "Discriminatory power" should not be confused with "accuracy" (e.g., ABO blood group typing is accurate but has low discriminatory power). The high discriminatory power of STRs is achieved because the statistic from each STR locus is multiplied together, the so-called "product rule" [84–88]. Current STR systems utilize genetically unlinked loci (STR loci are on different chromosomes, except CSF1PO and D5S818 which are sufficiently distant as to be genetically independent). Hardy-Weinberg disproportion, which may occur from population or racial grouping substructure (subgrouping), selection (non-random mating), inbreeding (mating within kindred), or linkage disequilibrium (from incomplete mixing of different ancestral populations), was cause for early court challenges to statistical interpretations of DNA results. Some of the early purported large deviations turned out to be an artifact of lower resolution RFLP tests where a single band was interpreted as a homozygote rather than two overlapping heterozygous bands [89, 90]. A National Research Council (NRC) report, NRC I [91], was issued in part to address these statistical concerns. The NRC I report itself proved controversial, which led to the NRC II report [92], that has, in fact, largely settled most statistical forensic identification issues.

In the USA, a Random Match Probability (RMP) is usually calculated as the chance of a random match in the population or racial grouping. Under conditions of Hardy-Weinberg proportions and linkage equilibria, the statistical calculation for the probability of an occurrence of a given genotype would be p^2 in the case of a homozygote or $2pq$ in the case of a heterozygote, where p is the frequency of observed occurrence for the p allele and q is the frequency of for the q allele. Instead, to account for population substructure, the NRC II recommended for calculation of homozygote frequencies from population allelic data: $p^2+p(1-p)\theta$, where θ is 0.01 for the US population as a whole and US racial groupings (empirically determined); but a more conservative value of 0.03 may be used in cases of smaller, isolated, and more inbred groups; and since heterozygote frequencies are overestimated in cases of disequilibria then $2pq$ can be used to calculate them (see Table 54.3 for an example RMP calculation).

In Europe, a Likelihood Ratio (LR) is usually used, wherein the hypothesis of the prosecution that the defendant is guilty and was the source of the DNA (assumed to be 100 % or 1) is divided by the hypothesis of the defense that the specimen is from someone else (some random individual) or p^2 or $2pq$ ($LR = 1/p^2$ or $1/2pq$) a result greater than one would support the prosecution and a result smaller than one would support the defense (see Table 54.3 for an example LR calculation).

MtDNA and Y-chromosome markers yield haplotype population frequency data that do not involve the product rule, and instead the frequency of the observed haplotype in a database is considered (the counting method). There has been some discussion as to whether these haplotype frequencies can be multiplied against each other as well as the STR statistic to achieve a summary discriminatory figure. Interpretation may be problematic when confronted with mixtures or from significant apparent imbalances or allelic drop-in and drop-out (Fig. 54.13) when testing highly degraded or trace DNA specimens.

Table 54.3 Example of random match probability and likelihood ratio calculations by ethnic group

D3S1358[a]										
allele	<12	**12**	**13**	**14**	**15**	**16**	**17**	**18**	**19**	>**19**
Caucasian	0.000	0.000	0.246	14.039	24.631	23.153	21.182	16.256	0.493	0.000
African American	0.476	0.238	1.190	12.143	29.048	30.714	20.000	5.476	0.476	0.238
Hispanic	0.000	0.000	0.239	7.895	42.584	26.555	12.679	8.373	1.435	0.239
D5S818[a]										
allele	**7**	**8**	**9**	**10**	**11**	**12**	**13**	**14**	**15**	>**15**
Caucasian	0.000	0.000	3.077	4.872	41.026	35.385	14.615	0.769	0.256	0.000
African American	0.278	5.000	1.389	6.389	26.111	35.556	24.444	0.556	0.000	0.278
Hispanic	6.158	0.246	5.419	6.650	42.118	29.064	9.606	0.493	0.246	0.000

***D3S1358* 13,16**	**RMP (2*pq*)**	**LR (1/2*pq*)**
Caucasian	0.000570	1754.39
African American	0.003655	273.60
Hispanic	0.000635	1574.80
***D5S818* 14**	**RMP ($p2+p(1-p)0.01$)**	**LR (1/2*pq*)**
Caucasian	0.009982	100.180
African American	0.010031	99.691
Hispanic	0.010024	99.761
Combined statistic	**RMP**	**LR**
Caucasian	5.68974×10^{-6}	1.75755×10^{5}
African American	3.66633×10^{-5}	2.72752×10^{4}
Hispanic	6.36524×10^{-6}	1.57103×10^{5}

[a]Observed allele distributions in % (converted to proper fraction for calculations)
From: Budowle B, Moretti TR, Baumstark AL, Defebaugh DA, Keys KM. Population Data on Thirteen CODIS Core Short Tandem Repeat Loci in African Americans, U.S. Caucasians, Hispanics, Bahamians, Jamaicans, and Trinidadians. J For Sci 1999;44(6):1277–1286

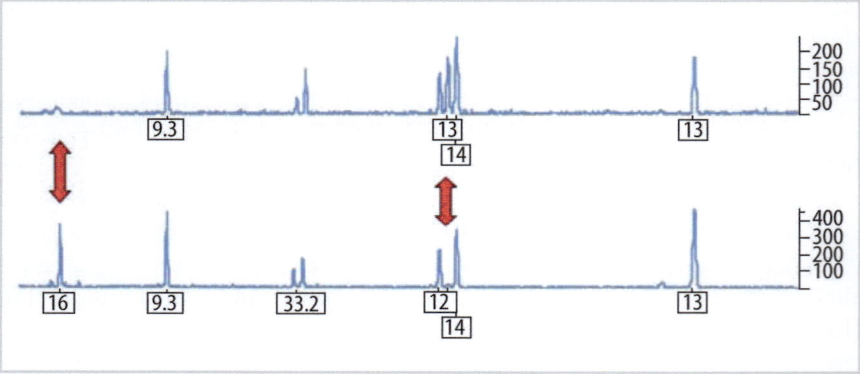

Figure 54.13 Allelic drop out from sample degradation or primer site polymorphism is one of the few interpretative pitfalls in the analysis of STRs. Allelic drop in can occur from contamination. This figure demonstrates a drop out of allele 16 and a drop in of allele 13 in the *upper* tracing compared to the *lower* tracing

Convicted Offender Databases

The DNA Identification Act of 1994 (US Public Law 103–322) authorized the creation of the FBI's National DNA Index System (NDIS). DNA profiles are uploaded using CODIS software, which may vary from state to state due to variations in state policy or statute [93]. Searches can be performed locally through a Local DNA Index System (LDIS) or State DNA Index System (SDIS), and across state lines through NDIS. Identifying information other than the DNA profile is not entered into the system. A match from an NDIS search results in the local crime laboratory of one state being put into contact with the local crime laboratory in another state to discuss case details. Uploading of DNA profiles triggers federal regulatory requirements on the use of the DNA specimens and profiles. The federal government has its own database for federal crimes as well. The number of profiles in the DNA databases has increased dramatically as state laws have expanded the convicted offender requirements from selected offenses to all felons, a broad array of misdemeanor crimes, and even arrestees. In 2012, the US Supreme Court, in *MD v King*, upheld the routine search of DNA databases when DNA samples are collected upon arrest [94]. Today, approximately ten million convicted offender profiles exist in the database. In recent years, "low stringency matches" have enabled searches for family members to assist investigations when no DNA profile of the perpetrator is in the database [95, 96].

Quality Assurance and Laboratory Issues

The FBI formed the Technical Working Group on DNA Analysis Methods (TWGDAM) to allow analysts from different laboratories to share information on the new DNA technology. The DNA Identification Act of 1994 gave the FBI regulatory oversight of DNA profiles entered into the national database [97]. The legislation called for a DNA Advisory Board (DAB) that produced recommended standards, based largely on guidelines of the TWGDAM, which were adopted with little change by the FBI director [98]. DAB requirements include minimal educational credits and experience of the testing personnel, proficiency testing twice a year per analyst, annual audits, and technical and administrative reviews of all tests. TWGDAM has since been renamed the Scientific Working Group on DNA Analysis Methods (SWGDAM) [99] and continues to recommend new standards to the FBI Director. The FBI conducts audits of laboratories to verify and enforce compliance with the standards, at least with respect to profiles that are generated and uploaded into NDIS.

The FBI/DAB standards require accreditation. The American Society of Crime Laboratory Directors/Laboratory Accreditation Board (ASCLD/LAB) and, more recently, the Forensic Quality Services (FQS) accredit laboratories. The accreditation requirements and audits are rigorous and are based on the International Organization for Standardization/International Electrotechnical Commission (ISO/IEC) Standard 17025. Standard reference materials from the National Institute of Standards and Technology (NIST) are available for autosomal STR analysis (SRM 2391b), Y-STRs (SRM 2395), mtDNA testing (SRM 2392), and DNA quantification (SRM 2372). Standards require annual comparisons with NIST-traceable standard materials [100]. In addition to these forensic science laboratory measures, judicial scrutiny provides further review of DNA findings in those cases that go to court.

Legal Issues

Shortly after forensic DNA tests were first introduced, defense attorneys attempted to directly attack this new scientific evidence. These early challenges are sometimes referred to as the "DNA wars" [101–104]. The first serious challenge to forensic DNA identity testing came in the 1989 case of *New York v Castro* [105] but legal admissibility of RFLP analysis was generally established in the 1991 case of *US v Yee* [106], and for PCR-based STR analysis in a series of cases in 2001 and again in 2005 [107–110]. Most prominent among the players were defense attorneys Peter Neufeld and Barry Scheck (subsequently part of the O.J. Simpson "dream team" and later founders of the Innocence Project), FBI lead scientist Dr. Bruce Budowle, and prosecutors Rockne Harmon and Woody Clark. The attacks were centered primarily on the issue of statistical interpretation. The early forensic DNA tests suffered from an inability to resolve discrete alleles. Moreover, the genetic independence of the loci was questioned based upon early Hardy–Weinberg disequilibrium calculations. Today, the "DNA wars" are largely over. The scientific basis of forensic DNA typing was never seriously questioned, but rather vitriolic challenges were launched at laboratory procedures and statistical interpretation. The admissibility of DNA evidence was not challenged in the 1995 O.J. Simpson trial despite the presence of a well-funded and experienced defense team; instead, the "weight" of the evidence was challenged, on the theory that police investigators had intentionally planted Mr. Simpson's blood. The most common challenges today are to sample collection, preservation of the evidence, chain of custody, documentation, and validation studies [111]. New genetic testing systems and technologies will undergo renewed judicial scrutiny and in particular, LCN DNA testing will generate anticipated challenges. While the challenges subside, the uses of DNA continue to grow. Police and prosecutors' office have created "cold case" units to try to close old cases with DNA evidence. Identification of the unidentified in medical examiner and coroner offices is also being pursued and is expected to close some old open cases as well. Indeed, the defense is now using forensic DNA identity tests after conviction to exonerate the previously convicted through the Innocence Project [112–114]. At the time of this writing there have been nearly 300 postconviction DNA exonerations.

References

1. Edwards HT, Gatsonis C, Berger MA, et al. Strengthening forensic science in the United States: a path forward. Washington, DC: National Academies Press; 2009.
2. Wilson DB, Weisburd D, McClure D. Use of DNA testing in police investigative work for increasing offender identification,

arrest, conviction, and case clearance. Published online at: http://ceps.anu.edu.au/events/criminal_investigations_workshop/papers/David%20Weisburd%20-%20Rethinking%20the%20Role%20of%20Detectives.pdf.
3. Weedn VW, Roby RK. Forensic DNA testing. Arch Pathol Lab Med. 1993;117:486–91.
4. Steadman GW. Survey of DNA Crime Laboratories, 1998. Bureau of Justice Statistics. NCJ 179104. February 2000:1–8.
5. Durose MR. Census of Publicly Funded Forensic Crime Laboratories, 2005. Bureau of Justice Statistics. NCJ 222181. July 29, 2008:1–12.
6. DNA Initiative: Advancing Criminal Justice Through DNA Technology website. http://www.dna.gov/. Accessed Mar 22, 2012.
7. Nelson M. Making Sense of DNA Backlogs, 2010 – Myths vs. Reality. National Institute of Justice. NCJ 232197. February 2011:1–20.
8. Gill P, Jeffreys AJ, Werrett DJ. Forensic application of DNA 'fingerprints'. Nature. 1985;318:577–9.
9. Kuperus WR, Hummel KH, Roney JM, et al. Crime scene links through DNA evidence: the practical experience from Saskatchewan casework. Can Soc For Sci J. 2003;36(1):19–28.
10. Parker B, Peterson J. Physical evidence utilization. In: Cohn SI, McMahon WB, editors. The administration of criminal justice, technology III. Chicago, IL: ITT Research Institute; 1970.
11. Foran DR, Gehring ME, Stallworth SE. The recovery and analysis of mitochondrial DNA from exploded pipe bombs. J For Sci. 2009;54:90–4.
12. Crime in the United States website, 2009 Summary. FBI. http://www2.fbi.gov/ucr/cius2009/about/crime_summary.html. Accessed Mar 22, 2012.
13. Crime in the United States website, 2007 Clearances. http://www2.fbi.gov/ucr/cius2007/offenses/clearances/index.html. Accessed Mar 22, 2012.
14. Kempf KL. Crime severity and criminal career progression. J Crim Law Criminol. 1988;79(2):524–40.
15. Zedlewski E, Murphy MB. DNA analysis for "minor" crimes: a major benefit for law enforcement. NIJ J. 2006;253:2–5.
16. Roman JK, Reid SE, Chalfin AJ, Knight CR. The DNA field experiment: a randomized trial of the cost-effectiveness of using DNA to solve property crimes. J Exp Criminol. 2009;5:345–69.
17. van Oorschot RAH, Jones MK. DNA fingerprints from fingerprints. Nature. 1997;387:767.
18. Gill P, Whitaker J, Flaxman C, Brown N, Buckleton J. An investigation of the rigor of interpretation rules for STRs derived from less than 100 pg of DNA. For Sci Int. 2000;112(1):17–40.
19. Caragine T, Mikulasovich R, Tamariz J. Validation of testing and interpretation protocols for low template DNA samples using AmpFlSTR Identifiler. Croat Med J. 2009;50:250–67.
20. Budowle B, Eisenberg AJ, van Daal A. Low copy number typing has yet to achieve "general acceptance". For Sci Int Genet. 2009;2(1):551–2. responses at For Sci Int Genet. 2011;5(1):3–11.
21. Castella V, Dimo-Simonin N, Brandt-Casadevall C, et al. Forensic identification of urine samples: a comparison between nuclear and mitochondrial DNA markers. Int J Legal Med. 2005;120(2):67–72.
22. Weedn VW, Baum H. DNA identification in mass fatality incidents. Am J For Med Pathol. 2011;32(4):393–7.
23. Sensabaugh G, Kaye DH. Non-human DNA evidence. Jurimetrics. 1998;39(1):1–16.
24. Budowle B, Schultze SE, Breeze RG, Keim PS, Morse SA, editors. Microbial forensics. 2nd ed. Burlington, MA: Academic; 2011.
25. Gast AP, Relman DA, et al. Review of the scientific approaches used during the FBI's investigation of the 2001 anthrax letters. Washington, DC: National Academies Press; 2001.
26. Tsongalis GJ, Wu AH, Silver H, Ricci A. Applications of forensic identity testing in the clinical laboratory. Am J Clin Pathol. 1999;112(1 Supp 1):S93–103.
27. Saks MJ, Koehler JJ. The coming paradigm shift in forensic identification science. Science. 2005;309(5736):892–5.
28. Southern EM. Detection of specific sequences among DNA fragments separated by gel electrophoresis. J Mol Biol. 1975;98(3):503–17.
29. Wyman AR, White R. A highly polymorphic locus in human DNA. Proc Natl Acad Sci U S A. 1980;77:6754–8.
30. Jeffreys AJ, Wilson V, Thein SL. Hypervariable "minisatellite" regions in human DNA. Nature. 1985;314:67–73.
31. Jeffreys AJ, Wilson V, Thein SL. Individual specific "fingerprints" of human DNA. Nature. 1985;316:76–9.
32. R. v. Pitchfork, EWCA Crim 963, Case No. 2008/04629/A1, 2009.
33. Wambaugh J. The blooding. New York, NY: Bantam Books; 1989.
34. Andrews v State, 533 So 841 (Fla Dist. Ct. App. 1988).
35. Commonwealth v Pestinikas, Ct of Common Pleas, Lackawanna Cnty, No. CR1019A-D/CR1020A-E, Dec. 2, 1988; 421 Pa Super. 371, 617 A2d 1339, 1343 (Pa Super. Ct. 1992).
36. Saiki RK, Gelfand DH, Stoffel S, et al. Primer-directed enzymatic amplification of DNA with a thermostable DNA polymerase. Science. 1988;239(4839):487–91.
37. Puers C, Hammond HA, Jin L, Caskey T, Schumm JW. Identification of repeat sequence heterogeneity at the polymorphic short tandem repeat locus HUMTHO1 [AATG]n and reassignment of alleles in population analysis by using a locus-specific ladder. Am J Hum Genet. 1993;53:953–8.
38. Lygo JE, Johnson PE, Holdaway DJ, et al. The validation of short tandem repeat (STR) loci for use in forensic casework. Int J Legal Med. 1994;107:77–89.
39. Clayton TM, Whitaker JP, Fisher DL, et al. Further validation of a quadruplex STR DNA typing system: a collaborative effort to identify victims of a mass disaster. For Sci Int. 1995;76(l):17–25.
40. Butler JM, Reeder DJ. Short Tandem Repeat DNA Internet DataBase website. http://www.cstl.nist.gov/strbase/
41. Butler JM. Genetics and genomics of core short tandem repeat Loci used in human identity testing. J For Sci. 2006;51(2):253–65.
42. Butler JM, Schoske R, Vallone PM, Redman JW, Kline MC. Allele frequencies for 15 autosomal STR loci on U.S. Caucasian, African American, and Hispanic populations. J For Sci. 2003;48(4):1–4.
43. Hares DR. Expanding the CODIS core loci in the United States. For Sci Int Genetics. 2012;6(1):e52–4.
44. Sullivan KM, Manucci A, Kimpton CP, Gill P. A rapid and quantitative DNA sex test: fluorescence-based PCR analysis of X-Y homologous gene amelogenin. Biotechniques. 1993;15:637–41.
45. Frances F, Portoles O, Gonzalez JI, et al. Amelogenin test: from forensics to biochemical genomics. Clin Chim Acta. 2007;386(1-2):53–6.
46. Foster EA, Jobling MA, Taylor PG, et al. Jefferson fathered slave's last child. Nature. 1998;396:27–8.
47. Butler JM, Reeder DJ. Short Tandem Repeat DNA Internet DataBase website, Y-Chromosome STRs. http://www.cstl.nist.gov/strbase/y_strs.htm
48. Syvanen A-C. Accessing genetic variation: genotyping single nuclear polymorphisms. Nat Rev Genet. 2001;2:930–42.
49. Sobrino B, Brion M, Carracedo A. SNPs in forensic genetics: a review on SNP typing methodologies. For Sci Int. 2005;154(2-3):181–94.
50. Kidd KK, Pakstis AJ, Speed WC, et al. Developing a SNP panel for forensic identification of individuals. For Sci Int. 2006;164(1):20–32.
51. Miller FJ, Rosenfeldt FL, Zhang C, et al. Precise determination of mitochondrial DNA copy number in human skeletal and cardiac

muscle by a PCR-based assay: lack of change of copy number with age. Nucleic Acids Res. 2003;31(11):e61.
52. Foran DR. 2006 The relative degradation of nuclear and mitochondrial DNA: an experimental approach. J For Sci. 2006;51:766–70.
53. Anderson S, Bankier AT, Barrell BG, et al. Sequence and organization of the human mitochondrial genome. Nature. 1981;290:457–65.
54. Andrews RM, Kubacka I, Chinnery PF, et al. Reanalysis and revision of the Cambridge reference sequence for human mitochondrial DNA. Nat Genet. 1999;23(2):147.
55. MITOMAP: A Human Mitochondrial Genome Database. http://www.mitomap.org, 2011.
56. Parsons TJ, Coble MD. Increasing the forensic discrimination of mitochondrial DNA testing through analysis of the entire mitochondrial DNA genome. Croat Med J. 2001;42(3):304–9.
57. Corach D, Sala A, Iannucci N, et al. Additional approaches to DNA typing of skeletal remains: the search for "missing" persons killed during the last dictatorship in Argentina. Electrophoresis. 1997;18:1608–12.
58. Holland MM, Fisher DL, Mitchell LG, et al. Mitochondrial DNA sequence analysis of human skeletal remains: identification of remains from the Vietnam War. J For Sci. 1993;38(3):542–53.
59. Holland MM, Parsons TJ. Mitochondrial DNA sequence analysis: validation and use for forensic casework. For Sci Rev. 1999;11:21–50.
60. State of Tenn. Hamilton Cnty No. 234768, E2008-02392-CCA-R3-PC, No. 03C01-9705-CR-00164, 1999 WL 233592 (Tenn Ct Crim App,1996).
61. Gill P, Ivanov PL, Kimpton C, et al. Identification of the remains of the Romanov family by DNA analysis. Nat Genet. 1994;6:130–5.
62. Ivanov PL, Wadhams MJ, Roby RK, Holland MM, Weedn VW, Parsons TJ. Mitochondrial DNA sequence heteroplasmy in the Grand Duke of Russia Georgij Romanov establishes the authenticity of Tsar Nicholas II. Nat Genet. 1996;12:417–20.
63. Parsons TJ, Muniec DS, Sullivan K. A high observed substitution rate in the human mitochondrial DNA control region. Nat Genet. 1997;15:363–8.
64. Budowle B, Allard MW, Wilson MR, Chakraborty R. Forensics and mitochondrial DNA: applications, debates, and foundations. Ann Rev Genom Hum Genet. 2003;4:119–41.
65. Pennisi E. Human genetic variation. Science. 2007;318:1842–3.
66. Walsh S, Liu F, Ballantyne KN, et al. IrisPlex:A sensitive DNA tool for accurate prediction of blue and brown eye colour in the absence of ancestry information. For Sci Int Genetics. 2011;5:170–80.
67. Walsh S, Lindenbergh A, Zuniga SB, et al. Developmental validation of the IrisPlex system: determination of blue and brown iris colour for forensic intelligence. For Sci Int Genetics. 2011;5:464–71.
68. Kayser M, Schneider PM. DNA-based prediction of human externally visible characteristics in forensics: motivations, scientific challenges, and ethical considerations. For Sci Int Genet. 2009;3:154–61.
69. Kosoy R, Nassir R, Tian C, et al. Ancestry informative marker sets for determining continental origin and admixture proportions in common populations in America. BMC Genet. 2009;10:39–52.
70. Phillips C, Salas A, Sanchez JJ, et al. Inferring ancestral origin using a single multiplex assay of ancestry-informative marker SNPs. For Sci Int Genetics. 2007;1:273–80.
71. Newsome M. The inconvenient science of racial DNA profiling. Wired. Oct 5, 2007. Available at: http://www.wired.com/science/discoveries/news/2007/10/dnaprint?currentPage=all
72. The Genographic Project website; https://genographic.nationalgeographic.com/genographic/index.html
73. Koops B-J, Schellekens M. Forensic DNA phenotyping: regulatory issues. Columbia Sci Technol Law Rev. 2008;9:158–202.
74. Jun J, Han SH, Jeong T-J, et al. Wildlife forensics using mitochondrial DNA sequences: species identification based on hairs collected in the field and confiscated tanned Felidae leathers. Gene Genom. 2011;33:721–6.
75. Melton T, Holland C. Routine forensic use of the mitochondrial 12S ribosomal RNA gene for species identification. J For Sci. 2007;52(6):1305–7.
76. Wells JD, Stevens JR. Application of DNA-based methods in forensic entomology. Annu Rev Entomol. 2008;53:103–20.
77. Nock CJ, Waters DLE, Edwards MA, et al. Chloroplast genome sequences from total DNA for plant identification. Plant Biotechnol J. 2011;9:328–33.
78. Hollingsworth PM, Graham SW, Little DP. Choosing and using a plant DNA barcode. PLoS One. 2011;6(5):e19254.
79. Coyle HM, Palmbach T, Juliano N, et al. An overview of methods for the identification and individualization of Marijuana. Croat Med J. 2003;44(3):315–21.
80. Lennard-Richard ML, Harper KA, Craig RL, et al. Evaluation of mRNA marker specificity for the identification of five human body fluids by capillary electrophoresis. For Sci Int Genetics. 2012;6(4):452–60.
81. Haas C, Muheim C, Kratzer A, et al. mRNA profiling for the identification of sperm and seminal plasma. For Sci Int Genet Suppl Ser. 2009;2:534–5.
82. NIJ Forensic DNA: Miniaturization and Automation website. http://www.nij.gov/topics/forensics/evidence/dna/research/miniaturization-automation.htm
83. Asplen C. Rapid DNA analysis is coming—rapidly. Forensic Mag. Dec 14, 2011. Available at: http://www.forensicmag.com/article/rapid-dna-analysis-coming-rapidly
84. Balding DJ. Weight-of-evidence for forensic DNA profiles. West Sussex, England: John Wiley & Sons; 2005.
85. Buckleton J, Triggs CM, Walsh SJ, editors. Forensic DNA evidence interpretation. Boca Raton, FL: CRC Press; 2005.
86. Evett IW, Weir BS. Interpreting DNA evidence: statistical genetics for forensic scientists. Sunderland, MA: Sinauer Associates; 1998.
87. Chakraborty R, Kidd KK. The utility of DNA typing in forensic casework. Science. 1991;254:1735–9.
88. Lander ES, Budowle B. DNA fingerprinting dispute laid to rest. Nature. 1994;371:735–8.
89. Devlin B, Risch N, Roeder K. No excess of homozygosity at DNA fingerprint loci. Science. 1990;249:1416–20.
90. Roeder K. DNA fingerprinting: a review of the controversy. Stat Sci. 1994;9(2):222–47.
91. McKusick VA, Lander ES, et al. DNA technology in forensic science (NRC I). Washington, DC: National Academy Press; 1992.
92. Crow JF, et al. The evaluation of forensic DNA evidence (NRC II). Washington, DC: National Academy Press; 1996.
93. Frequently Asked Questions (FAQs) on the CODIS Program and the National DNA Index System. FBI. http://www.fbi.gov/about-us/lab/codis/codis-and-ndis-fact-sheet
94. Maryland v King, 569 U.S. ___, 2013.
95. Bieber FR, Lazer D. Guilt by association. New Sci. 2004;184(2470):20.
96. Brown E. Study probes DNA search method that led to 'Grim Sleeper' suspect. Los Angeles Times, Aug 15, 2013, at: http://www.latimes.com/news/science/sciencenow/la-sci-sn-familial-dna-searches-california-20130814,0,5635600.story
97. Federal Legislation on Forensic DNA, NIJ website; http://www.dna.gov/statutes-caselaw/federal-legislation/
98. DNA Advisory Board Quality Assurance Standards for Forensic DNA Testing Laboratories, NIST website; http://www.cstl.nist.gov/strbase/dabqas.htm

99. Scientific Working Group on DNA Analysis Methods (SWGDAM) website; http://www.nfstc.org/pdi/Subject10/pdi_s10_m03_01_d.htm
100. Reeder DJ. Impact of DNA typing on standards and practice in the forensic community. Arch Pathol Lab Med. 1999;123:1063–5.
101. Coleman H, Swenson E. DNA in the courtroom: a trial watcher's guide. Seattle, WA: Genelex Press; 1994.
102. Aronson JD. Genetic witness: science, law, and controversy in the making of DNA profiling. New Brunswick, NJ: Rutgers Univ Press; 2007.
103. Lynch M, Cole SA, McNally R, Jordan K. Truth machine: the contentious history of DNA fingerprinting. Chicago, IL: The Univ of Chicago Press; 2008.
104. Calandro L, Reeder DJ, Cormier K. Evolution of DNA evidence for crime solving—a judicial and legislative history. Forensic Mag. January 6, 2005. Available at: http://www.forensicmag.com/article/evolution-dna-evidence-crime-solving-judicial-and-legislative-history?page=0,1
105. New York v Castro, 545 N.Y.S. 2d 985 (N.Y. Sup. Ct. 1989).
106. U.S. v Yee, 134 F.R.D. 161, 208 (N.D. Ohio 1991).
107. People v Hill, 107 Cal. Rptr. 2d 110, 89 Cal. App. 4th, 59-60 (Calif. 2001).
108. Lemour v State, 802 So. 2d 402 (Fla. Dist. Ct. App. 2001).
109. State v Butterfield, 27 P.3d 1133, 1144 (Utah 2001).
110. U.S. v Jenkins, 887 A.2d 1013, 1018 (D.C. 2005).
111. Kaye DH, Sensabaugh G. Reference guide on DNA identification evidence. Reference manual on scientific evidence. 3rd ed. Washington, DC: National Academies Press; 2011. p. 129–210.
112. Connors E, Lundregan T, Miller N, McEwen T. Convicted by juries, exonerated by science: case studies in the use of DNA evidence to establish innocence after trial. NCJ 161258. Washington, DC: National Institute of Justice; 1996.
113. Scheck B, Neufeld P, Dwyer J. Actual innocence: when justice goes wrong and how to make it right. New York, NY: Signet Books; 2001.
114. Innocence Project website (Benjamin Cardozo Law School); http://www.innocenceproject.org

Parentage and Relationship Testing

55

Robert W. Allen and Herbert F. Polesky*

Abstract

Parentage testing, also known as relatedness testing, is largely performed using polymerase chain reaction of short tandem repeats. The situations in which relatedness testing can be useful include parentage confirmation for legal cases, or for questions related to adoption, absent parents, or immigration. Sample collection methods depend on the purpose of the testing. Interpretation of the test results focus on exclusion or the likelihood of parentage when exclusion cannot be established, which requires use of standard probability calculations. Molecular testing of genetic systems can provide information to resolve questions of relatedness. Though these tests are powerful tools that can exclude almost all falsely accused parents, the tests alone do not prove absolutely that a relationship exists between two individuals.

Keywords

Identity testing • Parentage testing • Relatedness testing • Probability of parentage • Parentage index • Inclusion • Exclusion • Short tandem repeats

Historical Overview

Questions of parentage and other family relationships between individuals are not new. An early reference is found in the Bible (Kings 3:16–27), in which Solomon uses the threat of dividing the child to determine maternity. The application of scientific methods to this identification problem followed the discovery of the ABO blood group. Laws recognizing the possible exclusion of parentage by blood group testing were enacted by some states as early as 1935. Between 1940 and 1960, as additional blood group systems were defined and shown to follow Mendelian inheritance, more tests to exclude paternity were introduced. When appropriate reagents and methods were used, these red blood

***In Memoriam: Herb Polesky**

Herb Polesky authored this chapter in the first edition of this book and is coauthor of the chapter in this edition. Herb Polesky died in December 2011 while travelling with his wife Susan in Chile. Herb became active in the field of parentage testing early on and had the good fortune to contribute significantly to the field of Identity Testing as a whole, but especially to the application of DNA-based technology for questioned parentage. Work published by Herb and his collaborators early in the history of DNA testing is classic and moved DNA extraction methods into an era of development, culminating with the fast and efficient methods most laboratories use today. Herb also was instrumental in developing standards of practice, proficiency testing, and accreditation programs for both the American Association of Blood Banks and the College of American Pathologists. Finally, Herb was a teacher. He valued education and was always watchful for opportunities to weave the education process into an activity he was engaged in. While serving on the Histocompatibility and Identity Testing Committee of the College of American Pathologists, Herb endorsed and helped develop a Paper Challenge program which is still submitted to subscribing laboratories as part of their proficiency testing process. Challenges typically represent unusual cases that a laboratory may see occasionally and provide the pathologists and staff with a learning and teaching opportunity. Such is the legacy Herb Polesky leaves behind for the relationship testing field and those in it who knew and worked with him. He will be missed.

R.W. Allen, Ph.D. (✉)
School of Forensic Sciences, Center for Health Sciences, Oklahoma State University, 1111 West 17th St., Tulsa, OK 74107, USA
e-mail: Robert.w.allen@okstate.edu

D.G.B. Leonard (ed.), *Molecular Pathology in Clinical Practice*, DOI 10.1007/978-3-319-19674-9_55

cell (RBC) group marker systems were reliable; however, the relatively small number of marker alleles and their distribution in most populations limited the chance that a falsely accused man could be excluded. Subsequently, in the 1960s and 1970s, the discovery of polymorphic protein and red cell enzyme systems resulted in new markers that increased the power of the testing. The introduction of human leukocyte antigen (HLA)-A,B typing further expanded the possibility of excluding most falsely accused men [1].

Prior to the 1970s, the information from genetic marker testing was largely limited to providing evidence that a relationship did not exist. As more test systems were used, when testing failed to exclude, the probability of the alleged relationship between the tested individuals could be reliably calculated from the genetic information obtained. An amendment to the US Social Security Law (title IV D) in 1974 required that women requesting financial aid for dependent children identify the father. This change in the law increased the importance of providing estimates that tested individuals could be related in an alleged way.

Reports suggesting the use of DNA markers based on restriction fragment length polymorphisms (RFLP) for the determination of parentage first appeared in 1986 [2]. Over the next decade most laboratories performing relatedness testing applied DNA-based methods. The development of polymerase chain reaction (PCR) methods, that easily allowed testing of a minimal sample, led to a shift from testing by the classic marker systems (RBC antigens, HLA, etc.) to testing by only DNA marker systems [3]. The evolution of testing methods used by laboratories subscribing to the College of American Pathologists (CAP) parentage proficiency testing program between 1993 and 2003 is shown in Fig. 55.1. The doubling of the number of laboratories performing parentage testing over this time period correlated with a sharp increase in PCR testing and a decrease in all other testing methods. Today, virtually all parentage testing laboratories rely on PCR-based genetic testing methods. In the most recent report from the CAP, 91 laboratories subscribed to the parentage proficiency testing program.

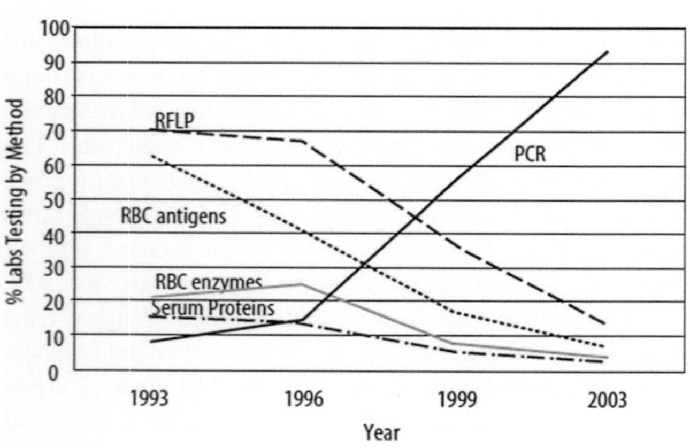

Figure 55.1 The evolution of testing methods offered by laboratories subscribing to the College of American Pathologists (CAP) parentage proficiency testing program between 1993 and 2003. There was a sharp increase in PCR testing with a concomitant drop in all other testing methods by 2003

Indications for Relatedness Testing

Parentage

Attempting to determine whether a man is or is not the biologic father of a child used to be the most frequent reason for performing relatedness testing. And although paternity testing may still represent the majority of tests performed, the expansion of testing into other biological relationships has occurred, largely due to the continued development of DNA markers with enhanced discriminatory power. As indicated above, child support programs are mandated to identify fathers of children born out of wedlock. In many situations the mother is unsure of who is the father. By establishing paternity, the mother is able to obtain financial support for the child from the father. Even when a child is born to a married couple, paternity is not a certainty. Family studies performed as part of medical trials have frequently reported that a small percentage of participants' children have extramarital genetic origins. Testing may be requested when a divorce is pending or when a father has doubts about his relationship to a child. Relatedness testing also is useful when it is suspected that babies have been mixed up in the nursery or to confirm the identity of a kidnapped child. Genetic marker tests can establish parentage of a child born to a surrogate mother or in some cases when assisted reproductive technologies, such as in vitro fertilization, are used.

Adoption and Absent Parents

A change in laws concerning availability of adoption records has increased requests for testing to identify biologic parents. Genetic evidence can confirm whether a relationship exists. Testing may be requested when individuals who were raised separately desire to establish whether they are siblings [4]. Similarly, testing may be useful to identify a person suspected of being an absent parent. In some cases, the establishment of parentage may be important with regard to resolution of inheritance claims. Proving membership in a Native American tribe is another reason for determining parentage.

Immigration

One rapidly expanding area for testing is in support of the immigration process in which claimed relationships to US residents must be proven genetically. The current US immigration quota system gives preference to relatives of US residents applying for immigrant status. Genetic testing evidence is considered in establishing the relationship between a US resident and a person desiring to immigrate to the USA. Often these cases involve putative children or parents with incomplete documentation of their relationship.

Forensic Parentage

The usual use of genetic testing in forensic cases is to compare DNA profile results generated from a reference sample from a suspect with the profile produced from a crime scene sample or a sample recovered from a victim. This testing generally involves determining whether the DNA profiles produced from the two samples match or not. In contrast, relatedness testing depends on the comparison of DNA profiles produced from samples from two or more individuals alleged to be related in some way and the goal of the testing is to assess whether or not alleles present in the tested individuals are identical by descent (i.e., inherited within a given family pedigree). Family relationship testing can be used to identify the perpetrator of a sexual assault resulting in conception, or for the identification of victims of naturally occurring or man-made disasters through establishing genetic relationships to surviving family members.

Sample Considerations

Samples

Relationship testing can be done using any sample from which DNA can be extracted and amplified. Most laboratories routinely use carefully collected buccal swabs. The advantages of buccal swabs include the ease of collection from infants, the ability to be collected by individuals with minimal training, and ease of sample shipping with a low risk for breakage or need of special shipping containers [3]. Additional sample types include whole blood, cord blood, tissue samples, and dried blood spotted on filter paper. Fetal DNA can be obtained from amniocytes, chorionic villus samples, and placental scrapings; however, it is important to rule out maternal contamination (see Chap. 57) when using these samples. The isolation of fetal cells from maternal peripheral blood samples also has been reported, but several laboratories using state-of-the-art single nucleotide polymorphism (SNP) testing platforms have reported successfully performing paternity testing with maternal blood during pregnancy, testing thousands of SNPs present in fetal DNA (inherited from the biological father and not present in the mother's DNA) [5].

Nuclear or mitochondrial DNA obtained from bones found at grave sites has been compared to samples from presumed relatives to identify individuals missing in action. Proof that the bones found in a mass grave site were those of Czar Nicholas II and his family was based on comparison with the mitochondrial DNA of living maternal relatives [6] (see Chap. 54).

Sample Collection

A testing facility must ensure that samples are identifiable and traceable from the time of collection through testing and reporting of results [7]. Samples need to be inspected and must meet acceptability criteria at all stages of testing. Collection of the samples must be done by individuals with no interest in the outcome of the testing, usually an employee or an agent of the laboratory; however, in some cases, submitted samples are collected "at home." Under these circumstances it is very important to have a second person witness and verify the collection procedure.

The American Association of Blood Banks (AABB) has developed very specific requirements for the information that must accompany samples used for parentage testing [8], including records of the name, alleged relationship, date of birth, and race or ethnic background of the individuals to be tested. Records must include information about the place, date, and person(s) collecting the sample. At the time of sample collection, the individual to be tested should be queried about a history of hematopoietic progenitor cell transplantation at any time in the past, as well as about transfusion in the past 3 months. If only DNA testing is to be done, it is unlikely that transfused donor DNA will be detected. In multiply transfused patients, DNA-based blood group testing is used to determine the blood group phenotype of the recipient when it is difficult to find compatible donor blood because of the presence of antibodies. For routine parentage testing, a photograph taken at the time of sample collection or a legible copy of a government photo ID, or both, should accompany the specimen.

Relationship Testing Methods

General Issues

RBC antigens, polymorphic red cell enzymes, serum proteins including Gm and Km, and serologic tests for HLA-A and HLA-B markers have been very useful systems for relatedness testing, although their use has all but disappeared in favor of DNA-based identity testing [9] (Fig. 55.1). The molecular methods used for testing parentage samples are identical to the methods for forensic testing described in Chap. 54; therefore, this discussion is limited to method-specific requirements and quality control issues, some of which are particular to parentage testing. As is true for all molecular tests, the reliability, reproducibility, and accuracy of the method should be evaluated prior to use. Any new method or system used by a testing facility should be validated in several ways beginning with learning most of what can be known about the system or assay through performing a literature review, by using the method in parallel with existing laboratory methods, by sample exchange with another laboratory, or by a combination of these approaches [8]. In addition, for amplification-based methods, inclusion of negative controls to monitor for sample contamination is important. Regardless of the method used, appropriate documentation of all sample handling and testing steps is critical for parentage testing as mandated by AABB standards.

RFLP Analysis

While the use of RFLP analysis demonstrated the possibilities associated with the use of DNA-based methods for parentage testing, this methodology is seldom, if ever, used in family relatedness testing currently. The RFLP methodology was powerful but suffered several limitations including sample requirements for the DNA used, the largely manual processing required, and the inability to precisely identify all of the sometimes hundreds of alleles associated with a particular marker. With the introduction of PCR amplification of DNA markers consisting of short tandem repeats (STRs) in the mid-1990s, many of the RFLP limitations disappeared, causing a natural progression of parentage testing laboratories to adopt PCR-STR technology over RFLP analysis.

Short Tandem Repeat Typing

PCR amplification of STR markers is the method most frequently used for relationship testing. Several commercial test kits are available for multiplex amplification of many STR markers. These kits usually include the 13 CODIS loci that form the foundation of felon databases that are routinely searched by forensic DNA laboratories hoping to link evidentiary DNA profiles to incarcerated or even arrested individuals who may have committed the specific crime or additional crimes [10]. For parentage testing, unlike for stain analysis used when comparing evidentiary stains to possible sources, there is no specific recommended panel of loci. Although the CODIS loci can be used, alternative or additional loci, or both, can be selected at the discretion of each laboratory as long as the final results achieve or exceed statistical significance (see section on "Reporting of Test Results," below) in almost all cases.

Typical STR typing results in a case of disputed paternity are shown in Fig. 55.2. Visible in the electropherogram are peaks of fluorescence corresponding to the collection of STR alleles for the different loci produced from genomic DNA extracted from each of the tested individuals (only those alleles amplified from STR loci with primers coupled to the green fluorescent dye JOE are shown for discussion purposes). Each allele in the profile is labeled with a numerical designation (seen as "al" with a number) that corresponds to the number of repeats of the 4 base pair (bp) repeated element. In the child's profile, those alleles inherited from the father whose identity is in question are indicated with an arrowhead and are identified through comparison of the profiles from mother (M) and child (C) (understanding that the mother's relationship with the child is unquestioned). The alleged father (AF#1) lacks the obligate alleles for the THO1 and D16S539 loci so is excluded, but AF#2 is included as evidenced by his sharing of at least one obligate allele with the child at each locus.

Identification of alleles for STR loci relies upon accurate size estimates (within 1 bp) of alleles amplified from a genomic DNA template by PCR. Primers that direct the amplification of STR alleles are coupled to one of three or four different fluorescent dyes so the amplified alleles can be detected by fluorescence. The color of the emission coupled with the size determination of the DNA fragment allows a computer to designate a tentative repeat size for each amplified product that is confirmed by comparing the amplicon in a sample to the collection of known allele repeat sizes for each STR locus (i.e., the allelic ladder) that is included with each electrophoretic run. Ultimately, the STR profile obtained from a sample may consist of up to 30 identified alleles (or more depending upon the STR kit used) obtained from 15 independent STR loci (or more) plus two fragments from the amelogenin locus that identify the sex of the sample donor (see Chap. 54 for explanation). Determination of correct allele sizes in STR amplifications is of critical importance. For this reason, a human control of known genotype is subjected to parallel testing with unknowns in each analysis to ensure the accuracy and reproducibility of the test system. Allele assignments can be made using computer software; however, verification of allele assignments should include the visual inspection of peaks by a knowledgeable individual. Regardless of the reading method, AABB standards as of this writing require that PCR results be interpreted twice, independently [6].

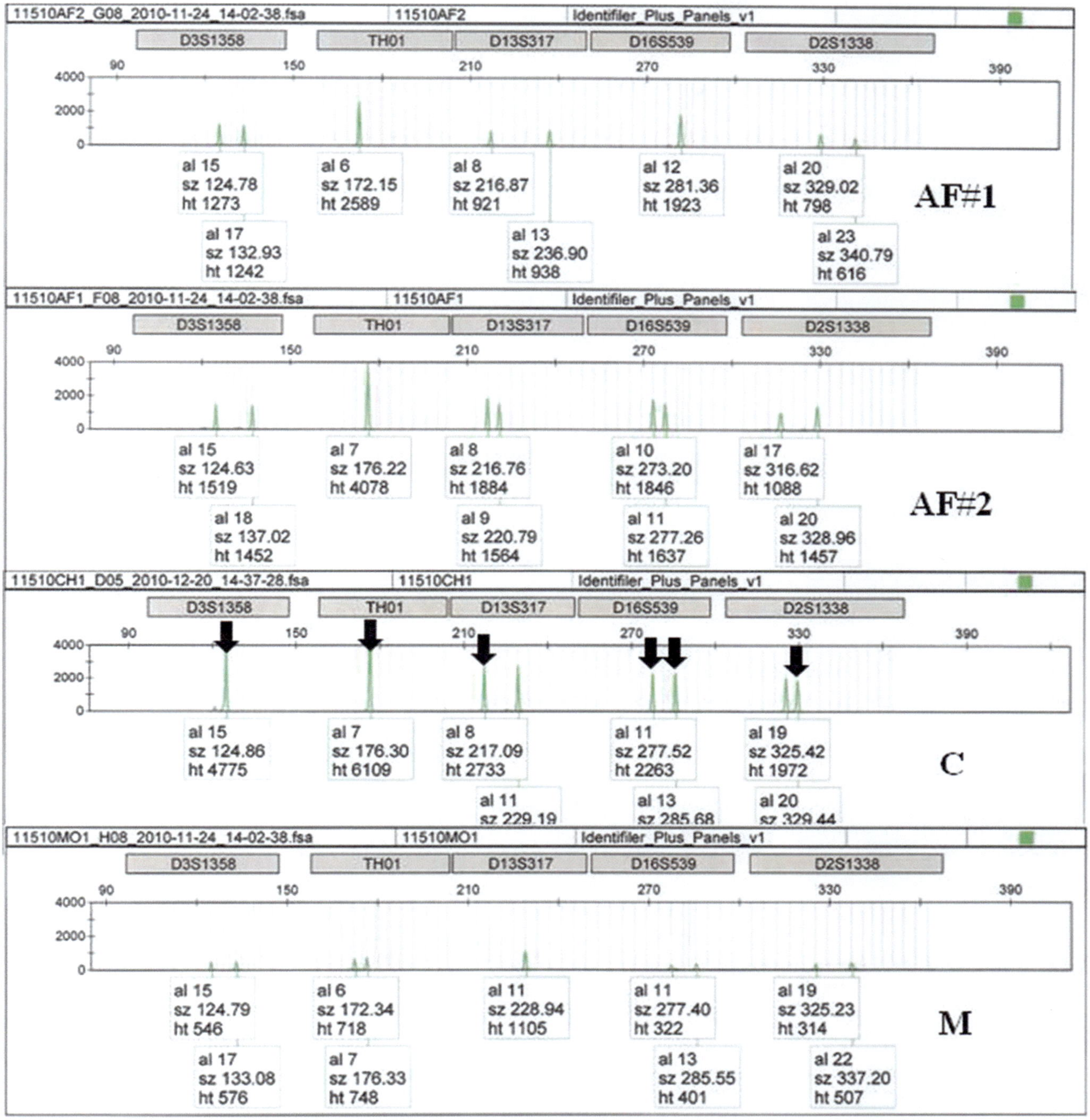

Figure 55.2 Typical STR typing results produced in a case of disputed parentage. DNA was extracted from a mother (M), a child (C), and two alleged fathers (AF#1 and AF#2) and amplified using the Identifiler® multiplex STR typing kit (Applied Biosystems, Inc., Foster City, CA). Amplified STR alleles were separated using capillary electrophoresis in an ABI 3130XL Genetic Analyzer and analyzed using GeneMapper software (Applied Biosystems). Only the results produced from the STR loci amplified from primers in the multiplex kit coupled to the green fluorescent dye JOE are shown in the figure and alleles are identified based upon the number of repeats in the tandem array. *Arrows* show the location of possible paternally inherited alleles in the child's sample. Alleged father 1 (AF#1) lacks obligate alleles for THO1 and D16S539 so is excluded, but alleged father #2 (AF#2) is included because he shares at least one obligate allele with the child at every locus shown

Nucleotide Sequence Determination

Nucleotide sequence determination can be used for relationship testing either by a traditional sequencing method or by a sequence-specific method, such as analysis of HLA alleles by sequence-specific oligonucleotide probes or sequence-specific primers [11, 12]. SNP analysis also can be applied using a variety of methods [13]. For all methods, inclusion of appropriate controls is important. Ideally, DNA sequencing should include analysis of both forward and reverse sequences. Comparison of results with a consensus sequence can be used for validation [8]. SSOP determination of HLA alleles should include a positive control probe that is complementary to a conserved sequence present in all alleles; likewise, the use of SSP requires that a positive internal amplification control of a nonpolymorphic sequence be included with each reaction. While SNP analysis can be highly automated, its use for relationship testing requires the analysis of a large number of loci to achieve statistical significance of the interpretation.

Next-generation DNA sequencing technology (NGS) has the potential to revolutionize the field of family relationship testing. Using NGS platforms, it is possible to determine the sequence of billions of nucleotides in a single sequencing run and, under the assumption that there is one SNP in every 1,000 bp of genomic DNA, there would be hundreds of thousands of SNPs in a single NGS test result. Among the SNPs detected, a significant proportion would differ between the mother and the child (i.e., those SNPs inherited from the father) and those remaining could be compared to an alleged father's reference sample to determine exclusion/inclusion in the case. The only question regarding the use of NGS technology is whether or not it can be priced competitively with classic STR testing performed by most laboratories.

Y Chromosomal and Mitochondrial DNA Markers

Polymorphisms residing on sex chromosomes are not routinely used for relatedness testing. However, the amelogenin locus is routinely amplified and is helpful to verify that male and female samples have not been switched. Mitochondrial DNA, which is maternally inherited, and Y chromosome markers (Y-STR) passed through the male lineage are useful for family and population reconstructions [14]. Sex-linked markers are especially useful when investigating questioned family relationships more distant than parent and child because of the conservation of haplotypes within the pedigree stemming from the lineage-specific inheritance pattern. For example, comparing the Y-chromosomal haplotypes of a male child and a male cousin of the untested alleged father who descended from a brother of the untested alleged father could establish with high certainty that the child whose paternity is in question does indeed belong to the male lineage within the pedigree. Autosomal STR markers would almost certainly fail to establish such a strong link. Sex-linked markers do have limitations, however. For example, in the scenario discussed above involving the Y-STR haplotypes, although the untested and deceased alleged father of the child could be the true father, his brother, or the cousin also possibly could be the father of the child. With sex-linked markers it is not possible to distinguish amongst all male or female members of the family. Some additional approach, such as those described below, must be taken with the sex-linked DNA results to make the distinction.

Interpretation of Parentage Results

Overview

Parentage testing seeks to determine whether a particular relationship exists between a set of individuals as evidenced by shared alleles inherited by the child from the parent (alleles designated as identical by descent). If the results of the testing provide sufficient evidence that the purported relationship does not exist, an exclusion is said to occur. When the results do not exclude a relationship, the situation is termed an inclusion, and a statistical analysis to calculate the probability or odds ratio that the relationship is true is performed using the test results. Several mathematical expressions are generally used to express the inclusionary results: paternity or parentage index (PI), combined paternity or parentage index (CPI), and the probability of paternity or parentage.

Exclusion

Test results from each of multiple independent systems are compared to establish whether the tested parties are related or unrelated. Table 55.1 shows examples of serological test results for several situations in which the test results indicate that a relationship does not exist. When an allele is found in a child that is not in the child's mother, it must have come from the biological father. Therefore, in a standard trio paternity case with a mother, father, and child, a direct exclusion for the system tested occurs when an alleged father does not have an allele that is found in the child but is not present in the child's mother (AF#1 in Fig. 55.2; Table 55.1). An indirect exclusion occurs when the exclusion is based on the observation that the child and the alleged father are homozygous for different alleles (Table 55.1). This type of exclusion is not conclusive, since it is possible that the child and alleged father actually share a null gene that is not detected.

Table 55.1 Examples of phenotypes that exclude parentage

Type of exclusion	Mother	Child	Tested man	Obligatory allele(s)
Direct	A	AB	C	b
	AB	AC	AD	c
Two-haplotype	A	A	BC	a
	AB	AB	CD	a or b
	AB	A	BC	a
	Unknown	AB	CD	a or b
Indirect[a]	A	A	B	a
	AB	B	A	b
	Unknown	B	A	b

The obligatory allele is based on the required paternal genetic contribution given the mother's and the child's phenotypes. If two alleles or two groups of linked markers are defined in one individual, but neither is present in the second tested person, the exclusion is defined as a "two-haplotype" exclusion

[a]Mutation must be considered if indirect exclusion is in a single system

Therefore, before an opinion of nonpaternity is rendered based on an indirect exclusion, a search is made for additional direct or indirect exclusions. Exclusions in two independent tests are sufficient to exclude an individual as the biological father of a child, as long as the chance of mutation has been considered.

Since mutations can occur, albeit rarely, in many of the DNA test systems, a single inconsistency in expected inheritance is also not adequate to reach a conclusion of nonparentage, particularly if the inconsistency is only one tandem repeat size different from the important allele in the alleged parent or child [7]. Mutation rates of commonly used loci are available, as well as statistical methods for incorporating the inconsistency into the final reported calculation [8]. To avoid misinterpretation, results should be reported as phenotype rather than as assumed genotype when a test indicates a single marker at a locus. In the parentage testing field, the term "phenotype" is used to represent the measurable genetic markers in a given individual at a specific locus. Although confusing to those more familiar with the term "genotype" in this setting, the terminology for parentage testing has its origins in RBC typing in which a person with type A blood is said to have the A phenotype but could have the AA or AO genotype. Therefore, to avoid the assumption of homozygosity, test results are reported as phenotypes, which may or may not reflect the genotype. While it is less common for a DNA-based genetic test result not to match the actual genotype, null alleles and primer-site polymorphisms have been reported. In addition to mutation, technical errors, sample mix ups, and reagent problems such as primer-binding site differences can lead to false exclusions. When an individual is excluded, his or her phenotype must be confirmed by repeating the test with an independent isolation of the DNA from the alleged parent and possibly also the child [7].

Maternity is presumed when samples are submitted for testing. However, occasionally a different child is substituted for the biologic child. When test results are completed on a trio (mother, child, and alleged father), the results on the mother and child should first be evaluated to determine that at each locus there is one common allele. This comparison is one of the ways that the laboratory can validate that the correct samples were tested. On rare occasions, inconsistencies between a mother and a child are observed. This finding can be due to a mutation and is not a maternal exclusion.

Inclusion

The most frequent use of relationship testing is to determine paternity. Each genetic system used in relationship testing should be well documented in the literature and must have been shown to follow Mendelian inheritance. Ideal genetic systems for relationship testing have multiple alleles, a low rate of mutation, and fairly uniform frequency distribution of alleles in the population [9]. The power of exclusion, which can be calculated for each locus based on the number of alleles in the population and their frequencies, represents the chance that an unrelated individual can be excluded by the locus. If a system has a few alleles that are common to most individuals, the chance that two unrelated individuals will share one or more alleles is high. If the system has multiple alleles, none of which occurs with a high frequency, then the power of exclusion is larger.

Based on Mendelian genetics, if a child has an allele that was not inherited from the mother, then it must have come from the biologic father. If the alleged father has that allele, then he is included among the group of men who could be the child's father (AF#2 in Fig. 55.2). The examination of alleles at multiple genetic loci is used to statistically reduce the number of men who could be the biologic father. AABB standards provide guidelines for the statistical significance that must be achieved to report the results, as described below.

Parentage Index

The PI expresses in mathematical terms how many times more likely it is that the tested individual is the biologic father of the child than a randomly selected man. Thus, the PI is an odds ratio comparing the probability that the child is the product of the mother and the alleged father vs the probability that the child is the product of the mother and a random man of the same racial background. At each of the multiple loci tested, the chance that the tested individual passed the obligatory allele is compared to the chance that the allele could have been contributed by a random individual [15]. A formula to calculate the PI can be derived using the laws of probability for each potential combination of alleles for a mother, child, and alleged-father trio at each locus, based on allele frequencies (Table 55.2). A PI must be calculated separately for each locus tested.

Since the PI calculations require allele frequencies by racial group, for each locus the frequency of all the possible alleles must be determined from the phenotypes of at least 100 unrelated individuals from the same racial group. The larger the available database, the smaller the error of the estimate. The ideal population frequency is one calculated from testing done by the specific laboratory. These data should be evaluated by comparison with published frequencies. When a laboratory has accumulated additional test data or introduces a new method, new values should be calculated and compared with existing frequencies. This is helpful in monitoring changes in the laboratory. For STR systems with discrete alleles, it is fairly easy to establish frequency tables that can be validated and compared with those of other facilities. RFLP markers occur over a continuum and are influenced by measurement variables. Thus, determining the frequency of each band requires the use of the delta value for the test system [9]. Computer programs and manual calculations must be periodically reviewed and validated. Cases may involve individuals from racial or ethnic groups for which there is only a limited sample from the testing laboratory. In these cases, published tables may be used [16]. Table 55.3 shows the variation in PI values by racial group for several STR markers using published allele frequencies.

Table 55.2 Phenotype results and formulas used to calculate the parentage index by allele combination

Mother	Child	Tested man	PI
A or AB	A	A	1/a
A or AB	A	AB or AC	0.5/a
B	AB	A	1/a
B	AB	AC or AB	0.5/a
AB	AB	AB or A	1/(a+b)
AB	AB	AC	0.5/(a+b)
BC	AB	AB or AD or AC	0.5/a
BC	AB	A	1/a

A, B, C, and D represent different alleles. A is always used to represent an obligatory paternal allele; *a* and *b* are frequencies of alleles A and B, respectively, in the same racial group as the tested man (alleged father)

Combined Parentage Index

Assuming each locus tested is inherited independently, a CPI is calculated by multiplying the PI values of all the individual loci to obtain a combined odds ratio, as specified by the third law of probability for completely independent events. AABB standards require that multiple independent genetic systems be tested that will provide a CPI of at least 100, which indicates that it is 100 times more likely that "this man," rather than "some random man," is the father of this child [7]. Table 55.4 is an example of a case meeting this requirement for the three ethnic groups shown.

Residual Paternity Index

The residual paternity index is a calculation that is useful when there are inconsistencies in inheritance for some systems. This index is calculated by multiplying the PI for all systems that fail to exclude. A high residual PI suggests that the true parent could be a relative of the tested individual. Since a father and son share at least one marker at each locus, and brothers have more markers in common with each other than either would with a random man, if the true father is related to the tested individual, the alleged father is less likely to be excluded in most systems. An avuncular index is used to calculate whether there is biological relationship between the alleged father's child and aunts or uncles of the alleged father [17]. A high residual PI also may occur if the single inconsistency is due to a mutation or if there has been a laboratory error in testing or recording results of a single system. If the inconsistency is considered to be a mutation, the PI for the system can be calculated using a value for the mutation frequency, if known [18]. In these cases the CPI often exceeds 100 even though the PI for the system with the mutation is very small.

Probability of Parentage

If the individual in question is included as the parent by the genetic testing, this information is combined with the nongenetic evidence to calculate the probability of parentage (*W*, expressed as a percentage) using Bayes' theorem:

$$W = \frac{(p)(\text{CPI})}{(p)(\text{CPI})+(1-p)} \times 100$$

Table 55.3 Calculation of the percentage index (PI) using allele frequencies for different racial groups

					paternity indices (by ethnic background)		
	M	Child	Man	X/Y	Caucasian	African American	Native American
CSF1PO	9, 11	9, 11	11	1/(a+b)	2.98	4.10	3.29
D5S818	10	10, 13	13	1/a	6.46	4.64	10.62
TH01	7, 8	8	8, 9	0.5/a	4.36	2.41	9.23
TPOX	8	8	8	1/a	1.86	2.77	2.63
Combined parentage index					156	127	848
Probability of paternity (%)					99.36	99.22	99.88

a, frequency for the obligatory paternal allele(s) in each population; *b*, frequency of the child's maternal allele when the mother and child are heterozygous for the same two alleles; M, mother; X/Y, odds ratio of tested man vs a random man being the father of this child (see Table 55.2)

Table 55.4 Detailed STR parentage test results for a Caucasian trio

	STR test results			Frequency of OG(s)	Calculations	
Locus	Mother	Child	Tested man		Formula X/Y	Locus PI
CSF1PO	10, 11	10, 12	10, 12	12=0.33	0.5/0.33	1.52
D3S1358	15	15	15	15=0.26	1/0.26	3.85
D5S818	10, 11	10, 12	11, 12	12=0.35	0.5/0.35	1.43
D7S820	8, 11	8, 11	8, 11	8=0.16 11=0.18	1/(0.16+0.18)	2.94
D8S1179	12, 13	13, 14	14	14=0.21	1/0.21	4.76
D21S11	28	28, 30	29, 30	30=0.25	0.5/0.25	2
FGA	22, 24	22, 23	23	23=0.15	1/0.15	6.67
TH01	9	7, 9	7	7=0.22	1/0.22	4.55
vwa31/A	18, 19	18, 19	17, 19	18=0.23 19=0.08	0.5/(0.23+0.08)	1.61
Combined parentage index						11,444
Probability of paternity						99.99 %

OG(s), obligatory paternal allele(s). Frequency of OG(s) refers to the allele frequency of the given OG allele in the Caucasian population. *X/Y*, odds ratio of tested man vs a random man being the father of this child. Formula *X/Y* can be found in Table 55.2. Locus PI is calculated for each locus, and then the individual locus PIs are multiplied together to obtain the combined Parentage Index (PI). The probability of paternity is calculated using Bayes' theorem and a neutral prior probability of 0.5

where p is the prior probability of nongenetic events and CPI is the combined parentage index [19]. The nongenetic information is referred to as the prior probability and includes information about access at the appropriate time, fertility, and so on. Since the nongenetic information is unknown to the testing facility, it is general practice to assign a neutral value of 0.5 (50 %) to perform this calculation. Alternatively, the probability of parentage can be calculated with prior probabilities of 0.1, 0.5, and 0.9 to give a range of probabilities. The number calculated, referred to as the posterior probability, is expressed as a percentage. If the CPI is 100, then the probability of parentage is 99 % when using a 50 % prior. The higher the value of the CPI, the closer the probability of parentage is to 100 %; however, 100 % can never be reached. If the genetic evidence indicates that no relationship exists (multiple exclusions), then the probability of parentage is reported as zero.

Random Man Not Excluded

Random man not excluded (RMNE) is a calculation that estimates the fraction of the population that would not be excluded by a test system based on the phenotypes of the mother and child [20]. The results of the tested man are not considered in determining this value. The RMNE value for several systems used as a battery of tests gives a power of exclusion for a random man that is compared to the mother–child pair. RMNE adds little or no additional information to the PI and is not routinely reported by most testing facilities.

Reconstruction Cases

In many circumstances it is possible to estimate the likelihood of a relationship when only some of the persons in the family are available for testing.

Motherless Cases

If only the man and child are tested, a PI can be calculated using formulas that compare the chance that the tested man will transmit the shared allele(s) to the child through a mating with a "random mother" with the chance that the allele(s) are from two unknown and random parents [21] (Table 55.5).

Fatherless Cases

Formulas are available to calculate the possibility of parentage when the mother, child in question, and unquestioned relatives of the unavailable father are tested [22]. A common situation, shown in Fig. 55.3, is to test one or both parents of a deceased man (i.e., the presumed grandparents). If the

Table 55.5 Phenotype results and formulas used to calculate the PI by allele combination in motherless cases

Child	Tested man	PI
A	A	1/a
A	AB	0.5/a
AB	A	0.5/a
AB	AB	(a+b)/4ab
AB	AC	0.25/a

A, B, and C represent different alleles; a and b are frequencies of alleles A and B, respectively

Figure 55.3 Reconstruction of a family with a deceased alleged father (?AF). (**a**) Phenotype results from two RFLP systems and three STR systems on members of the family shown in (**b**). (**b**) Pedigree of family relationships. The alleged father (?AF) is deceased. His presumed parents (?GF and ?GM) were tested, and the results are given in (**a**). Shown in *bold* are the obligatory paternal allele(s) (OG) that could be found in the alleged father if ?GF and ?GM are his parents. These results show that Child 1 (Ch 1) could be the product of a mating between the mother and the deceased man (?AF). Child 2 (Ch2) is excluded as being the child of ?AF and the mother in several systems (*shaded boxes*), since the OGs are not in the presumed parents of ?AF

a

System	Mother	Child 1	OG	Child 2	OG	?GF	?GM	Possible phenotype of ?AF
D2S44 *Hae* III	1.79, 2.09	1.59, 2.09	**1.59**	2.09, 2.56	2.56	1.59, 1.79	1.82	**1.59,1.82** 1.79,1.82
D10S28 *Hae* III	1.46, 4.08	4.08	**4.08**	1.46, 2.05	**2.05**	2.05, 3.44	1.71, 4.08	**1.71,2.05** 1.71,3.44 **2.05,4.08** **3.44,4.08**
D3S1358	15, 17	16, 17	**16**	15, 17	15, 17	16, 18	18	**16, 18** 18
D21S11	28, 29	28, 29	**28, 29**	28, 30	30	28	27, 29	**27, 28** **28, 29**
FGA	22	21, 22	**21**	20, 22	**20**	21, 22	20, 21	**20,21** **20,22** **21**

b

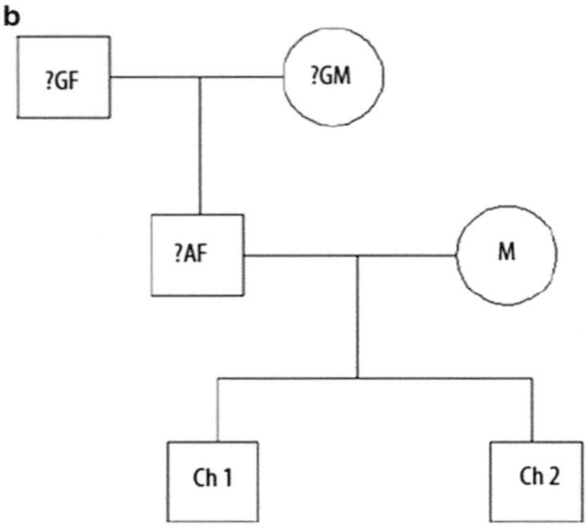

obligatory paternal allele in the child is not present in either of the child's presumed grandparents, the man is excluded. If it is present, then the PI can be determined. It is also possible to use tests of other children of the deceased man with or without testing their mother(s), his siblings, or other related individuals. In doing these reconstructions, one assumes that the surrogate individuals are biologically related to the father.

Kinship Analysis

Estimation of whether two tested individuals are full siblings, are half-siblings, or have some other relationship is possible using appropriate kinship coefficients [4, 23]. Although full siblings will share one or both alleles by descent in most systems, 25 % of the time they will not share a common allele. Molecular genetic markers also are very useful in determination of the zygosity of twins. Table 55.6 shows the testing results for a mother and three children. From this data it is possible to determine whether the children have the same or different fathers and thus are full or half siblings. For the case shown in Table 55.6, the data indicate the existence of multiple fathers.

Table 55.6 Relationship testing to determine sibship

Sample/ system	Mother	Child 1	Child 2	Child 3	Inferred paternal alleles
D3S1358	16	16	16	16	16
D5S818	11, 12	10, 11	12, 13	11	**10, 11, 13**
D7S820	12	11, 12	8, 12	9, 12	**8, 9, 11**
D8S1179	13, 15	13, 14	14, 15	10, 13	10, 14

The paternal alleles can be inferred from each child. The existence of more than two obligatory paternal alleles in loci D5S818 and D7S820 indicates the existence of multiple fathers of these children

Reporting of Test Results

Many of the reports of relatedness testing may become part of legal proceedings. In some cases, one of the tested parties may challenge the results, and thus it is very important to have careful documentation of all steps from sample collection to reporting of results. AABB standards define the required information for a report of parentage testing [7, 8]. The date of collection of each sample, the name of each person tested, and his or her relationship to the child should be stated in the report. The phenotype observed for each individual using standard nomenclature and the PI for each genetic system tested must be included. The report must explain whether a relationship can or cannot be excluded. The racial or ethnic background used for calculations, the combined parentage index, and the probability of parentage as a percentage must be stated. Any unusual findings such as mutations must be explained.

Conclusion

Testing of multiple genetic systems by validated molecular methods can provide information to resolve questions of relatedness. Though these tests are powerful tools that can exclude almost all falsely accused parents, they alone do not prove absolutely that a relationship exists between two individuals.

References

1. Miale JB, Jennings ER, Rettberg WAH, et al. Joint AMA-ABA guidelines: present status of serologic testing in problems of disputed parentage. Fam Law Q. 1976;10:247–85.
2. Baird M, Blazas I, Guisti A, et al. Allele frequency distribution of two highly polymorphic DNA sequences in three ethnic groups and its application to the determination of paternity. Am J Hum Genet. 1986;39:489–501.
3. Polesky HF. Impact of molecular (DNA) testing on determination of parentage. Arch Pathol Lab Med. 1999;123:1060–2.
4. Wenk RE, Traver M, Chiafari FA. Determination of sibship in any two persons. Transfusion. 1986;36:259–62.
5. Gary JW, LiaoAnn M, GronowskiZhen Z. Non-invasive prenatal testing using cell-free fetal DNA in maternal circulation. Clin Chim Acta. 2014;428:44–5023.
6. Ivanov PL, Gill P, Sullivan KM, et al. DNA-based identification of the last Russia's royal family. In: Proceedings from Fourth International Symposium on Human Identification. Madison, WI: Promega Corporation; 1993. p. 37–47.
7. AABB. Standards for relationship testing laboratories. 7th ed. Bethesda, MD: AABB; 2005.
8. American Association of Blood Banks. Guidance for standards for parentage testing laboratories. 5th ed. Bethesda, MD: American Association of Blood Banks; 2002.
9. Polesky HF. Parentage testing: use of DNA polymorphism and other genetic markers. In: Henry JB, editor. Clinical diagnosis and management by laboratory methods. Philadelphia, PA: WB Sanders; 2001. p. 1390–401.
10. Budowle B, Moretti TR, Niezgoda SJ, et al. CODIS and PCR based short tandem repeat loci: law enforcement tools. In: Second European Symposium on Human Identification, 1998. Madison, WI: Promega Corporation; 1998. p. 73–88.
11. Allen M, Lui L, Gyllensten U. A comprehensive polymerase chain reaction oligonucleotide typing system for the HLA class I A locus. Hum Immunol. 1994;40:25–32.
12. Bunce M, Fanning GC, Welsh KI. Comprehensive, serologically equivalent DNA typing for HLA-B by PCR using sequence-specific primers (PCAR-SSP). Tissue Antigens. 1995;45:81–90.
13. Nikiforov TT, Rendle RB, Goelet P, et al. Genetic bit analysis: a solid phase method for typing single nucleotide polymorphisms. Nucleic Acids Res. 1994;22:4167–75.
14. Roewer L. The use of the Y chromosome in forensic genetics—current practices and perspectives. In: Brinkmann B, Carracedo A, editors. Progress in forensic genetics, vol. 9. Amsterdam: Elsevier Science; 2001. p. 279–80.
15. Walker RH. Probability in the analysis of paternity test results. In: Silver H, editor. Paternity testing. Washington, DC: American Association of Blood Banks; 1978. p. 69–135.
16. Budowle B, Shea B, Niezgoda S, et al. CODIS STR loci data from 41 sample populations. J Forensic Sci. 2001;46:453–89.
17. Morris JW, Garber RA, d'Autremont J, et al. The avuncular index and the incest index. In: Mayr WR, editor. Advances in forensic haemogenetics, vol. 2. Berlin: Springer; 1988. p. 607–11.
18. Gjertson DW. The effect of an isolated single-locus inconsistency in the statistical evaluation of paternity. In: American Association of Blood Banks: guidance for standards for parentage testing laboratories. 5th ed. Bethesda, MD: American Association of Blood Banks; 2002. p. 143–4.
19. Essen-Moller E. The conclusive force of similarity in paternity proof: theoretical basis. Mitt Anthrop Ges (Wien). 1938;68:9–53.
20. Salmon D. The random man not excluded expression in paternity testing. In: Walker RH, editor. Inclusion probabilities in parentage testing. Arlington, VA: American Association of Blood Banks; 1983. p. 281–92.
21. Brenner CH. A note on paternity computation in cases lacking a mother. Transfusion. 1993;33:51–4.
22. Traver M. Numeric statements of the strength of the genetic evidence. In: American Association of Blood Banks: guidance for standards for parentage testing laboratories. 5th ed. Bethesda, MD: American Association of Blood Banks; 2002. p. 124–9.
23. Brenner CH. Symbolic kinship program. Genetics. 1997;145: 535–42.

Chimerism Testing in Allogeneic Hematopoietic Stem Cell Transplantation

56

Vivianna M. Van Deerlin and Ran Reshef

Abstract

Allogeneic hematopoietic stem cell transplantation (HSCT) is a well-established treatment option for a variety of malignant and nonmalignant diseases. Each year, more than 28,000 patients undergo allogeneic HSCT worldwide. Molecular analysis of chimerism levels is used to monitor the proportions of donor and recipient hematopoietic cells in patients after HSCT. Chimerism studies can help identify the source of hematopoiesis after engraftment, identify graft rejection in patients with poor hematologic recovery, and assist in the diagnosis and prediction of relapse and clinical graft-vs-host disease (GVHD). The most commonly applied method is PCR amplification of short tandem repeats (STR), a type of genetic polymorphism. The interpretation of chimerism results depends on the context in which the testing was done, i.e., the type of transplant, conditioning intensity, timing of testing post-transplant and results of concurrent blood counts and bone marrow morphology. While the methodology is technically straightforward, the implementation, analysis, and interpretation of results can be complicated. The clinical importance of chimerism results warrants the effort required by the laboratory for validation and performance of the test. In this chapter we review the clinical utility of chimerism analysis and laboratory aspects of testing, including methods, reagents, approaches to pre- and post-transplant testing, analysis and interpretation, pitfalls and limitations, reporting, and data management.

Keywords

Chimerism • Mixed chimerism • Engraftment • Donor • Recipient • Graft-vs-host disease • Bone marrow transplant • Reduced-intensity transplant • Stem cell transplant • Short tandem repeats • STR locus • Identity testing

V.M. Van Deerlin, M.D., Ph.D. (✉)
Pathology and Laboratory Medicine, Molecular Pathology Laboratory, Perelman School of Medicine at the University of Pennsylvania, 3400 Spruce St., 7.103 Founders Pavilion, Philadelphia, PA, 19104, USA
e-mail: vivianna@upenn.edu

R. Reshef, M.D.
Department of Medicine, Hematology & Oncology Division, Perelman School of Medicine at the University of Pennsylvania, Philadelphia, PA, USA

Introduction

Allogeneic hematopoietic stem cell transplantation (HSCT) is a well-established treatment option for a variety of malignant and nonmalignant diseases. Molecular analysis of chimerism levels is used to monitor the proportions of donor and recipient hematopoietic cells in patients after HSCT. Chimerism studies can identify the source of hematopoiesis after engraftment, identify graft rejection in patients with poor hematologic recovery, and assist in the diagnosis and prediction of relapse and graft-vs-host disease (GVHD). The most commonly applied method is PCR amplification of

D.G.B. Leonard (ed.), *Molecular Pathology in Clinical Practice*, DOI 10.1007/978-3-319-19674-9_56

Table 56.1 Terminology of post-transplant chimerism analysis

Term	Definition	Significance
Complete or full donor chimerism	Only donor detected	Suggests complete hematopoietic engraftment, but low levels of recipient cells may not be detected depending on the method used to assess
Mixed chimerism	Both donor and recipient detected	May indicate increased risk of relapse; dynamic change most important (increasing, decreasing, or stable); for RI-HSCT, mixed chimerism is expected initially
Subset chimerism	Mixed chimerism in a cellular subpopulation, e.g., T cells	Patterns of T cell and natural killer (NK) cell chimerism may be predictive of GVHD or graft loss in RI-HSCT recipients
Split chimerism	Recipient detectable only in some cell lineages	May indicate relapse or risk of relapse; important to correlate with clinical picture and original disease cell lineage
Microchimerism	<1 % recipient detected	Associated with solid organ transplantation; unclear significance in setting of allogeneic HSCT

RI-HSCT reduced intensity hematopoietic cell transplation

short tandem repeats (STR), a type of genetic polymorphism. The interpretation of chimerism results depends on the context in which the testing was done, i.e., the type of transplant, conditioning intensity, timing of testing post-transplant and results of concurrent blood counts and bone marrow morphology. In this chapter we review the clinical utility of chimerism analysis and laboratory aspects of testing including methods and analysis.

Terminology

A chimera is a mythological creature consisting of the head of a lion, the body of a goat, and the tail of a serpent. In medicine, a chimera is an individual whose cells derive from two or more genetically distinct individuals. While this can occur naturally by fetal-maternal transfer, in the context of HSCT, chimerism is the desired outcome, with the entire hematopoietic system genetically of donor origin. A variety of terms are used to describe post-transplant chimerism (Table 56.1). "Complete chimerism" (also referred to as "full donor chimerism") indicates that only donor hematopoietic cells are identified. In contrast, when both recipient and donor cells are present in a cellular subset, this is referred to as "mixed chimerism." The threshold that differentiates complete chimerism from mixed chimerism depends on the sensitivity of the assay used; that is, if the sensitivity of the assay is 5 %, then 95 % donor may not be a significantly different result from 100 % donor. Similarly, a technical result of complete chimerism does not indicate absolute absence of donor cells; only that it is below the limit of detection of the assay. Detection of < 1 % donor is sometimes referred to as "microchimerism," a term that arose from the solid organ transplant field, where passenger cells within the graft can persist in the recipient's blood.

Hematopoietic Stem Cell Transplantation

Each year, more than 28,000 patients undergo allogeneic HSCT worldwide. Allogeneic HSCT is accomplished by the infusion of either bone marrow or granulocyte colony stimulating factor (G-CSF)-mobilized peripheral blood stem cells from a related or unrelated donor. The stem cell infusion is preceded by the administration of a conditioning regimen (chemotherapy and/or radiotherapy), designed to eradicate residual malignant cells and induce sufficient immunosuppression to facilitate engraftment. Allogeneic HSCT permits the administration of myeloablative doses of chemotherapy and radiation, and offers important antitumor immunity through donor-derived T and NK cells. The genetic disparity between the donor and the recipient results in a therapeutic antitumor effect, often called the graft-vs-tumor (GVT) response, but also results in immune-mediated damage to normal recipient tissues, causing a clinical syndrome called GVHD. Reduced intensity HSCT (RI-HSCT) involves the administration of non-myeloablative doses of chemotherapy and radiation in order to reduce the toxicity associated with aggressive conditioning. The lower toxicity of RI-HSCT allows its use in patients deemed ineligible for myeloablative transplants due to age, comorbidities, or prior therapies. RI-HSCT eradicates malignant cells through a powerful GVT effect and not through chemotherapy or radiation.

Clinical Utility of Chimerism Analysis

Chimerism is a dynamic process following allogeneic HSCT, and its kinetics depend on the intensity of the conditioning regimen, sensitivity of different cell types to chemotherapy and radiation, the recipient's prior therapies, composition of the graft, and other factors. Therefore, identification of longitudinal changes (increasing or decreasing mixed chimerism over time) is most useful clinically. The interpretation of chimerism testing depends on clinical context, type of transplant, and time after transplant. For example, the presence of "10 % residual recipient cells" may have completely different implications on day 21 vs day 100 after HSCT, or if the patient had a myeloablative or a reduced-intensity conditioning regimen prior to transplant. Similarly, the presence of "25 % donor cells" in a patient with aplastic appearing bone marrow is interpreted differently from a patient who has evidence for relapsed leukemia occupying the marrow. Here we describe the common clinical situations and various clinical outcomes that can be evaluated with chimerism testing.

Patterns of Engraftment

Recovery of normal hematopoiesis after HSCT occurs gradually after the stem cell infusion. In typical hematologic recovery, granulocytes recover first (within 10–24 days) and platelets and red blood cells ensue. Complete blood counts fail to reveal the origin of recovering hematopoiesis, which can be donor-or recipient-derived, and is very often mixed in the early phases after HSCT. Chimerism analysis is usually done in the first 100 days after the stem cell infusion to verify and document adequate engraftment of donor cells [1]. In myeloablative HSCT, if careful sequential studies are done, an early phase of mixed chimerism is usually observed, rapidly followed by conversion to complete donor chimerism (Fig. 56.1a). In cases of graft failure, transient mixed chimerism transitions back to predominantly recipient chimerism, followed by disappearance of donor cells (Fig. 56.1b). Therefore, chimerism studies are useful in the evaluation of poor hematological recovery, which may be the result of engraftment failure, infection, GVHD, or ABO incompatibility. In RI-HSCT, mixed chimerism may persist for long periods of time without indicating engraftment failure.

The kinetics of the transition from mixed to complete chimerism reflect the complexity of immune interactions between donor and recipient cells as well as differences in the HSCT process for different clinical situations. The major determinants of engraftment timing and levels of mixed chimerism include the type of conditioning regimen used (myeloablative vs reduced-intensity), graft type (bone marrow vs peripheral blood stem-cells vs umbilical cord blood [UCB]), graft source (related vs unrelated donor), human leukocyte antigen (HLA) compatibility, numbers of CD34+ and CD3+ cells in the graft, prior chemotherapy, degree of lymphodepletion prior to transplant, type of disease (acute myelogenous leukemia [AML], lymphoma, chronic myelogenous

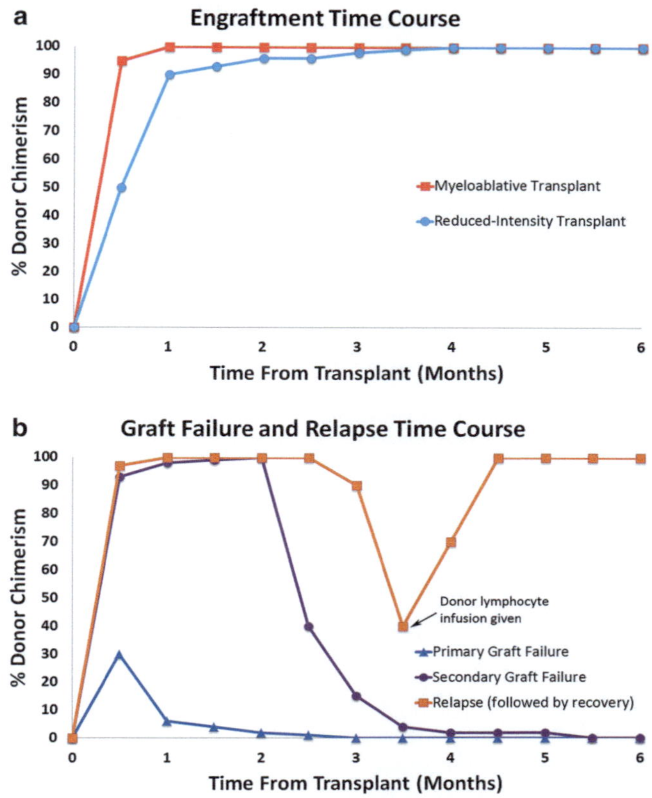

Figure 56.1 Comparisons of typical time courses of engraftment (**a**) and graft failure (**b**) after bone marrow transplant. The example of relapse (**b**) shows recovery of donor engraftment after infusion of donor lymphocytes

leukemia [CML], etc.), and the use of T cell depletion [2–11]. Acute GVHD is associated with accelerated engraftment, but the causal relationship is unclear. Faster engraftment may trigger GVHD by not allowing sufficient time for the immune system to develop tolerance [2, 3, 12, 13].

In RI-HSCT, higher levels of donor chimerism, and sometimes even early full chimerism, are more common in patients who had intensive chemotherapy prior to transplant, likely secondary to lymphodepletion, which leads to homeostatic expansion of donor cells and therefore faster engraftment [5, 14]. Strategies have been developed to intensify pre-transplant lymphodepletion in order to accelerate engraftment [11]. Chimerism analysis enables close monitoring in these cases.

In UCB transplants, slow engraftment and engraftment failure are common due to low numbers of CD34+ cells and HLA incompatibility. Chimerism is tested in these cases to monitor the engraftment process. Chimerism measurements as early as 14 days post-transplant can be helpful in predicting the risk for graft failure [15]. In order to overcome the barriers of slow engraftment and high incidence of graft failure after UCB transplants, a commonly used approach is the concurrent transplantation of two different UCB units, which accelerates engraftment and reduces the risk for graft failure [16, 17]. After double cord transplant, chimerism analysis often detects DNA from both UCB units at the same time, with occasional residual recipient cells, especially after reduced-intensity conditioning. The usual course is that both units contribute to early hematopoiesis, but by 21–100 days post-transplant, one of the units predominates, and eventually the minor unit can no longer be detected [17, 18]. The factors determining which unit "wins" include the CD3+ and CD34+ cell doses, the order of infusion, and the degree of HLA match [16, 19, 20]. Interestingly, cases have been reported where reversal of dominance occurs a long time after the transplant, even after documentation of full chimerism with one of the donors [20, 21]. Evaluation of chimerism in the setting of two donors is more complicated than with a single donor.

Evaluation of Graft Failure

Graft failure presents as either failure to achieve adequate engraftment and recovery of blood counts (primary graft failure) or loss of normal blood counts after initial engraftment (secondary graft failure) (Fig. 56.1b). In the evaluation of graft failure, it is important to differentiate between graft rejection, defined as the absence of donor-derived hematopoiesis (usually <5 % donor chimerism) in a patient with a hypocellular marrow, and poor graft function, where donor cells are present but production of blood elements is reduced. Poor graft function may result from a low dose of CD34+ cells in the graft, presence of recipient-derived anti-HLA antibodies against the donor cells, use of bone marrow or UCB as opposed to peripheral blood stem cells, infection, and factors in the bone marrow environment [22, 23]. A poorly functioning graft may respond to infusion of additional stem cells. Graft rejection is more likely to be the result of immunologic rejection of the graft, and can be treated with modulation of immunosuppressive therapies, donor lymphocyte infusions, or a second HSCT [24]. In all cases of graft failure, an evaluation of a bone marrow biopsy is mandatory to exclude a relapsed malignancy. The combination of bone marrow histology and chimerism levels in bone marrow and blood are useful to help interpret the clinical picture.

Mixed chimerism does not always predict graft failure, and is very common after RI-HSCT. However, it is known that predominant donor chimerism precedes hematologic recovery. A persistently low level of donor chimerism in whole blood, T cells, or NK cells after transplant is associated with subsequent graft failure [1, 5, 25, 26]. Serial monitoring every 1–4 weeks can identify a downward trend which predicts graft failure. Serial monitoring is also useful to measure responses to treatments of graft failure, such as withdrawal of immunosuppression, infusion of additional stem cells or additional lymphocytes, or a second transplant from a different donor.

Association with GVHD

In some studies, early conversion to full donor chimerism was associated with increased incidence of GVHD, while mixed chimerism seemed to be protective against acute and/or chronic GVHD [25, 27–29]. Mechanistically, co-existence of recipient and donor cells may facilitate peripheral tolerance induction, but mixed chimerism is not fully protective against GVHD, and conversion to full donor chimerism is not required for initiation of GVHD [5, 30–32]. Studies of T cell subset chimerism are potentially more informative than whole blood, and show that high donor T cell chimerism is associated with GVHD [5, 9].

Chimerism and Relapse in Myeloablative Transplants

The utility of chimerism testing for prediction of disease relapse depends on several factors. Attempts to associate mixed chimerism with relapse and survival outcomes resulted in conflicting results, possibly related to differences in diseases and conditioning regimens studied, and the use of T cell depletion strategies in some studies. In myeloablative HSCT for CML, the presence of mixed chimerism or mixed T-cell chimerism within 90 days after transplant correlates with disease relapse and a poor outcome, but this seems to depend on the conditioning regimen [33], and has questionable value in diseases other than CML [7]. The timing of testing is critical; studies in CML have shown that not only mixed chimerism but also residual copies of *BCR–ABL1* transcript are not predictive of relapse in the first 90 days after HSCT [34]. Therefore, in most clinical scenarios, early testing of mixed chimerism (day 30) should be reserved for evaluation of possible graft failure and not disease relapse [1].

Beyond the first 90 days post-transplant, many studies have demonstrated an association between persistence of recipient cells with relapse and worse survival [30, 35, 36]. More importantly, studies that looked at the dynamic changes in chimerism levels showed that a persistent or rapid trend of dropping chimerism levels often heralds relapse [31, 37–40], whereas stable mixed chimerism is not clearly associated with poor outcomes [27, 40–42]. One of the major limitations of these reports is that they included primarily patients with chronic phase CML, which rarely requires HSCT today [33, 36, 43–45]. In acute leukemias, trends seem to be more important than single measurements, and frequent monitoring is more likely to predict relapse successfully than less frequent testing since the kinetics of chimerism prior to relapse can show an abrupt change [45–47].

Chimerism in RI-HSCT

In RI-HSCT, early evaluation of chimerism may have a more important role than for myeloablative HSCT. The low intensity conditioning regimen, combined with post-transplant immunosuppression, allows the establishment of mixed chimerism in most patients [48, 49]. With time, mixed chimerism may transition to complete chimerism, or remain stable and serve as a platform for subsequent immunotherapies such as donor lymphocyte infusions (DLI) [50]. After RI-HSCT, the initial recovery of neutrophil counts, traditionally named "engraftment," represents a mixed recovery of autologous hematopoiesis and engrafted donor cells, which quickly transition into complete myeloid chimerism (Fig. 56.1a) [5, 51]. Other lineages also recover gradually, but often remain in a mixed chimeric state for prolonged periods of time. Multiple factors determine the kinetics and the degree of donor chimerism achieved after RI-HSCT, and higher levels are achieved with a more intensive conditioning regimen, use of chemotherapy prior to transplant, use of G-CSF mobilized peripheral blood stem cells as opposed to bone marrow, and pre-transplant lymphopenia [5, 52]. The critical role of lymphodepletion prior to transplant in inducing full donor chimerism has led to the development of chemotherapy regimens that efficiently deplete recipient lymphocytes prior to RI-HSCT for lymphoma [11].

Is the degree of donor chimerism associated with outcomes of RI-HSCT? Early studies showed that full T cell chimerism precedes full myeloid chimerism and suggested that full chimerism precedes GVT and GVH responses [51, 53]. Other studies have found that low levels of T and NK cell chimerism predict graft rejection and lack of antitumor activity; high levels of T cell chimerism are associated with GVHD, while high levels of NK cell chimerism predict improved progression free survival [5, 26]. Some of these correlations might be specific to certain diseases and certain conditioning regimens [4, 6]. Recently, large retrospective studies have demonstrated the prognostic value of early (day 30 and day 100) measurement of donor chimerism in predicting relapse and survival after related or unrelated donor transplants, regardless of disease [52, 54]. Similarly, full donor T-cell chimerism on day 100 after double UCB transplants with reduced intensity conditioning seems to predict a lower incidence of relapse [55]. These studies strengthen the rationale for chimerism testing in the setting of RI-HSCT.

Failure to achieve full chimerism after both myeloablative and RI-HSCT can be overcome by DLI, which often successfully induces transformation from mixed to full chimerism and enhances the GVT response [56, 57]. Monitoring whole blood or T cell chimerism after HSCT has been used to guide and monitor preemptive DLI strategies in patients with mixed chimerism, considered to be at high risk for rejection and disease relapse [35, 46, 51, 53, 58–62]. Randomized studies have not been conducted to provide solid evidence for the benefit of this approach, but it is clear that DLI can induce favorable antitumor responses in several diseases [37, 58, 62]. Cytokine therapy also has been used to enhance engraftment and increase donor chimerism levels [63].

Chimerism vs Minimal Residual Disease

Minimal residual disease (MRD) detection can be performed by amplification of disease-specific markers such as *BCR–ABL1* transcripts. The analytic sensitivity of MRD analysis (generally between one cell in 1,000 and one cell in 1,000,000) is greater than that of standard methods for chimerism analysis (generally 1–5 %). In addition, MRD detection with a disease-specific marker detects only the malignant cells, while chimerism analysis detects all recipient cells without distinguishing between malignant and normal host cells. Chimerism testing is useful because it offers a universal way to detect residual recipient cells without the need to have a known disease-specific cytogenetic or molecular marker. A way to augment the sensitivity of chimerism analysis for early detection of relapse is by enriching the sample for cells that carry a phenotypic marker similar to the patient's malignancy, i.e., enriching for CD19+ cells in a patient who underwent HSCT for B-lymphoblastic leukemia [64, 65]. Cells also can be enriched for either an abnormal phenotype or CD34 positivity (a surface marker of immaturity, which is carried by most acute leukemias) [66, 67]. Potentially the best way to predict disease relapse is to combine chimerism testing with other MRD assays, if available, to increase the predictive value of both tests [37, 68, 69].

Guidelines for Chimerism Testing in HSCT

The American Society for Blood and Marrow Transplantation published a set of guidelines for the testing of chimerism after allogeneic HSCT (Table 56.2) [53]. These guidelines support the use of STR or variable number tandem repeat (VNTR) analysis of peripheral blood samples as the standard method to analyze chimerism and specify that lineage specific chimerism is useful following non-myeloablative and reduced-intensity conditioning.

Table 56.2 Comparison of chimerism analysis in myeloablative and RI-HSCT based on recommendations of the National Marrow Donor Program and the International Bone Marrow Transplant Registry 2001 Workshop

	Myeloablative HSCT	RI-HSCT (Non-myeloablative)
Recommended sample	Peripheral blood	Peripheral blood and cell lineage subpopulations
Frequency of analysis	3, 6, and 12 months after HSCT; after complete chimerism, based on change in clinical condition	Every 2–4 weeks
Significance	Mixed chimerism, particularly increasing mixed chimerism, may help predict relapse; significance depends on disease and cell lineage of chimerism	Early patterns of chimerism may predict either GVHD or graft loss
Method	Tandem repeat loci sensitive for detection of recipient allele(s)	Tandem repeat loci sensitive for detection of both recipient and donor allele(s)

GVHD graft-vs-host disease, *RI-HSCT* reduced intensity hematopoietic stem cell transplantation

Other Applications of Chimerism Analysis

HSCT for Nonmalignant Conditions

RI-HSCT is commonly used to treat nonmalignant conditions, where mixed chimerism is sufficient to reverse a clinical phenotype such as congenital immunodeficiency, enzyme deficiency, or hemoglobinopathy. In these situations chimerism studies are helpful in predicting the clinical benefit. For example, in HSCT for congenital immunodeficiency, the increase in T cell chimerism correlates with immune reconstitution [70], and in HSCT for hemoglobinopathies, establishment of 25 % donor chimerism is sufficient to reverse the clinical phenotype of sickle cell anemia and thalassemia, and usually correlates with transfusion independence [71, 72]. Factors that are associated with stable mixed chimerism include younger donor age, sibling donor, and the type of conditioning regimen used. Acute GVHD occurs more often in patients who achieve full donor chimerism [73].

Donor-Derived Clonal Disorders

Donor-derived malignancies are rare after HSCT and solid organ transplants [74]. These malignancies can easily be confused with relapsed disease in a patient after HSCT, and therefore chimerism testing is important to identify the origin of the malignant clone. When the donor is still alive, this may require advising the donor about appropriate screening procedures. Similarly, chimerism analysis allows determination of the origin of proliferating lymphocytes in post-transplant lymphoproliferative disorders.

Transfusion-Associated and Solid Organ Transplant-Associated GVHD

GVHD is rarely associated with the transfusion of cellular blood products containing viable passenger lymphocytes as well as solid organ transplants. In both cases, immunosuppressed individuals are unable to eradicate donor-derived competent T cells. The result is a severe form of GVHD that primarily attacks the bone marrow, leading to aplasia, which is frequently fatal if not identified early. In these cases of transfusion-associated GVHD, prior donor DNA is usually not available, but analysis of the recipient's blood will reveal foreign DNA [75]. Chimerism studies can show mixed chimerism in these patients, and cases of >50 % T cell donor chimerism have been described [76]. This topic is described further in Chap. 57.

Methods

Fluorescence In Situ Hybridization

Fluorescence in situ hybridization (FISH) analysis for the X and Y chromosomes (XY-FISH) can be used for chimerism analysis by hybridization of interphase preparations with two differentially labeled probes for sequences on the X and Y chromosomes, respectively [77]. Classic karyotyping methods could be used for detection of X and Y chromosomes but would be labor-intensive, slow, and limited by the number of cells able to be analyzed. For example, to attain a sensitivity of 1 %, more than 300 cells would need to be evaluated. FISH allows the rapid screening of a large number of cells. The method can yield quantitative results by rapidly counting between 500 and 1,000 cells. A sensitivity of approximately 0.1 % or lower can be achieved [59]. Standardization of XY-FISH has made it suitable for clinical use [78]. However, the major limitation of XY-FISH is the applicability only for sex-mismatched transplants.

Tandem Repeats

Tandem repeats are a class of polymorphism consisting of a variable number of tandemly repeated core sequences [79]. Tandem repeats are classified according to the number of

Table 56.3 Comparison of methods of chimerism analysis

Method	Sensitivity	Advantages	Disadvantages
Karyotyping	5–10 %	Monitors chromosomal abnormalities as well	Requires dividing cells; low sensitivity; high false-positive rate
RFLP	5–10 %	Highly informative	Requires Southern blot analysis; alleles not distinct
Red blood cell phenotyping	0.04–3 %	Simple	Not very informative; can be affected by transfusion; not useful for rapidly proliferating diseases
STR-PCR	1–5 %	Highly informative; quantitative	Only moderate sensitivity; multiplex amplification may decrease sensitivity
FISH for X and Y chromosomes	0.1–0.5 %	Sensitive; feasible to screen large numbers of cells for quantitative result	Only for sex-mismatched transplants
SNP Analysis	0.01–1 %	Highly sensitive; quantitative	Less quantitative with higher chimerism; need to evaluate many SNPs to find informative SNP
Y-chromosome PCR	0.001–0.1 %	Sensitive; highly informative in sex-mismatched transplants	Only for sex-mismatched transplants with male recipient and female donor
Cell sorting + STR-PCR	0.0001–0.1 %	Informative; sensitive; cell lineage information important	Requires large volume of blood; technically demanding

RFLP restriction fragment length polymorphisms, *SNP* single nucleotide polymorphism, *STR-PCR* short tandem repeat polymerase chain reaction, *XY-FISH* X and Y chromosome fluorescence in situ hybridization

nucleotides in each core sequence. Minisatellites have core sequences of approximately 8–80 base pairs (bp) and are also known as VNTR. In contrast, microsatellites, also known as STR loci, have core sequences of up to 7 bp [80]. Allelic variation at each VNTR and STR locus arises from the number of core repeats present. STR alleles have between 3 and 40 tandem core repeats; each STR locus typically has 10–20 different allelic variants. Variant alleles with imperfect repeats also occur [80].

STR loci and some VNTR loci are amenable to PCR amplification using primers that flank the repeating sequence. After amplification, the number of repeats is calculated from the size of the PCR product, or, more simply, the products are compared to an "allelic ladder" constructed to contain the majority of known repeat size alleles in the human population at a particular locus [80]. PCR amplification of tetranucleotide (four bp in each core repeat) and pentanucleotide (five bp in each core repeat) STR loci has become the predominant method for DNA-based human identification [81]. Comprehensive information about STR loci and their application in human identification is available from a Web site sponsored by the National Institute of Standards and Technology (http://www.cstl.nist.gov/div831/strbase, accessed 4/12/2015).

Amplification of STR loci has become the most frequently applied technology for the study of chimerism after HSCT for several reasons [82, 83]. By examining multiple STR loci, which is made easier by multiplex PCR, it is possible to find at least one STR locus for each donor–recipient pair that can be used to distinguish the donor from the recipient; thus, STR-PCR is essentially universally informative, except in identical twins. In addition, STR-PCR can be used to quantitatively discriminate mixtures of DNA based on relative amplification of alleles. The sensitivity of STR-PCR for chimerism analysis can achieve a limit of detection of about 1 % chimerism if performed following recommended guidelines [84]. STR alleles are relatively similar in size due to the small repeat unit; thus, compared with VNTR alleles, which have larger differences, STR-PCR theoretically is better for quantification because preferential amplification of smaller alleles is less likely to occur. The advent of capillary electrophoresis (CE) and automated fluorescent detection has made the analysis of PCR products technically straightforward. In addition, the availability of commercial reagents for STR-PCR simplifies assay development.

Y Chromosome Analysis

Amplification of Y chromosome-specific sequences can be used for assessment of chimerism in sex-mismatched HSCT involving a male patient and a female donor, which represents approximately 25 % of all HSCT cases. Because the targeted sequences are present only on the Y chromosome, the method is very sensitive. Sensitivities as high as 1 male in 100,000 female cells (<0.001 %) have been reported, although the clinical relevance of chimerism detection at such high levels of sensitivity is not clear [45, 85]. Use of quantitative real-time PCR has the advantage of being not only sensitive but also quantitative for very low levels of mixed chimerism, useful for detecting an increasing or decreasing signal over time. Amplification of the amelogenin gene, which is present on both the X and Y chromosomes, but is 6 bp longer on the Y chromosome homolog, is used for sex typing in forensic analysis and also has utility for chimerism analysis [80]. The major disadvantage of all Y chromosome PCR methods is the limited application to only a subset of sex-mismatched transplants.

Single Nucleotide Polymorphism Analysis

Single nucleotide polymorphisms (SNPs) are primarily biallelic variants at a single nucleotide position. SNPs occur on average every 1.3 kilobases (kb) in the human genome. Since SNPs are sequence polymorphisms rather than length polymorphisms, their utility for chimerism analysis is based on the frequency of heterozygosity in the particular population under study. With only three potential genotypes for most SNP loci (AA, AB, BB), the chance of distinguishing two individuals is much lower than for STR loci, which have 10–20 alleles per locus. Consequently multiple SNPs must be analyzed to successfully distinguish all donors and recipients. One investigator statistically calculated the number of SNPs required to identify an informative locus in 96.5 % of cases to be 25 SNPs [86]. In one study using a panel of 51 SNPs, an informative locus was found in 100 % of cases; however, this study used a microarray-based system to enable high-throughput testing [87]. While the number of loci necessary is a disadvantage, an advantage of SNP detection over tandem repeat amplification is that SNPs are less susceptible to preferential amplification of alleles based on length, and stutter peaks (described later) are not a concern.

While there are many methods for analysis of SNPs, real-time PCR technology is commonly used for SNP-based chimerism analysis [82, 88]. Real-time PCR permits sensitive detection of mixed chimerism using SNPs at a level of approximately 0.1 %. Although real-time PCR is quantitative, the coefficient of variation (CV) at chimerism levels above 5 % is as high as 30–50 %, compared with a CV of about 5 % for STR-PCR methods [77]. Thus, while SNP real-time PCR is more sensitive and quantitative, particularly at low levels of mixed chimerism, the variability of the quantitation when the level of recipient is above 5 % does not permit accurate determination of dynamic change in mixed chimerism levels [82]. Real-time PCR SNP analysis of mixed chimerism is a promising method; yet, despite years of evaluation and new technologies for analysis, SNPs have not supplanted STRs for chimerism analysis [82].

Laboratory Testing

PCR amplification of STR loci is currently the most commonly accepted and most widely used method for assessment of mixed chimerism after HSCT [53, 84, 89]. Therefore, the remainder of this chapter details the use and interpretation of PCR testing of STR loci for analysis of mixed chimerism in a clinical laboratory.

STR Amplification Reagents

Chimerism analysis requires the identification of at least one informative STR locus that distinguishes recipient from donor cells prior to transplant, in order to be able to monitor recipient cells, donor cells, or both in the recipient after transplant. A variety of commercial reagents are available for amplification of STR loci. The majority of commercially available STR amplification reagents are designed for forensic analysis in which a maximum amount of information is desired from frequently limited samples. Multiplex PCR, in which multiple loci are amplified simultaneously by including more than one set of PCR primers in the reaction, is ideal for this purpose. The STR locus-specific PCR products from the multiplexed reactions are distinguished by the expected size range of the products for each locus (designed to be non-overlapping) and by the use of different fluorophores for each locus in a multiplexed set, allowing amplification of loci with overlapping product sizes. High-order multiplex primer sets have been designed that amplify 16 or more STR loci. The two major suppliers of forensic STR primer sets are Promega Corporation (Madison, WI) and Life Technologies (Foster City, CA), each with a variety of multiplex combinations, some designed for detection with specific methods or instruments. At the time of writing of this chapter, enforcement of a patent held by Promega currently prohibits the use of the Life Technologies STR reagents for chimerism analysis in the setting of HSCT and other clinical and research applications. Primer sequences are also available online and in publications for laboratories to develop and validate their own assays; however, the optimization of multiplex amplification is time-consuming and complex.

Selecting a STR Marker Panel

All STR loci are not created equal. Some are more informative than others based on allele frequencies and rates of heterozygosity. The possible constellations of alleles can be grouped into several categories [90, 91]. Some loci have a higher proportion of ideal allele constellations that improve the ability to detect low levels of recipient in a donor background. The Penta E locus was found to have the highest percent of ideal allele constellations in a study that evaluated 27 loci in 203 recipient–donor pairs [90]. Interestingly, in our laboratory's experience using 15 STR loci for pre-transplant analysis and then selecting a single optimal locus, Penta E was the most commonly selected single locus. In contrast, CSF1PO was the least selected locus and it had the lowest frequency of ideal allele constellations in the study by Thiede et al. [90]. In Europe, the EuroChimerism consortium was established to facilitate harmonization of chimerism diagnostics between European centers because of their assertion that existing forensic commercial primer sets are not ideal for chimerism [92]. This group recommended an STR marker panel specifically for chimerism analysis to maximize informativity, reliability, and sensitivity. Nevertheless, in our experience over 15 years, 12–15 commercially available forensic loci have been used successfully in an active transplant program to perform chimerism analysis. Even though several loci have been informative more often than others, the less informative loci have all been used for some recipient–donor pairs, indicating that they all have potential value; this is especially true in a two-donor transplant case where several loci are usually needed to monitor chimerism.

Detection Method

Amplified STR products can be detected in numerous ways, as described for forensic analysis in Chap. 54. By far the most frequently used method in clinical laboratories for analysis of STR amplification products is fluorescent detection by CE, which has the advantage that a gel does not need to be poured and analysis of samples is rapid [80]. CE can be performed with a single capillary instrument or with a multi-capillary instrument; for example, with 16 or 24 capillaries. The advantage of multiple parallel capillary systems is that analysis can be performed more rapidly than with a single capillary instrument. Capillary arrays with 96 or more capillaries are available; however, their instrument and reagent costs are greater, and thus they are only cost-effective for very high-volume testing. CE instruments that can detect multiple fluorophores permit not only multiplex amplification of loci resulting in PCR products overlapping in size, but also inclusion of a size marker for accurate sizing of the fragments. Of note, not all fluorophores are detected by all CE instruments; therefore it is important to check for compatibility before selecting reagents.

Pre-transplant Testing

The goal of pre-transplant analysis is to identify the informative loci that can be used to monitor chimerism after HSCT. This is accomplished by determining the STR alleles of the recipient and the donor(s) at each STR locus in the marker panel used by the laboratory, and then selecting at least one locus with one or more different donor and/or recipient alleles in a constellation pattern conducive to sensitive and accurate monitoring of post-transplant chimerism.

Samples

Usually peripheral blood samples from the donor and recipient are used to extract DNA for pre-transplant analysis. Analysis of an additional buccal cell sample from the recipient not only serves as a quality control to confirm the identity of the recipient sample in the laboratory, but also as a control for balanced amplification of alleles in a non-hematopoietic lineage. If there is allelic imbalance in the blood sample at a particular locus, comparison with the buccal sample amplification pattern can help determine if the effect is constitutional, stochastic, or due to disease (Fig. 56.2). A locus with significant unbalanced amplification of alleles in either sample should be avoided.

On occasion, a recipient is transplanted prior to the STR evaluation of a pre-transplant sample. In this case, a post-transplant blood sample will not be useful for identification of the recipient's genotype. Buccal cells are the most commonly used source of recipient DNA if blood is not an option, although any other available historical tissue that is appropriately preserved can be used. While post-transplant buccal samples will be of mostly recipient genetic origin, they will frequently contain a minority of admixed donor DNA, thereby generating a mixed chimeric pattern [93]. Since the recipient's alleles usually predominate, they can be deduced if the donor alleles are known. A saliva or mouthwash sample is not equivalent to a buccal cell sample since saliva generally contains significantly more leukocytes. In one study, the median amount of donor DNA in the buccal swabs was 21 % whereas it was 74 % in the mouthwash samples [94]. If only donor alleles are detected in a buccal swab DNA sample (and the donor is not an identical twin sibling), complete "engraftment" of buccal epithelial cells should be considered. Several cases of buccal cell "engraftment" after HSCT have been reported [95].

Identification of Informative Loci

To identify ideal informative loci for each recipient–donor pair usually many loci must be examined. This is particularly true when the individuals are related and share many alleles by inheritance. Multiplex amplification increases the speed and decreases the labor associated with the analysis of multiple loci. Of the loci found to be informative, not all will be appropriate for chimerism analysis. This is because the goal is not to differentiate the individuals as in forensic identity testing but to detect small amounts of recipient or donor alleles in a mixed specimen [90].

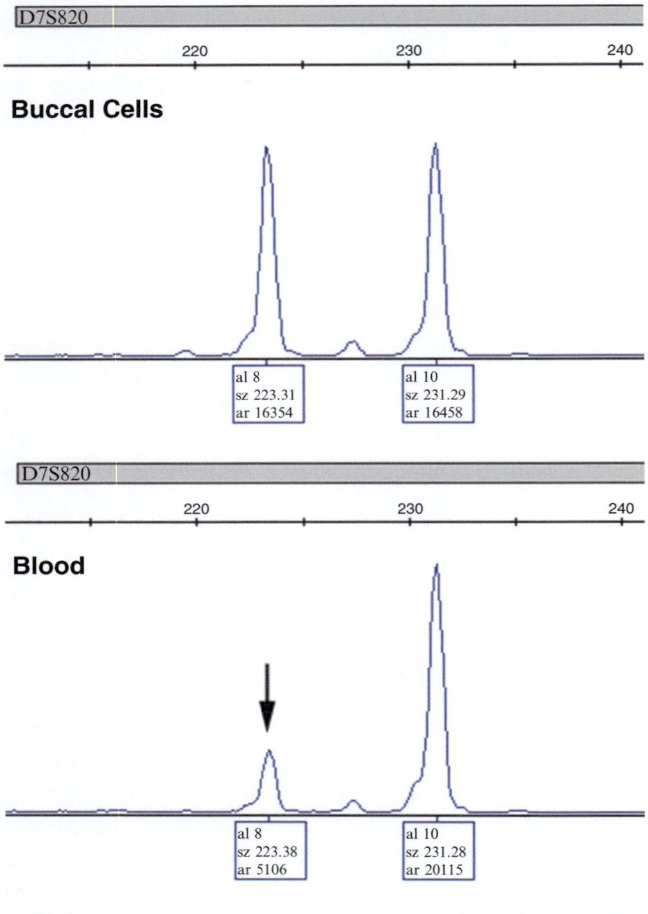

Figure 56.2 Amplification of the D7S820 locus in DNA obtained from buccal cells and blood in a patient with myelodysplastic syndrome. The blood, which contained disease, shows that one allele (8, *vertical arrow*) has only 25 % of the peak area of the other allele peak (10). The fact that the alleles are not imbalanced in the buccal cells suggests that this is due to a chromosomal abnormality related to the disease and not a constitutional polymorphism affecting amplification of allele 8. Thus, D7S820 should be excluded from calculations of chimerism due to underestimation of the % recipient if the disease relapses

The main factor limiting the utility of some informative alleles is the presence of a stutter peak which is one repeat smaller ($n-1$) and, to a much lesser extent, one repeat larger ($n+1$) or two repeats smaller ($n-2$) than each major allele peak [96]. When tandem repeats are amplified, stutter peaks are thought to result from slippage of the polymerase, causing mispairing of the template, which is shifted by one repeat unit, resulting in an additional PCR product predominantly one repeat smaller than the expected PCR product. The intensity of the $n-1$ stutter peak is usually approximately 2–11 % of the area of the corresponding STR allele [96]. The amount of stutter is influenced by the locus (some loci tend to have more stutter than others), the core repeat unit length (smaller core repeats have more stutter than larger repeats), and the allele size (larger repeat alleles have more stutter than smaller repeat alleles) [80].

For chimerism analysis, optimal informative loci have one or two recipient-specific allele(s) that do not co-localize with a donor allele or stutter peak (Fig. 56.3) [97]. Ideally, the recipient-specific allele should be at least two repeats larger or three repeats smaller than the donor allele(s) to avoid the stutter locations [89]. Having two unique recipient alleles that meet these criteria (recipient is heterozygous) may provide confirmation that a recipient DNA is present; however, at low levels of chimerism a heterozygous allele may be below the limit of detection compared to a homozygous peak. In addition, due to the theoretical possibility for preferential amplification of shorter fragments, the sensitivity for detection of a minor recipient-cell population may be greater if the informative recipient allele(s) have fewer repeats than the donor allele(s) [89]. Because of the many possible combinations of alleles between recipients and donors, each recipient–donor pair presents a unique situation, and each must be evaluated on a case-by-case basis to determine which loci can be used and which should be excluded due to artifacts (like stutter) that will reduce sensitivity and accuracy. These are only guidelines for the selection of informative loci; how useful or accurate a particular locus will be post-transplant ultimately is determined empirically by use in the post-transplant setting. In some instances, an optimal locus cannot be identified. In this case, post-transplant analysis still can be performed using a suboptimal locus with the caveat that the sensitivity of detection will be decreased because of co-localization of the recipient-specific allele with a stutter or other background peak. As described in the analysis section, chimerism calculations can be adjusted with caution to take stutter contributions into account.

Another factor to consider when selecting informative loci is whether there are specific alleles for both the recipient and the donor (Fig. 56.3). While this is not essential for myeloablative HSCT, for which the combined donor and recipient allele pattern of included loci must be optimized to enhance detection of a small percentage of recipient DNA in a donor background, it is very important for non-myeloablative HSCT, since any level of mixed chimerism (low donor or low recipient) may be seen. If no such locus can be found, then at least two loci should be selected, one optimized for detection of recipient allele(s) and the other for donor allele(s). As the level of mixed chimerism in the patient changes from low to high donor chimerism or vice versa in case of disease relapse, the loci used may need to be changed to optimize sensitivity (Fig. 56.4). The use of more than one informative locus to generate an average chimerism result will minimize the effect of artifacts and maximize analytic sensitivity. However, even if multiple loci are used the set of loci included in the average should be reevaluated if the percent of recipient DNA is very high.

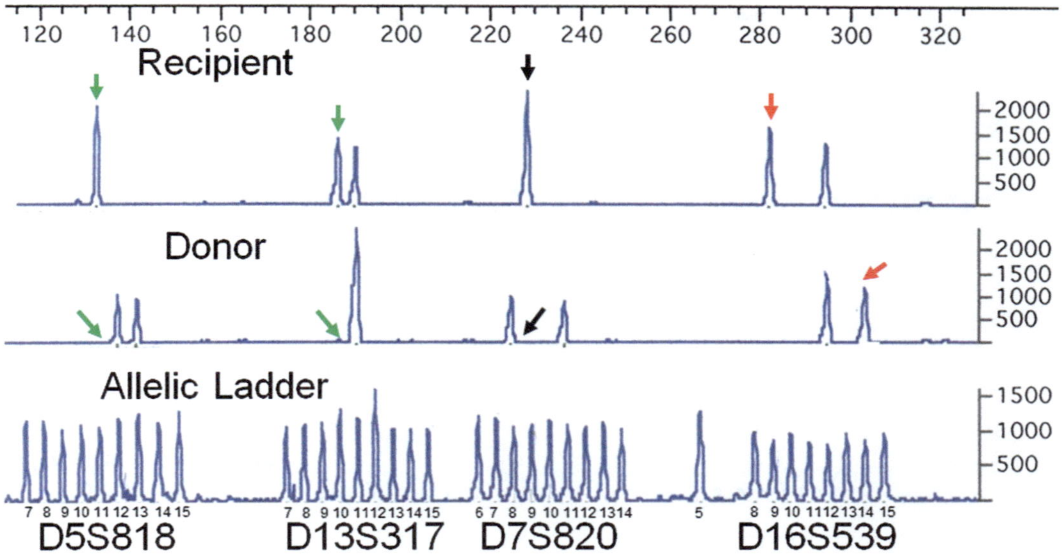

Figure 56.3 Identification of informative loci using PCR amplification of STR loci and CE analysis. The STR alleles at four loci (GammaSTR, Promega Corporation) are compared for a recipient–donor pair to identify the best informative locus. The number of repeats in each allele is determined by comparison to the allelic ladder for which the sizes are indicated. While all four loci are informative for distinguishing the recipient from the donor, the D16S539 locus is best because the recipient-specific allele (*red vertical arrow*) is separated from the nearest donor allele by at least two repeats. In contrast, for the D5S818 and D13S317 loci, the recipient-specific allele (*green vertical arrows*) co-localizes with a donor stutter peak, the location of which is indicated by the *diagonal green arrows*. The D7S820 recipient-specific allele (*black vertical arrow*) is acceptable, but, if present, an $n+1$ stutter (*black diagonal arrow*) from the smaller size donor allele may interfere with detection. The allele combination at the D16S539 locus also has the advantage of a unique donor allele (*red diagonal arrow*). *PCR* polymerase chain reaction, *STR* short tandem repeat, *CE* capillary electrophoresis

HSCT with Two Donors

A patient with a failed first transplant may undergo a second transplant with a new donor. The first donor may or may not be detectable in the recipient blood at the time of the second transplant. In addition, UCB transplants typically involve at least two donors. All these situations complicate the assessment of chimerism because all the individuals need to be able to be detected and distinguished. Generally one or more STR loci can be identified that have a unique allele for each individual. Prior to transplant an algorithm can be developed on a case-by-case basis to assess and calculate the percent of recipient, donor 1, and donor 2 [84, 98].

Post-transplant Testing

The goal of post-transplant analysis is to monitor chimerism after HSCT. This is accomplished by determining the percentage of recipient and the donor(s) alleles present in peripheral blood, lineage-specific cellular subsets, or bone marrow after HSCT.

Sample Types

Peripheral blood, lineage-specific cellular subsets, or bone marrow from the recipient after transplant can be analyzed for chimerism or to confirm engraftment. For RI-HSCT typically peripheral blood and a T-cell subset are evaluated in parallel at all time-points. CD3+ T-cells and other lineages such as myeloid and NK cells, can be obtained by manual or automated cell selection procedures [26, 99]. A commonly used procedure is the use of magnetic beads that bind to tetrameric antibody complexes recognizing CD3 or other lineage-specific markers (for example, StemCell Technologies, Vancouver, Canada). The unbound cells can be washed away and the cells of interest remain bound to the magnetic particles ready for DNA extraction. A purity of >99 % can be achieved for some subset types; however, the age of the sample is a critical preanalytic factor to control. Technical recommendations from the United Kingdom National External Quality Assessment Service for Leukocyte Immunophenotyping Chimerism Working Group (UK-CWG) suggest that lineage-specific cell separation should ideally be performed within 24 h of sample collection [84]. Additionally, each new lot of separation reagents should be assessed for production of high-purity subsets. This can be done using flow cytometry. Alternatively, commercial assays are available to assess purity of some cell subsets (for example PeloBiotech, Planegg, Germany or Accumol, Calgary, Canada). If using flow cytometry, it is important to be aware that certain individuals express one or more soluble serum factors that can cause cross-linking with the magnetic particles. This may result in visible aggregates in the enriched

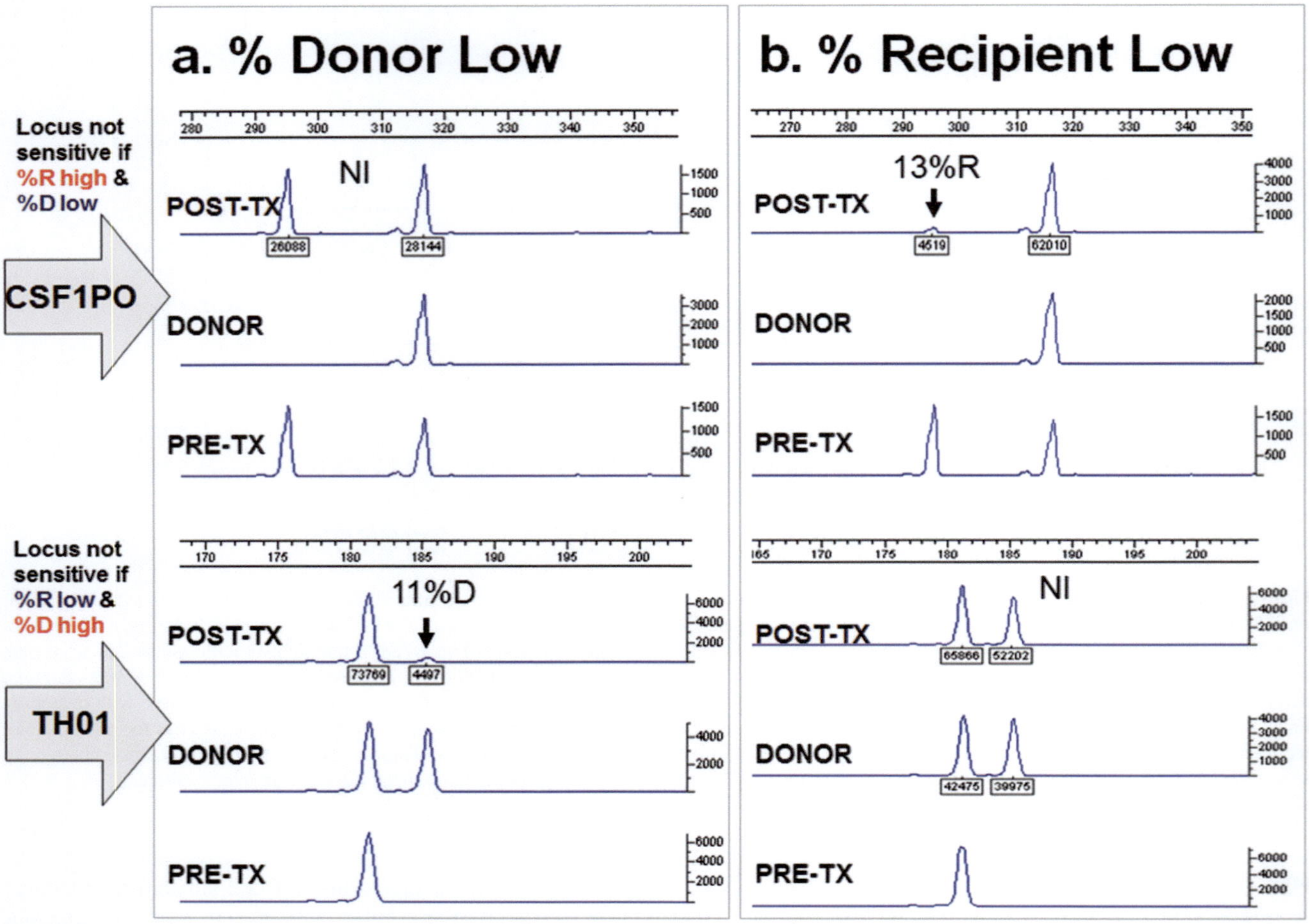

Figure 56.4 If the recipient or donor is homozygous and that allele is shared with the donor or recipient, respectively, this locus will not be equally informative at all levels of chimerism. Electropherograms at two loci (CSF1PO and TH01) are shown for two post-transplant time points (**a** and **b**) for a recipient–donor pair. For each time point, the donor and pre-transplant recipient (PRE-TX) alleles are shown as well as a post-transplant (POST-TX) sample showing mixed chimerism. For this recipient–donor pair, when the percentage of donor DNA is low (**a**), the CSF1PO locus is not informative (NI) for detection of donor because a small change in donor would be smaller than the measurement error of chimerism due to variable amplification of the two alleles. In contrast, the TH01 locus (*bottom* of panel **a**), which has a donor-specific allele is informative and sensitive for detection of donor (11 % donor). Similarly, when the percentage of donor DNA is increased (**b**), the situation is reversed. The CSF1PO locus is informative and sensitive for detection of low amounts of recipient (13 %R). On the other hand, the TH01 locus is not informative (NI) because, as with the CSF1PO locus when the donor was low, the potential variable amplification of the alleles (measurement error) could lead to a false-positive or a false-negative result. When the minor component (recipient or donor) is approximately 25 % or less, loci with this constellation of alleles should be excluded from use. In the ChimerMarker software (SoftGenetics). The use of loci with this constellation of alleles is called "deconvolution;" deconvolution should only be used when absolutely necessary if using this software because it does not distinguish between the two types of deconvolution

cell fraction following positive selection. These aggregates may appear as distinct, high side-scatter populations on forward-scatter vs side-scatter plots during flow cytometry analysis of the enriched fraction. This population consists solely of particles, with no cells or platelets present.

Approaches to Testing

In selecting the approach to use for post-transplant testing one must balance several factors: laboratory workflow, cost, accuracy, and analytic sensitivity. While sensitivity is theoretically optimized when a small number of loci are tested (single locus or low-number multiplex), laboratory workflow is more efficient with a high-order multiplex (fewer controls to run, less time determining which reagents to run for each patient, all reactions can be set up at the same time). Although cost of reagents is higher with high-order multiplex reactions, the improved efficiency of laboratory workflow may balance this factor, making it worthwhile to consider a reagent such as PowerPlex 16 (Promega Corp.) to simplify both pre- and post-transplant analysis.

A further advantage of using PowerPlex 16 for post-transplant testing is that accuracy may be theoretically improved if more than one locus is averaged (see section "Analysis and Interpretation" below). Indeed, the UK-CWG recommends reporting the mean of three or more markers where possible [84]. Changes made by the manufacturer in the conditions and reagents for PowerPlex 16 in recent years have improved the analytic sensitivity for detection of DNA mixtures of low percent (<5 %), making it amenable to use for post-transplant testing.

The alternative to using PowerPlex 16 is selecting from one of several lower-order multiplexes such as GammaSTR, CTTv, and CS7 (Promega Corp.). In this scenario, all loci are tested pre-transplant (PowerPlex 16 and CS7) [83]. One or more loci are selected and the primer set containing the locus/loci is selected for all post-transplant testing. Use of a primer set containing more than one optimal informative locus is preferable. This method has a lower reagent cost for the post-transplant analysis, but is more labor-intensive than using PowerPlex 16 for the technologists since they have to determine which primer set to use for each patient and set up the reactions separately.

Optimizing and Assessing Sensitivity

Irrespective of the primer set used, the sensitivity of chimerism analysis can be optimized. As mentioned earlier, the amount of DNA is important for sensitivity because it directly reflects the number of cells being analyzed. Since most commercial STR reagents are designed for forensic analysis of limited samples, the amount of input DNA indicated in the forensic protocols (usually <1 ng) may be less than optimal for chimerism analysis. Each laboratory should determine the maximum amount of DNA (usually 10–25 ng) that can be used without increasing the nonspecific background and spurious peaks that make interpretation difficult. The number of PCR cycles can be optimized to balance analytic sensitivity without exceeding the linear range of the detection method to ensure accurate quantification [84, 97]. The injection time for CE instruments, which is the time of applied voltage during which sample migrates into the capillary and is essentially equivalent to the amount of product loaded on a gel, also must be optimized (Fig. 56.5). Appropriate injection times are specific to each instrument. In some cases, very small recipient-specific peaks may be detected even though the predominant donor alleles are off-scale and not within

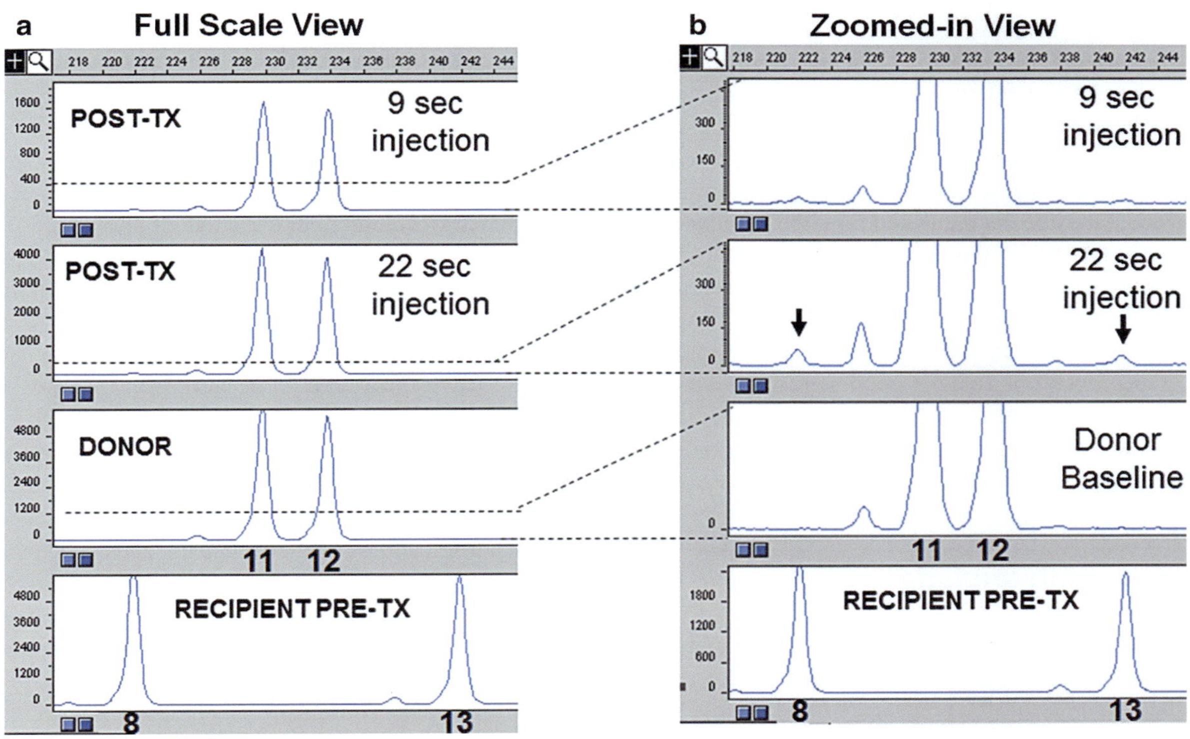

Figure 56.5 Optimizing sensitivity of PCR amplification of STR loci with CE analysis. The post-transplant (POST-TX) analysis of a recipient–donor pair at the D7S820 locus is shown at two injection times (9 and 22 s) on an ABI 3100 CE instrument (**a**). The donor and recipient pre-transplant (PRE-TX) alleles are shown. Because the recipient-specific peaks are small (*arrows*), the *y*-axis is expanded (zoomed-in view) to examine the baseline in greater detail (**b**). The zoomed-in view shows the presence of recipient-specific alleles in the 22-s injection, but they are not as clearly visible in the 9-s injection. To evaluate the post-transplant sample, a comparison is made to the donor baseline at the same *y*-axis scale, which in this case does not show a non-specific peak. *PCR* polymerase chain reaction, *STR* short tandem repeat, *CE* capillary electrophoresis

the linear range for quantification. The off-scale donor allele peak areas or heights would be under-representative of the actual amount of donor PCR product in the sample, but the percent recipient, if detected, can be reported as less than the limit of detection.

Unlike standard molecular pathology assays, assessment of the lower limit of detection (LOD) cannot be assessed for every possible sample, because each locus in each recipient–donor pair is a new situation. Mixing and artificial dilution experiments of a few sample pairs can be done to determine an average LOD (<1–10 % is typical), but the actual level of sensitivity may be higher or lower in different samples and even for different loci in the same sample. This variability may be explained not only by differences in methodology (number of loci co-amplified, input DNA, detection method) but also by differences in sensitivity for each recipient–donor pair based on each locus and its constellation of alleles [97]. Except in rare patient-specific scenarios, analytic sensitivities for chimerism analysis should generally be about 1 %. However, not all samples or loci will be equally analytically sensitive for the detection of low levels of mixed chimerism. If a locus is poorly amplified, then ability to detect low levels of donor or recipient will be compromised. If the yield of DNA is low due to low cellularity, this may affect the LOD for all loci tested. The total fluorescence at a locus should be high enough that a minor component of 1 % is detectable above background [92, 100]. The relevant peak areas or heights needed for 1 % sensitivity depend on whether the alleles are homozygous or heterozygous. In the simplest scenario where the recipient and donor are both homozygous for different alleles, if the detection threshold (the lowest peak that can accurately be distinguished from the baseline) using a specific instrument is 50 relative fluorescence units (RFU), then the sum of the unique donor allele peak areas must be 5,000 RFU in order to detect the recipient at 1 %. Any locus in a multiplex set for which the constellation of recipient and donor alleles does not achieve good sensitivity should be excluded from the average calculation, if more than one locus is averaged. If all loci tested have a compromised LOD, then a note stating this should be included in the report.

Analysis and Interpretation

CE results from post-transplant STR analysis are analyzed to determine whether recipient specific allele(s) are present, and if they are present, the percentage of recipient (%R) is calculated. Although analysis is focused on optimizing detection of the recipient component because it is usually the minor component, the percent donor (%D) or (100 – %R) is the value generally reported since clinicians base most patient management decisions on the level of donor in the patient. Absence of recipient-specific alleles or 100 % donor is consistent with complete engraftment at the level of sensitivity of the assay. Dynamic comparisons should be made only across the same type of sample, for example, peripheral blood, bone marrow, or cell lineage.

How Many Loci to Use?

The use of multiplex primer sets simplifies many aspects of chimerism testing as described above and enables the use of more than one locus to calculate chimerism. But is it necessary or advisable to use more than one locus? The use of a single locus or multiple loci each has advantages and disadvantages. An advantage of using a single locus is that manual calculation is relatively easy, so software to facilitate calculations is not needed. In contrast, since manual calculation of multiple loci is not time efficient, use of automated software for analysis is optimal. Commercial software packages are available (for example ChimerMarker, SoftGenetics, State College, PA) to simplify analysis of multiple loci. An advantage of using the mean of multiple loci is that the effect of any amplification artifact is minimized. In addition, this approach may prevent unrecognized chromosomal abnormalities such as loss of heterozygosity (Fig. 56.2) or extra copies of chromosomes from impacting the accuracy of chimerism results [82]. Furthermore, our experience indicates that using multiple loci increases the probability that low level recipient will be detected at one of the analyzed loci, whether it is stochastic or due to a locus-specific effect. These advantages would tend to greatly favor using multiple loci. For these reasons, as mentioned above, the UK-CWG recommends a minimum of three loci, if possible [84].

According to the Participant Summary Reports from the College of American Pathologists (CAP) Monitoring Engraftment (ME) proficiency testing survey, 75 % of participating laboratories use two or more loci to calculate chimerism; 10 % always use 14 or more loci. However, in one survey it was noted that 21 % of laboratories reported <100 % donor for a sample with a target value of 100 % donor. This may be due to reliance by some laboratories on automated software to average the results of multiple loci without regard to the appropriateness of each locus included. The more loci that are included without careful review of the contribution of background signals or artifacts in the calculation of chimerism, the less likely that a result of 100 % recipient or donor will be reported. Thus, the main drawback of using multiple loci in the chimerism calculation is the potential pitfall of automated analysis of data near 100 % recipient or donor. Near 100 % donor, the qualitative result of detected or not detected is more important than the quantitative value. Accuracy near 100 % ideally requires a manual review of the electropherograms with comparison to the donor baseline. Manual review of multiple loci for cases with >95 % donor

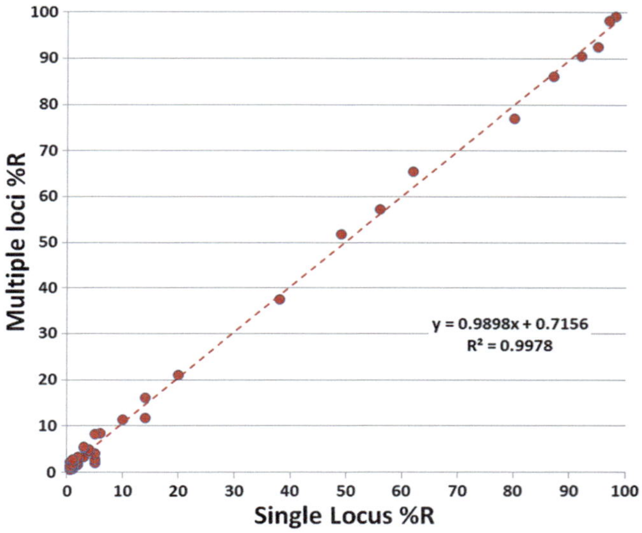

Figure 56.6 Comparison of the percent recipient (%R) result calculated using a single optimal locus to the mean result of all informative loci (mean 9, range 3–14, loci used) amplified with PowerPlex 16 reagents (Promega Corp.). Data are from 43 patients. The trend line (*red dashed line*) shows excellent correlation indicating that in most cases a single locus is approximately equivalent to the average of multiple loci. (Acknowledgement to Dr. Gregary Bocsi for assistance in data analysis.)

is possible, but could be cumbersome if the laboratory has a high volume of testing. Thus, automated analysis with chimerism software has many advantages, but must be done with careful attention to the interpretation. The ideal solution is to review all the loci at the time of the pre-transplant analysis to select the markers to include for post-transplant analysis using a pure donor sample and to analyze it as if it were a post-transplant sample. Any loci which do not yield a result of 0%R (100%D), as well as loci which are suboptimal due to co-localization of the recipient alleles in stutter locations, should be excluded from post-transplant analyses. A similar analysis can be performed with a pure recipient sample, if available, to select the markers best able to assess a result of 100%R (0%D).

Selecting a single optimal informative locus to calculate chimerism, on average, achieves an overall result essentially equivalent to the mean of multiple loci. We have demonstrated this in our laboratory experimentally (Fig. 56.6) and by review of data from the CAP ME proficiency survey for the last 2 years with over 70 participating laboratories. The key is the selection of an optimal locus using criteria described above to minimize the contribution of stutter peaks and other artifacts. That is not to say that a single locus will *always* perfectly match the mean of multiple loci, but on average, data suggest it will (Fig. 56.6). This is in part because the locus was selected to be optimal (including excluding chromosomal abnormalities at the locus in the diagnostic sample if possible) and because manual review enables identification and avoidance of artifacts. A single locus in a particular recipient–donor pair may have a significant bias compared to the true value at middle ranges (25–75 %) of chimerism due to a variety of factors; however, generally the locus will be consistently biased with each test for a specific recipient–donor pair. Thus, dynamic changes assessed over time will not be significantly affected by bias at a single locus used to follow the patient. In addition, a single locus, by virtue of the fact that it was selected to be optimal for the detection of low recipient, will generally provide a good assessment of complete engraftment (100 % donor) and low %R with manual review. Consequently, a single locus can achieve results similar to those of multiple loci, but has the advantage of being easier to analyze and more accurate qualitatively compared to an automated calculation of multiple loci without careful review of which loci to exclude. A schema for issuing a report on varying numbers of loci has been published taking into account variability between locus results [100].

In summary, both single and multiple loci are acceptable methods of calculating chimerism and both have some issues that must be evaluated before reporting results [82]. For multiple loci, the focus should be on the qualitative results near 100 % recipient or donor by careful selection of which loci to exclude. For a single locus, careful consideration of the patient's cytogenetic results to avoid loci on chromosomes affected by the malignancy and any artifacts that could affect the quantitative results is warranted. When a single locus is used, there is always the option, if a multiplex primer set was used, to review additional loci to confirm a questionable result before reporting.

Calculations

Single Donor

If both donor- and recipient-specific allele(s) are clearly identified in the post-transplant sample, then the percentage of recipient and donor DNA in the sample can be calculated [83, 92, 97]. For each allele peak, the intensity of the fluorescent signal, indicated by the peak area or height, is proportional to the amount of PCR product. CE instrument software can calculate the area or height of any peak recognized as an allele-specific signal. Either peak areas or heights can be used for chimerism analysis calculations as long as the same measure is used consistently and validated by the individual laboratory. In this chapter, peak area is used.

The percentage of recipient-specific DNA can be calculated as the quotient of the recipient specific peak area(s) to the sum of the recipient and donor specific peak areas, as shown in Fig. 56.7a, b. If the donor and recipient are both heterozygous and do not share any alleles, then the peak areas of both recipient alleles are added together for the numerator

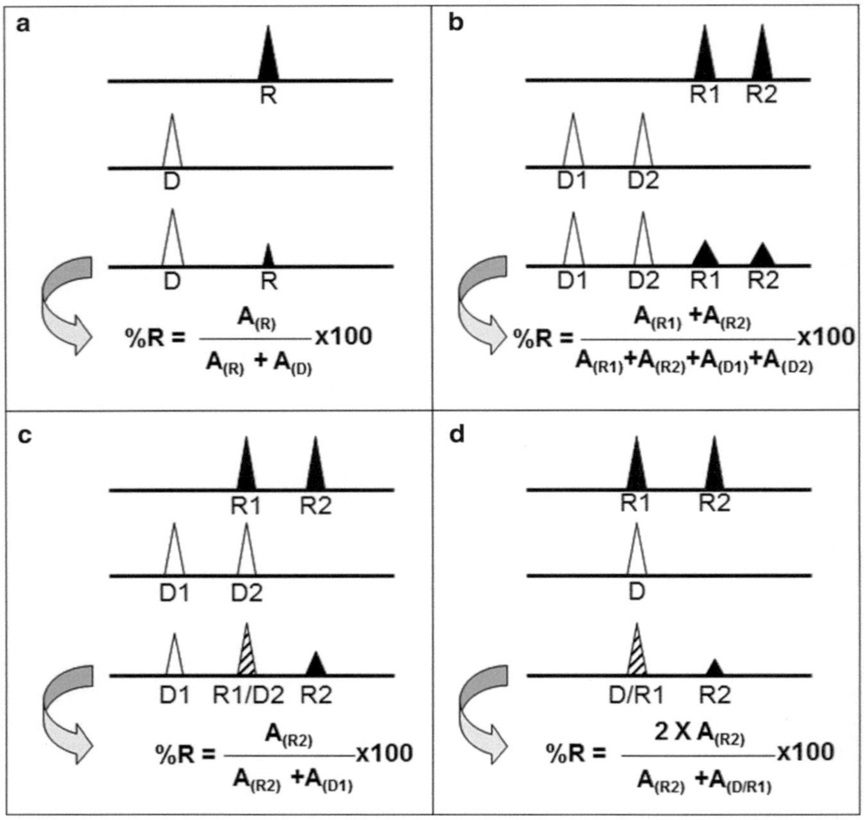

Figure 56.7 Formulas for calculation of percent recipient. Four representative scenarios (**a**–**d**) for combinations of informative recipient (R) and donor (D) alleles are shown. Recipient alleles are *black*, donor alleles are *white*, and shared peaks are striped. When heterozygous alleles are present, the numbers *1* and *2* indicate each allele. For each scenario, the third line in each box is a hypothetical post-transplant sample showing a mixed chimeric pattern. The calculation for the pattern shown in panel (**d**), also known as deconvolution, should only be used when the heterozygous individual (R in this example) is also the minor component. The formula that would be used to calculate the percent recipient is given, in which "A" represents the peak area of the appropriate peak designated by the *subscript*

and the areas of all four peaks (two donor and two recipient) are added for the denominator (Fig. 56.7b). When the recipient and donor share an allele, the %R is calculated based only on the unique alleles. The peak area of the shared allele does not enter into the calculation because it stays constant; that is, 100 % of the cells in the sample (donor and recipient) will have the shared allele (Fig. 56.7c). When the donor is homozygous for an allele and the recipient is heterozygous for the same donor allele and a second unique allele, as shown in Fig. 56.7d, the recipient area of the shared allele can be estimated by the area of the unique recipient allele. Thus, the %R is calculated as two times the unique recipient allele peak area divided by the sum of all peak areas (Fig. 56.7d). In this latter scenario, as the %R increases above 50–75 %, use of an alternate locus for the calculation should be considered because the constellation of alleles is not sensitive or accurate for detection of low %D (Fig. 56.4). In all cases, the fraction is converted to a percentage by multiplying by 100, and the %D is calculated as 100 minus the %R. Given that this method is inherently semiquantitative, rounding to the nearest percent to report the result is acceptable.

If recipient specific allele peak(s) are not visible initially, then close examination of the baseline in the region of the expected recipient-specific alleles is critical to identify small recipient peak(s) for each informative locus being analyzed. Depending on the analysis software being used, the scale of the *y*-axis can be adjusted to "zoom in" on the baseline (Fig. 56.5). Comparison of the post-transplant sample baseline at the location of the recipient alleles to the corresponding baseline of a donor sample is useful to assess for nonspecific peaks. Any peaks, including any bleed-through peaks from another fluorophore that happen to co-localize with the recipient alleles, that are present in the donor background in the location of a recipient-specific allele will not be mistaken for a recipient signal. When evaluating the donor baseline, the peak area(s) of the relevant donor-specific peaks should be compared to the peak area(s) in the post-transplant specimen. The peak area comparison is only valid if the areas of all the alleles are similar, because the level of background nonspecific signal is directly related to the adjacent peak areas. In cases of graft loss, comparison of the post-transplant sample baseline at the location of the donor alleles to the corresponding baseline of a pre-transplant recipient DNA sample can distinguish low levels of donor from nonspecific background signals in the recipient. For this reason, the use of recipient and donor DNA baseline controls is important. Historical recipient and donor baseline electropherogram traces are easy to use if a chimerism analysis software is used; however, it is important to make sure that the amplification levels of the donor baseline sample was optimal (not too high and not too low) so that it is representative of artifacts and stutter background. If using historical recipient and donor baselines for comparison to post-transplant analyses, the pre-transplant samples should be retested if any significant reagent changes occur.

Two Donors

Calculation of chimerism is more complicated when two donors are involved since up to six alleles could theoretically be detected in one sample and many allelic configurations are possible [98]. There are three main questions to assess in a double-donor post-transplant analysis:

1. Is any recipient (R) DNA present?
2. Is any donor 1 (D1) present?
3. Is any donor 2 (D2) present?

Selection of informative loci before transplant is directed at finding alleles at one or more loci to answer these questions. While early in the transplant both donors may be detectable, usually one donor eventually predominates with loss of the other donor, so that only one donor is detectable after engraftment. If, for example, D1 DNA predominates, the questions being asked in post-transplant testing change to become more like a single donor case:

1. Is any R DNA detectable?
2. Is any D2 DNA detectable?

Even after D2 becomes undetectable, it can still reemerge, so it is important to check for the detection of D2 to ensure that the chimerism percentages are calculated correctly. The clinical significance of which donor is detected varies depending on the type of transplant and the clinical situation. The approach is to find at least one allele at one locus that can unequivocally identify the presence of R. If R is absent, then the same or another locus should be used to determine if any D2 (or D1 as appropriate) is detected (Fig. 56.8). A qualitative assessment of detected alleles is a helpful first step that will then define the next steps to calculate the %D1 and %D2. If only D1 allele(s) and no recipient allele(s) are detected, then this will be reported as 100 % D1 and 0 % D2.

If either the minor donor component and/or R are detected then a calculation must be done. The concept is the same as for single donors: 100 % = %R + %D1 + %D2. If no alleles are shared among the three individuals the calculation is straightforward:

$$\%R = (Ra1 + Ra2) / (Ra1 + Ra2 + D1a1 + D1a2 + D2a1 + D2a2) \times 100$$

where a1 = allele 1 and a2 = allele 2 [98].

If Ra1 or Ra2 is shared with D1 or D2 the formula can be modified using 2 × Ra1 or 2 × Ra2 with the same denominator (using the shared peak area in place of the individual areas as shown in Fig. 56.8). Alternatively, when one or more allele(s) are shared it is sometimes easiest to do the calculation in a stepwise manner calculating each component separately using different loci. A detailed algorithm for calculating chimerism with shared alleles has been published [98]. In addition, ChimerMarker software (SoftGenetics) has an analysis mode for assessment of two donor chimerism (Fig. 56.8). From the pre-transplant evaluation, a case-specific analysis algorithm should be developed for which alleles and loci can be used to answer each of the questions above. The loci used can be subsequently refined and simplified after transplant as engraftment of one donor predominates.

Potential Pitfalls and Limitations

Assessment of Errors

There are several sources of error in the calculation of chimerism [101]. Measurement error estimates the relative deviation of DNA measurements from optimal at a single locus in a post-transplant sample. This is analogous to allelic imbalance which represents the ratio of heterozygous alleles at a single locus. Optimally, the measurement should be 1, indicating no imbalance between either donor–recipient allele pair. Percent measurement error (%ME) is only relevant for constellations of alleles in which the recipient and donor are both heterozygous.

$$\%ME = \frac{A - B}{C} \times 100$$

%ME is calculated with A as the sum of the two smaller allele peak areas (A = R1 + D1) and B is the sum of the two larger allele peak areas (B = R2 + D2) and C = the larger of A or B.

A high %ME indicates a greater likelihood that the calculation at a particular locus will be inaccurate so the locus should either be excluded, or the data used with caution.

Locus error provides a measure of how the %D chimerism calculation (CHM) at a particular locus (CHM_{locus}) is performing compared to the mean chimerism value using all loci (CHM_{mean}). Suboptimal amplification of one or more alleles, stutter contributions which are not accounted for, and nonideal constellations of recipient and donor alleles are all potential sources of high percent locus error (%LE). Since the mean may be smaller or larger than the value at a particular locus, the absolute value of the difference is taken to calculate %LE as shown in the formula below. %LE is only relevant if more than a single locus is being used in the chimerism analysis.

$$\%LE = \frac{|CHM_{mean} - CHM_{locus}|}{CHM_{mean}} \times 100$$

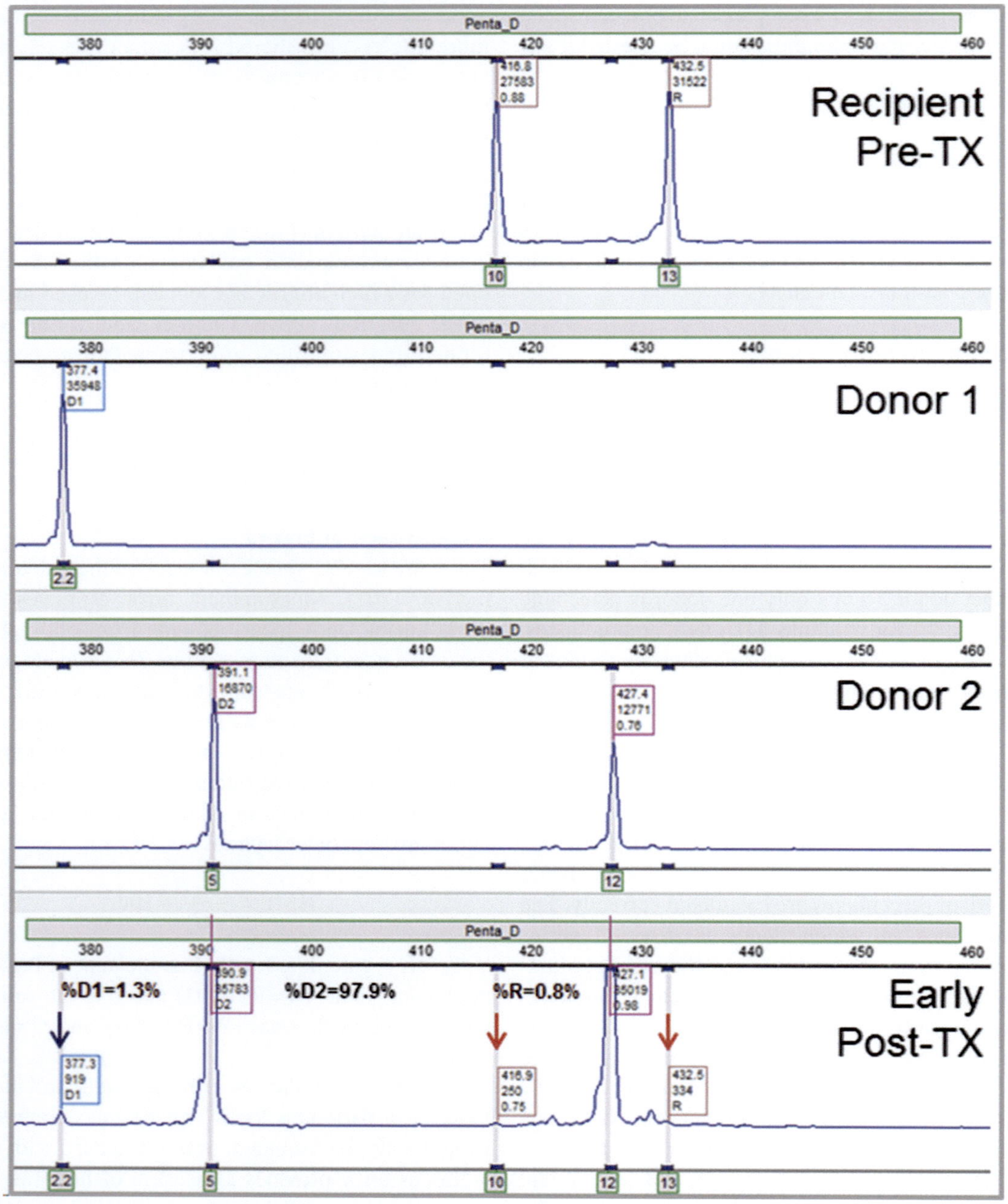

Figure 56.8 Two-donor chimerism analysis using ChimerMarker software (SoftGenetics). Electropherograms of a pre-transplant recipient (Pre-TX) and two donors (Donor 1 and 2) at the Penta D locus (CS7, Promega Corp.) from an ABI 3130 CE instrument (Life Technologies). ChimerMarker software labels each peak with a color-coded box with the peak size in base pairs, the peak area, and either the origin (R, D1, or D2) or the ratio of the sister peaks (to demonstrate how equally the two alleles amplified). An early post-transplant sample (Early Post-TX) within 30 days after transplant is shown in which predominantly Donor 2 has engrafted, but minor contributions of Donor 1 (*blue arrow*) and recipient (*red arrows*) are detected. Post-transplant chimerism was calculated using the following peak areas from the post-transplant sample: %R = (250 + 334)/(919 + 35,783 + 250 + 35,019 + 334) = 584/72,305 = 0.8 %, %D1 = 919/72,305 = 1.3 %, %D2 = 100.0 − 2.1 = 97.9 %. In a subsequent chimerism analysis only Donor 2 was detectable. *CE* capillary electrophoresis

Any locus with a %LE greater than 10 % should be evaluated to determine if there is an obvious cause for the variability, and therefore a reason for excluding the locus from the final calculation. In general, a higher %LE may be noted and tolerated at low levels of chimerism.

The coefficient of variation (CV) is another measure of the overall variability of the chimerism results. The %CV is calculated from the overall mean chimerism value and the standard deviation (σ) of all the included locus values.

$$\%CV = \frac{\sigma}{\text{mean}} \times 100$$

As with other error measurements, %CV is only a guide to flag potential problems and not as an absolute exclusionary criterion. For example, in Fig. 56.9 in the T cell subset, the %CV is low because the two included loci (Penta E and Penta D) have similar results; however, in the peripheral blood with a lower %R, the %CV is very high because one locus was not sensitive enough to detect the chimerism (Penta D), but 1.5 % chimerism was detected in the other (Penta E). Thus, in this case there is an explanation for the high percent CV which can be ignored.

The margin of error (MOE) is calculated using a T-table value obtained according to degree of freedom (Tscore) and the confidence interval (for example 90 %) multiplied by the standard error (SE) of the mean [102]. The standard error of the mean is calculated as $\sigma / \sqrt{N}$ where N=number of informative markers.

$$\text{MOE} = \text{SE} \times \text{Tscore}$$

A large MOE compared to the chimerism result is suggestive of greater variability in the data, in which case the results should be interpreted with caution.

If using chimerism software such as ChimerMarker (SoftGenetics), these error measurements are calculated and abnormal results are flagged automatically (Fig. 56.9). However, if the source of a high error measure is an artifact which could be manually corrected, the disadvantage of using analysis software is the relative inability to change the chimerism formula for specific analyses. In such cases, loci with artifacts can be excluded from the calculations, which is possible if a high-order multiplex with 16 loci is being used.

Stutter Adjustment

Loci for chimerism analysis should be selected to avoid recipient alleles that co-localize with a donor stutter peak ($n-1$ repeat, $n-2$ repeats, or $n+1$ repeat). If the recipient and donor are related, identification of ideal informative loci can be challenging. If using multiple loci, those loci in which a stutter peak would alter the calculation can be excluded. Comparison of the post-transplant recipient peak to the stutter peak in the donor baseline sample can help to determine whether the recipient signal is real if there is no unique recipient allele not affected by stutter. If for any reason it is necessary to use or include a locus in which a stutter peak would significantly alter the results, such as shown in Fig. 56.10a, several adjustment methods can be applied (see below), although the sensitivity for detection of low level recipient chimerism may be affected. The choice of adjustment method depends on the specific situation and the constellation of the donor and recipient alleles. In addition, these are only relevant for manual calculations, i.e., not if automated chimerism software is used.

Heterozygous Allele Estimate

When a heterozygous recipient has a unique informative allele and a second one that co-localizes with a donor stutter peak, the accuracy of quantification is affected rather than the sensitivity. The area of the peak co-localizing with the stutter is greater than the recipient contribution due to the additional stutter signal. To avoid an overestimate of the percent recipient, the peak area of the unique allele can be used as an estimate of the second recipient allele. Therefore, the area of the unique allele is multiplied by two (instead of including the area of the peak that co-localizes with the stutter peak) and used in the appropriate formula (Fig. 56.10b). This method also can be used to avoid other background artifacts affecting one recipient allele.

Donor Baseline Calculation

The donor baseline is a good control for the post-transplant sample if donor chimerism is high and if the levels of amplification (peak areas) are similar. While the peak areas cannot be directly compared between electropherograms, the percent contribution of the stutter peak to the chimerism result can be used. Thus, a calculation can be made for the donor stutter peak from the donor baseline sample analysis (using the same formula that would be used for the recipient if the stutter were not present), and this value can be subtracted from the chimerism result (Fig. 56.10c) [96]. Calculated differences of 1 % or less should not be used as the sole evidence for detected recipient; rather, if questionable, they can be reported as no recipient detected if they are below the LOD of the assay. Differences greater than 10 % clearly indicate presence of recipient DNA, because the contribution of recipient PCR product will be incremental and thereby additive to the stutter peak area. Differences between 1 and 10 % must be assessed on a case-by-case basis. To be clearly present, the recipient contribution must be greater than the standard deviation of the stutter percentage. In these cases, finding an alternate locus to use is the best option.

Stutter Percent Calculation

The stutter percentage (i.e., the percentage of the stutter peak relative to its main allele peak) is usually consistent within a narrow range for each locus, although it varies within a locus by allele size. An alternative method to perform stutter adjustment is to use the stutter percentage to calculate a correction for the area as shown in Fig. 56.10d [96]. The stutter percentage can either be determined on a case-by-case basis using the actual donor baseline sample or an average stutter percent can be determined for each locus using many samples and allele sizes. Once the stutter percentage is determined, the major allele peak area is multiplied by this value to determine what the expected area of the stutter peak would be. This calculated stutter value is then subtracted from the actual peak area in the stutter location. This adjusted peak area is used in the final chimerism calculation.

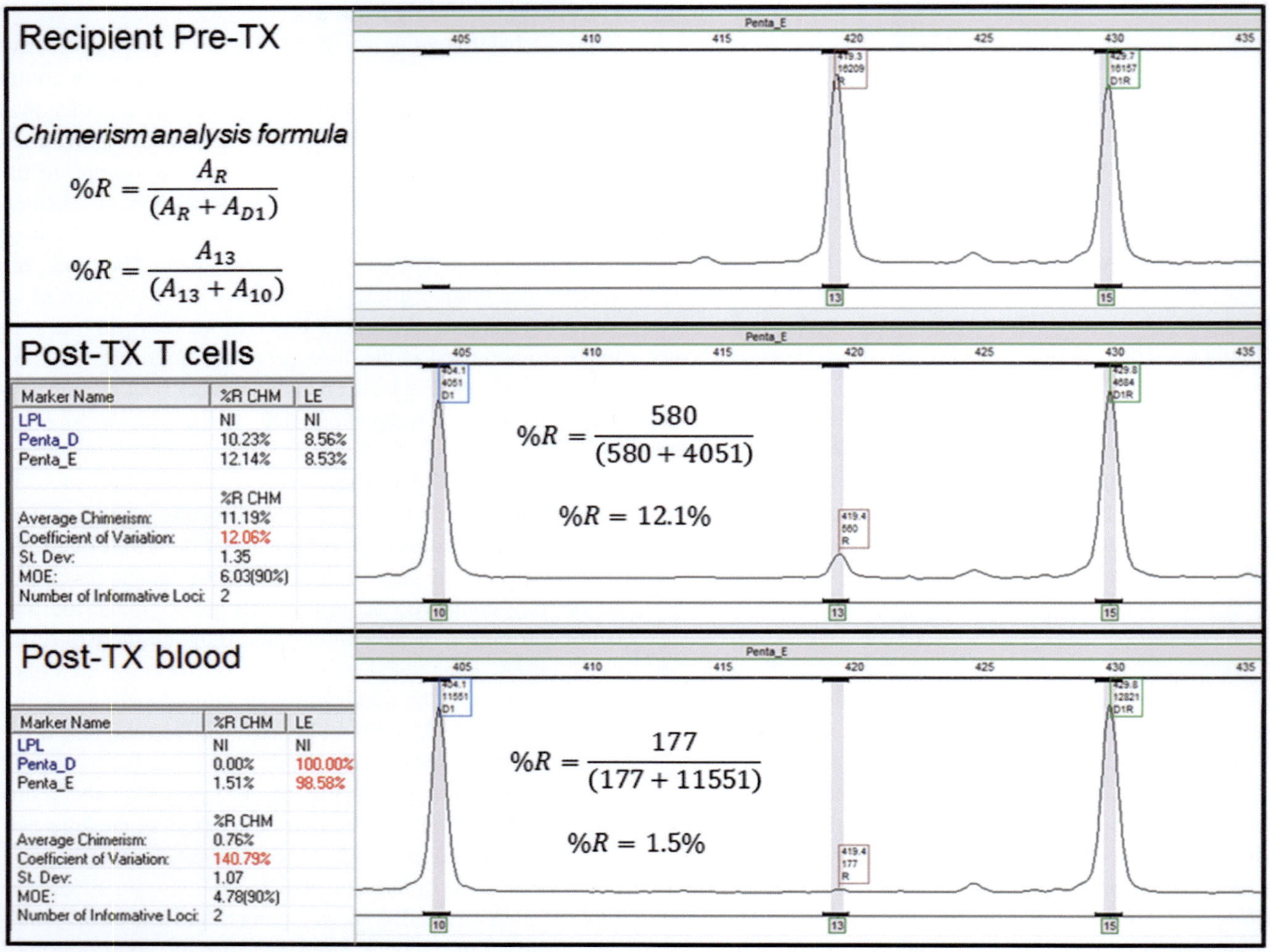

Figure 56.9 Single donor chimerism analysis in T cell subset and unfractionated peripheral blood using ChimerMarker software (SoftGenetics). Electropherograms (ABI 3130, Life Technologies) of recipient pre-transplant (Pre-TX) and two post-transplant (Post-TX) samples at the Penta E locus are shown. The recipient (R) is heterozygous for alleles 13 and 15 and the donor (D1 by convention of the software to designate the first donor) is heterozygous for alleles 10 and 15. Thus, allele 15 is shared between the recipient and donor (D1R). Each peak is labeled by the ChimerMarker software with a *color coded box* at the *top* with the peak size in base pairs, the peak area, and the source of the peak (R, D1, or D1R). The allele size in repeats is given at the *bottom* of each peak in a *green box*. The post-transplant samples are predominantly of donor origin with D1 and D1R peaks present. At the left of each post-transplant sample is a screen shot of the ChimerMarker single donor chimerism analysis results. Of the seven loci amplified (CS7, Promega Corp.), four were excluded before analysis for nonoptimal allele configurations, so the results of these loci are not shown. Of the remaining three shown, one (LPL) is not informative (NI). In addition to calculating the percent recipient chimerism (%R CHM) for each informative locus in each sample and the average chimerism (average of all informative loci), several measures of error are given: locus error (LE), coefficient of variation (CV), standard deviation (St. Dev), and margin of error at 90 % confidence interval (MOE). The formula for calculating the chimerism at the Penta E locus is given at the top left and the corresponding manual calculation with the actual areas in the electropherogram panels for both post-transplant samples. A similar calculation was done at the Penta D locus (electropherograms not shown) by the software, given in the result tables at left. For the T cell sample (*middle left panel*), the percent LE is low [1(average chimerism) − (locus % R chimerism)/average chimerism) × 100]. In contrast, in the post-transplant blood sample (*bottom left panel*) which has a much lower level of recipient chimerism, the recipient-specific allele is not detected at the Penta D locus, indicating that this locus is less sensitive than Penta E. Although the Penta E may be a false positive, this is unlikely because recipient is present in the T-cells which were originally isolated from the same blood sample. Therefore, the result of 0 % at the Penta D locus is indicative of lower analytic sensitivity at this locus. In this post-transplant blood sample, therefore, the LE and CV are very high, but these values are irrelevant because there is an explanation for the apparent variability. The average chimerism is reported, rounded to the nearest integer, as %D (or 100 - %R) which is 99 % for blood and 89 % for T cells

a

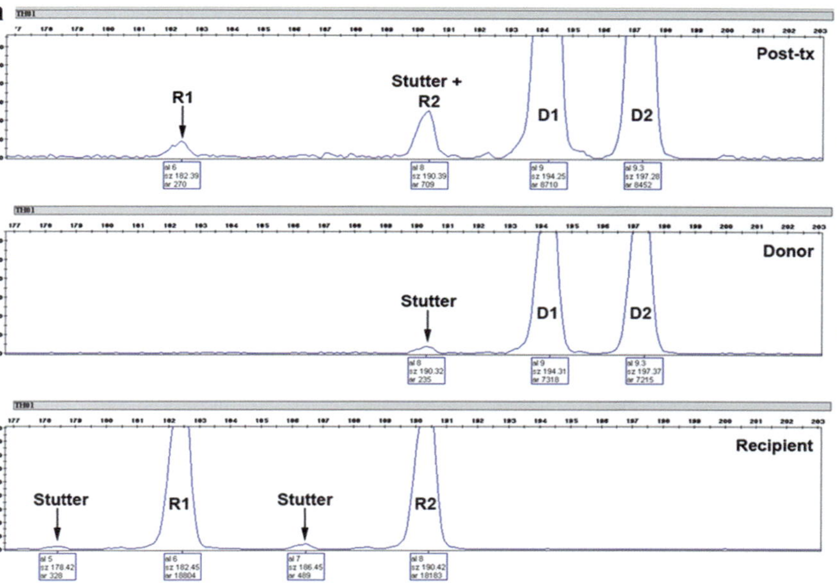

b Heterozygous allele estimate

$$\%R = \frac{2 * A_{R1}}{2 * A_{R1} + A_{D1} + A_{D2}} * 100$$

$$= \frac{2 * 270}{(2 * 270) + 8710 + 8452} * 100 = \boxed{3.1\%}$$

c Donor baseline calculation

Formula $\%R = \frac{A_{R1} + A_{R2}}{A_{R1} + A_{R2} + A_{D1} + A_{D2}} * 100$

Donor baseline $= \frac{0 + 235}{0 + 235 + 7318 + 7215} * 100 = 1.6\%$

Post-transplant $= \frac{270 + 709}{270 + 709 + 8710 + 8452} * 100 = 5.4\%$

Corrected $Corrected\%CHM = 5.4\% - 1.6\% = \boxed{3.8\%}$

d Stutter percent calculation

Donor baseline $\%Stutter = \frac{A_{R2}}{A_{D1}} * 100$

Post-transplant $= \frac{235}{7318} * 100 = 3.2\%$

Stutter contribution $Stutter\ area = \%stutter * A_{D1}$

$= 3.2\% * 8710 = 280$

Peak area correction $CorrectedA_{R2} = A_{R2(actual)} - A_{R2(stutter)}$

$= 709 - 280 = 429$

$$Corrected\%R = \frac{270 + 429}{270 + 429 + 8710 + 8452} * 100 = \boxed{3.9\%}$$

Figure 56.10 Example of chimerism analysis affected by a co-localized stutter peak. (**a**) Electropherograms of a recipient, donor, and post-transplant sample (post-tx) at the TH01 locus (CTTv, Promega Corp.) are shown. Below each peak the *box* indicates the repeat number (al), size in base pairs (sz), and area (ar). Stutter peaks ($n-1$) are indicated for the donor and recipient. In the post-transplant sample recipient allele 2 (R2) co-localizes with the stutter peak from donor allele 1 (Stutter + R2). Using all the peak areas in a standard chimerism formula would overestimate the percent recipient if an adjustment is not performed. Several adjustments to the chimerism calculation for stutter are shown in b, c, and d. For all three alternative methods, the final percent recipient (%R) result is given. (**b**) The heterozygous allele estimate method (b) assumes that the contribution of the R2 allele to the stutter + R2 peak area is similar to the area of R1. Thus, two times the area of R1 is used in the formula instead of the area of R1 plus the area of R2. (**c**) The donor baseline calculation method (c) uses the donor electropherogram to calculate the stutter contribution to the chimerism calculation by using the same chimerism formula used for post-transplant samples (formula). The corresponding peak areas from the donor baseline and the post-transplant electropherograms are used to calculate chimerism. The value from the donor baseline only represents the stutter contribution. Since this value is a percent and not an area it can be subtracted from the total post-transplant chimerism calculation to obtain the corrected chimerism (Corrected %CHM). (**d**) A stutter percent calculation is shown. In this example, the area of the stutter peak relative to the area of D1 is calculated as a percent (%Stutter). A standard average percent for the laboratory can be substituted if desired. Using the D1 peak area in the post-transplant sample, the %Stutter is used to calculate the contribution of stutter to the Stutter + R2 peak. The corrected area of R2 is used in the formula from (c) to calculate the final corrected percent chimerism. All three methods yield similar results for this case

Chromosomal Abnormalities

Chromosomal abnormalities are common in hematologic malignancies and may affect identity testing results if the locus used for chimerism analysis is present on the aberrant chromosome. Chromosomal abnormalities may be identified by cytogenetic analysis. If loci used for chimerism analysis are on the aberrant chromosome(s), the locus/loci should be avoided for chimerism analysis in the specific donor–recipient pair. On occasion unusual amplification patterns may provide evidence of abnormalities such as unequal amplification due to extra chromosomes or chromosomal deletions (Fig. 56.2). Chromosomal abnormalities also can arise after treatment. Such abnormalities have been reported and may produce unexpected or unusual post-transplant allele patterns and chimerism analysis results that are not consistent with the clinical status of the patient [103]. The use of multiple loci to calculate chimerism can minimize the potential impact of chromosomal abnormalities.

Doublet Peaks

Non-template addition of an extra nucleotide, usually an adenosine (A), at the 3′ end of PCR products is a known occurrence with DNA polymerases, particularly Taq [80]. This adenylation results in a PCR product that is 1 bp longer than the DNA template sequence. The degree of adenylation is dependent on the sequence of the template strand. Incomplete addition of A nucleotides can occur if too much DNA template is used. Addition of the A can be favored with a final incubation step at 60 °C at the end of the PCR reaction. If not all the PCR products have an extra A, this will lead to the appearance of split, or doublet, peaks. Usually this affects all the allele peaks at a particular locus. It is best to optimize reaction conditions to prevent incomplete adenylation, but if not possible and the peak areas of such doublet peaks are used to calculate the percent recipient, the areas of both parts of each peak should be summed and used for manual calculations (Fig. 56.11).

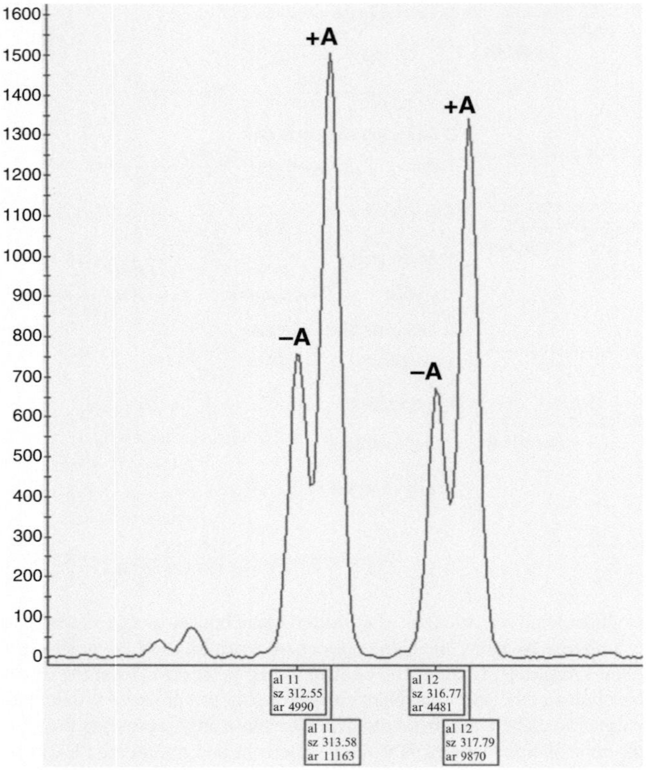

Figure 56.11 Non-template addition of an extra nucleotide, usually an adenosine (A), results in a PCR product that is 1 bp longer than the DNA template sequence. Heterozygous alleles of 11 and 12 repeats are shown, each with +A/–A doublet peaks

Reports

General molecular reporting guidelines should be followed for the reporting of chimerism results [104]. If pre-transplant testing is done, a report should be issued indicating that at least one informative locus that distinguishes recipient from donor DNA was identified. This pre-transplant report serves to inform the clinicians that the pre-transplant samples have been obtained and the pre-transplant analysis was successful. Post-transplant reports should report the %D rounded to the nearest integer for each specimen type tested; ideally peripheral blood and lineage-specific cellular subsets should be reported together in a single report to allow for easy visualization and longitudinal comparison by the clinicians. For two donor transplants the identification numbers for each donor should be provided along with the percent of each donor chimerism as well as the overall total percent donor chimerism. If the result of any sample or cellular subset had a compromised limit of detection, this should be noted in the report. The report is a method of communication between the laboratory and the clinicians; therefore, each laboratory should determine the information and format that are most valuable to their clinicians. In cases where mixed chimerism is detected or only donor (complete engraftment) is detected the report interpretation will reflect these results. However, there are a few possible results where a nonstandard interpretation is needed (see below).

Bone Marrow Specimens

When normocellular bone marrow is tested for chimerism, the finding of 1–3 % recipient DNA is very frequent. This is because there are non-hematopoietic cells, for example stromal cells, in the marrow. Thus, while mixed chimerism is commonly detected in bone marrow, low level chimerism is not likely to be clinically significant. Histologic and clinical correlation is always important. In particular, when the marrow is hypocellular the %R can be artificially elevated because the relative contribution of non-hematopoietic cells to the total DNA is high. In this situation an interpretive statement such as the following is recommended: "In the context of the concurrent bone marrow histologic evaluation demonstrating a hypocellular marrow, this chimerism result may not accurately reflect the percent of recipient hematopoietic cells due to the potential relative overrepresentation of non-hematopoietic elements in the bone marrow aspirate." This scenario should be considered whenever a bone marrow is tested and the donor chimerism is decreased (recipient increased) and there is no evidence of relapse.

Discordant Chimerism Result Between Blood and T-Cell Subset

When peripheral blood DNA is tested alongside a T cell subset, the detection of recipient DNA in T cells should by default imply that recipient DNA is present in whole blood. Occasionally recipient DNA is detected in T cells only and not in whole blood because T cells are only a subset of all nucleated blood cells so the overall level of chimerism in blood may be below the analytical sensitivity of the assay. This commonly occurs when the %R in the T cells is low and/or when the T cells represent a small proportion of all nucleated cells, which is a common scenario in the first few months after HSCT. The interpretation in the report should reflect this false-negative result rather than report complete donor engraftment. The opposite is not true. If recipient DNA is detected in the peripheral blood, but not the T cells then this simply means that the cells of recipient origin are not of T cell lineage. Interpretation of both "discordant" results should be made in the context of clinical and histologic correlation. For example, low levels of recipient T cells usually indicate incomplete donor engraftment, but persistence or reemergence of recipient T cells in a patient with a T cell malignancy may indicate residual disease or relapse.

Data Management and Quality Control

Chimerism analysis poses several unique clerical and data management issues for the clinical laboratory. The laboratory must have a mechanism to match donor and recipient pre-transplant samples and track the results of pre-transplant testing for use in post-transplant testing. Subsequently, the results of repeated post-transplant testing for each patient needs to be easily accessible for review with each new sample and for longitudinal assessment of engraftment trends. Specimen and result tracking can be accomplished with a well-organized paper folder system or electronically using software such as ChimerMarker (SoftGenetics). Longitudinal assessment of a patient's chimerism results enables critical evaluation of the significance of changes over time for each sample type (blood, T-cells, bone marrow, etc.) [100].

Quality control is inherent to chimerism analysis because identity testing is performed on each sample. A pre-transplant buccal sample in addition to the recipient blood can confirm that the recipient and donor DNA samples are properly identified. Quality control at the DNA level for specimen switching is inherent for all post-transplant samples since the expected genotypes are known and the patients are repeatedly tested over time so that any unexpected result, such as different alleles, is immediately noted and investigated. If multiplex primer sets are used for post-transplant sample amplification, it is important to consider whether a small peak seen in one fluorophore is a true peak rather than a bleed-through from another fluorophore window. Proficiency testing for chimerism analysis is available from the CAP in the ME survey.

Conclusion

The monitoring of chimerism after HSCT has become routine to confirm engraftment and detect and monitor mixed chimerism. The use of chimerism analysis and its clinical utility are different for myeloablative and RI-HSCT. Chimerism analysis has clinical utility in guiding the use of therapeutic interventions such as DLI to treat or prevent relapse or graft loss. Although many methods have been applied, PCR amplification of STR loci is the method of choice because it is informative, quantitative, relatively rapid, and sensitive. While the methodology is technically straightforward, the implementation, analysis, and reporting of results are more complicated. The clinical importance of chimerism results warrants the effort required by the laboratory for validation and performance of the test.

References

1. Dubovsky J, Daxberger H, Fritsch G, et al. Kinetics of chimerism during the early post-transplant period in pediatric patients with malignant and non-malignant hematologic disorders: implications for timely detection of engraftment, graft failure and rejection. Leukemia. 1999;2059(13):60–9.
2. Mackinnon S, Barnett L, Bourhis JH, Black P, Heller G, O'Reilly RJ. Myeloid and lymphoid chimerism after T-cell-depleted bone marrow transplantation: evaluation of conditioning regimens using the polymerase chain reaction to amplify human minisatellite regions of genomic DNA. Blood. 1992;80:3235–41.
3. Chalmers EA, Sproul AM, Mills KI, et al. Effect of radiation dose on the development of mixed haemopoietic chimerism following T cell-depleted allogeneic bone marrow transplantation. Bone Marrow Transplant. 1992;10:425–30.
4. Valcarcel D, Martino R, Caballero D, et al. Chimerism analysis following allogeneic peripheral blood stem cell transplantation with reduced-intensity conditioning. Bone Marrow Transplant. 2003;31:387–92.
5. Baron F, Baker JE, Storb R, et al. Kinetics of engraftment in patients with hematologic malignancies given allogeneic hematopoietic cell transplantation after nonmyeloablative conditioning. Blood. 2004;104:2254–62.
6. Mohty M, Avinens O, Faucher C, Viens P, Blaise D, Eliaou JF. Predictive factors and impact of full donor T-cell chimerism after reduced intensity conditioning allogeneic stem cell transplantation. Haematologica. 2007;92:1004–6.
7. Offit K, Burns JP, Cunningham I, et al. Cytogenetic analysis of chimerism and leukemia relapse in chronic myelogenous leukemia patients after T cell-depleted bone marrow transplantation. Blood. 1990;75:1346–55.
8. van Leeuwen JE, van Tol MJ, Joosten AM, et al. Persistence of host-type hematopoiesis after allogeneic bone marrow transplantation for leukemia is significantly related to the recipient's age and/or the conditioning regimen, but it is not associated with an increased risk of relapse. Blood. 1994;83:3059–67.
9. Mickelson DM, Sproat L, Dean R, et al. Comparison of donor chimerism following myeloablative and nonmyeloablative allogeneic hematopoietic SCT. Bone Marrow Transplant. 2011;46:84–9.
10. Sugita J, Tanaka J, Hashimoto A, et al. Influence of conditioning regimens and stem cell sources on donor-type chimerism early after stem cell transplantation. Ann Hematol. 2008;87:1003–8.
11. Salit RB, Fowler DH, Wilson WH, et al. Dose-adjusted EPOCH-rituximab combined with fludarabine provides an effective bridge to reduced-intensity allogeneic hematopoietic stem-cell transplantation in patients with lymphoid malignancies. J Clin Oncol. 2012;30:830–6.
12. Frassoni F, Strada P, Sessarego M, et al. Mixed chimerism after allogeneic marrow transplantation for leukaemia: correlation with dose of total body irradiation and graft-versus-host disease. Bone Marrow Transplant. 1990;5:235–40.
13. Mohr B, Koch R, Thiede C, Kroschinsky F, Ehninger G, Bornhauser M. CD34+ cell dose, conditioning regimen and prior chemotherapy: factors with significant impact on the early kinetics of donor chimerism after allogeneic hematopoietic cell transplantation. Bone Marrow Transplant. 2004;34:949–54.
14. Carvallo C, Geller N, Kurlander R, et al. Prior chemotherapy and allograft CD34+ dose impact donor engraftment following nonmyeloablative allogeneic stem cell transplantation in patients with solid tumors. Blood. 2004;103:1560–3.
15. Moscardo F, Sanz J, Senent L, et al. Impact of hematopoietic chimerism at day +14 on engraftment after unrelated donor umbilical cord blood transplantation for hematologic malignancies. Haematologica. 2009;94:827–32.

16. Barker JN, Weisdorf DJ, DeFor TE, et al. Transplantation of 2 partially HLA-matched umbilical cord blood units to enhance engraftment in adults with hematologic malignancy. Blood. 2005;105:1343–7.
17. Ballen KK, Spitzer TR, Yeap BY, et al. Double unrelated reduced-intensity umbilical cord blood transplantation in adults. Biol Blood Marrow Transplant. 2007;13:82–9.
18. Gutman JA, Turtle CJ, Manley TJ, et al. Single-unit dominance after double-unit umbilical cord blood transplantation coincides with a specific CD8+ T-cell response against the nonengrafted unit. Blood. 2010;115:757–65.
19. Ramirez P, Wagner JE, Defor TE, et al. Factors predicting single-unit predominance after double umbilical cord blood transplantation. Bone Marrow Transplant. 2012;47(6):799–803.
20. Haspel RL, Kao G, Yeap BY, et al. Preinfusion variables predict the predominant unit in the setting of reduced-intensity double cord blood transplantation. Bone Marrow Transplant. 2008;41: 523–9.
21. Yen HJ, Chiou TJ, Hung GY, et al. Long-term mixed full-donor chimerism with dominance reversion after a double-unit cord blood transplant. Eur J Haematol. 2008;80:366–7.
22. Mattsson J, Ringden O, Storb R. Graft failure after allogeneic hematopoietic cell transplantation. Biol Blood Marrow Transplant. 2008;14:165–70.
23. Spellman S, Bray R, Rosen-Bronson S, et al. The detection of donor-directed, HLA-specific alloantibodies in recipients of unrelated hematopoietic cell transplantation is predictive of graft failure. Blood. 2010;115:2704–8.
24. Wolff SN. Second hematopoietic stem cell transplantation for the treatment of graft failure, graft rejection or relapse after allogeneic transplantation. Bone Marrow Transplant. 2002;29:545–52.
25. Hill RS, Petersen FB, Storb R, et al. Mixed hematologic chimerism after allogeneic marrow transplantation for severe aplastic anemia is associated with a higher risk of graft rejection and a lessened incidence of acute graft-versus-host disease. Blood. 1986;67:811–6.
26. Matthes-Martin S, Lion T, Haas OA, et al. Lineage-specific chimaerism after stem cell transplantation in children following reduced intensity conditioning: potential predictive value of NK cell chimaerism for late graft rejection. Leukemia. 2003;17:1934–42.
27. Svenberg P, Mattsson J, Ringden O, Uzunel M. Allogeneic hematopoietic SCT in patients with non-malignant diseases, and importance of chimerism. Bone Marrow Transplant. 2009;44:757–63.
28. Balon J, Halaburda K, Bieniaszewska M, et al. Early complete donor hematopoietic chimerism in peripheral blood indicates the risk of extensive graft-versus-host disease. Bone Marrow Transplant. 2005;35:1083–8.
29. van Besien K, Dew A, Lin S, et al. Patterns and kinetics of T-cell chimerism after allo transplant with alemtuzumab-based conditioning: mixed chimerism protects from GVHD, but does not portend disease recurrence. Leuk Lymphoma. 2009;50:1809–17.
30. Lamba R, Abella E, Kukuruga D, et al. Mixed hematopoietic chimerism at day 90 following allogenic myeloablative stem cell transplantation is a predictor of relapse and survival. Leukemia. 2004;18:1681–6.
31. Zeiser R, Spyridonidis A, Wasch R, et al. Evaluation of immunomodulatory treatment based on conventional and lineage-specific chimerism analysis in patients with myeloid malignancies after myeloablative allogeneic hematopoietic cell transplantation. Leukemia. 2005;19:814–21.
32. Alpdogan O, van den Brink MR. Immune tolerance and transplantation. Semin Oncol. 2012;39:629–42.
33. Mackinnon S, Barnett L, Heller G, O'Reilly RJ. Minimal residual disease is more common in patients who have mixed T-cell chimerism after bone marrow transplantation for chronic myelogenous leukemia. Blood. 1994;83:3409–16.
34. Radich JP, Gehly G, Gooley T, et al. Polymerase chain reaction detection of the BCR-ABL fusion transcript after allogeneic marrow transplantation for chronic myeloid leukemia: results and implications in 346 patients. Blood. 1995;85:2632–8.
35. Horn B, Soni S, Khan S, et al. Feasibility study of preemptive withdrawal of immunosuppression based on chimerism testing in children undergoing myeloablative allogeneic transplantation for hematologic malignancies. Bone Marrow Transplant. 2009;43: 469–76.
36. Roman J, Serrano J, Jimenez A, et al. Myeloid mixed chimerism is associated with relapse in bcr-abl positive patients after unmanipulated allogeneic bone marrow transplantation for chronic myelogenous leukemia. Haematologica. 2000;85:173–80.
37. Thiede C, Bornhauser M, Oelschlagel U, et al. Sequential monitoring of chimerism and detection of minimal residual disease after allogeneic blood stem cell transplantation (BSCT) using multiplex PCR amplification of short tandem repeat-markers. Leukemia. 2001;15:293–302.
38. Bader P, Kreyenberg H, Hoelle W, et al. Increasing mixed chimerism defines a high-risk group of childhood acute myelogenous leukemia patients after allogeneic stem cell transplantation where preemptive immunotherapy may be effective. Bone Marrow Transplant. 2004;33:815–21.
39. Miflin G, Stainer CJ, Carter GI, Byrne JL, Haynes AP, Russell NH. Comparative serial quantitative measurements of chimaerism following unmanipulated allogeneic transplantation of peripheral blood stem cells and bone marrow. Br J Haematol. 1999;107:429–40.
40. Ortega M, Escudero T, Caballin MR, Olive T, Ortega JJ, Coll MD. Follow-up of chimerism in children with hematological diseases after allogeneic hematopoietic progenitor cell transplants. Bone Marrow Transplant. 1999;24:81–7.
41. Choi SJ, Lee KH, Lee JH, et al. Prognostic value of hematopoietic chimerism in patients with acute leukemia after allogeneic bone marrow transplantation: a prospective study. Bone Marrow Transplant. 2000;26:327–32.
42. Schattenberg A, De Witte T, Salden M, et al. Mixed hematopoietic chimerism after allogeneic transplantation with lymphocyte-depleted bone marrow is not associated with a higher incidence of relapse. Blood. 1989;73:1367–72.
43. Huss R, Deeg HJ, Gooley T, et al. Effect of mixed chimerism on graft-versus-host disease, disease recurrence and survival after HLA-identical marrow transplantation for aplastic anemia or chronic myelogenous leukemia. Bone Marrow Transplant. 1996;18:767–76.
44. Gardiner N, Lawler M, O'Riordan J, DeArce M, Humphries P, McCann SR. Persistent donor chimaerism is consistent with disease-free survival following BMT for chronic myeloid leukaemia. Bone Marrow Transplant. 1997;20:235–41.
45. Bader P, Beck J, Frey A, et al. Serial and quantitative analysis of mixed hematopoietic chimerism by PCR in patients with acute leukemias allows the prediction of relapse after allogeneic BMT. Bone Marrow Transplant. 1998;21:487–95.
46. Bader P, Klingebiel T, Schaudt A, et al. Prevention of relapse in pediatric patients with acute leukemias and MDS after allogeneic SCT by early immunotherapy initiated on the basis of increasing mixed chimerism: a single center experience of 12 children. Leukemia. 1999;13:2079–86.
47. Bader P, Kreyenberg H, Hoelle W, et al. Increasing mixed chimerism is an important prognostic factor for unfavorable outcome in children with acute lymphoblastic leukemia after allogeneic stem-cell transplantation: possible role for pre-emptive immunotherapy? J Clin Oncol. 2004;22:1696–705.
48. Giralt S, Thall PF, Khouri I, et al. Melphalan and purine analog-containing preparative regimens: reduced-intensity conditioning for patients with hematologic malignancies undergoing allogeneic progenitor cell transplantation. Blood. 2001;97:631–7.

49. Slavin S, Nagler A, Naparstek E, et al. Nonmyeloablative stem cell transplantation and cell therapy as an alternative to conventional bone marrow transplantation with lethal cytoreduction for the treatment of malignant and nonmalignant hematologic diseases. Blood. 1998;91:756–63.
50. Sykes M, Preffer F, McAfee S, et al. Mixed lymphohaemopoietic chimerism and graft-versus-lymphoma effects after non-myeloablative therapy and HLA-mismatched bone-marrow transplantation. Lancet. 1999;353:1755–9.
51. Childs R, Clave E, Contentin N, et al. Engraftment kinetics after nonmyeloablative allogeneic peripheral blood stem cell transplantation: full donor T-cell chimerism precedes alloimmune responses. Blood. 1999;94:3234–41.
52. Reshef R, Hexner EO, Loren AW, et al. Early donor chimerism levels predict relapse and survival after allogeneic stem-cell transplantation with reduced intensity conditioning. Biol Blood Marrow Transplant. 2014;20:1758–66.
53. Antin JH, Childs R, Filipovich AH, et al. Establishment of complete and mixed donor chimerism after allogeneic lymphohematopoietic transplantation: recommendations from a workshop at the 2001 Tandem Meetings of the International Bone Marrow Transplant Registry and the American Society of Blood and Marrow Transplantation. Biol Blood Marrow Transplant. 2001; 7:473–85.
54. Koreth J, Kim HT, Nikiforow S, et al. Donor chimerism early after reduced-intensity conditioning hematopoietic stem cell transplantation predicts relapse and survival. Biol Blood Marrow Transplant. 2014;20:1516–21.
55. Peterlin P, Delaunay J, Guillaume T, et al. Complete donor T cell chimerism predicts lower relapse incidence after standard double umbilical cord blood reduced-intensity conditioning regimen allogeneic transplantation in adults. Biol Blood Marrow Transplant. 2015;21:180–4.
56. Mapara MY, Kim YM, Wang SP, Bronson R, Sachs DH, Sykes M. Donor lymphocyte infusions mediate superior graft-versus-leukemia effects in mixed compared to fully allogeneic chimeras: a critical role for host antigen-presenting cells. Blood. 2002;100: 1903–9.
57. Spitzer TR, McAfee S, Sackstein R, et al. Intentional induction of mixed chimerism and achievement of antitumor responses after nonmyeloablative conditioning therapy and HLA-matched donor bone marrow transplantation for refractory hematologic malignancies. Biol Blood Marrow Transplant. 2000;6:309–20.
58. Peggs KS, Kayani I, Edwards N, et al. Donor lymphocyte infusions modulate relapse risk in mixed chimeras and induce durable salvage in relapsed patients after T-cell-depleted allogeneic transplantation for Hodgkin's lymphoma. J Clin Oncol. 2011;29:971–8.
59. Bader P, Niethammer D, Willasch A, Kreyenberg H, Klingebiel T. How and when should we monitor chimerism after allogeneic stem cell transplantation? Bone Marrow Transplant. 2005;35:107–19.
60. Dey BR, McAfee S, Colby C, et al. Impact of prophylactic donor leukocyte infusions on mixed chimerism, graft-versus-host disease, and antitumor response in patients with advanced hematologic malignancies treated with nonmyeloablative conditioning and allogeneic bone marrow transplantation. Biol Blood Marrow Transplant. 2003;9:320–9.
61. Massenkeil G, Nagy M, Lawang M, et al. Reduced intensity conditioning and prophylactic DLI can cure patients with high-risk acute leukaemias if complete donor chimerism can be achieved. Bone Marrow Transplant. 2003;31:339–45.
62. Mohamedbhai SG, Edwards N, Morris EC, Mackinnon S, Thomson KJ, Peggs KS. Predominant or complete recipient T-cell chimerism following alemtuzumab-based allogeneic transplantation is reversed by donor lymphocytes and not associated with graft failure. Br J Haematol. 2012;156:516–22.
63. Shatry A, Levy RB. In situ activation and expansion of host tregs: a new approach to enhance donor chimerism and stable engraftment in major histocompatibility complex-matched allogeneic hematopoietic cell transplantation. Biol Blood Marrow Transplant. 2009;15:785–94.
64. Zetterquist H, Mattsson J, Uzunel M, et al. Mixed chimerism in the B cell lineage is a rapid and sensitive indicator of minimal residual disease in bone marrow transplant recipients with pre-B cell acute lymphoblastic leukemia. Bone Marrow Transplant. 2000;25:843–51.
65. Mattsson J, Uzunel M, Tammik L, Aschan J, Ringden O. Leukemia lineage-specific chimerism analysis is a sensitive predictor of relapse in patients with acute myeloid leukemia and myelodysplastic syndrome after allogeneic stem cell transplantation. Leukemia. 2001;15:1976–85.
66. Lion T, Daxberger H, Dubovsky J, et al. Analysis of chimerism within specific leukocyte subsets for detection of residual or recurrent leukemia in pediatric patients after allogeneic stem cell transplantation. Leukemia. 2001;15:307–10.
67. Bornhauser M, Oelschlaegel U, Platzbecker U, et al. Monitoring of donor chimerism in sorted CD34+ peripheral blood cells allows the sensitive detection of imminent relapse after allogeneic stem cell transplantation. Haematologica. 2009;94:1613–7.
68. Serrano J, Roman J, Sanchez J, et al. Molecular analysis of lineage-specific chimerism and minimal residual disease by RT-PCR of p210(BCR-ABL) and p190(BCR-ABL) after allogeneic bone marrow transplantation for chronic myeloid leukemia: increasing mixed myeloid chimerism and p190(BCR-ABL) detection precede cytogenetic relapse. Blood. 2000;95: 2659–65.
69. Kroger N, Zagrivnaja M, Schwartz S, et al. Kinetics of plasma-cell chimerism after allogeneic stem cell transplantation by highly sensitive real-time PCR based on sequence polymorphism and its value to quantify minimal residual disease in patients with multiple myeloma. Exp Hematol. 2006;34:688–94.
70. Haddad E, Le Deist F, Aucouturier P, et al. Long-term chimerism and B-cell function after bone marrow transplantation in patients with severe combined immunodeficiency with B cells: a single-center study of 22 patients. Blood. 1999;94:2923–30.
71. Andreani M, Manna M, Lucarelli G, et al. Persistence of mixed chimerism in patients transplanted for the treatment of thalassemia. Blood. 1996;87:3494–9.
72. Hsieh MM, Kang EM, Fitzhugh CD, et al. Allogeneic hematopoietic stem-cell transplantation for sickle cell disease. N Engl J Med. 2009;361:2309–17.
73. Stikvoort A, Gertow J, Sundin M, Remberger M, Mattsson J, Uhlin M. Chimerism patterns of long-term stable mixed chimeras posthematopoietic stem cell transplantation in patients with non-malignant diseases: follow-up of long-term stable mixed chimerism patients. Biol Blood Marrow Transplant. 2013;19:838–44.
74. Sala-Torra O, Hanna C, Loken MR, et al. Evidence of donor-derived hematologic malignancies after hematopoietic stem cell transplantation. Biol Blood Marrow Transplant. 2006;12:511–7.
75. Schoniger-Hekele M, Muller C, Kramer L, et al. Graft versus host disease after orthotopic liver transplantation documented by analysis of short tandem repeat polymorphisms. Digestion. 2006;74:169–73.
76. Shin CR, Nathan J, Alonso M, et al. Incidence of acute and chronic graft-versus-host disease and donor T-cell chimerism after small bowel or combined organ transplantation. J Pediatr Surg. 2011; 46:1732–8.
77. Thiede C. Diagnostic chimerism analysis after allogeneic stem cell transplantation: new methods and markers. Am J Pharmacogenomics. 2004;4:177–87.
78. Dewald G, Stallard R, Al Saadi A, et al. A multicenter investigation with interphase fluorescence in situ hybridization using X- and Y-chromosome probes. Am J Med Genet. 1998;76:318–26.
79. Bennett P. Demystified … microsatellites. Mol Pathol. 2000;53: 177–83.

80. Butler JM. Forensic DNA typing: biology, technology, and genetics of STR markers. 2nd ed. New York: Academic; 2005.
81. Butler JM. Genetics and genomics of core short tandem repeat loci used in human identity testing. J Forensic Sci. 2006;51: 253–65.
82. Gineikiene E, Stoskus M, Griskevicius L. Recent advances in quantitative chimerism analysis. Expert Rev Mol Diagn. 2009; 9:817–32.
83. Van Deerlin VM, Leonard DG. Bone marrow engraftment analysis after allogeneic bone marrow transplantation. Clin Lab Med. 2000;20:197–225.
84. Clark JR, Scott SD, Jack AL, Lee H, Mason J, Carter GI, Pearce L, Jackson T, Clouston H, Sproul A, Keen L, Molloy K, Folarin N, Whitby L, Snowden JA, Reilly JT, Barnett D. Monitoring of chimerism following allogeneic haematopoietic stem cell transplantation (HSCT): technical recommendations for the use of short tandem repeat (STR) based techniques, on behalf of the United Kingdom National External Quality Assessment Service for Leucocyte Immunophenotyping Chimerism Working Group. Br J Haematol. 2015;168(1):26–37.
85. Fehse B, Chukhlovin A, Kuhlcke K, et al. Real-time quantitative Y chromosome-specific PCR (QYCS-PCR) for monitoring hematopoietic chimerism after sex-mismatched allogeneic stem cell transplantation. J Hematother Stem Cell Res. 2001;10:419–25.
86. Oliver DH, Thompson RE, Griffin CA, Eshleman JR. Use of single nucleotide polymorphisms (SNP) and real-time polymerase chain reaction for bone marrow engraftment analysis. J Mol Diagn. 2000;2:202–8.
87. Fredriksson M, Barbany G, Liljedahl U, Hermanson M, Kataja M, Syvanen AC. Assessing hematopoietic chimerism after allogeneic stem cell transplantation by multiplexed SNP genotyping using microarrays and quantitative analysis of SNP alleles. Leukemia. 2004;18:255–66.
88. Alizadeh M, Bernard M, Danic B, et al. Quantitative assessment of hematopoietic chimerism after bone marrow transplantation by real-time quantitative polymerase chain reaction. Blood. 2002;99: 4618–25.
89. Lion T. Summary: reports on quantitative analysis of chimerism after allogeneic stem cell transplantation by PCR amplification of microsatellite markers and capillary electrophoresis with fluorescence detection. Leukemia. 2003;17:252–4.
90. Thiede C, Bornhauser M, Ehninger G. Evaluation of STR informativity for chimerism testing—comparative analysis of 27 STR systems in 203 matched related donor recipient pairs. Leukemia. 2004;18:248–54.
91. Watzinger F, Lion T, Steward C, Eurochimerism C. The RSD code: proposal for a nomenclature of allelic configurations in STR-PCR-based chimerism testing after allogeneic stem cell transplantation. Leukemia. 2006;20:1448–52.
92. Lion T, Watzinger F, Preuner S, et al. The EuroChimerism concept for a standardized approach to chimerism analysis after allogeneic stem cell transplantation. Leukemia. 2012;26(8):1821–8.
93. Berger B, Parson R, Clausen J, Berger C, Nachbaur D, Parson W. Chimerism in DNA of buccal swabs from recipients after allogeneic hematopoietic stem cell transplantations: implications for forensic DNA testing. Int J Legal Med. 2013;127(1):49–54.
94. Thiede C, Prange-Krex G, Freiberg-Richter J, Bornhauser M, Ehninger G. Buccal swabs but not mouthwash samples can be used to obtain pretransplant DNA fingerprints from recipients of allogeneic bone marrow transplants. Bone Marrow Transplant. 2000;25:575–7.
95. Rennert H, Leonard DG, Cushing M, Azurin C, Shore T. Avoiding pitfalls in bone marrow engraftment analysis: a case study highlighting the weakness of using buccal cells for determining a patient's constitutional genotype after hematopoietic stem cell transplantation. Cytotherapy. 2013;15:391–5.
96. Chen DP, Tseng CP, Tsai SH, Wu TL, Chang PY, Sun CF. Systematic analysis of stutters to enhance the accuracy of chimerism testing. Ann Clin Lab Sci. 2008;38:264–72.
97. Nollet F, Billiet J, Selleslag D, Criel A. Standardisation of multiplex fluorescent short tandem repeat analysis for chimerism testing. Bone Marrow Transplant. 2001;28:511–8.
98. Kristt D, Gesundheit B, Stein J, et al. Quantitative monitoring of multi-donor chimerism: a systematic, validated framework for routine analysis. Bone Marrow Transplant. 2010;45:137–47.
99. Tobiasson M, Olsson R, Hellstrom-Lindberg E, Mattsson J. Early detection of relapse in patients with myelodysplastic syndrome after allo-SCT. Bone Marrow Transplant. 2011;46(5): 719–26.
100. Kristt D, Stein J, Yaniv I, Klein T. Assessing quantitative chimerism longitudinally: technical considerations, clinical applications and routine feasibility. Bone Marrow Transplant. 2007;39:255–68.
101. Kristt D, Klein T. Reliability of quantitative chimerism results: assessment of sample performance using novel parameters. Leukemia. 2006;20:1169–72.
102. ChimerMarker User Manual. SoftGenetics LLC; 2011.
103. Zhou M, Sheldon S, Akel N, Killeen AA. Chromosomal aneuploidy in leukemic blast crisis: a potential source of error in interpretation of bone marrow engraftment analysis by VNTR amplification. Mol Diagn. 1999;4:153–7.
104. Gulley ML, Braziel RM, Halling KC, et al. Clinical laboratory reports in molecular pathology. Arch Pathol Lab Med. 2007;131: 852–63.

Specimen Identification Through DNA Analysis

57

Gregary Bocsi, Andrew Ricci, Gregory J. Tsongalis, and Vivianna M. Van Deerlin

Abstract

Specimen identification through DNA analysis is an approach to solve several conundrums that may arise during the course of routine laboratory testing. In this chapter methods for specimen identification by DNA analysis are described, including specimen selection and specimen preparation, genotyping approaches, and result interpretation. Clinical applications for these methods are discussed, and example cases demonstrate how the methods can be applied to solve relevant problems such as identification of misidentified specimens, unexpected tissue in a specimen, maternal contamination of a prenatal diagnostic specimen, diagnosis of donor-associated malignancies, graft-vs-host disease, as well as gestational trophoblastic disease.

Keywords

Identity testing • Specimen identification • Specimen misidentification • Hydatidiform mole • Molar pregnancy • Gestational trophoblastic disease • Graft-vs-host disease • Donor-associated malignancy • Floater • Macrodissection • Microdissection

Introduction

In 1995, television viewers around the world followed a criminal trial, *People of the State of California v. Orenthal James Simpson*, which introduced many viewers to some of the nuances of DNA testing. More recently, the film and television industries have incorporated identity testing or DNA analysis in many productions, further familiarizing the lay public with the concept of "DNA testing" for identification purposes. In 1997, one of the first case reports on the use of forensic DNA analysis for specimen identification was published [1]. While analysis of identity through DNA typing has its origins in parentage testing and forensic identity testing, similar techniques have also found clinical utility in pathology laboratories for a variety of sample identification applications [2–5]. Such applications include identification of the origin of mislabeled specimens [2], exclusion of a potential source for a surreptitious histologic "floater" in an anatomic pathology specimen [2, 4, 6], diagnosis of hydatidiform moles [7, 8], detection of maternal

G. Bocsi, D.O.
Department of Pathology, University of Colorado School of Medicine, Aurora, CO, USA

A. Ricci, M.D.
Department of Pathology, Hartford Hospital, Hartford, CT, USA

G.J. Tsongalis, Ph.D.
Department of Pathology, Geisel School of Medicine at Dartmouth, Lebanon, NH, USA

Norris Cotton Cancer Center, Dartmouth-Hitchcock Medical Center, Lebanon, NH, USA

V.M. Van Deerlin, M.D., Ph.D. (✉)
Pathology and Laboratory Medicine, Molecular Pathology Laboratory, Perelman School of Medicine, University of Pennsylvania, Philadelphia, PA, USA
e-mail: vivianna@upenn.edu

D.G.B. Leonard (ed.), *Molecular Pathology in Clinical Practice*, DOI 10.1007/978-3-319-19674-9_57

cell contamination in prenatal specimens [9, 10], identification of cell lines or research specimens [11], diagnosis of graft-vs-host disease (GVHD) [12], and identification of the origin of tumor cells in a transplant recipient [13].

Specimen misidentification is not a rare event in clinical practice. For prostate biopsies, the combined rate of type 1 (complete transposition between patients) and type 2 (contamination of a patient's tissue with that of other patients) errors has been estimated as 0.93 % or nearly 1 in 100 [14]. Recently, DNA testing helped to resolve biopsy misidentifications in a large multicenter clinical trial (The Reduction by Dutasteride of Prostate Cancer Events clinical trial) [15], and The Dark Report (http://www.darkreport.com/) has reported that a large Urology Group in New England approached a commercial laboratory to perform DNA testing on cheek swabs to confirm patient identity on *all* patients with a positive prostate biopsy [16]. On occasion a patient who questions a new cancer diagnosis requests DNA identification analysis of the tumor to confirm that the diagnostic specimen originated from the patient's body. A full description of the scientific principles and technologies for identity testing appears in Chap. 54. The practice of specimen identification through DNA analysis is well-established, but the cost-effectiveness of the use of these techniques must be determined on a case-by-case basis. This chapter focuses on identity testing issues and result interpretation specific to patient identification and related applications of identity testing in the clinical laboratory.

Methods for Specimen Identification

DNA typing exploits the polymorphic differences in DNA between individuals to resolve questions of identity. The first polymerase chain reaction (PCR) based DNA typing system to become commercially available was the AmpliType PM + DQA1 system from Applied Biosystems (formerly Perkin Elmer, Foster City, CA). This kit typed multiple loci simultaneously using a reverse dot blot procedure with an array of immobilized allele specific probes in a dot blot pattern on a strip of nylon membrane. The AmpliType PM+DQA1 amplification and typing kit was used routinely by many forensic laboratories, and it was applied to cases of clinical specimen identification as it could be used with many different specimen types [1, 17–19]. In recent decades, short tandem repeat (STR)-based methods have supplanted reverse dot blot methods, in part due to their greater discriminatory power. Single nucleotide polymorphism (SNP) analysis and mitochondrial DNA polymorphism analysis have some applications.

Short Tandem Repeat Analysis

Among methods of specimen identity testing, STR analysis has become the method of choice in most laboratories due to the convenience of several commercial assays, accessibility of equipment and genotyping software to assist with the analyses, and availability of technical resources and experience to facilitate the interpretation of results. The forensics community took the lead in defining panels of STRs (also known as microsatellites) leading to the development of the Combined DNA Index System (CODIS) loci originally selected by the US Federal Bureau of Investigation (FBI) for criminal identification investigations [20]. These loci have proven extremely useful because they exhibit not only polyallelism but also wide distribution of the different alleles across various racial and ethnic groups. Combined, these features allow STR-based testing to offer a great degree of discriminatory power for specimen identification.

For both forensic analysis and specimen identification, the ability to work with minute samples is important, as illustrated by the application of microdissection in resolution of tissue section "floater" cases (see below). STR-based methods employing PCR amplification of specific STR regions of the genome are applicable to small samples, permitting the interrogation of nucleic acids extracted even from samples with only a few cells as well as from partially degraded samples such as from formalin-fixed, paraffin-embedded (FFPE) tissue. Many STR polymorphisms are present in the human genome, and specific subsets are commercially available for identity testing purposes.

Multiplex primer sets are commercially available for amplification of STR loci (http://www.cstl.nist.gov/strbase/multiplx.htm) [20]. Such primers co-amplify multiple STR loci in a single reaction. Fluorescent labeling of the PCR primers at overlapping loci with different fluorophores allows multiplexing of STR loci which may have alleles that fall in the same size range. After amplification of the STR loci, fragment size analysis, usually by capillary electrophoresis, enables precise determination of the size of the polymorphisms at each locus for a specimen [2]. In general, two specimens are considered different when the alleles differ for at least one locus. The calculated probability that two individuals will share a set of STR alleles by chance depends upon the number of loci tested, as well as the ethnicity of the individual. Different alleles at as few as eight loci can quickly push the probability of two specimens matching by chance to less than 1 in 100,000,000, well below the number of patient specimens encountered in an entire year in a histology laboratory. Detailed information on STRs is available at http://www.cstl.nist.gov/strbase/.

Single Nucleotide Polymorphism Analysis

SNPs are the most common genetic variants in the human genome and occur approximately every 100–300 bases.

Each individual has an allelic profile at these sites. Several studies related to specimen identification have been published using SNP profiling by real-time PCR as an alternative to STR analysis [21, 22]. SNP analysis has advantages over STR analysis, including a lower cost per reaction, smaller target sequence which is more amenable to amplification in degraded specimens, and no requirement for capillary electrophoresis equipment. A disadvantage of SNP analysis is a lower power of discrimination for each marker thus requiring use of a larger number of markers. Which SNPs to detect and their population frequencies must be carefully considered. Currently, SNP analysis is not frequently used for specimen identification except in degraded specimens.

Mitochondrial DNA Polymorphism Analysis

Mitochondria contain a circular genome that is distinct from the nuclear genome. Within this genome are two noncoding regions, hypervariable regions I and II, which vary in their sequences and contain known polymorphisms. Indeed, for unrelated individuals, the mitochondrial DNA sequence will differ at multiple nucleotide positions. However, maternal relatives share mitochondrial sequences except for the presence of new mutations. Mitochondrial DNA polymorphism analysis therefore can be used both to exclude the possibility that an unknown sample matches a reference sample or that the sample is derived from a maternal relative of the reference sample. Because mitochondrial genomes are naturally amplified due to the presence of multiple mitochondria per cell and the circular DNA is more resistant to degradation, sequencing of mitochondrial DNA may prove useful as an alternative to STR typing of archival specimens with low DNA content and high DNA degradation [23, 24]. Mitochondrial DNA polymorphism analysis is not commonly used for clinical laboratory specimen identity analysis.

Clinical Applications

DNA analysis of polymorphic markers used in forensic identity and relationship testing can aid in the identification of specimens that are essential to proper management of a patient when the possibility of specimen misidentification has arisen. As the cost of STR-based identity testing decreases, it has been suggested that routine verification of the source of certain cancer-positive diagnostic specimens (e.g., prostate biopsies), may become a cost-effective approach for preventing medical errors resulting from a misidentified patient sample [25].

Specimen Identification

For patient safety and quality assurance purposes, clinical specimens are required to be labeled with two patient identifiers to assure the proper identification of the patient specimen and to associate each specimen with a correct patient. Examples of identifying information include patient name, date of birth, medical record number, demographic data, date/time of specimen collection, and laboratory identifiers such as a unique accession number. Despite written policies, training of personnel, and the careful attention of personnel collecting and handling specimens, sample mislabeling or switches occasionally occur. Tissue specimens may be mislabeled, co-mingled, or interchanged at the time of collection (i.e., multiple biopsies from the same or different patients) or during the various stages of tissue processing such as labeling of the blocks containing the tissue or the glass slides with sections of the tissue [1, 3, 15, 17, 26]. In a Q-probe study performed by the College of American Pathologists (CAP), mislabeling occurred in approximately 1 per 1,000 cases [26]. Sometimes, a patient will not believe a tissue diagnosis made on a sample submitted under the patient's name and will challenge a physician to prove that the tested and reported specimen was truly the patient's specimen.

Mislabeled or unlabeled clinical specimens remain familiar identification issues in clinical laboratories. According to regulatory standards, these improperly labeled or unlabeled specimens should not be tested by a clinical laboratory. The strict adherence to this standard varies by specific circumstances. On occasion, when the clinician can definitively document the identity of such a specimen and the specimen is irreplaceable, a laboratory makes an exception. Ideally, though, one rejects a mislabeled specimen in favor of a new, equivalent specimen. Unfortunately, some specimens are difficult or impossible to replace. For example, a replacement blood sample is rather easily obtained in most circumstances, unless the specimen was a timed or pretreatment specimen. On the other hand, in the anatomic pathology laboratory, tissue specimen recollection may be difficult or impossible and typically results in increased morbidity for a patient who must undergo a repeat procedure. Occasionally, the specimen itself may be so unique that it suggests its likely source. In the right circumstances, available DNA identity testing methods can confirm or exclude the source of a sample.

Histologic "Floaters"

Unfortunate occurrences that become critical challenges for the anatomic pathologist are tissue fragments referred to as "floaters." These tissue contaminants do not originate from the patient's specimen but become intermingled with it at some point between specimen collection and pathologist interpretation. Indeed, these small fragments of loose tissue may be "carried over" from one case to another during various tissue handling or processing steps in the laboratory. During gross dissection, a tissue fragment from one dissecting field can be brought to another by a scalpel blade, forceps, or improper cleaning between grossing of specimens from different patients. Later, during histologic processing (i.e., fixation, dehydration, impregnation, sectioning, or staining), a tissue fragment may literally or figuratively float away from its source and become associated with another specimen. Such specimen contamination may occur despite rigorous quality control procedures. In one study, cross contamination to blank slides occurred in 8 % of cases (most commonly during the staining process) [27].

In many cases, during the course of careful histological examination of a slide, an anatomic pathologist is able to confidently identify when an unexpected fragment of tissue is present and dismiss it from diagnostic consideration. This is more easily accomplished when the "floater" does not resemble the histology of the remaining tissue, is positively recognized as coming from another case, is physically distinct from the main mass of tissue on the slide, or presents incongruous histology [2, 4]. However, when the "floater" is a type of cell or tissue compatible with the expected specimen or is closely intermingled with the expected cells or tissue, it is difficult to exclude the possibility that it is part of the sample originating from the patient. In addition, a "floater" may be a few cells or a cluster of cells that are difficult to evaluate and definitively classify. A common scenario is a tissue section that includes a small number of malignant cells suspected to be "floaters" by a pathologist. The pathologist cannot simply ignore such cells, but definitive interpretation and reporting of their significance is not straightforward. In the past, when diagnostic certainty could not be assured because of potential "floater" contamination, clinical recommendations were limited to a cautionary note such as "advise close follow-up and short term rebiopsy if possible" or a similar disclaimer. Using identity testing methods and processing techniques to carefully separate regions of tissue on a slide, the relevance of a potential "floater" to the diagnosis can be resolved.

Identifying Donor Cells in a Transplant Recipient

Chapter 56 details the utility of identity testing in the setting of hematopoietic stem cell transplantation (HSCT). Identifying cells of donor origin in a transplant recipient can be useful in additional settings, such as a new post-transplant neoplasm or suspected graft-vs-host disease in the recipient.

Donor-Transmitted Malignancies

Donor origin cancer, including malignancies transmitted with the graft as well as tumors that develop within a graft, have been estimated to occur in 0.02–0.06 % of recipients [28–30]. Donor-transmitted malignancies are more common in solid organ transplants than in HSCT [13]. When a transplant recipient develops a malignancy in the transplanted organ or in another location, identification of the origin of the tumor (recipient or donor) is important for patient management and for identification of other individuals who may be at risk because they received other tissues or organs from the same donor. Donors with a history of cancer are usually excluded; however, in some cases the cancer is remote or is not recognized at the time of tissue donation.

To assess the origin of a tumor sample one must have DNA from the recipient, the donor, and the tumor; the tumor being of "unknown" identity. The STR allele genotypes of these samples are compared. Usually the explanted paraffin-embedded tissue, if available, is a good source of recipient DNA; alternatively, recipient buccal cells may be used. Donor DNA or blood may be banked in an HLA laboratory or a donor tissue sample may be available (e.g., donor gallbladder is usually available in liver transplant cases). Alternatively, the transplanted organ can serve this function with the caveat that recipient white blood cells may be admixed, which can complicate the assignment of donor alleles. Assessment of the tumor specimen depends on whether the tumor is in the transplanted organ or in another location because this will determine the expected origin of the DNA of the adjacent normal tissue. The tumor specimen (either a biopsy or excision) should be evaluated as a paraffin-embedded tissue (unless it is a blood-based malignancy) in order to separate tumor from adjacent normal tissue, if possible. When the tumor is within the transplanted organ, the presence of recipient-origin white blood cells will complicate the interpretation. In such cases, a judgment must be made based on the relative abundance of donor and recipient DNA; therefore, it is preferable to isolate the tumor for DNA extraction by macrodissection or microdissection. A tumor that is not in the transplanted organ is easier to interpret as the presence of donor DNA is not expected, and the presence of a significant amount of donor DNA will indicate a tumor of donor origin. Assessment of recipient blood to rule out the presence of circulating donor DNA is a helpful control.

In a sex mismatched transplant, origin of a tumor can be inferred by traditional karyotyping when one has a viable tissue specimen with proliferating cells. Fluorescent in situ hybridization (FISH) can play a role in the evaluation of sex mismatched transplant recipients if the available sample is fresh frozen tissue, a cytologic preparation, or formalin-fixed paraffin-embedded tissue as the presence of two X chromosomes vs one X and one Y chromosome in the tumor cells can exclude a donor of the opposite sex as the source.

Limitations of FISH include nuclear truncation artifacts, hybridization failures, and a reliance on single regions of chromosomes that may be altered in a malignancy.

Graft-vs-Host Disease

Graft-vs-host disease (GVHD) results when donor T cells recognize alloantigens expressed on host antigen-presenting cells and initiate an attack on host epithelial cells, damaging host tissue in a variety of possible anatomic locations including the skin, mouth, eyes, gastrointestinal tract, or liver. As such, skin, gastrointestinal tract, or liver abnormalities in the setting of an organ transplant or even certain types of blood transfusion can point to the possible diagnosis of GVHD. A National Institutes of Health working group recognized two main categories of GVHD: acute and chronic [31]. Diagnostic manifestations in the skin, mouth, eyes, female genitalia, esophagus, lungs, and connective tissues exist for both categories. Although not always mandatory for the diagnosis of GVHD, a biopsy can confirm the diagnosis.

While the donor T cells are nonneoplastic, they may be abundant in GVHD. Although low levels of donor T cell chimerism may be observed in the peripheral blood of liver transplant recipients during the first month after transplantation [32], a study of liver transplant associated GVHD found T cell macrochimerism [33] of at least 4 % in the peripheral blood of patients with histologically diagnosed GVHD after transplant. Hence, DNA-based identity testing of a specimen with T cells can confirm donor origin and provide support for a diagnosis of GVHD.

Specimens for confirmation of GVHD are similar to specimens for assessment of a donor-associated malignancy, with selection of a recipient specimen, the "unknown" specimen suspected of containing the inflammatory cells of GVHD (usually blood or epithelium), and a donor specimen. Results supporting a diagnosis of GVHD would consist of the presence of donor DNA at a significant level in a specimen where only recipient DNA is expected, whereas detection of only recipient DNA indicates that GVHD is less likely. A negative result (no donor DNA detected) requires careful interpretation when only minimal inflammatory cells are present in the "unknown" specimen, as this can represent a false-negative result.

Maternal Cell Contamination of Prenatal Specimens

Clinical laboratories performing prenatal diagnostic testing of chorionic villus sampling (CVS) or amniocentesis specimens, or of products of conception face the risk of inaccurate prenatal diagnosis due to the presence of maternal cells in the specimen. If the specimen is mistakenly thought to contain only fetal cells, contaminating maternal cells may lead to a misdiagnosis even when the level of contamination is seemingly modest (1–2 %) [34]. Even with only approximately 10 % of fetal cell preparations complicated by maternal cell contamination, the problem is so well recognized that maternal cell contamination assessment has been recommended for all prenatal specimens [35, 36]. Despite the recommendation, all laboratories performing prenatal genetic testing do not exclude maternal cell contamination for every prenatal specimen [37].

Sometimes there is frank maternal blood in an amniotic fluid sample, but low levels of contamination usually go unnoticed. Interestingly, culture conditions favor growth of amniocytes over contaminating maternal cells, resulting in less maternal cell contamination of amniotic fluid cultures compared to direct amniotic fluid specimens [38]. CVS specimens present a higher risk of maternal cell contamination because completely separating the fetal cells from the maternal decidua is difficult to accomplish by gross dissection.

STR analysis can be used to test DNA isolated from a fetal specimen with comparison to maternal DNA tested in parallel to determine if maternal alleles are present and if so, to approximate the percentage of maternal DNA [9, 10]. The percent contaminating maternal DNA is significant depending on the prenatal testing method and its sensitivity. A relatively insensitive method may not be affected by 10 % or less maternal contamination; however a very sensitive method could result in an incorrect interpretation due to the unintended presence of maternal DNA. Therefore, the significance of the level of maternal contamination is assessed in the context of the intended use of the prenatal specimen. Recommendations by the American College of Medical Genetics, the Clinical Laboratory Standards Institute, and the Clinical Molecular Genetics Society confirm the importance of maternal cell contamination testing in prenatal diagnosis. Detailed preanalytical, technical, interpretive, and reporting guidelines for maternal cell contamination testing are available [36].

Evaluation of Hydatidiform Moles

Aberrant fertilization of a normal or abnormal egg by one or more sperm can lead to the formation of a hydatidiform mole. A hydatidiform mole can be classified as either complete or partial. Complete hydatidiform moles occur when one (90 %) or two (10 %) sperm fertilize an anucleate ovum, and the proliferating gestational tissue is entirely paternally derived (i.e., androgenetic diploidy). A complete hydatidiform mole can be either homozygous, when a single sperm fertilizes an empty ovum and that sperm's haploid genetic material is duplicated, or heterozygous when two sperm fertilize an empty ovum. Partial hydatidiform moles arise from the fertilization of a single egg by two sperm and are triploid with both maternal and paternal genetic material (i.e., diandric triploid; usually 69XXX or 69XXY).

Differentiation of a hydatidiform mole from a non-molar specimen, as well as the type of hydatidiform mole, is important for clinical management of the patient because complete hydatidiform moles have a higher risk of developing into choriocarcinoma than do partial moles. Reliable diagnosis of hydatidiform moles based solely on morphology is challenging especially after early evacuation of a complete mole and in many instances of partial moles [39]. Ancillary techniques such as DNA ploidy analysis, immunohistochemistry, conventional karyotyping, and interphase FISH can inform the diagnosis, but have limitations [40]. Partial moles are triploid, so can be distinguished from a non-molar specimen by DNA ploidy analysis. In contrast, complete moles with a higher risk of choriocarcinoma are diploid and harder to distinguish from a non-molar specimen by DNA ploidy analysis. STR analysis definitively distinguishes complete moles, partial moles, and non-molar specimens.

As with other applications of identity testing in the clinical laboratory, STR analysis is the most commonly applied approach to compare the genotypes of the hydropic chorionic villi to those of the decidua (or maternal blood) to determine the genetic origin of the villi. For identity testing, chorionic villi are microdissected from maternal decidua. Significant contamination with decidua tissue will complicate analysis since a complete mole has no maternal DNA while a partial mole does. The maternal DNA for comparison can be obtained from maternal blood if available, or alternatively from microdissected decidua. Additional testing of paternal DNA, while not required, can help confirm the informative alleles in the molar tissue. Analysis of complete moles will identify only non-maternally derived homozygous or heterozygous alleles at multiple loci in the hydropic villi consistent with fertilization of an empty ovum [7, 8]. Analysis of partial moles will show three different alleles at multiple loci, one of maternal origin and two of paternal origin consistent with the fertilization of a normal egg by two sperm. Non-molar specimens are usually diploid with one maternal and one paternal allele (biparental diploidy). In many cases, if the maternal and molar tissue is adequately separated, visual inspection of the results of STR analysis can be diagnostic of a complete or partial hydatidiform mole.

Specimen Considerations

Specimen Selection and Documentation

The critical initial step in identity testing is selection of appropriate specimens to test, which are determined in consideration of the purpose for the testing and the questions needing to be answered. At a minimum there will be an unknown sample and a known sample. In some cases additional known samples for comparison from one or more individuals may be required (Table 57.1).

Table 57.1 Specimens frequently used for identity testing

Type of analysis	Typically tested specimens
Specimen identification	Unknown specimen
	Specimen confirmed to be from the known individual(s)
Histologic floater	Macrodissected floater tissue
	Main tissue on slide separated from floater tissue
	If available, additional specimen confirmed to have tissue from the known individual helps confirm the origin of the main tissue in the block
Pathogenic donor cells in a transplant recipient	Post-transplant tissue with suspected donor cells present
	Specimen with only recipient cells (e.g., pre-transplant blood, tissue, or buccal cells)
	Specimen with only donor cells
Maternal contamination of a prenatal diagnostic specimen	Prenatal specimen or products of conception
	Maternal specimen
Gestational trophoblastic disease	Gestational specimen with suspicious features, microdissected to enrich for gestational cells (villi)
	Maternal specimen (blood or carefully microdissected decidua)
	Paternal specimen (optional)

For specimen identification testing, the "unknown" DNA from the specimen is compared to "known" DNA from a specimen verified to be from the individual, such as a blood sample or a tissue block from a previous procedure. For mislabeled specimens, additional documentation of specimen handling and processing is useful. In contrast, for the identification of suspected floaters that are not consistent with the remainder of the specimen section, "unknown" DNA from microdissected floater tissue will be tested and compared to "known" DNA from an area of tissue containing tissue consistent with what is expected for the specimen. In this scenario it may also be prudent to analyze a verified alternative sample from the same individual as the current specimen in question as a further confirmation that the "known" DNA did, in fact, originate from the individual whose sample was contaminated by the floater. Confirmation of the actual source of the floater is unnecessary in most cases. In a case of two possibly switched samples, both are "unknown" and can be compared with two "known" samples from the two potential source individuals.

Analysis of maternal cell contamination of a fetal specimen requires a known maternal blood sample in addition to the "unknown" fetal sample. Similarly, diagnosis of a hydatidiform mole requires analysis of both chorionic villi and a known maternal sample. In the typical post-transplant scenario, analysis of the "unknown" tumor specimen is compared with the analysis of "known" specimens from the donor and recipient.

These are only general examples, some of which are illustrated in the cases described later. In fact, identity testing for sample identification is useful in a host of situations, each requiring careful specimen selection on a case by case basis to ensure that the tested specimens reflect the best choices from the available specimens, and that the results of testing those specimens will enable resolution of the clinical question.

Tissue Processing

While specimen handling and processing are major issues for certain types of molecular genetic testing, the use of smaller polymorphic markers allows identity testing to be performed on specimens that would be less than ideal for other clinical molecular tests. Frequently, identity testing for sample identification involves the use of FFPE tissue specimens, which is the routine method for preserving tissue for histopathology in nearly all histology laboratories. Commercial reagents simplify extraction of adequate DNA for identity testing from FFPE tissue sections. However, not all fixatives or chemical treatments used in the histology laboratory are compatible with PCR amplification. Specimens exposed to fixatives containing heavy metals (for example B5 fixative) are not recommended due to inhibition of enzymatic reactions in PCR. Similarly, decalcification solutions are usually acidic as are some fixatives (e.g., Carnoy's, Zenker's, and Bouin's fixatives), which degrade the DNA and render the specimens unsuitable for PCR amplification. Therefore, it is very important to review the tissue processing during selection of tissue blocks for identity testing to avoid incompatible treatments. In extraordinary cases when the only specimen available is suboptimal but the testing will have a significant impact on patient management, testing of the compromised specimen can be considered. In such cases, if there is some amplification of the DNA, it may only be for loci with the smallest PCR target sizes. In some situations, sufficient information may be obtained to provide a limited interpretation, at the risk of over-interpreting potential artifacts that can occur at low DNA concentrations. If critical, testing using SNPs or mitochondrial DNA can be considered since those methods are more tolerant of degraded specimens.

Some staining methods may produce added damage to the nucleic acids. Most hematoxylin and eosin (H&E) stained tissue sections are acceptable [6, 41]. However, because reagents for histochemistry or immunohistochemistry may substantially degrade the nucleic acids or inhibit PCR and the effects of such potential interferences may not have been thoroughly examined during assay validation, due caution should accompany interpretation of STR analysis of previously stained material.

Selection of Tissue for Testing

Identity testing of tissue specimens begins with review of all available material by an anatomic pathologist. After assessing the quantity and distribution of the available material, the best method of isolating DNA from the submitted material is chosen. Available methods range from extraction of DNA from an entire tissue section to extracting DNA from small, isolated areas within a tissue section by macrodissection or microdissection. Regardless of the final method used, the goal of tissue selection is to obtain the appropriate specimens for comparison.

Testing All Tissue Within a Block

When the identity of all of the tissue in a block is in question, several (e.g., three) 10 μm thick section rolls from the FFPE tissue block can be cut and placed directly into microcentrifuge tubes for DNA extraction. This saves time and eliminates the effort of preparing a slide and then scraping the tissue off the slide for DNA extraction.

Testing Areas of Interest Within a Single Block

When different portions of tissue in the same block potentially originate from different sources, macrodissection or microdissection of the tissue from representative slides (see below) is appropriate to separate the tissues for subsequent comparison. Macrodissection after appropriate training and practice can be regularly employed using readily available tools [42]. Microdissection techniques permit more precise selection of cells for testing, but require more expertise and expensive equipment.

When the only slide containing the area of interest has been previously stained and coverslipped, xylenes can be used to remove the coverslip (with a risk of losing the desired cells) for DNA extraction from the stained tissue [6, 41]. Importantly, the scenario of tissue present on only a single level is suggestive of a true "floater" and may not merit further testing because tissue that is truly a part of the specimen is typically present on more than one level of a block.

Macrodissection

For macrodissection, an anatomic pathologist first identifies and outlines representative cellular, nucleated, non-necrotic areas of interest on a stained slide using a permanent marking pen (see Fig. 57.1a). Then, unstained

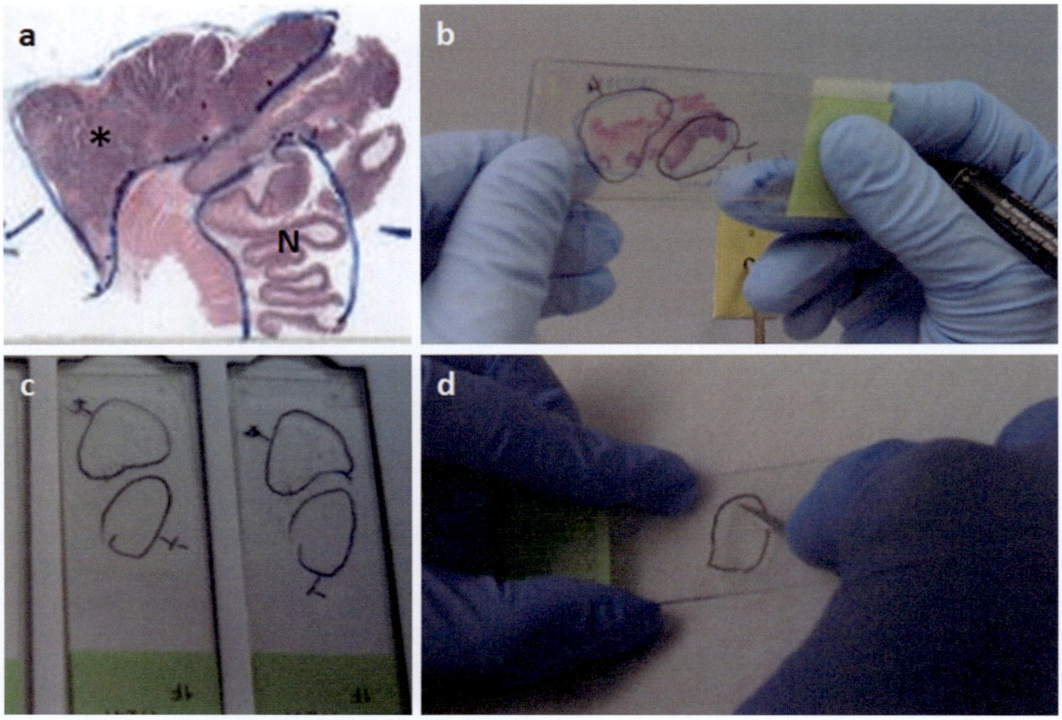

Figure 57.1 Macrodissection can be used to enrich for tumor and/or normal tissue from histologic tissue sections for identity testing, depending on the question being asked. Regions of interest on an H&E stained slide are indicated by an anatomic pathologist by circling the tissue areas of interest using a permanent marking pen, as shown in (**a**) (*, tumor; N, normal). This functions as a guide slide for marking regions of interest on unstained slides of sections adjacent to the tissue on the guide slide (**b**). A final H&E stained slide cut after the unstained sections is used to confirm that the tissue of interest is present on all the unstained slides. The marked tissue from the unstained slides (**c**) can then be individually scraped with a scalpel to isolate the tissue of interest (**d**)

4–10 μm sections are cut and placed onto glass slides (e.g., 5–15 slides are prepared). The first slide, "cut off the top," and the last slide "cut off the bottom" are stained with H&E to demonstrate the distribution of the areas of interest across the intervening unstained slides. Identifying the distinct areas of interest is necessary when the tissue on a slide is not homogenous. Regions representing "floaters," benign, malignant, or other relevant tissues and cells on a slide are delineated with a diamond etching pen (on the non-tissue-containing surface of the slide) or a permanent marking pen on a coverslipped slide (Fig. 57.1a, b). Alternatively, a permanent marking pen can be used to mark areas of interest directly on a faced FFPE block, and this marked area can be manually separated from the remainder of the block. The marked slides are used as guides for identifying and marking the areas of interest on the unstained slides that will be used for dissection and extraction of DNA (Fig. 57.1c). Macrodissection is done by eye or using a low power dissecting microscope and the equivalent circled tissue regions are scraped off the unstained slides (Fig. 57.1d).

Microdissection

Diamond etching pens and permanent marking pens are useful for delineating distinct areas on a slide, and in most cases of identity testing they are satisfactory for marking relevant areas to be collected for DNA extraction and comparison. When greater precision is required, microdissection techniques (i.e., use of a higher power microscope to assist dissection) may be used to isolate discrete cells or clusters of cells from a complex tissue section.

Laser Capture Microdissection

Laser capture microdissection (LCM) permits reliable procurement of pure cell populations from tissue sections. The principle advantage of LCM is the ability to isolate clusters of cells or even single cells of interest as a pure population free from contaminating stromal, inflammatory, and other surrounding cell types. Its precision can also complicate analysis by limiting the choice of analysis methods to those that are amplification-based because the amount of material isolated often is minute. Due to the increased expertise and cost associated with the LCM systems, many laboratories are unable to use LCM routinely for identity testing.

LCM systems such as the ArcturusXT™ LCM System (Life Technologies, Grand Island, NY), Leica LMD6500 and LMD7000 (Leica Microsystems Inc., Buffalo Grove, IL), or PALM MicroBeam (Carl Zeiss AG, Oberkochen, Germany) are available. Each system has unique technologies and techniques for separating the selected areas of interest from tissue sections. In general, the systems include an inverted microscope, an infrared laser, control systems for the laser and the microscope stage, and a digital imaging system to permit the user to view and capture images of the microdissected fragments [43]. The systems differ mostly in terms of the slides and other consumables they require to separate and collect the cells.

Chemical Microdissection

An alternative to LCM is The PinPoint Slide DNA Isolation System™ (Zymo Research, Orange, CA) [17]. With this system a solution is applied to the microscopic area of interest. The solution dries into a thin film that captures the underlying cells. The film is lifted with a scalpel and transferred into a tube for DNA extraction. This method is more time consuming than macrodissection of marked slides and requires a specific kit, but because the area of interest is precisely selected by an anatomic pathologist, the possibility that an incorrect area will be used for analysis is reduced.

Interpretation of Results

Specimen Identification

Sample identification determines whether two samples originated from the same or different individuals. Comparison of a tissue or other specimen with an identified specimen from the potential source patient, such as peripheral blood, can be used to verify the source of the specimen in question. Interpretation of the results involves comparison of the alleles (STR or sequence polymorphisms) between the samples. The identification of non-matching alleles, preferably in two or more loci, provides evidence to exclude a potential individual as the source of the sample, or at least to conclude that both samples did not originate from the same individual. The possibility of microsatellite instability, loss of heterozygosity, or chromosomal abnormalities should be considered when malignant tissues are being compared to normal samples using STR analysis, as described further below. If an exact allele match is observed between two samples, then the likelihood that they are from the same person is high, and the matching probability can be determined from published data or manufacturer data for the loci used. The following case is an example of identity testing for sample identification.

Table 57.2 Case 1 genotypes confirming that specimens were switched

	Alleles (repeats)			
Locus	Confirmed A	Confirmed B	Unknown A	Unknown B
D3S1358	17,18	15,16	15,16	17,18
TH01	6,9.3	7,9	7,9	6,9.3
D21S11	28,30	30,32.2	30,32.2	28,30
D18S51	14,16	14,15	14,15	14,16
PentaE	7,11	11,16	11,16	7,11
D5S818	12,13	11,13	11,13	12,13
D13S317	9	10,11	10,11	9
D7S820	12,13	10,11	10,11	12,13
D16S539	11	9,10	9,10	11
CSF1PO	10,11	11	11	10,11
vWA	14,17	15,18	15,18	14,17
TPOX	8	8,11	8,11	8

Case 1

Two blocks of tissue (Unknown A and Unknown B) obtained from two different individuals were suspected of being switched and mislabeled. An alternate, confirmed sample from each individual (Confirmed A and Confirmed B) was available. DNA was extracted from all four specimens and each was amplified at 12 STR loci. Comparison of the genotypes indicated that the unknown samples had been switched (Table 57.2). Blocks Unknown A and Unknown B were relabeled to accurately reflect their true source, thereby avoiding the diagnoses of the two individuals being switched.

A "confirmed" specimen is partially a subjective designation due to the possibility of specimen misidentification. As such, in interpretive reports language such as "…block number 1 is identified as originating from patient '1' and block number 2 is identified as originating from patient '2'…" makes it clear that even for specimens with presumably confirmed identity there remains the possibility of preanalytical errors resulting in a specimen misidentification.

Analysis of Floaters

To assess the origin of an extraneous, frequently small, tissue fragment (floater) in a tissue section, the genotype of the majority of the tissue on the slide is compared with that of the floater. As with other forms of identity testing, differences in two or more markers should be identified in order to exclude the patient as the source of the floater. Generally it is not necessary or cost-effective to identify the source of the extraneous tissue; however, if desired, possible source cases with similar histology that were processed during the same time period can be tested. As always, histopathologic review of the case to verify the nature of the submitted material and to select the appropriate tissues for analysis is essential before initiating identity testing. The histopathologic review also informs the analysis, as macrodissection is frequently

Table 57.3 Case 2 genotypes confirming the presence of a floater

	Alleles (repeats)		
Locus	Suspected floater	Suspected source of floater	Benign block containing floater
vWA	11,18	11,18	16,17
TH01	10	10	6
TPOX	8,11	8,11	9,11
CSF1PO	11,12	11,12	10
LPL	11,12	11,12	10,12
F13B	6,10	6,10	9,10
FESFPS	10,12	10,12	11,12
F13A01	3.2,7	3.2,7	5,6
D5S818	10,13	10,13	11
D13S317	9,10	9,10	9,10
D7S820	11,12	11,12	10
D16S539	10,12	10,12	12
Amelogenin	X,Y	X,Y	X,Y

imperfect and a minor component of the predominant tissue's genotype may be detected in what is intended to be only floater tissue. When mixed genotyping result are obtained, correlation with the histologic picture usually will show intermingled "known" and "floater" cells in the specimen with the mixed genotype result.

Case 2

An isolated fragment of adenocarcinoma was identified in a single block of prostate needle biopsies. The remaining five blocks were completely benign. A "floater" was suspected and the possible source was another prostate biopsy case processed immediately prior to the case with the suspected floater. The adenocarcinoma floater was macrodissected, as well as the majority tissue from the benign case with the floater and the prior case with adenocarcinoma. The three tissue DNAs were tested at 12 STR loci and the results confirmed that the tissue fragment was a "floater" (Table 57.3). As expected, testing of the amelogenin locus confirmed that both samples were from male patients.

Cells of Possible Donor Origin in Transplant Recipients

Case 3

GVHD was suspected in a patient who was critically ill and pancytopenic one month after an orthotopic liver transplant. A bone marrow biopsy showed that his bone marrow was aplastic. Identity testing was requested to determine whether donor cells were circulating in the recipient, which would support a diagnosis of GVHD [44]. Twenty STR loci were amplified using recipient DNA (FFPE tissue from the explanted native liver), donor DNA (FFPE tissue from the donor gallbladder that was removed and processed at the time of transplant), and three recipient-derived specimens: peripheral blood, CD3-positive cells (T cells) isolated from peripheral blood, and bone marrow. The results confirmed the presence of donor cells in each specimen. The relative amounts of recipient and donor DNA were calculated from the allele peak areas of four representative loci (Fig. 57.2), which demonstrated 62 % donor alleles in the recipient's bone marrow and supported the diagnosis of GVHD. GVHD after solid organ transplant has been reported, and in several cases macrochimerism (>1 % donor DNA) was observed. Thus, the finding of significant donor DNA in this case was consistent with the clinical impression of GVHD [45]. The percent of donor DNA in the blood may be tracked over time using this same method.

Case 4

Six months after receiving a double lung transplant, a patient was diagnosed with metastatic squamous cell carcinoma in a subcarinal lymph node. Identity testing was requested to ascertain whether the squamous cell carcinoma was of recipient or donor origin and to guide treatment of the patient and other potential recipients of organs from the same donor. Identity testing using 12 STR loci was performed using DNA from an FFPE cell block from an a fine needle aspiration (FNA) of the subcarinal lymph node with squamous cell carcinoma, an FFPE tissue section from the native right lung, and a stored peripheral blood specimen from the donor. Test results showed that the lymph node with the squamous cell carcinoma DNA had the same alleles as DNA extracted from the recipient's native lung specimen at 11 informative STR loci (Fig. 57.3 and Table 57.4). In interpretation of the test results, consideration was given to the surgical pathologist's note that the FNA only contained 5–10 % tumor cells. The relative amounts of neoplastic and nonneoplastic cells can help in interpretation of relative peak heights in an electropherogram and must be compared with an assay's ability to detect low levels of a minor DNA component. There was no evidence of donor allele peaks in the FNA specimen's electropherogram and the assay was validated to detect at least a 5 % component of DNA. In this context, the results were interpreted as consistent with a recipient origin of the squamous cell carcinoma cells in the lymph node.

Maternal Cell Contamination of a Prenatal Specimen

Case 5

A 37 year old pregnant woman underwent CVS. A limited amount of villi were collected, cultured, and karyotyped with a result of 46, XX. Identity testing was requested to determine whether the karyotype reflected only chromosomes

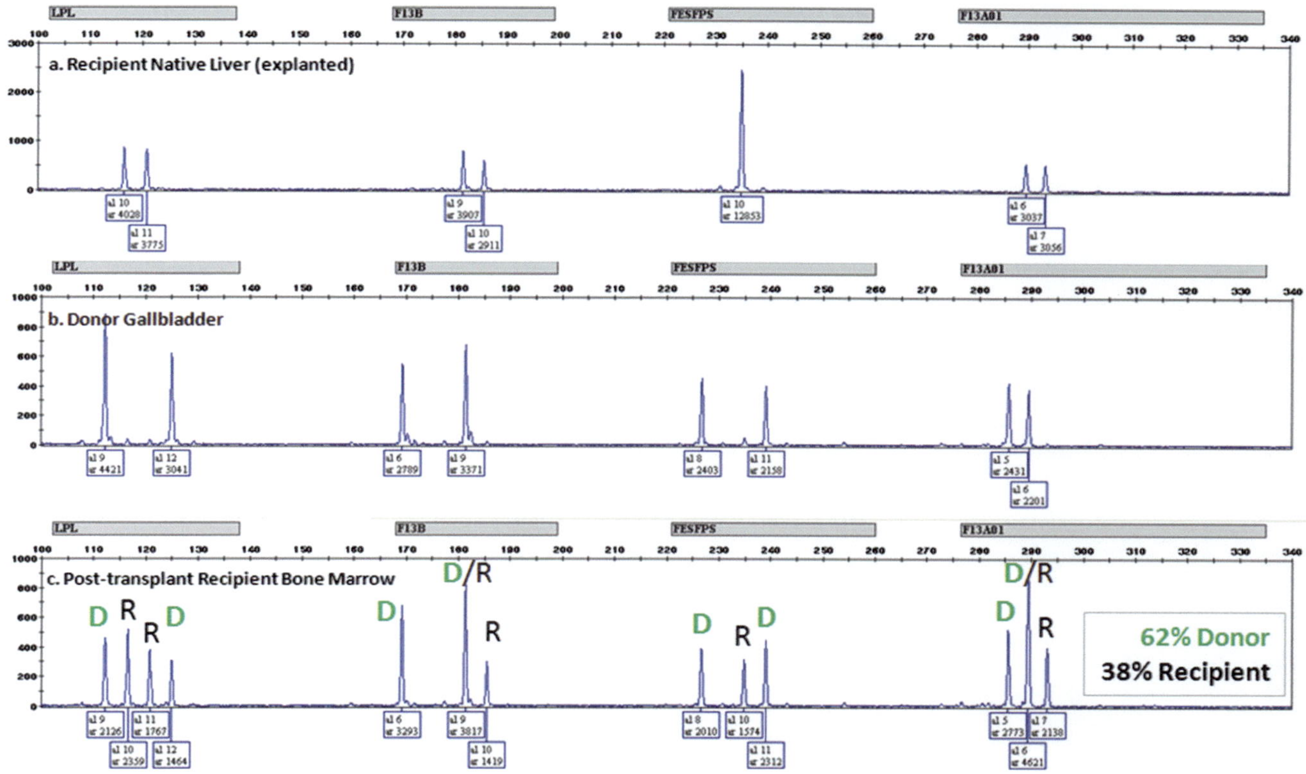

Figure 57.2 Electropherograms from Case 3. Amplification results for four STR loci are shown for DNA extracted from recipient native liver tissue (**a**), donor gallbladder tissue (**b**), and post-transplant recipient bone marrow (**c**). The bone marrow specimen shows the presence of both donor (green D) and recipient (R) alleles at all four loci. Alleles shared by the donor and recipient are indicated (D/R). The percent of donor DNA is calculated from the peak areas as described in Chap. 56. In this sample, the donor DNA was 62 %. This result was interpreted as macrochimerism supportive of a diagnosis of GVHD. *al* allele, *ar* area of peak, *GVHD* graft-vs-host disease, *STR* short tandem repeat

of the fetus or contaminating maternal cells. Identity testing using 12 STR loci and the amelogenin locus was performed using DNA from the cultured chorionic villus sample and DNA from a peripheral blood sample from the mother. The identity testing results demonstrate that the CVS contained fetal DNA with evidence of Mendelian inheritance, as well as low-level maternal contamination. The relative amounts of maternal and fetal DNA were calculated from the allele peak areas at informative loci with approximately 4 % maternal DNA present (Fig. 57.4).

Analysis of Hydatidiform Mole

Identity testing is used to characterize hydatidiform moles as complete or partial moles, as well as homozygous or heterozygous complete moles.

Case 6

A 25-year-old pregnant woman underwent a dilation and evacuation procedure after a missed abortion. The surgical pathologist who examined the specimen noted degenerated hydropic chorionic villi suggestive of a molar pregnancy. Tissue was submitted for cytogenetics and the resulting karyotype was 46, XX. Her physician was concerned about persistent trophoblastic disease or early choriocarcinoma based on serial measurements of human chorionic gonadotropin (hCG) in the patient's blood. Most cases of complete mole or choriocarcinoma have 46 chromosomes which are all of paternal origin. The genetic origin of the villi from the products of conception was questioned and DNA genotyping analysis was requested. Macrodissection was used to isolate the hydropic chorionic villi from the remaining tissue on the section (selected regions shown in Fig. 57.5).

Identity testing at 12 STR loci was performed on DNA from three specimens: macrodissected hydropic chorionic villi (Fig. 57.5) and maternal and paternal peripheral blood specimens. The chorionic villus genotype (Fig. 57.6 and Table 57.5) showed a mixed pattern attributable to incomplete separation of abnormal villus tissue from adjacent normal decidua by macrodissection, which is a common problem due to the difficulty in separating villus tissue from decidua using macrodissection rather than microdissection. Although the pattern appears triploid (three alleles

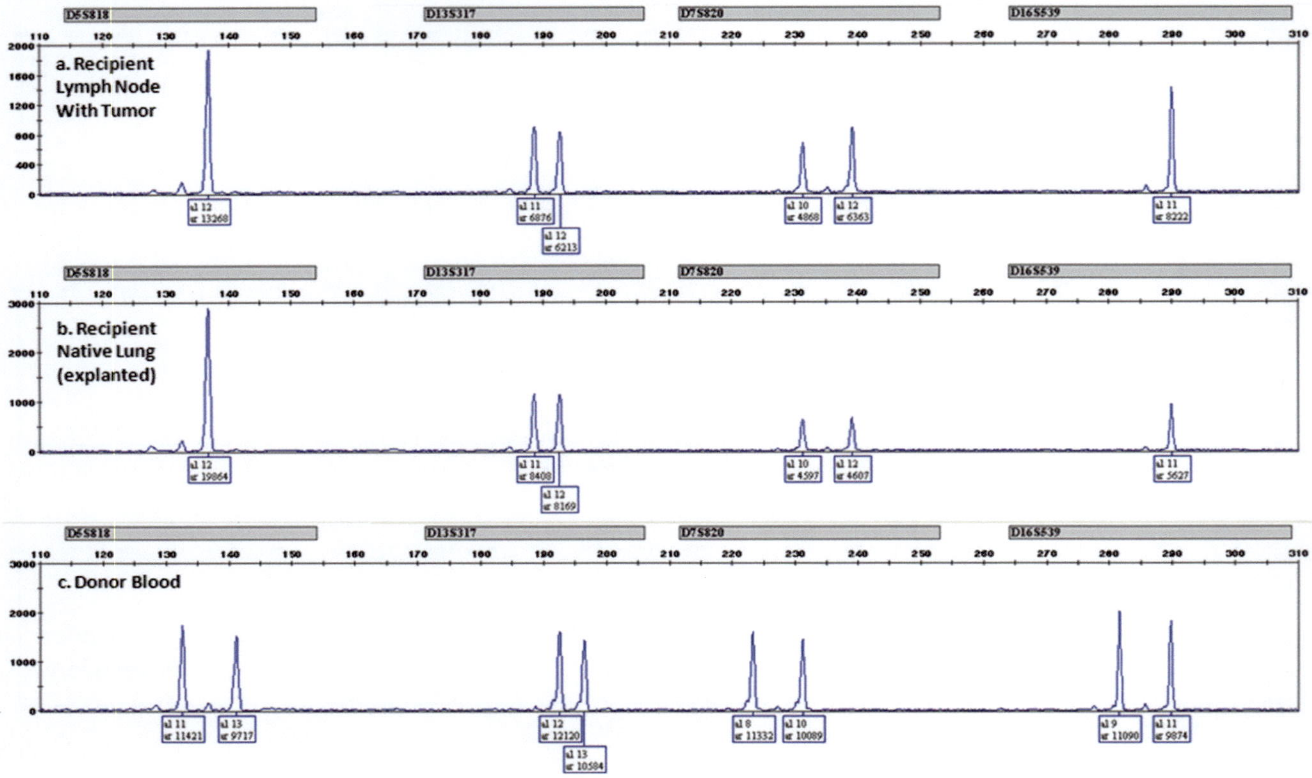

Figure 57.3 Electropherograms from Case 4. Amplification results for four STR loci are shown for DNA isolated from tumor-containing specimen (**a**), recipient native lung (**b**), and donor blood (**c**). Results indicate no evidence of donor-specific alleles in the tumor-containing specimen (**a**) at the level of sensitivity of the assay (5 %), supporting a recipient origin for the tumor. *al* allele, *ar* area of peak, *STR* short tandem repeat

Table 57.4 Case 4 genotypes demonstrating a match between the tumor and the recipient and confirming the tumor originates from recipient not donor cells

	Alleles (repeats)		
Locus	Tumor	Recipient	Donor
VWA	15, 19	15, 19	15, 18
TH01	7, 9.3	7, 9.3	7
TPOX	8, 11	8, 11	8, 11
CSF1PO	12	12	8, 9
LPL	12	12	10
F13B	8	8	7, 10
FESFPS	10	10	8
F13A01	4, 7	4, 7	3.2, 6
D5S818	12	12	11, 13
D13S317	11, 12	11,12	12, 13
D7S820	10, 12	10, 12	8, 10
D16S539	11	11	9, 11
Amelogenin	X	X	X

at some loci), each locus has a predominant allele peak matching a single paternal allele and smaller adjacent peaks attributable to contaminating maternal alleles. This case demonstrates the importance of careful microdissection, as well as careful interpretation of the results in the context of the histology. A higher level of maternal contamination would be difficult to interpret. Based on a comparison with the paternal genotype, the dominant allelic pattern in the hydropic villi sample is most consistent with paternal isodisomy in which only a single paternally derived allele is present at each informative locus. The reported histologic features and identity testing interpretation support the diagnosis of a complete hydatidiform mole.

Identity Testing Results for Neoplastic Tissue with Mutations

The presence of a genotype mismatch at two or more loci is usually sufficient to conclude that two samples are from two different individuals. However, when one of the tissues is neoplastic, the differences at a single locus or few loci may be due to mutations in the tumor tissue. Nucleotide polymorphisms are often conserved between the normal and tumor tissue from the same patient, but microsatellite instability (MSI), loss of heterozygosity (LOH), and chromosomal alterations occur in tumors and should be considered

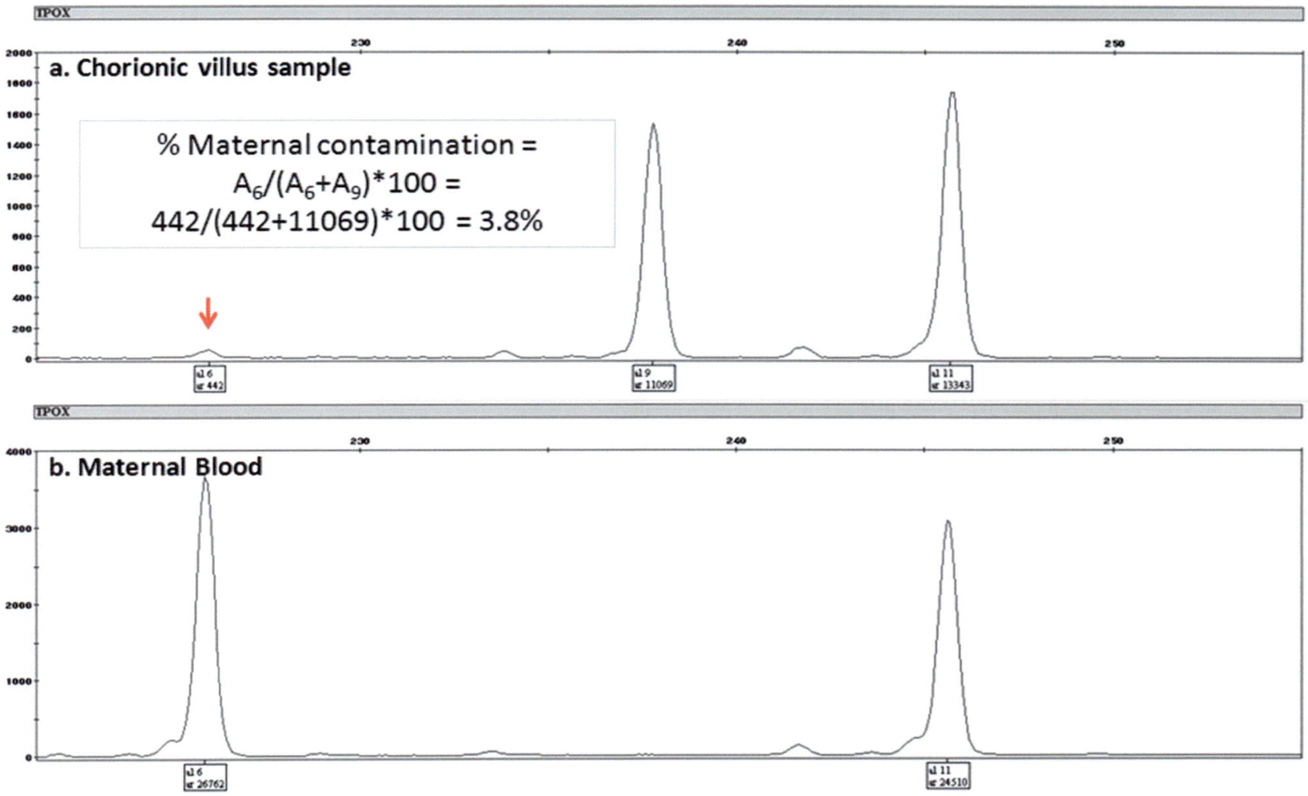

Figure 57.4 Electropherograms from Case 5. Amplification result for the TPOX locus is shown for DNA from chorionic villus sample (CVS) (**a**) and maternal blood (**b**). The CVS specimen shows a small amount (3.8 %) of maternal contamination indicated by the presence of the maternal allele of 6 repeats (*red arrow*). Mother and fetus share the 11 repeat allele. The percent of maternal contamination can be calculated using the peak areas as described in Chap. 56. *al* allele, *ar* area of peak

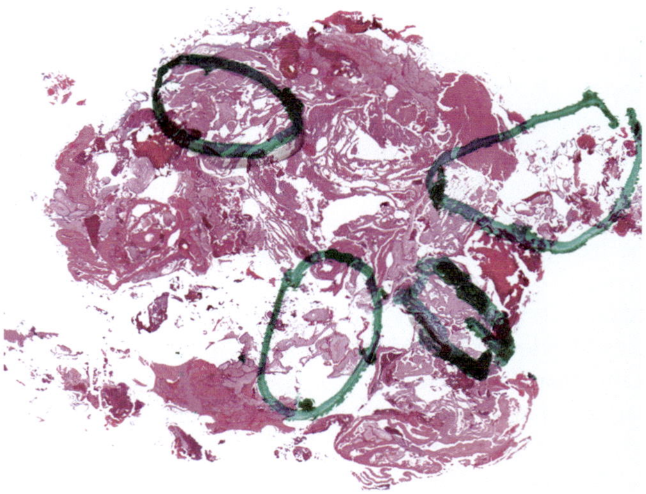

Figure 57.5 H&E-stained FFPE tissue section of a chorionic villus sample from a suspected molar pregnancy. Regions of hydropic villi were circled (*green circles*) with a marking pen to create a guide slide used as a reference for macrodissection of tissue on adjacent unstained slides. DNA was extracted from the macrodissected tissue for identity testing (fig. 57.6)

as a possible cause for allelic differences. MSI in a tumor results when errors in DNA replication of microsatellites (simple repetitive sequences) are unable to be repaired by DNA mismatch repair (MMR) proteins, either due to mismatch repair gene mutation or promoter hypermethylation. Since identity testing relies on polymorphic STR sequences, MSI at a locus being tested is a theoretical confounding factor in the interpretation of identity testing results. LOH at a tested locus is also possible. If a deletion or other mutational event involving a tested allele renders the tumor cells either hemizygous or homozygous at that allele compared to the heterozygous benign cells, then that discrepancy may mistakenly be interpreted as an indication that the tumor did not originate from the patient. Loci known to be frequently compromised by MSI, LOH, or chromosomal alterations and loci compromised in a specific tumor should not be utilized for an identity testing application. Therefore, when analyzing neoplastic tissue, examination of a number of loci rather than relying on the results at a single locus is necessary, and a cytogenetic karyotype, if available, can be used to assist with interpretation.

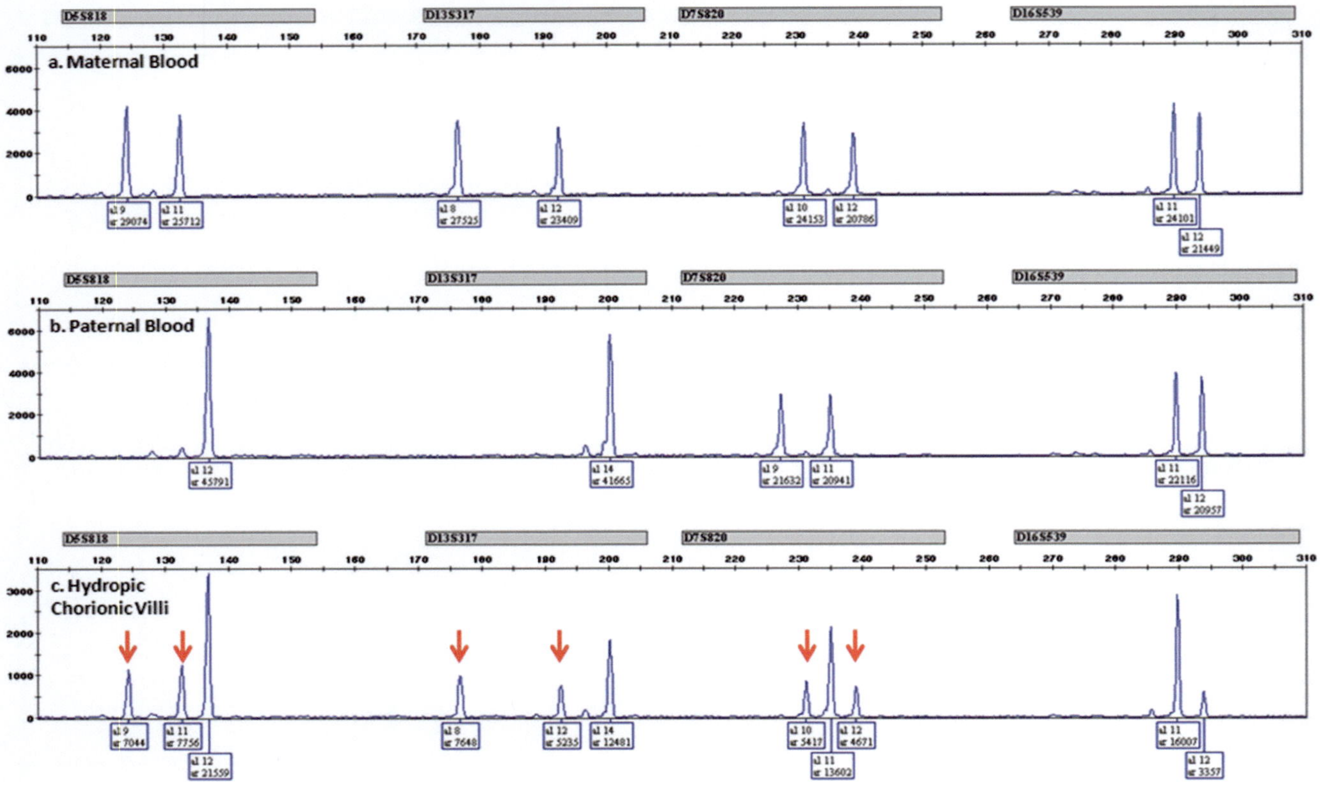

Figure 57.6 Electropherograms from Case 6. Amplification results for four STR loci are shown for DNA extracted from maternal blood (**a**), paternal blood (**b**), and macrodissected hydropic chorionic villi (**c**). The dominant alleles in the villus sample are composed of only a single paternal allele most consistent with paternal isodisomy. In addition, at all informative loci, both maternal alleles (*red arrows*) are present as a result of incomplete macrodissection with inclusion of maternal decidua. This result was interpreted as a complete hydatidiform mole. *al* allele, *ar* area of peak

Table 57.5 Case 6 alleles identified at each locus tested with bracketed alleles present at lower amplitude and derived from contaminating maternal tissue due to incomplete macrodissection of the villi from the decidua

	Alleles (repeats)		
Locus	Villi	Maternal	Paternal
VWA	17 [19]	17, 19	16, 17
TH01	6 [8]	6, 8	6, 9.3
TPOX	8	8	8, 11
CSF1PO	12 [11]	11	12
LPL	10 [12]	10, 12	10, 12
F13B	8 [10]	10	8, 10
FESFPS	8 [10, 12]	10, 12	8, 10
F13A01	5 [6, 7]	6, 7	5, 6
D5S818	12 [9, 11]	9, 11	12
D13S317	14 [8, 12]	8, 12	14
D7S820	11 [10, 12]	10, 12	9, 11
D16S539	11 [12]	11, 12	11, 12
Amelogenin	X	X	XY

Conclusion

Identity testing methods are well established for use in a variety of scenarios encountered in a clinical laboratory. Beyond the routine use for monitoring engraftment for HSCT, the applications described in this chapter demonstrate wide-ranging applicability of identity testing for clinical specimen identification. These applications include suspected specimen misidentifications, histologic floaters, or concern over the attribution of a diagnosis for a patient. Identity testing also has a demonstrable diagnostic role in the classification of hydatidiform moles, assessment of maternal cell contamination in prenatal specimens, determination of the origin of a tumor in a transplant recipient, and diagnosis of GVHD. In a vast majority of cases, polymorphic DNA marker analysis combined with clinical information and histologic correlation provides the answer to questions which are otherwise difficult to resolve.

References

1. Tsongalis GJ, Berman MM. Application of forensic identity testing in a clinical setting. Specimen identification. Diagn Mol Pathol. 1997;6:111–4.
2. Pfeifer JD, Zehnbauer B, Payton J. The changing spectrum of DNA-based specimen provenance testing in surgical pathology. Am J Clin Pathol. 2011;135:132–8.
3. Abeln EC, van Kemenade FD, van Krieken JH, Cornelisse CJ. Rapid identification of mixed up bladder biopsy specimens using polymorphic microsatellite markers. Diagn Mol Pathol. 1995;4:286–91.
4. Hunt JL, Swalsky P, Sasatomi E, Niehouse L, Bakker A, Finkelstein SD. A microdissection and molecular genotyping assay to confirm the identity of tissue floaters in paraffin-embedded tissue blocks. Arch Pathol Lab Med. 2003;127:213–7.
5. Shibata D, Kurosu M, Noguchi TT. Fixed human tissues: a resource for the identification of individuals. J Forensic Sci. 1991;36: 1204–12.
6. Hunt JL. Molecular pathology in anatomic pathology practice: a review of basic principles. Arch Pathol Lab Med. 2008;132: 248–60.
7. Keep D, Zaragoza MV, Hassold T, Redline RW. Very early complete hydatidiform mole. Hum Pathol. 1996;27:708–13.
8. Murphy KM, McConnell TG, Hafez MJ, Vang R, Ronnett BM. Molecular genotyping of hydatidiform moles: analytic validation of a multiplex short tandem repeat assay. J Mol Diagn. 2009;11:598–605.
9. Antoniadi T, Yapijakis C, Kaminopetros P, et al. A simple and effective approach for detecting maternal cell contamination in molecular prenatal diagnosis. Prenat Diagn. 2002;22:425–9.
10. Winsor EJ, Akoury H, Chitayat D, Steele L, Stockley TL. The role of molecular microsatellite identity testing to detect sampling errors in prenatal diagnosis. Prenat Diagn. 2010;30:746–52.
11. Barallon R, Bauer SR, Butler J, et al. Recommendation of short tandem repeat profiling for authenticating human cell lines, stem cells, and tissues. In Vitro Cell Dev Biol Anim. 2010;46: 727–32.
12. Saad R. Discovery, development, and current applications of DNA identity testing. Proc (Bayl Univ Med Cent). 2005;18:130–3.
13. Gandhi MJ, Strong DM. Donor derived malignancy following transplantation: a review. Cell Tissue Bank. 2007;8:267–86.
14. Pfeifer JD, Liu J. Rate of occult specimen provenance complications in routine clinical practice. Am J Clin Pathol. 2013;139:93–100.
15. Marberger M, McConnell JD, Fowler I, et al. Biopsy misidentification identified by DNA profiling in a large multicenter trial. J Clin Oncol. 2011;29:1744–9.
16. Michel R. Laboratory compliance watch: In-practice histology lab splits biopsies; ID's patient with DNA. The Dark Report 2011 October 12:10.
17. Tsongalis GJ, Wu AH, Silver H, Ricci Jr A. Applications of forensic identity testing in the clinical laboratory. Am J Clin Pathol. 1999;112:S93–103.
18. Tsongalis GJ, Anamani DE, Wu AH. Identification of urine specimen donors by the PM+DQA1 amplification and typing kit. J Forensic Sci. 1996;41:1031–4.
19. Linfert DR, Wu AH, Tsongalis GJ. The effect of pathologic substances and adulterants on the DNA typing of urine. J Forensic Sci. 1998;43:1041–5.
20. Butler JM. Genetics and genomics of core short tandem repeat loci used in human identity testing. J Forensic Sci. 2006;51:253–65.
21. Huijsmans CJ, Heilmann FG, van der Zanden AG, Schneeberger PM, Hermans MH. Single nucleotide polymorphism profiling assay to exclude serum sample mix-up. Vox Sang. 2007;92:148–53.
22. Huijsmans R, Damen J, van der Linden H, Hermans M. Single nucleotide polymorphism profiling assay to confirm the identity of human tissues. J Mol Diagn. 2007;9:205–13.
23. Budowle B, Wilson MR, DiZinno JA, et al. Mitochondrial DNA regions HVI and HVII population data. Forensic Sci Int. 1999;103:23–35.
24. Alonso A, Alves C, Suarez-Mier MP, et al. Mitochondrial DNA haplotyping revealed the presence of mixed up benign and neoplastic tissue sections from two individuals on the same prostatic biopsy slide. J Clin Pathol. 2005;58:83–6.
25. Pfeifer JD, Singleton MN, Gregory MH, Lambert DL, Kymes SM. Development of a decision-analytic model for the application of STR-based provenance testing of transrectal prostate biopsy specimens. Value Health. 2012;15:860–7.
26. Paxton A. Unmasking specimen ID errors every step of the way. CAP Today 2010.
27. Platt E, Sommer P, McDonald L, Bennett A, Hunt J. Tissue floaters and contaminants in the histology laboratory. Arch Pathol Lab Med. 2009;133:973–8.
28. Birkeland SA, Storm HH. Risk for tumor and other disease transmission by transplantation: a population-based study of unrecognized malignancies and other diseases in organ donors. Transplantation. 2002;74:1409–13.
29. Desai R, Collett D, Watson CJ, Johnson P, Evans T, Neuberger J. Cancer transmission from organ donors-unavoidable but low risk. Transplantation. 2012;94:1200–7.
30. Kauffman HM, McBride MA, Cherikh WS, Spain PC, Delmonico FL. Transplant tumor registry: donors with central nervous system tumors1. Transplantation. 2002;73:579–82.
31. Filipovich AH, Weisdorf D, Pavletic S, et al. National Institutes of Health consensus development project on criteria for clinical trials in chronic graft-versus-host disease: I. Diagnosis and staging working group report. Biol Blood Marrow Transplant. 2005;11:945–56.
32. Verdonk RC, Haagsma EB, Jongsma T, et al. A prospective analysis of the natural course of donor chimerism including the natural killer cell fraction after liver transplantation. Transplantation. 2011;92:e22–4.
33. Taylor AL, Gibbs P, Sudhindran S, et al. Monitoring systemic donor lymphocyte macrochimerism to aid the diagnosis of graft-versus-host disease after liver transplantation. Transplantation. 2004;77: 441–6.
34. Frederickson RM, Wang HS, Surh LC. Some caveats in PCR-based prenatal diagnosis on direct amniotic fluid versus cultured amniocytes. Prenat Diagn. 1999;19:113–7.
35. Stojilkovic-Mikic T, Mann K, Docherty Z, Mackie OC. Maternal cell contamination of prenatal samples assessed by QF-PCR genotyping. Prenat Diagn. 2005;25:79–83.
36. Nagan N, Faulkner NE, Curtis C, Schrijver I. Laboratory guidelines for detection, interpretation, and reporting of maternal cell contamination in prenatal analyses a report of the association for molecular pathology. J Mol Diagn. 2011;13:7–11.
37. Schrijver I, Cherny SC, Zehnder JL. Testing for maternal cell contamination in prenatal samples: a comprehensive survey of current diagnostic practices in 35 molecular diagnostic laboratories. J Mol Diagn. 2007;9:394–400.
38. Winsor EJ, Silver MP, Theve R, Wright M, Ward BE. Maternal cell contamination in uncultured amniotic fluid. Prenat Diagn. 1996;16: 49–54.
39. Genest DR. Partial hydatidiform mole: clinicopathological features, differential diagnosis, ploidy and molecular studies, and gold standards for diagnosis. Int J Gynecol Pathol. 2001;20:315–22.
40. Hui P. Molecular diagnosis of gestational trophoblastic disease. Expert Rev Mol Diagn. 2010;10:1023–34.
41. Morikawa T, Shima K, Kuchiba A, et al. No evidence for interference of h&e staining in DNA testing: usefulness of DNA extraction from H&E-stained archival tissue sections. Am J Clin Pathol. 2012;138:122–9.

42. Hunt JL, Finkelstein SD. Microdissection techniques for molecular testing in surgical pathology. Arch Pathol Lab Med. 2004;128: 1372–8.
43. Fend F, Kremer M, Quintanilla-Martinez L. Laser capture microdissection: methodical aspects and applications with emphasis on immuno-laser capture microdissection. Pathobiology. 2000;68: 209–14.
44. Wang XQ, Lo CM, Chen L, et al. Hematopoietic chimerism in liver transplantation patients and hematopoietic stem/progenitor cells in adult human liver. Hepatology. 2012;56:1557–66.
45. Schoniger-Hekele M, Muller C, Kramer L, et al. Graft versus host disease after orthotopic liver transplantation documented by analysis of short tandem repeat polymorphisms. Digestion. 2006;74: 169–73.

Section VII

HLA Typing

Section Editor: Debra G.B. Leonard

Molecular HLA Typing

58

Malek Kamoun, Jill A. Hollenbach, Steven J. Mack, and Thomas M. Williams

Abstract

This chapter describes the molecular genetics of the HLA genes, which reside within a genetic complex referred to as the major histocompatibility complex (MHC). The MHC contains the most polymorphic coding sequences in the human genome. HLA molecules provide the molecular basis for immunologic self-recognition, and many HLA genes encode proteins that function within immune regulatory networks.

This chapter describes (1) methods used for population genetic analyses including estimation of allele and haplotype frequencies and disease association studies; (2) the clinical utility of HLA typing for solid organ and bone marrow/hematopoietic cell transplantation, autoimmune diseases, and other disorders; (3) available assays for HLA typing, definition of typing resolution, and interpretation and reporting of test results.

Keywords

HLA • Haplotype • Genetics • Genome • Histocompatibility • Linkage disequilibrium • MHC • Polymorphisms • Transplantation

Molecular Genetics of the Human Major Histocompatibility Complex

Histocompatibility antigens were first described by Snell, using inbred strains of mice. Later, Dausset, Payne, Van Rood, and others discovered that in humans antibodies to white blood cell antigens can be induced after pregnancy or transfusion. These antibodies provided the tools to define the human leukocyte antigens (HLA) ([1–3] and references therein). Recently, using molecular methods, researchers have defined thousands of different HLA alleles. The HLA genes reside within a genetic complex referred to as the major histocompatibility complex (MHC). The MHC comprises about 4 megabases (Mb) on the short arm of chromosome 6 (6p21.3). The MHC contains the most polymorphic coding sequences in the human genome. HLA genetic diversity accounts for more than 10 % of all genetic diversity observed in the human genome. HLA molecules provide the molecular basis for immunologic self-recognition, and many HLA genes encode proteins that function within immune regulatory networks.

A number of genes in the MHC, arranged in order from the telomeric to the centromeric end, are displayed in Table 58.1. The MHC can be divided into three major regions, each of which controls the production of molecules that have distinct biologic functions [4]. The class I region includes the HLA-A, HLA-B, HLA-C, and related loci; the

M. Kamoun, M.D., Ph.D. (✉)
Pathology and Laboratory Medicine, Penn Medicine, Philadelphia, PA, USA
e-mail: malekkam@mail.med.upenn.edu

J.A. Hollenbach, Ph.D., M.P.H.
Center for Genetics, Children's Hospital Oakland Research Institute, Oakland, CA, USA

S.J. Mack, Ph.D.
Children's Hospital Oakland Research Institute, Oakland, CA, USA

T.M. Williams, M.D. (Deceased)

D.G.B. Leonard (ed.), *Molecular Pathology in Clinical Practice*, DOI 10.1007/978-3-319-19674-9_58

Table 58.1 Names for genes in the HLA class I and class II regions, ordered from telomeric to centromeric location on chromosome 6

Name	Molecular characteristics
HLA-F	Class I-like molecule
HLA-G	Class I-like molecule
HLA-H	Class I pseudogene
HLA-A	Class I α chain
HLA-J	Class I pseudogene
HLA-E	Class I-like molecule
HLA-C	Class I α chain
HLA-B	Class I α chain
MICA	MHC class I-like molecule
MICB	MHC class I-like molecule
HLA-DRA	DR α chain
HLA-DRB9	DRB pseudogene, isolated fragment
HLA-DRB3	DR β3 chain determining DR52 and Dw24, Dw25, Dw26 specificities
HLA-DRB2	Pseudogene with DR β-like sequences
HLA-DRB1	DR β 1 chain determining specificities DR1, DR2, DR3, DR4, DR5, etc.
HLA-DQA1	DQ α chain as expressed
HLA-DQB1	DQ β chain as expressed
HLA-DQB3	DQ β-chain-related sequence, not known to be expressed
HLA-DQA2	DQ α-chain-related sequence, not known to be expressed
HLA-DQB2	DQ β-chain-related sequence, not known to be expressed
HLA-DOB	DO β chain
TAP2	ABC (ATP-binding cassette) transporter (associated with antigen presentation)
LMP7	Proteosome-related sequence (role in loading class I molecules with peptides)
TAP1	ABC transporter (associated with antigen presentation)
LMP2	Proteosome-related sequence (role in loading class I molecules with peptides)
HLA-DMB	DM β chain (control peptide loading by class II molecules)
HLA-DMA	DM α chain (control peptide loading by class II molecules)
HLA-DPA1	DP α chain as expressed
HLA-DPB1	DP β chain as expressed
HLA-DPA2	DP α-chain-related pseudogene
HLA-DPB2	DP β-chain-related pseudogene

class II region includes the HLA-DR, HLA-DQ, and HLA-DP loci; and the class III region contains genes that encode a variety of proteins including molecules of the complement system (C2, C4, and Bf) and tumor necrosis factors (TNFs). Class I and class II loci encode two distinct classes of highly polymorphic cell surface molecules whose function is to capture and display various antigenic peptides to CD8+ and CD4+ T lymphocytes, respectively. The class II region also includes the genes for the TAP1 and TAP2 peptide transporter, the *LMP* genes that encode proteosome subunits, and the genes encoding the DMα and DMβ chains ([4] and references therein).

HLA Polymorphism

HLA genes are codominantly expressed, and most individuals are heterozygous at the classical (i.e., presenting peptides for inspection by T cells) HLA class I and class II loci. The nomenclature for the alleles of the HLA system is decided by an international nomenclature committee. Antigen names are composed of a letter designating the HLA protein encoded by a locus or loci and a number, for example, A2, B7, Cw4, DR17, and DQ3. Allele names are based on nucleotide sequence variation among alleles identified using DNA-based techniques (discussed below). The number of alleles at the HLA class I and class II loci and a listing of their serologically defined specificities and allele equivalents are available online at several Web sites (for instance, the Anthony Nolan Trust Web site at http://www.anthonynolan.org/clinicians-and-researchers/anthony-nolan-research-institute/hla-informatics-group and also at http://hla.alleles.org or the ImMunoGeneTics (IMGT)/HLA Database Web site at http://www.ebi.ac.uk/imgt/hla/).

Pattern of HLA Polymorphism

Most of the sequence diversity for the HLA class I loci is localized to the second and third exons and, for the class II loci, to the second exon of each gene. HLA diversity is generated through the selection of alleles with nonsynonymous substitutions encoding amino acid differences within the peptide-binding site. This contrasts with the bias against substitutions within the introns and other binding domains. Linear sequences identifying residues critical to the expression of allospecificities are found in the helices of the α1 and α2 domains as well as external portions of the β-pleated sheet. Other polymorphic amino acid residues that are important for peptide binding but not defined by alloantibodies are identified by DNA-based techniques [5–7].

The pattern of allelic sequence diversity for both the class I and class II loci is unusual; most alleles differ from their closest neighbor by multiple substitutions, with some alleles differing in the second and third exons by as much as 15 %. This pattern is suggestive of segmental exchange of nucleotide motifs between alleles of the same locus. There are also a few examples of interlocus gene conversion, and most are the result of HLA-B and HLA-C recombination. Thus, different HLA alleles of a locus are patchwork (i.e., mosaic) combinations of polymorphisms. The extensive allelic diversity at HLA loci is thought to have been generated by polymorphic sequence motifs generated by gene duplication and recombinational mechanisms such as gene conversion-like events, which have shuffled these polymorphic sequence motifs. Point mutations also contribute to this allelic diversity [6, 7]. One consequence of this pattern of patchwork polymorphism is that the sharing of specific epitopes on the HLA molecules leads to antigenic cross-reactivity. Due to epitope sharing, HLA antigens may be arranged in cross-reactive groups or CREGs [2, 3]. CREGs are important in that they allow for greater latitude in donor–recipient HLA matching and at the same time may be used to predict potential problems with graft outcome. A problematic consequence of the combinatorial nature of HLA alleles is that a given pattern of sequence motifs may be consistent with more than a single genotype. This problem of ambiguity in DNA-based typing is discussed below.

HLA Haplotypes

The term "haplotype" applies to any set of genetic polymorphisms at contiguous loci. These neighboring polymorphisms are co-transmitted on a single parental chromosome in the absence of recombination. A haplotype can be defined at any level of polymorphism. Alleles at different HLA loci are often described as being transmitted as a multi-locus haplotype (e.g., the A1-B8-DR3 haplotype), but the sequence variants associated with specific HLA allele names are in fact haplotypes of individual polymorphisms at a given locus. An individual inherits one haplotype from each parent. In any family having more than one sibling, there is a 1 in 4 chance that the two siblings will be HLA identical and a 1 in 2 chance that they will share one haplotype. Given the number of existing alleles, the number of possible haplotypes is astronomical. However, due to linkage disequilibrium (LD), the number of haplotypes found in a population is more restricted [7, 8].

The organization of HLA-DQ and HLA-DP loci is conserved within humans and other primates, whereas the number of HLA-DR genes varies in different haplotypes. Within the HLA-DR region, the DRB1 gene encodes the DRβ1 chain, which determines the DR private specificities DR1, DR2, DR3,DR4, DR5, and so on. The DRB3, DRB4, and DRB5 genes encode the DRβ3, DRβ4, and DRβ5 chains, which determine the DR52, DR53, and DR51 specificities, respectively (Fig. 58.1).

Genetic recombination or crossing over in the HLA region is a relatively rare event, occurring for the most part no more than 1 % per meiosis between HLA-A and HLA-B and between HLA-B and HLA-DR. Recombination also can occur between HLA-A and HLA-C and between HLA-B and HLA-C (0.6 % and 0.2 %, respectively). Such recombination can have important clinical implications for transplantation.

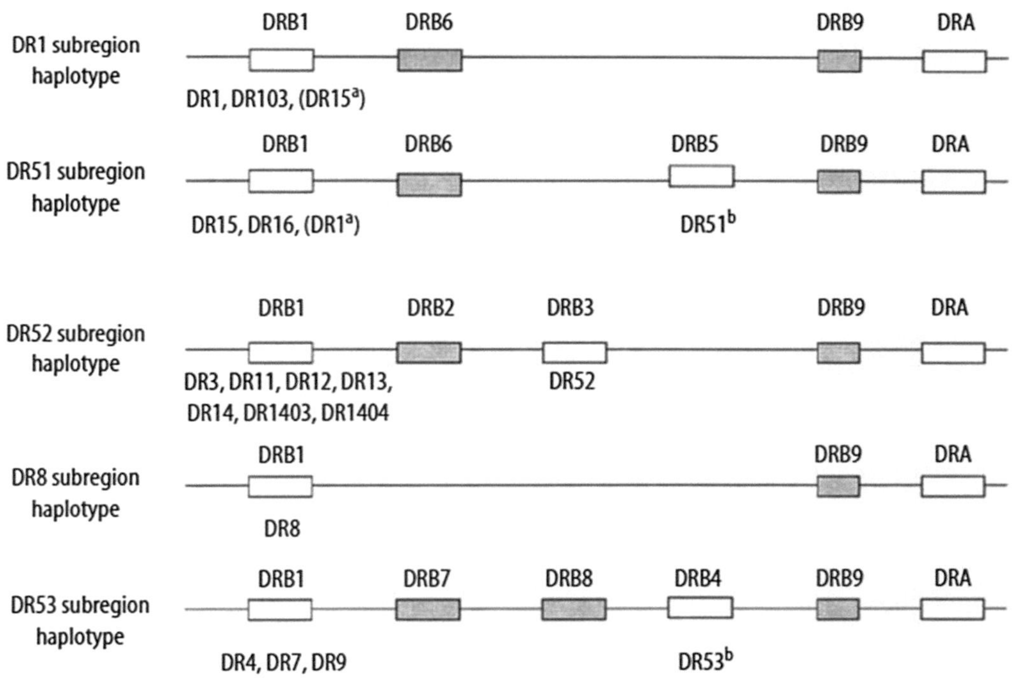

Figure 58.1 HLA-DR region and encoded allotypes. Pseudogenes are indicated by *shaded boxes*. Expressed genes are indicated by *open boxes*. The serologic specificity encoded by a gene is given underneath each expressed gene box. [a] Rarely observed haplotypes. [b] The DR51 and DR53 specificities may not be expressed on certain haplotypes (Adapted from Little AM, Parham P. Polymorphism and evolution of HLA class I and II genes and molecules. *Rev Immunogenet.* 1999;1:105–123)

Linkage Disequilibrium or Gametic Association

LD is an important feature of the HLA system. Gametic associations are regularly found between certain alleles of HLA-A and HLA-B, HLA-C and HLA-B, HLA-B and HLA-DR, and HLA-DR and HLA-DQ. In some so-called extended haplotypes, significant LD extends over 3 Mb from HLA-A at the telomeric end of the HLA region to HLA-DP at the centromeric end, including HLA class III genes ([8] and references therein). It is this LD that allows the identification of bone marrow or stem cell donors in population registries who are matched with a given patient at multiple loci (see "Histocompatibility Assessment in Unrelated Donors").

HLA Gene Frequencies in Human Populations

Although a very large number of alleles (e.g., >1,600 for HLA-B) can be found in the global population, a much smaller number (e.g., 30–50 for HLA-DRB1) is present in most individual populations. Importantly, different populations tend to have different frequency distributions of alleles and exhibit different patterns of LD. This variability exists among both racial and ethnic groups.

Clinical Utility of HLA Typing

Solid Organ Transplantation

Kidney and Pancreas

Over 570,000 patients had end-stage renal disease (ESRD) at the end of 2010. Treatment modalities include hemodialysis, peritoneal dialysis, and kidney transplantation. Kidney transplant is the most effective treatment for patients with ESRD. However, despite a waiting list of over 90,000 patients, only 10,622 deceased donor kidneys were transplanted in 2010. The median time a patient with blood type "O" listed in 2003 waited for a deceased donor graft was >5 years. Longer time on dialysis is one of the strongest risk factors for inferior transplant outcomes. The pursuit of kidney donation from living donors is essential to addressing the long and ever-growing waiting list (Scientific Registry of Transplant Recipients, 2011; http://www.srtr.org/).

Many transplant candidates have potential living donors, but approximately one-third of these potential donations do not lead to a transplant because of blood group type or crossmatch incompatibility. Kidney paired donation (KPD), also referred to as kidney exchange or live-donor paired exchange, provides an opportunity for donors to indirectly donate to their intended recipient, thereby ensuring living donor kidney transplantation without the barrier of incompatibility. Congress defined and supported KPD by passing the Charlie Norwood Living Organ Donation Act, signed in 2007. Support and interest in KPD has markedly grown in the last decade. However, KPD remains grossly underutilized. Nearly all the initial donor exchange transplants in the USA have been performed through independent, regional KPD registries. The logistics of maintaining a multicenter database, crossmatching potential pairs, and timing the transplants have become increasingly complex, raising concerns regarding programmatic efficiency and efficacy (reviewed in Ref. 9).

HLA Matching of Living Related Donors

Transplants are performed using donor–recipient pairs sharing HLA-A, HLA-B, and HLA-DR antigens from one or two haplotypes. The analysis of HLA matching for kidney graft survival over the period of 1985–1999 is based primarily on serologic typing data. The half-life survival for a graft from an HLA-identical sibling is 23 years, compared to a one-haplotype-related donor, which has a half-life of 12.8 years [6, 10].

HLA Matching of Cadaveric Donors

Data excerpted from the United Network for Organ Sharing (UNOS) transplant registry [9] indicate that HLA serologic matching appears to have an effect on long-term graft survival of kidneys from cadaveric donors. Although the 1-year graft survival is not very different in cases involving a complete match from those who are completely mismatched, after 5 years the gap in percent survival widens significantly, suggesting that the immunosuppressive drugs are potent in avoiding early graft loss due to acute rejections. However, as the drug dosages are tapered over time, the HLA-matching effect becomes significant. Patients receiving organs with zero mismatches for HLA-A, HLA-B, or HLA-DR antigens achieve a graft survival half-life of 11.3 years compared to a half-life of 6.3 years for grafts that were completely mismatched for these antigens. HLA matching is especially beneficial in second transplants and in patients with preformed antibodies. The effect of HLA-A, HLA-B, and HLA-DR matching remains significant even with the most recent forms of immunosuppression [10].

UNOS HLA-Matching Algorithm for Allocation of Cadaveric Kidneys and Pancreases

The selection of a recipient for any given random cadaveric donor is based on an HLA-matching algorithm defined by UNOS (http://www.unos.org). The current allocation policy considers the degree of HLA matching at HLA-A, HLA-B, and HLA-DR. The organs are distributed locally first, and if no match is found, they are offered regionally, and then nationally, until a recipient is found. Nationwide organ sharing is mandatory for pediatric and sensitized candidates with zero HLA-A, HLA-B, and HLA-DR mismatches; local and regional organ sharing is based on one or two HLA-DR mismatches. All other match grades are allocated without regard to mismatching. The main purpose of this algorithm is to try to transplant more minority patients while at the same time not reducing overall graft outcome.

Transplantation of Other Solid Organs

HLA typing for heart and lung transplant patients and their potential donors is an important step for donor selection by virtual crossmatching. Virtual crossmatching is accomplished by avoiding HLA class I and class II antibody specificities identified by screening patients' sera prior to transplant. HLA typing in these patients usually includes low-resolution HLA-A, HLA-B, HLA-C, HLA-DRB1, HLA-DRB3, HLA-DRB4, HLA-DRB5, and HLA-DQB for patients and their donors. In cases where anti-DQA, anti-DP, or allele-specific antibodies are present, HLA typing of donors and recipients also may include HLA-DQA, HLA-DP, or allele-level typing as needed.

The effect of HLA-A, HLA-B, and HLA-DR matching on the survival of heart and lung transplants is statistically significant. In addition, donor-specific antibodies to HLA antigens are associated with graft failure and poor survival. Antibody-mediated rejection appears in about 10–20 % of heart transplant patients, correlating with factors of poor outcome such as increased incidence for hemodynamic compromise rejection, greater development of cardiac allograft vasculopathy, and higher incidence of mortality. The effect of HLA matching for liver transplants is less clear.

Hematopoietic Cell Transplantation

HLA Typing Requirements

Typically, HLA typing for hematopoietic cell transplantation (HCT) initially would include low-resolution typing for HLA-A, HLA-B, HLA-C, HLA-DRB1, HLA-DRB3, HLA-DRB4, HLA-DRB5, and HLA-DQB1 loci. Allele-level typing is subsequently performed in the final identification of suitable donors for HCT. Three different categories of donors usually are considered in the following order of preference: HLA genotypically identical siblings, HLA-mismatched relatives, and matched or mismatched unrelated donors.

Histocompatibility Assessment in HLA-Matched Relatives

The goal when screening for an HLA-matched sibling donor is to identify which of any siblings have inherited the same HLA haplotype from their parents. This requires typing all siblings and, if possible, both parents for HLA-A, HLA-B, HLA-DRB1, and HLA-DQB1. Given the current average family size in the USA of 2.7 siblings, the approximate probability that a patient will have an HLA match within the family is 30–35 %. For those patients who do not have an HLA-matched sibling within the family, an HLA-mismatched relative who shares one haplotype can be considered. However, the clinical data clearly indicate that with increasing disparity for HLA-A, HLA-B, HLA-DRB1, or HLA-DQB1 loci, there is increased risk of graft-vs-host disease (GVHD) following HCT.

Histocompatibility Assessment in Unrelated Donors

When a matched sibling donor does not exist for a patient requiring allogeneic HCT (70 % of cases), searching for extended family members or donors from unrelated bone marrow registries would be the next option. Registries of volunteer bone marrow donors as well as cord blood exist in most developed countries. The largest of these is the National Marrow Donor Program (NMDP) in the USA (http://www.marrow.org).

The probability of finding a matched donor at HLA-A, HLA-B, HLA-DRB1, and HLA-DQB1 depends on the ethnic origin of the patient and the composition and size of the donor registry being searched. Identifying a patient's haplotypes can help predict the probability of finding matched donors and assist in developing a search strategy, because some alleles and haplotypes are more common than others, and they are distributed at different frequencies in different racial and ethnic groups. When searching for a donor, for some alleles, an allele-level match is more likely to be found among persons of a particular ethnicity [11–14]. The NMDP matching algorithm HapLogic℠ is based on this principle: identifying the donors or cord blood units (CBUs) with the highest potential to match the patient. This allows transplant physicians searching the Be The Match Registry® (operated by the NMDP) to identify more quickly and efficiently the best immunogenetically matched donor or CBU for their patients. The transplant center is responsible for selecting an unrelated donor or CBU for a patient. The NMDP recommends that, when possible, patients and adult donors (marrow or peripheral blood stem cells) should be fully matched (8 of 8 loci) at high resolution for HLA-A, HLA-B, HLA-C, and HLA-DRB1. Matching for CBUs is less stringent, and the NMDP recommends fully matched (6 of 6) CBUs at HLA-A, HLA-B (antigen level), and HLA-DRB1 (allele level). This does not imply that availability of a partially matched donor or CBU is a contraindication to transplant. Instead, a less-than-optimal match is another risk factor to be considered in developing the patient's treatment plan.

Likelihood of Finding an Unrelated Donor or Cord Blood Unit

Today, patients are more likely to find an unrelated donor or CBU than previously possible. Through the NMDP, three potential hematopoietic cell options for patients in need of an unrelated donor can be available: marrow, peripheral blood stem cells (PBSC), or umbilical cord blood. A patient's likelihood of finding a potential unrelated donor or CBU has increased with the continuing growth and increasing diversity of the Be The Match Registry. As of 2012, the registry includes nine million potential marrow or PBSC donors and nearly 145,000 CBUs. Through international connections, the NMDP searches more than 18.5 million potential donors as of 2012 and nearly 550,000 CBUs. Nearly all (>95 %) patients are able to find at least one potential 4 of 6 HLA-matched CBU on the Be The Match Registry, the largest in the USA, and the majority will find a potential 5 of 6 match. However, patients belonging to racial groups that are not well represented in the registries have a considerably decreased probability of matched donor identification [12].

Relative Impact of HLA Disparities

HLA compatibility affects not only the ability to achieve sustained engraftment following HCT but also the risk of developing acute and chronic GVHD [6, 13, 15]. Posttransplant risk of graft failure, GVHD, and mortality can be affected by quantitative and qualitative characteristics of donor and recipient HLA mismatching. Moreover, studies have reached different conclusions regarding the relative contributions of HLA class I and class II mismatching because of population-based differences in the specific HLA-mismatch combinations between patients and donors ([13] and references therein). In an analysis of HCT for chronic myelogenous leukemia (CML), the risk of graft failure is affected primarily by donor disparity for HLA class I including HLA-C. The incidence of rejection correlates with the number of donor-incompatible alleles. The incidence of graft rejection is 0.7 % for zero, 8 % for a single, and 19 % for multiple class I allele incompatibilities. Donor disparity for class II does not increase the risk of rejection [6, 13].

The level of matching is more critical for HCT than for solid organ transplantation because of the risk of GVHD. GVHD is a major cause of mortality in HCT and is more frequent than allograft rejection. Analysis of HLA and GVHD focuses on mismatches in the host recognized by donor T cells. Generally, host disparity for class II is thought to convey greater risk for GVHD than class I disparity. In an analysis of HCT for CML, patients with a single class II mismatch at HLA-DR or HLA-DQ have a hazard ratio of 1.8 compared to HLA matches. Single class I mismatches are well tolerated with respect to GVHD; however, combined mismatching at class I and class II confers a hazard ratio of 2.0. Allele mismatches for HLA-A, HLA-B, HLA-C, HLA-DRB1, and HLA-DQB1 also are a significant factor for survival. Patients mismatched for more than one class I allele and those mismatched at both class I and class II alleles have a significantly lower survival than patients and donors fully matched for HLA-A, HLA-B, HLA-C, HLA-DRB1, and HLA-DQB1. A single class I mismatch or single class II mismatch does not appear to affect survival [6, 13, 15]. It is likely that different modes of patients' immunosuppression after transplant would have an impact on the relative risk associated with various HLA loci. Criteria for "permissible" mismatching in HCT are center dependent. However, very few centers would perform HCT across more than one HLA mismatch at HLA-A, HLA-B, HLA-DR, or HLA-DQ. Interestingly, recent studies have shown that GVHD rates and survival outcomes in pediatric and adult patients receiving cord blood transplants with up to two HLA antigen mismatches (i.e., a 4 of 6 match) are similar to those for 6 of 6 HLA-matched unrelated donor marrow transplants, as long as the recipient received an optimal CD34 cell dose adjusted for the recipient's body weight [16–19].

HLA and Disease Association

Population Genetic Analyses

The extensive polymorphism observed for HLA loci requires a rigorous approach to data analysis [20]. The complex patterns of LD commonly observed for HLA data can make it difficult to identify specific causal genetic variants. Disease association studies of highly polymorphic HLA data may require the consideration of multiple units of analysis, including amino acid, allele, genotype, and haplotype levels, as well as consideration of gene–gene or gene–environment interactions. The selection of the appropriate statistical tests is critical and will be dependent on the nature of the data set as well as the specific research hypotheses being tested; there is no single analytical approach that can be applied to all data.

Population genetic analyses of gene (allele) frequencies, tests for fit Hardy–Weinberg equilibrium (HWE) expectations, and estimations of haplotype frequencies are the primary steps in analyzing immunogenetic data and provide additional means to assess underlying population substructure, as well as additional units of analysis on which association analyses will be performed. Basic methods for these analyses are described below.

Calculation of Gene (Allele) Frequencies

In the age of molecular typing techniques, HLA gene (allele) frequencies (GF) no longer need to be estimated from phenotype data. In most cases, GF for HLA data can be obtained via direct counting, where the number of observations for a given allele is divided by the number of chromosomes ($2n$, where n = sample size) under study.

Hardy–Weinberg Testing

The Hardy–Weinberg (HW) model is useful for primary quality control (QC) verification of the integrity of genotype data, as molecular genotyping errors can result in both individual genotype deviations and overall (locus-level) deviations from HWE. In addition, HW testing also is useful for detecting sampling errors (see below) in population samples. Confidence in the accuracy of HW testing therefore is crucial for confidence in subsequent analyses, as many analytical methods (e.g., LD and haplotype estimation) are predicated on an assumption of HWE in the data set.

In a HW test, observed genotype counts are compared to those expected under HWE proportions (HWEP), as calculated from a table of all possible genotypes generated using an appropriate statistical method [21]. The relationship between the allele and genotype frequencies under HWEP is given as

$$f\left(A_iA_i\right)=p_i^2 \quad \text{and} \quad f\left(A_iA_j\right)=2p_ip_j,$$

where *pi* is the allele frequency of allele *Ai* and *pj* is the allele frequency of allele *Aj*. Populations in HWE will not depart significantly from these allele and genotype frequencies.

Tests of overall locus-level HWEP compute a *p*-value to estimate the significance of observed deviations across all genotypes. Significant deviation of observed genotype counts from expected HWEP can result from factors that include sampling errors (the sampling of admixed, stratified, substructured, or some other form of blended populations), inbreeding or other nonrandom mating, natural selection, and genotyping errors. Tests for deviation from HWEP have low power, and significant deviation from HWEP is *not* common. Genotyping errors (e.g., failure to detect a specific allele, resulting in an excess of homozygotes) are the first consideration when significant deviations from HWEP are detected (especially when such deviations are detected only at a single locus in a multi-locus analysis), rather than the operation of selection, admixture, or nonrandom mating, unless the data are suspected to be from an unusual population.

Haplotype Estimation

Haplotype-level analyses are important to studies of the etiology of human disease, selective forces acting on populations, and optimal bone marrow donor registry (BMDR) size. Multi-locus analyses can be used to identify associations between markers and disease loci that are not evident with single-locus analyses. Haplotypes are used for disease association mapping, quantitative trait locus (QTL) mapping, and imputing underlying genetic markers.

Study design and subject recruitment depend on which of the alternative approaches of identifying haplotypes by segregation analysis in families or estimating haplotypes from population samples of phase-unknown unrelated individuals will be applied. Estimated haplotypes and haplotype frequencies (HFs) play a central role in most genetic studies [21].

It is important to understand that haplotype estimation always results in population-level frequency estimates, rather than haplotype assignments for individuals. Due to the limitations of current haplotype estimation methods, estimated haplotypes observed fewer than three times in a population should be considered unreliable.

Analysis in Disease Association Studies

The case–control study is the most common study design in HLA disease association studies. Case–control studies can be very sensitive to population stratification within sample cohorts. This issue is particularly important for HLA data, as HLA allele frequency distributions can vary considerably between human populations. If study subjects are not chosen with scrupulous attention to homogeneity of ancestral background, population-based genetic differences between cases and controls may be misinterpreted as disease associations.

The results of the basic population-level analyses outlined above can be used in case–control association analyses. Depending on the study hypothesis, the units of analysis may include gene, carrier, genotype, and/or haplotype frequencies in cases and controls. Assurance that the control population genotypic distributions conform to expected HWEP is critical.

Contingency Tables

A contingency table is used to test the independence of frequency distributions for categorical variables. Tests for heterogeneity between specific groups (e.g., cases and controls) for HLA data can be performed using contingency table testing and a standard Chi-square (χ^2) measure.

A contingency table always is constructed utilizing raw counts, rather than frequency data. The preferred approach in this type of analysis for highly polymorphic HLA data is to first examine heterogeneity in overall allele frequency distributions in cases vs controls for a particular locus, using a $2\times k$ row by column ($r\times c$) contingency table. If overall heterogeneity is detected at the locus level, the contributions of individual alleles to the overall deviation can be examined in a series of 2×2 tests.

When significance of the association of all individual alleles is assessed with the a priori knowledge of overall heterogeneity at the locus, it is not necessary to correct for multiple comparisons in subsequent 2×2 tests; however, if no overall heterogeneity has been detected, analysis of 2×2 tests requires corrections for multiple comparisons (usually via the Bonferroni method), with a correction factor minimally equivalent to the number of alleles tested.

Low-frequency alleles pose a particular challenge in traditional χ^2 association tests in disease studies. The χ^2 test can lead to false acceptance or rejection of the null hypothesis when the expected genotype counts in a contingency table are small. It is not unusual for 30 or more HLA alleles to be observed at a locus, with a wide range of frequencies, and the preferred approach is to combine low-frequency alleles into a single "binned" category, by combining alleles with an expected value of less than five in cases or controls prior to calculation of the χ^2 statistic. The χ^2 statistic for a contingency table analysis of case–control data for a genetic association is calculated as

$$\chi^2 = \sum \frac{(O_i - E_i)^2}{E_i}$$

where

O_i = the observed count of allele i

E_i = the expected count of allele i

The expected count for each cell in the $r \times c$ table is calculated as

$$\frac{(\text{row total allele } i) \times (\text{column total})}{2n}$$

where

column total = sum of the counts in the column

row total = number of observations of allele i in all subjects

n = number of individuals (cases + controls)

$2n$ = number of chromosomes (cases + controls)

The degrees of freedom (df) for the χ^2 analysis are the number of alleles with expected values in cases and controls of five or greater, plus the combined category, minus 1 (i.e., $k-1$). A p-value is obtained by comparing the test statistic to the χ^2 distribution for the appropriate df.

Odds Ratio and Relative Risk

Odds ratios (ORs) are used in disease association studies to describe the strength of association between two variables and reflect the ratio of odds of an outcome (e.g., disease) in one group (e.g., individuals with a particular allele) to the odds of this outcome in another group (individuals without that allele). Relative risk (RR) is a different measure that describes the risk of having the outcome of interest relative to exposure (e.g., positive or negative for a particular allele). RR is more applicable to prospective studies, while OR is preferred for retrospective studies.

OR and RR values are only meaningful when presented with a corresponding confidence interval (CI). The standard probability level is generally 95 %, meaning that there is a 95 % chance that the OR or RR value of interest is in that range. Because the null hypothesis of both tests is that OR or RR = 1, a CI that includes 1 is not considered statistically significant.

Logistic Regression

Logistic regression (LR) analyses also can be used in case–control studies. LR is a form of generalized linear modeling for data with a binary outcome variable, such as case–control data. LR provides a means to develop association models that include the contribution of numerous covariables. LR is a critical tool in the analysis of complex multivariate data sets.

LR analysis always is performed using software, but extreme care must be taken in the coding of HLA data, as most LR software is not designed to handle high levels of polymorphism common in these data sets. A regression analysis produces a model that includes all of the variables that are useful in predicting the (binary) outcome variable. LR provides an OR for each variable involved in predicting outcome and can be particularly useful in HLA studies that must consider a large number of cofactors.

HLA Typing for Autoimmune Diseases and Other Disorders

Specific alleles of HLA molecules are associated with certain diseases. Associations have been shown to be of two types: those with disease association with class I antigens and those with strong associations with class II antigens (Table 58.2). Importantly, as shown in Table 58.2, the following HLA disease associations are of diagnostic importance. The best known is the association of HLA-B27 with ankylosing spondylitis (AS) and associated spondyloarthropathies (reviewed in Ref. 23). More than 90 % of AS patients are B*27, which is found in 5–10 % of the general population. An increased incidence of B*27 also is seen in patients with Rieter syndrome and anterior uveitis.

Celiac disease (CD) is caused by an immune response to gluten in genetically predisposed individuals. Although patients with CD may be asymptomatic, infants and young children commonly present with diarrhea, failure to thrive, and abdominal pain and distention. The prevalence of CD in the general population is estimated to be higher than 1 %. Approximately 95 % of patients with CD have the HLA-DQ2 heterodimer encoded by the DQA1*05 and DQB1*02 alleles, which are found in 20–30 % of the general population. Close to 5–10 % of CD patients have the DQ8 heterodimer encoded by the DQA1*03 and DQB1*0302 alleles, which are present in 10 % of the general population. High-risk HLA class II haplotypes include DR3/DR3. DR3/DR7, DR11/DR3, or DR11/DR7 carrying DQA and DQB susceptibility alleles in cis/trans associations [24–26]. Since 25–40 % of the general population has either DQ2 or DQ8, the presence of either heterodimer is not diagnostic of CD; the primary use of HLA-DQ typing is to rule out CD and genetic susceptibility for CD. Determining genetic susceptibility can avoid continual serologic testing and initiation of a gluten-free diet, especially in individuals in high-risk groups.

Narcolepsy is a chronic sleep disorder characterized by daytime sleepiness and dysosomnia. Narcolepsy is associated with DRB1*15 and DQB1*06:02. The DQB1*06:02 allele is found in over 90 % of patients with narcolepsy–cataplexy and is found in about 20 % of the general population [27–29].

Table 58.2 Examples of HLA testing for autoimmune diseases

Disease	HLA test	Comment
Ankylosing spondylitis (AS)	HLA-B*27	B27 is found in >95 % of patients with AS but also is found in 7 % of the white population. The presence of B27 is not diagnostic. The absence of B27 tends to exclude AS.
Celiac disease	HLA-DQ2 (DQA1*05/DQB1*02) and DQ8	More than 97 % of celiac patients carry either HLA-DQ2 (DQA1*05/DQB1*02) or HLA-DQ8 (DQA1*03/DQB1*0302) or both. However, 39 % of the general US population carry these HLA-DQ variants.
Narcolepsy	HLA-DR2, DQB1*06:02	DR2 (DRB1*1501-DQB1*0602) is present in nearly all patients with narcolepsy but also is found in ~20 % of the general population. The presence of DQB1*0602 is not diagnostic of narcolepsy, but the absence of DQB1*0602 tends to exclude narcolepsy.
Birdshot retinochoroidopathy	HLA-A*29	>95 % of patients carry HLA-A*29
Behcet's disease	HLA-B*51	50–80 % of patients carry HLA-B*51

Table 58.3 Examples of HLA testing for hypersensitivity reactions to drugs

Drug	Clinical indication	HLA specificity
Abacavir	Antiviral	B*57:01
Carbamazepine	Antiepileptic	B*15:02
Carbamazepine	Antiepileptic	A*31:01[a]
Allopurinol	Hyperuricemia	B*58:01

[a]Japanese population established by genome-wide association studies

Birdshot retinochoroidopathy (BSCR) is a rare disease, characterized by a posterior uveitis with multiple hypopigmented choroidal and retinal lesions. >95 % of patients carry A*29 [30, 31].

Behcet's disease is a chronic inflammatory autoimmune disease characterized by oral aphthous lesions, genital ulcers, and other symptoms and occurs more frequently in the Middle East and Asia. Behcet's is strongly associated with B*51 (50–80 % of patients carry B*51) [32, 33].

HLA Typing for Drug Hypersensitivity Reactions

Hypersensitivity reactions to drugs typically occur within the first few weeks after drug intake, but in the case of a reexposure, symptoms can be seen within hours, suggesting a delayed-type hypersensitivity reaction. Cutaneous adverse drug reactions include Stevens–Johnson syndrome (SJS), toxic epidermal necrolysis (TEN), and drug-induced hypersensitivity syndrome (DIHS). SJS is considered to be a minor form of TEN. These reactions usually are manifested by painful blistering skin rashes that may cause the skin to slough off. Lesions also may involve the mucous membranes. Complications may include internal organ lesions and sepsis and may cause death. The amount of skin sloughing determines morbidity. In either case, urgent medical care is necessary. SJS and TEN also can be caused by other factors such as infections or can be idiopathic.

Abacavir is a nucleoside analog reverse transcriptase inhibitor used to treat HIV patients. In Caucasians, B*57:01 is associated with hypersensitivity to abacavir [34, 35]. B*57:01 is found most frequently in Caucasians (4 %) and less frequently in African (1 %), Asian (0.9 %), or Hispanic (<0.1 %) populations.

Carbamazepine (CBZ) is an anticonvulsant known to be associated with cutaneous adverse drug reactions (cADRs), including SJS, TEN, and DIHS. B*15:02 is associated with these disorders in Asians [36–38]. Studies from Europe have shown that B*15:02 is not a universal marker for SJS/TEN. The prevalence of B*15:02 is high among Chinese (5–15 %), Malays (12–15 %), and Thais (8–27 %), but low among Japanese, Korean, Sri Lankan, and most ethnic groups in India. At the request of the US Food and Drug Administration (FDA), the makers of this drug have agreed to include the recommendation that all Asians be genotyped for this HLA allele before the drug is prescribed. In addition, a recent GWAS study showed that A*31:01 has 60.7 % sensitivity and 87.5 % specificity as a risk predictor for CBZ-induced cADRs. Although DIHS is clinically distinguished from SJS and TEN, these data indicate that they share a common genetic factor as well as a common pathophysiological mechanism [39].

Allopurinol is used to treat hyperuricemia. B*58:01 was found to be highly associated with hypersensitivity to allopurinol-induced SJS and TEN in Asian populations [40, 41]. It is not clear if similar association exists in Caucasians and Africans.

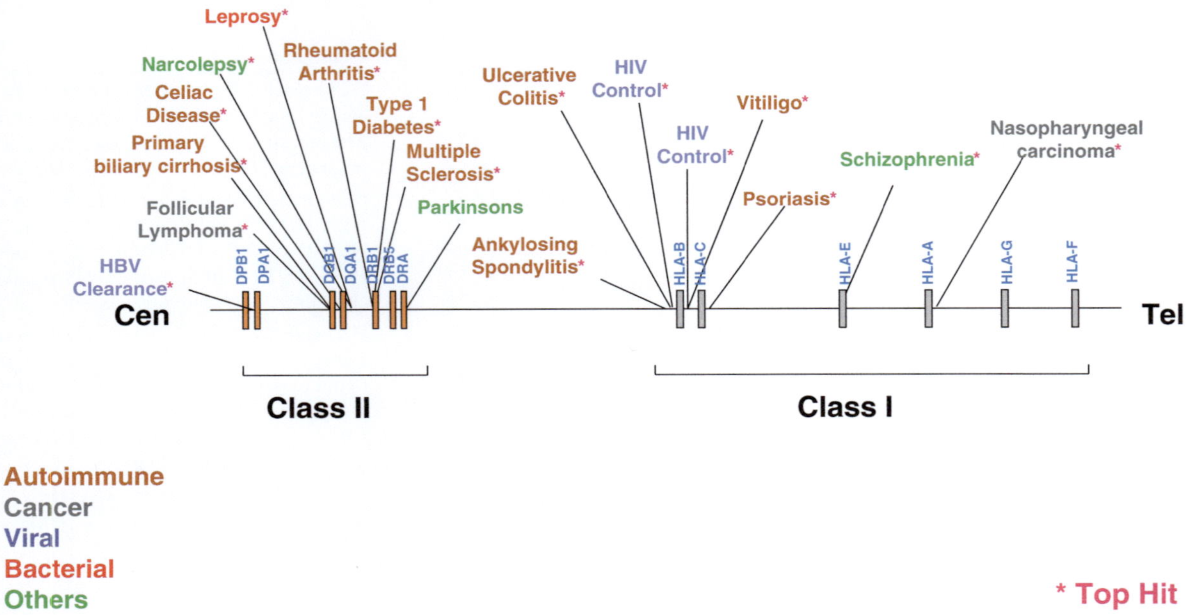

Figure 58.2 Genome-wide association studies within the MHC (This figure was kindly provided by Dr. Mary Carrington, National Institutes of Health, USA). *CEN* centromere, *TEL* telomere

Genome-Wide Association Studies Within the MHC

Genome-wide association studies have confirmed the preeminence of the human MHC in terms of the magnitude of the effect, statistical confidence, and the number of associations with autoimmune, infectious, inflammatory, and adverse drug effects (Fig. 58.2). Importantly, the MHC has the greatest genome-wide effect on control of human immunodeficiency virus (HIV) viral load; over 300 genome-wide significant single nucleotide polymorphism (SNPs) within the MHC were identified and none elsewhere. Stepwise regression analyses have narrowed these associations to four independent MHC SNP markers associated with host control of HIV viral load [42]. Specific amino acids in the HLA-B peptide-binding groove, which were previously described, as well as an independent HLA-C effect, explain the SNP associations and reconcile the previously reported protective and risk alleles.

Mechanisms for the Association of HLA Alleles with Autoimmune Diseases

The biological mechanisms underlying the associations between HLA antigens and various diseases remain mostly unknown. HLA-associated diseases are caused by interplay of multiple genes and environmental factors, in which HLA genes most often confer the strongest genetic predisposition. Based on results of a genome-wide search for susceptibility genes, HLA accounts for more than 50 % of the genetic risk in type 1 diabetes [23, 43]. Susceptibility to rheumatoid arthritis (RA) is strongly associated with the DRB1*04:01, *04:04, *04:05, and *04:08 alleles. On the other hand, DRB1*04:02, *04:03, and *04:07 are not associated with RA and may instead confer protection. A possible role of pocket 4 (residues 67, 70, 71, and 74) of the β chain of DR4 molecules has been suggested.

In type 1 diabetes, both susceptibility and protection are associated primarily with some class II HLA molecules. Association is strongest with heterozygosity for HLA-DR3- and HLA-DR4-bearing haplotypes. Data support that HLA-associated predisposition to type 1 diabetes is mainly determined by a complex multi-locus effect including HLA-DQ and HLA-DR alleles [22, 42]. This may explain differences among populations with respect to susceptibility associated with particular HLA-DQ or HLA-DR molecules. The HLA-DQ molecule associated with susceptibility often shares an amino acid other than aspartic acid at position 57 on the HLA-DQβ chain that is located in pocket 9 of the peptide-binding cleft. On the other hand, those HLA-DQ molecules associated with protection carry aspartic acid at this position (reviewed in Ref. 23).

Fine Mapping of Causal MHC Variants Associated with Complex Disease Traits

The mechanisms through which DNA sequence polymorphism operates remain unknown. The location of primary signal is confounded by multiplicity of DNA polymorphisms, frequencies in the population, and LD that may extend over several megabases in the MHC. Diseases often are found to be associated with common ancestral HLA haplotypes encompassing a very large number of MHC genes, many of which are candidates for complex disease association. Disease susceptibility appears to result from complex multilocus effects spanning the entire HLA class I, class II, and class III regions with evidence of shared loci [44–46]. Recent studies showed that a 3′ untranslated region (UTR) HLA-C variant associates strongly with control of HIV [47], potentially adding to the effects of genetic variation encoding the peptide-binding region of the HLA class I loci and indicating that both structural and regulatory variants are important and may be operating in tandem. Narrowing the HLA associations and identifying the causal HLA genes would require deep sequencing of MHC haplotypes using new technologies applied to large disease cohorts in different populations of distinct ancestry.

Other Applications

HLA-matching algorithms have been used for patients receiving repeated infusions of platelet concentrate who become refractory due to the generation of antibodies to HLA class I antigens expressed on the surface of platelets. Other important applications include vaccine clinical trials for patients with melanoma and HIV infection, in which vaccines rely on defined HLA-restricted epitopes. Identification of the appropriate HLA type is an important step in identifying patients who could benefit from these therapies.

Available Assays

Virtually all methods used widely in clinical molecular laboratories have been applied to the problem of identifying HLA alleles (Ref. [6] and references therein). Strategies based on allele-specific DNA amplification, oligonucleotide probe hybridization, and DNA sequencing have become the most common methods. Each of these methods relies on isolation of genomic DNA from the tested individual with polymerase chain reaction (PCR) amplification of relevant regions of an HLA gene. Samples for testing are usually peripheral blood but may be any nucleated cell or tissue. Laboratories typically amplify at least exons 2 and 3 of class I genes and exon 2 of class II genes, but may prepare larger amplification products that include exons 4 and 5 of class I genes for DNA sequencing. Amplification primers may be located within exons or introns. Intronic primers allow complete analysis of exons and inspection of exon–intron junctions for splice-site mutations. Primers must be chosen with care to achieve locus-specific amplification since the HLA loci are the products of gene duplication and divergence and retain substantial homology. Further, many HLA loci have closely related pseudogenes that do not encode functional polypeptides but may result in nonspecific PCR products. Each of the methods discussed below generates a large amount of data for each patient that must be compared to extensive lists of potential alleles, hybridization probe "hit" patterns, or allele sequence libraries to assign an allele type. While this may be done manually, most laboratories use software packages that must be updated frequently to include newly recognized alleles.

Resolving Power of Methods

Laboratories tailor HLA-typing assays to the specific clinical applications discussed above. For example, assays helpful in evaluation of narcolepsy may test only for presence or absence of DQB1*06:02. Matching unrelated donors and recipients for HCT requires allele-level (high resolution) typing at several class I and II loci. Conversely, low-resolution typing at the allele-group or serologic-equivalent level is typically performed for renal transplantation. Choice of the methods discussed below depends on typing volume, turnaround time requirements, and the resolution needed.

Sequence-Specific Primer Polymerase Chain Reaction

The sequence-specific primer polymerase chain reaction (SSP-PCR) method employs pairs of PCR primers chosen so that their 3′-most nucleotide or nucleotides are complementary to a polymorphic position that distinguishes an allele or allele group from other alleles ([6] and references therein). If the individual possesses the allele(s) of interest, the PCR will lead to a product whose size and presence is typically identified by agarose gel electrophoresis or can be detected in real time [6, 47]. If one or both primers are not complementary to their targets at their 3′ ends, the reaction will fail. By choosing many pairs of primers in independent reactions to cover all allele groups, laboratories can perform allele typing. Laboratories include a second set of generic primers for a control gene in each reaction, as a DNA amplification control. Because of the large number of allele groups, about 100 PCRs are necessary to perform a low-resolution HLA-A, HLA-B, and HLA-DRB1 typing for a single patient. Additional reactions are required if allele-level typing is desired. Thus SSP-PCR typing requires considerable thermal cycler resources. SSP-PCR is suitable for low to moderate typing volumes in laboratories. Since it can be performed in a few hours, SSP-PCR can be used to identify HLA alleles in time-sensitive situations such as in deceased donors prior to renal transplantation.

Sequence-Specific Oligonucleotide Probe Hybridization

For sequence-specific oligonucleotide probe hybridization (SSO), PCR products amplified from the relevant regions of a particular HLA gene are hybridized to a large panel of oligonucleotide probes that include the known polymorphisms ([6] and references therein). Hybridization and washing conditions of high stringency allow detection of single-nucleotide differences. Most laboratories detect bound probes colorimetrically or by chemiluminescence. The reactivity of the entire panel is analyzed against expected results for particular alleles or groups of alleles to assign an allele type. Forward SSO is useful for large-scale, batched testing, with the PCR products from many individuals immobilized on a membrane, with subsequent hybridization with a single probe. By preparing many membranes, the laboratory can test the entire panel of probes. Reverse SSO assays employ multiple probes immobilized on a membrane strip for hybridization to the PCR products from a single individual [6]. Whereas reverse dot-blot and SSO methods typically employ enzyme labels and colorimetric substrates that require subsequent development, other SSO methods employ microspheres. Up to 100 different populations of microspheres can be mixed together and distinguished by their unique fluorescence signatures when analyzed by a fluoroanalyzer. Thus, all variants in the PCR products are analyzed simultaneously, and the entire assay is carried out in a single vessel with the addition of a single reagent. Reverse SSO assays can be challenging to optimize since all probes must attain specificity under identical hybridization conditions. Reverse SSO reagents are available commercially. This type of method is very attractive for rapid, low- to mid-volume testing. SSO testing can yield low-resolution results or allele-level results using larger panels of probes.

DNA Sequencing

DNA sequencing of PCR products is a method increasingly attractive for allele-level typing because of the large numbers of alleles known to exist at several of the HLA loci. In theory, any known or new allele should be detected by this method if defined by polymorphisms within the nucleotide sequence amplified by the two PCR primers. Recombinant DNA polymerases for sequencing reactions, improved fluorescent dyes for dideoxynucleotides, powerful analysis software, and capillary electrophoresis instruments have made DNA sequencing technically easier and less labor-intensive for complex clinical molecular tests such as HLA typing [48]. Careful selection of PCR primers to ensure roughly equal amplification of the two alleles present in an individual is a crucial requirement for this method. Otherwise heterozygous peaks in the electropherograms will not be reliably identified and result in a false homozygous genotype. DNA sequencing requires less modification in response to new alleles than other methods and is a powerful and general way of performing allele-level typing.

The very large number of alleles and the patchwork patterns of polymorphisms clustered within a few exons make setting the phase of linked polymorphisms difficult and results in "ambiguous" typing results, i.e., data that are consistent with many different possible genotype assignments. Resolving these ambiguities with current techniques can be cumbersome, time-consuming, and expensive. One approach to reducing genotype ambiguity and achieving high-resolution HLA typing is to use the massively parallel clonal sequencing strategies of next-generation sequencing (NGS) systems. Current typing methods, including Sanger sequencing, yield ambiguous typing results because of incomplete genomic coverage and inability to set phase for HLA allele determination. When coupled with new softwares, NGS systems can provide very high-resolution HLA genotyping. High-throughput genotyping can be achieved by use of primers with multiplex identifier tags to allow pooling of the amplicons generated from different individuals prior to sequencing. NGS combines the advantage of long-range amplification and the power of high-throughput sequencing platforms. Overall, this technology has the capacity to deliver low-cost, high-throughput, and accurate HLA typing by multiplexing thousands of samples in a single sequencing run. Several strategies have been used; the first is an amplicon sequencing approach focused primarily on the exons of HLA class I and class II genes including HLA-A, HLA-B, HLA-C, DPB1, DQA1, DQB1, DRB1, DRB3, DRB4, and DRB5 (DRB3/4/5). Another strategy uses a long-range PCR of the entire HLA class I gene followed by fragmentation, shotgun sequencing, and assembly for a few samples on the first available NGS platform, the Roche GS 454 system (support for the GS 454 system is being phased out). Later, the Illumina (MiSeq) and Ion Torrent (PGM, Proton) platforms have been used for both of these approaches [49, 50]. A third strategy uses the Pacific Biosciences single-molecule real-time (SMRT) system to provide sequencing of entire long-range HLA PCR products, potentially generating complete allele-level genotypes for both HLA class I and class II genes [51].

In the targeted amplicon sequencing strategy, NGS permits phasing of polymorphisms within the amplicon but does not phase distinct amplicons. Genotyping ambiguity due to phasing can be eliminated using a bioinformatic approach wherein genotyping software considers all possible combinations of allelic amplicon sequences at various exons and compares these to the IMGT/HLA Database. However, this approach assumes that a potential genotype assignment with novel alleles that are absent from the database is extremely rare. Strategies that use a long-range PCR of the entire HLA gene can set phase for linked polymorphisms by shotgun assembly of overlapping short sequence reads and paired-end reads of fragments derived from the long-range amplicon. Phase can be set directly by long-read sequencing on the PacBio platform of the entire long-range HLA amplicon.

The use of clonal sequencing such as NGS has produced a large amount of novel HLA sequences including noncoding sequence. Polymorphisms located in these noncoding sequences (synonymous substitutions and intronic and flanking sequence) may have important biological function influencing gene expression. In addition, these polymorphisms can distinguish otherwise identical HLA haplotypes and contribute to disease association and population genetic analyses.

Other Methods

Nontargeted HLA typing: High-resolution HLA typing can be inferred from whole-genome sequences or whole-exome sequences using bioinformatics and software algorithms. Furthermore, the entire 4–5 Mb HLA region has been targeted by hybrid capture with probe panels. HLA types can also be imputed from SNP genotyping data. Typically, the HLA region SNPs used for HLA imputation are not in the HLA genes themselves. The imputation algorithms are based on LD between the SNPs and the sequence variants in the exons of HLA class I and class II genes. The accuracy of these imputation algorithms is highest when the training samples and the test samples come from similar ethnic populations. In general, the HLA typing performance of these imputation systems is high (>98 % concordance) at the single-field level and somewhat less accurate at the two-field level.

Early in the development of DNA-based HLA typing, restriction fragment length polymorphism (RFLP) analysis was employed. This approach declined in importance as laboratories realized that the complexity and number of HLA alleles outstripped the power of RFLP analysis. Reference strand conformation analysis is a method employing the analysis of heteroduplexes prepared by mixing PCR products from the tested individual with those prepared from a reference allele. The migration of the heteroduplexes is assessed on an acrylamide gel and compared to a library of migration profiles [6]. HLA alleles are likely to have unique migration patterns, especially when tested with several reference alleles. This is a fairly rapid method and is a simple and elegant way to assess whether a donor and a recipient are identical at a locus. Rare alleles not represented in the library with known migration patterns are difficult to identify.

Interpretation and Reporting of Test Results

HLA Nomenclature

HLA nomenclature and convention of HLA allele naming are shown in Table 58.4 and illustrated in Fig. 58.3. The alleles of each of the HLA genes are numbered based on the original serologic nomenclature. HLA alleles are designated by a superscripted asterisk after the locus of origin and a number corresponding to the particular allele (e.g., HLA-A*02:01). The parallel testing using serologic and DNA genotyping of HLA alleles has led to the use of one nomenclature for the description of low-resolution typing where the HLA assignment might include more than one possible related allele (e.g., HLA-A A2) and a nomenclature reflecting the high-resolution allelic typing. Thus, different HLA allele subtypes (e.g., for A2) can appear indistinguishable when tested by serology or with a limited panel of nucleic acid probes, so a generic or low-resolution typing is obtained. The naming of new HLA alleles is decided by an international nomenclature committee; however, the workshop prefix "w" and other designations often precede formal naming by the international nomenclature committee. As a result, the literature can be confusing for the uninitiated. Another feature of the nomenclature is the Bw4 and Bw6 specificities.

Table 58.4 Nomenclature of HLA alleles

Nomenclature	Indication
HLA	The HLA region and prefix for an HLA gene
HLA-DRB1	A particular HLA locus, i.e., DRB1
*HLA-DRB1*13*	A group of alleles that encode the DR13 antigen or sequence homology to other DRB1*13 alleles
*HLA-DRB1*13:01*	A specific HLA allele with a unique protein sequence
*HLA-DRB1*13:01:02*	An allele that differs by a synonymous mutation from DRB1*13:01:01
*HLA-DRB1*13:01:01:02*	An allele that contains a mutation outside the coding region from DRB1*13:01:01:01
*HLA-A*24:09N*	A "null" allele, an allele that is not expressed
*HLA-A*30:14L*	An allele encoding a protein with significantly reduced or "low" cell surface expression
*HLA-A*24:02:01:02L*	An allele encoding a protein with significantly reduced or "low" cell surface expression, where the mutation is found outside the coding region
*HLA-B*44:02:01:02S*	An allele encoding a protein that is expressed as a "secreted" molecule only
*HLA-A*32:11Q*	An allele that has a mutation that has previously been shown to have a significant effect on cell surface expression, but where this has not been confirmed and its expression remains "questionable"

Table adapted from a table kindly provided by Prof Steven Marsh, Anthony Nolan Research Institute, London, United Kingdom (www.hla.alleles.org)

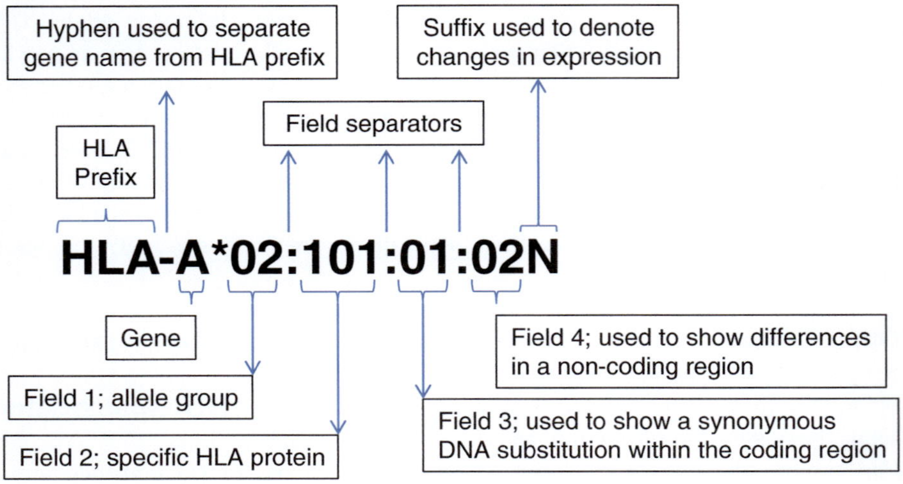

Figure 58.3 Convention for HLA allele naming (This figure was adapted from one kindly provided by Prof Steven Marsh, Anthony Nolan Research Institute, London, United Kingdom [www.hla.alleles.org])

All HLA-B alleles encode one of two possible epitopes located on the alpha 1 helix that were originally defined by serology as Bw4 and Bw6 specificities. The "w" prefix is retained in this case to distinguish them from true HLA alleles. Annual HLA nomenclature reports with frequent updates are available at several Web sites (HLA Informatics Group, http://www.anthonynolan.org/clinicians-and-researchers/anthony-nolan-research-institute/hla-informatics-group, or IMGT/HLA Database, http://www.ebi.ac.uk/imgt/hla/).

Due to the complexity of the HLA system, a common language for histocompatibility terms is used to avoid misunderstanding and for accurately reporting HLA typing results. In early 2010, representatives from clinical, registry, and histocompatibility organizations joined together as the Harmonization of Histocompatibility Typing Terms Working Group to define a consensual language for laboratories, physicians, and registries to communicate histocompatibility typing information. The Working Group defined terms for HLA typing resolution, HLA matching, and a format for reporting HLA assignments [52]. These recommendations are summarized below.

Definitions of Typing Resolution

The following definitions of typing resolution are currently recommended; however, the field of HLA biology continues to evolve; thus, changes in terminology are likely to occur in the future.

Allelic Resolution

The DNA-based typing result is consistent with a single allele as defined in a given version of the World Health Organization (WHO) HLA Nomenclature Report as described on the reference Web site (http://hla.alleles.org). An allele is defined as a unique nucleotide sequence for a gene as defined by the use of all of the fields in a current allele name. Examples include A*01:01:01:01 and A*02:07 (designations based on the international ImMunoGeneTics [IMGT]/HLA Database version 3.1.0, July 2010) (Fig. 58.3 and Table 58.4.).

High Resolution

A high-resolution typing result is defined as a set of alleles that encode the same protein sequence for the region of the HLA molecule called the antigen-binding site and that excludes alleles that are not expressed as cell surface proteins.

Low Resolution

A DNA-based typing result at the level of the digits comprising the first field in the DNA-based nomenclature. Examples include A*01 and A*02. If the resolution corresponds to a serologic equivalent, this typing result also should be called low resolution.

Other Levels of Resolution

If high resolution cannot be obtained, or if the laboratory's agreement with the entity requesting the testing limits the typing efforts to a subset of alleles, the laboratory may report its results at a level of resolution that falls between high resolution and low resolution. Examples include consideration of only those alleles that are expected to be found in the local population or that are designated as common and well defined. A third example is typing that assigns a G group code for reporting ambiguous allele typings. HLA alleles that have identical nucleotide sequences across the exons encoding the peptide-binding domains (exons 2 and 3 for HLA class I and exon 2 only for HLA class II alleles) are designated by an uppercase "G" which follows the first 3 fields of the allele designation of the lowest numbered allele in the group. The group designation contains three fields (e.g., A*02:01:01G). A computer-readable file of these codes, hla_nom_g.txt, is available to download at http://hla.alleles.org/alleles/g_groups.html.

Replacement of the Term "Confirmatory Typing"

Verification Typing

Verification HLA typing is performed on an independent sample (or, for a CBU, from an attached segment or from the unit itself) with the purpose of verifying concordance of the typing assignment with the initial HLA typing assignment for that unit. Concordance does not require identical levels of resolution for the two sets of typing but requires the two assignments to be consistent with one another.

Extended Typing

Extended HLA typing is performed to add additional information to an existing HLA assignment. The purpose of this additional HLA typing (1) may include assignments at additional HLA loci (e.g., to type HLA-C for an HLA-A-, HLA-B-, HLA-DRB1-typed volunteer donor) and/or (2) may include increased resolution at any previously typed HLA locus (e.g., to type an individual with HLA-B serologic assignments to identify the HLA-B alleles). For some cases, extended typing will fulfill requirements for verification typing at a particular locus. In these cases, a combined term "verification/extended typing" can be used.

Format for Reporting HLA Assignments

HLA typing assignments must be clearly understood by the end user. HLA laboratories should have a written agreement with each transplantation entity requesting HLA typing regarding the specifications for the typing. The agreement should include the loci to be tested, the level of resolution of the typing, and the format in which typing results will be reported. The typing assignments must conform with WHO nomenclature for factors of the HLA system (http://www.hla.alleles.org) and comply with other applicable international conventions (e.g., multiple allele code definitions as designated by the NMDP).

Unresolved Alternative Assignments

Best practice for reporting is to include all uncertainty in the typing assignment relevant to the level of resolution. This means that genotypes and/or alleles that have not been excluded should be listed in the report as not having been excluded. If it is not possible to provide a list of all unresolved alternatives on the report, the laboratory should indicate that alternative assignments exist and provide a rationale for the HLA assignment that is selected for inclusion in the report.

Reporting a String of Alleles

Slashes should be used to separate a string of alternative alleles (e.g., A*02:01/02:02/02:07/02:20 to mean A*02:01 or A*02:02 or A*02:07 or A*02:20). Based on resolution requirements, allele names might be truncated from the right; for example, A*02:01 is understood to include all silent substitutions, differences outside the coding region, and expression codes that begin with the digits 02:01.

Matching

Directionality of Match

The laboratory may wish to refer to directionality of the mismatch in cases where the patient or a potential donor is homozygous at a locus or has a nonexpressed allele. If the patient is homozygous and one of the HLA assignments is identical to an assignment of the heterozygous donor (e.g., patient A*01:01:01:01, potential donor A*01:01:01:01, A*23:01), the mismatch may be referred to as a mismatch in the host-vs-graft vector direction. If the potential donor is homozygous and one of the HLA assignments is identical to an assignment of the heterozygous patient, the mismatch may be referred to as a mismatch in the graft-vs-host vector direction.

Matching Within a Family

HLA Haplotypes Identical by Descent

This phrase may be used when (1) parental HLA assignments are available, (2) all four haplotypes are unequivocally defined in the family, (3) the HLA assignments of the parents are clearly distinguishable from one another, and (4) the assignments include HLA class I and class II loci to the extent that potential recombinations have been ruled out. The patient and potential donor who share both haplotypes may be described as HLA identical by descent.

HLA Identical for All Loci Tested

This phrase may be used to refer to matching of related donors who appear to share the HLA loci tested with the patient based on segregation within the family. This phrase would refer to matching in which not all HLA loci are tested (e.g., HLA-A, HLA-B, HLA-C, DRB1 typed, but not DQB1 or DPB1), so the possibility of recombination is not excluded.

Families Where Segregation to Confirm Identity by Descent Is Not Possible

When it is not possible to unequivocally define haplotypes, the phrases used to describe matching should be those used for an unrelated donor.

Matching of Patient to Unrelated Donor or Matching Within a Family Where Identity by Descent Cannot Be Ascertained

The report should indicate the number of loci tested, the potential identity of the assignments (e.g., 8/8, 7/8, or 9/10), and the level of resolution used to determine the potential identity (e.g., high resolution or low resolution).

Correlation of Serologic and Nucleic Acid-Based HLA Typing

The HLA Dictionary provides a list of WHO-assigned serologic designations and the actual serology test results for many alleles. For most of these alleles, the serologic types are known to correspond to the first field of the molecular type. For those molecular types for which no WHO assignment or serologic typing results are available, use of the one-field low-resolution type for conversion is appropriate. Most of the time, molecular typing gives clear results that can readily be interpreted, even when serologic typing is ambiguous. However, for many new alleles, the serologic equivalents have yet to be defined.

Conversion of HLA Molecular Types for UNOS Matching and Data Entry into UNet

For cadaveric kidney transplantation, matching at the antigen level still is considered the standard method by which donor kidneys are allocated through UNOS. UNOS provides a list of antigens that may be entered through UNet; this list forms the basis of the HLA-matching algorithm for cadaveric kidney and pancreas allocation (http://www.unos.org/). The list of antigens and criteria are reviewed annually. While molecular class I typing is more robust and more accurate than serologic typing, a definition of equivalent "antigens" is needed for the purpose of proper organ allocation. When allelic nomenclature was initiated, it was intended to reflect the existing serological nomenclature. Thus, for most types, low-resolution (one-field) class I molecular typing provides the appropriate serologic equivalent. However, as new alleles were discovered, names of alleles were derived based on nucleotide sequence similarities that did not always result in similar serology. Thus, in many cases, derivation of a serologic designation based on an interpretation of a molecular HLA type is difficult. The low-resolution molecular types B*15 and B*40 represent complex examples. The use of the B15, B40, or other broad antigen designation can cause incorrect donor–recipient "matching" and can render molecular typing less specific and less accurate than serologic typing for the purpose of organ allocation. Because of these complexities, UNOS has developed guidelines for assigning antigen equivalents (http:/www. unos.org/). UNOS standards require laboratories to report the correct serologic equivalents for the UNOS application to ensure the most appropriate allocation and to allow screening for unacceptable antigens.

Another problematic issue involves the molecular detection of serologically null alleles (see next section). For instance, a patient with the null variant of A24 could make an antibody to A24. A donor with A24 should not be considered to be a zero mismatch for a recipient with an A24 null allele. Ideally, null alleles should be identified either by use of parallel serologic typing or by use of molecular kits that identify null alleles. All confirmed null alleles should be entered as blanks.

Null Alleles

Most HLA alleles are defined by polymorphisms that are essentially missense mutations leading to amino acid substitutions. Null alleles are variants that result in reduced or absent expression of mature class I and II proteins on the plasma membrane. Null alleles generally result from either alterations at exon–intron boundaries that cause aberrant RNA splicing or nonsense mutations that lead to truncated polypeptides. Most of the null alleles occur within the HLA-A and HLA-B loci; however, they are found at other class I and II loci as well. The nucleic acid sequences that characterize some of these null alleles may not be in the genetic region normally targeted by DNA typing; thus, without serologic information, these null alleles may go undetected. However, once a null allele is identified by serology and characterized by nucleic acid sequencing to identify the reason for the lack of expression, the null allele readily can be detected in subsequent individuals by DNA testing procedures alone. Testing strategies that do not distinguish between a null allele and its closely related expressed counterpart can lead to clinically significant errors. Fortunately, the allele frequencies of most null alleles appear to be less than 0.001. However, exceptions occur: DRB4*01:03:01:02N is relatively common and C*04:09N is associated with the HLA-B*44:03 carrying haplotype in some ethnic groups. Laboratories providing HLA typing for NMDP transplant programs must distinguish common null alleles according to the NMDP policy: http://bioinformatics.nmdp.org/Policies/Policies.aspx.

New Alleles

Laboratories performing clinical HLA typing will encounter patients and donors who appear to have heretofore unknown alleles. New alleles can be observed at relatively high rates, particularly in indigenous populations [7] that have previously been poorly characterized for HLA polymorphism. New alleles may be suspected when SSP-PCR assays result in unexpected negative or positive reactions or reactions with products of unexpected size. Similarly, unusual SSO patterns for the panel of oligonucleotide probes used may indicate that a new allele is present. DNA sequencing assay results will indicate the presence of a nucleotide or nucleotides that have not previously been observed at a particular position in a library of known alleles. Finally, typings that indicate that an individual is heterozygous for two alleles that are each uncommon are sometimes alternatively explained by the presence of a known common allele and a new allele whose sequence is not present in a laboratory's library of known sequences. Since typing strategies often rely on heterozygous PCR products, determining which of the two identified alleles is new may not be possible. Thus, a method of isolating suspected new alleles in a hemizygous form via traditional cloning techniques, allele-specific amplification, or single-allele amplification is necessary for unambiguous characterization. The sequences of potential new alleles should be communicated to GenBank to obtain accession numbers and then to the IMGT/HLA Database (http://www.ebi.ac.uk/imgt/hla/). The WHO HLA Nomenclature Committee will review the data submitted and assign the allele a unique number. The IMGT will display an authoritative sequence for the allele and information about the ethnicity and HLA alleles identified at other loci in the individual with the new allele. With the use of clonal sequencing such as NGS, the identification of allelic diversity is rapidly growing and the IMGT database is becoming populated with entire gene sequences. Consequently, the number of rare sequence variants and the proportion of non-"common and well-defined" alleles are expected to expand dramatically.

HLA Typing Problems

Ambiguities

Two major sources of ambiguity in HLA typing are polymorphisms outside the gene regions targeted by testing and the lack of information about phase in heterozygous individuals. Many laboratories choose tests designed to analyze exon 2 of class II genes and exons 2 and 3 of class I genes, since these regions include most of the known polymorphisms and encode domains that interact with bound peptides; however, polymorphisms occur in other exons as well. When a method does not test for a possible polymorphism, the typing is necessarily ambiguous. The laboratory should discuss with clients whether an ambiguity is likely to be clinically relevant, although the impact on transplant outcome of many known polymorphisms in other exons is unknown.

The second major reason for ambiguous typings derives from the fact that heterozygous typing data often is entirely consistent with two, three, or more possible pairs of alleles rather than just one allele pair. If the PCR products prepared include the sequences of both alleles in an individual and contain several heterozygous possibilities, identification of the cis/trans relationships of the heterozygosities may not be possible. These ambiguous heterozygous combinations can be solved in several ways. Allele-specific amplification leading to PCR products from one of the two alleles will resolve ambiguities. Family studies will resolve heterozygosity ambiguities, if appropriate relatives are available for testing. Traditional cloning techniques are a general solution but are time-consuming and labor-intensive. Single-allele amplification is a general and rapid, but expensive solution.

Recombination

The fact that recombination within the MHC sometimes occurs during meiosis is discussed above. When recombination appears to have occurred within a family, interpretation of results can be difficult. Before concluding that recombination explains the results seen, laboratories should consider the possibilities of typing error and false paternity as alternatives.

False Paternity

HLA typing is a form of identity testing and may reveal false paternity when members of a family are tested. Some transplantation clinicians do not want to disclose to families before testing that discovery of false paternity is possible. The ethical considerations associated with this issue are complex. When results are consistent with false paternity, the findings can be discussed with the ordering healthcare provider verbally and the conclusion of nonpaternity not stated explicitly in the report.

Laboratory Issues

Quality Control

Controls

Laboratories find assembling a comprehensive array of positive controls for over 3,000 known class I and II alleles difficult or impossible. Most laboratories acquire examples of the more common alleles for use in quality control over time in the course of clinical and research typing. The NMDP and the American Society for Histocompatibility and Immunogenetics (ASHI) maintain a cell repository of a subset of known alleles (http://www.ashi-hla.org/). If controls for an allele cannot be obtained, alternative approaches include testing reagents such as SSO probes with related targets that have an identical sequence at a site of interest. Since HLA alleles in aggregate form a combinatorial array of possible sequences in the polymorphic regions, there are generally many opportunities to use surrogate alleles as positive controls.

Contamination

Potential contamination of pre-PCR work areas and reagents with extraneous genomic DNA or previously amplified PCR products is a problem clinical histocompatibility laboratories face in common with other clinical molecular laboratories. Appropriate measures to prevent contamination have been widely described (see Chapter 62; such information is available at the ASHI Web site [http://www.ashi-hla.org/]). Testing for contamination arising from PCR products prepared in SSP-PCR may be difficult. The products prepared in the many reactions necessary to type an individual vary in size and composition so that a general way to test for their presence may be difficult to devise.

Certifications of Laboratories and Professionals

Clinical histocompatibility laboratories are high-complexity laboratories that must be licensed under CLIA.

Laboratories may be inspected and accredited by the College of American Pathologists (CAP) or by the ASHI, UNOS, NMDP, and CLIA, all have designated ASHI with deemed status for purposes of accreditation of clinical histocompatibility laboratories. Laboratories are generally directed by individuals with Ph.D. or M.D. degrees or both. ASHI administers a program to assess the qualifications of doctoral-level individuals to direct ASHI-accredited laboratories. Directors can be certified by examination administered by the American Board for Histocompatibility and Immunogenetics (ABHI). The ABHI also certifies laboratory staff as histocompatibility technologists and specialists (http://www.ashi-hla.org/). The National Credentialing Agency and the American Society for Clinical Pathology have certification programs in molecular pathology for technologists.

Proficiency Testing

Three proficiency testing programs for HLA typing are available in the USA. The CAP, the ASHI, and the Southeastern Organ Procurement Foundation offer comprehensive programs to assess the ability of laboratories to correctly identify HLA alleles. Proficiency testing samples are typically peripheral blood samples for which laboratories can perform low-resolution or allele-level typing at one or several of the HLA class I and class II loci. These organizations also offer challenges for other histocompatibility laboratory tests such as crossmatching. Results from a number of years of DNA-based HLA allele identification proficiency testing challenges have demonstrated that participating laboratories generally achieve 90–100 % consensus. The University of California, Los Angeles (UCLA), has offered an international cell exchange program for many years. Laboratories are challenged to correctly type samples that often include unusual or recently described alleles. An important attribute of the UCLA cell exchange program is its ability to allow correlation of serologic and DNA-based results for a tested sample.

References

1. Snell GD. The nobel lectures in immunology. Lecture for the nobel prize for physiology or medicine, 1980: studies in histocompatibility. Scand J Immunol. 1992;36:513–26.
2. Amos DB. Fundamental antigens of HLA. Hum Immunol. 1991;30:236–46.
3. Van Rood JJ. HLA and I. Annu Rev Immunol. 1993;11:1–28.
4. Rhodes DA, Trowsdale J. Genetics and molecular genetics of the MHC. Rev Immunogenet. 1999;1:21–31.
5. Madden DR. The three-dimensional structure of peptide-MHC complexes. Annu Rev Immunol. 1995;13:587–622.
6. Erlich HA, Opelz G, Hansen J. HLA DNA typing and transplantation. Immunology. 2001;14:347–56.
7. Little AM, Parham P. Polymorphism and evolution of HLA class I and II genes and molecules. Rev Immunogenet. 1999;1:105–23.
8. Dawkins R, Leelayuwat C, Silvana G, et al. Genomics of the major histocompatibility complex: haplotypes, duplication, retroviruses and disease. Immunol Rev. 1999;167:275–304.
9. Gentry SE, Montgomery RA, Segev DL. Kidney paired donation: fundamentals, limitations, and expansions. Am J Kidney Dis. 2011;57(1):144–51.
10. United Network for Organ Sharing (UNOS). *2000 Annual Report, the U.S. Scientific Registry of Transplant Recipients and the Organ Procurement and Transplantation Network. Transplant data 1992-2001.* U.S. Department of Health and Human Services, Health Resources and Services Administration. 2005. Available at: http://www.unos.oi-g/
11. Hurley CK, Wagner JE, Setterholm MI, Confer DL. Advances in HLA: Practical implications for selecting adult donors and cord blood units. Biol Blood Marrow Transplant. 2006;12:28–33.
12. Beatty PG, Mori M, Milford E. Impact of racial genetic polymorphism on the probability of finding an HLA-matched donor. Transplantation. 1995;60:778–83.
13. Petersdorf EW, Anasetti C, Martin PJ, et al. Tissue typing in support of unrelated hematopoietic cell transplantation. Tissue Antigens. 2003;61:1–11.
14. Bray RA, Hurley CK, Kamani NR, et al. National Marrow Donor Program HLA matching guidelines for unrelated adult donor hematopoietic cell transplants. Biol Blood Marrow Transplant. 2008;14:45–53.

15. Lee S, Klein J, Haagenson M, et al. High-resolution donor-recipient HLA matching contributes to the success of unrelated donor marrow transplantation. Blood. 2007;110:4576–83.
16. Rocha V, Gluckman E. Clinical use of umbilical cord blood hematopoietic stem cells. Biol Blood Marrow Transplant. 2006;12:34–41.
17. Kamani N, Spellman S, Hurley CK, et al. State of the art review: HLA matching and outcome of unrelated donor umbilical cord blood transplants. Biol Blood Marrow Transplant. 2008;14:1–6.
18. Barker JN, Weisdorf DJ, DeFor TE, et al. Transplantation of 2 partially HLA-matched umbilical cord blood units to enhance engraftment in adults with hematologic malignancy. Blood. 2005;105:1343–7.
19. Majhail NS, Brunstein CG, Wagner JE. Double umbilical cord blood transplantation. Curr Opin Immunol. 2006;18:571–5.
20. Hollenbach JA, et al. A community standard for immunogenomic data reporting and analysis: proposal for a STrengthening the REporting of Immunogenomic Studies statement. Tissue Antigens. 2011;78(5):333–44.
21. Guo SW, Thompson EA. Performing the exact test of Hardy-Weinberg proportion for multiple alleles. Biometrics. 1992;48(2): 361–72.
22. Excoffier L, Slatkin M. Maximum-likelihood estimation of molecular haplotype frequencies in a diploid population. Mol Biol Evol. 1995;12(5):921–7.
23. Thorsby E. Invited anniversary review: HLA associated diseases. Hum Immunol. 1997;53:1–11.
24. Zubillaga P, Vidales MC, Zubillaga I, et al. HLA-DQA1 and HLA-DQB1 genetic markers and clinical presentation in celiac disease. J Pediatr Gastroenterol Nutr. 2002;34:548–54.
25. Sollid LM, Lie BA. Celiac disease genetics: current concepts and practical applications. Clin Gastroenterol Hepatol. 2005;3:843–51.
26. Bonamico M, Ferri M, Mariani P, et al. Serologic and genetic markers of celiac disease: a sequential study in the screening of first degree relatives. J Pediatr Gastroenterol Nutr. 2006;42:150–4.
27. Mignot E, Lin L, Rogers W, et al. Complex HLA-DR and -DQ interactions confer risk of narcolepsy-cataplexy in three ethnic groups. Am J Hum Genet. 2001;68:686–99.
28. Chabas D, Taheri S, Renier C, Mignot E. The genetics of narcolepsy. Annu Rev Genomics Hum Genet. 2003;4:459–83.
29. Hong SC, Lin L, Lo B, et al. DQB1*0301 and DQB1*0601 modulate narcolepsy susceptibility in Koreans. Hum Immunol. 2007;68: 59–68.
30. Bloch-Michel E, Frau E. Birdshot retinochoroidopathy and HLA-A29+ and HLA-A29- idiopathic retinal vasculitis: comparative study of 56 cases. Can J Ophthalmol. 1991;26:361–6.
31. Levinson RD, Rajalingam R, Park MS, et al. Human leukocyte antigen A29 subtypes associated with birdshot retinochoroidopathy. Am J Ophthalmol. 2004;138:631–4.
32. Ahn JK, Park YG. Human leukocyte antigen B27 and B51 double-positive Behçet uveitis. Arch Ophthalmol. 2007;125:1375–80.
33. Durrani K, Papaliodis GN. The genetics of Adamantiades-Behcet's disease. Semin Ophthalmol. 2008;23:73–9.
34. Mallal S, Nolan D, Witt C, et al. Association between presence of HLA-B*5701, DR7 and HLA-DQ3 and hypersensitivity to HIV-1 reverse transcriptase inhibitor abacavir. Lancet. 2002;359: 727–32.
35. Martin AM, Nolan D, Gaudieri S, et al. Predisposition to abacavir hypersensitivity conferred by HLA B*5701 and a haplotypic HSp70-Hom variant. Proc Natl Acad Sci U S A. 2004;101: 4180–5.
36. Ferrell PB, McLeod HL. Carbamazepine, HLA-B*1502 and risk of Stevens-Johnson syndrome and toxic epidermal necrolysis: USFDA recommendations. Pharmacogenomics. 2008;9:1543–6.
37. Hung SI, Chung WH, Jee SH, et al. Genetic susceptibility to carbamazepine-induced cutaneous adverse drug reactions. Pharmacogenet Genomics. 2006;16:297–306.
38. Lim KS, Kwan P, Tan CT. Association of HLA-B*1502 allele and carbamazepine-induced severe adverse cutaneous drug reaction among Asians, a review. Neurol Asia. 2008;13:15–21.
39. Ozeki T, Mushiroda T, Yowang A, et al. Genome-wide association study identifies HLA-A*3101 allele as a genetic risk factor for carbamazepine-induced cutaneous adverse drug reactions in Japanese population. Hum Mol Genet. 2011;20(5):1034–41.
40. Hung SI, Chung WH, Liou LB, et al. HLA-B*5801 allele as a genetic marker for severe cutaneous adverse reactions caused by allopurinol. *Proc Natl Acad Sci USA*. 2005;102:4134-9. Hum Mol Genet. 2011;20(5):1034–41.
41. Tassaneeyakul W, Jantararoungtong T, Chen P, et al. Strong association between HLA-B*5801 and allopurinol-induced Stevens-Johnson syndrome and toxic epidermal necrolysis in a Thai population. Pharmacogenet Genomics. 2009;19:704–9.
42. The International HIV Controllers Study. The major genetic determinants of HIV-1 control affect HLA class I peptide presentation. Science. 2010;330:1551–7.
43. Morahan G, Mehta M, James I, et al. Tests for genetic interactions in type 1 diabetes: linkage and stratification analyses of 4,422 affected sib-pairs. Diabetes. 2011;60:1030–40.
44. International MHC and Autoimmunity Genetics Network. Mapping of multiple susceptibility variants within the MHC region for 7 immune-mediated diseases. Proc Natl Acad Sci U S A. 2009;106: 18680–5.
45. Shiina T, Hosomichi K, Inoko H, Kulski JK. The HLA genomic loci map: expression, interaction, diversity and disease. J Hum Genet. 2009;54:15–39.
46. Vandiedonck C, Knight JC. The human Major Histocompatibility Complex as a paradigm in genomics research. Brief Funct Genomic Proteomic. 2009;8:379–94.
47. Kulkarni S, Savan R, Qi Y, et al. Differential microRNA regulation of HLA-C expression and its association with HIV control. Nature. 2011;472:495–8.
48. Wu J, Bassinger S, Griffith BB, et al. Analysis of HLA class I alleles via direct sequencing of PCR products. In: Hahn AB, Land GA, Strohman RM, eds. American Society for Histocompatibility and Immunogenetics. *ASHI Laboratory Manual.* 4th ed. 2000.
49. Holcomb CL, Höglund B, Anderson MW, et al. A multi-site study using high-resolution HLA genotyping by next generation sequencing. Tissue Antigens. 2011;77(3):206–17.
50. Wang C, Krishnakumar S, Wilhelmy J, et al. High-throughput, high-fidelity HLA genotyping with deep sequencing. Proc Natl Acad Sci U S A. 2012;109(22):8676–81.
51. Erlich HA. HLA typing using next generation sequencing: an overview. Hum Immunol (2015), in press. http://dx.doi.org/10.1016/j.humimm.2015.03.001
52. Nunes E, Heslop H, Fernandez-Vina M, et al. Definitions of histocompatibility typing terms. Blood. 2011;118:180–3.

Section VIII

Evolving Clinical Molecular Technologies

Section Editor: Debra G.B. Leonard

Next-Generation Sequencing: Principles for Clinical Application

59

Karl V. Voelkerding, Emily M. Coonrod, Jacob D. Durtschi, and Rebecca L. Margraf

Abstract

High-throughput, massively parallel DNA sequencing, more commonly termed "next-generation sequencing," is an innovation in sequencing that emerged during the past decade. Next-generation sequencing (NGS) is not a single technology, but rather several different technologies that share a common feature of massively parallel sequencing of clonally amplified or single DNA molecules in a flow cell or chip. Inherent to NGS technologies are unique sequencing chemistries that differ from the Sanger dideoxynucleotide chain termination chemistry. NGS can generate, in a single instrument run, hundreds of millions to gigabases of nucleotide sequence data depending upon platform configuration, chemistry, and flow cell or chip capacity. This chapter describes principles of NGS and considerations for its application to clinical molecular tests. Although several NGS technologies have been commercialized, technologies finding greatest adoption into clinical laboratories are emphasized. Current clinical testing applications including multigene panels and exome and genome sequencing for candidate and causal gene identification are discussed. While the examples are primarily based on analyses for inherited disorders, the principles described are applicable to oncology and infectious diseases, with certain modifications mostly specific to the specimen characteristics and sensitivity requirements for these other applications.

Keywords

Massively parallel sequencing • Next-generation sequencing • Clinical molecular tests • Multigene panels • Exome • Genome • Inherited disorders

K.V. Voelkerding, M.D. (✉)
Department of Pathology, ARUP Institute for Clinical and Experimental Pathology, University of Utah, Salt Lake City, UT, USA
e-mail: voelkek@aruplab.com

E.M. Coonrod, Ph.D.
Program in Personalized Health, Dean's Office Research Unit, University of Utah, Salt Lake City, UT, USA

J.D. Durtschi, B.S.
Bioinformatics, Institute for Clinical and Experimental Pathology, Salt Lake City, UT, USA

R.L. Margraf, Ph.D.
ARUP Laboratories, Institute for Clinical and Experimental Pathology, Salt Lake City, UT, USA

Introduction

High-throughput, massively parallel DNA sequencing, more commonly termed "next-generation sequencing," is an innovation in sequencing that emerged during the past decade. Next-generation sequencing (NGS) is not a single technology, but rather several different technologies that share a common feature of massively parallel sequencing of clonally amplified or single DNA molecules in a flow cell or chip. Inherent to NGS technologies are unique sequencing chemistries that differ from the Sanger dideoxynucleotide chain termination chemistry. NGS can generate, in a single instrument run, hundreds of millions to gigabases of nucleotide sequence

D.G.B. Leonard (ed.), *Molecular Pathology in Clinical Practice*, DOI 10.1007/978-3-319-19674-9_59

data depending upon platform configuration, chemistry, and flow cell or chip capacity. This chapter describes principles of NGS and considerations for its application to clinical molecular tests. Although several NGS technologies have been commercialized, technologies finding greatest adoption into clinical laboratories are emphasized. Current clinical testing applications including multigene panels and exome and genome sequencing for candidate and causal gene identification are discussed. While the examples are primarily based on analyses for inherited disorders, the principles described are applicable to oncology and infectious diseases, with certain modifications mostly specific to the specimen characteristics and sensitivity requirements for these other applications. To address the space limitations of a chapter, the authors refer the reader to references and reviews that provide greater detail where appropriate.

Instrumentation

Conceptualization and instrument prototyping for the first NGS instruments began in the late 1990s and early 2000s. In 2005, the first commercial NGS platform, designated the GS-20, was launched by 454 Life Sciences, a company founded by Jonathan Rothberg. Shortly thereafter, the first NGS publication, authored by Margulies and colleagues, reported sequencing the entire 580,069 bp genome of *Mycoplasma genitalium* at 96 % coverage and 99.96 % accuracy in a single GS-20 run [1]. In 2007, Roche Applied Sciences acquired 454 Life Sciences and introduced the second version 454 instrument, the GS FLX. As the initial commercialized NGS technology, a review of 454 technical principles is historically important and illustrative as its workflow is relevant to other NGS technologies.

The first step for sequencing on the 454 is to generate a "library" of overlapping DNA fragments from genomic DNA. The most popular fragmentation method employs an acoustic wave-based technology commercialized by Covaris (Woburn, Massachusetts) in which a tube of genomic DNA in solution is placed in the Covaris water bath chamber and subjected to bursts of ultrasonic frequencies (>400 KHz) transmitted via very short wavelengths (~3 mm). Burst intensity and duration can be independently programmed resulting in a tunable fragment size distribution suitable for NGS (typically a few hundred base pairs (bp) in length depending on NGS platform requirements). After DNA fragmentation, fragment ends have overhangs which are enzymatically repaired to blunt ends prior to ligation to 454-specific adapter oligonucleotides required for downstream processes (see Fig. 59.1).

Once generated, the overlapping fragment library is subjected to a clonal amplification step using emulsion PCR (ePCR). Under limiting dilution concentrations, the library is denatured and hybridized to individual beads whose surfaces contain capture oligonucleotides with sequences complementary to the adapter oligonucleotides. The beads are then mixed with PCR buffer components and biotinylated primers in conjunction with oil and surfactant under limiting dilution conditions to create individual water-in-oil microvesicles containing single beads with hybridized library fragments. The emulsion is subjected to PCR during which clonal expansion of single DNA molecules bound to individual

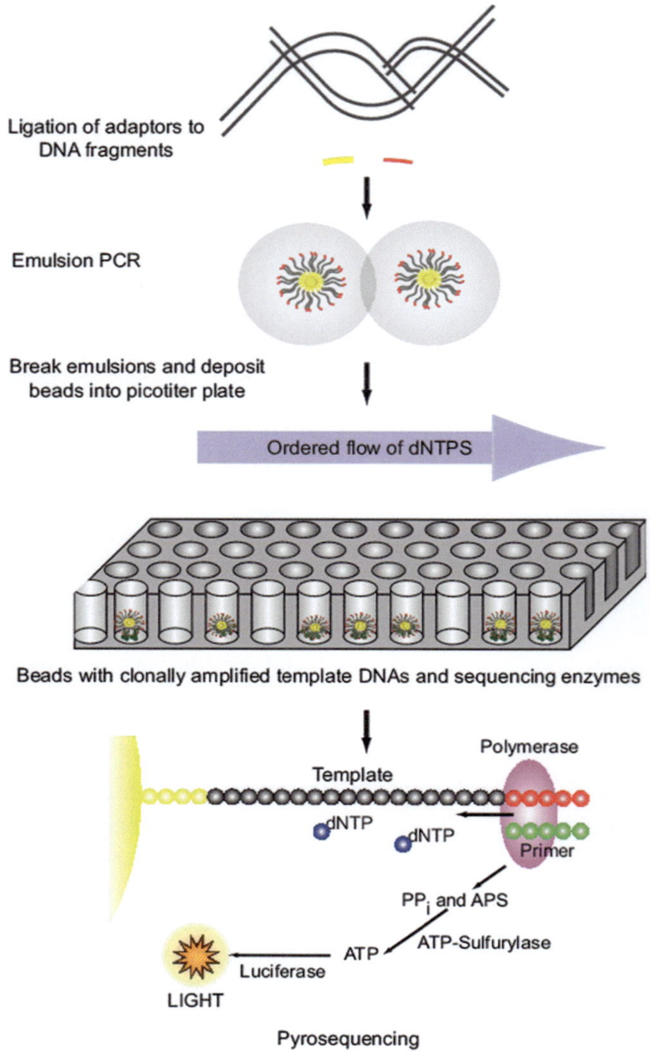

Figure 59.1 Roche 454 GS FLX sequencing. Template DNA is fragmented, end repaired, ligated to adapters, and clonally amplified by emulsion PCR. After amplification, the beads are deposited into picotiter-plate wells with sequencing enzymes. The picotiter plate functions as a flow cell where iterative pyrosequencing is performed. A nucleotide-incorporation event results in pyrophosphate (PPi) release and luminescence localized to the plate wells. *APS* adenosine 5′-phosphosulfate. From Karl V. Voelkerding, Shale A. Dames, and Jacob D. Durtschi. Next-Generation Sequencing: From Basic Research to Diagnostics. Clinical Chemistry 2009; v. 55, p. 641–658. Reproduced with permission from the American Association for Clinical Chemistry

beads occurs. After amplification, the emulsion is disrupted, and beads containing clonally amplified template DNA are enriched by a streptavidin hybridization step, removing the majority of beads without clonal amplicons.

The 454 technology introduced the concept of sequencing clonal amplicons in a flow cell. Specifically, the 454 flow cell is referred to as a "picotiter" plate and is made from a fused fiber-optic bundle into which millions of individual wells are etched into the surface. Beads containing clonal amplicons are deposited into individual picotiter wells that contain enzymatic components for pyrosequencing with luminescence signal generation. When loaded into the GS FLX instrument, the picotiter plate functions as a flow cell wherein iterative pyrosequencing is performed by successive microfluidic addition of polymerase and dNTPS (i.e., A followed by C, then G, then T, etc.). A nucleotide-incorporation event in a well containing a clonally amplified template results in pyrophosphate release, and the luminescence generated in the well is transmitted through the fiber-optic picotiter plate and recorded by a charge-coupled device (CCD) camera. With each dNTP reagent flow, wells are imaged and analyzed for signal-to-noise parameters. The collected data is algorithmically translated into a linear sequence output. One of the recognized strengths of the 454 technology is the progressive increase in sequencing read lengths that have been achieved, beginning with 100 base length reads on the GS-20 that have now been extended up to 1,000 bases.

In 2006, the second NGS technology, termed Solexa, was introduced onto the market. Review of this technology is essential as it is now the dominant NGS method [2]. In 1997, Shankar Balasubramanian and David Klenerman conceived of an approach to sequence single DNA molecules attached to microspheres, and in 1998 they founded Solexa. The goal of sequencing single DNA molecules was not achieved, and Solexa elected to pursue sequencing of clonally amplified templates. By 2006, the Solexa Genome Analyzer was commercialized and Illumina acquired Solexa.

The Genome Analyzer utilized a flow cell comprised of an optically transparent slide with eight individual microfluidic lanes on which oligonucleotide anchors are bound to the slide surface. As with the 454 method, genomic template DNA first is converted into a randomly overlapping fragment library using either Covaris fragmentation followed by enzymatic end repair and Illumina adapter ligation, or via Nextera transposition (described below). As shown in Fig. 59.2, the fragment library is denatured and, under limiting dilution conditions, is added to the flow cell and immobilized by hybridization to the oligonucleotide anchors. In contrast to ePCR, DNA templates are amplified by an isothermal "bridge" amplification method mediated by formamide denaturation that relies upon captured DNA strands "arching" over and hybridizing to an adjacent anchor

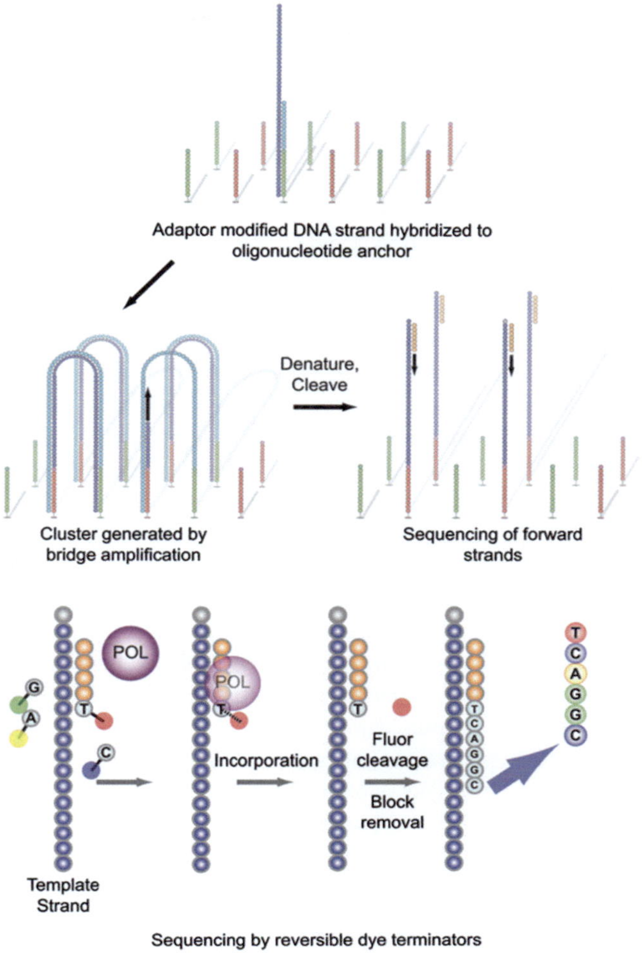

Figure 59.2 Cluster generation and sequencing on the Illumina platform. Denatured, adapter-modified DNA library fragments are hybridized, under limiting dilution concentrations, to complementary oligonucleotide anchors immobilized on the flow cell surface. Bridge amplification generates clonal clusters, which are subsequently cleaved to form single strands. Sequencing primer is annealed, and four uniquely fluorophore-labeled reversible dye terminators and polymerase (POL) are added during each sequencing cycle. Prior to initiation of the next sequencing cycle, the fluorescence signal of the incorporated base is optically recorded, and the fluorophore and termination block is cleaved and washed away. Sequencing is progressive and cyclical, and the read length is dependent on the number of sequencing cycles. From Karl V. Voelkerding, Shale A. Dames, and Jacob D. Durtschi. Next-Generation Sequencing: From Basic Research to Diagnostics. Clinical Chemistry 2009; v. 55, p. 641–658. Reproduced with permission from the American Association for Clinical Chemistry

oligonucleotide. Multiple amplification cycles result in conversion of single-molecule DNA templates to clonally amplified arching clusters with each cluster containing approximately 1,000 clonal DNA molecules. For sequencing, clusters are denatured, and then a chemical cleavage reaction and wash are conducted, leaving only forward strands for single end sequencing. Sequencing of the forward strands is initiated by hybridizing a primer complementary to adapter sequences followed by addition of polymerase and a mixture of four uniquely labeled, fluorescent "reversible" chain terminating nucleotides. The dye-labeled nucleotides are incorporated according to sequence complementarity in each strand in a clonal cluster. After incorporation, excess reagents are washed away, the clusters are optically interrogated, and fluorescence is recorded. With subsequent chemical steps, the chain termination moiety and fluorescent labels are removed and washed away, allowing for a next sequencing cycle to be performed. Initial read lengths with Solexa/Illumina were 36 bases but are currently 300 bases. In addition, Illumina developed a "turnaround chemistry" that allows sequencing of clonal clusters in the opposite strand direction, resulting in bi-directional sequencing of templates.

Recently, Illumina acquired an alternative library preparation method termed Nextera (developed by Epicentre, Madison, Wisconsin) [3]. This approach fragments DNA and introduces adapter sequences in a process termed "tagmentation." A transposase enzyme is complexed with a transposon, which is modified to contain Illumina-specific adapter sequences. DNA is fragmented to a desired size distribution by optimization of the enzyme concentration and incubation time, and then adapter sequences are inserted at the cut site. The Illumina adapter-tagged fragments are then PCR amplified with tailed primers containing sequences for annealing on the Illumina flow cell, sequencing, and optional indexing (or barcoding) to uniquely label all fragments of each library. Indexing multiple libraries allows for pooling to leverage instrument capacity and reduce per sample costs. Most library preparation methods currently require an input of one to several micrograms of genomic DNA, whereas the Nextera technology requires only 50 nanograms of input genomic DNA, which is a sufficient quantity to assure adequate library complexity.

The introduction of the 454/Roche and Solexa/Illumina technologies began a paradigm shift in the biomedical research community. Many complex genomic studies that were previously either cost prohibitive or not technically feasible by the Sanger sequencing were now possible using NGS. Additional NGS technologies were subsequently commercialized including clonal amplicon-based sequencing by ligation (SOLiD/Life Technologies) and fluorescence-based single-molecule sequencing methods introduced by Helicos and Pacific Biosciences. As of this writing, several NGS technologies that were commercialized are either being phased out (454/Roche) or have been abandoned (SOLiD and Helicos), primarily due to insufficient market share. The research community has continued to use the Pacific Biosciences platform due to its ability to generate several thousand base length reads, a feature that has gained traction in the microbial genome sequencing community. However, a relatively high sequence read error rate (~10 %) and an approximate $750,000 platform cost have thus far precluded its entry into clinical use. In 2014, the first single-molecule sequencing technology utilizing engineered protein nanopores was introduced by Oxford Nanopore Technologies. The nanopores are embedded in a membrane in a buffer with an applied electrical field. As strands of DNA pass through the nanopore, they cause a nucleotide base-dependent change in current which is registered and algorithmically converted to sequence. In its first commercial iteration, the Oxford Nanopore platform is handheld in size (MinION), and its first applications have been focused on microbial genome sequencing. The sequence read lengths are on the order of several thousand bases; however, they display substantial error rates (>5 %). At present, considerable effort is ongoing to develop bioinformatic algorithms capable of processing and analyzing sequencing reads generated by the MinION. For more detail on Pacific Biosciences and Oxford Nanopore, the reader is referred to other reviews describing these methods [4–6].

The most recently commercialized and clinically adopted NGS technology, termed Ion Torrent Thermo Fisher Scientific (Waltham, MA) (launched in 2011), also was developed by Jonathan Rothberg (founder of 454) [7]. The sample preparative workflow is quite similar to the 454 technology in that template DNA is converted to an overlapping fragment library and clonally amplified on beads. The flow cell is a chip manufactured from semiconductor material with a high-density micron-scale well pattern etched into its surface. Underlying the well layer is a proprietary ion-sensing technology comprised of a sensing layer and a pattern of photolithographic generated transistors and circuits that can monitor ionic changes in individual wells. Sequencing of clonally amplified library fragments is conducted by an iterative, sequential flow introduction of the four natural nucleotides and polymerase. In contrast to measuring pyrophosphate release, hydrogen ion liberated during nucleotide incorporation and phosphodiester bond formation is registered by the ion sensing mechanism. If three identical adjacent bases on a template are being sequenced (e.g., a TTT homopolymer), the approximate tripling of hydrogen ion liberated generates an approximately tripled ion signal and is interpreted as a three-identical-base incorporation. Currently, the Ion Torrent technology is capable of generating 400 base length reads. In comparison to 454 and Illumina, sequencing speeds are significantly faster with Ion Torrent because there is no requirement for generating luminescence or monitoring fluorescence with subsequent chemical reversal of chain termination. Table 59.1 shows a comparison of 454, Illumina, and Ion Torrent platforms including chemistry, current read lengths, error propensity, and error rates. For additional comparative details, the reader is referred to recent reviews [5, 8–10]. Next discussed are fundamentals of NGS bioinformatics.

Table 59.1 NGS platforms and specifications

Platform	Template preparation	Chemistry	Read length[a]	Run time[b]	Throughput[c]	Primary errors	Error rates[d]
Roche 454							
GS Junior	ePCR	Pyrosequencing	400	10 h	35 Mb	Indel	~1
GS FLX+	ePCR	Pyrosequencing	700–1,000	23 h	700 Mb	Indel	~1
Illumina							
MiSeq	Bridge amplification	Reversible dye terminators	36–250	4–40 h	600 Mb–8 Gb	Substitution	~0.5–1
HiSeq 2000	Bridge amplification	Reversible dye terminators	100	11 days	600 Gb	Substitution	~0.5–1
HiSeq2500 Rapid Run Mode	Bridge amplification	Reversible dye terminators	150	27 h	120 Gb	Substitution	~0.5–1
Ion Torrent							
PGM	ePCR	Hydrogen ion sensing	100–200	2.5–4.5 h	500 Mb–1 Gb	Indel	~0.5–2
Proton	ePCR	Hydrogen ion sensing	200	~4+ h	Up to 10 Gb	Indel	~0.5–2

ePCR emulsion PCR, *Gb* gigabases, *h* hour, *Mb* megabases
[a]Read length in bases
[b]Run time varies with read length and single vs paired-end sequencing
[c]Throughput varies with read length and single vs paired-end sequencing
[d]Percentage of errors per base within single reads at maximum read length as reported by vendor and literature

Bioinformatics and Data Analysis

Sequence Reads and Base Quality Scores

For the 454 and Illumina methods, NGS raw data is comprised of luminescent or fluorescent images, respectively, recorded after each iterative sequencing step. Each platform has its own algorithm for image processing, image compilation, signal-to-noise ratio assessment, and conversion into linear sequence. Nucleotide bases are assigned individual "quality" scores which share a conceptual analogy to Phred scores introduced in 1998 for estimating accuracy and quality of the Sanger sequence data [11, 12]. A Phred score provides quality values, q, using a mathematical scale converting the estimated probability of an incorrect call, e, to a log scale:

$$q = -10 \cdot \log_{10}(e)$$

Miscall probabilities of 0.1 (10 %), 0.01 (1 %), and 0.001 (0.1 %) yield increasing confidence Phred scores of 10, 20, and 30, respectively. Factors that contribute to lower quality bases in NGS include nonoptimal signal-to-background noise levels, cross talk between signals from adjacent beads or clusters, and a phenomenon termed dephasing due to unequal extension of individual reads in a clonal cluster or on a bead surface [13]. The signal output from Ion Torrent is a change in pH, and obtaining optimal signal-to-background pH ratios requires careful control of reagent pH. As with the 454 and Illumina methods, Ion Torrent signals are converted to linear sequence with quality scores assigned to individual bases. While each platform has a unique signal-to-sequence processing algorithm, instrument-specific sequence files are convertible to a common text-based file format termed FASTQ that contains sequence reads and individual base quality scores.

Sequence Mapping, Alignment, and Variant Calling

FASTQ-formatted sequence reads are used for two major computational purposes: assembly and alignment. Assemblies are performed when no reference genome exists for the sequenced DNA, an example being a previously uncharacterized pathogen. Assembly algorithms search for overlapping sections of sequence reads and join them together to generate longer length "contigs" that serve as a scaffold for genome assembly and subsequent alignments. To achieve more complete assemblies, longer sequence read lengths and sequencing from both ends of library fragments (termed paired-end read sequencing) are desirable. For most clinical applications, however, reference genomes exist (e.g., the human genome reference or a previously sequenced pathogen), and the primary computation is alignment of reads to the reference sequence. The unique features of NGS, notably shorter read lengths and massive read numbers, have spurred the development of many new alignment, variant calling, and annotation algorithms. While the reader is referred to a recent review on the topic of NGS bioinformatics [14] for greater details, major process steps are described next (shown in Fig. 59.3).

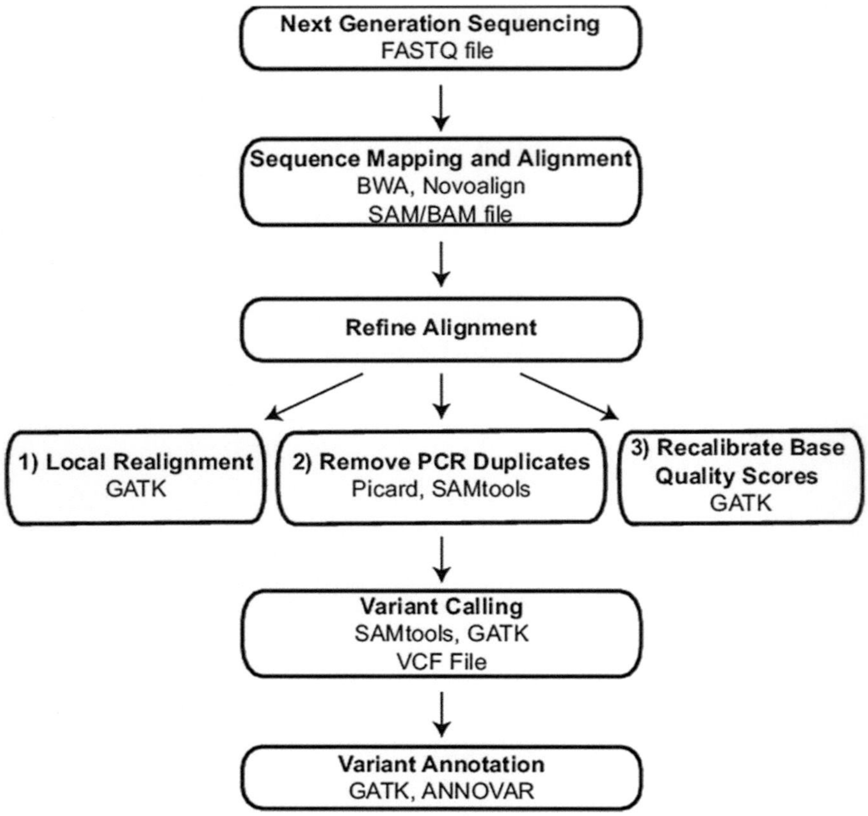

Figure 59.3 Exome and genome bioinformatic processing steps. Sequential steps required to generate an annotated variant list from exome and genome raw sequencing data are indicated in *bold*. For each step, programs used in the authors' laboratory are listed along with the file type that is generated, where applicable. *BWA* Burrows-Wheeler Aligner, *GATK* Genome Analysis Toolkit, *VCF* Variant Call Format. Reprinted from Coonrod EM et al. (2013). Developing Genome and Exome Sequencing for Candidate Gene Identification in Inherited Disorders. Arch Pathol Lab Med. Volume 137(3): 415–433 with permission from Archives of Pathology & Laboratory Medicine. Copyright 2013. College of American Pathologists

Alignment is the process of determining the best match between the sequencing reads and the reference sequence. Due to the large number of sequence reads that must be processed, NGS alignment algorithms typically employ one of two approaches to decrease computational time, and these include a data compression method referred to as a Burrows-Wheeler Transform (BWT) and a method based on the concept of a hash table. The BWT approach is integral to the popular open-source Burrows-Wheeler Aligner (BWA) algorithm that has become a standard for sequence alignment [15–17]. For hash table-based alignment, a first step is conversion of the reference sequence or the sequence reads into a population of shorter length sequences (termed an index), in which each sequence is given a read identifier that can be computationally tracked. By using indexes of shorter length (referred to as "seeds"), alignments proceed more rapidly [14]. An example of a popular aligner that utilizes a hash table function to create an index from the reference genome is NovoAlign (Novacraft, Selangor, Malaysia) [18]. For both BWT and hash table-based aligners, key criteria for initial mapping and alignment are established, including the number of nucleotide mismatches permitted across a given read or seed length and whether gaps in alignment are allowed to accommodate insertions and deletions (indels). With initial criteria applied, a first mapped and aligned read data set is generated. This data set is known to contain inaccuracies, and therefore additional algorithms are used to yield a more refined and accurate final set of alignments as described below.

Most alignment algorithms can provide results in a sequence alignment/map (SAM) file format, which contains information about read position and orientation in relationship to the reference sequence and confidence in the alignment. A binary version of SAM is the BAM format, and the SAM/BAM formats are the most commonly used file formats for storing and secondary manipulation of read alignments. After initial alignment, SAM/BAM files are used as inputs into secondary algorithms that refine and increase alignment accuracy prior to identifying differences between the sequencing reads and the reference sequence, a process referred to as variant calling. Popular open-source software for refining alignments and calling variants are the Genome Analysis Toolkit (GATK) [19] and SAMtools [20]. Algorithms within the GATK program are the most widely used for refining Illumina reads. Three major refinement steps are (1) marking and removal of reads with the same start and end points, referred to as PCR duplicates; (2) local realignment to improve accuracy in identifying indels; and (3) recalibration of base quality scores. PCR duplicates arise from sequencing identical fragments generated by PCR during library preparation. PCR nucleotide errors can be introduced

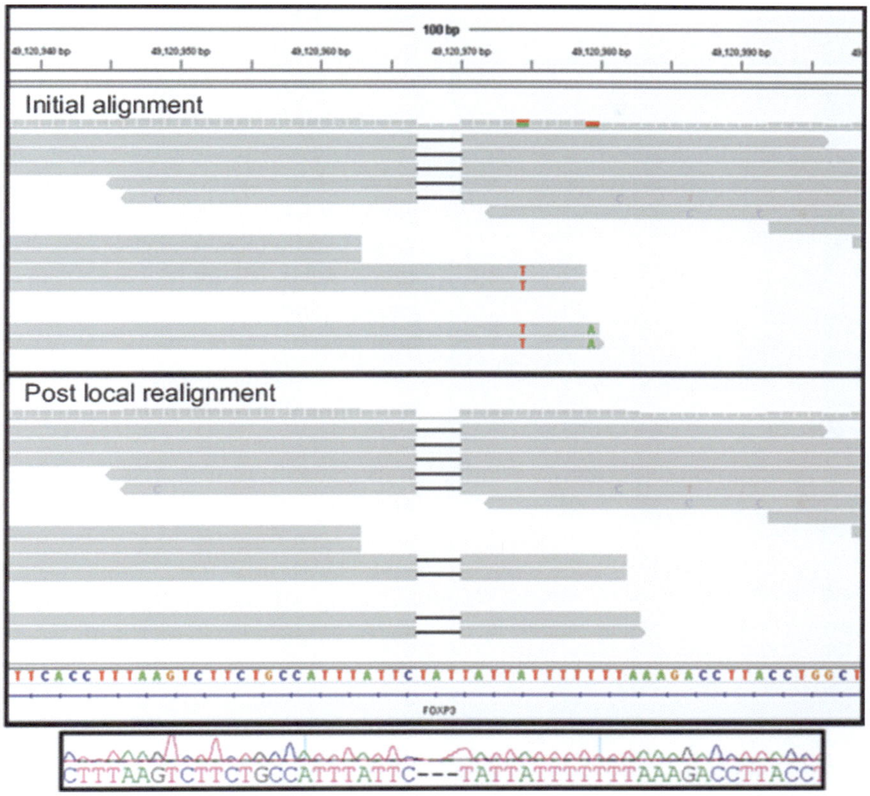

Figure 59.4 Generating refined alignments. Local realignment of an indel from a genome sequenced on the Illumina HiSeq 2000 and visualized in the Integrative Genomics Viewer is shown. The *upper panel* shows results from initial mapping and alignment of reads with an apparent 3 base pairs (bp) deletion in the *FOXP3* gene on the X chromosome of a male. In the *upper panel*, four reads contain the deletion (depicted by *black bars* within the read) and four reads do not contain the deletion. In the four reads that do not contain the deletion, six flanking single-nucleotide variants (SNVs) are present (T variant in *red* and A variant in *green*). The initial alignment suggests heterozygosity for the deletion on the X chromosome, but this is unlikely given that the sequence reads are derived from a male. The lower panel shows results after local realignment in which all reads contain the 3 bp deletion. In addition, flanking, false-positive SNVs are no longer present. The Sanger sequencing trace shown below confirms the deletion and zygosity of the g.49120967_49120971delTAT deletion. Reprinted from Coonrod EM et al. (2013). Developing Genome and Exome Sequencing for Candidate Gene Identification in Inherited Disorders. Arch Pathol Lab Med. Volume 137(3): 415–433 with permission from Archives of Pathology & Laboratory Medicine. Copyright 2013. College of American Pathologists

and propagated through unequal amplification of fragment library templates, and these errors can manifest as false-positive variants. During removal of PCR duplicates, only a single read with overall highest base qualities is retained for analysis. The purpose of recalibrating base quality scores is to compensate for the fact that the Phred-like quality scores generated by the Illumina platform have been demonstrated to deviate from the true error rate. Figure 59.4 shows an example of how local realignment improved the accuracy of detecting a 3 bp deletion in the *FOXP3* gene. The mapped and aligned reads are visualized in the open-source Integrative Genomics Viewer (IGV) [21, 22]. Subsequent to initial and refined alignment steps, variants are called and tabulated in the Variant Call Format (VCF) File that contains variant chromosomal position, reference base, and the alternate base(s) (e.g., single-nucleotide variant (SNV), indel).

Coverage and Variant Calling

By virtue of NGS libraries being comprised of randomly overlapping fragments, multiple reads align to the reference in a staggered fashion. This multiplicity provides quantitative information reflected in the number of reads aligned to the reference sequence at a given location and is designated as read coverage depth. Another feature of randomly fragmented libraries is that fragments are sequenced in both directions to yield forward and reverse strand sequences, and ideally their percentages should be approximately equal. If a variant is present, then the percentage of reads that contain the variant can be expressed as an "allelic read percentage," and the number of forward and reverse sequence strands containing the variant can be enumerated. Figure 59.5 shows a representative example of a heterozygous

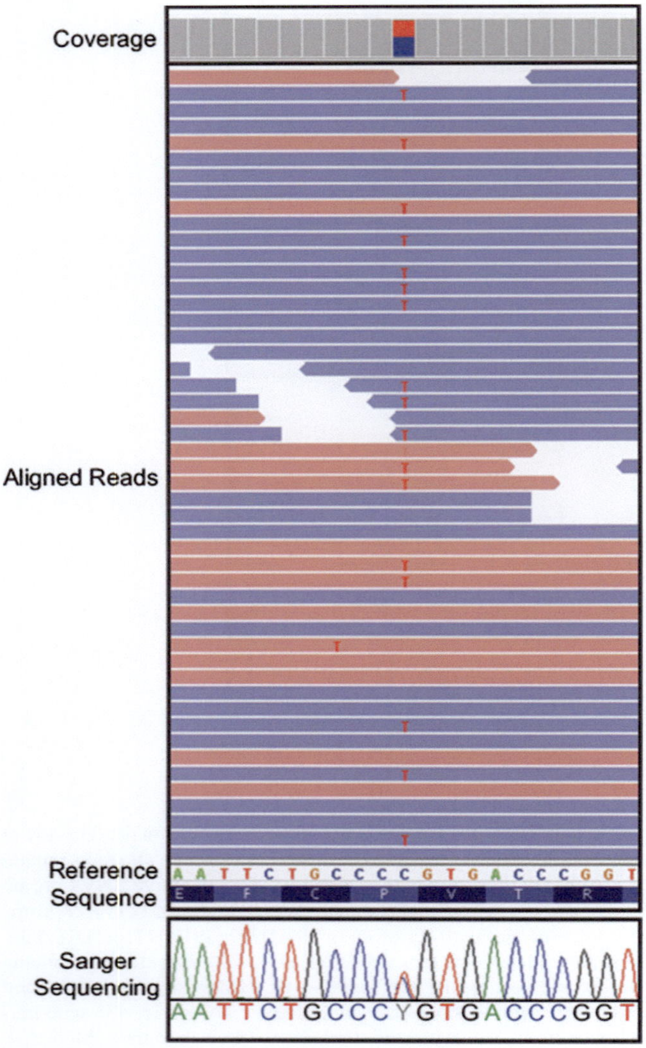

Figure 59.5 Example view of mapped and aligned Illumina reads in a genome browser. A screenshot of the *ZRSR2* gene from the Integrative Genomics Viewer is shown. Relative height of the gray boxes at the top indicates read coverage depth (Coverage). Mapped and aligned reads in the forward direction are shaded *red*, while reads aligning in the reverse direction are shaded blue (Aligned Reads). Variants from the reference are highlighted by a unique color. Forty-nine of 245 reads from exome sequence generated using the NimbleGen SeqCap in-solution exome capture and run on the Illumina HiSeq 2000 are shown. A cytosine to thymine (C>T) variant change is present with the T variant highlighted in *red* in the aligned reads. The heterozygous change also is indicated in the coverage portion of the viewer, and in this case because the variant is a heterozygote, the box is split into two colors, *red* for the variant nucleotide (T) and *blue* for the reference nucleotide (C). This T variant is present in 46 % of reads, while the other 54 % of reads contain a C at this position. The T variant is present in both forward and reverse reads. The reference nucleotide sequence (Reference Sequence) is shown below the aligned reads along with the amino acid translation of the sequence. This region was sequenced by the Sanger sequencing to confirm the heterozygous (C>T) variant. The trace from this sequence is shown at the bottom (Sanger Sequencing)

SNV and illustrates the concepts of coverage and allelic read percentage. Several points and caveats are important when considering coverage and variant calling. First, greater variant calling accuracy is achieved when there is a consensus among aligned reads that agrees with predictions for the variant. For example, a sample with a heterozygous SNV would ideally display a 50/50 ratio of reads containing variant and reference nucleotides, and forward and reverse strand reads would be equivalently represented in both variant- and reference-containing reads. By extension, a homozygous variant would be expected to be present in 100 % of aligned sequences with equal representation of forward and reverse strands. In practice, a wider range of allelic read percentages for true heterozygous and homozygous variants is observed. Further, forward and reverse strand read percentages divergent from expected are commonly seen (referred to as "read strand bias"). These read strand biases arise from technical and bioinformatic sources including differential PCR amplification of library fragments, sequencing errors in difficult-to-sequence regions, and misalignment of related sequences (e.g., pseudogenes or highly homologous genes).

Second, the minimum number of reads required to call a variant has not been standardized and varies depending on application needs and sequencing platform accuracy (i.e., lower sequencing error rates require fewer reads to accurately establish a variant call). In the 1000 Genomes Project [23], coverage as low as four- to six-fold has been used in a large-scale screening mode, whereas in other research studies 20- to 30-fold coverage has been empirically found to offer a balance between sensitivity, specificity, and sequencing costs for detection of constitutional variants [24–26]. By extension, clinical laboratories are typically requiring a minimum of 20- to 30-fold coverage for the detection of constitutional variants and are often designing diagnostic assays so that much higher coverages are routinely obtained in an effort to increase variant detection and improve variant call confidence.

Third, coverage depth across sequenced regions is variable, and factors that contribute to this are differential ligation of adapters to fragments during library preparation and differential amplification during clonal expansion [27]. NGS assays can be designed to achieve sufficient sequencing to meet clinically necessary minimum coverage for areas prone to lower coverage.

Fourth, whereas the above noted 50/50 and 100 % ratios are pertinent to identifying constitutional heterozygous and homozygous variants, respectively, they do not apply when identifying somatic variants in cancer samples comprised of a mixture of tumor and normal cell populations (where allelic read percentages for true somatic variants of interest can be quite low), as well as for tumor heterogeneity in which not all tumor cells have acquired the same variants. To identify low allelic read percentage somatic variants, increased read coverage in the several hundred- up to thousand-fold range are being applied empirically for clinical testing [28, 29]. In sum, multiple variables ultimately need to be considered in variant calling, and more sophisticated algorithms are beginning to emerge for the detection of variants in both constitutional and somatic testing applications. For example, the open-source GATK program factors in coverage depth, read bias, recalibrated base quality scores, and variant prior and posterior probabilities based on comparison to control samples. In combination, these factors are used by GATK to generate statistical measures that predict variant accuracy and generate a "refined" VCF file.

Annotation

A final step is to input the VCF file information into an "annotation" program that ascribes additional features to variants. Open-source software that contain annotation functions are ANNOVAR [30, 31], GATK, and snpEff [32], among others. Annotation outputs can include many features, but those that are common are chromosomal location of base change from reference, whether the variant is in a gene and its respective location (e.g., exon, intron, splice site), the consequence of the change to a codon (e.g., synonymous vs nonsynonymous, missense vs frameshift), and zygosity (e.g., homozygous or heterozygous). Often incorporated into annotation software programs are algorithms that predict the functional impact of variants on proteins such as Sorting Intolerant from Tolerant (SIFT) [33, 34], PolyPhen-2 [35], and MutationTaster [36, 37].

Clinical Applications

The impact of NGS on biomedical research has been transformative. Similarly, the ongoing translation of NGS into the clinical laboratory represents a significant shift. In this section, two major clinical applications of NGS are discussed: (1) disorder- or disease-based multigene panel sequencing, and (2) exome and genome sequencing for candidate and causal gene identification.

Multigene Panel Sequencing via Targeted Enrichment

Investigations into the genetic basis of a growing number of inherited disorders have revealed that a clinical phenotype can be due to multiple causative genes with a broad mutational spectrum. Examples include X-linked mental retardation, mitochondrial disorders (secondary to mutations in both the mitochondrial genome and nuclear genes), congenital hearing loss, cardiomyopathies, and primary immune deficiencies [8, 10, 38–41]. A comprehensive diagnostic approach can require the analysis of a few dozen to over one hundred genes. Similarly, molecular analyses of hematopoietic and solid malignancies continue to identify a growing number of genes relevant to diagnostic stratification, prognosis, and therapeutic response [42–44]. The technical complexity of multiple gene analysis is very challenging with the Sanger sequencing, whereas it can be addressed by targeted enrichment of multiple genes followed by NGS.

In general, enrichment strategies can be categorized as either amplification-based or oligonucleotide-array-capture-based [45, 46]. For amplification-based enrichment, single locus or multiplex PCR remains a mainstay method. Resequencing of exons by targeted PCR enrichment has been demonstrated for a number of genes wherein amplicons are generated from a sample, pooled in equimolar ratios, then ligated to adapter oligonucleotides to generate an NGS library (without overlapping fragments). This approach integrates well with the longer read length technologies (e.g., Roche 454). Another strategy for target enrichment is to use overlapping long-range PCR with 5–10 kilobase amplicons, which are then pooled, fragmented, and converted into a library. Multiple samples can be sequenced together if index or barcode sequences are incorporated into adapter sequences. After sequencing, indexed reads are assigned to their respective sample of origin by bioinformatic algorithms, which is sometimes referred to as "deconvolution" [47–49]. To automate PCR amplification of many targets, a highly parallel PCR microdroplet technology has been commercialized by RainDance Technologies (Lexington, MA) [50, 51]. In this technology, individual primer pairs for targets are designed (for amplicon lengths of 200–600 bp), synthesized, and sequestered in individual, stable, emulsion microdroplets. Up to a few thousand primer pairs can constitute a microdroplet primer population. For targeted amplification, genomic DNA is first fragmented into a size range of 2,000–4,000 bp and then randomly distributed into a separate microdroplet population. On an automated microfluidic platform, individual primer pair and genomic DNA microdroplets are merged by exposure to a voltage potential so that one microdroplet containing fragmented genomic DNA is associated with one microdroplet containing an individual primer pair. The fused microdroplets are collected into a single microfuge tube and thermocycled to achieve highly parallel PCR amplification. After amplification, the droplets are disrupted and the pooled amplification products are converted into a library for NGS. An additional PCR-based enrichment approach, Fluidigm (South San Francisco, CA), commercialized their Access Array platform based on a microfluidic chip that contains nanoliter-scale reaction chambers separated by valves. Forty-eight samples can be loaded onto the chip, and each sample can be distributed into 48 chambers with unique or multiplex primer pairs for subsequent PCR. After amplification, valves are reversed and samples are returned to their original wells and processed for NGS.

Oligonucleotide array capture methods constitute the second major enrichment strategy [52–59]. With array methods, genomic DNA, or genomic DNA converted into an NGS library, is hybridized to oligonucleotides complementary to target regions of interest. After hybridization, the enriched material is eluted from the array and processed for NGS. Originally, capture oligonucleotides were formatted on solid surface arrays, but this approach has been supplanted by in-solution formats offered by Roche NimbleGen (Madison, WI), Agilent (Santa Clara, CA), Illumina, and most recently Integrated DNA Technologies (IDT, Coralville, IA). In-solution oligonucleotide array capture procedures require several hours to days of hybridization depending on methodology, and an important array design consideration is the specificity of capture probes and the potential for co-capture and enrichment of nontarget sequences, notably from closely related genes and pseudogene analogs which can lead to false-positive variants in alignments. The inherent coverage variability in NGS libraries can be compounded by uneven and inadequate capture using in-solution probes, sometimes necessitating oligonucleotide array redesign.

A novel hybrid between capture and amplification approaches termed HaloPlex (Halo Genomics, Uppsala, Sweden and acquired by Agilent Technologies) is being adopted for clinical use. In this method, genomic DNA is digested with different combinations of restriction endonucleases and then hybridized to biotinylated oligonucleotide probes whose right and left sides are complementary to the fragment ends. The probes also contain a sequencing motif and index. Probe hybridization yields a genomic DNA circular structure that is isolated by incubation with magnetic streptavidin beads and then closed by ligation. Ligated circles are amplified by PCR yielding a library ready for sequencing.

Each enrichment method has advantages and disadvantages. For clinical applications, the choice of enrichment technology will depend on target size, content, and laboratory workflow preferences. Array capture is better suited for enrichment of larger target regions up to the scale of the human exome but is prone to co-capture of highly homologous sequences. Although amplification-based strategies are not as scalable, their increased target enrichment specificity may be preferable or required depending on target content. As an example of in-solution array capture data, Fig. 59.6 shows two genes, *FOXP3* and *HLA–DOB*, and their respective

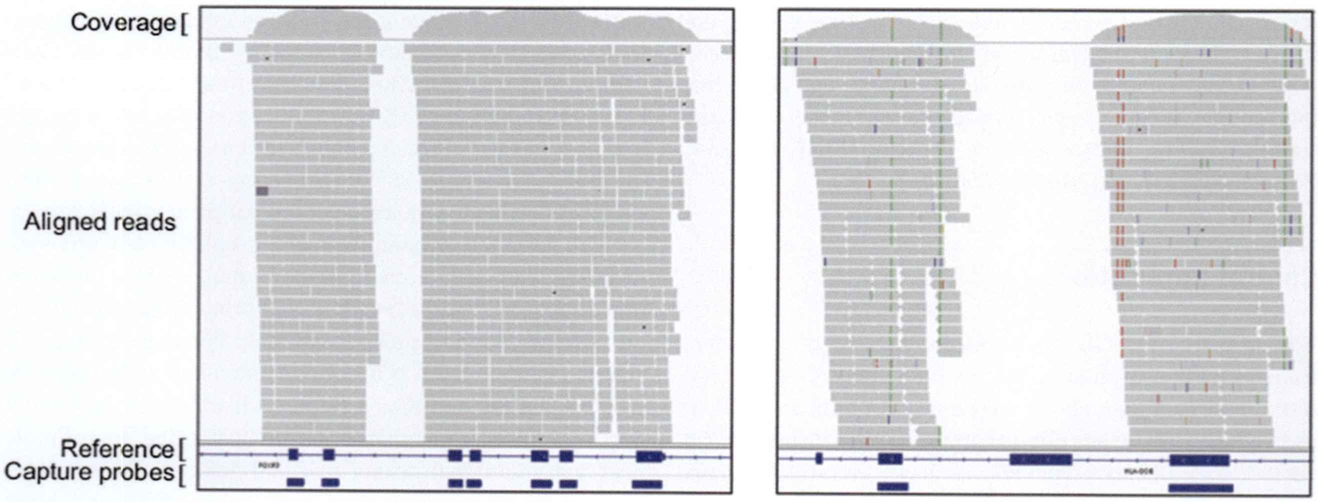

Figure 59.6 Exome read coverage and targeted regions. Paired-end exome sequencing reads are shown for two example genomic loci in the Integrated Genomics Viewer. *Boxes* along the bottom show the positions of the capture probes for the NimbleGen SeqCap in-solution capture design (Capture Probes). The reference sequence is shown above the capture probes, and exons are represented by *blue boxes* (Reference). Changes to the reference sequence are shown by vertical multicolored hatch marks throughout the coverage and aligned read regions (Aligned Reads). *Left panel* shows capture probes and coverage of seven exons from the *FOXP3* gene located on the X chromosome. *Right panel* shows capture probes and coverage of two of four exons from the *HLA–DOB* gene located on chromosome 6. *HLA–DOB* belongs to a larger gene family with highly homologous sequences, making the design of unique capture probes difficult. As a result, only two exons shown here contain unique probes, are captured efficiently, and can be aligned to the reference sequence, thus highlighting that problematic genomic regions are not included in capture probe design. Reprinted from Coonrod EM et al. (2013). Developing Genome and Exome Sequencing for Candidate Gene Identification in Inherited Disorders. Arch Pathol Lab Med. Volume 137(3): 415–433 with permission from Archives of Pathology & Laboratory Medicine. Copyright 2013. College of American Pathologists

capture results. The left panel shows capture probes and coverage of seven exons from the *FOXP3* gene located on the X chromosome. The right panel shows capture probes and coverage of two of four exons from the *HLA–DOB* gene located on chromosome 6. *HLA–DOB* belongs to a large gene family with highly homologous sequences, making the design of unique capture probes difficult for all exons.

Currently, the majority of clinical NGS testing is comprised of multigene panels for inherited disorders and oncology applications (discussed further in the Considerations for Clinical Implementation of NGS). The adoption of multigene panels has been greatly facilitated by lower cost platforms, notably the Illumina MiSeq and the Ion Torrent PGM. In parallel, exome sequencing (and to a lesser degree genome sequencing) is being increasingly applied to identify causal and candidate genes in patients with disorders suggestive of a genetic etiology. We next discuss exome and genome sequencing, and the Illumina technology is highlighted as it has been used in the majority of clinical exome and genome publications.

Exome and Genome Sequencing for Candidate and Causal Gene Identification

In the scenario of a suspected inherited disorder, the overarching goal of exome or genome sequencing is to generate a list of variants from which a presumptively rare and pathogenic variant (or variants depending on mode of inheritance) can be identified. The complexity of this goal is reduced if a family with more than one affected member or even a trio of both parents and the affected child can be tested, as this allows segregation analyses of putative pathologic variants to be performed. While complex, the reported success of exome and genome sequencing for identifying candidate and causal genes in patients and families whose disorders strongly suggest a genetic etiology is 25–40 % [60–63]. Technical and bioinformatic considerations are presented before describing how to "search" for candidate genes.

As shown in Fig. 59.7, initial preparatory steps are the same for exome and genome libraries and include genomic DNA fragmentation and conversion of fragments into an oligonucleotide adapter-tagged library. For exome sequencing, in-solution capture with probes complementary to coding regions is performed as described above to yield an exome-enriched library. Several commercial vendors offer in-solution exome capture probe reagents including Agilent which uses RNA probes and Roche NimbleGen and Illumina which use single-stranded DNA oligonucleotide probes. While there is considerable overlap in the performance characteristics of these three approaches, each differs in targeted capture areas and capture probe sequence composition [64–66].

Prior to Illumina sequencing, the genome or exome library concentration needs to be determined to guide the preparation of an appropriate dilution for loading onto the flow cell. Quantitative PCR (qPCR) is performed on the library using amplification primers complementary to the adapter oligonucleotide sequences that bind to the flow cell surface capture oligonucleotides. A qPCR standard curve is generated using artificial templates of known concentrations that also contain the same primer target sequences complementary to the flow cell surface capture oligonucleotides. The library concentration is determined by comparing the PCR crossing threshold of the library to those of the standard curve templates. The use of PCR primers complementary to adapter sequences that bind to flow cell surface oligonucleotides specifically assesses the number of library molecules that should form clusters. Based on the library concentration determined by qPCR, a dilution is prepared with the goal of achieving optimal cluster density formation.

The bioinformatic steps for generating annotated variants from Illumina exome or genome sequencing data are similar to those described above. After sequencing, FASTQ read files are aligned to the human genome reference sequence using BWA followed by refined alignment and variant calling with GATK. Annotation is performed with either GATK or ANNOVAR. The process of alignment and variant calling generates, for a genome, approximately 3–3.5 million positions that differ from the human reference sequence. In comparison, approximately 15,000–30,000 differences from the reference will be observed in the coding regions in a genome or exome data set depending on bioinformatic filtering parameters. Within these ranges, the greatest number of variants from the human genome reference is observed in individuals of African and African-American descent, an intermediate number are observed in individuals of Asian descent, and the fewest variants are observed in Caucasians of European descent. At this time, genome sequencing costs approximately three times more than exome sequencing. Operationally, analyses of either genome or exome data typically focus on coding region variants and variants in close proximity to coding regions because this currently is the most "interpretable" portion of the genome. In considering the use of exome vs genome sequencing, exome sequencing does not provide as comprehensive an analysis of coding regions as genome sequencing. This reflects the difficulty of designing specific capture probes for all coding regions due to the variability of capture efficiency and the presence of cross homologous sequences. Figure 59.8a shows a comparative example of these differences for the *RET* gene in exome and genome data sets. The genome data shows comprehensive coverage across the gene region, whereas the exome data has sequencing reads only in locations enriched by capture probes. Figure 59.8b illustrates in exome sequencing of the *ABCF1* gene that some exon regions do not have

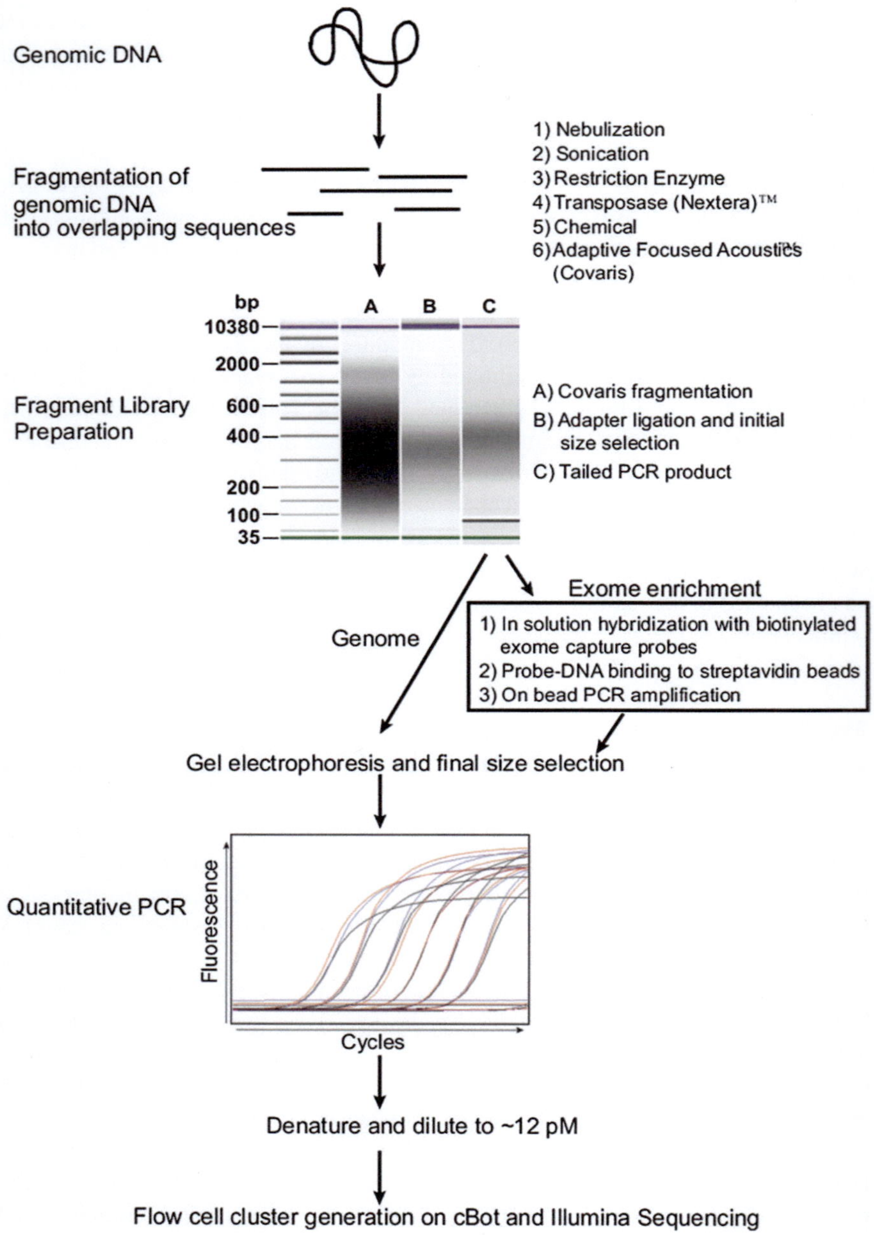

Figure 59.7 Sample preparation for genome and exome sequencing. Workflow diagram for converting genomic DNA into a genome or exome library for sequencing using the Illumina platform is shown. Options (*1–6*) for fragmenting DNA are shown at *top right*. Library preparative steps (*A–C*) as assessed on the Agilent BioAnalyzer are indicated. Steps for exome enrichment after polymerase chain reaction (PCR) amplification of adapter ligated library fragments are *boxed*. Example quantitative PCR traces are shown. Reprinted from Coonrod EM et al. (2013). Developing Genome and Exome Sequencing for Candidate Gene Identification in Inherited Disorders. Arch Pathol Lab Med. Volume 137(3): 415–433 with permission from Archives of Pathology & Laboratory Medicine. Copyright 2013. College of American Pathologists

probes and therefore are not covered (Fig. 59.8b), while the genome sequencing data is complete across this region. Another technical consideration of exome sequencing that impacts data analysis is that coding regions with high or low GC content are captured less efficiently under single temperature hybridization conditions. This variability of capture was described by Clark et al. [65] and is inherent to all three commercially available exome capture reagents. The effect of GC content is particularly pronounced for the first exon of human genes, which on average have higher GC content. This can lead to reduced coverage of first exons in exome data sets as illustrated for the *MAZ* gene in Fig. 59.9 where read coverage for exon 1 is greatly reduced compared to other exons although a capture probe is included for this exon. While these limitations exist, exome sequencing is routinely performed at higher coverage depths compared to genome sequencing (due to cost considerations). The increased coverage depth can allow for identification of coding region variants missed in lower coverage genome sequencing data [26, 65].

The operational premise used in most candidate gene discovery analyses is that one is looking for a rare variant(s) that encodes a pathologic change (with high phenotypic penetrance) in the form of a missense, nonsense, frameshift, or splicing mutation. Depending on the presumed inheritance pattern, either single variants (e.g., dominant, X-linked, or a

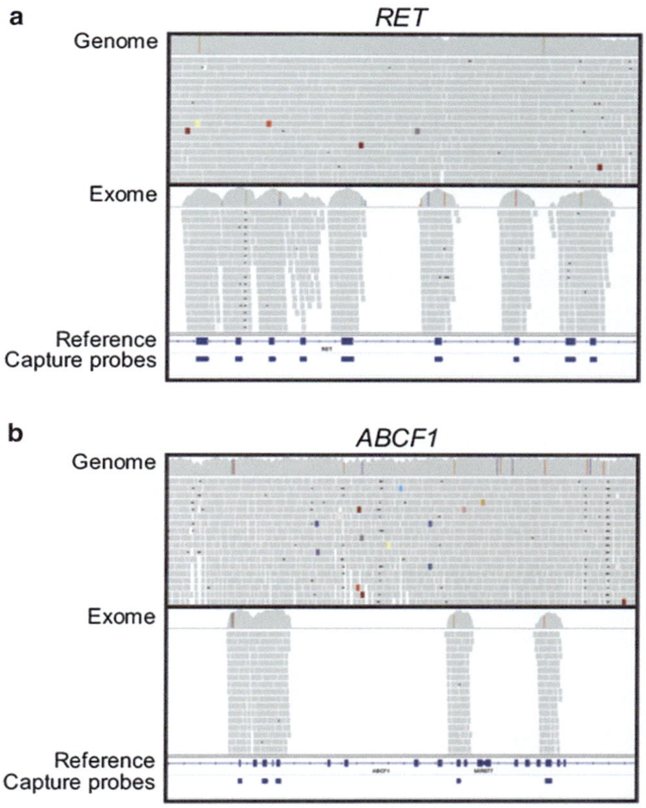

Figure 59.8 Comparison of genome and exome data. Screenshots of *RET* (**a**) and *ABCF1* (**b**) sequence alignments in the Integrative Genomics Viewer. In both **a** and **b**, *top panels* show genome read coverage and aligned reads (Genome), and *bottom panels* show exome read coverage and aligned reads (Exome). Reference exon positions and locations of corresponding NimbleGen capture probes are depicted as *dark blue boxes* (labeled Reference and Capture Probes, respectively). NimbleGen SeqCap EZ Human Exome Library version 2.0 reagents were used for exome enrichment, and the genome and exome samples were sequenced on the Illumina HiSeq 2000. These comparative results highlight the increased amount of sequencing information generated by genome sequencing (i.e., noncoding in addition to coding sequences) compared to exome sequencing. In addition, shown are differences between the well-captured gene, *RET*, and the suboptimally captured gene, *ABCF1*, using the exome sequencing approach. In this example, all exons in *RET* have exon capture probes and sequence information, whereas several exons in the *ABCF1* gene do not have exon capture probes. In contrast, all exons in both genes are sequenced with the genome sequencing approach. Reprinted from Coonrod EM et al. (2013). Developing Genome and Exome Sequencing for Candidate Gene Identification in Inherited Disorders. Arch Pathol Lab Med. Volume 137(3): 415–433 with permission from Archives of Pathology & Laboratory Medicine. Copyright 2013. College of American Pathologists

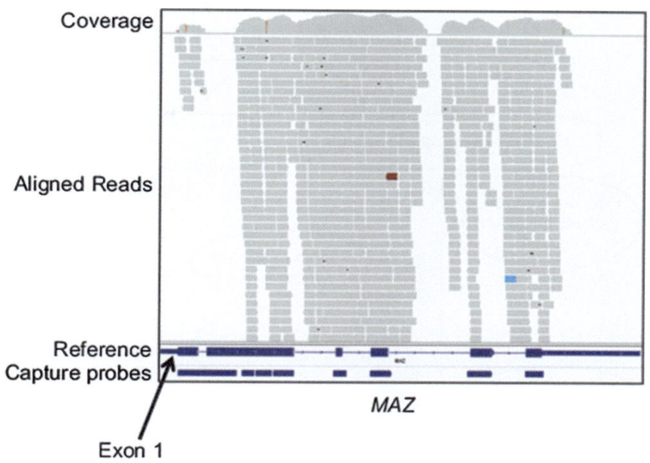

Figure 59.9 Effect of GC content on exome capture. Integrative Genomics Viewer screenshot of exome sequencing results for the *MAZ* gene using NimbleGen SeqCap EZ Human Exome Library version 2.0 capture probe enrichment and Illumina HiSeq 2000 sequencing. Read coverage (Coverage) and aligned reads (Aligned Reads) are shown with reference exon positions and locations of corresponding NimbleGen capture probes depicted as *dark blue boxes* and labeled Reference and Capture Probes, respectively. The capture probe track shows that a probe has been generated to capture exon 1, but the read viewer shows only nine reads aligned to exon 1 compared to the greater read depth observed for the other *MAZ* exons. This indicates suboptimal capture during probe hybridization. Reprinted from Coonrod EM et al. (2013). Developing Genome and Exome Sequencing for Candidate Gene Identification in Inherited Disorders. Arch Pathol Lab Med. Volume 137(3): 415–433 with permission from Archives of Pathology & Laboratory Medicine. Copyright 2013. College of American Pathologists

new `e novo] mutation) or combinations of variants (e.g., recessive homozygous or compound heterozygous) are being sought in the form of SNVs or indels. Copy-number variations or other structural changes may be disease causing, and improving their identification in exome and genome data is an active area of investigation. Prior to searching for causative variants, other data such as linkage or identity by descent in families may have identified areas of the genome for focused analysis. Due to the enormity of either exome or genome data sets, bioinformatic tools are required to narrow down variant lists to a smaller subset of variants in candidate genes. In this evolving area, two main categories of bioinformatic approaches are used: heuristic filtering methods and statistical prediction algorithms or a combination thereof. A schematic of these two approaches is shown in Fig. 59.10.

A heuristic is a series of logic steps applied to arrive at a solution. In the context of candidate gene identification, the heuristic is typically guided by the premise of a rare variant that co-segregates with disease; therefore, one first assumption is that the causative variant is not represented in databases of "control" genomes, such as dbSNP [67], the 1000 Genomes Project, or in-house control databases. When applied as a filter, variants present in these databases are removed and typically reduce an exome variant list by about 95 % from 15,000 to 20,000 variants to approximately 1,000 variants. Caveats with this filter are that some known rare pathogenic variants and more common variants linked to disease by genome-wide association studies are present in dbSNP and a subset of the 1000 Genomes Project subjects are likely carriers for a genetic disease or may have late-onset

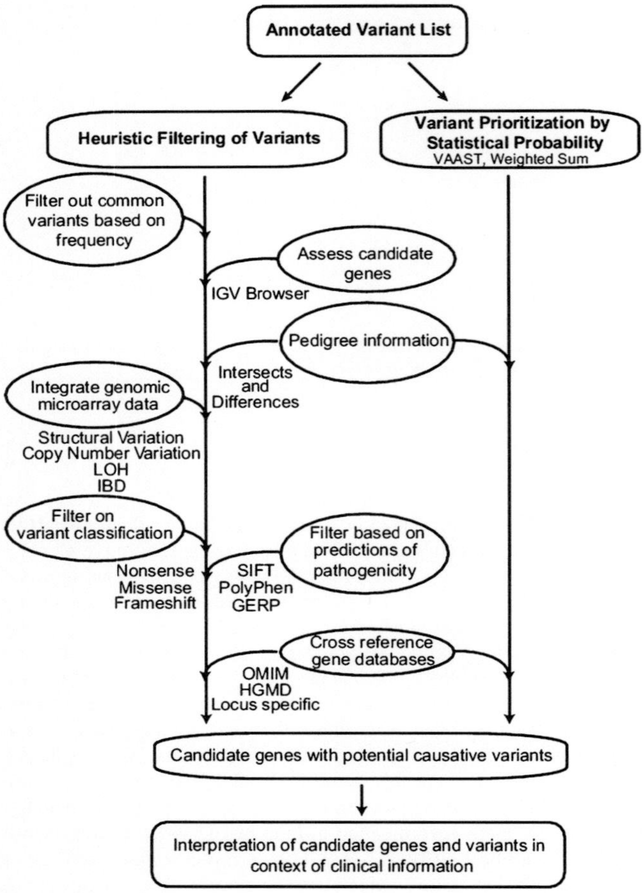

Figure 59.10 Heuristic and statistical probability approaches for candidate gene discovery. Shown is a schematic of sequential bioinformatic steps used by the authors for candidate gene discovery from exome and genome sequencing data. Annotated variant lists from genome or exome sequencing can be analyzed with heuristic filtering approaches, statistical probability approaches, or a combination of both to generate candidate gene lists. Multiple process steps are involved in heuristic filtering, as depicted. The process steps that incorporate pedigree information and cross-referencing of gene databases are critical components of both heuristic and statistical probability approaches. The additional steps involved in heuristic filtering are described in the text. *GERP* Genomic Evolutionary Rate Profiling, *HGMID* Human Gene Mutation Database, *IBD* identity by descent, *IGV* Integrative Genomics Viewer, *LOH* loss of heterozygosity, *OMIM* Online Mendelian Inheritance in Man, *PolyPhen* Polymorphism Phenotyping, *SIFT* Sorting Intolerant from Tolerant, *VAAST* Variant Annotation, Analysis, and Selection Tool. Reprinted from Coonrod EM et al. (2013). Developing Genome and Exome Sequencing for Candidate Gene Identification in Inherited Disorders. Arch Pathol Lab Med. Volume 137(3): 415–433 with permission from Archives of Pathology & Laboratory Medicine. Copyright 2013. College of American Pathologists

genetic diseases. Variants can alternatively be filtered into frequency bins such as 0–1 % and 1–5 % based on minor allele frequency (MAF) within the context of dbSNP, the 1000 Genomes Project, or in-house control databases. This approach assumes that variants with higher MAF values are less likely to be pathogenic but could lead to missing a deleterious compound heterozygous set of variants with different MAF values. Although most known highly penetrant, disease-causing variants are present at a frequency of <1 % in the population, deleterious variants can be present at higher frequencies [68].

The goal of the following filtering steps is to further reduce the list of potential candidate genes and their associated variants (Fig. 59.10). There are several options for filtering depending on the scenario, including (1) examining only genes previously implicated in the patient's disease phenotype, (2) identifying intersects (i.e., shared variants) and differences between affected and unaffected individuals based on pedigree information, (3) incorporating linkage or identity by descent (IBD) information from genomic microarray analyses, and (4) applying filters based on assumptions about the candidate gene and variant (e.g., zygosity, variant classification, or predictions of pathogenicity) (Fig. 59.10). To predict the functional effect of a DNA variant on the encoded protein, programs such as SIFT, Genomic Evolutionary Rate Profiling (GERP) [69, 70], and PolyPhen are often used and the results incorporated into the filtering and/or prioritization process. Once a candidate gene has been identified, cross-referencing the literature and consulting databases including the Human Gene Mutation Database (HGMD) [71], Online Mendelian Inheritance in Man (OMIM) [72], and locus-specific databases (e.g., http://www.arup.utah.edu/database/) may identify a previously described genotype-phenotype correlation for the specific variant or loss of gene function.

Heuristic filtering methods have proven successful in identifying the majority of reported candidate and causative genes. They do not, however, provide any measure of statistical uncertainty for a specific variant or candidate gene. Recently, a probabilistic candidate gene algorithm termed the Variant Annotation, Analysis, and Selection Tool (VAAST) has been described [73]. Using a multiparameter likelihood equation, VAAST compares allele frequencies between cases, controls, and background data sets in conjunction with modeling variant severity by amino acid substitution analysis to provide a list of variants, each associated with a VAAST ranking score and a p-value. The p-value is a measure of the probability that a variant is statistically significant in a case as compared to the control data set. Successful application of VAAST was recently reported in the discovery of a causative variant in a previously uncharacterized, rare, dominant, X-linked Mendelian disorder causing infant boys to have an "aged appearance" and cessation of growth after birth called Ogden syndrome (OMIM# 300855) [74]. In the future, additional algorithmic approaches for candidate gene identification are expected to emerge and will likely increasingly incorporate stratification based on population genetics data and cross correlation with evolving genotype-phenotype databases.

Follow-up medical, genetic, and/or functional studies are important to establish causality of a candidate gene with predicted deleterious variants. Correlation of known effects of gene function or loss with clinical symptoms and phenotype in the medical record can support the causality of the variant; however, correlation often requires discussion with the ordering physician(s), the patient, or their family regarding specific symptoms not described in the clinical record but known to result from the functional gene loss. In some cases, additional laboratory testing of the patient informed by the candidate gene can support causality. There are several different categories of variants that may be uncovered during a search for candidate genes. First, the gene and variant may have been previously associated with the patient phenotype. Second, the gene may have been previously implicated in the disease phenotype while the variant is novel. Screening for this variant in patients with similar signs and symptoms along with unaffected controls can be powerful for establishing causality. Third, the gene may not have been previously implicated in the patient phenotype but is supported by its known biological function. Here it is essential to understand the frequency of the variant in an ethnically matched data set and to screen for variants in the gene in unaffected individuals and patients with similar signs and symptoms.

Considerations for Clinical Implementation of NGS

A growing number of clinical laboratories are performing or developing clinical NGS-based tests. Multigene panels are driving this translation, and a literature base describing the development, validation, and implementation of NGS multigene panels is emerging. Overall, these reports describe encouraging performance characteristics for different multigene targets (e.g., retinal disorders, Lynch syndrome, *BRCA1* and *BRCA2*, and congenital hearing loss) using different enrichment approaches and sequencing platforms while also highlighting test limitations [38, 75–81]. Based on these initial reports and expected improvements in sequencing chemistries and options for data analysis, NGS is becoming a routine method in the clinical molecular laboratory. In this final section, we present several additional considerations based on our observations and those reported in the literature.

Clinical molecular tests based on NGS technologies should incorporate core principles shared with other clinical laboratory tests. Assay design, development, and optimization, followed by validation and subsequent quality control and assurance monitoring, are cornerstones. For multigene panel tests, panel content, choice of enrichment method, and platform compatibility are initial considerations. One continual challenging aspect is the rapidly growing knowledge base of genes involved in a particular phenotype posing the proverbial "moving target" problem to gene panel design. One approach is the design of panels to include only genes for which there is substantial evidence for their causal association with the disease phenotype. Alternatively, the panel can be expanded to include genes whose role in a given disease is biologically plausible but currently not proven. In this approach, only genes with the highest evidence for phenotypic association are reported clinically, while information is collected on less well-established gene-disease relationships for future use.

Major vendors offer free target enrichment design using chromosomal coordinates for the genes of interest, the sequencing platform, and the read length information to generate an in silico design report. The designs contain lists of primers and/or probes for the genes of interest and a bioinformatic projection of how comprehensively the targets will be enriched. Design success can vary significantly between target genes and enrichment methods. Critical to the success of these designs is the vendors' reporting on the potential for co-amplification or co-capture of nontarget, highly homologous sequences such as pseudogenes. In conjunction, the laboratory should independently determine if target genes have homologs or pseudogenes using homology search tools such as BLAST. While the presence of a highly homologous gene or pseudogene is not an absolute contraindication for inclusion in a multigene panel test, the laboratory needs to be aware that bioinformatic analysis of the corresponding functional target gene may be confounded by the pseudogene or homolog, especially when using an in-solution oligonucleotide capture method.

The next step is to assess the performance of the enrichment method in the laboratory. Pilot testing will define metrics such as actual target coverage in comparison to in silico predictions. Gene regions with inadequate coverage may be addressed by deeper sequencing or by redesign of the enrichment method. For regions that are recalcitrant to sequencing by NGS, the laboratory can develop an alternative analytical approach, such as targeted Sanger sequencing. In addition to determining coverage adequacy, assessment of sequence read qualities and allelic read percentage ranges provides method performance assessments. Plotting allelic read percentages for variants and performing confirmatory Sanger sequencing on a subset provide an evidence base by which the laboratory can establish allelic read percentage ranges for heterozygous and homozygous variant calls. The presence of co-captured homologs or pseudogenes can manifest as regions of poor sequence mapping and alignment or as variants with lower allelic read percentages. Interference by homologs and pseudogenes needs to be empirically determined because they can contribute to assay background noise. The range of allelic read percentages tends to be broader for in-solution capture-based enrichment methods compared to those that are amplification based.

Feedback from variant confirmation methods can guide the adjustment of technical wet bench approaches and bioinformatic parameters. For example, false-positive results may be due to co-capture of highly homologous sequences, sequencing errors, or alignment and variant calling errors. False-negative results may arise from inadequate coverage or alignment and variant calling errors. Therefore, confirmatory studies must be sufficiently comprehensive to define the sensitivity and specificity of the test, which is a significant but essential undertaking. If false-positive results are due to bioinformatic parameters, then these may be reduced by increasing the stringency of alignment and variant calling or utilizing different algorithms. The Sanger sequencing for confirmation of specific variants may reveal variants (NGS false negatives) in flanking regions not detected by NGS due to inadequate coverage or less permissive alignment and variant calling parameters.

Once basic technical performance characteristics of a targeted enrichment panel have been established, validation is undertaken using a series of samples. This is optimally done with the same reagent lots for sequencing, and the bioinformatic analysis parameters should be consistent. Traditionally, laboratories validating single-gene Sanger sequencing assays have tested samples with pathologic mutations present in the gene of interest. However, even at the single-gene level, obtaining samples with mutations for rare disorders can be challenging. This challenge is magnified when validating a multigene panel; therefore, a more practical approach to validating NGS-based tests is to perform a methods-based validation to determine the ability to accurately detect the types of variants for which the assay is designed (e.g., SNVs and indels). The combination of multiple gene targets and multiple samples typically yields a diversity of variants in most targeted genes with the caveat that some genes or gene regions are highly conserved and have fewer variants.

An open question is what constitutes an adequate validation for an NGS-based clinical test, and an important practical limitation for laboratories is the current significant cost of enrichment and sequencing reagents. In this context, reports describing the development and performance of NGS multigene panels have used sample numbers ranging from a dozen to over 80 with a mix of normal and variant-containing samples. One approach to reduce validation costs is the use of barcoding or indexing of samples, followed by pooling and data deconvolution. While a conceptually attractive approach from an operational and cost perspective, key caveats require attention. The use of sufficiently distinct combinations of indexes is critical to allow for unambiguous bioinformatic deconvolution and original sample assignment. Nucleotide errors can be introduced into indexes by PCR amplification during library or enrichment protocols, and these can lead to misassignment of sequence reads during deconvolution, which would manifest as variants with lower allelic read percentages than expected. Thus, pilot studies with confirmatory analyses should be performed to determine if the pooling and deconvolution approach yields equivalent results to those observed with single sample sequencing.

Following validation and implementation, ongoing monitoring of the assay performance through an ongoing quality assurance program is essential. Important metrics to accrue are false-positive and false-negative rates, which are determined through continuous or periodic confirmatory studies. An ongoing operational and cost challenge for laboratories is the evolution of NGS reagents and platform hardware and software that necessitate revalidation. This is anticipated to be a continual feature of NGS for some time.

While multigene panels are more common, several clinical laboratories now offer diagnostic exome and genome sequencing. In essence, exome sequencing is a large-scale multigene panel, and the considerations and caveats described above are directly applicable. Commercial exome enrichment reagents contain largely overlapping capture probe content. An important caveat is that current capture probe sets do not target the entire human coding region and in practice approximately 85 % of the coding region is enriched. During pilot experiments, the laboratory needs to define the coding regions that are adequately captured and sequenced. Conversely, the laboratory should define coding regions that are not represented or consistently display low coverage and those which are challenging or not feasible to interpret due to various factors including co-capture and alignment of highly homologous sequences or genome regions otherwise prone to sequencing errors. It is attractive to consider using exome sequencing as an "all-purpose" enrichment method followed by selective analysis of genes guided by phenotype. However, due to the incomplete coverage of the exome, this is feasible for some, but not all, sets of genes [80].

In contrast to exome sequencing, genome sequencing improves coding region coverage and approximately 95 % of coding regions are sequenced. Although co-enrichment of highly homologous regions is not inherent to genome sequencing, these regions and low-complexity intronic and intergenic regions pose the same bioinformatic challenges noted for multigene panels and exomes. As the cost of genome sequencing declines, genome sequencing may become the method of choice and thereby supplant panels and exome sequencing. From a practical standpoint, the actual preparation of a genome library is technically more straightforward than multigene panel and exome sequencing. Computationally, analysis of genome-scale data requires a much greater computational hardware infrastructure for expeditious alignment and variant calling and for data storage. In practice, most groups (including ours) that perform genome sequencing for candidate gene discovery efforts focus their analyses on coding regions. As our understanding of the contribution of noncoding variants to human disease increases, the ability to expand analyses into noncoding regions afforded by genome sequencing will be advantageous. For further details on the use of NGS in the clinical molecular laboratory, the reader is referred to several reviews [64, 82–84]. These reviews describe the successful application of NGS approaches to clarifying diagnoses, adjusting patient treatment based on the patient's genotype, and identifying novel causative variants associated with a variety of diseases.

Results Reporting and Informed Consent

The implementation of NGS into clinical practice has posed new questions with respect to appropriate test utilization, informed consent, and the reporting of genetic testing results [85–87]. While the conceptual framework for pretesting consent and genetic counseling and posttesting reporting and counseling has been in place and practiced for many years, studies have determined that patients and family members struggle with fully understanding the meaning of genetic testing results, even for single-gene tests [88, 89]. In this context, active discussions are ongoing within professional societies involved in genetic testing to address the question of how to assure the adequacy of the consent process and how and what results to deliver from multigene panel and exome and genome sequencing [90]. As multigene panel testing is largely performed for the purpose of determining if a mutation(s) is present in a gene previously associated with a disease, it is qualitatively similar to single-gene testing. However, multigene panel testing is inherently accompanied by an increase in the number of variants requiring classification and potentially reported, all of which adds substantially to the interpretive load in the clinical laboratory setting. As described earlier, clinical exome and genome sequencing are being applied primarily to elucidate genetic causes in the setting of enigmatic diagnostic scenarios, and the reader is referred to a policy statement on the clinical use of exome and genome sequencing published by the American College of Medical Genetics and Genomics (ACMG) [91]. The policy statement provides guidance on indications for diagnostic testing, reporting, and pre- and posttesting considerations including informed consent and counseling. When exome and genome sequencing are applied in a phenotype or symptom-guided approach, bioinformatic analyses are focused to yield a list of candidate genes and associated variants which, in some cases, contain the causal diagnostic variant(s). When applied in this manner, noncandidate genes throughout the genome that do not appear in the candidate gene list are typically not evaluated. However, the total variant file from exome or genome sequencing for each individual contains multiple variants in genes that are predicted to result in loss of gene function or otherwise affect gene function [92, 93].

A subset of functional variants may not be directly pertinent to patient management, and these are termed "secondary" or "incidental" variant findings [94]. An ongoing area of research and discussion is whether or not to evaluate for and disclose all or some subset of secondary deleterious variants [95, 96]. Strategies have been proposed to categorize secondary findings, and example categories include variants that are associated with (1) cancer predisposition, (2) non-oncologic early- or late-onset disease, (3) recessive disease (in the setting of reproductive decisions), and (4) drug metabolism [97]. Opinions regarding the reporting of secondary findings vary among authors, and the reader is referred to the ACMG [91] recommendations on the return of results from genome-scale sequencing which includes a list of genes for which the return of incidental findings are recommended. The most recent revision includes the recommendation that patients should have the option to opt out of receiving incidental findings.

Indeed, the complexity of primary and secondary findings that exome and genome sequencing generate necessitates and highlights the importance and challenge of informed consent in the genomics era. A tiered consent process can be envisioned in which patients will be informed of the types of information generated by exome and genome sequencing. Patients may elect to receive only information pertinent to their presenting symptoms, or they also may request to receive all or some portion of their secondary findings. Another scenario would allow for patients to request secondary findings at a later date. In the pediatric setting, consent scenarios also would need to account for primary and secondary findings in children that are relevant to siblings and biological parents. The consequence of this complexity is that the field of molecular pathology is entering into an unprecedented era of result reporting that will encompass not only diagnostic findings but risk prediction for patients and family members. While not a new concept in genetic testing, the magnitude of this endeavor will strain current healthcare delivery models. Going forward, the successful broader implementation of genome-scale testing therefore will require sophisticated consent and reporting approaches that accommodate individual patient wishes and provide genome-scale information to patients in accessible and understandable formats.

Conclusions

Next-generation sequencing has entered the clinical laboratory and in the years ahead will transform many areas of clinical molecular pathology. In the span of a single chapter, it has not been possible to describe all aspects and applications of NGS. In response to the growing adoption of NGS, professional societies and organizations have begun to develop guidelines and standards for the clinical use of NGS.

Recently, the College of American Pathologists (CAP) published NGS-specific laboratory accreditation requirements for clinical molecular laboratories [98]. As noted above, the ACMG has published a policy statement addressing the clinical use of genome sequencing. It is anticipated that additional guidelines will be developed for multiple areas of clinical applications of NGS and the CAP is actively developing the first NGS-based proficiency testing for clinical laboratories. These and other ongoing efforts by professional societies and organizations reflect the current and expected impact of NGS on the practice of medicine. As a technology, NGS is a convergence of innovations in sequencing chemistries, microfluidics, and optics. Like the polymerase chain reaction, NGS is a transformative technology, and the wealth of data generated poses a tremendous challenge for medicine and a unique opportunity for the field of molecular pathology to play a major role in its successful implementation to improve patient care.

References

1. Margulies M, Egholm M, Altman WE, Attiya S, Bader JS, Bemben LA, Berka J, Braverman MS, Chen YJ, Chen Z, Dewell SB, Du L, Fierro JM, Gomes XV, Godwin BC, He W, Helgesen S, Ho CH, Irzyk GP, Jando SC, Alenquer ML, Jarvie TP, Jirage KB, Kim JB, Knight JR, Lanza JR, Leamon JH, Lefkowitz SM, Lei M, Li J, Lohman KL, Lu H, Makhijani VB, McDade KE, McKenna MP, Myers EW, Nickerson E, Nobile JR, Plant R, Puc BP, Ronan MT, Roth GT, Sarkis GJ, Simons JF, Simpson JW, Srinivasan M, Tartaro KR, Tomasz A, Vogt KA, Volkmer GA, Wang SH, Wang Y, Weiner MP, Yu P, Begley RF, Rothberg JM. Genome sequencing in microfabricated high-density picolitre reactors. Nature. 2005;437:376–80.
2. Bentley DR, Balasubramanian S, Swerdlow HP, Smith GP, Milton J, Brown CG, Hall KP, Evers DJ, Barnes CL, Bignell HR, Boutell JM, Bryant J, Carter RJ, Keira Cheetham R, Cox AJ, Ellis DJ, Flatbush MR, Gormley NA, Humphray SJ, Irving LJ, Karbelashvili MS, Kirk SM, Li H, Liu X, Maisinger KS, Murray LJ, Obradovic B, Ost T, Parkinson ML, Pratt MR, Rasolonjatovo IM, Reed MT, Rigatti R, Rodighiero C, Ross MT, Sabot A, Sankar SV, Scally A, Schroth GP, Smith ME, Smith VP, Spiridou A, Torrance PE, Tzonev SS, Vermaas EH, Walter K, Wu X, Zhang L, Alam MD, Anastasi C, Aniebo IC, Bailey DM, Bancarz IR, Banerjee S, Barbour SG, Baybayan PA, Benoit VA, Benson KF, Bevis C, Black PJ, Boodhun A, Brennan JS, Bridgham JA, Brown RC, Brown AA, Buermann DH, Bundu AA, Burrows JC, Carter NP, Castillo N, Chiara ECM, Chang S, Neil Cooley R, Crake NR, Dada OO, Diakoumakos KD, Dominguez-Fernandez B, Earnshaw DJ, Egbujor UC, Elmore DW, Etchin SS, Ewan MR, Fedurco M, Fraser LJ, Fuentes Fajardo KV, Scott Furey W, George D, Gietzen KJ, Goddard CP, Golda GS, Granieri PA, Green DE, Gustafson DL, Hansen NF, Harnish K, Haudenschild CD, Heyer NI, Hims MM, Ho JT, Horgan AM, Hoschler K, Hurwitz S, Ivanov DV, Johnson MQ, James T, Huw Jones TA, Kang GD, Kerelska TH, Kersey AD, Khrebtukova I, Kindwall AP, Kingsbury Z, Kokko-Gonzales PI, Kumar A, Laurent MA, Lawley CT, Lee SE, Lee X, Liao AK, Loch JA, Lok M, Luo S, Mammen RM, Martin JW, McCauley PG, McNitt P, Mehta P, Moon KW, Mullens JW, Newington T, Ning Z, Ling Ng B, Novo SM, O'Neill MJ, Osborne MA, Osnowski A, Ostadan O, Paraschos LL, Pickering L, Pike AC, Chris Pinkard D, Pliskin DP, Podhasky J, Quijano VJ, Raczy C, Rae VH, Rawlings SR, Chiva Rodriguez A, Roe PM, Rogers J, Rogert Bacigalupo MC, Romanov N, Romieu A, Roth RK, Rourke NJ, Ruediger ST, Rusman E, Sanches-Kuiper RM, Schenker MR, Seoane JM, Shaw RJ, Shiver MK, Short SW, Sizto NL, Sluis JP, Smith MA, Ernest Sohna Sohna J, Spence EJ, Stevens K, Sutton N, Szajkowski L, Tregidgo CL, Turcatti G, Vandevondele S, Verhovsky Y, Virk SM, Wakelin S, Walcott GC, Wang J, Worsley GJ, Yan J, Yau L, Zuerlein M, Mullikin JC, Hurles ME, McCooke NJ, West JS, Oaks FL, Lundberg PL, Klenerman D, Durbin R, Smith AJ. Accurate whole human genome sequencing using reversible terminator chemistry. Nature. 2008;456:53–9.
3. Adey A, Morrison HG, Asan XX, Kitzman JO, Turner EH, Stackhouse B, MacKenzie AP, Caruccio NC, Zhang X, Shendure J. Rapid, low-input, low-bias construction of shotgun fragment libraries by high-density in vitro transposition. Genome Biol. 2010;11:R119.
4. Metzker ML. Sequencing technologies—the next generation. Nat Rev Genet. 2010;11:31–46.
5. Glenn TC. Field guide to next-generation DNA sequencers. Mol Ecol Resour. 2011;11:759–69.
6. Bayley H. Nanopore sequencing: from imagination to reality. Clin Chem. 2015;61:25–31.
7. Rothberg JM, Hinz W, Rearick TM, Schultz J, Mileski W, Davey M, Leamon JH, Johnson K, Milgrew MJ, Edwards M, Hoon J, Simons JF, Marran D, Myers JW, Davidson JF, Branting A, Nobile JR, Puc BP, Light D, Clark TA, Huber M, Branciforte JT, Stoner IB, Cawley SE, Lyons M, Fu Y, Homer N, Sedova M, Miao X, Reed B, Sabina J, Feierstein E, Schorn M, Alanjary M, Dimalanta E, Dressman D, Kasinskas R, Sokolsky T, Fidanza JA, Namsaraev E, McKernan KJ, Williams A, Roth GT, Bustillo J. An integrated semiconductor device enabling non-optical genome sequencing. Nature. 2011;475:348–52.
8. Ghosh S, Krux F, Binder V, Gombert M, Niehues T, Feyen O, Laws HJ, Borkhardt A. Array-based sequence capture and next-generation sequencing for the identification of primary immunodeficiencies. Scand J Immunol. 2012;75:350–4.
9. Loman NJ, Misra RV, Dallman TJ, Constantinidou C, Gharbia SE, Wain J, Pallen MJ. Performance comparison of benchtop high-throughput sequencing platforms. Nat Biotechnol. 2012;30:434–9.
10. Hu H, Wrogemann K, Kalscheuer V, Tzschach A, Richard H, Haas SA, Menzel C, Bienek M, Froyen G, Raynaud M, Van Bokhoven H, Chelly J, Ropers H, Chen W. Mutation screening in 86 known X-linked mental retardation genes by droplet-based multiplex PCR and massive parallel sequencing. Hugo J. 2009;3:41–9.
11. Ewing B, Green P. Base-calling of automated sequencer traces using phred. II. Error probabilities. Genome Res. 1998;8:186–94.
12. Ewing B, Hillier L, Wendl MC, Green P. Base-calling of automated sequencer traces using phred. I. Accuracy assessment. Genome Res. 1998;8:175–85.
13. Ledergerber C, Dessimoz C. Base-calling for next-generation sequencing platforms. Brief Bioinform. 2011;12:489–97.
14. Li H, Homer N. A survey of sequence alignment algorithms for next-generation sequencing. Brief Bioinform. 2010;11:473–83.
15. Li H, Durbin R. Fast and accurate short read alignment with Burrows-Wheeler transform. Bioinformatics. 2009;25:1754–60.
16. Li H, Durbin R. Fast and accurate long-read alignment with Burrows-Wheeler transform. Bioinformatics. 2010;26:589–95.
17. http://bio-bwa.sourceforge.net. Accessed 15 Jan 2015.
18. http://www.novocraft.com/products/novoalign/. Accessed 28 Jan 2015.
19. http://www.broadinstitute.org/gatk/. Accessed 20 Jan 2015.
20. http://samtools.sourceforge.net. Accessed 20 Jan 2015.
21. Robinson JT, Thorvaldsdottir H, Winckler W, Guttman M, Lander ES, Getz G, Mesirov JP. Integrative genomics viewer. Nat Biotechnol. 2011;29:24–6.
22. http://www.broadinstitute.org/igv. Accessed 15 Jan 2015.

23. Durbin RM. A map of human genome variation from population-scale sequencing. Nature. 2010;467:1061–73.
24. Brockman W, Alvarez P, Young S, Garber M, Giannoukos G, Lee WL, Russ C, Lander ES, Nusbaum C, Jaffe DB. Quality scores and SNP detection in sequencing-by-synthesis systems. Genome Res. 2008;18:763–70.
25. Dohm JC, Lottaz C, Borodina T, Himmelbauer H. Substantial biases in ultra-short read data sets from high-throughput DNA sequencing. Nucleic Acids Res. 2008;36, e105.
26. Ajay SS, Parker SC, Abaan HO, Fajardo KV, Margulies EH. Accurate and comprehensive sequencing of personal genomes. Genome Res. 2011;21:1498–505.
27. Hernandez D, Francois P, Farinelli L, Osteras M, Schrenzel J. De novo bacterial genome sequencing: millions of very short reads assembled on a desktop computer. Genome Res. 2008;18:802–9.
28. Marchetti A, Del Grammastro M, Filice G, Felicioni L, Rossi G, Graziano P, Sartori G, Leone A, Malatesta S, Iacono M, Guetti L, Viola P, Mucilli F, Cuccurullo F, Buttitta F. Complex mutations & subpopulations of deletions at exon 19 of EGFR in NSCLC revealed by next generation sequencing: potential clinical implications. PLoS One. 2012;7, e42164.
29. Wagle N, Berger MF, Davis MJ, Blumenstiel B, Defelice M, Pochanard P, Ducar M, Van Hummelen P, Macconaill LE, Hahn WC, Meyerson M, Gabriel SB, Garraway LA. High-throughput detection of actionable genomic alterations in clinical tumor samples by targeted, massively parallel sequencing. Cancer Discov. 2012;2:82–93.
30. Wang K, Li M, Hakonarson H. ANNOVAR: functional annotation of genetic variants from high-throughput sequencing data. Nucleic Acids Res. 2010;38, e164.
31. http://www.openbioinformatics.org/annovar/. Accessed 4 Apr 2012.
32. http://snpeff.sourceforge.net/. Accessed 28 Jan 2015.
33. Ng PC, Henikoff S. Predicting deleterious amino acid substitutions. Genome Res. 2001;11:863–74.
34. http://sift.jcvi.org/. Accessed 20 Jan 2015.
35. Sunyaev S, Ramensky V, Koch I, Lathe 3rd W, Kondrashov AS, Bork P. Prediction of deleterious human alleles. Hum Mol Genet. 2001;10:591–7.
36. Schwarz JM, Rodelsperger C, Schuelke M, Seelow D. MutationTaster evaluates disease-causing potential of sequence alterations. Nat Methods. 2010;7:575–6.
37. http://www.mutationtaster.org/index.html. Accessed 6 Sep 2012.
38. De Keulenaer S, Hellemans J, Lefever S, Renard JP, De Schrijver J, Van de Voorde H, Tabatabaiefar MA, Van Nieuwerburgh F, Flamez D, Pattyn F, Scharlaken B, Deforce D, Bekaert S, Van Criekinge W, Vandesompele J, Van Camp G, Coucke P. Molecular diagnostics for congenital hearing loss including 15 deafness genes using a next generation sequencing platform. BMC Med Genomics. 2012;5:17.
39. Gowrisankar S, Lerner-Ellis JP, Cox S, White ET, Manion M, LeVan K, Liu J, Farwell LM, Iartchouk O, Rehm HL, Funke BH. Evaluation of second-generation sequencing of 19 dilated cardiomyopathy genes for clinical applications. J Mol Diagn. 2010; 12:818–27.
40. Vasta V, Ng SB, Turner EH, Shendure J, Hahn SH. Next generation sequence analysis for mitochondrial disorders. Genome Med. 2009;1:100.
41. Voelkerding KV, Dames SA, Durtschi JD. Next-generation sequencing: from basic research to diagnostics. Clin Chem. 2009; 55:641–58.
42. Bejar R, Stevenson K, Abdel-Wahab O, Galili N, Nilsson B, Garcia-Manero G, Kantarjian H, Raza A, Levine RL, Neuberg D, Ebert BL. Clinical effect of point mutations in myelodysplastic syndromes. N Engl J Med. 2011;364:2496–506.
43. Cronin M, Ross JS. Comprehensive next-generation cancer genome sequencing in the era of targeted therapy and personalized oncology. Biomark Med. 2011;5:293–305.
44. Dohner H, Estey EH, Amadori S, Appelbaum FR, Buchner T, Burnett AK, Dombret H, Fenaux P, Grimwade D, Larson RA, Lo-Coco F, Naoe T, Niederwieser D, Ossenkoppele GJ, Sanz MA, Sierra J, Tallman MS, Lowenberg B, Bloomfield CD. Diagnosis and management of acute myeloid leukemia in adults: recommendations from an international expert panel, on behalf of the European LeukemiaNet. Blood. 2010;115:453–74.
45. Mamanova L, Coffey AJ, Scott CE, Kozarewa I, Turner EH, Kumar A, Howard E, Shendure J, Turner DJ. Target-enrichment strategies for next-generation sequencing. Nat Methods. 2010;7:111–8.
46. Garber K. Fixing the front end. Nat Biotechnol. 2008;26:1101–4.
47. Binladen J, Gilbert MT, Bollback JP, Panitz F, Bendixen C, Nielsen R, Willerslev E. The use of coded PCR primers enables high-throughput sequencing of multiple homolog amplification products by 454 parallel sequencing. PLoS One. 2007;2, e197.
48. Craig DW, Pearson JV, Szelinger S, Sekar A, Redman M, Corneveaux JJ, Pawlowski TL, Laub T, Nunn G, Stephan DA, Homer N, Huentelman MJ. Identification of genetic variants using bar-coded multiplexed sequencing. Nat Methods. 2008;5:887–93.
49. Stiller M, Knapp M, Stenzel U, Hofreiter M, Meyer M. Direct multiplex sequencing (DMPS)–a novel method for targeted high-throughput sequencing of ancient and highly degraded DNA. Genome Res. 2009;19:1843–8.
50. Kirkness EF. Targeted sequencing with microfluidics. Nat Biotechnol. 2009;27:998–9.
51. Tewhey R, Warner JB, Nakano M, Libby B, Medkova M, David PH, Kotsopoulos SK, Samuels ML, Hutchison JB, Larson JW, Topol EJ, Weiner MP, Harismendy O, Olson J, Link DR, Frazer KA. Microdroplet-based PCR enrichment for large-scale targeted sequencing. Nat Biotechnol. 2009;27:1025–31.
52. Summerer D. Enabling technologies of genomic-scale sequence enrichment for targeted high-throughput sequencing. Genomics. 2009;94:363–8.
53. Summerer D, Wu H, Haase B, Cheng Y, Schracke N, Stahler CF, Chee MS, Stahler PF, Beier M. Microarray-based multicycle-enrichment of genomic subsets for targeted next-generation sequencing. Genome Res. 2009;19:1616–21.
54. Bau S, Schracke N, Kranzle M, Wu H, Stahler PF, Hoheisel JD, Beier M, Summerer D. Targeted next-generation sequencing by specific capture of multiple genomic loci using low-volume microfluidic DNA arrays. Anal Bioanal Chem. 2009;393:171–5.
55. Hodges E, Xuan Z, Balija V, Kramer M, Molla MN, Smith SW, Middle CM, Rodesch MJ, Albert TJ, Hannon GJ, McCombie WR. Genome-wide in situ exon capture for selective resequencing. Nat Genet. 2007;39:1522–7.
56. Porreca GJ, Zhang K, Li JB, Xie B, Austin D, Vassallo SL, LeProust EM, Peck BJ, Emig CJ, Dahl F, Gao Y, Church GM, Shendure J. Multiplex amplification of large sets of human exons. Nat Methods. 2007;4:931–6.
57. Albert TJ, Molla MN, Muzny DM, Nazareth L, Wheeler D, Song X, Richmond TA, Middle CM, Rodesch MJ, Packard CJ, Weinstock GM, Gibbs RA. Direct selection of human genomic loci by microarray hybridization. Nat Methods. 2007;4:903–5.
58. Okou DT, Steinberg KM, Middle C, Cutler DJ, Albert TJ, Zwick ME. Microarray-based genomic selection for high-throughput resequencing. Nat Methods. 2007;4:907–9.
59. Fisher S, Barry A, Abreu J, Minie B, Nolan J, Delorey TM, Young G, Fennell TJ, Allen A, Ambrogio L, Berlin AM, Blumenstiel B, Cibulskis K, Friedrich D, Johnson R, Juhn F, Reilly B, Shammas R, Stalker J, Sykes SM, Thompson J, Walsh J, Zimmer A, Zwirko Z, Gabriel S, Nicol R, Nusbaum C. A scalable, fully automated process for construction of sequence-ready human exome targeted capture libraries. Genome Biol. 2011;12:R1.
60. Biesecker LG, Mullikin JC, Facio FM, Turner C, Cherukuri PF, Blakesley RW, Bouffard GG, Chines PS, Cruz P, Hansen NF, Teer JK, Maskeri B, Young AC, Manolio TA, Wilson AF, Finkel T,

Hwang P, Arai A, Remaley AT, Sachdev V, Shamburek R, Cannon RO, Green ED. The ClinSeq Project: piloting large-scale genome sequencing for research in genomic medicine. Genome Res. 2009;19:1665–74.
61. Gilissen C, Hoischen A, Brunner HG, Veltman JA. Unlocking Mendelian disease using exome sequencing. Genome Biol. 2011;12:228.
62. Lee H, Deignan JL, Dorrani N, Strom SP, Kantarci S, Quintero-Rivera F, Das K, Toy T, Harry B, Yourshaw M, Fox M, Fogel BL, Martinez-Agosto JA, Wong DA, Chang VY, Shieh PB, Palmer CG, Dipple KM, Grody WW, Vilain E, Nelson SF. Clinical exome sequencing for genetic identification of rare Mendelian disorders. JAMA. 2014;312:1880–7.
63. Yang Y, Muzny DM, Xia F, Niu Z, Person R, Ding Y, Ward P, Braxton A, Wang M, Buhay C, Veeraraghavan N, Hawes A, Chiang T, Leduc M, Beuten J, Zhang J, He W, Scull J, Willis A, Landsverk M, Craigen WJ, Bekheirnia MR, Stray-Pedersen A, Liu P, Wen S, Alcaraz W, Cui H, Walkiewicz M, Reid J, Bainbridge M, Patel A, Boerwinkle E, Beaudet AL, Lupski JR, Plon SE, Gibbs RA, Eng CM. Molecular findings among patients referred for clinical whole-exome sequencing. JAMA. 2014;312:1870–9.
64. Coonrod EM, Margraf RL, Voelkerding KV. Translating exome sequencing from research to clinical diagnostics. Clin Chem Lab Med. 2011;50(7):1161–8.
65. Clark MJ, Chen R, Lam HY, Karczewski KJ, Euskirchen G, Butte AJ, Snyder M. Performance comparison of exome DNA sequencing technologies. Nat Biotechnol. 2011;29:908–14.
66. Majewski J, Schwartzentruber J, Lalonde E, Montpetit A, Jabado N. What can exome sequencing do for you? J Med Genet. 2011;48(9):580–9.
67. http://www.ncbi.nlm.nih.gov/projects/SNP/. Accessed 4 Apr 2012.
68. Marth GT, Yu F, Indap AR, Garimella K, Gravel S, Leong WF, Tyler-Smith C, Bainbridge M, Blackwell T, Zheng-Bradley X, Chen Y, Challis D, Clarke L, Ball EV, Cibulskis K, Cooper DN, Fulton B, Hartl C, Koboldt D, Muzny D, Smith R, Sougnez C, Stewart C, Ward A, Yu J, Xue Y, Altshuler D, Bustamante CD, Clark AG, Daly M, Depristo M, Flicek P, Gabriel S, Mardis E, Palotie A, Gibbs R. The functional spectrum of low-frequency coding variation. Genome Biol. 2011;12:R84.
69. Davydov EV, Goode DL, Sirota M, Cooper GM, Sidow A, Batzoglou S. Identifying a high fraction of the human genome to be under selective constraint using GERP++. PLoS Comput Biol. 2010;6, e1001025.
70. http://mendel.stanford.edu/SidowLab/downloads/gerp/. Accessed 4 April 2012.
71. http://www.hgmd.cf.ac.uk/ac/index.php. Accessed 28 Jan 2015.
72. http://www.ncbi.nlm.nih.gov/omim. Accessed 15 Jan 2015.
73. Yandell M, Huff C, Hu H, Singleton M, Moore B, Xing J, Jorde LB, Reese MG. A probabilistic disease-gene finder for personal genomes. Genome Res. 2011;21(9):1529–42.
74. Rope AF, Wang K, Evjenth R, Xing J, Johnston JJ, Swensen JJ, Johnson WE, Moore B, Huff CD, Bird LM, Carey JC, Opitz JM, Stevens CA, Jiang T, Schank C, Fain HD, Robison R, Dalley B, Chin S, South ST, Pysher TJ, Jorde LB, Hakonarson H, Lillehaug JR, Biesecker LG, Yandell M, Arnesen T, Lyon GJ. Using VAAST to identify an X-linked disorder resulting in lethality in male infants due to N-terminal acetyltransferase deficiency. Am J Hum Genet. 2011;89(1):28–43.
75. Audo I, Bujakowska KM, Leveillard T, Mohand-Said S, Lancelot ME, Germain A, Antonio A, Michiels C, Saraiva JP, Letexier M, Sahel JA, Bhattacharya SS, Zeitz C. Development and application of a next-generation-sequencing (NGS) approach to detect known and novel gene defects underlying retinal diseases. Orphanet J Rare Dis. 2012;7:8.
76. Neveling K, Collin RW, Gilissen C, van Huet RA, Visser L, Kwint MP, Gijsen SJ, Zonneveld MN, Wieskamp N, de Ligt J, Siemiatkowska AM, Hoefsloot LH, Buckley MF, Kellner U, Branham KE, den Hollander AI, Hoischen A, Hoyng C, Klevering BJ, van den Born LI, Veltman JA, Cremers FP, Scheffer H. Next-generation genetic testing for retinitis pigmentosa. Hum Mutat. 2012;33:963–72.
77. Ozcelik H, Shi X, Chang MC, Tram E, Vlasschaert M, Di Nicola N, Kiselova A, Yee D, Goldman A, Dowar M, Sukhu B, Kandel R, Siminovitch K. Long-range PCR and next-generation sequencing of BRCA1 and BRCA2 in breast cancer. J Mol Diagn. 2012; 14:467–75.
78. Valencia CA, Rhodenizer D, Bhide S, Chin E, Littlejohn MR, Keong LM, Rutkowski A, Bonnemann C, Hegde M. Assessment of target enrichment platforms using massively parallel sequencing for the mutation detection for congenital muscular dystrophy. J Mol Diagn. 2012;14:233–46.
79. Pritchard CC, Smith C, Salipante SJ, Lee MK, Thornton AM, Nord AS, Gulden C, Kupfer SS, Swisher EM, Bennett RL, Novetsky AP, Jarvik GP, Olopade OI, Goodfellow PJ, King MC, Tait JF, Walsh T. ColoSeq provides comprehensive lynch and polyposis syndrome mutational analysis using massively parallel sequencing. J Mol Diagn. 2012;14:357–66.
80. Consugar MB, Navarro-Gomez D, Place EM, Bujakowska KM, Sousa ME, Fonseca-Kelly ZD, Taub DG, Janessian M, Wang DY, Au ED, Sims KB, Sweetser DA, Fulton AB, Liu Q, Wiggs JL, Gai X, Pierce EA. Panel-based genetic diagnostic testing for inherited eye diseases is highly accurate and reproducible, and more sensitive for variant detection, than exome sequencing. Genet Med. 2014.
81. Simen BB, Yin L, Goswami CP, Davis KO, Bajaj R, Gong JZ, Peiper SC, Johnson ES, Wang ZX. Validation of a next-generation-sequencing cancer panel for Use in the clinical laboratory. Arch Pathol Lab Med. 2015;139(4):508–17.
82. Ku CS, Naidoo N, Pawitan Y. Revisiting Mendelian disorders through exome sequencing. Hum Genet. 2011;129:351–70.
83. Zhang W, Cui H, Wong LJ. Application of next generation sequencing to molecular diagnosis of inherited diseases. Top Curr Chem. 2014;336:19–45.
84. Coonrod EM, Durtschi JD, Margraf RL, Voelkerding KV. Developing genome and exome sequencing for candidate gene identification in inherited disorders: an integrated technical and bioinformatics approach. Arch Pathol Lab Med. 2013;137:415–33.
85. Biesecker LG. Opportunities and challenges for the integration of massively parallel genomic sequencing into clinical practice: lessons from the ClinSeq project. Genet Med. 2012;14:393–8.
86. Biesecker LG, Burke W, Kohane I, Plon SE, Zimmern R. Next-generation sequencing in the clinic: are we ready? Nat Rev Genet. 2012;13:818–24.
87. Moorthie S, Hall A, Wright CF. Informatics and clinical genome sequencing: opening the black box. Genet Med. 2012;165:165–71.
88. Condit CM. Public understandings of genetics and health. Clin Genet. 2010;77:1–9.
89. Lanie AD, Jayaratne TE, Sheldon JP, Kardia SL, Anderson ES, Feldbaum M, Petty EM. Exploring the public understanding of basic genetic concepts. J Genet Couns. 2004;13:305–20.
90. Kaphingst KA, Facio FM, Cheng MR, Brooks S, Eidem H, Linn A, Biesecker BB, Biesecker LG. Effects of informed consent for individual genome sequencing on relevant knowledge. Clin Genet. 2012;82:408–15.
91. http://www.acmg.net/. Accessed 24 Dec 2012.
92. MacArthur DG, Balasubramanian S, Frankish A, Huang N, Morris J, Walter K, Jostins L, Habegger L, Pickrell JK, Montgomery SB, Albers CA, Zhang ZD, Conrad DF, Lunter G, Zheng H, Ayub Q, DePristo MA, Banks E, Hu M, Handsaker RE, Rosenfeld JA, Fromer M, Jin M, Mu XJ, Khurana E, Ye K, Kay M, Saunders GI, Suner MM, Hunt T, Barnes IH, Amid C, Carvalho-Silva DR, Bignell AH, Snow C, Yngvadottir B, Bumpstead S, Cooper DN, Xue Y, Romero IG, Wang J, Li Y, Gibbs RA, McCarroll SA, Dermitzakis

ET, Pritchard JK, Barrett JC, Harrow J, Hurles ME, Gerstein MB, Tyler-Smith C. A systematic survey of loss-of-function variants in human protein-coding genes. Science. 2012;335:823–8.

93. Westbrook MJ, Wright MF, Van Driest SL, McGregor TL, Denny JC, Zuvich RL, Clayton EW, Brothers KB. Mapping the incidentalome: estimating incidental findings generated through clinical pharmacogenomics testing. Genet Med. 2013;15(5):325–31.
94. Johnston JJ, Rubinstein WS, Facio FM, Ng D, Singh LN, Teer JK, Mullikin JC, Biesecker LG. Secondary variants in individuals undergoing exome sequencing: screening of 572 individuals identifies high-penetrance mutations in cancer-susceptibility genes. Am J Hum Genet. 2012;91:97–108.
95. Green RC, Berg JS, Berry GT, Biesecker LG, Dimmock DP, Evans JP, Grody WW, Hegde MR, Kalia S, Korf BR, Krantz I, McGuire AL, Miller DT, Murray MF, Nussbaum RL, Plon SE, Rehm HL, Jacob HJ. Exploring concordance and discordance for return of incidental findings from clinical sequencing. Genet Med. 2012;14:405–10.
96. Lemke A, Bick D, Dimmock D, Simpson P, Veith R. Perspectives of clinical genetics professionals toward genome sequencing and incidental findings: a survey study. Clin Genet. 2012;84(3):230–6.
97. Berg JS, Adams M, Nassar N, Bizon C, Lee K, Schmitt CP, Wilhelmsen KC, Evans JP. An informatics approach to analyzing the incidentalome. Genet Med. 2013;15(1):36–44.
98. Aziz N, Zhao Q, Bry L, Driscoll DK, Funke B, Gibson JS, Grody WW, Hegde MR, Hoeltge GA, Leonard DG, Merker JD, Nagarajan R, Palicki LA, Robetorye RS, Schrijver I, Weck KE, Voelkerding KV. College of American Pathologists' laboratory standards for next-generation sequencing clinical tests. Arch Pathol Lab Med. 2015;139(4):481–93.

Next-Generation Sequencing for the Analysis of Cancer Specimens

60

John D. Pfeifer

Abstract

Massively parallel sequencing (also known as next-generation sequencing, or NGS), which provides genomic data at low cost and high accuracy, is ideally suited for clinical testing of cancer specimens. NGS results may inform the cancer diagnosis or choice of therapy. The genomes of cancer cells carry somatic (often referred to as acquired) alterations, which fall into four general classes: single nucleotide variants (SNVs), small insertions and deletions (indels), copy number variants (CNVs), and structural variants (SVs). The genetic complexity of cancers underscores the importance of NGS to evaluate the full spectrum of sequence variations in dozens to thousands of genes in a single test. Amplification-based as well as hybrid capture-based methods for NGS testing can be used for the analysis of cancer specimens, and assays that target a panel of genes (from several genes, to several hundred genes), the exome, or the genome have been developed. Although each type of assay carries with it specific test design considerations, all NGS assays share a set of preanalytic, analytic, and postanalytic/reporting issues that must be addressed during test validation and routine clinical use. In addition, the analytic portion of an NGS test consists of three individual components (i.e., the sequencing platform; the wet bench procedures; and the bioinformatics pipeline), which creates some unique quality management issues.

Keywords

Next-generation sequencing • Massively parallel sequencing • Cancer • Single nucleotide variants • Insertions • Deletions • Indels • Structural variants • Copy number variants • Library preparation • Clinical molecular testing • Preanalytical • Analytical • Postanalytical

Introduction

Massively parallel sequencing (also known as next-generation sequencing, or NGS), which provides genomic data at low cost and high accuracy, is ideally suited for clinical testing of cancer specimens. NGS is increasingly being used for clinical testing of cancer specimens because NGS can comprehensively evaluate multiple genetic loci when only a limited quantity of DNA is available for testing. The ability to provide comprehensive analysis is important given the increasing number of targeted chemotherapy drugs (which requires analysis of an ever increasing number of genes), while ever smaller tissue specimens are available for testing. The smaller specimens are a result of trends to shift from large excisional biopsies to needle or aspiration biopsies for diagnosis.

The genetic complexity of cancers underscores the important role for NGS in evaluating the full spectrum of sequence variations in dozens to thousands of genes in a single test. The genomes of all cancer cells carry somatic

J.D. Pfeifer, M.D., Ph.D. (✉)
Department of Pathology, Washington University School of Medicine, Campus Box 8118, 660 South Euclid Ave., St. Louis, MO, 63110, USA
e-mail: Pfeifer@path.wustl.edu

D.G.B. Leonard (ed.), *Molecular Pathology in Clinical Practice*, DOI 10.1007/978-3-319-19674-9_60

or acquired DNA alterations, which fall into four general classes, single nucleotide variants (SNVs), small insertions and deletions (indels, which are generally less than a few dozen bases long), copy number variants (CNVs), and structural variants (SVs, such as translocations). Some of the mutations are so-called "driver mutations" because they confer selective clonal growth or survival advantage and are causally involved in oncogenesis. Other mutations are so-called "passenger mutations" since they do not contribute to development or progression of the cancer but are secondary changes with little diagnostic or therapeutic importance, usually due to the genomic instability of many cancers.

Identifying somatic driver mutations in cancer has several direct clinical applications. First, the specific pattern of mutations can be diagnostic in cases in which traditional histopathologic examination is not definitive, as for example in the setting of a tumor of unknown primary origin [1]. Second, somatic mutations can be used to predict how a patient may respond to a drug with respect to toxicity or efficacy. For example, alterations in exon 19 of *EGFR* in patients with non-small-cell lung cancer (NSCLC) are responsive to treatment with gefitinib [2]. Similarly, the majority of patients with NSCLC or lung adenocarcinoma who carry inversions in *ALK* or a translocation involving *ROS1* respond to treatment with crizotinib [3, 4]. Other somatic mutations predict resistance to therapy with tyrosine kinase inhibitors (TKIs), such as *KRAS* mutations in lung cancer [5]. Third, somatic mutations can provide prognostic information on the risk of disease progression or relapse. For example, an internal tandem duplication of *FLT3* is associated with poor prognosis in acute myeloid leukemia (AML), while mutations in nucleophosmin (*NPM1*) are associated with a favorable prognosis in AML [6].

Amplification-based as well as hybrid capture-based NGS methods can be used for the analysis of cancer specimens. Assays that target a panel of genes (from several genes, to several hundred genes), the exome, or the genome have been used clinically for cancer analysis. However, as with all laboratory tests, the clinical utility of the different assay designs is extremely dependent on the clinical setting. In general, since clinical utility has been defined for only a few thousand different mutations in a few hundred genes, sequence analysis of the exome or genome in a clinical setting is currently unjustified. In addition, due to the tissue and tumor heterogeneity of cancer specimens, detection of cancer mutations requires a high depth of coverage that cannot currently be accomplished with exome or genome NGS. Therefore, currently, the most common NGS tests for cancer focus on panels of genes with well documented roles in diagnosis, prognosis, or prediction of response to therapy.

Assay Design Considerations

Several practical and operational considerations of assay design determine the eventual utility of an NGS assay used in the clinical analysis of cancer specimens. The more general aspects of assay design are discussed in Chap. 61. The details that are specific to the analysis of somatic mutations in tissue specimens from cancer patients are discussed in this chapter.

Amplification-Based Methods

Amplification-based NGS methods rely on exponential amplification of the target region utilizing sequence-specific primers. When compared with hybrid capture-based methods, amplification methods have a simpler workflow, with reduced hands-on time and more rapid turnaround time (TAT), and so are more frequently used in clinical settings. Highly multiplexed microfluidic and microdroplet methods, e.g., RainDance Technologies (Billerica, MA) or Fluidigm (South San Francisco, CA), have substantial upfront hardware costs. Several amplification enrichment systems have been optimized for compatibility with benchtop sequencing instruments (e.g., Ion Torrent, Illumina MiSeq), which makes amplification-based technology accessible to any size laboratory for clinical use. However, amplification-based approaches have several limitations. First, there are significant limits on the size of the target region that can be sequenced because of practical issues with the number of PCR reactions that can be multiplexed in a single amplification. Second, only a subset of variant types can be detected; in general SNVs and small indels can be identified, while detection of CNVs and SVs is extremely challenging. Third, as with any amplification-based test, there is the potential for amplification bias, polymerase sequencing errors, contamination, and primer binding artifacts. Fourth, amplification-based NGS requires prior knowledge of the sequences and the nature of the mutations to be targeted; the assay lacks the potential for identifying novel disease-associated mutations outside the targeted regions.

Commercial Amplification-Based Tests

While many clinical NGS labs have internally developed amplification-based NGS tests [7–9], commercially available assays are commonly used in the clinical setting. The AmpliSeq hot spot panel (Life Technologies, Grand Island, NY) and the TruSeq hot spot panel (Illumina, San Diego, CA) are in clinical use.

AmpliSeq assays (Life Technologies) [10] use a proprietary ultra-high multiplex PCR technology to generate thousands of amplicons for massively parallel sequencing. Only approximately 10 ng of input DNA are required and the assays work well with different types of tumor samples, including archived formalin-fixed, paraffin-embedded (FFPE) tissue samples. The amplicons generated from AmpliSeq kits are ready for sequencing using the Ion PGM system (Life Technologies). The TAT from receiving samples to reporting results can be as short as 3–5 days. While the traditional assays involve only a limited set of loci in a panel of genes (Table 60.1), a new kit (Ion AmpliSeq Exome, Life Technologies) amplifies the exome in 12 primer pools using as little as 50 ng DNA [11]. Figure 60.1 shows the results of a representative assay performed on an Ion Torrent PGM platform with a 316 Chip v2 and using the AmpliSeq™ Cancer Panel v2 (Life Technologies).

TruSeq and related assays (Illumina) [12] also target a limited set of loci in a panel of genes (Table 60.2). The assays require 150–250 ng DNA based on the sample type, and have a TAT of 3–5 days.

Hybrid Capture-Based Methods

NGS using targeted hybridization (hybrid) capture is a sensitive and specific method to detect somatic alterations in cancer samples. With appropriate assay design, hybrid capture enables detection of all four classes of genomic alterations in cancer specimens with very high analytic sensitivity and specificity, a very low limit of detection, and very high reproducibility. Given the genomic heterogeneity that is a fundamental characteristic of cancer, particularly in solid tumors, the efficient and cost-effective targeting of multiple classes of mutations in a large number of genes in a single assay is

Table 60.1 The genes covered by Ion AmpliSeq™ Cancer Hotspot Panel v2

ABL1	*EGFR*	*GNAQ*	*KRAS*	*PTPN11*
AKT1	*ERBB2*	*GNAS*	*MET*	*RB1*
ALK	*ERBB4*	*HNF1A*	*MLH1*	*RET*
APC	*EZH2*	*HRAS*	*MPL*	*SMAD4*
ATM	*FBXW7*	*IDH1*	*NOTCH1*	*SMARCB1*
BRAF	*FGFR1*	*IDH2*	*NPM1*	*SMO*
CDH1	*FGFR2*	*JAK2*	*NRAS*	*SRC*
CDKN2A	*FGFR3*	*JAK3*	*PDGFRA*	*STK11*
CSF1R	*FLT3*	*KDR*	*PIK3CA*	*TP53*
CTNNB1	*GNA11*	*KIT*	*PTEN*	*VHL*

The size of the total targeted region of the panel is approximately 22 kb. A total of 207 primer pairs are amplified in a single tube to generate 207 different amplicons. The amplicon lengths range from 111 to 187 bp (average 154 bp)

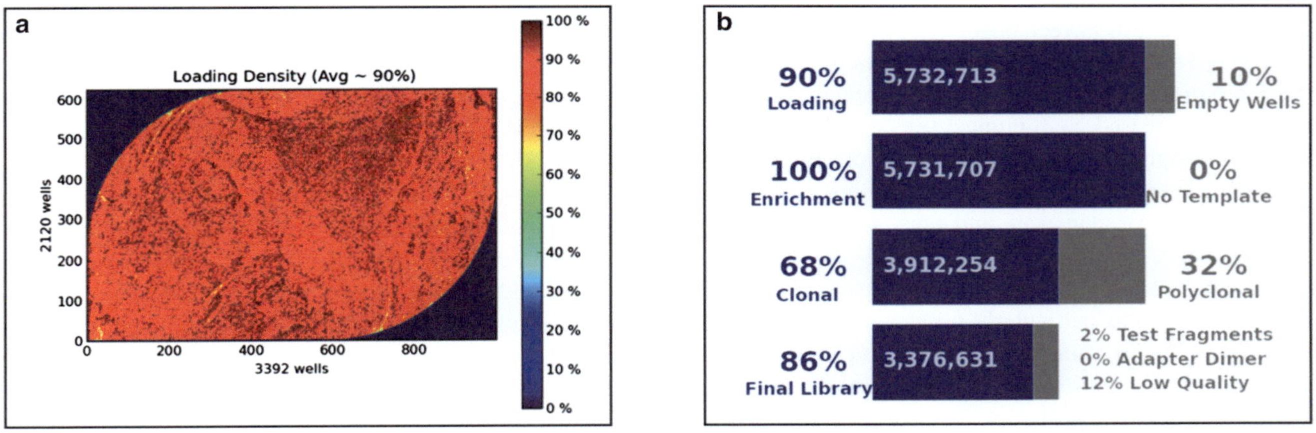

c

Variant Caller Reports	Mapped Reads	Reads On-Target	Bases On-Target	Read Depth	1x Coverage	20x Coverage	100x Coverage	Variants Detected
IonXpress_005	869,360	98.76%	92.09%	3,941.92	100.000%	100.000%	100.000%	16
IonXpress_006	966,818	98.51%	92.09%	4,355.44	100.000%	100.000%	100.000%	14
IonXpress_007	859,803	98.20%	91.37%	3,918.21	100.000%	100.000%	100.000%	15
IonXpress_008	644,058	98.88%	92.01%	2,859.55	100.000%	100.000%	100.000%	12

Figure 60.1 Performance specifics of a next-generation sequencing run performed on the Ion Torrent PGM platform with a 316 Chip v2 with AmpliSeq Cancer Panel v2 (Life Technologies). (**a**) Ion sphere particle (ISP) density indicates the distribution of the sequencing particles across the chip surface; (**b**) ISP summary table; (**c**) Variant Caller Report indicating test metrics. See Ref. 145 for details. Reprinted by permission from Elsevier Inc., *Clinical Genomics: A guide to clinical next generation sequencing.* Kulkarni S and Pfeifer J, Eds.

Table 60.2 Genes covered by the Illumina TruSeq Amplicon Cancer Panel

ABL1	*EGFR*	*GNAS*	*MLH1*	*RET*
AKT1	*ERBB2*	*HNF1A*	*MPL*	*SMAD4*
ALK	*ERBB4*	*HRAS*	*NOTCH1*	*SMARCB1*
APC	*FBXW7*	*IDH1*	*NPM1*	*SMO*
ATM	*FGFR1*	*JAK2*	*NRAS*	*SRC*
BRAF	*FGFR2*	*JAK3*	*PDGFRA*	*STK11*
CDH1	*FGFR3*	*KDR*	*PIK3CA*	*TP53*
CDKN2A	*FLT3*	*KIT*	*PTEN*	*VHL*
CSF1R	*GNA11*	*KRAS*	*PTPN11*	
CTNNB1	*GNAQ*	*MET*	*RB1*	

The panel targets mutation hotspots in 48 genes that are almost identical to those of the AmpliSeq™ Cancer Hotspot Panel (Table 60.1). The panel includes 212 amplicons ranging from 170 to 190 bp in length. The total genomic region covered is about 35 kb

required. Hybrid capture methodologies have the flexibility to target a wide range of genes from one gene to the exome. Currently available liquid capture kits (e.g., Ref. 13) have a target size of 1 kb to 24 Mb.

However, hybrid capture NGS tests have several disadvantages. DNA library preparation generally takes 3–5 days (compared with 1 day for amplification-based enrichment library preparation), with a large proportion of this time allocated to probe hybridization (typically 24–48 h incubation time for the hybridization step itself). Therefore, clinical hybrid capture tests have a longer TAT. Although automation can be used to decrease TAT, the equipment is expensive and thus requires a substantial initial capital investment. Hybridization-based NGS clinical tests also frequently suffer from design restrictions, including problems producing high quality sequence data from DNA regions with high GC content, repetitive sequences, and gene family members that share sequence homology (pseudogenes). The bioinformatics and interpretive component of hybrid-capture based testing has emerged as particularly problematic, since the ease with which massive amounts of sequence can be generated on the current generation of platforms can easily overwhelm a laboratory's ability to analyze the data.

Assay Scope

Targeted Gene Panels

Gene panels for acquired mutations in cancer specimens focus on genes that are considered clinically actionable based on evidence for their diagnostic, predictive, and/or prognostic value. The gene panels may be quite narrow (e.g., only a few dozen genes) based on the specific cancer being evaluated, such as colon adenocarcinoma, lung adenocarcinoma, or gastrointestinal stromal tumor [14–16], or much broader (e.g., hundreds of genes) based on recurrently mutated genes across multiple cancer types [17, 18].

Smaller and larger gene panels each have distinct advantages and disadvantages. For clinical testing, limiting the number of targeted genes avoids an excessive number of distracting variants of unknown significance (VUSs), decreases incidental findings, and decreases TAT. Assays with a smaller target region make it cost effective to sequence at greater depth even with multiplexed samples, providing greater analytical sensitivity for detecting mutations with low variant allele frequencies (VAFs) and a lower cost. Another important advantage of small panels that target only loci with well-established clinical relevance is higher rates of reimbursement, a difference that is critical in the clinical setting where testing is funded by insurance payers rather than research grants or philanthropy. In contrast, large gene panels are more likely to include genes relevant to clinical trials or drug development, and so have much more utility in investigational settings. In the end, gene panel design is determined by examining factors such as clinical need, expected sample volume, practicality of running multiple small disease-directed panels vs a single more general cancer based panel, and sources of revenue.

Exomes and Genomes

Exome and genome sequencing often are applied to the study of cancer as a discovery tool in the investigative setting. Exome or genome sequencing is helpful for detection of CNVs and is especially well suited to detection of structural variants (SV), which often involve noncoding DNA breakpoints. However, the use of exome and whole genome in routine clinical practice has several limitations. First, because of the high depth of coverage (about 1,000×) required for sensitive and specific identification of somatic variants in cancer samples due to admixing of benign and malignant cells within the tumor, clonal heterogeneity of the tumor cells, and variation in coverage across different regions of DNA, the cost of exome or genome sequencing is often prohibitive in clinical practice. Second, the utility of sequencing genes without established clinical significance for cancer patient management is an issue. Beyond the genes evaluated by focused panels, there are relatively few loci for which sufficient evidence of clinical significance exists to support interpretation of functional or therapeutic consequences for the variants identified; thus, most variants identified are VUSs and do not meaningfully contribute to patient management. Third, intensive bioinformatics analysis is required to manage the vast amounts of data generated by such large scale sequencing.

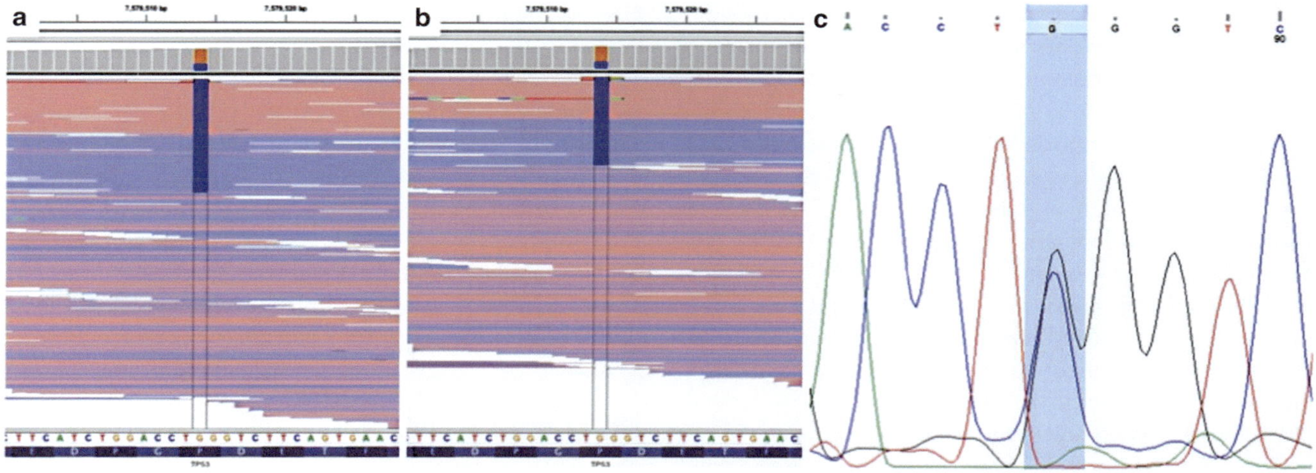

Figure 60.2 Ambiguity of variant allele frequencies (VAFs). Next-generation sequencing (NGS) was performed on two separate tumor samples from one patient; a *TP53* variant was identified in both samples (chr17:7579514G.C). The patient's oropharyngeal squamous cell carcinoma (SCC) contained the variant with a VAF of 0.30 (**a**). The same variant was present in the lung SCC with a VAF of 0.32 (**b**). Sanger sequencing was performed on nonneoplastic tissue from the same patient, which demonstrated that the variant was heterozygous in the germline (**c**), and copy number analysis at this position showed no copy number alterations (not shown). Thus, based on the VAF alone, this variant may have been incorrectly interpreted as a somatic mutation that was shared between the two tumors. Reprinted by permission from Elsevier Inc., *Clinical Genomics: A guide to clinical next generation sequencing*. Kulkarni S and Pfeifer J, Eds.

Determination of Somatic Status with or Without Paired Tumor-Normal Tissue Analyses

Determination of Somatic Status Without Paired Normal Tissue

Many factors complicate predictions regarding the germline vs somatic status of a variant, as well as estimates of the percentage of tumor cells that harbor the variant, for sequence changes identified from a cancer sample when a normal tissue sample from the same patient is not available or tested for comparison. Most approaches to this problem rely on the VAF, which is essentially the percentage of sequence reads that have the variant. However, when evaluating the VAF for variants identified from cancer samples, it is important to remember that tumor samples in general, and solid tumor samples in particular, are inherently heterogeneous, consisting not only of the tumor cells but also of associated inflammatory cells, stromal cells, endothelial cells, and normal parenchymal cells (as discussed in more detail below). Since the relative proportion of these various cell types is highly variable between different tumor samples, and even between different areas of the same tumor, the VAF from the cancer specimen is an uncertain guide as to whether a variant is a somatic mutation present in the majority of the tumor cells, only a small subclone of the tumor cells, or even a germline variant. For example, a heterozygous mutation present in a sample that consists almost entirely of tumor cells could have the same VAF (i.e., 0.5, often indicated as 50 %) as a homozygous mutation present in half of the tumor cells, or as a germline variant (Fig. 60.2). Interpretation of VAFs is further complicated by a complex interplay of various classes of mutation affecting the same locus. For example, a SNV in a gene that is amplified in a small subclone of the tumor could produce the same VAF as a heterozygous mutation present in the majority of tumor cells. The use of VAFs as a basis for evaluating the percentage of tumor cells that contain a variant, or to infer the somatic vs germline status for an identified variant, is further complicated by analytic factors inherent to capture and/or amplification techniques that introduce technical sources of bias.

Paired Tumor-Normal Analysis

For NGS analysis of cancer specimens, paired tumor-normal testing can sometimes provide insight into the significance of a VUS obtained from tumor tissue. However, the laboratory decision to perform paired tumor-normal testing, whether ad hoc based on the NGS findings in a particular case or as the routine approach for all cases, depends on a number of factors including the cost, the size of the target region, and the anticipated clinical use of the sequence results. In general, for NGS assays focused on a limited panel of genes designed to identify mutations that are the targets of specific drug therapies, paired tumor-normal testing provides little additional information that impacts patient care. However, for very large gene panels, exome, and genome sequencing, paired tumor-normal testing is an integral part of NGS analysis, essentially in order to filter out germline variants. Unfortunately, current reimbursement paradigms do not support clinical sequencing of non-tumor samples for comparison to tumor samples.

Even before acquired mutations are considered, bioinformatics analysis of exome and genome sequence results of tumor specimens is complicated by the fact that an average person has from 140 to 420 non-silent (non-synonymous SNV, gain or loss of stop codon, frameshift or in-frame indel, or change in splice site) germline variants not present in any significant proportion of other individuals (i.e., they are variants with a minor allele frequency of <0.5 %) [19]. Nonetheless, these variants are not expected to contribute directly to carcinogenesis and thus likely represent benign variation seen in healthy humans [20]. In addition, the number of "novel" germline variants increases dramatically for individuals from ethnicities that are less well genetically characterized, based solely on inadequate sampling of rare benign polymorphisms in those populations. Since benign polymorphisms are generally indistinguishable from tumor-associated mutations in cancer samples if matched normal tissue is not available for comparison, these polymorphisms in the patient's background germline genetic profile cannot be separated from tumor-associated acquired mutations.

With respect to acquired somatic mutations, the number of somatic mutations in a tumor sample is highly variable between cancer types. Some cancers have <1 mutation per megabase (Mb) of coding DNA sequence, with others having >100 mutations per Mb [21–29]. Unlike targeted NGS analysis of relatively limited and well-described hot spot mutations and cancer genes, exome targeting captures 30–75 Mb of sequence (depending on the reagent used for capture) and identifies hundreds of nonsynonymous coding sequence variants from each cancer sample. In so-called "hypermutator phenotype" tumors characterized by unusually high rates of somatic mutation, over 1,000 somatic mutations can be identified [21, 26]. For example, lung squamous cell carcinoma, which has one of the highest described somatic mutation rates, harbors an average of 228 non-silent protein coding sequence mutations, 165 structural rearrangements, and 323 copy number changes per tumor [22]. Inclusion of the noncoding (e.g., intronic or untranslated region) sequence identified by genome sequencing hugely increases the number of variants identified; for example, a median of over 18,000 SNVs alone are found by genome sequencing of lung adenocarcinoma [27].

Comparison of tumor tissue to normal (or more accurately, non-neoplastic) tissue from the same patient is extremely valuable for determining whether an identified variant is a germline variant or a somatic mutation, and for decreasing the overall number of variants that need to be evaluated and interpreted. The simplest bioinformatics approach for paired tumor-normal NGS testing involves subtracting variants identified in the normal sample, producing a set of variants that appears to be enriched in the tumor. The subtraction approach relies on a pure normal sample, verified by tissue histology or some other method, to avoid "subtracting" variants present in even a low level of contaminating tumor cells.

One caveat to removal of germline variants from subsequent analyses is worth note, namely that some germline variants are very relevant in cancer and will be removed by this analytical method. For example, germline variants in *BRCA1* or *BRCA2* drive oncogenesis in families with hereditary breast cancer, and germline variants in *TP53* cause cancer in families with Li–Fraumeni syndrome [30, 31]. However, ideally, standard clinical evaluation should identify those patients at risk for a hereditary cancer syndrome.

Library Complexity

The number of independent DNA template molecules (sometimes referred to as genome equivalents) sequenced in an NGS assay has a profound impact on the sensitivity and specificity of variant detection. While it is possible to perform NGS analysis using only picogram quantities of DNA [32–34], this technical feat is accomplished by simply increasing the number of amplification cycles during library preparation. However, the information content in 1,000 sequence reads derived from one genome is quite different than the information content present in 1,000 sequence reads from 1,000 different genomes. Thus, library complexity and sequence depth (see below) are independent parameters in NGS assay design.

One common way to measure library complexity is through quantitation of the number of unique, on-target reads. Sequence reads with different 5′ and 3′ termini are usually unique and thus arise from DNA from more than one genome (and more than one cell); thus, it is straightforward to estimate the complexity of a DNA library produced by a hybrid capture method since the sequence reads have different 5′ and 3′ termini reflecting the population of DNA fragments captured during the hybridization step. However, it is uncertain whether sequence reads with identical 5′ and 3′ termini have an origin from different genomes (cells) or merely represent PCR amplification bias; thus, direct measurement of the complexity in a DNA library produced by an amplification method is difficult since all the sequence reads from one amplicon will have identical 5′ and 3′ termini regardless of the population of DNA fragments from which they originated.

Accurate calculation (or even estimation) of complexity from morphologic assessment of patient specimens is difficult since all the steps of library preparation involve inefficiencies that interact in complicated ways. Cancer specimens that are highly cellular and contain a high percentage of viable tumor cells typically produce an adequately complex DNA library. Small paucicellular specimens have the potential for generating low complexity DNA libraries likely to produce biased sequence results. The complicated intratumoral heterogeneity of malignancies (see below) dictates that DNA library complexity should be maximized to achieve optimal NGS sequencing results.

Depth of Coverage

Depth of coverage is defined as the number of aligned reads that contain a given nucleotide position, and sufficient depth of coverage is critical in clinical NGS assays for identification of sequence variants with the required level of sensitivity and specificity. Many factors influence the required depth of coverage. The first variable is the sequence complexity of the target region. Target regions with homology to multiple regions of the genome, a higher number of repetitive sequence elements, pseudogenes, and increased GC content generally have decreased coverage due to technical aspects of the sequencing process [35, 36]. Second, the method used for targeted enrichment can impact coverage depth with amplification methods often providing higher depth (although the complexity of the sequence data may be uncertain, as discussed above). Third, in a multiplexed clinical test where multiple samples are sequenced simultaneously, the size of the target region (e.g., 400 kb for a typical panel of genes, vs 30–75 Mb for an exome, vs over 3 Gb for a genome) will impact the depth of coverage that can be reasonably achieved for each sample because of the defined sequencing capacity of the chip used to generate the sequence reads.

The relationship between depth of coverage and the reproducibility of variant detection from a given sample is straightforward: a higher number of high-quality sequence reads lends confidence to the base called at a particular location, whether the base call from the sequenced sample is the same as the reference base (no variant identified) or is a non-reference base (variant identified), and thus increases assay sensitivity and specificity [35–38]. However, the depth of coverage required to make accurate variant calls also is dependent upon the type of variant being evaluated, and whether the variant is germline or acquired. In general, a lower depth of coverage is acceptable for constitutional testing where germline alterations are more easily identified since they are in either a heterozygous or homozygous state, and all DNA has the same sequence, except for mosaicism. A minimum of 30× coverage with balanced reads (forward and reverse reads equally represented) is usually sufficient for germline testing [39, 40]. However, much higher read depths are necessary to confidently identify somatic variants in tumor specimens due to tissue and tumor heterogeneity (see below); an overall coverage of approximately 1,000× is optimal [7]. For NGS of mitochondrial DNA, an average coverage of >20,000 is required to reliably detect heteroplasmic variants present at 1.5 % [41].

The need for high read depths reflects the complexity involved in somatic variant detection. As discussed below in more detail, tumor biopsy specimens represent a heterogeneous mixture of tissue encompassing malignant cells, as well as supporting stromal cells, inflammatory cells, and uninvolved tissue; malignant cells harboring somatic variation can become diluted out in this admixture. Of additional consideration, intratumoral heterogeneity creates tumor subclones so that only a small proportion of the total tumor cell population may have a given mutation. Thus, the read depth of the assay should be sufficiently high to compensate for this variation.

Preanalytic Issues

Specimen Requirements

The amount of specimen DNA required for clinical NGS testing can be from a variety of patient sample sources including peripheral blood, bone marrow aspirates, buccal swabs, surgical resections, needle biopsies, and fine needle aspirations (FNAs). For solid tumors the most frequently available specimen type is FFPE tumor tissue. Fortunately, FFPE specimens as well as fresh tumor samples are both amenable to NGS analysis by current NGS technologies. However, DNA from FFPE will be a suboptimal substrate for use with emerging approaches that make it possible to determine the sequence of over a thousand bases per individual DNA template molecule, which will improve the analysis of currently difficult regions such as pseudogenes or repetitive sequences.

While it is well established that formaldehyde reacts with DNA and proteins to form covalent crosslinks, engenders oxidation and deamination reactions, and leads to the formation of cyclic based derivatives [42–46], with higher depths of coverage, the rate of sequence artifacts from FFPE samples is quite small compared with paired fresh samples from the same tumor, and is in fact several orders of magnitude below the cutoff for reporting variants in routine clinical practice [47]. Similarly, several studies have demonstrated that, for both amplification and hybrid capture methods, alcohol fixation does not induce sequence artifacts at a clinically significant rate [48, 49]. The lack of a significant rate of NGS sequence artifacts has been shown for both ethanol-fixed specimens (of the type used in Papanicolaou stains) as well as methanol-fixed specimens (of the type used in Romanowsky stains such as Diff-Quik), which allows the increasingly common use of cytology specimens for clinical NGS tests. Since exposure to acid efficiently hydrolyzes phosphate diester links (and also damages nucleotides leading to abasic sites) in both DNA and RNA, acid decalcification renders tissue samples unacceptable for NGS analysis [50]. When decalcification is required, calcium chelating agents such as EDTA should be used since they have no significant impact on nucleic acids.

Histopathologic Review

Prior to DNA extraction from the tumor specimen, the specimen slides corresponding to the tumor used for NGS testing should be reviewed by an anatomic pathologist to ensure the presence of viable (non-necrotic) malignant tissue, and to assess the quality and quantity of the material submitted for testing. The pathologic assessment is an important quality control step since it permits evaluation of possible analytic confounders, including the percentage of nonneoplastic tissue, necrosis, cautery artifact, and so on, and thus helps ensure that the specimen is adequate for the validated assay. More specifically, if a cutoff of 10 % VAF is used for clinical reporting of a variant, then areas with more than 20 % tumor cellularity should be used to ensure that heterozygous variants present in all the tumor cells will likely be detected. Obtaining an estimation of the percentage of tumor cells present in the tissue section relative to total number of cells is useful during interpretation of the sequencing data in regard to VAF. Unfortunately, although a pathologist's review of cancer samples is required to select the regions of tumor with high cellularity and viability, the estimates of percent tumor cells present are unreliable [51, 52].

It is important to recognize that the percentage of nonneoplastic tissue (also known as tissue heterogeneity) is different from intratumoral heterogeneity. Tissue heterogeneity refers to the fact that no tumor specimen is composed of 100 % neoplastic cells. Instead, cancer samples contain a varying proportion of nonneoplastic cells including stromal cells (benign parenchymal cells and fibroblasts), inflammatory cells (primarily neutrophils, lymphocytes, and macrophages), and endothelial cells (of blood vessels and lymphatics). Intratumoral heterogeneity is a term used to refer to the fact that malignant neoplasms usually demonstrate clonal heterogeneity [53, 54]. Consequently, even with a relatively pure tumor sample identified by histopathologic review, the number, type, and frequency of sequence variants detected in that sample may or may not be an accurate reflection of the range and frequency of the variants elsewhere in the tumor.

DNA Extraction

Total DNA yield from a cancer specimen is commonly measured by either spectrophotometry or fluorometry. Metrics including A_{260}/A_{280} and A_{260}/A_{230} are commonly used to estimate nucleic acid purity, and agarose gel electrophoresis can be performed to ensure the presence of high molecular weight genomic DNA. However, the presence of high molecular weight DNA is not necessarily mandatory for NGS, as demonstrated by the fact that both amplification-based and hybrid capture-based methods work well with FFPE samples that contain damaged nucleic acids due to formalin-fixation during routine processing [47]. While sample processing is generally standardized within a laboratory, many variables can significantly impact nucleic acid quality, such as fixation time, storage conditions, and acid decalcification, and in turn can affect subsequent library preparation and sequencing. The use of acid decalcification is especially problematic since acid exposure rapidly destroys nucleic acids [50]; decalcification with a chelating agent (EDTA) is preferred [55].

Analytic Issues

NGS tests require three components, specifically: the sequencing instrument; the laboratory procedures including extraction of nucleic acids and DNA library preparation; and the bioinformatics processes for base calling, reference genome alignment, variant identification, variant annotation, and variant interpretation. The general features of all three of these components as they apply to NGS analysis of cancer specimens are similar to those for constitutional testing, and are covered in Chap. 61. However, some additional issues must be considered in the analysis of tumor samples, specifically in the bioinformatics analysis.

As with all NGS testing, after the sequencing reads are generated from the DNA extracted from a tumor specimen, bioinformatics tools are used to align the reads against a reference genome and identify differences between the tumor DNA sequence and the reference sequence. Given the intrinsic genomic instability of malignancies, and often complicated intratumoral heterogeneity due to the presence of various tumor subclones, maximum clinical utility of NGS testing of cancer specimens can only be achieved using a bioinformatics pipeline designed to detect all four classes of genomic variants (SNVs, indels, CNVs, and SVS) at allele frequencies that are physiologically relevant. The four main classes of variants each require different computational approaches for sensitive and specific identification (assuming the assay is designed to permit their detection) [56], and since various bioinformatics pipelines are known to yield different variant calls for the different classes of variants, and even for specific variants, optimization of the bioinformatics pipeline used for a clinical NGS test is imperative [57].

Single Nucleotide Variations

SNVs occur when a single nucleotide (e.g., A, T, C, or G) is altered in the DNA sequence; note that single base pair insertions and deletions are technically not SNVs but rather indels. SNVs are by far the most common class of sequence variant, and the high density of polymorphic SNVs segregating in the human population (about 1 SNV is present per 800 bases between a single diploid individual and the reference genome) makes them ideal markers for genetic mapping [58]. Inherited SNVs are generally classified as single nucleotide polymorphisms (SNPs) if they are present at a moderately high frequency in the population (greater than 1 %), although many inherited SNVs exist at lower population allele frequencies yet are nonetheless benign polymorphisms with no known disease association. While SNPs are polymorphisms that have no direct (or clearly established indirect) association with a specific disease, SNVs that are correlated with disease often are referred to as single base pair mutations or point mutations. The biologic impact of SNVs in protein-coding regions depends on whether the change is synonymous (silent) or nonsynonymous (of which the two types are missense mutations and nonsense mutations). In noncoding regions, as well as some coding regions, SNVs may affect RNA processing or gene regulation [59–62]. Nonetheless, selection pressure reduces the overall frequency of single base pair substitutions in coding DNA and in associated regulatory sequences, with the result that the overall SNV rate in protein-coding DNA is much less than that of noncoding DNA. In addition, clinical testing does not usually consider the noncoding regions of the genome, although these regions are being studied and clearly can cause disease.

The platforms and bioinformatics pipelines of NGS are well suited to the detection of SNVs, although the error rates of different platforms must be considered during platform selection and assay design (Fig. 60.3). In fact, the earliest clinical applications of NGS were designed to detect

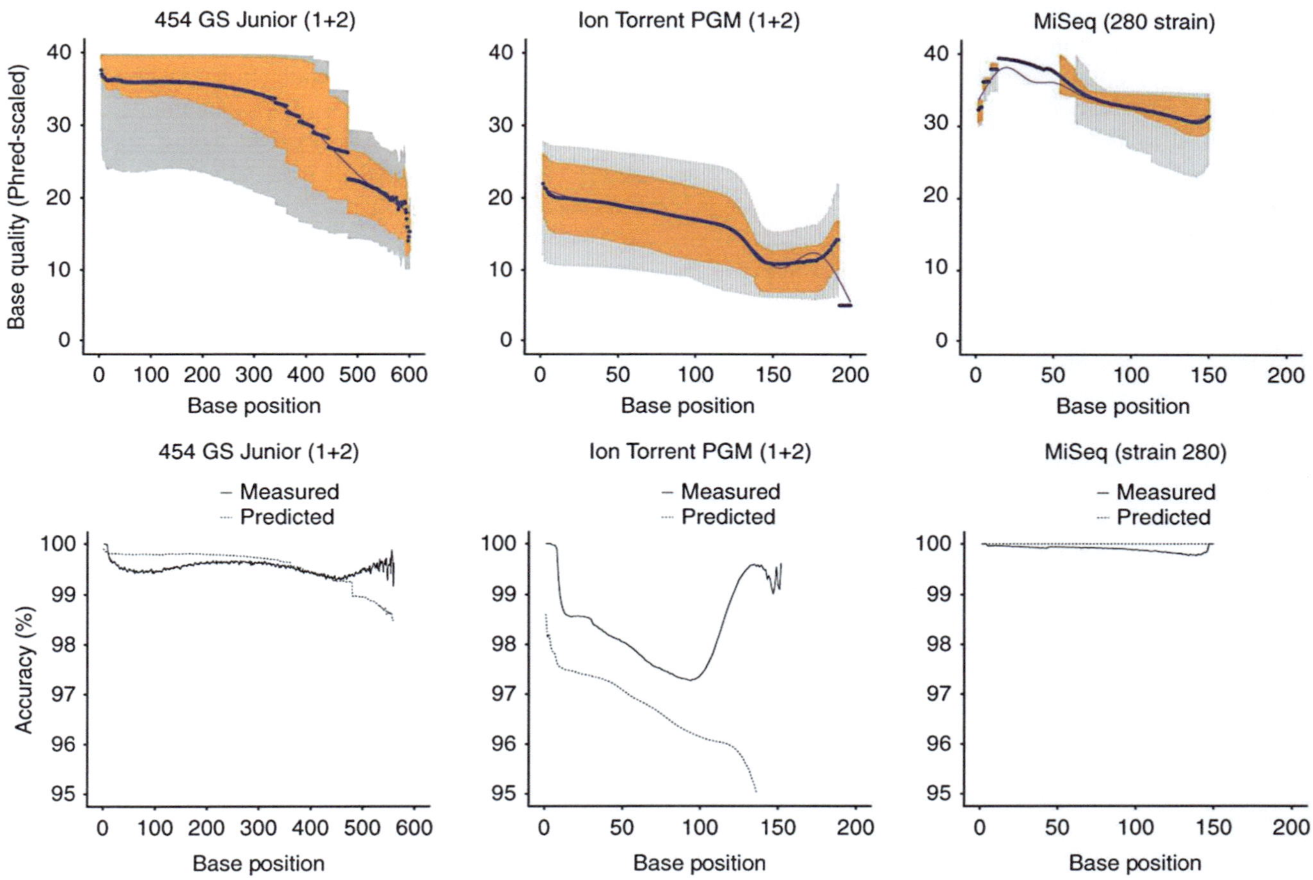

Figure 60.3 Comparison of three major platforms currently used in clinical NGS assays. Since the platforms vary with respect to their chemistry, it is not surprising that they each have different intrinsic error rates which affect the performance for single nucleotide variant (SNV) detection. In one comprehensive study evaluating sequencing platform differences [141], the MiSeq instrument (Illumina) had the lowest substitution error rate (about 0.1 substitutions per 100 bases). The Ion Torrent PGM (Life Technologies) had a substitution error rate over ten-fold greater, which steadily decreased across the read length; however, increased accuracy could be achieved by "clipping" read ends determined to be of low quality [142]. The substitution error rate of the 454GS Junior (454 Life Sciences, A Roche Company, Branford, CT) was intermediate between the MiSeq and Ion Torrent PGM. In terms of indel detection, admittedly only one of many factors that must be considered in selecting an NGS platform, the reversible dye terminator approach of the MiSeq has a lower indel error rate (<0.001 indels per 100 bases sequenced) compared with pH detection of the Ion Torrent PGM (1.5 indels per 100 bases), for reasons discussed in the text [143]. From Loman NJ, Misra RV, Dallman TJ et al. (2012) Performance comparison of benchtop high-throughput sequencing platforms. Nat Biotechnol 30:434-9. Reprinted by permission from Nature Publishing Group

SNVs in inherited and acquired diseases, and for this reason the bioinformatics pipelines required for sensitive and specific detection of single base substitutions are among the most advanced in clinical NGS. The expanding catalog of clinically relevant point mutations has been an especially important driver of development of NGS assays [21, 63, 64]. Indeed, to date, NGS tests have been successfully implemented in several clinical laboratories for detecting SNVs [7–9, 14, 16, 17].

From a bioinformatics perspective, many popular NGS analysis programs for SNV detection are designed for constitutional genome analysis where variants occur in 0 % (wild type), 50 % (heterozygous), or 100 % (homozygous) of the reads. These prior probabilities are often built into the algorithms, and consequently, SNVs with VAFs falling too far outside the expected range for homozygous and heterozygous variants are often ignored as false positives. Thus, sensitive and specific bioinformatics approaches for somatically acquired SNVs require either significant revision of the software packages designed for constitutional testing or new algorithms altogether. Some bioinformatics tools are optimized for very sensitive detection of SNVs in NGS data, but these tools require high coverage depth for acceptable performance and rely on spiked in control samples used to calibrate run-dependent error models [37], features that must be accounted for in assay design. The published comparative performance of the various bioinformatics tools for SNV detection provides some guidance to clinical laboratories for design and implementation of NGS assays for somatic mutations [37, 65].

A number of on-line tools can be used to predict the impact of a SNV and evaluate whether a SNV has a documented disease association. However, given the lack of standardized annotation formats, and variability in the level of review that was performed to establish the associations between a specific genotype and a specific phenotype, putative associations must be carefully reviewed in the context of the published medical literature.

Insertions and Deletions

By definition, indels are an insertion and/or deletion of one or more nucleotides into genomic DNA and include events less than 1 kb in length, although most indels are only several bp to several dozen base pair (bp) in length. Of note, many indels are not necessarily the direct result of DNA damage, per se, but instead originate from DNA polymerase errors or incorrect DNA repair following a genomic insult. As a result, indels may be complex (e.g., include both inserted and deleted bases) and often involve areas with repetitive sequences, factors that can make identification difficult. Indels can have widely variable consequences, including altered gene transcription, altered RNA splicing, in frame mutations (synonymous, missense, and nonsense mutations), frameshift mutations (that can be silent, or result in production of a protein with altered structure and function), and change the length of repetitive regions which can lead to the clinical phenomenon known as anticipation (more severe and earlier onset disease with each generation).

Indel detection is very important in clinical NGS of cancer specimens since indels are implicated as the driving mechanism for many oncologic diseases. Additionally, indels are a common mechanism of kinase activation in cancer, a feature exploited clinically by targeted therapy with kinase inhibitors. While the sequencing techniques and bioinformatics tools used for NGS analysis both influence the sensitivity and specificity of indel detection, several specific factors inherent to indels as a mutation class also complicate their detection, including size, DNA sequence context (including the fact that indels commonly occur in repetitive DNA sequences), and variant annotation. The bioinformatics tools optimized for detection of SNVs or other classes of mutation are not optimized to detect indels, and therefore specific tools for indel detection are required.

Since alignment of indel-containing sequence reads is technically challenging, significant improvement in bioinformatics detection of indels can be achieved simply by using algorithms specifically designed for the task. One such specialized approach is called local realignment, which essentially tweaks the local alignment of bases within each mapped read so as to minimize the number of base mismatches [66].

Probabilistic modeling based on mapped sequence reads can be used to identify indels that are up to approximately 15 % the length of an individual sequence read, but not longer. This level of sensitivity is suitable for the detection of many clinically relevant indels like *EGFR* exon 19 activating indels. However, probabilistic methods do not provide an acceptable sensitivity for detection of other insertions such as *FLT3* internal tandem duplications (ITDs) that range from 15 bp to over 300 bp in length [67], the presence of which is used clinically to predict prognosis and guide treatment in patients with cytogenetically normal AML [68].

Split-read analysis approaches to indel detection utilize algorithms that focus on split and soft-clipped reads (sometimes called one-end anchored reads) to identify possible breakpoints in NGS sequence data. The reads can either be analyzed using a pattern-growth algorithm whereby unmapped reads are broken into smaller pieces and realigned separately to identify possible indels, and/or by de novo assembly whereby unmapped reads are reassembled into a contiguous sequence (contig) based on their overlaps with each other [67, 69]. Importantly, evaluation of split and soft-clipped reads allows for the identification of the full size spectrum of indels, and the approach is not subject to the same read length constraints as probabilistic methods [67].

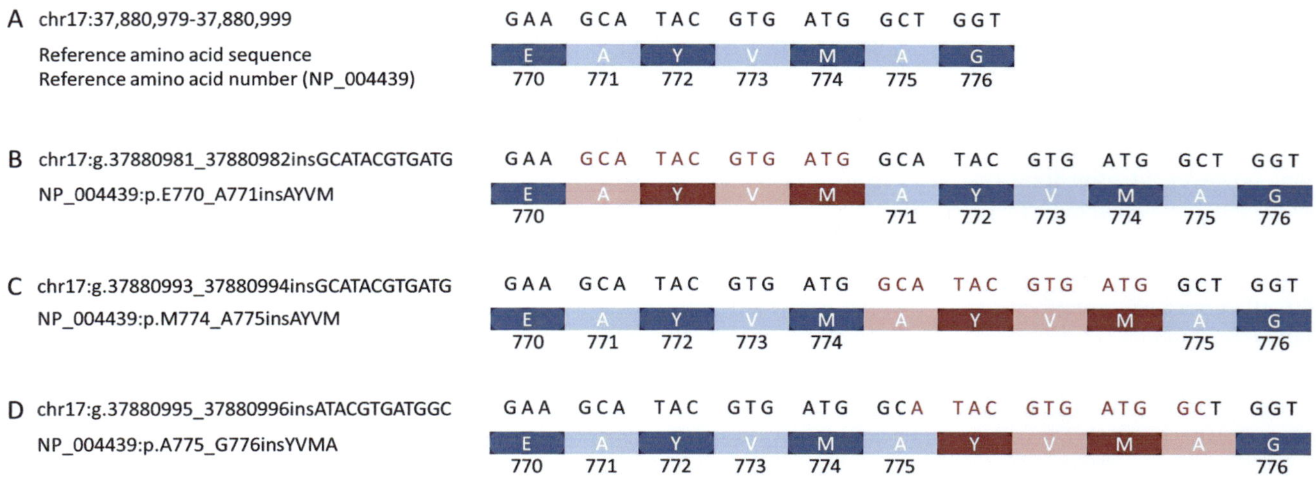

Figure 60.4 Redundant annotations for indels. The most common activating *ERBB2* indel in lung cancer results from duplication of 12 nucleotides in exon 20, resulting in insertion of four amino acids in the protein sequence, but can be annotated in multiple ways. The reference genomic nucleotide sequence and resulting amino acid sequence at the beginning of exon 20, with amino acid numbering according to the NP_00439 isoform of the ERBB2/HER2 protein, are shown (**a**). Three possible annotations for the activating *ERBB2* indel are shown (**b, c,** and **d**; inserted nucleotides and amino acids shown in *red*, reference shown in *blue*). In (**b** and **c**), the inserted nucleotide sequence is the same (GCATACGTGATG), but the site of insertion is different. In (**b**), the insertion is made at the beginning of the reference AYVM sequence, with the genomic annotation chr17:g.37880981_377880982ins12 and protein annotation NP_004439:p.E770_A771insAYVM. In (**c**), the insertion is made after the reference AYVM sequence, shifting the indel annotations to chr17:g.37880993_37880994ins12 and NP_004439:p.M774_A775insAYVM. However, the resulting nucleotide and amino acid sequences are exactly the same in (**b**) and (**c**). However, the same insertion also can be annotated with what seems to be a completely different inserted sequence (**d**). Note that the amino acid before and after the reference YVM is an alanine. However, the reference A771 is encoded by the genomic sequence GCA, whereas the reference A775 is encoded by the genomic sequence GCT. Insertion of the sequence ATACGTGATGGC, splitting the GC and T that normally encode A775 (i.e., genomic annotation chr17:g.37880995_37880996insATACGTGATGGC) keeps an A at amino acid number 775 (though now encoded by GCA instead of the reference GCT). The inserted nucleotides result in insertion of amino acids YVMA between reference amino acid positions 775 and 776 (i.e., protein annotation NP_00439:p.A775_G776insYVMA). The inserted A (just prior to G776) is derived from the last two inserted nucleotides (GC) and the T that was split off from what was originally A775. Although at first glance the various annotations listed in parts (**b**), (**c**), and (**d**) seem different, all result in the same final nucleotide and amino acid sequence. Of note, none of these possible annotations is technically correct based on the Human Genome Variation Society recommendations for mutation nomenclature [144], in which the variant is most appropriately annotated as a duplication (dup): chr17:g.378800982_37880993dup and NP_004439:p.A771_M774dup. Reprinted by permission from Elsevier Inc., *Clinical Genomics: A guide to clinical next generation sequencing.* Kulkarni S and Pfeifer J, Eds.

Indel Annotation

A major issue with clinical indel detection is annotation (i.e., how the size, composition, and genomic location of the indel is written). As discussed above, indels often occur in repetitive sequences, and thus multiple possible annotations can describe the same resulting sequence (see Fig. 60.4). Left-alignment prior to indel calling can decrease this problem by combining the multiple possible annotations into a single left-aligned annotation [66]. Importantly, left-alignment does not necessarily facilitate comparison of the identified indel to existing databases and literature in which indels are often not annotated in left-aligned format. In fact, left-alignment may preclude correlation of a potentially relevant indel with existing databases during interpretation.

Reference Standards

Since highly optimized indel detection by NGS is relatively new, gold standards for detection and annotation are not yet established. However, the lack of consensus indel calls across various technical approaches and variant annotations make establishing a reference standard difficult. Efforts to develop indel standards are underway, which will markedly increase the ease and clinical utility of clinical NGS testing results [70], but until these efforts are complete, it will be difficult to assess the sensitivity and specificity of clinical NGS assays for indel detection.

Copy Number Variations

CNV refers to structural changes resulting in gain or loss of genomic DNA in a chromosomal region. Individual CNVs may be inherited in the germline, or acquired as somatic mutations as in cancer genomes, such as *MYCN* gene amplification in neuroblastoma. Unlike SNVs, CNVs vary greatly in size and structure, ranging from thousands (by most definitions, CNVs are at least 1 kb long) to millions of nucleotides in length, and often involve complex

DNA rearrangements. While less common than SNVs, CNVs account for the majority of nucleotide differences between any two genomes because of the large size of individual CNVs [71].

NGS provides a comprehensive method for CNV screening; however, identification of CNVs from the short read sequence data generated by current NGS platforms presents significant bioinformatics challenges for both amplification and hybrid capture methods. As discussed in detail in Chap. 59, all current NGS platforms generate relatively short individual read sequences; the individual reads are combined via alignment to a reference genome to identify variants. However, detection of CNVs is conceptually different from identification of SNVs or indels since the individual sequence reads arising from CNVs often do not have sequence changes at the base pair (bp) level. Instead, the reads from within a region of a CNV are simply underrepresented or overrepresented in the collection of individual sequence reads when a deletion or amplification has occurred, respectively. Thus, the bioinformatics approaches to CNV identification rely on detection of an altered number of reads from a particular genetic region, or detection of sequence changes at the margins of the deletion or amplification, or both.

Relative Depth of Coverage

Since a diploid human genome contains two copies of the majority of genomic regions in every cell, a CNV results in a proportional change in the relative DNA content within the region encompassed by the CNV. Assuming deep enough sequencing coverage, the relative change in DNA content will be reflected in the number of reads mapping within the region of the CNV. The relative depth of coverage for a region must be interpreted with respect to an external baseline reference, which is generally accomplished by normalization to the "average" read depth across the same sample [72–74].

SNP Allele Frequency

Analysis of allele frequency at commonly occurring SNVs can be a useful indicator of CNVs or loss of heterozygosity (LOH) in NGS data [75]. Since single SNVs are often not informative for the presence of CNVs or LOH, the analysis usually combines information from multiple SNPs within the CNV region. An amplified CNV region will contain a shift of the allelic ratio away from 50:50 for heterozygous SNVs, with a predominance of the amplified allele nucleotide. For LOH, all SNVs in the region will be homozygous for the retained allele nucleotide, with a loss of any heterozygous SNVs. SNV allele frequency results can provide complementary information to more sensitive methods such as depth of coverage.

Discordant Mate Pair Methods

Mate pair libraries refer to sequence generated from the ends of DNA fragments in the range of 2–5 kb long. Since current NGS platforms only generate sequence reads up to several hundred bp long, only the ends of the DNA fragments are sequenced, generating what are termed paired ends [76, 77]. The paired ends are mapped back to the reference genome using standard alignment algorithms, and the distance between mapped reads is considered proportional to the length of sequence contained in the original fragment. While mate pair mapping can be used to improve variant detection for several classes of mutations, including CNVs, it is most useful for detecting structural variants. Those paired ends that map with an intervening distance significantly greater or less than predicted by the fragment size are referred to as discordant, and the presence of discordant reads indicates the presence of a structural variant.

Split Read Mapping

Direct evidence of a CNV can be obtained from the sequences of DNA fragments that overlap the breakpoints of the CNV. These reads in the presence of a CNV or SV are referred to as split reads, and can be used to anchor the breakpoints of a CNV [78, 79]. Split read mapping allows identification of the precise genomic coordinates of a CNV, to the resolution of single nucleotides. Split read mapping requires sequence reads that are long enough to permit partial read alignment on both sides of the breakpoint, a technical issue that has been largely resolved by the longer read lengths offered by current NGS platforms.

Structural Variants

Identification of structural variants (SVs), including translocations and other chromosomal rearrangements, is critically important in the analysis of cancer specimens for diagnosis, to predict prognosis, and to direct therapy, for both hematologic malignancies and solid tumors. In the clinical laboratory, detection of rearrangements is typically performed by routine cytogenetics or interphase/metaphase fluorescence in-situ hybridization (FISH), but NGS methods also are capable of detecting SVs with high sensitivity and specificity, and offer several advantages over conventional methods such as FISH and cytogenetics. For example, in the case of *MLL* rearrangements characteristic of acute leukemia, where over 100 known fusion partners have been identified, NGS testing has the potential to identify all known and unknown partner genes, while similar testing by fusion FISH probes would be cost prohibitive. Similarly, translocation identification by NGS allows for single base resolution of the chromosomal breakpoints, which allows for the identification of noncanonical breakpoints that may not respond to chemotherapy. At best, FISH and conventional cytogenetics can only localize breakpoints within 100–300 kb.

Genome sequencing is an unbiased approach for the identification of SVs similar to conventional cytogenetics. In theory, all rearrangements can be detected by genome sequencing as the sequence data cover both introns and exons, but in routine clinical practice genome sequencing is not practical for identification of rearrangements due to the high cost. SVs also can be detected using hybrid capture exome sequencing; however, intronic regions, where rearrangements are known to occur, must be directly targeted, and therefore the use of exome capture reagents in general will not identify SVs and custom capture panels that include intronic probes are required. NGS of RNA (known as RNAseq, which can be performed on the transcriptome or limited to specific targeted regions via hybrid capture-based approaches) can be used to identify SVs [80, 81], but obviously is limited to those settings in which the rearrangement produces a chimeric fusion transcript. Amplification NGS methods require a priori knowledge of the SV architecture and exact breakpoints so that appropriate primers can be used; since this information is rarely known in advance, amplification NGS approaches have very limited utility for SV detection from DNA.

SV detection in NGS methods is challenging but possible. The challenges arise from the mechanisms by which SVs are generated. The breakpoints for interchromosomal and intrachromosomal rearrangements most often are located in noncoding (e.g., intronic or intergenic) DNA sequences, often in highly repetitive regions, and therefore are difficult both to capture and to map to the reference genome. In addition, SV breakpoints often contain superimposed sequence variation ranging from small indels to fragments from several chromosomes [82, 83]. NGS sequence reads spanning complex rearrangements with multiple contributing chromosomes are difficult to map to the reference genome because only small DNA sequences (in general only tens of bases long) map to each of the contributing chromosomes [84].

Bioinformatics Approaches to SV Detection

Numerous software tools are available for SV detection which utilize the orientation, spacing, and depth of mapped NGS sequence reads. Most algorithms rely on discordant mate pairs and split reads, with a few also considering read depth. When implementing NGS for translocation detection, multiple tools should be evaluated to determine which one has optimal performance characteristics for the particular assay under consideration, since, depending on the design of capture probes and specific sequence of the target regions, different translocation detection tools may have large differences in sensitivity or specificity.

As noted above, discordant mate pair reads are paired-end reads that do not map to the reference genome as expected, and split reads are single end reads that map to the genome discontinuously. In the setting of SV detection, paired-end reads that map to different chromosomes, to the same chromosome but in the incorrect orientation, or in the proper orientation but too far apart or too close together can be used to detect genomic rearrangements. Because bioinformatics approaches based on discordant mate pair reads alone are subject to a high false-positive rate, some algorithms for SV detection make use of split reads. Similarly, due to the short read lengths currently available from NGS data, bioinformatics analysis of split reads for the detection of SVs is most reliable when evaluated in concert with paired-end data, since the position of the split read can be determined with higher confidence when its mate can be uniquely mapped to the genome, serving as an anchor. Depending on the choice of mapping software, "soft-clipped" reads may serve to indicate the presence of split reads (soft clips are produced by some alignment software when one member of a mate pair can be uniquely mapped to the genome but its mate cannot; if the mate can be partially aligned, in the correct orientation and with an insert size within the expected range, the unmapped remainder of the sequence is considered to be "soft-clipped") [85]. Soft-clipped reads often can be used to provide single base accuracy for the localization of rearrangements [86, 87], a significant advantage in that such precise localization of gene rearrangement breakpoints facilitates orthogonal validation by PCR.

Orthogonal Validation

As with any laboratory test, clinical NGS tests to detect sequence variants in cancer specimens require confirmation of test results by orthogonal methods during assay development and validation [7–9, 14, 16, 17, 88, 89], as well as to confirm unexpected or puzzling results that arise in routine clinical use. Test validation in general includes three steps, namely establishment of the analytic sensitivity and specificity of the test, definition of the range of detectable mutations and the limits of detection of the assay, and demonstration of detection of variants in cancers which are known to have the mutation. Given that the bioinformatics associated with base calling, reference genome alignment, and variant identification, annotation, and interpretation are such a key component of an NGS test, the bioinformatics methods must be validated as a part of overall test validation.

While each orthogonal validation method has advantages and disadvantages, several issues are common to all methods in the setting of NGS tests of tumor specimens. First, although the lower limit of sensitivity of optimized conventional approaches is similar to that of routine NGS tests for SNVs, enhanced NGS bioinformatics analysis methods enable detection of variants present at a frequency of < 1 %, a level of sensitivity significantly better than can be achieved by conventional techniques. Second, some of the discrepancies between SNVs detected by NGS assays and an orthogonal validation method may actually represent tissue heterogeneity and/or intratumoral heterogeneity rather than technical errors. Third, orthogonal validation used as confirmatory testing of positive results but not of negative results can raise the issue of discrepant analysis (also known as discordant analysis or review bias) that may poorly estimate test performance [90–92]. This last issue is especially problematic since some current guidelines recommend the use of confirmatory testing for positive results [93–95] without associated testing of negative results (i.e., wild type results).

Conventional orthogonal validation approaches that have been used to confirm SNVs in NGS test results include Sanger sequencing, restriction fragment length polymorphism (RFLP) analysis, allele specific PCR, and SNP arrays. Similar approaches are well suited to confirm the presence of indels identified by NGS. Common technologies used for orthogonal CNV validation are quantitative real-time PCR (qPCR), interphase FISH, and array-based comparative genomic hybridization. The optimal choice depends on the size and scope of CNVs being validated. Classical cytogenetics, metaphase FISH, and interphase FISH are commonly used to confirm the presence of SVs identified by NGS.

Annotation

Use of NGS for clinical testing of cancer specimens is a paradigm shift that has profound implications for variant annotation. Unlike focused testing for genes with well-established clinical correlations, NGS involves analysis of numerous genes for which the spectrum of variation has not been well characterized and for which often only limited evidence is available for a disease association. Essentially, many of the evidence gathering and analysis activities traditionally performed for diagnosis, prognosis, or prediction of response to therapy have migrated from their classical position prior to testing (in the clinic), to a position where they follow the testing (interpretation of test results). This poses challenges to interpretation of whether the variant has a plausible contribution to the cancer phenotype (whether for diagnosis, prognosis, or response to a specific therapy). The annotation of the clinical significance of an identified sequence variant is therefore often a difficult and time-consuming process of gathering and interpreting the relevant scientific and medical evidence. The major factors that complicate annotation of sequence variants include the lack of clinical standards for interpreting primary NGS results, inconsistencies in reporting clinical variants in commonly used file formats, and a lack of systematized communication among clinical (and research) laboratories and the scientific literature.

Fortunately, an increasing number of resources are being created to support the task of interpretation of variants identified by NGS. First, common variants not associated with disease must be filtered out. Large-scale efforts such as HapMap and the 1000 Genomes Project that characterize genetic variation in diverse population groups support assessments of the frequency of human variation; ClinVar, dbSNP, and Variation Viewer support searching and filtering functions related to allele frequencies, and dbSNP provides files of common variants not known to be disease-related. Then, the disease associations of the variant must be considered. Many centralized reference databases, such as those at NCBI, are designed for representing relationships between variants and phenotypes; for example, dbGaP is a catalog of variation–disease associations, ClinVar supports clinical interpretation of variants, and MedGen harmonizes phenotype terminologies and supports computational access to phenotype data.

It is important to recognize that the assessment of pathogenicity reported by many databases is not determined by the database itself, but instead reflects what is submitted. For example sources of data in ClinVar include genetic testing laboratories, semiautomatic data flows from OMIM and GeneReviews, locus-specific databases, research studies, and community projects [96]. The annotation of sequence variations also hinges on standardized classification systems [97–99]; however, for most genes, reliable functional assessments are not possible due to insufficient classification methods. Currently, the clinical significance of pathogenicity is performed using tiered levels ranging from benign to uncertain significance to pathogenic (see reporting section below).

One particularly useful resource under development is the Clinical Genome Resource (ClinGen), an NIH-funded program envisioned to become a centralized resource of clinically annotated genes and variants to improve the understanding of genomic variation. Data are to be collected from numerous clinical and research testing results. Expert curation efforts and development of standards will help standardize clinical assessment of variants in the ClinVar database, develop a consensus process for identifying clinically relevant variants, develop machine learning algorithms to improve accuracy and throughput for variant interpretation, and disseminate and explore integration with electronic health records.

Variants of Unknown Significance

The issues associated with annotation of variants are so important because, even with gene panels, exome, or genome NGS tests optimized for clinically relevant sensitivity and specificity, the majority of variants identified currently fall into the category of VUSs. By definition, for a VUS, insufficient existing evidence exists to support a definitive annotation regarding the effect of the variant on protein function, cell function, tumor behavior, and/or response to treatment. VUSs are particularly abundant in the sequence of tumor specimens due to the intrinsic genetic instability of most malignancies.

Several general categories of VUSs are defined. A sequence change affecting the coding region of a well-established gene in a particular tumor type, but not following the pattern of somatic mutation typical for that gene, would be a VUS. For example, constitutive activation of ABL1 in myeloid neoplasms typically occurs via translocation with a resulting BCR-ABL fusion protein kinase [100, 101]; however, a novel nonsynonymous SNV in *ABL1* would be a VUS since its effect on ABL1 kinase function cannot be extrapolated from literature about BCR-ABL activity or response to targeted kinase inhibition. Another category of VUSs is previously undescribed variants occurring in DNA sequences that do not encode amino acids, including splice sites and regulatory regions (promoters, enhancers, UTRs), or even more broadly acting regulatory elements like microRNAs or long noncoding RNAs. As examples, variants in the splice acceptor site may result in exon skipping, which may or may not have a significant impact on the protein's function [20], and variants occurring in regulatory regions can have unanticipated and widespread consequences in terms of gene expression or cell function.

A number of different statistical approaches can be applied to predict the likely impact of a nonsynonymous mutation on the function of a gene product. Some widely used prediction algorithms (e.g., SIFT, PROVEAN, PolyPhen) rely on evolutionary conservation of a particular base or amino acid, frequency of a given variant in the normal population, and/or location of a variant within the protein structure to determine whether an identified variant is likely to alter the function of a gene [102–106], although predicting the effect of a mutation on protein function is rarely straightforward [107]. Other approaches cluster somatically mutated genes by the functional pathways in which they are involved, usually in the setting of exome or genome analysis of cancer samples [108–111]; this pathway analysis approach facilitates understanding of shared biological implications of VUSs occurring in otherwise seemingly unrelated genes. Driver mutation analysis is an approach focused on identification of the variants in genes important for tumor growth, survival, or metastasis, as opposed to the passenger variants in genes that merely represent collateral damage in genetically unstable tumor cells [112]. Finally, clonal architecture analysis seeks to glean information about VUSs based on recognition of the rich clonal genetic diversity present in many morphologically homogenous tumors; for example, exome and genome sequencing studies of AML samples both at initial diagnosis and relapse have clearly shown that environmental selective pressures (e.g., the administration of chemotherapy) cause expansion or development of tumor clones with a relatively limited repertoire of escape mutations [113].

All these approaches for assigning functional significance to VUSs in a clinical setting must be viewed with caution. Even rational criteria such as biological plausibility should not stand alone, since identification of a novel variant in a known disease-associated gene, with a predicted functional impact similar to other disease-associated mutations in that gene, or in a pathway with other disease-associated genes, typically does not constitute sufficient evidence of causality. A false-positive assignment of a VUS as pathogenic can have profound clinical consequences including misdiagnosis, inappropriate care (including the delivery of radiation therapy and/or chemotherapy, both of which carry potentially very harmful side effects), and cessation of further testing that may uncover the true genetic features of the tumor.

Postanalytic Issues and Reporting

As discussed in detail in Chap. 59, professional organizations have recommended specific guidelines for reporting constitutional variants; for ease of interpretation, most clinical laboratories classify variants identified in constitutional testing into five categories, as follows: (1) pathogenic, (2) likely pathogenic, (3) uncertain significance, (4) likely benign, and (5) benign [114, 115]. This five-level classification scheme has recently been proposed as the standard for interpretation of variants in inherited disorders through a joint recommendation of the American College of Medical Genetics and Genomics (ACMG) and the Association of Molecular Pathology (AMP) and is expected to be formally adopted following member comment and organizational approval.

In contrast, no consensus guidelines have been published for reporting somatic or acquired variants, although several work groups are currently addressing this issue. Most laboratories currently classify sequence variations with regard to the disease and in relation to the actionability of the given variant with respect to prognosis, diagnosis, or therapeutic selection using the same five categories as for reporting constitutional variants [7]. Since predicted responsiveness to targeted therapy is often the primary reason for NGS testing in the cancer setting, variants expected to be sensitive or resistant to a given therapy should be documented; driver and passenger variants should be reported even in the absence of a direct role in choice of therapy. When a variant is identified that is known to be associated with a familial cancer predisposition syndrome (and when paired tumor-normal analysis is not performed), formal genetic counseling and germline analysis should be recommended in the report since it can be difficult to ascertain the etiology of a given variant as germline or somatic based on the VAF from NGS analysis of a tumor sample alone.

Quality Management and Other Regulatory Issues

NGS is subject to the same regulatory standards as other clinical molecular tests, and, like other laboratory tests, has a test cycle that includes a preanalytic phase, an analytic phase, and a postanalytic phase. However, the fact that the analytic portion of a NGS test consists of three components (i.e., the sequence platform; the laboratory procedures that are involved in DNA sequence generation; and the bioinformatics associated with base calling, reference genome alignment, variant identification, variant annotation, and variant interpretation) creates some unique quality management issues [88]. Because NGS is a relatively new type of DNA sequence analysis, different laboratories have developed different models for the associated quality control and quality assurance activities to meet appropriate regulatory guidelines and best practice standards, although the methods most useful in routine clinical testing have not been established. The more general aspects of a quality management system are covered in Chap. 62; the focus here is on those aspects unique to NGS testing of tumors.

Preanalytic Issues

The preanalytic phase of testing is traditionally the most difficult aspect of quality management since most of the preanalytic variables that impact laboratory testing are outside traditional laboratory boundaries. Because of the many unique aspects of NGS testing, the situation is even more complex for the analysis of tumor tissue. The first factor is time of specimen fixation, and the specific fixative used. Although, as discussed above, FFPE tissue is an acceptable substrate for NGS testing, the chemical changes in DNA that result from formalin fixation affect the quantity of intact DNA that can be recovered from tissue, and can have very subtle impacts on the actual sequence itself because of deamination reactions that result from formalin exposure; these changes become more significant the longer the period of exposure to formalin. Also, ethanol and methanol fixation (e.g., cytology specimens) create subtle differences in the quantity of nucleic acids that can be recovered.

Specimen size is the second important preanalytic factor. Most amplification-based NGS approaches require a minimum DNA input in the range of 10 ng. While hybrid capture methods have been described that utilize as little as 10 ng of DNA, concerns about library complexity lead most clinical laboratories to require 100–200 ng of DNA as a minimum for hybrid capture NGS testing.

Third, the tissue sample must be appropriate. In the setting of oncology testing, this variable is far more nuanced than the simple requirement that the tissue contains high neoplastic cellularity and viability. Questions occur regarding the most appropriate site to sample in a patient with recurrent disease. Given that clonal heterogeneity is often present within the primary tumor, and that tissue metastases often represent divergent tumor clones [53, 54, 116], the tumor site sampled can have a profound effect on test results, and potentially patient care.

Fourth, in patients who have had an allogeneic bone marrow transplant, it can be difficult to collect tissue with sufficient levels of the patient's tumor cells to allow for the detection and interpretation of variants present at low allele frequencies.

Analytic Issues

Most laboratory tests involve the measurement of continuous variables, and consequently measures of test calibration, analytic variability, and other performance measures required for assay validation usually rely on statistical methods. For example, sophisticated QC approaches based on the Gaussian (normal) distribution have been developed to detect imprecision or systematic bias [117], and Levey-Jennings plots are used to detect variability that cannot be explained by a Gaussian distribution [118, 119]. However, DNA sequencing requires fundamentally different QC approaches to evaluate the integrity of the test results because DNA sequence is a discontinuous, nominal variable [120]. For NGS tests, an estimate of the probability of correctness may be substituted for a quantitative estimate of uncertainty, and several methods have been proposed to address this issue [66, 121–123].

Proficiency Testing

The Clinical Laboratory Improvement Amendments of 1988 (CLIA) regulations mandates proficiency testing (PT) for external quality assessment (EQA) as part of the laboratory accreditation process [124–126], although the precise rules and regulations that govern proficiency testing continue to evolve. Numerous organizations are accredited by CLIA to provide PT programs, but NGS testing of cancer specimens has many analytes for which EQA surveys are not available, and in this setting, laboratories must implement alternative PT assessment procedures. These alternative assessment procedures include split sample analysis with other laboratories, assessment of split samples with an established method in the laboratory using previously assayed material, blinded exchange of samples with another laboratory, retesting of de-identified patient samples, analysis of DNA from cell lines with previously determined genotypes, or analysis of synthetic DNA of known genotype [127, 128].

Many PT programs are based on an individual analyte, and are appropriately termed analyte-specific or disease-specific PT programs. The utility of disease-specific approaches for DNA analysis has been well documented [129–131]; however, given the number of genes and range of mutations that are routinely evaluated by NGS tests, clinical laboratories cannot follow an analyte-specific PT approach. For this reason, methods-based proficiency testing (MBPT) paradigms have been developed which are centered on the method of analysis rather than the specific analyte being tested [126, 132]. The Centers for Medicare and Medicaid Services (CMS) that oversees the CLIA inspection and accreditation process understands that analyte-specific PT is not possible for the many different mutations that can occur in the many different genes that are analyzed by NGS tests, and therefore supports the concept of MBPT.

MBPT has some distinct advantages for PT of NGS tests. First, MBPT is scalable in that comparisons are possible between laboratories testing for dozens (if not hundreds or thousands) of different genes. MBPT also allows evaluation of proficiency in detection of a wide range of variants, rather than one specific mutation type. Laboratories that participate in MBPT challenges are not penalized for an inability to detect a sequence variant that lies in a region outside the scope of their validated test, or types of sequence variants that are not validated for their NGS test. However, at present, MBPT cannot be used for PT when developed internally by an individual laboratory; MBPT is only acceptable when administered by an external PT provider.

While the emphasis to date has been on comprehensive PT assessments that evaluate all three aspects of an NGS test (the sequence platform, the wet bench procedures involved in DNA sequence data generation, and the bioinformatics associated with variant identification), a novel type of PT termed in silico PT has recently been developed to specifically address the bioinformatics component of NGS tests [126, 128]. In silico PT is a response to the fact that clinical NGS bioinformatics methods are not standardized across laboratories, and thus bioinformatics analysis of NGS sequence reads is a major source of variability between laboratories performing an NGS test on the same nucleic acid sequence. For in silico PT, sequence files from an NGS test are manipulated by computerized algorithms that introduce relevant sequence variants [133]. The resulting in silico data files (also referred to as simulated data files) mimic the complexity of clinical samples and thus are ideal for MBPT for several reasons. First, they challenge every step in the bioinformatics analysis from alignment through variant detection, annotation, and interpretation. Second, simulated data files can include all four major classes of variants, either alone or in combination, for any set of genetic loci. Third, the variant allele frequency can be manipulated to test the sensitivity and specificity of variant detection.

FDA Oversight

In the USA, the US Food and Drug Administration (FDA) regulates the manufacture of equipment, devices, and assay reagent kits used in clinical testing (which in the context of NGS includes the sequencing instruments, the kits used for DNA extraction, library preparation, and specific tests) and the bioinformatics methods to analyze the sequence data [134–136]. The US FDA defines tests that are developed and used within the same clinical laboratory, and that are not provided to other clinical laboratories, as laboratory developed tests (LDTs). In addition, the laboratory that develops an LDT must inform the medical professional who requested the test, in a statement appended to the test report, that, "This test was developed and its performance characteristics determined by {Name of the Laboratory}. It has not been cleared or approved by the US Food and Drug Administration" [137]. Because the number of US FDA cleared or approved NGS platforms, tests, and bioinformatics tools is currently very small, virtually all current clinical NGS assays are LDTs.

In 2010 the US FDA announced its intention to begin oversight of LDTs, and in response professional societies have proposed regulations to help guide FDA into best methods for ensuring appropriate oversight and validation of clinical molecular procedures including NGS tests [138, 139]. As part of the continuing evolution of regulatory oversight of LDTs, the US FDA issued revised guidance in 2013 on the distribution of in vitro diagnostic products labeled for research use only or investigational use only [140]. In this context it is noteworthy that clinical NGS testing is emblematic of the regulatory issues surrounding many LDTs developed for genetic analysis of tumors in that the rapid pace of advancements in understanding the molecular basis of cancer is driving adoption of clinical testing, but the demand and pace of change for clinical testing is far outstripping the pace at which clinical laboratories and vendors can complete the regulatory requirements required for US FDA clearance or approval as an in vitro diagnostic.

Conclusions

The rapid pace of advancements in understanding the genetic basis of cancer is driving adoption of genetic testing of cancer tissue specimens for diagnosis, to provide prognostic information, and to guide therapy. NGS methods have been adopted for clinical testing because they provide rapid, accurate, and cost effective approaches for sequence analysis of the large genome regions that are increasingly used to stratify patients into different prognostic and treatment response groups. However, since NGS is a new method of sequence analysis that has only recently been introduced into clinical laboratories, sequencing platforms, techniques, assay designs, bioinformatics approaches, and regulatory paradigms are still evolving. In this changing regulatory environment, different laboratories have developed different quality management systems to ensure that NGS tests are performed to the same rigorous standards as more conventional clinical tests that focus on the analysis of nucleic acids, such as DNA sequence analysis by Sanger sequencing, microarray analysis, conventional cytogenetics, and metaphase or interphase FISH.

References

1. Sehn JK, Hagemann IS, Pfeifer JD, et al. Diagnostic utility of targeted next-generation sequencing in problematic cases. Am J Surg Pathol. 2014;38:534–41.
2. Lynch TJ, Bell DW, Sordella R, et al. Activating mutations in the epidermal growth factor receptor underlying responsiveness of non-small-cell lung cancer to Gefitinib. N Engl J Med. 2004; 350:2129–39.
3. Camidge DR, Bang YJ, Kwak EL, et al. Activity and safety of crizotinib in patients with ALK-positive non-small-cell lung cancer: updated results from a phase 1 study. Lancet Oncol. 2012;13: 1011–9.
4. Bergethon K, Shaw AT, Ou SH, et al. ROS1 rearrangements define a unique molecular class of lung cancers. J Clin Oncol. 2012;30: 863–70.
5. Campos-Parra AD, Zuloaga C, Manriquez ME, et al. KRAS mutation as the biomarker of response to chemotherapy and EGFR-TKIs in patients with advanced Non-small cell lung cancer: clues for its potential Use in second-line therapy decision making. Am J Clin Oncol. 2015;38:33–40.
6. Estey EH. Acute myeloid leukemia: (2013) update on risk-stratification and management. Am J Hematol. 2013;88:318–27.
7. Singh RR, Patel KP, Routbort MJ, et al. Clinical validation of a next-generation sequencing screen for mutational hotspots in 46 cancer-related genes. J Mol Diagn. 2014;15:607–22.
8. Simen BB, Yin L, Goswami CP, et al. Validation of a next-generation–sequencing cancer panel for Use in the clinical laboratory. Arch Pathol Lab Med. 2015;139(4):508–17.
9. Lin MT, Mosier SL, Tiess M, et al. Clinical validation of KRAS, BRAF, and EGFR mutation detection using next-generation sequencing. Am J Clin Pathol. 2014;141:856–66.
10. http://www.lifetechnologies.com
11. Ion AmpliSeq™ Exome Solution flyer, http://tools.invitrogen.com/content/sfs/brochures/Ion-AmpliSeq-Exome-Kit-Product-Flyer.pdf
12. http://www.illumina.com/applications/cancer/cancer-sequencing-methods/targeted-cancer-sequencing.html
13. http://www.genomics.agilent.com/en/NGS-Target-Enrichment/;jsessionid=V6dpJmZJVvr3yqNBMgvQc4vnQvLtWvhDnsWwdWLZPCQh5jpGYrwy!1469574312?pgid=AG-PG-11
14. Pritchard CC, Salipante SJ, Koehler K, et al. Validation and implementation of targeted capture and sequencing for the detection of actionable mutation, copy number variation, and gene rearrangement in clinical cancer specimens. J Mol Diagn. 2014;16:56–67.
15. Pritchard CC, Smith C, Salipante SJ, et al. ColoSeq provides comprehensive lynch and polyposis syndrome mutational analysis using massively parallel sequencing. J Mol Diagn. 2012;14:357–66.
16. Cottrell CE, Al-Kateb H, Bredemeyer AJ, et al. Validation of a next-generation sequencing assay for clinical molecular oncology. J Mol Diagn. 2014;16:89–105.
17. Frampton GM, Fichtenholtz A, Otto GA. Development and validation of a clinical cancer genomic profiling test based on massively parallel DNA sequencing. Nat Biotechnol. 2013;31:1023–3115.
18. http://foundationone.com/learn.php - 2.
19. Abecasis GR, Auton A, Brooks LD, et al. An integrated map of genetic variation from 1,092 human genomes. Nature. 2012;491: 56–65.
20. Strachan T, Read AP. Human genetic variability and its consequences, Human molecular genetics. 4th ed. New York: Garland Science; 2011. p. 405–40.
21. Govindan R, Ding L, Griffith M, et al. Genomic landscape of non-small cell lung cancer in smokers and never-smokers. Cell. 2012;150:1121–34.
22. Network CGAR. Comprehensive genomic characterization of squamous cell lung cancers. Nature. 2012;489:519–25.
23. Network CGAR. Integrated genomic analyses of ovarian carcinoma. Nature. 2011;474:609–15.
24. Network CGA. Comprehensive molecular characterization of human colon and rectal cancer. Nature. 2012;487:330–7.
25. Network CGAR. Comprehensive molecular characterization of clear cell renal cell carcinoma. Nature. 2013;499:43–9.
26. Kandoth C, McLellan MD, Vandin F, et al. Mutational landscape and significance across 12 major cancer types. Nature. 2013;502:333–9.
27. Imielinski M, Berger AH, Hammerman PS, et al. Mapping the hallmarks of lung adenocarcinoma with massively parallel sequencing. Cell. 2012;150:1107–20.
28. Network CGAR. Comprehensive genomic characterization defines human glioblastoma genes and core pathways. Nature. 2008;455:1061–8.
29. Network CGAR. Comprehensive molecular portraits of human breast tumours. Nature. 2012;490:61–70.
30. Marcus JN, Watson P, Page DL, et al. Hereditary breast cancer: pathobiology, prognosis, and BRCA1 and BRCA2 gene linkage. Cancer. 1996;77:697–709.
31. Malkin D, Li FP, Strong LC, et al. Germ line p53 mutations in a familial syndrome of breast cancer, sarcomas, and other neoplasms. Science. 1990;250:1233–8.
32. Nawy T. Single-cell sequencing. Nature Methods. 2014;11. doi:10.1038/nmeth.2771
33. Heitzer E, Auer M, Gasch C, et al. Complex tumor genomes inferred from single circulating tumor cells by array-CGH and next-generation sequencing. Cancer Res. 2013;73:2965–75.
34. Macaulay IC, Voet T. Single cell genomics: advances and future perspectives. PLoS Genet. 2014;10, e1004126. doi:10.1371/journal.pgen.1004126.
35. Clark MJ, Chen R, Lam HY, et al. Performance comparison of exome DNA sequencing technologies. Nat Biotechnol. 2011; 29:908–14.
36. Sims D, Sudbery I, Ilott NE. Sequencing depth and coverage: key considerations in genomic analyses. Nat Rev Genet. 2014;15: 121–32.
37. Spencer DH, Tyagi M, Vallania F, et al. Performance of common analysis methods for detecting low-frequency single nucleotide variants in targeted next-generation sequence data. J Mol Diagn. 2014;16:75–88.
38. Lohr JG, Stojanov P, Carter SL, et al. Widespread genetic heterogeneity in multiple myeloma: implications for targeted therapy. Cancer Cell. 2014;25:91–101.

39. Asan XY, Jiang H, Tyler-Smith C, et al. Comprehensive comparison of three commercial human whole-exome capture platforms. Genome Biol. 2011;12:R95.
40. Parla JS, Iossifov I, Grabill I, et al. A comparative analysis of exome capture. Genome Biol. 2011;12:R97.
41. Cui H, Li F, Chen D, et al. Comprehensive next-generation sequence analyses of the entire mitochondrial genome reveal new insights into the molecular diagnosis of mitochondrial DNA disorders. Genet Med. 2013;15:388–94.
42. Pfeifer JD. Molecular genetic testing in surgical pathology (Chapters 2 and 5). Philadelphia: Lippincott Williams & Wilkins; 2006. p. 29–57. 86-110.
43. Auerbach C, Moutschen-Dahmen M, Moutschen J. Genetic and cytogenetical effects of formaldehyde and related compounds. Mutat Res. 1977;39:317–61.
44. Bresters D, Schipper M, Reesink H, et al. The duration of fixation influences the yield of HCV cDNAPCR products from formalin-fixed, paraffin-embedded liver tissue. J Virol Methods. 1994;48: 267–72.
45. Feldman MY. Reactions of nucleic acids and nucleoproteins with formaldehyde. Prog Nucleic Acid Res Mol Biol. 1973;13:1–49.
46. Karlsen F, Kalantari M, Chitemerere M, et al. Modifications of human and viral deoxyribonucleic acid by formaldehyde fixation. Lab Invest. 1994;71:604–11.
47. Spencer DH, Sehn JK, Abel HJ, et al. Comparison of clinical targeted next-generation sequence data from formalin-fixed and fresh-frozen tissue specimens. J Mol Diagn. 2013;15:623–33.
48. Karnes H, Duncavage ED, Bernadt CT. Targeted next-generation sequencing using fine-needle aspirates from adenocarcinomas of the lung. Cancer Cytopathol. 2014;122:104–13.
49. Kanagal-Shamanna R, Portier BP, Singh RR, et al. Next-generation sequencing-based multi-gene mutation profiling of solid tumors using fine needle aspiration samples: promises and challenges for routine clinical diagnostics. Mod Pathol. 2013;27:314–27.
50. Williams NH. DNA hydrolysis: mechanism and reactivity. In: Zenkova MA, editor. Nucleic acids and molecular biology. Berlin: Springer-Verlag; 2004. p. 3–18.
51. Smits AJ, Kummer JA, de Bruin PC, et al. The estimation of tumor cell percentage for molecular testing by pathologists is not accurate. Mod Pathol. 2014;27:168–74.
52. Viray H, Li K, Long T, et al. A prospective, multi-institutional diagnostic trial to determine pathologist accuracy in estimation of percentage of malignant cells. Arch Pathol Lab Med. 2014; 137:1545–9.
53. Renovanz M, Kim EL. Intratumoral heterogeneity, its contribution to therapy resistance and methodological caveats to assessment. Front Oncol. 2014;4:142.
54. Gerlinger M, Rowan A, Horswell S, et al. Intratumor heterogeneity and branched evolution revealed by multiregion sequencing. N Engl J Med. 2012;366:883–92.
55. Wickham CL, Sarsfield P, Joyner MV, et al. Formic acid decalcification of bone marrow trephines degrades DNA: alternative use of EDTA allows the amplification and sequencing of relatively long PCR products. Mol Pathol. 2000;53:336.
56. Duncavage EJ, Abel HJ, Szankasi P, et al. Targeted next generation sequencing of clinically significant gene mutations and translocations in leukemia. Mod Pathol. 2012;25:795–804.
57. O'Rawe J, Jiang T, Sun G, Wu Y, et al. Low concordance of multiple variant-calling pipelines: practical implications for exome and genome sequencing. Genome Med. 2013;5:28.
58. Abecasis GR, Altshuler D, Auton A, et al. A map of human genome variation from population-scale sequencing. Nature. 2010;467:1061–73.
59. Mendell JT, Dietz HC. When the message goes awry: disease-producing mutations that influence mRNA content and performance. Cell. 2001;107:411–4.
60. Li X, Park WJ, Pyeritz RE, Jabs EW. Effect on splicing of a silent FGFR2 mutation in Crouzon syndrome. Nat Genet. 1995;9: 232–3.
61. Krawczak M, Reiss J, Cooper DN. The mutational spectrum of single base-pair substitutions in mRNA splice junctions of human genes: causes and consequences. Hum Genet. 1992;90:41–54.
62. Martin DI, Tsai SF, Orkin SH. Increased γ-globin expression in a nondeletion HPFH mediated by an erythroid-specific DNA-binding factor. Nature. 1989;338:435–8.
63. Miki Y, Swensen J, Shattuck-Eidens D, et al. A strong candidate for the breast and ovarian cancer susceptibility gene BRCA1. Science. 1994;266:66–71.
64. D'Arcangelo M, Cappuzzo F. K-ras mutations in non-small cell lung cancer: prognostic and predictive value. ISRN Mol Biol. 2012. doi:10.5402/2012/837306.
65. Vallania FL, Druley TE, Ramos E, et al. High-throughput discovery of rare insertions and deletions in large cohorts. Genome Res. 2010;20:1711–8.
66. DePristo MA, Banks E, Poplin R, et al. A framework for variation discovery and genotyping using next-generation DNA sequencing data. Nat Genet. 2011;43:491–8.
67. Spencer DH, Abel HJ, Lockwood CM, et al. Detection of FLT3 internal tandem duplication in targeted, short-read-length, next-generation sequencing data. J Mol Diagn. 2013;15:81–93.
68. Kottaridis PD, Gale RE, Frew ME, et al. The presence of a FLT3 internal tandem duplication in patients with acute myeloid leukemia AML) adds important prognostic information to cytogenetic risk group and response to the first cycle of chemotherapy: analysis of 854 patients from the United Kingdom Medical Research Council AML 10 and 12 trials. Blood. 2001;98:1752–9.
69. Koboldt DC, Zhang Q, Larson DE, et al. VarScan 2: somatic mutation and copy number alteration discovery in cancer by exome sequencing. Genome Res. 2012;22:568–76.
70. Lubin IM, Aziz N, Babb L, et al. The clinical next-generation sequencing variant file: advances, opportunities, and challenges for the clinical laboratory. Submitted
71. Conrad DF, Pinto D, Redon R, Feuk L, et al. Origins and functional impact of copy number variation in the human genome. Nature. 2010;464:704–12.
72. Krumm N, Sudmant PH, Ko A, et al. Copy number variation detection and genotyping from exome sequence data. Genome Res. 2012;22(8):1525–32.
73. Benjamini Y, Speed TP. Summarizing and correcting the GC content bias in high-throughput sequencing. Nucleic Acids Res. 2012;40, e72.
74. Amarasinghe KC, Li J, Halgamuge SK. CoNVEX: copy number variation estimation in exome sequencing data using HMM. BMC Bioinformatics. 2013;14 Suppl 2:S2.
75. Korn JM, Kuruvilla FG, McCarroll SA, et al. Integrated genotype calling and association analysis of SNPs, common copy number polymorphisms and rare CNVs. Nat Genet. 2008;40:1253–60.
76. Medvedev P, Fiume M, Dzamba M, et al. Detecting copy number variation with mated short reads. Genome Res. 2010;20:1613–22.
77. Murphy SJ, Cheville JC, Zarei S, et al. Mate pair sequencing of whole-genome-amplified DNA following laser capture microdissection of prostate cancer. DNA Res. 2012;19:395–406.
78. Chen K, Wallis JW, McLellan MD, et al. BreakDancer: an algorithm for high-resolution mapping of genomic structural variation. Nat Methods. 2009;6:677–81.
79. Wang K, Bucan M. Copy number variation detection via high-density SNP genotyping. Cold Spring Harb Protoc. 2008. doi:10.1101/pdb.top46.
80. Maher CA, Kumar-Sinha C, Cao X. Transcriptome sequencing to detect gene fusions in cancer. Nature. 2009;458:97–101.
81. Cabanski CR, Magrini V, Griffith OL. cDNA hybrid capture improves transcriptome analysis on low-input and archived samples. J Mol Diagn. 2014;16:440–51.

82. Nambiar M, Raghavan SC. How does DNA break during chromosomal translocations? Nucleic Acids Res. 2011;39:5813–25.
83. Roukos V, Misteli T. The biogenesis of chromosome translocations. Nat Cell Biol. 2014;16:293–300.
84. Abel HJ, Al-Kateb H, Cottrell CE, et al. Detection of gene rearrangements in targeted clinical next-generation sequencing. J Mol Diagn. 2014;16:405–17.
85. Li H, Durbin R. Fast and accurate long-read alignment with burrows-wheeler transform. Bioinformatics. 2010;26:589–95.
86. Wang J, Mullighan CG, Easton J, et al. Crest maps somatic structural variation in cancer genomes with base-pair resolution. Nat Methods. 2011;8:652–4.
87. Suzuki S, Yasuda T, Shiraishi Y, et al. Clipcrop: a tool for detecting structural variations with single-base resolution using soft-clipping information. BMC Bioinformatics. 2011;12 Suppl 14:S7.
88. Gargis AS, Kalman L, Berry MW, et al. Assuring the quality of next-generation sequencing in clinical laboratory practice. Nat Biotechnol. 2012;30:1033–6.
89. Rehm HL, Bale SJ, Bayrak-Toydemir P, et al. ACMG clinical laboratory standards for next-generation sequencing. Genet Med. 2013;15:733–47.
90. Lipman HB, Astles JR. Quantifying the bias associated with use of discrepant analysis. Clin Chem. 1998;44:108–15.
91. Hadgu A. Discrepant analysis is an inappropriate and unscientific method. J Clin Microbiol. 2000;38:4301–2.
92. Miller WC. Bias in discrepant analysis: when two wrongs don't make a right. J Clin Epidemiol. 1998;51:219–31.
93. CLSI. Molecular methods for clinical genetics and oncology testing; approved guideline, CLSI document MM01-A3. 3rd ed. Wayne: Clinical Laboratory Standards Institute; 2012.
94. American College of Medical Genetics. ACMG standards and guidelines for clinical genetic laboratories. 2008. http://www.acmg.net/AM/Template.cfm?Section=Laboratory_Standards_and_Guidelines&Template=/CM/HTML
95. NCCLS. Nucleic acid sequencing methods in diagnostic laboratory medicine; approved guideline. NCCLS 2004. document MM9-A [ISBN 1-56238-558-5]. NCCLS, 940 West Valley Road, Suite 1400, Wayne, Pennsylvania 19087-1898 USA.
96. http://www.ncbi.nlm.nih.gov/clinvar/docs/datasources/
97. Thompson BA, Spurdle AB, Plazzer JP, et al. Application of a 5-tiered scheme for standardized classification of 2,360 unique mismatch repair gene variants in the InSiGHT locus-specific database. Nat Genet. 2014;46:107–15.
98. Plon SE, Eccles DM, Easton D, et al. Sequence variant classification and reporting: recommendations for improving the interpretation of cancer susceptibility genetic test results. Hum Mutat. 2008;29:1282–91.
99. Greenblatt MS, Brody LC, Foulkes WD, et al. Locus-specific databases and recommendations to strengthen their contribution to the classification of variants in cancer susceptibility genes. Hum Mutat. 2008;29:1273–81.
100. Kantarjian H, Sawyers C, Hochhaus A, et al. Hematologic and cytogenetic responses to Imatinib mesylate in chronic myelogenous leukemia. N Engl J Med. 2002;346:645–52.
101. Melo JV. The diversity of BCR-ABL fusion proteins and their relationship to leukemia phenotype. Blood. 1996;88:2375–84.
102. Grantham R. Amino acid difference formula to help explain protein evolution. Science. 1974;185:862–4.
103. Davydov EV, Goode DL, Sirota M. Identifying a high fraction of the human genome to be under selective constraint using GERP++. PLoS Comput Biol. 2010;6:e1001025.
104. Kumar P, Henikoff S, Ng PC. Predicting the effects of coding non-synonymous variants on protein function using the SIFT algorithm. Nat Protoc. 2009;4:1073–81.
105. Choi Y, Sims GE, Murphy S. Predicting the functional effect of amino acid substitutions and indels. PLoS One. 2012;7, e46688.
106. Adzhubei IA, Schmidt S, Peshkin L, et al. A method and server for predicting damaging missense mutations. Nat Methods. 2010;7:248–9.
107. Tchernitchko D, Goossens M, Wajcman H. In silico prediction of the deleterious effect of a mutation: proceed with caution in clinical genetics. Clin Chem. 2004;50:1974–8.
108. Vaske CJ, Benz SC, Sanborn JZ, et al. Inference of patient-specific pathway activities from multi-dimensional cancer genomics data using PARADIGM. Bioinformatics. 2010;26:i237–45.
109. Wendl MC, Wallis JW, Lin L, et al. PathScan: a tool for discerning mutational significance in groups of putative cancer genes. Bioinformatics. 2011;27:1595–602.
110. Schaefer CF, Anthony K, Krupa S, et al. PID: the pathway interaction database. Nucleic Acids Res. 2009;37(Database issue): D674–9.
111. Kanehisa M, Goto S, Sato Y, Furumichi M, et al. KEGG for integration and interpretation of large-scale molecular data sets. Nucleic Acids Res. 2012;40(Database issue):D109–14.
112. Greenman C, Stephens P, Smith R, et al. Patterns of somatic mutation in human cancer genomes. Nature. 2007;446:153–8.
113. Ding L, Ley TJ, Larson DE, et al. Clonal evolution in relapsed acute myeloid leukaemia revealed by whole-genome sequencing. Nature. 2012;481:506–10.
114. Kearney H, Thorland E, Brown K, et al. American College of Medical Genetics standards and guidelines for interpretation and reporting of postnatal constitutional copy number variants. Genet Med. 2011;13:680–5.
115. Richards CS, Bale S, Bellissimo DB, et al. ACMG recommendations for standards for interpretation and reporting of sequence variations: Revisions 2007. Genet Med. 2008;10:294–300.
116. Yachida S, Jones S, Bozic I, et al. Distant metastasis occurs late during the genetic evolution of pancreatic cancer. Nature. 2010;467:1114–7.
117. Ryan TP. Statistical methods for quality control. New York: Wiley; 1989.
118. Levey S, Jennings ER. The use of control charts in the clinical laboratory. Am J Clin Pathol. 1950;20:1059–66.
119. Westgard JO, Barry PL, Hunt MR. A multi-rule Shewhart chart for quality control in clinical chemistry. Clin Chem. 1981;27:493–501.
120. Pyzdek T. What every engineer should know about quality control. New York: Marcel Dekker Inc.; 1989.
121. McKenna A, Hanna M, Banks E, et al. The genome analysis toolkit: a MapReduce framework for analyzing next-generation DNA sequencing data. Genome Res. 2010;20:1297–303.
122. Danecek P, Auton A, Abecasis G, et al. The variant call format and VCFtools. Bioinformatics. 2011;27:2156–8.
123. Ajay SS, Parker SCJ, Abaan HO, et al. Accurate and comprehensive sequencing of personal genomes. Genome Res. 2011;21: 1498–505.
124. Public Law 100-578 (1988) Clinical Laboratory Improvement Amendments of 1988. Stat 42 USC 201, HR 5471, October 31, 1988
125. US Department of Health and Human Services: Clinical Laboratory Improvement Amendments of 1988; Final Rules and Notice. 42 CFR Part 493. The Federal Register. 57;7188-288, 1992
126. Schrijver I, Aziz N, Jennings LJ, et al. Methods-based proficiency testing in molecular genetic pathology. J Mol Diagn. 2014;16: 283–7.
127. CLSI: Assessment of Laboratory Tests When Proficiency Testing Is Not Available; Approved Guideline, ed 2. CLSI document GP29–A2: Clinical and Laboratory Standards Institute, Wayne, PA 2008)
128. Kalman LV, Lubin IM, Barker S, et al. Current landscape and new paradigms of proficiency testing and external quality assessment for molecular genetics. Arch Pathol Lab Med. 2013; 137:983–8.

129. Palomaki GE, Richards CE. Assessing the analytic validity of molecular testing for Huntington disease using data from an external proficiency testing survey. Genet Med. 2012;14:69–75.
130. Weck KE, Zehnbauer B, Datto M, et al. Molecular genetic testing for fragile X syndrome: laboratory performance on the College of American Pathologists proficiency surveys 2001–2009. Genet Med. 2012;14:306–12.
131. Feldman GL, Schrijver I, Lyon E, et al. Results of the College of American Pathology/American College of Medical Genetics and Genomics external proficiency testing from 2006 to 2013 for three conditions prevalent in the Ashkenazi Jewish population. Genet Med. 2014;16:695–702.
132. Richards CS, Palomaki GE, Lacbawan FL, et al. Three-year experience of a CAP/ACMG methods-based external proficiency testing program for laboratories offering DNA sequencing for rare inherited disorders. Genet Med. 2014;16:25–32.
133. Frampton M, Houlston R. Generation of artificial FASTQ files to evaluate the performance of next generation sequencing pipelines. PLoS One. 2012;7, e49110.
134. The Medical Device Amendments of 1976 MDA. 21 USC. 1360c et seq. 1976
135. Federal Food, Drug and Cosmetic Act of 1994 FD&C, 21 USC 301-395 1994
136. Javitt GH. In search of a coherent framework: options for FDA oversight of genetic tests. Food Drug Law J. 2007;62:617–52.
137. Department of Health and Human Services Food and Drug Administration. Medical devices classification reclassification restricted devices analyte specific reagents final rule. Fed Regist. 1997;62(225):62243–45 [21CFR809, 21CFR864].
138. Ferreira-Gonzalez A, Emmadi R, Day SP, et al. Revisiting oversight and regulation of molecular-based laboratory-developed tests: a position statement of the Association for Molecular Pathology. J Mol Diagn. 2014;16:3–6.
139. Association for molecular pathology statement recommendations for in-house development and operation of molecular diagnostic tests. Am J Clin Pathol. 1999;111:449–63
140. https://www.federalregister.gov/articles/2014/10/03/2014-23596/framework-for-regulatory-oversight-of-laboratory-developed-tests-draft-guidance-for-industry-food
141. Loman NJ, Misra RV, Dallman TJ, et al. Performance comparison of benchtop high-throughput sequencing platforms. Nat Biotechnol. 2012;30:434–9.
142. Li H, Handsaker B, Wysoker A, et al. The sequence alignment/Map format and SAMtools. Bioinformatics. 2009;25:2078–9.
143. Jünemann S, Sedlazeck FJ, Prior K, et al. Updating benchtop sequencing performance comparison. Nat Biotechnol. 2013;31:294–6.
144. http://www.hgvs.org/mutnomen/disc
145. http://mendel.iontorrent.com/ion-docs/Classic-Ion-Sphere-Particle-Summary.html

Clinical Applications of Proteomics

61

Delphine Rolland and Kojo S.J. Elenitoba-Johnson

Abstract

This chapter provides an overview of potential and current clinical applications of proteomics. Although the clinical applications of protein microarrays are discussed in this chapter, we particularly emphasize the potential utilization of mass spectrometry-based approaches for diagnosis, biomarker detection, and quantitation.

Keywords

Protein microarray • Mass spectrometry • Proteomics • Biomarkers

Overview

The term "proteomics" was first used in the mid-1990s to describe large-scale characterization of the entire protein complement of a cell, tissue, or organism. The goal of proteomics is to obtain a more global and integrated view of biology by studying protein expression, localization, interaction, modification, and function. In fact, proteomics has been widely applied in various areas of science, ranging from the deciphering of molecular pathogenesis of diseases and the characterization of novel drug targets, to the discovery of potential diagnostic and prognostic biomarkers. Although the largest application of proteomic analysis remains scientific research, such technologies have already been introduced into clinical laboratories and are poised for broader routine use in the future.

D. Rolland, Pharm.D., Ph.D.
Department of Pathology, University of Michigan Medical School, 2037 BSRB, 109 Zina Pitcher Place, Ann Arbor, MI, 48109, USA

K.S.J. Elenitoba-Johnson, M.D. (✉)
Department of Pathology and Laboratory Medicine, Perelman School of Medicine of the University of Pennsylvania, 609A Stellar-Chance Laboratories, 422 Curie Boulevard, Philadelphia, PA, 19104–6100, USA
e-mail: Kojo.Elenitobas-Johnson@uphs.upenn.edu

Protein Microarrays

Principle of Protein Microarrays

Technologies well established for DNA/RNA applications have been adapted for protein-based research resulting in the creation of protein microarrays. Currently, protein microarray formats include two major classes, forward-phase arrays and reverse-phase arrays, depending on whether the sample is captured from solution phase or bound to the solid phase (Fig. 61.1).

Forward-phase microarrays are the most frequently used formats allowing the simultaneous analysis of multiple parameters per sample. Specific proteins of interest are selectively trapped from complex protein mixtures (serum, plasma, cell lysate, or cell culture supernatant) by well-defined capture or "bait" molecules (usually antibodies but full-length functional proteins or protein active domains could be used) that are immobilized onto a solid surface. Each spot of the array contains one type of immobilized antibody or bait molecule. Each array is incubated with one sample and the bound analytes are visualized either by direct labeling of the analytes or via labeled secondary antibodies. Standard detection methods include fluorescence, chemiluminescence, and colorimetry. A planar microarray-based

D.G.B. Leonard (ed.), *Molecular Pathology in Clinical Practice*, DOI 10.1007/978-3-319-19674-9_61

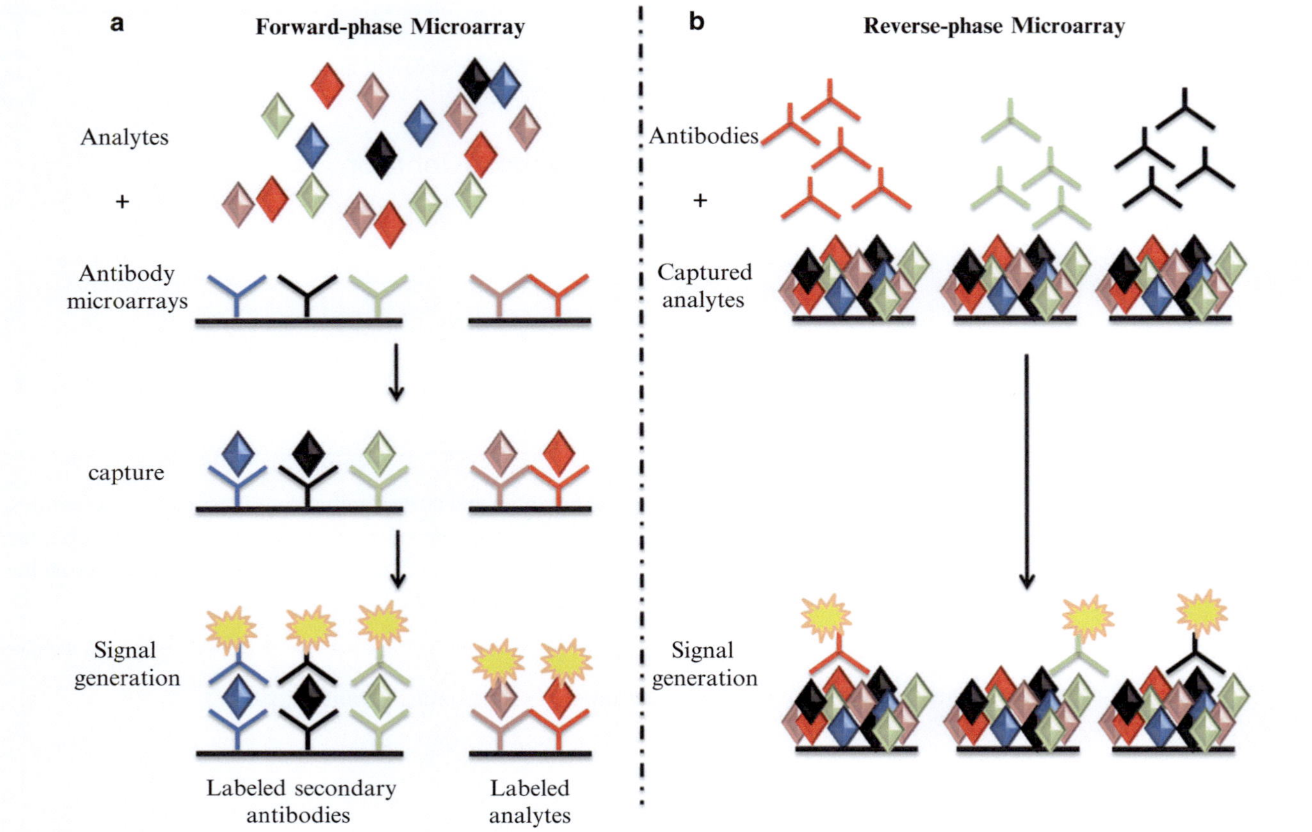

Figure 61.1 Comparison of forward-phase and reverse-phase protein microarrays. (**a**) Forward-phase microarray. Capture antibodies are first immobilized on the slide surface. These immobilized antibodies are used to capture the antigens they recognize from a test sample. (**b**) Reverse-phase microarray. Complex samples are immobilized on the surface and targeted by antibodies overlaid on them

system can generate high-density protein microarrays to screen a large number of analytes in a single experiment. The concept of planar microarray-based systems has been successfully miniaturized and operationalized into a bead-based microarray system where each bead is coupled to a specific bait molecule. This bead-based microarray system provides an interesting alternative since it is more flexible, robust, and advanced with respect to automation to screen thousands of samples within a short time.

For reversed-phase microarrays, a multitude of different samples (tissues or cell lysates) are immobilized as spots in rows on a solid support such that the array contains numerous spots representing the proteome of different patient samples or cell lysates. Then, each microarray is incubated with one highly specific detection molecule or antibody, measuring a single analyte with direct comparison of the analyte across multiple samples. This approach allows sets of proteins to be detected in large collections of tissue or cell samples.

Clinical Applications of Protein Microarrays

To date, many commercial forward-phase microarrays are available to investigate different classes of proteins such as cytokines and chemokines, cancer biomarkers or molecules involved in signaling pathways. Interestingly, several clinical protein microarrays have been cleared by the US Food and Drug Administration (FDA) or CE-marked for use in the European Union. So far, the main applications of these protein microarrays are diagnosis of infectious diseases or immune diseases. For example, the AtheNA Muli-Lyte® Test System (Zeus Scientific, Raritan, NJ, USA) can be used for the diagnosis of the infection by *Borrelia burgdorferi* by multiplex sandwich immunoassay for the quantitative detection of distinct IgG antibody to Vlse-1 and distinct IgM antibody to pepC10. Another example is the Bio-Plex™ 2200 ANA Screen (Bio-Rad Laboratories, Hercules, CA) which detects autoantibodies in serum or plasma as an aid in the diagnosis of systemic rheumatic diseases such as systemic

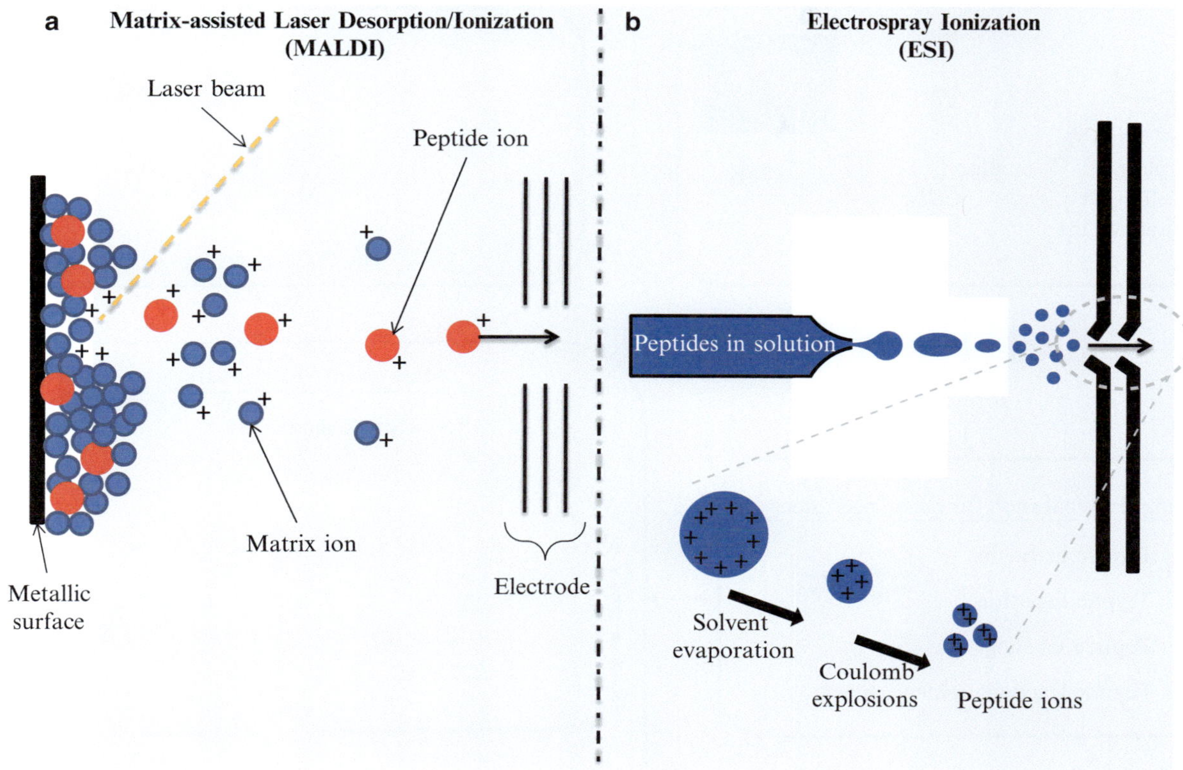

Figure 61.2 Principles of operation of Matrix-Assisted Laser Desorption Ionization (MALDI) and Electrospray Ionization (ESI). (**a**) MALDI. The protein/peptide sample is co-crystallized with a matrix, then the vaporization and ionization of the protein/peptide sample is achieved by a laser pulse-irradiation of the surface. The matrix material heavily absorbs UV laser light, leading to the ablation of the upper layer of the matrix. This process generates ions that are usually accelerated into a mass analyzer for analysis. (**b**) ESI. The liquid containing the analyte is dispersed by electrospray into a fine aerosol. Via Coulomb explosions, large charged droplets are sequentially blown apart to form smaller droplets. Upon reaching a certain size limit, only the discrete peptide sample ions enter the mass analyzer

lupus erythematosus, mixed connective tissue disease, undifferentiated connective tissue disease, Sjogren's syndrome, scleroderma, dermatomyositis, polymyositis, rheumatoid arthritis, CREST syndrome, and Raynaud's disease.

Mass Spectrometry-Based Proteomic Analysis

Introduction to Mass Spectrometry

Instrumentation

Since the first description of a mass spectrometry (MS) experiment in the early 1900s by Thomson [1], MS-based approaches have come a long way from being narrowly applied in analytical chemistry to a key device for clinical testing. The description in the late 1980s of two different soft ionization methods named Matrix-Assisted Laser Desorption/Ionization (MALDI) [2, 3] and ElectroSpray Ionization (ESI) [4] (Fig. 61.2) significantly accelerated MS-based interrogation of large biologically important molecules. The principle of operation of MALDI-based proteomics involves the co-crystallization of a protein/peptide sample on a designated matrix medium (Fig. 61.2a). The vaporization and ionization of the protein/peptide sample is achieved by pulse-irradiation of the surface with a laser. This process generates ions that are accelerated into the mass analyzer for analysis, filtering, and detection. By comparison, the ESI process involves the transfer of ions from solution to gaseous phase at atmospheric pressure (Fig. 61.2b). The application of a very high voltage across a sample solution at very low flow rates in a capillary needle causes ions to accumulate at the narrow tip of the needle where they are then drawn out as the sample solution is pushed out of the needle creating charged droplets that are accelerated in an electric field. Via the Coulomb explosion, large charged droplets are sequentially blown apart to form smaller droplets upon reaching a certain limit leaving only the discrete peptide sample ions to enter the mass analyzer.

After ionization the sample reaches the mass analyzer which separates ions by their mass-to-charge (m/z) ratios. Ion motion in the mass analyzer can be manipulated by electric or magnetic fields to direct ions to a detector which

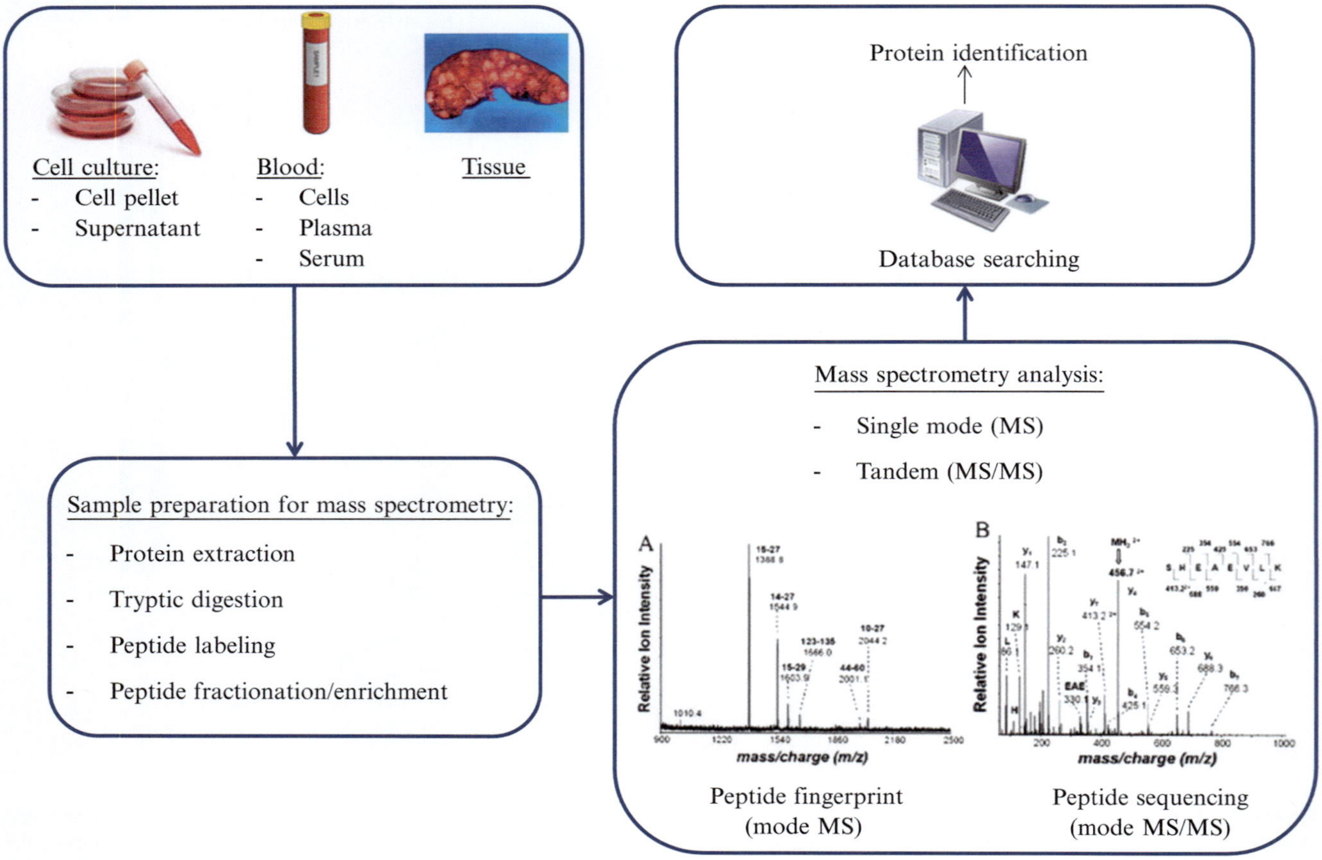

Figure 61.3 Workflow for mass spectrometry proteomics

registers the number of ions at each individual *m/z* value. Different types of mass analyzers are available: time-of-flight (TOF), ion trap, and quadrupoles. These mass analyzers differ considerably in sensitivity, resolution, mass accuracy, and the possibility to obtain fragment peptide ions which results in mass spectra with high content of information (MS/MS spectra). The choice of the combination of the ion source with the mass analyzer and the detector depends on the specific application.

Classical Workflow for Mass Spectrometry Proteomics

Mass spectrometry-based proteomic analyses can be divided into top-down or bottom-up processes. In top-down proteomics, intact proteins or polypeptides are directly analyzed by mass spectrometry. On the other hand, bottom-up proteomics entails digestion of complex protein mixtures into peptides using a proteolytic enzyme (typically trypsin). Resulting peptides are separated by liquid chromatography (LC) and analyzed by tandem mass spectrometry (MS/MS). Proteins are identified by matching experimental spectra with those from theoretical spectra of translated genomic databases generated by in silico cleavage using specific enzymes (Fig. 61.3).

Quantitative Mass Spectrometry-Based Proteomics

Quantitative measurement of protein concentrations is one of the key advancements in MS-based proteomics. Global quantitation of protein levels can be achieved by stable isotope labeling of proteins/peptides, use of heavy peptides as standards, and label-free quantitation (Fig. 61.4). Isotope labels can be introduced metabolically (i.e., in vivo), chemically, or enzymatically (i.e., in vitro). Since the metabolic labeling (stable isotope labeling with amino acids in cell culture, [SILAC]) requires maintaining cells in culture for several passages (usually six or seven passages) in the presence of stable isotopes of amino acids (heavy Arg, Lys, Leu, or Ile), its direct application to clinically relevant scenarios is less likely. The in vitro methods for labeling include isotope-coded affinity tagging (ICAT) and isobaric tags for relative and absolute quantitation (iTRAQ). These methods may be adaptable to clinical scenarios since cell viability is not required for labeling. In the original ICAT labeling method, cysteine residues were specifically derivatized with a reagent containing either zero or eight deuterium atoms as well as a biotin group for affinity purification of cysteine-derivatized peptides and subsequent mass spectrometry analysis. The iTRAQ method is another in vitro labeling reagent which targets the

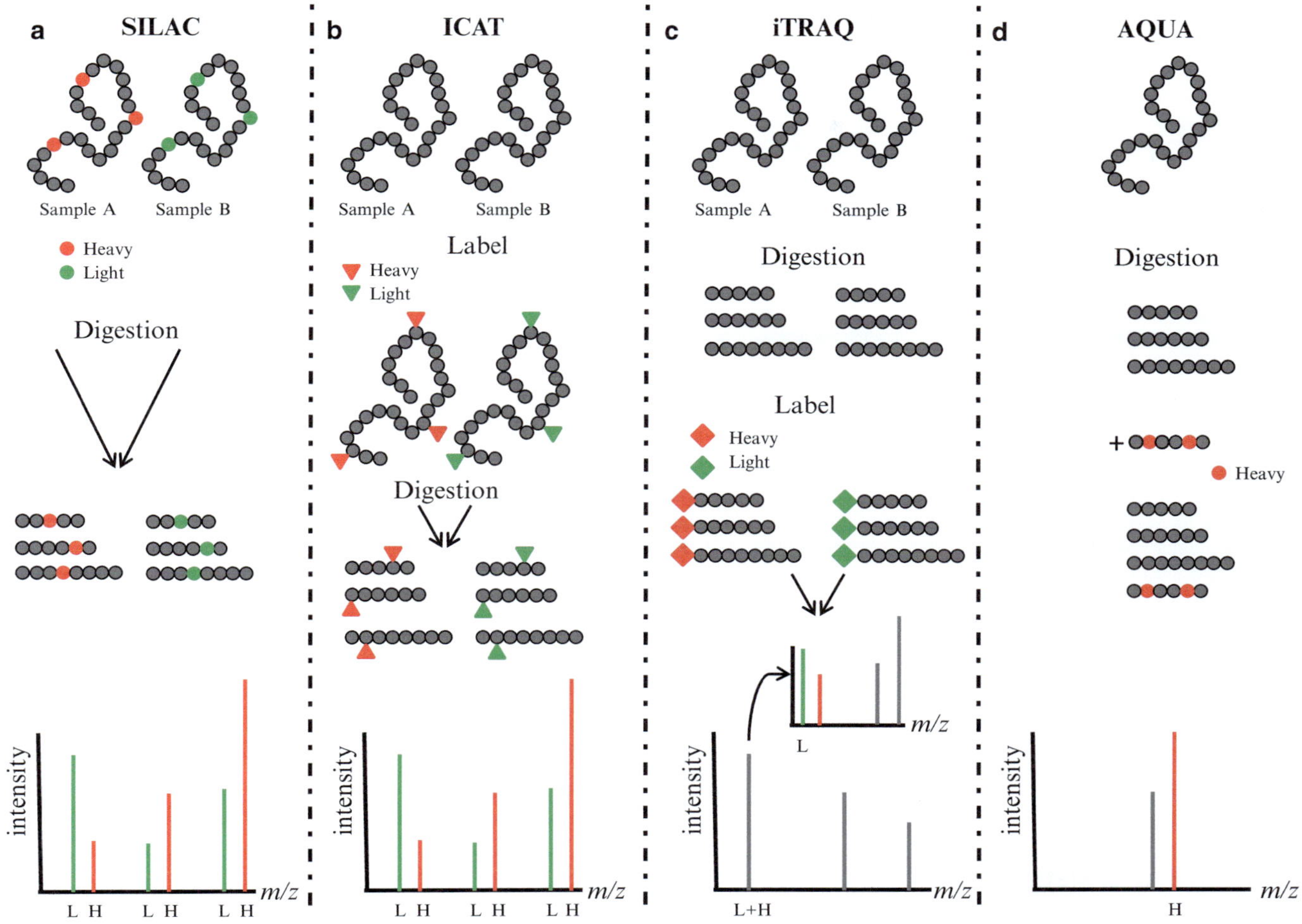

Figure 61.4 Quantitative proteomics. (**a**) In stable isotope labeling with amino acids in cell culture (SILAC), two cell cultures are differentially labeled with heavy amino acids containing stable isotopes (heavy, H) and normal amino acids (light, L). Lysates from labeled cells are digested, mixed, and analyzed by mass spectrometry. Differentially labeled peptides having the same amino acid sequence are detected in MS spectra and the relative abundance of the peptides can be compared. (**b**) In isotope-coded affinity tagging (ICAT), proteins are labeled at cysteine residues with reagent containing either 0 (light, L) or 8 (heavy, H) deuterium atoms. After digestion, labeled peptides are combined and analyzed by mass spectrometry. Peptides with the same amino acid sequence are detected in MS spectra and the relative abundance of the peptides can be compared. (**c**) In isobaric tags for relative and absolute quantitation (iTRAQ), peptides are labeled using isobaric amine-specific tandem tags. The iTRAQ reagent consists of a reporter region with 1 Da difference and a balance region that adjusts the molecular weight of the labeled parent ions. Each tag generates a unique reporter in MS/MS spectra and the relative abundance of peptides can be compared. (**d**) In absolute quantification (AQUA), an isotope-labeled peptide is spiked at a known amount into the sample preparation. The abundance of peptide can be compared with the abundance of the spiked peptide

N-terminus amino acid of peptides with a varying mass. The AQUA (absolute quantification) quantitative approach uses isotope-labeled synthetic peptides as standards spiked at a known amount into a sample preparation. The quantitation is achieved by comparing the mass spectrometric signal of the synthetic peptide to the endogenous peptide in the sample. Label-free quantitation methods are gaining in popularity and are increasingly being employed as an alternative to label-based approaches. These techniques do not use isotopic labeling, but instead directly compare signal intensities across different mass spectrometry runs using either the signal intensity of peptide precursors or the number of fragment spectra identifying peptides of a given protein.

Selected Reaction Monitoring (SRM)

Selected reaction monitoring (SRM), formerly referred to as multiple reaction monitoring mass spectrometry, utilizes two rounds of mass selection by quadrupole mass analyzers to discriminate specific ion peptides within a complex sample based on *m/z* ratios (Fig. 61.5) [5]. Following sample processing with trypsin and separation by nano-LC, ionized peptide precursors of predetermined interest are selected in the first quadrupole (Q1). After Q1 selection, only ions with the predefined *m/z* value are transmitted to the second quadrupole (Q2) where a collision-assisted dissociation causes peptide fragmentation. Detection and quantitation of the

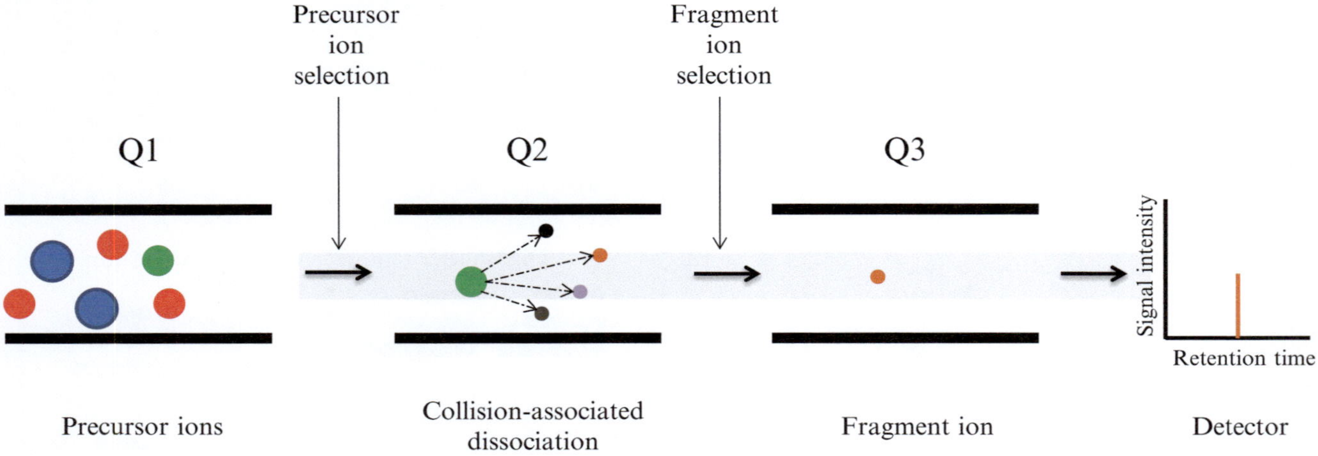

Figure 61.5 Selected Reaction Monitoring (SRM) analysis on triple quadrupole mass spectrometer. Several analytes are co-eluted from the chromatographic system. The ionized peptide precursors with a specific *m/z* are selected in the first quadrupole (Q1). Only ions with the predefined *m/z* value are transmitted to the second quadrupole (Q2) where a collision-assisted dissociation causes peptide fragmentation. Detection and quantitation of the target analyte is achieved following the selective transmission in the third quadrupole (Q3) of a predefined product ion

target analyte is achieved following the selective transmission in the third quadrupole (Q3) of a predefined product ion (a fragment of the precursor peptide). Ultimately, SRM allows the quantitation of a large set of target proteins in complex biological samples.

Protein Posttranslational Modification Study by Mass Spectrometry

Phosphoproteomics

Reversible protein phosphorylations at serine, threonine, and tyrosine residues represent fundamental and highly evolutionarily conserved types of protein posttranslational modifications which control essential cellular processes, including metabolism, growth, cell cycle, motility and differentiation [6, 7]. The Human Genome Project revealed that more than 520 protein kinases and 130 protein phosphatases exert tight and reversible control on protein phosphorylation. Perturbations in protein phosphorylation underlie many human diseases, including diabetes, cardiovascular diseases [8], immune disorders, [9] and cancers [10]. Recently, there has been increased interest in tyrosine kinases (TKs) due to the remarkably successful introduction of specific inhibitors, the TKIs, for the treatment of cancers. Indeed, many TKIs have been approved by the US FDA as routine therapeutic options for certain human cancers [11].

In order to identify aberrant protein phosphorylations via mass spectrometry analysis, an enrichment of the phosphoproteome is required prior to further analysis. This is mostly due to the low phosphorylation stoichiometry of phosphoproteins and the limited dynamic range of mass spectrometers. Several methods are well-described for phosphopeptide or phosphoprotein enrichments such as strong cation exchange chromatography (SCX), immobilized metal affinity chromatography (IMAC), metal oxide affinity chromatography (MOAC) [12], and immunoaffinity purification (IAP) using high affinity anti-phosphotyrosine antibodies [13]. The first three methods are used for global phosphorylation enrichment and will enrich for proteins that are phosphorylated at tyrosine, serine, or threonine residues. With the identification and quantification of phosphorylated peptides extracted from samples, intracellular signaling networks can be generated to highlight pathophysiological mechanisms. The better understanding of biological processes involved in the initiation or maintenance of a deleterious phenotype would be helpful to target specifically activated pathways as therapeutic options.

Glycoproteomics

Glycosylation represents the most common of all known posttranslational modification and, like the majority of cell surface proteins, receptor TKs are also glycoproteins with Asn (N)-linked oligosaccharides (N-glycans). Since glycopeptides often constitute a minor portion of a complex peptide mixture, several procedures have been developed to reduce the sample complexity and enrich glycoprotein content. One way to reduce the complexity is to perform lectin affinity chromatography to enrich for glycopeptides. In 2003, Zhang et al. suggested a new method for the selective isolation of N-glycosyl peptides [14]. This method involves glycoprotein oxidation which converts the *cis*-diol groups of carbohydrates to aldehydes. These aldehydes then can be derivatized with hydrazide groups immobilized on a solid support to form covalent hydrazone bonds. After proteolytic digestion with trypsin, N-glycopeptides is released by using peptide N-glycosidases (PNGase). The identification and quantification of N-glycopeptides leads to characterization of proteins that are mainly expressed at the plasma membrane and therefore could be useful as potential diagnostic biomarkers.

Clinical Applications of Qualitative Mass Spectrometry Proteomic Analysis

Typing of Amyloidosis

MS-based proteomics has been combined with tissue microdissection for the diagnosis and typing of amyloidosis [15, 16]. With this approach, specific clinical variants of amyloidosis are identified based on correlation with the predominating protein components within the amyloid deposits in the tissue specimens. In this regard, MS-based proteomics has been used to accurately define AL amyloidosis (lambda/kappa light chain), heavy chain amyloidosis, AA amyloidosis, fibrinogen-a-amyloidosis, LECT2 amyloidosis, and other types. The accuracy and sensitivity of this approach continues to drive its potential to supplant Congo-red staining as the primary technique for the identification of amyloid.

MALDI-TOF and Clinical Microbial Identification

Classically, microbiological diagnoses are based on microscopic and biochemical characteristics, growth preference on specific media, metabolic traits and antimicrobial susceptibilities. The first attempt to identify bacteria using mass spectrometry was done more than 30 years ago [17]; however, only recently have MALDI-TOF devices become available for utilization by non-mass spectrometry specialists in a clinical laboratory setting. In practice, the sample can be applied onto the target plate either by deposition of a protein solution when an extraction step has been performed, or by touching the colony of interest with a sterile pipette tip and directly applying a small amount of sample onto the surface of the target plate. Samples are overlaid by a suitable matrix and then analyzed by MALDI-TOF-MS. A characteristic spectrum is recorded and constitutes a specific sample fingerprint, which is unique for a given species. For species-level identification, the size range generally used is 2–20 kDa, which was found to be very stable and with a strong signal-to-noise ratio. The computer software automatically compares the collected spectra with a reference databank containing a wide variety of medically relevant isolates. A retrospective study of 1,116 routine isolates representing the main bacterial groups encountered in the clinical microbiology laboratory showed 95.2 % correct identification by MALDI-TOF [18]. In 2010, Van Veen et al. prospectively analyzed 980 isolates and found an overall concordance between MALDI-TOF and conventional methods of 92 % at the species level and an addition of 6.8 % for specimen identified only at the genus level [19]. The main advantages of MALDI-TOF are the speed of testing, with results available up to 20 h earlier than by conventional testing, and the cost-effectiveness of the method.

Imaging Mass Spectrometry

Imaging mass spectrometry is the use of MALDI-TOF-MS for profiling and imaging proteins directly from thin tissue sections [20]. This application provides specific information on the local molecular composition, relative abundance, and spatial distribution of peptides and proteins in the analyzed section (Fig. 61.6). A tissue section is uniformly coated with a matrix solution by air spraying within which the tissue section becomes physically bound and co-crystallized. The co-crystallized area is then subjected to MALDI ionization using a discrete Cartesian pattern of laser shot spots. The distance between the spots is fixed and depends on the chosen resolution, typically 10–100 μm. From the intensity of a given *m*/*z* value monitored in each spectrum, a two-dimensional ion density image is reconstructed using specialized software. When full images are not required, but rather data are needed from discrete targeted areas within the tissue, a histology-directed profiling approach can be employed. Several studies have shown the potential of imaging MS in molecular diagnosis of prostate cancer [21], prediction of the response to neoadjuvant chemotherapy and radiation or HER2 status in breast cancer [22, 23], classification and survival prediction for lung cancer, [24] and determination of molecular tumor margins [25]. However, since imaging mass spectrometry is based on MALDI-TOF-MS, the principal drawbacks of this application are the fact that almost 90 % of the observed signals are below *m*/*z* 30,000 and a poor resolution of signal above *m*/*z* 50,000.

Clinical Applications of SRM Mass Spectrometry

The prostate-specific antigen (PSA) is a well-established biomarker which has been used in the diagnosis and surveillance of prostate cancer. In 2009, Fortin et al. published a

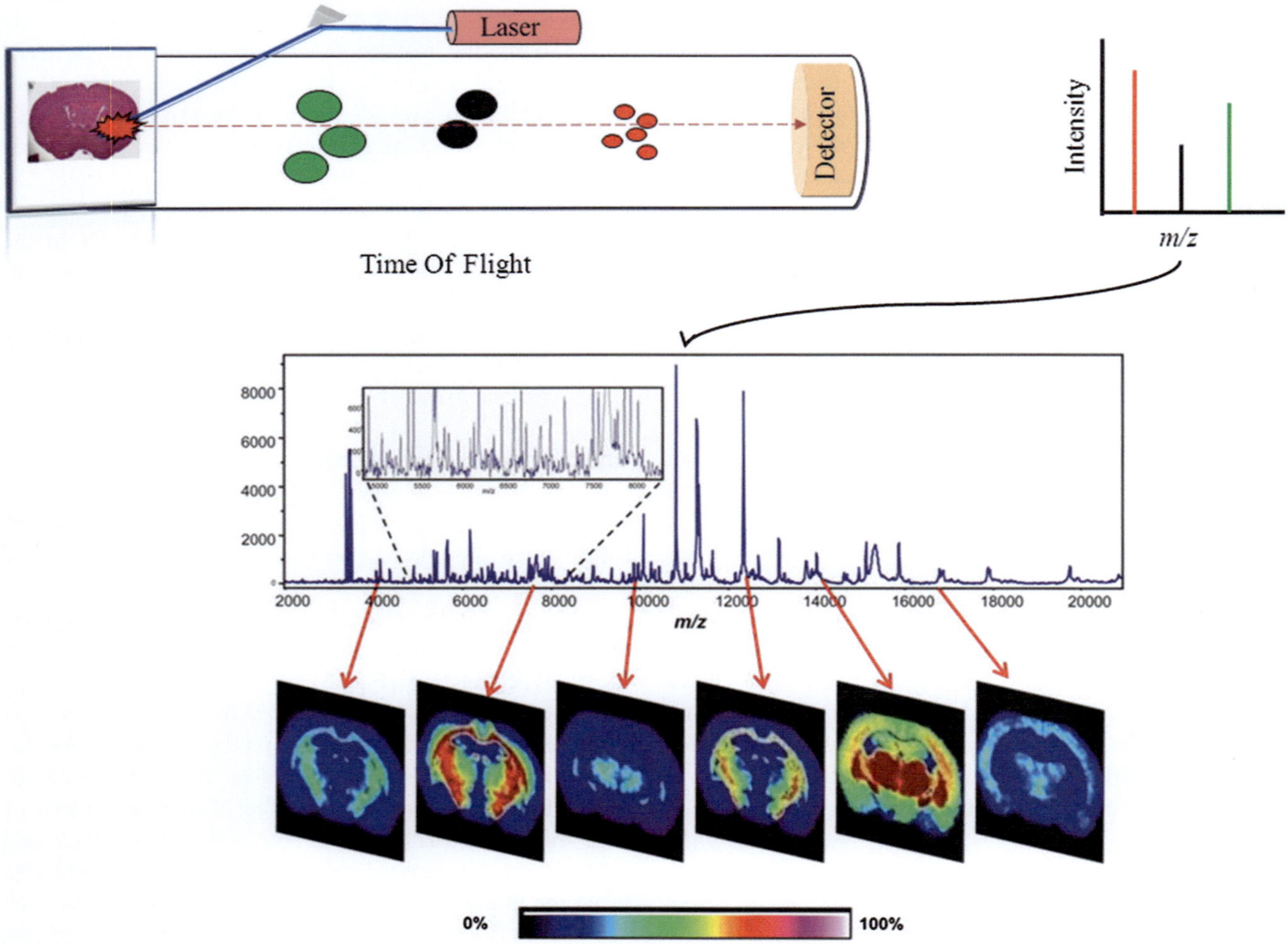

Figure 61.6 Imaging mass spectrometry. Tissue sections are mounted on a metal plate, coated with matrix, and placed in the mass spectrometer (MALDI-TOF). The laser desorbs and ionizes analytes from the tissue and their *m/z* values are determined using a time-of-flight analyzer. By scanning over the tissue and measuring the peak intensities over thousands of spots, mass spectrometric images are generated at specific molecular weight values

sensitive SRM assay to detect PSA in the sera of patients with either benign prostate hyperplasia or prostate cancer [26]. They demonstrated a limit of detection of the PSA peptide LSEPAELTDAVK of 1.5 ng/ml by SRM MS. The PSA levels measured by SRM MS were validated using the VIDAS TPSA ELISA test (bioMérieux) with a reliable correlation between these two technologies ($r^2=0.99$). Several other studies established SRM MS as a useful method to detect and quantify different biomarkers such as the C-reactive protein (CRP) [27] and the inter-α trypsin inhibitor heavy chain 4 (ITIH4) [28]. Recently a proof-of-principle study published by Wang et al. demonstrated the potential of SRM MS for clinical application [29]. They were able to design an assay to profile and quantify the high-frequency KRAS missense mutation in colorectal and pancreatic tumors.

Concluding Remarks

Proteomic approaches are increasingly being employed in the clinical laboratory, and include nonneoplastic and neoplastic applications. Routine implementation of proteomic techniques in the clinical laboratory is anticipated to occur in the next few years.

References

1. Thomson JJ. Cathode rays. Philos Mag. 1897;44:293.
2. Tanaka K, Waki H, et al. Protein and polymer analysis up to m/z 100 000 by ionization time-flight mass spectrometry. Rapid Commun Mass Spectrom. 1988;2:151–3.

3. Karas M, Bachamann D, et al. Matrix-assisted ultraviolet laser desorption of non-volatile compounds. Int J Mass Spectrom Ion Proc. 1989;78:53–68.
4. Fenn JB, Mann M, et al. Electrospray ionization for mass spectrometry of large biomolecules. Science. 1989;246(4926):64–71.
5. Lange V, Picotti P, et al. Selected reaction monitoring for quantitative proteomics: a tutorial. Mol Syst Biol. 2008;4:222.
6. Hunter T. Signaling—2000 and beyond. Cell. 2000;100(1):113–27.
7. Schlessinger J. Cell signaling by receptor tyrosine kinases. Cell. 2000;103(2):211–25.
8. Zahedi RP, Lewandrowski U, et al. Phosphoproteome of resting human platelets. J Proteome Res. 2008;7(2):526–34.
9. Matsuo K, Arito M, et al. Arthritogenicity of annexin VII revealed by phosphoproteomics of rheumatoid synoviocytes. Ann Rheum Dis. 2011;70(8):1489–95.
10. Blume-Jensen P, Hunter T. Oncogenic kinase signalling. Nature. 2001;411(6835):355–65.
11. Druker BJ, Guilhot F, et al. Five-year follow-up of patients receiving imatinib for chronic myeloid leukemia. N Engl J Med. 2006; 355(23):2408–17.
12. Larsen MR, Thingholm TE, et al. Highly selective enrichment of phosphorylated peptides from peptide mixtures using titanium dioxide microcolumns. Mol Cell Proteomics. 2005;4(7):873–86.
13. Rush J, Moritz A, et al. Immunoaffinity profiling of tyrosine phosphorylation in cancer cells. Nat Biotechnol. 2005;23(1):94–101.
14. Zhang H, Li XJ, et al. Identification and quantification of N-linked glycoproteins using hydrazide chemistry, stable isotope labeling and mass spectrometry. Nat Biotechnol. 2003;21(6):660–6.
15. Vrana JA, Gamez JD, et al. Classification of amyloidosis by laser microdissection and mass spectrometry-based proteomic analysis in clinical biopsy specimens. Blood. 2009;114(24):4957–9.
16. Figueroa JJ, Peter Bosch E, et al. Amyloid-like IgM deposition neuropathy: a distinct clinico-pathologic and proteomic profiled disorder. J Peripher Nerv Syst. 2012;17(2):182–90.
17. Anhalt JP, Fenselau C. Identification of bacteria using mass spectrometry. Anal Chem. 1975;47(2):219–25.
18. Eigner U, Holfelder M, et al. Performance of a matrix-assisted laser desorption ionization-time-of-flight mass spectrometry system for the identification of bacterial isolates in the clinical routine laboratory. Clin Lab. 2009;55(7–8):289–96.
19. van Veen SQ, Claas EC, et al. High-throughput identification of bacteria and yeast by matrix-assisted laser desorption ionization-time of flight mass spectrometry in conventional medical microbiology laboratories. J Clin Microbiol. 2010;48(3):900–7.
20. Stoeckli M, Chaurand P, et al. Imaging mass spectrometry: a new technology for the analysis of protein expression in mammalian tissues. Nat Med. 2001;7(4):493–6.
21. Schwamborn K, Krieg RC, et al. Identifying prostate carcinoma by MALDI-imaging. Int J Mol Med. 2007;20(2):155–9.
22. Bauer JA, Chakravarthy AB, et al. Identification of markers of taxane sensitivity using proteomic and genomic analyses of breast tumors from patients receiving neoadjuvant paclitaxel and radiation. Clin Cancer Res. 2010;16(2):681–90.
23. Rauser S, Marquardt C, et al. Classification of HER2 receptor status in breast cancer tissues by MALDI imaging mass spectrometry. J Proteome Res. 2010;9(4):1854–63.
24. Groseclose MR, Massion PP, et al. High-throughput proteomic analysis of formalin-fixed paraffin-embedded tissue microarrays using MALDI imaging mass spectrometry. Proteomics. 2008;8(18): 3715–24.
25. Oppenheimer SR, Mi D, et al. Molecular analysis of tumor margins by MALDI mass spectrometry in renal carcinoma. J Proteome Res. 2010;9(5):2182–90.
26. Fortin T, Salvador A, et al. Clinical quantitation of prostate-specific antigen biomarker in the low nanogram/milliliter range by conventional bore liquid chromatography-tandem mass spectrometry (multiple reaction monitoring) coupling and correlation with ELISA tests. Mol Cell Proteomics. 2009;8(5): 1006–15.
27. Kuhn E, Wu J, et al. Quantification of C-reactive protein in the serum of patients with rheumatoid arthritis using multiple reaction monitoring mass spectrometry and 13C-labeled peptide standards. Proteomics. 2004;4(4):1175–86.
28. van den Broek I, Sparidans RW, et al. Quantitative assay for six potential breast cancer biomarker peptides in human serum by liquid chromatography coupled to tandem mass spectrometry. J Chromatogr B Analyt Technol Biomed Life Sci. 2010; 878(5–6):590–602.
29. Wang Q, Chaerkady R, et al. Mutant proteins as cancer-specific biomarkers. Proc Natl Acad Sci U S A. 2011;108(6):2444–9.

Section IX

Laboratory Management

Section Editor: Debra G.B. Leonard

Molecular Pathology Laboratory Management

62

Hanna Rennert and Debra G.B. Leonard

Abstract

Clinical molecular pathology tests identify or measure molecular and genetic markers for an individual patient. These markers confirm a diagnosis, predict prognosis, guide treatment, and monitor response to therapy. The rapid turnaround time, reliability, and high accuracy of molecular pathology tests have reduced the occurrence and cost of health care services, enhanced patient outcome, and improved disease management, making molecular pathology one of the fastest-growing sectors of clinical pathology, with more than 2,500 tests currently available in the National Institutes of Health Genetic Testing Registry (NIH GTR) (Rubinstein et al., Nucleic Acids Res 41(Database issue): D925–D935, 2013). The vast majority of these tests are developed and performed as laboratory developed tests (LTDs), which to date have limited oversight by the US Food and Drug Administration. Regulatory and quality oversight of all clinical testing in the USA is provided by the Clinical Laboratory Improvement Act of 1988 and its implementation through the Centers for Medicare and Medicaid Services. The operation of a clinical molecular pathology laboratory requires integration of medical, scientific, and clinical molecular pathology expertise, resources including facilities, equipment, and personnel, and skills in organization, administration, management, and communication. Quality service is achieved by adherence to clinical laboratory regulations and standards, from specimen collection and processing to reporting of patient results. This chapter reviews fundamental knowledge important for the management and operation of a clinical molecular pathology laboratory.

Keywords

Molecular pathology laboratory management • Molecular pathology laboratory operations • CLIA • US FDA • New York State Department of Health • Standards • Regulation • Facilities • Personnel management • Specimen handling

Introduction

Clinical molecular pathology tests identify or measure molecular and genetic markers for an individual patient. These markers confirm a diagnosis, predict prognosis, guide treatment, and monitor response to therapy. The rapid turnaround time (TAT), reliability, and high accuracy of molecular pathology tests have reduced the occurrence and cost of health care services, enhanced patient outcome, and improved disease management, making molecular pathology one of the

H. Rennert, Ph.D., F.A.C.M.G. (✉)
Department of Pathology and Laboratory Medicine,
Weill Cornell Medical College, New York Presbyterian Hospital,
New York, NY, USA
e-mail: har2006@med.cornell.edu

D.G.B. Leonard, M.D., Ph.D.
Department of Pathology and Laboratory Medicine,
University of Vermont College of Medicine and
University of Vermont Medical Center, Burlington, VT, USA
e-mail: debra.leonard@med.uvm.edu

D.G.B. Leonard (ed.), *Molecular Pathology in Clinical Practice*, DOI 10.1007/978-3-319-19674-9_62

fastest-growing sectors of clinical pathology, with more than 2,500 tests currently available in the National Institutes of Health Genetic Testing Registry (NIH GTR) [1]. The vast majority of these tests are developed and performed as laboratory developed tests (LTDs), which to date have limited oversight by the US Food and Drug Administration (FDA). Regulatory and quality oversight of all clinical testing in the USA is provided by the Clinical Laboratory Improvement Act of 1988 (CLIA) and its implementation through the Centers for Medicare and Medicaid Services (CMS). The operation of a clinical molecular pathology laboratory requires integration of medical, scientific, and clinical molecular pathology expertise, resources including facilities, equipment, and personnel, and skills in organization, administration, management, and communication. Quality service is achieved by adherence to clinical laboratory regulations and standards, from specimen collection and processing to reporting of patient results. This chapter reviews fundamental knowledge important for the management and operation of a clinical molecular pathology laboratory.

The Role of the Molecular Pathology Laboratory

Molecular pathology laboratories perform tests for different clinical purposes, including genetics, cancer, infectious diseases, identity testing, and human leukocyte antigen (HLA) typing. Although all applications share the use of nucleic acids as the main analyte, the different types of testing require different management considerations (Table 62.1). Considerations relevant for each type of test performed in molecular pathology are reviewed.

Table 62.1 Special considerations in molecular pathology by clinical application

Application	Considerations
Genetics	Ethical issues (presymptomatic and prenatal testing)
	Consequences for family members
	Informed consent requirements
	Requirements for family-related information (ethnicity, pedigree, specimens)
	Time sensitivity (prenatal diagnosis)
	Complex risk-assessment calculations
Oncology	Many types of samples
	Extensive use of paraffin-embedded tissue and fine needle aspirate samples (familiarity with limitations)
	Small biopsy specimens
	Need for diagnostic samples for optimal interpretation of minimal residual disease test results
Infectious diseases	High-volume testing
	Use of automated platforms
	High cost of commercial in vitro diagnostic test kits
	Increased need for quantitative testing with a wide dynamic range and low detection limit
Identity testing	Chain-of-custody documentation for specimens
	Special patient identification requirements
	Complex calculations
	Special accreditation requirements for paternity and forensic testing
	Special qualifications required for laboratory director
HLA testing	Time sensitivity (<24 h turnaround time)
	Complex analyses
	Special accreditation requirements for the laboratory and laboratory director

HLA Human leukocyte antigen

Genetic Disorders

All diseases have a genetic contribution, whether it is a specific genetic disease or an increased likelihood for developing a medical condition. Genetic disorders are primarily caused by mutations present in every cell of an individual. Molecular testing for neoplasia or an infectious disease requires a sample of the tumor or the infected tissue, respectively, while molecular testing for a genetic disease can be performed on most accessible tissue types, the simplest being a blood or buccal cell specimen. In addition, because genetic testing examines germline mutations, it has important implications not only for the individual but also for family members that may have inherited the same mutation. Genetic testing also raises ethical concerns, including informed consent, potential for employment or insurance discrimination based on test results, and beginning-of-life issues with prenatal or preimplantation testing. Genetic test results often are not definitive, requiring complex risk-assessment calculations for interpretation. The American College of Medical Genetics (ACMG) and the American Society of Human Genetics (ASHG) have published guidelines and recommendations for many of the more common single-gene disorders (Table 62.2).

Genetic Testing

Molecular genetic testing is currently used for the following major clinical purposes: diagnostic, carrier, prenatal/preimplantation, presymptomatic, and population screening [2]. Diagnostic testing is performed on affected individuals for establishing or confirming a clinical diagnosis. In general, for diagnostic genetic testing, the patient should have symptoms consistent with the disorder to justify performing the test. Genetic tests may be useful to diagnose an early atypical clinical presentation, or when other diagnostic procedures are more expensive, complex, or will not provide a definite diagnosis. For example, molecular testing for the absence of

Table 62.2 Professional organizations providing standards and guidelines for molecular pathology laboratories

Organization	Standards and guidelines
Centers for Medicare and Medicaid Services (CMS; http://www.hcfa.gov)	Mandatory federal guidelines for regulating laboratory testing via the Clinical Laboratory Improvement Amendments of 1988 (CLIA) and the Laboratory Improvement Amendments of 2003 (CLIA) "Final Rules"
New York State Department of Health (NYS DOH)	Comprehensive test approval policy and submission guidelines
The Clinical Laboratory Evaluation Program (CLEP)	Assay approval in genetic testing—molecular
	Assay approval in oncology
	Approval of microbiology nucleic acid amplification assays
	Next-generation sequencing (NGS) guidelines for somatic genetic variant detection
American College of Medical Genetics and Genomics (ACMG; http://www.acmg.net)	Standards and guidelines for clinical genetic laboratories
	Gene patents and accessibility of genetic testing
	Policy regarding genetic testing of minors
	Storage and use of genetic materials
	Recommended standards for interpretation of sequence variations
	Recommendations and guidelines regarding genetic testing for certain diseases including fragile X syndrome, apolipoprotein testing for Alzheimer disease, Prader Willi–Angelman syndrome, Canavan disease, cystic fibrosis, Huntington disease, venous thromboembolism (factor V Leiden and prothrombin), congenital hearing loss, colon cancer, and breast and ovarian cancer
American Society of Human Genetics (ASHG; http://www.ashg.org)	Educational resources in human genetics
	Legislation for genetic information nondiscrimination
American Society for Histocompatibility and Immunogenetics (ASHI; http://www.ashi-hla.org)	Standards for molecular histocompatibility and immunogenetic testing
Association for Molecular Pathology (AMP; http://www.amp.org/)	Educational resources in molecular pathology
	Reports and guidelines for clinical testing and diagnostic genome sequencing
Clinical and Laboratory Standards Institute (http://www.clsi.org) (formerly National Committee for Clinical laboratory Standards, NCCLS)	Molecular diagnostic methods for genetic diseases (MM1-A2); approved guidelines 2nd edition (2006)
	Immunoglobulin and T-cell receptor gene rearrangement assays (MM2-A); approved guideline (2002)
	Molecular diagnostic methods for infectious diseases (MM3-A2); approved guideline 2nd edition (2006)
	Nucleic acid-amplification assays for hematopathology (MM5-A); approved guideline (2003)
	Quantitative molecular diagnostics for infectious diseases (MM6-A)
	Nucleic acid sequencing methods in diagnostic laboratory medicine; approved guideline (2004)
	Fluorescence in situ hybridization (FISH) methods for medical genetics; approved guideline (2004)
	Proficiency testing (external quality assessment) for molecular methods; approved guideline (2005)
	Collection, transport, preparation, and storage of specimens for molecular methods, approved guideline (2005)
	Use of external DNA controls in gene expression assays; approved guideline (2006)
	Diagnostic nucleic acid microarrays (2006)
	Verification and validation of multiplex nucleic acid assays; proposed guideline (2007)
	Interpretive criteria for identification of bacteria and fungi by DNA target sequencing (2008)
	Quality management for molecular genetic testing
	Establishing molecular testing in clinical laboratory environment (2011)
The College of American Pathologists (CAP; http://www.cap.org)	Recommendations for in-house development and performance of molecular tests (2012)
	Molecular pathology checklist for laboratory accreditation
	Molecular Testing Guideline for Selection of Lung Cancer Patients for EGFR and ALK Tyrosine Kinase Inhibitors (jointly with the Association for the Study of Lung Cancer [IASLC], and the Association for Molecular Pathology [AMP]) (2013)
	Molecular Markers for Colorectal Cancer (jointly with the American Society for Clinical Pathology [ASCP], and the AMP) (2015)

(continued)

Table 62.2 (continued)

Organization	Standards and guidelines
US Food and Drug Administration (FDA; http://www.fda.gov)	Guidelines for industry registration and listing of analyte-specific reagents (ASRs)
	Guidelines for laboratory development and reporting of tests using ASR
	Premarket review templates for in-house-developed genetic tests
	Guidelines for industry for manufacturing and validating molecular tests for the detection of HIV-1 and hepatitis C virus (HCV)
	Draft guidance for industry, clinical laboratories, and US FDA staff for in vitro diagnostic multivariate index assays (IVDMIAs)
National Institutes of Health (NIH; http://www.nih.gov)	Promoting safe and effective genetic testing in the Unites States: final report of the task force in genetic testing
Secretary's Advisory Committee on Genetics, Health and Society (SACGHS; http://wwwAod.nih.gov/oba/sacghs.htm) (formerly Secretary's Advisory Committee on Genetic Testing, SACGT)	Recommendations to the secretary of Health and Human Services on all aspects of the development and use of genetic tests
Clinical Laboratory Improvement Advisory Committee (CLIAC; http://www.phppo.cdc.gov/cliac/default.asp)	Setting new CLIA regulations for genetic testing
	Guidelines and recommendations for laboratory testing of HCV and HIV
Centers for Disease Control and Prevention (CDC; http://www.cdc.gov)	Data collection of genetic testing and results

the survival motor neuron 1 (*SMN1*) gene for spinal muscular atrophy (SMA) in hypotonic newborns is a simple procedure performed on peripheral blood lymphocytes (PBL), replacing the need for a more painful and complex muscle biopsy. Carrier testing is used to detect recessive mutations in healthy individuals to identify the risk of having an affected child, and can be used for individuals with a family history of a genetic disorder, or for population-based pregnancy screening. Testing of an affected family member can identify the specific mutation present in a family, thus allowing directed testing for other family members and improving the accuracy of the risk assessment for individuals with a negative test result.

Prenatal testing refers to the detection of disease mutations in a fetus, using fetal cells obtained by amniocentesis or chorionic villus sampling (CVS). To overcome some of the problems associated with pregnancy termination for an affected fetus, some laboratories offer preimplantation genetic diagnosis (PGD) in the setting of in vitro fertilization for couples with a family history of a specific genetic disease. PGD is performed on a single blastomere from an early embryo, allowing selection of only unaffected embryos for implantation.

Presymptomatic testing is used primarily for the identification of adult-onset dominant disorders prior to the onset of clinical symptoms, in which the offspring of an affected parent has a 50 % chance of inheriting the disease. This category includes neurological diseases such as Huntington disease and some types of cancer. Presymptomatic testing is the most problematic and challenging in terms of its psychological effect on the individual and hence requires extensive protocols for pre- and post-genetic test counseling. Population screening is also a type of presymptomatic testing and focuses on the most prevalent mutations, often with different sensitivity of mutation detection for different ethnic populations.

Genetic Counseling, Informed Consent, and Ethical Considerations

Genetic testing requires special attention to informed consent issues, the appropriateness of the testing, and the urgency of testing. Many laboratories choose to require documentation of informed consent for the specific genetic test being requested prior to performing the genetic test. In some states, such as New York, documentation by the laboratory of informed consent for genetic testing is required by law (Civil Rights Law §79-l). Non-consensual genetic testing and non-consensual disclosure of genetic test results are only permitted in certain cases, such as the New York Newborn Screening Program. Informed consent can be documented by obtaining a copy of the completed informed consent form signed by the patient and the health care provider who discussed the risks and benefits of testing with the patient, or by confirmation by the physician on the laboratory requisition form that informed consent is on record in his or her medical office. Until informed consent is documented, the laboratory can extract and store the appropriate nucleic acid, but only after confirmation of informed consent can the laboratory perform testing.

The clinical molecular laboratory also should review the clinical and test order information provided on the requisition form to determine whether the test is appropriate for the patient and his or her demographics and clinical history. For example, carrier testing of a minor should be deferred until the minor is an adult, and should prompt a discussion with the referring clinician. Similarly, a request for testing of an asymptomatic individual for a dominant disease requires confirmation of adequate presymptomatic genetic counseling. For prenatal test requests, gestational age should be assessed to assure that the test result is available to allow for termination of the pregnancy, if this is the family's choice. Finally, the laboratory should understand and communicate to health care providers the sensitivities and limitations of the tests performed.

Despite the tremendous advances in understanding of the human genome, the benefit of genetic testing for the patient is not always clear. Testing may be warranted, even if the results are inconclusive or preventive strategies or treatments are not available [3], because of the usefulness of a diagnosis for the patient and their family. The availability of individual genetic information raises critical ethical, legal, and social issues because genetic testing examines the patient's genetic makeup, rather than acquired (somatic) genome abnormalities or infectious agents, with implications for other family members. After intensive lobbying by many advocacy organizations including health professionals and industry leaders, the federal Genetic Information Nondiscrimination Act of 2008, also referred to as GINA, was passed and signed into law on May 21, 2008 [4]. This federal legislation prevents health insurers and employers from using information to determine eligibility, set premiums, or hire and fire employees, and ensures that genetic information is used for the benefit of the patient. The law also encourages individuals to take advantage of genetic screening, counseling, testing, and new therapies that will result from the scientific advances in the field of genetics. All entities that are subject to GINA must, at a minimum, comply with all applicable GINA requirements, and may also need to comply with more protective state laws.

Molecular genetic testing often requires interpretation using complex risk-assessment calculations [5]. Health care professionals must correctly interpret laboratory test results and be able to accurately convey the test results and interpretation to the patient, and the patient's family, as appropriate. Accurate communication of results to patients and families, however, can be complex and time-consuming and therefore may be performed by genetic counselors or physicians trained in medical genetics, rather than physicians without genetics expertise. The benefits of this approach are illustrated by a study in which one-third of physicians misinterpreted a negative genetic test result for familial adenomatous polyposis (FAP) and inappropriately suggested that the patients discontinue recommended aggressive surveillance [6]. Moreover, despite tremendous advances in genetic testing technologies, understanding of genetic test results still tends to be poor in the general public and in individuals undergoing genetic testing to assess disease risk [7–9]. For these reasons, most genetic tests should be ordered through health care professionals trained in genetics to ensure that the benefits and risks of testing have been explained to the patient during the informed consent process [10, 11]. This also ensures that genetic testing is voluntary. Although obtaining consent is primarily the responsibility of the referring clinician, the clinical molecular laboratory should consider requiring documentation of informed consent [2]. New York state law allows the health care professional to attest that consent has been received and kept in the patient medical record prior to testing. Proposed changes by the Centers for Disease Control and Prevention (CDC) to CLIA regulations specific for genetic testing include a requirement for laboratories to document informed consent prior to performing a genetic test [12]. However, since the CDC issued its Notice of Intent to add informed consent documentation to CLIA more than 10 years ago, the number of clinical genetic tests has increased substantially, but the proposed changes have not been finalized.

Confidentiality

Although GINA is a strong and essential first step in the fight against genetic discrimination and misuse of medical information, the sensitivity of and need for special protections for genetic test results is unclear. Some consider that genetic test results need the highest protections of health information, even beyond that provided by the Health Insurance Portability and Accountability Act of 1996 (HIPAA) [13]. The protections include only communicating genetic test results to the referring physician or genetic counselor [2], and even potentially not placing genetic test reports into the health care record of patients to avoid discrimination. Others consider the medical significance of genetic test results warrants these results being available in the health care record and feel that "genetic exceptionalism" is wrong and may prevent appropriate medical care. HIPAA requires that release of any patient information, especially to non-health care entities, must be authorized by the patient and documented. To ensure the confidentiality of genetic test results, some patients choose to personally pay for genetic testing rather than use health insurance, and clinical molecular laboratories should develop processes for handling such payments. The US Department of Health and Human Services (DHHS) has issued guidelines for ensuring the privacy of patients' health information as part of HIPAA [13]. Breach of patients' confidentiality for any type of health care information, not just for genetic information, can result in litigation against the individual and/or the institution.

Cancer

Hematopoietic Neoplasms

Molecular hematopathology refers to molecular testing for leukemias, lymphomas, multiple myeloma, and myelodysplastic conditions to identify somatic DNA alterations [14]. These DNA changes are present only in the affected population of hematopoietic cells and are not a part of the genetic makeup of the individual. The recent development in polymerase chain reaction (PCR) methods, particularly quantitative real-time PCR (qPCR), has provided greater diagnostic sensitivity and specificity for diagnostic testing, as well as for monitoring of disease during and after therapy. Likewise, the ability to perform molecular tests with very small amounts of nucleic acid has enabled the use of a wide range of sample types, including formalin-fixed, paraffin-embedded (FFPE) tissue specimens. For molecular testing, formalin fixation is optimal. In contrast to genetic tests, which need be performed only once for an individual, molecular oncology tests often are performed repeatedly for initial diagnosis and during and after treatment to monitor for residual disease. If testing is not performed at the time of diagnosis, later testing of the diagnostic specimen may be useful to confirm a molecular marker for minimal residual disease (MRD) testing. Molecular hematopathology results, whenever possible, are interpreted in the context of histopathology, flow cytometry, and clinical findings.

Solid Tumors

As the molecular rearrangements and mutations that cause specific solid tumor types are identified, the detection of these mutations is used for diagnosis, prognosis, therapy selection, and MRD assessment [15]. Many of these molecular rearrangements were identified through molecular characterization of specific chromosomal translocations identified by cytogenetic analysis of solid tumors, including bone and soft tissue sarcomas such as alveolar rhabdomyosarcoma, Ewing sarcoma, and synovial sarcoma. The expression of the fusion transcripts for the more common translocations can be detected by reverse transcription-polymerase chain reaction (RT-PCR) testing. The preferred specimen for sarcoma testing is frozen tissue because the optimal analyte is RNA, but in general, the majority of molecular diagnostic tests are performed on FFPE tissue specimens with DNA as the principal analyte. Specific somatic changes in solid tumors also can provide prognostic information. For example, genetic analysis for loss of heterozygosity on chromosomes 1p and 19q in oligodendroglioma tumors correlates with a better outcome [16]. Recently the development of new drugs targeted to specific genetic changes, such as anti-tyrosine kinase inhibitors (TKIs), has enabled the development of new tests such as *EGFR*, *KRAS*, and *BRAF* mutation testing that predict response to the targeted therapies. The tests, coupled to certain therapies, are called companion diagnostic tests and are used for evaluating the patient's tumor molecular profile prior to therapy initiation [17, 18]. The major laboratory issues specific to solid tumor testing today include: (1) the use of FFPE tissue specimens for mutation analysis, as formalin fixation greatly reduced the quality and integrity of DNA; (2) the careful selection of a FFPE tissue block with predominantly tumor cells or the use of macrodissection to reduce the nonmalignant cell population used for testing; and (3) working with small tissue specimens such as needle biopsies and fine needle aspiration specimens (FNAs). As next-generation sequencing (NGS) methods are increasingly used for solid tumor testing, TAT becomes an issue with oncologists needing the test results for selection and initiation of treatment, as well as the interpretation of large amount of data and variants of uncertain significance (VUS).

Infectious Diseases

As molecular techniques have become routine, more and more microorganisms are detected or characterized by molecular testing [16]. Molecular tests are especially suitable for infectious agents that are difficult to culture and for drug-resistance testing to provide more rapid diagnostic results. Molecular methods also are useful for viral quantitation as a part of monitoring response to therapy, such as human immunodeficiency virus type 1 (HIV-1), hepatitis C virus (HCV), and cytomegalovirus (CMV) infections. Because some infectious disease tests are high volume and have been clearly shown to improve patient management through therapy, automated instrumentation has been developed, and commercial test kits, including US FDA-cleared or -approved assays for many pathogen types are available. However, these commercial infectious disease test kits are expensive, and although improved patient outcomes due to early diagnosis and treatment may outweigh laboratory expenses, such savings for all infectious diseases have not been demonstrated.

Identity Testing and HLA Typing

Identity tests use polymorphic DNA markers to establish the identity of an individual or to determine an inheritance pattern [19]. Molecular identity testing is used for medical applications including analysis of bone marrow engraftment following bone marrow transplantation, and maternal cell contamination studies for prenatal genetic testing, as well as for paternity testing and forensic identity testing. Paternity and forensic identity testing, in particular, require additional considerations, including special accreditation (reviewed in

Table 62.1), director qualifications, verification of the identity of the person being tested, chain-of-custody documentation for the specimen, and expertise in complex probability calculations, reporting of results, and legal proceedings. HLA typing is time-sensitive, requires 24-h laboratory staffing, and involves complex analysis of the test results. Laboratories performing HLA typing require special accreditation by the American Society for Histocompatibility and Immunogenetics (ASHI) (Table 62.2).

Regulatory Agencies

All laboratories performing clinical testing must comply with numerous regulations. With the advent of CLIA [20], all laboratories are required to implement minimum quality and personnel standards. Proof of meeting these standards (accreditation), which may be done through voluntary accreditation programs offered by professional organizations, is critical to providing high-quality laboratory services. Clinical molecular laboratories are faced with special challenges due to the complex technical issues and ethical considerations involved in DNA-based testing. Several regulatory agencies are currently developing guidelines and standards for molecular pathology tests (Table 62.2). Some of these regulatory agencies and regulations are discussed below.

CLIA and CLIA'03

All clinical laboratories are regulated by CLIA. The US Congress passed CLIA to establish quality standards for all clinical laboratory testing to ensure the accuracy, reliability, and timeliness of patient test results [21]. CLIA is "test-site neutral," meaning that the same regulations apply to any location performing testing. Every laboratory examining "material derived from the human body for the purpose of providing information for the diagnosis, prevention, or treatment of any disease" is subject to CLIA. Final regulations to implement the law were published in 1992 in the Federal Register [22]. In 2003, new, extensively revised CLIA regulations were published and have been called CLIA'03, also termed the "Final Rules." The changes include major reorganization and consolidation of the regulations by basing requirements on the flow of a patient sample through the laboratory, updating the requirements to accommodate new technologies, and introducing a new quality control concept termed equivocal quality control (EQC), which empowers manufacturers to design instruments with internal quality assessment systems [23]. By this concept, laboratory directors alone, not manufacturers or regulators, must decide to adopt or eschew ECQ in their laboratory.

The CMS, formerly known as the Health Care Financing Administration (HCFA), in conjunction with the CDC, were originally charged with developing and enforcing the CLIA regulations. CMS continues to oversee much of these regulatory activities, including laboratory registration, on-site inspection, training, and accreditation.

CLIA certificates are based on the complexity of the test methods being performed by a clinical laboratory and are divided into three main categories: waived, moderate complexity, and high complexity. The level of complexity is determined by assigning a numerical score for each test or methodology based on numerous criteria including the knowledge, training, and experience required to perform the test, complexity of reagent and material preparation, characteristics of the operational steps, availability of calibrators, controls, and proficiency testing, equipment and test system troubleshooting, and interpretation of results. Under the CLIA'03 regulations, however, all quality control and quality assessment requirements now apply equally to high- and moderate-complexity laboratories, although some of the personnel qualifications remain more stringent for high-complexity laboratories [23]. These criteria are considered to be key elements in performing clinical testing and can be found on the US FDA Web site (http://www.fda.gov/).

Molecular pathology tests are considered high-complexity tests and as such must comply with CLIA requirements. Some of the requirements for high-complexity tests include qualifications of personnel performing and overseeing the testing, procedure manual specifications, method performance verification specifications, proficiency testing, quality assurance, patient test management, and inspection. CLIA, however, does not provide specific guidelines for molecular testing, and, therefore, each clinical molecular laboratory is responsible for the development of a test and quality management program according to CLIA criteria.

Voluntary Accreditation Organizations

CLIA regulations allow CMS to approve nonprofit, professional organizations that have laboratory testing and inspection standards equivalent to or more stringent than the CLIA regulations to inspect clinical laboratories in place of CLIA inspection. The two major organizations providing CLIA inspections are the Joint Commission on Accreditation of Healthcare Organizations (the Joint Commission), which accredits more than 80 % of the US health care organizations, and the Laboratory Accreditation Program of the College of American Pathologists (LAP-CAP). The majority of clinical molecular laboratories are inspected and accredited by LAP-CAP. Other CLIA accrediting organizations include AABB, American Association for Laboratory Accreditation, American Osteopathic Association, ASHI, and COLA. When a test site meets the accrediting agency's requirements, as assessed by inspection, the laboratory, in essence, is meeting CLIA requirements and receives a CLIA certificate.

The College of American Pathologists

LAP-CAP accredits only clinical laboratories and not entire health care organizations. LAP-CAP does not base its requirements for accreditation on the different CLIA complexity levels of testing; instead it requires that all testing laboratories adhere to the same guidelines. LAP-CAP lists its requirements and guidelines in checklists, each consisting of a series of laboratory guideline questions. All laboratories must follow the Laboratory General checklist as well as the specific laboratory checklists relevant to the testing performed in the clinical laboratory, such as microbiology, blood bank, and other laboratory specialty sections. In addition to general requirements concerning personnel qualifications, quality control, test performance verification, and operation-related guidelines similar to CLIA, the Molecular Pathology checklist also includes test- and application-specific guidelines. The Molecular Pathology checklist also contains specific standards for tests using NGS methods, and addresses both the testing steps to generate the sequence data, the bioinformatics steps used for sequence analysis and variant calling, and the reporting of results. LAP-CAP requires laboratories to have a procedure manual for each test or process that complies with the GP2-3A standards of the Clinical and Laboratory Standards Institute (CLSI; formerly National Committee for Clinical Laboratory Standards, NCCLS) [24]. Clinical laboratories accredited by the CAP, as required by CLIA, also, for each test performed, must participate in a proficiency testing program when available, or perform internal proficiency checks when an external proficiency testing program is not available. Currently CAP inspections are performed every 2 years and are unannounced, with a self-inspection on alternate years.

The New York State Department of Health

The New York State Department of Health (NYSDOH) provides regulatory oversight of all clinical laboratories performing testing of any type on any specimen from a New York resident. The Clinical Laboratory Evaluation Program (CLEP) at Wadsworth Center in Albany, NY, seeks to ensure the accuracy and reliability of results of laboratory tests on specimens obtained within the state through on-site inspections, proficiency testing, and evaluation of the qualifications of personnel of state permit-holding clinical laboratories. NYS Public Health Law Article 5, Title V, requires the licensure of clinical laboratories by establishing minimum qualifications for directors, and by requiring that the performance of all procedures employed by the clinical laboratories meet minimum standards accepted and approved by the NYSDOH. The New York State Clinical Laboratory Technology Practice Act that became effective in 2008 requires that all clinical laboratory technologists and technicians, cytotechnologists, and histological technicians meet specific training requirements and be licensed by the state. However, because of the high complexity of molecular and cytogenetic testing and the lack of adequately trained staff through medical technology training programs, a limited license in molecular pathology or cytogenetics is provided for training under the direction of the laboratory director with qualification for a full license based on training and experience within a molecular laboratory. The clinical laboratory license requirements have been established for laboratories located in or accepting laboratory specimens originating from NYS. CLEP currently issues annual permits to over 1,000 laboratories in NYS. In addition, CLEP provides, on a biennial basis, approximately 3,100 certificates of qualification (CoQs) to individuals to serve as directors and assistant directors of clinical laboratories, which requires either specific training or experience to oversee testing of specific types across the clinical laboratory. A NYSDOH license is issued by testing category, following an on-site inspection. The clinical laboratory must have someone with a CoQ for each category of testing being performed. Finally, NYSDOH requires any test which is not US FDA-approved or -cleared and performed according to the manufacturer's instructions to be approved by the NYSDOH. This test review and approval is frequently required of clinical molecular laboratories because fewer of the tests are US FDA-approved or -cleared. Specific NGS test validation guidelines and requirements have been developed by the NYSDOH. More information about CLEP, NYSDOH regulatory oversight programs, and test approval policies can be found on NYSDOH Web site (http://www.wadsworth.org/).

The US Food and Drug Administration

The US FDA oversees regulation of medical devices under the 1938 Federal Food, Drug, and Cosmetics Act and subsequent amendments. Unless specifically exempted, medical devices must "be properly labeled and packaged, be cleared for marketing by the US FDA, meet their labeling claims, and be manufactured under Good Manufacturing Practices (GMP), which is a mandated quality assurance system."

These rules concerning the design, manufacturing, marketing, and surveillance of medical devices can be found in the Code for Federal Regulations (CFR). The US FDA also oversees some of the functions related to laboratory operations, including classification of tests as required by CLIA and review of clinical laboratory test kits or systems.

The US FDA and Genetic Testing

The recent growth of genetic testing, mostly developed and performed by individual clinical molecular laboratories without US FDA review, has raised public concerns about the quality and clinical usefulness of these tests. The Secretary's Advisory Committee on Genetic Testing (SACGT) was established in 1998 to advise the secretary of the DHHS on medical, scientific, ethical, legal, and social issues raised by the development and use of genetic testing. The SACGT, in conjunction with the Clinical Laboratory Improvement Advisory Committee (CLIAC), recommended that the US FDA provide regulatory oversight of laboratory-developed genetic tests. The vast majority of genetic testing is performed using laboratory developed assays rather than by commercial US FDA-approved or -cleared test kits, raising concerns about the quality and clinical usefulness of these tests. As the first step in developing a review process for LDTs, the US FDA developed a "test review template" for gathering data on the use, performance, interpretation, and reporting of LDTs [25]. Although this template was well received by SACGT, the US FDA was concerned that LTDs were part of medical practice, which is not regulated by the US FDA, and did not develop a review mechanism for LDTs at that time. The successor committee to the SACGT, the Secretary's Advisory Committee on Genetics, Health, and Society (SACGHS), was formed in 2001 and served for 10 years. The SACGHS studied the regulatory oversight of genetic LDTs, and their report provides an overview of the oversight system [26]. Both the Association for Molecular Pathology (AMP) and the CAP have developed proposals for the oversight and strengthening of LDT regulation, after the US FDA announced in 2009 an intention to abandon its regulatory policy of enforcement discretion toward some LDTs. The US FDA has published preliminary guidelines for the oversight of LDTs which will be based on the complexity of the test, with the most high-risk tests requiring US FDA review.

Analyte-Specific Reagents

Although the majority of the US FDA regulations for clinical assays target commercially developed in vitro diagnostic test kits intended for clinical use, the US FDA issued regulations for commercial reagents used in LDTs in 1997 [27, 28]. Although these regulations are not specific for molecular tests, many tests in the clinical molecular laboratory are developed, validated, and performed without the use of US FDA-approved test kits. These tests are distinct from research assays that have unproven clinical utility and cannot be used for patient care. In 1997, the US FDA developed regulations for manufacturers of reagents used in LDTs, as well as the clinical laboratories using such reagents in their LDTs. These reagents, termed "analyte-specific reagents" (ASRs), serve as the key component for LDTs including molecular pathology tests, and include primers or probes that hybridize to specific DNA sequences. The manufacturers of ASRs are prohibited from making statements about the analytic or clinical performance or the recommended use of the reagents, and validation of tests using ASRs is the responsibility of the laboratory. The laboratory must include a disclaimer in the patient report stating, "This test was developed and its performance characteristics determined by (laboratory name). It has not been cleared or approved by the US Food and Drug Administration." The result of the ASR regulations has been an increase in the availability of commercial reagents for molecular pathology tests; however, in the past few years the US FDA has been moving towards in vitro diagnostics (IVDs) and eliminating ASRs whenever possible [29].

Elements of Laboratory Design

Successful laboratory operation requires optimal utilization of space, appropriate equipment, qualified personnel, adequate laboratory information system (LIS) support, and financial management.

Facilities

The power of molecular testing is achieved by the use of PCR as the main diagnostic procedure. A serious problem in the clinical use of PCR is false-positive amplification due to PCR contamination. Because the products of PCR amplification, called an amplicons, can serve as the substrate for the generation of additional PCR products, and because PCR amplification produces a very large number of amplicons, the potential contamination of subsequent amplifications of the same target sequence with amplicons resulting in inaccurate results is immense without the use of proper controls. This kind of contamination has been termed "carryover" to differentiate it from contamination by genomic DNA. This potential for PCR product contamination requires special precautions. Therefore, the single most important step in designing laboratory space for molecular pathology testing is meticulous attention to the physical separation of the pre-PCR and post-PCR work areas to minimize PCR contamination [30].

The pre-PCR area, also referred to as a "clean room" or "pre-amplification area," is used for the pre-PCR steps of sample receiving and processing, including extraction of nucleic acids and setting up of amplification reactions. The post-PCR area, also considered a "dirty room" or "post-amplification area," is used for PCR amplification and analysis of PCR products. The pre-PCR laboratory ideally contains separate work areas for nucleic acid extractions and PCR setup to minimize cross-contamination of patient nucleic acid samples. Additionally, a containment unit, such as a biosafety cabinet, may be used for setting up PCR reactions. These cabinets usually are equipped with ultraviolet light for reducing DNA contamination of the work area at the end of reaction setup. Some clinical molecular laboratories prefer to further separate the various steps of the pre- and post-PCR areas into separate rooms.

If possible, the air system for the pre-PCR and post-PCR areas should be independent. Otherwise, air filters can be installed in the inflow to the pre-PCR room air system, which can be cleaned routinely. An additional measure to limit PCR contamination is to maintain the pre- PCR and post-PCR rooms at different air pressures. The pre-PCR area is maintained at positive pressure, reducing the entrance of airborne contaminants and PCR products, while the post-PCR room is maintained at negative pressure, reducing contaminants that exit the room. If installation of a pressure system is not possible, then the two work areas can be located at a relative distance from each other.

To comply with universal blood-borne pathogen precautions, nucleic acid extraction from patient specimens can be performed in a closed safety cabinet. Specimens known to contain infectious agents, such as HIV-1 and HCV, can be processed in a separate biological safety hood. If organic solvents such as phenol, chloroform, or xylenes are used, a chemical fume hood should be available in the work area. Within the pre-PCR laboratory, RNA extractions should be physically separated from DNA extraction if the DNA extraction procedure uses RNase, which can degrade RNA. All work areas should be cleaned daily with 10 % bleach solution. In addition to pre-PCR and post-PCR areas, the clinical molecular laboratory also may have a neutral reagent preparation area (unless reagents are separately prepared in both rooms) and a data management room for the processing, review, and reporting of test results, which also may be performed in the post-PCR area.

To maximize use of space, equipment, technical expertise, and trained technologists, all types of molecular pathology testing (genetics, infectious disease, cancer, and identity testing) can be consolidated into a single laboratory. Implementing a core molecular pathology laboratory can reduce labor costs by approximately 30 % [31] as well as reduce equipment costs and space requirements due to duplication of these resources in several laboratories. As more infectious disease testing systems have become available, molecular infectious disease testing is more commonly performed in the microbiology laboratory rather than a molecular laboratory, although this is institution-specific.

PCR Contamination Control

In addition to physical separation of the pre-PCR and post-PCR areas, specific procedures are recommended for use of PCR in the clinical laboratory. To ensure that PCR products are not transferred from the post-PCR to the pre-PCR area, each should contain separate supplies and equipment. Pipettes, instruments, and supplies should not be transferred from the post-PCR to the pre-PCR area. This separation of supplies and equipment also dictates the workflow in the laboratory. PCR samples are first set up in the pre-PCR area and then transferred to the post-PCR area for PCR amplification and post-PCR analysis. Worksheets, once moved to the post-PCR area for post-PCR analysis, can no longer be taken back into the pre-PCR area and must be processed and filed in the post-PCR area or a neutral area.

Reagents and solutions for sample preparation and PCR work should be prepared with type I water, which is defined by specific ion, pH, and contaminant limitation requirements. All reagents, except primers, deoxynucleotide triphosphates (dNTPs), and enzymes, should be purchased as sterile reagents or sterilized to prevent bacterial growth. Reagents, including autoclaved type I water and 10 mM Tris–1 mM EDTA buffer (TE) used to dissolve DNA, should be stored as small aliquots to minimize the number of samplings from the same aliquot. Similarly, oligonucleotides used for PCR amplification should be synthesized and purified in a clean environment. To minimize the number of sample transfers and the chance of sporadic contamination and errors, PCR reagents, including primers, dNTPs and buffers, can be combined into a "premixture master mix" (MM), divided into aliquots that are appropriately labeled, and stored at −20 °C [30]. Before using for clinical testing, a new lot of MM must be tested to ensure that it specifically amplifies the target sequence without producing PCR products in the negative "minus DNA" controls, as is done for new lots of any reagents in the clinical laboratory. A "minus DNA" negative control not containing any specimen DNA is tested last in each run to ensure the lack of DNA or amplicon contamination in the PCR reagents.

Although carryover of amplified sequences contributes to the majority of false positives, cross-contamination can occur between samples, especially from specimens containing a high level of the target sequence such as occurs with infectious disease specimens. Consequently, precautions must be taken not only during the setup of PCR amplification reactions but also in all aspects of sample handling, from sample collection to sample extraction. For good laboratory practice, gloves should be changed frequently, at least when entering or reentering the pre-PCR area and whenever the technologist notes the gloves to have been contaminated. Technologists should wear protective clothes to prevent operator-borne spread of contaminating DNA products, with separate protective clothes (i.e., laboratory coats) for the pre-PCR and post-PCR areas.

To minimize aerosolization of PCR products, PCR tubes should be pulse-centrifuged before opening. Microcentrifuge tube caps should be opened using both hands, and not flicked open with the thumb of the same hand, to prevent aerosolization. Because cross-contamination of pipettors can lead to false-positive results, and to minimize aerosolization, aerosol barrier tips are used for all pre-PCR steps. MM and other non-sample components should be added to the reaction tubes before the specimen DNA is added; DNA should be added last and each tube capped before the technologist proceeds to the addition of specimen DNA to the next sample. Positive and negative control DNA or RNA should be the last reaction tubes to be set up, after the patient sample reactions are set up and closed.

Another approach to minimize carryover of PCR products is to synthesize all PCR products with deoxyuridine triphosphate (dUTP) in place of deoxythymidine triphosphate (dTTP). Prior to amplification, the PCR reactions are treated with uracil-N-glycosylase (UNG), which will degrade uracil-containing amplicons, allowing amplification only from thymidine-containing target DNA [32]. Some commercial test kits incorporate this process into the kits.

Finally, automation of DNA extraction as well as PCR setup by the use of automated, robotic nucleic acid extractors and liquid handlers has greatly facilitated standardization of testing, reducing PCR contamination, and increasing overall testing accuracy and reliability of results. Real-time PCR technology, in particular, provided additional tools for PCR contamination control by combining PCR amplification with amplicon analysis and thus eliminating aerosolization of PCR products due to manipulation of PCR products [33].

Equipment

The equipment used for clinical molecular testing is rarely manufactured for clinical use. Most equipment is designed for research purposes and adapted for clinical use [30]. Nucleic acid extractions may be performed manually, although for higher volume testing, automated extraction instruments are available with improved reproducibility and reduced technologist time for the clinical laboratory. PCR can be set up manually in biosafety cabinets; for higher-volume testing, robotic liquid handling systems are available. Robotic systems, however, have reagent dead volumes that increase reagent wastage. Thermal cyclers are standard equipment in the molecular pathology laboratory, and the number required depends on the work volume. Post-PCR analysis is highly variable, and is based on the types of PCR product analysis being performed.

Other specialized equipment for post-PCR analysis includes automated sequencers or capillary electrophoresis instruments, chemiluminescent or colorimetric plate readers, and real-time PCR instruments. However, numerous clinical tests have been approved by the US FDA. These assays use commercial kits and specialized equipment for automated extraction and viral load quantitation, usually supplied by the test kit manufacturer [34]. Recently, with the advent of NGS technology, high-throughput sequencing instruments have been developed for simultaneous analysis of thousands of genes to exomes to genomes [35, 36]. Guidelines and checklists for NGS test validation and performance have been developed by both the CAP and NYSDOH [37]. Because of the high level of testing complexity and the concern of PCR contamination, researchers or personnel not trained in clinical molecular testing requirements and processes should not use the clinical molecular equipment.

Automated platforms for molecular tests are becoming available and are more significant for the clinical laboratory as test volumes increase. Automated systems include extraction systems, as well as real-time thermal cyclers that combine PCR amplification and detection. Automated systems are routinely and widely used for viral load testing, such as for HIV-1 and HCV viral load testing. Automated instrumentation can greatly reduce TAT, human error, and technologist time.

Because nonclinical instruments are used for clinical testing, they require rigorous surveillance and prompt technical support by manufacturers who are not always aware of the critical clinical testing issues. In addition, these instruments require ongoing maintenance. Most maintenance procedures are defined by the manufacturer and include temperature checks of the PCR wells for thermal cyclers and calibration of pipettors. In the absence of manufacturer's guidelines, the laboratory should set up its own maintenance program in consultation with the manufacturer.

Laboratory Personnel

Personnel Qualifications

Effective laboratory operation requires well-trained staff and a good management team. CLIA regulations specify that for high-complexity testing, individuals for the positions of director, technical supervisor, and testing staff must have specific qualifications. The director, as named on the CLIA certificate, is required to be a licensed doctor of medicine, osteopathy, or podiatry or have a doctoral degree in one of the biological, chemical, physical, or medical sciences, and have 2 years of experience supervising a high-complexity laboratory. In NY, laboratories holding or applying for a NYSDOH clinical laboratory permit must also have a director or assistant director holding a CoQ for each testing category. To qualify for a CoQ, an individual must comply with CLIA requirements, in addition to having board certification in the appropriate specialty and working experience, with at least 2 years in current methodology in each category sought and in general laboratory management documented in the form of recommendation letters. The laboratory director is responsible for the overall operation and administration of the laboratory either personally or through oversight of assistant directors. Overall operation and administration of the laboratory includes the development, validation, and implementation of new tests, current procedure manuals, quality control, and training programs for staff, and teaching residents.

The technical supervisor establishes the quality standards of the laboratory by selecting and monitoring methods and instruments and documenting the competency of laboratory personnel, while the general supervisor provides day-to-day supervision of testing, personnel, and reporting of results. The qualifications for these positions range from a licensed doctor to an individual holding a bachelor's degree in science plus specific training or experience or both. The laboratory also may have clinical consultants, who must hold a medical or doctoral degree in a relevant discipline with appropriate experience in molecular testing. The Genetic Testing Good Laboratory Practices Workgroup of CLIAC, created in 1998, reviewed personnel qualifications and recommended including specific genetic experience and board certification for supervisors who oversee genetic testing [25].

Testing personnel who perform high-complexity testing must have an associate's degree in laboratory science or medical laboratory technology, or education and training equivalent to an associate's degree. Laboratory technologists are responsible for all tasks associated with the daily operation of the laboratory, including specimen receiving and processing, testing, identifying problems and troubleshooting, maintaining equipment, and documenting quality control procedures. In addition, they are required to work according to established procedures in adherence with the quality control standards implemented in the laboratory to comply with CLIA, CAP, or other regulations. Because very few molecular tests are approved by the US FDA, molecular pathology technologists perform much of the development of new tests, as well as validation of commercial molecular kits used for clinical molecular testing.

Because of the high level of desired expertise, technologists also need to be encouraged to attend educational courses to obtain the appropriate background in molecular pathology and the skills required for performing these tests. For the same reason, it is also crucial for the senior management of the laboratory to acknowledge the staff, encourage personal growth, and create new mechanisms for promotion. Although some of these recommendations represent the authors' personal views and may present a burden in the stringent financial environment of many health care institutions, the cost of training new technologists is higher than that of creating an environment that promotes job satisfaction and employee retention.

Genetic Counselors

The role of the genetic counselor is to assess the need for genetic testing through obtaining a medical and family history, inform patients about the risks and benefits of specific genetic tests, order the tests, and communicate the results to the patient and their family, as appropriate. Although the genetic counselor is traditionally a part of the clinical medical genetics service, an increasing number of test sites have genetic counselors on their staff as a link between the patient and health care providers with the laboratory.

Resident and Fellow Training in Molecular Pathology

Pathology residency training programs are required to provide molecular pathology training to their residents. Because the molecular biology knowledge and practical molecular experience of pathology residents is highly variable, the AMP Training and Education Committee generated general molecular pathology training goals for pathology resident training programs. These goals include basic knowledge in human genetics and molecular biology which are relevant to all aspects of molecular testing, specific technology information, as well as knowledge of specific molecular pathology tests [38]. Because molecular pathology training time can be brief (1–3 months), training may need to be accomplished through didactic lectures that encompass the tests performed in the laboratory as well as basic concepts in molecular pathology and technology, rather than more extensive practical experience.

Education of molecular pathology fellows requires broader training, resources, and time. The increasing importance of this field for clinical practice and the desire to undergo formal molecular pathology training led to the development of fellowship training programs and professional certification by several professional boards, specifically the American Board of Medical Genetics (ABMG) and the American Board of Pathology (ABP). Official training programs in clinical molecular genetics, established by the ABMG, and in molecular genetic pathology (MGP; jointly established by the ABMG and the ABP) are accredited by the Accreditation Committee on Graduate Medical Education (ACMGE). Official accreditation of either type of training program requires filing of a program application and review and on-site formal inspection by an ACMGE representative [39]. The goal of these fellowship training programs is to provide structured education for qualified individuals seeking to integrate molecular genetic pathology into their clinical practice experience in all current aspects of the field, including basic science, diagnostic laboratory procedures, laboratory management, and consultation. To be eligible for the board examination, fellows should have a strong background in molecular biology and molecular genetics as well as practical experience, and should be able to use this information for diagnosis and management of genetic disorders for clinical molecular genetics board certification, as well as infectious diseases, malignancies, identity testing, and HLA typing for MGP board certification. Guidelines for competency-based fellowship training in MGP as well as for the development of a new MGP program have been developed by the AMP Training and Education Committee and Directors of MGP Programs [40].

Residents and fellows can contribute significantly to the daily operation of the laboratory, including review of test results under the supervision of the laboratory director, acquisition of clinical information, and communication of test results. In addition, they can assist with the development and implementation of new tests, according to the skill level of the trainee and as time permits. In return, they gain new expertise that may be an advantage when seeking employment.

Staff Training and Accreditation Programs

Appropriate technical staff training is vital to the successful operation of a molecular pathology laboratory [39]. Accreditation programs in medical genetics and molecular pathology ensure that members of the laboratory staff are well trained for performing their assigned roles. Individuals who want to practice clinical molecular pathology have several career pathway options, depending on their initial education.

Individuals who hold a medical or doctoral degree and are interested in directing a molecular pathology laboratory can be certified by the ABMG. ABMG is a member of the American Board of Medical Specialists (ABMS) that provides certification for all medical specialties. Eligibility for certification in clinical molecular genetics by the ABMG requires a doctoral degree (M.D. or Ph.D.) and 2 years of training in an accredited medical genetics program, plus completion of a logbook that documents the trainees' involvement in at least 150 clinical molecular genetic cases, which must be signed by the director of the training program. Certification requires passing a general examination in medical genetics as well as a subspecialty examination in clinical molecular genetics. The examinations are offered every 2 years.

In 1999, the ABMS approved a new MGP subspecialty offered jointly by the ABMG and the ABP. Candidates for this certification must hold a medical degree, have board certification in either medical genetics or pathology (either anatomic or clinical pathology, or both), have a valid license to practice medicine in the USA, and have completed a year of training in an accredited MGP fellowship training program. The first MGP examination was given in 2001, and is now given twice per year. MGP training programs are accredited based on standards developed jointly by the ABP and the ABMG. Diplomates of the ABMG and/or ABMG/ABP are certified for a period of 10 years, after which they are required to participate in a Maintenance of Certification (MOC) program. Participation in MOC begins as soon as certification is granted. The procedures and requirements are described on the ABMG and ABP websites under MOC. MOC is required for all new diplomates to maintain their board certification and individual MOC information is public.

The American Board of Clinical Chemistry (ABCC) has a certification program in molecular diagnosis, offered for the first time in 2000. This certification is offered biannually to individuals who hold doctoral degrees and practice in any one of several clinical laboratory specialties.

Certification in molecular biology is offered to medical and molecular biology technologists by the National Credentialing Agency for Laboratory Personnel, Inc. (NCA). The examination is given biannually and is useful for clinical molecular laboratory staff, particularly the senior technical staff who become certified laboratory specialists in molecular biology. The American Society of Clinical Pathology certifies technical staff as a technologist in molecular pathology, based on qualification for and passing an examination.

Financial Management

Molecular pathology testing is a market with growing gross revenue, which requires an understanding of the influence of finances on the technical aspects of the laboratory. Because many clinical molecular pathology laboratories are part of health care systems, molecular pathology test payment often is subject to limiting managed care contracts and reduced reimbursements, and as such, are often viewed as cost centers. Molecular pathology laboratory management should develop cost-effective business plans that present molecular pathology testing in the context of the clinical programs the testing supports, if the testing is not independently cost-effective, such that hospital administration views the laboratory as a revenue center.

Cost Analysis

In the current restrictive medical economic environment, the decision to perform a specific test must include business (financial) as well as medical considerations. The evaluation process for deciding to implement a new test or deciding to discontinue a current test should include a cost analysis. The amount charged for a test is determined mostly by the costs of performing the test and the value of the test in the market (demand). A cost analysis should account for all expenses associated with performing a given test, both direct and indirect. In a structured approach, a standard template can be developed and used to set a price for any new test, based on the cost for each step of the testing process, plus standard indirect costs.

Cost analysis involves two main types of expenses: direct expenses and indirect expenses [41]. The direct expenses enumerate all costs directly related to the testing, including equipment, reagents, consumables, salary, and benefits. The calculation of reagent costs is based on the known volume of reagent used and the cost per volume, including reagents for controls, dead volumes, and wasted reagents due to expiration or other causes. For manual, low-volume testing, the largest component of direct cost is labor, which can comprise up to 90 % of the total direct test cost. Laboratory labor cost calculations are generally done using the hands-on technologist time needed to perform the test multiplied by an average hourly salary rate plus the appropriate benefit rate. For example, the cost for a PCR-based test should take into consideration the time required for specimen accessioning and storage, DNA extraction, PCR setup, post-PCR analysis (if required), technical interpretation, and entry of results into the LIS, to determine the average hours of technologist time per testing run, which is divided by the number of samples tested at the same time to reach the labor cost per test.

Indirect costs include overhead, such as licensing fees, royalties or licensing fees, supervisory and administrative salaries, equipment maintenance fees, building services (such as electricity, phones, heating, etc.), marketing, and LIS support requirements. These costs are more difficult to determine and are not usually a part of the routine cost analysis for academic laboratories. Accurate determination of laboratory costs is important for assessing profitability.

Billing

Billing for molecular pathology tests follows the same guidelines as billing for other pathology laboratory services, requiring a Current Procedural Terminology (CPT) code for the test performed and an International Classification of Diseases (ICD- 9-CM) diagnostic code to determine the necessity for the test. The ICD-9 code, which is required for payment, should be provided by the requesting physician when a test is ordered, while the pathologist is responsible for using the appropriate CPT codes for billing of test services. Traditional CPT coding of molecular pathology tests, other than most molecular infectious disease tests which have single test-specific CPT codes, have described a molecular procedure rather than a specific method, and billing was based on a combination of several combined CPT codes for the various procedural steps that are performed as part of a molecular test. For tests requiring professional interpretation, the professional component was coded using an interpretation and report CPT code with a modifier code to differentiate the professional billing from the technical component, reported with a "TC." Under the old system, CPT codes were not test specific, could be billed multiple times for a single test as appropriate for the testing method, and created difficulties for payers to understand the test performed and the medical purpose of the test. By describing the work done but not the specific test, the previous molecular procedure-based CPT codes created a non-transparent system. To this end, the American Medical Association (AMA) created a series of new CPT codes for molecular tests that are test specific and the molecular procedure-based codes are no longer in use. A copy of the final rule can be found on the Federal Register Web site [42].

The molecular test CPT billing codes as of 2013 are a two-tiered system. Tier 1 represents more than 95 % of the molecular test volume performed in the USA, while Tier 2 contains nine levels based on test complexity for less commonly performed and more specialized tests. These codes are on the Clinical Laboratory Fee Schedule (CLFS) of CMS, rather than the Physician Fee Schedule (PFS) as requested by the CAP. Self-assignment of codes for tests is not allowed. A new not-otherwise-specified (NOS) code is available for unspecified analytes or emerging tests. The CPT codes will be maintained by a molecular pathology advisory panel (MPAP) advising the AMA CPT Editorial Panel. Code proposals also are reviewed by the Pathology Coding Caucus before submission to the AMA for review and approval. New CPT codes for genomic and multi-gene tests have been approved for use as of January 2015. A complete list of the CPT codes can be found in the *Physician's Current Procedural Manual*, published by the AMA [43]. Pathogen-specific codes for molecular infectious disease tests, such as HIV-1, HCV, and hepatitis B virus (HBV) viral loads, for which all steps of the procedure (extraction, amplification, detection, and reagents) are covered by a single CPT code, have remained the same.

Reimbursement for molecular pathology tests is dictated, to a large extent, by the reimbursement policies of CMS, which historically are used as a guideline for payment by third-party payers such as insurance companies. US FDA approval is not necessary for billing of molecular pathology tests, but payment now or in the future may be linked to US FDA approval of a test, especially with the new guidelines for US FDA oversight of LDTs.

Patents

Another consideration prior to the implementation of a new test is the patent status of the test. Patents can cover instruments and reagents, but also can cover a specific method of testing for an analyte, any method of testing for an analyte, or a mutation-gene-disease association in general. The most common royalty payments for molecular pathology laboratories are payments for the use of the PCR method and *Taq* polymerase, licensed by Roche Diagnostics, Inc. Many diagnostic tests use PCR. Royalty payments for use of *Taq* polymerase ranged from 9–15 % of the amount billed or reimbursed for a test, and generally are higher for commercial laboratories than for academic laboratories. Although the original patent expired on March 2005, legal arguments in the industry over the use of *Taq* polymerase are still ongoing.

Of special concern are patenting and licensing of patents for mutations in specific genes associated with disease. Examples of such patents include apolipoprotein E genotyping for Alzheimer disease, T- and B-cell receptor gene rearrangement testing, and the hereditary breast cancer genes, *BRCA1* and *BRCA2*. Patenting of genes and gene-disease associations poses a significant risk to the molecular pathology laboratory because many clinically relevant DNA sequences are patented, and the terms of use offered by the holders vary considerably; in some instances, a laboratory will be unable to perform a test because the patent is exclusively licensed to another laboratory [44]. Thus, a laboratory considering implementation of a new molecular test first may conduct searches of existing patents and patent applications to see whether the new test infringes on existing or pending patents. Typically, such searches, if performed, are done by patent attorneys employed by the medical center where the laboratory is located. Internet resources provided by the US Patent and Trademark Office (http://www.uspto.gov) allow laboratories to perform searches directly. If a patent exists that covers any part of the molecular test to be implemented, the laboratory or medical center must negotiate an agreement for clinical testing with the patent holder or licensee, if the patent holder will grant a license. Licensing agreements may include royalty payments that increase the cost of the test, and limitations on the use of the test or the volume of testing the laboratory can perform. For this reason, many molecular pathology leaders argue that patented genetic tests should be broadly licensed at affordable costs to allow any qualified clinical laboratory to perform the tests. Professional societies of pathologists, such as CAP and AMP, have criticized patents on disease genes and exclusive licenses to perform DNA diagnostic tests. In the 2009 lawsuit against Myriad, doctors and pathologists presented arguments that the patents on the *BRCA1* and *BRCA2* genes and the gene-disease association prevented patients from receiving second opinions on their test results and prevented laboratories from performing diagnostic tests on patient samples and interpreting the results. Although initially the US District Court for the Southern District of New York ruled that all the challenged claims were not patentable subject matter, the case was appealed to the US Court of Appeals for the Federal Circuit, which overturned the previous decision in part, ruling that isolated DNA which does not exist alone in nature *can* be patented. As of December 2012 isolated genes remained patentable in the USA; however, on November 30, 2012, the US Supreme Court agreed to hear the case, which eventually led to a unanimous decision of the US Supreme Court that genes are not patentable. In the same decision, the Court decided that complementary DNA (cDNA), which is DNA copied from RNA, is not found in nature and is made by man and therefore is patent-eligible matter. This continues to allow patent enforcements against clinical molecular laboratories, although patent cases have not supported the patent eligibility of cDNA to date.

Laboratory Information Systems

Most molecular pathology laboratories require a computer information system to handle the large volume of data that is both received and reported. Selecting and installing a LIS is a lengthy and labor-intensive process, usually performed by the department or institution rather than by the laboratory. The application software allows users to perform tasks that are specific to the laboratory operations [45]. These tasks include registering patients, accessioning specimens, ordering laboratory tests, reporting test results, and tracking quality control data (Fig. 62.1). In addition, the LIS facilitates use of appropriate templates for reporting of results. The primary function of the LIS is the management of the database of patients and laboratory test results. The most-used system is a relational database management system, which links all the data in tables related to one another by common elements. This kind of structure allows the technologist, for example, to quickly produce a list of only those patient specimens that are going be tested for a particular test. When two or more tables contain the same primary field (patient identifier), information can be retrieved from multiple tables. For example, to monitor engraftment after allogeneic bone marrow transplant, the entire list of test results and dates of testing can be obtained for any specific patient. Because departmental LIS systems have not traditionally been designed to meet the specific information requirements of

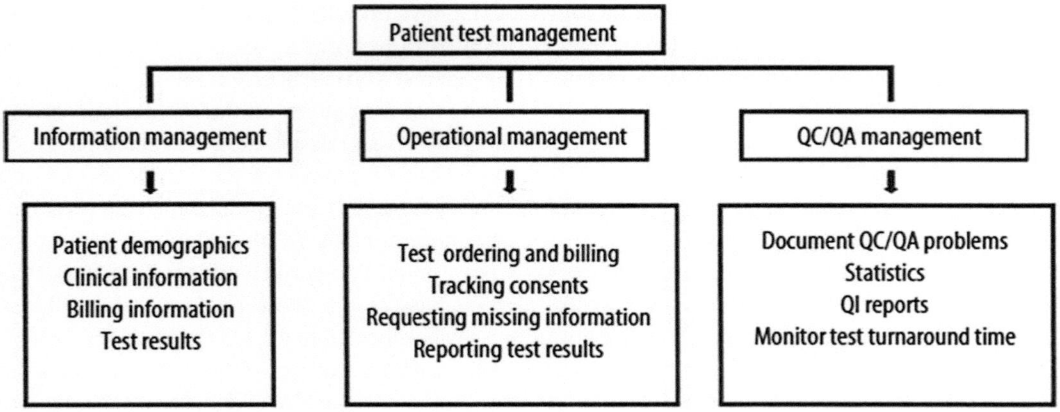

Figure 62.1 Organizational chart for LIS-based molecular pathology testing management

the molecular pathology laboratory, many molecular pathology laboratories also use networked personal computers (PCs) for data management. These PCs are mostly used as tools for running standard applications, such as word processing, spreadsheets, and other specialized applications, such as DNA sequence analysis and genetic risk-assessment applications. Since, however, molecular pathology laboratories have unique data management requirements, a separate patient database may be maintained in the laboratory as an electronic searchable database. Several systems have developed that accommodate the unique workflow and complex data capture needs of the molecular pathology laboratory. These systems, such as Millennium Helix™ (CERNER, Kansas City, MO), have been designed specifically for molecular testing for infectious diseases and molecular genetics by supporting the documentation of mutation results, numeric results associated with short tandem repeat markers, and viral load results. The *Unified Case Manager*™ in Helix, for example, allows the ability to create individual worksheets associated with the case and to view the succession of activities associated with the case. The application also contains bioinformatics coded values from the *Clinical Bioinformatics Ontology*™ (CBO) that enables the use of standard vocabulary for describing molecular and cytogenetic concepts.

To reduce transcription errors and eliminate the labor-intensive work of retyping patient information and test results, the LIS can interface with laboratory instruments for direct transfer of test results for each patient. This has been successfully implemented for specific instruments, such as the COBAS AmpliPrep system (Roche Diagnostics Pleasanton, CA) for HIV-1, HCV, and HBV viral load testing. The results, collated with the patient and specimen identification, are automatically transferred to the LIS, followed by performance and verification by laboratory personnel and report release and transfer to the electronic medical record system for clinical use. For instruments where a direct link is not available the use of a "flat file" of test data can assist in transfer of data from the instrument to the LIS using patient accession numbers.

To improve laboratory operations, many quality control activities can be performed using the LIS, including monitoring of TAT, control results, and statistics. Procedures and other documentation can be maintained and managed by the laboratory computer as well. Security and access control are crucial components of the LIS. Access control (passwords) and patient confidentiality (limiting access to only those who need specific information) are some of the tools required to maintain patient information security. Finally, NGS data pose a special challenge. The large volumes of data produced by NGS platforms, in addition to the requirements for documentation, data storage, interpretation of sequencing variations, as well as appropriate algorithms for reporting of results, require special software and system considerations.

Test Management

Choice of Test Menu

The menu of tests performed by molecular pathology laboratories varies significantly and is determined by three principal factors: clinical requirement and usefulness, laboratory competency, and test costs. Other factors that affect the decision about adding a new test include the prevalence of the disease, the mutation(s) causing the disease, the number of different mutations associated with the disease, availability of ASR or US FDA-approved or -cleared test kits, the complexity of testing, equipment requirements, and existence of patents that apply to the test. Each of these items requires serious consideration and support on behalf of the laboratory and the institution.

The clinical requirement for and usefulness of a test are defined by the significance of the test result for disease diagnosis or prognosis and clinical management. For example, HIV-1 viral load testing is widely used because it provides immediate information regarding the patient response to treatment and prognosis. Likewise, population-based genetic screening for cystic fibrosis (CF), now offered to all individuals and couples of childbearing age, provides immediate information about a couple's risk of having a child affected by CF [46].

"Competency" refers to the availability of knowledgeable and skilled laboratory personnel who can perform, supervise, troubleshoot, and correctly interpret molecular tests. For example, RT-PCR-based tests require knowledge not only of PCR but also of RNA processing in the clinical laboratory.

Test costs are another important factor for selection of tests to offer. Generally, when the cost of a test is low and the volume is high, a test will have a profit margin. A common issue is deciding whether to perform the test or use a reference laboratory for a specific test. This usually requires a break-even analysis to determine the point (threshold) at which there is no profit or loss for performing the test, taking into consideration the cost of the test, the expected revenue, and the expected volume of testing. Rare or urgent tests may be more expensive since tests are run individually rather than as batched analyses, as can be done in a reference laboratory, with combined testing from many sites. However, the need for very rapid test results for critically urgent patient care decisions may require that testing be performed locally rather than by a reference laboratory. In contrast, high-volume tests are likely to be profitable when performed by a laboratory.

The prevalence of the disease or mutation in the population affects the testing volume and therefore the number of laboratories that perform a specific test. The laboratory, however, may choose to test for less-common diseases or mutations if it receives a sufficient specimen volume to make the testing cost-effective. For example, some laboratories offer comprehensive testing for neurological diseases when there is specific clinical expertise at their medical center, or with inclusion of clinical samples referred to the laboratory from other sites in the USA or internationally.

The number of different mutations in one or more genes accounting for a disease is a consideration for testing. In general, the greater the number of mutations in a single gene or the number of different genes that can cause a disease, the more complex and labor-intensive testing becomes. Therefore, for common disorders, such as CF, commercial kits are available that detect at least 25 of the more common mutations in the *CFTR* gene, requiring substantially less time for test development than laboratory-developed methods or complete *CFTR* gene analysis by sequencing.

The complexity of testing and the availability of needed equipment are two important considerations. Tests requiring lengthy procedures, such as Sanger sequencing, or complex analyses (SMA carrier testing, for example) are less likely to be performed by many laboratories, especially if the test volume is low or commercial test kits are not available. The use of ASRs or US FDA-approved IVD test kits, particularly for viral load testing, is preferred by many laboratories because the kit simplifies the laboratory workflow and facilitates testing standardization and quality assurance in the laboratory and across laboratories, even though the IVD test kits are often more expensive than laboratory-developed tests.

Finally, patents that cover the disease mutations, genes, or testing methods or reagents for a test can be a consideration when deciding to implement and perform a test. Patent or license exclusivity may be enforced, licensing or sublicensing fees may be too costly, or other conditions of licensing may not be reasonable for the laboratory, such that the laboratory is not legally allowed or chooses not to implement and perform a test covered by one or more patents. This may be even more significant for complex genetic disease tests that require testing of multiple genes, each of which may be covered by patents, although the US Supreme Court decision that genes are not patent-eligible matter has reduced the patent burden for clinical molecular pathology laboratories.

Choice of Test Methods

Several factors influence the selection of the testing method, including the mutation type, the degree of mutation heterogeneity, the anticipated test volume, the available resources, such as equipment and expertise, and patent issues. The majority of clinical tests target specific mutations or sequences. The greater the number of sequence variations that need to be detected by a test, the more difficult and labor-intensive the test becomes. The most-frequently used method in molecular pathology laboratories is nucleic acid amplification, usually by PCR. Some of the more common factors affecting the choice of methods from nucleic acid extraction through PCR and post-PCR analysis are discussed.

Nucleic acid extraction is a principal part of most molecular tests. Numerous extraction methods are currently available. Some of the issues to consider in choosing an extraction method for DNA or RNA are yield, quality of the nucleic acid required for the subsequent testing steps, storage, processing speed, and costs. Laboratories may use more than one method for DNA or RNA purification. Some of the more common methods currently utilized are desalting methods and silica-gel membrane columns. Columns are particularly convenient for processing of small volumes of blood for a large number of samples and are available for either DNA or RNA isolation. Many of these extraction methods can be automated, allowing batching of multiple samples in a single run.

The most common method in the molecular pathology laboratory is PCR, which has enabled the implementation of hundreds of clinical molecular tests. The method is particularly suitable for detection of point mutations and other small sequence variations, for detection of chromosomal rearrangements, for detection or quantification of pathogens by amplification, or for sequence analysis. Variations of PCR include RT-PCR for amplification of RNA sequences, multiplex PCR for the simultaneous amplification of two or more sequences, and qPCR for quantification of specific sequences (see Chap. 2).

While PCR amplification is the most commonly used method for nucleic acid amplification in clinical molecular laboratories, many methods are used to analyze the resulting PCR products. The simplest method for analysis of PCR products is gel electrophoresis to visualize and determine the size of the PCR products that have been synthesized with comparison to a sizing standard that has been run on the same gel. A second common method for analysis of PCR products is digestion with a restriction enzyme followed by analysis of the DNA fragments by gel electrophoresis. PCR products can be hybridized to allele-specific oligonucleotide (ASO) probes complementary to either the normal or mutant allele. However, these methods are more labor intensive and expensive and are currently rarely used in clinical molecular laboratories.

Small length changes and genetic rearrangements present in PCR products can be detected by size variations using agarose or acrylamide gel electrophoresis with ethidium bromide staining, or by a fluorescent-dependent detection method using either a plate- or capillary-based automated sequencer. Automated analyzers are especially useful for the simultaneous analysis of numerous PCR products labeled either with a single or multiple fluorophores, or when quantitation of a PCR product is required. Recently, automated microarray based multiplexing molecular platforms have been developed that can be used to assess disease signatures for several clinical applications, including infectious diseases, women's health, cancer, and pharmacogenetics, using a variety of methods for target detection.

In the last decade, a significant portion of PCR testing has been transitioned to real-time PCR, which monitors the generation of the PCR product throughout the amplification process. This approach can be used for either point mutation detection or quantitation, eliminating the need for time-consuming post-PCR analysis and decreasing risk of PCR contamination. This application became the method of choice for many clinical molecular tests, particularly viral load testing as well as genetic tests such as Factor V Leiden and Prothrombin mutation analysis for thrombophilia risk.

When the disease gene is known but the mutations are unknown, mutation-scanning methods are used. The most common scanning methods are single-strand conformation polymorphism (SSCP) and denaturing high pressure liquid chromatography (DHPLC), both of which detect single base pair variations with high sensitivity. Alternatively, Sanger sequencing can be used for direct mutation detection and is currently considered the gold standard for mutation detection. NGS technologies are a powerful strategy sequence analysis of a large number of individuals for multiple genetic targets by bar coding of DNA samples and batching them together in a NGS run. This strategy has significantly decreased the cost of sequencing, providing greater sequence output per run at lower costs with faster TAT.

Clinical Information Requirements

Clinical information is essential for determining the appropriateness of the ordered test and is critical for interpretation of results. Clinical information usually is obtained from the requisition form or an electronic test order system. A complete requisition contains patient demographic information to allow for identification of the patient, the ordering health care provider's name and contact information, the type of sample, the name of the ordered test(s), relevant clinical information, and any other information essential for appropriate interpretation of test results. For some genetic disorders, such as CF, ethnic background is particularly important because disease prevalence can vary significantly with ethnic background, while a pedigree is required for linkage analysis studies and risk assessments. Laboratories should document informed consent for genetic tests (as discussed above in the "Genetic Testing" section), which may be required by state regulation, such as in NY. For cancer or infectious disease testing, indication of the purpose for testing (diagnosis or minimal residual disease assessment) is needed for appropriate interpretation of the test result.

Specimen Requirements

Molecular pathology testing can be performed using many patient sample types. A list of the more common specimen types, applications, handling, and storage requirements is presented in Table 62.3. The most common sample for genetic testing is peripheral blood (PB); buccal cells may be acceptable for some genetic tests. Prenatal testing is performed on cultured or direct amniotic cells and CVS specimens. A maternal sample may be required for prenatal testing to rule out maternal cell contamination of the fetal specimen, usually by identity testing of the fetal and maternal samples, to ensure that the test result reflects the fetal genotype rather

Table 62.3 Specimen types and handling for molecular pathology testing

Specimen type	Test type	Requirements	Shipment	Storage
Blood	Genetics, cancer, identity, HLA typing, virology	EDTA (0.5–10 ml)[a]	RT	4 °C
Bone marrow	Cancer, identity testing	EDTA (0.5–1 ml)	RT	4 °C
Plasma	Infectious diseases	EDTA (2 ml)	Dry ice	−80 °C
Cerebrospinal fluid	Cancer, infectious diseases	None (0.5–2 ml)	Dry ice	−80 °C
Sputum	Cancer, infectious diseases	None (0.5–2 ml)	RT	4 °C
Amniotic fluid (<15 weeks gestation)	Genetics	None (10–15 ml)	RT	4 °C
CVS	Genetics	5–15 mg	RT	4 °C
Cultured amniocytes or CVS	Genetics	2 T25 flasks	RT	4 °C
Buccal cells	Genetics, cancer, identity	2 swabs	RT	4 °C
Fresh tissue	Cancer, identity	50–100 mg	Dry ice	−80 °C
FFPE tissue or cells	Cancer, identity	2–10 5 μm sections	RT	RT
DNA	Genetics, cancer, identity, HLA typing	<1–100 μg	RT	4 °C
RNA	Genetics, cancer	<1–20 μg	Dry ice	−80 °C

CVS chorionic villus sampling, *DNA* deoxyribonucleic acid, *EDTA* ethylene diamine tetraacetic acid, *FFPE* formalin-fixed paraffin-embedded, *HLA* human leukocyte antigen, *RT* room temperature
[a]Sample volume requirements may vary based on application and age of patient

than the maternal genotype. Samples for molecular oncology and infectious disease testing may include PB, bone marrow, tissues, and other body fluid (cerebral spinal fluid, sputum, etc.). FFPE tissue specimens are used predominantly for DNA-based testing, such as gene rearrangement studies for lymphomas and mutation detection in solid tumors, while fresh or frozen tissue generally is used for RNA-based testing, such as the detection of specific fusion transcripts in cancers. Sample requirements and collection and shipment information for molecular tests should be provided by the laboratory to ensure that samples are collected, handled, shipped, and stored appropriately before shipment, during transit, and during storage in the laboratory before sample processing.

Laboratory Operations

Workflow includes the steps of testing from specimen collection to reporting of results. This process can be divided into preanalytic, analytic, and postanalytic phases. The preanalytic phase consists of collecting, transporting, accessioning, and storage of the sample(s) prior to testing, as well as test ordering. The analytic phase is the process of performing the test. The postanalytic phase consists of all steps after the test is performed, including analysis of the test result, generation of the test report, and communication of the results. Although the preanalytic phase is difficult to control since the steps are performed by individuals outside the laboratory, most errors occur in the analytic phase because of the multistep, predominantly manual nature of molecular testing.

Preanalytic Phase

Samples are usually transported to a central receiving area of the laboratory or directly to the molecular pathology laboratory, either by a local hospital transport system or by courier or mail if the samples are sent from remote sites. Upon arrival, samples are accessioned into the LIS and assigned a unique identifier or accession number, allowing the sample to be tracked in the laboratory and hospital database. Information entered during accessioning includes patient demographics, ordered test(s), specimen type, and time and date of specimen collection and receipt by the laboratory. If available, bar-coded labels can be attached to the requisition form and specimen container, and can be used throughout the testing process for tracking of the specimen through the testing process.

The clinical information and specimen type are reviewed for appropriateness of the test requested. Missing clinical information can be obtained by contacting the health care provider or through the electronic medical record system. Genetic test requests are reviewed for ethical considerations.

Some sample types require additional processing prior to nucleic acid extraction. For example, FFPE tissue blocks are sectioned and slides are prepared and reviewed by a pathologist to assess the percentage of tumor cells in the tissue block and sections. CVS tissue is examined by a qualified cytogeneticist to remove contaminating maternal tissue prior to DNA extraction. Similarly, prenatal cultured cells are examined for confluence; low numbers of cells may not produce sufficient DNA for some analyses. For HIV-1 and HCV viral load tests, for example, the plasma must be separated from the blood cells within 4–6 h of collection and the plasma is stored frozen until processing begins (Table 62.3).

Analytic Phase

For laboratory efficiency and cost-effectiveness, testing is performed on batches of specimens, and the frequency of testing depends on test volume and urgency of clinical need of the test results. The first step in molecular testing is nucleic acid extraction. DNA or RNA can be extracted from the patient specimens using either laboratory-developed methods or commercial nucleic acid extraction kits, and the nucleic acid stored appropriately (see Table 62.3). Most tests use PCR, which is set up in the pre-PCR area of the laboratory. To verify sample identity throughout all the steps of testing and prevent possible mix-up and cross-contamination, a worksheet can be used to indicate sample identifiers and numerical locations in the run, as well as reagent information such as lot numbers and expiration dates. Barcode labels can be used for tracking the specimens through the testing process. The same worksheet can be used later for documentation of test results for patient samples and controls. Patient sample reactions should be set up first, followed by the controls, as discussed in the "PCR Contamination Control" section.

Regardless of the procedure used, certain principles are essential. Specimen and reagent identifications should be checked with every manipulation performed. Expiration dates and identification of reagents should be checked before each use. New lots of reagents must be tested against old lots prior to clinical use. Test results should be documented, either by photographing the gel or by printing out the data from the instrument, unless the results are electronic and are stored in the laboratory database or LIS. Proper labeling and identification of the samples on photographs or data sheets is essential to prevent interpretation errors.

Postanalytic Phase

After tests are performed, the results are analyzed, the test results and interpretation are entered into the laboratory computer manually or by electronic transfer from an instrument, and the results are reported in the LIS and communicated verbally to the health care provider, if appropriate. To reduce errors, results should be interpreted by two independent reviewers, which may include a technologist previously certified to perform a technical interpretation of the specific test through the laboratory's training program, a resident or fellow, or the laboratory director or appropriate designee. Results must comply with the established criteria for result analysis and interpretation as defined in the test procedure manual. Control results are reviewed for accuracy before analysis of patient test results. For PCR-based tests analyzed by electrophoresis, the water/no-template control should not have bands other than primer dimers, and control samples must demonstrate expected results. For quantitative assays, control results must fall within the established cycle threshold (C_T) assay ranges. Patient test results are interpreted as positive or negative, or a quantitative result is obtained by comparison with the assay controls and by comparison to size markers or quantitation standards, as appropriate for the specific test method. Unexpected results are assessed for errors in the analytic process. The identified problems are corrected and testing of all or selected specimens is repeated. Results should be recorded manually or electronically transferred to the assay worksheet by the technologist who performed the assay, signed, dated, and entered in the computer using a report template, if available. Entered reports should then be reviewed and released by a second interpreter. For complex testing, such as HIV-1 genotyping, or test results requiring professional interpretation, the second interpreter should be a qualified professional. For efficient workflow, use of report templates for the most common test results and interpretations, with revisions for specific specimens, facilitates test reporting.

The information required for test reports is defined in the CAP Molecular Pathology checklist and includes patient demographics, test methods, mutation(s) tested, and a clinical interpretation in an easy-to-interpret format. Although the CAP, in compliance with CLIA, does not require supervisory review of all test results, good practice is for all manual assays to be reviewed and approved by the laboratory director or qualified designee before reporting. A final report is generated only after results are verified and electronically signed by the laboratory director or a qualified designee. When laboratory director review is not deemed necessary, such as for tests performed using automated equipment, two separate technologists trained to perform the assay, or the same technologist in duplicate, should review the results after manual entry into the LIS to ensure accurate transcription into the LIS prior to release of the reports. Results most often are communicated by printed report or an electronic information system, but direct discussion of urgent or complex test results may be useful for the clinician. Verbal communication or faxing of test results should be performed in compliance with HIPAA regulations to protect patient confidentiality.

Quality Management Systems

The molecular pathology laboratory must establish, maintain, and document the quality performance of all aspects of laboratory operations and test performance, including quality control (QC), quality assessment also known as quality assurance (QA), and quality improvement (QI) programs that are adequate and appropriate for the validity of the procedures performed. The next few sections focus on the principal aspects of these programs.

Quality Control Program

The QC program focuses on the analytic validity of the testing process with the purpose of assessing and ensuring the reliability of patient results. According to CLIA, "The laboratory must establish and follow written QC procedures for monitoring and evaluating the quality of the analytic testing process of each method to assure the accuracy and reliability of patient test results and reports" [22]. Specific requirements include adherence to the manufacturer's instructions for instrument operation and test performance, having a current procedure manual, performing and documenting QC test results, maintaining records of all QC activities, and verifying performance specifications. Test sites, especially high-complexity laboratories, may choose to impose more, but not less, stringent QC requirements for the testing process. Molecular pathology tests are largely manual, laboratory-developed, multistep assays, requiring a variety of commercial or laboratory-produced reagents. QC procedures should be designed to detect and reduce errors in the entire testing process. Special attention should be given to the most common types of errors that occur during testing, such as use of expired reagents, improper preparation and storage of reagents and controls, clerical errors, and sample misidentification. Some of the key components of the QC program are discussed below.

Test Validation (Verification of Test Performance Characteristics)

Major differences are defined by CLIA for the implementation of a US FDA-approved or -cleared test compared to the implementation of a LDT. If the test is performed using a US FDA-approved or -cleared IVD test kit, the laboratory needs only to verify the performance characteristics of the test for the population of patients seen at that specific laboratory site. Implementation of a LDT requires collection of more extensive analytic data to establish the performance characteristics of the test. The performance characteristics that need to be evaluated include accuracy, precision, sensitivity, specificity, reportable range, population-specific reference ranges, and any other applicable test characteristics. Laboratories can use the manufacturer's criteria as long as the director determines that these are appropriate for the laboratory's population of patients. To assist in this process, CLIA also recommends that performance characteristics of a new test be compared to a known "gold standard" testing method. This is not always practical, since molecular methods often are developed because of the inadequacy of the currently available test methods. The test method also should be validated for all types of specimens that will be accepted for testing, as well as for interfering substances that may be present in the specimen types.

Establishing the test accuracy requires determining that the test yields appropriate positive, negative, or quantitative results, based on samples with known characteristics as determined by an independent test method. Samples used to determine accuracy can be obtained from several sources, including proficiency surveys or other laboratories performing the test by the same or a different test method. For example, validation results for new RT-PCR procedures for the diagnosis of certain translocations in leukemia can be supported by cytogenetic results for the same specimens.

Establishing the precision of an assay requires demonstrating that the assay results are reproducible. Testing well characterized control specimens and a variety of patient specimens multiple times in separate runs and comparing the results can demonstrate the precision of a test. For quantitative tests, precision is tested over the range of reportable values.

Analytic sensitivity refers to the lowest amount of analyte (nucleic acid) detected or quantified by a test. Analytic sensitivity is determined as the proportion of patient samples that contain the target nucleic acid sequence that tests positive using the test. For qualitative tests, the analytic sensitivity represents the smallest amount of analyte that is reliably detected by the test. For quantitative tests, limit of quantification (LOQ) is used, which is different than the limit of detection (LOD) that simply implies the lower limit of analyte detected by the assay. LOQ is the lowest amount of analyte that can be reliably and accurately quantified. Sensitivity should be determined for quantitative tests such as viral load assays, qualitative assays for pathogen detection, or for MRD monitoring to establish the utility and limitations of the test.

Analytic specificity measures the degree to which the test reacts with nucleic acids other than the intended sequence. It is measured as the proportion of patient samples that do not contain the target nucleic acid that test negative by the test. The analytic specificity of a test can be determined by analyzing a series of positive and negative samples and calculating the detection rate of the true negative samples, as defined by samples that do not contain the target of the test. Distinguishing among closely related pathogens, however, requires a precise design of primers specific for the target microorganism. Nonspecific signals can be produced by nonoptimal amplification conditions or inhibitors, which can be overcome by high-quality DNA extraction procedures and optimization of assay conditions.

The development of a new test usually is driven by new molecular information combined with a clinical need for a better test. Once the laboratory director decides that a new molecular test will be implemented, the methodology for the test, controls, test validation samples, specimen types, costs, and other factors are determined. The method for the assay is chosen based on the type of test information required, clinical utility, current use of the test platform in the laboratory, ease of test performance, and clinically required test characteristics and TAT. Once the test method is chosen, the specific test parameters are designed. Each step of the assay is optimized, including nucleic acid extraction, amplification, detection, and interpretation of results. For laboratories that develop many assays, standard starting conditions and optimization criteria facilitate test implementation. For example, PCR assays can initially use standard reagent concentrations and amplification conditions, followed by fine optimization of the PCR conditions as needed. Once the optimal assay conditions are established, the analytic validation of the assay is performed on clinical specimens and/or controls using those testing conditions.

Initial optimization and performance of the assay must include establishing the controls to be used for testing. Appropriate controls are often commercially available from organizations such as Coriell Institute for Medical Research (Camden, NJ) and the American Type Culture Collection (ATCC; Manassas, VA) as frozen immortalized cell lines or DNA containing the pathogen genome or mutation of interest. Standardized reference panels for viral load testing are available for many viral targets, including HIV-1, HCV, HBV, CMV, and Epstein–Barr virus. In the absence of purchased controls, patient samples tested by a different method or provided by another laboratory may be used.

The last step of the test evaluation requires clinical validation of the new test. Clinical validation determines the probability that a sample from a patient with the disease or disease risk will test positive (clinical sensitivity), and that a sample from a patient without the disease or disease risk will test negative (clinical specificity). A final step of the clinical validation may be to obtain a panel of mixed positive and negative patient samples without the known test results from another laboratory that performs the same test. After the testing, results are compared to the results obtained by the other laboratory and documented. Any discrepancies should be resolved by a different test method or a third laboratory.

Analytic Validity Assessment

The principal focus of current CLIA regulations for test validation is assessment of the analytic validity of the tests. To address this, CAP published recommendations on how to perform analytic and clinical validation studies in a series of checklists also used for laboratory accreditation. NY law (Subsection 58-1.10(g) of Part 58 of Title 10 (Health) of the Official Compilation of Codes, Rules and Regulations) specifically requires that all validation data of new testing are submitted to the state for review and approval prior to clinical use of the test, using guidance documents and checklists in the specific categories of testing. Validation studies must be submitted by NYSDOH prior to use of the test for clinical purposes, but testing can begin once data is submitted and before NYSDOH approval is obtained [47]. Recently, the CLIAC Genetic Testing Good Laboratory Practices Workgroup published a report that provided a series of recommendations for ensuring the quality of genetic testing [48]. The recommendations were made to CLIAC, an advisory entity providing recommendations to the DHHS on approaches required to ensure genetic testing quality since 1997.

Test Procedure Manual

Test procedure manuals are essential for clinical molecular laboratory function and are required by CLIA. The manual should be simple, easy to follow, and functional, but should provide sufficient detail to act as a reference for all aspects of testing for laboratory personnel performing the test and for training purposes. The manual, in a written or electronic format, must be current and available to all laboratory personnel. Manuals for high-complexity tests include written policies for sample collection, equipment performance evaluation, QC program, and standard operating procedures (SOP) for test performance. An example of the contents of a test procedure manual is shown in Table 62.4. The procedures are usually written by laboratory technologists or a supervisor, and then reviewed, edited, and approved by the laboratory director or designee. Any changes to an established procedure manual are documented in writing or electronically and approved by the director. Any laboratory staff members that perform a specific test must review the procedure manual annually, with documentation of the review. All procedure manuals must be reviewed annually by the laboratory director or their designee, as documented in writing.

The necessary elements of a test procedure manual are detailed in the CLIA guidelines, which follow closely the items described in CLSI GP2-A3, Clinical Laboratory Technical Procedure Manuals [24]. An example of a complete laboratory procedure manual is presented in Table 62.5. Manufacturer's product inserts or operation manuals can be used as a component of a test procedure manual, but additional information specific to the testing as performed by the laboratory must be provided.

Controls

Every clinical test requires use of appropriate controls. Controls are used to document reproducibility and to ensure that the test is working properly and results are reliable. Several types of controls are used for molecular tests: positive,

Table 62.4 Contents of a standard test procedure (an example of a PCR-RFLP test)

Item	Content
Background	Theoretical information concerning the disorder and the test
Principle of the assay	Description of how the restriction enzyme detects the specific mutation
Summary of the assay	Characteristics of the restriction-based assay used
Clinical significance	Use of the test for patient care
Strategy for analysis	Overview of the testing steps (i.e., extraction, PCR amplification, digestion, gel electrophoresis)
Specimen collection or acquisition	Description of acceptable specimen type, storage, shipment, and required clinical information
Criteria for rejected samples	Description of unacceptable samples (i.e., specific specimen types, improper labeling, damage)
Equipment and supplies	List of equipment necessary for testing (i.e., PCR machine, gel electrophoresis)
Reagents	List of reagents used for each test step (e.g., PCR, restriction enzyme digestion, gel electrophoresis equipment)
Assay procedure	Description of the testing steps, including general considerations, sample preparation, pre-PCR preparation and setup, thermal cycling, PCR cleanup, PCR product digestion, gel preparation and electrophoresis, gel documentation
Analysis of results	Description of expected results, control results, criteria for gel analysis and interpretation, documentation of results in the LIS and laboratory database, if used
Turnaround time and schedule for retaining specimen	Expected turnaround time for the specific test, specimen and DNA storage, and schedule for retaining the specimen and DNA
References	Literature or commercial-based information
Addenda	E.g., the worksheet for the specific test, the manufacturer's product insert

negative, sensitivity, inhibition, water/no-template, and QC controls. Combinations of these controls are used as appropriate based on the method and purpose of the test. A positive control is defined as a sample that contains the target sequence and produces a positive result when tested. Sources of positive controls include positive patient samples and commercially available cell lines or nucleic acids. A negative control is a sample that does not contain the target sequence and produces a negative result when tested. Sensitivity controls are needed for assays that require a specified level of analytical sensitivity. The sensitivity control is particularly important for MRD tests for cancer and viral load tests to define the lower limit of detection of the specific test. In general, a sensitivity control is included in each run of the test, since the sensitivity of each test run should be documented and not be assumed to be the same as during validation of the test. A no-template control or water control is a control reaction containing all reagents but no template nucleic acid, which tests for contamination of the PCR reagents with sample nucleic acid or amplicons and should not produce any PCR products except for primer dimers. An inhibition control (addition of external target nucleic acid or amplification of another template sequence to check for PCR amplification and absence of PCR inhibitors) is used only when the lack of production of a PCR product is interpreted as a negative result for the test. A QC control is a patient sample that was previously tested and is included for repeat testing on a new run. These samples function to assess the accuracy of the patient specimen results in the current test run, as well as to monitor for interassay variability. A QA sample which is a patient sample tested in two consecutive runs also may be included in each test run. The QA typically monitors for sporadic errors and testing accuracy of individual samples.

The controls should be processed in the same manner as the patient samples during testing; however, their use and storage should be well defined in the test procedure manual to avoid degradation. Controls should be validated for acceptability and approved by the laboratory director or designee before use in clinical testing. Failure of controls to perform as expected should be investigated, with findings and corrective action documented. Some QC results, for example, viral load testing, should be tracked over time and analyzed on standard Levey–Jennings plots. Deviations and adverse trends indicate that something is changing in the analytic system, and requires investigation and corrective action.

Preventive Equipment Maintenance

All instruments used in the clinical molecular laboratory require written standard procedures for normal operation, performance evaluation, and preventive maintenance. Function checks should be performed on a regular schedule to check critical characteristics and detect malfunctions before test results are affected. In the absence of manufacturer's guidelines, the laboratory should establish a mainte-

Table 62.5 Complete molecular pathology laboratory procedure manual: examples of required information, guidelines, and protocols

General information
Staff and contact information
Test information
Requisition forms (genetics, oncology, infectious diseases, identity testing)
Information for clients (shipping, sample type, billing information, consent form, test-specific fax cover-sheets)
Licenses and permits (CLIA certification and CAP accreditation form)
Reagent handling for molecular testing guidelines
Probe and primer documentation
General laboratory operating procedures
Quality control, quality assurance, and quality improvement programs
Specimen-receiving procedure
Prevention of PCR contamination
Logging-of-primers procedure
Autoclaving of solutions procedure
Use of PCR biosafety chambers
Programming of PCR thermal cyclers
Sequencing using a capillary electrophoresis instrument
Equipment-maintenance procedures
Centrifuges, balance, pH meter, and spectrophotometer: checks and cleanup
Water check procedure
Timer check procedure
Thermometer validation
Temperature-check procedure
Maintenance and validation of PCR thermal cyclers
Nucleic acid extraction procedures
Large-scale DNA extraction from blood by desalting method
Small-scale DNA extraction from blood by column
Fresh- and frozen-tissue DNA extraction
Paraffin-embedded-tissue DNA extraction
Prenatal (amniocytes and CVS) DNA extraction
RNA extraction from blood by column
Nucleic acid quantitation
Test-specific procedure manuals
Genetics
Factor V Leiden analysis
Myotonic dystrophy PCR and Southern analysis
Cystic fibrosis mutation analysis
Spinal muscular atrophy direct testing
Spinal muscular atrophy carrier testing (dosage analysis)
Spinal muscular atrophy linkage analysis
Oncology
IGH gene PCR for detection of B-cell clonality
T-cell receptor PCR for detection of T-cell clonality
BCL2 gene PCR for detection of M-bcr and m-bcr breakpoints
PML–RARA RT-PCR for detection of t(15;17) in APL
BCR–ABL RT-PCR for detection of t(9;22) in CML and ALL
RT-PCR for detection of translocations in sarcomas
Identity Testing
Bone marrow engraftment analysis by genotyping of STR markers
Parentage and identity testing
Maternal cell contamination analysis
Infectious Diseases
HIV-1 viral load assay
HCV viral load assay
HBV viral load assay
Microbial molecular identification analysis

ALL acute lymphoblastic leukemia, *APL* acute promyelocytic leukemia, *BCL2* B-cell lymphoma protein 2, *CML* chronic myelogenous leukemia, *HBV* hepatitis B virus, *HCV* hepatitis C virus, *IGH*, immunoglobulin heavy chain, *m-bcr* minor breakpoint cluster *region*, *M-bcr* major breakpoint cluster region, *PML–RARA* promyelocytic leukemia-retinoic acid receptor alpha, *STR* short tandem repeat

nance procedure that appropriately reflects the use of the instrument and assesses its performance characteristics over time. Of particular importance are thermal cyclers, because any change in their performance will have a direct impact on many tests. Thermal cyclers should be routinely monitored for cycle time reproducibility, verification of temperature accuracy, and efficiency of heating and cooling rates. These performance checks are usually incorporated into the instrument's software and are a part of the manufacturer's recommendations for instrument maintenance. Temperature logs for each temperature-dependent piece of equipment, including an acceptable temperature range, are required by CLIA. Temperatures of refrigerators, freezers, and incubators must be documented daily if used for reagent storage. Other instruments, such as water baths, should be documented each day of use. An equipment maintenance and performance evaluation log should be maintained for every laboratory instrument and should be kept for the duration of the clinical use of the instrument. The log should document any maintenance, assessment checks, problems, and any maintenance or repairs performed by the laboratory or manufacturer.

Quality Assessment Program

CLIA requires each laboratory to have an active QA program to assess various aspects of the technical and nontechnical performance of the molecular pathology laboratory. CLIA requires establishment of guidelines and procedures designated not only "to evaluate the ongoing and overall quality of the testing process," but also to evaluate "the effectiveness of its policies and procedures," followed by requirements to "identify and correct problems, assure reliable and prompt reporting of test reports, and assure the adequacy and competence of the staff" [22]. In CLIA'03, "quality assurance" was renamed "quality assessment," recognizing that quality cannot always be assured but it can be evaluated or assessed [23]. The laboratory QA program must monitor and evaluate both the ongoing and the overall quality of the total testing process through error detection, corrective actions and their review, and the integration of improvements in procedures. To meet the CLIA requirements, the clinical molecular laboratory must have a QA program that includes numerous laboratory practices, including personnel training and performance evaluation, proficiency testing, inspections, correlation of molecular results with clinical data, and a QC program. Elements monitored by the QA program, such as TAT, rejected specimens, and various indicators of test quality, do not relate directly to the analytic validity of the testing process and thus are not a part of the QC program. A complete list of these indicators can be found in the LAP-CAP Molecular Pathology checklist. Table 62.6 lists some of the major components for which the LAP-CAP requires ongoing surveillance and documentation.

Table 62.6 Examples of QC and QA topics that require documentation and corrective action

QC and QA of testing
Ongoing evaluation of proficiency test results
Detection and correction of clerical and analytic errors
Recording of failed nucleic acid isolations
Recording of failed hybridization reactions
Monitoring of test turnaround time
Discrepancies between preliminary and final reported results
Discrepancies between the molecular pathology laboratory and other laboratory findings Performance of statistics and appropriate comparative studies on all molecular pathology tests
Logging of unusual, difficult, and instructive cases
Laboratory-developed assay validation
Performing validation to confirm analytic test performance characteristics
Documenting validation studies for establishing assay performance characteristics
Documenting analytic characteristics including accuracy, sensitivity, specificity, and precision
Demonstrating and documenting clinical validity
Procedure manual
Annual review of all policies and procedures by the laboratory director or designee
Review of all new policies, procedures, and changes to existing procedures
Knowledge of testing procedures for the tests performed by each technologist in the laboratory
Information for all DNA probes, PCR primers, and other nucleic acid reagents used for testing
Paternity and forensic identity
Chain-of-custody (proof of identity)
Genetic characteristics (heterogeneity, recombination rates, etc.) of the DNA markers used
Documentation of release of information
Specimen handling
Disposition of unacceptable specimens
Sample condition, inadequate volumes, and evidence of tampering
Reagents
Validation of reagents used for tests
Characteristics of the specific reagents used in each assay
Controls
Failed control results or when results exceed defined tolerance limits
Instruments
Ongoing evaluation of results of instrument maintenance and function (temperatures, instrument characteristics, cleanliness)
Function checks for detection of problems and malfunctions
Repairs and services
Temperature checks for temperature-dependent equipment
Personnel
Continuing medical laboratory education
Safety
Radioactive area surveys and wipe tests
Radioactive waste disposal

Although CLIA requires that clinical laboratories continually evaluate and improve their work in all areas, some requirements are particularly important from an institutional perspective. CLIA mandates that test results obtained from different testing methods performed under the same certificate be compared, documented, and reviewed for the detection of errors that can affect patient care. This means that molecular oncology test results, for example, should be compared with the results obtained by other laboratories, such as the flow cytometry and cytogenetics laboratories, for the same patient.

Training

Personnel performing high-complexity molecular testing must meet established qualifications in education, training, experience, job performance, and competency. Training includes competency in performance of the test methodology, calculations, independent judgment, quality control of the method, and knowledge of the instruments. These training requirements cannot be based simply on academic requirements or experience. The on-site training must be sufficient to ensure that staff members have the skills necessary for performing every step of the analytic process including assay method, preventive maintenance, and quality control measures, as well as recognition of a problem in test performance should it occur.

To this end, a training program ensuring that technologists are properly trained to perform laboratory procedures must be used. As the first step, technologists can be trained by observing a technologist who knows how to perform the procedure and by reading the procedure manual. Then, the technologist should test two to three blind sets of specimens in addition to known controls, with or without observation depending upon the level of experience of the technologist, to ensure that the technologist understands the test and performs it correctly. Monitoring of the training test runs ensures the accuracy of the technologist's performance. Finally, the results of training runs must be documented and approved by the laboratory director or designee.

A part of ongoing training is annual competency evaluation. This allows the laboratory director or designee to review different aspects of the technologist's performance, including technical skills, control of PCR contamination, equipment operation, procedure knowledge, and laboratory safety. The overall performance of each technologist is documented, and corrective or additional training measures are implemented, as needed.

Training also includes continuing education programs, which assist laboratory personnel in attaining new technical skills and knowledge required to keep up with changes in procedures, instruments, and new tests, as well as improve their ability to perform new assays, troubleshoot, and handle new problems.

Proficiency Testing

Proficiency testing plays a key role in assessing the internal quality of work in CLIA-regulated high-complexity testing clinical laboratories. CLIA requires the laboratory to successfully participate in a CMS-approved proficiency testing program for all analytes tested. The CAP provides approved proficiency testing programs in several relevant fields, including genetics, infectious diseases, oncology, and identity testing (Table 62.7). Proficiency testing must be performed at least once per year. In the absence of an external proficiency testing program for a specific test, the laboratory can set up a sample exchange proficiency testing program with another laboratory performing the same test. Proficiency samples must be tested in the same manner as patient samples, by the same technologists performing the clinical testing, using the same interpretation procedures. Laboratories failing two of three consecutive testing events for any test must submit a plan of corrective action with documentation that the test is now performing accurately to the CAP or other proficiency testing agency.

Laboratory Inspection

Molecular pathology laboratories must be inspected by an external inspection team every 2 years for compliance with CLIA regulations. LAP-CAP inspections are performed by a team of inspectors from an institution other than that of the laboratories being inspected, and the inspection team assesses the quality indicators for continued quality performance as listed in the LAP-CAP checklists [49]. The checklists address laboratory procedures including specimen processing and testing, reagents, controls, instrumentation, personnel, physical facilities, and laboratory safety. Inspection also assesses for PCR contamination control, participation and performance in proficiency testing programs, and documentation of the QC and QA program activities (Table 62.6). Failure to comply with specific checklist items is documented as a "Phase I" or "Phase II" deficiency. Most items on the molecular pathology checklist are Phase II, with a serious potential to affect patient care. Phase II deficiencies require immediate attention and correction, documented in writing, to the CAP. Phase I deficiencies are less serious but also require documentation of corrective action. On alternate years, the laboratory is required to perform a self-inspection.

Recently, as part of ongoing efforts to strengthen the laboratory accreditation process, to promote public confidence in the LAP-CAP, and to help assure regulators that CAP-accredited laboratories meet or exceed CLIA requirements, the CAP has made significant changes in its LAP processes, including unannounced inspections rather than scheduled inspections beginning in January 2006. This means that laboratories will not know the exact date of the inspection and the identity of the inspection team members prior to the inspection. Instead, the laboratories will be provided with a 90-day window of the anniversary of their last inspection, 45 days prior to and 45 days after their last inspection, pending CMS approval, in which the inspection will occur. By implementing this process for routine inspections, CAP expects to help ensure that laboratories are in continuous compliance and that they are providing quality patient testing at all times.

Alternatively, laboratories can be inspected directly by CLIA, the Joint Commission, or one of the other accrediting organizations for clinical laboratories under the CLIA program. The CLIA inspection regulations are found in Subpart

Table 62.7 CAP proficiency surveys for molecular pathology testing

Category/name	Survey	Type of testing
Genetics		
MGL	Molecular genetics	Molecular testing for various genetic diseases or genes
PGX	Pharmacogenetics	Molecular testing for various genes
SEC	DNA sequence interpretation	DNA sequence electropherogram analysis and reporting
CY, CYBK, CYM	Cytogenetics	Analysis of online images or prints of metaphase cells
CYCGH	Cytogenomic microarray analysis	Analysis of DNA for constitutional or neoplastic abnormality
Oncology		
MO	Molecular oncology	Molecular analysis of leukemia and lymphomas
BRAF	HNPCC	Molecular analysis of PET for HNPCC
EGFR	Solid tumors-other	Molecular analysis of PET for NSCLC Adenocarcinoma
KIT	Solid tumors-other	Molecular analysis of PET for GIST
KRAS	Solid tumors-other	Molecular analysis of PET metastatic, colorectal carcinoma
MSI	Microsatellite instability	Molecular analysis of PET colorectal carcinoma by DNA amplification of microsatellites
SARC	Sarcoma translocation	Molecular analysis of various sarcoma translocations by RT-PCR
GLI	Glioma	Molecular analysis of PET for glioma by PCR
MHO	Molecular hematologic oncology	Molecular analysis of DNA, cells, and PET, for genotyping myeloid and lymphoid malignancies
MRD	Minimum residual disease	Analysis of BCR/ABL1 and PML/RARA transcripts
CYF, CYH, CYI, CYJ, CYK, CYL	Fluorescence in situ hybridization	Analysis of FISH using amplification and chromosome-specific DNA probes
Identity		
ME	Monitoring engraftment	Monitoring for bone marrow and stem cell engraftment
PAR, PARF	Parentage testing	DNA testing by PCR and RFLP
ML, DL, DML	HLA molecular typing	Molecular typing of class I and class II HLA markers
FID, FIDM	Forensic sciences—nuclear and mitochondrial DNA	Nuclear and mitochondrial DNA analysis for numerous polymorphic loci
DNA, DNAF	Forensic sciences—DNA database	Analysis of polymorphic loci for the DNA database program
Infectious disease		
ID, IDO	Nucleic acid amplification identification	Analysis of infectious pathogens analyzed by advanced amplification methods (NASBA, bDNA, LCR, PCR)
HIV, HV2, HIVG	HIV viral load	Quantitative analysis of HIV by nucleic acid amplification and genotyping, respectively
HBVL, HCVN	Hepatitis B and C viral load	Quantitative analysis of HBV and HCV by nucleic acid amplification and HCV genotyping, respectively
VLS2	CMV, EBV, BK, HHV6, ADV, viral load	Quantitative analysis by nucleic acid amplification
HPV	Human papillomavirus	Qualitative analysis of HPV by nucleic acid testing
HC5, HC6	*C. trachomatis*, herpes, and *N. gonorrhoeae*	Pathogen analysis by nucleic acid probe methods and nucleic acid amplification methods, respectively
NAT	Nucleic acid testing	Qualitative analysis of infectious pathogens designated for blood donor centers
ISH	In situ hybridization	In situ hybridization testing for various viral nucleic acid targets

bDNA branched DNA technology, *FISH* fluorescence in situ hybridization, *HCV* hepatitis C virus, *HLA* human leukocyte antigen, *HPV* human papillomavirus, *LCR* ligase chain reaction, *NASBA* nucleic acid sequence-based amplification, *PCR* polymerase chain reaction, *PET* paraffin-embedded tissue, *RFLP* restriction fragment length polymorphism, *RT-PCR* reverse transcription-polymerase chain reaction

Q of the *Code of Federal Regulations*, which addresses both basic and specific inspection requirements [50]. CLIA inspections under the Joint Commission are conducted by CMS. The CMS policy for laboratory inspections includes announced initial and biennial recertification inspections and unannounced complaint and follow-up inspections. The CMS inspection focuses more on outcomes than on laboratory process. The goals of this outcome-oriented survey are not only to determine the laboratory's regulatory compliance but also to assist laboratories in improving patient care by emphasizing those aspects that have a direct impact on the laboratory's overall test performance.

Accreditation by the Joint Commission meets the conditions required by federal law and regulations. Consequently, laboratories that are accredited by the Joint Commission in lieu of direct federal oversight and that meet the CLIA requirements for laboratories are not subject to routine inspection by state survey agencies to determine their compliance with federal requirements [51]. To be eligible, the Joint Commission must apply standards and criteria that are equal to or more stringent than the requirements established by DHHS. The Joint Commission accreditation process is more stringent than federal certification requirements in that the Joint Commission accredits a health care organization (for example, a hospital) as a whole, not just the laboratory. As such, an organization that loses the Joint Commission accreditation for reasons other than poor laboratory performance also would lose the ability to legally test human specimens under the laboratory's existing certificate of accreditation, if the Joint Commission accreditation is being used to meet the CLIA requirements. The Joint Commission also began conducting unannounced inspections in 2006.

Summary

In this chapter, many of the issues and considerations that are important for the successful management of a molecular pathology laboratory have been discussed. Although these issues are addressed separately, many are interconnected. If even one function is weak, the success of testing is compromised. Molecular pathology is a rapidly growing field of anatomic pathology and laboratory medicine. The most significant challenges facing the management team of a clinical molecular pathology laboratory are continuous acquaintance with rapidly developing new technologies, new approaches for data analysis (bioinformatics), changing regulations, and evolving testing considerations for a variety of clinical applications, as well as understanding basic business concepts in marketing and finance. Keeping pace with these challenges ensures that the clinical molecular pathology laboratory will be an even greater driving force of medical practice in the 21st century and beyond.

References

1. Rubinstein WS, et al. The NIH genetic testing registry: a new, centralized database of genetic tests to enable access to comprehensive information and improve transparency. Nucleic Acids Res. 2013;41(Database issue):D925–35.
2. Grody WW, et al. Molecular diagnostic methods for genetic diseases; approved guidelines. MM1-A2. CLSI Vol 26 No 27, 2000: Wayne PA, 2000.
3. Casey DK. Genes, dreams and reality. The promises and risks of the new genetics. Judicature. 1999;83:105–11.
4. Genetic Information Nondiscrimination Act of 2008 (S 306). https://www.federalregister.gov/articles/2010/11/09/2010-28011/regulations-under-the-genetic-information-nondiscrimination-act-of-2008. Part 1635, p. 68911–39.
5. Grody WW, et al. Molecular diagnosis of genetic diseases. In: Clinical diagnosis and management by laboratory methods Henry JB, editor. Philadelphia: WB Saunders; 2001. p. 1372–81.
6. Giardiello FM, et al. The use and interpretation of commercial APC gene testing for familial adenomatous polyposis. N Engl J Med. 1997;336(12):823–7.
7. Condit CM. Public understandings of genetics and health. Clin Genet. 2010;77(1):1–9.
8. Klitzman RL. Misunderstandings concerning genetics among patients confronting genetic disease. J Genet Couns. 2010;19(5):430–46.
9. Reiff M, et al. "What does it mean?": uncertainties in understanding results of chromosomal microarray testing. Genet Med. 2012;14(2):250–8.
10. Promoting Safe and Effective Genetic Testing Final Report of the Task Force on Genetic Testing National Human Genome Research Institute. Bethesda, MD: National Human Genome Research Institute; 1997.
11. Ekberg M. Maximizing the benefits and minimizing the risks associated with prenatal genetic testing. Health Risk Soc. 2007;9:67–81.
12. U.S. Department of Health and Human Services, Centers for Disease Control and Prevention. Notice of intent genetic testing under the Clinical Laboratory Improvement Amendments. Fed Regist. 2000 65(87):25928–34.
13. Health Insurance Portability and Accountability Act of 1996. Public Law 104-191. 104th Congress (1996). http://aspe.hhs.gov/admnsimp/p1104191.htm.
14. Gulley ML. Leukemias and lymphomas. In: Leonard DGB, editor. Diagnostic molecular pathology. Philadelphia: WB Saunders; 2003. p. 113–27.
15. Barr FG, Ladanyi M. Sarcomas. In: Leonard DGB, editor. Diagnostic molecular pathology. Philadelphia: WB Saunders; 2003. p. 53–76.
16. Fallon KB, et al. Prognostic value of 1p, 19q, 9p, 10q, and EGFR-FISH analyses in recurrent oligodendrogliomas. J Neuropathol Exp Neurol. 2004;63(4):314–22.
17. Maemondo M, et al. Gefitinib or chemotherapy for non-small-cell lung cancer with mutated EGFR. N Engl J Med. 2010;362(25):2380–8.
18. Ellison G, et al. EGFR mutation testing in lung cancer: a review of available methods and their use for analysis of tumour tissue and cytology samples. J Clin Pathol. 2013;66(2):79–89.
19. Deerlin V. Identity testing: applications of DNA typing in anatomic pathology. In: Leonard DGB, editor. Diagnostic molecular pathology. Philadelphia: WB Saunders; 2003. p. 163–88.
20. US Department of Health and Human Services. Clinical Laboratory Improvement Amendments (CLIA) of 1988. Public Law 100-578. 100th Congress (1988). http://www.cms.hhs.gov/clia.
21. Ehrmeyer SS, Lawessig HR. Compliance issues—the regulations. In: Harmening DM, editor. Laboratory management principles and processes. Upper Saddle River, NJ: Prentice-Hall; 2003. p. 225–43.
22. US Department of Health and Human Services. Medicare and CLIA programs. Regulations implementing the Clinical Laboratory Improvement of 1988 (CLIA). Fed Regist. 1992;57:7002–186.
23. US Department of Health and Human Services. Medicare and CLIA programs. Regulations implementing the Clinical Laboratory Improvement of 1988 (CLIA). Fed Regist. 2003;68:3639–714.
24. Hoeltge GA, et al. Clinical laboratory technical procedure manuals approved guidelines, 3 Edition. National Committee for Clinical Laboratory Standards 2A3P; 1996;16(15): Wayne, PA.

25. Kaul KL, et al. Oversight of genetic testing: an update. J Mol Diagn. 2001;3(3):85–91.
26. Secretary's Advisory Committee on Genetics, Health and Society (SACGHS). U.S. system of oversight of genetic testing: a response to the charge of the Secretary of Health and Human Services. Washington, DC: Department of Health & Human Services; 2008. p. 276.
27. Food and Drug Administration. Medical devices: classification/reclassification: restricted devices: analyte specific reagents. Fed Regist. 1997;62:62243–60.
28. Takes PA, Murray G. The analyte specific reagent rule: a new set of regulations for labs, manufacturers. Clin Lab News. 1998;24:10.
29. Flannery E, Danzis S. FDA plan to regulate laboratory developed tests as devices. J Medical Device Regulation. 2010; 7(3): 63–6.
30. Ferreira-Gonzales A. Establishing a molecular diagnostics laboratory. In: Henry JB, editor. Clinical diagnosis and management by laboratory methods. Philadelphia: WB Saunders; 2001. p. 1333–9.
31. Dadoun R. Impact on human resources: Core Laboratory versus laboratory information system versus modular robotics. Clin Lab Manage Rev. 1998;12(4):248–55.
32. Udaykumar, Epstein JS, Hewlett IK. A novel method employing UNG to avoid carry-over contamination in RNA-PCR. Nucleic Acids Res. 1993;21(16):3917–8.
33. Espy MJ, et al. Real-time PCR in clinical microbiology: applications for routine laboratory testing. Clin Microbiol Rev. 2006;19(1):165–256.
34. Burd EM. Validation of laboratory-developed molecular assays for infectious diseases. Clin Microbiol Rev. 2010;23(3):550–76.
35. ten Bosch JR, Grody WW. Keeping up with the next generation: massively parallel sequencing in clinical diagnostics. J Mol Diagn. 2008;10(6):484–92.
36. Natrajan R, Reis-Filho JS. Next-generation sequencing applied to molecular diagnostics. Expert Rev Mol Diagn. 2011;11(4): 425–44.
37. Comprehensive test approval policy and submission guidelines. Oncology molecular assays. NGS guidelines for somatic genetic variant detection. New York State Department of Health. Clinical laboratory standards of practice. Albany, NY: New York State Department of Health; 2014.
38. Dumler S, Fink LM, Frank TS, et al. Goals and objectives for molecular pathology education in residency programs. J Mol Diagn. 1999;1:5–15.
39. Killeen AA, et al. Certification in molecular pathology in the United States (Training and Education Committee, The Association for Molecular Pathology). J Mol Diagn. 2002;4(4):181–4.
40. Talbert ML, et al. Competency-based education for the molecular genetic pathology fellow: a report of the association for molecular pathology training and education committee. J Mol Diagn. 2009; 11(6):497–507.
41. Griffey PA, Fundamentals of financial management In: Laboratory Management: Principles and Processes. Harmening DM, editor. Upper Saddle River, N.T: Prentice-Hall; 2003: 163–179.
42. Centers for Medicare & Medicaid Services. Medicare program; revisions to payment policies under the physician fee schedule, DME face-to-face encounters, elimination of the requirement for termination of non-random prepayment complex medical review and other revisions to Part B for CY 2013. 42 CFR Parts 410, 414, 415, 421, 423, 425, 486 and 495.
43. American Medical Association. 2015 CPT. Current Procedural Terminology (Professional Edition). Chicago: American Medical Association; 2015.
44. Cho MK, et al. Effects of patents and licenses on the provision of clinical genetic testing services. J Mol Diagn. 2003;5(1):3–8.
45. Gomah ME, et al. Modeling complex workflow in molecular diagnostics: design specifications of laboratory software for support of personalized medicine. J Mol Diagn. 2010;12(1):51–7.
46. Grody WW, et al. Laboratory standards and guidelines for population-based cystic fibrosis carrier screening. Genet Med. 2001;3(2):149–54.
47. New York State Department of Health. Clinical laboratory standards of practice. Albany, NY: New York State Department of Health; 2012.
48. Chen B, et al. Good laboratory practices for molecular genetic testing for heritable diseases and conditions. MMWR Recomm Rep. 2009;58(RR-6):1–37. quiz CE-1-4.
49. College of American Pathologists. Molecular Pathology checklist. Northfield, IL: Laboratory Accreditation Program—College of American Pathologists; 2005.
50. Department of Health and Human Services, Centers for Disease Control and Prevention. Subpart Q—inspection. Fed Regist. 1998;63:986–7.
51. Department of Health and Human Services. CLIA Program: approval of the Joint Commission on Accreditation of Healthcare Organizations as an accrediting organization. Fed Regist. 1995;60:130–2.

Index

D.G.B. Leonard (ed.), *Molecular Pathology in Clinical Practice*, DOI 10.1007/978-3-319-19674-9

G

I

J

K

L

Q

R

T

U

V

W

MIX
Papier aus verantwortungsvollen Quellen
Paper from responsible sources
FSC® C105338

If you have any concerns about our products,
you can contact us on
ProductSafety@springernature.com

In case Publisher is established outside the EU,
the EU authorized representative is:
Springer Nature Customer Service Center GmbH
Europaplatz 3, 69115 Heidelberg, Germany

Printed by Libri Plureos GmbH
in Hamburg, Germany